CONTENTS

D1430892

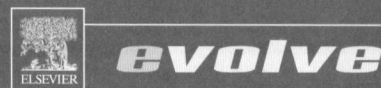

evolve

•• To access your Student Resources, visit:
http://evolve.elsevier.com/SaundersNDH

Evolve ® Student Learning Resources for *Saunders Nursing Drug Handbook 2007* offer the following features:

- **Quarterly Drug Updates and Alerts**
  Abbreviated monographs on new drugs and updated information on new indications and new dosages for existing drugs. Important information about drugs recently withdrawn from the market, new drug safety information, and other news to help you provide the best possible care.

- **Do Not Confuse Table**
  A complete listing of drug names that sound or look alike and are often confused.

- **Less Frequently Used Drugs**
  Find vital information about drugs used less often in everyday practice.

- **WebLinks**
  Access links to places of interest on the web.

- **Interactive Drug Calculator**

- **Sign-up page for the Elsevier ePharmacology Update newsletter**
  An informative, full-color, quarterly newsletter written by Evelyn Salerno, PharmD, the Elsevier ePharmacology Update provides current and well-documented information on new drugs, drug warnings, medication errors, and more. Available to students and instructors.

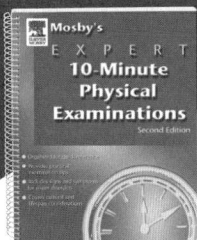

Saunders

Nursing Drug Handbook

2007

BARBARA B. HODGSON, RN, OCN
Cancer Institute
St. Joseph's Hospital
Tampa, Florida

ROBERT J. KIZIOR, BS, RPh
Education Coordinator
Department of Pharmacy
Alexian Brothers Medical Center
Elk Grove Village, Illinois

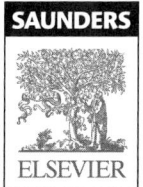

SAUNDERS

ELSEVIER

SAUNDERS
ELSEVIER

11830 Westline Industrial Drive
St. Louis, Missouri 63146

ISBN-13: 978-1-4160-3612-8
ISBN-10: 1-4160-3612-1

SAUNDERS NURSING DRUG HANDBOOK 2007
Copyright © 2007, 2006, 2005, 2004, 2003, 2002,
2001, 2000, 1999, 1998, 1997, 1996, 1995, 1994,
1993 by Saunders, an imprint of Elsevier Inc.

NOTICE

Knowledge and best practice in this field are constantly changing. As new research and
experience broaden our knowledge, changes in practice, treatment and drug therapy may
become necessary or appropriate. Readers are advised to check the most current information
provided (i) on procedures featured or (ii) by the manufacturer of each product to be
administered, to verify the recommended dose or formula, the method and duration of
administration, and contraindications. It is the responsibility of the practitioner, relying on their
own experience and knowledge of the patient, to make diagnoses, to determine dosages and
the best treatment for each individual patient, and to take all appropriate safety precautions.
To the fullest extent of the law, neither the Publisher nor the Authors assume any liability
for any injury and/or damage to persons or property arising out of or related to any use of the
material contained in this book.

ISBN-13: 978-1-4160-3612-8
ISBN-10: 1-4160-3612-1

Executive Vice President, Nursing & Health Professions: Sally Schrefer
Publishing Executive: Barbara Nelson Cullen
Executive Editor: Cynthia Tryniszewski
Developmental Editor: Gina Hopf
Publishing Services Manager: Melissa Lastarria
Project Manager: Kelly E.M. Steinmann
Designer: Paula Ruckenbrod

Printed in the United States of America.

Last digit is the print number: 9 8 7 6 5 4 3 2 1

I dedicate this work to my daughter Lauren, a true friend, for her unconditional love; my daughter Kathryn, always supportive, always encouraging; and my son, Keith, a source of great pride to us all. This is also dedicated to my sons-in-law, Jim and Andy, who have added so very much to my family, and to the smallest members of my growing family, my granddaughter, Paige Olivia, and my grandsons, Logan James, Ryan James, and Dylan Boyd. I couldn't love you more.

BARBARA HODGSON, RN, OCN

To all health care professionals, who in the expectation of little glory or material reward dedicate themselves to the art and science of healing.

ROBERT KIZIOR, BS, RPh

AUTHOR BIOGRAPHIES

Barbara Hodgson, RN, OCN

Born and raised in Michigan, Barbara was married and raising a young family in Chicago when she decided to fulfill a lifelong dream and become a nurse. After graduation, she started her own business as author and publisher of **Medcards, The Total Medication Reference Guide,** the first of its kind. These drug cards were designed to assist nursing students in understanding drug information to give knowledgeable care to their patients.

In 1981, she met co-author Robert (Bob) Kizior, who was teaching a pharmacology class. After class, Barbara approached him and asked if he would be interested in working on **Medcards** with her. He agreed, and together they became so successful that a few years later Barbara was able to fulfill another dream and move to Florida.

By 1987, Barbara was approached by W.B. Saunders and asked to author the **Saunders Nursing Drug Handbook.** Since then, Barbara and Bob have worked together on this handbook and on two more drug resources, the **Saunders Electronic Nursing Drug Cards** and the **Saunders Drug Handbook for Health Professions.**

Barbara specializes in oncology at the Cancer Institute, St. Joseph's Hospital, in Tampa, Florida. Barbara's daughter Lauren, her son-in-law, Jim, and her son, Keith, are emergency nurses. Her daughter Kathryn is a research biologist.

Barbara's favorite interests are spending time with her very busy, tight-knit family and, when she has a rare moment, getting her hands full of dirt working in her garden.

Robert (Bob) Kizior, BS, RPh

Bob graduated from the University of Illinois School of Pharmacy and is licensed to practice in the state of Illinois. He has worked as a hospital pharmacist for more than 35 years at Alexian Brothers Medical Center in Elk Grove Village, Illinois—a suburb of Chicago. Bob is the Education Coordinator for the Department of Pharmacy, where he participates in educational programs for pharmacists, nurses, physicians, and patients. He plays a major role in conducting Drug Utilization Reviews and is a member of the Infection Control Committee and the Bariatric Committee. His hospital experience is diverse and includes participation in clinical pharmacy initiatives on inpatient units and in the surgical pharmacy satellite. Bob is a former adjunct faculty member at William Rainey Harper Community College in Palatine, Illinois. It was there that Bob first met Barbara and commenced their long-standing professional association.

An avid fan of Big Ten college athletics, Bob also has eclectic tastes in music that range from classical, big band, rock 'n' roll, and jazz to country and western. Bob spends much of his free time reviewing the professional literature to stay current on new drug information. He and his wife, Marcia, and their two Labrador retrievers—Zak and Callie—enjoy escape weekends at their year-round lake house in central Wisconsin.

CONSULTANTS

Katherine B. Barbee, MSN, ANP,
  F-NP-C
Kaiser Permanente
Washington, District of Columbia

Lisa Brown
Jackson State Community College
Jackson, Tennessee

Marla J. DeJong, RN, MS, CCRN,
  CEN, Capt.
Wilford Hall Medical Center
Lackland Air Force Base, Texas

Diane M. Ford, RN, MS, CCRN
Andrews University
Berrien Springs, Michigan

Denise D. Hopkins, PharmD
College of Pharmacy
University of Arkansas
Little Rock, Arkansas

Barbara D. Horton, RN, MS
Arnot Ogden Medical Center School
  of Nursing
Elmira, New York

Mary Beth Jenkins, RN, CCRN,
  CAPA
Elliott One Day Surgery Center
Manchester, New Hampshire

Kelly W. Jones, PharmD, BCPS
McLeod Family Medicine Center
McLeod Regional Medical Center
Florence, South Carolina

Autumn E. Korson
Western Michigan University Bronson
  School of Nursing
Kalamazoo, Michigan

Linda Laskowski-Jones,
  MS, RN, CS, CCRN, CEN
Christiana Care Health System
Newark, Delaware

Jessica K. Leet, RN, BSN
Cardinal Glennon Children's Hospital
St. Louis, Missouri

Denise Macklin, BSN, RNC,
  CRNI
President, Professional Learning
  Systems, Inc.
Marietta, Georgia

Nancy L. McCartney
Valencia Community College
Orlando, Florida

Judith L. Myers, MSN, RN
Health Sciences Center
St. Louis University School of Nursing
St. Louis, Missouri

Kimberly R. Pugh, MSEd, RN, BS
Nurse Consultant
Baltimore, Maryland

Regina T. Schiavello, BSN, RNC
Wills Eye Hospital
Philadelphia, Pennsylvania

Gregory M. Susla, PharmD,
  FCCM
National Institutes of Health
Bethesda, Maryland

Elizabeth Taylor
Tennessee Wesleyan College of Nursing
Fort Saunders Regional
Knoxville, Tennessee

REVIEWERS

PREFACE

Nurses are faced with the ever-challenging responsibility of ensuring safe and effective drug therapy for their patients. Not surprisingly, the greatest challenge for nurses is keeping up with the overwhelming amount of new drug information, including the latest FDA-approved drugs and changes to already approved drugs, such as new uses, dosage forms, warnings, and much more. Nurses must integrate this information into their patient care quickly and in an informed manner.

Saunders Nursing Drug Handbook 2007 is designed as an easy-to-use source of current drug information to help the busy nurse meet these challenges. What separates this book from others is that it guides the nurse through patient care to better practice and better care.

This handbook contains the following:

1. **An IV Compatibility Chart.** This handy chart is updated this edition and bound into the handbook to prevent accidental loss.
2. **The Classification Section.** The action and uses for some of the most common clinical and pharmacotherapeutic classes are presented. Two classifications are new to this edition, medications that treat Parkinson's disease and smoking cessation agents. Unique to this handbook, each class provides an at-a-glance table that compares all the generic drugs within the classification according to product availability, dosages, side effects, and other characteristics. Its orange full-page color tab ensures you can't miss it!
3. **An attractive four-color atlas of medications.** This section contains photographs of 158 of the most commonly used oral medications. The medications, both brand and generic, are shown in their different dosage forms. Just look for the glossy orange full-page color tab to help you identify those medications presented to you sans prescription bottle or order. A 🖋 appears in the individual drug entries when there is a corresponding illustration in the atlas.
4. **An alphabetical listing of drug entries by generic name.** Orange letter thumb tabs help you page through this section quickly. New to this edition is the FDA "Tall Man" lettering presentation of those drugs that, for patient safety, should be written with emphasis on certain syllables to avoid confusing them with similarly sounding/looking medications. Tall Man lettering is shown in slim orange capitalized letters (e.g., *aceta**ZOLAMIDE**). High Alert drugs with an orange flag ⚑ are considered dangerous by the Joint Commission on Accreditation of Healthcare Organizations (JCAHO) and the Institute for Safe Medication Practices (ISMP) because if they are administered incorrectly, they may cause life-threatening or permanent harm to the patient. The entire High Alert generic drug entry sits on an orange-shaded background so it's easy to spot! To make scanning pages easier, each new entry begins with a shaded box containing the generic name, pronunciation, trade name(s) fixed-combination(s), and classification(s).

5. **Herbal entries.** Included in this edition are 18 of the most commonly used herbs, each indicated with an orange leaf 🍃 . In this edition, each herb is cross-referenced to the Herbal Therapies and Interactions (Appendix G) so that you have the most comprehensive view of herbal therapies related to patient care.

6. **Trade name cross-references in the A to Z section of the book.** We have over 400 of the top trade name drugs with cross-references within the A to Z section! These entries are shaded in gray for easy identification.

7. **A comprehensive reference section.** The reference section is updated and expanded with a new appendix on cytochrome P450 (CYP) enzymes. Other appendixes include vital information on calculation of doses, controlled drugs, drip rates for critical care medications, drugs of abuse, equi-analgesic dosing, FDA pregnancy categories, herbal therapies and interactions, lifespan and cultural aspects of drug therapy, normal laboratory values, orphan drugs, poison antidotes, recommended childhood and adult immunizations, signs and symptoms of electrolyte imbalance, sound-alike and look-alike drugs, Spanish phrases often used in clinical settings, and techniques of medication administration.

8. **Drugs by Disorder.** You'll find Drugs by Disorder in the front of the book for easy reference. It lists common disorders and the drugs often used for treatment.

9. **The index.** The comprehensive index is located at the back of the book on light orange pages. Undoubtedly the best tool to help you navigate the handbook, the comprehensive index is organized by showing generic drug names in **bold**, trade names in regular type, classifications in *italics*, drugs with expanded information on the Internet with an Evolve icon ⓔ, and the page number of the main drug entry listed first and in **bold**.

10. **A mini CD.** Saunders Nursing Drug Handbook 2007 has a mini CD-ROM packaged in the back of the book. The software features 340 monographs for most commonly used medications. Users can customize and print these drug entries.

A DETAILED GUIDE TO THE SAUNDERS NURSING DRUG HANDBOOK

An intensive review by Consultants and Reviewers helped us to revise the **Saunders Nursing Drug Handbook** so that it is most useful in educational and clinical practice. The main objective of the handbook is to provide essential drug information in a user-friendly format. The bulk of the handbook contains an alphabetical listing of drug entries by generic name.

To maintain the portability of this handbook and meet the challenge of keeping content current, we have also included additional information for some medications on an EVOLVE Internet site. EVOLVE also includes drug alerts (e.g., medications removed from the market) and drug updates (e.g., new drugs, updates on existing entries). Information is periodically added, allowing the nurse to keep abreast of current drug information. The drug entries with EVOLVE enhancement are indicated with an ⓔ next to the generic drug name.

You'll also notice that some entries for infrequently used medications are condensed to reflect only the absolutely essential points the nurse should know when called upon to administer them.

We have incorporated the IV Incompatibilities heading ▒. The drugs listed in this section are not compatible with the generic drug when administered direct by IV push, via Y-site, or via IV piggyback. We have highlighted the intravenous drug administration and handling information with a special heading icon ⬚ and have broken it down by Reconstitution, Rate of Administration, and Storage.

We present entries in an order that follows the logical thought process the nurse undergoes whenever a drug is ordered for a patient:

- What is the drug?
- How is the drug classified?
- What does the drug do?
- What is the drug used for?
- Under what conditions should you **not** use the drug?
- How do you administer the drug?
- How do you store the drug?
- What is the dose of the drug?
- What should you monitor the patient for once he or she has received the drug?
- What do you assess the patient for?
- What interventions should you perform?
- What should you teach the patient?

The following are included within the drug entries:

Generic Name, Pronunciation, Trade Names. Each entry begins with the generic name and pronunciation, followed by the U.S. and Canadian trade names. Exclusively Canadian trade names are followed by an orange maple leaf ✦. Trade names that were most prescribed in the year 2005 are underlined in this section.

Do Not Confuse With. Drug names that sound similar to the generic and/or trade names are listed under this heading to help you avoid potential medication errors.

Fixed-Combination Drugs. Where appropriate, fixed-combinations, or drugs made up of two or more generic medications, are listed with the generic drug.

Pharmacotherapeutic and Clinical Classification Names. Each full entry includes both the pharmacotherapeutic and clinical classifications for the generic drug. When available, the page number of the classification description in the front of the book is provided in this section as well.

Action/Therapeutic Effect. This section describes how the drug is predicted to behave, with the expected therapeutic effect(s) under a separate heading.

Pharmacokinetics. This section includes the absorption, distribution, metabolism, excretion, and half-life of the medication. The half-life is bolded in orange for easy access.

Uses/Off-Label. The listing of uses for each drug includes both the FDA uses and off-label uses. The off-label heading is shown in bold orange for emphasis.

Precautions. This heading incorporates a discussion on when the generic drug is contraindicated or should be used with caution. The cautions warn the nurse of specific situations in which a drug should be closely monitored.

Lifespan Considerations ⌛ includes the pregnancy category and lactation data, as well as age-specific information concerning children and the elderly.

Interactions. This heading enumerates drug, food, and herbal interactions with the generic drug. As the number of medications a patient receives increases, awareness of drug interactions becomes more important. Also included is information on therapeutic and toxic blood levels in addition to the altered lab values that show what effects the drug may have on lab results.

Product Availability. Each drug monograph gives the form and availability of the drug.

Administration/Handling. Instructions for administration are given for each route of administration (e.g., IV, IM, PO, rectal). Special handling such as refrigeration is also included where applicable. The routes in this section are always presented in the order IV, IM, Subcutaneous, PO, with subsequent routes in alphabetical order (e.g., Ophthalmic, Otic, Topical). **IV administration** ⬆ is broken down by reconstitution, rate of administration (how fast the IV should be given), and storage (including how long the medication is stable once reconstituted).

IV Compatibilities/IV Incompatibilities ▧ give the nurse the most comprehensive compatibility information possible when administering medications by direct IV push, via a Y-site, or via IV piggyback.

Indications/Routes/Dosage. Each full entry provides specific dosing guidelines for adults, the elderly, children, and patients with renal and/or hepatic impairment. Dosages are clearly indicated for each approved indication and route.

Side Effects. Side effects are defined as those responses that are usually predictable with the drug, are **not** life-threatening, and may or may not require discontinuation of the drug. Unique to this handbook, side effects are grouped by frequency listed from highest occurrence percentage to lowest so that the nurse can focus on patient care without wading through myriad signs and symptoms of side effects.

Adverse Reactions/Toxic Effects. Adverse reactions and toxic effects are very serious and often life-threatening undesirable responses that require prompt intervention from a health care provider.

Nursing Considerations. Nursing considerations are organized as care is organized. That is:

- What needs to be assessed or done before the first dose is administered? (Baseline Assessment)
- What interventions and evaluations are needed during drug therapy? (Intervention/Evaluation)
- What explicit teaching is needed for the patient and family? (Patient/Family Teaching)

Saunders Nursing Drug Handbook is an easy-to-use source of current drug information for nurses, students, and other health care providers. It is our hope that this handbook will help you provide quality care to your patients.

We welcome any comments you may have that would help us to improve future editions of the handbook. Please contact us via the publisher at *http://evolve.elsevier.com/SaundersNDH.*

Barbara B. Hodgson, RN, OCN
Robert J. Kizior, BS, RPh

ACKNOWLEDGMENTS

I offer a special heartfelt thank you to my co-author, Bob Kizior, for his continuing, superb work. Without Bob's effort in this major endeavor, this book would not have reached the par excellence it has achieved. I thank my siblings, Jane Sperry and Milt, Bruce, Rich, Vance, and Greg Boyd, who have encouraged me through the years; Jim Witmer, BSN, CCRN, CEN, for the many hours he spent assisting me in this huge endeavor and the consistent support he offered; and Andrew Ross, who enlightens my family so dearly.

Barbara Hodgson, RN, OCN

BIBLIOGRAPHY

Briggs G, Freeman R, Yaffe S: *Drugs in Pregnancy and Lactation,* ed 6, Greenwood Village, Colorado, 2003, Micromedex.
Drug Facts and Comparisons, St. Louis, 2005, Facts and Comparisons.
Lacy CF, Armstrong LL, Goldman MP, et al: *Lexi-Comp's Drug Information Handbook,* ed 13, Hudson, Ohio, 2005, Lexi-Comp.
Mosby's Drug Consult 2005, ed 15, St. Louis, 2005, Mosby.
Natural Medicines Comprehensive Database, 2006.
Rakel RE, Bope ET: *Conn's Current Therapy,* ed 2, Philadelphia, 2005, WB Saunders.
Takemoto CR, Hodding JH, Kraus DM: *Lexi-Comp's Pediatric Dosage Handbook,* ed 12, Hudson, Ohio, 2004, Lexi-Comp.
Trissel LA: *Handbook of Injectable Drugs,* ed 12, Bethesda, 2004, American Society of Health-System Pharmacist.
USPDI Drug Information for the Health Care Professional, 2005.

ILLUSTRATION CREDITS

Kee JL, Hayes ER, McCuiston LE (eds): *Pharmacology: A Nursing Process Approach,* ed 5, Philadelphia, 2006, WB Saunders.
Mosby's GenRx, ed 12, St. Louis, 2004, Mosby.

DRUGS BY DISORDER

Note: Not all medications appropriate for a given condition are listed, nor are those not listed inappropriate.

Generic names appear first, followed by brand names in parentheses.

Allergy
Beclomethasone (Beclovent, Vanceril)
Betamethasone (Celestone)
Brompheniramine (Dimetane)
Budesonide (Pulmicort, Rhinocort)
Chlorpheniramine (Chlor-Trimeton)
Clemastine (Tavist)
Cyproheptadine (Periactin)
Desloratadine (Clarinex)
Dexamethasone (Decadron)
Dimenhydrinate (Dramamine)
Diphenhydramine (Benadryl)
Epinephrine (Adrenalin)
Fexofenadine (Allegra)
Flunisolide (AeroBid, Nasalide)
Fluticasone (Flovent)
Hydrocortisone (Solu-Cortef)
Loratadine (Claritin)
Prednisolone (Prelone)
Prednisone (Deltasone)
Promethazine (Phenergan)
Triamcinolone (Kenalog)

Alzheimer's disease
Donepezil (Aricept)
Galantamine (Reminyl)
Memantine (Namenda)
Rivastigmine (Exelon)
Tacrine (Cognex)

Angina
Amlodipine (Norvasc)
Atenolol (Tenormin)
Diltiazem (Cardizem, Dilacor)
Isosorbide (Imdur, Isordil)
Metoprolol (Lopressor)
Nadolol (Corgard)
Nicardipine (Cardene)
Nifedipine (Adalat, Procardia)
Nitroglycerin

Propranolol (Inderal)
Timolol (Blocadron)
Verapamil (Calan, Isoptin)

Anxiety
Alprazolam (Xanax)
Buspirone (BuSpar)
Diazepam (Valium)
Doxepin (Sinequan)
Hydroxyzine (Atarax, Vistaril)
Lorazepam (Ativan)
Oxazepam (Serax)

Arrhythmias
Acebutolol (Sectral)
Adenosine (Adenocard)
Amiodarone (Cordarone, Pacerone)
Digoxin (Lanoxin)
Diltiazem (Cardizem, Dilacor)
Disopyramide (Norpace)
Dofetilide (Tikosyn)
Esmolol (Brevibloc)
Ibutilide (Corvert)
Lidocaine
Mexiletine (Mexitil)
Moricizine (Ethmozine)
Phenytoin (Dilantin)
Procainamide (Procan, Pronestyl)
Propafenone (Rythmol)
Propranolol (Inderal)
Quinidine
Sotalol (Betapace)
Tocainide (Tonocard)
Verapamil (Calan, Isoptin)

Arthritis, rheumatoid (RA)
Abatacept (Orencia)
Adalimumab (Humira)
Anakinra (Kineret)
Aspirin

Auranofin (Ridaura)
Aurothioglucose (Solganal)
Azathioprine (Imuran)
Betamethasone (Celestone)
Capsaicin (Zostrix)
Celecoxib (Celebrex)
Cyclosporine (Sandimmune)
Diclofenac (Cataflam, Voltaren)
Diflunisal (Dolobid)
Etanercept (Enbrel)
Hydroxychloroquine (Plaquenil)
Infliximab (Remicade)
Leflunomide (Arava)
Methotrexate
Penicillamine (Cuprimine)
Prednisone (Deltasone)

Asthma
Albuterol (Proventil, Ventolin)
Aminophylline (Theophylline)
Beclomethasone (Beclovent, Vanceril)
Budesonide (Pulmicort)
Cromolyn (Crolom, Intal)
Dexamethasone (Decadron)
Epinephrine (Adrenalin)
Flunisolide (AeroBid)
Fluticasone (Flovent)
Formoterol (Foradil)
Hydrocortisone (Solu-Cortef)
Ipratropium (Atrovent)
Levalbuterol (Xopenex)
Metaproterenol (Alupent)
Methylprednisolone (Solu-Medrol)
Mometasone (Asmanex)
Montelukast (Singulair)
Nedocromil (Tilade)
Prednisolone (Prelone)
Prednisone (Deltasone)
Salmeterol (Serevent)
Terbutaline (Brethine)
Theophylline (SloBid)
Zafirlukast (Accolate)

Attention deficit hyperactivity disorder (ADHD)
Atomoxetine (Strattera)
Bupropion (Wellbutrin)
Desipramine (Norpramin)
Dexmethylphenidate (Focalin)
Dextroamphetamine (Dexedrine)

Imipramine (Tofranil)
Methylphenidate (Ritalin)
Mixed amphetamine (Adderall)
Modafinil (Provigil)

Benign prostatic hypertrophy (BPH)
Alfuzosin (UroXatral)
Doxazosin (Cardura)
Finasteride (Proscar)
Tamsulosin (Flomax)
Terazosin (Hytrin)

Bladder hyperactivity
Darifenacin (Enablex)
Solifenacin (VESIcare)
Tolterodine (Detrol)
Trospium (Sanctura)

Bronchospasm
Albuterol (Proventil, Ventolin)
Bitolterol (Tornalate)
Epinephrine (Adrenalin)
Levalbuterol (Xopenex)
Metaproterenol (Alupent)
Salmeterol (Serevent)
Terbutaline (Brethine)
Theophylline (SloBid)

Cancer
Abarelix (Plenaxis)
Aldesleukin (Proleukin)
Alemtuzumab (Campath)
Alitretinoin (Panretin)
Altretamine (Hexalen)
Anastrozole (Arimidex)
Arsenic trioxide (Trisenox)
Asparaginase (Elspar)
Azacitadine (Vidaza)
BCG (TheraCys, Tice BCG)
Bevacizumab (Avastin)
Bexarotene (Targretin)
Bicalutamide (Casodex)
Bleomycin (Blenoxane)
Bortezomib (Velcade)
Busulfan (Myleran)
Capecitabine (Xeloda)
Carboplatin (Paraplatin)
Carmustine (BiCNU)
Cetuximab (Erbitux)
Chlorambucil (Leukeran)

Cisplatin (Platinol)
Cladribine (Leustatin)
Clofarabine (Clolar)
Cyclophosphamide (Cytoxan)
Cytarabine (Ara-C, Cytosar)
Dacarbazine (DTIC)
Dactinomycin (Cosmegen)
Daunorubicin (Cerubidine, DaunoXome)
Denileukin (Ontak)
Docetaxel (Taxotere)
Doxorubicin (Adriamycin, Doxil)
Epirubicin (Ellence)
Ertotinib (Tarceva)
Estramustine (Emcyt)
Etoposide (VePesid)
Fludarabine (Fludara)
Fluorouracil
Flutamide (Eulexin)
Fulvestrant (Faslodex)
Gefitnib (Iressa)
Gemcitabine (Gemzar)
Gemtuzumab (Mylotarg)
Goserelin (Zoladex)
Hydroxyurea (Hydrea)
Ibritumomab (Zevalin)
Idarubicin (Idamycin)
Ifosfamide (Ifex)
Imatinib (Gleevec)
Interferon alfa-2a (Roferon A)
Interferon alfa-2b (Intron A)
Irinotecan (Camptosar)
Letrozole (Femara)
Leuprolide (Lupron)
Lomustine (CeeNU)
Mechlorethamine (Mustargen)
Megestrol (Megace)
Melphalan (Alkeran)
Mercaptopurine (Purinethol)
Methotrexate
Mitomycin (Mutamycin)
Mitotane (Lysodren)
Mitoxantrone (Novantrone)
Nelarabine (Arranon)
Nilutamide (Nilandron)
Oxaliplatin (Eloxatin)
Paclitaxel (Taxol)
Pemetrexed (Alimta)
Pentostatin (Nipent)
Plicamycin (Mithracin)
Procarbazine (Matulane)

Rituximab (Rituxan)
Sorafenib (Nexavar)
Streptozocin (Zanosar)
Tamoxifen (Nolvadex)
Temozolomide (Temodar)
Teniposide (Vumon)
Thioguanine
Thiotepa (Thioplex)
Topotecan (Hycamtin)
Toremifene (Fareston)
Tositumomab (Ber)
Trastuzumab (Herceptin)
Tretinoin (Vesanoid)
Valrubicin (Valstar)
Vinblastine (Velban)
Vincristine (Oncovin)
Vinorelbine (Navelbine)

Cerebrovascular accident (CVA)
Aspirin
Clopidogrel (Plavix)
Heparin
Nimodipine (Nimotop)
Ticlopidine (Ticlid)
Warfarin (Coumadin)

Chronic obstructive pulmonary disease (COPD)
Albuterol (Proventil, Ventolin)
Aminophylline (Theophylline)
Budesonide (Pulmicort)
Epinephrine (Adrenalin)
Formoterol (Foradil)
Levalbuterol (Xopenex)
Metaproterenol (Alupent)
Salmeterol (Serevent)
Theophylline (SloBid)
Tiotropium (Spiriva)

Congestive heart failure (CHF)
Amlodipine (Norvasc)
Bumetanide (Bumex)
Captopril (Capoten)
Carvedilol (Coreg)
Digoxin (Lanoxin)
Dobutamine (Dobutrex)
Dopamine (Intropin)
Enalapril (Vasotec)
Eprosartan (Teveten)
Fosinopril (Monopril)

Furosemide (Lasix)
Hydralazine (Apresoline)
Isosorbide (Isordil)
Lisinopril (Prinivil, Zestril)
Losartan (Cozaar)
Metoprolol (Lopressor)
Milrinone (Primacor)
Moexipril (Univasc)
Nitroglycerin
Nitroprusside (Nipride)
Quinapril (Accupril)
Ramipril (Altace)

Constipation
Bisacodyl (Dulcolax)
Docusate (Colace)
Lactulose (Kristalose)
Methylcellulose (Citrucel)
Milk of magnesia (MOM)
Psyllium (Metamucil)
Senna (Senokot)

Crohn's disease
Cyclosporine (Neoral)
Hydrocortisone (Cortenema)
Infliximab (Remicade)
Mesalamine (Asacol, Pentasa)
Olsalazine (Dipentum)
Sulfasalazine (Azulfidine)

Deep vein thrombosis (DVT)
Dalteparin (Fragmin)
Enoxaparin (Lovenox)
Heparin
Tinzaparin (Innohep)
Warfarin (Coumadin)

Depression
Amitriptyline (Elavil, Endep)
Bupropion (Wellbutrin)
Citalopram (Celexa)
Clomipramine (Anafranil)
Desipramine (Norpramin)
Doxepin (Sinequan)
Escitalopram (Lexapro)
Fluoxetine (Prozac)
Imipramine (Tofranil)
Maprotiline (Ludiomil)
Mirtazapine (Remeron)
Nefazodone

Nortriptyline (Aventyl, Pamelor)
Paroxetine (Paxil)
Phenelzine (Nardil)
Sertraline (Zoloft)
Tranylcypromine (Parnate)
Trazodone (Desyrel)
Venlafaxine (Effexor)

Diabetes mellitus
Acarbose (Precose)
Chlorpropamide (Diabinese)
Exenatide (Byetta)
Glimepiride (Amaryl)
Glipizide (Glucotrol)
Glyburide (Micronase)
Insulin
Metformin (Glucophage)
Miglitol (Glyset)
Nateglinide (Starlix)
Pioglitazone (Actos)
Pramlintide (Symlin)
Repaglinide (Prandin)
Rosiglitazone (Avandia)

Diarrhea
Bismuth subsalicylate (Pepto-Bismol)
Diphenoxylate and atropine (Lomotil)
Kaolin-pectin (Kaopectate)
Loperamide (Imodium)
Octreotide (Sandostatin)
Rifaximin (Xifaxan)

Duodenal, gastric ulcer
Cimetidine (Tagamet)
Esomeprazole (Nexium)
Famotidine (Pepcid)
Lansoprazole (Prevacid)
Misoprostol (Cytotec)
Nizatidine (Axid)
Omeprazole (Prilosec)
Pantoprazole (Protonix)
Rabeprazole (Aciphex)
Ranitidine (Zantac)
Sucralfate (Carafate)

Edema
Amiloride (Midamor)
Bumetanide (Bumex)
Chlorthalidone (Hygroton)
Ethacrynic acid (Edecrin)

Furosemide (Lasix)
Hydrochlorothiazide (HydroDIURIL)
Indapamide (Lozol)
Metolazone (Zaroxolyn)
Spironolactone (Aldactone)
Torsemide (Demadex)
Triamterene (Dyrenium)

Epilepsy
Acetazolamide (Diamox)
Carbamazepine (Tegretol)
Clonazepam (Klonopin)
Clorazepate (Tranxene)
Diazepam (Valium)
Fosphenytoin (Cerebyx)
Gabapentin (Neurontin)
Lamotrigine (Lamictal)
Levetiracetam (Keppra)
Lorazepam (Ativan)
Oxcarbazepine (Trileptal)
Phenobarbital
Phenytoin (Dilantin)
Primidone (Mysoline)
Tiagabine (Gabitril)
Topiramate (Topamax)
Valproic acid (Depakene, Depakote)
Zonisamide (Zonegran)

Esophageal reflux, esophagitis
Cimetidine (Tagamet)
Esomeprazole (Nexium)
Famotidine (Pepcid)
Lansoprazole (Prevacid)
Nizatidine (Axid)
Omeprazole (Prilosec)
Pantoprazole (Protonix)
Rabeprazole (Aciphex)
Ranitidine (Zantac)

Fever
Acetaminophen (Tylenol)
Aspirin
Ibuprofen (Advil, Motrin)
Naproxen (Aleve, Anaprox, Naprosyn)

Fibromyalgia
Acetaminophen (Tylenol)
Amitriptyline (Elavil)
Carisoprodol (Soma)
Cyclobenzaprine (Flexeril)
Duloxetine (Cymbalta)

Fluoxetine (Prozac)
Pregabalin (Lyrica)
Tramadol (Ultram)
Venlafaxine (Effexor)

Gastritis
Cimetidine (Tagamet)
Famotidine (Pepcid)
Nizatidine (Axid)
Ranitidine (Zantac)

Gastroesophageal reflux disease (GERD)
Cimetidine (Tagamet)
Esomeprazole (Nexium)
Famotidine (Pepcid)
Lansoprazole (Prevacid)
Metoclopramide (Reglan)
Nizatidine (Axid)
Omeprazole (Prilosec)
Pantoprazole (Protonix)
Rabeprazole (Aciphex)
Ranitidine (Zantac)

Glaucoma
Acetazolamide (Diamox)
Apraclonidine (Iopidine)
Betaxolol (Betoptic)
Bimatoprost (Lumigan)
Brimonidine (Alphagan)
Brinzolamide (Azopt)
Carbachol
Carteolol (Ocupress)
Dipivefrin (Propine)
Dorzolamide (Trusopt)
Echothiophate iodide (Phospholine)
Latanoprost (Xalatan)
Levobunolol (Betagan)
Metipranolol (OptiPranolol)
Pilocarpine (Isopto Carpine)
Timolol (Timoptic)
Travoprost (Travatan)
Unoprostone (Rescula)

Gout
Allopurinol (Zyloprim)
Colchicine
Indomethacin (Indocin)
Probenecid (Benemid)
Sulindac (Clinoril)

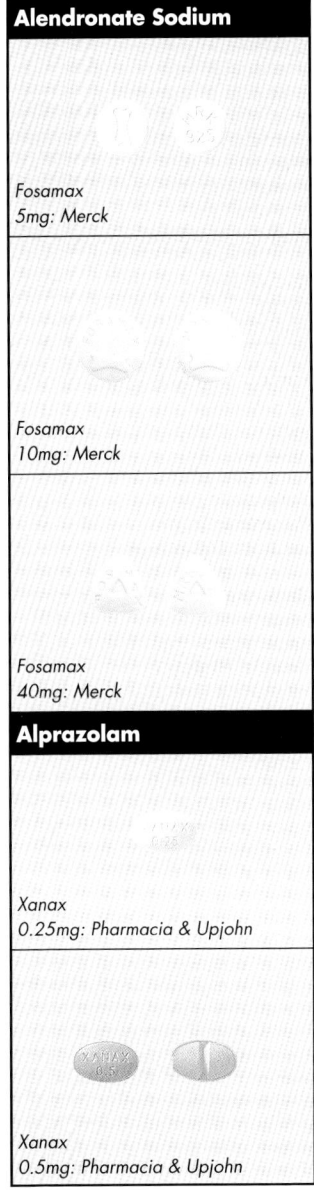

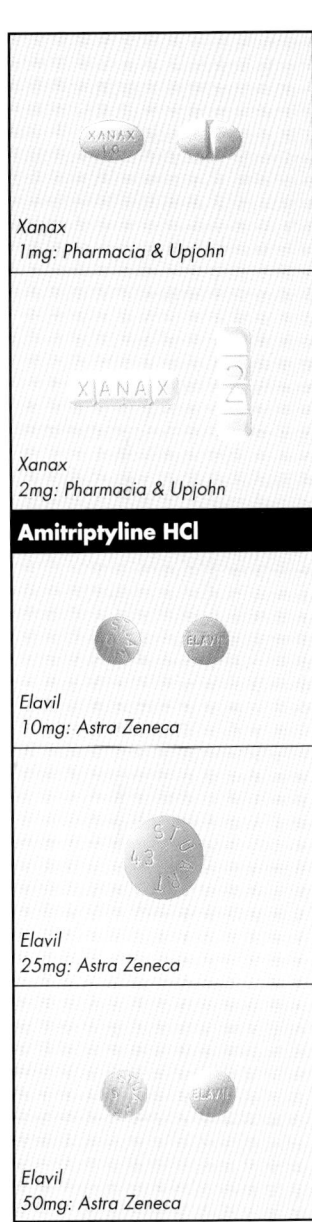

Alendronate Sodium

Fosamax
5mg: Merck

Fosamax
10mg: Merck

Fosamax
40mg: Merck

Alprazolam

Xanax
0.25mg: Pharmacia & Upjohn

Xanax
0.5mg: Pharmacia & Upjohn

Xanax
1mg: Pharmacia & Upjohn

Xanax
2mg: Pharmacia & Upjohn

Amitriptyline HCl

Elavil
10mg: Astra Zeneca

Elavil
25mg: Astra Zeneca

Elavil
50mg: Astra Zeneca

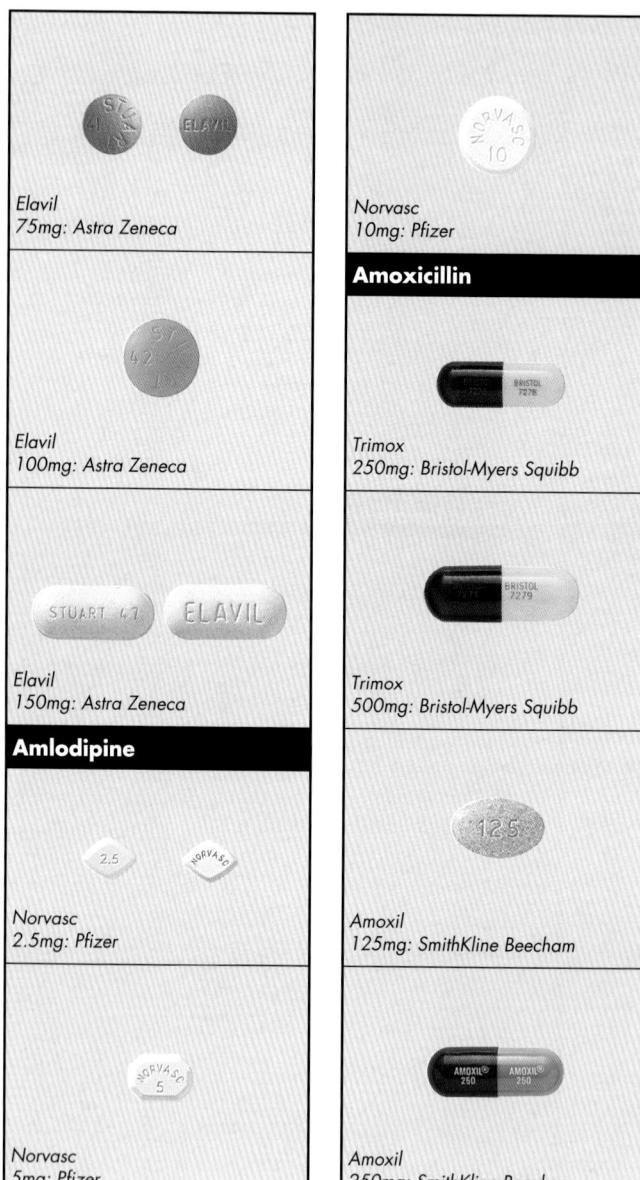

Elavil
75mg: Astra Zeneca

Elavil
100mg: Astra Zeneca

Elavil
150mg: Astra Zeneca

Amlodipine

Norvasc
2.5mg: Pfizer

Norvasc
5mg: Pfizer

Norvasc
10mg: Pfizer

Amoxicillin

Trimox
250mg: Bristol-Myers Squibb

Trimox
500mg: Bristol-Myers Squibb

Amoxil
125mg: SmithKline Beecham

Amoxil
250mg: SmithKline Beecham

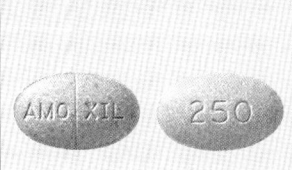

Amoxil
250mg: SmithKline Beecham

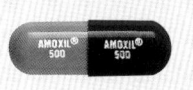

Amoxil
500mg: SmithKline Beecham

Amoxicillin; Clavulanate

Augmentin
125/31.25mg: SmithKline Beecham

Augmentin
200mg: SmithKline Beecham

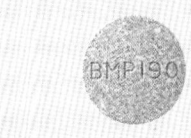

Augmentin
250/62.5mg: SmithKline Beecham

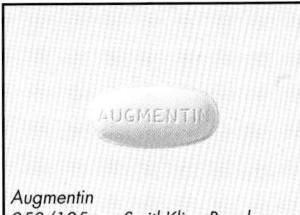

Augmentin
250/125mg: SmithKline Beecham

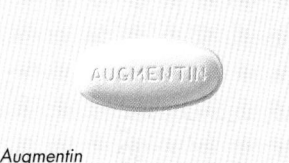

Augmentin
500/125mg: SmithKline Beecham

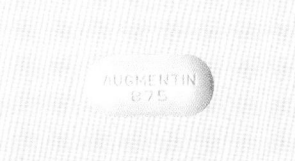

Augmentin
875/125mg: SmithKline Beecham

Atenolol; Chlorthalidone

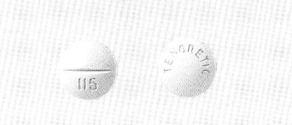

Tenoretic
50/25mg: Astra Zeneca

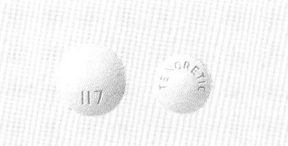

Tenoretic
100/25mg: Astra Zeneca

Atorvastatin Calcium

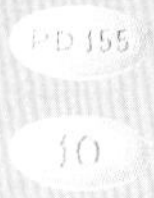

Lipitor
10mg: Parke-Davis

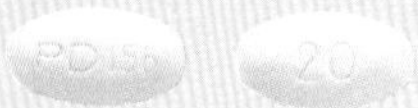

Lipitor
20mg: Parke-Davis

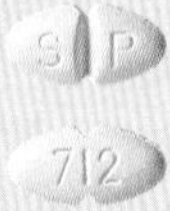

Lipitor
40mg: Parke-Davis

Azithromycin

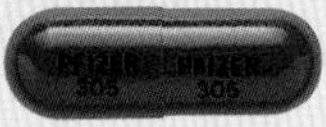

Zithromax
250mg: Pfizer

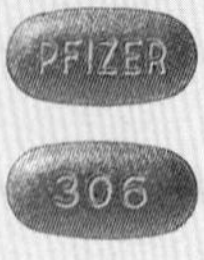

Zithromax
250mg: Pfizer

Bupropion HCl

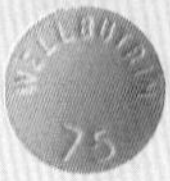

Wellbutrin
75mg: Glaxo Wellcome

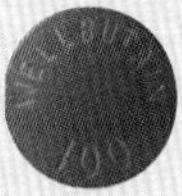

Wellbutrin
100mg: Glaxo Wellcome

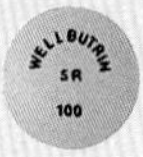

Wellbutrin SR
100mg: Glaxo Wellcome

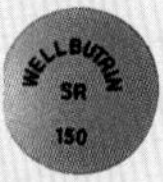

Wellbutrin SR
150mg: Glaxo Wellcome

Celecoxib

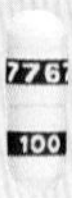

Celebrex
100mg: Searle

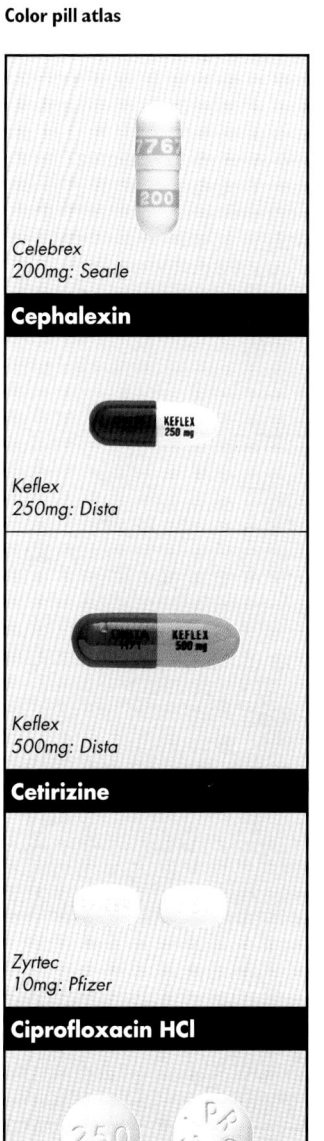

Celebrex
200mg: Searle

Cephalexin

Keflex
250mg: Dista

Keflex
500mg: Dista

Cetirizine

Zyrtec
10mg: Pfizer

Ciprofloxacin HCl

Cipro
250mg: Miles

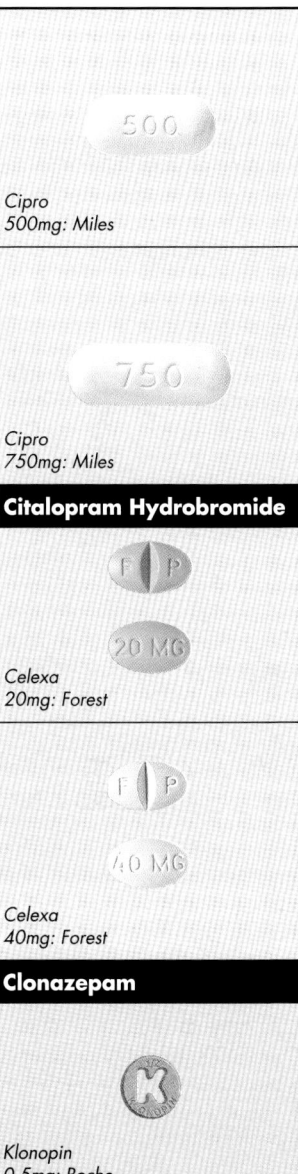

Cipro
500mg: Miles

Cipro
750mg: Miles

Citalopram Hydrobromide

Celexa
20mg: Forest

Celexa
40mg: Forest

Clonazepam

Klonopin
0.5mg: Roche

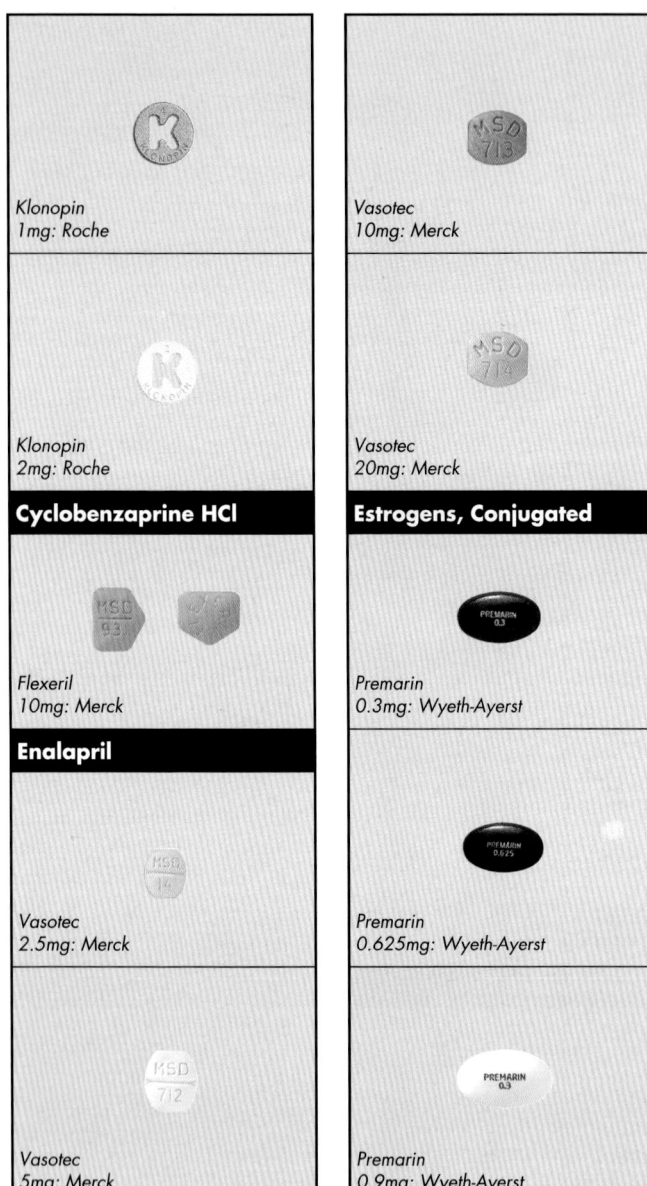

Klonopin
1mg: Roche

Klonopin
2mg: Roche

Cyclobenzaprine HCl

Flexeril
10mg: Merck

Enalapril

Vasotec
2.5mg: Merck

Vasotec
5mg: Merck

Vasotec
10mg: Merck

Vasotec
20mg: Merck

Estrogens, Conjugated

Premarin
0.3mg: Wyeth-Ayerst

Premarin
0.625mg: Wyeth-Ayerst

Premarin
0.9mg: Wyeth-Ayerst

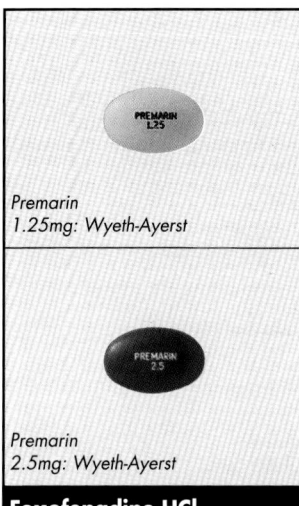

Premarin
1.25mg: Wyeth-Ayerst

Premarin
2.5mg: Wyeth-Ayerst

Fexofenadine HCl

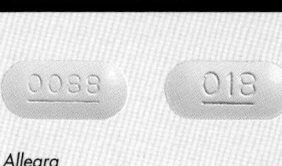

Allegra
180mg: Aventis

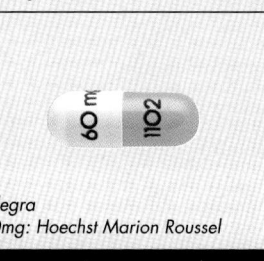

Allegra
60mg: Hoechst Marion Roussel

Fluconazole

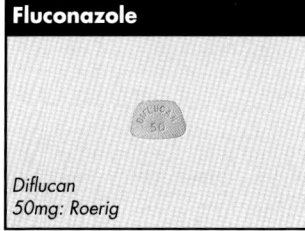

Diflucan
50mg: Roerig

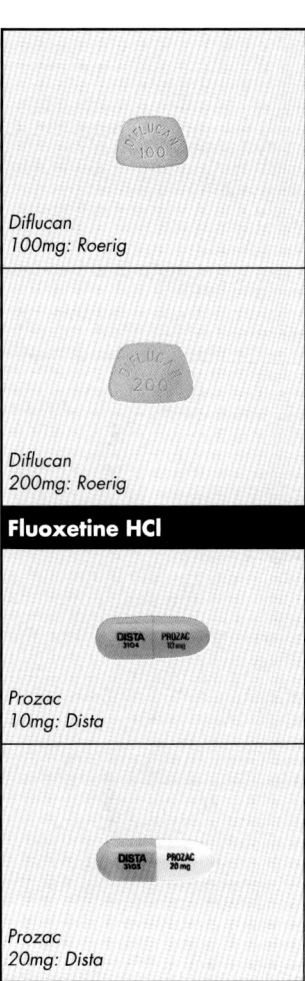

Diflucan
100mg: Roerig

Diflucan
200mg: Roerig

Fluoxetine HCl

Prozac
10mg: Dista

Prozac
20mg: Dista

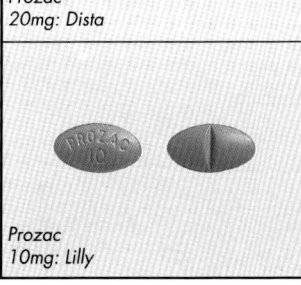

Prozac
10mg: Lilly

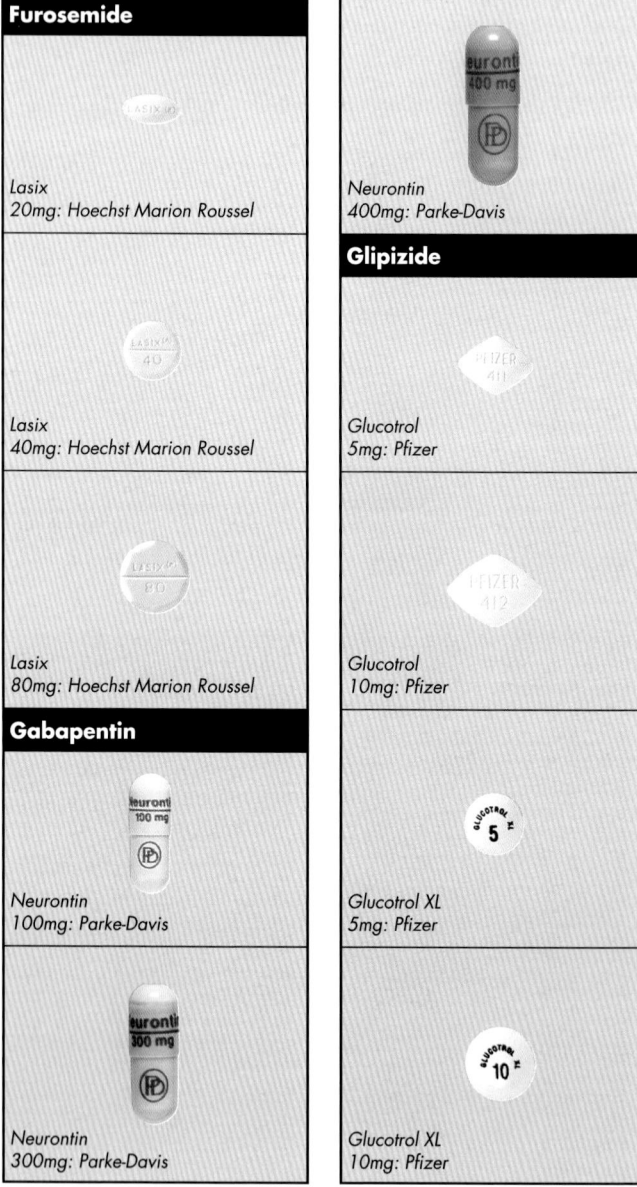

Furosemide

Lasix
20mg: Hoechst Marion Roussel

Lasix
40mg: Hoechst Marion Roussel

Lasix
80mg: Hoechst Marion Roussel

Gabapentin

Neurontin
100mg: Parke-Davis

Neurontin
300mg: Parke-Davis

Neurontin
400mg: Parke-Davis

Glipizide

Glucotrol
5mg: Pfizer

Glucotrol
10mg: Pfizer

Glucotrol XL
5mg: Pfizer

Glucotrol XL
10mg: Pfizer

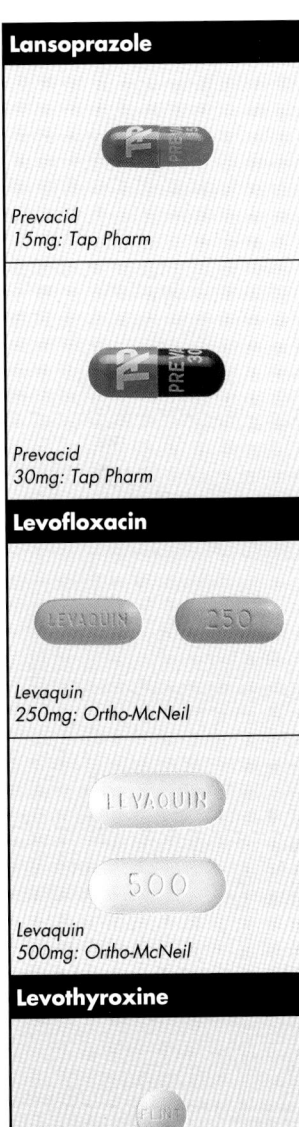

Hydrochlorothiazide

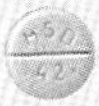

HydroDIURIL
25mg: Merck

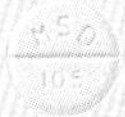

HydroDIURIL
50mg: Merck

Ibuprofen

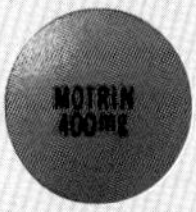

Motrin
400mg: Pharmacia & Upjohn

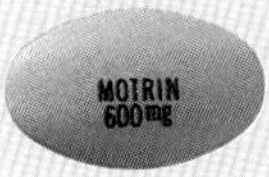

Motrin
600mg: Pharmacia & Upjohn

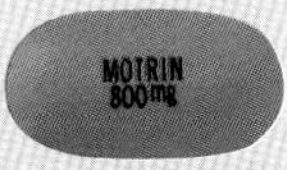

Motrin
800mg: Pharmacia & Upjohn

Lansoprazole

Prevacid
15mg: Tap Pharm

Prevacid
30mg: Tap Pharm

Levofloxacin

Levaquin
250mg: Ortho-McNeil

Levaquin
500mg: Ortho-McNeil

Levothyroxine

Synthroid
0.025mg: Knoll

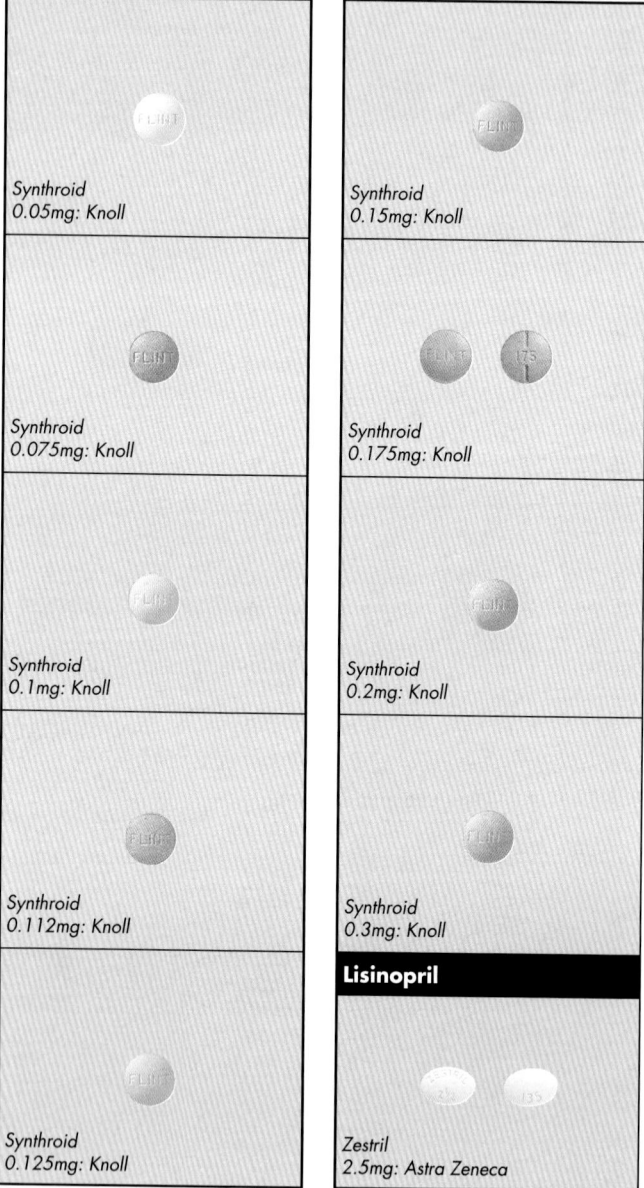

Synthroid
0.05mg: Knoll

Synthroid
0.075mg: Knoll

Synthroid
0.1mg: Knoll

Synthroid
0.112mg: Knoll

Synthroid
0.125mg: Knoll

Synthroid
0.15mg: Knoll

Synthroid
0.175mg: Knoll

Synthroid
0.2mg: Knoll

Synthroid
0.3mg: Knoll

Lisinopril

Zestril
2.5mg: Astra Zeneca

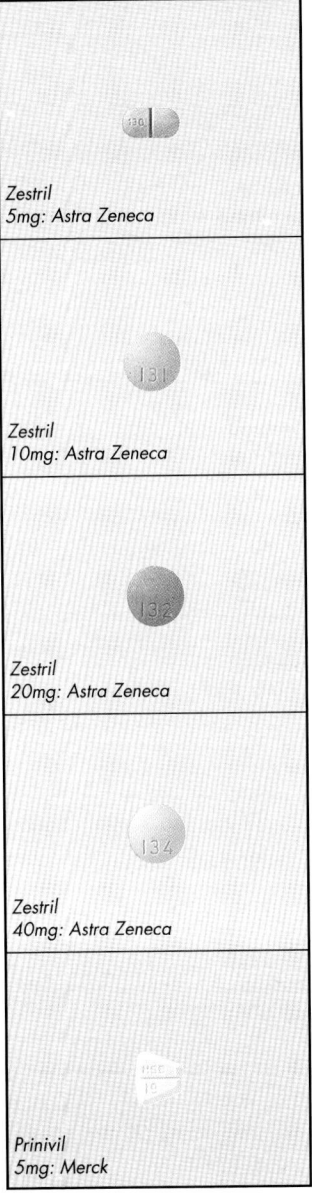

Zestril
5mg: Astra Zeneca

Zestril
10mg: Astra Zeneca

Zestril
20mg: Astra Zeneca

Zestril
40mg: Astra Zeneca

Prinivil
5mg: Merck

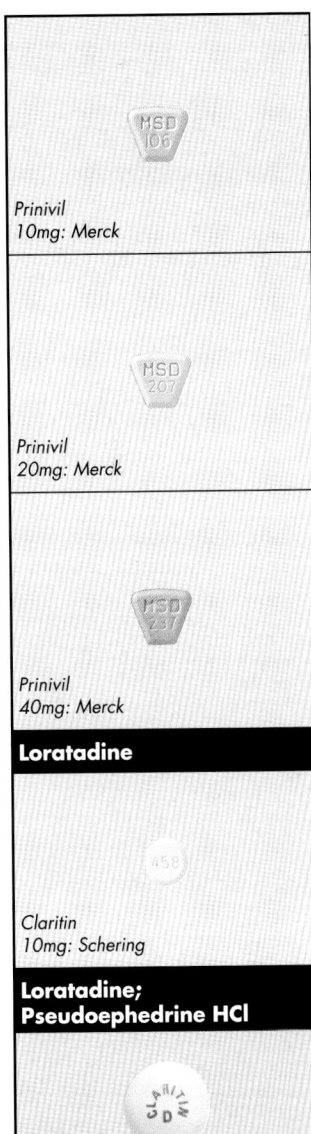

Prinivil
10mg: Merck

Prinivil
20mg: Merck

Prinivil
40mg: Merck

Loratadine

Claritin
10mg: Schering

**Loratadine;
Pseudoephedrine HCl**

Claritin D
5/120mg: Schering

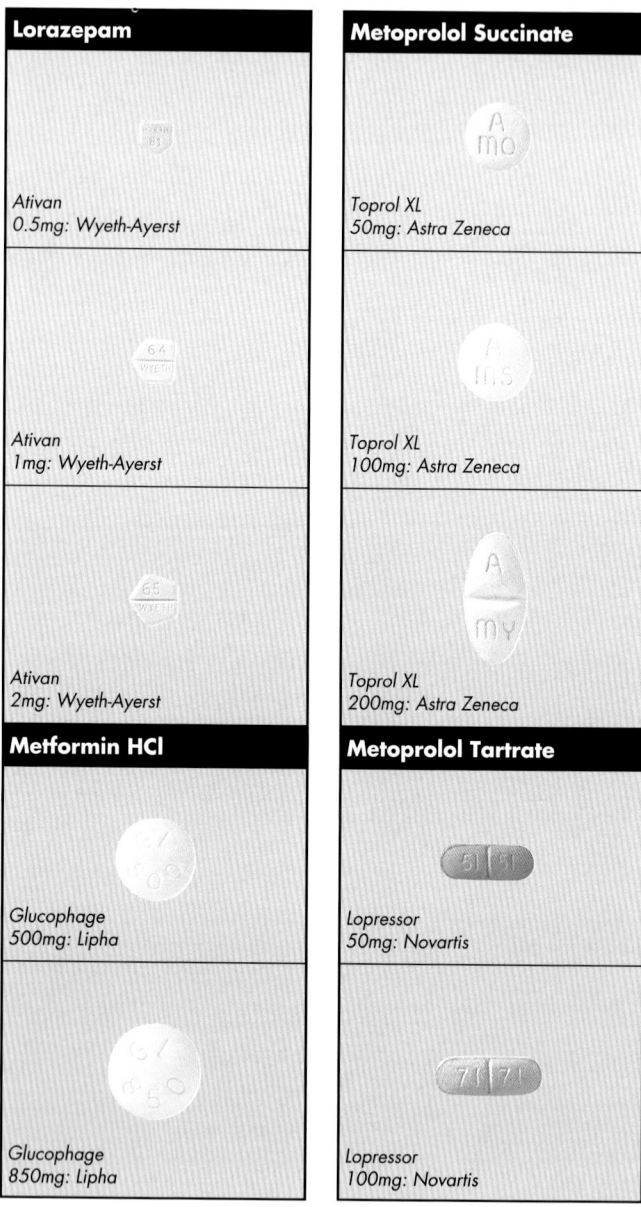

Lorazepam

Ativan
0.5mg: Wyeth-Ayerst

Ativan
1mg: Wyeth-Ayerst

Ativan
2mg: Wyeth-Ayerst

Metformin HCl

Glucophage
500mg: Lipha

Glucophage
850mg: Lipha

Metoprolol Succinate

Toprol XL
50mg: Astra Zeneca

Toprol XL
100mg: Astra Zeneca

Toprol XL
200mg: Astra Zeneca

Metoprolol Tartrate

Lopressor
50mg: Novartis

Lopressor
100mg: Novartis

Montelukast Sodium

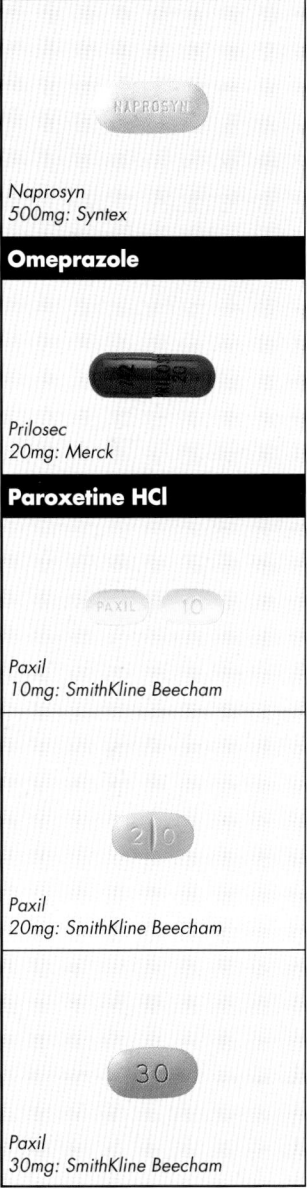

Singulair
4mg: Merck

Singulair
5mg: Merck

Singulair
10mg: Merck

Naproxen

Naprosyn
250mg: Syntex

Naprosyn
375mg: Syntex

Naprosyn
500mg: Syntex

Omeprazole

Prilosec
20mg: Merck

Paroxetine HCl

Paxil
10mg: SmithKline Beecham

Paxil
20mg: SmithKline Beecham

Paxil
30mg: SmithKline Beecham

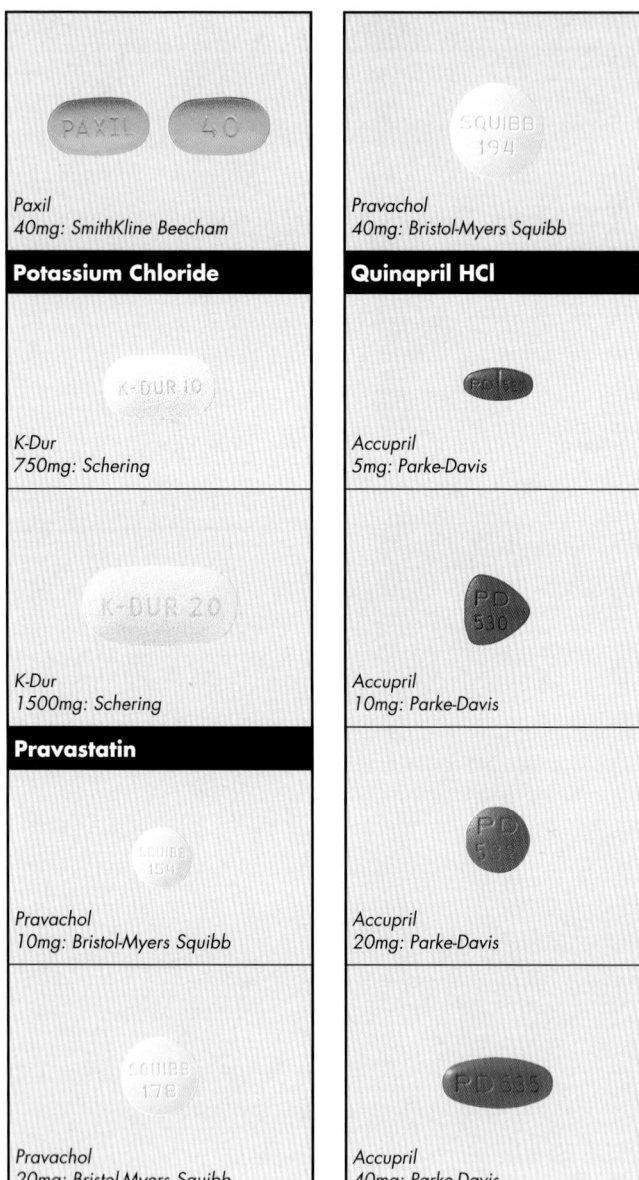

Paxil
40mg: SmithKline Beecham

Pravachol
40mg: Bristol-Myers Squibb

Potassium Chloride

Quinapril HCl

K-Dur
750mg: Schering

Accupril
5mg: Parke-Davis

K-Dur
1500mg: Schering

Accupril
10mg: Parke-Davis

Pravastatin

Pravachol
10mg: Bristol-Myers Squibb

Accupril
20mg: Parke-Davis

Pravachol
20mg: Bristol-Myers Squibb

Accupril
40mg: Parke-Davis

Ranitidine HCl

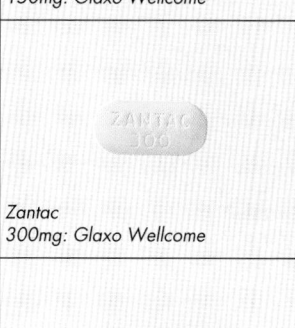

Zantac
150mg: Glaxo Wellcome

Zantac
150mg: Glaxo Wellcome

Zantac
300mg: Glaxo Wellcome

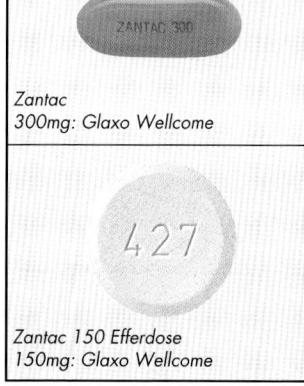

Zantac
300mg: Glaxo Wellcome

Zantac 150 Efferdose
150mg: Glaxo Wellcome

Sertraline HCl

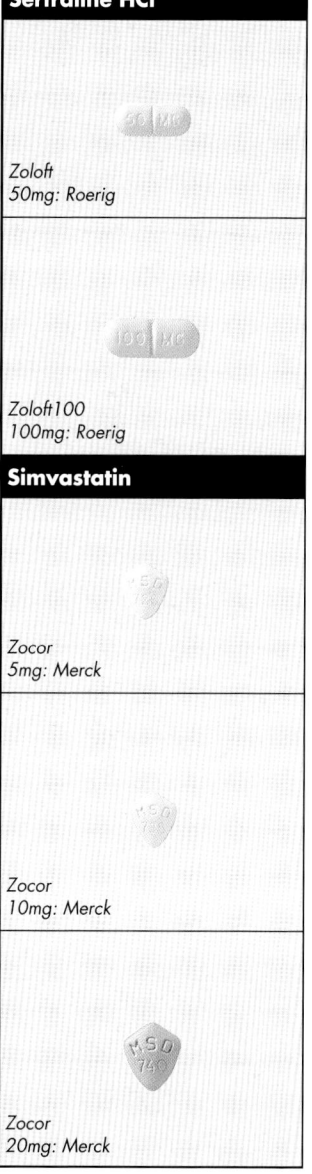

Zoloft
50mg: Roerig

Zoloft100
100mg: Roerig

Simvastatin

Zocor
5mg: Merck

Zocor
10mg: Merck

Zocor
20mg: Merck

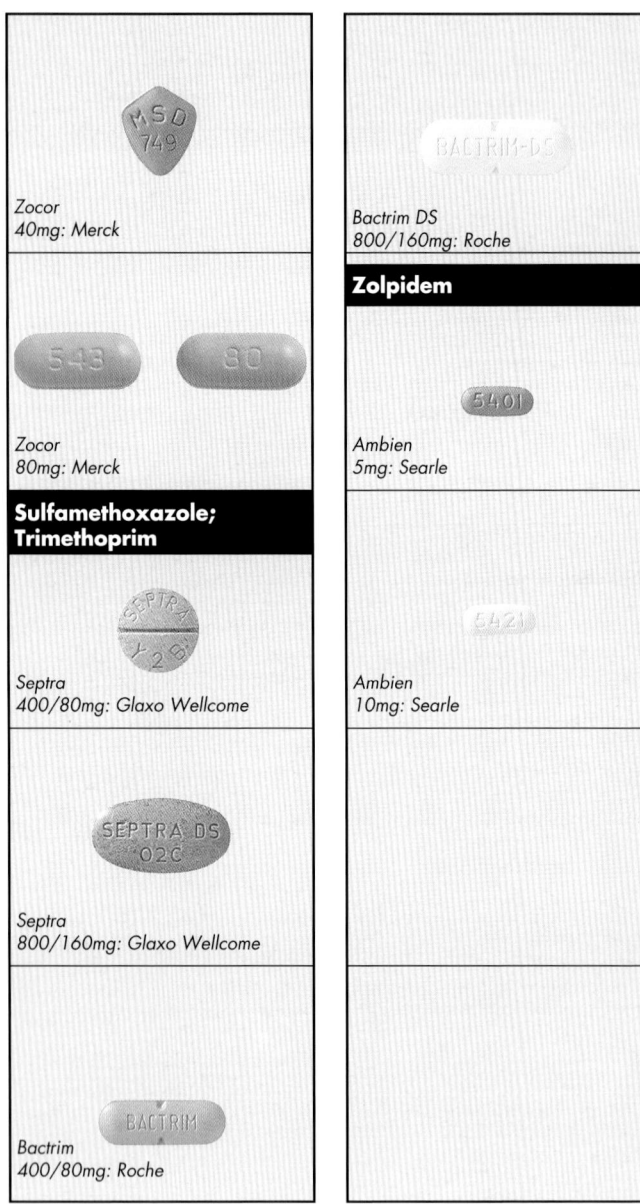

Zocor
40mg: Merck

Zocor
80mg: Merck

Sulfamethoxazole; Trimethoprim

Septra
400/80mg: Glaxo Wellcome

Septra
800/160mg: Glaxo Wellcome

Bactrim
400/80mg: Roche

Bactrim DS
800/160mg: Roche

Zolpidem

Ambien
5mg: Searle

Ambien
10mg: Searle

Human immunodeficiency virus (HIV)
Abacavir (Ziagen)
Amprenavir (Agenerase)
Atazanavir (Reyataz)
Delavirdine (Rescriptor)
Didanosine (Videx)
Efavirenz (Sustiva)
Emtricitabine (Emtriva)
Enfuvirtide (Fuzeon)
Indinavir (Crixivan)
Lamivudine (Epivir)
Lopinavir/ritonavir (Kaletra)
Nelfinavir (Viracept)
Nevirapine (Viramune)
Ritonavir (Norvir)
Saquinavir (Fortovase, Invirase)
Stavudine (Zerit)
Tenofovir (Viread)
Tipranavir (Aptivus)
Zalcitabine (Hivid)
Zidovudine (AZT, Retrovir)

Hypercholesterolemia
Atorvastatin (Lipitor)
Cholestyramine (Questran)
Colesevelam (Welchol)
Colestipol (Colestid)
Ezetimibe (Zetia)
Fenofibrate (Tricor)
Fluvastatin (Lescol)
Gemfibrozil (Lopid)
Lovastatin (Mevacor)
Niacin (Niaspan)
Pravastatin (Pravachol)
Rosuvastatin (Crestor)
Simvastatin (Zocor)

Hyperphosphatemia
Aluminum salts
Calcium salts
Lanthanum (Fosrenol)
Sevelamer (Renagel)

Hypertension
Amiloride (Midamor)
Amlodipine (Norvasc)
Atenolol (Tenormin)
Benazepril (Lotensin)
Bisoprolol (Zebeta)

Candesartan (Atacand)
Captopril (Capoten)
Clonidine (Catapres)
Diltiazem (Cardizem, Dilacor)
Doxazosin (Cardura)
Enalapril (Vasotec)
Eplerenone (Inspra)
Eprosartan (Teveten)
Felodipine (Plendil)
Fosinopril (Monopril)
Hydralazine (Apresoline)
Hydrochlorothiazide (HydroDIURIL)
Indapamide (Lozol)
Irbesartan (Avapro)
Isradipine (DynaCirc)
Labetalol (Normodyne, Trandate)
Lisinopril (Prinivil, Zestril)
Losartan (Cozaar)
Methyldopa (Aldomet)
Metolazone (Diulo, Zaroxolyn)
Metoprolol (Lopressor)
Minoxidil (Loniten)
Moexipril (Univasc)
Nadolol (Corgard)
Nicardipine (Cardene)
Nifedipine (Adalat, Procardia)
Nitroglycerin
Nitroprusside (Nipride)
Olmesartan (Benicar)
Perindopril (Aceon)
Pindolol (Visken)
Prazosin (Minipress)
Propranolol (Inderal)
Quinapril (Accupril)
Ramipril (Altace)
Spironolactone (Aldactone)
Telmisartan (Micardis)
Terazosin (Hytrin)
Timolol (Blocadren)
Trandolapril (Mavik)
Valsartan (Dovan)
Verapamil (Calan, Isoptin)

Hypertriglyceridemia
Atorvastatin (Lipitor)
Fenofibrate (Tricor)
Fluvastatin (Lescol)
Gemfibrozil (Lopid)
Lovastatin (Mevacor)
Niacin (Niaspan)

Pravastatin (Pravachol)
Rosuvastatin (Crestor)
Simvastatin (Zocor)

Hyperuricemia
Allopurinol (Zyloprim)
Colchicine
Probenecid (Benemid)

Hypotension
Norepinephrine (Levophed)
Phenylephrine (Neo-Synephrine)

Hypothyroidism
Levothyroxine (Levoxyl, Synthroid)
Liothyronine (Cytomel)
Thyroid

Idiopathic thrombocytopenic purpura (ITP)
Azathioprine (Imuran)
Cyclophosphamide (Cytoxan)
Danazol (Danocrine)
Dexamethasone (Decadron)
Prednisone

Insomnia
Diphenhydramine (Benadryl)
Estazolam (ProSom)
Eszopiclone (Lunesta)
Flurazepam (Dalmane)
Ramelteon (Rozerem)
Temazepam (Restoril)
Triazolam (Halcion)
Zaleplon (Sonata)
Zolpidem (Ambien)

Migraine headaches
Almotriptan (Axert)
Amitriptyline (Elavil, Endep)
Dihydroergotamine
Eletriptan (Relpax)
Ergotamine (Ergomar)
Frovatriptan (Frovan)
Naratriptan (Amerge)
Propranolol (Inderal)
Rizatriptan (Maxalt)
Sumatriptan (Imitrex)
Zolmitriptan (Zomig)

Multiple sclerosis (MS)
Glatiramer (Copaxone)
Interferon beta-1a (Avonex, Rebif)
Interferon beta-1b (Betaseron)
Mitoxantrone (Novantrone)
Natalizumab (Tysabri)

Myocardial infarction (MI)
Alteplase (Activase)
Aspirin
Atenolol (Tenormin)
Captopril (Capoten)
Clopidogrel (Plavix)
Dalteparin (Fragmin)
Diltiazem (Cardizem, Dilacor)
Enalapril (Vasotec)
Enoxaparin (Lovenox)
Heparin
Lidocaine
Lisinopril (Prinivil, Zestril)
Metoprolol (Lopressor)
Morphine
Nitroglycerin
Propranolol (Inderal)
Quinapril (Accupril)
Ramipril (Altace)
Reteplase (Retavase)
Streptokinase
Timolol (Blocadren)
Verapamil (Calan, Isoptin)
Warfarin (Coumadin)

Nausea
Aprepitant (Emend)
Chlorpromazine (Thorazine)
Dexamethasone (Decadron)
Dimenhydrinate (Dramamine)
Dolasetron (Anzemet)
Dronabinol (Marinol)
Droperidol (Inapsine)
Granisetron (Kytril)
Hydroxyzine (Vistaril)
Lorazepam (Ativan)
Meclizine (Antivert)
Metoclopramide (Reglan)
Ondansetron (Zofran)
Palonosetron (Aloxi)
Prochlorperazine (Compazine)
Promethazine (Phenergan)
Trimethobenzamide (Tigan)

Obsessive-compulsive disorder (OCD)
Citalopram (Celexa)
Clomipramine (Anafranil)
Fluoxetine (Prozac)
Fluvoxamine Paroxetine (Paxil)
Sertraline (Zoloft)

Osteoporosis
Alendronate (Fosamax)
Calcitonin (Miacalcin)
Calcium salts
Conjugated estrogens (Premarin)
Estradiol (Estrace)
Ibandronate (Boniva)
Raloxifene (Evista)
Risedronate (Actonel)
Teriparatide (Forteo)
Vitamin D

Paget's disease
Alendronate (Fosamax)
Calcitonin (Miacalcin)
Etidronate (Didronel)
Pamidronate (Aredia)
Risedronate (Actonel)
Tiludronate (Skelid)

Pain, mild to moderate
Acetaminophen (Tylenol)
Aspirin
Celecoxib (Celebrex)
Codeine
Diclofenac (Cataflam, Voltaren)
Diflunisal (Dolobid)
Etodolac (Lodine)
Flurbiprofen (Ansaid)
Ibuprofen (Advil, Motrin)
Ketorolac (Toradol)
Naproxen (Anaprox, Naprosyn)
Propoxyphene (Darvon)
Salsalate (Disalcid)
Tramadol (Ultram)

Pain, moderate to severe
Butorphanol (Stadol)
Fentanyl (Sublimaze)
Hydromorphone (Dilaudid)
Meperidine (Demerol)
Methadone (Dolophine)

Morphine (MS Contin)
Nalbuphine (Nubain)
Oxycodone (OxyFast, Roxicodone)
Ziconotide (Prialt)

Panic attack disorder
Alprazolam (Xanax)
Clonazepam (Klonopin)
Paroxetine (Paxil)
Sertraline (Zoloft)

Parkinsonism
Amantadine (Symmetrel)
Apomorphine (Apokyn)
Bromocriptine (Parlodel)
Carbidopa/levodopa (Sinemet)
Diphenhydramine (Benadryl)
Entacapone (Comtan)
Pergolide (Permax)
Pramipexole (Mirapex)
Ropinirole (Requip)
Selegiline (Eldepryl)
Tolcapone (Tasmar)

Peptic ulcer disease
Cimetidine (Tagamet)
Esomeprazole (Nexium)
Famotidine (Pepcid)
Lansoprazole (Prevacid)
Misoprostol (Cytotec)
Nizatidine (Axid)
Omeprazole (Prilosec)
Pantoprazole (Protonix)
Rabeprazole (Aciphex)
Ranitidine (Zantac)
Sucralfate (Carafate)

Pneumonia
Amoxicillin (Amoxil)
Amoxicillin/clavulanate (Augmentin)
Ampicillin (Polycillin)
Azithromycin (Zithromax)
Cefaclor (Ceclor)
Cefpodoxime (Vantin)
Ceftriaxone (Rocephin)
Cefuroxime (Kefurox, Zinacef)
Clarithromycin (Biaxin)
Co-trimoxazole (Bactrim, Septra)
Dirithromycin (Dynabac)
Erythromycin
Gentamicin (Garamycin)

Loracarbef (Lorabid)
Piperacillin/tazobactam (Zosyn)
Tobramycin (Nebcin)
Vancomycin (Vancocin)

Pneumonia, *Pneumocystis carinii*
Atovaquone (Mepron)
Clindamycin (Cleocin)
Co-trimoxazole (Bactrim, Septra)
Pentamidine (Pentam)
Trimethoprim (Proloprim)

Pruritus
Amcinonide (Cyclocort)
Brompheniramine (Dimetane)
Cetirizine (Zyrtec)
Chlorpheniramine (Dimetane)
Clemastine (Tavist)
Clobetasol (Temovate)
Cyproheptadine (Periactin)
Desloratadine (Clarinex)
Desonide (Tridesilon)
Desoximetasone (Topicort)
Diphenhydramine (Benadryl)
Fluocinolone (Synalar)
Fluocinonide (Lidex)
Halobetasol (Ultravate)
Hydrocortisone (Cort-Dome, Hytone)
Hydroxyzine (Atarax, Vistaril)
Prednisolone (Prelone)
Prednisone (Deltasone)
Promethazine (Phenergan)

Psychosis
Aripiprazole (Abilify)
Chlorpromazine (Thorazine)
Clozapine (Clozaril)
Fluphenazine (Prolixin)
Haloperidol (Haldol)
Lithium (Lithobid)
Olanzapine (Zyprexa)
Perphenazine (Trilafon)
Quetiapine (Seroquel)
Risperidone (Risperdal)
Thioridazine (Mellaril)
Thiothixene (Navane)
Ziprasidone (Geodon)

Pulmonary arterial hypertension
Bosentan (Tracleer)
Epoprostenol (Flolan)

Iloprost (Ventavis)
Sildenafil (Revatio)
Treprostinil (Remodulin)

Respiratory distress syndrome (RDS)
Beractant (Survanta)
Calfactant (Infasurf)
Poractant alfa (Curosurf)

Schizophrenia
Aripiprazole (Abilify)
Chlorpromazine (Thorazine)
Clozapine (Clozaril)
Fluphenazine (Prolixin)
Haloperidol (Haldol)
Lithium (Lithobid)
Olanzapine (Zyprexa)
Perphenazine (Trilafon)
Quetiapine (Seroquel)
Risperidone (Risperdal)
Thioridazine (Mellaril)
Thiothixene (Navane)
Ziprasidone (Geodon)

Smoking cessation
Bupropion (Zyban)
Clonidine (Catapres)
Nicotine (Nicoderm, Nicotrol)

Thrombosis
Dalteparin (Fragmin)
Enoxaparin (Lovenox)
Heparin
Tinzaparin (Innohep)
Warfarin (Coumadin)

Thyroid disorders
Levothyroxine (Levoxyl, Synthroid)
Liothyronine (Cytomel)
Thyroid

Transient ischemic attack (TIA)
Aspirin
Clopidogrel (Plavix)
Ticlopidine (Ticlid)
Warfarin (Coumadin)

Tremor
Atenolol (Tenormin)
Chlordiazepoxide (Librium)
Diazepam (Valium)

Lorazepam (Ativan)
Metoprolol (Lopressor)
Nadolol (Corgard)
Propranolol (Inderal)

Tuberculosis (TB)
Ethambutol (Myambutol)
Isoniazid (INH)
Pyrazinamide
Rifabutin (Mycobutin)
Rifampin (Rifadin)
Rifapentine (Priftin)
Streptomycin

Urticaria
Cetirizine (Zyrtec)
Cimetidine (Tagamet)
Clemastine (Tavist)
Cyproheptadine (Periactin)
Diphenhydramine (Benadryl)
Hydroxyzine (Atarax, Vistaril)
Loratadine (Claritin)
Promethazine (Phenergan)
Ranitidine (Zantac)

Vertigo
Dimenhydrinate (Dramamine)
Diphenhydramine (Benadryl)
Meclizine (Antivert)
Scopolamine (Trans-Derm Scop)

Vomiting
Aprepitant (Emend)
Chlorpromazine (Thorazine)
Dexamethasone (Decadron)
Dimenhydrinate (Dramamine)
Dolasetron (Anzemet)
Dronabinol (Marinol)
Droperidol (Inapsine)
Granisetron (Kytril)
Hydroxyzine (Vistaril)
Lorazepam (Ativan)
Meclizine (Antivert)
Metoclopramide (Reglan)
Ondansetron (Zofran)
Palonosetron (Aloxi)
Prochlorperazine (Compazine)
Promethazine (Phenergan)
Trimethobenzamide (Tigan)

Zollinger-Ellison syndrome
Aluminum salts
Cimetidine (Tagamet)
Esomeprazole (Nexim)
Famotidine (Pepcid)
Lansoprazole (Prevacid)
Omeprazole (Prilosec)
Pantoprazole (Protonix)
Rabeprazole (Aciphex)
Ranitidine (Zantac)

Drug Classification Contents

anesthetics: general
anesthetics: local
anesthetics: local topical
angiotensin-converting enzyme (ACE)
   inhibitors
angiotensin II receptor antagonists
antacids
antianxiety
antiarrhythmics
antibiotics
antibiotic: aminoglycosides
antibiotic: cephalosporins
antibiotic: fluoroquinolones
antibiotic: macrolides
antibiotic: penicillins
anticoagulants/antiplatelets/
   thrombolytics
anticonvulsants
antidepressants
antidiabetics
antidiarrheals
antifungals: topical
antiglaucoma agents
antihistamines
antihyperlipidemics
antihypertensives
antimigraine (triptans)
antipsychotics
antivirals
beta-adrenergic blockers
bronchodilators
calcium channel blockers

cancer chemotherapeutic agents
cardiac glycosides (inotropic agents)
cholinergic agonists/anticholinesterase
corticosteroids
corticosteroids: topical
diuretics
fertility agents
H_2 antagonists
hematinic preparations
hormones
human immunodeficiency virus
   (HIV) infection
immunosuppressive agents
laxatives
neuromuscular blockers
nitrates
nonsteroidal anti-inflammatory drugs
   (NSAIDs)
nutrition: enteral
nutrition: parenteral
obesity management
opioid analgesics
oral contraceptives
parkinson's disease treatment
proton pump inhibitors
sedative-hypnotics
skeletal muscle relaxants
smoking cessation agents
sympathomimetics
thyroid
vitamins

Anesthetics: General

USES

IV anesthetic agents are used to induce general anesthesia. The general anesthetic state consists of unconsciousness, amnesia, analgesia, immobility, and attenuation of autonomic responses to noxious stimuli.

Volatile inhalation agents produce all the components of the anesthetic state but are administered through the lungs via an anesthesia machine. Agents for use include desflurane, sevoflurane, isoflurane, enflurane, and halothane.

General anesthetics are medications producing unconsciousness and a lack of response to all painful stimuli.

ACTION

IV anesthetic agents: Most agents produce CNS depression by action on the GABA receptor complex. GABA is the primary inhibitory neurotransmitter in the CNS. Ketamine produces dissociation between the thalamus and the limbic system.

Volatile inhalation agents: Not fully understood but may disrupt neuronal transmission throughout the CNS. These agents may either block excitatory or enhance inhibitory transmission through axons or synapses.

ANESTHETICS: GENERAL

Name	Availability	Uses	Dosage Range	Side Effects
Etomidate (Amidate)	I: 2 mg/ml	IV induction	0.2–0.6 mg/kg	Myoclonus, pain on injection, nausea, vomiting, respiratory depression
Ketamine (p. 653) (Ketalar)	I: 10 mg/ml, 50 mg/ml, 100 mg/ml	Analgesia, sedation, IV induction	1–4.5 mg/kg	Delirium, euphoria, nausea, vomiting
Methohexital (Brevital)	Powder for injection: 500 mg	IV induction, sedation	50–120 mg	Cardiovascular depression, myoclonus, nausea, vomiting, respiratory depression

Midazolam (p. 772) (Versed)	**I:** 1 mg/ml, 5 mg/ml	Anxiolytic, amnesic, sedation	1–5 mg titrated slowly	Respiratory depression
Propofol (p. 976) (Diprivan)	**I:** 10 mg/ml	Sedation IV induction Maintenance	0.5 mg/kg 2–2.5 mg/kg 100–200 mcg/ kg/min	Cardiovascular depression, delirium, euphoria, pain on injection, respiratory depression
Thiopental (Pentothal)	**Powder for injection:** 2.5% (25 mg/ml)	IV induction	Titrate vs. patient response. **Average:** 50–75 mg	Cardiovascular depression, nausea, vomiting, respiratory depression

I, Injection.

Anesthetics: Local

USES

Local anesthetics suppress pain by blocking impulses along axons. Suppression of pain does not cause generalized depression of the entire nervous system. Local anesthetics may be given topically and by injection (local infiltration, peripheral nerve block [axillary], IV regional [bier block], epidural, and spinal).

ACTION

Most local anesthetics fall into one of two groups: esters or amides. Both provide anesthesia and analgesia by reversibly binding to and blocking sodium (Na) channels. This slows the rate of depolarization of the nerve action potential; thus, propagation of the electrical impulses needed for nerve conduction is prevented.

(continued)

Anesthetics: Local   *(continued)*

ANESTHETICS: LOCAL

Name	Uses	Onset (min)	Duration (hours)	Side Effects
Esters				
Chloroprocaine (Nesacaine)	Local infiltrate, nerve block, spinal	6–12	0.25–0.5	Excitation (e.g., seizures) followed by decreased level of consciousness (drowsiness to unconsciousness), bradycardia, heart block, decreased myocardial contractile force, hypotension, hypersensitivity reaction
Procaine (Novocaine)	Local infiltrate, nerve block, spinal	2–5	0.25–1	Same as above
Tetracaine	Topical, spinal	15	2–3	Same as above
Amides				
Bupivacaine (Marcaine, Sensorcaine)	Local infiltrate, nerve block, epidural, spinal	5	2–4	Same as above
Etidocaine (Duranest)	Local infiltrate, nerve block, epidural	3–5	5–10	Same as above
Levobupivacaine (Chirocaine)	Nerve block, epidural	—	—	Same as above

Lidocaine (p. 688)	Local infiltrate, nerve block, spinal, epidural, topical, IV regional	Less than 2	0.5–1	Same as above
Mepivacaine (Carbocaine, Polocaine)	Local infiltrate, nerve block, epidural	3–5	0.75–1.5	Same as above
Ropivacaine (Naropin)	Local infiltrate, nerve block, epidural, spinal	1–15	2–6	Same as above

Note: Most side effects are manifestations of excessive plasma concentrations.

Anesthetics: Local Topical

ANESTHETICS: LOCAL TOPICAL

Name	Indications	Peak Effect (min)	Duration (min)
Amides			
Dibucaine (Nupercainal)	Skin	Less than 5	15–45
Lidocaine (p. 688)	Skin, mucous membranes	2–5	15–45

(continued)

ANESTHETICS: LOCAL TOPICAL (continued)

Name	Indications	Peak Effect (min)	Duration (min)
Esters			
Benzocaine	Skin, mucous membranes	Less than 5	15–45
Cocaine (p. 280) ©	Mucous membranes	2–5	30–60
Tetracaine (Pontocaine)	Skin, mucous membranes	3–8	30–60

Angiotensin-Converting Enzyme (ACE) Inhibitors

USES

Treatment of hypertension (HTN), adjunctive therapy for congestive heart failure (CHF).

ACTION

Antihypertensive: Exact mechanism unknown. May be related to competitive inhibition of angiotensin I converting enzyme (ACE) activity causing decreased conversion of angiotensin I to angiotensin II, a potent vasoconstrictor. Reduces peripheral arterial resistance.

Congestive heart failure: Decreases peripheral vascular resistance (afterload), pulmonary capillary wedge pressure (preload), improves cardiac output, exercise tolerance.

ACE INHIBITORS

Name	Availability	Uses	Dosage Range (per day)	Side Effects
Benazepril (p. 125) (Lotensin)	**T:** 5 mg, 10 mg, 20 mg, 40 mg	HTN	**HTN:** 5–80 mg	Headaches, dizziness, fatigue, cough
Captopril (p. 180) (Capoten)	**T:** 12.5 mg, 25 mg, 50 mg, 100 mg	HTN CHF	**HTN:** 50–450 mg **CHF:** 12.5–450 mg	Insomnia, headaches, dizziness, fatigue, GI complaints, cough, rash
Enalapril (p. 408) (Vasotec)	**T:** 2.5 mg, 5 mg, 10 mg, 20 mg **IV:** 1.25 mg/ml	HTN CHF	**HTN:** 10–40 mg; **(IV:** 1.25 mg q6h) **CHF:** 5–20 mg	Chest pain, hypotension, headaches, fatigue, dizziness
Fosinopril (p. 517) (Monopril)	**T:** 10 mg, 20 mg, 40 mg	HTN CHF	**HTN:** 10–80 mg **CHF:** 20–40 mg	Hypotension, nausea, vomiting, cough
Lisinopril (p. 695) (Prinivil, Zestril)	**T:** 2.5 mg, 5 mg, 10 mg, 20 mg, 40 mg	HTN CHF	**HTN:** 10–40 mg **CHF:** 5–20 mg	Chest pain, hypotension, headaches, dizziness, fatigue, diarrhea
Moexipril (p. 789) (Univasc)	**T:** 7.5 mg, 15 mg	HTN	**HTN:** 7.5–30 mg	Dizziness, fatigue, diarrhea, cough
Perindopril (Aceon)	**T:** 2 mg, 4 mg, 6 mg	HTN	**HTN:** 4–16 mg	Hypotension, dizziness, fatigue, syncope, cough
Quinapril (p. 994) (Accupril)	**T:** 5 mg, 10 mg, 20 mg, 40 mg	HTN CHF	**HTN:** 10–80 mg **CHF:** 10–40 mg	Chest pain, hypotension, headaches, dizziness, fatigue, diarrhea, nausea, vomiting, cough
Ramipril (p. 1005) (Altace)	**C:** 1.25 mg, 2.5 mg, 5 mg, 10 mg	HTN CHF	**HTN:** 2.5–20 mg **CHF:** 1.25–10 mg	Hypotension, headaches, dizziness, cough
Trandolapril (p. 1160) (Mavik)	**T:** 1 mg, 2 mg, 4 mg	HTN CHF	**HTN:** 1–4 mg **CHF:** 1–4 mg	Dizziness, dyspepsia, cough, asthenia, syncope, myalgia

C, Capsules; *CHF,* congestive heart failure; *HTN,* hypertension; *IV,* intravenous; *T,* tablets.

Angiotensin II Receptor Antagonists

USES

Treatment of hypertension (HTN) alone or in combination with other antihypertensives.

ACTION

Angiotensin II receptor antagonists (AIIRA) block vasoconstrictor and aldosterone-secreting effects on angiotensin II by selectively blocking the binding of angiotensin II to AT_1 receptors in vascular smooth muscle and adrenal gland, causing vasodilation and a decrease in aldosterone effects.

ANGIOTENSIN II RECEPTOR ANTAGONISTS

Name	Availability	Uses	Dosage Range (per day)	Side Effects
Candesartan (p. 176) (Atacand)	T: 4 mg, 8 mg, 16 mg, 32 mg	HTN	2–32 mg	Headaches, upper respiratory tract infections, pain, dizziness
Eprosartan (p. 426) (Teveten)	T: 400 mg, 600 mg	HTN	400–800 mg	Headaches, upper respiratory tract infections, myalgia
Irbesartan (p. 636) (Avapro)	T: 75 mg, 150 mg, 300 mg	HTN	75–300 mg	Headaches, upper respiratory tract infections
Losartan (p. 711) (Cozaar)	T: 25 mg, 50 mg, 100 mg	HTN	25–100 mg	Dizziness, headaches, upper respiratory tract infections, diarrhea, fatigue, cough
Olmesartan (p. 863) (Benicar)	T: 5 mg, 20 mg, 40 mg	HTN	20–40 mg	Headaches, upper respiratory tract infection, flu-like symptoms, dizziness, bronchitis, rhinitis, back pain, pharyngitis, sinusitis, diarrhea, peripheral edema
Telmisartan (p. 1100) (Micardis)	T: 40 mg, 80 mg	HTN	20–80 mg	Upper respiratory tract infections, dizziness, back pain, sinusitis, diarrhea
Valsartan (p. 1194) (Diovan)	T: 80 mg, 160 mg	HTN	80–320 mg	Dizziness, headaches, upper respiratory tract infections, diarrhea, fatigue

HTN, Hypertension; *T,* tablets.

Antacids

USES

Relief of symptoms associated with hyperacidity (e.g., heartburn, acid indigestion, sour stomach), hyperacidity associated with gastric/duodenal ulcers, treatment of pathologic gastric hypersecretion associated with Zollinger-Ellison syndrome, symptomatic treatment of gastroesophageal reflux disease (GERD), prevention and treatment of upper GI stress-induced ulceration and bleeding (especially in ICU).

Aluminum carbonate and hydroxide in conjunction with a low-phosphate diet to reduce elevated phosphate in patients with renal insufficiency. Calcium for calcium deficiency, magnesium for magnesium deficiency.

ACTION

Act primarily in the stomach to neutralize gastric acid (increase pH). Antacids do not have a direct effect on acid output. The ability to increase pH depends on the dose, dosage form used, presence or absence of food in the stomach, and acid-neutralizing capacity (ANC). ANC is the number of mEq of hydrochloric acid that can be neutralized by a particular weight or volume of antacid.

Reduce elevated phosphate by binding with phosphate in the intestine to form an insoluble complex, which is then eliminated.

ANTACIDS

Antacid	Brand Names	Availability	Dosage Range	Side Effects
Aluminum				
Hydroxide (p. 45)	Amphojel, Alu-Tab, Dialume	**T:** 300 mg, 500 mg, 600 mg **C:** 500 mg	500–1,500 mg 3–6 times/day	Chalky taste, mild constipation, abdominal cramps *Long-term use:* Neurotoxicity in dialysis patients, hypercalcemia, osteoporosis *Large doses:* Fecal impaction, peripheral edema

(continued)

ANTACIDS	(continued)			
Antacid	Brand Names	Availability	Dosage Range	Side Effects
Calcium				
Carbonate (p. 172)	Tums, Maalox, Antacid	**T (chewable):** 500 mg, 750 mg, 1,000 mg	500–1,500 mg as needed	Chalky taste *Large doses:* Fecal impaction, peripheral edema, metabolic alkalosis *Long-term use:* Difficult/painful urination
Magnesium				
Hydroxide (p. 717)	Milk of Magnesia	**T (chewable):** 311 mg **L:** 400 mg/5 ml, 800 mg/5 ml	**T:** 622–1,244 mg up to 4 times/day **L:** 2.5–7.5 ml up to 4 times/day	Chalky taste, diarrhea, laxative effect, electrolyte imbalance (dizziness, irregular heartbeat, fatigue)
Oxide (p. 717)	Mag-Ox 400, Maox 420	**T:** 400 mg, 420 mg, 500 mg	400–800 mg/ day	Same as above

C, Capsules; *L,* liquid; *T,* tablets.

Antianxiety

USES

Treatment of anxiety including generalized anxiety disorder (GAD), panic disorder, obsessive-compulsive disorder (OCD), social anxiety disorder (SAD), post-traumatic stress disorder (PTSD), and acute stress disorder. In addition, some benzodiazepines are used as hypnotics, anticonvulsants to prevent delirium tremors during alcohol withdrawal and as adjunctive therapy for relaxation of skeletal muscle spasms. Midazolam, a short-acting benzodiazepine, is used for preoperative sedation and relief of anxiety for short diagnostic/endoscopic procedures (see individual monograph for midazolam).

ACTION

Benzodiazepines are the largest and most frequently prescribed group of antianxiety agents. The exact mechanism is unknown but may increase the inhibiting effect of gamma-aminobutyric acid (GABA), which inhibits nerve impulse transmission by binding to specific benzodiazepine receptors in various areas of the central nervous system (CNS).

◀ **ALERT** ▶ Refer to individual entries of non-benzodiazepine drugs for more information on uses and actions.

ANTIANXIETY AGENTS

Name	Availability	Uses	Dosage Range (per day)	Side Effects
Benzodiazepine				
Alprazolam (p. 39) (Xanax)	**T:** 0.25 mg, 0.5 mg, 1 mg, 2 mg **S:** 0.5 mg/5 ml, 1 mg/ml	Anxiety, panic disorder	0.75–10 mg	Drowsiness, weakness or fatigue, ataxia, slurred speech, confusion, lack of coordination, impaired memory, paradoxical agitation, dizziness, nausea
Chlordiazepoxide (p. 237) @ (Librium, Libritabs)	**C:** 5 mg, 10 mg, 25 mg **T:** 10 mg, 25 mg **I:** 100 mg	Anxiety, alcohol withdrawal	5–300 mg	Same as above
Clorazepate (p. 275) @ (Tranxene)	**C:** 3.75 mg, 7.5 mg, 15 mg **SD:** 11.25 mg, 22.5 mg	Anxiety, alcohol withdrawal, anticonvulsant	7.5–90 mg	Same as above
Diazepam (p. 345) (Valium)	**T:** 2.5 mg, 5 mg, 10 mg **S:** 5 mg/5 ml, 5 mg/ml **I:** 5 mg/ml	Anxiety, alcohol withdrawal, anticonvulsant, muscle relaxant	2–40 mg	Same as above

(continued)

ANTIANXIETY AGENTS *(continued)*

Name	Availability	Uses	Dosage Range (per day)	Side Effects
Benzodiazepine *(continued)*				
Lorazepam (p. **709**) (Ativan)	**T:** 0.5 mg, 1 mg, 2 mg **S:** 2 mg/ml **I:** 2 mg/ml, 4 mg/ml	Anxiety	0.5–10 mg	Same as above
Oxazepam (p. **878**) (Serax)	**C:** 10 mg, 15 mg, 30 mg **T:** 15 mg	Anxiety, alcohol withdrawal	30–120 mg	Same as above
Nonbenzodiazepine				
Buspirone (p. **163**) (BuSpar)	**T:** 5 mg, 10 mg, 15 mg, 30 mg	Anxiety	7.5–60 mg	Dizziness, lightheadedness, headaches, nausea, restlessness
Hydroxyzine (p. **591**) (Atarax, Vistaril)	**T:** 10 mg, 25 mg, 50 mg, 100 mg	Anxiety, rhinitis, pruritus, urticaria, nausea or vomiting	100–400 mg	Drowsiness; dry mouth, nose, and throat
Paroxetine (p. **897**) (Paxil)	**S:** 10 mg/5 ml **T:** 10 mg, 20 mg, 30 mg, 40 mg **T(CR):** 12.5 mg, 25 mg, 37.5 mg	Anxiety, depression, obsessive-compulsive disorder, panic disorder	10–50 mg	Drowsiness; dry mouth, nose, and throat; dizziness; diarrhea; diaphoresis; constipation; vomiting; tremors
Trazodone (p. **1165**) (Desyrel)	**T:** 50 mg, 100 mg, 150 mg, 300 mg	Anxiety, depression	100–400 mg	Drowsiness, dizziness, headaches, dry mouth, nausea, vomiting, unpleasant taste
Venlafaxine (p. **1201**) (Effexor)	**C:** 37.5 mg, 75 mg, 150 mg	Anxiety, depression	37.5–225 mg	Drowsiness, nausea, headaches, dry mouth

C, Capsules; *CR*, controlled-release; *I*, injection; *S*, solution; *SD*, single dose; *T*, tablets.

Antiarrhythmics

USES

Prevention and treatment of cardiac arrhythmias, such as premature ventricular contractions, ventricular tachycardia, premature atrial contractions, paroxysmal atrial tachycardia, atrial fibrillation and flutter.

ACTION

The antiarrhythmics are divided into four classes based on their effects on certain ion channels and/or receptors located on the myocardial cell membrane. Class I is further divided into three subclasses (IA, IB, IC) based on electrophysiologic effects.

Class I: Block cardiac sodium channels and slow conduction velocity, prolonging refractoriness and decreasing automaticity of sodium-dependent tissue.

Class IA: Block sodium and potassium channels.

Class IB: Shorten the repolarization phase.

Class IC: No effect on repolarization phase, but slow conduction velocity.

Class II: Slow the sinus and atrioventricular (AV) nodal conduction.

Class III: Block cardiac potassium channels, prolonging the repolarization phase of electrical cells.

Class IV: Inhibit the influx calcium through its channels, causing slower conduction through the sinus and AV nodes.

ANTIARRHYTHMICS

Name	Availability	Uses	Dosage Range	Side Effects
Class IA				
Disopyramide (p. 371) @ **(Norpace SR, Norpace CR)**	**C:** 100 mg, 150 mg **C(ER):** 100 mg, 150 mg	AF, WPW, PSVT, PVCs, VT	400–800 mg/day	Dry mouth, blurred vision, urinary retention, CHF, proarrhythmia

(continued)

ANTIARRHYTHMICS	(continued)			
Name	Availability	Uses	Dosage Range	Side Effects
Class IA	*(continued)*			
Procainamide (p. 964) (Pronestyl, Procan-SR)	**T:** 250 mg, 375 mg, 500 mg **C:** 250 mg, 375 mg, 500 mg **T (SR):** 250 mg, 500 mg, 750 mg, 1,000 mg **I:** 100 mg/ml, 500 mg/ml	AF, WPW, PVCs, VT	**A (PO):** 250–500 mg q3h; **(ER):** 250–750 mg q6h	Hypotension, fever, agranulocytosis, SLE, headaches, proarrhythmia
Quinidine (p. 996) (Quinidex, Quinaglute)	**T:** 200 mg, 300 mg **T (ER):** 300 mg, 324 mg **I:** 80 mg/ml	AF, WPW, PVCs VT	**A:** 200–600 mg q2–4h; **(ER):** 300–600 mg q8h	Diarrhea, hypotension, nausea, vomiting, cinchonism, fever, thrombocytopenia, proarrhythmia
Class IB				
Lidocaine (p. 688) (Xylocaine)	**I:** 300 mg for IM **IV Infusion:** 2 mg/ml, 4 mg/ml	PVCs, VT, VF	**IV:** 50–100 mg bolus, then 1–4 mg/min infusion	Drowsiness, agitation, muscle twitching, seizures, paraesthesias, proarrhythmia
Mexiletine (Mexitil)	**C:** 150 mg, 200 mg, 250 mg	PVCs, VT, VF	**A:** 600–1,200 mg/day	Drowsiness, agitation, muscle twitching, seizures, paraesthesias, proarrhythmia, nausea, vomiting
Tocainide (p. 1146) (Tonocard)	**T:** 400 mg, 600 mg	PVCs, VT, VF	**A:** 1,200–1,800 mg/day	Drowsiness, agitation, muscle twitching, seizures, paraesthesias, proarrhythmia, nausea, vomiting, diarrhea, agranulocytosis

Class IC

Flecainide (Tambocor)	**T:** 50 mg, 100 mg, 150 mg	AF, PSVT, life-threatening ventricular arrhythmias	**A:** 200–400 mg/day	Dizziness, tremors, lightheadedness, flushing, blurred vision, metallic taste, proarrhythmia
Moricizine (Ethmozine)	**T:** 200 mg, 250 mg, 300 mg	Life-threatening ventricular arrhythmias	**A:** 600–900 mg/day	Nausea, dizziness, perioral numbness, euphoria
Propafenone (p. 975) (Rythmol)	**T:** 150 mg, 225 mg, 300 mg	PAF, WPW, life-threatening ventricular arrhythmias	**A:** 450–900 mg/day	Dizziness, blurred vision, altered taste, nausea, exacerbation of asthma, proarrhythmia

Class II (Beta-Blockers)

Acebutolol (p. 10) (Sectral)	**C:** 200 mg, 400 mg	AF, A flutter, PSVT, PVCs	**A:** 600–1,200 mg/day	Bradycardia, hypotension, depression, nightmares, fatigue, sexual dysfunction
Esmolol (p. 438) (Brevibloc)	**I:** 10 mg/ml, 250 mg/ml	AF, A flutter, PSVT, PVCs	**A:** 50–200 mcg/kg/min	Hypotension
Propranolol (p. 980) (Inderal)	**T:** 10 mg, 20 mg	AF, A flutter, PSVT, PVCs	**A:** 10–30 mg 3–4 times/day	Bradycardia, hypotension, depression, nightmares, fatigue, sexual dysfunction

(continued)

ANTIARRHYTHMICS *(continued)*

Name	Availability	Uses	Dosage Range	Side Effects
Class III				
Amiodarone (p. 57) (Cordarone, Pacerone)	**T:** 200 mg, 400 mg **I:** 50 mg/ml	AF, PAF, PSVT, life-threatening ventricular arrhythmias	**A (PO):** 800–1,600 mg/day for 1–3 wk, then 600–800 mg/day **(IV):** 150 mg bolus, then IV infusion	Blurred vision, photophobia, constipation, ataxia, proarrhythmia
Dofetilide Ⓔ (Tikosyn)	**C:** 125 mcg, 250 mcg, 500 mcg	AF, A flutter	**A:** Individualized	Torsades de pointes, hypotension
Ibutilide Ⓔ (Corvert)	**I:** 0.1 mg/ml	AF, A flutter	**A (greater than 60 kg):** 1 mg over 10 min **(less than 60 kg):** 0.01 mg/kg over 10 min	Torsades de pointes
Sotalol (p. 1072) (Betapace)	**T:** 80 mg, 120 mg, 160 mg, 240 mg	AF, PAF, PSVT, life-threatening ventricular arrhythmias	**A:** 160–640 mg/day	Fatigue, dizziness, dyspnea, bradycardia, proarrhythmia
Class IV (Calcium Channel Blockers)				
Diltiazem (p. 360) (Cardizem)	**I:** 25 mg/ml vials, **Infusion:** 1 mg/ml	AF, A flutter, PSVT	**A (IV):** 20–25 mg bolus, then infusion of 5–15 mg/hr	Hypotension, bradycardia, dizziness, headaches
Verapamil (p. 1203) (Isoptin)	**I:** 5 mg/2 ml	AF, A flutter, PSVT	**A (IV):** 5–10 mg	Hypotension, bradycardia, dizziness, headaches, constipation

A, Adults; *AF,* atrial fibrillation; *A flutter,* atrial flutter; *C,* capsules; *CHF,* congestive heart failure; *CR,* controlled-release; *ER,* extended-release; *I,* injection; *PAF,* paroxysmal atrial fibrillation; *PSVT,* paroxysmal supraventricular tachycardia; *PVCs,* premature ventricular contractions; *SLE,* systemic lupus erythematosus; *SR,* sustained-release; *T,* tablets; *VF,* ventricular fibrillation; *VT,* ventricular tachycardia; *WPW,* Wolff-Parkinson-White syndrome.

Antibiotics

USES

Treatment of wide range of gram-positive or gram-negative bacterial infections, suppression of intestinal flora before surgery, control of acne, prophylactically to prevent rheumatic fever, prophylactically in high-risk situations (e.g., some surgical procedures or medical conditions) to prevent bacterial infection.

ACTION

Antibiotics (antimicrobial agents) are natural or synthetic compounds that have the ability to kill or suppress the growth of microorganisms.

One means of classifying antibiotics is by their antimicrobial spectrum. Narrow-spectrum agents are effective against few microorganisms (e.g., aminoglycosides are effective against gram-negative aerobes), whereas broad-spectrum agents are effective against a wide variety of microorganisms (e.g., fluoroquinolones are effective against gram-positive cocci and gram-negative bacilli).

Antimicrobial agents may also be classified based on their mechanism of action.

- Agents that inhibit cell wall synthesis or activate enzymes that disrupt the cell wall, causing a weakening in the cell, cell lysis, and death. Include penicillins, cephalosporins, vancomycin, imidazole antifungal agents.

- Agents that act directly on the cell wall, affecting permeability of cell membranes, causing leakage of intracellular substances. Include antifungal agents amphotericin and nystatin, polymyxin, colistin.

- Agents that bind to ribosomal subunits, altering protein synthesis and eventually causing cell death. Include aminoglycosides.

- Agents that affect bacterial ribosome function, altering protein synthesis and causing slow microbial growth. Do not cause cell death. Include chloramphenicol, clindamycin, erythromycin, tetracyclines.

- Agents that inhibit nucleic acid metabolism by binding to nucleic acid or interacting with enzymes necessary for nucleic acid synthesis. Inhibit DNA or RNA synthesis. Include rifampin, metronidazole, quinolones (e.g., ciprofloxacin).

- Agents that inhibit specific metabolic steps necessary for microbial growth, causing a decrease in essential cell components or synthesis of nonfunctional analogues of normal metabolites. Include trimethoprim, sulfonamides.

- Agents that inhibit viral DNA synthesis by binding to viral enzymes necessary for DNA synthesis, preventing viral replication. Include acyclovir, vidarabine.

Antibiotics   *(continued)*

SELECTION OF ANTIMICROBIAL AGENTS

The goal of therapy is to achieve antimicrobial action at the site of infection sufficient to inhibit the growth of the microorganism. The agent selected should be the most active against the most likely infecting organism, least likely to cause toxicity or allergic reaction. Factors to consider in selection of an antimicrobial agent include the following:

- Sensitivity pattern of the infecting microorganism
- Location and severity of infection (may determine route of administration)
- Patient's ability to eliminate the drug (status of renal and hepatic functions)
- Patient's defense mechanisms (includes both cellular and humoral immunity)
- Patient's age, pregnancy status, genetic factors, allergies, CNS disorder, preexisting medical problems

CATEGORIZATION OF ORGANISMS BY GRAM STAINING

Gram-Positive Cocci	Gram-Negative Cocci	Gram-Positive Bacilli	Gram-Negative Bacilli
Aerobic	**Aerobic**	**Aerobic**	**Aerobic**
Staphylococcus aureus	*Neisseria gonorrhoeae*	*Listeria monocytogenes*	*E. coli*
Staphylococcus epidermidis	*Neisseria meningitidis*	*Bacillus anthracis*	*Klebsiella pneumoniae*
Streptococcus pneumoniae	*Moraxella catarrhalis*	*Corynebacterium diphtheriae*	*Proteus mirabilis*
Streptococcus pyogenes		**Anaerobic**	*Serratia marcescens*
Viridans streptococci		*Clostridium difficile*	*Pseudomonas aeruginosa*
Enterococcus faecalis		*Clostridium perfringens*	*Enterobacter* spp.
Enterococcus faecium		*Clostridium tetani*	*Haemophilus influenzae*
Anaerobic		*Actinomyces* spp.	*Legionella pneumophila*
Peptostreptococcus spp.			**Anaerobic**
Peptococcus spp.			*Bacteroides fragilis*
			Fusobacterium spp.

Antibiotic: Aminoglycosides

USES

Treatment of serious infections when other less toxic agents are not effective, are contraindicated, or require adjunctive therapy (e.g., with penicillins or cephalosporins). Used primarily in the treatment of infections caused by gram-negative microorganisms, such as those caused by *Proteus, Klebsiella, Pseudomonas,* *Escherichia coli, Serratia, and Enterobacter.* Inactive against most gram-positive microorganisms. Not well absorbed systemically from GI tract (must be administered parenterally for systemic infections). Oral agents are given to suppress intestinal bacteria.

ACTION

Bactericidal. Transported across bacterial cell membrane; irreversibly binds to specific receptor proteins of bacterial ribosomes. Interfere with protein synthesis, preventing cell reproduction and eventually causing cell death.

ANTIBIOTIC: AMINOGLYCOSIDES

Name	Availability	Dosage Range	Side Effects
Amikacin (p. 50) (Amikin)	**I:** 250 mg/ml, 50 mg/ml	**A:** 15 mg/kg/day **C:** 15 mg/kg/day	Nephrotoxicity, neurotoxicity, ototoxicity (both auditory and vestibular), hypersensitivity (skin itching, redness, rash, swelling)
Gentamicin (p. 542) (Garamycin)	**I:** 40 mg/ml, 10 mg/ml	**A:** 3–5 mg/kg/day **C:** 6–7.5 mg/kg/day	Same as amikacin
Neomycin (p. 823)	**T:** 500 mg	**A:** 1 g for 3 doses as preop	Nausea, vomiting, diarrhea
Netilmicin (Netromycin)	**I:** 100 mg/ml	**A:** 3–6.5 mg/kg/day **C:** 5.5–8 mg/kg/day	Same as amikacin

(continued)

ANTIBIOTIC: AMINOGLYCOSIDES *(continued)*

Name	Availability	Dosage Range	Side Effects
Streptomycin	**I:** 1 g	**A:** 15 mg/kg/day **C:** 20–40 mg/kg/day **Maximum:** 1 g	Same as amikacin Peripheralneuritis (numbness), optic neuritis (any vision loss)
Tobramycin (p. 1144) (Nebcin)	**I:** 40 mg/ml,10 mg/ml	**A:** 3–5 mg/kg/day **C:** 6–7.5 mg/kg/day	Same as amikacin

A, Adults; *C (dosage),* children; *I,* injection; *T,* tablets.

Antibiotic: Cephalosporins

USES

Broad-spectrum antibiotics, which, like penicillins, may be used in a number of diseases, including respiratory diseases, skin and soft tissue infection, bone/joint infections, GU infections, prophylactically in some surgical procedures.

First-generation cephalosporins have good activity against gram-positive organisms and moderate activity against gram-negative organisms, including *Escherichia coli, Klebsiella pneumoniae, Proteus mirabilis.*

Second-generation cephalosporins have increased activity against gram-negative organisms.

Third-generation cephalosporins are less active against gram-positive organisms but more active against the Enterobacteriaceae with some activity against *Pseudomonas aeruginosa.*

Fourth-generation cephalosporins have good activity against gram-positive organisms (e.g., *Staphylococcus aureus*) and gram-negative organisms (e.g., *Pseudomonas aeruginosa*).

ACTION

Cephalosporins inhibit cell wall synthesis or activate enzymes that disrupt the cell wall, causing cell lysis and cell death. May be bacteriostatic or bactericidal. Most effective against rapidly dividing cells.

ANTIBIOTIC: CEPHALOSPORINS

Name	Availability	Dosage Range	Side Effects
First-Generation			
Cefadroxil (p. 197) (Duricef)	**C:** 500 mg **T:** 1 g **S:** 125 mg/5 ml, 250 mg/5 ml, 500 mg/5 ml	**A:** 1–2 g/day **C:** 30 mg/kg/day	Abdominal cramps/pain, fever, nausea, vomiting, diarrhea, headaches, oral/vaginal candidiasis
Cefazolin (p. 198) (Ancef, Kefzol)	**I:** 500 mg, 1 g, 2 g	**A:** 0.75–6 g/day **C:** 25–100 mg/kg/day	Same as above
Cephalexin (p. 228) (Keftab)	**C:** 250 mg, 500 mg **T:** 250 mg, 500 mg, 1 g	**A:** 1–4 g/day **C:** 25–100 mg/kg/day	Same as above
Second-Generation			
Cefaclor (p. 195) (Ceclor)	**C:** 250 mg, 500 mg **T (ER):** 375 mg, 500 mg **S:** 125 mg/5 ml, 187 mg/5 ml, 250 mg/5 ml, 375 mg/5 ml	**A:** 250–500 mg q8h **C:** 20–40 mg/kg/day	Same as cefadroxil May have serum sickness–like reaction
Cefotetan (p. 209) (Cefotan)	**I:** 1 g, 2 g	**A:** 1–6 g/day	Same as cefadroxil May cause unusual bleeding/ecchymoses
Cefoxitin (p. 211) (Mefoxin)	**I:** 1 g, 2 g	**A:** 3–12 g/day	Same as cefadroxil
Cefpodoxime (p. 213) (Vantin)	**T:** 100 mg, 200 mg **S:** 50 mg/5 ml, 100 mg/5 ml	**A:** 200–800 mg/day **C:** 10 mg/kg/day	Same as cefadroxil
Cefprozil (p. 215) (Cefzil)	**T:** 250 mg, 500 mg **S:** 125 mg/5 ml, 250 mg/5 ml	**A:** 0.5–1 g/day **C:** 30 mg/kg/day	Same as above

(continued)

ANTIBIOTIC: CEPHALOSPORINS   *(continued)*

Name	Availability	Dosage Range	Side Effects
Second-Generation *(continued)*			
Cefuroxime (p. 224) (Ceftin, Kefurox, Zinacef)	**T:** 125 mg, 250 mg, 500 mg **S:** 125 mg/5 ml, 250 mg/5 ml **I:** 750 mg, 1.5 g	**A (PO):** 0.25–1 g/day; **(IM/IV):** 2.25–9 g/day **C (PO):** 250–500 mg/day; **(IM/IV):** 50–100 mg/kg/day	Same as above
Loracarbef (p. 706) (Lorabid)	**C:** 200 mg, 400 mg **S:** 100 mg/5 ml, 200 mg/5 ml	**A:** 200–800 mg/day **C:** 15–30 mg/kg/day	Same as above
Third-Generation			
Cefdinir (p. 200) (Omnicef)	**C:** 300 mg **S:** 125 mg/5 ml	**A:** 600 mg/day **C:** 14 mg/kg/day	Same as above
Cefditoren (p. 202) (Spectracef)	**T:** 200 mg	**A:** 400–800 mg/day	Same as above
Cefotaxime (p. 207) (Claforan)	**I:** 500 mg, 1 g, 2 g	**A:** 2–12 g/day **C:** 100–200 mg/kg/day	Same as above
Ceftazidime (p. 216) (Fortaz, Tazicef, Tazidime)	**I:** 500 mg, 1 g, 2 g	**A:** 0.5–6 g/day **C:** 90–150 mg/kg/day	Same as above

Ceftibuten (p. 218) (Cedax)	**C:** 400 mg **S:** 90 mg/5 ml, 180 mg/5 ml	**A:** 400 mg/day **C:** 9 mg/kg/day	Same as above
Ceftizoxime (p. 220) (Cefizox)	**I:** 500 mg, 1 g, 2 g	**A:** 1–12 g/day **C:** 150–200 mg/kg/day	Same as above
Ceftriaxone (p. 222) (Rocephin)	**I:** 250 mg, 500 mg, 1 g, 2 g	**A:** 1–4 g/day **C:** 50–100 mg/kg/day	Same as above

Fourth-Generation

| Cefepime (p. 203) (Maxipime) | **I:** 500 mg, 1 g, 2 g | **A:** 1–6 g/day | Same as above |

A, Adults; *C,* capsules; *C (dosage),* children; *ER,* extended-release; *I,* injection; *S,* suspension; *T,* tablets.

Antibiotic: Fluoroquinolones

USES

Fluoroquinolones act against a wide range of gram-negative and gram-positive organisms. They are used primarily in the treatment of lower respiratory infections, skin/skin structure infections, UTIs, and sexually transmitted diseases.

ACTION

Bactericidal. Inhibit DNA gyrase in susceptible micro-organisms, interfering with bacterial DNA replication and repair.

Antibiotic: Fluoroquinolones   *(continued)*

ANTIBIOTIC: FLUOROQUINOLONES

Name	Availability	Dosage Range	Side Effects
Ciprofloxacin (p. 252) (Cipro)	**T:** 250 mg, 500 mg, 750 mg **S:** 5 g/100 ml **I:** 200 mg, 400 mg	**A (PO):** 250–750 mg q12h; **(IV):** 200–400 mg q12h	Dizziness, headaches, nervousness, drowsiness, insomnia, abdominal pain, nausea, diarrhea, vomiting, phlebitis (parenteral)
Enoxacin (Penetrex)	**T:** 200 mg, 400 mg	**A:** 200–400 mg q12h	Same as above
Gatifloxacin (p. 532) (Tequin)	**T:** 200 mg, 400 mg **I:** 200 mg, 400 mg	**A:** 200–400 mg q12h	Same as above
Gemifloxacin (p. 539) (Factive)	**T:** 320 mg	**A:** 320 mg/day	Same as above
Levofloxacin (p. 684) (Levaquin)	**T:** 250 mg, 500 mg, 750 mg **I:** 250 mg, 500 mg, 750 mg	**A (PO/IV):** 250–750 mg/day as single dose	Same as above
Lomefloxacin (p. 700) (Maxaquin)	**T:** 400 mg	**A:** 400 mg/day	Same as above
Moxifloxacin (p. 797) (Avelox)	**T:** 400 mg **I:** 400 mg	**A:** 400 mg/day	Same as above; may prolong QT interval
Norfloxacin (p. 851) (Noroxin)	**T:** 400 mg	**A:** 400 mg q12h	Same as above
Ofloxacin (p. 858) (Floxin)	**T:** 200 mg, 300 mg, 400 mg	**A:** 200–400 mg q12h	Same as above

A, Adults; *I,* injection; *S,* suspension; *T,* tablets.

Antibiotic: Macrolides

USES

Macrolides act primarily against gram-positive microorganisms and gram-negative cocci. Azithromycin and clarithromycin appear to be more potent than erythromycin. Macrolides are used in the treatment of pharyngitis/tonsillitis, sinusitis, chronic bronchitis, pneumonia, uncomplicated skin/skin structure infections.

ACTION

Bacteriostatic or bactericidal. Reversibly bind to the P site of the 50S ribosomal subunit of susceptible organisms, inhibiting RNA-dependent protein synthesis.

ANTIBIOTIC: MACROLIDES

Name	Availability	Dosage Range	Side Effects
Azithromycin (p. 113) (Zithromax)	**T:** 250 mg, 600 mg **S:** 100 mg/5 ml, 200 mg/5 ml, 1-g packet **I:** 500 mg	**A (PO):** 500 mg once, then 250 mg days 2–5; **(IV):** 500 mg/day **C (PO):** 10 mg/kg once, then 5 mg/kg/day on days 2–5	**PO:** Nausea, diarrhea, vomiting, abdominal pain **IV:** Pain, redness, swelling at injection site
Clarithromycin (p. 261) (Biaxin)	**T:** 250 mg, 500 mg **T (XL):** 500 mg **S:** 125 mg/5 ml	**A:** 250–500 mg q12h **C:** 7.5 mg/kg q12h	Headaches, loss of taste, nausea, vomiting, diarrhea, abdominal pain/discomfort
Dirithromycin (p. 370) (Dynabac)	**T:** 250 mg	**A, C (older than 12 yr):** 500 mg/day as a single daily dose	Dizziness, nausea, vomiting, diarrhea, abdominal pain, headaches, weakness

(continued)

ANTIBIOTIC: MACROLIDES		*(continued)*	
Name	Availability	Dosage Range	Side Effects
Erythromycin (p. 434) **(Ery-Tab, PCE, Eryc, EES,** **EryPed, Erythrocin)**	**T:** 200 mg, 250 mg, 333 mg, 400 mg, 500 mg **C:** 250 mg **S:** 125 mg/5 ml, 200 mg/5 ml, 250 mg/5 ml, 400 mg/5 ml, 100 mg/2.5 ml	**A (PO):** 250–500 mg q6h **C (PO):** 30–50 mg/kg/day **A, C (IV):** 15–20 mg/kg/day **Maximum:** 4 g/day	**PO:** Nausea, vomiting, diarrhea, abdominal pain **IV:** Inflammation, phlebitis at injection site

A, Adults; *C,* capsules; *C (dosage),* children; *I,* injection; *S,* suspension; *T,* tablets; *XL,* long acting.

Antibiotic: Penicillins

USES

Penicillins may be used to treat a large number of infections, including pneumonia and other respiratory diseases, UTIs, septicemia, meningitis, intra-abdominal infections, gonorrhea and syphilis, bone/joint infection.

Penicillins are classified based on an antimicrobial spectrum:

Natural penicillins are very active against gram-positive cocci but ineffective against most strains of *Staphylococcus aureus* (inactivated by enzyme penicillinase).

Penicillinase-resistant penicillins are effective against penicillinase-producing *Staphylococcus aureus* but are less effective against gram-positive cocci than the natural penicillins.

Broad-spectrum penicillins are effective against gram-positive cocci and some gram-negative bacteria (e.g., *Haemophilus influenzae, Escherichia coli, Proteus mirabilis*).

Extended-spectrum penicillins are effective against *Pseudomonas aeruginosa, Enterobacter, Proteus* species, *Klebsiella,* and some other gram-negative microorganisms.

ACTION

Penicillins inhibit cell wall synthesis or activate enzymes, which disrupt the bacterial cell wall, causing cell lysis and cell death. May be bacteriostatic or bactericidal. Most effective against bacteria undergoing active growth and division.

ANTIBIOTIC: PENICILLINS

Name	Availability	Dosage Range	Side Effects
Natural			
Penicillin G benzathine (p. 909) (Bicillin)	**I:** 600,000 units, 1.2 million units, 2.4 million units	**A:** 1.2 million units/day **C:** 0.3–1.2 million units/day	Mild diarrhea, nausea, vomiting, headaches, sore mouth/tongue, vaginal itching/discharge, allergic reaction (including anaphylaxis, skin rash, hives, itching)
Penicillin G potassium (p. 910) (Pfizerpen)	**I:** 1, 2, 3, 5 million-unit vials	**A:** 2–24 million units/day **C:** 100–250,000 units/kg/day	Same as above
Penicillin G procaine (Wycillin)	**I:** 600,000 units, 1.2 million units, 2.4 million units	**A, C:** 0.6–1.2 million units/day	Same as above; increased risk of mental disturbances
Penicillin V potassium (p. 912) (V-Cillin-K)	**T:** 250 mg, 500 mg **S:** 125 mg/5 ml, 250 mg/5 ml	**A:** 0.5–2 g/day **C:** 25–50 mg/kg/day	Same as above
Penicillinase-Resistant			
Cloxacillin (Tegopen)	**C:** 250 mg, 500 mg **S:** 125 mg/5 ml	**A:** 1–2 g/day **C:** 50–100 mg/kg/day	Same as penicillin G benzathine; increased risk of hepatic toxicity
Dicloxacillin (Dynapen, Pathocil)	**C:** 125 mg, 250 mg, 500 mg **S:** 62.5 mg/5 ml	**A:** 1–2 g/day **C:** 12.5–25 mg/kg/day	Same as above Increased risk of hepatic toxicity
Nafcillin (p. 809) (Unipen)	**C:** 250 mg **I:** 500 mg, 1 g, 2 g	**A (PO):** 1–6 g/day; **(IV):** 2–6 g/day **C (PO):** 25–50 mg/kg/day; **(IV):** 50 mg/kg/day	Same as penicillin G benzathine; increased risk of interstitial nephritis
Oxacillin (Bactocill)	**C:** 250 mg, 500 mg **S:** 250 mg/5 ml **I:** 250 mg, 500 mg, 1 g, 2 g	**A (PO/IV):** 2–6 g/day **C (PO/IV):** 50–100 mg/kg/day	Same as above; increased risk of hepatictoxicity, interstitial nephritis

(continued)

ANTIBIOTIC: PENICILLINS   (continued)

Name	Availability	Dosage Range	Side Effects
Broad-Spectrum			
Amoxicillin (p. 63) (Amoxil, Trimox)	**T:** 125 mg, 250 mg, 500 mg, 875 mg **C:** 250 mg, 500 mg **S:** 50 mg/ml, 125 mg/5 ml, 250 mg/5 ml	**A:** 0.75–1.5 g/day **C:** 20–40 mg/kg/day	Same as above
Amoxicillin/clavulanate (p. 65) (Augmentin)	**T:** 250 mg, 500 mg, 875 mg **T (chewable):** 125 mg, 200 mg, 250 mg, 400 mg **S:** 125 mg/5 ml, 200 mg/5 ml, 250 mg/5 ml, 400 mg/5 ml	**A:** 0.75–1.5 g/day **C:** 20–40 mg/kg/day	Same as above
Ampicillin (p. 70) (Principen)	**C:** 250 mg, 500 mg **S:** 125 mg/5 ml, 250 mg/5 ml **I:** 125 mg, 250 mg, 500 mg, 1 g, 2 g	**A:** 1–12 g/day **C:** 50–200 mg/kg/day	Same as above
Ampicillin/sulbactam (p. 73) (Unasyn)	**I:** 1.5 g, 3 g	**A:** 6–12 g/day **C:** 100–200 mg/kg/day	Same as above
Extended-Spectrum			
Carbenicillin (Geocillin)	**T:** 382 mg	**A:** 382–764 mg 4 times/day	Same as above
Piperacillin/tazobactam (p. 936) (Zosyn)	**I:** 2.25 g, 3.375 g, 4.5 g	**A:** 2.25–4.5 g q6–8h **C:** 200–400 mg/kg/day	Same as above
Ticarcillin/clavulanate (p. 1127) (Timentin)	**I:** 3.1 g	**A:** 3.1 g q4–6h **C:** 200–300 mg/kg/day	Same as above

A, Adults; *C,* capsules; *C (dosage),* children; *I,* injection; *S,* suspension; *T,* tablets.

Anticoagulants/Antiplatelets/Thrombolytics

USES

Treatment and prevention of venous thromboembolism, acute MI, acute cerebral embolism; reduce risk of acute MI; reduce total mortality in patients with unstable angina; prevent occlusion of saphenous grafts following open heart surgery; prevent embolism in select patients with atrial fibrillation, prosthetic heart valves, valvular heart disease, cardiomyopathy. Heparin also used for acute/chronic consumption coagulopathies (disseminated intravascular coagulation).

ACTION

Anticoagulants: Inhibit blood coagulation by preventing the formation of new clots and extension of existing ones *but do not dissolve formed clots.* Anticoagulants are subdivided into two common classes: *Heparin:* Indirectly interferes with blood coagulation by blocking the conversion of prothrombin to thrombin and fibrinogen to fibrin. *Coumarin:* Acts indirectly to prevent synthesis in the liver of vitamin K–dependent clotting factors.

Antiplatelets: Interfere with platelet aggregation. Effects are irreversible for life of platelet. Medications in this group act by different mechanisms and are used in combinations to provide desired effect.
Thrombolytics: Act directly or indirectly on fibrinolytic system to dissolve clots (converting plasminogen to plasmin, an enzyme that digests fibrin clot).

ANTICOAGULANTS/ANTIPLATELETS/THROMBOLYTICS

Name	Availability	Uses	Side Effects
Anticoagulants			
Argatroban (p. 84)	**I:** 100 mg/ml	Prevent/treat VTE in patients with HIT or at risk for HIT undergoing PCI	Bleeding
Bivalirudin (p. 144) (Angiomax)	**I:** 250-mg vials	Patients with unstable angina undergoing PTCA	Bleeding
Dalteparin (p. 310) (Fragmin)	**I:** 2,500 units, 5,000 units, 7,500 units, 10,000 units	Hip surgery; abdominal surgery; unstable angina or non-Q-wave myocardial infarction	Bleeding, hematoma
Desirudin @ (Iprivask)	**I:** 15-mg vials	Prevent VTE in patients undergoing hip replacement surgery	Bleeding, hematoma

(continued)

ANTICOAGULANTS/ANTIPLATELETS/THROMBOLYTICS *(continued)*

Name	Availability	Uses	Side Effects
Anticoagulants *(continued)*			
Enoxaparin (p. 411) (Lovenox)	I: 30 mg, 40 mg, 60 mg, 80 mg, 100 mg, 120 mg, 150 mg	Hip surgery; knee surgery; abdominal surgery; unstable angina or non–Q-wave myocardial infarction; acute illness	Bleeding, thrombocytopenia, hematoma
Fondaparinux (p. 509) (Arixtra)	I: 2.5 mg	Hip surgery; knee surgery	Bleeding, thrombocytopenia, hematoma
Heparin (p. 570)	I: 1,000 units/ml, 2,500 units/ml, 5,000 units/ml, 7,500 units/ml, 10,000 units/ml, 20,000 units/ml	Prevent/treat VTE	Bleeding, thrombocytopenia, skin rash
Lepirudin (p. 674) (Refludan)	I: 50-mg vials	Prevent VTE in patients with HIT	Bleeding
Tinzaparin (p. 1137) (Innohep)	I: 20,000 units/ml vials	Treatment of VTE (with warfarin)	Bleeding, thrombocytopenia
Warfarin (p. 1221) (Coumadin)	PO: 1 mg, 2 mg, 2.5 mg, 3 mg, 4 mg, 5 mg, 6 mg, 7.5 mg, 10 mg; I: 2 mg/ml	Prevent/treat VTE in patients; prevent systemic embolism in patients with heart valve replacement, valve heart disease, myocardial infarction, atrial fibrillation	Bleeding, skin necrosis

HIT, Heparin-induced thrombocytopenia; *I,* injection; *PCI,* percutaneous coronary intervention; *PTCA,* percutaneous transluminal coronary angioplasty; *TIA,* transient ischemic attack; *VTE,* venous thromboembolism.

Name	Availability	Uses	Side Effects
Antiplatelets			
Abciximab (p. 5) (ReoPro)	I: 2 mg/ml	Adjunct to PCI to prevent acute cardiac ischemic complications (with heparin and aspirin)	Bleeding, hypotension, nausea, vomiting, back pain, allergic reactions, thrombocytopenia
Aspirin (p. 93)	PO: 81 mg, 165 mg, 325 mg, 500 mg, 650 mg	TIA in males; myocardial infarction prophylaxis; cardiac vascular disease	Tinnitus, dizziness, hypersensitivity, dyspepsia, minor bleeding, gastro-intestinal ulceration
Clopidogrel (p. 274) (Plavix)	PO: 75 mg	Reduce risk in patients with unstable angina, non–Q-wave myocardial infarction, recent myocardial infarction, CVA	Bleeding
Dipyridamole (p. 369) (Persantine)	PO: 25 mg, 50 mg, 75 mg	Prevent postoperative thromboembolic complications following cardiac valve replacement	Dizziness, gastrointestinal distress
Eptifibatide (p. 427) (Integrilin)	I: 0.75 mg/ml, 2 mg/ml	Treatment of acute coronary syndrome	Bleeding, hypotension
Ticlopidine (p. 1129) (Ticlid)	PO: 250 mg	Reduce risk stroke in patients with CVA precursors, TIA	Neutropenia, agranulocytosis, thrombocytopenia, aplastic anemia, increased serum cholesterol/ triglycerides, rash, diarrhea, nausea, vomiting, gastrointestinal pain
Tirofiban (p. 1141) (Aggrastat)	I: 50 mcg/ml, 250 mcg/ml	Treatment of acute coronary syndrome	Bleeding, thrombocytopenia

CVA, Cerebrovascular attack; *I*, injection; *PCI*, percutaneous coronary intervention; *PO*, oral; *TIA*, transient ischemic attack.

(continued)

ANTICOAGULANTS/ANTIPLATELETS/THROMBOLYTICS   *(continued)*

Name	Availability	Indications	Side Effects
Thrombolytics			
Alteplase (p. 42) (Activase)	I: 50 mg, 100 mg	Acute myocardial infarction, acute ischemic stroke, pulmonary embolism	Bleeding, cholesterol embolism, arrhythmias
Reteplase (p. 1012) (Retavase)	I: 10.4 units	Acute myocardial infarction	Bleeding, cholesterol embolism, arrhythmias
Streptokinase (p. 1079)	I: 250,000 units, 750,000 units, 1.5 million units	Myocardial infarction; venous thromboembolism; arterial thromboembolism	Bleeding, cholesterol embolism, arrhythmias, hypotension
Tenecteplase (p. 1105) (TNKase)	I: 50 mg	Acute myocardial infarction	Bleeding, cholesterol embolism, arrhythmias

I, Injection.

Anticonvulsants

USES

Anticonvulsants are used to treat seizures. Seizures can be divided into two broad categories: partial seizures and generalized seizures. Partial seizures begin focally in the cerebral cortex, undergoing limited spread. Simple partial seizures do not involve loss of consciousness but may evolve secondarily into generalized seizures. Complex partial seizures involve impairment of consciousness.

Generalized seizures may be convulsive or noncovulsive and usually produce immediate loss of consciousness.

ACTION

Anticonvulsants can prevent or reduce excessive discharge of neurons with seizure foci or decrease the spread of excitation from seizure foci to normal neurons. The exact mechanism is unknown but may be due to (1) suppressing sodium influx; (2) suppressing calcium influx; or (3) increasing the action of GABA, which inhibits neurotransmitters throughout the brain.

ANTICONVULSANTS

Name	Availability	Uses	Dosage Range	Side Effects
Carbamazepine (p. 182) (Tegretol)	**S:** 100 mg/5 ml **T (chewable):** 100 mg **T:** 200 mg **T (ER):** 100 mg, 200 mg, 400 mg **C (ER):** 200 mg, 300 mg	Complex partial, tonic-clonic, mixed seizures; trigeminal neuralgia	**A:** 800–1,200 mg/day **C:** 400–800 mg/day	Dizziness, diplopia, leukopenia
Clonazepam (p. 270) (Klonopin)	**T:** 0.5 mg, 1 mg, 2 mg	Petit mal, akinetic, myoclonic, absence seizures	**A:** 1.5–20 mg/day	CNS depression, sedation, ataxia, confusion, depression

(continued)

ANTICONVULSANTS (continued)

Name	Availability	Uses	Dosage Range	Side Effects
Diazepam (p. 345) (Valium)	**T:** 2 mg, 5 mg, 10 mg; **I:** 5 mg/ml; **R:** 2.5 mg, 5 mg, 10 mg, 20 mg	Adjunctive therapy status epilepticus	**A (PO):** 4–40 mg/day; **(IM/IV):** 5–30 mg; **C (PO):** 3–10 mg/day; **(IM/IV):** 1–10 mg	CNS depression, sedation, confusion, mental depression, respiratory depression
Fosphenytoin (p. 519) (Cerebyx)	**I:** 50 mg PE/ml	Status epilepticus, seizures occurring during neurosurgery	**A:** 15–20 mg PE/kg bolus, then 4–6 mg PE/kg/day maintenance	Burning, itching, paraesthesia, nystagmus, ataxia
Gabapentin (p. 526) (Neurontin)	**C:** 100 mg, 300 mg, 400 mg	Partial seizures with and without secondary generalization	**A:** 900–1,800 mg/day	CNS depression, fatigue, somnolence, dizziness, ataxia
Lamotrigine (p. 666) (Lamictal)	**T:** 25 mg, 100 mg, 150 mg, 200 mg	Partial seizures	**A:** 100–500 mg/day	Dizziness, ataxia, somnolence, diplopia, nausea, rash
Oxcarbazepine (p. 879) (Trileptal)	**T:** 150 mg, 300 mg, 600 mg	Partial seizures	**A:** 900–1,800 mg/day	
Phenobarbital (p. 921)	**T:** 30 mg, 60 mg, 100 mg; **I:** 65 mg, 130 mg	Tonic-clonic, partial seizures; status epilepticus	**A (PO):** 100–300 mg/day; **(IM/IV):** 200–600 mg. **C (PO):** 3–5 mg/kg/day, **(IM/IV):** 100–400 mg	CNS depression, sedation, paradoxical excitement and hyperactivity, rash
Phenytoin (p. 927) (Dilantin)	**C:** 100 mg; **T: (chewable):** 50 mg; **S:** 125 mg/5 ml; **I:** 50 mg/ml	Tonic-clonic, psychomotor seizures	**A (PO):** 300–600 mg/day; **IV:** 150–250 mg; **C (PO):** 4–8 mg/kg/day; **(IV):** 10–15 mg/kg	Nystagmus, ataxia, hypertrichosis, gingival hyperplasia, rashes, osteomalacia, lymphadenopathy

Primidone (p. 961) (Mysoline)	**T:** 50 mg; 250 mg **S:** 250 mg/5 ml	Complex, partial, akinetic, tonic-clonic seizures	**A:** 750–2,000 mg/day **C:** 10–25 mg/kg/day	CNS depression, sedation, paradoxical excitement and hyperactivity, rash, dizziness, ataxia
Tiagabine (p. 1126) (Gabitril)	**T:** 4 mg, 12 mg, 16 mg, 20 mg	Partial seizures	**A:** Initially, 4 mg up to 56 mg **C:** Initially, 4 mg up to 32 mg	Dizziness, asthenia, nervousness, anxiety, tremors, abdominal pain
Topiramate (p. 1149) (Topamax)	**T:** 25 mg, 100 mg, 200 mg	Partial seizures	**A:** 25–400 mg/day **C:** 1–9 mg/kg/day	Impaired concentration, speech impairment, fatigue
Valproic acid (p. 1191) (Depakene, Depakote)	**C:** 250 mg **S:** 250 mg/5 ml **Sprinkles:** 125 mg **T:** 125 mg, 250 mg, 500 mg **T (ER):** 500 mg **I:** 100 mg/ml	Complex partial, absence seizures	**A, C:** 15–60 mg/kg/day	Nausea, vomiting, tremors, thrombocytopenia, hair loss, hepatic dysfunction
Zonisamide (p. 1237) (Zonegran)	**C:** 100 mg	Partial seizures	**A:** 500 mg/day	Somnolence, dizziness, anorexia, headaches, nausea

A, Adults; *C (dosage),* children; *C,* capsules; *ER,* extended-release; *I,* injection; *R,* rectal; *S,* suspension; *T,* tablets.

Antidepressants

USES

Used primarily for the treatment of depression. Imipramine is also used for childhood enuresis. Clomipramine is used only for obsessive-compulsive disorder (OCD). Monoamine oxidase inhibitors (MAOIs) are rarely used as initial therapy except for patients unresponsive to other therapy or when other therapy is contraindicated.

ACTION

Antidepressants are classified as tricyclics, MAOIs, or second-generation antidepressants (further subdivided into selective serotonin reuptake inhibitors [SSRIs] and atypical antidepressants). Depression may be due to reduced functioning of monoamine neurotransmitters (e.g., norepinephrine, serotonin [5-HT], dopamine) in the CNS (decreased amount and/or decreased effects at the receptor sites). Antidepressants block metabolism, increase amount/effects of monoamine neurotransmitters, and act at receptor sites (change responsiveness/sensitivities of both presynaptic and postsynaptic receptor sites).

ANTIDEPRESSANTS

Name	Availability	Uses	Dosage Range (per day)	Side Effects
Tricyclics				
Amitriptyline (p. 60) (Elavil)	**T:** 10 mg, 25 mg, 59 mg, 75 mg, 100 mg, 150 mg	Depression	40–300 mg	Drowsiness, blurred vision, constipation, confusion, postural hypotension, cardiac conduction defects, weight gain, seizures
Clomipramine (p. 269) (Anafranil)	**C:** 25 mg, 50 mg, 75 mg	OCD	25–250 mg	Same as above
Desipramine (p. 328) (Norpramin)	**T:** 10 mg, 25 mg, 50 mg, 75 mg, 100 mg, 150 mg	Depression	25–100 mg	Same as above

Drug	Forms	Indication	Dose	Side Effects
Doxepin (p. 386) (Sinequan)	**C:** 10 mg, 25 mg, 50 mg, 75 mg, 100 mg, 150 mg **OC:** 10 mg/ml	Depression	25–300 mg	Same as above
Imipramine (p. 608) (Tofranil)	**T:** 10 mg, 25 mg, 50 mg **C:** 75 mg, 100 mg, 125 mg, 150 mg	Depression, enuresis	30–300 mg	Same as above
Nortriptyline (p. 852) @ (Aventyl, Pamelor)	**C:** 10 mg, 25 mg, 50 mg, 75 mg **S:** 10 mg/5 ml	Depression	25–100 mg	Same as above
Protriptyline (Vivactil)	**T:** 5 mg, 10 mg	Depression	15–60 mg	Same as above

Monoamine Oxidase Inhibitors

Drug	Forms	Indication	Dose	Side Effects
Phenelzine (p. 919) @ (Nardil)	**T:** 15 mg	Depression	15–90 mg	Sedation, hypertensive crisis, weight gain, orthostatic hypotension
Tranylcypromine (p. 1162) @ (Parnate)	**T:** 10 mg	Depression	30–60 mg	Same as above

Selective Serotonin Reuptake Inhibitors

Drug	Forms	Indication	Dose	Side Effects
Citalopram (p. 257) (Celexa)	**T:** 20 mg, 40 mg **S:** 10 mg/5 ml	Depression	25–60 mg	Insomnia or sedation, nausea, agitation, headaches
Escitalopram (p. 437) (Lexapro)	**T:** 5 mg, 10 mg, 20 mg	Depression	10–20 mg	Insomnia or sedation, nausea, agitation, headaches
Fluoxetine (p. 495) (Prozac)	**C:** 10 mg, 20 mg, 40 mg **T:** 10 mg **S:** 20 mg/5 ml	Depression, OCD, bulimia	10–80 mg	Akathisia, sexual dysfunction, skin rash, hives, itching, decreased appetite, asthenia, diarrhea, drowsiness, headaches, diaphoresis, insomnia, nausea, tremors
Fluvoxamine (p. 507) @ (Luvox)	**T:** 25 mg, 50 mg, 100 mg	OCD	100–300 mg	Sexual dysfunction, fatigue, constipation, dizziness, drowsiness, headaches, insomnia, nausea, vomiting

(continued)

ANTIDEPRESSANTS *(continued)*

Selective Serotonin Reuptake Inhibitors *(continued)*

Name	Availability	Uses	Dosage Range (per day)	Side Effects
Paroxetine (p. 897) (Paxil)	**T:** 10 mg, 20 mg, 30 mg, 40 mg **S:** 10 mg/5 ml	Depression, OCD, panic attack, social anxiety disorder	20–50 mg	Asthenia, constipation, diarrhea, diaphoresis, insomnia, nausea, sexual dysfunction, tremors, vomiting, urinary frequency or retention
Sertraline (p. 1050) (Zoloft)	**T:** 25 mg, 50 mg, 100 mg **S:** 20 mg/ml	Depression, OCD, panic attack	50–200 mg	Sexual dysfunction, dizziness, drowsiness, anorexia, diarrhea, nausea, dry mouth, abdominal cramps, decreased weight, headaches, increased diaphoresis, tremors, insomnia

Atypical

Name	Availability	Uses	Dosage Range (per day)	Side Effects
Bupropion (p. 161) (Wellbutrin)	**T:** 75 mg, 100 mg **SR:** 100 mg, 150 mg	Depression	150–450 mg	Insomnia, irritability, seizures
Duloxetine (p. 397) (Cymbalta)	**C:** 20 mg, 30 mg, 60 mg	Depression, neuropathic pain	40–60 mg	Nausea, dry mouth, constipation, decreased appetite, fatigue, diaphoresis
Mirtazapine (p. 781) (Remeron)	**T:** 15 mg, 30 mg, 45 mg	Depression	15–45 mg	Sedation, dry mouth, weight gain, agranulocytosis, hepatic toxicity
Nefazodone ℗	**T:** 50 mg, 100 mg, 150 mg, 200 mg, 250 mg	Depression	200–600 mg	Sedation, orthostatic hypotension, nausea
Trazodone (p. 1165) (Desyrel)	**T:** 50 mg, 100 mg, 150 mg, 300 mg	Depression	50–600 mg	Sedation, orthostatic hypotension, priapism
Venlafaxine (p. 1201) (Effexor)	**T:** 25 mg, 37.5 mg, 50 mg, 75 mg, 100 mg **T (ER):** 37.5 mg, 75 mg, 150 mg	Depression, anxiety	75–375 mg	Increased blood pressure, agitation, sedation, insomnia, nausea

C, Capsules; *ER,* extended-release; *OC,* oral concentrate; *OCD,* obsessive-compulsive disorder; *S,* suspension; *SR,* sustained-release; *T,* tablets.

Antidiabetics

USES

Insulin: Treatment of insulin-dependent diabetes (type 1) and non–insulin-dependent diabetes (type 2). Also used in acute situations such as ketoacidosis, severe infections, major surgery in otherwise non–insulin-dependent diabetics. Administered to patients receiving parenteral nutrition. Drug of choice during pregnancy.

Sulfonylureas: Control hyperglycemia in type 2 diabetes not controlled by weight and diet alone. Chlorpropamide also used in adjunctive treatment of neurogenic diabetes insipidus.

Alpha-glucosidase inhibitors: Adjunct to diet to lower blood glucose in patients with type 2 diabetes mellitus whose hyperglycemia cannot be managed by diet alone.

Biguanides: Adjunct to diet to lower blood glucose in patients with type 2 diabetes mellitus whose hyperglycemia cannot be managed by diet alone.

Thiazolinediones: Adjunct in patients with type 2 diabetes currently on insulin therapy.

ACTION

Insulin: A hormone synthesized and secreted by beta cells of Langerhans' islet in the pancreas. Controls storage and utilization of glucose, amino acids, and fatty acids by activated transport systems/enzymes. Inhibits breakdown of glycogen, fat, protein. Insulin lowers blood glucose by inhibiting glycogenolysis and gluconeogenesis in liver; stimulates glucose uptake by muscle, adipose tissue. Activity of insulin is initiated by binding to cell surface receptors.

Sulfonylureas: Stimulate release of insulin from beta cells; increase sensitivity of insulin to peripheral tissue. Endogenous insulin must be present for oral hypoglycemics to be effective.

Alpha-glucosidase inhibitors: Work locally in small intestine, slowing carbohydrate breakdown and glucose absorption.

Biguanides: Decrease hepatic glucose output; enhance peripheral glucose uptake.

Thiazolinediones: Decrease insulin resistance.

Antidiabetics *(continued)*

Antidiabetics

INSULIN

Name	Onset	Peak	Duration	Side Effects
Rapid Acting				
Insulin aspart (p. 619) (Novolog)	½ hr	1–3 hr	3–5 hr	Hypoglycemia, weight gain, lipodystrophy, local skin reactions
Glulisine (p. 619) (Apidra)	¼ hr	1 hr	3–5 hr	Same as above
Lispro (p. 619) (Humalog)	¼ hr	½–1 ½ hr	4–5 hr	Same as above
Regular (p. 619) (Humulin R, Novolin R)	½–1 hr	2–4 hr	5–7 hr	Same as above
Intermediate Acting				
NPH (p. 619) (Humulin N, Novolin N)	2–4 hr	6–14 hr	14–18 hr	Same as above
Long Acting				
Detemir (p. 620) (Levemir)	—	2–5 hr	24 hr	Same as above
Glargine (p. 620) (Lantus)	4 hr	—	24+ hr	Same as above

ORAL AGENTS

Name	Availability	Dosage Range	Side Effects
Sulfonylureas			
Acetohexamide **(Dymelor)**	**T:** 250 mg, 500 mg	0.25–1.5 g/day	Hypoglycemia, weight gain, skin rash, hemolytic anemia, GI distress, cholestasis
Chlorpropamide **(Diabinese)**	**T:** 100 mg, 250 mg	100–500 mg/day	Same as above
Glimepiride (p. 549) **(Amaryl)**	**T:** 1 mg, 2 mg, 4 mg	1–8 mg/day	Same as above
Glipizide (p. 551) **(Glucotrol)**	**T:** 5 mg, 10 mg **T (XL):** 5 mg	**T:** 2.5–40 mg/day **XL:** 5–20 mg/day	Same as above
Glyburide (p. 555) **(DiaBeta, Micronase)**	**T:** 1.25 mg, 2.5 mg, 5 mg **PT:** 1.5 mg, 3 mg	**T:** 1.25–20 mg/day **PT:** 1–12 mg/day	Same as above
Tolazamide **(Tolinase)**	**T:** 100 mg, 250 mg, 500 mg	0.2–1 g/day	Same as above
Tolbutamide **(Orinase)**	**T:** 250 mg, 500 mg	0.5–3 g/day	Same as above
Alpha Glucosidase Inhibitors			
Acarbose (p. 8) **(Precose)**	**T:** 25 mg, 50 mg, 100 mg	75–300 mg/day	Flatulence, diarrhea
Miglitol © **(Glyset)**	**T:** 25 mg, 50 mg, 100 mg	75–300 mg/day	Same as above

(continued)

ANTIDIABETICS	*(continued)*		
ORAL AGENTS *(continued)*			
Name	Availability	Dosage Range	Side Effects
Biguanides			
Metformin (p. 744) (Glucophage)	**T:** 500 mg, 850 mg **XR:** 500 mg	**T:** 0.5–2.5 g/day **XR:** 1,500–2,000 mg/day	Nausea, vomiting, diarrhea, loss of appetite, metallic taste, metabolic acidosis (rare)
Meglitinides			
Nateglinide (p. 818) (Starlix)	**T:** 60 mg, 120 mg	60–120 mg 3 times/day	Hypoglycemia, weight gain
Repaglinide (p. 1010) (Prandin)	**T:** 0.5 mg, 1 mg, 2 mg	0.5–1 mg with each meal (**Maximum:** 16 mg/day)	Same as above
Thiazolidinediones			
Pioglitazone (p. 934) (Actos)	**T:** 15 mg, 30 mg, 45 mg	15–45 mg/day	Mild anemia, mild to moderate edema, weight gain
Rosiglitazone (p. 1035) (Avandia)	**T:** 2 mg, 4 mg, 8 mg	4–8 mg/day	Same as above
Miscellaneous			
Exenatide (p. 458) (Byetta)	**I:** 5 mcg, 10 mcg	**A,E:** 5–10 mcg 2 times/day	Diarrhea, dizziness, dyspnea, headaches, nausea, vomiting
Pramlintide (p. 950) (Symlin)	**I:** 0.6 mg/ml	**A,E:** 15–60 mcg immediately prior to meals	Allergic reaction, hypoglycemia, abdominal pain, anorexia, arthralgia, headaches, nausea, vomiting

PT, Prestab; *T,* tablets; *XL,* extended-release; *XR,* extended-release.

Antidiarrheals

USES

Acute diarrhea, chronic diarrhea of inflammatory bowel disease, reduction of fluid from ileostomies.

ACTION

Systemic agents: Act at smooth muscle receptors (enteric) disrupting peristaltic movements, decreasing GI motility, increasing transit time of intestinal contents.

Local agents: Adsorb toxic substances and fluids to large surface areas of particles in the preparation. Some of these agents coat and protect irritated intestinal walls. May have local anti-inflammatory action.

ANTIDIARRHEALS

Name	Availability	Type	Dosage Range
Bismuth subsalicylate (p. 141) (Pepto-Bismol)	**T:** 262 mg **C:** 262 mg **L:** 130 mg/15 ml, 262 mg/15 ml, 524 mg/15 ml	Local	**A:** 2 T or 30 ml **C (9-12 yr):** 1 T or 15 ml **C (6-8 yr):** $^2/_3$ T or 10 ml **C (3-5 yr):** $^1/_3$ T or 5 ml
Diphenoxylate (with atropine) (p. 367) (Lomotil)	**T:** 2.5 mg **L:** 2.5 mg/5 ml	Systemic	**A:** 5 mg 4 times/day **C:** 0.3-0.4 mg/kg/day in 4 divided doses (L)
Kaolin (with pectin) (p. 651) (Kaopectate)	Suspension	Local	**A:** 60-120 ml after each bowel movement **C (6-12 yr):** 30-60 ml **C (3-5 yr):** 15-30 ml
Loperamide (p. 703) (Imodium)	**C:** 2 mg **T:** 2 mg **L:** 1 mg/5 ml, 1 mg/ml	Systemic	**A:** Initially, 4 mg (**Maximum:** 16 mg/day) **C (9-12 yr):** 2 mg 3 times/day **C (6-8 yr):** 2 mg 2 times/day **C (2-5 yr):** 1 mg 3 times/day (L)

A, Adults; *C,* capsules; *C (dosage),* children; *L,* liquid; *T,* tablets.

Antifungals: Topical

USES

Treatment of tinea infections, cutaneous candidiasis (moniliasis) due to *Candida albicans*.

ACTION

Exact mechanism unknown. May deplete essential intracellular components by inhibiting transport of potassium, other ions into cells; alter membrane permeability, resulting in loss of potassium, other cellular components.

ANTIFUNGALS: TOPICAL

Name	Availability	Dosage Range	Side Effects
Butenafine (Mentax)	**C:** 1%	2 times/day	Burning, stinging, itching, contact dermatitis, erythema
Ciclopirox (Loprox)	**C:** 1% **L:** 1%	2 times/day	Irritation, pruritus, redness
Clioquinol (Vioform)	**C:** 3% **O:** 3%	2–3 times/day	Irritation, stinging, swelling
Clotrimazole (p. 277) (Lotrimin, Mycelex)	**C:** 1% **L:** 1% **S:** 1%	2 times/day	Erythema, stinging, blistering, edema, itching
Econazole (Spectazole)	**C:** 1%	1–2 times/day	Burning, stinging, irritation, erythema
Ketoconazole (p. 654) @ (Nizoral)	**C:** 2%	1–2 times/day	Irritation, itching, stinging
Miconazole (p. 771) (Micatin, Monistat)	**C:** 2% **P:** 2%	2 times/day	Irritation, burning, allergic contact dermatitis

Nystatin (p. 854) (Mycostatin, Niistat)	**C:** 100,000 g **O:** 100,000 g **P:** 100,000 g	Irritation
Oxiconazole (Oxistat)	**C:** 1% **L:** 1%	2–3 times/day	Pruritus, burning, stinging, irritation, pain, tingling
Sertaconazole © (Ertaczo)	**C:** 2%	1–2 times/day	Dry skin, burning, pruritus, erythema
Terbinafine (p. 1109) (Lamisil)	**C:** 1% **G:** 10 mg	2 times/day	Irritation, burning, pruritus, dryness
Tolnaftate (Tinactin)	**C:** 1% **G:** 1% **S:** 1%	1–2 times/day	Mild irritation
Triacetin (Fungoid)	**C:** 1% **S:** 1%	2 times/day	Irritation
Undecylenic acid (Desenex, Cruex, Caldesene)	**C, O, P**	3 times/day	None significant
		As needed	

C, Cream; *G*, gel; *L*, lotion; *O*, ointment; *P*, powder; *S*, solution.

Antiglaucoma Agents

USES	ACTION	
Reduction of elevated intraocular pressure (IOP) in patients with open-angle glaucoma and ocular hypertension.	Medications that decrease IOP by increasing outflow of aqueous humor:	• *Miotics (direct acting):* Cholinergic agents or miotics stimulate ciliary muscles, leading to increases in contraction of the iris sphincter muscle.

Antiglaucoma Agents *(continued)*

ACTION *(continued)*

- *Miotics (indirect acting):* Primarily inhibit cholinesterase, allowing accumulation of acetylcholine, prolonging parasympathetic activity.
- *Sympathomimetics:* Increase the rate of fluid flow out of the eye and decrease the rate of aqueous humor production.

Medications that decrease IOP by decreasing aqueous humor production:

- *Alpha₂-agonists:* Activate receptors in ciliary body, inhibiting aqueous secretion and increasing uveoscleral aqueous outflow.
- *Beta-blockers:* Reduce production of aqueous humor.

- *Carbonic anhydrase inhibitors:* Reduce fluid flow into the eye by inhibiting enzyme carbonic anhydrase.
- *Prostaglandins:* Increase outflow of aqueous fluid through uveoscleral route.

ANTIGLAUCOMA AGENTS

Name	Availability	Dosage Range	Side Effects
Miotics			
Carbachol (Isopto-Carbachol)	**S:** 0.75%, 1.5%, 2.25%, 3%	1 drop 2 times/day	Ciliary or accommodative spasm, blurred vision, reduced night vision, diaphoresis, increased salivation, urinary frequency, nausea, diarrhea
Echothiophate (Phospholine Iodide)	**S:** 0.03%, 0.06%, 0.125%, 0.25%	1 drop 2 times/day	Headaches, accommodative spasm, diaphoresis, vomiting, nausea, diarrhea, tachycardia
Physostigmine (p. 932)	**O:** 0.25%	Apply up to 3 times/day	Blurred vision, eye pain
Pilocarpine Ⓔ (Isopto Carpine)	**S:** 0.25%, 0.5%, 1%, 2%, 3%, 4%, 5%, 6%, 8%, 10%	1–2 drops 3–4 times/day	Same as carbachol

Sympathomimetics

Dipivefrin (Propine)	S: 0.1%	1 drop q12h	Ocular congestion, burning, stinging
Epinephrine (p. 416)	S: 0.5%, 1%, 2%	1 drop 1–2 times/day	Mydriasis, blurred vision, tachycardia, hypertension, tremors, headaches, anxiety

Alpha₂-Agonists

Apraclonidine (Iopidine)	S: 0.5%	1–2 drops 3 times/day	Hypersensitivity reaction, change in visual acuity, lethargy
Brimonidine (Alphagan)	S: 0.2%	1–2 drops 2–3 times/day	Hypersensitivity reaction, headaches, drowsiness, fatigue

Prostaglandins

Bimatoprost (Lumigan)	S: 0.03%	1 drop daily in evening	Ocular hyperemia, eyelash growth, pruritus
Latanoprost (Xalatan)	S: 0.005%	1 drop daily in evening	Burning, stinging, iris pigmentation
Travoprost (Travatan)	S: 0.004%	1 drop daily in evening	Ocular hyperemia, eye discomfort, foreign body sensation, pain, pruritus
Unoprostone (Rescula)	S: 0.15%	1 drop 2 times/day	Iris pigmentations

Beta-Blockers

Betaxolol (p. 132) (Betoptic-S)	Suspension: 0.25% S: 0.5%	1–2 drops 1–2 times/day	Transient irritation, burning, tearing, blurred vision
Carteolol @ (Ocupress)	S: 1%	1 drop 2 times/day	Mild, transient ocular stinging, burning, discomfort

(continued)

ANTIGLAUCOMA AGENTS   *(continued)*

Name	Availability	Dosage Range	Side Effects
Beta-Blockers *(continued)*			
Levobetaxolol (Betaxon)	**S:** 0.5%	1 drop 2 times/day	Transient irritation, burning, tearing, blurred vision
Levobunolol (Betagan)	**S:** 0.25%, 0.5%	1 drop 1–2 times/day	Local discomfort, conjunctivitis, brow ache, tearing, blurred vision, headaches, anxiety
Metipranolol (OptiPranolol)	**S:** 0.3%	1 drop 2 times/day	Transient irritation, burning, stinging, blurred vision
Timolol (p. 1133) (Istalol, Timoptic)	**S:** 0.25%, 0.5% **G:** 0.25%, 0.5%	**S:** 1 drop 2 times/day (Istalol): 1 drop daily **G:** 1 drop daily	Same as above
Carbonic Anhydrase Inhibitors			
Acetazolamide (p. 14) (Diamox)	**T:** 125 mg, 250 mg **C:** 500 mg	0.25–1 g/day	Diarrhea, loss of appetite, metallic taste, nausea, paraesthesia
Brinzolamide (Azopt)	**Suspension:** 1%	1 drop 3 times/day	Blurred vision, bitter taste
Dorzolamide (Trusopt)	**S:** 2%	1 drop 2–3 times/day	Burning, stinging, blurred vision, bitter taste

C, Capsules; *G,* gel; *O,* ointment; *S,* solution; *T,* tablets.

Antihistamines

USES

Symptomatic relief of upper respiratory allergic disorders. Allergic reactions associated with other drugs respond to antihistamines, as do blood transfusion reactions. Used as a second-choice drug in treatment of angioneurotic edema. Effective in treatment of acute urticaria and other dermatologic conditions. May also be used for preop sedation, Parkinson's disease, and motion sickness.

ACTION

Antihistamines (H₁ antagonists) inhibit vasoconstrictor effects and vasodilator effects on endothelial cells of histamine. They block increased capillary permeability, formation of edema/wheal caused by histamine. Many antihistamines can bind to receptors in CNS, causing primarily depression (decreased alertness, slowed reaction times, somnolence) but also stimulation (restlessness, nervousness, inability to sleep). Some may counter motion sickness.

ANTIHISTAMINES

Name	Availability	Dosage Range	Side Effects
Azatadine (Optimine)	T: 1 mg	A: 1–2 mg q12h C: 0.05 mg/kg/day	Dry mouth, urinary retention, blurred vision, sedation, dizziness, paradoxical excitement
Brompheniramine (Dimetane)	T: 4 mg T (SR): 4 mg, 6 mg S: 2 mg/5 ml	A: 4–8 mg q4–6h or T (SR): 8–12 mg q12–24h C: 0.5 mg/kg/day	Dry mouth, urinary retention, blurred vision
Cetirizine (p. 229) (Zyrtec)	T: 5 mg, 10 mg S: 5 mg/5 ml	A: 5–10 mg/day C (6–12 yr): 5–10 mg/day C (2–5 yr): 2.5–5 mg/day	Minimal CNS and anticholinergic side effects

(continued)

ANTIHISTAMINES *(continued)*

Name	Availability	Dosage Range	Side Effects
Chlorpheniramine (Chlor-Trimeton)	**T:** 4 mg **T (chewable):** 2 mg **T (SR):** 8 mg, 12 mg **S:** 2 mg/5 ml	**A:** 2–4 mg q4–6h or **SR:** 8–12 mg q12–24h **C:** 0.35 mg/kg/day	Same as brompheniramine
Clemastine (p. 263) (Tavist)	**T:** 1.34 mg, 2.68 mg **S:** 0.67 mg/5 ml	**A:** 1.34–2.68 mg q8–12h **C (6–12 yr):** 0.67–1.34 mg q8–12h	Same as azatadine
Cyproheptadine (p. 303) @ (Periactin)	**T:** 4 mg **S:** 2 mg/5 ml	**A:** 4 mg q8h **C:** 0.25 mg/kg/day	Same as azatadine
Dexchlorpheniramine (Polaramine)	**T:** 2 mg **S:** 2 mg/5 ml	**A:** 2 mg q4–6h **C:** 0.5–1 mg q4–6h	Same as brompheniramine
Dimenhydrinate (Dramamine)	**T:** 50 mg **L:** 12.5 mg/5 ml	**A:** 50–100 mg q4–6h **C:** 12.5–50 mg q6–8h	Same as azatadine
Diphenhydramine (p. 365) (Benadryl)	**T:** 25 mg, 50 mg **C:** 25 mg, 50 mg **L:** 6.25 mg/5 ml, 12.5 mg/5 ml	**A:** 25–50 mg q6–8h **C (6–11 yr):** 12.5–25 mg q4–6h **C (2–5 yr):** 6.25 mg q4–6h	Same as azatadine
Fexofenadine (p. 477) (Allegra)	**T:** 30 mg, 60 mg, 180 mg	**A:** 60 mg q12h or 180 mg/day; **C (6–11 yr):** 30 mg q12h	Same as cetirizine
Hydroxyzine (p. 591) (Atarax, Vistaril)	**T:** 10 mg, 25 mg, 50 mg, 100 mg **C:** 25 mg, 50 mg, 100 mg **S:** 10 mg/5 ml, 25 mg/5 ml	**A:** 25 mg q6–8h **C:** 2 mg/kg/day	Same as azatadine

| **Loratadine (p. 707)** (Claritin) | **T:** 10 mg **S:** 1 mg/ml | **A:** 10 mg/day **C (6–12 yr):** 10 mg/day | Same as cetirizine |
| **Promethazine (p. 972)** (Phenergan) | **T:** 12.5 mg, 25 mg, 50 mg **S:** 6.25 mg/5 ml, 25 mg/5 ml | **A:** 25 mg at bedtime or 12.5 mg q8h **C:** 0.5 mg/kg at bedtime or 0.1 mg/kg q6–8h | Same as azatadine |

A, Adults; *C*, capsules; *C (dosage)*, children; *L*, liquid; *S*, syrup; *SR*, sustained-release; *T*, tablets.

Antihyperlipidemics

USES

Cholesterol management.

ACTION

Bile acid sequestrants: Bind bile acids in the intestine; prevent active transport and reabsorption and enhance bile acid excretion. Depletion of hepatic bile acid results in the increased conversion of cholesterol to bile acids.

HMG-CoA reductase inhibitors (statins): Inhibit HMG-CoA reductase, the last regulated step in the synthesis of cholesterol. Cholesterol synthesis in the liver is reduced.

Niacin (nicotinic acid): Reduces hepatic synthesis of triglycerides and secretion of VLDL by inhibiting the mobilization of free fatty acids from peripheral tissues.

Fibric acid: Increases the oxidation of fatty acids in the liver, resulting in reduced secretion of triglyceride-rich lipoproteins and increases lipoprotein lipase activity and fatty acid uptake.

Cholesterol absorption inhibitor: Acts in the gut wall to prevent cholesterol absorption through the intestinal villi.

Antihyperlipidemics *(continued)*

ANTIHYPERLIPIDEMICS

Name	Availability	Primary Effect	Dosage Range (per day)	Side Effects
Bile Acid Sequestrants				
Cholestyramine (p. 242) (Questran, Prevalite)	**P:** 4 g	Decreases LDL	4–8 g	GI complaints (constipation, bloating, abdominal pain, gas), reduced absorption of other drugs
Colesevelam (p. 284) (Welchol)	**T:** 625 mg	Decreases LDL	4–6 **T**	Same as cholestyramine
Colestipol (Colestid)	**T:** 1 g **G:** 5 g	Decreases LDL	**T:** 2–16 g **G:** 5–30 g	Same as cholestyramine
HMG-CoA Reductase Inhibitors (Statins)				
Atorvastatin (p. 101) (Lipitor)	**T:** 10 mg, 20 mg, 40 mg, 80 mg	Decreases LDL, TG Increases HDL	10–80 mg	Headaches, dizziness, nausea, vomiting, diarrhea, myalgia, increased LFTs, rhabdomyolysis
Fluvastatin (p. 505) (Lescol)	**C:** 20 mg, 40 mg **T (ER):** 80 mg	Decreases LDL, TG Increases HDL	20–80 mg	Same as above
Lovastatin (p. 713) (Mevacor)	**T:** 10 mg, 20 mg, 40 mg	Decreases LDL, TG Increases HDL	10–80 mg	Same as above
Pravastatin (p. 952) (Pravachol)	**T:** 10 mg, 20 mg, 40 mg	Decreases LDL, TG Increases HDL	10–40 mg	Same as above

Rosuvastatin (p. 1037) (Crestor)	**T:** 5 mg, 10 mg, 20 mg, 40 mg	Decreases LDL, TG Increases HDL	5–40 mg	Same as above
Simvastatin (p. 1056) (Zocor)	**T:** 5 mg, 10 mg, 20 mg, 40 mg, 80 mg	Decreases LDL, TG Increases HDL	5–80 mg	Same as above
Niacin				
Nicotinic acid (p. 829) *Crystalline* (Niacor)	**T:** 500 mg	Decreases LDL, TG Increases HDL	Up to 6 g	Flushing, hepatic toxicity, increased serum glucose, GI distress, gout
Nicotinic acid (p. 829) *Long-acting* (Niaspan)	**T (ER):** 500 mg, 750 mg, 1,000 mg	Decreases LDL, TG Increases HDL	Up to 2,000 mg	Same as above
Fibric Acid				
Fenofibrate (p. 467) (Tricor)	**T:** 48 mg, 145 mg	Decreases TG	67–200 mg	Diarrhea, nausea, constipation, abdominal pain, back pain, headaches
Gemfibrozil (p. 538) (Lopid)	**T:** 600 mg	Decreases TG	1,200 mg	Dyspepsia, abdominal pain, diarrhea, nausea, vomiting, fatigue
Cholesterol Absorption Inhibitor				
Ezetimibe (p. 460) (Zetia)	**T:** 10 mg	Decreases LDL, TG	10 mg	Headache, viral infection, arthralgia, upper respiratory tract infections

C, Capsules; *ER,* extended-release; *G,* granules; *HDL,* high-density lipoprotein; *LDL,* low-density lipoprotein; *LFTs,* liver function tests; *P,* powder; *T,* tablets; *TG,* triglycerides.

Antihypertensives

USES

Treatment of mild to severe hypertension.

ACTION

Many groups of medications are used in the treatment of hypertension. In addition to the alpha-adrenergic central agonists, peripheral antagonists, and vasodilators listed in the following table, refer to the classifications of diuretics, beta-adrenergic blockers, calcium channel blockers, and ACE inhibitors or to individual drug monographs.

Alpha-agonists (central action): Stimulate alpha$_2$-adrenergic receptors in the cardiovascular centers of the CNS, reducing sympathetic outflow and producing an antihypertensive effect.

Alpha-antagonists (peripheral action): Block alpha$_1$-adrenergic receptors in arterioles and veins, inhibiting vasoconstriction and decreasing peripheral vascular resistance, causing a fall in B/P.

Vasodilators: Directly relax arteriolar smooth muscle, decreasing vascular resistance. Exact mechanism unknown.

ANTIHYPERTENSIVES

Name	Availability	Dosage Range	Side Effects
Alpha-Agonists: Central Action			
Clonidine (p. 272) (Catapres)	**T:** 0.1 mg, 0.2 mg, 0.3 mg **P:** 0.1 mg/hr, 0.2 mg/hr, 0.3 mg/hr	**PO:** 0.2–0.8 mg/day **Topical:** 0.1–0.6 mg/wk	Sedation, dry mouth, constipation, sexual dysfunction, bradycardia
Guanabenz (Wytensin)	**T:** 4 mg, 8 mg	**PO:** 8–32 mg/day	Same as above
Guanfacine (Tenex)	**T:** 1 mg, 2 mg	**PO:** 1–3 mg/day	Same as above
Methyldopa (p. 753) © **(Aldomet)**	**T:** 125 mg, 250 mg, 500 mg	**PO:** 0.5–3 g/day	Same as above Impaired memory, depression, nasal congestion

Alpha-Agonists: Peripheral Action

Doxazosin (p. 385) (Cardura) @	**T:** 1 mg, 2 mg, 4 mg, 8 mg	**PO:** 2–16 mg/day	Dizziness, vertigo, headaches
Prazosin (p. 953) (Minipress)	**C:** 1 mg, 2 mg, 5 mg	**PO:** 6–20 mg/day	Dizziness, lightheadedness, headaches, drowsiness
Terazosin (p. 1108) (Hytrin)	**C:** 1 mg, 2 mg, 5 mg, 10 mg	**PO:** 1–20 mg/day	Dizziness, headaches, asthenia

Vasodilators

Hydralazine (p. 575) (Apresoline)	**T:** 10 mg, 25 mg, 50 mg, 100 mg	**PO:** 40–300 mg/day	Anorexia, nausea, diarrhea, vomiting, headaches, palpitations
Minoxidil (p. 780) (Loniten)	**T:** 2.5 mg, 10 mg	**PO:** 10–40 mg/day	Rapid/irregular heartbeat, hypertrichosis, peripheral edema

C, Capsules; *P,* patch; *T,* tablets.

Antimigraine (Triptans)

USES

Treatment of migraine headaches with or without aura in adults 18 yr and older.

ACTION

Triptans are selective agonists of the serotonin (5-HT) receptor that inhibit neuropeptide release and vasodilation, causing vasoconstriction.

Antimigraine (Triptans) *(continued)*

TRIPTANS

Name	Availability	Dosage Range	Contraindications	Side Effects
Almotriptan (p. 37) (Axert)	**T:** 6.25 mg, 12.5 mg	6.25–12.5 mg; may repeat after 2 hr	Ischemic heart disease, angina pectoris, arrhythmias, previous MI, uncontrolled hypertension	Drowsiness, dizziness, fatigue, hot flashes, chest pain/discomfort, paraesthesia, nausea, vomiting
Eletriptan (p. 405) (Relpax)	**T:** 20 mg, 40 mg	**A:** 20–40 mg. May repeat after 2 hr	Same as above	Asthenia, nausea, dizziness, somnolence
Frovatriptan (p. 521) (Frova)	**T:** 2.5 mg	2.5 mg; may repeat after 2 hr; no more than 3 **T**/day	Same as above	Hot/cold sensations, dizziness, fatigue, headaches, chest pain, skeletal pain, dry mouth, dyspepsia, flushing
Naratriptan (p. 816) (Amerge)	**T:** 1 mg, 2.5 mg	2.5 mg; may repeat once after 4 hr	Same as above	Atypical sensations, pain, nausea
Rizatriptan (p. 1032) (Maxalt, Maxalt-MLT)	**T:** 5 mg, 10 mg **DT:** 5 mg, 10 mg	5 or 10 mg; may repeat after 2 hr	Same as above	Atypical sensations, pain, nausea, dizziness, somnolence, asthenia, fatigue
Sumatriptan (p. 1087) (Imitrex)	**T:** 25 mg, 50 mg **NS:** 5 mg, 20 mg **I:** 4 mg, 6 mg	**PO:** 25–100 mg; may repeat q2h **NS:** 5–20 mg; may repeat after 2 hr **Subcutaneous:** 4–6 mg; may repeat after 1 hr	Ischemic heart disease, angina pectoris, arrhythmias, previous MI, uncontrolled hypertension	*Oral:* Atypical sensations, pain, malaise, fatigue *Injection:* Atypical sensations, flushing, chest pain/discomfort, injection site reaction, dizziness, vertigo *Nasal:* Discomfort, nausea, vomiting, altered taste

| Zolmitriptan (p. 1234) (Zomig) | T: 2.5 mg, 5 mg DT: 2.5 mg, 5 mg | 2.5–5 mg; may repeat after 2 hr | Same as above | Atypical sensations, pain, nausea, dizziness, asthenia, somnolence |

DT, Disintegrating tablets; *I,* injection; *NS,* nasal spray; *T,* tablets.

Antipsychotics

USES

Antipsychotics are primarily used in managing psychotic illness (especially in patients with increased psychomotor activity). They are also used to treat the manic phase of bipolar disorder, behavioral problems in children, nausea and vomiting, intractable hiccups, anxiety and agitation, as adjunct in treatment of tetanus, and to potentiate effects of narcotics.

ACTION

Effects of these agents occur at all levels of the CNS. Antipsychotic mechanism unknown but may antagonize dopamine action as a neurotransmitter in basal ganglia and limbic system. Antipsychotics may block postsynaptic dopamine receptors, inhibit dopamine release, increase dopamine turnover.

These medications can be divided into the phe-nothiazines and nonphenothiazines (miscellaneous). In addition to their use in symptomatic treatment of psychiatric illness, some have antiemetic, antinausea, antihistamine, anticholinergic, and/or sedative effects.

ANTIPSYCHOTICS

| Name | Availability | Dosage | Relative Side Effects Profile | | | |
			EPS	Anticholinergic	Sedation	Hypotension
Aripiprazole (p. 86) (Abilify)	T: 5 mg, 10 mg, 15 mg	15–30 mg/day	Low	Low	Low	Low

(continued)

ANTIPSYCHOTICS *(continued)*

Name	Availability	Dosage	Relative Side Effects Profile			
			EPS	Anticholinergic	Sedation	Hypotension
Chlorpromazine (p. 240) ⓔ (Thorazine)	**T:** 10 mg, 25 mg, 50 mg, 100 mg, 200 mg **SR:** 30 mg, 75 mg, 100 mg **OC:** 30 mg/ml, 100 mg/ml	50–2,000 mg/day	Moderate	Moderate	High	High
Clozapine (p. 278) ⓔ (Clozaril) ⓔ	**T:** 25 mg, 100 mg	75–900 mg/day	Rare	High	High	High
Fluphenazine (p. 497) (Prolixin)	**T:** 1 mg, 2.5 mg, 5 mg, 10 mg **I:** 25 mg/ml **OC:** 5 mg/ml	**PO:** 2–40 mg/day **I:** 12.5–75 mg q2wk	High	Low	Low	Low
Haloperidol (p. 568) (Haldol)	**T:** 0.5 mg, 1 mg, 2 mg, 5 mg, 10 mg, 20 mg **I:** 5 mg/ml **OC:** 2 mg/ml	2–40 mg/day	High	Low	Low	Low
Loxapine (Loxitane)	**C:** 5 mg, 10 mg, 25 mg, 50 mg **OC:** 25 mg/ml **I:** 50 mg/ml	20–250 mg/day	High	Low	Moderate	Moderate
Mesoridazine (p. 741) (Serentil)	**T:** 10 mg, 25 mg, 50 mg, 100 mg **I:** 25 mg/ml **OC:** 25 mg/ml	100–400 mg/day	Low	High	High	High
Olanzapine (p. 860) (Zyprexa)	**T:** 2.5 mg, 5 mg, 7.5 mg, 10 mg, 15 mg, 20 mg **DT:** 5 mg, 10 mg **I:** 10 mg	10–20 mg/day	Low	Low	Moderate	Low

Quetiapine (p. 993) (Seroquel)	T: 25 mg, 100 mg, 200 mg, 300 mg	100–800 mg/day	Rare	Low	Moderate	Moderate
Risperidone (p. 1026) (Risperdal)	T: 0.25 mg, 0.5 mg, 1 mg, 2 mg, 3 mg, 4 mg OC: 1 mg/ml I: 25 mg, 37.5 mg, 50 mg	2–6 mg/day IM: 25–50 mg q2wk	Low	Low	Low	Moderate
Thioridazine (p. 1121) (Mellaril)	T: 10 mg, 15 mg, 25 mg, 50 mg, 100 mg, 150 mg, 200 mg OC: 30 mg/ml, 100 mg/ml	50–800 mg/day	Low	High	High	High
Thiothixene (p. 1124) (Navane)	C: 1 mg, 2 mg, 5 mg	5–60 mg/day	High	Low	Low	Low
Trifluoperazine (p. 1176) (Stelazine)	T: 1 mg, 2 mg, 5 mg, 10 mg I: 5 mg/ml OC: 2 mg/ml	5–80 mg/day	High	Low	Low	Low
Ziprasidone (p. 1231) (Geodon)	C: 20 mg, 40 mg, 60 mg, 80 mg I: 20 mg	40–160 mg/day	Low	Low	Low to moderate	Low to moderate

C, Capsules; *DT,* disintegrating tablets; *EPS,* extrapyramidal symptoms; *I,* injection; *OC,* oral concentrate; *SR,* sustained-release; *T,* tablets.

Antivirals

USES

Treatment of HIV infection. Treatment of cytomegalovirus (CMV) retinitis in patients with AIDS, acute herpes zoster (shingles), genital herpes (recurrent), mucosal and cutaneous herpes simplex virus (HSV), chickenpox, and influenza A viral illness.

ACTION

Effective antivirals must inhibit virus-specific nucleic acid/protein synthesis. Possible mechanisms of action of antivirals used for non-HIV infection may include interference with viral DNA synthesis and viral replication, inactivation of viral DNA polymerases, incorporation and termination of the growing viral DNA chain, prevention of release of viral nucleic acid into the host cell, or interference with viral penetration into cells.

Antivirals   *(continued)*

ANTIVIRALS

Name	Availability	Uses	Side Effects
Abacavir (p. 1) (Ziagen)	**T:** 300 mg **OS:** 20 mg/ml	HIV infection	Nausea, vomiting, loss of appetite, diarrhea, headaches, fatigue
Acyclovir (p. 17) (Zovirax)	**T:** 400 mg, 800 mg **C:** 200 mg **I:** 50 mg/ml	Mucosal/cutaneous HSV-1 and HSV-2, varicella-zoster (shingles), genital herpes, herpes simplex, encephalitis, chickenpox	Malaise, anorexia, nausea, vomiting, lightheadedness
Adefovir (p. 21) (Hepsera)	**T:** 10 mg	Chronic hepatitis B	Asthenia, headaches, abdominal pain, nausea, diarrhea, flatulence, dyspepsia
Amantadine (p. 46) (Symmetrel)	**C:** 100 mg **S:** 50 mg/5 ml	Influenza A	Anxiety, dizziness, lightheadedness, headaches, nausea, loss of appetite
Amprenavir (p. 75) (Agenerase)	**C:** 50 mg, 150 mg **OS:** 15 mg/ml	HIV infection	Hyperglycemia, rash, abdominal pain, nausea, vomiting, diarrhea
Cidofovir (p. 245) (Vistide)	**I:** 75 mg/ml	CMV retinitis	Decreased urination, fever, chills, diarrhea, nausea, vomiting, headaches, loss of appetite
Delavirdine (p. 324) (Rescriptor)	**T:** 100 mg, 200 mg	HIV infection	Diarrhea, fatigue, rash, headaches, nausea
Didanosine (p. 352) (Videx)	**T:** 25 mg, 50 mg, 100 mg, 150 mg, 200 mg **C:** 125 mg, 200 mg **Powder for suspension:** 100 mg, 167 mg, 250 mg	HIV infection	Peripheral neuropathy, anxiety, headaches, rash, nausea, diarrhea, dry mouth

Name (page)	Dosage Forms	Uses	Side Effects
Efavirenz (p. 403) (Sustiva)	**C:** 50 mg, 100 mg, 200 mg	HIV infection	Diarrhea, dizziness, headaches, insomnia, nausea, vomiting, drowsiness
Famciclovir (p. 462) (Famvir)	**T:** 125 mg, 250 mg, 500 mg	Herpes zoster, genital herpes	Headaches
Foscarnet (p. 514) (Foscavir)	**I:** 24 mg/ml	CMV retinitis, HSV infections	Decreased urination, abdominal pain, nausea, vomiting, dizziness, fatigue, headaches
Ganciclovir (p. 529) (Cytovene)	**C:** 250 mg, 500 mg **I:** 500 mg	CMV retinitis, CMV disease	Sore throat, fever, unusual bleeding/ecchymoses
Indinavir (p. 614) (Crixivan)	**C:** 200 mg, 400 mg	HIV infection	Blood in urine, weakness, nausea, vomiting, diarrhea, headaches, insomnia, altered taste
Lamivudine (p. 664) (Epivir)	**T:** 100 mg, 150 mg **OS:** 5 mg/ml, 10 mg/ml	HIV infection	Nausea, vomiting, abdominal pain, paraesthesia
Lopinavir/ritonavir (p. 704) (Kaletra)	**C:** 133/33 mg **OS:** 80/20 mg	HIV infection	Diarrhea, nausea
Nelfinavir (p. 822) (Viracept)	**T:** 250 mg **Powder:** 50 mg/g	HIV infection	Diarrhea
Oseltamivir (p. 874) (Tamiflu)	**C:** 75 mg **S:** 12 mg/ml	Influenza	Diarrhea, nausea, vomiting
Ribavirin (p. 1016) (Virazole)	**Aerosol:** 6 g	Lowers respiratory infections in infants, children due to respiratory syncytial virus (RSV)	Anemia
Ritonavir (p. 1028) (Norvir)	**C:** 100 mg **OS:** 80 mg/ml	HIV infection	Weakness, diarrhea, nausea, decreased appetite, vomiting, altered taste

(continued)

ANTIVIRALS	*(continued)*		
Name	Availability	Uses	Side Effects
Saquinavir (p. 1041) (Invirase)	**C:** 200 mg	HIV infection	Weakness, diarrhea, nausea, oral ulcers, abdominal pain
Stavudine (p. 1077) (Zerit)	**C:** 15 mg, 20 mg, 30 mg, 40 mg **OS:** 1 mg/ml	HIV infection	Paraesthesia, decreased appetite, chills, fever, rash
Tenofovir (p. 1106) (Viread)	**T:** 300 mg	HIV infection	Diarrhea, nausea, pharyngitis, headaches
Valacyclovir (p. 1187) (Valtrex)	**T:** 500 mg	Herpes zoster, genital herpes	Headaches, nausea
Valganciclovir (p. 1189) (Valcyte)	**T:** 450 mg	CMV retinitis	Anemia, abdominal pain, diarrhea, headaches, nausea, vomiting, paraesthesia
Zalcitabine (p. 1225) (Hivid)	**T:** 0.375 mg, 0.75 mg	HIV infection	Paraesthesia, arthralgia, rash, nausea, vomiting
Zanamivir (p. 1228) (Relenza)	**Inhalation:** 5 mg	Influenza	Cough, diarrhea, dizziness, headaches, nausea, vomiting
Zidovudine (p. 1229) (Retrovir)	**T:** 300 mg **C:** 100 mg **S:** 50 mg/5 ml	HIV infection	Unusual fatigue, fever, chills, headaches, nausea, muscle pain

C, Capsules; *I,* injection; *OS,* oral solution; *S,* syrup; *T,* tablets.

Beta-Adrenergic Blockers

USES

Management of hypertension, angina pectoris, arrhythmias, hypertrophic subaortic stenosis, migraine headaches, MI (prevention), glaucoma.

ACTION

Beta-adrenergic blockers competitively block $beta_1$-adrenergic receptors, located primarily in myocardium, and $beta_2$-adrenergic receptors, located primarily in bronchial and vascular smooth muscle. By occupying beta-receptor sites, these agents prevent naturally occurring or administered epinephrine/norepinephrine from exerting their effects. The results are basically opposite to those of sympathetic stimulation.

Effects of $beta_1$-blockade include slowing heart rate, decreasing cardiac output and contractility; effects of $beta_2$-blockade include bronchoconstriction, increased airway resistance in patients with asthma or chronic obstructive pulmonary disease (COPD). Beta-blockers can affect cardiac rhythm/automaticity (decrease sinus rate, SA/AV conduction; increase refractory period in AV node). Decrease systolic and diastolic BP; exact mechanism unknown but may block peripheral receptors, decrease sympathetic outflow from CNS, or decrease renin release from kidney. All beta-blockers mask tachycardia that occurs with hypoglycemia. When applied to the eye, reduce intraocular pressure and aqueous production.

BETA-ADRENERGIC BLOCKERS

Name	Availability	Selectivity	Dosage Range	Side Effects
Acebutolol (p. 10) (Sectral)	**C:** 200 mg, 400 mg	Beta₁	200–1,200 mg/day	Lightheadedness, fatigue, weakness, decreased sexual function, insomnia
Atenolol (p. 97) (Tenormin)	**T:** 25 mg, 50 mg, 100 mg	Beta₁	50–100 mg/day	Same as above
Betaxolol (p. 132) (Kerlone)	**T:** 10 mg, 20 mg	Beta₁	10–20 mg/day	Same as above

(continued)

BETA-ADRENERGIC BLOCKERS   *(continued)*

Name	Availability	Selectivity	Dosage Range	Side Effects
Bisoprolol (p. 142) (Zebeta)	**T:** 5 mg, 10 mg	Beta$_1$	2.5–20 mg/day	Same as above
Carteolol (Cartrol)	**T:** 2.5 mg, 5 mg	Beta$_1$, beta$_2$	2.5–10 mg/day	Same as above
Carvedilol (p. 190) (Coreg)	**T:** 3.125 mg, 6.25 mg, 12.5 mg, 25 mg	Beta$_1$, beta$_2$, alpha$_1$	12.5–50 mg/day	Same as above
Esmolol (p. 438) (Brevibloc)	**I:** 10 mg/ml, 250 mcg/ml	Beta$_1$	50–200 mcg/kg/min	Same as above
Metoprolol (p. 764) (Lopressor)	**T:** 50 mg, 100 mg/ml **I:** 1 mg/ml	Beta$_1$	50–450 mg/day	Same as above, increased risk of CNS effects
Nadolol (p. 806) (Corgard)	**T:** 20 mg, 40 mg, 80 mg, 120 mg, 160 mg	Beta$_1$, beta$_2$	40–320 mg/day	Same as above
Penbutolol (Levatol)	**T:** 20 mg	Beta$_1$, beta$_2$	10–40 mg/day	Same as above
Pindolol (Visken)	**T:** 5 mg, 10 mg	Beta$_1$, beta$_2$	10–60 mg/day	Same as above
Propranolol (p. 980) (Inderal)	**T:** 10 mg, 20 mg, 40 mg, 60 mg, 80 mg, 90 mg **C (SR):** 60 mg, 80 mg, 120 mg, 160 mg **S:** 4 mg/ml, 8 mg/ml **I:** 1 mg/ml	Beta$_1$, beta$_2$	80–320 mg/day	Same as above, increased risk of CNS effects

| Sotalol (p. 1072) (Betapace) | T: 80 mg, 120 mg, 160 mg, 240 mg | Beta₁, beta₂ | 160–640 mg/day | Same as above |
| Timolol (p. 1133) (Blocadren) | T: 5 mg, 10 mg, 20 mg | Beta₁, beta₂ | 10–60 mg/day | Same as above |

C, Capsules; *I,* injection; *S,* solution; *SR,* sustained-release; *T,* tablets.

Bronchodilators

USES

Relief of bronchospasm occurring during anesthesia and in bronchial asthma, bronchitis, emphysema.

ACTION

Inhaled corticosteroids: Exact mechanism unknown. May act as anti-inflammatories, decrease mucus secretion.

Beta₂-adrenergic agonists: Stimulate beta-receptors in lung, relax bronchial smooth muscle, increase vital capacity, decrease airway resistance.

Anticholinergics: Inhibit cholinergic receptors on bronchial smooth muscle (block acetylcholine action).

Leukotriene modifiers: Decrease effect of leukotrienes, which increase migration of eosinophils, producing mucus/edema of airway wall, causing bronchoconstriction.

Methylxanthines: Directly relax smooth muscle of bronchial airway, pulmonary blood vessels (relieve bronchospasm, increase vital capacity). Increase cyclic 3,5-adenosine monophosphate.

Bronchodilators *(continued)*

BRONCHODILATORS

Anticholinergics

Name	Availability	Dosage Range	Side Effects
Ipratropium (p. 634) (Atrovent)	**Neb:** 0.02% **MDI:** 18 mcg/actuation **Nasal:** 0.03%, 0.06%	**A (Neb):** 0.02% q3–4h **A (MDI):** 2 puffs 4 times/day **A (Nasal):** 2 sprays 2–4 times/day	Palpitations, nervousness, dizziness, headaches, pain, nausea, dry mucous membranes, dyspnea
Tiotropium (p. 1138) (Spiriva)	**Inhalation powder:** 18 mcg	**A:** Once/day	Dry mouth, tachycardia, constipation, blurred vision, urinary difficulty/ retention, upper respiratory tract infections

Beta-Agonists

Name	Availability	Dosage Range	Side Effects
Albuterol (p. 26) (Proventil, Ventolin, Volmax)	**T:** 2 mg, 4 mg **T (SR):** 4 mg, 8 mg **S:** 2 mg/5 ml **MDI (Neb):** 0.5%, 2.5 mg/3 ml, 1.25 mg/3 ml, 0.63 mg/3 ml	**A, C (MDI):** 2 puffs q4–6h as needed **A, C (Rotacaps):** 1–2 caps q4–6h as needed **A (Neb):** 2.5 mg q4–6h as needed **C (Neb):** 0.1–0.15 mg/kg q4–6h as needed **A [T (SR)]:** 4–8 mg q12h **C [T (SR)]:** 4 mg q12h	Tremors, tachycardia, palpitations, hypokalemia
Formoterol (p. 511) (Foradil)	**C:** 12 mcg	**A:** 1 capsule q12h	Same as above
Levalbuterol (p. 681) (Xopenex)	**Neb:** 0.63 mg/3 ml, 1.25 mg/3 ml	**A:** 0.63 mg q6–8h as needed	Same as above

Metaproterenol (p. 742) (Alupent, Metaprel)	MDI (Neb): 5% S: 10 mg/5 ml T: 10 mg, 20 mg		Same as above
Pirbuterol (Maxair)	MDI	A, C: 2 puffs q4–6h as needed	Same as above
Salmeterol (p. 1039) (Serevent)	MDI C: 50 mcg	A (MDI): 2 puffs q12h C: 1–2 puffs q12h A, C (C): 1 inhalation q12h	Same as above
Terbutaline (p. 1110) (Brethine, Bricanyl)	MDI T: 2.5 mg, 5 mg	A: 2.5 mg 3–4 times/day C: 0.05 mg/kg/dose 3 times/day	Same as above

Inhaled Anti-Inflammatory Agents

Beclomethasone (p. 123) (Beclovent, Vanceril, Qvar)	MDI	1–2 inhalations 2–4 times/day	Oropharyngeal candidiasis, dysphonia, hoarseness, cough
Budesonide (p. 157) (Pulmicort)	MDI Neb	MDI (A): 1–4 inhalations 2 times/day D (older than 6 yr): 1–2 inhalations 2 times/day	Same as above
Cromolyn (p. 293) (Intal)	MDI Neb	MDI: C (older than 5 yr): 2 inhalations up to 4 times/day Neb: C (older than 2 yr): 20 mg 4 times/day	Cough, urticaria, bronchospasm
Flunisolide (p. 491) (AeroBid)	MDI	A: 2–4 inhalations 2 times/day C (6–15 yr): 1–2 inhalations 2 times/day	Same as beclomethasone
Fluticasone (p. 503) (Flovent)	MDI Rotadisk	MDI: A, C (older than 12 yr): 2 inhalations 2 times/day Rotadisk: A, C (older than 4 yr): 1 inhalation 2 times/day	Same as beclomethasone

(continued)

BRONCHODILATORS *(continued)*

Name	Availability	Dosage Range	Side Effects
Inhaled Anti-Inflammatory Agents *(continued)*			
Mometasone (p. 791) (Asmanex)	**MDI**	1 puff 2 times/day or 2 puffs once daily up to 4 puffs/day	Pharyngitis, sinusitus, upper respiratory tract infection, allergic rhinitis, dyspepsia, headache, fatigue
Nedocromil (p. 819) (Tilade)	**MDI**	**A, C (older than 6 yr):** 2 inhalations 4 times/day	Altered taste, headaches, nausea
Triamcinolone (p. 1170) (Azmacort)	**MDI**	**A:** 2 inhalations 3–4 times/day or 4–8 inhalations 2 times/day **C:** 1–2 inhalations 3–4 times/day or 2–6 inhalations 2 times/day	Same as beclomethasone
Leukotriene Modifiers			
Montelukast (p. 793) (Singulair)	**T:** 4 mg, 5 mg, 10 mg	**A:** 10 mg/day **C (6–14 yr):** 5 mg/day **C (2–5 yr):** 4 mg/day	Dyspepsia, increased hepatic function tests
Zafirlukast (p. 1224) (Accolate)	**T:** 10 mg, 20 mg	**A, C (12 yr and older):** 20 mg 2 times/day **C (5–11 yr):** 10 mg 2 times/day	Same as above

A, Adults; *C (dosage),* children; *MDI,* metered dose inhaler; *Neb,* nebulization; *S,* syrups; *SR,* sustained-release; *T,* tablet.

Calcium Channel Blockers

USES

Treatment of essential hypertension, treatment of and prophylaxis of angina pectoris (including vasospastic, chronic stable, unstable), prevention/control of supraventricular tachyarrhythmias, prevention of neurologic damage due to subarachnoid hemorrhage.

ACTION

Calcium channel blockers inhibit the flow of extracellular Ca^{2+} ions across cell membranes of cardiac cells, vascular tissue. They relax arterial smooth muscle, decrease the rate of sinus node pacemaker, slow AV conduction, decrease heart rate, produce negative inotropic effect (rarely seen clinically due to reflex response). Calcium channel blockers decrease coronary vascular resistance, increase coronary blood flow, reduce myocardial oxygen demand. Degree of action varies with individual agent.

CALCIUM CHANNEL BLOCKERS

Name	Availability	Dosage Range	Side Effects
Amlodipine (p. 62) (Norvasc)	**T:** 2.5 mg, 5 mg, 10 mg	2.5–10 mg/day	Abdominal pain, flushing, headaches
Diltiazem (p. 360) (Cardizem)	**T:** 30 mg, 60 mg, 90 mg **T (SR):** 120 mg, 180 mg, 240 mg **C (SR):** 60 mg, 90 mg, 120 mg, 180 mg, 240 mg, 300 mg, 360 mg **I:** 5 mg/ml	**PO:** 120–360 mg/day **I:** 20–25 mg IV bolus, then 5–15 mg/hr infusion	Dizziness, drowsiness
Felodipine (p. 465) (Plendil)	**T:** 2.5 mg, 5 mg, 10 mg	5–10 mg/day	Peripheral edema, headaches
Isradipine (p. 647) (DynaCirc)	**T:** 5 mg, 10 mg **C:** 2.5 mg, 5 mg	5–20 mg/day	Headaches
Nicardipine (p. 831) (Cardene)	**C:** 20 mg, 30 mg **C (ER):** 30 mg, 45 mg, 60 mg **I:** 2.5 mg/ml	**PO:** 60–120 mg/day	Flushing, feeling of warmth
Nifedipine (p. 835) (Adalat, Procardia)	**C:** 10 mg, 20 mg **T (ER):** 30 mg, 60 mg, 90 mg	30–120 mg/day	Peripheral edema, dizziness, flushed face, headaches, nausea
Nimodipine (p. 838) (Nimotop)	**C:** 30 mg	60 mg q4h for 21 days	Nausea
Verapamil (p. 1203) (Calan, Isoptin)	**T:** 40 mg, 80 mg, 120 mg **T (SR):** 120 mg, 180 mg, 240 mg	120–480 mg/day	Constipation, nausea

C, Capsules; *ER,* extended-release; *I,* injection; *SR,* sustained-release; *T,* tablets.

Cancer Chemotherapeutic Agents

USES

Treatment of a variety of cancers; may be palliative or curative. Treatment of choice in hematologic cancers. Often used as adjunctive therapy (e.g., with surgery or irradiation); most effective when tumor mass has been removed or reduced by radiation. Often used in combinations to increase therapeutic results, decrease toxic effects. Certain agents may be used in nonmalignant conditions: polycythemia vera, psoriasis, rheumatoid arthritis, or immunosuppression in organ transplantation (used only in select cases that are severe and unresponsive to other forms of therapy). Refer to individual monographs.

ACTION

Most antineoplastics inhibit cell replication by interfering with the supply of nutrients or genetic components of the cell (DNA or RNA). Some antineoplastics, referred to as *cell cycle–specific* (CCS), are particularly effective during a specific phase of cell reproduction (e.g., antimetabolites and plant alkaloids). Other antineoplastics, referred to as *cell cycle–nonspecific*, act independently of a specific phase of cell division (e.g., alkylating agents and antibiotics). Some hormones are also classified as antineoplastics. Although not cytotoxic, they act to depress cancer growth by altering the hormone environment. In addition, there are a number of miscellaneous agents acting through different mechanisms.

CANCER CHEMOTHERAPEUTIC AGENTS

Name	Availability	Side Effects
Abarelix (p. 2) (Plenaxis)	I: 100 mg	Fatigue, headaches, nausea, abdominal pain, hot flashes, menstrual disorders
Aldesleukin (p. 30) (Proleukin)	I: 22 million units **Powder**	Hypotension, sinus tachycardia, nausea, vomiting, diarrhea, renal impairment, anemia, rash, fatigue, agitation, pulmonary congestion, dyspnea, fever, chills, oliguria, weight gain, dizziness
Alemtuzumab (p. 30) (Campath)	I: 30 mg/3 ml	Rigors, fever, fatigue, hypotension, neutropenia, anemia, sepsis, dyspnea, bronchitis, pneumonia, urticaria

Drug	Dosage Form	Adverse Effects
Alitretinoin (p. 34) (Panretin)	**Gel:** 0.1%	Burning, pain, edema, dermatitis, rash, skin disorders
Altretamine (Hexalen)	**C:** 50 mg	Nausea, vomiting, myelosuppression, peripheral neuropathy, altered mood, ataxia, dizziness, nervousness, vertigo
Aminoglutethimide (Cytadren)	**T:** 250 mg	Orthostatic hypotension, hypothyroidism, vomiting, anorexia, rash, drowsiness, headaches, fever, myalgia
Anastrozole (p. 78) (Arimidex)	**T:** 1 mg	Peripheral edema, chest pain, nausea, vomiting, diarrhea, constipation, abdominal pain, anorexia, pharyngitis, vaginal hemorrhage, anemia, leukopenia, rash, weight gain, diaphoresis, increased appetite, pain, headaches, dizziness, depression, paraesthesias, hot flashes, increased cough, dry mouth, asthenia, dyspnea, phlebitis
Arsenic trioxide (p. 87) (Trisenox)	**I:** 10 mg/ml	AV block, GI hemorrhage, hypertension, hypoglycemia, hypokalemia, hypomagnesemia, neutropenia, oliguria, prolonged QT interval, seizures, sepsis, thrombocytopenia
Asparaginase (p. 91) (Elspar)	**I:** 10,000 units	Anorexia, nausea, vomiting, hepatic toxicity, pancreatitis, nephrotoxicity, clotting factor abnormalities, malaise, confusion, lethargy, EEG changes, respiratory distress, fever, hyperglycemia, depression, stomatitis, allergic reactions, drowsiness
Azacitadine (p. 109) (Vidaza)	**I:** 100 mg	Edema, hypokalemia, weight loss, myalgia, cough, dyspnea, upper respiratory tract infection, back pain, pyrexia, weakness
BCG (Tice BCG, TheraCys)	**I:** 50 mg, 81 mg	Nausea, vomiting, anorexia, diarrhea, dysuria, hematuria, cystitis, urinary urgency, anemia, malaise, fever, chills
Bevacizumab (p. 135) (Avastin)	**I:** 25 mg/ml	Increased blood pressure, fatigue, blood clots, diarrhea, decreased WBCs, headaches, decreased appetite, stomatitis
Bexarotene (p. 137) (Targretin)	**C:** 75 mg **Gel:** 1%	Anemia, dermatitis, fever, hypercholesterolemia, infection, leukopenia, peripheral edema
Bicalutamide (p. 138) (Casodex)	**T:** 50 mg	Gynecomastia, hot flashes, breast pain, nausea, diarrhea, constipation, nocturia, impotence, pain, muscle pain, asthenia, abdominal pain

(continued)

CANCER CHEMOTHERAPEUTIC AGENTS *(continued)*

Name	Availability	Side Effects
Bleomycin (p. 146) (Blenoxane)	I: 15 units, 30 units	Nausea, vomiting, anorexia, stomatitis, hyperpigmentation, alopecia, pruritus, hyperkeratosis, urticaria, pneumonitis progression to fibrosis, weight loss, rash
Bortezomib (p. 148) (Velcade)	I: 3.5 mg	Anxiety, dizziness, headaches, insomnia, peripheral neuropathy, pruritus, rash, abdominal pain, decreased appetite, constipation, diarrhea, dyspepsia, nausea, vomiting, arthralgia, dyspnea, asthenia, edema, pain
Busulfan (p. 164) (Myleran)	T: 2 mg	Nausea, vomiting, hyperuricemia, myelosuppression, skin hyperpigmentation, alopecia, anorexia, weight loss, diarrhea, stomatitis
Capecitabine (p. 178) (Xeloda)	T: 150 mg, 300 mg	Nausea, vomiting, diarrhea, stomatitis, bone marrow depression, palmoplantar erythrodysesthia syndrome, dermatitis, fatigue, anorexia
Carboplatin (p. 186) (Paraplatin)	I: 50 mg, 150 mg, 450 mg	Nausea, vomiting, nephrotoxicity, bone marrow suppression, alopecia, peripheral neuropathy, hypersensitivity, ototoxicity, asthenia, diarrhea, constipation
Carmustine (p. 188) (BiCNU)	I: 100 mg	Anorexia, nausea, vomiting, bone marrow depression, pulmonary fibrosis, pain at injection site, diarrhea, skin discoloration
Cetuximab (p. 231) (Erbitux)	I: 2 mg/ml	Dyspnea, hypotension, acne-like rash, dry skin, weakness, fatigue, fever, constipation, abdominal pain
Chlorambucil (p. 235) (Leukeran)	T: 2 mg	Bone marrow suppression, dermatitis, nausea, vomiting, hepatic toxicity, anorexia, diarrhea, abdominal discomfort, rash
Cisplatin (p. 255) (Platinol-AQ)	I: 50 mg, 100 mg	Nausea, vomiting, nephrotoxicity, bone marrow depression, neuropathies, ototoxicity, anaphylactic-like reactions, hyperuricemia, hypomagnesemia, hypophosphatemia, hypokalemia, hypocalcemia, pain at injection site
Cladribine (p. 260) (Leustatin)	I: 1 mg/ml	Nausea, vomiting, diarrhea, bone marrow depression, chills, fatigue, rash, fever, headaches, anorexia, diaphoresis

Drug	Doses	Side Effects
Cyclophosphamide (p. 298) (Cytoxan)	**I:** 100 mg, 200 mg, 500 mg, 1 g, 2 g **T:** 25 mg, 50 mg	Nausea, vomiting, hemorrhagic cystitis, bone marrow depression, alopecia, interstitial pulmonary fibrosis, amenorrhea, azoospermia, diarrhea, darkening skin/fingernails, headaches, diaphoresis
Cytarabine (p. 304) (Cytosar, Ara-C)	**I:** 100 mg, 500 mg, 1 g, 2 g	Anorexia, nausea, vomiting, stomatitis, esophagitis, diarrhea, bone marrow depression, alopecia, rash, fever, neuropathies, abdominal pain
Dacarbazine (p. 307) (DTIC)	**I:** 200 mg	Nausea, vomiting, anorexia, hepatic necrosis, bone marrow depression, alopecia, rash, facial flushing, photosensitivity, flulike syndrome, confusion, blurred vision
Daunorubicin (p. 319) (Cerubidine)	**I:** 20 mg	CHF, nausea, vomiting, stomatitis, mucositis, diarrhea, hematuria, bone marrow depression, alopecia, fever, chills, abdominal pain
Daunorubicin (p. 319) (DaunoXome)	**I:** 50 mg	Nausea, diarrhea, abdominal pain, anorexia, vomiting, stomatitis, myelosuppression, rigors, back pain, headaches, neuropathy, depression, dyspnea, fatigue, fever, cough, allergic reactions, diaphoresis
Denileukin (p. 327) (Ontak)	**I:** 300 mcg/2 ml	Hypersensitivity reaction, back pain, dyspnea, rash, chest pain, tachycardia, asthenia, flulike syndrome, chills, nausea, vomiting, infection
Docetaxel (p. 375) (Taxotere)	**I:** 20 mg, 80 mg	Hypotension, nausea, vomiting, diarrhea, mucositis, bone marrow suppression, rash, paraesthesia, hypersensitivity, fluid retention, alopecia, asthenia, stomatitis, fever
Doxorubicin (p. 388) (Adriamycin)	**I:** 10 mg, 20 mg, 50 mg, 75 mg, 150 mg, 200 mg	Cardiotoxicity, including CHF, arrhythmias, nausea, vomiting, stomatitis, esophagitis, GI ulceration, diarrhea, anorexia, hematuria, bone marrow depression, alopecia, hyperpigmentation of nail beds and skin, local inflammation at injection site, rash, fever, chills, urticaria, lacrimation, conjunctivitis
Doxorubicin (p. 388) (Doxil)	**I:** 20 mg, 50 mg	Neutropenia, palmoplantar erythrodysesthesia syndrome, cardiomyopathy, CHF
Epirubicin (p. 419) (Ellence)	**I:** 2 mg/ml	Anemia, leukopenia, neutropenia, infection, mucositis
Erlotinib (p. 431) (Tarceva)	**T:** 25 mg, 100 mg, 150 mg	Diarrhea, rash, nausea, vomiting

(continued)

CANCER CHEMOTHERAPEUTIC AGENTS   *(continued)*

Name	Availability	Side Effects
Estramustine (p. 444) (Emcyt)	C: 140 mg	Increased risk of thrombosis, gynecomastia, nausea, vomiting, diarrhea, thrombocytopenia, peripheral edema
Etoposide (p. 455) (VePesid)	I: 20 mg/ml C: 50 mg	Nausea, vomiting, anorexia, bone marrow depression, alopecia, diarrhea, somnolence, peripheral neuropathies
Exemestane (p. 457) (Aromasin)	T: 25 mg	Dyspnea, edema, hypertension, mental depression
Fludarabine (p. 486) (Fludara)	I: 50 mg	Nausea, diarrhea, stomatitis, bleeding, anemia, bone marrow depression, skin rash, weakness, confusion, visual disturbances, peripheral neuropathy, coma, pneumonia, peripheral edema, anorexia
Fluorouracil (p. 493)	I: 50 mg/ml Cream: 1%, 5% Solution: 1%, 2%, 5%	Nausea, vomiting, stomatitis, GI ulceration, diarrhea, anorexia, bone marrow depression, alopecia, skin hyperpigmentation, nail changes, headaches, drowsiness, blurred vision, fever
Flutamide (p. 502) (Eulexin)	C: 125 mg	Hot flashes, nausea, vomiting, diarrhea, hepatitis, impotence, decreased libido, rash, anorexia
Fulvestrant (p. 522) (Faslodex)	I: 250 mg/5 ml, 125 mg/2.5 ml syringes	Asthenia, pain, headaches, injection site pain, flulike symptoms, fever, nausea, vomiting, constipation, anorexia, diarrhea, peripheral edema, dizziness, depression, anxiety, rash, increased cough, UTI
Gefitinib (p. 535) (Iressa)	T: 250 mg	Diarrhea, rash, acne, nausea, dry skin, vomiting, pruritus, anorexia
Gemcitabine (p. 536) (Gemzar)	I: 200 mg, 1 g	Increased serum hepatic function tests, nausea, vomiting, diarrhea, stomatitis, hematuria, myelosuppression, rash, mild paresthesias, dyspnea, fever, edema, flulike symptoms, constipation
Gemtuzumab (p. 541) (Mylotarg)	I: 5 mg/20 ml	Anemia, hematuria, hepatic toxicity, pneumonia, herpes simplex, nausea, vomiting, dyspnea, headaches, hypotension, hypoxia, mucositis, myelosuppression, peripheral edema, tachycardia, thrombocytopenia

Goserelin (p. 561) (Zoladex)	**I:** 3.6 mg, 10.8 mg	Hot flashes, sexual dysfunction, erectile dysfunction, gynecomastia, lethargy, pain, lower urinary tract symptoms, headaches, nausea, depression, diaphoresis
Hydroxyurea (p. 589) (Hydrea)	**C:** 500 mg	Anorexia, nausea, vomiting, stomatitis, diarrhea, constipation, bone marrow depression, fever, chills, malaise
Ibritumomab (p. 596) (Zevalin)	Injection kit	Neutropenia, thrombocytopenia, anemia, infection, asthenia, abdominal pain, fever, pain, headaches, nausea, peripheral edema, allergic reaction, GI hemorrhage, apnea
Idarubicin (p. 600) (Idamycin PFS)	**I:** 5 mg, 10 mg, 20 mg	CHF, arrhythmias, nausea, vomiting, stomatitis, bone marrow depression, alopecia, rash, urticaria, hyperuricemia, abdominal pain, diarrhea, esophagitis, anorexia
Ifosfamide (p. 602) (Ifex)	**I:** 1 g, 3 g	Nausea, vomiting, hemorrhagic cystitis, bone marrow depression, alopecia, lethargy, somnolence, confusion, hallucinations, hematuria
Imatinib (p. 605) (Gleevec)	**C:** 100 mg	Nausea, fluid retention, hemorrhage, musculoskeletal pain, arthralgia, weight gain, pyrexia, abdominal pain, dyspnea, pneumonia
Interferon alfa-2a (p. 622) (Roferon-A)	**I:** 3 million units, 6 million units, 9 million units, 18 million units	Anorexia, nausea, diarrhea, bone marrow depression, pruritus, myalgia, dizziness, headaches, paraesthesias, fatigue, fever, chills, dyspnea, flulike symptoms, vomiting, coughing, altered taste
Interferon alfa-2b (p. 624) (Intron-A)	**I:** 3 million units, 5 million units, 10 million units, 18 million units, 25 million units, 50 million units	Mild hypotension, hypertension, tachycardia with high fever, nausea, diarrhea, altered taste, weight loss, thrombocytopenia, bone marrow depression, rash, pruritus, myalgia, arthralgia associated with flulike syndromes
Irinotecan (p. 637) (Camptosar)	**I:** 40 mg, 100 mg	Diarrhea, nausea, vomiting, abdominal cramps, anorexia, stomatitis, increased AST, severe myelosuppression, alopecia, diaphoresis, rash, weight loss, dehydration, increased serum alkaline phosphatase, headaches, insomnia, dizziness, dyspnea, cough, asthenia, rhinitis, fever, back pain, chills

(continued)

CANCER CHEMOTHERAPEUTIC AGENTS *(continued)*

Name	Availability	Side Effects
Letrozole (p. 676) **(Femara)**	**T:** 2.5 mg	Hypertension, nausea, vomiting, constipation, diarrhea, abdominal pain, anorexia, rash, pruritus, musculoskeletal pain, arthralgia, fatigue, headaches, dyspnea, coughing, hot flashes
Leuprolide (p. 679) **(Lupron)**	**I:** 3.75 mg, 5 mg, 7.5 mg, 11.25 mg, 15 mg, 22.5 mg, 30 mg	Hot flashes, gynecomastia, nausea, vomiting, constipation, anorexia, dizziness, headaches, insomnia, paraesthesias, bone pain
Lomustine (p. 701) **(CeeNU)**	**C:** 10 mg, 40 mg, 100 mg	Anorexia, nausea, vomiting, stomatitis, hepatic toxicity, nephrotoxicity, bone marrow depression, alopecia, confusion, slurred speech
Mechlorethamine **(Mustargen)**	**I:** 10 mg/ml	Severe nausea and vomiting, metallic taste, diarrhea, bone marrow depression, alopecia, phlebitis, vertigo, tinnitus, hyperuricemia, infertility, azoospermia, anorexia, headaches, drowsiness, fever
Megestrol (p. 727) **(Megace)**	**T:** 20 mg, 40 mg **Suspension:** 40 mg/ml	Deep vein thrombosis, Cushing-like syndrome, alopecia, carpal tunnel syndrome, weight gain, nausea
Melphalan (p. 730) **(Alkeran)**	**T:** 2 mg	Anorexia, nausea, vomiting, bone marrow depression, diarrhea, stomatitis
Mercaptopurine **(Purinethol)**	**T:** 50 mg	Anorexia, nausea, vomiting, stomatitis, hepatic toxicity, bone marrow depression, hyperuricemia, diarrhea, rash
Methotrexate (p. 749)	**T:** 2.5 mg, 5 mg, 7.5 mg, 10 mg, 15 mg **I:** 5 mg, 50 mg, 100 mg, 200 mg, 250 mg	Nausea, vomiting, stomatitis, GI ulceration, diarrhea, hepatic toxicity, renal failure, cystitis, bone marrow suppression, alopecia, urticaria, acne, photosensitivity, interstitial pneumonitis, fever, malaise, chills, anorexia
Mitomycin-C (p. 784) **(Mutamycin)**	**I:** 20 mg, 40 mg	Anorexia, nausea, vomiting, stomatitis, diarrhea, renal toxicity, bone marrow depression, alopecia, pruritus, fever, hemolytic uremic syndrome, weakness
Mitotane **(Lysodren)**	**T:** 500 mg	Anorexia, nausea, vomiting, diarrhea, skin rashes, depression, lethargy, somnolence, dizziness, adrenal insufficiency, blurred vision, impaired hearing

Mitoxantrone (p. 786) (Novantrone)	I: 20 mg, 25 mg, 30 mg	CHF, tachycardia, EKG changes, chest pain, nausea, vomiting, stomatitis, mucositis, myelosuppression, rash, alopecia, urine discoloration (bluish green), phlebitis, diarrhea, cough, headaches, fever
Nelarabine (p. 820) (Arranon)	I: 5 mg/ml	Anemia, neutropenia, thrombocytopenia, nausea, vomiting, diarrhea, fatigue, fever, dyspnea, severe neurologic events (e.g., convulsions), peripheral neuropathy)
Nilutamide (p. 837) (Nilandron)	T: 50 mg	Hypertension, angina, hot flashes, nausea, anorexia, increased hepatic enzymes, dizziness, dyspnea, visual disturbances, impaired adaptation to dark, constipation, decreased libido
Oxaliplatin (p. 875) (Eloxatin)	I: 50 mg, 100 mg	Fatigue, neuropathy, abdominal pain, dyspnea, diarrhea, nausea, vomiting, anorexia, fever, edema, chest pain, anemia, thrombocytopenia, thromboembolism, altered serum hepatic function tests
Paclitaxel (p. 887) (Taxol)	I: 30 mg, 100 mg	Hypertension, bradycardia, EKG changes, nausea, vomiting, diarrhea, mucositis, bone marrow depression, alopecia, peripheral neuropathies, hypersensitivity reaction, athralgia, myalgia
Pegaspargase (Oncaspar)	I: 750 international units/ml	Hypotension, anorexia, nausea, vomiting, hepatic toxicity, pancreatitis, depression of clotting factors, malaise, confusion, lethargy, EEG changes, respiratory distress, hypersensitivity reaction, fever, hyperglycemia, stomatitis
Pemetrexed (p. 905) (Alimta)	I: 500 mg	Anorexia, constipation, diarrhea, neuropathy, anemia, chest pain, dyspnea, rash, fatigue
Pentostatin (Nipent)	I: 10 mg	Nausea, vomiting, hepatic disorders, elevated serum hepatic function tests, leukopenia, anemia, thrombocytopenia, rash, fever, upper respiratory infection, fatigue, hematuria, headaches, myalgia, arthralgia, diarrhea, anorexia
Plicamycin (Mithracin)	I: 2.5 mg	Anorexia, nausea, vomiting, stomatitis, diarrhea, clotting factor disorders, facial flushing, mental depression, confusion, fever, hypocalcemia, hypophosphatemia, hypokalemia, headaches, dizziness, rash
Procarbazine (p. 966) (Matulane)	C: 50 mg	Nausea, vomiting, stomatitis, diarrhea, constipation, bone marrow depression, pruritus, hyperpigmentation, alopecia, myalgia, paraesthesias, confusion, lethargy, mental depression, fever, hepatic toxicity, arthralgia, respiratory disorders

(continued)

CANCER CHEMOTHERAPEUTIC AGENTS *(continued)*

Name	Availability	Side Effects
Rituximab (p. 1030) (Rituxan)	**I:** 100 mg, 500 mg	Hypotension, arrhythmias, peripheral edema, nausea, vomiting, abdominal pain, leukopenia, thrombocytopenia, neutropenia, rash, pruritus, urticaria, angioedema, myalgia, headaches, dizziness, throat irritation, rhinitis, bronchospasm, hypersensitivity reaction
Sorafenib (p. 1071) (Nexavar)	**T:** 200 mg	Fatigue, alopecia, nausea, vomiting, anorexia, constipation, diarrhea, neuropathy, dyspnea, cough, asthenia, pain
Streptozocin (Zanosar)	**I:** 1 g	May lead to insulin-dependent diabetes, nausea, vomiting, nephrotoxicity, renal tubular acidosis, bone marrow depression, lethargy, diarrhea, confusion, depression
Tamoxifen (p. 1095) (Nolvadex)	**T:** 10 mg, 20 mg	Skin rash, nausea, vomiting, anorexia, menstrual irregularities, hot flashes, pruritus, vaginal discharge or bleeding, bone marrow depression, headaches, tumor or bone pain, ophthalmic changes, weight gain, confusion
Temozolomide (p. 1103) (Temodar)	**C:** 5 mg, 20 mg, 100 mg, 250 mg	Amnesia, fever, infection, leukopenia, neutropenia, peripheral edema, seizures, thrombocytopenia
Teniposide (Vumon)	**I:** 50 mg/5 ml	Hypotension with rapid infusion, diarrhea, nausea, vomiting, mucositis, bone marrow depression, alopecia, anemia, rash, hypersensitivity reaction
Thioguanine	**T:** 40 mg	Anorexia, stomatitis, bone marrow depression, hyperuricemia, nausea, vomiting, diarrhea
Thiotepa (p. 1123)	**I:** 15 mg	Anorexia, nausea, vomiting, mucositis, bone marrow depression, amenorrhea, reduced spermatogenesis, fever, hypersensitivity reactions, pain at injection site, headaches, dizziness, alopecia
Topotecan (p. 1151) (Hycamtin)	**I:** 4 mg	Nausea, vomiting, diarrhea, constipation, abdominal pain, stomatitis, anorexia, neutropenia, leukopenia, thrombocytopenia, anemia, alopecia, headaches, dyspnea, paraesthesia
Toremifene (p. 1153) (Fareston)	**T:** 60 mg	Elevated serum hepatic function tests, nausea, vomiting, constipation, skin discoloration, dermatitis, dizziness, hot flashes, diaphoresis, vaginal discharge or bleeding, ocular changes, cataracts, anxiety

Tositumomab (p. 1156) (Bexxar)	**I:** 14 mg/ml	Headaches, rash, pruritus, abdominal pain, anorexia, diarrhea, nausea, vomiting, arthralgia, myalgia, cough, dyspnea, asthenia, chills, fever, infection
Trastuzumab (p. 1164) (Herceptin)	**I:** 440 mg	CHF, heart murmur (S3 gallop), nausea, vomiting, diarrhea, abdominal pain, anorexia, rash, peripheral edema, back or bone pain, asthenia, headaches, insomnia, dizziness, cough, dyspnea, rhinitis, pharyngitis
Tretinoin (p. 1168) (Vesanoid)	**C:** 10 mg	Flushing, nausea, vomiting, diarrhea, constipation, dyspepsia, mucositis, leukocytosis, dry skin/mucous membranes, rash, itching, alopecia, dizziness, anxiety, insomnia, headaches, depression, confusion, intracranial hypertension, agitation, dyspnea, shivering, fever, visual changes, earaches, hearing loss, bone pain, myalgia, arthralgia
Valrubicin (p. 1193) (Valstar)	**I:** 200 mg/5 ml	Dysuria, hematuria, urinary frequency/incontinence, urinary urgency
Vinblastine (p. 1206) (Velban)	**I:** 10 mg	Nausea, vomiting, stomatitis, constipation, bone marrow depression, alopecia, peripheral neuropathy, loss of deep tendon reflexes, paraesthesias, diarrhea
Vincristine (p. 1208) (Oncovin)	**I:** 1 mg, 2 mg, 3 mg	Nausea, vomiting, stomatitis, constipation, pharyngitis, polyuria, bone marrow depression, alopecia, numbness, paraesthesias, peripheral neuropathy, loss of deep tendon reflexes, headaches, abdominal pain
Vinorelbine (p. 1210) (Navelbine)	**I:** 10 mg, 50 mg	Elevated serum hepatic function tests, nausea, vomiting, constipation, ileus, anorexia, stomatitis, bone marrow suppression, alopecia, vein discoloration, venous pain, phlebitis, interstitial pulmonary changes, asthenia, fatigue, diarrhea, peripheral neuropathy, loss of deep tendon reflexes

C, Capsules; *I*, injection; *T*, tablets.

Cardiac Glycosides (Inotropic Agents)

USES

CHF, atrial fibrillation, atrial flutter, paroxysmal atrial tachycardia, treatment of cardiogenic shock with pulmonary edema.

ACTION

Direct action on myocardium causes increased force of contraction, resulting in increased stroke volume and cardiac output. Depression of SA node, decreased conduction time through AV node, and decreased electrical impulses due to vagal stimulation slow heart rate. Improved myocardial contractility is probably due to improved transport of calcium, sodium, and potassium ions across cell membranes.

CARDIAC GLYCOSIDES (INOTROPIC AGENTS)

Name	Availability	Dosage Range	Side Effects
Digoxin (p. 356) (Lanoxin)	**C:** 0.05 mg, 0.1 mg, 0.2 mg **T:** 0.125 mg, 0.25 mg **E:** 0.05 mg/ml **I:** 0.1 mg/ml, 0.25 mg/ml	**PO/IV:** 0.125–0.375 mg/day	Arrhythmias, blurred vision, confusion, hallucinations, nausea, vomiting, diarrhea, abdominal pain
Inamrinone	**I:** 5 mg/ml	**IV:** 0.75 mg/kg bolus, then 5–10 mcg/kg/min infusion	Arrhythmias, hypotension
Milrinone (p. 776) (Primacor)	**I:** 1 mg/ml	**IV:** 50 mcg/kg bolus, then 0.375–0.75 mcg/kg/min infusion	Arrhythmias, hypotension, headaches

C, Capsules; *E,* elixir; *I,* injection; *T,* tablets.

Cholinergic Agonists/Anticholinesterase

USES

Paralytic ileus and atony of urinary bladder. Myasthenia gravis (weakness, marked fatigue of skeletal muscle). Terminates, reverses effects of neuromuscular blocking agents.

ACTION

Cholinergic agonists: Referred to as *muscarinics* or *parasympathetics* and consist of two basic drug groups: choline esters and cholinomimetic alkaloids. Primary action mimics actions of acetylcholine at postganglionic parasympathetic nerves. Primary properties include the following:
Cardiovascular system: Vasodilation; decreased cardiacrate; decreased conduction in SA, AV nodes; decreased force of myocardial contraction.
Gastrointestinal: Increased tone, motility of GI smooth muscle, increased secretory activity of GI tract.
Urinary tract: Increased contraction of detrusor muscle of urinary bladder, resulting in micturition.
Eye: Miosis, contraction of ciliary muscle.

Anticholinesterase (anti-ChE), also known as *cholinesterase inhibitors:* Inactivates cholinesterase, which prevents acetylcholine breakdown, causing acetylcholine to accumulate at cholinergic receptor sites. These agents can be considered indirect-acting cholinergic agonists. Primary properties include action of cholinergic agonists just noted. *Skeletal neuromuscular junction:* Effects are dose dependent. At therapeutic doses, increases force of skeletal muscle contraction; at toxic doses, reduces muscle strength.

CHOLINERGIC AGONISTS/ANTICHOLINESTERASE

Name	Availability	Uses	Dosage Range	Side Effects
Bethanechol (p. 134) (Urecholine)	**T:** 5 mg, 10 mg, 25 mg, 50 mg **I:** 5 mg/ml	Nonobstructive urinary retention	**PO:** 10–50 mg 3–4 times/day **Subcutaneous:** 2.5–5 mg 3–4 times/day	Increased urinary frequency, salivation, belching, nausea, dizziness

(continued)

CHOLINERGIC AGONISTS/ANTICHOLINESTERASE   *(continued)*

Name	Availability	Uses	Dosage Range	Side Effects
Edrophonium (Tension)	**I:** 10 mg/ml	Diagnosis of myasthenia gravis, reverses tubocurarine	**IV:** 10 mg over 30 sec up to 40 mg	Bradycardia, nausea, vomiting, diarrhea, urinary frequency
Neostigmine (p. 825) (Prostigmin)	**T:** 15 mg **I:** 0.25 mg/ml, 0.5 mg/ml, 1 mg/ml	Symptomatic control of myasthenia gravis, neuromuscular blocker	**PO:** 15–365 mg/day **Subcutaneous, IM:** 0.5 mg **IV:** 0.5–2 mg	Diarrhea, diaphoresis, nausea, vomiting, abdominal cramps
Pyridostigmine (p. 989) (Mestinon)	**T:** 60 mg **T (ER):** 180 mg **S:** 60 mg/5 ml **I:** 5 mg/ml	Treats myasthenia gravis, reverses tubocurarine	**PO:** 60–1,500 mg/day **IM:** 0.5–1.5 mg/kg **IV:** 0.1–0.25 mg/kg	Diarrhea, diaphoresis, nausea, vomiting, abdominal cramps

ER, Extended release; *I,* injection; *S,* suspension; *T,* tablets.

Corticosteroids

USES

Replacement therapy in adrenal insufficiency, including Addison's disease. Symptomatic treatment of multiorgan disease/conditions. Rheumatoid arthritis, osteoarthritis, severe psoriasis, ulcerative colitis, lupus erythematosus, anaphylactic shock, acute excacerbation of asthma, status asthmaticus, organ transplant.

ACTION

Suppress migration of polymorphonuclear leukocytes (PML) and reverse increased capillary permeability by their anti-inflammatory effect. Suppress immune system by decreasing activity of lymphatic system.

CORTICOSTEROIDS

Name	Availability	Route of Administration	Side Effects
Beclomethasone (p. 123) (Beclovent, Beconase, Vanceril)	**Inhalation, nasal:** 42 mcg/spray, 84 mcg/spray	Inhalation, intranasal	**I:** Cough, dry mouth/throat, headaches, throat irritation **Nasal:** Headaches, sore throat, intranasal ulceration
Betamethasone (p. 130) (Celestone, Diprosone)	**I:** 4 mg/ml	IV, intralesional, intra-articular	Nausea, vomiting, increased appetite, weight gain, insomnia
Budesonide (p. 157) (Rhinocort, Pulmicort)	**Nasal:** 32 mcg/spray	Intranasal	**Nasal:** Headaches, sore throat, intranasal ulceration
Cortisone (p. 288) (Cortone)	**T:** 5 mg, 10 mg, 25 mg	PO	Same as betamethasone
Dexamethasone (p. 334) (Decadron)	**T:** 0.5 mg, 1 mg, 4 mg, 6 mg **OS:** 0.5 mg/5 ml **I:** 4 mg/ml	PO, parenteral	Same as betamethasone
Fludrocortisone (p. 488) (Florinef)	**T:** 0.1 mg	PO	Same as betamethasone
Flunisolide (p. 491) (AeroBid, Nasalide)	**Inhalation, nasal:** 25 mcg/spray	Inhalation, intranasal	Same as beclomethasone
Fluticasone (p. 503) (Flonase, Flovent)	**Inhalation:** 44 mcg, 110 mg/220 mcg **Nasal:** 50 mg, 100 mcg	Inhalation, intranasal	Same as beclomethasone
Hydrocortisone (p. 581) (Solu-Cortef)	**T:** 5 mg, 10 mg, 25 mg **I:** 100 mg, 250 mg, 500 mg, 1 g	PO, parenteral	Same as betamethasone

(continued)

CORTICOSTEROIDS	*(continued)*		
Name	Availability	Route of Administration	Side Effects
Methylprednisolone (p. 758) (Solu-Medrol)	**T:** 4 mg **I:** 40 mg, 125 mg, 500 mg, 1 g, 2 g	PO, parenteral	Same as betamethasone
Prednisolone (p. 955) (Prelone)	**T:** 5 mg **OS:** 5 mg/5 ml, 15 mg/5 ml	PO	Same as betamethasone
Prednisone (p. 957) (Deltasone)	**T:** 1 mg, 2.5 mg, 5 mg, 10 mg, 20 mg, 50 mg	PO	Same as betamethasone
Triamcinolone (p. 1170) (Azmacort, Kenalog)	**T:** 4 mg, 8 mg **Inhalation:** 100 mcg	PO, inhalation	Same as betamethasone **I:** Cough, dry mouth/throat, headaches, throat irritation

I, Injection; *OS,* oral suspension; *T,* tablets.

Corticosteroids: Topical

USES

Provide relief of inflammation/pruritus associated with corticosteroid-responsive disorders (e.g., contact dermatitis; eczema, insect bite reactions, first- and second-degree localized burns/sunburn).

ACTION

Diffuse across cell membranes, form complexes with cytoplasm. Complexes stimulate protein synthesis of inhibitory enzymes responsible for anti-inflammatory effects (e.g., inhibit edema, erythema, pruritus, capillary dilation, phagocytic activity).

Topical corticosteroids can be classified based on potency:

Low potency: Modest anti-inflammatory effect, safest for chronic application, facial and intertriginous application, with occlusion, for infants/young children.

Medium potency: For moderate inflammatory conditions (e.g., chronic eczematous dermatoses).

May use for facial and intertriginous application for only limited time.

High potency: For more severe inflammatory conditions (e.g., lichen simplex chronicus, psoriasis). May use for facial and intertriginous application for short time only. Used in areas of thickened skin due to chronic conditions.

Very high potency: Alternative to systemic therapy for local effect (e.g., chronic lesions caused by psoriasis). Increased risk of skin atrophy. Used for short periods on small areas. Avoid occlusive dressings.

CORTICOSTEROIDS: TOPICAL

Name	Availability	Potency	Side Effects
Alclometasone (Aclovate)	**C, O:** 0.05%	Low	Skin atrophy, contact dermatitis, stretch marks on skin, enlarged blood vessels in the skin, hair loss, pigment changes, secondary infections

(continued)

CORTICOSTEROIDS: TOPICAL	*(continued)*		
Name	Availability	Potency	Side Effects
Amcinonide (Cyclocort)	**C, O, L:** 0.1%	High	Same as above
Betamethasone dipropionate (p. 130) (Diprosone)	**C, O, G, L:** 0.05%	High	Same as above
Betamethasone valerate (p. 130) (Valisone)	**C:** 0.01%, 0.05%, 0.1% **O:** 0.1% **L:** 0.1%	High	Same as above
Clobetasol (Temovate)	**C, O:** 0.05%	High	Same as above
Desonide (Tridesilon)	**C, O, L:** 0.05%	Low	Same as above
Desoximetasone (Topicort)	**C:** 0.25%, 0.5% **O:** 0.25% **G:** 0.05%	High	Same as above
Dexamethasone (p. 334) (Decadron)	**C:** 0.1%	Medium	Same as above
Fluocinolone (Synalar)	**C:** 0.01%, 0.025%, 0.2% **O:** 0.025%	High	Same as above
Fluocinonide (Lidex)	**C, O, G:** 0.05%	High	Same as above
Flurandrenolide (Cordran)	**C, O, L:** 0.025%, 0.05%	Medium	Same as above
Fluticasone (p. 503) (Cutivate)	**C:** 0.05% **O:** 0.005%	Medium	Same as above

Halobetasol (Ultravate)	C, O: 0.05%	High	Same as above
Hydrocortisone (p. 581) (Hytone)	C, O: 0.5%, 1%, 2.5%	Medium	Same as above
Mometasone (p. 791) (Elocon)	C, O, L: 0.1%	Medium	Same as above
Prednicarbate (Dermatop)	C: 0.1%	—	Same as above
Triamcinolone (p. 1170) (Aristocort, Kenalog)	C, O, L: 0.025%, 0.1%, 0.5%	Medium	Same as above

Diuretics

USES

Thiazides: Management of edema resulting from a number of causes (e.g., CHF, hepatic cirrhosis); hypertension either alone or in combination with other antihypertensives. *Loop:* Management of edema associated with CHF, cirrhosis of the liver, and renal disease. Furosemide used in treatment of hypertension alone or in combination with other antihypertensives. *Potassium-sparing:* Adjunctive treatment with thiazides, loop diuretics in treatment of CHF and hypertension.

Diuretics   *(continued)*

ACTION

Diuretics act to increase the excretion of water/sodium and other electrolytes via the kidneys. Exact mechanism of antihypertensive effect unknown; may be due to reduced plasma volume or decreased peripheral vascular resistance. Subclassifications of diuretics are based on their mechanism and site of action.

Thiazides: Act at the cortical diluting segment of nephron, block reabsorption of Na, Cl, and water; promote excretion of Na, Cl, K, and water. *Loop:* Act primarily at the thick ascending limb of Henle's loop to inhibit Na, Cl, and water absorption.

Potassium-sparing: Spironolactone blocks aldosterone action on distal nephron (causes K retention, Na excretion). Triamterene, amiloride act on distal nephron, decreasing Na reuptake, reducing K secretion.

DIURETICS

Name	Availability	Dosage Range	Side Effects
Chlorothiazide (Diuril)	**T:** 250 mg, 500 mg **S:** 250 mg/5 ml **I:** 500 mg	5–20 mg/day	Confusion, fatigue, muscle cramps, abdominal discomfort
Thiazides			
Chlorthalidone © (Hygroton)	**T:** 15 mg, 25 mg, 50 mg, 100 mg	25–200 mg/day	Same as above
Hydrochlorothiazide (p. 576) (HydroDIURIL)	**T:** 25 mg, 50 mg, 100 mg **C:** 12.5 mg **Solution:** 50 mg/15 ml	25–100 mg/day	Same as above
Indapamide (p. 612) (Lozol)	**T:** 1.25 mg, 2.5 mg	2.5–5 mg/day	Same as above
Metolazone (p. 762) (Diulo, Zaroxolyn)	**T:** 2.5 mg, 5 mg, 10 mg	2.5–10 mg/day	Same as above

Loop

Bumetanide (p. 159) (Bumex)	T: 0.5 mg, 1 mg, 2 mg I: 0.25 mg/ml	5–10 mg/day	Orthostatic hypotension
Ethacrynic acid ℮ (Edecrin)	T: 25 mg, 50 mg I: 50-mg vial	50–200 mg/day	Same as above
Furosemide (p. 523) (Lasix)	T: 20 mg, 40 mg, 80 mg OS: 10 mg/ml, 40 mg/5 ml I: 10 mg/ml	HTN: 40–80 mg/day Edema: Up to 600 mg/day	Same as above
Torsemide (p. 1154) (Demadex)	T: 5 mg, 10 mg, 20 mg, 100 mg I: 10 mg/ml	Edema: 10–200 mg/day HTN: 5–10 mg/day	Constipation, dizziness, headaches, abdominal discomfort

Potassium-sparing

Amiloride (p. 52) (Midamor)	T: 5 mg	5–20 mg/day	Hyperkalemia
Spironolactone (p. 1074) (Aldactone)	T: 25 mg, 50 mg, 100 mg	25–100 mg/day	Hyperkalemia, nausea, vomiting, abdominal cramps, diarrhea
Triamterene (p. 1173) (Dyrenium)	C: 50 mg, 100 mg	Up to 300 mg/day	Same as amiloride

C, Capsules; *HTN,* hypertension; *I,* injection; *OS,* oral solution; *S,* suspension; *T,* tablets.

Fertility Agents

Infertility is defined as a decreased ability to reproduce as opposed to *sterility*, the inability to reproduce. Infertility may be due to reproduction dysfunction of the male, female, or both.

Female infertility can be due to disruption of any phase of the reproductive process. The most critical phases include follicular maturation, ovulation, transport of the ovum through the fallopian tubes, fertilization of the ovum, nidation, and growth/development of the conceptus. Causes of infertility include the following:

Anovulation, failure of follicular maturation: Absence of adequate hormonal stimulation; ovarian follicles do not ripen, and ovulation will not occur.

Unfavorable cervical mucus: Normally the cervical glands secrete large volumes of thin, watery mucus, but if the mucus is unfavorable (scant, thick, or sticky), sperm is unable to pass through to the uterus.

Hyperprolactinemia: Excessive prolactin secretion may cause amenorrhea, galactorrhea, and infertility.

Luteal phase defect: Progesterone secretion by the corpus luteum is insufficient to maintain endometrial integrity.

Endometriosis: Endometrial tissue is implanted in abnormal locations (e.g., uterine wall, ovary, extragenital sites).

Androgen excess: May decrease fertility (the most common condition is polycystic ovary).

Male infertility is due to decreased density or motility of sperm or semen of abnormal volume or quality. The most obvious manifestation of male infertility is impotence (inability to achieve erection). Whereas in female infertility an identifiable endocrine disorder can be found, most cases of male infertility are not associated with an identifiable endocrine disorder.

ACTION

Antiestrogens: Nonsteroidal estrogen antagonist that increases follicle-stimulating hormone (FSH) and luteinizing hormone (LH) levels by blocking estrogen-negative feedback at the hypothalamus.

Gonadotropins: Produce ovulation induction in women with hypogonadotropic hypogonadism and polycystic ovarian syndrome (PCOS). Ovaries must be able to respond normally to FSH and LH stimulation.

Gonadotropin-releasing hormone (GnRH) agonists: Causes down-regulation of endogenous FSH and LH levels. GnRH agonists stimulate release of pituitary gonadotropins. Suppression of endogenous LH can decrease number of oocytes released prematurely, improve oocyte quality, and increase pregnancy rates.

Gonadotropin-releasing hormone (GnRH) antagonists: Suppress endogenous LH surges during ovarian stimulation. GnRH antagonists avoid initial flare-up seen with GnRH agonists, shortening the number of days needed for LH suppression and allowing ovarian stimulation to begin within the spontaneous cycle.

MEDICATIONS TO INDUCE OVULATION

Name	Category	Availability	Uses	Side Effects
Cetrorelix (Cetrotide)	GnRH antagonist	**I:** 0.25 mg, 3 mg	Inhibition of premature LH surges in women undergoing ovarian hyperstimulation	OHSS (ovarian hyperstimulation syndrome): Abdominal pain, indigestion, bloating, decreased urine output, nausea, vomiting, diarrhea, rapid weight gain, shortness of breath, peripheral/dependent edema, Headaches, pain/redness at injection site

(continued)

MEDICATIONS TO INDUCE OVULATION (continued)

Name	Category	Availability	Uses	Side Effects
Chorionic gonadotropin (p. 244) (APL, Pregnyl, Profasi, Profasi HP)	Gonadotropin	**I:** 5,000 units, 10,000 units, 20,000 units	In conjunction with clomiphene, human menotropins or urofollitropin to stimulate ovulation	OHSS (ovarian hyperstimulation syndrome): Abdominal pain, indigestion, bloating, decreased urine output, nausea, vomiting, diarrhea, rapid weight gain, shortness of breath, peripheral/dependent edema Ovarian enlargement, ovarian cyst formation
Clomiphene (Clomid, Milophene, Serophene)	Antiestrogen	**T:** 50 mg	Anovulation, oligo-ovulation with intact pituitary/ovarian response and endogenous estrogen	Ovarian cyst formation, ovarian enlargement visual disturbances, premenstrual syndrome, hot flashes
Follitropin alpha (Gonal-F)	Gonadotropin	**I:** 37.5 international units FSH, 75 international units FSH, 150 international units FSH	In conjunction with human chorionic gonadotropin to stimulate ovarian follicular development in patients with ovulatory dysfunction not due to primary ovarian failure (e.g., anovulation, oligo-ovulation)	OHSS (ovarian hyperstimulation syndrome): Abdominal pain, indigestion, bloating, decreased urine output, nausea, vomiting, diarrhea, rapid weight gain, shortness of breath, peripheral/dependent edema Flulike symptoms, upper respiratory tract infections, bleeding between menstrual periods, nausea, ovarian enlargement, ovarian cysts, acne, breast pain/tenderness

Follitropin beta (Follistem)	Gonadotropin	**I:** 75 international units FSH	In conjunction with human chorionic gonadotropin to stimulate ovarian follicular development in patients with ovulatory dysfunction not due to primary ovarian failure (e.g., anovulation, oligo-ovulation)	OHSS (ovarian hyperstimulation syndrome): Abdominal pain, indigestion, bloating, decreased urine output, nausea, vomiting, diarrhea, rapid weight gain, shortness of breath, peripheral/dependent edema Flulike symptoms, breast tenderness, dry skin, rash, dizziness, fever, headaches, nausea, unusual fatigue
Ganirelex (Antagon)	GnRH antagonist	**I:** 250 mcg/0.5 ml	Inhibition of premature LH surges in women undergoing ovarian hyperstimulation	OHSS (ovarian hyperstimulation syndrome): Abdominal pain, indigestion, bloating, decreased urine output, nausea, vomiting, diarrhea, rapid weight gain, shortness of breath, peripheral/dependent edema Headaches, nausea, pain/redness at injection site
Goserelin (p. 561) (Zoladex)	GnRH agonist	**Implant:** 3.6 mg	Endometriosis, adjunct to menotropins for ovulation induction	Hot flashes, amenorrhea, blurred vision, edema, headaches, nausea, vomiting, breast tenderness, weight gain
Leuprolide (p. 679) (Lupron)	GnRH agonist	5 mg/ml for subcutaneous injection	Endometriosis, adjunct to menotropins/human chorionic gonadotropin for ovulation induction	Hot flashes, amenorrhea, blurred vision, edema, headaches, nausea, vomiting, breast tenderness, weight gain

(continued)

MEDICATIONS TO INDUCE OVULATION *(continued)*

Name	Category	Availability	Uses	Side Effects
Menotropins (Humegon, Pergonal)	Gonadotropin	75 units FSH, 75 units LH activity; 150 units FSH, 150 units LH activity	In conjunction with chorionic gonadotropin for ovulation stimulation in patients with ovulatory dysfunction due to primary ovarian failure	OHSS (ovarian hyperstimulation syndrome): Abdominal pain, indigestion, bloating, decreased urine, nausea, vomiting, diarrhea, rapid weight gain, shortness of breath, edema of lower legs, ovarian enlargement, ovarian cyst formation
Nafarelin (p. 808) (Synarel)	GnRH	2 mg/ml nasal spray	Endometriosis, adjunct to menotropins/human chorionic gonadotropin for ovulation induction	Loss of bone mineral density, breast enlargement, bleeding between regular menstrual periods, acne, mood swings, seborrhea, hot flashes
Urofollitropin (Fertinex, Metrodin)	Gonadotropin	75 units FSH activity, 150 units FSH activity	In conjunction with human chorionic gonadotropin for ovulation stimulation in patients with polycystic ovary syndrome who have elevated LH:FSH ratio and have failed clomiphene therapy	OHSS (ovarian hyperstimulation syndrome): Abdominal pain, indigestion, bloating, decreased urine, nausea, vomiting, diarrhea, rapid weight gain, shortness of breath, swelling of lower legs, ovarian enlargement, ovarian cyst formation, pain/redness at injection site, breast tenderness, nausea vomiting, diarrhea

I, Injection; *T,* tablets.

H₂ Antagonists

USES

Short-term treatment of duodenal ulcer (DU), active benign gastric ulcer (GU), maintenance therapy of DU, pathologic hypersecretory conditions (e.g., Zollinger-Ellison syndrome), gastroesophageal reflux disease (GERD), and prevention of upper GI bleeding in critically ill patients.

ACTION

Inhibit gastric acid secretion by interfering with histamine at the histamine H_2 receptors in parietal cells. Also inhibit acid secretion caused by gastrin. Inhibition occurs with basal (fasting), nocturnal, food-stimulated, or fundic distention secretion. H_2 antagonists decrease both the volume and H_2 concentration of gastric juices.

H₂ ANTAGONISTS

Name	Availability	Dosage Range	Side Effects
Cimetidine (p. 248) (Tagamet)	**T:** 200 mg, 300 mg, 400 mg, 800 mg **L:** 300 mg/5 ml **I:** 150 mg/ml	**Treatment of DU:** 800 mg/at bedtime, 400 mg 2 times/day or 300 mg 4 times/day **Maintenance of DU:** 400 mg/at bedtime **Treatment of GU:** 800 mg/at bedtime or 300 mg 4 times/day **GERD:** 1,600 mg/day **Hypersecretory:** 1,200–2,400 mg/day	Headaches, fatigue, dizziness, confusion, diarrhea, gynecomastia

(continued)

H2 ANTAGONISTS *(continued)*

Name	Availability	Dosage Range	Side Effects
Famotidine (p. 463) (Pepcid)	**T:** 10 mg, 20 mg, 40 mg **T (chewable):** 10 mg **DT:** 20 mg, 40 mg **Gelcap:** 10 mg **OS:** 40 mg/5 ml **I:** 10 mg/ml	**Treatment of DU:** 40 mg/day **Maintenance of DU:** 20 mg/day **Treatment of GU:** 40 mg/day **GERD:** 40–80 mg/day **Hypersecretory:** 80–640 mg/day	Headaches, dizziness, diarrhea, constipation, abdominal pain, tinnitus
Nizatidine (p. 847) (Axid)	**T:** 75 mg **C:** 150 mg, 300 mg	**Treatment of DU:** 300 mg/day **Maintenance of DU:** 150 mg/day	Fatigue, urticaria, abdominal pain, constipation, nausea
Ranitidine (p. 1007) (Zantac)	**T:** 75 mg, 150 mg, 300 mg **C:** 150 mg, 300 mg **Syrup:** 15 mg/ml **Granules:** 150 mg **I:** 0.5 mg/ml, 25 mg/ml	**Treatment of DU:** 300 mg/day **Maintenance of DU:** 150 mg/day **Treatment of GU:** 300 mg/day **GERD:** 300 mg/day **Hypersecretory:** 0.3–6 g/day	Blurred vision, constipation, nausea, abdominal pain

C, Capsules; *DT,* disintegrating tablets; *I,* injection; *L,* liquid; *OS,* oral suspension; *T,* tablets.

Hematinic Preparations

USES

Prevention or treatment of iron deficiency resulting from improper diet, pregnancy, impaired absorption, or prolonged blood loss.

ACTION

Iron supplements are provided to ensure adequate supplies for the formation of hemoglobin, which is needed for erythropoiesis and O_2 transport.

HEMATINIC (IRON) PREPARATIONS

Name	Availability	Elemental Iron	Side Effects
Ferrous fumarate (p. 474) (Femiron, Feostat)	**T:** 63 mg, 200 mg, 324 mg **S:** 100 mg/5 ml **D:** 45 mg/0.6 ml	33	Constipation, nausea, vomiting, diarrhea, abdominal pain/cramps
Ferrous gluconate (p. 474) (Fergon)	**T:** 240 mg, 325 mg	12	Same as above
Ferrous sulfate (p. 474) (Fer-In-Sol)	**T:** 325 mg **Syrup:** 90 mg/5 ml **E:** 220 mg/5 ml **D:** 75 mg/0.6 ml	20	Same as above
Ferrous sulfate exsiccated (p. 474) (Slow-Fe)	**T:** 187 mg, 200 mg **T (SR):** 160 mg **C (ER):** 160 mg	30	Same as above

C, Caplets; *D,* drops; *E,* elixir; *ER,* extended-release; *S,* suspension; *SR,* sustained-release; *T,* tablets.

Hormones

USES

Functions of the body are regulated by two major control systems: the nervous system and the endocrine (hormone) system. Together they maintain homeostasis and control different metabolic functions in the body.

Hormones are concerned with control of different metabolic functions in the body (e.g., rates of chemical reactions in cells, transporting substances through cell membranes, cellular metabolism [growth/secretions]). By definition, a hormone is a chemical substance secreted into body fluids by cells and has control over other cells in the body.

Hormones can be local or general:

- *Local hormones* have specific local effects (e.g., acetylcholine, which is secreted at parasympathetic and skeletal nerve endings).

Hormones *(continued)*

- *General hormones* are mostly secreted by specific endocrine glands (e.g., epinephrine/norepinephrine are secreted by the adrenal medulla in response to sympathetic stimulation), transported in the blood to all parts of the body, causing many different reactions.

Some general hormones affect all or almost all cells of the body (e.g., thyroid hormone from the thyroid gland increases the rate of most chemical reactions in almost all cells of the body); other general hormones affect only specific tissue (e.g., ovarian hormones are specific to female sex organs and secondary sexual characteristics of the female).

ACTION

Endocrine hormones almost never directly act intracellularly affecting chemical reactions. They first combine with hormone receptors either on the cell surface or inside the cell (cell cytoplasm or nucleus). The combination of hormone and receptors alters the function of the receptor, and the receptor is the direct cause of the hormone effects. Altered receptor function may include the following:

Altered cell permeability, which causes a change in protein structure of the receptor, usually opening or closing a channel for one or more ions. The movement of these ions causes the effect of the hormone.

Activation of intracellular enzymes immediately inside the cell membrane (e.g., hormone combines with receptor that then becomes the activated enzyme adenyl cyclase, which causes formation of cAMP).

◄ ALERT ► cAMP has effects inside the cell. It is not the hormone but cAMP that causes these effects.

Regulation of hormone secretion is controlled by an internal control system, the negative feedback system:

- Endocrine gland oversecretes.
- Hormone exerts more and more of its effect.
- Target organ performs its function.
- Too much function in turn feeds back to endocrine gland to decrease secretory rate.

The endocrine system contains many glands and hormones. A summary of the important glands and their hormones secreted are as follows:

The pituitary gland (hypophysis) is a small gland found in the sella turcica at the base of the brain. The pituitary is divided into two portions physiologically: the anterior pituitary (adenohypophysis) and the posterior pituitary (neurohypophysis). Six important hormones are secreted from the anterior pituitary and two from the posterior pituitary.

Anterior pituitary hormones:

- Growth hormone
- Adrenocorticotropin (corticotropin)
- Thyroid-stimulating hormone (thyrotropin)
- Follicle-stimulating hormone (FSH)

ACTION (cont.)

- Luteinizing hormone (LH)
- Prolactin

Posterior pituitary hormones:

- Antidiuretic hormone (vasopressin)
- Oxytocin

Almost all secretions of the pituitary hormones are controlled by hormonal or nervous signals from the hypothalamus. The hypothalamus is a center of information concerned with the well-being of the body, which in turn is used to control secretions of the important pituitary hormones just listed. Secretions from the posterior pituitary are controlled by nerve signals originating in the hypothalamus; anterior pituitary hormones are controlled by hormones secreted within the hypothalamus. These hormones are as follows:

- Thyrotropin-releasing hormone (TRH) releasing thyroid-stimulating hormone
- Corticotropin-releasing hormone (CRH) releasing adrenocorticotropin
- Growth hormone-releasing hormone (GHRH) releasing growth hormone and growth hormone inhibitory hormone (GHIH) (same as somato-statin)

- Gonadotropin-releasing hormone r(GnRH) releasing the two gonadotropic hormones LH and FSH
- Prolactin inhibitory factor (PIF) causing inhibition of prolactin and prolactin-releasing factor

Anterior Pituitary Hormones

All anterior pituitary hormones (except growth hormone) have as their principal effect stimulating target glands.

Growth Hormone (GH)

Growth hormone affects almost all tissues of the body. GH (somatropin) causes growth in almost all tissues of the body (increases cell size, increases mitosis with increased number of cells, and differentiates certain types of cells). Metabolic effects include increased rate of protein synthesis, mobilization of fatty acids from adipose tissue, decreased rate of glucose utilization.

Thyroid-Stimulating Hormone (TSH)

Thyroid-stimulating hormone controls secretion of the thyroid hormones. The thyroid gland is located immediately below the larynx on either side of and anterior to the trachea and secretes two significant hormones, thyroxine (T_4) and triiodothyroxine (T_3), which have a profound effect on increasing the metabolic rate of the body. The thyroid gland also secretes calcitonin, an important hormone for calcium metabolism. Calcitonin promotes deposition of calcium in the bones, which decreases calcium concentration in the extracellular fluid.

Adrenocorticotropin

Adrenocorticotropin causes the adrenal cortex to secrete adrenocortical hormones. The adrenal glands lie at the superior poles of the two kidneys. Each gland is composed of two distinct parts: the adrenal medulla and the cortex. The adrenal medulla, related to the sympathetic nervous system, secretes the hormones epinephrine and norepinephrine. When stimulated, they cause constriction of blood vessels, increased activity of the heart, inhibitory effects on the GI tract, and dilation of the pupils. The adrenal cortex secretes corticosteroids, of which there are two major types: mineralocorticoids and glucocorticoids. Aldosterone, the principal mineralocorticoid, primarily

Hormones *(continued)*

ACTION *(cont.)*

affects electrolytes of the extracellular fluids. Cortisol, the principal glucocorticoid, affects glucose, protein, and fat metabolism.

LUTEINIZING HORMONE (LH)

Luteinizing hormone plays an important role in ovulation and causes secretion of female sex hormones by the ovaries and testosterone by the testes.

FOLLICLE-STIMULATING HORMONE (FSH)

Follicle-stimulating hormone causes growth of follicles in the ovaries before ovulation and promotes formation of sperm in the testes.

Ovarian sex hormones are estrogens and progestins. Estradiol is the most important estrogen; progesterone is the most important progestin.

Estrogens mainly promote proliferation and growth of specific cells in the body and are responsible for development of most of the secondary sex characteristics. Primarily cause cellular proliferation and growth of tissues of sex organs/other tissue related to reproduction. Ovaries, fallopian tubes, uterus, vagina increase in size. Estrogen initiates growth of breast and milk-producing apparatus, external appearance.

Progesterone stimulates secretion of the uterine endometrium during the latter half of the female sexual cycle, preparing the uterus for implantation of the fertilized ovum. Decreases the frequency of uterine contractions (helps prevent expulsion of the implanted ovum). Progesterone promotes development of breasts, causing alveolar cells to proliferate, enlarge, and become secretory in nature.

Testosterone is secreted by the testes and formed by the interstitial cells of Leydig. Testosterone production increases under the stimulus of the anterior pituitary gonadotropic hormones. It is responsible for distinguishing characteristics of the masculine body (stimulates the growth of male sex organs and promotes the development of male secondary sex characteristics, e.g., distribution of body hair, effect on voice, protein formation, and muscular development).

PROLACTIN

Prolactin promotes the development of breasts and secretion of milk.

POSTERIOR PITUITARY HORMONES

ANTIDIURETIC HORMONE (ADH) (VASOPRESSIN)

Antidiuretic hormone can cause antidiuresis (decreased excretion of water by the kidneys). In the presence of ADH the permeability of the renal-collecting ducts and tubules to water increases, which allows water to be absorbed, conserving water in the body. ADH in higher concentrations is a very potent vasoconstrictor, constricting arterioles everywhere in the body, increasing BP.

OXYTOCIN

Oxytocin contracts the uterus during the birthing process, esp. toward the end of the pregnancy, helping expel the baby. Oxytocin also contracts myoepithelial cells in the breasts, causing milk to be expressed from the alveoli into the ducts so that the baby can obtain it by suckling.

ACTION *(cont.)*

PANCREAS

The pancreas is composed of two tissue types: *acini* (secrete digestive juices in the duodenum) and *islets of Langerhans* (secrete insulin/glucagons directly into the blood). The islets of Langerhans contain three cells: alpha, beta, and delta. Alpha cells secrete glucagon, beta cells secrete insulin, and delta cells secrete somatostatin.

Insulin promotes glucose entry into most cells, thus controlling the rate of metabolism of most carbohydrates. Insulin also affects fat metabolism.

Glucagon effects are opposite those of insulin, the most important of which is increasing blood glucose concentration by releasing it from the liver into the circulating body fluids.

Somatostatin (same chemical as secreted by the hypothalamus) has multiple inhibitory effects: depresses secretion of insulin and glucagon, decreases GI motility, decreases secretions/absorption of the GI tract.

Human Immunodeficiency Virus (HIV) Infection

USES

Antiretroviral agents are used in the treatment of HIV infection.

ACTION

There are currently five classes of antiretroviral agents used in the treatment of HIV disease. *Nucleoside reverse transcriptase inhibitors* (NRTIs) compete with natural substrates for formation of proviral DNA by reverse transcriptase inhibiting viral replication.

Nucleotide reverse transcriptase inhibitors (NtRTIs) inhibit reverse transcriptase by competing with the natural substrate deoxyadenosine triphosphate and by DNA chain termination.

Nonnucleoside reverse transcriptase inhibitors (NNRTIs) directly bind to reverse transcriptase and blocks the RNA-dependent and DNA-dependent DNA polymerase activities by causing a disruption of the enzyme's catalytic site.

Protease inhibitors (PIs) bind to the active site of HIV-1 protease and prevent the processing of viral gag and gag-pol polyprotein precursors resulting in immature, noninfectious viral particles.

Fusion inhibitors interfere with the entry of HIV-1 into cells by inhibiting fusion of viral and cellular membranes.

Human Immunodeficiency Virus (HIV) Infection *(continued)*

ANTIRETROVIRAL AGENTS FOR TREATMENT OF HIV INFECTION

Name	Availability	Dosage Range	Side Effects
Nucleoside Analogues			
Abacavir (p. 1) (Ziagen)	**T:** 300 mg **OS:** 20 mg/ml	**A:** 300 mg 2 times/day	Nausea, vomiting, malaise, rash, fever, headaches, asthenia, fatigue
Abacavir/lamivudine (Epzicom)	**T:** 600 mg abacavir/ 300 mg lamivudine	**A:** once/day	Allergic reaction, insomnia, headaches, depression, dizziness, fatigue, diarrhea, fever, abdominal pain, anxiety
Didanosine (p. 352) (Videx)	**T:** 25 mg, 50 mg, 100 mg, 150 mg, 200 mg **C:** 125 mg, 200 mg, 250 mg, 400 mg **OS:** 100 mg, 167 mg, 250 mg	**T (weighing more than 60 kg):** 200 mg 2 times/day; **(weighing less than 60 kg):** 125 mg 2 times/day **OS (weighing more than 60 kg):** 250 mg 2 times/day; **(weighing less than 60 kg):** 167 mg 2 times/day	Peripheral neuropathy, pancreatitis, diarrhea, nausea, vomiting, headaches, insomnia, rash, hepatitis, seizures
Emtricitabine (p. 406) (Emtriva)	**C:** 200 mg	**A:** 200 mg/day	Headaches, insomnia, depression, diarrhea, nausea, vomiting, rhinitis, asthenia, rash
Emtricitabine/tenofovir (Truvada)	**T:** 200 mg emtricitabine/ 300 mg tenofovir	**A:** once/day	Dizziness, diarrhea, headaches, rash, belching/flatulence, skin discoloration

Name	Forms	Dosage	Side Effects
Lamivudine (p. 664) (Epivir)	**T:** 100 mg, 150 mg **OS:** 5 mg/ml, 10 mg/ml	**A:** 150 mg 2 times/day **C:** 4 mg/kg 2 times/day	Diarrhea, malaise, fatigue, headaches, nausea, vomiting, abdominal pain, peripheral neuropathy, arthralgia, myalgia, skin rash
Stavudine (p. 1077) (Zerit)	**C:** 15 mg, 20 mg, 30 mg, 40 mg **OS:** 1 mg/ml	**A:** 40 mg 2 times/day (20 mg 2 times/day if peripheral neuropathy occurs)	Peripheral neuropathy, anemia, leukopenia, neutropenia
Zalcitabine (p. 1225) (Hivid)	**T:** 0.375 mg, 0.75 mg	**A (weighing more than 60 kg):** 0.75 mg 3 times/day; **(weighing less than 60 kg):** 0.375 mg 3 times/day	Peripheral neuropathy, stomatitis, granulocytopenia, leukopenia
Zidovudine (p. 1229) (Retrovir)	**C:** 100 mg **T:** 300 mg **Syrup:** 50 mg/5 ml, 10 mg/ml	**A:** 500–600 mg/day (100 mg 5 times/day or 300 mg 2 times/day)	Anemia, granulocytopenia, myopathy, nausea, malaise, fatigue, insomnia
Zidovudine/lamivudine (AZT/3TC) (Combivir)	**C:** 300 mg AZT/150 mg 3TC	**A:** 1 capsule 2 times/day	Bone marrow suppression, peripheral neuropathy, pancreatitis
Zidovudine/lamivudine/ abacavir (AZT/3TC/ABC) (Trizivir)	**C:** 300 mg AZT/150 mg 3TC/ 300 mg ABC	**A:** 1 capsule 2 times/day	Bone marrow suppression, peripheral neuropathy, anaphylactic reaction
Nucleotide Analogues			
Tenofovir (p. 1106) (Viread)	**T:** 300 mg	**A:** 300 mg/day	Nausea, vomiting, diarrhea

(continued)

ANTIRETROVIRAL AGENTS FOR TREATMENT OF HIV INFECTION *(continued)*

Name	Availability	Dosage Range	Side Effects
Nonnucleoside Analogues			
Delavirdine (p. 324) (Rescriptor)	T: 100 mg, 200 mg	**A:** 200 mg 3 times/day for 14 days, then 400 mg 3 times/day	Rash, nausea, headaches, elevations in serum hepatic function tests
Efavirenz (p. 403) (Sustiva)	C: 50 mg, 100 mg, 200 mg	**A:** 600 mg/day **C:** 200–600 mg/day based on weight	Headaches, dizziness, insomnia, fatigue, rash, nightmares
Nevirapine (p. 828) (Viramune)	T: 200 mg	**A:** 200 mg/day for 14 days, then 200 mg 2 times/day	Rash, nausea, fatigue, fever, headaches, abnormal serum hepatic function tests
Protease Inhibitors			
Amprenavir (p. 75) (Agenerase)	C: 50 mg, 150 mg OS: 15 mg/ml	**A:** 1,200 mg 2 times/day **C (4–16 yr, weighing less than 50 kg):** 20 mg/kg 2 times/day or 15 mg/kg 3 times/day	Rash, diarrhea, headaches, nausea, vomiting, numbness, abdominal pain, fatigue
Atazanavir (p. 95) (Reyataz)	C: 100 mg, 150 mg, 200 mg	**A:** 400 mg/day	Headaches, diarrhea, abdominal pain, nausea, rash
Fosamprenavir (p. 513) (Lexiva)	T: 700 mg	**A:** 1,400–2,800 mg/day	Headaches, fatigue, rash, nausea, diarrhea, vomiting, abdominal pain
Indinavir (p. 614) (Crixivan)	C: 200 mg, 400 mg	**A:** 800 mg q8h	Nephrolithiasis, hyperbilirubinemia, abdominal pain, asthenia, fatigue, flank pain, nausea, vomiting, diarrhea, headaches, insomnia, dizziness, altered taste

Lopinavir/ritonavir (p. 704) (Kaletra)	**C:** 133/33 mg **OS:** 80/20 mg	**A:** 400/100 mg/day **C (4-12 yr):** 10-13 mg/kg 2 times/day	Diarrhea, nausea, vomiting, abdominal pain, headaches, rash
Nelfinavir (p. 822) (Viracept)	**T:** 250 mg **Oral Powder:** 50 mg/g	**A:** 750 mg q8h **C:** 20-25 mg/kg q8h	Diarrhea, fatigue, asthenia, headaches, hypertension, impaired concentration
Ritonavir (p. 1028) (Norvir)	**C:** 100 mg **OS:** 80 mg/ml	**A:** Titrate up to 600 mg 2 times/day	Nausea, vomiting, diarrhea, altered taste sensation, fatigue, elevated serum hepatic function tests and triglyceride levels
Saquinavir (p. 1041) (Invirase)	**C:** 200 mg	**A:** 600 mg 3 times/day	Diarrhea, elevations in serum hepatic function tests, hypertriglycerides, cholesterol, abnormal fat accumulation, hyperglycemia
Tipranavir (p. 1140) (Aptivus)	**C:** 250 mg	**A:** 500 mg (with 200 mg ritonavir) 2 times/day	Diarrhea, nausea, fatigue, headaches, vomiting

Fusion Inhibitors

Enfuvirtide (p. 410) (Fuzeon)	**I:** 108 mg (90 mg when reconstituted)	**Subcutaneous:** 90 mg 2 times/day	Insomnia, depression, peripheral neuropathy, decreased appetite, constipation, asthenia, cough

A, Adults; *C,* capsules; *C (dosage),* children; *I,* injection; *OS,* oral solution; *T,* tablets.

Immunosuppressive Agents

USES

Improvement of both short- and long-term allograft survivals.

ACTION

Basiliximab: An interleukin-2 (IL-2) receptor antagonist inhibiting IL-2 binding. This prevents activation of lymphocytes and the response of the immune system to antigens is impaired.

Cyclosporine: Inhibits production and release of IL-2.

Daclizumab: An IL-2 receptor antagonist inhibiting IL-2 binding.

Mycophenolate: A prodrug that reversibly binds and inhibits inosine monophosphate dehydrogenase (IMPD), resulting in inhibition of purine nucleotide synthesis, inhibiting DNA and RNA synthesis and subsequent synthesis of T and B cells.

Sirolimus: Inhibits IL-2–stimulated T-lymphocyte activation and proliferation, which may occur through formation of a complex.

Tacrolimus: Inhibits IL-2–stimulated T-lymphocyte activation and proliferation, which may occur through formation of a complex.

IMMUNOSUPPRESSIVES

Name	Availability	Dosage	Side Effects
Basiliximab (p. 121) (Simulect)	**I:** 20 mg	20 mg for 2 doses	Abdominal pain, asthenia, cough, dizziness, dyspnea, dysuria, edema, hypertension, infection, tremors
Cyclosporine (p. 300) (Neoral, Sandimmune)	**C:** 25 mg, 50 mg, 100 mg, **S:** 100 mg/ml **I:** 50 mg/ml	7–10 mg/kg/day	Hypertension, hyperkalemia, nephrotoxicity, coarsening of facial features, hirsutism, gingival hyperplasia, nausea, vomiting, diarrhea, hepatic toxicity, hyperuricemia, hypertriglycerides/cholesterol, tremors, paraesthesia, seizures, risk of infection/malignancy
Daclizumab (p. 308) (Zenapax)	**I:** 25 mg/5 ml	1 mg/kg (**Maximum:** 100 mg)	Dyspnea, fever, hypertension, nausea, peripheral edema, tachycardia, tremors, vomiting, weakness, wound infection

Mycophenolate (p. 802) (CellCept)	**C:** 250 mg **I:** 500 mg **S:** 200 mg/ml **T:** 500 mg	1 g 2 times/day	Diarrhea, vomiting, leukopenia, neutropenia, infections
Sirolimus (p. 1058) (Rapamune)	**S:** 1 mg/ml **T:** 1 mg	2–10 mg/day	Dyspnea, leukopenia, thrombocytopenia, hyperlipidemia, abdominal pain, acne, arthralgia, fever, diarrhea, constipation, headaches, vomiting, weight gain
Tacrolimus (p. 1091) (Prograf)	**C:** 0.5 mg, 1 mg, 5 mg **I:** 5 mg/ml	0.1–0.15 mg/kg/day	Nephrotoxicity, neurotoxicity, hyperglycemia, nausea, vomiting, photophobia, infections, hypertension, hyperlipidemia

C, Capsules; *I,* injection; *S,* oral solution or suspension; *T,* tablets.

Laxatives

USES

Short-term treatment of constipation; colon evacuation before rectal/bowel examination; prevention of straining (e.g., after anorectal surgery, MI); to reduce painful elimination (e.g., episiotomy, hemorrhoids, anorectal lesions); modification of effluent from ileostomy, colostomy; prevention of fecal impaction; removal of ingested poisons.

ACTION

Laxatives ease or stimulate defecation. Mechanisms by which this is accomplished include (1) attracting, retaining fluid in colonic contents due to hydrophilic or osmotic properties; (2) acting directly or indirectly on mucosa to decrease absorption of water and NaCl; or (3) increasing intestinal motility, decreasing absorption of water and NaCl by virtue of decreased transit time.

Bulk-forming: Act primarily in small/large intestine. Retain water in stool, may bind water, ions in colonic lumen (soften feces, increase bulk); may increase colonic bacteria growth (increases fecal mass). Produce soft stool in 1–3 days.

Lubricant: Mineral oil is the only agent in this group. Promotes stool passage by coating the fecal surface with an oil layer that retains fecal fluid and prevents absorption of fecal water by the colon.

Hyperosmotic agents: Acts in colon. Similar to saline laxatives. Osmotic action may be enhanced in distal ileum/colon by bacterial metabolism to lactate, other organic acids. This decrease in pH increases motility, secretion. Produces soft stool in 1–3 days.

Saline: Acts in small/large intestine, colon (sodium phosphate). Poorly, slowly absorbed; causes hormone cholecystokinin release from duodenum (stimulates fluid secretion, motility); possesses osmotic properties; produces watery stool in 2–6 hr (small doses produce semifluid stool in 6–12 hr).

Stimulant: Acts in colon. Enhances accumulation of water/electrolytes in colonic lumen, enhances intestinal motility. May act directly on intestinal mucosa. Produces semifluid stool in 6–12 hr.

◀ ALERT ▶ Bisacodyl suppository acts in 15–60 min.

Surfactants: Act in small/large intestine. Hydrate and soften stools by their surfactant action, facilitating penetration of fat and water into stool. Produce soft stool in 1–3 days.

LAXATIVES

Name	Onset of Action	Uses
Bulk-forming		
Methylcellulose (p. 752) (Citrucel)	12–24 hr up to 3 days	First line for postpartum women; elderly; patients with diverticulosis, irritable bowel syndrome, hemorrhoids. Safe for chronic use
Polycarbophil (p. 941) (Fibercon, Mitrolan)	Same as above	Same as above
Psyllium (p. 987) (Metamucil, Konsyl)	Same as above	Same as above
Surfactant		
Docusate calcium (p. 377) (Surfak)	Same as above	Aids in passage of hard, painful feces, prevents straining
Docusate sodium (p. 377) (Colace)	1–3 days	Same as above
Lubricant		
Mineral oil (Kondremul)	6–8 hr	Prevents straining
Saline		
Magnesium citrate (p. 717) (Citrate of Magnesia)	30 min–3 hr	Bowel evacuation for colonic procedures/exams, fecal impaction, hepatic coma
Magnesium hydroxide (p. 717)	Same as above	Same as above

(continued)

LAXATIVES *(continued)*

Name	Onset of Action	Uses
Saline *(continued)*		
Sodium phosphate (Fleets Phospho-Soda)	5–15 min	Same as above
Hyperosmotic		
Glycerin	less than 30 min	Short-term relief of constipation
Lactulose (p. 663) (Constilac)	1–3 days	Hepatic comas
Polyethylene glycol-electrolyte solution (p. 942) (GoLYTELY)	30–60 min	Bowel evacuation for colonic procedures/exams
Stimulant		
Bisacodyl (p. 139) (Dulcolax)	**PO:** 6–12 hr **Rectal:** 15–60 min	Same as above
Casanthranol	6–12 hr	Same as above
Cascara sagrada (p. 192)	6–12 hr	Bowel evacuation for colonic procedures/exams
Castor oil	6–12 hr	Same as above
Senna (p. 1049) (Senokot)	6–12 hr	Same as above

Neuromuscular Blockers

USES

Adjunct in surgical anesthesia to relax skeletal muscle (especially abdominal wall) for surgery (allows lighter level of anesthesia; valuable in orthopedic procedures). Neuromuscular blocking agents of short duration often used to facilitate endotracheal intubation, laryngoscopy, bronchoscopy, and esophagoscopy in combination with general anesthetics. Provide muscle relaxation in patients undergoing mechanical ventilation, muscle relaxation in diagnosis of myasthenia gravis. Prevent convulsive movements during electroconvulsive therapy.

ACTION

Paralysis results from the blocking of the normal neuromuscular transmission. Succinylcholine, a depolarizing agent, attaches to the acetylcholine (ACh) receptor on the motor end plate, causing depolarization. It prevents the binding of ACh to the receptor. Nondepolarizing agents also bind to the receptor at the motor end plate but competitively block ACh from attaching to the receptor. These agents also block presynaptic channels that cause the release of ACh.

NEUROMUSCULAR BLOCKERS

Name	Class	Intubation Dose	ICU Dose	Side Effects
Atracurium (Tracrium)	Short	0.4–0.5 mg/kg	0.4–0.5 mg/kg bolus, then 4–12 mcg/kg/min	Flushed skin, hives
Cisatracurium (Nimbex)	Intermediate	0.15–2 mg/kg	0.10–0.2 mg/kg bolus, then 2.5–3 mcg/kg/min	Skin rash, flushing
Doxacurium (Nuromax)	Long	0.05 mg/kg	0.025–0.05 mg/kg bolus, then 0.3–0.5 mg/kg/min	Injection site reaction, urticaria

(continued)

NEUROMUSCULAR BLOCKERS			(continued)	
Name	Class	Intubation Dose	ICU Dose	Side Effects
Mivacurium (Mivacron)	Short	0.15–0.2 mg/kg	0.15–0.25 mg/kg bolus, then 9–10 mcg/kg/min	Flushing, hypotension, dizziness, muscle spasm
Pancuronium (Pavulon)	Long	0.06–0.1 mg/kg	0.05–0.1 mg/kg bolus, then 1–2 mcg/kg/hr	Increased BP, increased salivation, pruritus
Rocuronium (Zemuron)	Intermediate	0.45–1.2 mg/kg	0.15–0.25 mg/kg bolus, then 10–12 mcg/kg/min	Pain at injection site, hypertension or hypotension
Succinylcholine (Anectine, Quelicin)	Ultrashort	1–2 mg/kg	NA	Increased intracranial pressure, increased intraocular pressure, postop muscle pain, weakness, increased salivation, bradycardia, cardiac arrhythmias
Tubocurarine	Intermediate	0.5–0.6 mg/kg	NA	Decreased BP
Vecuronium (Norcuron)	Intermediate	0.08–0.1 mg/kg	0.08–0.1 mg/kg bolus, then 0.8–1.2 mcg/kg/min	Skeletal muscle weakness with prolonged use

Nitrates

USES

Sublingual: Acute relief of angina pectoris.

Oral, topical: Long-term prophylactic treatment of Angina pectoris.

Intravenous: Adjunctive treatment in CHF associated with acute MI. Produce controlled hypotension during surgical procedures; control BP in perioperative hypertension, angina unresponsive to organic nitrates or beta-blockers.

ACTION

Relax most smooth muscles, including arteries and veins. Effect is primarily on veins (decrease left/right ventricular end-diastolic pressure). In angina, nitrates decrease myocardial work and O_2 requirements (decrease preload by venodilation and after-load by arteriodilation). Nitrates also appear to redistribute blood flow to ischemic myocardial areas, improving perfusion without increase in coronary blood flow.

Nitrates *(continued)*

NITRATES

Name	Availability	Dosage Range	Side Effects
Isosorbide (p. 644) (Isordil)	**T:** 5 mg, 10 mg, 20 mg, 30 mg, 40 mg **T (ER):** 30 mg, 40 mg, 60 mg, 120 mg **SL:** 2.5 mg, 5 mg **T (chewable):** 5 mg, 10 mg **C (SR):** 40 mg	**SL:** 2.5–10 mg q2–3h **PO:** 10–40 mg q6h **PO (SR):** 40–80 mg q8–12h	Flushing, headaches, nausea, vomiting, orthostatic hypotension, restlessness, tachycardia
Nitroglycerin (p. 842) (Minitran, Nitro-Bid, Nitro-Dur, Nitrostat)	**SL:** 0.4 mg **T (SR):** 2.6 mg, 6.5 mg, 9 mg **C (SR):** 2.5 mg, 6.5 mg, 9 mg, 13 mg **Topical:** 2% ointment **Trans:** 0.1 mg/hr, 0.2 mg/hr, 0.3 mg/hr, 0.4 mg/hr, 0.6 mg/hr, 0.8 mg/hr **I:** 0.5 mg/ml, 5 mg/ml **Infusion:** 100 mcg/ml, 200 mcg/ml	**SL:** 0.4 mg up to 3 times q15min **SR:** 2.5–26 mg 3–4 times/day **Trans:** 0.1–0.8 mg/hr **T:** 1–2 inches up to 4–5 inches q4h	Same as above

C, Capsules; *ER*, extended-release; *I*, injection; *SL*, sublingual; *SR*, sustained-release; *T*, tablets; *Trans*, transdermal.

Nonsteroidal Anti-Inflammatory Drugs (NSAIDs)

USES

Provide symptomatic relief from *pain/inflammation* in the treatment of musculoskeletal disorders (e.g., rheumatoid arthritis, osteoarthritis, ankylosing spondylitis), *analgesic* for low to moderate pain, *reduction in fever* (many agents not suited for routine/prolonged therapy due to toxicity). By virtue of its action on platelet function, aspirin is used in treatment or prophylaxis of diseases associated with hypercoagulability (reduces risk of stroke/heart attack).

ACTION

Exact mechanism for anti-inflammatory, analgesic, antipyretic effects unknown. Inhibition of enzyme cyclo-oxygenase, the enzyme responsible for prostaglandin synthesis, appears to be a major mechanism of action. May inhibit other mediators of inflammation (e.g., leukotrienes). Direct action on hypothalamus heat-regulating center may contribute to antipyretic effect.

NSAIDs

Name	Availability	Dosage Range	Side Effects
Aspirin (p. 93)	**T:** 81 mg, 160 mg, 325 mg **Supplement:** 300 mg, 600 mg	**P (A):** 325–650 mg q4h as needed **C:** Up to 60–80 mg/kg/day **Arthritis:** 3.2–6 g/day **JRA:** 60–110 mg/kg/day **RF (A):** 5–8 g/day **C:** 75–100 mg/kg/day **TIA:** 1,300 mg/day **MI:** 81–325 mg/day	GI discomfort, dizziness, headaches

(continued)

NSAIDs	*(continued)*		
Name	Availability	Dosage Range	Side Effects
Celecoxib (p. 226) (Celebrex)	**C:** 100 mg, 200 mg	**OA:** 200 mg/day **RA:** 100–200 mg 2 times/day **FAP:** 400 mg 2 times/day	Diarrhea, back pain, dizziness, heartburn, headaches, nausea, abdominal pain
Diclofenac (p. 347) (Voltaren)	**T:** 25 mg, 50 mg, 75 mg, 100 mg	**Arthritis:** 100–200 mg/day	Indigestion, constipation, diarrhea, nausea, headaches, fluid retention, abdominal cramps
Diflunisal (p. 354) (Dolobid)	**T:** 250 mg, 500 mg	**Arthritis:** 0.5–1 g/day **P:** 0.5 g q8–12h	Headaches, abdominal cramps, indigestion, diarrhea, nausea
Etodolac (p. 453) (Lodine)	**T:** 400 mg, 500 mg **T (ER):** 400 mg, 500 mg, 600 mg **C:** 200 mg, 300 mg	**Arthritis:** 600–800 mg/day **P:** 200–400 mg q6–8h	Indigestion, dizziness, headaches, bloated feeling, diarrhea, nausea, weakness, abdominal cramps
Fenoprofen (p. 470) (Nalfon)	**C:** 200 mg, 300 mg **T:** 600 mg	**Arthritis:** 300–600 mg 3–4 times/day **P:** 200 mg q4–6h as needed	Nausea, indigestion, nervousness, constipation, shortness of breath, heartburn
Flurbiprofen (p. 500) (Ansaid)	**T:** 50 mg, 100 mg	**Arthritis:** 200–300 mg/day	Indigestion, nausea, fluid retention, headaches, abdominal cramps, diarrhea
Ibuprofen (p. 598) (Motrin, Advil)	**T:** 100 mg, 200 mg, 400 mg, 600 mg, 800 mg **T (chewable):** 50 mg, 100 mg **C:** 200 mg **S:** 100 mg/5 ml, 100 mg/2.5 ml **Drops:** 40 mg/ml	**Arthritis:** 1.2–3.2 g/day **P:** 400 mg q4–6h as needed **Fever:** 200 mg q4–6h as needed **JA:** 30–40 mg/kg/day	Dizziness, abdominal cramps, abdominal pain, heartburn, nausea
Indomethacin (p. 615) (Indocin)	**C:** 25 mg, 50 mg **C (SR):** 75 mg **S:** 25 mg/5 ml **Supplement:** 50 mg	**Arthritis:** 50–200 mg/day **Bursitis/tendonitis:** 75–150 mg/day **GA:** 150 mg/day	Fluid retention, dizziness, headaches, abdominal pain, indigestion, nausea

Drug	Dosage Forms	Dosage	Side Effects
Ketoprofen (p. 656) (Orudis)	**T:** 12.5 mg **C:** 25 mg, 50 mg, 75 mg **C (ER):** 100 mg, 150 mg, 200 mg	**Arthritis:** 150–300 mg/day **P:** 25–50 mg q6–8h as needed	Headaches, nervousness, abdominal pain, bloated feeling, constipation, diarrhea, nausea
Ketorolac (p. 658) (Toradol)	**T:** 10 mg **I:** 15 mg/ml, 30 mg/ml	**P (PO):** 10 mg q4–6h as needed; **(IM/IV):** 60–120 mg/day	Fluid retention, abdominal pain, diarrhea, dizziness, headaches, nausea
Meloxicam (p. 729) (Mobic)	**C:** 7.5 mg	**Arthritis:** 7.5–15 mg/day	Heartburn, indigestion, nausea, diarrhea, headaches
Nabumetone (p. 805) (Relafen)	**T:** 500 mg, 750 mg	**Arthritis:** 1–2 g/day	Fluid retention, dizziness, headaches, abdominal pain, constipation, diarrhea, nausea
Naproxen (p. 814) (Anaprox, Naprosyn)	**T:** 200 mg, 250 mg, 375 mg, 500 mg **T (CR):** 375 mg **S:** 125 mg/5 ml	**Arthritis:** 250–550 mg/day **P:** 250 mg q6–8h **JA:** 10 mg/kg/day **GA:** 750 mg once, then 250 mg q8h	Tinnitus, fluid retention, shortness of breath, dizziness, drowsiness, headaches, abdominal pain, constipation, heartburn, nausea
Oxaprozin (p. 877) (Daypro)	**C:** 600 mg	**Arthritis:** 600–1,800 mg/day	Constipation, diarrhea, nausea, indigestion
Piroxicam (p. 938) @ (Feldene)	**C:** 10 mg, 20 mg	**Arthritis:** 20 mg/day	Abdominal pain, stomach pain, nausea
Sulindac (p. 1086) (Clinoril)	**T:** 150 mg, 200 mg	**Arthritis:** 300 mg/day **GA:** 400 mg/day	Dizziness, abdominal pain, constipation, diarrhea, nausea
Tolmetin @ (Tolectin)	**T:** 200 mg, 600 mg **C:** 400 mg	**Arthritis:** 600–1,800 mg/day **JA:** 15–30 mg/kg/day	Fluid retention, dizziness, headaches, weakness, abdominal pain, diarrhea, indigestion, nausea, vomiting

A, Adults; *C,* capsules; *C (dosage),* children; *CR,* controlled-release; *ER,* extended-release; *FAP,* familial adenomatous polyposis; *GA,* gouty arthritis; *I,* injection; *JA,* juvenile arthritis; *JRA,* juvenile rheumatoid arthritis; *MI,* myocardial infarction; *OA,* osteoarthritis; *P,* pain; *RA,* rheumatoid arthritis; *RF,* rheumatic fever; *S,* suspension; *T,* tablets; *TIA,* transient ischemic attack.

Nutrition: Enteral

Enteral nutrition (EN), also known as *tube feedings*, provides food/nutrients via the GI tract using special formulas, delivery techniques, and equipment. All routes of EN consist of a tube through which liquid formula is infused.

INDICATIONS

Tube feedings are used in patients with major trauma, burns; those undergoing radiation and/or chemotherapy; patients with hepatic failure, severe renal impairment, physical or neurologic impairment; preop and postop to promote anabolism; prevention of cachexia, malnutrition.

ROUTES OF ENTERAL NUTRITION DELIVERY

Nasogastric (NG):
INDICATIONS: Most common for short-term feeding in patients unable or unwilling to consume adequate nutrition by mouth. Requires at least a partially functioning GI tract.
ADVANTAGES: Does not require surgical intervention and is fairly easily inserted. Allows full use of digestive tract. Decreases abdominal distention, nausea, vomiting that may be caused by hyperosmolar solutions.
DISADVANTAGES: Temporary. May be easily pulled out during routine nursing care. Has potential for pulmonary aspiration of gastric contents, risk of refluxesophagitis, regurgitation.
Nasoduodenal (ND), Nasojejunal (NJ):
INDICATIONS: Patients unable or unwilling to consume adequate nutrition by mouth. Requires atleast a partially functioning GI tract.
ADVANTAGES: Does not require surgical intervention and is fairly easily inserted. Preferred for patients at risk of aspiration. Valuable for patients with gastroparesis.

ROUTES OF ENTERAL NUTRITION DELIVERY *(cont.)*

DISADVANTAGES: Temporary. May be pulled out during routine nursing care. May be dislodged by coughing, vomiting. Small lumen size increases risk of clogging when medication is administered via tube, more susceptible to rupturing when using infusion device. Must be radiographed for placement, frequently extubated.

GASTROSTOMY:

INDICATIONS: Patients with esophageal obstruction or impaired swallowing; patients in whom NG, ND, or NJ not feasible; when long-term feeding indicated.

ADVANTAGES: Permanent feeding access. Tubing has larger bore, allowing noncontinuous (bolus) feeding (300–400 ml over 30–60 min q3–6h). May be inserted endoscopically using local anesthetic (procedure called *percutaneous endoscopic gastrostomy* [PEG]).

DISADVANTAGES: Requires surgery; may be inserted in conjunction with other surgery or endoscopically (see **ADVANTAGES**). Stoma care required. Tube may be inadvertently dislodged. Risk of aspiration, peritonitis, cellulitis, leakage of gastric contents.

JEJUNOSTOMY:

INDICATIONS: Patients with stomach or duodenal obstruction, impaired gastric motility; patients in whom NG, ND, or NJ not feasible; when long-term feeding indicated.

ADVANTAGES: Allows early postop feeding (small bowel function is least affected by surgery). Risk of aspiration reduced. Rarely pulled out inadvertently.

DISADVANTAGES: Requires surgery (laparotomy). Stoma care required. Risk of intraperitoneal leakage. Can be dislodged easily.

INITIATING ENTERAL NUTRITION

With continuous feeding, initiation of isotonic (about 300 mOsm/L) or moderately hypertonic feeding (up to 495 mOsm/L) can be given full strength, usually at a slow rate (30–50 ml/hr) and gradually increased (25 ml/hr q6–24h). Formulas with osmolality greater than 500 mOsm/L are generally started at half strength and gradually increased in rate, then concentration. Tolerance is increased if the rate and concentration are not increased simultaneously.

Nutrition: Enteral *(continued)*

SELECTION OF FORMULAS

Protein: Has many important physiologic roles and is the primary source of nitrogen in the body. Provides 4 kcal/g protein. Sources of protein in enteral feedings: sodium caseinate, calcium caseinate, soy protein, dipeptides.

Carbohydrate (CHO): Provides energy for the body and heat to maintain body temperature. Provides 3.4 kcal/g carbohydrate. Sources of CHO in enteral feedings: corn syrup, cornstarch, maltodextrin, lactose, sucrose, glucose.

Fat: Provides concentrated source of energy. Referred to as *kilocalorie dense* or *protein sparing*. Provides 9 kcal/g fat. Sources of fat in enteral feedings: corn oil, safflower oil, medium-chain triglycerides.

Electrolytes, vitamins, trace elements: Contained in formulas (not found in specialized products for renal/hepatic insufficiency). All products containing protein, fat, carbohydrate, vitamin, electrolytes, trace elements are nutritionally complete and designed to be used by patients for long periods.

COMPLICATIONS

MECHANICAL: Usually associated with some aspect of the feeding tube.

Aspiration pneumonia: Caused by delayed gastric emptying, gastroparesis, gastroesophageal reflux, or decreased gag reflex. May be prevented or treated by reducing infusion rate, using lower fat formula, feeding beyond pylorus, checking residuals, using small-bore feeding tubes, elevating head of bed 30°–45° during and for 30–60 min after intermittent feeding, and regularly checking tube placement.

Esophageal, mucosal, pharyngeal irritation, otitis: Caused by using large-bore NG tube. Prevented by use of small bore whenever possible.

Irritation, leakage at ostomy site: Caused by drainage of digestive juices from site. Prevented by close attention to skin/stoma care.

Tube, lumen obstruction: Caused by thickened formula residue, formation of formula-medication complexes. Prevented by frequently irrigating tube with clear water (also before and after giving formulas/medication), avoiding instilling medication if possible.

GASTROINTESTINAL: Usually associated with formula, rate of delivery, unsanitary handling of solutions or delivery system.

Diarrhea: Caused by low-residue formulas, rapid delivery, use of hyperosmolar formula, hypoalbuminemia, malabsorption, microbial contamination, or rapid GI transit time. Prevented by using fiber supplemented formulas, decreasing rate of delivery, using dilute formula and gradually increasing strength.

Cramps, gas, abdominal distention: Caused by nutrient malabsorption, rapid delivery of refrigerated formula. Prevented by delivering formula by continuous methods, giving formulas at room temperature, decreasing rate of delivery.

Nausea, vomiting: Caused by rapid delivery of formula, gastric retention. Prevented by reducing rate of delivery, using dilute formulas, selecting low-fat formulas.

COMPONENTS OF PN *(cont.)*

Electrolytes: Major electrolytes (calcium, magnesium, potassium, sodium; also acetate, chloride, phosphate). Doses of electrolytes are individualized, based on many factors (e.g., renal/hepatic function, fluid status).

Vitamins: Essential components in maintaining metabolism and cellular function; widely used in PN.

Trace elements: Necessary in long-term PN administration. Trace elements include zinc, copper, chromium, manganese, selenium, molybdenum, iodine.

Miscellaneous: Additives include insulin, albumin, heparin, and histamine$_2$ blockers (e.g., cimetidine, ranitidine, famotidine). Other medication may be included, but compatibility for admixture should be checked on an individual basis.

ROUTE OF ADMINISTRATION

PN is administered via either peripheral or central vein.

Peripheral: Usually involves 2–3 L/day of 5%–10% dextrose with 3%–5% amino acid solution along with IV fat emulsion. Electrolytes, vitamins, trace elements are added according to patient needs. Peripheral solutions provide about 2,000 kcal/day and 60–90 g protein/day.

ADVANTAGES: Lower risks vs. central mode of administration.

DISADVANTAGES: Peripheral veins may not be suitable (especially in patients with illness of long duration): more susceptible to phlebitis (due to osmolalities over 600 mOsm/L); veins may be viable only 1–2 wk; large volumes of fluid are needed to meet nutritional requirements, which may be contraindicated in many patients.

Central: Usually utilizes hypertonic dextrose (concentration range of 15%–35%) and amino acid solution of 3%–7% with IV fat emulsion. Electrolytes, vitamins, trace elements are added according to patient needs. Central solutions provide 2,000–4,000 kcal/day. Must be given through large central vein with high blood flow, allowing rapid dilution, avoiding phlebitis/thrombosis (usually through per-cutaneous insertion of catheter into subclavian vein then advancement of catheter to superior vena cava).

ADVANTAGES: Allows more alternatives/flexibility in establishing regimens; allows ability to provide full nutritional requirements without need of daily fat emulsion; useful in patients who are fluid restricted (increased concentration), those needing large nutritional requirements (e.g., trauma, malignancy), or those for whom PN indicated more than 7–10 days.

DISADVANTAGES: Risk with insertion, use, maintenance of central line; increased risk of infection, catheter-induced trauma, and metabolic changes.

Nutrition: Parental (continued)

MONITORING

May vary slightly from institution to institution.

Baseline: CBC, platelet count, prothrombin time, weight, body length/head circumference (in infants), serum electrolytes, glucose, BUN, creatinine, uric acid, total protein, cholesterol, triglycerides, bilirubin, alkaline phosphatase, LDH, AST, albumin, other tests as needed.

Daily: Weight, vital signs (TPR), nutritional intake (kcal, protein, fat), serum electrolytes (potassium, sodium chloride), glucose (serum, urine), acetone, BUN, osmolarity, other tests as needed.

2-3 times/wk: CBC, coagulation studies (PT, PTT), serum creatinine, calcium, magnesium, phosphorus, acid-base status, other tests as needed.

Weekly: Nitrogen balance, total protein, albumin, prealbumin, transferrin, hepatic function tests AST, ALT), serum alkaline phosphatase, LDH, bilirubin, Hgb, uric acid, cholesterol, triglycerides, other tests as needed.

COMPLICATIONS

Mechanical: Malfunction in system for IV delivery (e.g., pump failure; problems with lines, tubing, administration sets, catheter). Pneumothorax, catheter misdirection, arterial puncture, bleeding, hematoma formation may occur with catheter placement.

Infectious: Infections (patients often more susceptible to infections), catheter sepsis (e.g., fever, shaking chills, glucose intolerance where no other site of infection is identified).

Metabolic: Includes hyperglycemia, elevated cholesterol and triglycerides, abnormal serum hepatic function tests.

Fluid, electrolyte, acid-base disturbances: May alter serum potassium, sodium, phosphate, magnesium levels.

Nutritional: Clinical effects seen may be due to lack of adequate vitamins, trace elements, essential fatty acids.

DRUG THERAPY/ADMINISTRATION METHODS:

Compatibility of other intravenous medications patients may be administered while receiving parenteral nutrition is an important concern.

Intravenous medications usually are given as a separate admixture via piggyback to the parenteral nutrition line, but in some instances may be added directly to the parenteral nutrition solution. Because of the possibility of incompatibility when adding medication directly to the parenteral nutrition solution, specific criteria should be considered:

- Stability of the medication in the parenteral nutrition solution
- Properties of the medication, including pharmacokinetics that determine if the medication is appropriate for continuous infusion
- Documented chemical and physical compatibility with the parenteral nutrition solution

In addition, when medication is given via piggyback using the parenteral nutrition line, important criteria should include:

- Stability of the medication in the parenteral nutrition solution
- Documented chemical and physical compatibility with the parenteral nutrition solution

Obesity Management

USES

Adjunct to diet and physical activity in the treatment of chronic, relapsing obesity.

ACTIONS

Two categories of medications are used for weight control.

Appetite suppressants: Stimulate the central nervous system to decrease cause a feeling of fullness or satiety.

Digestion inhibitors: Reversible lipase inhibitors that block the breakdown and absorption of dietary fats, reappetite and ducing calorie intake.

ANOREXIANTS

Name	Type	Availability	Dosage	Side Effects
Benzphetamine (Didrex)	AS	**T:** 50 mg	25–50 mg 1–3 times/day	Headaches, insomnia, nervousness, anxiety, irritability, dry mouth, constipation, euphoria, palpitations, hypertension
Diethylpropion (Tenuate)	AS	**T:** 25 mg, 75 mg	25 mg 3 times/day or 75 mg once/day	Headaches, insomnia, nervousness, anxiety, irritability, dry mouth, constipation, euphoria, palpitations, hypertension
Mazindol (Sanorex)	AS	**T:** 1 mg, 2 mg	1–3 mg/day with meals	Palpitations, restlessness, dizziness, headaches, depression, weakness, abdominal pain
Orlistat (p. 873) (Xenical)	DI	**C:** 120 mg	120 mg 3 times/day before meals	Flatulence, rectal incontinence, oily stools

(continued)

ANOREXIANTS (continued)

Name	Type	Availability	Dosage	Side Effects
Phendimetrazine (Bontril)	AS	**C:** 105 mg **T:** 35 mg	17.5–70 mg 2–3 times/day or 105 mg once/day	Headaches, insomnia, nervousness, anxiety, irritability, dry mouth, constipation, euphoria, palpitations, hypertension
Phenmetrazine (Preludin)	AS	**T:** 75 mg	75 mg once/day	Palpitations, hypertension, nervousness, headaches, dizziness, dry mouth, euphoria, constipation
Phenteramine (Ionamin)	AS	**C:** 15 mg, 30 mg, 37.5 mg	15–37.5 mg once/day	Headaches, insomnia, nervousness, anxiety, irritability, dry mouth, constipation, euphoria, palpitations, hypertension
Sibutramine (Meridia)	AS	**C:** 5 mg, 10 mg, 15 mg	Initially, 10 mg/day, then increase to 15 mg/day or decrease to 5 mg/day	Hypertension, increased heart rate, headaches, dry mouth, loss of appetite, insomnia, constipation

AS, Appetite suppressant; *C,* capsules; *DI,* digestion inhibitor; *T,* tablets.

Opioid Analgesics

USES

Relief of moderate to severe pain associated with surgical procedures, MI, burns, cancer, or other conditions. May be used as an adjunct to anesthesia, either as a preop medication or intraoperatively as a supplement to anesthesia. Also used for obstetric analgesia. Codeine and hydrocodone have an antitussive effect. Opium tinctures, such as paregoric, are used for severe diarrhea. Methadone relieves severe pain but is used primarily as part of heroin detoxification.

ACTION

Opioids refer to all drugs having actions similar to morphine and to receptors combining with these agents. Major effects are on the CNS (produce analgesia, drowsiness, mood changes, impaired concentration, analgesia without loss of consciousness, nausea and vomiting) and GI tract (decrease HCl secretion; diminish biliary, pancreatic, and intestinal secretions; diminish propulsive peristalsis). Also affects respiration (depressed) and cardiovascular system (peripheral vasodilation, decrease peripheral resistance, inhibit baroreceptor reflexes).

OPIOID ANALGESICS

Names	Equianalgesic Dose	Onset (min)	Peak (min)	Duration (hours)	Dosage Range
			Analgesic Effect		
Butorphanol (p. 167) (Stadol)	**IM:** 2 mg **IV:** —	**IM:** 10–30 **IV:** 2–3	**IM:** 30–60 **IV:** 30	**IM:** 3–4 **IV:** 2–4	**IM:** 1–4 mg q3–4h **IV:** 0.5–2 mg q3–4h
Codeine (p. 281)	**IM:** 15–30 mg **PO:** 15–30 mg	**IM:** 10–30 **PO:** 30–45	**IM:** 30–60 **PO:** 60–120	**IM/PO:** 4–6	**IM/PO (A):** 15–60 mg q4–6h; **(C):** 0.5 mg/kg q4–6h

(continued)

Opioid Analgesics	*(continued)*				
Names	Equianalgesic Dose	Onset (min)	Peak (min)	Duration (hours)	Dosage Range
Fentanyl (p. 471) (Sublimaze)	**IM:** 0.1–0.2 mg **IV:** —	**IM:** 7–15 **IV:** 1–2	**IM:** 20–30 **IV:** 3–5	**IM:** 1–2 **IV:** 0.5–1	**IM:** 50–100 mcg q1–2h
Hydrocodone (p. 579)	**PO:** 5–10 mg	10–30	30–60	4–6	5–10 mg q4–6h
Hydromorphone (p. 584) (Dilaudid)	**PO:** 7.5 mg **IM:** 1.5 mg	**PO:** 0–30 **IM:** 15 **IV:** 10–15	**PO:** 90–120 **IM:** 30–60 **IV:** 15–30	**PO:** 4–5 **IM:** 4–5 **IV:** 4	**PO:** 1–4 mg q3–6h **IM:** 1–4 mg q3–6h **IV:** 0.5–1 mg q3h **R:** 3 mg q4–8h
Levorphanol (Levo-Dromoran)	**PO:** 4 mg **IM:** 2 mg	**PO:** 10–60 **IM:** —	**PO:** 90–120 **IM:** 60	4–5	**PO:** 2–4 mg q4h **IM:** 2–3 mg q4h
Meperidine (p. 734) (Demerol)	**PO:** 300 mg **IM:** 75 mg **IV:** —	**PO:** 15 **IM:** 10–15 **IV:** 1	**PO:** 60–90 **IM:** 30–60 **IV:** 5–7	2–4	**PO, IM (A):** 50–150 mg q3–4h; **(C):** 1–1.8 mg/kg q3–4h
Methadone (p. 746) (Dolophine)	**PO:** 10–20 mg **IM:** 10 mg	**PO:** 30–60 **IM:** 10–20 **IV:** —	**PO:** 90–120 **IM:** 60–120 **IV:** 15–30	**PO:** 4–6 **IM:** 4–5 **IV:** 3–4	**IM, PO:** 2.5–10 mg q3–4h
Morphine (p. 794) (Roxanol, MS Contin)	**PO:** 30 mg **IM:** 10 mg **IV:** —	**PO:** 30–60 **IM:** 10–30 **IV:** —	**PO:** 90 **IM:** 30–60 **IV:** 20	**PO:** 4 **IM/IV:** 4–5	**PO:** 10–30 mg q4h **IM:** 5–20 mg q4h **IV:** 0.05–0.1 mg/kg q4h
Nalbuphine (p. 811) (Nubain)	**IM:** 10 mg **IV:** —	**IM:** 2–15 **IV:** 2–3	**IM:** 60 **IV:** 30	**IM:** 3–6 **IV:** 3–4	**IM/IV:** 10–20 mg q3–6h
Oxycodone (p. 883) (Roxicodone)	**PO:** 20–30 mg	30	60	3–4	5–15 mg or 5 ml q4–6h **(ER):** q12h (dose titrated)
Propoxyphene (p. 978) (Darvon)	**PO:** 65 mg	15–60	60–120	4–6	**PO:** 100 mg q4–6h

Oral Contraceptives

ACTION

Combination oral contraceptives decrease fertility primarily by inhibition of ovulation. In addition, they can promote thickening of the cervical mucus, thereby creating a physical barrier for the passage of sperm. Also, they can modify the endometrium, making it less favorable for nidation.

CLASSIFICATION

Oral contraceptives either contain both an estrogen and a progestin (combination oral contraceptives) or contain only a progestin (progestin-only oral contraceptives). The combination oral contraceptives have four subgroups:

Monophasic: Daily estrogen and progestin dosage remains constant.

Biphasic: Estrogen remains constant, but the progestin dosage increases during the second half of the cycle.
Triphasic: Progestin changes for each phase of the cycle.
Estrophasic: Progestin remains constant, and the estrogen dose gradually increases through the monthly cycle.

ORAL CONTRACEPTIVES

Brand Names	Estrogen (mcg)	Progestin (mg)	Brand Names	Estrogen (mcg)	Progestin (mg)
Monophasic			**Monophasic**		
Genora 1/50	50 mestranol	1 norethindrone	**NuvaRing**	2.7 ethinyl estradiol	11.7 etonogestrel
Nelova 1/50M			**Modicon**		
Norethin 1/50M			**Nelova 0.5/35E**		
Norinyl 1+50			**Ovcon-35**	35 ethinyl estradiol	0.4 norethindrone
Ortho-Novum 1/50			**Ortho-Cyclen**	35 ethinyl estradiol	0.25 norgestimate
Ovcon-50	50 ethinyl estradiol	1 norethindrone	**Demulen 1/35**	35 ethinyl estradiol	1 ethynodiol diacetate
Demulen 1/50	50 ethinyl estradiol	1 ethynodiol diacetate	**Loestrin 21 1.5/30**	30 ethinyl estradiol	1.5 norethindrone acetate
Ovral	50 ethinyl estradiol	0.5 norgestrel	**Loestrin Fe 1.5/30**		
Genora 1/35	35 ethinyl estradiol	1 norethindrone	**Lo/Ovral**	30 ethinyl estradiol	0.3 norgestrel
Nelova 1/35E			**Desogen**	30 ethinyl estradiol	0.15 desogestrel
Norethin 1/35E			**Ortho-Cept**		
Norinyl 1+35			**Levlen**	30 ethinyl estradiol	0.15 levonorgestrel
Ortho-Novum 1/35			**Levora**		
Brevicon	35 ethinyl estradiol	0.5 norethindrone	**Nordette**		
Genora 0.5/35			**Yasmin**	30 ethinyl estradiol	3 drospirenone
Ortho Evra	0.02 ethinyl estradiol	0.15 norelgestromin	**Loestrin 21 1/20**	20 ethinyl estradiol	1 norethindrone acetate

	Phase 1	Phase 2	Phase 3
Biphasic			
Jenest-28	0.5 mg norethindrone 35 mcg ethinyl estradiol	1 mg norethindrone 35 mcg ethinyl estradiol	
Nelova 10/11	0.5 mg norethindrone 35 mcg ethinyl estradiol	1 mg norethindrone 35 mcg ethinyl estradiol	
Ortho-Novum 10/11	0.5 mg norethindrone 35 mcg ethinyl estradiol	1 mg norethindrone 35 mcg ethinyl estradiol	
Triphasic			
Ortho-Novum 7/7/7	0.5 mg norethindrone 35 mcg ethinyl estradiol	0.75 mg norethindrone 35 mcg ethinyl estradiol	1 mg norethindrone 35 mcg ethinyl estradiol
	Phase 1	Phase 2	Phase 3
Ortho Tri-Cyclen	0.18 mg norgestimate 35 mcg ethinyl estradiol	0.215 mg norgestimate 35 mcg ethinyl estradiol	0.25 mg norgestimate 35 mcg ethinyl estradiol
Tri-Levlen Triphasil	0.05 mg levonorgestrel 30 mcg ethinyl estradiol	0.075 mg levonorgestrel 40 mcg ethinyl estradiol	0.125 mg levonorgestrel 30 mcg ethinyl estradiol
Tri-Norinyl	0.5 mg norethindrone 35 mcg ethinyl estradiol	1 mg norethindrone 35 mcg ethinyl estradiol	0.5 mg norethindrone 35 mcg ethinyl estradiol
Estrophasic			
Estrostep	1 mg norethindrone 20 mcg ethinyl estradiol	1 mg norethindrone 30 mcg ethinyl estradiol	1 mg norethindrone 35 mcg ethinyl estradiol
Progestin only			
Micronor Nor Q D Ovrette	0.35 mg norethindrone 0.075 mg norgestrel		

NEW CONTRACEPTIVE OPTIONS

Name	Ingredients	Cycle Duration
Oral Contraceptive		
Micrette, Kariva	20 mcg ethinyl estradiol 0.15 mg desogestrel 10 mcg placebo, ethinyl estradiol	28-day cycle (21 days active, 2 days placebo, 5 days ethinyl estradiol 10 mcg)
Nortrel 7/7/7	35 mcg ethinyl estradiol norethindrone 0.5 mg (7 days), 0.75 mg (7 days), 1 mg (7 days), 7 days placebo	28-day cycle (21 days active, 7 days placebo)
Ortho Tri-Cyclen Lo	25 mcg ethinyl estradiol 180 mcg norgestimate (7 days), 215 mcg (7 days), 250 mcg (7 days), 7 days placebo	28-day cycle (21 days active, 7 days placebo)
Yasmin 28	30 mcg ethinyl estradiol 3 mg drospirenone	28-day cycle (21 days active, 7 days placebo)
Extended Contraceptive Regimen		
Seasonale	30 mcg ethinyl estradiol 150 mcg levonorgestrel	91-day cycle (84 days active, 7 days placebo)
Intrauterine System		
Mirena	52 mg levonorgestrel; total releasing 20 mcg/day	Device inserted into uterus once every 5 yr
Vaginal Ring		
Nuva-Ring	15 mcg ethinyl estradiol 120 mcg/day etonorgestrel	28-day cycle; self-inserted vaginal ring releasing active for 21 days
Transdermal Patch		
Ortho-Evra	20 mcg ethinyl estradiol 150 mcg norelgestromin released per day	28-day cycle patch applied once/wk for 3 wk in the 4-wk cycle
Injectable		
Lunelle	5 mg ethinyl cypionate 25 mg medroxyprogesterone	28-day cycle administered IM once q28days

Parkinson's Disease Treatment

USES	ACTION
To slow or stop clinical progression of Parkinson's disease and to improve patient function and quality of life in those with Parkinson's disease, a progressive neurodegenerative disorder.	Normal motor function is dependent on the synthesis and release of dopamine by neurons projecting from the substantia nigra to the corpus striatum. In Parkinson's disease, there is disruption of this pathway resulting in diminished levels of the neurotransmitter dopamine. Medication is aimed at providing improved function using the lowest effective dose.

TYPES OF MEDICATIONS FOR PARKINSON'S DISEASE

DOPAMINE PRECURSOR

Levodopa/carbidopa:

Levodopa: Dopamine precursor supplementation to enhance dopaminergic neurotransmission. A small amount of levodopa crosses the blood-brain barrier and is decarboxylated to dopamine which is then available to stimulate dopaminergic receptors.

Carbidopa: Inhibits peripheral decarboxylation of levodopa, decreasing its conversion to dopamine in peripheral tissues which results in an increased availability of levodopa for transport across the blood-brain barrier.

COMT INHIBITORS

Reversible inhibitor of catechol-O-methyltransferase (COMT). COMT is responsible for catalyzing levodopa. In the presence of a decarboxylase inhibitor (carbidopa), COMT becomes the major metabolizing enzyme for levodopa in the brain and periphery. By inhibiting COMT, higher plasma levels of levodopa are attained, resulting in more dopaminergic stimulation in the brain and lessening the symptoms of Parkinson's disease.

DOPAMINE RECEPTOR AGONISTS

Apomorphine: Stimulates dopamine receptors in the brain.

Bromocroptine: Stimulates postsynaptic dopamine type 2 receptors in the neostriatum of the central nervous system (CNS).

Pergolide: Directly stimulates post-synaptic dopamine receptors (at both D1 and D2 receptor sites) in the nigrostriatal system. Independent of presynaptic dopamine synthesis or stores.

Pramipexole: Stimulates dopamine receptors in the striatum of the CNS.

Ropinirole: Stimulates postsynaptic dopamine D2 type receptors within the caudate putamen in the brain.

MAO B INHIBITORS

Selegiline: Increases dopaminergic activity due to irreversible inhibition of monoamine oxidase type B (MAO B). MAO B is involved in the oxidative deamination of dopamine in the brain.

Parkinson's Disease Treatment

MEDICATIONS FOR THE TREATMENT OF PARKINSON'S DISEASE

Name	Type	Dosage	Side Effects
Apomorphine (p. 81) (Apokyn)	Dopamine agonist	2 mg, initially up to 2–6 mg given 3–5 times/day as needed	Drowsiness, increased salivation, headache, vomiting, orthostatic hypotension
Bromocriptine (p. 155) (Parlodel)	Dopamine agonist	2.5 mg 3 times/day initially up to maximum of 90 mg/day divided into 2 or 3 doses/day	Hypotension, nausea, livedo reticularis, edema, confusion, hallucinations
Carbidopa/levodopa (p. 184) (Sinemet)	Dopamine precursor	25/100 mg 3 times/day initially up to 200/2,000 mg divided into 3–6 doses/day	Hypotension, nausea, confusion, dyskinesia
Entacapone (p. 413) (Comtan)	COMT inhibitor	200 mg with each dose of levodopa (maximum 8 tablets or 1,600 mg/day)	Urine discoloration (benign), diarrhea
Pergolide (p. 917) (Permax)	Dopamine agonist	0.05–0.25 mg 3 times/day initially up to 0.75–5 mg/day	Hypotension, nausea, livedo reticularis, edema, confusion, hallucinations
Pramipexole (p. 948) (Mirapex)	Dopamine agonist	0.125 mg 3 times/day initially up to 1.5–4.5 mg/day in divided doses	Nausea, hypotension, sedation, hallucinations
Ropinirole (p. 1034) (Requip)	Dopamine agonist	0.25 mg 3 times/day up to 9–24 mg/day in 3 divided doses	Nausea, hypotension, sedation, hallucinations
Selegiline (p. 1047) (Eldepryl)	MAO B inhibitor	10 mg/day (5 mg at breakfast and lunch)	Nausea, dizziness, faintness, abdominal discomfort
Tolcapone (Tasmar)	COMT inhibitor	100 mg 3 times/day up to 200 mg 3 times/day	Urine discoloration (benign), diarrhea, liver toxicity (liver monitoring required)

Proton Pump Inhibitors

USES

Treatment of various gastric disorders, including gastric and duodenal ulcers, GERD, pathologic hypersecretory conditions.

ACTION

Suppress gastric acid secretion by specific inhibition of the hydrogen-potassium-adenosine triphosphatase (H^+/K^+ ATPase) enzyme system, which transports the acid at the gastric parietal cells. These agents do not have anticholinergic or histamine receptor antagonistic properties.

PROTON PUMP INHIBITORS

Name	Availability	Indications	Usual Dosage	Side Effects
Esomeprazole (p. 440) (Nexium)	C: 20 mg, 40 mg I: 20 mg	H. pylori eradication, gastroesophageal reflux disease (GERD), erosive esophagitis	20–40 mg/day	Headaches, diarrhea, abdominal pain, nausea
Lansoprazole (p. 668) (Prevacid)	C: 15 mg, 30 mg I: 30 mg	Duodenal ulcer, gastric ulcer, NSAID-associated gastric ulcer, hypersecretory conditions, H. pylori eradication, gastroesophageal reflux disease (GERD), erosive esophagitis	15–30 mg/day	Diarrhea, skin rash, itching, headaches
Omeprazole (p. 868) (Prilosec)	C: 10 mg, 20 mg, 40 mg	Duodenal ulcer, gastric ulcer, hypersecretory conditions, H. pylori eradication, gastroesophageal reflux disease (GERD), erosive esophagitis	20–40 mg/day	Headaches, diarrhea, abdominal pain, nausea
Pantoprazole (p. 895) (Protonix)	T: 20 mg, 40 mg I: 40 mg	Erosive esophagitis, hypersecretory conditions	40 mg/day	Diarrhea, headaches

| Rabeprazole (p. 1002) (Aciphex) | **T:** 20 mg | Duodenal ulcer, hypersecretory conditions, *H. pylori* eradication, gastroesophageal reflux disease (GERD), erosive esophagitis | 20 mg/day | Headaches |

C, Capsules; *I,* Injection; *T,* tablets.

Sedative-Hypnotics

USES

Treatment of insomnia, e.g., difficulty falling asleep initially, frequent awakening, awakening too early.

ACTION

Benzodiazepines are the most widely used agents and largely replace barbiturates due to greater safety, lower incidence of drug dependence. Benzodiazepines nonselectively bind to at least three receptor subtypes accounting for sedative, anxiolytic, relaxant, and anticonvulsant properties. Benzodiazepines enhance the effect of the inhibitory neuro-transmitter gamma-aminobutyric acid (GABA), which inhibits impulse transmission in the CNS reticular formation in brain. Benzodiazepines decrease sleep latency, number of nocturnal awakenings, and time spent in awake stage of sleep; increase total sleep time. The *nonbenzodiazepines* zaleplon and zolpidem preferentially bind with one receptor subtype, reducing sleep latency and nocturnal awakenings and increasing total sleep time.

HYPNOTICS/SEDATIVES

Name	Availability	Dosage Range	Side Effects
Benzodiazepines			
Estazolam (ProSom)	**T:** 1 mg, 2 mg	**A:** 1–2 mg **E:** 0.5–1 mg	Daytime sedation, memory and psychomotor impairment, tolerance, withdrawal reactions, rebound insomnia, dependence

(continued)

HYPNOTICS/SEDATIVES *(continued)*

Name	Availability	Dosage Range	Side Effects
Benzodiazepines			
Eszopiclone (p. 447) (Lunesta)	**T:** 1 mg, 2 mg, 3 mg	**A:** 2–3 mg **E:** 1–2 mg	Headaches, unpleasant taste, dry mouth, dizziness, nervousness, nausea
Flurazepam (p. 499) (Dalmane)	**C:** 15 mg, 30 mg	**A/E:** 15–30 mg	Same as above
Quazepam (Doral)	**T:** 7.5 mg, 15 mg	**A:** 7.5–15 mg **E:** 7.5 mg	Same as above
Ramelteon (p. 1004) (Rozerem)	**T:** 8 mg	**A:** 8 mg	Headaches, dizziness, fatigue, diarrhea, upper respiratory tract infection.
Temazepam (p. 1102) (Restoril)	**C:** 7.5 mg, 15 mg, 30 mg	**A:** 15–30 mg **E:** 7.5–15 mg	Same as above
Triazolam (p. 1175) (Halcion)	**T:** 0.125 mg, 0.25 mg	**A:** 0.125–0.25 mg **E:** 0.125 mg	Same as above
Nonbenzodiazepines			
Zaleplon (p. 1227) (Sonata)	**C:** 5 mg, 10 mg	**A:** 5–10 mg **E:** 5 mg	Headaches, dizziness, myalgia, somnolence, asthenia, abdominal pain
Zolpidem (p. 1236) (Ambien)	**T:** 5 mg, 10 mg	**A:** 10 mg **E:** 5 mg	Dizziness, daytime drowsiness, headaches, confusion, depression, hangover, asthenia

A, Adults; *C,* capsules; *E,* elderly; *T,* tablets.

Skeletal Muscle Relaxants

USES

Central acting muscle relaxants: Adjunct to rest, physical therapy for relief of discomfort associated with acute, painful musculoskeletal disorders, i.e., local spasms from muscle injury.

Baclofen, dantrolene, diazepam: Treatment of spasticity characterized by heightened muscle tone, spasm, loss of dexterity caused by multiple sclerosis, cerebral palsy, spinal cord lesions, CVA.

ACTION

Central acting muscle relaxants: Exact mechanism unknown. May act in CNS at various levels to depress polysynaptic reflexes; sedative effect may be responsible for relaxation of muscle spasm.

Baclofen, diazepam: May mimic actions of gamma-aminobutyric acid on spinal neurons; does not directly affect skeletal muscles.

Dantrolene: Acts directly on skeletal muscle, relieving spasticity.

SKELETAL MUSCLE RELAXANTS

Name	Availability	Dosage Range	Side Effects
Baclofen (p. 119) (Lioresal)	**T:** 10 mg, 20 mg	**A:** 40–80 mg/day	Drowsiness, dizziness, weakness, confusion, nausea
Carisoprodol (Rela)	**T:** 350 mg	**A:** 350 mg 4 times/day	Drowsiness
Chlorzoxazone (Parafon Forte DSC)	**T:** 250 mg, 500 mg **Caplets:** 250 mg, 500 mg	**A:** 250–750 mg 3–4 times/day **C:** 125–500 mg 3–4 times/day	Drowsiness, dizziness
Cyclobenzaprine (p. 297) (Flexeril)	**T:** 10 mg	**A:** 10 mg 3 times/day	Drowsiness, dizziness, dry mouth, blurred vision
Dantrolene (p. 313) (Dantrium)	**C:** 25 mg, 50 mg, 100 mg	**A:** 25 mg/day increased slowly to 400 mg/ day or less	Drowsiness, dizziness, fatigue, diarrhea

(continued)

SKELETAL MUSCLE RELAXANTS *(continued)*

Name	Availability	Dosage Range	Side Effects
Diazepam (p. 345) (Valium)	**T:** 2 mg, 5 mg, 10 mg	**A:** 2–10 mg 3–4 times/day **E:** 2–2.5 mg initially **C:** 1–2.5 mg 3–4 times/day	Ataxia, dizziness, drowsiness, slurred speech
Methocarbamol (Robaxin)	**T:** 500 mg, 750 mg	**A:** 500–1,000 mg 4 times/day	Altered vision, drowsiness, dizziness
Orphenadrine (Norflex)	**T:** 100 mg	**A:** 100 mg 2 times/day	Drowsiness
Tizanidine (p. 1143) (Zanaflex)	**T:** 2 mg, 4 mg	**A:** 4–8 mg/dose; 24–36 mg/day	Drowsiness, dizziness, weakness, dry mouth, heartburn

A, Adults; *C,* capsules; *C (dosage),* children; *E,* elderly; *T,* tablets.

Smoking Cessation Agents

Tobacco smoking is associated with the development of lung cancer and chronic obstructive pulmonary disease (COPD). Smoking is not just harmful to the smoker but also family members, coworkers and others breathing cigarette smoke.

Quitting smoking decreases the risk of developing lung cancer, other cancers, heart disease, stroke and respiratory illnesses. Several medications have proven useful as smoking cessation aids. Nausea and lightheadedness are possible signs of overdose of nicotine warranting a reduction in dosage.

Name	Brand	Availability	Dosage	Comments
Nicotine gum (p. 833)	Nicorette	2 mg/square, 4 mg/square	1 piece when urge to smoke up to 30 pieces/day. **Usual:** 10–12 pieces/day	2 mg recommended for patients smoking less than 25 cigarettes/day. 4 mg recommended for patients smoking 25 or more cigarettes/day. Chew until a peppery or minty taste emerges and then "park" between cheek and gums to facilitate nicotine absorption through oral mucosa. Chew slowly and intermittently and parked for about 30 min or taste dissipates to avoid jaw ache and achieve maximum benefit. 15 min before and during chewing only water should be taken
Nicotine patch (p. 833)	Nicoderm CQ, Nicotrol	**Nicoderm CQ:** 7 mg/24 hr, 14 mg/24 hr, 21 mg/24 hr. **Nicotrol:** 15 mg/16 hr	Continue treatment with patch for minimum of 6–8 wk.	The 16 and 24 hr patches are of comparable efficacy. Begin with a lower patch dose in patients smoking 10 or fewer cigarettes/day. Place new patch on a relatively hair-free location, usually between the neck and waist, in the morning. If insomnia occurs, remove the 24 hr patch prior to bedtime or use the 16 hr patch. May cause localized erythema, pruritus, rash or urticaria Rotate patch site to diminish skin irritation.

(continued)

Name	Brand	Availability	Dosage	Comments
Nicotine lozenge (p. 833)	Commit	2 mg, 4 mg	**Wk 1-6:** 1 q1-2h **Wk 7-9:** 1 q2-4h **Wk 10-12:** 1 q4-8h	Use at least 9 lozenges/day first 6 wk. Only 1 lozenge at a time, 5 per 6 hr and 20 per 24 hr. Do not chew or swallow.
Nicotine nasal spray (p. 833)	Nicotrol NS	10 mg/ml delivers 0.5 mg/spray	A dose consists of one 0.5 mg delivery to each nostril. Initial dose is 1-2 sprays per hr, increasing as needed. **Minimum:** 8 doses/day **Maximum:** 40 doses/day	Usual duration is 3-6 mo. Do not sniff, swallow or inhale through the nose while administering nicotine doses (may increase irritating effect). Tilt head back slightly for best results.
Bupropion (p. 161)	Zyban	150 mg tablets	150 mg once daily for 3 days then 150 mg 2 times/day for 7-12 wk or longer with or without nicotine replacement	Contraindicated in patients with a seizure disorder, current or prior diagnosis of bulimia or anorexia nervosa, use of a monoamine oxidase (MAO) inhibitor within previous 14 days, or taking another medication containing bupropion. Most common side effects are insomnia, dry mouth, tremor, rash. Stop smoking during the second week of treatment and use counseling/support services along with the medication.
Clonidine (p. 272)	Catapres	**Tablets:** 0.1mg, 0.2 mg **Patch:** 0.1 mg/24 hr, 0.2 mg/24 hr, 0.3 mg/24 hr	Dosage varied from 0.1-0.75 mg/day and duration from 3-10 wk.	Abrupt discontinuation can result in nervousness, agitation, headache, tremor accompanied or followed by rapid rise in blood pressure. Most common side effects include dry mouth, drowsiness, dizziness, sedation and constipation.

Nortriptyline (p. 852)	Pamelor	**Tablets:** 25 mg, 50 mg, 75 mg, 100 mg	Initially 25 mg/day, increasing gradually to target dose of 75–100 mg/day. Duration up to 12 wk.	Therapy initiated 10–28 days before the quit date to allow steady state of nortriptyline at target dose. Most common side effects include sedation, dry mouth, blurred vision, urinary retention, lightheadedness, shaky hands.

Sympathomimetics

USES

Stimulation of alpha₁ receptors: Induce vasoconstriction primarily in skin and mucous membranes nasal decongestion; combine with local anesthetics to delay anesthetic absorption; increases BP in certain hypotensive states; produce mydriasis, facilitating eye exams, ocular surgery.
Stimulation of beta₁-receptors: Treatment of cardiac arrest, heart failure, shock, AV block.
Stimulation of beta₂-receptors: Treatment of asthma.
Stimulation of dopamine receptors: Treatment of shock.

ACTION

The sympathetic nervous system (SNS) is involved in maintaining homeostasis (involved in regulation of heart rate, force of cardiac contractions, BP, bronchial airway tone, carbohydrate, fatty acid meters (primarily norepinephrine, epinephrine, and dopamine), which act on adrenergic receptors. These receptors include beta₁, beta₂, alpha₁, alpha₂, and dopaminergic. Sympathomimetics differ widely in their actions based on their specificity to affect these receptors.

- *Alpha₁:* Causes mydriasis, constriction of arterioles, veins.
- *Alpha₂:* Inhibits transmitter release.
- *Beta₁:* Increases rate, force of contraction, conduction velocity of heart; releases renin from kidney.
- *Beta₂:* Dilates arterioles, bronchi; relaxes uterus.
- *Dopaminergic:* Dilates kidney vasculature.

Sympathomimetics *(continued)*

SYMPATHOMIMETICS

Name	Availability	Receptor Specificity	Uses	Dosage Range
Dobutamine (p. 373) (Dobutrex)	**I:** 12.5 mg/ml, 500 mg/ 250 ml	Beta₁, beta₂, alpha₁	Inotropic support in cardiac decompensation	**IV infusion:** 2.5–10 mcg/kg/min
Dopamine (p. 382) (Intropin)	**I:** 40 mg, 80 mg, 160-ml vials, 800 mcg/ml, 1,600 mcg/ml	Beta₁, alpha₁, dopaminergic	Vasopressor, cardiac stimulant	**Dopaminergic:** 0.5–3 mcg/kg/min **Beta 1:** 2–10 mcg/ kg/min **Alpha 1:** more than 10 mcg/kg/min
Ephedrine	**I:** 50 mg/ml	Alpha, beta₁, beta₂	Acute hypotensive states, especially with spinal anesthesia	**IV:** 5–25 mg
Epinephrine (p. 416) (Adrenalin)	**I:** 0.1 mg/ml, 1 mg/ml	Beta₁, beta₂, alpha₁	Cardiac arrest, anaphylactic shock	**Vasopressor:** 1–10 mcg/min **Cardiac arrest:** 1 mg q3–5min during resuscitation
Norepinephrine (p. 848) (Levophed)	**I:** 1 mg/ml	Beta₁, alpha₁	Vasopressor	**IV:** 0.5–1 mcg/min up to 2–12 mcg/min
Phenylephrine (p. 925) (Neo-Synephrine)	**I:** 10 mg/ml	Alpha₁	Vasopressor	**IV:** Initially, 10–180 mcg/min, then 40–60 mcg/min

I, Injection.

Thyroid

USES

Treatment of hypothyroidism, a common endocrine disorder in which the thyroid fails to release sufficient amounts of thyroid hormones.

ACTION

Thyroid hormones are necessary for proper metabolism, growth, and homeostasis. Thyroid hormone regulates energy and heat production; facilitates development of the central nervous system, growth, and puberty. Regulates the synthesis of proteins that are important in hepatic, cardiac, neurological, and muscular functions.

THYROID

Name	Availability	Dosage Average	Side Effects
Levothyroxine (p. 686) (Levoxyl, Synthroid)	**T:** 25 mcg, 50 mcg, 75 mcg, 88 mcg, 100 mcg, 112 mcg, 125 mcg, 137 mcg, 150 mcg, 175 mcg, 200 mcg, 300 mcg	75–100 mcg/day	Side effects are due to excessive amounts of medication, including diarrhea, heat intolerance, palpitations, tremors, tachycardia, vomiting, weight loss, increased BP.
Liothyronine (p. 693) @ (Cytomel)	**T:** 5 mcg, 25 mcg, 50 mcg	25–50 mcg/day	Same as above
Liotrix (Thyrolar)	**T:** ¼ grain, ½ grain, 1 grain, 2 grain, 3 grain	½–1 grain/day	Same as above
Thyroid	**T:** 15 mg, 30 mg, 60 mg, 90 mg, 120 mg, 180 mg, 240 mg, 300 mg	60–120 mg/day	Same as above

T, Tablets.

Vitamins

INTRODUCTION

Vitamins are organic substances required for growth, reproduction, and maintenance of health and are obtained from food or supplementation in small quantities (vitamins cannot be synthesized by the body or the rate of synthesis is too slow/inadequate to meet metabolic needs). Vitamins are essential for energy transformation and regulation of metabolic processes. They are catalysts for all reactions using proteins, fats, carbohydrates for energy, growth, and cell maintenance.

WATER SOLUBLE

Water-soluble vitamins include vitamin C (ascorbic acid), B_1 (thiamine), B_2 (riboflavin), B_3 (niacin), B_5 (pantothenic acid), B_6 (pyridoxine), folic acid, B_{12} (cyanocobalamin). Water-soluble vitamins act as coenzymes for almost every cellular reaction in the body. B-complex vitamins differ from one another in both structure and function but are grouped together because they first were isolated from the same source (yeast and liver).

FAT SOLUBLE

Fat-soluble vitamins include vitamins A, D, E, and K. They are soluble in lipids and are usually absorbed into the lymphatic system of the small intestine and then into the general circulation. Absorption is facilitated by bile. These vitamins are stored in the body tissue when excessive quantities are consumed. May be toxic when taken in large doses (see sections on individual vitamins).

VITAMINS

Name	Uses	RDA	Side Effects
Vitamin A (p. 1213)	Required for normal growth, bone development, vision, reproduction, maintenance of epithelial tissue	**M:** 1,000 mcg **F:** 800 mcg	**High dosages:** Hepatic toxicity, cheilitis, facial dermatitis, photosensitivity, mucosal dryness
Vitamin B₁ (p. 1120) (Thiamine)	Important in red blood cell formation, carbohydrate metabolism, neurologic function, myocardial contractility, growth, energy production	**M:** 1.5 mg **F:** 1.1 mg	**Large parenteral doses:** May cause pain on injection
Vitamin B₂ (Riboflavin)	Necessary for function of coenzymes in oxidation-reduction reactions, essential for normal cellular growth, assists in absorption of iron and pyridoxine	**M:** 1.7 mg **F:** 1.3 mg	Orange-yellow discoloration in urine

Vitamin B₃ (p. 829) (Niacin)	Coenzyme for many oxidation-reduction reactions	**M:** 19 mg **F:** 15 mg	**High dosage (over 500 mg):** Nausea, vomiting, diarrhea, gastritis, hepatic toxicity, skin rash, facial flushing, headaches
Vitamin B₅ (Pantothenic acid)	Precursor to coenzyme A, important in synthesis of cholesterol, hormones, fatty acids	**M:** 4–7 mg **F:** 4–7 mg	Occasional GI disturbances (e.g., diarrhea)
Vitamin B₆ (p. 991) (Pyridoxine)	Enzyme cofactor for amino acid metabolism, essential for erythrocyte production, Hgb synthesis	**M:** 2 mg **F:** 1.6 mg	**High dosages:** May cause sensory neuropathy
Vitamin B₁₂ (p. 295) (Cyanocobalamin)	Coenzyme in cells, including bone marrow, CNS, and GI tract, necessary for lipid metabolism, formation of myelin	**M:** 2 mcg **F:** 2 mcg	Skin rash, diarrhea, pain at injection site
Vitamin C (p. 89) (Ascorbic acid)	Cofactor in various physiologic reactions, necessary for collagen formation, acts as an antioxidant	**M:** 60 mg **F:** 60 mg (increased with smoking, pregnancy, lactation)	**High dosages:** May cause calcium oxalate crystalluria, esophagitis, diarrhea
Vitamin D (p. 1214) (Calciferol)	Necessary for proper formation of bone, calcium, mineral homeostasis, regulation of parathyroid hormone, calcitonin, phosphate	**M:** 200–400 units **F:** 200–400 units	Hypercalcemia, kidney stones, renal failure, hypertension, psychosis, diarrhea, nausea, vomiting, anorexia, fatigue, headaches, altered mental status
Vitamin E (p. 1216) (Tocopherol)	Antioxidant	**M:** 10 mg **F:** 8 mg	**High dosages:** GI disturbances, malaise, headaches

F, Females; *M,* males.

abacavir

ah-bah-**kay**-veer

(Ziagen)

FIXED-COMBINATION(S)

Epzicom: abacavir/lamivudine (antiretroviral): 600 mg/300 mg. **Trizivir:** abacavir/lamivudine (antiretroviral)/zidovudine (antiretroviral): 300 mg/150 mg/300 mg.

• CLASSIFICATION

PHARMACOTHERAPEUTIC: Antiretroviral agent. **CLINICAL:** Antiviral (see p. 60C).

ACTION

An antiretroviral that inhibits the activity of HIV-1 reverse transcriptase by competing with the natural substrate dGTP and by its incorporation into viral DNA. Therapeutic Effect: Inhibits viral DNA growth.

PHARMACOKINETICS

Rapidly and extensively absorbed after PO administration. Protein binding: 50%. Widely distributed, including to cerebrospinal fluid (CSF) and erythrocytes. Metabolized in the liver to inactive metabolites. Primarily excreted in urine. Unknown if removed by hemodialysis. Half-life: 1.5 hr.

USES

Treatment of HIV infection, in combination with other agents.

PRECAUTIONS

CONTRAINDICATIONS: Moderate or severe hepatic impairment. **CAUTIONS:** Liver disease.

⧗ LIFESPAN CONSIDERATIONS: **Pregnancy/Lactation:** Unknown if excreted in breast milk. Do not breast-feed while taking abacavir (may increase potential for HIV transmission, adverse effects).

Pregnancy Category B. **Children:** No safety issues noted in those 3 mo–13 yr. **Elderly:** No information available.

INTERACTIONS

DRUG: **Alcohol:** May increase abacavir blood concentration and half-life. HERBAL: **St. John's wort:** May decrease abacavir blood concentration and effect. FOOD: None known. LAB VALUES: May increase blood glucose and serum GGT, AST, ALT, and triglyceride levels.

AVAILABILITY (Rx)

TABLETS: 300 mg. ORAL SOLUTION: 20 mg/ml.

ADMINISTRATION/HANDLING

PO

• May give without regard to food.
• Oral solution may be refrigerated. Do not freeze.

INDICATIONS/ROUTES/DOSAGE

HIV INFECTION (IN COMBINATION WITH OTHER ANTIRETROVIRALS)

PO: ADULTS: 300 mg twice a day or 600 mg once daily. CHILDREN: (3 mo–16 yr) 8 mg/kg twice a day. **Maximum:** 300 mg twice a day.

DOSAGE IN HEPATIC IMPAIRMENT

Mild impairment: 200 mg twice a day. **Moderate to severe impairment:** Not recommended.

SIDE EFFECTS

ADULT: **FREQUENT:** Nausea (47%), nausea with vomiting (16%), diarrhea (12%), decreased appetite (11%). **OCCASIONAL:** Insomnia (7%). CHILDREN: **FREQUENT:** Nausea with vomiting (39%), fever (19%), headache, diarrhea (16%), rash (11%). **OCCASIONAL:** Decreased appetite (9%).

ADVERSE REACTIONS/ TOXIC EFFECTS

A hypersensitivity reaction may be life-threatening. Signs and symptoms include fever, rash, fatigue, intractable nausea and vomiting, severe diarrhea, abdominal pain, cough, pharyngitis, and dyspnea. Life-threatening hypotension may occur. Lactic acidosis and severe hepatomegaly may occur.

NURSING CONSIDERATIONS

BASELINE ASSESSMENT

Question for possibility of pregnancy. Obtain baseline laboratory testing, especially liver function tests, before beginning therapy and at periodic intervals during therapy. Offer emotional support.

INTERVENTION/EVALUATION

Assess for nausea, vomiting. Determine pattern of bowel activity and stool consistency. Assess eating pattern; monitor for weight loss. Monitor lab values carefully, particularly liver function.

PATIENT/FAMILY TEACHING

• Do not take any medications, including OTC drugs, without consulting physician. • Small, frequent meals may offset anorexia, nausea. • Abacavir is not a cure for HIV infection, nor does it reduce risk of transmission to others.

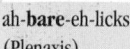

abarelix

ah-**bare**-eh-licks
(Plenaxis)

CLASSIFICATION

PHARMACOTHERAPEUTIC: Gonadotropin-releasing hormone antagonist. **CLINICAL:** Sex hormone.

ACTION

A luteinizing hormone-releasing hormone (LHRH) antagonist that inhibits gonadotropin and androgen production by blocking gonadotropin releasing-hormone (GnRH) receptors in the pituitary. **Therapeutic Effect:** Suppresses luteinizing hormone, follicle stimulating hormone secretion, reducing the secretion of testosterone by the testes.

PHARMACOKINETICS

Slowly absorbed following intramuscular administration. Distributed extensively. Protein binding: 96%–99%. **Half-life:** 13.2 days.

USES

Treatment of men with advanced symptomatic prostate cancer in whom luteinizing hormone release hormone (LHRH) agonist therapy is not appropriate, who refuse surgical castration, and have 1 or more of the following: 1) risk of neurologic compromise due to metastases, 2) ureteral or bladder outlet obstruction, or 3) severe bone pain from bone metastases.

PRECAUTIONS

CONTRAINDICATIONS: Female patients, children, pregnancy. **CAUTIONS:** Patients with prolonged QT interval, patients weighing more than 225 lb (103 kg).

LIFESPAN CONSIDERATIONS: Pregnancy/Lactation: Embryolethal. Mothers should avoid breast-feeding. **Pregnancy Category X. Children:** Not indicated for use in pediatric patients. **Elderly:** No age-related precautions noted.

INTERACTIONS

DRUG: Amiodarone, procainamide, quinidine, sotalol: May increase risk of cardiotoxicity. **HERBAL:** None known. **FOOD:** None known. **LAB VALUES:** May increase serum transaminase, serum AST, ALT, and serum triglyceride levels. May slightly decrease blood hemoglobin concentrations. May decrease bone mineral density.

AVAILABILITY (Rx)

POWDER FOR INJECTION: 113 mg kit containing 10 ml 0.9% NaCl, 18-gauge

---

needle, 22-gauge needle (provides 100 mg/2 ml when reconstituted).

ADMINISTRATION/HANDLING

IM

Reconstitution • Before reconstitution, shake vial gently. Withdraw 2.2 ml 0.9% NaCl, and inject diluent quickly. • Shake immediately for approximately 15 sec. Let vial stand for 2 min. • Tap vial to reduce foaming and swirl vial occasionally. • Shake again for approximately 15 sec. • Allow vial to stand for 2 min.

Rate of administration • Following reconstitution, administer within 1 hr. • Administer at dorsogluteal or ventrogluteal region of buttock. • Following administration, monitor patient for 30 min (cumulative risk for allergic reaction increases with each injection).

Storage • Store at room temperature.

INDICATIONS/ROUTES/DOSAGE

PROSTATE CANCER

IM: ADULTS, ELDERLY: 100 mg on days 1, 15, 29 and q4wk thereafter. Treatment failure can be detected by obtaining serum testosterone concentration prior to abarelix administration, day 19 and q8wk thereafter.

SIDE EFFECTS

FREQUENT (79%–30%): Hot flashes, sleep disturbances, breast enlargement. **OCCASIONAL (20%–11%):** Breast pain, nipple tenderness, back pain, constipation, peripheral edema, dizziness, upper respiratory tract infection, diarrhea. **RARE (10%):** Fatigue, nausea, dysuria, micturition frequency, urinary retention, urinary tract infection.

ADVERSE REACTIONS/ TOXIC EFFECTS

◀ **ALERT** ▶ Immediate-onset systemic allergic reaction characterized by hypotension, urticaria, pruritus, periorbital and/or circumoral edema, shortness of breath, wheezing, and syncope may occur.

Prolongation of the QT interval may occur. Esophageal spasm, tongue swelling, wheezing, shortness of breath, and hypotension occur rarely.

NURSING CONSIDERATIONS

BASELINE ASSESSMENT

Inform patient of treatment duration and required monitoring procedures. Obtain serum transaminase levels before treatment and periodically thereafter.

INTERVENTION/EVALUATION

Monitor patient for at least 30 min each time abarelix is given. Assess for systemic allergic reaction. Measure serum testosterone concentration before administration beginning on day 29 and q8wk thereafter. Monitor periodic serum prostate-specific antigen (PSA) levels.

PATIENT/FAMILY TEACHING

• Inform physician or nurse immediately if rash, hives, itching, tingling, flushing occurs (skin reaction may occur immediately after injection or several days later).

---

abatacept

ah-**bah**-tah-cept
(Orencia)

◆ **CLASSIFICATION**

PHARMACOTHERAPEUTIC: Selective T-cell co-stimulation modulator. **CLINICAL:** Rheumatoid arthritis agent.

ACTION

Inhibits T-lymphocyte activation, necessary in the inflammatory cascade leading to joint inflammation and destruction

---

of rheumatoid arthritis. **Therapeutic Effect:** Induces major clinical response to adult patients with moderate to severely active rheumatoid arthritis.

PHARMACOKINETICS

Higher clearance with increasing body weight. Age, gender does not affect clearance. **Half-life:** 13–16 days.

USES

Reduces signs and symptoms, progression of structural damage in adults with moderate to severe rheumatoid arthritis unresponsive to other disease-modifying antirheumatic drugs.

PRECAUTIONS

CONTRAINDICATIONS: None known. **CAUTIONS:** Chronic, latent, or localized infection, chronic obstructive pulmonary disease (COPD), elderly.

🕱 **LIFESPAN CONSIDERATIONS: Pregnancy/Lactation:** Crosses placenta; unknown if distributed in breast milk. **Pregnancy Category C. Children:** Safety and efficacy not established. **Elderly:** Cautious use due to increased risk of serious infection and malignancy.

INTERACTIONS

DRUG: Tumor necrosis factor (TNF) antagonists (infliximab, etanercept, adalimumab: Concurrent therapy produces increased incidence of serious infection. **HERBAL:** None known. **FOOD:** None known. **LAB VALUES:** None known.

AVAILABILITY (Rx)

POWDER FOR INJECTION: 250 mg in 15 ml vial.

ADMINISTRATION/HANDLING
🖳 IV

Reconstitution • Reconstitute powder in each vial with 10 ml sterile water for injection using the silicone-free syringe provided with each vial and an 18–21 gauge needle. • Rotate solution gently to avoid foaming until powder is completely dissolved. • From a 100 ml 0.9% NaCl infusion bag, withdraw and discard an amount equal to the volume of the reconstituted vials (for 2 vials remove 20 ml, for 3 vials remove 30 ml, for 4 vials remove 40 ml). • Slowly add the reconstituted solution from each vial into the infusion bag using the same syringe provided with each vial. • The concentration in the infusion bag will be 5, 7.5 or 10 mg abatacept per ml of infusion, depending on the number of vials of abatacept used.

Rate of administration • Infuse over 30 min using a low-protein binding filter.

Storage • Any reconstitution that has been prepared by using siliconized syringes will develop translucent particles and must be discarded. • Solution should appear clear and colorless to pale yellow. Discard if solution is discolored or contains precipitate. • Solution is stable for up to 14 hr after reconstitution. • Reconstituted solution may be stored at room temperature or refrigerated.

▨ IV INCOMPATIBILITIES

Do not infuse concurrently in same IV line as other agents.

INDICATIONS/ROUTES/DOSAGE
RHEUMATOID ARTHRITIS

IV: BODY WEIGHT 101 KG OR MORE: 1 gram (4 vials) given as a 30-min infusion. Following initial therapy, give at 2 wk and 4 wk after first infusion, then q3wk thereafter. BODY WEIGHT 60–100 KG: 750 mg (3 vials) given as a 30-min infusion. Following initial therapy, give at 2 wk and 4 wk after first infusion, then q3wk thereafter. BODY WEIGHT 59 KG OR LESS: 500 mg (2 vials) given as a 30-min infusion. Following initial therapy, give at 2 wk and 4 wk after first infusion, then q3wk thereafter.

SIDE EFFECTS

FREQUENT (18%): Headache. **OCCASIONAL (9%–6%):** Dizziness, cough, back pain, hypertension, nausea.

ADVERSE REACTIONS/ TOXIC EFFECTS

Upper respiratory tract infection, nasopharyngitis, sinusitis, UTI, influenza, bronchitis occur in 5% of patients. Serious infections manifested as pneumonia, cellulites, diverticulitis, acute pyelonephritis occurs in 3% of patients. Hypersensitivity reaction (rash, uriticaria, hypotension, dyspnea) occurs rarely.

NURSING CONSIDERATIONS

BASELINE ASSESSMENT

Assess onset, type, location, duration of pain/inflammation. Inspect appearance of affected joint for immobility, deformities, skin condition.

INTERVENTION/EVALUATION

Assess for therapeutic response: relief of pain, stiffness, swelling, improved joint mobility, reduced joint tenderness, improved grip strength. Monitor COPD patients for worsening of respiratory symptoms; discontinuing drug therapy may be necessary.

PATIENT/FAMILY TEACHING

• Consult physician or nurse if infection occurs. • Do not receive live virus vaccine during treatment or within 3 mo of its discontinuation.

abciximab ▷

ab-**six**-ih-mab
(c7E3 Fab, <u>ReoPro</u>)

CLASSIFICATION

PHARMACOTHERAPEUTIC: Glycoprotein IIb/IIIa receptor inhibitor.
CLINICAL: Antiplatelet; antithrombotic (see p. 31C).

ACTION

A glycoprotein IIb/IIIa receptor inhibitor that rapidly inhibits platelet aggregation by preventing the binding of fibrinogen to GP IIb/IIIa receptor sites on platelets. Therapeutic Effect: Prevents closure of treated coronary arteries. Prevents acute cardiac ischemic complications.

PHARMACOKINETICS

Rapidly cleared from plasma. Initial-phase half-life is less than 10 min; second-phase half-life is 30 min. Platelet function generally returns within 48 hr.

USES

Adjunct to aspirin and heparin therapy to prevent cardiac ischemic complications in patients undergoing percutaneous coronary intervention (PCI) and those with unstable angina not responding to conventional medical therapy when PCI is planned within 24 hr.

PRECAUTIONS

CONTRAINDICATIONS: Active internal bleeding, arteriovenous malformation or aneurysm, cerebrovascular accident (CVA) with residual neurologic defect, history of CVA (within the past 2 yr) or oral anticoagulant use within the past 7 days unless PT is less than 1.2 × control, history of vasculitis, hypersensitivity to murine proteins, intracranial neoplasm, prior IV dextran use before or during percutaneous transluminal coronary angioplasty (PTCA), recent surgery or trauma (within the past 6 wks), recent (within the past 6 wks or less) GI or GU bleeding, thrombocytopenia (less than 100,000 cells/mcl), and severe uncontrolled hypertension. **CAUTIONS:** Patients who weigh less than 75 kg; those older than 65 yr; those with history of GI disease; those receiving thrombolytics, heparin, aspirin, percutaneous transluminal coronary angioplasty (PTCA) less than 12 hr of onset of symptoms for acute MI, prolonged PTCA (longer than 70 min), failed PTCA.

⏳ LIFESPAN CONSIDERATIONS: **Pregnancy/Lactation:** Unknown if distributed in breast milk. **Pregnancy Category C. Children:** Safety and efficacy not established. **Elderly:** Increased risk of major bleeding.

INTERACTIONS

DRUG: **Anticoagulants, including heparin:** May increase risk of hemorrhage. **Platelet aggregation inhibitors (such as aspirin, dextran, thrombolytic agents):** May increase risk of bleeding. HERBAL: None known. FOOD: None known. LAB VALUES: Increases activated clotting time (ACT), aPTT, and PT. Decreases platelet count.

AVAILABILITY (Rx)

INJECTION: 2 mg/ml (5-ml vial).

ADMINISTRATION/HANDLING

💧 IV

Reconstitution ● Use 0.2- to 0.22-micron filter; filtering may be done during preparation or at administration. ● Bolus dose may be given undiluted. ● Withdraw desired dose and further dilute in 250 ml of 0.9% NaCl or D₅W (e.g., 10 mg in 250 ml equals concentration of 40 mcg/ml).

Rate of administration ● See Indications/Routes/Dosage.

Administration precautions ● Give in separate IV line; do not add any other medication to infusion. ● For bolus injection and continuous infusion, use sterile, nonpyrogenic, low protein-binding 0.2- or 0.22-micron filter. ● While vascular sheath is in position, maintain patient on complete bed rest with head of bed elevated at 30°. ● Maintain affected limb in straight position. ● After sheath removal, apply femoral pressure for 30 min, either manually or mechanically, then apply pressure dressing.

Storage ● Store vials in refrigerator. Solution appears clear, colorless. Do not shake. Discard any unused portion left in vial or if preparation contains *any* opaque particles.

🔲 IV INCOMPATIBILITY

Administer in separate line; no other medication should be added to infusion solution.

INDICATIONS/ROUTES/DOSAGE
PERCUTANEOUS CORONARY INTERVENTION (PCI)
IV BOLUS: ADULTS: 0.25 mg/kg 10–60 min before angioplasty or atherectomy, then 12-hr IV infusion of 0.125 mcg/kg/min. **Maximum:** 10 mcg/min.

PCI (UNSTABLE ANGINA)
IV BOLUS: ADULTS: 0.25 mg/kg, followed by 18- to 24-hr infusion of 10 mcg/min, ending 1 hr after procedure.

SIDE EFFECTS

FREQUENT: Nausea (16%), hypotension (12%). **OCCASIONAL (9%):** Vomiting. **RARE (3%):** Bradycardia, confusion, dizziness, pain, peripheral edema, urinary tract infection.

ADVERSE REACTIONS/ TOXIC EFFECTS

Major bleeding complications may occur. If complications occur, stop the infusion immediately. Hypersensitivity reaction may occur. Atrial fibrillation or flutter, pulmonary edema, and complete AV block occur occasionally.

NURSING CONSIDERATIONS

BASELINE ASSESSMENT

Heparin should be discontinued 4 hr before arterial sheath removal. Maintain patient on bed rest for 6–8 hr following sheath removal or drug discontinuation, whichever is later. Check platelet count, PT, aPTT before infusion (assess for preexisting blood abnormalities), 2–4 hr following treatment, and at 24 hr or before discharge, whichever is first. Check insertion site, distal pulse of affected limb while femoral artery sheath is in place, and then routinely for 6 hr following femoral artery sheath removal. Minimize need for injections, blood draws, intubations, catheters.

INTERVENTION/EVALUATION

Stop abciximab and/or heparin infusion if any serious bleeding occurs that is uncontrolled by pressure. Assess skin for ecchymosis, petechiae, particularly femoral arterial access, also catheter insertion, arterial and venous puncture, cutdown, needle sites. Handle patient carefully and as infrequently as possible to prevent bleeding. Do not obtain BP in lower extremities (possible deep vein thrombi). Assess for decrease in BP, increase in pulse rate, complaint of abdominal or back pain, severe headache, evidence of GI hemorrhage. Monitor ACT, PT, aPTT, platelet counts. Question for increase in discharge during menses. Assess urine output for hematuria. Monitor for any occurring hematoma. Use care in removing any dressing, tape.

Abelcet, see
amphotericin B

Abilify, see *aripiprazole*

acamprosate calcium

ah-**camp**-pro-sate
(Campral)

◆CLASSIFICATION

CLINICAL: Alcohol abuse deterrent.

ACTION

An alcohol abuse deterrent that appears to interact with glutamate and gamma-aminobutyric acid neurotransmitter systems centrally, restoring their balance. **Therapeutic Effect:** Reduces alcohol dependence.

PHARMACOKINETICS

Slowly absorbed from the GI tract. Steady-state plasma concentrations are reached within 5 days. Does not undergo metabolism. Excreted in urine. **Half-life:** 20–33 hr.

USES

Maintenance of alcohol abstinence in patients with alcohol dependence who are abstinent at treatment initiation.

PRECAUTIONS

CONTRAINDICATIONS: Severe renal impairment (creatinine clearance of 30 ml/min or less). **CAUTIONS:** Mental depression, renal impairment.

⚖ LIFESPAN CONSIDERATIONS:: **Pregnancy/Lactation:** Unknown if distributed in breast milk. **Pregnancy Category C. Children:** Safety and efficacy not established. **Elderly:** Age-related decreased renal function may require dosage adjustment.

INTERACTIONS

DRUG: **Antidepressants:** May cause weight gain or loss. **Naltrexone:** May increase acamprosate blood concentration. HERBAL: None known.

FOOD: None known. **LAB VALUES:** None known.

AVAILABILITY (Rx)
TABLETS: 333 mg.

ADMINISTRATION/HANDLING
PO
• Do not crush, break enteric-coated tablets. • Give without regard to meals; however, giving with food may aid in compliance of patients who regularly eat three meals daily.

INDICATIONS/ROUTES/DOSAGE
MAINTENANCE OF ALCOHOL ABSTINENCE IN ALCOHOL-DEPENDENT PATIENTS WHO ARE ABSTINENT AT INITIATION OF TREATMENT
PO: ADULTS, ELDERLY: Two tablets 3 times a day.
DOSAGE IN RENAL IMPAIRMENT
For patients with creatinine clearance of 30–49 ml/min, dosage is decreased to one tablet 3 times a day.

SIDE EFFECTS
FREQUENT (17%): Diarrhea. **OCCASIONAL (6%–4%):** Insomnia, asthenia, fatigue, anxiety, flatulence, nausea, depression, pruritus. **RARE (3%–1%):** Dizziness, anorexia, paresthesia, diaphoresis, dry mouth.

ADVERSE REACTIONS/ TOXIC EFFECTS
Acute renal failure has been reported.

NURSING CONSIDERATIONS

BASELINE ASSESSMENT
Obtain BUN, serum creatinine before treatment. Assess motor responses (agitation, trembling, tension), autonomic responses (cold and clammy hands, diaphoresis).

INTERVENTION/EVALUATION
Monitor pattern of bowel activity and stool consistency. Assess sleep pattern and provide environment conducive to sleep (quiet environment, low lighting). Offer emotional support to anxious patient. Assist with ambulation if dizziness occurs.

PATIENT/FAMILY TEACHING
• Inform patient that medication does not eliminate or diminish withdrawal symptoms. • Avoid tasks that require alertness, motor skills until response to drug is established. • Advise patient that medication helps maintain abstinence only when used as a part of a treatment program that includes counseling and support.

acarbose

ah-**car**-bose
(Prandase ✿, Precose)
Do not confuse Precose with PreCare.

◆ CLASSIFICATION
PHARMACOTHERAPEUTIC: Alpha glucosidase inhibitor. **CLINICAL:** Antidiabetic: Oral (see p. 41C).

ACTION
An alpha glucosidase inhibitor that delays glucose absorption and digestion of carbohydrates, resulting in a smaller rise in blood glucose concentration after meals. **Therapeutic Effect:** Lowers postprandial hyperglycemia.

USES
Adjunctive therapy to diet in treatment of patients with type 2 diabetes. May be used alone or in combination with other antidiabetic agents.

PRECAUTIONS
CONTRAINDICATIONS: Chronic intestinal diseases associated with marked disorders of digestion or absorption,

cirrhosis, colonic ulceration, conditions that may deteriorate as a result of increased gas formation in the intestine, diabetic ketoacidosis, hypersensitivity to acarbose, inflammatory bowel disease, partial intestinal obstruction or pre-disposition to intestinal obstruction, significant renal dysfunction (serum creatinine level greater than 2 mg/dl). **CAUTIONS:** Fever, infection, surgery, trauma (may cause loss of glycemic control). **Pregnancy Category B.**

INTERACTIONS

DRUG: **Beta blockers:** May increase the risk of hypoglycemia, hyperglycemia, or hypertension. **Digestive enzymes, intestinal absorbents (such as charcoal):** Reduces effects of acarbose. **Fluoroquinolones:** May cause changes in blood glucose and increase the risk of hypoglycemia or hyperglycemia. **Sulfonylureas:** May increase the risk of hypoglycemia. **Warfarin:** May increase the risk of bleeding. HERBAL: **Bitter melon, eucalyptus, fenugreek, ginseng, guar gum, St. John's wort:** May increase the risk of hypoglycemia. **Glucosamine, licorice:** May decrease the effectiveness of acarbose. FOOD: None known. LAB VALUES: May increase AST levels.

AVAILABILITY (Rx)

TABLETS: 25 mg, 50 mg, 100 mg.

ADMINISTRATION/HANDLING

PO
• Give with the first bite of each main meal.

INDICATIONS/ROUTES/DOSAGE

DIABETES MELLITUS
PO: ADULTS, ELDERLY: Initially, 25 mg 3 times a day with first bite of each main meal. May increase at 4- to 8-wk intervals. **Maximum:** For patients weighing more than 60 kg, 100 mg 3 times a day; for patients weighing 60 kg or less, 50 mg 3 times a day.

SIDE EFFECTS

Side effects diminish in frequency and intensity over time. **FREQUENT:** Transient GI disturbances: flatulence (77%), diarrhea (33%), abdominal pain (21%).

ADVERSE REACTIONS/ TOXIC EFFECTS

None known.

NURSING CONSIDERATIONS

BASELINE ASSESSMENT

Check blood glucose level. Discuss lifestyle to determine extent of learning, emotional needs.

INTERVENTION/EVALUATION

Monitor blood glucose, glycosylated hemoglobin, transaminase values, food intake. Assess for hypoglycemia (cool wet skin, tremors, dizziness, anxiety, headache, tachycardia, numbness in mouth, hunger, diplopia) or hyperglycemia (polyuria, polyphagia, polydipsia, nausea, vomiting, dim vision, fatigue, deep rapid breathing). Be alert to conditions that alter glucose requirements: fever, increased activity/stress, surgical procedure.

PATIENT/FAMILY TEACHING

• Do not skip or delay meals. • Check with physician when glucose demands are altered (e.g., fever, infection, trauma, stress, heavy physical activity). • Avoid alcoholic beverages. • Weight control, exercise, hygiene (including foot care), nonsmoking are essential parts of therapy.

Accupril, *see quinapril*

Accutane, *see isotretinoin*

acebutolol 🏴

ah-see-**beaut**-oh-lol

(Apo-Acebutolol 🍁, Monitan 🍁, Novo-Acebutolol 🍁, Rhotral 🍁, Sectral)

Do not confuse Sectral with Factrel or Septra.

◆CLASSIFICATION

PHARMACOTHERAPEUTIC: Beta₁-adrenergic blocker. **CLINICAL:** Antihypertensive, antiarrhythmic (see pp. 15C, 63C).

ACTION

A beta₁-adrenergic blocker that competitively blocks beta₁-adrenergic receptors in cardiac tissue. Reduces the rate of spontaneous firing of the sinus pacemaker and delays AV conduction. Therapeutic Effect: Slows heart rate, decreases cardiac output, decreases BP, and exhibits antiarrhythmic activity.

PHARMACOKINETICS

Route	Onset	Peak	Duration
PO (hypotensive)	1–1.5 hr	2–8 hr	24 hr
PO (antiarrhythmic)	1 hr	4–6 hr	10 hr

Well absorbed from the GI tract. Protein binding: 26%. Undergoes extensive first-pass liver metabolism to active metabolite. Eliminated via bile, secreted into GI tract via intestine, and excreted in urine. Removed by hemodialysis. Half-life: 3–4 hr; metabolite, 8–13 hr.

USES

Management of mild to moderate hypertension. Used alone or in combination with other antihypertensives. Management of cardiac arrhythmias (primarily premature ventricular contractions [PVCs]). OFF-LABEL: Treatment of anxiety, chronic angina pectoris, hypertrophic cardiomyopathy, MI, pheochromocytoma, syndrome of mitral valve prolapse, thyrotoxicosis, tremors.

PRECAUTIONS

CONTRAINDICATIONS: Cardiogenic shock, heart block greater than first degree, overt heart failure, severe bradycardia. **CAUTIONS:** Impaired renal/hepatic function, peripheral vascular disease, hyperthyroidism, diabetes, inadequate cardiac function, bronchospastic disease.

⏳ LIFESPAN CONSIDERATIONS: **Pregnancy/Lactation:** Readily crosses placenta; distributed in breast milk. May produce bradycardia, apnea, hypoglycemia, hypothermia during delivery, low birth-weight infants. **Pregnancy Category B (D if used in second or third trimester). Children:** No age-related precautions noted. Dosage not established. **Elderly:** Age-related peripheral vascular disease requires caution.

INTERACTIONS

DRUG: **Diuretics, other antihypertensives:** May increase hypotensive effect of acebutolol. **Sympathomimetics, xanthines:** May mutually inhibit effects of acebutolol; may mask symptoms of hypoglycemia and prolong hypoglycemic effect of **insulin** and **oral hypoglycemics.** HERBAL: None known. FOOD: None known. LAB VALUES: May increase antinuclear antibody titer and serum alkaline phosphatase, serum bilirubin, BUN, serum creatinine, LDH, lipoproteins, serum potassium, AST, ALT, triglyceride, and uric acid levels.

AVAILABILITY (Rx)

CAPSULES: 200 mg, 400 mg.

ADMINISTRATION/HANDLING

◀ ALERT ▶ Do not abruptly withdraw acebutolol as this may produce angina or MI.

PO
• May be given without regard to meals.

INDICATIONS/ROUTES/DOSAGE

MILD TO MODERATE HYPERTENSION
PO: ADULTS: Initially, 400 mg/day in 12 divided doses. Range: Up to 1,200 mg/day in 2 divided doses. Maintenance: 400–800 mg/day.

VENTRICULAR ARRHYTHMIAS
PO: ADULTS: Initially, 200 mg q12h. Increase gradually to 600–1,200 mg/day in 2 divided doses. ELDERLY: Initially, 200–400 mg/day. **Maximum:** 800 mg/day.

ANGINA
PO: ADULTS: 600–1,600 mg in 2–3 divided doses.

DOSAGE IN RENAL IMPAIRMENT
Dosage is modified based on creatinine clearance.

Creatinine Clearance	% of Usual Dosage
Less than 50 ml/min	50
Less than 25 ml/min	25

SIDE EFFECTS

FREQUENT: Hypotension manifested as dizziness, nausea, diaphoresis, headache, cold extremities, fatigue, constipation, or diarrhea. **OCCASIONAL:** Insomnia, urinary frequency, impotence or decreased libido. **RARE:** Rash, arthralgia, myalgia, confusion (especially in the elderly), altered taste.

ADVERSE REACTIONS/ TOXIC EFFECTS

Overdose may produce profound bradycardia and hypotension. Abrupt withdrawal may result in diaphoresis, palpitations, headache, and tremors. Acebutolol administration may precipitate CHF or MI in patients with heart disease; thyroid storm in those with thyrotoxicosis; or peripheral ischemia in those with existing peripheral vascular disease. Hypoglycemia may occur in patients with previously controlled diabetes. Signs of thrombocytopenia, such as unusual bleeding or bruising, occur rarely.

NURSING CONSIDERATIONS

BASELINE ASSESSMENT
Assess BP, apical pulse immediately before drug administration. If pulse is 60 beats/min or less or systolic BP is less than 90 mm Hg, withhold medication, contact physician. **Antianginal:** Record onset, type (sharp, dull, squeezing), radiation, location, intensity and duration of anginal pain, and precipitating factors (exertion, emotional stress).

INTERVENTION/EVALUATION
Monitor BP for hypotension, respiration for shortness of breath. Assess pulse for quality, rate, rhythm. Monitor EKG for cardiac arrhythmias, shortening of QT interval, prolongation of PR interval. Assess frequency/consistency of stools. Assess for evidence of CHF: dyspnea (particularly on exertion or lying down), night cough, peripheral edema, distended neck veins, decreased urine output, weight gain. Assess for nausea, diaphoresis, headache, fatigue.

PATIENT/FAMILY TEACHING
• Do not abruptly discontinue medication. • Compliance with therapy regimen is essential to control hypertension, arrhythmias. • Report shortness of breath, excessive fatigue, weight gain, prolonged dizziness, headache. • Do not use nasal decongestants, OTC cold preparations (stimulants) without physician approval. • Restrict salt, alcohol intake.

acetaminophen

ah-see-tah-**min**-oh-fen

(Abenol ✤, Apo-Acetaminophen ✤, Atasol ✤, Feverall, Mapap, Tempra, Tylenol)

✤ Canadian trade name   ℮ see **evolve**   ▶ High Alert drug

Do not confuse with Fiorinal, Hycodan, Indocin, Percodan, or Tuinal.

FIXED-COMBINATION(S)

Anexsia: acetaminophen/hydrocodone: 500 mg/5 mg, 650 mg/7.5 mg, 660 mg/10 mg. **Balacet 325:** acetaminophen/propoxyphene napsylate: 325 mg/100 mg. **Capital with Codeine, Tylenol with Codeine:** acetaminophen/codeine: 120 mg/12 mg per 5 ml. **Darvocet-N:** acetaminophen/propoxyphene: 325 mg/50 mg, 650 mg/100 mg. **Fioricet:** acetaminophen/caffeine/butalbital: 325 mg/40 mg/50 mg. **Hycet:** acetaminophen/hydrocodone: 325 mg/7.5 mg per 15 ml. **Lortab:** acetaminophen/hydrocodone: 500 mg/2.5 mg; 500 mg/5 mg; 500 mg/7.5 mg. **Lortab Elixir:** acetaminophen/hydrocodone: 167 mg/2.5 mg per 5 ml. **Norco:** acetaminophen/hydrocodone: 325 mg/10 mg. **Percocet, Roxicet:** acetaminophen/oxycodone: 325 mg/5 mg. **Tylenol with Codeine:** acetaminophen/codeine: 300 mg/15 mg, 300 mg/30 mg, 300 mg/60 mg. **Tylox:** acetaminophen/oxycodone: 500 mg/5 mg. **Ultracet:** acetaminophen/tramadol: 325 mg/37.5 mg. **Vicodin:** acetaminophen/hydrocodone: 500 mg/5 mg. **Vicodin ES:** acetaminophen/hydrocodone: 750 mg/7.5 mg. **Vicodin HP:** acetaminophen/hydrocodone: 660 mg/10 mg. **Zydone:** acetaminophen/hydrocodone: 400 mg/5 mg; 400 mg/7.5 mg; 400 mg/10 mg.

◆CLASSIFICATION

PHARMACOTHERAPEUTIC: Central analgesic. **CLINICAL:** Non-narcotic analgesic, antipyretic.

ACTION

A central analgesic whose exact mechanism is unknown, but appears to inhibit prostaglandin synthesis in the CNS and, to a lesser extent, block pain impulses through peripheral action. Acetaminophen acts centrally on hypothalamic heat-regulating center, producing peripheral vasodilation (heat loss, skin erythema, sweating). **Therapeutic Effect:** Results in antipyresis. Produces analgesic effect.

PHARMACOKINETICS

Route	Onset	Peak	Duration
PO	15–30 min	1–1.5 hr	4–6 hr

Rapidly, completely absorbed from GI tract; rectal absorption variable. Protein binding: 20%–50%. Widely distributed to most body tissues. Metabolized in liver; excreted in urine. Removed by hemodialysis. **Half-life:** 1–4 hr (half-life is increased in those with hepatic disease, elderly, neonates; decreased in children).

USES

Relief of mild to moderate pain, fever.

PRECAUTIONS

CONTRAINDICATIONS: Active alcoholism, liver disease, or viral hepatitis, all of which increase the risk of hepatotoxicity. **CAUTIONS:** Sensitivity to acetaminophen, severe impaired renal function, phenylketonuria, G6PD deficiency.

⌛ **LIFESPAN CONSIDERATIONS: Pregnancy/Lactation:** Crosses placenta; distributed in breast milk. Routinely used in all stages of pregnancy, appears safe for short-term use. **Pregnancy Category B. Children/Elderly:** No age-related precautions noted.

INTERACTIONS

DRUG: Alcohol (chronic use), hepatotoxic medications (e.g., phenytoin),

liver enzyme inducers (e.g., cimetidine): May increase risk of hepatotoxicity with prolonged high dose or single toxic dose. **Warfarin:** May increase the risk of bleeding with regular use. **HERBAL:** None known. **FOOD:** None known. **LAB VALUES:** May increase serum bilirubin, PT (may indicate hepatotoxicity), AST, and ALT. Therapeutic serum level: 10–30 mcg/ml; toxic serum level: greater than 200 mcg/ml.

AVAILABILITY (OTC)

CAPLETS (GENAPAP, TYLENOL): 500 mg. **CAPLETS (EXTENDED-RELEASE [MAPAP, TYLENOL ARTHRITIS PAIN]):** 650 mg. **CAPSULES (MAPAP):** 500 mg. **ELIXIR:** 160 mg/5 ml. **LIQUID (ORAL [TYLENOL EXTRA STRENGTH]):** 500 mg/15 ml. **SOLUTION (ORAL DROPS [GENAPAP INFANT]):** 80 mg/0.8 ml. **SUPPOSITORY (RECTAL):** 80 mg (Feverall), 120 mg (Acephen, Feverall), 325 mg (Acephen, Feverall), 650 mg (Acephen, Feverall). **TABLETS (GENAPAP, MAPAP, TYLENOL):** 325 mg, 500 mg. **TABLETS (CHEWABLE [GENAPAP, MAPAP, TYLENOL]):** 80 mg.

ADMINISTRATION/HANDLING
PO
• Give without regard to meals.
• Tablets may be crushed.

RECTAL
• Moisten suppository with cold water before inserting well up into rectum.

INDICATIONS/ROUTES/DOSAGE
ANALGESIA AND ANTIPYRESIS
PO: ADULTS, ELDERLY, CHILDREN 13 YR AND OLDER: 325–650 mg q4–6h or 1 g 3–4 times/day. **Maximum:** 4 g/day. CHILDREN 12 YR AND YOUNGER: 10–15 mg/kg/dose q4–6h as needed. **Maximum:** 5 doses/24 hr. NEONATES: 10–15 mg/kg/dose q6–8h as needed.
RECTAL: ADULTS: 650 mg q4–6h. **Maximum:** 6 doses/24 hr. CHILDREN: 10–20 mg/kg/dose q4–6h as needed.

NEONATES: 10–15 mg/kg/dose q6–8h as needed.

DOSAGE IN RENAL IMPAIRMENT

Creatinine Clearance	Frequency
10–50 ml/min	q6h
Less than 10 ml/min	q8h

SIDE EFFECTS
RARE: Hypersensitivity reaction.

ADVERSE REACTIONS/ TOXIC EFFECTS

Acetaminophen toxicity is the primary serious reaction. Early signs and symptoms of acetaminophen toxicity include anorexia, nausea, diaphoresis, and generalized weakness within the first 12–24 hr. Later signs of acetaminophen toxicity include vomiting, right upper quadrant tenderness, and elevated liver function tests within 48–72 hr after ingestion. The antidote to acetaminophen toxicity is acetylcysteine.

NURSING CONSIDERATIONS

BASELINE ASSESSMENT
If given for analgesia, assess onset, type, location, duration of pain. Effect of medication is reduced if full pain response recurs prior to next dose. **Fixed-Combination:** Obtain vital signs before giving medication. If respirations are 12/min or less (20/min or less in children), withhold medication, contact physician.

INTERVENTION/EVALUATION
Assess for clinical improvement and relief of pain, fever. Therapeutic serum level: 10–30 mcg/ml; toxic serum level: greater than 200 mcg/ml.

PATIENT/FAMILY TEACHING
• Consult physician for use in children younger than 2 yr; oral use longer than 5 days (children), longer than 10 days (adults), or fever longer than 3 days.

• Severe/recurrent pain or high/continuous fever may indicate serious illness.

*acetaZOLAMIDE

ah-seat-ah-**zole**-ah-myd
(Apo-Acetazolamide ♣, Diamox, Diamox Sequels)
Do not confuse with acetohexamide, Trimox.

◆CLASSIFICATION

PHARMACOTHERAPEUTIC: Carbonic anhydrase inhibitor. **CLINICAL:** Antiglaucoma, anticonvulsant, diuretic, urinary alkalinizer (see p. 48C).

ACTION

Reduces formation of hydrogen and bicarbonate ions by inhibiting the enzyme carbonic anhydrase. **Therapeutic Effect:** Increases excretion of sodium, potassium, bicarbonate, and water in kidney; decreases formation of aqueous humor in eye; retards abnormal discharge from CNS neurons.

USES

Treatment of glaucoma, control of intraocular pressure (IOP) before surgery, adjunct in management of seizures, edema, decreases incidence/severity of symptoms associated with acute altitude sickness. **OFF-LABEL:** Lowers IOP in treatment of malignant glaucoma, treatment of toxicity of weakly acidic medications, prevents uric acid/renal calculi by alkalinizing the urine.

PRECAUTIONS

CONTRAINDICATIONS: Hypersensitivity to sulfonamides, severe renal disease, adrenal insufficiency, hypochloremic acidosis. **CAUTIONS:** History of hypercalcemia, diabetes mellitus, gout, concurrent digoxin therapy, obstructive pulmonary disease. **Pregnancy Category C.**

INTERACTIONS

DRUG: **Amphetamines:** May increase the effects or toxicity of these drugs. **Digoxin:** Levels of this drug may be increased due to hypokalemia. **Methenamine:** May decrease the effects of this drug. HERBAL: None known. FOOD: None known. LAB VALUES: May increase serum ammonia, bilirubin, glucose, chloride, uric acid, calcium; may decrease serum bicarbonate, potassium.

AVAILABILITY (Rx)

CAPSULES (SUSTAINED-RELEASE [Diamox Sequels]): 500 mg. **TABLETS (Diamox):** 125 mg, 250 mg. **INJECTION:** 500 mg.

▦ IV INCOMPATIBILITY

Diltiazem.

IV COMPATIBILITIES

Cimetidine, ranitidine.

INDICATIONS/ROUTES/DOSAGE

GLAUCOMA
IV: ADULTS, ELDERLY: 250–500 mg; may repeat in 2–4 hr, then continue with oral therapy. CHILDREN: 5–10 mg/kg q6h. **Maximum:** 1 g a day.
PO: ADULTS, ELDERLY: 250 mg 1–4 times a day.
PO (EXTENDED-RELEASE): ADULTS, ELDERLY: 500 mg twice a day. CHILDREN: 8–30 mg/kg/day in divided doses q8h.

EDEMA
PO, IV: ADULTS: 250–375 mg a day. CHILDREN: 5 mg/kg/dose once daily.

EPILEPSY
PO: ADULTS, ELDERLY, CHILDREN: 8–30 mg/kg/day in up to 4 divided doses. Sustained-release formulation not recommended for epilepsy.

ALTITUDE SICKNESS
PO: ADULTS: 250 mg q8–12h or 500 mg

---

* "Tall Man" lettering   ✐ see color pill atlas   ✐ herb   underlined – top prescribed drug

extended-release capsule q12–24h. Begin 24–48 hr before and continue during ascent and for at least 48 hr following arrival at high altitude.

SIDE EFFECTS

FREQUENT: Fatigue, diarrhea, increased urination/frequency, decreased appetite/weight, altered taste (metallic), nausea, vomiting, paresthesia, circumoral numbness. **OCCASIONAL**: Depression, drowsiness. **RARE**: Headache, photosensitivity, confusion, tinnitus, severe muscle weakness, loss of taste.

ADVERSE REACTIONS/ TOXIC EFFECTS

Long-term therapy may result in acidotic state. Nephrotoxicity/hepatotoxicity occurs occasionally, manifested as dark urine/stools, pain in lower back, jaundice, dysuria, crystalluria, renal colic/calculi. Bone marrow depression may be manifested as aplastic anemia, thrombocytopenia, thrombocytopenic purpura, leukopenia, agranulocytosis, hemolytic anemia.

NURSING CONSIDERATIONS

BASELINE ASSESSMENT
Glaucoma: Assess affected pupil for dilation, response to light. **Epilepsy:** Obtain history of seizure disorder (length, intensity, duration of seizure, presence of aura, level of consciousness [LOC]).

INTERVENTION/EVALUATION
Monitor for acidosis (headache, lethargy progressing to drowsiness, CNS depression, Kussmaul's respiration).

PATIENT/FAMILY TEACHING
• Report presence of tingling/tremor in hands or feet, unusual bleeding or bruising, unexplained fever, sore throat, flank pain.

---

*acetoHEXAMIDE

(Dymelor)
See Antidiabetics (p. 41C)

---

acetylcysteine (*N*-acetylcysteine)   @

ah-sea-tyl-**sis**-teen

(Acetadote, Mucomyst, Parvolex ✤)

Do not confuse acetylcysteine with acetylcholine.

◆CLASSIFICATION

PHARMACOTHERAPEUTIC: Respiratory inhalant, intratracheal. **CLINICAL:** Mucolytic, antidote.

ACTION

An intratracheal respiratory inhalant that splits the linkage of mucoproteins, reducing the viscosity of pulmonary secretions. Therapeutic Effect: Facilitates the removal of pulmonary secretions by coughing, postural drainage, mechanical means. Protects against acetaminophen overdose-induced hepatotoxicity.

USES

Inhalation: Adjunctive treatment for abnormally viscid mucous secretions present in acute and chronic bronchopulmonary disease and pulmonary complication of cystic fibrosis, tracheostomy care. **Injection, oral:** Antidote in acute acetaminophen toxicity. OFF-LABEL: Prevention of renal damage from dyes given during certain diagnostic tests (such as CT scans).

PRECAUTIONS

CONTRAINDICATIONS: None known. **CAUTIONS:** Bronchial asthma, elderly, debilitated with severe respiratory insufficiency. **Pregnancy Category B.**

INTERACTIONS

DRUG: Carbamazepine: May increase the risk of subtherapeutic carbamazepine levels. **Nitroglycerin:** May enhance hypotension and nitroglycerin-induced headache. **HERBAL:** None known. **FOOD:** None known. **LAB VALUES:** None known.

AVAILABILITY (Rx)

INJECTION (ACEDOTE): 20% (200 mg/ml). **INHALATION SOLUTION (MUCO-MYST):** 10% (100 mg/ml), 20% (200 mg/ml).

ADMINISTRATION/HANDLING

 IV

• Give 3 infusions of different strengths: first dose (150 mg/kg) in 200 ml D$_5$W and infused over 15 min, second dose (50 mg/kg) in 500 ml D$_5$W and infused over 4 hr, third dose (100 mg/kg) in 1,000 ml D$_5$W and infused over 16 hr.

PO

• Give as a 5% solution. • Dilute 20% solution 1:3 with cola, orange juice, other soft drink. • Give within 1 hr of preparation.

INHALATION

• May administer either undiluted or diluted with 0.9% NaCl.

INDICATIONS/ROUTES/DOSAGE

ADJUNCTIVE TREATMENT OF VISCID MUCUS SECRETIONS FROM CHRONIC BRONCHOPULMONARY DISEASE AND FOR PULMONARY COMPLICATIONS OF CYSTIC FIBROSIS

NEBULIZATION

◄ **ALERT** ► Bronchodilators should be given 15 min before acetylcysteine. ADULTS, ELDERLY, CHILDREN: 3–5 ml (20% solution) 3–4 times a day or 6–10 ml (10% solution) 3–4 times a day. Range: 1–10 ml (20% solution) q2–6h or 2–20 ml (10% solution) q2–6h. INFANTS: 1–2 ml (20%) or 2–4 ml (10%) 3–4 times a day.

TREATMENT OF VISCID MUCUS SECRETIONS IN PATIENTS WITH A TRACHEOSTOMY

INTRATRACHEAL: ADULTS, CHILDREN: 1–2 ml of 10% or 20% solution instilled into tracheostomy q1–4h.

ACETAMINOPHEN OVERDOSE

PO (ORAL SOLUTION 5%): ADULTS, ELDERLY, CHILDREN: Loading dose of 140 mg/kg, followed in 4 hr by maintenance dose of 70 mg/kg q4h for 17 additional doses (unless acetaminophen assay reveals nontoxic level). Repeat dose if emesis occurs within 1 hr of administration. Continue until all doses are given, even if acetaminophen plasma level drops below toxic range.

IV: ADULTS, ELDERLY, CHILDREN: 150 mg/kg infused over 15 min, then 50 mg/kg infused over 4 hr, then 100 mg/kg infused over 16 hr. See administration and handling.

PREVENTION OF RENAL DAMAGE FROM DYES USED DURING CERTAIN DIAGNOSTIC TESTS

PO (ORAL SOLUTION 5%): ADULTS, ELDERLY: 600 mg twice a day for 4 doses starting the day before the procedure.

SIDE EFFECTS

FREQUENT: Inhalation: Stickiness on face, transient unpleasant odor. **OCCASIONAL: Inhalation:** Increased bronchial secretions, throat irritation, nausea, vomiting, rhinorrhea. **RARE: Inhalation:** Rash. **Oral:** Facial edema, bronchospasm, wheezing.

ADVERSE REACTIONS/TOXIC EFFECTS

Large doses may produce severe nausea and vomiting.

NURSING CONSIDERATIONS

BASELINE ASSESSMENT

Mucolytic: Assess pretreatment respirations for rate, depth, rhythm.

INTERVENTION/EVALUATION

If bronchospasm occurs, treatment should be discontinued and physician notified; bronchodilator may be added to therapy. Monitor rate, depth, rhythm, type of respiration (abdominal, thoracic). Check sputum for color, consistency, amount.

PATIENT/FAMILY TEACHING

• A slight, disagreeable odor from solution may be noticed during initial administration but disappears quickly. • Explain importance of adequate hydration. • Teach proper coughing and deep breathing.

Aciphex, *see rabeprazole*

Actiq, *see fentanyl*

Activase, *see alteplase*

Actonel, *see risedronate*

Actos, *see pioglitazone*

---

acyclovir

aye-**sigh**-klo-veer

(Apo-Acyclovir ✢, Avirax ✢, Zovirax)

Do not confuse Zovirax with Zostrix, Zyvox.

CLASSIFICATION

PHARMACOTHERAPEUTIC: Synthetic nucleoside. **CLINICAL:** Antiviral (see p. 60C).

ACTION

A synthetic nucleoside that converts to acyclovir triphosphate, becoming part of the DNA chain. Therapeutic Effect: Interferes with DNA synthesis and viral replication. Virustatic.

PHARMACOKINETICS

Poorly absorbed from the GI tract; minimal absorption following topical application. Protein binding: 9%–36%. Widely distributed. Partially metabolized in liver. Excreted primarily in urine. Removed by hemodialysis. Half-life: 2.5 hr (increased in impaired renal function).

USES

Oral and/or parenteral: Treatment of herpes infections including genital (initial, recurrent), simplex (mucotaneous, neonatal, encephalitis), zoster (chickenpox, immunocompromised patients, shingles). **Topical:** Treatment of initial herpes simplex (genital, mucutaneous). OFF-LABEL: **Oral, parenteral:** Prophylaxis of herpes simplex and herpes zoster infections, infectious mononucleosis. **Topical:** Treatment adjunct for herpes zoster infections.

PRECAUTIONS

CONTRAINDICATIONS: Use in neonates when acyclovir is reconstituted with bacteriostatic water containing benzyl alcohol. **CAUTIONS:** Renal/hepatic impairment, dehydration, fluid/electrolyte imbalance, concurrent use of nephrotoxic agents, neurologic abnormalities.

⌛ LIFESPAN CONSIDERATIONS: Pregnancy/Lactation: Crosses placenta;

distributed in breast milk. **Pregnancy Category B. Children:** Safety and efficacy in children younger than 2 yr not established (younger than 1 yr for IV use). **Elderly:** Age-related decrease in renal function may require decreased dosage.

INTERACTIONS

DRUG: **Nephrotoxic medications (such as aminoglycosides):** May increase the nephrotoxicity of acyclovir. **Probenecid:** May increase acyclovir half-life. **Varicella virus vaccine:** May decrease varicella virus vaccine effectiveness. HERBAL: None known. FOOD: None known. LAB VALUES: May increase BUN and serum creatinine concentrations.

AVAILABILITY (Rx)

CAPSULES: 200 mg. TABLETS: 400 mg, 800 mg. INJECTION SOLUTION: 50 mg/ml. ORAL SUSPENSION: 200 mg/5 ml. POWDER FOR INJECTION: 500 mg, 1,000 mg. OINTMENT: 5%.

ADMINISTRATION/HANDLING

 IV

Reconstitution • Add 10 ml sterile water for injection to each 500-mg vial (50 mg/ml). Do not use bacteriostatic water for injection containing benzyl alcohol or parabens (will cause precipitate). • Shake well until solution is clear. • Further dilute with at least 100 ml D₅W or 0.9 NaCl. Final concentration should be 7 mg/ml or less.

Rate of administration • Infuse over at least 1 hr (renal tubular damage may occur with too rapid rate). • Maintain adequate hydration during infusion and for 2 hr following IV administration.

Storage • Store vials at room temperature • Solutions of 50 mg/ml stable for 12 hr at room temperature; may form precipitate when refrigerated. Potency not affected by precipitate and redissolution. • IV infusion (piggyback)

stable for 24 hr at room temperature. Yellow discoloration does not affect potency.

PO
• May give without regard to food. • Do not crush/break capsules. • Store capsules at room temperature.

TOPICAL
• Avoid eye contact. • Use finger cot/rubber glove to prevent autoinoculation.

IV INCOMPATIBILITIES

Aztreonam (Azactam), cefepime (Maxipime), diltiazem (Cardizem), dobutamine (Dobutrex), dopamine (Intropin), levofloxacin (Levaquin), meropenem (Merrem IV), ondansetron (Zofran), piperacillin and tazobactam (Zosyn), total parenteral nutrition (TPN).

IV COMPATIBILITIES

Allopurinol (Alloprim), amikacin (Amikin), ampicillin, cefazolin (Ancef), cefotaxime (Claforan), ceftazidime (Fortaz), ceftriaxone (Rocephin), cimetidine (Tagamet), clindamycin (Cleocin), famotidine (Pepcid), fluconazole (Diflucan), gentamicin, heparin, hydromorphone (Dilaudid), imipenem (Primaxin), lorazepam (Ativan), magnesium sulfate, methylprednisolone (SoluMedrol), metoclopramide (Reglan), metronidazole (Flagyl), morphine, multivitamins, potassium chloride, propofol (Diprivan), ranitidine (Zantac), vancomycin.

INDICATIONS/ROUTES/DOSAGE

GENITAL HERPES (INITIAL EPISODE)
IV: ADULTS, ELDERLY, CHILDREN 12 YR AND OLDER: 5 mg/kg q8h for 5 days.
PO: ADULTS, ELDERLY, CHILDREN 12 YR AND OLDER: 200 mg q4h 5 times a day.

GENITAL HERPES (RECURRENT)
Less than 6 episodes per year: PO: ADULTS, ELDERLY, CHILDREN 12 YR AND OLDER: 200 mg q4h 5 times a day for 5 days. **6 episodes or more per year: PO:** ADULTS, ELDERLY, CHILDREN 12 YR AND

OLDER: 400 mg 2 times a day or 200 mg 3–5 times a day for up to 12 months.

HERPES SIMPLEX MUCOCUTANEOUS

IV: ADULTS, ELDERLY, CHILDREN 12 YR AND OLDER: 5 mg/kg/dose q8h for 7 days. CHILDREN YOUNGER THAN 12 YR: 10 mg/kg q8h for 7 days.

HERPES SIMPLEX NEONATAL

IV: CHILDREN YOUNGER THAN 4 MO: 10 mg/kg q8h for 10 days.

HERPES SIMPLEX ENCEPHALITIS

IV: ADULTS, ELDERLY, CHILDREN 12 YR AND OLDER: 10 mg/kg q8h for 10 days. CHILDREN 3 MO–YOUNGER THAN 12 YR: 20 mg/kg q8h for 10 days.

HERPES ZOSTER (CAUSED BY VARICELLA)

IV: ADULTS, ELDERLY, CHILDREN 12 YR AND OLDER: 10 mg/kg q8h for 7 days. CHILDREN YOUNGER THAN 12 YR: 20 mg/kg q8h for 7 days.

HERPES ZOSTER (SHINGLES)

PO: ADULTS, ELDERLY, CHILDREN 12 YR AND OLDER: 800 mg q4h 5 times a day for 7–10 days.

TOPICAL: ADULTS, ELDERLY: Apply to affected area 3–6 times a day for 7 days.

VARICELLA (CHICKENPOX)

PO: ADULTS, ELDERLY, CHILDREN OLDER THAN 12 YR OR CHILDREN 2–12 YR, WEIGHING 40 KG OR MORE: 800 mg 4 times a day for 5 days. CHILDREN 2–12 YR, WEIGHING LESS THAN 40 KG: 20 mg/kg 4 times a day for 5 days. **Maximum:** 800 mg/dose. CHILDREN YOUNGER THAN 2 YR: 80 mg/kg/day.

DOSAGE IN RENAL IMPAIRMENT

Dosage and frequency are modified based on severity of infection and degree of renal impairment.

PO: Normal dose 200 mg q4h.

Creatinine clearance greater than 10 ml/min: Give usual dose and at normal interval, 200 mg q4h.

Creatinine clearance 10 ml/min and less: 200 mg q12h.

PO: Normal dose 400 mg q12h.

Creatinine clearance greater than 10 ml/min: Give usual dose and at normal interval, 400 mg q12h.

Creatinine clearance 10 ml/min and less: 200 mg q12h.

PO: Normal dose 800 mg q4h.

Creatinine clearance greater than 25 ml/min: Give usual dose and at normal interval, 800 mg q4h.

Creatinine clearance 10–25 ml/min: 800 mg q8h.

Creatinine clearance less than 10 ml/min: 800 mg q12h.

IV:

Creatinine Clearance	Dosage Percent	Dosage Interval
Greater than 50 ml/min	100	8 hr
25–50 ml/min	100	12 hr
10–24 ml/min	100	24 hr
Less than 10 ml/min	50	24 hr

SIDE EFFECTS

FREQUENT: Parenteral (9%–7%): Phlebitis or inflammation at IV site, nausea, vomiting. **Topical (28%):** Burning, stinging. **OCCASIONAL: Parenteral (3%):** Pruritus, rash, urticaria. **Oral (12%–6%):** Malaise, nausea. **Topical (4%):** Pruritus. **RARE: Oral (3%–1%):** Vomiting, rash, diarrhea, headache. **Parenteral (2%–1%):** Confusion, hallucinations, seizures, tremors. **Topical (less than 1%):** Rash.

ADVERSE REACTIONS/ TOXIC EFFECTS

Rapid parenteral administration, excessively high doses, or fluid and electrolyte imbalance may produce renal failure exhibited by such signs and symptoms as abdominal pain, decreased urination, decreased appetite, increased thirst, nausea, and vomiting. Toxicity has not been reported with oral or topical use.

NURSING CONSIDERATIONS

BASELINE ASSESSMENT

Question for history of allergies, particularly to acyclovir. Assess herpes

---

 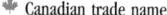

simplex lesions before treatment to compare baseline with treatment effect.

INTERVENTION/EVALUATION

Assess IV site for phlebitis (heat, pain, red streaking over vein). Evaluate cutaneous lesions. Ensure adequate ventilation. Manage chickenpox and disseminated herpes zoster with strict isolation. Provide analgesics and comfort measures; especially exhausting to elderly. Encourage fluids.

PATIENT/FAMILY TEACHING

• Drink adequate fluids. • Do not touch lesions with fingers to prevent spreading infection to new site. • **Genital Herpes:** Continue therapy for full length of treatment. • Space doses evenly. • Use finger cot/rubber glove to apply topical ointment. • Avoid sexual intercourse during duration of lesions to prevent infecting partner. • Acyclovir does not cure herpes infections. • Pap smear should be done at least annually due to increased risk of cervical cancer in women with genital herpes.

Adalat, see *nifedipine*

---

adalimumab

ah-dah-**lim**-you-mab
(Humira)

◆**CLASSIFICATION**

PHARMACOTHERAPEUTIC: Monoclonal antibody. **CLINICAL:** Rheumatoid arthritis agent.

ACTION

A monoclonal antibody that binds specifically to tumor necrosis factor (TNF) alpha, blocking its interaction with cell surface TNF receptors. **Therapeutic Effect:** Reduces inflammation, tenderness, and swelling of joints; slows or prevents progressive destruction of joints in rheumatoid arthritis.

PHARMACOKINETICS

Half-life: 10–20 days.

USES

Reduces signs, symptoms, progression of structural damage and improves physical function in adults with moderate to severe rheumatoid arthritis unresponsive to other disease-modifying antirheumatic drugs. First line treatment of moderate to severe rheumatoid arthritis, treatment of psoriatic arthritis.

PRECAUTIONS

CONTRAINDICATIONS: Active infections. **CAUTIONS:** History of sensitivity to monoclonal antibodies, cardiovascular disease, pregnancy, preexisting or recent onset CNS demyelinating disorders, elderly.

⧗ **LIFESPAN CONSIDERATIONS: Pregnancy/Lactation:** Unknown if excreted in breast milk. **Pregnancy Category B. Children:** Safety and efficacy not established. **Elderly:** Cautious use due to increased risk of serious infection and malignancy.

INTERACTIONS

DRUG: Methotrexate: Reduces the absorption of adalimumab by 29%–40%, but dosage adjustment is unnecessary if given concurrently. **HERBAL:** None known. **FOOD:** None known. **LAB VALUES:** May increase levels of blood cholesterol, other lipids, and serum alkaline phosphatase.

AVAILABILITY (Rx)

INJECTION: 40 mg/0.8 ml in prefilled syringes.

ADMINISTRATION/HANDLING
SUBCUTANEOUS
• Refrigerate. Do not freeze. • Discard unused portion. • Rotate injection sites. Give new injection at least 1 inch from an old site and never into area where skin is tender, bruised, red, or hard.

INDICATIONS/ROUTES/DOSAGE
RHEUMATOID ARTHRITIS, PSORIATIC ARTHRITIS
SUBCUTANEOUS: ADULTS, ELDERLY: 40 mg every other week. Dose may be increased to 40 mg/wk in those not taking methotrexate.

SIDE EFFECTS
FREQUENT (20%): Injection site, erythema, pruritus, pain, and swelling. **OCCASIONAL (12%–9%):** Headache, rash, sinusitis, nausea. **RARE (7%–5%):** Abdominal or back pain, hypertension.

ADVERSE REACTIONS/ TOXIC EFFECTS
Rare reactions include hypersensitivity reactions, malignancies, respiratory tract infections, bronchitis, UTIs, and more serious infections (such as pneumonia, tuberculosis, cellulitis, pyelonephritis, and septic arthritis).

NURSING CONSIDERATIONS
BASELINE ASSESSMENT
Assess onset, type, location, duration of pain or inflammation. Inspect appearance of affected joints for immobility, deformities, skin condition. If patient is to self-administer, instruct subcutaneous injection technique, including areas of the body acceptable for injection sites.

INTERVENTION/EVALUATION
Monitor lab values, particularly alkaline phosphatase. Assess for therapeutic response: relief of pain, stiffness, swelling, increased joint mobility, reduced joint tenderness, improved grip strength.

PATIENT/FAMILY TEACHING
• Injection site reaction generally occurs in first month of treatment and decreases in frequency during continued therapy. • Do not receive live vaccines during treatment.

adefovir dipivoxil

add-eh-**foe**-vir
(Hepsera)

FIXED-COMBINATION(S)
Epzicom: abacavir/lamivudine (antiretroviral): 600 mg/300 mg. **Trizivir:** abacavir/lamivudine (antiretroviral)/zidovudine (antiretroviral): 300 mg/150 mg/300 mg.

◆CLASSIFICATION
PHARMACOTHERAPEUTIC: Antiviral. **CLINICAL:** Hepatitis B agent.

ACTION
An antiviral that inhibits the enzyme DNA polymerase, causing DNA chain termination after its incorporation into viral DNA. **Therapeutic Effect:** Prevents cell replication of viral DNA.

PHARMACOKINETICS
Binds to proteins after PO administration. Protein binding: less than 4%. Excreted in urine. **Half-life:** 7 hr (increased in impaired renal function).

USES
Treatment of chronic hepatitis B in adults with evidence of active viral replication and evidence of persistent elevations of serum AST or ALT or active disease.

PRECAUTIONS
CONTRAINDICATIONS: None known. **CAUTIONS:** Patients with known risk

factors for hepatic disease, impaired renal function, elderly.

⧗ **LIFESPAN CONSIDERATIONS: Pregnancy/Lactation:** Unknown if drug crosses placenta or is distributed in breast milk. **Pregnancy Category C. Children:** Safety and efficacy not established. **Elderly:** Age-related renal impairment, decreased cardiac function requires cautious use.

INTERACTIONS

DRUG: Ibuprofen: Increases adefovir plasma concentration. **HERBAL:** None known. **FOOD:** None known. **LAB VALUES:** May increase serum amylase, creatinine, AST and ALT levels.

AVAILABILITY (Rx)

TABLETS: 10 mg.

ADMINISTRATION/HANDLING

PO
• Give without regard to food.

INDICATIONS/ROUTES/DOSAGE

CHRONIC HEPATITIS B IN PATIENTS WITH NORMAL RENAL FUNCTION
PO: ADULTS, ELDERLY: 10 mg once a day.

CHRONIC HEPATITIS B IN PATIENTS WITH IMPAIRED RENAL FUNCTION
PO: ADULTS, ELDERLY WITH CREATININE CLEARANCE 20–49 ML/MIN: 10 mg q48h. ADULTS, ELDERLY WITH CREATININE CLEARANCE 10–19 ML/MIN: 10 mg q72h. ADULTS, ELDERLY ON HEMODIALYSIS: 10 mg every 7 days following dialysis.

SIDE EFFECTS

FREQUENT (13%): Asthenia. **OCCASIONAL (9%–4%):** Headache, abdominal pain, nausea, flatulence. **RARE (3%):** Diarrhea, dyspepsia.

ADVERSE REACTIONS/ TOXIC EFFECTS

Nephrotoxicity (characterized by increased serum creatinine and decreased serum phosphorus levels) is a treatment-limiting toxicity of adefovir therapy. Lactic acidosis and severe hepatomegaly occur rarely, particularly in female patients.

NURSING CONSIDERATIONS

BASELINE ASSESSMENT

Obtain baseline renal function lab values before therapy begins and routinely thereafter. Those with preexisting renal insufficiency or during treatment may require dose adjustment. HIV antibody testing should be performed before therapy begins (unrecognized or untreated HIV infection may result in emergence of HIV resistance).

INTERVENTION/EVALUATION

Monitor I&O, serum creatinine; AST, ALT, and alkaline phosphatase levels. Closely monitor for adverse reactions in those taking other medications that are excreted renally or with other drugs known to affect renal function.

Adenoscan, see
adenosine

adenosine

ah-**den**-oh-seen
(Adenocard, Adenoscan)

◆**CLASSIFICATION**

PHARMACOTHERAPEUTIC: Cardiac agent, diagnostic aid. **CLINICAL:** Antiarrhythmic.

ACTION

A cardiac agent that slows impulse formation in the SA node and conduction time through the AV node. Adenosine also acts as a diagnostic aid in myocardial perfusion imaging or stress echocardiography. **Therapeutic Effect:** Depresses left ventricular function and restores normal sinus rhythm.

USES

Treatment of paroxysmal supraventricular tachycardia, including those associated with accessory bypass tracts (Wolff-Parkinson-White syndrome). Adjunct in diagnosis in myocardial perfusion imaging or stress echocardiography.

PRECAUTIONS

CONTRAINDICATIONS: Atrial fibrillation or flutter, second- or third-degree AV block or sick sinus syndrome (with functioning pacemaker), ventricular tachycardia. **CAUTIONS:** Heart block, arrhythmias at time of conversion, asthma, hepatic/renal failure. **Pregnancy Category C.**

INTERACTIONS

DRUG: Carbamazepine: May increase degree of heart block caused by adenosine. **Dipyridamole:** May increase effect of adenosine. **Methylxanthines (e.g., caffeine, theophylline):** May decrease effect of adenosine. **HERBAL:** None known. **FOOD:** None known. **LAB VALUES:** None known.

AVAILABILITY (Rx)

INJECTION (ADENOCARD): 3 mg/ml in 2 ml, 4 ml syringes. **INJECTION (ADENOSCAN):** 3 mg/ml in 20 ml, 30 ml vials.

ADMINISTRATION/HANDLING

 IV

Rate of administration • Administer very rapidly (over 1–2 sec) undiluted directly into vein, or if using IV line, use closest port to insertion site. If IV line is infusing any fluid other than 0.9% NaCl, flush line first. • After rapid bolus injection, follow with rapid 0.9% NaCl flush.

Storage • Store at room temperature. Solution appears clear. • Crystallization occurs if refrigerated; if crystallization occurs, dissolve crystals by warming to room temperature. Discard unused portion.

IV INCOMPATIBILITIES

Any drug or solution other than 0.9% NaCl or D_5W.

INDICATIONS/ROUTES/DOSAGE

PAROXYSMAL SUPRAVENTRICULAR TACHYCARDIA (PSVT)
RAPID IV BOLUS: ADULTS, ELDERLY, CHILDREN WEIGHING 50 KG AND MORE: Initially, 6 mg given over 1–2 sec. If first dose does not convert within 1–2 min, give 12 mg; may repeat 12-mg dose in 1–2 min if no response has occurred. CHILDREN WEIGHING LESS THAN 50 KG: Initially 0.1 mg/kg (**maximum:** 6 mg). If ineffective, may give 0.2 mg/kg (**maximum:** 12 mg).

DIAGNOSTIC TESTING
IV INFUSION: ADULTS: 140 mcg/kg/min for 6 min.

SIDE EFFECTS

FREQUENT (18%–12%): Facial flushing, dyspnea. **OCCASIONAL (7%–2%):** Headache, nausea, light-headedness, chest pressure. **RARE (1% or less):** Numbness or tingling in arms; dizziness; diaphoresis; hypotension; palpitations; chest, jaw, or neck pain.

ADVERSE REACTIONS/ TOXIC EFFECTS

May produce short-lasting heart block.

NURSING CONSIDERATIONS

BASELINE ASSESSMENT
Identify arrhythmia per cardiac monitor and assess apical pulse.

INTERVENTION/EVALUATION
Assess cardiac performance per continuous EKG. Monitor BP, apical pulse

(rate, rhythm, quality). Auscultate patient's breath sounds for clarity. Monitor respiratory rate. Monitor I&O; assess for fluid retention. Check electrolytes.

Advair, *see fluticasone*

Advair diskus, *see fluticasone and salmeterol*

Aggrenox, *see dipyridamole and aspirin*

---

albumin, human

al-**byew**-min

(Albuminar-5, Albuminar-25, Albutein, Buminate, Flexbumin, Plasbumin)

Do not confuse albumin with albuterol.

◆CLASSIFICATION

PHARMACOTHERAPEUTIC: Plasma protein fraction. **CLINICAL:** Blood derivative.

ACTION

A plasma protein fraction that acts as a blood volume expander. **Therapeutic Effect:** Provides temporary increase in blood volume; reduces hemoconcentration and blood viscosity.

PHARMACOKINETICS

Route	Onset	Peak	Duration
IV	15 min (in well-hydrated patient)	N/A	N/A

Distributed throughout extracellular fluid. **Half-life:** 15–20 days.

USES

Treatment of hypovolemia, hypoproteinemia. Adjunct in treatment of severe burns, neonatal hyperbilirubinemia, adult respiratory distress syndrome (ARDS), cardiopulmonary bypass, ascites, acute nephrosis or nephrotic syndrome, hemodialysis, pancreatitis, intra-abdominal infections, acute hepatic failure.

PRECAUTIONS

CONTRAINDICATIONS: Heart failure, history of allergic reaction to albumin level, hypervolemia, normal serum albumin, pulmonary edema, severe anemia. **CAUTIONS:** Hypertension, normal serum albumin concentration, low cardiac reserve, pulmonary disease, hepatic/renal failure.

⧖ LIFESPAN CONSIDERATIONS: **Pregnancy/Lactation:** Unknown if drug crosses placenta or is distributed in breast milk. **Pregnancy Category C. Children/Elderly:** No age-related precautions noted.

INTERACTIONS

DRUG: None known. **HERBAL:** None known. **FOOD:** None known. **LAB VALUES:** May increase serum alkaline phosphatase concentration.

AVAILABILITY (Rx)

INJECTION: 5% (Albuminar-5, Albutein, Buminate, Plasbumin), 25% (Albuminar-25, Flexbumin).

ADMINISTRATION/HANDLING

IV

Reconstitution • A 5% solution may be made from 25% solution by adding 1 volume 25% to 4 volumes 0.9% NaCl or D_5W (NaCl preferred). Do not use sterile water for injection (life-threatening hemolysis, acute renal failure can result).

Rate of administration • Give by IV infusion. Rate is variable, depends on

---

use, blood volume, concentration of solute. 5%: usually given at 5–10 ml/min; 25%: usually at 2–3 ml/min. 5% administered undiluted; 25% may be administered undiluted or diluted with 0.9% NaCl or D$_5$W. NaCl preferred.
• May give without regard to patient blood group or Rh factor.

Storage • Store at room temperature. Appears as clear, brownish, odorless, moderate viscous fluid. • Do not use if solution has been frozen, appears turbid, contains sediment, or if not used within 4 hr of opening vial.

▥ IV INCOMPATIBILITIES

Lipids, midazolam (Versed), vancomycin (Vancocin), verapamil (Isoptin).

IV COMPATIBILITIES

Diltiazem (Cardizem), lorazepam (Ativan).

INDICATIONS/ROUTES/DOSAGE

HYPOVOLEMIA

IV: ADULTS, ELDERLY: Initially, 25 g; may repeat in 15–30 min. **Maximum:** 250 g within 48 hr. CHILDREN: 0.5–1 g/kg/dose (10–20 ml/kg/dose of 5% albumin) **Maximum:** 6 g/kg/day.

HYPOPROTEINEMIA

IV: ADULTS, ELDERLY, CHILDREN: 0.5–1 g/kg/dose (10–20 ml/kg/dose of 5% albumin). Repeat in 1–2 days.

BURNS

IV: ADULTS, ELDERLY, CHILDREN: Initially, give large volumes of crystalloid infusion to maintain plasma volume. After 24 hr, give 25 g, then adjust dosage adjusted to maintain plasma albumin concentration of 2–2.5 g/100 ml.

CARDIOPULMONARY BYPASS

IV: ADULTS, ELDERLY: 5% or 25% albumin with crystalloid to maintain plasma albumin concentration of 2.5 g/100 ml.

ACUTE NEPHROSIS, NEPHROTIC SYNDROME

IV: ADULTS, ELDERLY: 25 g of 25% injection, with diuretic once a day for 7–10 days.

HEMODIALYSIS

IV: ADULTS, ELDERLY: 100 ml (25 g) of 25% albumin.

HYPERBILIRUBINEMIA, ERYTHROBLASTOSIS FETALIS

IV: INFANTS: 1 g/kg 1–2 hr before transfusion.

SIDE EFFECTS

OCCASIONAL: Hypotension. **RARE:** High dose in repeated therapy: altered vital signs, chills, fever, increased salivation, nausea, vomiting, urticaria, tachycardia.

ADVERSE REACTIONS/TOXIC EFFECTS

Fluid overload may occur, marked by increased BP, and distended neck veins. Neurological changes that may occur include headache, weakness, blurred vision, behavioral changes, incoordination, and isolated muscle twitching. Pulmonary edema may also occur, evidenced by rapid breathing, rales, wheezing, and coughing.

NURSING CONSIDERATIONS

BASELINE ASSESSMENT

Obtain BP, pulse, respirations immediately before administration. Adequate hydration required before albumin is administered.

INTERVENTION/EVALUATION

Monitor BP for hypotension/hypertension. Assess frequently for evidence of fluid overload, pulmonary edema (see Adverse Reactions/Toxic Effects). Check skin for flushing, urticaria. Monitor I&O ratio (watch for decreased output). Assess for therapeutic response (increased BP, decreased edema).

Albuminar, *see albumin*

---

albuterol

ale-**beut**-er-all

(AccuNeb, Asmavent ✹, Novosalmol ✹, Proventil, Proventil HFA, Proventil Repetabs, Ventolin, Ventolin HFA, Volmax, Vospire ER)

Do not confuse albuterol with Albutein or atenolol, or Proventil with Prinivil.

FIXED-COMBINATION(S)

Combivent: albuterol/ipratropium (a bronchodilator): 103 mcg/18 mcg per actuation. **Duoneb:** albuterol/ipratropium 3 mg/0.5 mg.

◆ CLASSIFICATION

PHARMACOTHERAPEUTIC: Sympathomimetic (adrenergic agonist). **CLINICAL:** Bronchodilator (see p. 66C).

ACTION

A sympathomimetic that stimulates beta$_2$-adrenergic receptors in the lungs, resulting in relaxation of bronchial smooth muscle. Therapeutic Effect: Relieves bronchospasm and reduces airway resistance.

PHARMACOKINETICS

Route	Onset	Peak	Duration
PO	15–30 min	2–3 hr	4–6 hr
PO (extended-release)	30 min	2–4 hr	12 hr
Inhalation	5–15 min	0.5–2 hr	2–5 hr

Rapidly, well absorbed from the GI tract; gradually absorbed from the bronchi after inhalation. Metabolized in the liver. Primarily excreted in urine. Half-life: 2.7–5 hr (PO); 3.8 hr (inhalation).

USES

Relief of bronchospasm due to reversible obstructive airway disease, exercise-induced bronchospasm.

PRECAUTIONS

CONTRAINDICATIONS: History of hypersensitivity to sympathomimetics. **CAUTIONS:** Hypertension, cardiovascular disease, hyperthyroidism, diabetes mellitus.

⧗ **LIFESPAN CONSIDERATIONS: Pregnancy/Lactation:** Appears to cross placenta; unknown if distributed in breast milk. May inhibit uterine contractility. **Pregnancy Category C. Children:** Safety and efficacy not established in children younger than 2 yr (syrup) or younger than 6 yr (tablets). **Elderly:** May be more sensitive to tremor or tachycardia due to age-related increased sympathetic sensitivity.

INTERACTIONS

DRUG: **Beta blockers:** Antagonize effects of albuterol. **Digoxin:** May increase the risk of arrhythmias. **MAOIs, tricyclic antidepressants:** May potentiate cardiovascular effects. HERBAL: None known. FOOD: None known. LAB VALUES: May increase blood glucose level. May decrease serum potassium level.

AVAILABILITY (Rx)

SYRUP: 2 mg/5 ml. **TABLETS (PROVENTIL, VENTOLIN):** 2 mg, 4 mg. **TABLETS (EXTENDED-RELEASE):** 4 mg (Proventil Repetabs, Volmax, VoSpire ER), 8 mg (Volmax, VoSpire ER). **INHALATION AEROSOL (PROVENTIL, VENTOLIN):** 90 mcg/spray. **INHALATION SOLUTION (ACCUNEB):** 0.75 mg/3 ml (0.63 mg/3 ml albuterol), 1.5 mg/3 ml (1.25 mg/3 ml albuterol). **INHALATION SOLUTION:** 0.083% (Proventil), 0.5% (Proventil, Ventolin).

ADMINISTRATION/HANDLING

PO
• Do not crush/break extended-release tablets. • May give without regard to food.

INHALATION
- Shake container well before inhalation.
- Wait 2 min before inhaling second dose (allows for deeper bronchial penetration). • Rinse mouth with water immediately after inhalation (prevents mouth/throat dryness).

NEBULIZATION
- Dilute 0.5 ml of 0.5% solution to final volume of 3 ml with 0.9% NaCl to provide 2.5 mg. • Administer over 5–15 min. • Nebulizer should be used with compressed air or O_2 at rate of 6–10 L/min.

INDICATIONS/ROUTES/DOSAGE

ACUTE BRONCHOSPASM
INHALATION: ADULTS, ELDERLY, CHILDREN OLDER THAN 12 YR: 4–8 puffs q20min up to 4 hr, then q1–4h as needed. CHILDREN 12 YR AND YOUNGER: 4–8 puffs q20min for 3 doses, then q1–4h as needed.
NEBULIZATION: ADULTS, ELDERLY, CHILDREN OLDER THAN 12 YR: 2.5–5 mg q20min for 3 doses, then 2.5–10 mg q1–4h or 10–15 mg/hr continuously. CHILDREN 12 YR AND YOUNGER: 0.15 mg/kg q20min for 3 doses (minimum: 2.5 mg), then 0.15–0.3 mg/kg q1–4h as needed.

BRONCHOSPASM
PO: ADULTS, CHILDREN OLDER THAN 12 YR: 2–4 mg 3–4 times a day. **Maximum:** 8 mg 4 times a day. ELDERLY: 2 mg 3–4 times a day. **Maximum:** 8 mg 4 times a day. CHILDREN 6–12 YR: 2 mg 3–4 times a day. **Maximum:** 24 mg/day. CHILDREN 2–5 YR: 0.1–0.2 mg/kg/dose 3 times a day. **Maximum:** 12 mg/day.
PO (EXTENDED-RELEASE): ADULTS, CHILDREN OLDER THAN 12 YR: 4–8 mg q12h.
NEBULIZATION: ADULTS, ELDERLY, CHILDREN OLDER THAN 12 YR: 2.5 mg 3–4 times a day over 5–15 min. CHILDREN 12 YR AND YOUNGER: 0.05 mg/kg q4–6h. Minimum: 1.25 mg/dose. **Maximum:** 2.5 mg/dose.

CHRONIC BRONCHOSPASM
INHALATION: ADULTS, ELDERLY, CHILDREN 4 YR AND OLDER: 1–2 puffs q4–6h. **Maximum:** 12 puffs per day.

EXERCISE-INDUCED BRONCHOSPASM
INHALATION: ADULTS, ELDERLY, CHILDREN OLDER THAN 12 YR: 2 puffs 15–30 min before exercise. CHILDREN 12 YR AND YOUNGER: 1–2 puffs 5 min before exercise.

SIDE EFFECTS
FREQUENT: Headache (27%); nausea (15%); restlessness, nervousness, tremors (20%); dizziness (less than 7%); throat dryness and irritation, pharyngitis (less than 6%); BP changes, including hypertension (5%–3%); heartburn, transient wheezing (less than 5%). **OCCASIONAL (3%–2%):** Insomnia, asthenia, altered taste. **Inhalation:** Dry, irritated mouth or throat; cough; bronchial irritation. **RARE:** Somnolence, diarrhea, dry mouth, flushing, diaphoresis, anorexia.

ADVERSE REACTIONS/ TOXIC EFFECTS
Excessive sympathomimetic stimulation may produce palpitations, extrasystole, tachycardia, chest pain, a slight increase in BP followed by a substantial decrease, chills, diaphoresis, and blanching of skin. Too-frequent or excessive use may lead to decreased bronchodilating effectiveness and severe, paradoxical bronchoconstriction.

NURSING CONSIDERATIONS

BASELINE ASSESSMENT
Offer emotional support (high incidence of anxiety due to difficulty in breathing and sympathomimetic response to drug).

INTERVENTION/EVALUATION
Monitor rate, depth, rhythm, type of respiration; quality and rate of pulse; EKG; serum potassium, ABG determinations. Assess lung sounds for wheezing (bronchoconstriction) and rales.

PATIENT/FAMILY TEACHING
- Instruct on proper use of inhaler.
- Increase fluid intake (decreases lung

secretion viscosity). • Do not take more than 2 inhalations at any one time (excessive use may produce paradoxical bronchoconstriction or a decreased bronchodilating effect). • Rinsing mouth with water immediately after inhalation may prevent mouth/throat dryness. • Avoid excessive use of caffeine derivatives (chocolate, coffee, tea, cola, cocoa).

---

alclometasone

(Aclovate)
See Corticosteroids: topical (p. 85C)

---

aldesleukin ⚑

all-des-**lyew**-kin
(Interleukin-2, IL-2, <u>Proleukin</u>)
See Interleukin-2, pp. 70C, 630.

---

alefacept

ale-fah-cept
(Amevive)

◆CLASSIFICATION

PHARMACOTHERAPEUTIC: Immunologic agent. **CLINICAL:** Immunosuppressive.

ACTION

An immunologic agent that interferes with the activation of T-lymphocytes by binding to the lymphocyte antigen, thus reducing the number of circulating T-lymphocytes. **Therapeutic Effect:** Prevents T cells from becoming overactive, which may help reduce symptoms of chronic plaque psoriasis.

PHARMACOKINETICS

Half-life: 270 hr.

USES

Treatment of adults with moderate to severe chronic plaque psoriasis who are candidates for systemic therapy or phototherapy.

PRECAUTIONS

CONTRAINDICATIONS: History of systemic malignancy, concurrent use of immunosuppressive agents or phototherapy. Do not administer to patients infected with HIV (reduces CD4 + T lymphocyte count, which may accelerate disease progression or increase disease complications). **CAUTIONS:** Those at high risk for malignancy, chronic infections, history of recurrent infection, elderly.

⧗ **LIFESPAN CONSIDERATIONS: Pregnancy/Lactation:** Unknown if drug crosses placenta or is distributed in breast milk. **Pregnancy Category B. Children:** Safety and efficacy not established. **Elderly:** Cautious use due to higher incidence of infections and certain malignancies.

INTERACTIONS

DRUG: None known. **HERBAL:** None known. **FOOD:** None known. **LAB VALUES:** Decreases serum T-lymphocyte levels. May increase serum AST and ALT levels.

AVAILABILITY (Rx)

POWDER FOR INJECTION: 7.5 mg for IV administration, 15 mg for IM administration.

ADMINISTRATION/HANDLING

◀ ALERT ▶ For both IM and IV administration, withdraw 0.6 ml of the supplied diluent and with the needle pointed at the side-wall of the vial, slowly inject the diluent into the vial of alefacept. Avoid excessive foaming by swirling gently to dissolve.

IV

Reconstitution • Reconstitute 7.5 mg with 0.6 ml of supplied diluent (sterile water for injection); 0.5 ml of reconstituted solution contains 7.5 mg alefacept.

Rate of administration • Prepare 2 syringes with 3 ml 0.9% NaCl for pre- and post-administration flush. • Prime the winged infusion set with 3 ml 0.9% NaCl and insert the set into the vein. • Attach the medication-filled syringe to the infusion set and give over no more than 5 sec. • Flush with 3 ml 0.9% NaCl.

Storage • Store unopened vials at room temperature. • Following reconstitution, use immediately, or if refrigerated, within 4 hr. • Discard unused portion within 4 hr of reconstitution. • Reconstituted solution should be clear and colorless to slightly yellow. • Do not use if discolored or cloudy or if undissolved material remains.

IM

Reconstitution • Reconstitute 15 mg with 0.6 ml of supplied diluent (sterile water for injection); 0.5 ml of reconstituted solution contains 15 mg alefacept. • Inject the full 0.5 ml of solution. • Use a different IM site for each new injection. Give new injections at least 1 inch from the old site. Avoid areas where the skin is tender, bruised, red, or hard.

Storage • Store unopened vials at room temperature. • Following reconstitution, use immediately, or if refrigerated, within 4 hr. • Discard unused portion within 4 hr of reconstitution. • Reconstituted solution should be clear and colorless to slightly yellow. • Do not use if discolored or cloudy or if undissolved material remains.

▧ IV INCOMPATIBILITIES

Don't mix alefacept with any other medications. Don't reconstitute it with any diluent other than that supplied by the manufacturer.

INDICATIONS/ROUTES/DOSAGE
PLAQUE PSORIASIS
IV: ADULTS, ELDERLY: 7.5 mg once weekly for 12 wk.
IM: ADULTS, ELDERLY: 15 mg once weekly for 12 wk.

SIDE EFFECTS
FREQUENT (16%): Injection site pain and inflammation (with IM administration). **OCCASIONAL (5%):** Chills. **RARE (2% or less):** Pharyngitis, dizziness, cough, nausea, myalgia.

ADVERSE REACTIONS/ TOXIC EFFECTS
Rare reactions include hypersensitivity reactions, lymphopenia, malignancies, and serious infections requiring hospitalization (such as abscess, pneumonia, and postoperative wound infection). Coronary artery disease and MI occur in less than 1% of patients.

NURSING CONSIDERATIONS

BASELINE ASSESSMENT
Obtain baseline CD4+ T lymphocyte levels before treatment and weekly during the 12-wk dosing period.

INTERVENTION/EVALUATION
Closely monitor CD4+ T lymphocyte levels. Withhold dose if CD4+ T lymphocyte levels are below 250 cells/mcl. If the levels remain below 250 cells/mcl for 1 mo, discontinue treatment.

PATIENT/FAMILY TEACHING
• Regular monitoring of WBC count during therapy is necessary. • Promptly report any signs of infection or evidence of malignancy.

alemtuzumab

al-lem-**two**-zoo-mab
(Campath)

CLASSIFICATION

PHARMACOTHERAPEUTIC: Monoclonal antibody. **CLINICAL:** Antineoplastic (see p. 70C).

ACTION

Binds to CD52, a cell surface glycoprotein, found on the surface of all B- and T-lymphocytes, most monocytes, macrophages, natural killer cells, and granulocytes. **Therapeutic Effect:** Produces cytotoxicity reducing tumor size.

PHARMACOKINETICS

Half-life: About 12 days. Peak and trough levels rise during first few weeks of therapy and approach steady state by about week 6.

USES

Treatment of B-cell chronic lymphocytic leukemia (B-CLL) in patients who have been treated with alkylating agents and who have failed fludarabine (Fludara) therapy.

PRECAUTIONS

CONTRAINDICATIONS: Active systemic infections, history of hypersensitivity or anaphylactic reaction to alemtuzumab, other monoclonal antibodies, immunosuppression. **CAUTIONS:** None known.

LIFESPAN CONSIDERATIONS: Pregnancy/Lactation: Has potential to cause fetal B- and T-lymphocyte depletion. Discontinue breast-feeding during treatment and for at least 3 mo after last dose. **Pregnancy Category** C. **Children:** Safety and efficacy not established. **Elderly:** No age-related precautions noted.

INTERACTIONS

DRUG: Live virus vaccines: May potentiate viral replication, increase side effects, and decrease the patient's antibody response to the vaccine. **HERBAL:** None known. **FOOD:** None known. **LAB VALUES:** May decrease Hgb level, platelet count, and WBC count.

AVAILABILITY (Rx)

SOLUTION FOR INJECTION: 30 mg/ml.

ADMINISTRATION/HANDLING

◻ IV

◀ **ALERT** ▶ Single doses of alemtuzumab greater than 30 mg or cumulative doses greater than 90 mg/wk should not be administered (higher incidence of pancytopenia).
◀ **ALERT** ▶ Do not give by IV push or bolus.

Reconstitution • Withdraw needed amount from ampule into a syringe. • Using a low-protein binding, non–fiber-releasing 5-micron filter, inject into 100 ml 0.9% NaCl or D₅W. • Invert bag to mix; do not shake.

Rate of administration • Give the 100 ml solution as a 2-hr IV infusion.

Storage • Before dilution, refrigerate ampules. Do not freeze. • Use within 8 hr after dilution. Diluted solution may be stored at room temperature or refrigerated. • Discard if particulate matter is present or if solution is discolored.

▩ IV INCOMPATIBILITIES

Don't mix alemtuzumab with any other medications.

INDICATIONS/ROUTES/DOSAGE

CHRONIC LYMPHOCYTIC LEUKEMIA

IV: ADULTS, ELDERLY: Initially, 3 mg/day as a 2-hr infusion. When the 3-mg daily dose is tolerated (with only low-grade or no infusion-related toxicities), increase daily dose to 10 mg. When the 10 mg/day dose is tolerated, maintenance dose may be initiated. Maintenance: 30 mg/day 3 times a wk on alternate days (such as Monday, Wednesday, and Friday or Tuesday, Thursday, and Saturday) for up to 12 wk. The increase to 30 mg/day is usually achieved in 3–7 days.

SIDE EFFECTS

FREQUENT: Rigors, tremors (86%), fever (85%), nausea (54%), vomiting (41%), rash (40%), fatigue (34%), hypotension (32%), urticaria (30%), pruritus, skeletal pain, headache (24%), diarrhea (22%), anorexia (20%). **OCCASIONAL (less than 10%):** Myalgia, dizziness, abdominal pain, throat irritation, vomiting, neutropenia, rhinitis, bronchospasm, urticaria.

ADVERSE REACTIONS/ TOXIC EFFECTS

Neutropenia occurs in 85% of patients, anemia occurs in 80% of patients, and thrombocytopenia occurs in 72% of patients. A rash occurs in 40% of patients. Respiratory toxicity, manifested as dyspnea, cough, bronchitis, pneumonitis, and pneumonia, occurs in 26%–16% of patients. Serious, sometimes fatal bacterial, viral, fungal, and protozoan infections have been reported.

NURSING CONSIDERATIONS

BASELINE ASSESSMENT

Pretreatment with acetaminophen and diphenhydramine before each infusion may prevent infusion-related side effects. CBC, platelet count should be obtained frequently during and after therapy to assess for neutropenia, anemia, thrombocytopenia.

INTERVENTION/EVALUATION

Monitor for an infusion-related symptoms complex consisting mainly of rigors, fever, chills, hypotension, generally occurring within 30 min–2 hr of beginning of first infusion. Slowing infusion rate

resolves symptoms. Monitor for hematologic toxicity (fever, sore throat, signs of local infection, easy bruising, or unusual bleeding from any site), symptoms of anemia (excessive fatigue, weakness).

PATIENT/FAMILY TEACHING

• Avoid crowds, those with known infection. • Avoid contact with those who recently received live virus vaccine; do not receive vaccinations.

---

alendronate sodium

ah-**len**-drew-nate

(Fosamax)

Do not confuse Fosamax with Flomax.

◆ CLASSIFICATION

PHARMACOTHERAPEUTIC: Bisphosphonate. **CLINICAL:** Bone resorption inhibitor, calcium regulator.

ACTION

A bisphosphonate that inhibits normal and abnormal bone resorption, without retarding mineralization. **Therapeutic Effect:** Leads to significantly increased bone mineral density; reverses the progression of osteoporosis.

PHARMACOKINETICS

Poorly absorbed after oral administration. Protein binding: 78%. After oral administration, rapidly taken into bone, with uptake greatest at sites of active bone turnover. Excreted in urine. **Terminal half-life:** Greater than 10 yr (reflects release from skeleton as bone is resorbed).

USES

Treatment of osteoporosis in men. Treatment adjunct in glucocorticoid-induced osteoporosis, treatment and prevention of osteoporosis in postmenopausal women, treatment of Paget's disease. OFF-LABEL: Treatment of breast cancer.

PRECAUTIONS

CONTRAINDICATIONS: GI disease, including dysphagia, frequent heartburn, gastrointestinal reflux disease, hiatal hernia, and ulcers, inability to stand or sit upright for at least 30 min; renal impairment; sensitivity to alendronate. **CAUTIONS:** Hypocalcemia, vitamin D deficiency.

⧗ **LIFESPAN CONSIDERATIONS:** **Pregnancy/Lactation:** Possible incomplete fetal ossification, decreased maternal weight gain, delay in delivery. Excretion in breast milk unknown. Do not give to breast-feeding women. **Pregnancy Category C. Children:** Safety and efficacy not established. **Elderly:** No age-related precautions noted.

INTERACTIONS

DRUG: **Antacids, calcium supplements:** May interfere with the absorption of alendronate. **Aspirin, NSAIDs:** May increase GI disturbances. **IV ranitidine:** May double the bioavailability of alendronate. HERBAL: None known. FOOD: **Beverages other than plain water, dietary supplements, food:** May interfere with absorption of alendronate. LAB VALUES: Reduces serum calcium and serum phosphate concentrations. Significantly decreases serum alkaline phosphatase level in patients with Paget's disease.

AVAILABILITY (Rx)

TABLETS: 5 mg, 10 mg, 35 mg, 40 mg, 70 mg. **ORAL SOLUTION:** 70 mg/75 ml.

ADMINISTRATION/HANDLING

PO
• Give at least 30 min before first food, beverage, or medication of the day.
• Give with 6–8 oz plain water only

(mineral water, coffee, tea, juice will decrease absorption). • Instruct patient **not** to lie down or eat for at least 30 min after administering medication (plain water and not lying down allow medication to reach stomach quickly, minimizing esophageal irritation).

INDICATIONS/ROUTES/DOSAGE

OSTEOPOROSIS (IN MEN)
PO: ADULTS, ELDERLY: 10 mg once a day in the morning or 70 mg weekly.

GLUCOCORTICOID-INDUCED OSTEOPOROSIS
PO: ADULTS, ELDERLY: 5 mg once a day in the morning. POST-MENOPAUSAL WOMEN NOT RECEIVING ESTROGEN: 10 mg once a day in the morning.

POST-MENOPAUSAL OSTEOPOROSIS
PO (TREATMENT): ADULTS, ELDERLY: 10 mg once a day in the morning or 70 mg weekly.
PO (PREVENTION): ADULTS, ELDERLY: 5 mg once a day in the morning or 35 mg weekly.

PAGET'S DISEASE
PO: ADULTS, ELDERLY: 40 mg once a day in the morning for 6 mo.

SIDE EFFECTS

FREQUENT (8%–7%): Back pain, abdominal pain. **OCCASIONAL (3%–2%):** Nausea, abdominal distention, constipation, diarrhea, flatulence. **RARE (less than 2%):** Rash, severe bone, joint, muscle pain.

ADVERSE REACTIONS/ TOXIC EFFECTS

Overdose causes hypocalcemia, hypophosphatemia, and significant GI disturbances. Esophageal irritation occurs if alendronate is not given with 6–8 oz of plain water or if the patient lies down within 30 min of drug administration.

NURSING CONSIDERATIONS

BASELINE ASSESSMENT
Hypocalcemia, vitamin D deficiency must be corrected before therapy. Check

electrolytes (especially calcium and alkaline phosphatase serum levels).

INTERVENTION/EVALUATION

Monitor electrolytes (especially calcium and alkaline phosphatase serum levels).

PATIENT/FAMILY TEACHING

• Instruct patient that expected benefits occur only when medication is taken with full glass (6–8 oz) of plain water, first thing in the morning and at least 30 min before first food, beverage, or medication of the day is taken. Any other beverage (mineral water, orange juice, coffee) significantly reduces absorption of medication. • Do not lie down for at least 30 min after taking medication (potentiates delivery to stomach, reducing risk of esophageal irritation). • Consider weight-bearing exercises, modify behavioral factors (e.g., cigarette smoking, alcohol consumption).

alfentanil

(Alfenta)
See Opioid analgesics

alfuzosin hydrochloride

ale-few-**zoe**-sin
(Uroxatral, Xatra ✤)

CLASSIFICATION

PHARMACOTHERAPEUTIC: Alpha₁-adrenergic blocker. **CLINICAL:** Benign prostatic hyperplasia agent.

ACTION

An alpha₁ antagonist that targets receptors around bladder neck and prostate capsule. **Therapeutic Effect:** Relaxes smooth muscle and improves urinary flow and symptoms of prostatic hyperplasia.

PHARMACOKINETICS

Rapidly absorbed and widely distributed. Protein binding: 90%. Extensively metabolized in the liver. Primarily excreted in urine. **Half-life:** 3–9 hr.

USES

Treatment of signs and symptoms of benign prostatic hyperplasia.

PRECAUTIONS

CONTRAINDICATIONS: Hepatic disease, concomitant use of ketoconazole, itraconazole, ritonavir. **CAUTIONS:** Coronary artery disease, hepatic disease, orthostatic hypotension, general anesthesia.

⚠ LIFESPAN CONSIDERATIONS: **Pregnancy/Lactation:** Not indicated for use in this patient population. **Pregnancy Category B. Children:** Not indicated for use in this patient population. **Elderly:** No age-related precautions noted.

INTERACTIONS

DRUG: Cimetidine: May increase alfuzosin blood concentration. **Ketoconazole, itraconazole, ritonavir:** May increase alfuzosin serum levels. **Other alpha blockers, such as doxazosin, prazosin, tamsulosin, and terazosin:** May increase the alpha-blockade effects of both drugs. **HERBAL:** None known. **FOOD:** None known. **LAB VALUES:** None known.

AVAILABILITY (Rx)

TABLETS (EXTENDED-RELEASE): 10 mg.

ADMINISTRATION/HANDLING

PO
• Give after the same meal each day. • Do not chew or crush extended-release tablet.

INDICATIONS/ROUTES/DOSAGE

BENIGN PROSTATIC HYPERPLASIA

PO: ADULTS: 10 mg once a day, approximately 30 min after same meal each day.

SIDE EFFECTS

FREQUENT (7%–6%): Dizziness, headache, malaise. **OCCASIONAL (4%):** Dry mouth. **RARE (3%–2%):** Nausea, dyspepsia (such as heartburn, and epigastric discomfort), diarrhea, orthostatic hypotension, tachycardia, drowsiness.

ADVERSE REACTIONS/ TOXIC EFFECTS

Ischemia-related chest pain may occur rarely. Priapism has been reported.

NURSING CONSIDERATIONS

BASELINE ASSESSMENT

Question for sensitivity to alfuzosin, use of other alpha-blocking agents (prazosin, terazosin, doxazosin, tamsulosin). Obtain patient BP.

INTERVENTION/EVALUATION

Assist with ambulation if dizziness occurs. Report headache. Monitor for hypotension.

PATIENT/FAMILY TEACHING

• Take after the same meal each day. • Avoid tasks that require alertness, motor skills until response to drug is established. • Do not chew or crush extended-release tablet.

Alimta, *see pemetrexed*

---

alitretinoin 🏳

al-**lee**-tret-ih-nown
(Panretin)

Do not confuse Panretin with pancreatin.

CLASSIFICATION

PHARMACOTHERAPEUTIC: Second-generation retinoid. **CLINICAL:** Antineoplastic (see p. 71C).

ACTION

Binds to and activates all known retinoid receptors. Once activated, receptors act as transcription factors, regulating genes that control cellular differentiation and proliferation. Therapeutic Effect: Inhibits growth of Kaposi's sarcoma (KS) cells.

USES

Topical treatment of cutaneous lesions in those with AIDS-related KS. OFF-LABEL: Breast, cervical, ovarian, prostatic carcinomas; myelodysplastic syndrome; psoriasis.

PRECAUTIONS

CONTRAINDICATIONS: When systemic therapy is required (more than 10 new KS lesions in previous month), symptomatic pulmonary KS, symptomatic visceral involvement or symptomatic lymphedema in KS. **CAUTIONS:** None known. **Pregnancy Category D.**

INTERACTIONS

DRUG: **DEET (component of insect repellent):** Alitretinoin use increases risk of toxicity to products containing DEET. HERBAL: None known. FOOD: None known. LAB VALUES: None known.

AVAILABILITY (Rx)

GEL: 0.1%.

INDICATIONS/ROUTES/DOSAGE

KAPOSI'S SARCOMA

TOPICAL: ADULTS: Initially, apply twice a day to lesions. May increase to 3–4 times a day. Allow gel to dry 3–5 min before

---

covering with clothing. Do not use occlusive dressings.

SIDE EFFECTS

FREQUENT (greater than 5%): Rash (erythema, scaling, irritation, redness, dermatitis), pruritus, exfoliative dermatitis (flaking, peeling, desquamation, exfoliation), stinging, tingling, edema, skin disorders (scabbing, crusting, drainage).

ADVERSE REACTIONS/ TOXIC EFFECTS

Severe local skin reaction (intense erythema, edema, vesiculation) may limit treatment.

NURSING CONSIDERATIONS

PATIENT/FAMILY TEACHING

• Do not apply dressings over medication gel. • Do not apply gel to healthy skin surrounding lesions or on or near mucosal surfaces. • If severe irritation occurs, frequency of application can be reduced or discontinued for a few days until symptoms subside.

Allegra, *see fexofenadine*

Allegra-D, *see fexofenadine and pseudoephedrine*

---

allopurinol

al-low-**pure**-ih-nal
(Aloprim, Apo-Allopurinol ✦, Zyloprim)

Do not confuse Zyloprim with ZORprin.

◆CLASSIFICATION

PHARMACOTHERAPEUTIC: Xanthine oxidase inhibitor. **CLINICAL:** Antigout.

ACTION

A xanthine oxidase inhibitor that decreases uric acid production by inhibiting xanthine oxidase, an enzyme. **Therapeutic Effect:** Reduces uric acid concentrations in both serum and urine.

PHARMACOKINETICS

Route	Onset	Peak	Duration
PO, IV	2–3 days	1–3 wk	1–2 wk

Well absorbed from the GI tract. Widely distributed. Metabolized in the liver to active metabolite. Excreted primarily in urine. Removed by hemodialysis. **Half-life:** 1–3 hr; metabolite, 12–30 hr.

USES

Oral: Prevents attacks of gouty arthritis, nephropathy. Treatment of secondary hyperuricemia that may occur during cancer treatment. Prevents recurrent uric acid and calcium oxalate calculi. **Injection:** Management of elevated uric acid in cancer patients unable to tolerate oral therapy. **OFF-LABEL:** In mouthwash following fluorouracil therapy to prevent stomatitis.

PRECAUTIONS

CONTRAINDICATIONS: Asymptomatic hyperuricemia. **CAUTIONS:** Impaired renal, hepatic function, CHF, diabetes mellitus, hypertension.

⌛ LIFESPAN CONSIDERATIONS: **Pregnancy/Lactation:** Unknown if drug crosses placenta or is distributed in breast milk. **Pregnancy Category C. Children/Elderly:** No age-related precautions noted.

INTERACTIONS

DRUG: Amoxicillin, ampicillin: May increase incidence of rash. **Angiotensin-converting enzyme (ACE) inhibitors:** May cause hypersensitivity reactions. **Azathioprine, mercaptopurine:** May increase therapeutic effect and toxicity of azathioprine and mercaptopurine. **Oral anticoagulants:** May increase anticoagulant effect. **Thiazide diuretics:** May decrease the effect of allopurinol. **HERBAL:** None known. **FOOD:** None known. **LAB VALUES:** May increase BUN, serum creatinine, serum alkaline phosphatase, AST, and ALT levels.

AVAILABILITY (Rx)

TABLETS (ZYLOPRIM): 100 mg, 300 mg. **POWDER FOR INJECTION (ALOPRIM):** 500 mg.

ADMINISTRATION/HANDLING

 IV

Reconstitution • Reconstitute 500-mg vial with 25 ml sterile water for injection, giving a clear, almost colorless solution (concentration of 20 mg/ml). • Further dilute with 0.9% NaCl or D_5W (19 ml of added diluent yields 1 mg/ml, 9 ml yields 2 mg/ml, 2.3 ml yields maximum concentration of 6 mg/ml).

Rate of administration • Infuse over 30–60 min.

Storage • Store unreconstituted vials at room temperature. • May store reconstituted solution at room temperature and give within 10 hr. Do not use if precipitate forms or solution is discolored.

PO

• May give with or immediately after meals or milk. • Instruct patient to drink at least 10–12 eight-oz glasses of water/day. • Dosages greater than 300 mg/day to be administered in divided doses.

IV INCOMPATIBILITIES

Amikacin (Amikin), carmustine (BiCNU), cefotaxime (Claforan), chlorpromazine (Thorazine), cimetidine (Tagamet), clindamycin (Cleocin), cytarabine (Ara-C), dacarbazine (DTIC), diphenhydramine (Benadryl), doxorubicin (Adriamycin), doxycycline (Vibramycin), droperidol (Inapsine), fludarabine (Fludara), gentamicin (Garamycin), haloperidol (Haldol), hydroxyzine (Vistaril), idarubicin (Idamycin), imipenem-cilastatin (Primaxin), meperidine (Demerol), methylprednisolone (Solu-Medrol), metoclopramide (Reglan), ondansetron (Zofran), prochlorperazine (Compazine), promethazine (Phenergan), streptozocin (Zanosar), tobramycin (Nebcin), vinorelbine (Navelbine).

IV COMPATIBILITIES

Bumetanide (Bumex), calcium gluconate, furosemide (Lasix), heparin, hydromorphone (Dilaudid), lorazepam (Ativan), morphine, potassium chloride.

INDICATIONS/ROUTES/DOSAGE

CHRONIC GOUTY ARTHRITIS

PO: ADULTS, CHILDREN OLDER THAN 10 YR: Initially, 100 mg/day; may increase by 100 mg/day at weekly intervals. **Maximum:** 800 mg/day. Maintenance: 100–200 mg 2–3 times a day or 300 mg/day.

TO PREVENT URIC ACID NEPHROPATHY DURING CHEMOTHERAPY

◀ **ALERT** ▶ Maintenance dosage is based on serum uric acid levels. Discontinue following the period of tumor regression. **PO:** ADULTS: Initially, 600–800 mg/day starting 2–3 days before initiation of chemotherapy or radiation therapy. CHILDREN 6–10 YR: 100 mg 3 times a day or 300 mg once a day. CHILDREN LESS THAN 6 YR: 50 mg 3 times a day. **IV:** ADULTS: 200–400 mg/m^2/day beginning 24–48 hr before initiation of chemotherapy. CHILDREN: 200 mg/m^2/day. **Maximum:** 600 mg/day.

PREVENTION OF URIC ACID CALCULI
PO: ADULTS: 100–200 mg 1–4 times a day or 300 mg once a day.

RECURRENT CALCIUM OXALATE CALCULI
PO: ADULTS: 200–300 mg/day. ELDERLY: Initially, 100 mg/day, gradually increased until optimal uric acid level is reached.

DOSAGE IN RENAL IMPAIRMENT
Dosage is modified based on creatinine clearance.

Creatinine Clearance	Dosage Adjustment
10–20 ml/min	200 mg/day
3–9 ml/min	100 mg/day
Less than 3 ml/min	100 mg at extended intervals

SIDE EFFECTS
OCCASIONAL: Oral: Somnolence, unusual hair loss. **IV:** Rash, nausea, vomiting. **RARE:** Diarrhea, headache.

ADVERSE REACTIONS/ TOXIC EFFECTS
Pruritic maculopapular rash possibly accompanied by malaise, fever, chills, joint pain, nausea, and vomiting should be considered a toxic reaction. Severe hypersensitivity may follow appearance of rash. Bone marrow depression, hepatic toxicity, peripheral neuritis, and acute renal failure occur rarely.

NURSING CONSIDERATIONS

BASELINE ASSESSMENT
Instruct patient to drink 10–12 glasses (8 oz) of fluid daily while taking medication.

INTERVENTION/EVALUATION
Discontinue medication immediately if rash or other evidence of allergic reaction appears. Monitor I&O (output should be at least 2,000 ml/day). Assess CBC, uric acid and hepatic function serum levels. Assess urine for cloudiness, unusual color, odor. Assess for therapeutic response (reduced joint tenderness, swelling, redness, limited motion).

PATIENT/FAMILY TEACHING
• May take 1 wk or longer for full therapeutic effect. • Encourage drinking 10–12 glasses (8 oz) of fluid daily while taking medication. • Avoid tasks that require alertness, motor skills until response to drug is established.

almotriptan malate

al-moe-**trip**-tan
(Axert)
Do not confuse Axert with Antivert.

◆CLASSIFICATION
PHARMACOTHERAPEUTIC: Serotonin receptor agonist. **CLINICAL:** Antimigraine (see p. 56C).

ACTION
A serotonin receptor agonist that binds selectively to vascular receptors, producing a vasoconstrictive effect on cranial blood vessels. **Therapeutic Effect:** Produces relief of migraine headache.

PHARMACOKINETICS
Well absorbed after PO administration. Metabolized by the liver, excreted in urine. **Half-life:** 3–4 hr.

USES
Acute treatment of migraine headache with or without aura.

PRECAUTIONS
CONTRAINDICATIONS: Arrhythmias associated with conduction disorders,

hemiplegic or basilar migraine, ischemic heart disease (including angina pectoris, history of MI, silent ischemia, and Prinzmetal's angina), uncontrolled hypertension, use within 24 hr of ergotamine-containing preparation or another serotonin receptor antagonist, use within 14 days of MAOIs, Wolff-Parkinson-White syndrome. **CAUTIONS:** Mild to moderate renal or hepatic impairment, patient profile suggesting cardiovascular risks, controlled hypertension, history of cerebrovascular accident (CVA).

⏳ LIFESPAN CONSIDERATIONS: **Pregnancy/Lactation:** Unknown if distributed in breast milk. **Pregnancy Category C. Children:** Safety and efficacy not established in patients younger than 12 yr. **Elderly:** No age-related precautions noted.

INTERACTIONS

DRUG: **Ergotamine-containing medications:** May produce a vasospastic reaction. **Erythromycin, itraconazole, ketoconazole, MAOIs, ritonavir:** May increase the almotriptan plasma level. **Fluoxetine, fluvoxamine, paroxetine, sertraline:** May produce weakness, hyperreflexia, and incoordination. HERBAL: None known. FOOD: None known. LAB VALUES: None known.

AVAILABILITY (Rx)

TABLETS: 6.5 mg, 12.5 mg.

ADMINISTRATION/HANDLING
PO
• Swallow tablets whole. • Take with full glass of water.

INDICATIONS/ROUTES/DOSAGE
MIGRAINE HEADACHE
PO: ADULTS, ELDERLY: Initially, 6.25–12.5 mg as a single dose. If headache improves but then returns, dose may be repeated after 2 hr. **Maximum:** 2 doses/24 hr.

DOSAGE IN RENAL IMPAIRMENT
For adult and elderly patients, recommended initial dose is 6.25 mg and maximum daily dose is 12.5 mg.

SIDE EFFECTS
FREQUENT: Nausea, dry mouth, paresthesia, flushing. OCCASIONAL: Changes in temperature sensation, asthenia, dizziness.

ADVERSE REACTIONS/ TOXIC EFFECTS

Excessive dosage may produce tremor, red extremities, reduced respirations, cyanosis, seizures, and chest pain. Serious arrhythmias occur rarely, particularly in patients with hypertension or diabetes, obese patients, smokers, and those with a strong family history of coronary artery disease.

NURSING CONSIDERATIONS

BASELINE ASSESSMENT
Question for history of peripheral vascular disease. Question patient regarding onset, location, duration of migraine and possible precipitating symptoms.

INTERVENTION/EVALUATION
Evaluate for relief of migraine headache and resulting photophobia, phonophobia (sound sensitivity), nausea, vomiting.

PATIENT/FAMILY TEACHING
• Take a single dose as soon as symptoms of an actual migraine attack appear. • Medication is intended to relieve migraine, not to prevent or reduce number of attacks. • Lie down in quiet, dark room for additional benefit after taking medication. • Avoid tasks that require alertness, motor skills until response to drug is established. • If palpitations, pain or tightness in chest or throat, or pain or weakness of extremities occurs, contact physician immediately.

alprazolam

ale-**praz**-oh-lam

(Apo-Alpraz 🍁, Niravam, Novo-Alprazol 🍁, Xanax, Xanax XR)

Do not confuse alprazolam with lorazepam, or Xanax with Tenex or Zantac.

◆CLASSIFICATION

PHARMACOTHERAPEUTIC: Benzodiazepine (**Schedule IV**). **CLINICAL:** Antianxiety (see p. 11C).

ACTION

A benzodiazepine that enhances the action of the inhibitory neurotransmitter gamma-aminobutyric acid in the brain. Therapeutic Effect: Produces anxiolytic effect from its CNS depressant action.

PHARMACOKINETICS

Well absorbed from GI tract. Protein binding: 80%. Metabolized in the liver. Primarily excreted in urine. Minimal removal by hemodialysis. Half-life: 11–16 hr.

USES

Management of anxiety disorders associated with depression, panic disorder. OFF-LABEL: Management of premenstrual syndrome symptoms (mood disturbances, insomnia, and cramps), irritable bowel syndrome, treatment of agoraphobia, post-traumatic stress disorder, tremors, ethanol withdrawal, anxiety in children.

PRECAUTIONS

CONTRAINDICATIONS: Acute alcohol intoxication with depressed vital signs, acute angle-closure glaucoma, concurrent use of itraconazole or ketoconazole, myasthenia gravis, severe COPD. **CAUTIONS:** Impaired renal/hepatic function.

⏳ LIFESPAN CONSIDERATIONS: Pregnancy/Lactation: Crosses placenta; distributed in breast milk. Chronic ingestion during pregnancy may produce withdrawal symptoms, CNS depression in neonates. **Pregnancy Category D. Children:** Safety and efficacy not established. **Elderly:** Use small initial doses with gradual increase to avoid ataxia (muscular incoordination) or excessive sedation.

INTERACTIONS

DRUG: **Alcohol, other CNS depressants:** Potentiate effects of alprazolam and may increase sedation. **Fluvoxamine, itraconazole, ketoconazole, nefazodone:** May inhibit metabolism and increase serum concentrations of alprazolam. HERBAL: **Kava kava, valerian:** May increase CNS depressant effect of alprazolam. **St. John's wort:** May reduce effectiveness of alprazolam. FOOD: **Grapefruit, grapefruit juice:** May inhibit alprazolam's metabolism. LAB VALUES: None known.

AVAILABILITY (Rx)

ORAL SOLUTION (ALPRAZOLAM INTENSOL): 1 mg/ml. **TABLETS (XANAX):** 0.25 mg, 0.5 mg, 1 mg, 2 mg. **TABLETS (EXTENDED-RELEASE [XANAX XR]):** 0.5 mg, 1 mg, 2 mg, 3 mg. **TABLETS (ORALLY-DISINTEGRATING [NIRAVAM]):** 0.25 mg, 0.5 mg, 1 mg, 2 mg.

ADMINISTRATION/HANDLING

PO, IMMEDIATE-RELEASE

• May be given without regard to meals. • Tablets may be crushed.

PO, EXTENDED-RELEASE

• Administer once daily. • Do not crush, chew, break. Swallow whole.

PO, ORALLY DISINTEGRATING

• Place tablet on tongue, allow to dissolve. • Swallow with saliva.

INDICATIONS/ROUTES/DOSAGE

ANXIETY DISORDERS

PO (IMMEDIATE-RELEASE): ADULTS: Initially, 0.25–0.5 mg 3 times a day. May titrate q3–4 days. **Maximum:** 4 mg/day in divided doses. ELDERLY, DEBILITATED PATIENTS, PATIENTS WITH HEPATIC DISEASE OR LOW SERUM ALBUMIN: Initially, 0.25 mg 2–3 times a day. Gradually increase to optimum therapeutic response.

PO (ORALLY-DISINTEGRATING): ADULTS: 0.25–0.5 mg 3 times a day. **Maximum:** 4 mg/day in divided doses.

ANXIETY WITH DEPRESSION

PO: ADULTS: 2.5–3 mg/day in divided doses.

PANIC DISORDER

PO (IMMEDIATE-RELEASE): ADULTS: Initially, 0.5 mg 3 times a day. May increase at 3- to 4-day intervals. Range: 5–6 mg/day. **Maximum:** 10 mg/day. ELDERLY: Initially, 0.125–0.25 mg twice a day. May increase in 0.125-mg increments until desired effect attained.

PO (EXTENDED-RELEASE):

◄ ALERT ► To switch from immediate-release to extended–release form, give total daily dose (immediate–release) as a single daily dose of extended–release form. ADULTS: Initially, 0.5–1 mg once a day. May titrate at 3- to 4-day intervals. Range: 3–6 mg/day. **Maximum:** 10 mg/day. ELDERLY: Initially, 0.5 mg once daily.

PO (ORALLY-DISINTEGRATING): ADULTS: Initially, 0.5 mg 3 times a day. May increase at 3- to 4-day intervals. Range: 5–6 mg/day. **Maximum:** 10 mg/day.

PREMENSTRUAL SYNDROME

PO: ADULTS: 0.25 mg 3 times a day.

SIDE EFFECTS

FREQUENT: Ataxia; lightheadedness; transient, mild somnolence; slurred speech (particularly in elderly or debilitated patients). **OCCASIONAL:** Confusion, depression, blurred vision, constipation, diarrhea, dry mouth, headache, nausea. **RARE:** Behavioral problems such as anger, impaired memory, paradoxical reactions such as insomnia, nervousness, or irritability.

ADVERSE REACTIONS/ TOXIC EFFECTS

Abrupt or too rapid withdrawal may result in pronounced restlessness, irritability, insomnia, hand tremors, abdominal and muscle cramps, diaphoresis, vomiting, and seizures. Overdose results in somnolence, confusion, diminished reflexes, and coma. Blood dyscrasias have been reported rarely.

NURSING CONSIDERATIONS

BASELINE ASSESSMENT

Offer emotional support to anxious patient. Assess motor responses (agitation, trembling, tension), autonomic responses (cold/clammy hands, diaphoresis).

INTERVENTION/EVALUATION

For those on long-term therapy, perform liver/renal function tests, blood counts periodically. Assess for paradoxical reaction, particularly during early therapy. Evaluate for therapeutic response: calm facial expression, decreased restlessness, insomnia.

PATIENT/FAMILY TEACHING

• Drowsiness usually disappears during continued therapy. • If dizziness occurs, change positions slowly from recumbent to sitting position before standing. • Avoid tasks that require alertness, motor skills until response to drug is established. • Smoking reduces drug effectiveness. • Sour hard candy, gum, sips of tepid water may relieve dry mouth. • Do not abruptly withdraw medication after long-term therapy. • Avoid alcohol. • Do not take other medications without consulting physician.

alprostadil (prostaglandin E₁; PGE₁)

ale-**pros**-tah-dill

(Caverject, Edex, Edex Refill, Muse, Prostin VR Pediatric)

◆ CLASSIFICATION

PHARMACOTHERAPEUTIC: Prostaglandin. **CLINICAL:** Patent ductus arteriosus agent, anti-impotence.

ACTION

A prostaglandin that directly affects vascular and ductus arteriosus smooth muscle and relaxes trabecular smooth muscle. **Therapeutic Effect:** Causes vasodilation; dilates cavernosal arteries, allowing blood flow to and entrapment in the lacunar spaces of the penis.

USES

Temporarily maintains patency of ductus arteriosus until surgery is performed in those with congenital heart defects and dependent on patent ductus for survival (e.g., pulmonary atresia or stenosis). Treatment of erectile dysfunction due to neurogenic, vasculogenic, psychogenic causes; adjunct in diagnosis of erectile dysfunction. **OFF-LABEL:** Treatment of atherosclerosis, gangrene, pain due to severe peripheral arterial occlusive disease, treatment of pulmonary hypertension in infants, children.

PRECAUTIONS

CONTRAINDICATIONS: Conditions predisposing to anatomic deformation of penis, hyaline membrane disease, penile implants, priapism, respiratory distress syndrome. **CAUTIONS:** Severe hepatic disease, coagulation defects, leukemia, multiple myeloma, polycythemia, sickle cell disease, thrombocythemia. **Pregnancy Category C.**

INTERACTIONS

DRUG: Anticoagulants, including heparin, thrombolytics: May increase risk of bleeding. **Sympathomimetics:** May decrease effect of alprostadil. **Vasodilators:** May increase risk of hypotension. **HERBAL:** None known. **FOOD:** None known. **LAB VALUES:** May increase blood bilirubin levels. May decrease glucose, serum calcium, and serum potassium levels.

AVAILABILITY (Rx)

INJECTION (PROSTIN VR PEDIATRIC): 500 mcg/ml. **POWDER FOR INJECTION (CAVERJECT, EDEX):** 10 mcg, 20 mcg, 40 mcg. **URETHRAL PELLET (MUSE):** 125 mcg, 250 mcg, 500 mcg, 1,000 mcg.

ADMINISTRATION/HANDLING

URETHRAL PELLET

Storage: Refrigerate pellet unless used within 14 days.

 IV

Reconstitution • Dilute 500-mcg ampule with D₅W or 0.9% NaCl to volume dependent on infusion pump capabilities.

Rate of administration • Infuse for shortest time, lowest dose possible. • If significant decrease in arterial pressure is noted via umbilical artery catheter, auscultation, or Doppler transducer, decrease infusion rate immediately. • Discontinue infusion immediately if apnea or bradycardia occurs (overdosage).

Storage • Store parenteral form in refrigerator. • Must dilute before use. • Prepare fresh q24h. • Discard unused portions.

▦ IV INCOMPATIBILITIES

No information available.

INDICATIONS/ROUTES/DOSAGE

MAINTAIN PATENCY OF DUCTUS ARTERIOSUS

IV INFUSION: NEONATES: Initially, 0.05–0.1 mcg/kg/min. Maintenance: 0.01–0.4 mcg/kg/min. **Maximum:** 0.4 mcg/kg/min.

IMPOTENCE

PELLET, INTRACAVERNOSAL: ADULTS: Dosage is individualized.

SIDE EFFECTS

FREQUENT: Intracavernosal (4%–1%): Penile pain (37%), prolonged erection, hypertension, localized pain, penile fibrosis, injection site hematoma or ecchymosis, headache, respiratory infection, flu-like symptoms. **Intraurethral (3%):** Penile pain (36%), urethral pain or burning, testicular pain, urethral bleeding, headache, dizziness, respiratory infection, flu-like symptoms. **Systemic (greater than 1%):** Fever, flushing, bradycardia, hypotension, tachycardia, diarrhea. **OCCASIONAL: Intracavernosal (less than 1%):** Hypotension, pelvic pain, back pain, dizziness, cough, nasal congestion. **Intraurethral (less than 3%):** Fainting, sinusitis, back and pelvic pain. **Systemic (less than 1%):** Anxiety, lethargy, myalgia, arrhythmias, respiratory depression, anemia, bleeding, hematuria.

ADVERSE REACTIONS/ TOXIC EFFECTS

◀ **ALERT** ▶ Apnea is experienced by about 10%–12% of neonates with congenital heart defects.
Overdose is manifested as apnea, flushing of the face and arms, and bradycardia. Cardiac arrest and sepsis occur rarely. Seizures, apnea, sepsis, and thrombocytopenia occur rarely.

NURSING CONSIDERATIONS

INTERVENTION/EVALUATION

Patent Ductus Arteriosus: Monitor arterial pressure by umbilical artery catheter, auscultation, Doppler transducer. If significant decrease in arterial pressure occurs, decrease infusion rate immediately. Maintain continuous cardiac monitoring. Assess heart sounds, femoral pulse (circulation to lower extremities), respiratory status frequently. Monitor for symptoms of hypotension. Assess BP, arterial blood gases, temperature. If apnea or bradycardia occurs, discontinue infusion and notify physician. In infants with restricted systemic blood flow, efficacy should be measured by monitoring improvement of systemic blood pressure and blood pH.

PATIENT/FAMILY TEACHING

• **Patent Ductus Arteriosus:** Explain purpose of this palliative therapy to parents. • **Impotence:** Erection is to occur within 2–5 min. • Do not use if female is pregnant (unless using condom barrier). • Inform physician if erection lasts longer than 4 hr or becomes painful.

Altace, *see ramipril*

---

alteplase, recombinant   ⚐

all-teh-place
(Activase, Cathflo Activase)
Do not confuse alteplase or Activase with Altace.

◆CLASSIFICATION

PHARMACOTHERAPEUTIC: Tissue plasminogen activator (tPA). **CLINICAL:** Thrombolytic (see p. 32C).

ACTION

A tissue plasminogen activator that acts

as a thrombolytic by binding to the fibrin in a thrombus and converting entrapped plasminogen to plasmin. This process initiates fibrinolysis. **Therapeutic Effect:** Degrades fibrin clots, fibrinogen, and other plasma proteins.

PHARMACOKINETICS

Rapidly metabolized in the liver. Primarily excreted in urine. **Half-life:** 35 min.

USES

Treatment of acute MI, acute ischemic stroke, acute massive pulmonary embolism. Treatment of occluded central venous catheters. **OFF-LABEL:** Acute peripheral occlusive disease, basilar artery occlusion, cerebral infarction, deep vein thrombosis, femoropopliteal artery occlusion, mesenteric or subclavian vein occlusion, pleural effusion (parapneumonic).

PRECAUTIONS

CONTRAINDICATIONS: Active internal bleeding, AV malformation or aneurysm, bleeding diathesis, intracranial neoplasm, intracranial or intraspinal surgery or trauma, recent (within past 2 mo) cerebrovascular accident, severe uncontrolled hypertension. **CAUTIONS:** Recent (within 10 days) major surgery or GI bleeding, OB delivery, organ biopsy, recent trauma (CPR, left heart thrombus, endocarditis, severe hepatic/renal disease, pregnancy, elderly, cerebrovascular disease, diabetic retinopathy, thrombophlebitis, occluded AV cannula at infected site).

⏳ **LIFESPAN CONSIDERATIONS: Pregnancy/Lactation:** Use only when benefit outweighs potential risk to fetus. Unknown if drug crosses placenta or is distributed in breast milk. **Pregnancy Category C. Children:** Safety and efficacy not established. **Elderly:** Risk of bleeding with thrombolytic therapy increased, careful patient selection, monitoring recommended.

INTERACTIONS

DRUG: Anticoagulants, including **cefotetan, heparin, plicamycin, valproic acid:** May increase risk of hemorrhage. **Platelet aggregation inhibitors, including aspirin, NSAIDs, ticlopidine:** May increase risk of bleeding. **HERBAL: Arnica, astragalus, bilberry, black currant, cat's claw, chaparral, dong quai, evening primrose, fenugreek, feverfew, garlic, ginger, ginkgo biloba, kava kava, licorice, tan-shen:** May increase the risk of bleeding. **FOOD:** None known. **LAB VALUES:** Decreases plasminogen and fibrinogen levels during infusion, which decreases clotting time (and confirms the presence of lysis). Decreases Hgb and Hct.

AVAILABILITY (Rx)

POWDER FOR INJECTION: 2 mg (Cathflo Activase), 50 mg (Activase), 100 mg (Activase).

ADMINISTRATION/HANDLING

 IV

Reconstitution • Reconstitute immediately before use with sterile water for injection. • Reconstitute 100-mg vial with 100 ml sterile water for injection (50-mg vial with 50 ml sterile water) without preservative to provide a concentration of 1 mg/ml. May be further diluted with equal volume D_5W or 0.9% NaCl to provide a concentration of 0.5 mg/ml. • Avoid excessive agitation; gently swirl or slowly invert vial to reconstitute.

Rate of administration • Give by IV infusion via infusion pump. See individual dosages. • If minor bleeding occurs at puncture sites, apply pressure for 30 sec; if unrelieved, apply pressure dressing. • If uncontrolled hemorrhage occurs, discontinue infusion immediately (slowing rate of infusion may produce worsening hemorrhage). • Avoid undue pressure when drug is injected into catheter (can rupture catheter or expel clot into circulation).

Storage • Store vials at room temperature. • After reconstitution, solutions appear colorless to pale yellow. • Solution is stable for 8 hr after reconstitution. Discard unused portions.

❀ IV INCOMPATIBILITIES

Dobutamine (Dobutrex), dopamine (Intropin), heparin, nitroglycerin.

IV COMPATIBILITIES

Lidocaine, metoprolol (Lopressor), morphine, nitroglycerin, propranolol (Inderal).

INDICATIONS/ROUTES/DOSAGE

ACUTE MI

IV INFUSION: ADULTS WEIGHING GREATER THAN 67 KG: 100 mg over 90 min, starting with 15-mg bolus over 1–2 min, then 50 mg over 30 min, then 35 mg over 60 min. Or a 3-hour infusion, giving 60 mg over first hr (6–10 mg as bolus over 1–2 min), 20 mg over second hr, and 20 mg over third hr. ADULTS WEIGHING 67 KG OR LESS: 100 mg over 90 min, starting with 15-mg bolus, then 0.75 mg/kg over 30 min (**Maximum:** 50 mg), then 0.5 mg/kg over 60 min (**Maximum:** 35 mg). Or 3-hour infusion of 1.25 mg/kg giving 60% of dose over first hr (6%–10% as 1- to 2-min bolus), 20% over second hr, and 20% over third hr.

ACUTE PULMONARY EMBOLI

IV INFUSION: ADULTS: 100 mg over 2 hr. Institute or reinstitute heparin near end or immediately after infusion when aPTT or thrombin time (TT) returns to twice normal or less.

ACUTE ISCHEMIC STROKE

◂ ALERT ▸ Dose should be given within the first 3 hr of the onset of symptoms. **IV INFUSION:** ADULTS: 0.9 mg/kg over 60 min (load with 0.09 mg/kg [10% of 0.9 mg/kg dose] as IV bolus over 1 min).

CENTRAL VENOUS CATHETER CLEARANCE

IV: ADULTS, ELDERLY: 2 mg; may repeat after 2 hr.

SIDE EFFECTS

FREQUENT: Superficial bleeding at puncture sites, decreased BP. **OCCASIONAL:** Allergic reactions, such as rash or wheezing; bruising.

ADVERSE REACTIONS/ TOXIC EFFECTS

Severe internal hemorrhage may occur. Lysis of coronary thrombi may produce atrial or ventricular arrhythmias or stroke.

NURSING CONSIDERATIONS

BASELINE ASSESSMENT

Obtain baseline BP, apical pulse. Record weight. Evaluate 12-lead EKG, CPK, CPK-MB, electrolytes. Assess Hct, platelet count, thrombin (TT), aPTT, PT, fibrinogen level before therapy is instituted. Type and hold blood.

INTERVENTION/EVALUATION

Perform continuous cardiac monitoring for arrhythmias. Check BP, pulse, and respirations q15 min until stable, then hourly. Check peripheral pulses, heart and lung sounds. Monitor chest pain relief and notify physician of continuation or recurrence (note location, type, intensity). Assess for bleeding: overt blood, blood in any body substance. Monitor PTT per protocol. Maintain BP; avoid any trauma that might increase risk of bleeding (e.g., injections, shaving). Assess neurologic status.

altretamine (hexamethyl-melamine)

(Hexalen)
See Antineoplastics (p. 71C)

aluminum hydroxide

a-**loo**-mi-num hye-**drox**-ide
(Alternagel, Amphojel ✤, Basaljel
✤)

FIXED-COMBINATION(S)

With magnesium, an antacid (**Gaviscon, Maalox**); with magnesium
and simethicone, an antiflatulent
(**Gelusil, Maalox Plus, Mylanta,
Silain-Gel**).

◆ CLASSIFICATION

CLINICAL: Antacid (p. 9C).

ACTION

An antacid that reduces gastric acid
by binding with phosphate in the
intestine and is then excreted as aluminum carbonate in feces; decreased
serum phosphate levels may result
in increased absorption of calcium.
The drug also has astringent and
adsorbent properties. **Therapeutic
Effect:** Neutralizes or increases gastric
pH; reduces phosphate levels in
urine, preventing formation of phosphate
urinary calculi; reduces the serum phosphate level; decreases the fluidity of
stools.

USES

Treatment of hyperacidity, hyperphosphatemia.

PRECAUTIONS

CONTRAINDICATIONS: Children   age
6 yr and younger, intestinal obstruction. **CAUTIONS:** Impaired renal function,   gastric   outlet   obstruction,
elderly, dehydration, fluid restriction,
Alzheimer's disease, symptoms of appendicitis, GI/rectal bleeding, constipation, fecal impaction, chronic diarrhea.
**Pregnancy Category C (considered
safe except for chronic, high-dose
usage).**

INTERACTIONS

DRUG: Anticholinergics,   quinidine:
May decrease excretion of aluminum
hydroxide. **Iron preparations, isoniazid,   ketoconazole,   quinolones,
tetracyclines:** May decrease absorption of aluminum hydroxide. **Methenamine:** May decrease effects of the
methenamine. **Salicylate:** May increase
salicylate   excretion.   **HERBAL:** None
known.   **FOOD:** None   known.   **LAB
VALUES:** May   increase   the   serum
gastrin level and systemic and urinary
pH. May decrease the serum phosphate
level.

AVAILABILITY (OTC)

CAPSULES: 475   mg.   **SUSPENSION
(ALTERNAGEL):**   320 mg/5 ml, 600 mg/
5 ml.

ADMINISTRATION/HANDLING

PO
• Usually administered 1–3 hr after
meals. • Individualize dose (based on
neutralizing   capacity   of   antacids).
• Chewable tablets (fixed combinations): Thoroughly chew tablets before
swallowing (follow with glass of water
or milk). • If administering suspension,
shake well before use.

INDICATIONS/ROUTES/DOSAGE

ANTACID
PO: ADULTS, ELDERLY: 600–1,200   mg
between meals and at bedtime.

HYPERPHOSPHATEMIA
PO: ADULTS, ELDERLY: Initially, 300–600 mg
3 times a day with meals.   CHILDREN:
Initially, 50–150 mg/kg/day in divided
doses q4–6h. Titrate to maintain serum
phosphorus within normal range.

SIDE EFFECTS

FREQUENT: Chalky taste, mild constipation, abdominal cramps. **OCCASIONAL:**
Nausea, vomiting, speckling or whitish
discoloration of stools.

✤ Canadian trade name   @ see **evolve**   ▶ High Alert drug

ADVERSE REACTIONS/ TOXIC EFFECTS

Prolonged constipation may result in intestinal obstruction. Excessive or chronic use may produce hypophosphatemia manifested as anorexia, malaise, muscle weakness, or bone pain, which may result in osteomalacia and osteoporosis. Prolonged use may produce urinary calculi.

NURSING CONSIDERATIONS

BASELINE ASSESSMENT

Do not give other PO medication within 1–2 hr of antacid administration.

INTERVENTION/EVALUATION

Assess pattern of daily bowel activity and stool consistency. Monitor serum phosphate, calcium, uric acid, aluminum levels. Assess for relief of gastric distress.

PATIENT/FAMILY TEACHING

• **Chewable Tablets (fixed combinations):** Chew tablets thoroughly before swallowing (may be followed by water or milk). • Tablets may discolor stool. • Maintain adequate fluid intake.

---

amantadine hydrochloride

ah-**man**-tih-deen

(Endantadine ✤ , PMS-Amantadine ✤ , Symmetrel)

◆CLASSIFICATION

PHARMACOTHERAPEUTIC: Dopaminergic agonist. **CLINICAL:** Antiviral, antiparkinson agent (see p. 60C).

ACTION

A dopaminergic agonist that blocks the uncoating of influenza A virus, preventing penetration into the host and inhibiting M2 protein in the assembly of progeny virions. Amantadine also blocks the reuptake of dopamine into presynaptic neurons and causes direct stimulation of postsynaptic receptors. **Therapeutic Effect:** Antiviral and antiparkinsonian activity.

PHARMACOKINETICS

Rapidly and completely absorbed from the GI tract. Protein binding: 67%. Widely distributed. Primarily excreted in urine. Minimally removed by hemodialysis. **Half-life:** 11–15 hr (increased in the elderly, decreased in impaired renal function).

USES

Prevention, treatment of respiratory tract infections due to influenza virus, Parkinson's disease, drug-induced extrapyramidal reactions. **OFF-LABEL:** Treatment of ADHD, fatigue associated with multiple sclerosis.

PRECAUTIONS

CONTRAINDICATIONS: None known. **CAUTIONS:** History of seizures, orthostatic hypotension, CHF, peripheral edema, hepatic disease, recurrent eczematoid dermatitis, cerebrovascular disease, renal dysfunction, those receiving CNS stimulants.

⧗ **LIFESPAN CONSIDERATIONS: Pregnancy/Lactation:** Unknown if drug crosses placenta; distributed in breast milk. **Pregnancy Category C. Children:** No age-related precautions noted in those older than 1 yr. **Elderly:** May exhibit increased sensitivity to anticholinergic effects. Age-related decreased renal function may require dosage adjustment.

INTERACTIONS

DRUG: Alcohol: May increase CNS effects, including dizziness, confusion,

---

light-headedness, and orthostatic hypotension. **Anticholinergics, antihistamines, phenothiazine, tricyclic antidepressants:** May increase anticholinergic effects of amantadine. **Hydrochlorothiazide, triamterene:** May increase amantadine blood concentration and risk for toxicity. **HERBAL:** None known. **FOOD:** None known. **LAB VALUES:** None known.

AVAILABILITY (Rx)

CAPSULES: 100 mg. **SYRUP:** 50 mg/5 ml. **TABLETS:** 100 mg.

ADMINISTRATION/HANDLING

PO

• May give without regard to food.
• Administer nighttime dose several hours before bedtime (prevents insomnia).

INDICATIONS/ROUTES/DOSAGE

TREATMENT OF INFLUENZA A

PO: ADULTS, CHILDREN 13 YR AND OLDER: 100 mg twice a day. Initiate within 24–48 hr after onset of symptoms; discontinue as soon as possible based on clinical response. ELDERLY: 100 mg a day. CHILDREN 10–12 YR, WEIGHING 40 KG AND MORE: 100 mg twice a day. CHILDREN 10 YR AND OLDER, WEIGHING LESS THAN 40 KG: 5 mg/kg/day. **Maximum:** 150 mg/day. CHILDREN 1–9 YR: 5 mg/kg/day. **Maximum:** 150 mg/day.

PREVENTION OF INFUENZA A

PO: ADULTS, CHILDREN 13 YR AND OLDER: 100 mg twice a day.

PARKINSON'S DISEASE, EXTRAPYRAMIDAL SYMPTOMS

PO: ADULTS, ELDERLY: 100 mg twice a day. May increase up to 400 mg/day in divided doses.

DOSAGE IN RENAL IMPAIRMENT

Dose and frequency are modified based on creatinine clearance.

Creatinine Clearance	Dosage
30–50 ml/min	200 mg first day; 100 mg/day thereafter
15–29 ml/min	200 mg first day; 100 mg on alternate days
Less than 15 ml/min	200 mg every 7 days

SIDE EFFECTS

FREQUENT (10%–5%): Nausea, dizziness, poor concentration, insomnia, nervousness. **OCCASIONAL (5%–1%):** Orthostatic hypotension, anorexia, headache, livedo reticularis (reddish blue, netlike blotching of skin), blurred vision, urine retention, dry mouth or nose. **RARE:** Vomiting, depression, irritation or swelling of eyes, rash.

ADVERSE REACTIONS/ TOXIC EFFECTS

CHF, leukopenia, and neutropenia occur rarely. Hyperexcitability, seizures, and ventricular arrhythmias may occur.

NURSING CONSIDERATIONS

BASELINE ASSESSMENT

When treating infections caused by influenza A virus, obtain specimens for viral diagnostic tests before giving first dose (therapy may begin before results are known).

INTERVENTION/EVALUATION

Monitor I&O, renal function tests if ordered; check for peripheral edema. Evaluate food tolerance, vomiting. Assess skin for mottling or rash. Assess for dizziness. **Parkinson's Disease:** Assess for clinical reversal of symptoms (improvement of tremor of head/hands at rest, mask-like facial expression, shuffling gait, muscular rigidity).

PATIENT/FAMILY TEACHING

• Continue therapy for full length of treatment. • Doses should be evenly spaced. • Do not take any other medications without consulting physician. • Avoid alcoholic beverages. • Do not drive, use machinery, or engage in other activities that require mental acuity if experiencing dizziness, blurred vision. • Get up slowly from a sitting or lying position. • Inform physician of new symptoms, especially blotching, rash, dizziness, blurred vision, nausea/vomiting. • Take nighttime dose several hours before bedtime to prevent insomnia.

Amaryl, *see glimepiride*

Ambien, *see zolpidem*

AmBisome, *see amphotericin B*

---

amcinonide

(Cyclocort)
See Corticosteroids: topical (p. 86C)

---

amifostine

am-ih-**fos**-teen
(Ethyol)
Do not confuse Ethyol with ethanol.

◆ CLASSIFICATION
PHARMACOTHERAPEUTIC: Antineoplastic adjunct. **CLINICAL:** Protective agent.

ACTION
An antineoplastic adjunct and cytoprotective agent that is converted to an active metabolite by alkaline phosphatase in tissues. The active metabolite binds to and detoxifies metabolites of cisplatin. These actions occur more readily in normal tissues than in tumor tissue. **Therapeutic Effect:** Reduces the toxic effect of the chemotherapeutic agent cisplatin.

USES
Reduces cumulative renal toxicity associated with repeated administration of cisplatin in those with advanced ovarian cancer. Treatment of postop radiation-induced dry mouth in patients with head or neck cancer. **OFF-LABEL:** Prophylaxis of antineoplastic agent-induced bone marrow toxicity, cisplatin-induced neurotoxicity, protection of lung fibroblasts from damaging effects of chemotherapeutic agent paclitaxel, reduction of mucositis of radiation therapy or radiation therapy combined with chemotherapy, treatment of myelodysplastic syndrome.

PRECAUTIONS
CONTRAINDICATIONS: Sensitivity to aminothiol compounds or mannitol. **CAUTIONS:** Uncorrected dehydration or hypotensive patients, those receiving antihypertensive therapy that cannot be interrupted prior to 24 hr before amifostine treatment, preexisting cardiovascular or cerebrovascular conditions (i.e., ischemic heart disease, arrhythmias, CHF, history of stroke or transient ischemic attack [TIA]), patients receiving chemotherapy for

malignancies that are potentially curable (e.g., certain malignancies of germ cell origin). **Pregnancy Category C.**

INTERACTIONS

DRUG: Antihypertensive medications or drugs that may potentiate hypotension: May increase the risk of hypotension. **HERBAL:** None known. **FOOD:** None known. **LAB VALUES:** May reduce serum calcium levels, especially in patients with nephrotic syndrome.

AVAILABILITY (Rx)

POWDER FOR INJECTION: 500 mg in a 10-ml single-use vial.

ADMINISTRATION/HANDLING
 IV

Reconstitution • Reconstitute with 9.7 ml 0.9% NaCl. • Further dilute with 0.9% NaCl for a concentration of 5–40 mg/ml.

Rate of administration • Administer over 15 min (30 min before chemotherapy). • If hypotension requires interruption of therapy, place patient in Trendelenburg position; give a bolus infusion of normal saline using a separate IV line. • An antiemetic, dexamethasone 20 mg IV and serotonin 5-HT$_3$ (receptor antagonist) should be given before and concurrently with amifostine.

Storage • Reconstituted solution stable for 5 hr at room temperature, 24 hr if refrigerated. • Do not use if discolored or contains particulate matter.

IV INCOMPATIBILITIES
Don't mix amifostine in any solution other than 0.9% NaCl.

IV COMPATIBILITIES
Mannitol, potassium chloride.

INDICATIONS/ROUTES/DOSAGE
TO REDUCE CUMULATIVE RENAL TOXICITY FROM REPEATED ADMINISTRATION OF CISPLATIN IN PATIENTS WITH ADVANCED OVARIAN CANCER
IV: ADULTS: 910 mg/m^2 once a day as 15-min infusion, beginning 30 min before chemotherapy. A 15-min infusion is better tolerated than extended infusions. If the full dose can't be administered, dose for subsequent cycles should be 740 mg/m^2.

TREATMENT OF POSTOPERATIVE RADIATION-INDUCED XEROSTOMIA IN PATIENTS WITH HEAD AND NECK CANCER
IV: ADULTS: 200 mg/m^2 once a day as 3-min infusion, starting 15–30 min before radiation therapy.
SUBCUTANEOUS: ADULTS: 500 mg/day during radiation therapy.

SIDE EFFECTS

FREQUENT (62%): Transient reduction in BP (usually starts 14 min into infusion, lasts about 6 min and returns to normal in 5–15 min); severe nausea, vomiting. **OCCASIONAL (20%–10%):** Flushing or feeling of warmth or chills or feeling of coldness; dizziness, hiccups, sneezing, somnolence. **RARE (less than 1%):** Clinically relevant hypocalcemia, mild rash.

ADVERSE REACTIONS/ TOXIC EFFECTS

A pronounced drop in BP may require temporary cessation of amifostine and fluid resuscitation.

NURSING CONSIDERATIONS

BASELINE ASSESSMENT
Be sure patient is adequately hydrated before infusion. Patient should maintain supine position during the infusion. Interrupt infusion if systolic BP decreases significantly from baseline (for baseline

of less than 100, BP drop by 20 mm Hg; for baseline of 100–119, a drop by 25 mm Hg; for baseline of 120–139, a drop by 30 mm Hg; for baseline of 140–179, a drop by 40 mm Hg; for baseline of greater than 180, a drop by 50 mm Hg). If BP returns to normal within 5 min and patient appears asymptomatic, begin infusion again so that full dose can be administered.

INTERVENTION/EVALUATION

Carefully monitor patient for fluid balance, adequate hydration. Monitor serum calcium levels in those at risk of hypocalcemia (nephrotic syndrome). Monitor BP q5min during infusion.

---

amikacin sulfate

am-i-**kay**-sin

(Amikin, Amikin Pediatric)

Do not confuse amikacin or Amikin with Amicar.

◆ CLASSIFICATION

PHARMACOTHERAPEUTIC: Aminoglycoside. **CLINICAL:** Antibiotic (see p. 19C).

ACTION

An aminoglycoside antibiotic that irreversibly binds to protein on bacterial ribosomes. **Therapeutic Effect:** Interferes with protein synthesis of susceptible microorganisms.

PHARMACOKINETICS

Rapid, complete absorption after IM administration. Protein binding: 0%–10%. Widely distributed (doesn't cross the blood-brain barrier, low concentrations in CSF). Excreted unchanged in urine. Removed by hemodialysis. **Half-life:** 2–4 hr (increased in impaired

renal function and neonates; decreased in cystic fibrosis and burn or febrile patients).

USES

Treatment of susceptible infections due to Pseudomonas, other gram-negative organisms including biliary tract, bone and joint, CNS, intra-abdominal, skin and soft tissue and urinary tract infections. Treatment of bacterial pneumonia, septicemia.

PRECAUTIONS

CONTRAINDICATIONS: Hypersensitivity to amikacin, or other aminoglycosides (cross-sensitivity), or their components. **CAUTIONS:** Myasthenia gravis, parkinsonism, decreased renal function, 8th cranial nerve impairment (vestibulocochlear nerve).

⧖ **LIFESPAN CONSIDERATIONS: Pregnancy/Lactation:** Readily crosses placenta; small amounts distributed in breast milk. May produce fetal nephrotoxicity. **Pregnancy Category C. Children:** Neonates, premature infants may be more susceptible to toxicity due to immature renal function. **Elderly:** Higher risk of toxicity due to age-related renal impairment, increased risk of hearing loss.

INTERACTIONS

DRUG: Nephrotoxic medications, other aminoglycosides, ototoxic medications: May increase the risk of nephrotoxicity or ototoxicity. **Neuromuscular blockers:** May enhance neuromuscular blockade. **HERBAL:** None known. **FOOD:** None known. **LAB VALUES:** May increase serum bilirubin, BUN, serum creatinine, serum LDH, AST and ALT levels. May decrease serum calcium, magnesium, potassium, and sodium concentrations. Therapeutic peak serum level is greater than 30 mcg/ml; toxic trough serum level is greater than 10 mcg/ml.

AVAILABILITY (Rx)

INJECTION: 50 mg/ml (Amikin Pediatric), 62.5 mg/ml (Amikin), 250 mg/ml (Amikin).

ADMINISTRATION/HANDLING

 IV

Reconstitution • Dilute each 500 mg with 100 ml 0.9% NaCl or D$_5$W.

Rate of administration • Infuse over 30–60 min for adults, older children; over 60–120 min for infants, young children.

Storage • Store vials at room temperature. • Solutions appear clear but may become pale yellow (does not affect potency). • Intermittent IV infusion (piggyback) is stable for 24 hr at room temperature. • Discard if precipitate forms or dark discoloration occurs.

IM
• To minimize discomfort, give deep IM slowly. • Less painful if injected into gluteus maximus rather than in lateral aspect of thigh.

IV INCOMPATIBILITIES

Amphotericin, ampicillin, cefazolin (Ancef), heparin, propofol (Diprivan).

IV COMPATIBILITIES

Amiodarone (Cordarone), aztreonam (Azactam), calcium gluconate, cefepime (Maxipime), cimetidine (Tagamet), ciprofloxacin (Cipro), clindamycin (Cleocin), diltiazem (Cardizem), enalapril (Vasotec), esmolol (BreviBloc), fluconazole (Diflucan), furosemide (Lasix), levofloxacin (Levaquin), lorazepam (Ativan), magnesium sulfate, midazolam (Versed), morphine, ondansetron (Zofran), potassium chloride, ranitidine (Zantac), total parenteral nutrition (TPN), vancomycin.

INDICATIONS/ROUTES/DOSAGE

UTIs
IV, IM: ADULTS, ELDERLY: 250 mg q12h.

MODERATE TO SEVERE INFECTIONS
IV, IM: ADULTS, ELDERLY: 15 mg/kg/day in divided doses q8–12h. **Maximum:** 1.5 g/day. CHILDREN, INFANTS: 15–22.5 mg/kg/day in divided doses q8h. NEONATES: 7.5–10 mg/kg/dose q8–24h.

DOSAGE IN RENAL IMPAIRMENT
Dosage and frequency are modified based on the degree of renal impairment and serum drug concentration. After a loading dose of 5–7.5 mg/kg, the maintenance dose and frequency are based on serum creatinine levels and creatinine clearance.

SIDE EFFECTS

FREQUENT: IM: Pain, induration. **IV:** Phlebitis, thrombophlebitis. **OCCASIONAL:** Hypersensitivity reactions (rash, fever, urticaria, pruritus). **RARE:** Neuromuscular blockade (difficulty breathing, drowsiness, weakness).

ADVERSE REACTIONS/ TOXIC EFFECTS

Serious reactions may include nephrotoxicity (as evidenced by increased thirst, decreased appetite, nausea, vomiting, increased BUN and serum creatinine levels, and decreased creatinine clearance); neurotoxicity (manifested as muscle twitching, visual disturbances, seizures, and tingling); and ototoxicity (as evidenced by tinnitus, dizziness, and loss of hearing).

NURSING CONSIDERATIONS

BASELINE ASSESSMENT
Dehydration must be treated before aminoglycoside therapy. Establish patient's baseline hearing acuity before beginning therapy. Question for history of allergies, especially to aminoglycosides and sulfite. Obtain specimen for culture, sensitivity before giving the first dose (therapy may begin before results are known).

INTERVENTION/EVALUATION

Monitor I&O (maintain hydration), urinalysis (casts, RBC, WBC, decrease in specific gravity). Monitor results of serum peak/trough levels. Be alert to ototoxic, neurotoxic symptoms (see Adverse Reactions/Toxic Effects). Check IM injection site for pain, induration. Evaluate IV site for phlebitis (heat, pain, red streaking over vein). Assess for skin rash, superinfection (particularly genital/anal pruritus), changes of oral mucosa, diarrhea. When treating patients with neuromuscular disorders, assess respiratory response carefully. Therapeutic serum level: Peak: 20–30 mcg/ml; toxic serum level: greater than 30 mcg/ml; trough: 1–9 mcg/ml; toxic serum level: greater than 10 mcg/ml.

PATIENT/FAMILY TEACHING

• Continue antibiotic for full length of treatment. • Space doses evenly. • IM injection may cause discomfort. • Notify physician in event of any hearing, visual, balance, urinary problems even after therapy is completed. • Do not take other medication without consulting physician. • Lab tests are essential part of therapy.

---

amiloride hydrochloride

a-**mill**-oh-ride
(Midamor)

Do not confuse amiloride with amiodarone or amlodipine.

FIXED-COMBINATION(S)

Moduretic: amiloride/hydrothiazide (a diuretic): 5 mg/50 mg.

◆CLASSIFICATION

PHARMACOTHERAPEUTIC: Guanidine derivative. **CLINICAL:** Potassium-sparing diuretic, antihypertensive, antihypokalemic (see p. 89C).

ACTION

A guanidine derivative that acts as a potassium-sparing diuretic, antihypertensive, and antihypokalemic by directly interfering with sodium reabsorption in the distal tubule. **Therapeutic Effect:** Increases sodium and water excretion and decreases potassium excretion.

PHARMACOKINETICS

Route	Onset	Peak	Duration
PO	2 hr	6–10 hr	24 hr

Incompletely absorbed from the GI tract. Protein binding: Minimal. Primarily excreted in urine; partially eliminated in feces. **Half-life:** 6–9 hr.

USES

Treatment of hypertension. Management of edema in CHF, hepatic cirrhosis, nephrotic syndrome. **OFF-LABEL:** Treatment of edema associated with CHF, liver cirrhosis, and nephrotic syndrome; treatment of hypertension, reduces lithium-induced polyuria, slows pulmonary function reduction in cystic fibrosis.

PRECAUTIONS

CONTRAINDICATIONS: Acute or chronic renal insufficiency, anuria, diabetic nephropathy, patients on other potassium-sparing diuretics, serum potassium greater than 5.5 mEq/L. **CAUTIONS:** BUN greater than 30 mg/dl or serum creatinine greater than 1.5 mg/dl, elderly, debilitated, hepatic insufficiency, cardiopulmonary disease, diabetes mellitus.

⚖ **LIFESPAN CONSIDERATIONS: Pregnancy/Lactation:** Unknown if drug crosses placenta or is distributed in breast milk. **Pregnancy Category B (D if used in pregnancy-induced** hypertension). **Children:** No age-related precautions noted. **Elderly:** Increased risk of hyperkalemia, age-related decreased renal function may require caution.

INTERACTIONS

DRUG: **Angiotensin-converting enzyme (ACE) inhibitors, including captopril, and potassium-containing diuretics:** May increase potassium levels. **Anticoagulants, including heparin:** May decrease effect of anticoagulants, including heparin. **Lithium:** May decrease lithium clearance and increase risk of amiloride toxicity. **NSAIDs:** May decrease antihypertensive effect. **HERBAL:** None known. **FOOD:** None known. **LAB VALUES:** May increase BUN, calcium excretion, and glucose, serum creatinine, serum magnesium, serum potassium, and uric acid levels. May decrease serum sodium levels.

AVAILABILITY (Rx)

TABLETS: 5 mg.

ADMINISTRATION/HANDLING

PO
• Give with food to avoid GI distress.

INDICATIONS/ROUTES/DOSAGE

TO COUNTERACT POTASSIUM LOSS INDUCED BY OTHER DIURETICS
PO: ADULTS, CHILDREN WEIGHING MORE THAN 20 KG: 5–10 mg/day up to 20 mg. ELDERLY: Initially, 5 mg/day or every other day. CHILDREN WEIGHING 6–20 KG: 0.625 mg/kg/day. **Maximum:** 10 mg/day.

DOSAGE IN RENAL IMPAIRMENT

Creatinine Clearance	Dosage
10–50 ml/min	50% of normal
Less than 10 ml/min	avoid use

SIDE EFFECTS

FREQUENT (8%–3%): Headache, nausea, diarrhea, vomiting, decreased appetite. **OCCASIONAL (3%–1%):** Dizziness,

constipation, abdominal pain, weakness, fatigue, cough, impotence. **RARE (less than 1%):** Tremors, vertigo, confusion, nervousness, insomnia, thirst, dry mouth, heartburn, shortness of breath, increased urination, hypotension, rash.

ADVERSE REACTIONS/TOXIC EFFECTS

Severe hyperkalemia may produce irritability, anxiety, a feeling of heaviness in the legs, paresthesia of hands, face, and lips, hypotension, bradycardia, tented T waves, widening of QRS, and ST depression.

NURSING CONSIDERATIONS

BASELINE ASSESSMENT

Assess baseline serum electrolytes, particularly for low potassium. Assess renal/hepatic functions. Assess edema (note location, extent), skin turgor, mucous membranes for hydration status. Assess muscle strength, mental status. Note skin temperature, moisture. Obtain baseline weight. Initiate strict I&O. Obtain baseline 12-lead EKG. Note pulse rate/rhythm.

INTERVENTION/EVALUATION

Monitor BP, vital signs, electrolytes (particularly potassium), I&O, weight. Note extent of diuresis. Watch for changes from initial assessment; hyperkalemia may result in muscle strength changes, tremor, muscle cramps, change in mental status (orientation, alertness, confusion), cardiac arrhythmias. Monitor serum potassium level, particularly during initial therapy. Weigh daily. Assess lung sounds for rales, wheezing.

PATIENT/FAMILY TEACHING

• Expect increase in volume/frequency of urination. • Therapeutic effect takes several days to begin and can last for several days when drug is discontinued. • High-potassium diet/potassium supplements can be dangerous, especially if patient has renal/hepatic problems. • Avoid foods high in potassium such as whole grains (cereals), legumes, meat, bananas, apricots, orange juice, potatoes (white, sweet), raisins. • Contact physician if confusion, irregular heartbeat, nervousness, numbness of hands, feet, lips, difficulty breathing, unusual fatigue, or weakness in legs occur (hyperkalemia).

aminocaproic acid

a-mee-noe-ka-**proe**-ik
(Amicar)

Do not confuse Amicar with amikacin or Amikin.

◆CLASSIFICATION

PHARMACOTHERAPEUTIC: Systemic hemostatic. **CLINICAL:** Antifibrinolytic, antihemorrhagic.

ACTION

A systemic hemostatic that acts as an antifibrinolytic and antihemorrhagic by inhibiting the activation of plasminogen activator substances. **Therapeutic Effect:** Prevents formation of fibrin clots.

USES

Treatment of excessive bleeding from hyperfibrinolysis or urinary fibrinolysis as noted in anemia, abruptio placentae, cirrhosis, carcinoma of prostate, lung, stomach, cervix. **OFF-LABEL:** Control of bleeding in thrombocytopenia, control of oral bleeding in congenital and acquired coagulation disorders, prevention of recurrence of subarachnoid hemorrhage, prevention of hemorrhage in hemophiliacs following dental surgery, treatment of traumatic hyphema.

PRECAUTIONS

CONTRAINDICATIONS: Evidence of active intravascular clotting process, disseminated intravascular coagulation without concurrent heparin therapy, hematuria of upper urinary tract origin (unless benefit outweighs risk); newborns (parenteral form). **CAUTIONS:** Impaired cardiac, hepatic, renal disease, those with hyperfibrinolysis, premature neonates. **Pregnancy Category C.**

INTERACTIONS

DRUG: Anti-inhibitor coagulant complex, tretinoin: May increase the risk of thrombosis. **HERBAL:** None known. **FOOD:** None known. **LAB VALUES:** May elevate serum potassium level.

AVAILABILITY (Rx)

SYRUP: 250 mg/ml. **TABLETS:** 500 mg. **INJECTION:** 250 mg/ml.

ADMINISTRATION/HANDLING
IV

Reconstitution • Dilute each 1 g in up to 50 ml 0.9% NaCl, D_5W, Ringer's, or sterile water for injection (do not use sterile water for injection in patients with subarachnoid hemorrhage).

Rate of administration • Give only by IV infusion. • Infuse 5 g or less over first hr in 250 ml of solution; give each succeeding 1 g over 1 hr in 50–100 ml solution.

Administration precaution • Monitor for hypotension during infusion. • Rapid infusion may produce bradycardia, arrhythmias.

IV INCOMPATIBILITY
Sodium lactate.

INDICATIONS/ROUTES/DOSAGE
ACUTE BLEEDING
PO, IV INFUSION: ADULTS, ELDERLY: 4–5 g over first hr; then 1–1.25 g/hr. Continue for 8 hr or until bleeding is controlled.

✎ see color pill atlas   ⬤ herb   underlined – top prescribed drug

Maximum: 30 g/24 hr. CHILDREN: 3 g/m^2 over first hr; then 1 g/m^2/hr. **Maximum:** 18 g/m^2/24 hr.

DOSAGE IN RENAL IMPAIRMENT
Decrease dose to 25% of normal.

SIDE EFFECTS

OCCASIONAL: Nausea, diarrhea, cramps, decreased urination, decreased BP, dizziness, headache, muscle fatigue and weakness, myopathy, bloodshot eyes.

ADVERSE REACTIONS/ TOXIC EFFECTS

Too rapid IV administration produces tinnitus, rash, arrhythmias, unusual fatigue, and weakness. Rarely, a grand mal seizure occurs, generally preceded by weakness, dizziness, and headache.

NURSING CONSIDERATIONS

INTERVENTION/EVALUATION
Question for any change in muscle strength as noted by patient. Monitor for increased serum creatine kinase (CK), AST serum levels (skeletal myopathy). Monitor heart rhythm. Assess for decrease in BP, increase in pulse rate, abdominal/back pain, severe headache (may be evidence of hemorrhage). Assess peripheral pulses, skin for ecchymoses, petechiae. Question for increased discharge during menses. Check for excessive bleeding from minor cuts, scratches. Assess gums for erythema, gingival bleeding. Assess urine output for hematuria.

PATIENT/FAMILY TEACHING
• Report any sign of red/dark urine, black/red stool, coffee-ground vomitus, blood-tinged mucus from cough.

aminophylline (theophylline ethylenediamine) ℮

am-in-**ah**-phil-lin
(Phyllocontin)

theophylline

(Elixophyllin, Quibron-T, Quibron-T/SR, Slo-Bid Gyrocaps, Theo-24, Thoechron, Theodur, Theolair, T-Phyl, Uniphyl)

Do not confuse aminophylline with amitriptyline or ampicillin, or Slo-Bid with Dolobid.

♦ CLASSIFICATION

PHARMACOTHERAPEUTIC: Xanthine derivative. **CLINICAL:** Bronchodilator (see p. 65C).

ACTION

A xanthine derivative that acts as a bronchodilator by directly relaxing smooth muscle of the bronchial airways and pulmonary blood vessels. **Therapeutic Effect:** Relieves bronchospasm and increases vital capacity.

USES

Symptomatic relief, prevention of bronchial asthma, reversible bronchospasm due to chronic bronchitis, emphysema, or chronic obstructive pumonary disease (COPD). **OFF-LABEL:** Treatment of apnea in neonates.

PRECAUTIONS

CONTRAINDICATIONS: History of hypersensitivity to caffeine or xanthine. **CAUTIONS:** Impaired cardiac, renal, hepatic function; hypertension; hyperthyroidism; diabetes mellitus; peptic ulcer; glaucoma; severe hypoxemia; underlying seizure disorder. **Pregnancy Category C.**

INTERACTIONS

DRUG: Beta blockers: May decrease the effects of aminophylline. **Cimetidine, ciprofloxacin, erythromycin, norfloxacin:** May increase aminophylline blood concentration and risk of aminophylline toxicity. **Glucocorticoids:** May produce hypernatremia. **Phenytoin, primidone, rifampin:** May increase aminophylline metabolism. **Smoking:** May decrease aminophylline blood concentration. **HERBAL:** None known. **FOOD: Charcoal-broiled foods; high-protein, low-carbohydrate diet:** May decrease the theophylline blood level. **LAB VALUES:** None known.

AVAILABILITY (Rx)

CAPSULES (EXTENDED-RELEASE [THEO-24]): 100 mg, 200 mg, 300 mg, 400 mg. **ELIXIR (ELIXOPHYLLIN):** 80 mg/15 ml. **ORAL SOLUTION:** 80 mg/15 ml. **TABLETS (CONTROLLED-RELEASE):** 100 mg **(THEOCHRON)**, 200 mg **(THEOCHRON, T-PHYL)**, 300 mg **(QUIBRON-T/SR, THEOCHRON, THEOLAIR-SR)**, 400 mg **(UNIPHYL)**, 500 mg **(THEOLAIR-SR)**, 600 mg **(UNIPHYL)**. **INFUSION (THEOPHYLLINE):** 0.8 mg/ml, 1.6 mg/ml, 2 mg/ml, 3.2 mg/ml, 4 mg/ml. **INJECTION (AMINOPHYLLINE):** 25 mg/ml.

ADMINISTRATION/HANDLING
 IV

Dilution • Give loading dose diluted in 100–200 ml of D5W or 0.9% NaCl. • Prepare maintenance dose in larger volume parenteral infusion.

Rate of administration • Do not exceed flow rate of 1 ml/min (25 mg/min) for either piggyback or infusion. • Administer loading dose over 20–30 min. • Use infusion pump or microdrip to regulate IV administration.

Storage • Store at room temperature. • Discard if solution contains a precipitate.

PO
• Give with food to avoid GI distress.
• Do not crush/break extended-release forms.

IV INCOMPATIBILITIES
Amiodarone (Cordarone), ciprofloxacin (Cipro), dobutamine (Dobutrex), ondansetron (Zofran).

IV COMPATIBILITIES
Aztreonam (Azactam), ceftazidime (Fortaz), fluconazole (Diflucan), heparin, morphine, potassium chloride, total parenteral nutrition (TPN).

INDICATIONS/ROUTES/DOSAGE
ASTHMA
IV: ADULTS: Initially 5 mg/kg bolus over 20–30 min (to provide serum theophylline of 5–15 mg/ml), then 0.4 mg/kg/hr continuous infusion. ELDERLY: 5 mg/kg bolus, then 0.2 mg/kg/hr continuous infusion. CHILDREN 9–6 YR: Initially 5 mg/kg bolus, then 0.7 mg/kg/hr. CHILDREN 1–8 YR: Initially 5 mg/kg bolus, then 0.8 mg/kg/hr.

PO: ADULTS: Initially 5 mg/kg (use ideal body weight), then 300–600 mg/day in 3–4 divided doses. ELDERLY: Initially 5 mg/kg, then 2 mg/kg q8h.

PO (CONTROLLED-RELEASE 12-HOUR FORMULATIONS): ADULTS, CHILDREN WEIGHING 45 KG AND MORE: Initially 300 mg/day in 2 divided doses. May increase in 3 days to 400 mg/day in 2 divided doses. May increase in 3 days to 600 mg/day in 2 divided doses. CHILDREN WEIGHING LESS THAN 45 KG: Initially 12–24 mg/kg/day in divided doses (**Maximum:** 300 mg). May increase in 3 days to 16 mg/kg/day (**Maximum:** 400 mg). May increase in 3 days to 20 mg/kg/day (**Maximum:** 600 mg).

PO (EXTENDED-RELEASE 24-HOUR FORMULATIONS): ADULTS, CHILDREN WEIGHING 45 KG AND MORE: Initially 300–400 mg/day. May increase in 3 days to 400–600 mg/day. May then titrate according to blood level.

CHILDREN WEIGHING LESS THAN 45 KG: Initially 12–24 mg/kg/day (**Maximum:** 300 mg). May increase in 3 days to 16 mg/kg/day (**Maximum:** 400 mg). May increase in 3 days to 20 mg/kg/day (**Maximum:** 600 mg).

SIDE EFFECTS

FREQUENT: Altered smell (during IV administration), restlessness, tachycardia, tremor. **OCCASIONAL:** Heartburn, vomiting, headache, mild diuresis, insomnia, nausea.

ADVERSE REACTIONS/ TOXIC EFFECTS

Too-rapid IV administration may produce marked hypotension with accompanying faintness, light-headedness, palpitations, tachycardia, hyperventilation, nausea, vomiting, angina-like pain, seizures, ventricular fibrillation, and cardiac standstill.

NURSING CONSIDERATIONS

BASELINE ASSESSMENT

Offer emotional support (high incidence of anxiety due to difficulty in breathing and sympathomimetic response to drug). Peak serum concentration should be drawn 1 hr following IV dose, 1–2 hr after immediate-release dose, 3–8 hr after extended-release dose. Draw trough level just before next dose.

INTERVENTION/EVALUATION

Monitor rate, depth, rhythm, type of respiration; quality/rate of pulse. Assess lung sounds for rhonchi, wheezing, rales. Monitor ABGs. Observe lips, fingernails for cyanosis (blue or dusky color in light-skinned patients; gray in dark-skinned patients). Observe for clavicular retractions, hand tremor. Evaluate for clinical improvement (quieter, slower respirations, relaxed facial expression, cessation of clavicular retractions). Monitor theophylline serum levels (therapeutic serum level range: 10–20 mcg/ml).

PATIENT/FAMILY TEACHING

• Increase fluid intake (decreases lung secretion viscosity). • Avoid excessive caffeine derivatives (chocolate, coffee, tea, cola, cocoa). • Smoking, charcoal-broiled food, high-protein, low-carbohydrate diet may decrease serum theophylline level.

---

amiodarone hydrochloride

ah-me-**oh**-dah-roan

(<u>Cordarone</u>, Cordarone I.V., Pacerone)

Do not confuse amiodarone with amiloride or Cordarone with Cardura.

CLASSIFICATION

PHARMACOTHERAPEUTIC: Cardiac agent. **CLINICAL:** Antiarrhythmic (see p. 16C).

ACTION

A cardiac agent that prolongs duration of myocardial cell action potential and refractory period by acting directly on all cardiac tissue. Decreases AV and sinus node function. **Therapeutic Effect:** Suppresses arrhythmias.

PHARMACOKINETICS

Route	Onset	Peak	Duration
PO	3 days–3 wk	1 wk–5 mo	7–50 days after discontinuation

Slowly, variably absorbed from GI tract. Protein binding: 96%. Extensively metabolized in the liver to active metabolite. Excreted via bile; not removed by hemodialysis. **Half-life:** 26–107 days; metabolite, 61 days.

USES

Oral: Management of life-threatening recurrent ventricular fibrillation, hemodynamically unstable ventricular tachycardia (VT). **IV:** Management/prophylaxis of frequently occurring ventricular fibrillation, unstable ventricular tachycardia (VT) unresponsive to other therapy. **OFF-LABEL:** Control of hemodynamically stable VT, control of rapid ventricular rate due to accessory pathway conduction in pre-excited atrial arrhythmias, conversion of atrial fibrillation to normal sinus rhythm, in cardiac arrest with persistent VT or ventricular fibrillation, paroxysmal supraventricular tachycardia, polymorphic VT or wide complex tachycardia of uncertain origin, prevention of post-operative atrial fibrillation.

PRECAUTIONS

CONTRAINDICATIONS: Bradycardia-induced syncope (except in the presence of a pacemaker), second- and third-degree AV block, severe hepatic disease, severe sinus-node dysfunction. **CAUTIONS:** Thyroid disease, electrolyte imbalance, hepatic disease, hypotension, left ventricular dysfunction, photosensitivity, pulmonary disease.

⏳ **LIFESPAN CONSIDERATIONS: Pregnancy/Lactation:** Crosses placenta; distributed in breast milk. May adversely affect fetal development. **Pregnancy Category D. Children:** Safety and efficacy not established. **Elderly:** May be more sensitive to effects on thyroid function. May experience increased incidence ataxia, other neurotoxic effects.

INTERACTIONS

DRUG: Antiarrhythmics, fluoroquinolones, haloperidol: May increase cardiac effects. **Beta blockers, oral anticoagulants:** May increase effect of beta blockers and oral anticoagulants. **Digoxin, fosphenytoin, phenytoin:** May increase drug concentration and risk of toxicity of digoxin, fosphenytoin, and phenytoin. **Simvastatin:** May increase risk for myopathy, rhabdomyolysis. **HERBAL: St. John's wort:** May decrease effect. **FOOD: Grapefruit/grapefruit juice:** May decrease effect. **LAB VALUES:** May increase antinuclear antibody titers and AST, ALT, and serum alkaline phosphatase levels. May cause changes in EKG and thyroid function test results. Therapeutic serum level is 0.5–2.5 mcg/ml; toxic serum level has not been established.

AVAILABILITY (Rx)

TABLETS: 100 mg (Pacerone), 200 mg (Cordarone, Pacerone), 400 mg (Pacerone). **INJECTION (CORDARONE I.V.):** 50 mg/ml.

ADMINISTRATION/HANDLING

💉 **IV**

Reconstitution • Use glass or polyolefin containers for dilution. • Dilute loading dose (150 mg) in 100 ml D_5W (1.5 mg/ml). • Dilute maintenance dose (900 mg) in 500 ml D_5W (1.8 mg/ml). Concentrations greater than 3 mg/ml cause peripheral vein phlebitis.

Rate of administration • Does not need protection from light during administration. • Administer through central venous catheter (CVC) if possible, using in-line filter. • Bolus over 10 min (15 mg/min) not to exceed 30 mg/min; then 1 mg/min over 6 hr; then 0.5 mg/min over 18 hr. • Infusions longer than 1 hr, concentration not to exceed 2 mg/ml unless CVC used.

Storage • Store at room temperature. • Use in PVC containers within 2 hr of dilution; within 24 hr with glass or polyolefin containers.

PO
• Give with meals to reduce GI distress.
• Tablets may be crushed.

🌐 IV INCOMPATIBILITIES

Aminophylline (theophylline), cefazolin (Ancef), heparin, sodium bicarbonate.

IV COMPATIBILITIES

Dobutamine (Dobutrex), dopamine (Intropin), furosemide (Lasix), insulin (regular), labetalol (Normodyne), lidocaine, midazolam (Versed), morphine, nitroglycerin, norepinephrine (Levophed), phenylephrine (Neo-Synephrine), potassium chloride, vancomycin.

INDICATIONS/ROUTES/DOSAGE

LIFE-THREATENING RECURRENT VENTRICULAR FIBRILLATION OR HEMODYNAMICALLY UNSTABLE VENTRICULAR TACHYCARDIA

PO: ADULTS, ELDERLY: Initially, 800–1,600 mg/day in 2–4 divided doses for 1–3 wk. After arrhythmia is controlled or side effects occur, reduce to 600–800 mg/day for about 4 wk. Maintenance: 200–600 mg/day. CHILDREN: Initially, 10–20 mg/kg/day for 4–14 days, then 5 mg/kg/day for several wks. Maintenance: 2.5 mg/kg/day or lowest effective maintenance dose for 5 of 7 days/wk.

IV INFUSION: ADULTS: Initially, 1,050 mg over 24 hr; 150 mg over 10 min, then 360 mg over 6 hr; then 540 mg over 18 hr. May continue at 0.5 mg/min for up to 2–3 wk regardless of age or renal or left ventricular function.

SIDE EFFECTS

EXPECTED: Corneal microdeposits are noted in almost all patients treated for more than 6 mo (can lead to blurry vision). FREQUENT (greater than 3%): Parenteral: Hypotension, nausea, fever, bradycardia. Oral: Constipation, headache, decreased appetite, nausea, vomiting, paresthesias, photosensitivity, muscular incoordination. OCCASIONAL (less than 3%): Oral: Bitter or metallic taste; decreased libido; dizziness; facial flushing; blue-gray coloring of skin (face, arms, and neck); blurred vision; bradycardia; asymptomatic corneal deposits. RARE (less than 1%): Oral: Rash, vision loss, blindness.

ADVERSE REACTIONS/ TOXIC EFFECTS

Serious, potentially fatal pulmonary toxicity (alveolitis, pulmonary fibrosis, pneumonitis, acute respiratory distress syndrome) may begin with progressive dyspnea and cough with crackles, decreased breath sounds, pleurisy, CHF or hepatotoxicity. Amiodarone may worsen existing arrhythmias or produce new arrhythmias (called proarrhythmias).

NURSING CONSIDERATIONS

BASELINE ASSESSMENT

Obtain baseline pulmonary function tests, chest x-ray, hepatic enzyme tests, serum AST, ALT, alkaline phosphatase, 12-lead EKG. Assess BP, apical pulse immediately before drug is administered (if pulse is 60/min or less or systolic BP is less than 90 mm Hg, withhold medication, contact physician).

INTERVENTION/EVALUATION

Monitor for symptoms of pulmonary toxicity (progressively worsening dyspnea, cough). Dosage should be discontinued or reduced if toxicity occurs. Assess pulse for quality, rhythm, bradycardia. Monitor EKG for cardiac changes, (e.g., widening of QRS, prolongation of PR and QT intervals). Notify physician of any significant interval changes. Assess for nausea, fatigue, paresthesia, tremor. Monitor for signs of hypothyroidism (periorbital edema, lethargy, pudgy hands/feet, cool/pale skin, vertigo, night cramps) and hyperthyroidism (hot/dry skin, bulging eyes [exophthalmos], frequent urination, eyelid edema, weight loss, difficulty breathing). Monitor serum AST, ALT, alkaline phosphatase for evidence of hepatic toxicity. Assess skin, cornea for bluish discoloration in those who have been on drug therapy longer than 2 mo. Monitor liver function tests, thyroid test results. If elevated hepatic enzymes occur, dosage reduction or discontinuation is necessary. Monitor for therapeutic serum level (0.5–2.5 mcg/ml). Toxic serum level not established.

PATIENT/FAMILY TEACHING

• Protect against photosensitivity reaction on skin exposed to sunlight. • Bluish skin discoloration gradually disappears when drug is discontinued. • Report shortness of breath, cough. • Outpatients should monitor pulse before taking medication. • Do not abruptly discontinue medication. • Compliance with therapy regimen is essential to control arrhythmias. • Restrict salt, alcohol intake. • Recommend ophthalmic exams q6mo. • Report any vision changes.

amitriptyline hydrochloride

a-me-**trip**-tih-leen

(Apo-Amitriptyline ✦, Elavil)

Do not confuse amitriptyline with aminophylline or nortriptyline, or Elavil with Equanil or Mellaril.

FIXED-COMBINATION(S)

Etrafon, Triavil: amitriptyline/perphenazine (an antipsychotic): 10 mg/2 mg; 25 mg/2 mg; 10 mg/4 mg; 25 mg/4 mg. **Limbitrol:** amitriptyline/chlordiaz-epoxide (an antianxiety): 12.5 mg/5 mg; 25 mg/10 mg.

CLASSIFICATION

PHARMACOTHERAPEUTIC: Tricyclic. **CLINICAL:** Antidepressant, antineuralgic, antibulimic (see p. 36C).

ACTION

A tricyclic antidepressant that blocks the reuptake of neurotransmitters, including norepinephrine and serotonin, at presynaptic membranes, thus increasing their availability at postsynaptic receptor sites. Also has strong anticholinergic activity. **Therapeutic Effect:** Relieves depression.

PHARMACOKINETICS

Rapidly and well absorbed from the GI tract. Protein binding: 90%. Undergoes first-pass metabolism in the liver. Primarily excreted in urine. Minimal removal by hemodialysis. **Half-life:** 10–26 hr.

USES

Treatment of various forms of depression, exhibited as persistent, prominent dysphoria (occurring nearly every day for at least 2 wk) manifested by 4 of 8 symptoms: appetite change, sleep pattern change, increased fatigue, impaired concentration, feelings of guilt or worthlessness, loss of interest in usual activities, psychomotor agitation or retardation, suicidal tendencies. **OFF-LABEL:** Relief of neuropathic pain, such as that experienced by patients with diabetic neuropathy or postherpetic neuralgia; treatment of anxiety, bulimia nervosa, migraine, nocturnal enuresis, panic disorder, peptic ulcer.

PRECAUTIONS

CONTRAINDICATIONS: Acute recovery period after MI, use within 14 days of MAOIs. **CAUTIONS:** Prostatic hypertrophy, history of urinary retention or obstruction, glaucoma, diabetes mellitus, history of seizures, hyperthyroidism, cardiac/hepatic/renal disease, schizophrenia, increased intraocular pressure (IOP), hiatal hernia.

⧖ **LIFESPAN CONSIDERATIONS: Pregnancy/Lactation:** Crosses placenta; minimally distributed in breast milk. **Pregnancy Category C. Children:** More sensitive to increased dosage, toxicity, increased risk of suicidal ideation, worsening of depression. **Elderly:** Increased risk of toxicity. Increased sensitivity to anticholinergic effects. Cautions in those with cardiovascular disease.

INTERACTIONS

DRUG: Antithyroid agents: May increase the risk of agranulocytosis. **Cimetidine, valproic acid:** May increase amitriptyline blood concentration and risk of toxicity. **Clonidine, guanadrel:** May decrease the effects of these drugs. **CNS depressants (including alcohol, anticonvulsants, barbiturates, phenothiazines, and sedative-hypnotics):** May increase CNS and respiratory depression and the hypotensive effects of amitriptyline. **MAOIs:** May increase the risk of neuroleptic malignant syndrome, seizures, hypertensive crisis, and hyperpyresis. **Phenothiazines:** May increase the sedative and anticholinergic effects of amitriptyline. **Sympathomimetics:** May increase the risk of cardiac effects. **HERBAL:** None known. **FOOD:** None known. **LAB VALUES:** May alter blood glucose levels and EKG readings. Therapeutic serum drug level is 120–250 ng/ml; toxic serum drug level is greater than 500 ng/ml.

AVAILABILITY (Rx)

TABLETS (ELAVIL): 10 mg, 25 mg, 50 mg, 75 mg, 100 mg, 150 mg. **INJECTION (ELAVIL):** 10 mg/ml.

ADMINISTRATION/HANDLING

IM
• Give by IM only if PO administration is not feasible. • Crystals may form in injectable solution. Redissolve by immersing ampule in hot water for 1 min. • Give deep IM slowly.

PO
• Give with food or milk if GI distress occurs.

INDICATIONS/ROUTES/DOSAGE

DEPRESSION
PO: ADULTS: 25–100 mg/day as a single dose at bedtime or in divided doses. May gradually increase up to 300 mg/day. Titrate to lowest effective dosage. ELDERLY: Initially, 10–25 mg at bedtime. May increase by 10–25 mg at weekly intervals. Range: 25–150 mg/day. CHILDREN 6-12 YR: 1–5 mg/kg/day in 2 divided doses.
IM: ADULTS: 20–30 mg 4 times a day.

PAIN MANAGEMENT
PO: ADULTS, ELDERLY: 25–100 mg at bedtime.

SIDE EFFECTS

FREQUENT: Dizziness, somnolence, dry mouth, orthostatic hypotension, headache, increased appetite, weight gain, nausea, unusual fatigue, unpleasant taste. **OCCASIONAL:** Blurred vision, confusion, constipation, hallucinations, delayed micturition, eye pain, arrhythmias, fine muscle tremors, parkinsonian syndrome, anxiety, diarrhea, diaphoresis, heartburn, insomnia. **RARE:** Hypersensitivity, alopecia, tinnitus, breast enlargement, photosensitivity.

ADVERSE REACTIONS/ TOXIC EFFECTS

Overdose may produce confusion, seizures, severe somnolence, arrhythmias, fever, hallucinations, agitation, dyspnea, vomiting, and unusual fatigue or weakness. Abrupt discontinuation after prolonged therapy may produce headache, malaise, nausea, vomiting, and vivid dreams. Blood dyscrasias and cholestatic jaundice occur rarely.

NURSING CONSIDERATIONS

BASELINE ASSESSMENT
Observe and record behavior. Assess psychological status, thought content, sleep patterns, appearance, interest in environment. For those on long-term therapy, hepatic/renal function tests,

blood counts should be performed periodically.

INTERVENTION/EVALUATION

Supervise suicidal-risk patient closely during early therapy (as depression lessens, energy level improves, increasing suicide potential). Assess appearance, behavior, speech pattern, level of interest, mood. Monitor BP, pulse for hypotension, arrhythmias. Therapeutic serum level: Peak: 120–250 ng/ml; toxic serum level: greater than 500 ng/ml.

PATIENT/FAMILY TEACHING

• Change positions slowly to avoid hypotensive effect. Tolerance to postural hypotension, sedative and anticholinergic effects usually develop during early therapy. • Maximum therapeutic effect may be noted in 2–4 wk. • Sensitivity to sun may occur. • Report visual disturbances. • Do not abruptly discontinue medication. • Avoid tasks that require alertness, motor skills until response to drug is established. • Sips of tepid water may relieve dry mouth.

amlodipine

am-**low**-dih-peen
(Norvasc)

Do not confuse amlodipine with amiloride, or Norvasc with Navane or Vascor.

FIXED-COMBINATIONS

Caduet: amlodipine/atorvastatin (hydroxamethylglutaryl-CoA [HMG-CoA] reductase inhibitor): 5 mg/10 mg; 10 mg/10 mg; 5 mg/20 mg; 10 mg/20 mg; 5 mg/40 mg; 10 mg/40 mg; 5 mg/80 mg; 10 mg/80 mg. **Lotrel:** amlodipine/benazepril (an angiotensin-converting enzyme [ACE] inhibitor): 2.5 mg/10 mg; 5 mg/10 mg; 5 mg/20 mg; 10 mg/20 mg.

◆CLASSIFICATION

PHARMACOTHERAPEUTIC: Calcium channel blocker. **CLINICAL:** Antihypertensive, antianginal (see p. 69C).

ACTION

A calcium channel blocker that inhibits calcium movement across cardiac and vascular smooth-muscle cell membranes. **Therapeutic Effect:** Relieves angina by dilating coronary arteries, peripheral arteries, and arterioles. Decreases total peripheral vascular resistance and BP by vasodilation.

PHARMACOKINETICS

Route	Onset	Peak	Duration
PO	0.5–1 hr	6–12 hr	24 hr

Slowly absorbed from the GI tract. Protein binding: 93%. Undergoes first-pass metabolism in the liver. Excreted primarily in urine. Not removed by hemodialysis. **Half-life:** 30–50 hr (increased in the elderly and those with liver cirrhosis).

USES

Management of hypertension, chronic stable angina, vasospastic (Prinzmetal's or variant) angina. May be used alone or with other antihypertensives or antianginals.

PRECAUTIONS

CONTRAINDICATIONS: Severe hypotension. **CAUTIONS:** Impaired hepatic function, aortic stenosis, CHF.

⧗ **LIFESPAN CONSIDERATIONS: Pregnancy/Lactation:** Unknown if drug crosses placenta or is distributed in breast milk. **Pregnancy Category C. Children:** Safety and efficacy not established. **Elderly:** Half-life may be increased, more sensitive to hypotensive effects.

INTERACTIONS

DRUG: None known. **HERBAL:** None known. **FOOD: Grapefruit, grapefruit juice:** May increase amlodipine blood concentration and hypotensive effects. **LAB VALUES:** None known.

AVAILABILITY (Rx)

TABLETS: 2.5 mg, 5 mg, 10 mg.

ADMINISTRATION/HANDLING

PO
• May give without regard to food.
• Grapefruit juice may increase drug concentration.

INDICATIONS/ROUTES/DOSAGE

HYPERTENSION
PO: ADULTS: Initially, 5 mg/day as a single dose. **Maximum:** 10 mg/day. SMALL-FRAME, FRAGILE, ELDERLY: Initially, 2.5 mg/day as a single dose. CHILDREN 6–17 YR: 2.5–5 mg/day.

ANGINA (CHRONIC STABLE OR VASOSPASTIC)
PO: ADULTS: 5–10 mg/day as a single dose. ELDERLY, PATIENTS WITH HEPATIC INSUFFICIENCY: 5 mg/day as a single dose.

DOSAGE IN RENAL IMPAIRMENT
ADULTS, ELDERLY: (Hypertension) 2.5 mg/day. (Angina) 5 mg/day.

SIDE EFFECTS

FREQUENT (greater than 5%): Peripheral edema, headache, flushing. **OCCASIONAL (5%–1%):** Dizziness, palpitations, nausea, unusual fatigue or weakness (asthenia). **RARE (less than 1%):** Chest pain, bradycardia, orthostatic hypotension.

ADVERSE REACTIONS/ TOXIC EFFECTS

Overdose may produce excessive peripheral vasodilation and marked hypotension with reflex tachycardia.

NURSING CONSIDERATIONS

BASELINE ASSESSMENT
Assess baseline renal and liver function tests, BP, apical pulse.

INTERVENTION/EVALUATION
Assess BP (if systolic BP is less than 90 mm Hg, withhold medication, contact physician). Assess for peripheral edema behind medial malleolus (sacral area in bedridden patients). Assess skin for flushing. Question for headache, asthenia.

PATIENT/FAMILY TEACHING
• Do not abruptly discontinue medication. • Compliance with therapy regimen is essential to control hypertension. • Avoid tasks that require alertness, motor skills until response to drug is established. • Avoid concomitant ingestion of grapefruit juice.

---

amoxicillin

ah-mocks-ih-**sill**-in

(Amoxicot, <u>Amoxil</u>, Amoxil Pediatric Drops, Biomox, DisperMox, Moxilin, Novamoxin ✤, Polymox, Trimox, Wymox)

Do not confuse amoxicillin with amoxapine or DisperMox with Diamox or Trimox with Tylox.

◆CLASSIFICATION

PHARMACOTHERAPEUTIC: Penicillin. **CLINICAL:** Antibiotic (see p. 28C).

ACTION

A penicillin that inhibits bacterial cell wall synthesis. **Therapeutic Effect:** Bactericidal in susceptible microorganisms.

PHARMACOKINETICS

Well absorbed from the GI tract. Protein binding: 20%. Partially metabolized in the liver. Primarily excreted in urine. Removed by hemodialysis. **Half-life:** 1–1.3 hr (increased in impaired renal function).

USES

Treatment of susceptible infections due to *streptococci, E. coli, E. faecalis, P. mirabilis, H. influenceae, N. gonorrhoeae* including ear, nose and throat, lower respiratory tract, skin and skin structure and urinary tract infections, acute uncomplicated gonorrhea, *H. pylori*. OFF-LABEL: Treatment of Lyme disease and typhoid fever.

PRECAUTIONS

CONTRAINDICATIONS: Hypersensitivity to any penicillin, infectious mononucleosis. **CAUTIONS:** History of allergies (especially cephalosporins), antibiotic-associated colitis.

⧖ **LIFESPAN CONSIDERATIONS: Pregnancy/Lactation:** Crosses placenta, appears in cord blood, amniotic fluid. Distributed in breast milk in low concentrations. May lead to allergic sensitization, diarrhea, candidiasis, skin rash in infant. **Pregnancy Category B. Children:** Immature renal function in neonate/young infant may delay renal excretion. **Elderly:** Age-related renal impairment may require dosage adjustment.

INTERACTIONS

DRUG: **Allopurinol:** May increase incidence of rash. **Oral contraceptives:** May decrease effectiveness of oral contraceptives. **Probenecid:** May increase amoxicillin blood concentration and risk of toxicity. HERBAL: None known. FOOD: None known. LAB VALUES: May increase BUN and serum LDH, bilirubin, creatinine, AST, and ALT levels. May cause a positive Coombs' test.

AVAILABILITY (Rx)

CAPSULES: 250 mg (Amoxil, Biomox, Trimox, Wymox), 500 mg (Amoxil, Biomox, Trimox). **POWDER FOR RECONSTITUTION:** 50 mg/ml (Amoxil Pediatric Drops, Trimox), 125 mg/5 ml (Amoxil, Trimox), 200 mg/ml (Amoxil), 250 mg/ml (Amoxil, Biomox, Trimox), 400 mg/ml (Amoxil). **TABLETS (AMOXIL):** 500 mg, 875 mg. **TABLETS (CHEWABLE [AMOXIL]):** 125 mg, 200 mg, 250 mg, 400 mg. **TABLETS FOR ORAL SUSPENSION (DISPERMOX):** 200 mg, 400 mg.

ADMINISTRATION/HANDLING

◄ ALERT ► To reduce development of drug-resistant bacteria and maintain the effectiveness of amoxicillin and other antibacterial drugs, amoxicillin should be used only to treat or prevent infections that are proved or strongly suspected to be caused by bacteria.

PO
• Store capsules, tablets at room temperature • After reconstitution, oral solution is stable for 14 days at either room temperature or refrigerated. • Give without regard to meals. • Instruct patient to chew/crush chewable tablets thoroughly before swallowing. • **DisperMox:** Mix 1 tablet in 10 ml water. Do not chew or swallow tablets.

INDICATIONS/ROUTES/DOSAGE

SUSCEPTIBLE INFECTIONS
PO: ADULTS, ELDERLY: 250–500 mg q8h or 500–875 mg q12h. CHILDREN OLDER THAN 3 MO: 25–50 mg/kg/day in 3 divided doses. CHILDREN 3 MO AND YOUNGER: 30 mg/kg/day in 2 divided doses.

LOWER RESPIRATORY TRACT INFECTION
PO: ADULTS, ELDERLY: 500 mg q8h or 875 mg q12h.

H. PYLORI INFECTION
PO: ADULTS, ELDERLY: 1 g twice a day in combination with clarithromycin and lansoprazole for 14 days.

OTITIS MEDIA
PO: CHILDREN: 80–90 mg/kg/day in 2 or 3 divided doses.

GONORRHEA
PO: ADULTS, ELDERLY: 3 g as a single dose.

ENDOCARDITIS PROPHYLAXIS
PO: ADULTS, ELDERLY: 2 g 1 hr before procedure. CHILDREN: 50 mg/kg 1 hr

before procedure. **Maximum:** 2 g.

DOSAGE IN RENAL IMPAIRMENT

Dosage interval is modified based on creatinine clearance. **Creatinine Clearance 10–30 ml/min:** Usual dose q12h. **Creatinine Clearance less than 10 ml/min:** Usual dose q24h.

SIDE EFFECTS

FREQUENT: GI disturbances (mild diarrhea, nausea, or vomiting), headache, oral or vaginal candidiasis. **OCCASIONAL:** Generalized rash, urticaria.

ADVERSE REACTIONS/ TOXIC EFFECTS

Antibiotic-associated colitis and other superinfections may result from altered bacterial balance. Severe hypersensitivity reactions, including anaphylaxis and acute interstitial nephritis occur rarely.

NURSING CONSIDERATIONS

BASELINE ASSESSMENT

Question for history of allergies, especially penicillins, cephalosporins.

INTERVENTION/EVALUATION

Hold medication and promptly report rash or diarrhea (with fever, abdominal pain, mucus and blood in stool may indicate antibiotic-associated colitis). Be alert for superinfection: increased fever, sore throat, vomiting, diarrhea, black/hairy tongue, stomatitis, anal/genital pruritus.

PATIENT/FAMILY TEACHING

• Continue antibiotic for full length of treatment. Space doses evenly. • Take with meals if GI upset occurs. • Thoroughly chew the chewable tablets before swallowing. • Notify physician in event of rash, diarrhea, or other new symptom.

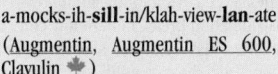

amoxicillin/ clavulanate potassium

a-mocks-ih-**sill**-in/klah-view-**lan**-ate (Augmentin, Augmentin ES 600, Clavulin ✤)

Do not confuse amoxicillin with amoxapine.

◆ CLASSIFICATION

PHARMACOTHERAPEUTIC: Penicillin. **CLINICAL:** Antibiotic (see p. 28C).

ACTION

Amoxicillin inhibits bacterial cell wall synthesis, while clavulanate inhibits bacterial beta-lactamase. **Therapeutic Effect:** Amoxicillin is bactericidal in susceptible microorganisms. Clavulanate protects amoxicillin from enzymatic degradation.

PHARMACOKINETICS

Well absorbed from the GI tract. Protein binding: 20%. Partially metabolized in the liver. Primarily excreted in urine. Removed by hemodialysis. **Half-life:** 1–1.3 hr (increased in impaired renal function).

USES

Treatment of susceptible infections due to *streptococci, E. coli, E. faecalis, P. mirabilis,* beta lactamase producing *H. influenzae, Klebsiella species, M. catarrhalis,* and *S. aureus* (not methicillin-resistant *Staphylococcus aureus* [MRSA]) including lower respiratory, skin and skin structure and urinary tract infections, otitis media, sinusitis. **OFF-LABEL:** Treatment of bronchitis and chancroid.

PRECAUTIONS

CONTRAINDICATIONS: Hypersensitivity to any penicillins, infectious mononucleosis. **CAUTIONS:** History of allergies, especially cephalosporins; antibiotic-associated colitis.

⧗ **LIFESPAN CONSIDERATIONS: Pregnancy/Lactation:** Crosses placenta, appears in cord blood, amniotic fluid. Distributed in breast milk in low concentrations. May lead to allergic sensitization, diarrhea, candidiasis, skin rash in infant. **Pregnancy Category B. Children:** Immature renal function in neonate/young infant may delay renal excretion. **Elderly:** Age-related renal impairment may require dosage adjustment.

INTERACTIONS

DRUG: Allopurinol: May increase incidence of rash. **Oral contraceptives:** May decrease effects of oral contraceptives. **Probenecid:** May increase amoxicillin and clavulanate blood concentration and risk of toxicity. **HERBAL:** None known. **FOOD:** None known. **LAB VALUES:** May increase serum AST and ALT levels. May cause a positive Coombs' test.

AVAILABILITY (Rx)

POWDER FOR ORAL SUSPENSION (AUGMENTIN): 125 mg–31.25 mg/5 ml, 200 mg–28.5 mg/5 ml, 250 mg–62.5 mg/5 ml, 400 mg–57 mg/5 ml, 600 mg–42.9 mg/5 ml. **TABLETS (AUGMENTIN):** 250 mg–125 mg, 500 mg–125 mg, 875 mg–125 mg. **TABLETS (EXTENDED-RELEASE [AUGMENTIN XR]):** 1,000 mg–62.5 mg. **TABLETS (CHEWABLE [AUGMENTIN]):** 125 mg–31.25 mg, 200 mg–28.5 mg, 250 mg–62.5 mg, 400 mg–57 mg.

ADMINISTRATION/HANDLING

PO

• Store tablets at room temperature. • After reconstitution, oral solution is stable for 14 days at room temperature or refrigerated. • Give without regard to meals. • Instruct patientt to chew/crush

chewable tablets thoroughly before swallowing.

INDICATIONS/ROUTES/DOSAGE

MILD TO MODERATE INFECTIONS
PO: ADULTS, ELDERLY: 500 mg q12h or 250 mg q8h.

SEVERE INFECTIONS, RESPIRATORY TRACT INFECTIONS
PO: ADULTS, ELDERLY: 875 mg q12h or 500 mg q8h.

COMMUNITY-ACQUIRED PNEUMONIA, SINUSITIS
PO: ADULTS, ELDERLY: 2 g (extended-release tablets) q12h for 7–10 days.

USUAL PEDIATRIC DOSAGE
PO: CHILDREN WEIGHING 40 KG AND LESS: 25–45 mg/kg/day (200 or 400 mg/5 ml powder or 200 or 400 chewable tablets) in 2 divided doses or 20–40 mg/kg/day (125 or 250 mg/5 ml powder or 125 or 250 mg chewable tablets) in 3 divided doses.

OTITIS MEDIA
PO: CHILDREN: 90 mg/kg/day (600 mg/5 ml suspension) in divided doses q12h for 10 days.

USUAL NEONATE DOSAGE
PO: NEONATES, CHILDREN YOUNGER THAN 3 MO: 30 mg/kg/day (125 mg/5 ml suspension) in divided doses q12h.

DOSAGE IN RENAL IMPAIRMENT
Dosage and frequency are modified based on creatinine clearance. **Creatinine clearance 10–30 ml/min:** 250–500 mg q12h. **Creatinine clearance less than 10 ml/min:** 250–500 mg q24h.

SIDE EFFECTS

FREQUENT: GI disturbances (mild diarrhea, nausea, vomiting), headache, oral or vaginal candidiasis. **OCCASIONAL:** Generalized rash, urticaria.

ADVERSE REACTIONS/ TOXIC EFFECTS

Antibiotic-associated colitis and other superinfections may result from altered bacterial balance. Severe hypersensitivity reactions, including anaphylaxis and acute interstitial nephritis occur rarely.

NURSING CONSIDERATIONS

BASELINE ASSESSMENT
Question for history of allergies, especially penicillins, cephalosporins.

INTERVENTION/EVALUATION
Hold medication and promptly report rash or diarrhea (with fever, abdominal pain, mucus and blood in stool may indicate antibiotic-associated colitis). Be alert for superinfection: increased fever, sore throat, vomiting, diarrhea, black/hairy tongue, ulceration or changes of oral mucosa, anal/genital pruritus.

PATIENT/FAMILY TEACHING
• Continue antibiotic for full length of treatment. • Space doses evenly. • Take with meals if GI upset occurs. • Thoroughly chew the chewable tablets before swallowing. • Notify physician in event of rash, diarrhea, or other new symptom.

Amoxil, *see amoxicillin*

---

amphotericin B ▶

am-foe-**tear**-ih-sin

(Abelcet, AmBisome, Amphocin, Amphotec, Fungizone, Fungizone for Tissue Culture)

◆CLASSIFICATION
CLINICAL: Antifungal, antiprotozoal.

ACTION
An antifungal and antiprotozoal that is generally fungistatic but may become fungicidal with high dosages or very susceptible microorganisms. This drug binds to sterols in the fungal cell membrane. Therapeutic Effect: Increases fungal cell-membrane permeability, allowing loss of potassium and other cellular components.

PHARMACOKINETICS
Protein binding: 90%. Widely distributed. Metabolic fate unknown. Cleared by nonrenal pathways. Minimal removal by hemodialysis. Amphotec and Abelcet are not dialyzable. Half-life: Fungizone, 24 hr (increased in neonates and children); Amphotec, 26–28 hr; Abelcet, 7.2 days; AmBisome, 100–153 hr.

USES
Abelcet: Treatment of invasive fungal infections refractory or intolerant to Fungizone. AmBisome: Empiric treatment for fungal infection in febrile neutropenic patients. *Aspergillus,* candida, or cryptococcus infections refractory to Fungizone or patient with renal impairment or toxicity with Fungizone. Treatment of visceral leishmaniasis. Amphotec: Treatment of invasive aspergillosis in patients with renal impairment or toxicity or prior treatment failure with Fungizone. Fungizone: Treatment of cryptococcosis, blastomycosis, systemic candidiasis, disseminated forms of moniliasis, coccidioidomycosis, and histoplasmosis, zygomycosis, sporotrichosis, aspergillosis. Topical: Treatment of cutaneous/mucocutaneous infections caused by *Candida albicans* (paronychia, oral thrush, perle'che, diaper rash, intertriginous candidiasis). OFF-LABEL: Febrile neutropenia, meningoencephalitis, paracoccidioidomycosis

PRECAUTIONS
CONTRAINDICATIONS: Hypersensitivity to amphotericin B or sulfites. CAUTIONS: Renal impairment, in combination with antineoplastic therapy. Give only

---

for progressive, potentially fatal fungal infection.

⧗ **LIFESPAN CONSIDERATIONS: Pregnancy/Lactation:** Crosses placenta; unknown if distributed in breast milk. **Pregnancy Category B. Children:** Safety and efficacy not established, but use the least amount for therapeutic regimen. **Elderly:** No age-related precautions noted.

INTERACTIONS

DRUG: Bone marrow depressants: May increase the risk of anemia. **Digoxin:** May increase the risk of digoxin toxicity from hypokalemia. **Nephrotoxic medications:** May increase the risk of nephrotoxicity. **Steroids:** May cause severe hypokalemia. **HERBAL:** None known. **FOOD:** None known. **LAB VALUES:** May increase BUN, serum alkaline phosphatase, serum creatinine, serum AST, and ALT levels. May decrease serum calcium, magnesium, and potassium levels.

AVAILABILITY (Rx)

CREAM (FUNGIZONE): 3%. **INJECTION (POWDER FOR RECONSTITUTION):** 50 mg (AmBisome, Amphocin, Amphotec, Fungizone), 100 mg (Amphotec). **INJECTION (SUSPENSION [ABELCET]):** 5 mg/ml.

ADMINISTRATION/HANDLING

IV

• Monitor BP, temperature, pulse, respirations; assess for adverse reactions q15min twice, then q30min for 4 hr after initial infusion. • Potential for thrombophlebitis may be less with use of pediatric scalp vein needles or (with physician order) adding dilute heparin solution. • Observe strict aseptic technique because no bacteriostatic agent or preservative is present in diluent.

Reconstitution
ABELCET
• Shake 20-ml (100-mg) vial gently until contents are dissolved. Withdraw required dose using 5-micron filter needle (supplied by manufacturer). • Inject dose into D_5W; 4 ml D_5W required for each 1 ml (5 mg) to final concentration of 1 mg/ml. Reduce dose by half for pediatric, fluid-restricted patients (2 mg/ml).
AMBISOME
• Reconstitute each 50-mg vial with 12 ml sterile water for injection to provide concentration of 4 mg/ml. • Shake vial vigorously for 30 sec. Withdraw required dose and empty syringe contents through a 5-micron filter into an infusion of D_5W to provide final concentration of 1–2 mg/ml.
AMPHOTEC
• Add 10 ml sterile water for injection to each 50-mg vial to provide concentration of 5 mg/ml. Shake gently. • Further dilute **only** with D_5W using specific amount recommended by manufacturer to provide concentration of 0.16–0.83 mg/ml.
FUNGIZONE
• Rapidly inject 10 ml sterile water for injection to each 50-mg vial to provide concentration of 5 mg/ml. Immediately shake vial until solution is clear. • Further dilute each 1 mg in at least 10 ml D_5W to provide a concentration of 0.1mg/ml.

Rate of administration
• Give by slow IV infusion. Infuse conventional amphotericin or Fungizone over 2–6 hr; Abelcet over 2 hr (shake contents if infusion longer than 2 hr); Amphotec over 2–4 hr; AmBisome over 1–2 hr.

Storage
ABELCET
• Refrigerate unreconstituted solution. Reconstituted solution is stable for 48 hr if refrigerated; 6 hr at room temperature.
AMBISOME
• Refrigerate unreconstituted solution. Reconstituted solution of 4 mg/ml is

stable for 24 hr. Concentration of 1–2 mg/ml is stable for 6 hr.

AMPHOTEC

• Store unreconstituted solution at room temperature. Reconstituted solution stable for 24 hr.

FUNGIZONE

• Refrigerate unreconstituted solution. • Reconstituted solution is stable for 24 hr at room temperature or 7 days if refrigerated. • Diluted solution 0.1 mg/ml or less to be used promptly. Do not use if cloudy or contains a precipitate.

▨ IV INCOMPATIBILITIES

Abelcet, AmBisome, Amphotec: Don't mix with any other drug, diluent, or solution. Fungizone: Allopurinol (Aloprim), amifostine (Ethyol), aztreonam (Azactam), calcium gluconate, cefepime (Maxipime), cimetidine (Tagamet), ciprofloxacin (Cipro), docetaxel (Taxotere), dopamine (Intropin), doxorubicin (Adriamycin), enalapril (Vasotec), etoposide (VP-16), filgrastim (Neupogen), fluconazole (Diflucan), fludarabine (Fludara), foscarnet (Foscavir), gemcitabine (Gemzar), magnesium sulfate, meropenem (Merrem IV), ondansetron (Zofran), paclitaxel (Taxol), piperacillin and tazobactam (Zosyn), potassium chloride, propofol (Diprivan), total parenteral nutrition (TPN), vinorelbine (Navelbine).

IV COMPATIBILITIES

None known; don't mix with other medications or electrolytes.

INDICATIONS/ROUTES/DOSAGE

CRYPTOCOCCOSIS; BLASTOMYCOSIS; SYSTEMIC CANDIDIASIS; DISSEMINATED FORMS OF MONILIASIS, COCCIDIOIDOMYCOSIS, AND HISTOPLASMOSIS; ZYGOMYCOSIS; SPOROTRICHOSIS; ASPERGILLOSIS

IV INFUSION (FUNGIZONE): ADULTS, ELDERLY: Dosage based on patient tolerance and severity of infection. Initially, 1-mg test dose is given over 20–30 min. If test dose is tolerated, 5-mg dose may be given the same day. Subsequently, dosage is increased by 5 mg q12–24h until desired daily dose is reached. Alternatively, if test dose is tolerated, 0.25 mg/kg is given on same day and 0.5 mg/kg on second day; then dosage is increased until desired daily dose reached. Total daily dose: 1 mg/kg/day up to 1.5 mg/kg every other day. **Maximum:** 1.5 mg/kg/day. CHILDREN: Test dose of 0.1 mg/kg/dose (**Maximum:** 1 mg) is infused over 20–60 min. If test dose is tolerated, initial dose of 0.4 mg/kg may be given on same day; dosage is then increased in 0.25-mg/kg increments as needed. Maintenance dose: 0.25–1 mg/kg/day.

INVASIVE FUNGAL INFECTIONS UNRESPONSIVE TO OR INTOLERANT OF FUNGIZONE

IV INFUSION (ABELCET): ADULTS, CHILDREN: 2.5–5 mg/kg at rate of 2.5 mg/kg/hr.

EMPIRIC TREATMENT OF FUNGAL INFECTIONS IN PATIENTS WITH FEBRILE NEUTROPENIA; ASPERGILLOSIS, CANDIDIASIS, OR CRYPTOCOCCOSIS IN PATIENTS WITH RENAL IMPAIRMENT AND THOSE WHO HAVE EXPERIENCED TOXICITY OR TREATMENT FAILURE WITH FUNGIZONE

IV INFUSION (AMBISOME): ADULTS, CHILDREN: 3–5 mg/kg over 1 hr.

INVASIVE ASPERGILLOSIS IN PATIENTS WITH RENAL IMPAIRMENT AND THOSE WHO HAVE EXPERIENCED TOXICITY OR TREATMENT FAILURE WITH FUNGIZONE

IV INFUSION (AMPHOTEC): ADULTS, CHILDREN: 3–4 mg/kg over 2–4 hr. **Maximum:** 7.5 mg/kg/day.

CUTANEOUS AND MUCOCUTANEOUS INFECTIONS CAUSED BY CANDIDA ALBICANS, SUCH AS PARONYCHIA, ORAL THRUSH, PERLÈCHE, DIAPER RASH, AND

INTERTRIGINOUS CANDIDIASIS
TOPICAL: ADULTS, ELDERLY, CHILDREN: Apply liberally to affected area and rub in 2–4 times a day.

SIDE EFFECTS
FREQUENT (greater than 10%): Abelcet: Chills, fever, increased serum creatinine level, multiple organ failure. **Ambisome:** Hypokalemia, hypomagnesemia, hyperglycemia, hypocalcemia, edema, abdominal pain, back pain, chills, chest pain, hypotension, diarrhea, nausea, vomiting, headache, fever, rigors, insomnia, dyspnea, epistaxis, increased hepatic or renal function test results. **Amphotec:** Chills, fever, hypotension, tachycardia, increased serum creatinine level, hypokalemia, bilirubinemia. **Fungizone:** Fever, chills, headache, anemia, hypokalemia, hypomagnesemia, anorexia, malaise, generalized pain, nephrotoxicity. **Topical:** Local irritation, dry skin. **RARE: Topical:** Rash.

ADVERSE REACTIONS/ TOXIC EFFECTS
Cardiovascular toxicity (as evidenced by hypotension, ventricular fibrillation, and anaphylaxis) occurs rarely. Altered vision and hearing, seizures, hepatic failure, coagulation defects, multiple organ failure, and sepsis may be noted.

NURSING CONSIDERATIONS

BASELINE ASSESSMENT
Question for history of allergies, especially to amphotericin B, sulfite. Avoid, if possible, other nephrotoxic medications. Obtain premedication orders to reduce adverse reactions during IV therapy (antipyretics, antihistamines, antiemetics, or small doses of corticosteroids given before or during amphotericin administration may control reactions).

INTERVENTION/EVALUATION
Monitor BP, temperature, pulse, respirations; assess for adverse reactions (fever, tremors, chills, anorexia, nausea, vomiting, abdominal pain) q15min twice, then q30min for 4 hr of initial infusion. If symptoms occur, slow infusion, administer medication for symptomatic relief. For severe reaction or without symptomatic relief orders, stop infusion and notify physician. Evaluate IV site for phlebitis (heat, pain, red streaking over vein). Monitor I&O, renal function tests for nephrotoxicity. Check serum potassium and magnesium levels, hematologic and hepatic function test results. **Topical:** Assess for itching, irritation, burning.

PATIENT/FAMILY TEACHING
• Prolonged therapy (weeks or months) is usually necessary. • Fever reaction may decrease with continued therapy. • Muscle weakness may be noted during therapy (due to hypokalemia). **Topical:** Application may cause staining of skin or nails; soap and water or dry cleaning will remove fabric stains. • Do not use other preparations or occlusive coverings without consulting physician. • Keep areas clean, dry; wear light clothing. • Separate personal items with direct contact to area.

ampicillin sodium

am-pi-**sill**-in **soe**-dee-um

(Apo-Ampi ✦, Novo-Ampicillin ✦, Nu-Ampi ✦, Polycillin, Principen)

Do not confuse ampicillin with aminophylline, Imipenem, or Unipen.

◆CLASSIFICATION
PHARMACOTHERAPEUTIC: Penicillin. **CLINICAL:** Antibiotic (see p. 28C).

ACTION

A penicillin that inhibits cell wall synthesis in susceptible microorganisms. **Therapeutic Effect:** Bactericidal.

PHARMACOKINETICS

Moderately absorbed from the GI tract. Protein binding: 28%. Widely distributed. Partially metabolized in the liver. Primarily excreted in urine. Removed by hemodialysis. **Half-life:** 1–1.5 hr (increased in impaired renal function).

USES

Treatment of susceptible infections due to *streptococci, S. pneumoniae, staphylococci* (non–penicillinase producing), *meningococci, Listeria,* some *Klebsiella, E. coli, H. influenzae, Salmonella, Shigella* including GI, GU and respiratory infections, meningitis, and endocarditis prophylaxis.

PRECAUTIONS

CONTRAINDICATIONS: Hypersensitivity to any penicillin, infectious mononucleosis. **CAUTIONS:** History of allergies, particularly cephalosporins, antibiotic-associated colitis.

LIFESPAN CONSIDERATIONS: Pregnancy/Lactation: Readily crosses placenta; appears in cord blood, amniotic fluid. Distributed in breast milk in low concentrations. May lead to allergic sensitization, diarrhea, candidiasis, skin rash in infant. **Pregnancy Category B. Children:** Immature renal function in neonates/young infants may delay renal excretion. **Elderly:** Age-related renal impairment may require dosage adjustment.

INTERACTIONS

DRUG: Allopurinol: May increase incidence of rash. **Oral contraceptives:** May decrease effectiveness of oral contraceptives. **Probenecid:** May increase ampicillin blood concentration and risk of ampicillin toxicity. **HERBAL:** None known. **FOOD:** None known. **LAB VALUES:** May increase AST and ALT levels. May cause a positive Coombs' test.

AVAILABILITY (Rx)

CAPSULES (PRINCIPEN): 250 mg, 500 mg. **POWDER FOR ORAL SUSPENSION:** 125 mg/5 ml **(POLYCILLIN, PRINCIPEN),** 250 mg/5 ml **(POLYCILLIN, PRINCIPEN),** 500 mg/5 ml **(POLYCILLIN). POWDER FOR INJECTION (POLYCILLIN):** 125 mg, 250 mg, 500 mg, 1 g, 2 g.

ADMINISTRATION/HANDLING

 IV

Reconstitution • For IV injection, dilute each vial with 5 ml sterile water for injection (10 ml for 1- and 2-g vials). • For intermittent IV infusion (piggyback), further dilute with 50–100 ml 0.9% NaCl or D_5W.

Rate of administration • For IV injection, give over 3–5 min (10–15 min for 1- to 2-g dose). • For intermittent IV infusion (piggyback), infuse over 20–30 min. • Due to potential for hypersensitivity/anaphylaxis, start initial dose at few drops per min, increase slowly to ordered rate; stay with patient first 10–15 min, then check q10min. • Change to PO as soon as possible.

Storage • The IV solution, diluted with 0.9% NaCl, is stable for 2–8 hr at room temperature or 3 days if refrigerated. • If diluted with D_5W, is stable for 2 hr at room temperature or 3 hr if refrigerated. • Discard if precipitate forms.

IM
• Reconstitute each vial with sterile water for injection or bacteriostatic water for injection (consult individual vial for specific volume of diluent). • Stable for 1 hr. • Give deeply in large muscle mass.

PO

- Store capsules at room temperature.
- Oral suspension, after reconstituted, is stable for 7 days at room temperature, 14 days if refrigerated. • Give orally 1 hr before or 2 hr after meals for maximum absorption.

▨ IV INCOMPATIBILITIES

Amikacin (Amikin), diltiazem (Cardizem), gentamicin, midazolam (Versed).

IV COMPATIBILITIES

Calcium gluconate, cefepime (Maxipime), dopamine (Intropin), famotidine (Pepcid), furosemide (Lasix), heparin, hydromorphone (Dilaudid), insulin (regular), levofloxacin (Levaquin), magnesium sulfate, morphine, multivitamins, potassium chloride, propofol (Diprivan), total parenteral nutrition (TPN) (if ampicillin sodium concentration is less than 40 mg/ml).

INDICATIONS/ROUTES/DOSAGE

USUAL DOSAGE

PO: ADULTS, ELDERLY: 250–500 mg q6h. CHILDREN: 50–100 mg/kg/day in divided doses q6h. **Maximum:** 3 g/day.
IV, IM: ADULTS, ELDERLY: 500 mg–3 g q4–6h. **Maximum:** 14 g/day. CHILDREN: 100–200 mg/kg/day in divided doses q6h. NEONATES: 50–100 mg/kg/day in divided doses q6–12h.

GI, GU INFECTIONS

IV, IM: ADULTS, ELDERLY: 500 mg q6h.
PO: ADULTS, ELDERLY: 500 mg q6h. CHILDREN: 100 mg/kg/day in 4 divided doses.

RESPIRATORY TRACT INFECTIONS

IV, IM: ADULTS, ELDERLY: 250–500 mg q6h.
PO: ADULTS, ELDERLY: 250 mg q6h.

ENDOCARDITIS PROPHYLAXIS

IV, IM: ADULTS, ELDERLY: 1–2 g (plus gentamicin) 30 min before procedure. CHILDREN: 50 mg/kg (plus gentamicin in high-risk patients), with follow up dose of 25–50 mg/kg 6–8 hr later.

MENINGITIS

IV: ADULTS, ELDERLY: 8–14 g/day in 4–6 divided doses. CHILDREN: 200–400 mg/kg/day in divided doses q6h. **Maximum:** 12 g/day. NEONATES: 100–200 mg/kg/day in divided doses q6–12h.

GONOCOCCAL INFECTIONS

PO: ADULTS: 3.5 g one time with 1 g probenecid.
IM: MALES: 500 mg for 2 doses.

PERIOPERATIVE PROPHYLAXIS

IV, IM: ADULTS, ELDERLY: 2 g 30 min before procedure. May repeat in 8 hr. CHILDREN: 50 mg/kg 30 min before procedure. May repeat in 8 hr.

DOSAGE IN RENAL IMPAIRMENT

Creatinine Clearance	% of Normal Dosage
10–30 ml/min	Give q6–12h
Less than 10 ml/min	Give q12h

SIDE EFFECTS

FREQUENT: Pain at IM injection site, GI disturbances (mild diarrhea, nausea, vomiting), oral or vaginal candidiasis.
OCCASIONAL: Generalized rash, urticaria, phlebitis or thrombophlebitis (with IV administration), headache.
RARE: Dizziness, seizures (especially with IV therapy).

ADVERSE REACTIONS/ TOXIC EFFECTS

Antibiotic-associated colitis and other superinfections may result from altered bacterial balance. Severe hypersensitivity reactions, including anaphylaxis and acute interstitial nephritis, occur rarely.

NURSING CONSIDERATIONS

BASELINE ASSESSMENT

Question for history of allergies, especially penicillins, cephalosporins.

INTERVENTION/EVALUATION

Hold medication and promptly report rash (although common with ampicillin, may indicate hypersensitivity) or diarrhea (with fever, abdominal pain, mucus and blood in stool may indicate antibiotic-associated colitis). Evaluate IV site for phlebitis (heat, pain, red streaking over vein). Check IM injection site for pain, induration. Monitor I&O, urinalysis, renal function tests. Assess for signs of superinfection: increased fever, sore throat, vomiting, diarrhea, anal/genital pruritus, oral ulcerations or pain, black/hairy tongue.

PATIENT/FAMILY TEACHING

• Space doses evenly. • Take antibiotic for full length of treatment. • More effective if taken 1 hr before or 2 hr after food/beverages. • Discomfort may occur with IM injection. • Notify physician of rash, diarrhea, or other new symptom.

ampicillin/ sulbactam sodium

amp-ih-**sill**-in/sull-**bak**-tam soe-dee-um

(Unasyn)

◆CLASSIFICATION

PHARMACOTHERAPEUTIC: Penicillin. **CLINICAL:** Antibiotic (see p. 28C).

ACTION

Ampicillin inhibits bacterial cell wall synthesis, while sulbactam inhibits bacterial beta-lactamase. **Therapeutic Effect:** Ampicillin is bactericidal in susceptible microorganisms. Sulbactam protects ampicillin from enzymatic degradation.

PHARMACOKINETICS

Protein binding: 28%–38%. Widely distributed. Partially metabolized in the liver. Primarily excreted in urine. Removed by hemodialysis. **Half-life:** 1 hr (increased in impaired renal function).

USES

Treatment of susceptible infections due to beta-lactamase producing orgainisms including *H. influenzae, E. coli, Klebsiella, Acinetobacter, Enterobacter, S. aureus,* and Bacteroides species including intra-abdominal, skin/skin structure, gynecologic infections.

PRECAUTIONS

CONTRAINDICATIONS: Hypersensitivity to any penicillin or sulbactam, infectious mononucleosis. **CAUTIONS:** History of allergies, particularly to cephalosporins, antibiotic-associated colitis.

⧖ **LIFESPAN CONSIDERATIONS: Pregnancy/Lactation:** Readily crosses placenta; appears in cord blood, amniotic fluid. Distributed in breast milk in low concentrations. May lead to allergic sensitization, diarrhea, candidiasis, skin rash in infant. **Pregnancy Category B. Children:** Safety and efficacy not established in children younger than 1 yr. **Elderly:** Age-related renal impairment may require dosage adjustment.

INTERACTIONS

DRUG: Allopurinol: May increase incidence of rash. **Oral contraceptives:** May decrease effectiveness of oral contraceptives. **Probenecid:** May increase ampicillin blood concentration and risk of ampicillin toxicity. **HERBAL:** None known. **FOOD:** None known. **LAB VALUES:** May increase serum LDH, alkaline phosphatase, creatinine, AST, and ALT levels. May cause a positive Coombs' test.

AVAILABILITY (Rx)

POWDER FOR INJECTION: 1.5 g (ampicillin 1 g/sulbactam 500 g), 3 g (ampicillin 2 g/sulbactam 1 g).

ADMINISTRATION/HANDLING

 IV

Reconstitution • For IV injection, dilute with 10–20 ml sterile water for injection. • For intermittent IV infusion (piggyback), further dilute with 50–100 ml D_5W or 0.9% NaCl.

Rate of administration • For IV injection, give slowly over minimum of 10–15 min. • For intermittent IV infusion (piggyback), infuse over 15–30 min. • Due to potential for hypersensitivity/anaphylaxis, start initial dose at few drops per min, increase slowly to ordered rate; stay with patient first 10–15 min, then check q10min. • Change to PO antibiotic as soon as possible.

Storage • When reconstituted with 0.9% NaCl, IV solution is stable for 8 hr at room temperature, 48 hr if refrigerated. Stability may be different with other diluents. • Discard if precipitate forms.

IM
• Reconstitute each 1.5-g vial with 3.2 ml sterile water for injection to provide concentration of 250 mg ampicillin/125 mg sublactam/ml. • Give deeply into large muscle mass within 1 hr after preparation.

IV INCOMPATIBILITIES

Diltiazem (Cardizem), idarubicin (Idamycin), ondansetron (Zofran), sargramostim (Leukine), total parenteral nutrition (TPN).

IV COMPATIBILITIES

Famotidine (Pepcid), heparin, insulin (regular), morphine.

INDICATIONS/ROUTES/DOSAGE

SKIN AND SKIN-STRUCTURE, INTRA-ABDOMINAL, AND GYNECOLOGIC

INFECTIONS

IV, IM: ADULTS, ELDERLY: 1.5 g (1 g ampicillin/500 mg sulbactam) to 3 g (2 g ampicillin/1 g sulbactam) q6h.

SKIN AND SKIN-STRUCTURE INFECTIONS

IV: CHILDREN 12 YR AND YOUNGER: 150–400 mg/kg/day in divided doses q6h.

DOSAGE IN RENAL IMPAIRMENT

Dosage and frequency are modified based on creatinine clearance and the severity of the infection.

Creatinine Clearance	Dosage
Greater than 30 ml/min	0.5–3 g q6–8h
15–29 ml/min	1.5–3 g q12h
5–14 ml/min	1.5–3 g q24h
Less than 5 ml/min	Not recommended

SIDE EFFECTS

FREQUENT: Diarrhea and rash (most common), urticaria, pain at IM injection site, thrombophlebitis with IV administration, oral or vaginal candidiasis.
OCCASIONAL: Nausea, vomiting, headache, malaise, urine retention.

ADVERSE REACTIONS/ TOXIC EFFECTS

Severe hypersensitivity reactions, including anaphylaxis, acute interstitial nephritis, and blood dyscrasias may occur. Antibiotic-associated colitis and other superinfections may result from altered bacterial balance. Overdose may produce seizures.

NURSING CONSIDERATIONS

BASELINE ASSESSMENT

Question for history of allergies, especially penicillins, cephalosporins.

INTERVENTION/EVALUATION

Hold medication and promptly report rash (although common with ampicillin, may indicate hypersensitivity) or diarrhea (with fever, mucus and blood in stool, abdominal pain may indicate antibiotic-associated colitis). Evaluate IV site for phlebitis (heat, pain, red streaking over vein). Check IM injection site for pain, induration. Monitor I&O, urinalysis, renal function tests. Assess for initial signs of superinfection: increased fever, sore throat onset, vomiting, diarrhea, anal/genital pruritus, ulceration or changes of oral mucosa.

PATIENT/FAMILY TEACHING

• Space doses evenly. • Take antibiotic for full length of treatment. • Discomfort may occur with IM injection. • Notify physician of rash, diarrhea, or other new symptoms.

---

amprenavir

am-**prehn**-eh-veer

(Agenerase)

Do not confuse Agenerase with asparaginase.

◆ CLASSIFICATION

PHARMACOTHERAPEUTIC: Antiviral. **CLINICAL:** Protease inhibitor (see pp. 70C, 104C).

ACTION

An antiretroviral that inhibits HIV-1 protease by binding to the enzyme's active site, thus preventing processing of viral precursors and resulting in the formation of immature, noninfectious viral particles. **Therapeutic Effect:** Impairs HIV replication and proliferation.

PHARMACOKINETICS

Rapidly absorbed after PO administration. Protein binding: 90%. Metabolized in the liver. Primarily excreted in feces. **Half-life:** 7.1–10.6 hr.

USES

Treatment of HIV-1 infection in combination with other antiretroviral agents.

PRECAUTIONS

CONTRAINDICATIONS: None known. **CAUTIONS:** Hepatic impairment, diabetes mellitus, hemophilia, hypersensitivity to sulfas, vitamin K deficiency due to anticoagulant/malabsorption.

⧗ **LIFESPAN CONSIDERATIONS: Pregnancy/Lactation:** Unknown if drug crosses placenta or is distributed in breast milk. **Pregnancy Category C. Children:** Safety and efficacy of capsules not established in those younger than 4 yr. **Elderly:** Age-related liver impairment may require decreased dosage.

INTERACTIONS

DRUG: Amiodarone, bepridil, ergotamine, lidocaine, midazolam, oral contraceptives, quinidine, triazolam, tricyclic antidepressants: May interfere with the metabolism of these drugs. **Antacids, didanosine:** May decrease amprenavir absorption. **Carbamazepine, phenobarbital, phenytoin, rifampin:** May decrease amprenavir blood concentration. **Clozapine, HMG-CoA reductase inhibitors (including statins), warfarin:** May increase the blood concentration of these drugs. HERBAL: **St. John's wort:** May decrease amprenavir blood concentration. FOOD: **High-fat meals:** May decrease amprenavir absorption. LAB VALUES: May increase blood cholesterol, serum glucose, and triglyceride levels.

AVAILABILITY (Rx)

CAPSULES: 50 mg. **ORAL SOLUTION:** 15 mg/ml.

ADMINISTRATION/HANDLING

PO

• May give without regard to food.

INDICATIONS/ROUTES/DOSAGE

HIV-1 INFECTION (IN COMBINATION WITH OTHER ANTIRETROVIRALS)

PO: ADULTS, CHILDREN 17 YR AND OLDER, CHILDREN 13–16 YR WEIGHING 50 KG AND MORE:

1,200 mg twice a day. CHILDREN 4–12 YR, CHILDREN 13–16 YR WEIGHING LESS THAN 50 KG: 20 mg/kg twice a day or 15 mg/kg 3 times a day. **Maximum:** 2,400 mg/day.

ORAL SOLUTION: ADULTS, CHILDREN 17 YR AND OLDER, CHILDREN 13–16 YR WEIGHING 50 KG AND MORE: 1,400 mg twice a day. CHILDREN 4–12 YR, CHILDREN 13–16 YR WEIGHING LESS THAN 50 KG: 22.5 mg/kg/day (1.5 ml/kg) oral solution twice a day or 17 mg/kg/day (1.1 ml/kg) 3 times a day. **Maximum:** 2,800 mg/day.

DOSAGE IN HEPATIC IMPAIRMENT

Dosage and frequency are modified based on the Child-Pugh score.

Child-Pugh Score	Capsules	Oral Solution
5–8	450 mg bid	513 mg bid
9–12	300 mg bid	342 mg bid

SIDE EFFECTS

FREQUENT: Diarrhea or loose stools (56%), nausea (38%), oral paresthesia (30%), rash (25%), vomiting (20%). **OCCASIONAL:** Peripheral paresthesia (12%), depression (4%).

ADVERSE REACTIONS/ TOXIC EFFECTS

Severe hypersensitivity reactions or Stevens-Johnson syndrome as evidenced by blisters, peeling of the skin, loosening of skin and mucous membranes, and fever may occur.

NURSING CONSIDERATIONS

BASELINE ASSESSMENT

Obtain baseline laboratory tests before beginning therapy and at periodic intervals during therapy. Offer emotional support.

INTERVENTION/EVALUATION

Assess for nausea, vomiting. Determine pattern of bowel activity and stool consistency. Assess eating pattern; monitor for weight loss. Assess for paresthesias. Assess skin for rash.

PATIENT/FAMILY TEACHING

• Avoid high-fat meals (decreases drug absorption). • Small, frequent meals may offset anorexia, nausea. • Amprenavir is not a cure for HIV infection, nor does it reduce risk of transmission to others.

anagrelide

ah-na-**greh**-lide
(Agrylin)

◆ CLASSIFICATION

PHARMACOTHERAPEUTIC: Hematologic agent. **CLINICAL:** Antiplatelet.

ACTION

A hematologic agent that reduces platelet production and prevents platelet shape changes caused by platelet aggregating agents. **Therapeutic Effect:** Inhibits platelet aggregation.

PHARMACOKINETICS

After oral administration, plasma concentration peak within 1 hr. Extensively metabolized. Primarily excreted in urine. **Half-life:** About 3 days.

USES

Treatment of essential thrombocythemia, reducing elevated platelet count and risk of thrombosis. Treatment of thrombocythemia due to myeloproliferative disorders.

PRECAUTIONS

CONTRAINDICATIONS: Severe hepatic impairment. **CAUTIONS:** Cardiac disease; renal or hepatic impairment.

⧗ **LIFESPAN CONSIDERATIONS: Pregnancy/Lactation:** Unknown if drug crosses placenta or is distributed in breast milk. May cause fetal harm.

Pregnancy Category C. Children: Safety and efficacy in those younger than 16 yr not established. **Elderly**: Age-related renal or hepatic impairment, cardiac disease requires caution.

INTERACTIONS

DRUG: None known. **HERBAL**: **Ginkgo biloba**: May increase the risk of bleeding. **FOOD**: None known. **LAB VALUES**: May increase hepatic enzymes levels (rare).

AVAILABILITY (Rx)

CAPSULES: 0.5 mg, 1 mg.

ADMINISTRATION/HANDLING

PO
• Give without regard to food.

INDICATIONS/ROUTES/DOSAGE

THROMBOCYTHEMIA
PO: ADULTS, ELDERLY: Initially, 0.5 mg 4 times a day or 1 mg twice a day. Adjust to lowest effective dosage, increasing by up to 0.5 mg/day or less in any 1 wk. **Maximum**: 10 mg/day or 2.5 mg/dose. CHILDREN: Initially, 0.5 mg/day. Range: 0.5 mg 1–4 times a day.

SIDE EFFECTS

FREQUENT (5% or more): Headache, palpitations, diarrhea, abdominal pain, nausea, flatulence, bloating, asthenia, pain, dizziness. **OCCASIONAL (less than 5%)**: Tachycardia, chest pain, vomiting, paresthesia, peripheral edema, anorexia, dyspepsia, rash. **RARE**: Confusion, insomnia.

ADVERSE REACTIONS/ TOXIC EFFECTS

Angina, heart failure, and arrhythmias occur rarely.

NURSING CONSIDERATIONS

BASELINE ASSESSMENT
Assess platelet count, Hgb, Hct, WBC before treatment, q2days during first wk of treatment, and weekly thereafter until therapeutic range is achieved. Ask if patient is breast-feeding, pregnant, or planning to become pregnant (may cause fetal harm).

INTERVENTION/EVALUATION
Monitor serum liver function, BUN, creatinine. Patients with suspected heart disease should be monitored closely. Assess skin for bruises, petechiae, also catheter insertion site, needle site, GI sites.

PATIENT/FAMILY TEACHING
• Platelet count responds within 7–14 days. • Not recommended in pregnancy. • Use contraceptives while taking anagrelide.

anakinra

an-a-**kin**-ra
(Kineret)

CLASSIFICATION

PHARMACOTHERAPEUTIC: Interleukin-1 receptor antagonist. **CLINICAL**: Anti-inflammatory.

ACTION

An interleukin-1 (IL-1) receptor antagonist that blocks the binding of IL-1, a protein that is a major mediator of joint disease and is present in excess amounts in patients with rheumatoid arthritis. **Therapeutic Effect**: Inhibits the inflammatory response.

PHARMACOKINETICS

No accumulation of anakinra in tissues or organs was observed after daily subcutaneous doses. Excreted in urine. **Half-life**: 4–6 hr.

USES

Treatment of signs and symptoms or slows the progression of structural damage of moderate to severely active rheumatoid arthritis in patients who have failed treatment with one or more disease modifying antirheumatic drugs.

PRECAUTIONS

CONTRAINDICATIONS: Known hypersensitivity to *Escherichia coli*-derived proteins, serious infection. **CAUTIONS:** Renal function impairment (risk of toxic reaction is increased), asthma (higher incidence of serious infection).

LIFESPAN CONSIDERATIONS: Pregnancy/Lactation: Unknown if distributed in breast milk. **Pregnancy Category B. Children:** Safety and efficacy not established. **Elderly:** Age-related renal impairment may require caution.

INTERACTIONS

DRUG: Live-virus vaccines: May cause the vaccines to be ineffective. **HERBAL:** None known. **FOOD:** None known. **LAB VALUES:** May increase the eosinophil count. May decrease WBC, platelet, and absolute neutrophil counts.

AVAILABILITY (Rx)

SOLUTION: 100-mg syringe.

ADMINISTRATION/HANDLING

SUBCUTANEOUS
• Store in refrigerator. Do not freeze or shake. • Do not use if particulate or discoloration is noted. • Give by subcutaneous injection.

INDICATIONS/ROUTES/DOSAGE

RHEUMATOID ARTHRITIS
SUBCUTANEOUS: ADULTS, ELDERLY: 100 mg/day, given at same time each day.

SIDE EFFECTS

OCCASIONAL: Injection site ecchymosis, erythema, and inflammation. **RARE:** Headache, nausea, diarrhea, abdominal pain.

ADVERSE REACTIONS/TOXIC EFFECTS

Infections, including upper respiratory tract infection, sinusitis, flu-like symptoms, and cellulitis, have been noted. Neutropenia may occur, particularly when anakinra is used in combination with tumor necrosis factor-blocking agents.

BASELINE ASSESSMENT
Do not give live vaccine concurrently (vaccination may not be effective in those receiving anakinra).

INTERVENTION/EVALUATION
Monitor neutrophil count before therapy begins, monthly for 3 mo while receiving therapy, and then quarterly for up to 1 yr. Assess for inflammatory reaction, especially during first 4 wk of therapy (uncommon after the first month of therapy).

PATIENT/FAMILY TEACHING
• Instruct patient on proper dosage and administration, correct procedure to administer subcutaneous dosage.
• Advise patient on importance of proper disposal of syringes and needles.

---

anastrozole

ah-**nas**-trow-zole
(Arimidex)
Do not confuse Arimidex with Imitrex.

◆CLASSIFICATION

PHARMACOTHERAPEUTIC: Aromatase inhibitor. **CLINICAL:** Antineoplastic hormone (see p. 71C).

ACTION

Decreases the circulating estrogen level by inhibiting aromatase, the

---

enzyme that catalyzes the final step in estrogen production. **Therapeutic Effect:** Inhibits the growth of breast cancers that are stimulated by estrogens.

PHARMACOKINETICS

Well absorbed into systemic circulation (absorption not affected by food). Protein binding: 40%. Extensively metabolized in the liver. Eliminated by biliary system and, to a lesser extent, kidneys. **Mean half-life:** 50 hr in postmenopausal women. Steady-state plasma levels reached in about 7 days.

USES

Treatment of advanced breast cancer in postmenopausal women who have developed progressive disease while receiving tamoxifen therapy. First-line therapy in advanced or metastatic breast cancer. Adjuvant treatment in early breast cancer.

PRECAUTIONS

CONTRAINDICATIONS: None known. **CAUTIONS:** None known.

⌛ **LIFESPAN CONSIDERATIONS: Pregnancy/Lactation:** Crosses placenta; may cause fetal harm. Unknown if excreted in breast milk. **Pregnancy Category D. Children:** Safety and efficacy not established. **Elderly:** No age-related precautions noted.

INTERACTIONS

DRUG: None known. **HERBAL:** None known. **FOOD:** None known. **LAB VALUES:** May elevate serum GGT level in patients with liver metastasis. May increase serum LDL, serum alkaline phosphate, AST, ALT, and total cholesterol levels.

AVAILABILITY (Rx)

TABLETS: 1 mg.

ADMINISTRATION/HANDLING

PO
- Give without regard to food.

INDICATIONS/ROUTES/DOSAGE

BREAST CANCER
PO: ADULTS, ELDERLY: 1 mg once a day.

SIDE EFFECTS

FREQUENT (16%–8%): Asthenia, nausea, headache, hot flashes, back pain, vomiting, cough, diarrhea. **OCCASIONAL (6%–4%):** Constipation, abdominal pain, anorexia, bone pain, pharyngitis, dizziness, rash, dry mouth, peripheral edema, pelvic pain, depression, chest pain, paresthesia. **RARE (2%–1%):** Weight gain, diaphoresis.

ADVERSE REACTIONS/TOXIC EFFECTS

Thrombophlebitis, anemia, leukopenia, and vaginal hemorrhage occur rarely.

NURSING CONSIDERATIONS

INTERVENTION/EVALUATION

Monitor for asthenia and dizziness and assist with ambulation if needed. Assess for headache. Offer antiemetic for nausea and vomiting. Monitor for onset of diarrhea; offer antidiarrheal medication.

PATIENT/FAMILY TEACHING

- Notify physician if nausea, asthenia, hot flashes become unmanageable.

Ancef, *see cefazolin*

AndroGel, *see testosterone*

Angiomax, *see bivalirudin*

---

antihemophilic factor (factor VIII, AHF)

an-tee-hee-moe-**fill**-ick **fak**-tor
(Alphanate, Hemofil M, Humanate P, Koate DVI, Monarc M, Monoclate-P)

Do not confuse Alphanate with Alfenta.

◆CLASSIFICATION

PHARMACOTHERAPEUTIC: Antihemophilic agent. **CLINICAL:** Hemostatic.

ACTION

An antihemophilic agent that assists in conversion of prothrombin to thrombin, essential for blood coagulation. Replaces missing clotting factor. **Therapeutic Effect:** Produces hemostasis; corrects or prevents bleeding episodes.

PHARMACOKINETICS

Half-Life: 12–17 hr.

USES

Prevention and treatment of bleeding in hemophilia A (factor VIII deficiency), prevention and treatment of bleeding in hemophilia A in patients with acquired Factor VIII inhibitors (not exceeding 10 Bethesda units/ml), treatment of spontaneous bleeding in patients with severe von Willebrand's disease. **OFF-LABEL:** Treatment of disseminated intravascular coagulation.

PRECAUTIONS

CONTRAINDICATIONS: None known. **CAUTIONS:** Hepatic disease, those with blood types A, B, AB.

⧗ **LIFESPAN CONSIDERATIONS: Pregnancy/Lactation:** Unknown if drug crosses placenta or is distributed in breast milk. **Pregnancy Category C. Children:** Safety and efficacy not established. **Elderly:** No age-related precautions noted.

INTERACTIONS

DRUG: None known. **HERBAL:** None known. **FOOD:** None known. **LAB VALUES:** None known.

AVAILABILITY (Rx)

INJECTION: Actual number of AHF units is listed on each vial.

ADMINISTRATION/HANDLING

 IV

Reconstitution • Warm concentrate and diluent to room temperature. • Using needle supplied by the manufacturer, add diluent to powder to dissolve, gently agitate or rotate. Do not shake vigorously. Complete dissolution may take 5–10min. • Use second filtered needle supplied by the manufacturer, and add to infusion bag.

Rate of administration • Administer IV at rate of approximately 2 ml/min. May give up to 10 ml/min.

Administration precautions • Check pulse rate before and after administration. If pulse rate increases, reduce or stop administration. • After administration, apply prolonged pressure on venipuncture site. • Monitor IV site for oozing q5–15 min for 1–2 hr following administration.

Storage • Refrigerate.

▦ IV INCOMPATIBILITIES

Do not mix with other IV solutions or medications.

INDICATIONS/ROUTES/DOSAGE

TREATMENT AND PREVENTION OF BLEEDING IN PATIENTS WITH HEMOPHILIA A FACTOR VIII DEFICIENCY, HYPOFIBRINOGENEMIA, VON WILLEBRAND'S DISEASE

IV: ADULTS, ELDERLY, CHILDREN: Dosage is highly individualized and is based on patient's weight, severity of bleeding, and coagulation studies.

SIDE EFFECTS

OCCASIONAL: Allergic reaction, including fever, chills, urticaria, wheezing, hypotension, nausea, feeling of chest tightness; stinging at injection site; dizziness; dry mouth; headache; altered taste.

ADVERSE REACTIONS/ TOXIC EFFECTS

There is a risk of transmitting viral hepatitis. Intravascular hemolysis may occur if large or frequent doses are used with blood group A, B, or AB.

NURSING CONSIDERATIONS

BASELINE ASSESSMENT

When monitoring BP, avoid overinflation of cuff. Remove adhesive tape from any pressure dressing very carefully and slowly.

INTERVENTION/EVALUATION

Following IV administration, apply prolonged pressure on venipuncture site. Monitor IV site for oozing q5–15 min for 1–2 hr following administration. Assess for allergic reaction. Report immediately any evidence of hematuria or change in vital signs. Assess for decreases in BP, increased pulse rate, complaint of abdominal or back pain, severe headache (may be evidence of hemorrhage). Question for increased discharge during menses. Assess skin for bruises, petechiae. Check for excessive bleeding from minor cuts, scratches. Assess gums for erythema, gingival bleeding. Assess urine for hematuria. Evaluate for therapeutic relief of pain, reduction of swelling, and restricted joint movement.

PATIENT/FAMILY TEACHING

• Use electric razor, soft toothbrush to prevent bleeding. • Report any sign of red or dark urine, black/red stool, coffee-ground vomitus, blood-tinged mucus from cough.

Anzemet, *see dolasetron*

Apokyn, *see apomorphine*

---

apomorphine hydrochloride

aye-poe-**more**-feen
(Apokyn)

◆ CLASSIFICATION

PHARMACOTHERAPEUTIC: Dopaminergics. **CLINICAL:** Antiparkinson.

ACTION

An antiparkinson agent that stimulates postsynaptic dopamine receptors in the brain. **Therapeutic Effect:** Relieves signs and symptoms of Parkinson's disease and improves motor function.

PHARMACOKINETICS

Rapidly absorbed after subcutaneous administration. Protein binding: 99.9%. Widely distributed. Rapidly eliminated from plasma. Not detected in urine or secretions. **Half-life:** 41–45 min.

USES

Acute, intermittent treatment of hypomobility, ("off" episodes) associated with advanced Parkinson's disease. Acute, intermittent treatment of hypomobility, ("off" episodes) associated with advanced Parkinson's disease.

PRECAUTIONS

CONTRAINDICATIONS: Concurrent use of 5-HT₃ antagonists (e.g. alosetron, dolasetron, granisetron, ondansetron, or palonosetron). **CAUTIONS:** Impaired hepatic or renal function, cardiac decompensation.

⧗ **LIFESPAN CONSIDERATIONS: Pregnancy/Lactation:** Unknown if drug is distributed in breast milk. **Pregnancy Category C. Children:** Safety and efficacy not established. **Elderly:** No age-related precautions noted, but hallucinations appear to occur more frequently.

INTERACTIONS

DRUG: Alosetron, dolasetron, granisetron, ondansetron, palonosetron: May produce profound hypotension and loss of consciousness. **Butyrophenones, metoclopramide, phenothiazines, thioxanthenes:** Decrease the effectiveness of apomorphine. **CNS depressants:** May increase CNS depressant effects. **HERBAL:** None known. **FOOD:** None known. **LAB VALUES:** May increase serum alkaline phosphatase level.

AVAILABILITY (Rx)

INJECTION: 10 mg/ml.

ADMINISTRATION/HANDLING

SUBCUTANEOUS

Storage • Store at room temperature.

INDICATIONS/ROUTES/DOSAGE

ACUTE, INTERMITTENT TREATMENT OF HYPOMOBILITY ("OFF" EPISODES) ASSOCIATED WITH ADVANCED PARKINSON'S DISEASE

SUBCUTANEOUS: ADULTS, ELDERLY: Initially, 0.2 ml (2 mg); may be increased in 0.1-ml (1-mg) increments every few days. **Maximum:** 0.6 ml (6 mg).

SIDE EFFECTS

OCCASIONAL (4%–3%): Injection site discomfort, arthralgia, somnolence, hypersalivation, pallor, yawning, headache, dizziness, diaphoresis, vomiting, orthostatic hypotension. **RARE (less than 2%):** Psychosis, stomatitis, altered taste, hallucinations.

ADVERSE REACTIONS/ TOXIC EFFECTS

Respiratory depression or CNS stimulation (characterized by tachypnea, bradycardia or persistent vomiting) may occur. Apomorphine use may cause or exacerbate preexisting dyskinesia.

NURSING CONSIDERATIONS

INTERVENTION/EVALUATION

Instruct patient to change positions slowly to prevent risk of orthostatic hypotension. Assist with ambulation if dizziness occurs. Assess for clinical improvement, reversal of symptoms (improvement of tremor of head/hands at rest, mask-like facial expression, shuffling gait, muscular rigidity).

PATIENT/FAMILY TEACHING

• Drowsiness, dizziness may be an initial response to drug. • Avoid tasks that require alertness, motor skills until response to drug is established. • Inform patient and family that hallucinations may occur, especially in the elderly.

---

apraclonidine

(Iopidine)
See Antiglaucoma agents (p. 47C)

---

aprepitant

ah-**prep**-ih-tant
(Emend, Emend 3-Day)

CLASSIFICATION

PHARMACOTHERAPEUTIC: Selective receptor antagonist. **CLINICAL:** Anti-nausea, antiemetic.

ACTION

A selective human substance P and neurokinin-1 (NK_1) receptor antagonist that inhibits chemotherapy-induced nausea and vomiting centrally in the chemoreceptor trigger zone. **Therapeutic Effect:** Prevents the acute and delayed phases of chemotherapy-induced emesis, including vomiting caused by high-dose cisplatin.

PHARMACOKINETICS

Crosses the blood-brain barrier. Extensively metabolized in the liver. Eliminated primarily by liver metabolism (not excreted renally). **Half-life:** 9–13 hr.

USES

Prevention of acute and delayed nausea and vomiting associated with initial and repeat courses of emetogenic cancer chemotherapy, including high-dose cisplatin.

PRECAUTIONS

CONTRAINDICATIONS: Breast-feeding, concurrent use of astemizole, cisapride, pimozide, or terfenadine. **CAUTIONS:** None known.

⌛ **LIFESPAN CONSIDERATIONS: Pregnancy/Lactation:** Unknown if drug crosses placenta or is distributed in breast milk. **Pregnancy Category B. Children:** Safety and efficacy not established. **Elderly:** No age-related precautions noted.

INTERACTIONS

DRUG: Alprazolam, docetaxel, etoposide, ifosfamide, imatinib, irinotecan, midazolam, paclitaxel, triazolam, vinblastine, vincristine, **vinorelbine:** May increase the plasma concentrations of these drugs. **Antifungals, clarithromycin, diltiazem, nefazodone, nelfinavir, ritonavir:** Increase aprepitant plasma concentration. **Carbamazepine, phenytoin, rifampin:** Decrease aprepitant plasma concentration. **Contraceptives:** May decrease the effectiveness of contraceptives. **Paroxetine:** May decrease the effectiveness of either drug. **Steroids:** Increases the blood levels and effects of steroids. **Warfarin:** May decrease the effectiveness of warfarin. **HERBAL:** None known. **FOOD:** None known. **LAB VALUES:** May increase BUN level and serum creatinine, AST, and ALT levels. May produce proteinuria.

AVAILABILITY (Rx)

CAPSULES (EMEND): 80 mg, 125 mg. **KIT (EMEND 3-DAY):** 125 mg-80 mg.

ADMINISTRATION/HANDLING

PO
• Give without regard to food.

INDICATIONS/ROUTES/DOSAGE

PREVENTION OF CHEMOTHERAPY-INDUCED NAUSEA AND VOMITING
PO: ADULTS, ELDERLY: 125 mg 1 hr before chemotherapy on day 1 and 80 mg once a day in the morning on days 2 and 3.

SIDE EFFECTS

FREQUENT (17%–10%): Fatigue, nausea, hiccups, diarrhea, constipation, anorexia. **OCCASIONAL (8%–4%):** Headache, vomiting, dizziness, dehydration, heartburn. **RARE (3% or less):** Abdominal pain, epigastric discomfort, gastritis, tinnitus, insomnia.

ADVERSE REACTIONS/ TOXIC EFFECTS

Neutropenia and mucous membrane disorders occur rarely.

NURSING CONSIDERATIONS

BASELINE ASSESSMENT

Assess for dehydration if excessive vomiting occurs (poor skin turgor, dry mucous membranes, longitudinal furrows in tongue). Provide emotional support.

INTERVENTION/EVALUATION

Monitor patient in environment. Assess bowel sounds for peristalsis. Assist with ambulation if dizziness occurs. Provide supportive measures. Monitor pattern of daily bowel activity and stool consistency. Record time of evacuation.

PATIENT/FAMILY TEACHING

• Relief from nausea and vomiting generally occurs shortly after drug administration. • Report persistent vomiting, headache.

Aptivus, *see tipranavir*

Aranesp, *see darbepoetin alfa*

Arava, *see leflunomide*

---

argatroban

our-ga-**trow**-ban
(Acova)

Do not confuse argatroban with Aggrestat or Organan.

• CLASSIFICATION

PHARMACOTHERAPEUTIC: Thrombin inhibitor. **CLINICAL:** Anticoagulant.

ACTION

A direct thrombin inhibitor that reversibly binds to thrombin-active sites. Inhibits thrombin-catalyzed or thrombin-induced reactions, including fibrin formation, activation of coagulant factors V, VIII, and XIII; also inhibits protein C formation; and platelet aggregation. **Therapeutic Effect:** Produces anticoagulation.

PHARMACOKINETICS

Following IV administration, distributed primarily in extracellular fluid. Protein binding: 54%. Metabolized in the liver. Primarily excreted in the feces, presumably through biliary secretion. **Half-life:** 39–51 min.

USES

Prophylaxis or treatment of thrombosis in heparin-induced thrombocytopenia (HIT). Prevention of HIT during percutaneous coronary procedures. **OFF-LABEL:** Cerebral thrombosis, MI.

PRECAUTIONS

CONTRAINDICATIONS: Overt major bleeding. **CAUTIONS:** Severe hypertension, immediately following lumbar puncture, spinal anesthesia, major surgery, patients with congenital or acquired bleeding disorders, ulcerations, hepatic impairment.

    LIFESPAN CONSIDERATIONS: Pregnancy/Lactation: Unknown if excreted in breast milk. **Pregnancy Category B. Children:** Safety and efficacy not established in those younger than 18 yr. **Elderly:** No age-related precautions noted.

INTERACTIONS

DRUG: Antiplatelet agents, thrombolytics, other anticoagulants: May increase the risk of bleeding. **HERBAL: Arnica, astragalus, bilberry, black currant, cat's claw, chaparral, dandelion, evening primrose, feverfew,**

garlic, ginger, **ginkgo biloba**, hawthorn, kava, licorice, tan-shen, vitamin A: May increase the risk of bleeding. **FOOD:** None known. **LAB VALUES:** Increases aPTT, International Normalized Ratio, and PT.

AVAILABILITY (Rx)

INJECTION: 100 mg/ml.

ADMINISTRATION/HANDLING

 IV

Reconstitution • Must be diluted 100-fold before infusion in 0.9% NaCl, D₅W, or lactated Ringer's solution to provide a final concentration of 1 mg/ml. • The solution must be mixed by repeated inversion of the diluent bag for 1 min. • After reconstitution, solution may show a brief haziness due to formation of microprecipitates that rapidly dissolve upon mixing.

Rate of administration • Rate of administration is based on body weight at 2 mcg/kg/min (e.g., 50-kg patient infuse at 6 ml/hr).

Storage • Discard if solution appears cloudy or an insoluble precipitate is noted. • Following reconstitution, stable for 24 hr at room temperature, 48 hr if refrigerated. • Avoid direct sunlight.

▨ IV INCOMPATIBILITIES

Do not mix with other medications or solutions.

INDICATIONS/ROUTES/DOSAGE

TO PREVENT AND TREAT HEPARIN-INDUCED THROMBOCYTOPENIA
IV INFUSION: ADULTS, ELDERLY: Initially, 2 mcg/kg/min administered as a continuous infusion. After initial infusion, dose may be adjusted until steady state aPTT is 1.5–3 times initial baseline value, not to exceed 100 sec.

PERCUTANEOUS CORONARY INTERVENTION
IV INFUSION: ADULTS, ELDERLY: Initially, 25 mcg/kg/min and administer bolus of

350 mcg/kg over 3–5 min. ACT (activated clotting time) checked in 5–10 min following bolus. If ACT is less than 300 sec, give additional bolus 150 mcg/kg, increase infusion to 30 mcg/kg/min. If ACT is greater than 450 sec, decrease infusion to 15 mcg/kg/min. Once ACT of 300–450 sec achieved, proceed with procedure.

DOSAGE IN HEPATIC IMPAIRMENT
ADULTS, ELDERLY: Initially, 0.5 mcg/kg/min.

SIDE EFFECTS

FREQUENT (8%–3%): Dyspnea, hypotension, fever, diarrhea, nausea, pain, vomiting, infection, cough.

ADVERSE REACTIONS/ TOXIC EFFECTS

Ventricular tachycardia and atrial fibrillation occur occasionally. Major bleeding and sepsis occur rarely.

NURSING CONSIDERATIONS

BASELINE ASSESSMENT

Check CBC, including platelet count, PT, PTT. Determine initial BP. Minimize need for numerous injection sites, blood draws, catheters.

INTERVENTION/EVALUATION

Assess for any sign of bleeding: bleeding at surgical site, hematuria, blood in stool, bleeding from gums, petechiae, ecchymuses, bleeding from injection sites. Handle patient carefully and as infrequently as possible to prevent bleeding. Do not obtain BP in lower extremities (possible deep vein thrombi). Assess for decreased BP, increased pulse rate, complaint of abdominal/back pain, severe headache (indicates evidence of hemorrhage). Monitor ACT, PT, aPTT, platelet count. Question for increase in discharge during menses. Assess urine output for hematuria. Observe for any occurring hematoma. Use care in removing any dressing, tape.

PATIENT/FAMILY TEACHING
• Use electric razor, soft toothbrush to prevent bleeding. • Report any sign of red/dark urine, black/red stool, coffee-ground vomitus, blood-tinged mucus from cough.

Aricept, *see donepezil*

Arimidex, *see anastrozole*

---

aripiprazole

air-ee-**pip**-rah-zole
(Abilify)

◆ CLASSIFICATION
PHARMACOTHERAPEUTIC: Dopamine agonist. **CLINICAL:** Antipsychotic agent.

ACTION
An antipsychotic agent that provides partial agonist activity at dopamine and serotonin (5-HT$_{1A}$) receptors and antagonist activity at serotonin (5-HT$_{2A}$) receptors. **Therapeutic Effect:** Diminishes schizophrenic behavior.

PHARMACOKINETICS
Well absorbed through the GI tract. Protein binding: 99% (primarily albumin). Reaches steady levels in 2 wk. Metabolized in the liver. Eliminated primarily in feces and, to a lesser extent, in urine. Not removed by hemodialysis. **Half-life:** 75 hr.

USES
Treatment of schizophrenia. Maintains stability in patients with schizophrenia.

Treatment of bipolar disorder. **OFF-LABEL:** Schizoaffective disorder.

PRECAUTIONS
CONTRAINDICATIONS: None known. **CAUTIONS:** Concurrent use of CNS depressants (including alcohol), cardio-vascular or cerebrovascular diseases (may induce hypotension), Parkinson's disease (potential for exacerbation), history of seizures or conditions that may lower seizure threshold (Alzheimer's disease), renal or hepatic impairment.

⌛ **LIFESPAN CONSIDERATIONS: Pregnancy/Lactation:** Unknown if drug crosses placenta. May be distributed in breast milk; avoid breast-feeding. **Pregnancy Category C. Children:** Safety and efficacy not established. **Elderly:** No age-related precautions noted.

INTERACTIONS
DRUG: Carbamazepine: May decrease the aripiprazole blood concentration. **Fluoxetine, ketoconazole, quinidine, paroxetine:** May increase the aripiprazole blood concentration. **HERBAL:** None known. **FOOD:** None known. **LAB VALUES:** None known.

AVAILABILITY (Rx)
TABLETS: 2 mg, 5 mg, 10 mg, 15 mg, 20 mg, 30 mg. **ORAL SOLUTION:** 1 mg/ml.

ADMINISTRATION/HANDLING
PO
• Give without regard to food.

INDICATIONS/ROUTES/DOSAGE
SCHIZOPHRENIA
PO: ADULTS, ELDERLY: Initially, 10–15 mg once a day. May increase up to 30 mg/day.

BIPOLAR DISORDER
PO: ADULTS, ELDERLY: 30 mg once a day. May decrease to 15 mg/day based on patient tolerance.

✔ see color pill atlas   🌿 herb   underlined – top prescribed drug

SIDE EFFECTS

FREQUENT (11%–5%): Weight gain, headache, insomnia, vomiting. **OCCASIONAL (4%–3%):** Light-headedness, nausea, akathisia, somnolence. **RARE (2% or less):** Blurred vision, constipation, asthenia or loss of energy and strength, anxiety, fever, rash, cough, rhinitis, orthostatic hypotension.

ADVERSE REACTIONS/ TOXIC EFFECTS

Extrapyramidal symptoms and neuroleptic malignant syndrome occur rarely. Prolonged QT interval occurs rarely.

NURSING CONSIDERATIONS

BASELINE ASSESSMENT

Assess behavior, appearance, emotional status, response to environment, speech pattern, thought content. Correct dehydration, hypovolemia.

INTERVENTION/EVALUATION

Periodically monitor weight. Monitor for extrapyramidal symptoms (abnormal movement), tardive dyskinesia (protrusion of tongue, puffing of cheeks, chewing/puckering of the mouth). Periodically monitor BP, pulse (particularly in those with preexisting cardiovascular disease). Assess for therapeutic response (greater interest in surroundings, improved self-care, increased ability to concentrate, relaxed facial expression).

PATIENT/FAMILY TEACHING

• Avoid alcohol. • Avoid tasks that require alertness, motor skills until response to drug is established.

Arixtra, *see fondaparinux*

Aromasin, *see exemestane*

Arranon, *see nelarbine*

---

arsenic trioxide

are-sih-nic try-**ox**-ide
(Trisenox)
Do not confuse Trisenox with Trimox.

◆ CLASSIFICATION

CLINICAL: Antineoplastic (see p. 71C).

ACTION

An antineoplastic that produces morphologic changes and DNA fragmentation in promyelocytic leukemia cells. **Therapeutic Effect:** Produces cell death.

PHARMACOKINETICS

Distributed in liver, kidneys, heart, lungs, hair, and nails. Metabolized in liver. Eliminated by kidneys. Does not have a half-life.

USES

Induction of remission and consolidations in patients with acute promyelocytic leukemia (APL) who are refractory to or have relapsed from retinoid and anthracycline chemotherapy.

PRECAUTIONS

CONTRAINDICATIONS: None known. **CAUTIONS:** Renal impairment, cardiac abnormalities.

 LIFESPAN CONSIDERATIONS: Pregnancy/Lactation: Distributed is breast milk. May cause fetal harm. **Pregnancy Category D. Children:** Safety and efficacy not established in children younger than 5 yr. **Elderly:** Age-related renal impairment may require dosage adjustment.

INTERACTIONS

DRUG: Amphotericin B, diuretics: May produce electrolyte imbalances. **Antiarrhythmics, thioridazine:** May prolong QT interval. **HERBAL:** None known. **FOOD:** None known. **LAB VALUES:** May decrease Hgb levels, serum calcium and magnesium levels, and platelet and WBC counts. May increase AST and ALT levels.

AVAILABILITY (Rx)

INJECTION: 1 mg/ml.

ADMINISTRATION/HANDLING

🔹 IV

‹ **ALERT** › A central venous line is not required for drug administration.

Reconstitution • After withdrawing drug from ampule, dilute with 100–250 ml D₅W or 0.9% NaCl.

Rate of administration • Infuse over 1–2 hr. Duration of infusion may be extended up to 4 hr.

Storage • Store at room temperature. • Diluted solution is stable for 24 hr at room temperature, 48 hr if refrigerated.

▦ IV INCOMPATIBILITIES

Don't mix arsenic trioxide with any other medications.

INDICATIONS/ROUTES/DOSAGE

ACUTE PROMYELOCYTIC LEUKEMIA

IV: ADULTS, ELDERLY, CHILDREN OLDER THAN 5 YR: Induction: 0.15 mg/kg/day until myelosuppression occurs. Do not exceed 60 induction doses. Beginning 3–6 wk after completion of induction therapy, 0.15 mg/kg/day for 25 doses over a period of up to 5 wk.

SIDE EFFECTS

EXPECTED (75%–50%): Nausea, cough, fatigue, fever, headache, vomiting, abdominal pain, tachycardia, diarrhea, dyspnea. **FREQUENT (43%–30%):** Dermatitis, insomnia, edema, rigors, prolonged QT interval, sore throat, pruritus, arthralgia, paresthesia, anxiety. **OCCASIONAL (28%–20%):** Constipation, myalgia, hypotension, epistaxis, anorexia, dizziness, sinusitis. **(15%–8%):** Ecchymosis, nonspecific pain, weight gain, herpes simplex, wheezing, flushing, diaphoresis, tremor, hypertension, palpitations, dyspepsia, eye irritation, blurred vision, asthenia, diminished breath sounds, crackles. **RARE:** Confusion, petechiae, dry mouth, oral candidiasis, incontinence, rhonchi.

ADVERSE REACTIONS/ TOXIC EFFECTS

Seizures, GI hemorrhage, renal impairment or failure, pleural or pericardial effusion, hemoptysis, and sepsis occur rarely. Prolonged QT interval, complete AV block, unexplained fever, dyspnea, weight gain, and effusion are evidence of arsenic toxicity. If arsenic toxicity is apparent, stop arsenic trioxide treatment and begin steroid treatment as ordered.

NURSING CONSIDERATIONS

BASELINE ASSESSMENT

Assess platelet count, Hgb, Hct, WBC before and frequently during treatment. Ask if patient is breast-feeding, pregnant, or planning to become pregnant (may cause fetal harm).

INTERVENTION/EVALUATION

Monitor liver function test results, CBC, serum values. Monitor for arsenic toxicity syndrome (fever, dyspnea, weight gain, confusion, muscle weakness, seizures).

PATIENT/FAMILY TEACHING

• Avoid crowds, those with known infection. • Avoid tasks that require alertness, motor skills, until response to drug is established. • Contact physician if high fever, vomiting, difficulty breathing, or rapid heart rate occur.

Arthrotec, *see*
diclofenac and misoprostil

artificial tears

(Eye Tears, Hypotears, Isopto Tears, Refresh Aquasite, Tears Naturale, Tears Plus, Ultra Fresh Eyes, Visine Tears, Viva Drops)

◆ CLASSIFICATION

PHARMACOTHERAPEUTIC: Ophthalmic lubricant.

ACTION

Stabilizes/thickens precorneal tear film, lengthening tear film breakup time. **Therapeutic Effect:** Protects and lubricates the eyes.

USES

Relief of dryness and irritation due to deficient tear production; ocular lubricant for artificial eyes; some products may be used with hard contact lenses. **OFF-LABEL:** Treatment of recurrent corneal erosions, decreased corneal sensitivity.

PRECAUTIONS

CONTRAINDICATIONS: Hypersensitivity to any component of preparation. **CAUTIONS:** None known. **Pregnancy Category A.**

INTERACTIONS

DRUG: None known. **HERBAL:** None known. **FOOD:** None known. **LAB VALUES:** None known.

INDICATIONS/ROUTES/DOSAGE

OPHTHALMIC LUBRICANT

ADULTS, ELDERLY: 1–2 drops 3–4 times a day as needed.

SIDE EFFECTS

OCCASIONAL: Eye irritation, blurred vision, stickiness of eyelashes.

ADVERSE REACTIONS/ TOXIC EFFECTS

None known.

NURSING CONSIDERATIONS

BASELINE ASSESSMENT

Determine extent of dryness, irritation.

INTERVENTION/EVALUATION

Monitor for increased irritation or discomfort. Assess therapeutic response.

PATIENT/FAMILY TEACHING

• Wash hands thoroughly before use.
• Do not touch the tip of the dropper or container to any surface.

Asacol, *see mesalamine*

ascorbic acid (vitamin C)

a-**skor**bic

(Ascor L 500, Cecon, Cee-500, Cenolate, Mega-C/A Plus, Vitamin C)

◆ CLASSIFICATION

CLINICAL: Vitamin (see p. 145C).

ACTION

Assists in collagen formation and tissue repair and is involved in oxidation reduction reactions and other metabolic reactions. **Therapeutic Effect:** Involved in carbohydrate use and metabolism, as well as synthesis of carnitine, lipids, and proteins. Preserves blood vessel integrity.

PHARMACOKINETICS

Readily absorbed from the GI tract. Protein binding: 25%. Metabolized in the liver. Excreted in urine. Removed by hemodialysis.

USES

Prevention and treatment of scurvy, acidification of urine, dietary supplement, prevention of and reduction in the severity of colds. **OFF-LABEL:** Chronic iron toxicity, control of idiopathic methemoglobinemia, macular degeneration, prevention of common cold, urine acidifier.

PRECAUTIONS

CONTRAINDICATIONS: None known. **CAUTIONS:** Those on sodium restriction, daily salicylate treatment, warfarin therapy; diabetes mellitus; history of renal stones.

⏳ **LIFESPAN CONSIDERATIONS: Pregnancy/Lactation:** Crosses placenta; excreted in breast milk. Large doses during pregnancy may produce scurvy in neonates. **Pregnancy Category A (C if used in doses above recommended daily allowance). Children/Elderly:** No age-related precautions noted.

INTERACTIONS

DRUG: Deferoxamine: May increase iron toxicity. **HERBAL:** None known. **FOOD:** None known. **LAB VALUES:** May decrease serum bilirubin level and urinary pH. May increase urine uric acid and urine oxalate levels.

AVAILABILITY (OTC)

CAPSULES (CONTROLLED-RELEASE): 500 mg. **LIQUID:** 500 mg/5 ml. **ORAL SOLUTION:** 500 mg/5 ml. **TABLETS:** 100 mg, 250 mg, 500 mg, 1 g. **TABLETS (CHEWABLE):** 100 mg, 250 mg, 500 mg. **TABLETS (CONTROLLED-RELEASE):** 500 mg, 1 g, 1,500 mg. **INJECTION:** 222 mg/ml (Mega-C/A Plus, Vitamin C), 250 mg/ml (Cenolate), 500 mg/ml (Ascor L 500, Cee-500, Cenolate, Vitamin C).

ADMINISTRATION/HANDLING
 IV

Rate of administration • May give undiluted or dilute in D$_5$W, 0.9% NaCl, lactated Ringer's solution. • For IV push, dilute with equal volume D$_5$W or 0.9% NaCl and infuse over 10 min. For IV solution, infuse over 4–12 hr.

Storage • Refrigerate. • Protect from freezing and light.

PO
• Give without regard to food.

🔲 IV INCOMPATIBILITIES

No information available for Y-site administration.

IV COMPATIBILITIES

Calcium gluconate, heparin.

INDICATIONS/ROUTES/DOSAGE
DIETARY SUPPLEMENT
PO: ADULTS, ELDERLY: 50–200 mg/day. CHILDREN: 35–100 mg/day.

ACIDIFICATION OF URINE
PO: ADULTS, ELDERLY: 4–12 g/day in 3–4 divided doses. CHILDREN: 500 mg q6–8h.

SCURVY
PO: ADULTS, ELDERLY: 100–250 mg 1–2 times a day. CHILDREN: 100–300 mg/day in divided doses.

PREVENTION AND REDUCTION OF SEVERITY OF COLDS
PO: ADULTS, ELDERLY: 1–3 g/day in divided doses.

SIDE EFFECTS

RARE: Abdominal cramps, nausea, vomiting, diarrhea, increased urination with doses exceeding 1 g. **Parenteral:** Flushing, headache, dizziness, sleepiness or insomnia, soreness at injection site.

ADVERSE REACTIONS/ TOXIC EFFECTS

Ascorbic acid may acidify urine, leading to crystalluria. Large doses of IV ascorbic acid may lead to deep vein thrombosis. Abrupt discontinuation after prolonged use of large doses may produce rebound ascorbic acid deficiency.

NURSING CONSIDERATIONS

INTERVENTION/EVALUATION

Assess for clinical improvement (improved sense of well-being and sleep patterns). Observe for reversal of deficiency symptoms (gingivitis, bleeding gums, poor wound healing, digestive difficulties, joint pain).

PATIENT/FAMILY TEACHING

• Abrupt vitamin C withdrawal may produce rebound deficiency. Reduce dosage gradually. • Foods rich in vitamin C include rose hips, guava, black currant jelly, Brussels sprouts, green peppers, spinach, watercress, strawberries, citrus fruits.

---

asparaginase

ah-spa-**raj**-in-ace
(Elspar, Kidrolase ✤)

Do not confuse asparaginase with pegaspargase.

⬧CLASSIFICATION

PHARMACOTHERAPEUTIC: Enzyme. **CLINICAL:** Antineoplastic (see p. 71C).

ACTION

An enzyme that inhibits DNA, RNA, and protein synthesis by breaking down asparagine, thus depriving tumor cells of this essential amino acid. Cell cycle–specific for G_1 phase of cell division. **Therapeutic Effect:** Toxic to leukemic cells.

PHARMACOKINETICS

Metabolized by the reticuloendothelial system through slow sequestration. **Half-life:** 39–49 hr IM; 8–30 hr IV.

USES

Treatment of acute lymphocytic leukemia (ALL), lymphoma in combination with other therapy. **OFF-LABEL:** Treatment of acute myelocytic leukemia, acute myelomonocytic leukemia, chronic lymphocytic leukemia, Hodgkin's disease, lymphosarcoma, melanosarcoma, and reticulum cell sarcoma.

PRECAUTIONS

CONTRAINDICATIONS: History of hypersensitivity to asparaginase, pancreatitis. **CAUTIONS:** Existing or recent chickenpox, herpes zoster, diabetes mellitus, gout, infection, hepatic/renal impairment, recent cytotoxic/radiation therapy. ⧗ **LIFESPAN CONSIDERATIONS:** Pregnancy/Lactation: If possible, avoid use during pregnancy, especially first trimester. Breast-feeding not recommended. **Pregnancy Category C. Children/Elderly:** No age-related precautions noted.

INTERACTIONS

DRUG: Antigout medications: May decrease the effects of these drugs. **Live-virus vaccines:** May potentiate virus replication, increase vaccine side effects, and decrease the patient's antibody response to the vaccine. **Methotrexate:** May block the effects of this drug. **Steroids, vincristine:** May increase the risk of neuropathy and disturbances of erythropoiesis; may enhance hyperglycemic effect of asparaginase. **HERBAL:** None known. **FOOD:** None known. **LAB VALUES:** May increase BUN, blood ammonia, and blood glucose levels; serum alkaline phosphatase, bilirubin, uric acid, AST, and ALT levels; platelet count, PT; activated partial thromboplastin time; and thrombin time. May decrease blood-clotting factors, (including antithrombin, plasma fibrinogen, and plasminogen) as well as serum albumin, calcium, and cholesterol levels.

AVAILABILITY (Rx)

POWDER FOR INJECTION: 10,000 international units.

ADMINISTRATION/HANDLING

◄ **ALERT** ► May be carcinogenic, mutagenic, teratogenic. Handle with extreme care during preparation/administration. Handle voided urine as infectious waste. Powder, solution may irritate skin on contact. Wash area for 15 min if contact occurs.

 IV

Reconstitution ◄ **ALERT** ► Administer intradermal test dose (2 international units) before initiating therapy or when longer than 1 wk has elapsed between doses.
• Observe patient for 1 hr for appearance of wheal or erythema.

Test Solution • Reconstitute 10,000 international units vial with 5 ml sterile water for injection or 0.9% NaCl. • Shake to dissolve. • Withdraw 0.1 ml, inject into vial containing 9.9 ml same diluent for concentration of 20 international units/ml. • Reconstitute 10,000 international units vial with 5 ml sterile water for injection or 0.9% NaCl to provide a concentration of 2,000 international units/ml. • Shake gently to ensure complete dissolution (vigorous shaking produces foam, some loss of potency).

Rate of administration • For IV injection, administer into tubing of freely running IV solution of D₅W or 0.9% NaCl over at least 30 min. • For IV infusion, further dilute with up to 1,000 ml D₅W or 0.9% NaCl.

Storage • Refrigerate powder for reconstitution. • Reconstituted solutions stable for 8 hrs if refrigerated. • Gelatinous fiber-like particles may develop (remove via 5-micron filter during administration).

IM

• Add 2 ml 0.9% NaCl injection to 10,000 international units vial to provide a concentration of 5,000 international units/ml. • Administer no more than 2 ml at any one site.

⊞ IV INCOMPATIBILITIES

None known.

INDICATIONS/ROUTES/DOSAGE

ACUTE LYMPHOCYTIC LEUKEMIA

IV: ADULTS, ELDERLY, CHILDREN: 1,000 units/kg/day for 10 days as combination therapy or 200 units/kg/day for 28 days as monotherapy.
IM: ADULTS, ELDERLY, CHILDREN: 6 to 6,000 units/m²/dose 3 times a week for 3 wk as combination therapy.

SIDE EFFECTS

FREQUENT: Allergic reaction (rash, urticaria, arthralgia, facial edema, hypotension, respiratory distress) pancreatitis (severe abdominal pain, nausea and vomiting). **OCCASIONAL:** CNS effects (confusion, drowsiness, depression, anxiety, and fatigue), stomatitis, hypoalbuminemia or uric acid nephropathy, (manifested as pedal or lower extremity edema), hyperglycemia. **RARE:** Hyperthermia (including fever or chills), thrombosis, seizures.

ADVERSE REACTIONS/TOXIC EFFECTS

Hepatotoxicity usually occurs within 2 wk of initial treatment. The risk of an allergic reaction, including anaphylaxis, increases after repeated therapy. Myelosuppression may be severe.

NURSING CONSIDERATIONS

BASELINE ASSESSMENT

Before giving medication, agents for adequate airway and allergic reaction (antihistamine, epinephrine, O₂, IV corticosteroid) should be readily available. Assess baseline CNS functions. CBC,

---

comprehensive serum chemistry should be performed before therapy begins and when 1 or more wk have elapsed between doses.

INTERVENTION/EVALUATION

Assess serum amylase concentration frequently during therapy. Discontinue medication at first sign of renal failure (oliguria, anuria), pancreatitis (abdominal pain, nausea, vomiting). Monitor for hematologic toxicity (fever, sore throat, signs of local infection, unusual bruising/bleeding), symptoms of anemia (excessive fatigue, weakness).

PATIENT/FAMILY TEACHING

• Increase fluid intake (protects against renal impairment). • Nausea may decrease during therapy. • Do not have immunizations without physician's approval (drug lowers body's resistance). • Avoid contact with those who have recently taken a live virus vaccine.

---

aspirin (acetylsalicylic acid, ASA) ⚑

ass-purr-in

(Asaphen E.C. ✤, Bayer, Bufferin, Ecotrin, Entaprin, Entrophen ✤, Halfprin, Novasen ✤, YSP Aspirin, Zero-Order Release, ZORprin)

Do not confuse aspirin or Ascriptin with Aricept, Afrin, or Asendin, or Ecotrin with Edecrin.

FIXED-COMBINATION(S)

Aggrenox: aspirin/dipyridamole (an antiplatelet agent): 25 mg/200 mg. **Fiorinal:** aspirin/butalbital/caffeine (a barbiturate): 325 mg/50 mg/40 mg. **Lortab/ASA:** aspirin/hydrocodone (an analgesic): 325

mg/5 mg. **Percodan:** aspirin/oxycodone (an analgesic): 325 mg/4.5 mg; 325 mg/2.25 mg. **Pravigard:** aspirin/pravastatin (a cholesterol lowering agent): 81 mg/20 mg, 81 mg/40 mg, 81 mg/80 mg, 325 mg/20 mg, 325 mg/40 mg, 325 mg/80 mg.

◆CLASSIFICATION

PHARMACOTHERAPEUTIC: Non-steroidal salicylate. **CLINICAL:** Anti-inflammatory, antipyretic, anticoagulant (see pp. 31C, 115C).

ACTION

A nonsteroidal salicylate that inhibits prostaglandin synthesis, acts on the hypothalamus heat-regulating center, and interferes with the production of thromboxane A, a substance that stimulates platelet aggregation. **Therapeutic Effect:** Reduces inflammatory response and intensity of pain; decreases fever; inhibits platelet aggregation.

PHARMACOKINETICS

Route	Onset	Peak	Duration
PO	1 hr	2–4 hr	4–6 hr

Rapidly and completely absorbed from GI tract; enteric-coated absorption delayed; rectal absorption delayed and incomplete. Protein binding: High. Widely distributed. Rapidly hydrolyzed to salicylate. **Half-life:** 15–20 min (aspirin); 2–3 hr (salicylate at low dose); more than 20 hr (salicylate at high dose).

USES

Treatment of mild to moderate pain, fever. Reduces inflammation including rheumatoid arthritis, juvenile arthritis, osteoarthritis, rheumatic fever. As platelet aggregation inhibitor in the prevention of transient ischemic attacks

---

(TIAs), cerebral thromboembolism, MI or reinfarction. OFF-LABEL: Acute ischemic stroke, complications of pregnancy (prophylaxis), MI (prophylaxis), prevention of thromboembolism, rheumatic fever, treatment of Kawasaki disease.

PRECAUTIONS

CONTRAINDICATIONS: Allergy to tartrazine dye, bleeding disorders, chickenpox or flu in children and teenagers, GI bleeding or ulceration, hepatic impairment, history of hypersensitivity to aspirin or NSAIDs. **CAUTIONS:** Vitamin K deficiency, chronic renal insufficiency, those with "aspirin triad" (rhinitis, nasal polyps, asthma).

⏳ **LIFESPAN CONSIDERATIONS: Pregnancy/Lactation:** Readily crosses placenta; distributed in breast milk. May prolong gestation and labor; decrease fetal birth weight; increase incidence of stillbirths, neonatal mortality, hemorrhage. Avoid use during last trimester (may adversely affect fetal cardiovascular system: premature closure of ductus arteriosus). **Pregnancy Category C (D if full dose used in third trimester of pregnancy). Children:** Caution in children with acute febrile illness (Reye's syndrome). **Elderly:** May be more susceptible to toxicity; lower dosages recommended.

INTERACTIONS

DRUG: Alcohol, NSAIDs: May increase the risk of adverse GI effects, including ulceration. **Antacids, urinary alkalinizers:** Increase the excretion of aspirin. **Anticoagulants, heparin, thrombolytics:** Increase the risk of bleeding. **Insulin, oral antidiabetics:** May increase the effects of these drugs (with large doses of aspirin). **Methotrexate, zidovudine:** May increase the risk of toxicity of these drugs. **Ototoxic medications, vancomycin:** May increase the risk of ototoxicity.

Platelet aggregation inhibitors, valproic acid: May increase the risk of bleeding. **Probenecid, sulfinpyrazone:** May decrease the effects of these drugs. **HERBAL:** None known. **FOOD:** None known. **LAB VALUES:** May alter serum alkaline phosphatase, uric acid, AST, and ALT levels. May prolong PT and bleeding time. May decrease serum cholesterol, serum potassium, and T_3 and T_4 levels.

AVAILABILITY (OTC)

CAPLETS (BAYER): 81 mg, 325 mg, 500 mg. **GELCAPS (BAYER):** 325 mg, 500 mg. **TABLETS:** 162 mg (Halfprin), 325 mg (Bayer), 500 mg (Bayer). **TABLETS (CHEWABLE [BAYER, ST. JOSEPH]):** 81 mg. **TABLETS (ENTERIC-COATED [BAYER, ECOTRIN, ST. JOSEPH]):** 81 mg, 325 mg, 500 mg, 650 mg. **SUPPOSITORIES:** 60 mg, 120 mg, 125 mg, 200 mg, 325 mg, 600 mg, 650 mg.

ADMINISTRATION/HANDLING

PO
• Do not crush or break enteric-coated tablet. • May give with water, milk, meals if GI distress occurs.

RECTAL
• Refrigerate suppositories. • If suppository is too soft, chill for 30 min in refrigerator or run cold water over foil wrapper. • Moisten suppository with cold water before inserting well into rectum.

INDICATIONS/ROUTES/DOSAGE

ANALGESIA, FEVER
PO, RECTAL: ADULTS, ELDERLY: 325–1,000 mg q4–6h. CHILDREN: 10–15 mg/kg/dose q4–6h. **Maximum:** 4 g/day.

ANTI-INFLAMMATORY
PO: ADULTS, ELDERLY: Initially, 2.4–3.6 g/day in divided doses; then 3.6–5.4 g/day. CHILDREN: Initially, 60–90 mg/kg/day in divided doses; then 80–100 mg/kg/day.

PLATELET AGGREGATION INHIBITOR
PO: ADULTS, ELDERLY: 80–325 mg/day.

KAWASAKI DISEASE
PO: CHILDREN: 80–100 mg/kg/day in divided doses.

SIDE EFFECTS

OCCASIONAL: GI distress (including abdominal distention, cramping, heartburn, and mild nausea); allergic reaction (including bronchospasm, pruritus, and urticaria).

ADVERSE REACTIONS/ TOXIC EFFECTS

High doses of aspirin may produce GI bleeding and gastric mucosal lesions. Dehydrated, febrile children may experience aspirin toxicity quickly. Reye's syndrome may occur in children with the chickenpox or the flu. Low-grade toxicity characterized is by tinnitus, generalized pruritus (possibly severe), headache, dizziness, flushing, tachycardia, hyperventilation, diaphoresis, and thirst. Marked toxicity is characterized by hyperthermia, restlessness, seizures, abnormal breathing patterns, respiratory failure, and coma.

NURSING CONSIDERATIONS

BASELINE ASSESSMENT

Do not give to children or teenagers who have flu or chickenpox (increases risk of Reye's syndrome). Do not use if vinegar-like odor is noted (indicates chemical breakdown). Assess type, location, duration of pain, inflammation. Inspect appearance of affected joints for immobility, deformities, skin condition. Therapeutic serum level for anti-arthritic effect: 20–30 mg/dl (toxicity occurs if levels are greater than 30 mg/dl).

INTERVENTION/EVALUATION

Monitor urinary pH (sudden acidification, pH from 6.5 to 5.5, may result in toxicity). Assess skin for evidence of ecchymosis. If given as antipyretic, assess temperature directly before and 1 hr after giving medication. Evaluate for therapeutic response: relief of pain, stiffness, swelling; increase in joint mobility; reduced joint tenderness; improved grip strength.

PATIENT/FAMILY TEACHING

• Do not crush or chew enteric-coated tablets. • Report ringing in ears (tinnitus) or persistent abdominal GI pain. • Therapeutic anti-inflammatory effect noted in 1–3 wk. • Behavioral changes, vomiting may be early signs of Reye's syndrome. Contact physician.

Astelin, *see azelastine*

Atacand, *see candesartan*

---

atazanavir sulfate

ah-tah-**zan**-ah-veer
(Reyataz)

Do not confuse Reyataz with Retavase.

CLASSIFICATION

PHARMACOTHERAPEUTIC: Antiretroviral. **CLINICAL:** Protease inhibitor.

ACTION

An antiviral that acts as an HIV-1 protease inhibitor, selectively preventing the processing of viral precursors found in cells infected with HIV-1. **Therapeutic Effect:** Prevents the formation of mature HIV cells.

PHARMACOKINETICS

Rapidly absorbed after PO administration. Protein binding: 86%. Extensively metabolized in the liver. Excreted primarily in urine and, to a lesser extent, in feces. **Half-life:** 5–8 hr.

USES

Treatment of HIV-1 infection in combination with other antiretroviral agents.

PRECAUTIONS

CONTRAINDICATIONS: Concurrent use with ergot derivatives, midazolam, pimozide, or triazolam; severe hepatic insufficiency. **EXTREME CAUTION:** Hepatic impairment. **CAUTIONS:** Preexisting conduction system disease (first-degree AV block or second- or third-degree AV block), diabetes mellitus, elderly, renal impairment.

⏳ **LIFESPAN CONSIDERATIONS: Pregnancy/Lactation:** Unknown if drug crosses placenta or distributed in breast milk. Lactic acidosis syndrome, hyperbilirubinemia, kernicterus have been reported. **Pregnancy Category B. Children:** Safety and efficacy not established in those younger than 3 mo. **Elderly:** Age-related hepatic impairment may require dose reduction.

INTERACTIONS

DRUG: Antacids, H$_2$ receptor antagonists, proton pump inhibitors, rifampin: May decrease atazanavir plasma concentrations. **Atorvastatin, calcium channel blockers, immunosuppressants, irinotecan, lovastatin, sildenafil, simvastatin, tricyclic antidepressants:** May increase atazanavir plasma concentrations. **HERBAL: St. John's wort:** May decrease atazanavir plasma concentration. **FOOD: High-fat meals:** May decrease atazanavir absorption. **LAB VALUES:** May increase serum amylase, bilirubin, lipase, AST, and ALT levels. May decrease blood Hgb level and neutrophil and platelet counts. May alter LDL and serum triglyceride levels.

AVAILABILITY (Rx)

CAPSULES: 100 mg, 150 mg, 200 mg.

ADMINISTRATION/HANDLING
PO
- Give with food.

INDICATIONS/ROUTES/DOSAGE
HIV-1 INFECTION
PO: ADULTS, ELDERLY (ANTIRETROVIRAL-NAIVE): 400 mg (2 capsules) once a day with food. ADULTS, ELDERLY (ANTIRETROVIRAL-EXPERIENCED): 300 mg and ritonavir (Norvir) 100 mg once a day.

HIV-1 INFECTION (CONCURRENT THERAPY WITH EFAVIRENZ)
PO: ADULTS, ELDERLY: 300 mg atazanavir, 100 mg ritonavir, and 600 mg efavirenz as a single daily dose with food.

HIV-1 INFECTION (CONCURRENT THERAPY WITH DIDANOSINE)
PO: ADULTS, ELDERLY: Give atazanavir with food 2 hr before or 1 hr after didanosine.

HIV-1 INFECTION (CONCURRENT THERAPY WITH TENOFOVIR)
PO: ADULTS, ELDERLY: 300 mg atazanavir and 100 mg ritonavir and 300 mg tenofovir given as a single daily dose with food.

HIV-1 INFECTION IN PATIENTS WITH MILD TO MODERATE HEPATIC IMPAIRMENT
PO ◄ **ALERT** ► Avoid use in patients with severe hepatic impairment.
ADULTS, ELDERLY: 300 mg once a day with food.

SIDE EFFECTS

FREQUENT (16%–14%): Nausea, headache. **OCCASIONAL (9%–4%):** Rash, vomiting, depression, diarrhea, abdominal pain, fever. **RARE (3% or less):** Dizziness, insomnia, cough, fatigue, back pain.

ADVERSE REACTIONS/ TOXIC EFFECTS

A severe hypersensitivity reaction (marked by angioedema and chest pain) and jaundice may occur.

NURSING CONSIDERATIONS

BASELINE ASSESSMENT

Obtain baseline laboratory tests, CBC, liver function tests, before beginning therapy and at periodic intervals during therapy. Offer emotional support.

INTERVENTION/EVALUATION

Assess for nausea, vomiting; assess eating pattern. Determine pattern of bowel activity, stool consistency. Assess skin for rash. Question for evidence of headache. Monitor for onset of depression.

PATIENT/FAMILY TEACHING

• Take with food. • Small, frequent meals may offset nausea, vomiting. • Atazanavir is not a cure for HIV infection, nor does it reduce risk of transmission to others.

---

atenolol

ay-**ten**-oh-lol

(Tenolin ✤, Tenormin)

Do not confuse atenolol with albuterol or timolol.

FIXED-COMBINATION(S)

Tenoretic: atenolol/chlorthalidone (a diuretic): 50 mg/25 mg; 100 mg/25 mg.

◆CLASSIFICATION

PHARMACOTHERAPEUTIC: Beta₁-adrenergic blocker. **CLINICAL:** Antihypertensive, antianginal, antiarrhythmic (see p. 63C).

ACTION

A beta₁-adrenergic blocker that acts as an antianginal, antiarrhythmic, and antihypertensive agent by blocking beta₁-adrenergic receptors in cardiac tissue. **Therapeutic Effect:** Slows sinus node heart rate, decreasing cardiac output and BP. Decreases myocardial oxygen demand.

PHARMACOKINETICS

Route	Onset	Peak	Duration
PO	1 hr	2–4 hr	24 hr

Incompletely absorbed from the GI tract. Protein binding: 6%–16%. Minimal liver metabolism. Primarily excreted unchanged in urine. Removed by hemodialysis. **Half-life:** 6–7 hr (increased in impaired renal function).

USES

Treatment of hypertension, alone or in combination with other agents; management of angina pectoris; reduces cardiovascular mortality in those with definite or suspected acute MI. **OFF-LABEL:** Acute alcohol withdrawal, arrhythmia (especially supraventricular and ventricular tachycardia), improved survival in diabetics with heart disease, mild to moderately severe CHF (adjunct); prevention of migraine, thyrotoxicosis, tremors; treatment of hypertrophic cardiomyopathy, pheochromocytoma, and syndrome of mitral valve prolapse.

PRECAUTIONS

CONTRAINDICATIONS: Cardiogenic shock, overt heart failure, second- or third-degree heart block, severe bradycardia. **CAUTIONS:** Renal/hepatic impairment, peripheral vascular disease, hyperthyroidism, diabetes, inadequate cardiac function, bronchospastic disease. ⧗ **LIFESPAN CONSIDERATIONS: Pregnancy/Lactation:** Readily crosses placenta; distributed in breast milk. Avoid use during first trimester. May produce bradycardia, apnea, hypoglycemia, hypothermia during delivery; low birth-weight infants. **Pregnancy Category D. Children:** No age-related precautions

---

noted. **Elderly:** Age-related peripheral vascular disease, renal impairment requires caution.

INTERACTIONS

DRUG: **Cimetidine:** May increase atenolol blood concentration. **Diuretics, other antihypertensives:** May increase hypotensive effect of atenolol. **Insulin, oral hypoglycemics:** May mask symptoms of hypoglycemia and prolong hypoglycemic effect of insulin and oral hypoglycemics. **NSAIDs:** May decrease antihypertensive effect of atenolol. **Sympathomimetics, xanthines:** May mutually inhibit effects. **HERBAL:** None known. **FOOD:** None known. **LAB VALUES:** May increase serum antinuclear antibody titer and BUN, serum creatinine, potassium, lipoprotein, triglyceride, and uric acid levels.

AVAILABILITY (Rx)

TABLETS: 25 mg, 50 mg, 100 mg. **INJECTION:** 5 mg/10 ml.

ADMINISTRATION/HANDLING

IV

Reconstitution • May give undiluted or dilute in 10–50 ml 0.9% NaCl or D_5W.

Rate of administration • Give IV push over 5 min. • Give IV infusion over 15 min.

Storage • Store at room temperature. • After reconstitution, parenteral form is stable for 48 hr at room temperature.

PO

• Give without regard to food. • Tablets may be crushed.

IV INCOMPATIBILITIES

Amphotericin complex (Abelcet, AmBisome, Amphotec).

INDICATIONS/ROUTES/DOSAGE

HYPERTENSION

PO: ADULTS: Initially, 25–50 mg once a day. May increase dose up to 100 mg once a day. ELDERLY: Usual initial dose, 25 mg a day. CHILDREN: Initially, 0.8–1 mg/kg/dose given once a day. Range: 0.8–1.5 mg/kg/day. **Maximum:** 2 mg/kg/day or 100 mg/day.

ANGINA PECTORIS

PO: ADULTS: Initially, 50 mg once a day. May increase dose up to 200 mg once a day. ELDERLY: Usual initial dose, 25 mg a day.

ACUTE MI

IV: ADULTS: Give 5 mg over 5 min; may repeat in 10 min. In those who tolerate full 10-mg IV dose, begin 50-mg tablets 10 min after last IV dose followed by another 50-mg oral dose 12 hr later. Thereafter, give 100 mg once a day or 50 mg twice a day for 6–9 days. Or, for those who do not tolerate full IV dose, give 50 mg orally twice a day or 100 mg once a day for at least 7 days.

DOSAGE IN RENAL IMPAIRMENT

Dosage interval is modified based on creatinine clearance.

Creatinine Clearance	Dosage Interval
15–35 ml/min	50 mg a day
Less than 15 ml/min	50 mg every other day

SIDE EFFECTS

Atenolol is generally well tolerated, with mild and transient side effects. **FREQUENT:** Hypotension manifested as cold extremities, constipation or diarrhea, diaphoresis, dizziness, fatigue, headache, and nausea. **OCCASIONAL:** Insomnia, flatulence, urinary frequency, impotence or decreased libido, depression. **RARE:** Rash, arthralgia, myalgia, confusion (especially in the elderly), altered taste.

ADVERSE REACTIONS/TOXIC EFFECTS

Overdose may produce profound bradycardia and hypotension. Abrupt atenolol withdrawal may result in diaphoresis, palpitations, headache, and tremors. Atenolol administration may precipitate CHF or MI in patients with cardiac disease; thyroid storm in those with thyrotoxicosis; and peripheral ischemia in those with existing peripheral vascular disease. Hypoglycemia may occur in patients with previously controlled diabetes. Thrombocytopenia, manifested as unusual bruising or bleeding, occurs rarely.

NURSING CONSIDERATIONS

BASELINE ASSESSMENT
Assess BP, apical pulse immediately before drug is administered (if pulse is 60/min or less, or systolic BP is less than 90 mm Hg, withhold medication, contact physician). **Antianginal:** Record onset, quality (sharp, dull, squeezing), radiation, location, intensity, duration of anginal pain, precipitating factors (exertion, emotional stress). Assess baseline renal/hepatic function tests.

INTERVENTION/EVALUATION
Monitor BP for hypotension, pulse for bradycardia, respiration for difficulty in breathing. Assess pattern of daily bowel activity and stool consistency. Assess for evidence of CHF: dyspnea (particularly on exertion or lying down), night cough, peripheral edema, distended neck veins. Monitor I&O (increased weight, decreased urine output may indicate CHF). Assess extremities for coldness. Assist with ambulation if dizziness occurs.

PATIENT/FAMILY TEACHING
• Do not abruptly discontinue medication. • Compliance with therapy essential to control hypertension, angina. • To reduce hypotensive effect, rise slowly from lying to sitting position and permit legs to dangle from bed momentarily before standing. • Avoid tasks that require alertness, motor skills until drug reaction is established. • Report dizziness, depression, confusion, rash, unusual bruising/bleeding. • Outpatients should monitor BP, pulse before taking medication (teach correct technique). • Restrict salt, alcohol intake. • Therapeutic antihypertensive effect noted in 1–2 wk.

Ativan, *see lorazepam*

atomoxetine
ah-toe-**mocks**-eh-teen
(<u>Strattera</u>)

CLASSIFICATION
PHARMACOTHERAPEUTIC: Norepinephrine reuptake inhibitor. **CLINICAL:** Psychotherapeutic agent.

ACTION
A norepinephrine reuptake inhibitor that enhances noradrenergic function by selective inhibition of the presynaptic norepinephrine transporter. **Therapeutic Effect:** Improves symptoms of attention-deficit hyperactivity disorder (ADHD).

PHARMACOKINETICS
Rapidly absorbed after PO administration. Protein binding: 98% (primarily to albumin). Eliminated primarily in urine and, to a lesser extent, in feces. Not removed by hemodialysis. **Half-life:** 4–5 hr in general population, 22 hr in 7% of Caucasians and 2% of African-Americans; (increased in moderate to severe hepatic insufficiency).

USES

Treatment of ADHD. OFF-LABEL: Treatment of depression.

PRECAUTIONS

CONTRAINDICATIONS: Angle-closure glaucoma, use within 14 days of MAOIs. **CAUTIONS:** Hypertension; tachycardia; cardiovascular disease; patients at risk for urinary retention, moderate or severe hepatic impairment.

⌛ LIFESPAN CONSIDERATIONS: **Pregnancy/Lactation:** Unknown if excreted in breast milk. **Pregnancy Category C. Children:** Safety and efficacy in patients younger than 6 yr have not been established. May produce suicidal thoughts in children and adolescents. **Elderly:** Age-related hepatic/renal impairment, cardiovascular or cerebrovascular disease may increase risk of effects.

INTERACTIONS

DRUG: **Fluoxetine, paroxetine, quinidine:** May increase atomoxetine blood concentration. **MAOIs:** May increase the risk of toxic effects. HERBAL: None known FOOD: None known. LAB VALUES: None known.

AVAILABILITY (Rx)

CAPSULES: 10 mg, 18 mg, 25 mg, 40 mg, 60 mg, 80 mg, 100 mg.

ADMINISTRATION/HANDLING

PO

• Give without regard to food.

INDICATIONS/ROUTES/DOSAGE

ADHD

PO: ADULTS, CHILDREN WEIGHING 70 KG AND MORE: 40 mg once a day. May increase after at least 3 days to 80 mg as a single daily dose or in divided doses. **Maximum:** 100 mg. CHILDREN WEIGHING LESS THAN 70 KG: Initially, 0.5 mg/kg/day. May increase after at least 3 days to 1.2 mg/kg/day. **Maximum:** 1.4 mg/kg/day or 100 mg.

DOSAGE IN HEPATIC IMPAIRMENT

Expect to administer 50% of normal atomoxetine dosage to patients with moderate hepatic impairment and 25% of normal dosage to those with severe hepatic impairment.

SIDE EFFECTS

FREQUENT: Headache, dyspepsia, nausea, vomiting, fatigue, decreased appetite, dizziness, altered mood. **OCCASIONAL:** Tachycardia, hypertension, weight loss, delayed growth in children, irritability. **RARE:** Insomnia, sexual dysfunction in adults, fever.

ADVERSE REACTIONS/ TOXIC EFFECTS

Urine retention or urinary hesitance may occur. In overdose, gastric emptying and repeated use of activated charcoal may prevent systemic absorption. Severe hepatic injury occurs rarely.

NURSING CONSIDERATIONS

BASELINE ASSESSMENT

Assess pulse, BP before therapy, following dose increases, and periodically while on therapy.

INTERVENTION/EVALUATION

Monitor urinary output; complaints of urinary retention or hesitancy may be a related adverse reaction. Assist with ambulation if dizziness occurs. Be alert to mood changes. Monitor fluid and electrolyte status in those with significant vomiting.

PATIENT/FAMILY TEACHING

• Avoid tasks that require alertness, motor skills until response to drug is established. • Take last dose early in evening to avoid insomnia. • Report palpitations, fever, vomiting, irritability.

atorvastatin

ah-tore-**vah**-stah-tin
(Lipitor)
Do not confuse Lipitor with Levatol.

FIXED-COMBINATION(S)

Caduet: atorvastatin/amlodipine (calcium channel blocker): 10 mg/5 mg, 10 mg/10 mg, 20 mg/5 mg, 20 mg/10 mg, 40 mg/5 mg, 40 mg/10 mg, 80 mg/5 mg, 80 mg/10 mg.

CLASSIFICATION

PHARMACOTHERAPEUTIC: Hydroxymethylglutaryl CoA (HMG-CoA) reductase inhibitor. **CLINICAL:** Antihyperlipidemic (see p. 52C).

ACTION

An antihyperlipidemic that inhibits hydroxamethylglutaryl-CoA (HMG-CoA) reductase, the enzyme that catalyzes the early step in cholesterol synthesis. **Therapeutic Effect:** Decreases LDL and VLDL cholesterol, and plasma triglyceride levels; increases HDL cholesterol concentration.

PHARMACOKINETICS

Poorly absorbed from the GI tract. Protein binding: greater than 98%. Metabolized in the liver. Minimally eliminated in urine. Plasma levels are markedly increased in chronic alcoholic hepatic disease, but are unaffected by renal disease. **Half-life:** 14 hr.

USES

Primary prevention of cardiovascular disease in high-risk patients. Reduces risk of stroke and heart attack in patients with Type 2 diabetes without evidence of heart disease but other risk factors. Reduces risk of stroke without evidence of heart disease but with multiple risk factors other than diabetes. Adjunct to diet therapy in management of hyperlipidemias (reduces elevations in total cholesterol, LDL C, apolipoprotein B and triglycerides in patients with primary hypercholesterolemia), homozygous familial hypercholesterolemia, and heterozygous familial hypercholesterolemia in patients 10–17 yr of age, females more than 1 yr post-menarche). **OFF-LABEL:** Secondary prevention of ischemia in patients with CHF.

PRECAUTIONS

CONTRAINDICATIONS: Active hepatic disease, lactation, pregnancy, unexplained elevated liver function test results. **CAUTIONS:** Anticoagulant therapy, history of hepatic disease, substantial alcohol consumption, major surgery, severe acute infection, trauma, hypotension, severe metabolic, endocrine, or electrolyte disorders, uncontrolled seizures.

⏳ **LIFESPAN CONSIDERATIONS: Pregnancy/Lactation:** Distributed in breast milk. Contraindicated during pregnancy. May produce skeletal malformation. **Pregnancy Category X. Children:** Safety and efficacy not established. **Elderly:** No age-related precautions noted.

INTERACTIONS

DRUG: Antacids, colestipol, propranolol: Decreases atorvastatin activity. **Cyclosporine, erythromycin, gemfibrozil, nicotinic acid:** Increases the risk of acute renal failure and rhabdomyolysis with these drugs. **Digoxin, itraconazole, oral contraceptives, warfarin:** May increase atorvastatin blood concentration, producing severe muscle inflammation, pain, and weakness. **HERBAL:** None known. **FOOD:** None known. **LAB VALUES:** May increase serum creatine kinase (CK) and transaminase concentrations.

AVAILABILITY (Rx)

TABLETS: 10 mg, 20 mg, 40 mg, 80 mg.

ADMINISTRATION/HANDLING

PO

- Give without regard to food.
- Do not break film-coated tablets.

INDICATIONS/ROUTES/DOSAGE

PREVENTION OF CARDIOVASCULAR DISEASE (CVD)

PO: ADULTS, ELDERLY: 10 mg once daily.

HYPERLIPIDEMIAS

PO: ADULTS, ELDERLY: Initially, 10–20 mg/day (40 mg in patients requiring greater than 45% reduction in LDL-C). Range: 10–80 mg/day.

HETEROZYGOUS HYPERCHOLESTEROLEMIA

PO: CHILDREN 10–17 YR: Initially, 10 mg/day. **Maximum:** 20 mg/day.

SIDE EFFECTS

COMMON: Atorvastatin is generally well tolerated. Side effects are usually mild and transient. **FREQUENT (16%):** Headache. **OCCASIONAL (5%–2%):** Myalgia, rash or pruritus, allergy. **RARE (less than 2%–1%):** Flatulence, dyspepsia.

ADVERSE REACTIONS/ TOXIC EFFECTS

Cataracts may develop, and photosensitivity may occur.

BASELINE ASSESSMENT

Question for possibility of pregnancy before initiating therapy (Pregnancy Category X). Assess baseline lab results: cholesterol, triglycerides, liver function tests.

INTERVENTION/EVALUATION

Monitor for headache. Assess for rash, pruritus, malaise. Monitor cholesterol and triglyceride lab values for therapeutic response.

PATIENT/FAMILY TEACHING

- Follow special diet (important part of treatment). • Periodic lab tests are essential part of therapy. • Do not take other medications without physician's knowledge.

atovaquone

a-**toe**-va-kwone
(Mepron)

♦CLASSIFICATION

PHARMACOTHERAPEUTIC: Systemic anti-infective. **CLINICAL:** Antiprotozoal.

ACTION

A systemic anti-infective that inhibits the mitochondrial electron-transport system at the cytochrome bc1 complex (Complex III), which interrupts nucleic acid and adenosine triphosphate synthesis. **Therapeutic Effect:** Antiprotozoal and antipneumocystic activity.

USES

Treatment or prevention of mild to moderate *Pneumocystis carinii* pneumonia (PCP) in those intolerant to trimetho-prim-sulfamethoxazole (TMP-SMZ).

PRECAUTIONS

CONTRAINDICATIONS: Development or history of potentially life-threatening allergic reaction to the drug. **CAUTIONS:** Elderly, patients with severe PCP, chronic diarrhea, malabsorption syndromes. **Pregnancy Category C.**

INTERACTIONS

DRUG: Rifampin: May decrease atovaquone blood concentration and increase rifampin blood concentration. **HERBAL:** None known. **FOOD:** None known. **LAB VALUES:** May increase serum alkaline phosphatase, amylase,

AST, and ALT levels. May decrease serum sodium levels.

AVAILABILITY (Rx)
ORAL SUSPENSION: 750 mg/5 ml.

INDICATIONS/ROUTES/DOSAGE
PNEUMOCYSTIS CARINII PNEUMONIA (PCP)
PO: ADULTS, CHILDREN OLDER THAN 12 YR: 750 mg twice a day with food for 21 days. CHILDREN 12 YR AND YOUNGER: 40 mg/kg/day in 2 divided doses. **Maximum:** 1,500 mg/day.

PREVENTION OF PCP
PO: ADULTS: 1,500 mg once a day with food. CHILDREN 4-24 MO: 45 mg/kg/day as single dose. **Maximum:** 1,500 mg/day. CHILDREN 1-3 MO AND OLDER THAN 24 MO: 30 mg/kg/day as single dose. **Maximum:** 1,500 mg/day.

SIDE EFFECTS
FREQUENT (greater than 10%): Rash, nausea, diarrhea, headache, vomiting, fever, insomnia, cough. **OCCASIONAL (less than 10%):** Abdominal discomfort, thrush, asthenia, anemia, neutropenia.

ADVERSE REACTIONS/ TOXIC EFFECTS
None known.

NURSING CONSIDERATIONS

INTERVENTION/EVALUATION
Assess for GI discomfort, nausea, vomiting. Check consistency and frequency of stools. Assess skin for rash. Monitor I&O, renal function tests, Hgb. Monitor elderly closely for decreased hepatic, renal, and cardiac function.

PATIENT/FAMILY TEACHING
• Continue therapy for full length of treatment. • Do not take any other medication unless approved by physician. • Notify physician in event of rash, diarrhea, or other new symptom.

atracurium
(Tracrium)
See Neuromuscular blockers (p. 111C)

atropine sulfate
ah-trow-peen
(AtroPen Auto Injector, Atropine-Care, Atropine Sulfate, Atropisol, Atrosulf-1, Isopto Atropine, Ocu-Tropine, Sal-Tropine)
Do not confuse atropine with Akarpine, or Atropisol with Aplisol.

FIXED-COMBINATION(S)
Donnatal: atropine/hyoscyamine (anticholinergic)/phenobarbital (sedative)/scopolamine (anticholinergic): 0.0194 mg/0.1037 mg/16.2 mg/0.0065 mg. **Lomotil:** atropine/diphenoxylate: 0.025 mg/2.5 mg.

CLASSIFICATION
PHARMACOTHERAPEUTIC: Acetylcholine antagonist. **CLINICAL:** Antiarrhythmic, antispasmodic, antidote, cycloplegic, antisecretory, anticholinergic.

ACTION
An acetylcholine antagonist that inhibits the action of acetylcholine by competing with acetylcholine for common binding sites on muscarinic receptors, which are located on exocrine glands, cardiac and smooth-muscle

ganglia, and intramural neurons. This action blocks all muscarinic effects. **Therapeutic Effect:** Decreases GI motility and secretory activity, and GU muscle tone (ureter, bladder); produces ophthalmic cycloplegia, and mydriasis.

PHARMACOKINETICS

AtroPen auto injector: Rapidly and well absorbed after IM administration. Much of the drug is destroyed by enzymatic hydrolysis, particularly in the liver. Partially excreted unchanged in urine.

USES

Treatment in cardiopulmonary (ACLS) resuscitation for treatment of sinus bradycardia accompanied by hemodynamic compromise (hypotension, altered mental status, frequent ventricular ectopy or ventricular asystole. Preop medication to prevent or reduce salivation, excessive secretions of respiratory tract. Prevention of cholinergic effects during surgery: cardiac arrhythmias, hypotension, reflex bradycardia. Blocks adverse muscarinic effects of anticholinesterase agents (e.g., neostigmine). **OFF-LABEL:** Malignant glaucoma.

PRECAUTIONS

CONTRAINDICATIONS: Bladder neck obstruction due to prostatic hypertrophy, cardiospasm, intestinal atony, myasthenia gravis in those not treated with neostigmine, narrow-angle glaucoma, obstructive disease of the GI tract, paralytic ileus, severe ulcerative colitis, tachycardia secondary to cardiac insufficiency or thyrotoxicosis, toxic megacolon, unstable cardiovascular status in acute hemorrhage. **EXTREME CAUTION:** Autonomic neuropathy, known or suspected GI infections, diarrhea, mild to moderate ulcerative colitis. **CAUTIONS:** Hyperthyroidism, hepatic or renal disease, hypertension, tachyarrhythmias, CHF, coronary artery disease, gastric ulcer, esophageal reflux or hiatal hernia associated with reflux esophagitis, infants,

elderly, systemic administration in those with chronic obstructive pulmonary disease (COPD). Ophthalmic: Spastic paralysis, brain damage, Down syndrome.
◄ **ALERT** ► Organophosphorous poison will generally mask minor atropine effects.

⌛ **LIFESPAN CONSIDERATIONS: Pregnancy/Lactation:** Crosses placenta; distributed in breast milk. **Pregnancy Category C. Children:** Increased susceptibility to atropine effects. **Elderly:** Increased susceptibility to atropine effects.

INTERACTIONS

DRUG: Antacids, antidiarrheals: May decrease absorption of atropine. **Anticholinergics:** May increase effects of atropine. **Ketoconazole:** May decrease absorption of ketoconazole. **Potassium chloride:** May increase severity of GI lesions (wax matrix). **Pralidoxime:** May increase the risk of atropinization (flushing, mydriasis, tachycardia, dryness of the mouth and nose) when used with the AtroPen auto injector. **HERBAL:** None known. **FOOD:** None known. **LAB VALUES:** None known.

AVAILABILITY (Rx)

INJECTION: 0.05 mg/ml, 0.1 mg/ml, 0.4 mg/0.5 ml, 0.4 mg/ml, 0.5 mg/ml, 1 mg/ml. **IM INJECTION (AtroPen):** 0.25 mg, 0.5 mg, 1 mg, 2 mg. **OPHTHALMIC OINTMENT:** 0.5%, 1%. **OPHTHALMIC SOLUTION:** 0.5% (Isopto Atropine), 1% (Atropisol, Isopto Atropine), 2% (Atropisol).

ADMINISTRATION/HANDLING
⌛ IV

• Administer the IV form rapidly (prevents paradoxical slowing of heart rate).

IM
• May be given subcutaneously or IM.

IM, Atro-Pen
◀ **ALERT** ▶ Primary protection against exposure to chemical nerve agents and insecticide poisonings is the wearing of protective garments including masks designed specifically for this use. Individuals should not rely solely upon antidotes such as atropine and pralidoxime to provide complete protection from chemical nerve agents and insecticide poisoning.

◀ **ALERT** ▶ The AtroPen should be used by persons who have adequate training in the recognition and treatment of nerve agent or insecticide intoxication.
• Store at room temperature. • Give as soon as symptoms of organophosphorous or carbamate poisoning appear. • Don't use more than three Atro-Pen auto injectors in each person at risk for nerve agent or organophosphate insecticide poisoning.

OPHTHALMIC
• Place a gloved finger on the patient's lower eyelid and pull it out until a pocket is formed between the eye and lower lid. • Hold the dropper above the pocket and place the prescribed number of drops (or ¼–½ inch of ointment) into the pocket. Close the eye gently. • For ophthalmic solution, apply digital pressure to the lacrimal sac for 1–2 min to minimize systemic absorption. • For ophthalmic ointment, close the patient's eye for 1–2 min. Instruct the patient to roll the eyeball to increase the contact area of the drug to the eye. • Remove excess solution or ointment around eye with tissue.

▒ IV INCOMPATIBILITY
Pentothal (Thiopental).

IV COMPATIBILITIES
Diphenhydramine (Benadryl), droperidol (Inapsine), fentanyl (Sublimaze), glycopyrrolate (Robinul), heparin, hydromorphone (Dilaudid), midazolam (Versed), morphine, potassium chloride, propofol (Diprivan).

INDICATIONS/ROUTES/DOSAGE
ASYSTOLE, SLOW PULSELESS ELECTRICAL ACTIVITY
IV: ADULTS, ELDERLY: 1 mg; may repeat q3–5min to total dose of 0.04 mg/kg.

PRE-ANESTHETIC
IV, IM, SUBCUTANEOUS: ADULTS, ELDERLY: 0.4–0.6 mg 30–60 min preop. CHILDREN WEIGHING 5 KG AND MORE: 0.01–0.02 mg/kg/dose to maximum of 0.4 mg/dose. CHILDREN WEIGHING LESS THAN 5 KG: 0.02 mg/kg/dose 30–60 min preop.

BRADYCARDIA
IV: ADULTS, ELDERLY: 0.5–1 mg q5min not to exceed 2 mg or 0.04 mg/kg. CHILDREN: 0.02 mg/kg with a minimum of 0.1 mg to a maximum of 0.5 mg in children and 1 mg in adolescents. May repeat in 5 min. **Maximum total dose:** 1 mg in children, 2 mg in adolescents.

CYCLOPLEGIC REFRACTION, POSTOPERATIVE MYDRIASIS, UVEITIS
OPHTHALMIC SOLUTION: ADULTS, ELDERLY: Instill 1 drop of 1% or 2% solution in affected eye(s) up to 4 times a day.
OPHTHALMIC OINTMENT: ADULTS, ELDERLY: Apply ointment several hours prior to examination when used for refraction.

POISONING BY SUSCEPTIBLE ORGANOPHOSPHOROUS NERVE AGENTS HAVING CHOLINESTERASE ACTIVITY, ORGANOPHOSPHOROUS OR CARBAMATE INSECTICIDES
IM: ADULTS, CHILDREN WEIGHING MORE THAN 90 LB: AtroPen 2 mg (green). CHILDREN WEIGHING 40–90 LB: AtroPen 1 mg (dark red). CHILDREN WEIGHING 15–39 LB: AtroPen 0.5 mg (blue). INFANTS WEIGHING LESS THAN 15 LB: AtroPen 0.25 mg (yellow).

SIDE EFFECTS
FREQUENT: Dry mouth, nose, and throat that may be severe; decreased sweating,

constipation, irritation at subcutaneous or IM injection site. **OCCASIONAL:** Swallowing difficulty, blurred vision, bloated feeling, impotence, urinary hesitancy. **Ophthalmic:** Mydriasis, blurred vision, photophobia, decreased visual acuity, tearing, dry eyes or dry conjunctiva, eye irritation, crusting of eyelid. **RARE:** Allergic reaction, including rash and urticaria; mental confusion or excitement, particularly in children, fatigue.

ADVERSE REACTIONS/ TOXIC EFFECTS

Overdosage may produce tachycardia, palpitations, hot, dry or flushed skin, absence of bowel sounds, increased respiratory rate, nausea, vomiting, confusion, somnolence, slurred speech, dizziness and CNS stimulation. Overdosage may also produce psychosis as evidenced by agitation, restlessness, rambling speech, visual hallucinations, paranoid behavior, and delusions, followed by depression. Increased intraocular pressure occurs rarely with the use of the ophthalmic form.

NURSING CONSIDERATIONS

BASELINE ASSESSMENT

Before giving medication, instruct patient to void (reduces risk of urinary retention). Determine if the patient is sensitive to atropine, homatropine, or scopolamine. Treatment with the Atro-Pen auto injector may be instituted without waiting for lab results.

INTERVENTION/EVALUATION

Monitor changes in BP, pulse, temperature. Observe for tachycardia if patient has cardiac abnormalities. Assess skin turgor, mucous membranes to evaluate hydration status (encourage adequate fluid intake unless NPO for surgery) bowel sounds for peristalsis. Be alert for fever (increased risk of hyperthermia). Monitor I&O, palpate bladder

for urinary retention. Assess stool frequency, consistency.

PATIENT/FAMILY TEACHING

• For preoperative use, explain that warm, dry, flushing feeling may occur.
• Remind patient to remain in bed and not eat or drink anything.

Atrovent, *see ipratropium*

Augmentin, *see amoxicillin/clavulanate potassium*

Augmentin ES-600, *see amoxicillin/clavulanate potassium*

Augmentin XR, *see amoxicillin/clavulanate potassium*

---

auranofin

aur-an-**oh**-fin
(Ridaura)

aurothioglucose

ah-row-thigh-oh-**glue**-cose
(Solganal)
Do not confuse Ridaura with Cardura.

◆**CLASSIFICATION**
PHARMACOTHERAPEUTIC: Gold compound. **CLINICAL:** Anti-rheumatic.

ACTION

Gold compounds that alter cellular mechanisms, collagen biosynthesis, enzyme systems, and immune responses. **Therapeutic Effect:** Suppress synovitis in the active stage of rheumatoid arthritis.

PHARMACOKINETICS

Auranofin (29% gold): Moderately absorbed from the GI tract. Protein binding: 60%. Rapidly metabolized. Primarily excreted in urine. **Half-life:** 21–31 days. **Aurothioglucose (50% gold):** Slowly and erratically absorbed after IM administration. Protein binding: 95%–99%. Primarily excreted in urine. **Half-life:** 3–27 days (increased with increased number of doses).

USES

Management of rheumatoid arthritis in those with insufficient therapeutic response to NSAIDs. **OFF-LABEL:** Treatment of discoid refractory lupus erythematosus, Felty's syndrome, pemphigus, psoriatic arthritis, systemic lupus erythematosus.

PRECAUTIONS

CONTRAINDICATIONS: Bone marrow aplasia, history of gold-induced pathologies (including blood dyscrasias, exfoliative dermatitis, necrotizing enterocolitis, and pulmonary fibrosis), severe blood dyscrasias. **CAUTIONS:** Renal/hepatic disease, marked hypertension, compromised cerebral/cardiovascular circulation. Blood dyscrasias, severe debilitation, history of sensitivity to gold compounds, Sjögren's syndrome in rheumatoid arthritis, systemic lupus erythematosus, eczema.

⌛ **LIFESPAN CONSIDERATIONS: Pregnancy/Lactation:** Crosses placenta; distributed in breast milk. Use only when benefits outweigh hazard to fetus. **Pregnancy Category C. Children:** No age-related precautions noted. **Elderly:** Age-related renal impairment may require caution.

INTERACTIONS

DRUG: Bone marrow depressants; hepatotoxic and nephrotoxic medications: May increase the risk of aurothioglucose toxicity. **Penicillamine:** May increase the risk of hematologic or renal adverse effects. **HERBAL:** None known. **FOOD:** None known. **LAB VALUES:** May decrease Hgb level, Hct, WBC and platelet counts. May increase urine protein level. May alter hepatic function test results.

AVAILABILITY (Rx)

CAPSULES (RIDAURA): 3 mg. **INJECTION (SOLGANAL):** 50-mg/ml suspension.

ADMINISTRATION/HANDLING

IM
• Give in upper outer quadrant of gluteus.

PO
• Give without regard to food.

INDICATIONS/ROUTES/DOSAGE

RHEUMATOID ARTHRITIS
PO: ADULTS, ELDERLY: 6 mg/day as a single or 2 divided doses. If there is no response in 6 mo, may increase to 9 mg/day in 3 divided doses. If response is still inadequate, discontinue. CHILDREN: 0.1 mg/kg/day as a single or 2 divided doses. Maintenance: 0.15 mg/kg/day. **Maximum:** 0.2 mg/kg/day.
IM: ADULTS, ELDERLY: Initially, 10 mg, followed by 25 mg for 2 doses, then 50 mg weekly until total dose of 0.8–1 g has been given. If patient has improved and shows no signs of toxicity, may give 50 mg q3–4wk for many months. CHILDREN: 0.25 mg/kg; may increase by 0.25 mg/kg each week. Maintenance: 0.75–1 mg/kg/dose. **Maximum:** 25 mg/dose for 20 doses, then repeated q2–4wk.

SIDE EFFECTS

FREQUENT: Auranofin: Diarrhea (50%), pruritic rash (26%), abdominal pain (14%), stomatitis (13%), nausea (10%). **Aurothioglucose:** Rash (39%), stomatitis (19%), diarrhea (13%).
OCCASIONAL: Aurothioglucose: Nausea, vomiting, anorexia, abdominal cramps.

ADVERSE REACTIONS/ TOXIC EFFECTS

Signs and symptoms of gold toxicity, the primary serious reaction, include decreased Hgb level, decreased granulocyte count (less than 150,000/mm^3), proteinuria, hematuria, stomatitis, blood dyscrasias (anemia, leukopenia [WBC count less than 4,000/mm^3], thrombocytopenia, and eosinophilia), glomerulonephritis, nephrotic syndrome, and cholestatic jaundice.

NURSING CONSIDERATIONS

BASELINE ASSESSMENT
Rule out pregnancy before beginning treatment. CBC, urinalysis, platelet count, renal/liver function tests should be performed before therapy begins.

INTERVENTION/EVALUATION
Monitor daily bowel activity and stool consistency. Assess urine tests for proteinuria, hematuria. Monitor CBC, blood chemistries, renal/liver function studies. Question for pruritus (may be first sign of impending rash). Assess skin daily for rash, purpura, ecchymoses. Assess oral mucous membranes, borders of tongue, palate, pharynx for ulceration, complaint of metallic taste sensation (sign of stomatitis). Evaluate for therapeutic response: relief of pain, stiffness, swelling, increase in joint mobility, reduced joint tenderness, improved grip strength.

PATIENT/FAMILY TEACHING
• Therapeutic response may be expected in 3–6 mo. • Avoid exposure to sunlight (gray to blue pigment may appear). • Contact physician if pruritus, rash, sore mouth, indigestion, or metallic taste occurs. • Maintain diligent oral hygiene.

Avalide, *see hydrochlorothiazide and irbesartan*

Avandia, *see rosiglitazone*

Avapro, *see irbesartan*

Avastin, *see bevacizumab*

Avelox, *see moxifloxacin*

Avodart, *see dutasteride*

Avonex, *see interferon beta 1a*

Axid, *see nizatidine*

---

azacitidine

ay-zah-**sigh**-tih-deen
(Vidaza)

CLASSIFICATION

PHARMACOTHERAPEUTIC: Antineo-plastic. **CLINICAL:** DNA demethyla-tion agent.

ACTION

An antineoplastic agent that exerts a cytotoxic effect on rapidly dividing cells by causing demethylation of DNA in abnormal hematopoietic cells in the bone marrow. **Therapeutic Effect:** Restores normal function to tumor-suppressor genes regulating cellular differentiation and proliferation.

PHARMACOKINETICS

Rapidly absorbed after subcutaneous administration. Metabolized by the liver. Eliminated in urine. **Half-life:** 4 hr.

USES

Treatment of myelodysplastic syndromes, specifically refractory anemia and myelo-monocytic leukemia.

PRECAUTIONS

CONTRAINDICATIONS: Advanced malig-nant hepatic tumors, hypersensitivity to mannitol. **CAUTIONS:** Hepatic disease, renal impairment.

⏳ **LIFESPAN CONSIDERATIONS: Preg-nancy/Lactation:** May be embryotoxic; may cause developmental abnormalities of the fetus. Mothers should avoid breast-feeding. **Pregnancy Category D. Children:** Safety and efficacy have not been established. **Elderly:** Age-related renal impairment may increase risk of renal toxicity.

INTERACTIONS

DRUG: Bone marrow suppressants: May increase myelosuppression.

HERBAL: None known. **FOOD:** None known. **LAB VALUES:** May decrease Hgb level, Hct, and WBC, RBC, and platelet counts. May increase serum creatinine and potassium levels.

AVAILABILITY (Rx)

POWDER FOR INJECTION: 100 mg.

ADMINISTRATION/HANDLING
SUBCUTANEOUS

Reconstitution • Reconstitute with 4 ml sterile water for injection. • Reconstituted solution will appear cloudy. • Solution must be used within 1 hr after reconstitution.

Rate of administration • Doses greater than 4 ml should be divided equally into 2 syringes. • Contents of syringe must be resuspended by inverting the syringe 2–3 times and rolling the syringe between the palms for 30 sec immediately before adminis-tration. • Rotate site for each injection (thigh, upper arm, abdomen). New injections should be administered at least 1 inch from the old site.

Storage • Store vials at room tem-perature. • Reconstituted solution may be stored for up to 1 hr at room tem-perature or up to 8 hr if refrigerated. • The solution may be allowed to return to room temperature and used within 30 min.

INDICATIONS/ROUTES/DOSAGE
REFRACTORY ANEMIA, CHRONIC MYELOMONOCYTIC LEUKEMIA
SUBCUTANEOUS: ADULTS, ELDERLY: 75 mg/m^2/day for 7 days every 4 wk. Dosage may be increased to 100 mg/m^2 if initial dose is insufficient and toxicity is manageable. Treatment recommended for at least 4 cycles.

SIDE EFFECTS

FREQUENT (71%–29%): Nausea, vomiting, fever, diarrhea, fatigue, injection site erythema, constipation, ecchymosis, cough, dyspnea, weakness. **OCCASIONAL (26%–16%):** Rigors, petechiae, injection site pain, pharyngitis, arthralgia, headache, limb pain, dizziness, peripheral edema, back pain, erythema, epistaxis, weight loss, myalgia. **RARE (13%–8%):** Anxiety, abdominal pain, rash, depression, tachycardia, insomnia, night sweats, stomatitis.

ADVERSE REACTIONS/ TOXIC EFFECTS

Hematologic toxicity, manifested as anemia, leukopenia, neutropenia, and thrombocytopenia, is a common adverse effect.

NURSING CONSIDERATIONS

BASELINE ASSESSMENT

Give emotional support to patient and family. Use strict asepsis and protect patient from infection. Obtain blood counts as needed to monitor response and toxicity but particularly before each dosing cycle.

INTERVENTION/EVALUATION

Monitor for hematologic toxicity (fever, sore throat, signs of local infections, unusual bruising or bleeding), symptoms of anemia (excessive fatigue, weakness). Assess response to medication; monitor and report nausea, vomiting, diarrhea. Avoid rectal temperatures, other traumas that may induce bleeding.

PATIENT/FAMILY TEACHING

• Do not have immunizations without physician's approval (drug lowers body's resistance). • Avoid crowds, persons with known infections. • Report signs of infection at once (fever, flu-like symptoms). • Contact physician if nausea or vomiting continues at home. • Advise men to use barrier contraception while receiving treatment.

---

azathioprine

ay-za-**thye**-oh-preen

(Azasan, Azathioprine Sodium, Imuran)

Do not confuse azathioprine with Azulfidine or azatadine, or Imuran with Elmiron or Imferon.

◆ CLASSIFICATION

PHARMACOTHERAPEUTIC: Immunologic agent. **CLINICAL:** Immunosuppressant.

ACTION

An immunologic agent that antagonizes purine metabolism and inhibits DNA, protein, and RNA synthesis. **Therapeutic Effect:** Suppresses cell-mediated hypersensitivities; alters antibody production and immune response in transplant recipients; reduces the severity of arthritis symptoms.

USES

Adjunct in prevention of rejection in kidney transplantation; treatment of rheumatoid arthritis in those unresponsive to conventional therapy. **OFF-LABEL:** Treatment of biliary cirrhosis, chronic active hepatitis, glomerulonephritis, inflammatory bowel disease, inflammatory myopathy, multiple sclerosis, myasthenia gravis, nephrotic syndrome, pemphigoid, pemphigus, polymyositis, systemic lupus erythematosus.

PRECAUTIONS

CONTRAINDICATIONS: Pregnant patients with rheumatoid arthritis. **CAUTIONS:** Immunosuppressed patients, those previously treated for rheumatoid arthritis with alkylating agents (cyclophosphamide, chlorambucil, melphalan), chickenpox (current or recent), herpes zoster, gout, hepatic/renal

---

impairment, infection. **Pregnancy Category D.**

INTERACTIONS

DRUG: Allopurinol: May increase activity and risk of toxicity of azathioprine. **Bone marrow depressants:** May increase myelosuppression. **Live-virus vaccines:** May potentiate virus replication, increase the vaccine's side effects, and decrease the patient's antibody response to the vaccine. **Other immunosuppressants:** May increase the risk of infection or neoplasms. **HERBAL:** None known. **FOOD:** None known. **LAB VALUES:** May decrease serum albumin, Hgb, and serum uric acid levels. May increase serum alkaline phosphatase, amylase, bilirubin, AST, and ALT levels.

AVAILABILITY (Rx)

TABLETS: 25 mg (Azasan), 50 mg (Azasan, Imuran), 75 mg (Azasan), 100 mg (Azasan). **INJECTION (IMURAN):** 100-mg vial.

ADMINISTRATION/HANDLING

 IV

Reconstitution • Reconstitute 100-mg vial with 10 ml sterile water for injection to provide concentration of 10 mg/ml. • Swirl vial gently to mix and dissolve solution. • May further dilute in 50 ml D₅W or 0.9% NaCl.

Rate of administration • Infuse over 30–60 min. Range: 5 min–8 hr.

Storage • Store parenteral form at room temperature. • After reconstitution, IV solution stable for 24 hr.

PO
• Give during or after food to reduce potential for GI disturbances. • Store oral form at room temperature.

▓ IV INCOMPATIBILITIES

Methyl and propyl parabens, phenol.

INDICATIONS/ROUTES/DOSAGE

ADJUNCT IN PREVENTION OF RENAL ALLOGRAFT REJECTION

PO, IV: ADULTS, ELDERLY, CHILDREN: 2–5 mg/kg/day on day of transplant, then 1–3 mg/kg/day as maintenance dose.

RHEUMATOID ARTHRITIS

PO: ADULTS: Initially, 1 mg/kg/day as a single dose or in 2 divided doses. May increase by 0.5 mg/kg/day after 6–8 wk at 4-wk intervals up to maximum of 2.5 mg/kg/day. Maintenance: Lowest effective dosage. May decrease dose by 0.5 mg/kg or 25 mg/day q4wk (while other therapies, such as rest, physiotherapy, and salicylates, are maintained). ELDERLY: Initially, 1 mg/kg/day (50–100 mg); may increase by 25 mg/day until response or toxicity.

DOSAGE IN RENAL IMPAIRMENT

Dosage is modified based on creatinine clearance.

Creatinine Clearance	Dose
10–50 ml/min	75% of usual dose
less than 10 ml/min	50% of usual dose

SIDE EFFECTS

FREQUENT: Nausea, vomiting, anorexia (particularly during early treatment and with large doses). **OCCASIONAL:** Rash. **RARE:** Severe nausea and vomiting with diarrhea, abdominal pain, hypersensitivity reaction.

ADVERSE REACTIONS/ TOXIC EFFECTS

Azathioprine use increases the risk of developing neoplasia (new abnormalgrowth tumors). Significant leukopenia and thrombocytopenia may occur, particularly in those undergoing kidney transplant rejection. Hepatotoxicity occurs rarely.

NURSING CONSIDERATIONS

BASELINE ASSESSMENT

Arthritis: Assess onset, type, location,

and duration of pain, fever, inflammation. Inspect appearance of affected joints for immobility, deformities, skin condition.

INTERVENTION/EVALUATION

CBC, platelet count, liver function studies should be performed weekly during first month of therapy, twice monthly during second and third months of treatment, then monthly thereafter. If rapid fall in WBC occurs, dosage should be reduced or discontinued. Assess particularly for delayed bone marrow suppression. Routinely watch for any change from normal. **Arthritis:** Evaluate for therapeutic response: relief of pain, stiffness, swelling, increase in joint mobility, reduced joint tenderness, improved grip strength.

PATIENT/FAMILY TEACHING

• Contact physician if unusual bleeding/bruising, sore throat, mouth sores, abdominal pain, fever occurs. • Therapeutic response in rheumatoid arthritis may take up to 12 wk. • Women of child-bearing age must avoid pregnancy.

---

azelastine

aye-zeh-**las**-teen

(Astelin, Optivar)

Do not confuse Optivar with Optiray.

• CLASSIFICATION

PHARMACOTHERAPEUTIC: Antihistamine. **CLINICAL:** Antiallergy.

ACTION

An antihistamine that competes with histamine for histamine receptor sites on cells in the blood vessels, GI tract, and respiratory tract. Therapeutic Effect: Relieves symptoms associated with seasonal allergic rhinitis such as increased mucus production and sneezing and symptoms associated with allergic conjunctivitis, such as redness, itching, and excessive tearing.

PHARMACOKINETICS

Route	Onset	Peak	Duration
Nasal spray	0.5–1 hr	2–3 hr	12 hr
Ophthalmic	N/A	3 min	8 hr

Well absorbed through nasal mucosa. Primarily excreted in feces. Half-life: 22 hr.

USES

Nasal: Treatment of symptoms of seasonal and perennial allergic rhinitis. **Ophthalmic:** Treatment of itching associated with allergic conjunctivitis.

PRECAUTIONS

CONTRAINDICATIONS: Breast-feeding women; history of hypersensitivity to antihistamines; neonates or premature infants; third trimester of pregnancy. **CAUTIONS:** Renal impairment.

⧗ LIFESPAN CONSIDERATIONS: Pregnancy/Lactation: Unknown if drug crosses placenta or is distributed in breast milk. Do not use during third trimester. **Pregnancy Category C. Children:** Safety and efficacy not established in those younger than 12 yr. **Elderly:** No age-related precautions noted.

INTERACTIONS

DRUG: **Alcohol, other CNS depressants:** May increase CNS depression. **Cimetidine:** May increase azelastine blood concentration. HERBAL: None known. FOOD: None known. LAB VALUES: May increase ALT levels. May suppress flare and wheal reactions

---

to antigen skin testing unless drug is discontinued 4 days before testing.

AVAILABILITY (Rx)

NASAL SPRAY (ASTELIN): 137 mcg/spray. **OPHTHALMIC SOLUTION (OPTIVAR):** 0.05%.

ADMINISTRATION/HANDLING

NASAL
• Instruct the patient to clear nasal passages as much as possible before use. • Tilt head slightly forward. • Insert spray tip into nostril, pointing toward nasal passage, away from nasal septum. • Spray into nostril while holding the other nostril closed. Have patient concurrently inhale through nose to permit medication as high into nasal passages as possible.

OPHTHALMIC
• Tilt patient's head back; place solution in conjunctival sac. • Have patient close eyes; press gently on lacrimal sac for 1 min.

INDICATIONS/ROUTES/DOSAGE

ALLERGIC RHINITIS
NASAL: ADULTS, ELDERLY, CHILDREN 12 YR AND OLDER: 2 sprays in each nostril twice a day. CHILDREN 5-11 YR: 1 spray in each nostril twice a day.

ALLERGIC CONJUNCTIVITIS
OPHTHALMIC: ADULTS, ELDERLY, CHILDREN 3 YR OR OLDER: 1 drop into affected eye twice a day.

SIDE EFFECTS

FREQUENT (20%-15%): Headache, bitter taste. **RARE:** Nasal burning, paroxysmal sneezing, somnolence. **Ophthalmic:** Transient eye burning or stinging, bitter taste, headache.

ADVERSE REACTIONS/ TOXIC EFFECTS

Epistaxis occurs rarely.

BASELINE ASSESSMENT
Question for hypersensitivity to antihistamines.

INTERVENTION/EVALUATION
Assess therapeutic response to medication.

azithromycin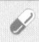

aye-zith-row-**my**-sin

(<u>Zithromax</u>, Zithromax TRI-PAK, <u>Zithromax Z-PAK</u>, Zmax)

Do not confuse azithromycin with erythromycin.

◆CLASSIFICATION

PHARMACOTHERAPEUTIC: Macrolide.
CLINICAL: Antibiotic (see p. 25C).

ACTION

A macrolide antibiotic that binds to ribosomal receptor sites of susceptible organisms, inhibiting RNA-dependent protein synthesis. **Therapeutic Effect:** Bacteriostatic or bactericidal, depending on the drug dosage.

PHARMACOKINETICS

Rapidly absorbed from the GI tract. Protein binding: 7%-50%. Widely distributed. Eliminated primarily unchanged by biliary excretion. **Half-life:** 68 hr.

USES

Treatment of susceptible infections due to *Chlamydia pneumoniae, C. trachomatis, H. influenza, Legionella, M. catarrhalis, Mycoplasma pneumoniae, N. gonorrhoeae, S. aureus. S. pneumoniae, S. pyogenes* including mild to moderate infections of upper respiratory tract (pharyngitis, tonsillitis), lower respiratory tract (acute bacterial exacerbations, chronic obstructive pulmonary disease [COPD], pneumonia), uncomplicated skin and skin-structure infections, sexually transmitted diseases (nongonococcal urethritis, cervicitis due to *Chlamydia trachomatis*), chancroid. Prevents disseminated *Mycobacterium avium* complex (MAC). Treatment of mycoplasma pneumonia. **Injection:** Community-acquired pneumonia, pelvic inflammatory disease (PID). **OFF-LABEL:** Chlamydial infections, gonococcal pharyngitis, uncomplicated gonococcal infections of the cervix, urethra, and rectum.

PRECAUTIONS

CONTRAINDICATIONS: Hypersensitivity to other macrolide antibiotics. **CAUTIONS:** Hepatic or renal dysfunction.

⧖ **LIFESPAN CONSIDERATIONS: Pregnancy/Lactation:** Unknown if distributed in breast milk. **Pregnancy Category B. Children:** Safety and efficacy not established in those younger than 16 yr for IV use and younger than 6 mo for oral use. **Elderly:** No age-related precautions in those with normal renal function.

INTERACTIONS

DRUG: Aluminum- or magnesium-containing antacids: May decrease azithromycin blood concentration. **Carbamazepine, cyclosporine, theophylline, warfarin:** May increase the serum concentrations of these drugs. **HERBAL:** None known. **FOOD:** None known. **LAB VALUES:** May increase serum creatine kinase (CK), AST, and ALT levels.

AVAILABILITY (Rx)

ORAL SUSPENSION (ZITHROMAX): 100 mg/5 ml, 200 mg/5 ml. **ORAL SUSPENSION (EXTENDED-RELEASE [ZMAX]):** 1 g single-dose packet, 2 g single-dose packet. **TABLETS:** 250 mg, 500 mg, 600 mg (Zithromax). Tri-Pak: 3 × 500 mg (Zithromax TRI-PAK). Z-Pak: 6 × 250 mg (Zithromax Z-PAK). **POWDER FOR INJECTION (ZITHROMAX):** 500 mg. **POWDER FOR RECONSTITUTION (ZITHROMAX):** 1 g.

ADMINISTRATION/HANDLING

 IV

Reconstitution ● Reconstitute each 500-mg vial with 4.8 ml sterile water for injection to provide concentration of 100 mg/ml. ● Shake well to ensure dissolution. ● Further dilute with 250 or 500 ml 0.9% NaCl or D_5W to provide final concentration of 2 mg with 250 ml diluent or 1 mg/ml with 500 ml diluent.

Rate of administration ● Infuse over 60 min.

Storage ● Store vials at room temperature. ● Following reconstitution, suspension is stable for 24 hr at room temperature or 7 days if refrigerated.
PO
● Give tablets without regard to food. ● May store suspension at room temperature. Stable for 10 days after reconstitution. ● Do not administer oral suspension with food. Give at least 1 hr before or 2 hr after meals. Zmax should be taken within 12 hr of reconstitution.

▨ IV INCOMPATIBILITIES

Ceftriaxone (Rocephin), ciprofloxacin (Cipro), famotidine (Pepcid), furosemide (Lasix), ketorolac (Toradol), levofloxacin (Levaquin), morphine, piperacillin/tazobactam (Zosyn), potassium chloride.

IV COMPATIBILITY

Diphenhydramine (Benadryl).

INDICATIONS/ROUTES/DOSAGE

ACUTE EXACERBATIONS OF COPD
PO: ADULTS, ELDERLY, CHILDREN 16 YR AND OLDER: 500 mg/day for 3 days or 500 mg on day 1, then 250 mg/day on days 2–5.

ACUTE BACTERIAL SINUSITIS
PO (ZMAX): ADULTS, ELDERLY: 2 g as a single dose.
PO: ADULTS, ELDERLY: 500 mg/day for 3 days. CHILDREN 6 MO AND OLDER: 10 mg/kg for 3 days. **Maximum:** 500 mg/day.

CERVICITIS
PO: ADULTS, ELDERLY: 1–2 g as single dose.

CHANCROID
PO: ADULTS, ELDERLY: 1 g as single dose.

MAC PREVENTION
PO: ADULTS, ELDERLY: 1,200 mg once weekly. CHILDREN: 20 mg/kg once weekly. **Maximum:** 1,200 mg/dose.

MAC TREATMENT
PO: ADULTS, ELDERLY: 600 mg/day with ethambutol 15 mg/kg/day. CHILDREN: 5–20 mg/kg/day for 1 mo or longer.

OTITIS MEDIA
PO: CHILDREN 6 MO AND OLDER: 30 mg/kg as single dose or 10 mg/kg/day for 3 days or 10 mg/kg on day 1 then 5 mg/kg on days 2–5.

PHARYNGITIS, TONSILLITIS
PO: ADULTS, ELDERLY, CHILDREN 16 YR AND OLDER: 500 mg on day 1, then 250 mg on days 2–5. CHILDREN 2–15 YR: 12 mg/kg daily for 5 days.

PNEUMONIA, COMMUNITY ACQUIRED
PO (ZMAX): ADULTS, ELDERLY: 2 g as a single dose.
PO: ADULTS, ELDERLY, CHILDREN 16 YR AND OLDER: 500 mg on day 1, then 250 mg on days 2–5 or 500 mg/day IV for 2 days, then 500 mg/day PO to complete course of therapy. CHILDREN 6 MO–15 YR: 10 mg/kg on day 1, then 5 mg/kg on days 2–5.

SKIN AND SKIN-STRUCTURE INFECTIONS
PO: ADULTS, ELDERLY, CHILDREN 16 YR AND OLDER: 500 mg on day 1, then 250 mg on days 2–5.

PELVIC INFLAMMATORY DISEASE (PID)
IV: ADULTS, ELDERLY: 500 mg/day for at least 2 days, then 250 mg/day to complete a 7-day course of therapy.

SIDE EFFECTS
OCCASIONAL: Nausea, vomiting, diarrhea, abdominal pain. **RARE:** Headache, dizziness, allergic reaction.

ADVERSE REACTIONS/ TOXIC EFFECTS
Antibiotic-associated colitis and other superinfections may result from altered bacterial balance. Acute interstitial nephritis and hepatotoxicity occur rarely.

NURSING CONSIDERATIONS

BASELINE ASSESSMENT
Question for history of hepatitis, allergies to azithromycin, erythromycins.

INTERVENTION/EVALUATION
Check for GI discomfort, nausea, vomiting. Determine pattern of bowel activity and stool consistency. Monitor liver function tests, assess for hepatotoxicity: malaise, fever, abdominal pain, GI disturbances. Evaluate for superinfection: genital or anal pruritus, sore mouth or tongue, moderate to severe diarrhea.

PATIENT/FAMILY TEACHING
• Continue therapy for full length of treatment. • Doses should be evenly spaced. • Take oral medication with 8 oz water at least 1 hr before or 2 hr after food or beverage.

Azmacort, *see*
triamcinolone

---

aztreonam

az-**tree**-oo-nam
(Azactam)

◆**CLASSIFICATION**

PHARMACOTHERAPEUTIC: Monobactam. **CLINICAL:** Antibiotic.

ACTION

A monobactam antibiotic that inhibits
bacterial cell wall synthesis. Therapeutic Effect: Bactericidal.

PHARMACOKINETICS

Completely absorbed after IM administration. Protein binding: 56%–60%.
Partially metabolized by hydrolysis.
Primarily excreted unchanged in urine.
Removed by hemodialysis. Half-life:
1.4–2.2 hr (increased in impaired
renal or hepatic function).

USES

Treatment of infections caused by susceptible gram-negative micro-organisms
*P. aeruginose, E. coli, S. marcescens,
K. pneumoniae, P. mirabilis, H. influenzae,* Enterobacter, Citrobacter species
including lower respiratory tract, skin/
skin structure, intra-abdominal, gynecologic, complicated/uncomplicated urinary tract infections; septicemia, cystic
fibrosis. OFF-LABEL: Treatment of
bone and joint infections.

PRECAUTIONS

CONTRAINDICATIONS: None known.
CAUTIONS: History of allergy, especially
antibiotics, hepatic/renal impairment.

⧗ LIFESPAN CONSIDERATIONS: Preg-
nancy/Lactation: Crosses placenta,
distributed in amniotic fluid; low concentration in breast milk. **Pregnancy
Category B.** **Children:** Safety and
efficacy not established in children
younger than 9 mo. **Elderly:** Age-related
renal impairment may require dosage
adjustment.

INTERACTIONS

DRUG: None known. HERBAL: None
known. FOOD: None known. LAB
VALUES: May increase serum alkaline
phosphatase, creatinine, LDH, AST, and
ALT levels. Produces a positive Coombs'
test.

AVAILABILITY (Rx)

**INJECTION POWDER FOR RECONSTITU-
TION:** 500 mg, 1 g, 2 g.

ADMINISTRATION/HANDLING

▢ IV

Reconstitution • For IV push, dilute
each gram with 6–10 ml sterile water for
injection. • For intermittent IV infusion,
further dilute with 50–100 ml D₅W or
0.9% NaCl.

Rate of administration • For IV
push, give over 3–5 min. • For IV
infusion, administer over 20–60 min.

Storage • Store vials at room temperature. • Solution appears colorless to
light yellow. • Following reconstitution,
solution is stable for 48 hr at room
temperature or 7 days if refrigerated.
• Discard if precipitate forms. Discard
unused portions.

IM
• Shake immediately, vigorously after
adding diluent. • Inject deeply into
large muscle mass. • Following reconstitution for IM injection, solution is
stable for 48 hr at room temperature
or 7 days if refrigerated.

▦ IV INCOMPATIBILITIES

Acyclovir (Zovirax), amphotericin (Fungizone), daunorubicin (Cerubidine),

---

ganciclovir (Cytovene), lorazepam (Ativan), metronidazole (Flagyl), vancomycin (Vancocin).

IV COMPATIBILITIES

Aminophylline, bumetanide (Bumex), calcium gluconate, cimetidine (Tagamet), diltiazem (Cardizem), dobutamine (Dobutrex), dopamine (Intropin), famotidine (Pepcid), furosemide (Lasix), heparin, hydromorphone (Dilaudid), insulin (regular), magnesium sulfate, morphine, potassium chloride, propofol (Diprivan), total parenteral nutrition (TPN).

INDICATIONS/ROUTES/DOSAGE

UTIs
IV, IM: ADULTS, ELDERLY: 500 mg–1 g q8–12h.
MODERATE TO SEVERE SYSTEMIC INFECTIONS
IV, IM: ADULTS, ELDERLY: 1–2 g q8–12h.
SEVERE OR LIFE-THREATENING INFECTIONS
IV: ADULTS, ELDERLY: 2 g q6–8h.
CYSTIC FIBROSIS
IV: CHILDREN: 50 mg/kg/dose q6–8h up to 200 mg/kg/day. **Maximum:** 8g/d.
MILD TO SEVERE INFECTIONS IN CHILDREN
IV: CHILDREN: 30 mg/kg q6–8h. **Maximum:** 120 mg/kg/day. NEONATES: 60–120 mg/kg/day q6–12h.
DOSAGE IN RENAL IMPAIRMENT
Dosage and frequency are modified based on creatinine clearance and the severity of the infection:

Creatinine Clearance	Dosage
10–30 ml/min	1–2 g initially, then ½ usual dose at usual intervals
Less than 10 ml/min	1–2 g initially, then ¼ usual dose at usual intervals

SIDE EFFECTS

OCCASIONAL (less than 3%): Discomfort and swelling at IM injection site, nausea, vomiting, diarrhea, rash. **RARE (less than 1%):** Phlebitis or thrombophlebitis at IV injection site, abdominal cramps, headache, hypotension.

ADVERSE REACTIONS/TOXIC EFFECTS

Antibiotic-associated colitis and other superinfections may result from altered bacterial balance. Severe hypersensitivity reactions, including anaphylaxis, occur rarely.

NURSING CONSIDERATIONS

BASELINE ASSESSMENT
Question for history of allergies, especially to aztreonam, other antibiotics.

INTERVENTION/EVALUATION
Evaluate for phlebitis (heat, pain, red streaking over vein), pain at IM injection site. Assess for GI discomfort, nausea, vomiting. Monitor stool frequency and consistency. Assess skin for rash. Be alert for superinfection: increased temperature, sore throat, vomiting, diarrhea, black/hairy tongue, ulceration or changes of oral mucosa, anal/genital pruritus.

PATIENT/FAMILY TEACHING
• Report nausea, vomiting, diarrhea, rash.

bacitracin

bah-cih-**tray**-sin

(AK-Tracin, Baci-IM, Baci-Rx, Bacitracin, Ocu-Tracin, Ziba-Rx)

Do not confuse bacitracin with Bactrim or Bactroban.

FIXED-COMBINATION(S)

With polymyxin B, an antibiotic **(Polysporin)**; with polymyxin B and neomycin, antibiotics **(Mycitracin, Neosporin)**.

CLASSIFICATION

PHARMACOTHERAPEUTIC: Anti-infective. **CLINICAL:** Antibiotic.

ACTION

An antibiotic that interferes with plasma membrane permeability and inhibits bacterial cell wall synthesis in susceptible bacteria. **Therapeutic Effect:** Bacteriostatic.

USES

Ophthalmic: Superficial ocular infections (conjunctivitis, keratitis, corneal ulcers, blepharitis). **Topical:** Minor skin abrasions, superficial infections. **Irrigation:** Treatment, prophylaxis of surgical procedures.

PRECAUTIONS

CONTRAINDICATIONS: None known. **CAUTIONS:** None known. **Pregnancy Category C.**

INTERACTIONS

DRUG: Nephrotoxic medications: May increase the risk of nephrotoxicity with IM bacitracin therapy. **HERBAL:** None known. **FOOD:** None known. **LAB VALUES:** IM injection form may produce albuninuria, cylindruria.

AVAILABILITY (Rx)

POWDER FOR IRRIGATION: 50,000 units. **POWDER FOR INJECTION (BACI-IM):** 50,000 units. **OPHTHALMIC OINTMENT (AK-TRACIN):** 500 units/g. **TOPICAL OINTMENT (OCU-TRACIN [OTC]):** 500 units/g.

ADMINISTRATION/HANDLING

OPHTHALMIC

• Place finger on lower eyelid. Pull out until a pocket is formed between eye and lower lid. • Place ¼–½ inch ointment in pocket. • Close the patient's eye for 1–2 min. • Instruct patient to roll the eyeball to increase the contact area of the drug to the eye. • Remove excess ointment around eye with tissue.

TOPICAL

• Do not use the topical preparation on deep or puncture wounds. • Wash affected area with soap and water and dry before application.

INDICATIONS/ROUTES/DOSAGE

SUPERFICIAL OCULAR INFECTIONS

OPHTHALMIC: ADULTS: ½-inch ribbon in conjunctival sac q3–4h.

SKIN ABRASIONS, SUPERFICIAL SKIN INFECTIONS

TOPICAL: ADULTS, CHILDREN: Apply to affected area 1–5 times a day.

SURGICAL TREATMENT AND PROPHYLAXIS

IRRIGATION: ADULTS, ELDERLY: 50,000–150,000 units, as needed.

PNEUMONIA AND EMPYEMA CAUSED BY STAPHYLOCOCCI

IM: INFANTS WEIGHING 2,500 G AND LESS: 900 units/kg/24 hours in 2 or 3 divided doses. **INFANTS WEIGHING MORE THAN 2,500 G:** 1,000 units/kg/24 hours in 2 or 3 divided doses.

SIDE EFFECTS

RARE: Ophthalmic: Burning, itching, redness, swelling, pain. **Topical:** Hypersensitivity reaction (allergic contact

---

dermatitis, burning, inflammation, pruritus). **IM injection:** Nausea, vomiting, pain at injection site, rash, azotemia, rising blood levels without any increase in dosage.

ADVERSE REACTIONS/ TOXIC EFFECTS

◀ **ALERT** ▶ Bacitracin used intramuscularly may cause renal failure due to tubular and glomerular necrosis. Its use should be restricted to infants with staphylococci pneumonia and empyema. Severe hypersensitivity reactions, including apnea and hypotension, occur rarely.

NURSING CONSIDERATIONS

INTERVENTION/EVALUATION

Topical: Evaluate for hypersensitivity reaction: itching, burning, inflammation. With preparations containing corticosteroids, consider masking effect on clinical signs. **Ophthalmic:** Assess eye for therapeutic response or increased redness, swelling, burning, itching (hypersensitivity reaction).

PATIENT/FAMILY TEACHING

• Continue therapy for full length of treatment. • Doses should be evenly spaced. • Report burning, itching, rash, increased irritation.

baclofen

bak-loe-fen

(Apo-Baclofen ✤, Lioresal, Liotec ✤, Novo-Baclofen ✤, Nu-Baclofen ✤)

Do not confuse baclofen with Bactroban or Beclovent.

◆ CLASSIFICATION

PHARMACOTHERAPEUTIC: Skeletal muscle relaxant. **CLINICAL:** Antispastic, analgesic in trigeminal neuralgia (see p. 137C).

ACTION

A direct-acting skeletal muscle relaxant that inhibits transmission of reflexes at the spinal cord level. **Therapeutic Effect:** Relieves muscle spasticity.

PHARMACOKINETICS

Well absorbed from the GI tract. Protein binding: 30%. Partially metabolized in the liver. Primarily excreted in urine. **Half-life:** 2.5–4 hr; intrathecal: 1.5 hr.

USES

Treatment of cerebral spasticity, reversible spasticity associated with multiple sclerosis, spinal cord lesions. **Intrathecal:** For those unresponsive to oral therapy or exhibiting intolerable side effects. **OFF-LABEL:** Treatment of bladder spasms, cerebral palsy, intractable hiccups or pain, Huntington's chorea, trigeminal neuralgia.

PRECAUTIONS

CONTRAINDICATIONS: Skeletal muscle spasm due to cerebral palsy, Parkinson's disease, rheumatic disorders, CVA, cough, intractable hiccups, neuropathic pain. **CAUTIONS:** Renal impairment, cerebrovascular accident (CVA), diabetes mellitus, epilepsy, preexisting psychiatric disorders.

⧖ **LIFESPAN CONSIDERATIONS: Pregnancy/Lactation:** Unknown if drug crosses placenta or is distributed in breast milk. **Pregnancy Category C. Children:** Safety and efficacy not established in those younger than 12 yr. **Elderly:** Increased risk of CNS toxicity (hallucinations, sedation, confusion, mental depression); age-related renal impairment may require decreased dosage.

INTERACTIONS

DRUG: Alcohol, other CNS depressants: May increase CNS depression. **HERBAL:** None known. **FOOD:** None known. **LAB VALUES:** May increase blood glucose level and serum alkaline phosphatase, AST, and ALT levels.

AVAILABILITY (Rx)

TABLETS: 10 mg, 20 mg. **INTRATHECAL INJECTION:** 50 mcg/ml, 500 mcg/ml, 2,000 mcg/ml.

ADMINISTRATION/HANDLING

PO
- Give without regard to food. • Tablets may be crushed.

INTRATHECAL
- IV, IM, subcutaneous, or epidural administration is not recommended.
- For screening, a 50 mcg/ml concentration should be used for injection.
- For maintenance therapy, solution should be diluted for patients who require concentrations other than 500 mcg/ml or 2,000 mcg/ml. • Baclofen should be diluted with sterile preservative-free sodium chloride for injection.

INDICATIONS/ROUTES/DOSAGE

SPASTICITY
PO: ADULTS: Initially, 5 mg 3 times a day. May increase by 15 mg/day at 3-day intervals. Range: 40–80 mg/day. **Maximum:** 80 mg/day. ELDERLY: Initially, 5 mg 2–3 times a day. May gradually increase dosage. CHILDREN: Initially, 10–15 mg/day in divided doses q8h. May increase by 5–15 mg/day at 3-day intervals. **Maximum:** 40 mg/day (children 2–7 yr); 60 mg/day (children 8 yr and older).

USUAL INTRATHECAL DOSAGE
ADULTS, ELDERLY, CHILDREN OLDER THAN 12 YR: 300–800 mcg/day. CHILDREN 12 YR AND YOUNGER: 100–300 mcg/day.

SIDE EFFECTS

FREQUENT (greater than 10%): Transient somnolence, asthenia, dizziness, lightheadedness, nausea, vomiting. **OCCASIONAL (10%–2%):** Headache, paresthesia, constipation, anorexia, hypotension, confusion, nasal congestion. **RARE (less than 1%):** Paradoxical CNS excitement or restlessness, slurred speech, tremor, dry mouth, diarrhea, nocturia, impotence.

ADVERSE REACTIONS/ TOXIC EFFECTS

Abrupt discontinuation of baclofen may produce hallucinations and seizures. Overdose results in blurred vision, seizures, myosis, mydriasis, severe muscle weakness, strabismus, respiratory depression, and vomiting.

NURSING CONSIDERATIONS

BASELINE ASSESSMENT
Record onset, type, location, duration of muscular spasm. Check for immobility, stiffness, swelling.

INTERVENTION/EVALUATION
Assess for paradoxical reaction. Assist with ambulation at all times. For those on long-term therapy, liver/renal function tests, blood counts should be performed periodically. Evaluate for therapeutic response: decreased intensity of skeletal muscle pain.

PATIENT/FAMILY TEACHING
- Drowsiness usually diminishes with continued therapy. • Avoid tasks that require alertness, motor skills until response to drug is established. • Do not abruptly withdraw medication after long-term therapy. • Avoid alcohol, CNS depressants.

Bactrim, see
co-trimoxazole

Bactroban, see *mupirocin*

Baraclude, *see entecavir*

basiliximab

bay-zul-**ix**-ah-mab
(Simulect)
Do not confuse basiliximab with daclizumab.

CLASSIFICATION
PHARMACOTHERAPEUTIC: Monoclonal antibody. **CLINICAL:** Immunosuppressive (see p. 106C).

ACTION
A monoclonal antibody that binds to and blocks the receptor of interleukin-2, a protein that stimulates the proliferation of T lymphocytes, which play a major role in organ transplant rejection. **Therapeutic Effect:** Prevents lymphocytic activity and impairs response of the immune system to antigens, which prevents acute renal transplant rejection.

PHARMACOKINETICS
Half-life: Adults, 4–10 days; children, 5–17 days.

USES
Adjunct with cyclosporine, corticosteroids in the prevention of acute organ rejection in patients receiving renal transplant.

PRECAUTIONS
CONTRAINDICATIONS: None known. **CAUTIONS:** Infection, history of malignancy.

⏳ **LIFESPAN CONSIDERATIONS:** Pregnancy/Lactation: Unknown if drug crosses placenta or is distributed in breast milk. **Pregnancy Category B.**

Children/Elderly: No age-related precautions noted.

INTERACTIONS
DRUG: None known. **HERBAL:** None known. **FOOD:** None known. **LAB VALUES:** May increase BUN and serum cholesterol, creatinine, and uric acid levels. May decrease platelet count and serum magnesium and phosphate levels. May increase or decrease blood glucose, Hct, Hbg level, and serum calcium and potassium levels.

AVAILABILITY (Rx)
POWDER FOR INJECTION: 20 mg.

ADMINISTRATION/HANDLING
 IV

Reconstitution • Reconstitute with 5 ml sterile water for injection. • Shake gently to dissolve. • Further dilute with 50 ml 0.9% NaCl or D₅W. • Gently invert to avoid foaming.

Rate of administration • Infuse over 20–30 min.

Storage • Refrigerate. • After reconstitution, use within 4 hr (24 hr if refrigerated). • Discard if precipitate forms.

IV INCOMPATIBILITIES
Specific information is not available. Don't infuse other drugs through the same IV line.

INDICATIONS/ROUTES/DOSAGE
PREVENTION OF ACUTE ORGAN REJECTION IN PATIENTS RECEIVING A KIDNEY TRANSPLANT
IV: ADULTS, ELDERLY, CHILDREN WEIGHING 35 KG OR MORE: 20 mg within 2 hr before transplant surgery and 20 mg 4 days after transplant. CHILDREN WEIGHING LESS THAN 35 KG: 10 mg within 2 hr before transplant surgery and 10 mg 4 days after transplant.

SIDE EFFECTS

FREQUENT (greater than 10%): GI disturbances (constipation, diarrhea, dyspepsia), CNS effects (dizziness, headache, insomnia, tremor), respiratory tract infection, dysuria, acne, leg or back pain, peripheral edema, hypertension. **OCCASIONAL (10%–3%):** Angina, neuropathy, abdominal distention, tachycardia, rash, hypotension, urinary disturbances (urinary frequency, genital edema, hematuria), arthralgia, hirsutism, myalgia.

ADVERSE REACTIONS/ TOXIC EFFECTS

Severe acute hypersensitivity reactions including anaphylaxis characterized by hypotension, tachycardia, cardiac failure, dyspnea, wheezing, bronchospasm, pulmonary edema, respiratory failure, urticaria, rash, pruritus, and/or sneezing, as well as capillary leak syndrome and cytokine release syndrome, have been reported.

NURSING CONSIDERATIONS

BASELINE ASSESSMENT

Obtain baseline BUN, creatinine, serum potassium, uric acid, glucose, calcium, phosphatase levels and vital signs, particularly BP, pulse rate. Breast-feeding not recommended.

INTERVENTION/EVALUATION

Diligently monitor CBC, all serum levels. Assess BP for hypertension/hypotension; pulse for evidence of tachycardia. Question for GI disturbances, CNS effects, urinary changes. Monitor for presence of wound infection, signs of infection (fever, sore throat, unusual bleeding or bruising).

PATIENT/FAMILY TEACHING

• Report difficulty in breathing or swallowing, tachycardia, rash, itching, swelling of lower extremities, weakness.
• Avoid pregnancy.

BCG, intravesical

(Immu Cyst ✢, Pacis, TheraCys, Tice BCG)

See Cancer Chemotherapeutic Agents (p. 71C)

becaplermin

beh-**cap**-lear-min
(Regranex)

Do not confuse Regranex with Repronex.

CLASSIFICATION

PHARMACOTHERAPEUTIC: Biologic response modifier. **CLINICAL:** Growth factor.

ACTION

Platelet-derived growth factor. **Therapeutic Effect:** Stimulates body to grow new tissue to heal open wounds.

USES

Treatment of lower extremity diabetic neuropathic ulcers extending into or beyond subcutaneous tissue.

PRECAUTIONS

CONTRAINDICATIONS: Skin neoplasms at site of application. **CAUTIONS:** Wounds showing exposed joints, tendons, ligaments, bones. **Pregnancy Category C.**

INTERACTIONS

DRUG: None known. **HERBAL:** None known. **FOOD:** None known. **LAB VALUES:** None known.

AVAILABILITY (Rx)

GEL: 0.01%.

ADMINISTRATION/HANDLING

• Refrigerate gel. • Measure gel on a clean, nonabsorbable surface. • Transfer to ulcer and spread as a thin, continuous layer onto the ulcer. • With a gauze pad moistened with 0.9% NaCl, cover ulcer for 12 hr; remove and wash any residual gel from ulcer and replace with new gauze pad moistened with 0.9% NaCl until time of next application.

INDICATIONS/ROUTES/DOSAGE

ULCERS

TOPICAL: ADULTS, ELDERLY: Apply once a day (spread evenly; cover with saline-moistened gauze dressing). After 12 hr, rinse ulcer, recover with saline gauze.

SIDE EFFECTS

OCCASIONAL (2%): Local rash near ulcer.

ADVERSE REACTIONS/ TOXIC EFFECTS

None known.

NURSING CONSIDERATIONS

INTERVENTION/EVALUATION

Do not allow tip of tube to come in contact with ulcer.

PATIENT/FAMILY TEACHING

• Dosage requires recalculation weekly or biweekly, depending on rate of change in width and length of ulcer.

beclomethasone dipropionate

be-kloe-**meth**-a-sone
(Beclodisk ✦, Becloforte inhaler ✦, Beconase AQ, Qvar)

Do not confuse Becloforte or Beconase with baclofen.

CLASSIFICATION

PHARMACOTHERAPEUTIC: Adrenocorticosteroid. **CLINICAL:** Anti-inflammatory, immunosuppressant (see pp. 67C, 83C).

ACTION

An adrenocorticosteroid that prevents or controls inflammation by controlling the rate of protein synthesis; decreasing migration of polymorphonuclear leukocytes and fibroblasts; and reversing capillary permeability. **Therapeutic Effect: Inhalation:** Inhibits bronchoconstriction, produces smooth muscle relaxation, decreases mucus secretion. **Intranasal:** Decreases response to seasonal and perennial rhinitis.

PHARMACOKINETICS

Rapidly absorbed from pulmonary, nasal, and GI tissue. Undergoes extensive first-pass metabolism in the liver. Protein binding: 87%. Primarily eliminated in feces. **Half-life:** 15 hr.

USES

Inhalation: Long-term control of bronchial asthma. Reduce need for oral corticosteroid therapy for asthma. **Intranasal:** Relief of seasonal/perennial rhinitis; prevention of nasal polyps from recurring after surgical removal; treatment of nonallergic rhinitis. **OFF-LABEL:** Prevention of seasonal rhinitis (nasal form).

PRECAUTIONS

CONTRAINDICATIONS: Hypersensitivity to beclomethasone, acute exacerbation of asthma, status asthmaticus. **CAUTIONS:** Cirrhosis, glaucoma, hypothyroidism, untreated systemic infections, osteoporosis, tuberculosis.

⌛ **LIFESPAN CONSIDERATIONS: Pregnancy/Lactation:** Unknown if drug crosses placenta or is distributed in breast milk. **Pregnancy Category C. Children:** Prolonged treatment/high dosages may decrease short-term growth rate, cortisol secretion. **Elderly:** No age-related precautions noted.

INTERACTIONS

DRUG: None known. **HERBAL:** None known. **FOOD:** None known. **LAB VALUES:** None known.

AVAILABILITY (Rx)

ORAL INHALATION (QVAR): 40 mcg per inhalation, 80 mcg/inhalation. **NASAL SPRAY (BECONASE AQ):** 42 mcg/inhalation.

ADMINISTRATION/HANDLING

INHALATION

• Shake container well, exhale completely, place mouthpiece between lips, inhale, hold breath as long as possible before exhaling. • Allow at least 1 min between inhalations. • Rinse mouth after each use to decrease dry mouth, hoarseness.

INTRANASAL

• Clear nasal passages as much as possible. • Insert spray tip into nostril, pointing toward nasal passages, away from nasal septum. • Spray into nostril while holding other nostril closed, concurrently inspire through nose to permit medication as high into nasal passages as possible.

INDICATIONS/ROUTES/DOSAGE

LONG-TERM CONTROL OF BRONCHIAL ASTHMA, REDUCES NEED FOR ORAL CORTICOSTEROID THERAPY FOR ASTHMA
ORAL INHALATION: ADULTS, ELDERLY CHILDREN 12 YR AND OLDER: 40–160 mcg twice a day. **Maximum:** 320 mcg twice a day. CHILDREN 5–11 YR: 40 mcg twice a day. **Maximum:** 80 mcg twice a day.

RHINITIS, PREVENTION OF RECURRENCE OF NASAL POLYPS
NASAL INHALATION: ADULTS, ELDERLY, CHILDREN 12 YR AND OLDER: 1 spray in each

nostril 2–4 times a day or 2 sprays twice a day. Maintenance: 1 spray 3 times a day. CHILDREN 6–12 YR: 1 spray 3 times a day.

SIDE EFFECTS

FREQUENT: Inhalation (14%–4%): Throat irritation, dry mouth, hoarseness, cough. **Intranasal:** Nasal burning, mucosal dryness. **OCCASIONAL: Inhalation (3%–2%):** Localized fungal infection (thrush). **Intranasal:** Nasal-crusting epistaxis, sore throat, ulceration of nasal mucosa. **RARE: Inhalation:** Transient bronchospasm, esophageal candidiasis. **Intranasal:** Nasal and pharyngeal candidiasis, eye pain.

ADVERSE REACTIONS/ TOXIC EFFECTS

An acute hypersensitivity reaction, as evidenced by urticaria, angioedema, and severe bronchospasm, occurs rarely. A transfer from systemic to local steroid therapy may unmask previously suppressed bronchial asthma condition.

NURSING CONSIDERATIONS

BASELINE ASSESSMENT

Question for hypersensitivity to any corticosteroids.

INTERVENTION/EVALUATION

In those receiving bronchodilators by inhalation concomitantly with inhalation of steroid therapy, advise to use bronchodilator several minutes before corticosteroid aerosol (enhances penetration of steroid into bronchial tree).

PATIENT/FAMILY TEACHING

• Do not change dose schedule or stop taking drug; must taper off gradually under medical supervision. • **Inhalation:** Maintain careful oral hygiene. • Rinse mouth with water immediately after inhalation (prevents mouth/throat dryness, fungal infection of mouth). • Contact physician/nurse if sore throat or mouth occurs.

- **Intranasal:** Contact physician if no improvement in symptoms or sneezing, nasal irritation occurs. • Clear nasal passages prior to use. • Improvement noted after several days.

Benadryl, see
diphenhydramine

benazepril

ben-**ayz**-ah-prill
(Lotensin)
Do not confuse benazepril with Benadryl, or Lotensin with Loniten or lovastatin.

FIXED-COMBINATION(S)

Lotensin HCT: benazepril/hydrochlorothiazide (a diuretic): 5 mg/625 mg; 10 mg/12.5 mg; 20 mg/12.5 mg; 20 mg/25 mg. **Lotrel:** benazepril/amlodipine (a calcium blocker): 2.5 mg/10 mg; 5 mg/10 mg; 5 mg/20 mg; 10 mg/20 mg.

CLASSIFICATION

PHARMACOTHERAPEUTIC: Angiotensin-converting enzyme (ACE) inhibitor. **CLINICAL:** Antihypertensive (see p. 7C).

ACTION

ACE inhibitor that decreases the rate of conversion of angiotensin I to angiotensin II, a potent vasoconstrictor. Reduces peripheral arterial resistance. **Therapeutic Effect:** Lowers BP.

PHARMACOKINETICS

Route	Onset	Peak	Duration
PO	1 hr	2–4 hr	24 hr

Partially absorbed from the GI tract. Protein binding: 97%. Metabolized in the liver to active metabolite. Primarily excreted in urine. Minimal removal by hemodialysis. **Half-life:** 35 min; metabolite 10–11 hr.

USES

Treatment of hypertension. Used alone or in combination with other antihypertensives. **OFF-LABEL:** Treatment of CHF.

PRECAUTIONS

CONTRAINDICATIONS: History of angioedema from previous treatment with ACE inhibitors, pregnancy. **CAUTIONS:** Renal impairment, sodium depletion, diuretic therapy, dialysis, hypovolemia, coronary or cerebrovascular insufficiency, hepatic impairment, diabetes mellitus.

⏳ LIFESPAN CONSIDERATIONS: **Pregnancy/Lactation:** Crosses placenta. Unknown if distributed in breast milk. May cause fetal, neonatal mortality or morbidity. **Pregnancy Category C (D if used in second or third trimester). Children:** Safety and efficacy not established. **Elderly:** May be more sensitive to hypotensive effects.

INTERACTIONS

DRUG: Alcohol, antihypertensives, diuretics: May increase the effects of benazepril. **Lithium:** May increase the lithium blood concentration and risk of lithium toxicity. **NSAIDs:** May decrease the effects of benazepril. **Potassium-sparing diuretics, potassium supplements:** May cause hyperkalemia. **HERBAL:** None known. **FOOD:** None known. **LAB VALUES:** May increase BUN, serum alkaline phosphatase, serum bilirubin, serum potassium, AST, and ALT levels. May decrease serum sodium levels. May cause positive ANA titer.

AVAILABILITY (Rx)

TABLETS: 5 mg, 10 mg, 20 mg, 40 mg.

ADMINISTRATION/HANDLING

• Give without regard to food.

INDICATIONS/ROUTES/DOSAGE

HYPERTENSION (MONOTHERAPY)

PO: ADULTS: Initially, 10 mg/day. Maintenance: 20–40 mg/day as single or in 2 divided doses. **Maximum:** 80 mg/day. ELDERLY: Initially, 5–10 mg/day. Range: 20–40 mg/day.

HYPERTENSION (COMBINATION THERAPY)

PO: ADULTS: Discontinue diuretic 2–3 days prior to initiating benazepril, then dose as noted above. If unable to discontinue diuretic, begin benazepril at 5 mg/day.

USUAL PEDIATRIC DOSAGE

PO: CHILDREN 6 YR AND OLDER: Initially, 0.2 mg/kg/day. Range: 0.1–0.6 mg/kg/day. **Maximum:** 40 mg/day.

DOSAGE IN RENAL IMPAIRMENT

For adult patients with creatinine clearance less than 30 ml/min, initially, 5 mg/day titrated up to maximum of 40 mg/day.

SIDE EFFECTS

FREQUENT (6%–3%): Cough, headache, dizziness. **OCCASIONAL (2%):** Fatigue, somnolence or drowsiness, nausea. **RARE (less than 1%):** Rash, fever, myalgia, diarrhea, loss of taste.

ADVERSE REACTIONS/ TOXIC EFFECTS

Excessive hypotension ("first-dose syncope") may occur in patients with CHF and in those who are severely salt or volume depleted. Angioedema (swelling of the face and lips) and hyperkalemia occur rarely. Agranulocytosis and neutropenia may be noted in those with collagen vascular disease, including scleroderma and systemic lupus erythematosus, and impaired renal function. Nephrotic syndrome may be noted in patients with history of renal disease.

NURSING CONSIDERATIONS

BASELINE ASSESSMENT

Obtain BP immediately before each dose, in addition to regular monitoring (be alert to fluctuations). If excessive reduction in BP occurs, place patient in supine position with legs elevated. In patients with renal impairment, autoimmune disease, or taking drugs that affect leukocytes or immune response, CBC should be performed before therapy begins and q2wk for 3 mo, then periodically thereafter.

INTERVENTION/EVALUATION

Assist with ambulation if dizziness occurs. Monitor BP, renal function, urinary protein, leukocyte count.

PATIENT/FAMILY TEACHING

• To reduce hypotensive effect, rise slowly from lying to sitting position, permit legs to dangle from bed momentarily before standing. • Full therapeutic effect may take 2–4 wk. • Skipping doses or noncompliance with drug therapy may produce severe, rebound hypertension.

Benicar, *see olmesartan*

benzocaine

(Americaine, Anbesol, Cetacaine, Chloraseptic Lozenges, Dermoplast, Hurricane, Orajel)
See Anesthetics: local

benzonatate

ben-**zoe**-na-tate
(Tessalon, Tessalon Perles)

◆CLASSIFICATION

PHARMACOTHERAPEUTIC: Non-narcotic antitussive. **CLINICAL:** Anti-cough.

ACTION

A non-narcotic antitussive that anesthetizes stretch receptors in respiratory passages, lungs, and pleura. **Therapeutic Effect:** Reduces cough production.

USES

Relief of nonproductive cough, including acute cough of minor throat/bronchial irritation.

PRECAUTIONS

CONTRAINDICATIONS: None known. **CAUTIONS:** Productive cough. **Pregnancy Category C.**

INTERACTIONS

DRUG: CNS depressants: May increase the effects of benzonatate. **HERBAL:** None known. **FOOD:** None known. **LAB VALUES:** None known.

AVAILABILITY (Rx)

CAPSULES (TESSALON): 100 mg, 200 mg.

ADMINISTRATION/HANDLING

PO
• Give without regard to food. • Swallow whole, do not chew/dissolve in mouth (may produce temporary local anesthesia/choking).

INDICATIONS/ROUTES/DOSAGE

ANTITUSSIVE
PO: ADULTS, ELDERLY, CHILDREN OLDER THAN 10 YR: 100 mg 3 times a day or q4h up to 600 mg/day.

SIDE EFFECTS

OCCASIONAL: Mild somnolence, mild dizziness, constipation, GI upset, skin eruptions, nasal congestion.

ADVERSE REACTIONS/ TOXIC EFFECTS

A paradoxical reaction, including restlessness, insomnia, euphoria, nervousness, and tremor, has been noted.

NURSING CONSIDERATIONS

BASELINE ASSESSMENT

Assess type, severity, frequency of cough; monitor amount, color, consistency of sputum.

INTERVENTION/EVALUATION

Initiate deep breathing/coughing exercises, particularly in patients with impaired pulmonary function. Monitor for paradoxical reaction. Increase fluid intake, environmental humidity to lower viscosity of lung secretions. Assess for clinical improvement and record onset of relief of cough.

PATIENT/FAMILY TEACHING

• Avoid tasks that require alertness, motor skills until response to drug is established. • Dry mouth, drowsiness, dizziness may be an expected response of drug.

benztropine mesylate

benz-**trow**-peen
(Apo-Benthropine ♣, Cogentin)
Do not confuse benztropine with bromocriptine.

◆CLASSIFICATION

PHARMACOTHERAPEUTIC: Anticholinergic. **CLINICAL:** Antiparkinson agent.

ACTION

An antiparkinson agent that selectively blocks central cholinergic receptors, helping to balance cholinergic and dopaminergic activity. **Therapeutic Effect:** Reduces the incidence and severity of akinesia, rigidity, and tremor.

PHARMACOKINETICS

Well absorbed following oral and IM administration. Oral onset of action: 1–2 hr, IM onset of action: minutes. The pharmacologic effects may not be apparent until 2 to 3 days after initiation of therapy and may persist for up to 24 hr after discontinuation of the drug. **Half-life:** Extended.

USES

Treatment of Parkinson's disease, drug-induced extrapyramidal reactions (except tardive dyskinesia).

PRECAUTIONS

CONTRAINDICATIONS: Angle-closure glaucoma, benign prostatic hyperplasia, children younger than 3 yr, GI obstruction, intestinal atony, megacolon, myasthenia gravis, paralytic ileus, severe ulcerative colitis. **CAUTIONS:** Treated open-angle glaucoma, heart disease, hypertension; patients with tachycardia, arrhythmias, prostatic hypertrophy, hepatic or renal impairment, obstructive diseases of the GI/GU tract, urinary retention.

⧗ **LIFESPAN CONSIDERATIONS: Pregnancy/Lactation:** Unknown if drug crosses placenta or is distributed in breast milk. **Pregnancy Category C. Children:** Safety and efficacy not established. **Elderly:** No age-related precautions noted, but there is a higher risk for adverse effects.

INTERACTIONS

DRUG: Alcohol, other CNS depressants: May increase sedation. **Amantadine, anticholinergics, MAOIs:** May increase the effects of benztropine. **Antacids, antidiarrheals:** May decrease the absorption and effects of benztropine. **Tricyclic antidepressants:** May cause excessive anticholinergic effects (dry mouth, constipation, sedation). **HERBAL:** None known. **FOOD:** None known. **LAB VALUES:** None known.

AVAILABILITY (Rx)

TABLETS: 0.5 mg, 1 mg, 2 mg. **INJECTION:** 1 mg/ml.

ADMINISTRATION/HANDLING
IM

● Therapy should be initiated with a low dose and increased gradually at five- or six-day intervals to the smallest therapeutic level for optimal relief.

PO

● Benztropine is usually taken at bedtime.

INDICATIONS/ROUTES/DOSAGE
PARKINSONISM

PO: ADULTS: 0.5–6 mg/day as a single dose or in 2 divided doses. Titrate by 0.5 mg at 5–6 day intervals. ELDERLY: Initially, 0.5 mg once or twice a day. Titrate by 0.5 mg at 5–6 day intervals. **Maximum:** 4 mg/day.

DRUG-INDUCED EXTRAPYRAMIDAL SYMPTOMS

PO, IM: ADULTS: 1–4 mg once or twice a day. CHILDREN OLDER THAN 3 YR: 0.02–0.05 mg/kg/dose once or twice a day.

ACUTE DYSTONIC REACTIONS

IV, IM: ADULTS: Initially, 1–2 mg; then 1–2 mg PO twice a day to prevent recurrence.

SIDE EFFECTS

FREQUENT: Somnolence, dry mouth, blurred vision, constipation, decreased sweating or urination, GI upset, photosensitivity. **OCCASIONAL:** Headache, memory loss, muscle cramps, anxiety, peripheral paresthesia, orthostatic hypotension, abdominal cramps. **RARE:** Rash, confusion, eye pain.

ADVERSE REACTIONS/ TOXIC EFFECTS

Overdose may produce severe anticholinergic effects, such as unsteadiness, somnolence, tachycardia, dyspnea, skin flushing, and severe dryness of the mouth, nose, or throat. Severe paradoxical reactions, marked by hallucinations, tremor, seizures, and toxic psychosis, may occur.

BASELINE ASSESSMENT

Assess mental status for confusion, disorientation, agitation, psychotic-like symptoms (medication frequently produces such side effects in those older than 60 yr).

INTERVENTION/EVALUATION

Be alert to neurologic effects: headache, drowsiness, mental confusion, agitation. Assess for clinical reversal of symptoms (improvement of tremor of head and hands at rest, mask-like facial expression, shuffling gait, muscular rigidity).

PATIENT/FAMILY TEACHING

• Avoid tasks that require alertness, motor skills until response to drug is established. • Dry mouth, drowsiness, dizziness may be an expected response to drug. • Avoid alcoholic beverages during therapy. • Drowsiness tends to diminish or disappear with continued therapy.

beractant

burr-**act**-ant

(Survanta Intratracheal)

Do not confuse Survanta with Sufenta.

◆ CLASSIFICATION

PHARMACOTHERAPEUTIC: Natural bovine lung extract. **CLINICAL:** Pulmonary surfactant.

ACTION

A natural bovine lung extract that reduces alveolar surface tension, stabilizing alveoli. **Therapeutic Effect:** Improves lung compliance and respiratory gas exchange.

PHARMACOKINETICS

Not absorbed systemically.

USES

Prevention and treatment (rescue) of respiratory distress syndrome (RDS—hyaline membrane disease) in premature infants. Oxygenation improves within minutes of administration.

PRECAUTIONS

CONTRAINDICATIONS: None known. **CAUTIONS:** Those at risk for circulatory overload. This drug is for use only in neonates. **Pregnancy Category:** This drug is not indicated for use in pregnant women.

INTERACTIONS

DRUG: None known. **HERBAL:** None known. **FOOD:** None known. **LAB VALUES:** None known.

AVAILABILITY (Rx)

INTRATRACHEAL SUSPENSION FOR INHALATION: 25-mg/ml vials.

ADMINISTRATION/HANDLING

INTRATRACHEAL

Administration • Instill through catheter inserted into infant's endotracheal tube. Do not instill into main stem bronchus. • Monitor for bradycardia, decreased O_2 saturation during administration. Stop dosing procedure if these effects occur; begin appropriate measures before reinstituting therapy.

Storage • Refrigerate vials. • Warm by standing vial at room temperature for 20 min or warm in hand 8 min. • If settling occurs, gently swirl vial (do not shake) to redisperse. • After warming, may return to refrigerator within 8 hr one time only. • Each vial should be injected with a needle only one time; discard unused portions. • Color appears off-white to light brown.

INDICATIONS/ROUTES/DOSAGE
PREVENTION AND RESCUE TREATMENT OF RDS OR HYALINE MEMBRANE DISEASE IN PREMATURE INFANTS
INTRATRACHEAL: INFANTS: 100 mg of phospholipids/kg birth weight (4 ml/kg). Give within 15 min of birth if infant weighs less than 1,250 g and has evidence of surfactant deficiency; give within 8 hr when RDS is confirmed by X-ray and requires mechanical ventilation. May repeat 6 hr or longer after preceding dose. **Maximum:** 4 doses in the first 48 hr of life.

SIDE EFFECTS
FREQUENT: Transient bradycardia, oxygen (O_2) desaturation, increased carbon dioxide (CO_2) retention. **OCCASIONAL:** Endotracheal tube reflux. **RARE:** Apnea, endotracheal tube blockage, hypotension or hypertension, pallor, vasoconstriction.

ADVERSE REACTIONS/ TOXIC EFFECTS
Life-threatening nosocomial sepsis may occur.

NURSING CONSIDERATIONS

BASELINE ASSESSMENT
Drug must be administered in highly supervised setting. Clinicians caring for neonate must be experienced with intubation, ventilator management. Offer emotional support to parents.

INTERVENTION/EVALUATION
Monitor infant with arterial or transcutaneous measurement of systemic O_2, CO_2. Assess lung sounds for rales, moist breath sounds.

betamethasone

bay-ta-**meth**-a-sone
(Abdeon, Alphatrex, Betaderm ✦, Beta-Phos/AC, Betatrex, Beta-Val, Betnesol ✦, Celestone, Celestone Phosphate, Celestone Soluspan, Diprolene, Luxiq, Maxivate)

FIXED-COMBINATION(S)
Lotrisone: betamethasone/clotrimazole (an antifungal): 0.05%/1%. **Taclonex:** betamethasone/calcipotriene (an anti-psoriatic): 0.064%/ 0.005%

CLASSIFICATION
PHARMACOTHERAPEUTIC: Adrenocorticosteroid. **CLINICAL:** Antiinflammatory, immunosuppressant (see pp. 83C, 86C).

ACTION
An adrenocortical steroid that controls the rate of protein synthesis, depresses the migration of polymorphonuclear leukocytes and fibroblasts, reduces capillary permeability and prevents or controls inflammation. Therapeutic Effect: Decreases tissue response to inflammatory process.

PHARMACOKINETICS
Rapidly and almost completely absorbed following PO administration. After topical application, limited absorption systemically. Metabolized in liver. Excreted in urine. Half-life: 36–54 hr.

USES
Systemic: Anti-inflammatory, immunosuppressant, corticosteroid replacement therapy. **Topical:** Relief of inflammatory and pruritic dermatoses. **Foam:** Relief of inflammation, itching associated with dermatosis.

✐ see color pill atlas   ✒ herb   underlined – top prescribed drug

PRECAUTIONS

CONTRAINDICATIONS: Hypersensitivity to betamethasone, systemic fungal infections. **CAUTIONS:** Hypothyroidism, cirrhosis, nonspecific ulcerative colitis, patients at increased risk for peptic ulcer.

⌛ **LIFESPAN CONSIDERATIONS: Pregnancy/Lactation:** Crosses placenta, distributed in breast milk. **Pregnancy Category C (D if used in first trimester). Children:** Prolonged treatment, high-dose therapy may decrease short-term growth rate, cortisol secretion. **Elderly:** Higher risk for developing hypertension, osteoporosis.

INTERACTIONS

DRUG: Amphotericin: May increase hypokalemia. **Digoxin:** May increase digoxin toxicity secondary to hypokalemia. **Diuretics, insulin, oral hypoglycemics, potassium supplements:** May decrease the effects of these drugs. **Hepatic enzyme inducers:** May decrease the effect of betamethasone. **Live-virus vaccines:** May decrease the patient's antibody response to vaccine, increase vaccine side effects, and potentiate virus replication. **HERBAL:** None known. **FOOD:** None known. **LAB VALUES:** May increase blood glucose levels and serum lipids, amylase, and sodium levels. May decrease serum calcium, potassium, and thyroxine levels.

AVAILABILITY (Rx)

TABLETS (CELESTONE): 0.6 mg. **CREAM:** 0.05% (Alphatrex, Diprolene, Maxivate), 0.1% (Betatrex, Beta-Val). **FOAM (LUXIQ):** 0.12%. **GEL (DIPROLENE):** 0.05%. **LOTION:** 0.05% (Alphatrex, Diprolene, Maxivate), 0.1% (Betatrex, Beta-Val). **OINTMENT:** 0.05% (Alphatrex, Diprolene, Maxivate), 0.1% (Betatrex). **SYRUP (CELESTONE):** 0.6 mg/5 ml. **INJECTION SOLUTION (ABDEON, CELESTONE PHOSPHATE):** 4 mg/ml. **INJECTION SUSPENSION (BETA-PHOS/AC, CELESTONE SOLUSPAN):** 3 mg acetate/3 mg betamethasone sodium phosphate.

ADMINISTRATION/HANDLING

◂ **ALERT** ▸ Dosage requirements are variable and must be individualized on the basis of the disease under treatment and response of the patient.

IM
• Do not administer the injectable suspension intravenously. • The IM dose is usually ⅓–½ the oral dose.

PO
• Protect syrup from light and tablets from excessive moisture. • Give with milk or food (decreases GI upset). • Give single doses before 9 AM; multiple doses should be given at evenly spaced intervals.

TOPICAL
• Gently cleanse area before application. • Use occlusive dressings only as ordered. • Apply sparingly and rub into area thoroughly. • When using aerosol, spray area 3 sec from 15-cm distance; avoid inhalation.

INDICATIONS/ROUTES/DOSAGE

ANTI-INFLAMMATION, IMMUNO-SUPPRESSION, CORTICOSTEROID REPLACEMENT THERAPY
PO: ADULTS, ELDERLY: 0.6–7.2 mg/day. CHILDREN: 0.0175–0.25 mg/kg/day in 3–4 divided doses.
IM: ADULTS, ELDERLY: 0.5–9 mg/day in 2 divided doses. CHILDREN: 0.0175–0.125 mg/kg/day in 3–4 divided doses.

RELIEF OF INFLAMMED AND PRURITIC DERMATOSES
TOPICAL: ADULTS, ELDERLY: 1–3 times a day. **Foam:** Apply twice a day.

SIDE EFFECTS

FREQUENT: Systemic: Increased appetite, abdominal distention, nervousness, insomnia, false sense of well-being. **Topical:** Burning, stinging, pruritus.

OCCASIONAL: Systemic: Dizziness, facial flushing, diaphoresis, decreased or blurred vision, mood swings. **Topical:** Allergic contact dermatitis, purpura or blood-containing blisters, thinning of skin with easy bruising, telangiectases or raised dark red spots on skin.

ADVERSE REACTIONS/ TOXIC EFFECTS

Overdose may cause systemic hypercorticism and adrenal suppression.

NURSING CONSIDERATIONS

BASELINE ASSESSMENT

Question for hypersensitivity to any of the corticosteroids, sulfite. Obtain baselines for height, weight, BP, glucose, electrolytes. Check results of initial tests (tuberculosis [TB] skin test, x-rays, EKG).

INTERVENTION/EVALUATION

Monitor BP, blood glucose, electrolytes. Apply topical preparation sparingly. Not for use on broken skin or in areas of infection. Do not apply to wet skin, face, inguinal areas.

PATIENT/FAMILY TEACHING

• Take with food, milk. • Take single daily dose in the morning. • Do not stop abruptly. • Apply topical preparations in a thin layer. • Do not receive smallpox vaccination during or immediately after therapy.

Betaseron, *see interferon beta 1b*

---

betaxolol ⓔ 🚩

bay-**tax**-oh-lol
(Betoptic, Betoptic-S, Kerlone)
Do not confuse betaxolol with bethanechol.

◆CLASSIFICATION

PHARMACOTHERAPEUTIC: Beta-adrenergic blocker. **CLINICAL:** Antihypertensive; antiglaucoma (see pp. 47C, 63C).

ACTION

An antihypertensive and antiglaucoma agent that blocks beta$_1$-adrenergic receptors in cardiac tissue. Reduces aqueous humor production. **Therapeutic Effect:** Slows sinus heart rate, decreases BP and reduces intraocular pressure (IOP).

USES

Ophthalmic: Treatment of chronic open-angle glaucoma, ocular hypertension. **Systemic:** Management of hypertension. **OFF-LABEL:** Treatment of angle-closure glaucoma during or after iridectomy, malignant glaucoma, secondary glaucoma; with miotics, to decrease IOP in acute and chronic angle-closure glaucoma.

PRECAUTIONS

CONTRAINDICATIONS: Cardiogenic shock, overt cardiac failure, second- or third-degree heart block, sinus bradycardia. **CAUTIONS:** Renal or hepatic impairment, peripheral vascular disease, hyperthyroidism, diabetes mellitus, inadequate cardiac function. **Pregnancy Category C (D if used in second or third trimester).**

INTERACTIONS

DRUG: Cimetidine: May increase betaxolol blood concentration. **Diuretics, other antihypertensives:** May increase hypotensive effect of betaxolol. **Insulin, oral hypoglycemics:** May prolong hypoglycemic effect of these drugs. **NSAIDs:** May decrease antihypertensive effect. **Sympathomimetics, xanthines:** May mutually inhibit hypotensive effects and may mask symptoms of hypoglycemia. **HERBAL:** None known. **FOOD:** None known. **LAB VALUES:** May increase serum antinuclear antibody titer and BUN, serum lipoprotein, creatinine, potassium, uric acid, and triglyceride levels.

AVAILABILITY (Rx)

TABLETS (KERLONE): 10 mg, 20 mg. **OPHTHALMIC SOLUTION (BETOPTIC):** 0.5%. **OPHTHALMIC SUSPENSION (BETOPTIC-S):** 0.25%.

ADMINISTRATION/HANDLING

PO
• Assess the patient's tolerance for betaxolol. • Obtain a standing systolic BP 1 hr after giving the drug. • Give without regard to meals.

OPHTHALMIC
• Shake suspension well before using. • Place a gloved finger on the lower eyelid and pull it out until pocket is formed between the eye and lower lid. • Hold the dropper above the pocket and place the prescribed number of drops into pocket. • Close eye gently so the medication will not be squeezed out of the sac. • Apply gentle digital pressure to the lacrimal sac at the inner canthus for 1 min after instillation to lessen the risk of systemic absorption.

INDICATIONS/ROUTES/DOSAGE

HYPERTENSION
PO: ADULTS: Initially, 5–10 mg/day. May increase to 20 mg/day after 7–14 days. ELDERLY: Initially, 5 mg/day.

CHRONIC OPEN-ANGLE GLAUCOMA AND OCULAR HYPERTENSION
OPHTHALMIC (SOLUTION): ADULTS, ELDERLY: 1 drop twice a day.
OPHTHALMIC (SUSPENSION): ADULTS, ELDERLY: 1–2 drops twice a day.

DOSAGE IN RENAL IMPAIRMENT
For adult and elderly patients who are on dialysis, initially give 5 mg/day; increase by 5 mg/day q2wk. **Maximum:** 20 mg/day.

SIDE EFFECTS

Betaxolol is generally well tolerated, with mild and transient side effects. **FREQUENT: Systemic:** Hypotension manifested as dizziness, nausea, diaphoresis, headache, fatigue, constipation or diarrhea, dyspnea. **Ophthalmic:** Eye irritation, visual disturbances. **OCCASIONAL: Systemic:** Insomnia, flatulence, urinary frequency, impotence or decreased libido. **Ophthalmic:** Increased light sensitivity, watering of eye. **RARE: Systemic:** Rash, arrhythmias, arthralgia, myalgia, confusion, altered taste, increased urination. **Ophthalmic:** Dry eye, conjunctivitis, eye pain.

ADVERSE REACTIONS/ TOXIC EFFECTS

Overdose may produce profound bradycardia, hypotension, and bronchospasm. Abrupt withdrawal may result in diaphoresis, palpitations, headache, and tremors. Betaxolol administration may precipitate CHF or MI in patients with cardiac disease; thyroid storm in those with thyrotoxicosis; and peripheral ischemia in those with existing peripheral vascular disease. Hypoglycemia may occur in patients with previously controlled diabetes. Ophthalmic overdose may produce bradycardia, hypotension, bronchospasm, and acute cardiac failure.

NURSING CONSIDERATIONS

BASELINE ASSESSMENT
PO: Assess baseline renal and liver hepatic function tests. Assess BP, apical pulse immediately before drug is administered (if pulse is 60/min or less or systolic BP is less than 90 mm Hg, withhold medication, contact physician).

INTERVENTION/EVALUATION
Monitor BP for hypotension. Assess pulse for quality, irregular rate,

bradycardia. Monitor daily pattern of bowel activity and stool consistency. Assist with ambulation if dizziness occurs. Assess for evidence of CHF: dyspnea (particularly on exertion or lying down), night cough, peripheral edema, distended neck veins, increase in weight, decrease in urine output. Assess for nausea, diaphoresis, headache, fatigue.

PATIENT/FAMILY TEACHING

• Do not abruptly discontinue medication. • Compliance with therapy regimen is essential to control glaucoma, hypertension. • To avoid hypotensive effect, rise slowly from lying to sitting position, wait momentarily before standing. • Avoid tasks that require alertness, motor skills until response to drug is established. • Report shortness of breath, excessive fatigue, prolonged dizziness, headache. • Do not use nasal decongestants, OTC cold preparations (stimulants) without physician approval. • Restrict salt, alcohol intake.

---

bethanechol chloride

be-**than**-e-kole
(Duvoid, Myotonachol ♣, Urecholine)

Do not confuse bethanechol with betaxolol.

◆CLASSIFICATION

PHARMACOTHERAPEUTIC: Cholinergic (see p. 81C).

ACTION

A cholinergic that acts directly at cholinergic receptors in the smooth muscle of the urinary bladder and GI tract. Increases detrusor muscle tone. **Therapeutic Effect:** May initiate micturition and bladder emptying. Improves gastric and intestinal motility.

PHARMACOKINETICS

Poorly absorbed following PO administration. Does not cross the blood-brain barrier. Metabolism, **Half-life:** Unknown.

USES

Treatment of nonobstructive urinary retention, retention due to neurogenic bladder. **OFF-LABEL:** Treatment of congenital megacolon, gastroesophageal reflux, postoperative gastric atony.

PRECAUTIONS

CONTRAINDICATIONS: Active or latent bronchial asthma, acute inflammatory GI tract conditions, anastomosis, bladder wall instability, cardiac or coronary artery disease, epilepsy, hypertension, hyperthyroidism, hypotension, mechanical GI or urinary tract obstruction or recent GI resection, parkinsonism, peptic ulcer, pronounced bradycardia, vasomotor instability. **CAUTIONS:** Presence of bacteremia, urinary retention.

⧗ **LIFESPAN CONSIDERATIONS: Pregnancy/Lactation:** Unknown if drug crosses placenta or is distributed in breast milk. **Pregnancy Category C. Children:** No age-related precautions noted. **Elderly:** No age-related precautions noted.

INTERACTIONS

DRUG: Cholinesterase inhibitors: May increase the effects and risk of toxicity of bethanechol. **Procainamide, quinidine:** May decrease the effects of bethanechol. **HERBAL:** None known. **FOOD:** None known. **LAB VALUES:** May increase serum amylase, lipase, and AST levels.

AVAILABILITY (Rx)

TABLETS: 5 mg (Urecholine), 10 mg (Duvoid, Urecholine), 25 mg (Duvoid,

Urecholine), 50 mg (Duvoid, Urecholine). **SUBCUTANEOUS SOLUTION:** 5 mg/ml (Urecholine).

INDICATIONS/ROUTES/DOSAGE

POSTOPERATIVE AND POSTPARTUM URINE RETENTION, ATONY OF BLADDER

PO: ADULTS, ELDERLY: 10–50 mg 3–4 times a day. Minimum effective dose determined by giving 5–10 mg initially, then repeating same amount at 1-hr intervals until desired response is achieved. CHILDREN: 0.6 mg/kg/day in 3–4 divided doses.

SUBCUTANEOUS: ADULTS, ELDERLY: Initially, 2.5–5 mg. Minimum effective dose determined by giving 2.5 mg (0.5 ml), repeating same amount at 15- to 30-min intervals up to a maximum of 4 doses. Minimum dose repeated 3–4 times a day. CHILDREN: 0.2 mg/kg/day in 3–4 divided doses.

SIDE EFFECTS

OCCASIONAL: Belching, changes in vision, blurred vision, diarrhea, frequent urinary urgency. **RARE: Subcutaneous:** Shortness of breath, chest tightness, bronchospasm.

ADVERSE REACTIONS/ TOXIC EFFECTS

Overdosage produces CNS stimulation, including insomnia, nervousness, and orthostatic hypotension, and cholinergic stimulation, such as headache, increased salivation and diaphoresis, nausea, vomiting, flushed skin, abdominal pain, and seizures.

NURSING CONSIDERATIONS

BASELINE ASSESSMENT

Violent cholinergic reaction if given IM or IV (circulatory collapse, severe hypotension, bloody diarrhea, shock, cardiac arrest). **Antidote:** 0.6–1.2 mg atropine sulfate.

INTERVENTION/EVALUATION

Assess for cholinergic reaction: GI discomfort or cramping, feeling of facial warmth, excessive salivation and diaphoresis, lacrimation, pallor, urinary urgency, blurred vision. Question for complaints of difficulty chewing, swallowing, progressive muscle weakness.

PATIENT/FAMILY TEACHING

• Report nausea, vomiting, diarrhea, diaphoresis, increased salivary secretions, irregular heartbeat, muscle weakness, severe abdominal pain, difficulty breathing.

bevacizumab

be-vah-**ciz**-you-mab
(Avastin)

◆CLASSIFICATION

PHARMACOTHERAPEUTIC: Monoclonal antibody. **CLINICAL:** Antineoplastic.

ACTION

An antineoplastic that binds to and inhibits vascular endothelial growth factor, a protein that plays a major role in the formation of new blood vessels to tumors. **Therapeutic Effect:** Inhibits metastatic disease progression.

PHARMACOKINETICS

Clearance varies by body weight, gender, and tumor burden. **Half-life:** 20 days (range, 11–50 days).

USES

Combination chemotherapy with 5-fluorouracil (5-FU) for first-line treatment of patients with metastatic carcinoma of the colon or rectum. **OFF-LABEL:** Adjunctive therapy in breast cancer, malignant mesothelioma, prostate cancer, renal cell carcinoma.

PRECAUTIONS

CONTRAINDICATIONS: GI perforation, hypertensive crisis, nephrotic syndrome, recent hemoptysis, serious bleeding, wound dehiscence requiring medical intervention. **CAUTIONS:** Hypertension, proteinuria, CHF, epistaxis, renal insufficiency.

⏳ **LIFESPAN CONSIDERATIONS: Pregnancy/Lactation:** Teratogenic. Potential for fertility impairment. May decrease maternal and fetal body weight; increase risk of skeletal fetal abnormalities. Do not breast-feed. **Pregnancy Category C. Children:** Safety and efficacy not established. **Elderly:** Higher incidence of severe adverse reactions in patients older than 65 yr.

INTERACTIONS

DRUG: None known. **HERBAL:** None known **FOOD:** None known. **LAB VALUES:** May decrease serum potassium, sodium, and Hgb levels; Hct; and WBC and platelet counts.

AVAILABILITY (Rx)

INJECTION: 25-mg/ml vial.

ADMINISTRATION/HANDLING

💧 IV

◀ **ALERT** ▶ Do not give by IV push or bolus.

Reconstitution • Withdraw amount of bevacizumab for a dose of 5 mg/kg and dilute in 100 ml 0.9% NaCl. • Discard any unused portion.

Rate of administration • Infuse IV over 90 min following chemotherapy. • If first infusion is well tolerated, second infusion may be administered over 60 min. • If 60-min infusion is well tolerated, all subsequent infusion may be administered over 30 min.

Storage • Refrigerate vials. • Diluted solution may be stored for up to 8 hr if refrigerated.

⬛ IV INCOMPATIBILITIES

Don't mix bevacizumab with dextrose solutions.

INDICATIONS/ROUTES/DOSAGE

FIRST-LINE TREATMENT OF METASTATIC CARCINOMA OF THE COLON OR RECTUM IN COMBINATION WITH 5-FU
IV: ADULTS, ELDERLY: 5 mg/kg once every 14 days.

SIDE EFFECTS

FREQUENT (73%–25%): Asthenia, vomiting, anorexia, hypertension, epistaxis, stomatitis, constipation, headache, dyspnea. **OCCASIONAL (21%–15%):** Altered taste, dry skin, exfoliative dermatitis, dizziness, flatulence, excessive lacrimation, skin discoloration, weight loss, myalgia. **RARE (8%–6%):** Nail disorder, skin ulcer, alopecia, confusion, abnormal gait, dry mouth.

ADVERSE REACTIONS/ TOXIC EFFECTS

UTIs, manifested as urinary frequency or urgency and proteinuria, occur frequently. CHF, deep vein thrombosis, GI perforation, wound dehiscence, hypertensive crisis, nephrotic syndrome, and severe hemorrhage are the most serious reactions that occur. Anemia, neutropenia, and thrombocytopenia occur occasionally. Hypersensitivity reactions occur rarely.

NURSING CONSIDERATIONS

BASELINE ASSESSMENT

Monitor BP regularly during treatment. Assess for proteinuria with urinalysis. For those with 2+ or greater urine dipstick reading, a 24-hr urine collection is advisable. Monitor CBC, serum potassium and sodium levels at regular intervals during therapy.

INTERVENTION/EVALUATION

Assess for asthenia (loss of strength, energy). Assist with ambulation if asthenia occurs. Monitor for fever, chills, abdominal pain. Offer antiemetic if nausea, vomiting occurs. Monitor pattern of daily bowel activity and stool consistency.

PATIENT/FAMILY TEACHING

• Do not have immunizations without physician's approval (lowers body's resistance). • Avoid contact with anyone who recently received a live virus vaccine. • Avoid crowds, those with infection. • Warn female patient of childbearing age of potential fetal risk if pregnancy occurs.

bexarotene　

becks-**aye**-row-teen
(Targretin, Targretin Topical)

◆CLASSIFICATION

PHARMACOTHERAPEUTIC: Retinoid.
CLINICAL: Antineoplastic (see p. 71C).

ACTION

This retinoid antineoplastic agent binds to and activates retinoid X receptor subtypes, which regulate the genes that control cellular differentiation and proliferation. Therapeutic Effect: Inhibits growth of tumor cell lines of hematopoietic and squamous cell origin and induces tumor regression.

PHARMACOKINETICS

Moderately absorbed from the GI tract. Protein binding: greater than 99%. Metabolized in the liver. Primarily eliminated through the hepatobiliary system. Half-life: 7 hr.

USES

Treatment of cutaneous T-cell lymphoma (CTCL) in those refractory to at least one prior systemic therapy. OFF-LABEL: Treatment of diabetes mellitus; head, neck, lung, and renal cell carcinomas; Kaposi's sarcoma.

PRECAUTIONS

CONTRAINDICATIONS: None known.
CAUTIONS: Hepatic impairment, diabetes mellitus, lipid abnormalities.
⏳ LIFESPAN CONSIDERATIONS: **Pregnancy/Lactation:** May cause fetal harm. Unknown if distributed in breast milk. **Pregnancy Category X. Children:** Safety and efficacy not established. **Elderly:** No age-related precautions noted.

INTERACTIONS

DRUG: **Antidiabetics:** May enhance the effects of these drugs. **Erythromycin, itraconazole, ketoconazole:** May increase bexarotene blood concentrations. **Phenytoin, rifampin:** May decrease bexarotene blood concentrations. HERBAL: None known. FOOD: **Grapefruit, grapefruit juice:** May increase bexarotene blood concentration and risk of toxicity. LAB VALUES: May increase serum cholesterol, triglyceride, and total and LDL cholesterol levels. May increase CA-125 assay value in patients with ovarian cancer. May decrease serum HDL cholesterol levels. May produce abnormal liver function test results.

AVAILABILITY (Rx)

CAPSULES (SOFT GELATIN [TARGRETIN]): 75 mg. **TOPICAL GEL (TARGRETIN TOPICAL):** 1%.

ADMINISTRATION/HANDLING

PO
• Give with food.

TOPICAL
- Generously coat lesions with gel.
- Allow to dry before covering. • Avoid applying gel to normal skin surrounding lesions or near mucosal surfaces.

INDICATIONS/ROUTES/DOSAGE

CUTANEOUS T-CELL LYMPHOMA REFRACTORY TO AT LEAST ONE PRIOR SYSTEMIC THERAPY

PO: ADULTS: 300 mg/m²/day. If no response and initial dose is well tolerated, may be increased to 400 mg/m²/day. If not tolerated, may decrease to 200 mg/m²/day, then to 100 mg/m²/day. **TOPICAL:** ADULTS: Initially, apply once every other day for first wk. May increase at weekly intervals to once daily, then twice a day, then 3 times a day up to 4 times a day.

SIDE EFFECTS

FREQUENT: Hyperlipidemia (79%), headache (30%), hypothyroidism (29%), asthenia (20%). **OCCASIONAL:** Rash (17%); nausea (15%); peripheral edema (13%); dry skin, abdominal pain (11%); chills, exfoliative dermatitis (10%); diarrhea (7%).

ADVERSE REACTIONS/ TOXIC EFFECTS

Pancreatitis, hepatic failure, and pneumonia occur rarely.

NURSING CONSIDERATIONS

BASELINE ASSESSMENT

Assess baseline lipid profile, WBC, liver function, thyroid function. Question about possibility of pregnancy (Pregnancy Category X). Warn women of childbearing age about potential fetal risk if pregnancy occurs. Instruct in need for use of 2 reliable forms of contraceptives concurrently during therapy and for 1 mo after discontinuation of therapy, even in infertile, premenopausal woman.

INTERVENTION/EVALUATION

Monitor serum cholesterol, triglycerides, liver and thyroid function tests, CBC.

PATIENT/FAMILY TEACHING

- Do not use medicated, drying, abrasive soaps; wash with gentle, bland soap. • Inform physician if pregnant or planning to become pregnant (Pregnancy Category X).

Biaxin, *see clarithromycin*

Biaxin XL, *see clarithromycin*

---

bicalutamide

by-kale-**yew**-tah-myd
(Casodex)

CLASSIFICATION

PHARMACOTHERAPEUTIC: Antiandrogen hormone. **CLINICAL:** Antineoplastic (see p. 71C).

ACTION

An antiandrogen antineoplastic agent that competitively inhibits androgen action by binding to androgen receptors in target tissue. **Therapeutic Effect:** Decreases growth of prostatic carcinoma.

PHARMACOKINETICS

Well absorbed from the GI tract. Protein binding: 96%. Metabolized in the liver to inactive metabolite. Excreted in urine and feces. Not removed by hemodialysis. **Half-life:** 5.8 days.

USES

Treatment of advanced metastatic prostatic carcinoma (in combination with luteinizing hormone-releasing hormone [LHRH] agonistic analogues—i.e., leuprolide). Treatment with both drugs must be started at same time.

PRECAUTIONS

CONTRAINDICATIONS: Women, especially women who may become pregnant. **CAUTIONS:** Moderate to severe hepatic impairment.

⌛ **LIFESPAN CONSIDERATIONS: Pregnancy/Lactation:** May inhibit spermatogenesis, not used in women. **Pregnancy Category X. Children:** Safety and efficacy not established. **Elderly:** No age-related precautions noted.

INTERACTIONS

DRUG: Warfarin: May increase warfarin's effects. **HERBAL:** None known. **FOOD:** None known. **LAB VALUES:** May increase BUN level and serum alkaline phosphatase, bilirubin, AST, and ALT levels. May decrease blood Hgb level and WBC count.

AVAILABILITY (Rx)

TABLETS: 50 mg.

ADMINISTRATION/HANDLING

PO

• Give without regard to food. • Take at same time each day.

INDICATIONS/ROUTES/DOSAGE

PROSTATIC CARCINOMA

PO: ADULTS, ELDERLY: 50–100 mg once a day in morning or evening, given concurrently with an LHRH analogue or after surgical castration.

SIDE EFFECTS

FREQUENT: Hot flashes (49%), breast pain (38%), muscle pain (27%), constipation (17%), asthenia (15%), diarrhea (10%), nausea (11%). **OCCASIONAL (9%–8%):** Nocturia, abdominal pain, peripheral edema. **RARE (7%–3%):** Vomiting, weight loss, dizziness, insomnia, rash, impotence, gynecomastia.

ADVERSE REACTIONS/TOXIC EFFECTS

Sepsis, CHF, hypertension, iron deficiency anemia, interstitial pneumonitis, and pulmonary fibrosis may occur. Severe hepatotoxicity occurs rarely within the first 3–4 mo of treatment. Cases of death due to severe hepatic injury have been reported.

NURSING CONSIDERATIONS

INTERVENTION/EVALUATION

Perform periodic liver function tests. If transaminases increase over 2 times the upper limit of normal, discontinue treatment. Monitor for diarrhea, nausea, vomiting.

PATIENT/FAMILY TEACHING

• Do not stop taking medication (both drugs must be continued). • Take medications at same time each day. • Explain possible expectancy of frequent side effects. • Contact physician for persistent nausea, vomiting.

bimatoprost

(Lumigan)
See Antiglaucoma agents (p. 47C)

bisacodyl

bise-ah-**co**-dahl

(Alophen, Apo-Bisacodyl ✦, Dulcolax, Fleet, Gentlax, Modane, Veracolate)

Do not confuse Veracolate with Accolate or Modane with Mudrane.

CLASSIFICATION

PHARMACOTHERAPEUTIC: GI stimulant. **CLINICAL:** Laxative (see p. 110C).

ACTION

A GI stimulant that has a direct effect on colonic smooth musculature by stimulating the intramural nerve plexi. **Therapeutic Effect:** Promotes fluid and ion accumulation in the colon increasing peristalsis and producing a laxative effect.

PHARMACOKINETICS

Route	Onset	Peak	Duration
PO	6–12 hr	N/A	N/A
Rectal	15–60 min	N/A	N/A

Minimal absorption following oral and rectal administration. Absorbed drug is excreted in urine; remainder is eliminated in feces.

USES

Treatment of constipation, colonic evacuation before examinations or procedures.

PRECAUTIONS

CONTRAINDICATIONS: Abdominal pain, appendicitis, intestinal obstruction, nausea, undiagnosed rectal bleeding, vomiting. **CAUTIONS:** Excessive use may lead to fluid, electrolyte imbalance.

⧗ **LIFESPAN CONSIDERATIONS: Pregnancy/Lactation:** Unknown if drug crosses placenta or is distributed in breast milk. **Pregnancy Category C. Children:** Avoid in children younger than 6 yr (usually unable to describe symptoms or more severe side effects). **Elderly:** Repeated use may cause weakness, orthostatic hypotension due to electrolyte loss.

INTERACTIONS

DRUG: Antacids, cimetidine, famotidine, ranitidine: May cause rapid dissolution of bisacodyl, producing abdominal cramping, and vomiting. **Oral medications:** May decrease transit time of concurrently administered oral medications, decreasing absorption of bisacodyl. **HERBAL:** None known. **FOOD: Milk:** May cause rapid dissolution of bisacodyl. **LAB VALUES:** None known.

AVAILABILITY (OTC)

TABLETS (ENTERIC-COATED [DULCOLAX, FLEET]): 5 mg. **RECTAL ENEMA (FLEET):** 10 mg/1.25 oz. **SUPPOSITORIES (DULCOLAX, FLEET):** 10 mg.

ADMINISTRATION/HANDLING

PO
• Give on empty stomach (faster action). • Offer 6–8 glasses of water a day (aids stool softening). • Administer tablets whole; do not chew or crush. • Avoid giving within 1 hr of antacids, milk, other oral medication.

RECTAL, ENEMA
• Shake enema and remove orange protective shield from tip before administering. • Position patient on left side with left knee slightly bent and the right leg drawn up, or in knee-chest position. • The diaphragm at base of tube prevents reflux and assures controlled flow of the enema solution. • The enema should be used at room temperature.

RECTAL, SUPPOSITORY
• If suppository is too soft, chill for 30 min in refrigerator or run cold water over foil wrapper. • Moisten suppository with cold water before inserting well into rectum.

INDICATIONS/ROUTES/DOSAGE

TREATMENT OF CONSTIPATION
PO: ADULTS, CHILDREN OLDER THAN 12 YR: 5–15 mg as needed. **Maximum:** 30 mg.

CHILDREN 3–12 YR: 5–10 mg or 0.3 mg/kg at bedtime or after breakfast. ELDERLY: Initially, 5 mg/day.

RECTAL, ENEMA: ADULTS, CHILDREN OLDER THAN 12 YR: One 1.25 oz bottle in a single daily dose.

RECTAL, SUPPOSITORY: ADULTS, CHILDREN OLDER THAN 12 YR: 10 mg to induce bowel movement. CHILDREN 2–12 YR: 5–10 mg as a single dose. CHILDREN YOUNGER THAN 2 YR: 5 mg. ELDERLY: 5–10 mg/day.

SIDE EFFECTS

FREQUENT: Some degree of abdominal discomfort, nausea, mild cramps, faintness. **OCCASIONAL:** Rectal administration: burning of rectal mucosa, mild proctitis.

ADVERSE REACTIONS/ TOXIC EFFECTS

Long-term use may result in laxative dependence, chronic constipation, and loss of normal bowel function. Prolonged use or overdose may result in electrolyte or metabolic disturbances (such as hypokalemia, hypocalcemia, and metabolic acidosis or alkalosis), as well as persistent diarrhea, vomiting, muscle weakness, malabsorption, and weight loss.

NURSING CONSIDERATIONS

INTERVENTION/EVALUATION

Encourage adequate fluid intake. Assess bowel sounds for peristalsis. Monitor pattern of daily bowel activity and stool consistency; record time of evacuation. Assess for abdominal disturbances. Monitor serum electrolytes in those exposed to prolonged, frequent, or excessive use of medication.

PATIENT/FAMILY TEACHING

• Institute measures to promote defecation: increase fluid intake, exercise, high-fiber diet. • Do not take antacids, milk, or other medication within 1 hr of taking medication (decreased effectiveness). • Report unrelieved constipation, rectal bleeding, muscle pain or cramps, dizziness, weakness.

bismuth subsalicylate

bis-muth sub-sal-**ih**-sah-late
(Bismed ❧, Colo-Fresh, Devrom, Kaopectate, Pepto-Bismol)

FIXED-COMBINATION(S)

Helidac: bismuth/metronidazole/ tetracycline: 262 mg/250 mg/ 500 mg.

◆CLASSIFICATION

PHARMACOTHERAPEUTIC: Antisecretory, antimicrobial. **CLINICAL:** Antidiarrheal, antinauseant, antiulcer (see p. 43C).

ACTION

An antinauseant and antiulcer agent that absorbs water and toxins in the large intestine and forms a protective coating in the intestinal mucosa. Also possesses antisecretory and antimicrobial effects. **Therapeutic Effect:** Prevents diarrhea. Helps treat *Helicobacter-pylori–* associated peptic ulcer disease.

USES

Treatment of diarrhea, indigestion, nausea. Adjunct in treatment of *H. pylori–*associated peptic ulcer disease. **OFF-LABEL.** Prevention of traveler's diarrhea.

PRECAUTIONS

CONTRAINDICATIONS: Bleeding ulcers, gout, hemophilia, hemorrhagic states, renal impairment. **CAUTIONS:** Elderly, diabetic patients. **Pregnancy Category C.**

INTERACTIONS

DRUG: Anticoagulants,   heparin, thrombolytics: May increase the risk of bleeding. **Aspirin, other salicylates:** May increase the risk of salicylate toxicity. **Insulin, oral antidiabetics:** Large dose may increase the effects of insulin and oral antidiabetics. **Tetracyclines:** May decrease the absorption of tetracyclines. **HERBAL:** None known. **FOOD:** None known. **LAB VALUES:** May alter serum alkaline phosphatase, AST, ALT, and uric acid levels. May decrease serum potassium level. May prolong PT.

AVAILABILITY (OTC)

CAPLETS (DEVROM): 200 mg. **LIQUID (KAOPECTATE,   PEPTO-BISMOL):** 262 mg/15 ml, 525 mg/15 ml. **TABLETS (COLO-FRESH):** 324 mg. **TABLETS (CHEWABLE):** 200 mg (Devrom), 262 mg (Pepto-Bismol).

ADMINISTRATION/HANDLING

• Shake the suspension well. • Chew or dissolve the chewable tablet before swallowing.

INDICATIONS/ROUTES/DOSAGE

DIARRHEA, GASTRIC DISTRESS

PO: ADULTS, ELDERLY: 2 tablets (30 ml) q30–60min. **Maximum:** 8 doses in 24 hr. CHILDREN 9–12 YR: 1 tablet or 15 ml q30–60min. **Maximum:** 8 doses in 24 hr. CHILDREN 6–8 YR: ⅔ tablet or 10 ml q30–60min. **Maximum:** 8 doses in 24 hr. CHILDREN 3–5 YR: ⅓ tablet or 5 ml q30–60min. **Maximum:** 8 doses in 24 hr.

H. PYLORI–ASSOCIATED DUODENAL ULCER, GASTRITIS

PO: ADULTS, ELDERLY: 525 mg 4 times a day, with 500 mg amoxicillin and 500 mg metronidazole, 3 times a day after meals, for 7–14 days.

CHRONIC INFANT DIARRHEA

PO: CHILDREN 2–24 MO: 2.5 ml q4h.

SIDE EFFECTS

FREQUENT: Grayish black stools. **RARE:** Constipation.

ADVERSE REACTIONS/ TOXIC EFFECTS

Debilitated patients and infants may develop impaction.

INTERVENTION/EVALUATION

Encourage adequate fluid intake. Assess bowel sounds for peristaltic activity. Monitor stool frequency, consistency.

PATIENT/FAMILY TEACHING

• Stool may appear gray/black. • Chew the chewable tablets thoroughly before swallowing.

bisoprolol fumarate

bye-**sew**-pro-lol
(Monocor ✸, Zebeta)
Do not confuse Zebeta with DiaBeta.

FIXED-COMBINATION(S)

Ziac: bisoprolol/hydrochlorothiazide (a diuretic): 2.5 mg/6.25 mg; 5 mg/6.25 mg; 10 mg/6.25 mg.

CLASSIFICATION

PHARMACOTHERAPEUTIC: Beta-adrenergic blocker. **CLINICAL:** Antihypertensive (see p. 64C).

ACTION

An antihypertensive that blocks beta$_1$-adrenergic receptors in cardiac tissue. **Therapeutic Effect:** Slows sinus heart rate and decreases BP.

PHARMACOKINETICS

Well absorbed from the GI tract. Protein binding: 26%–33%. Metabolized in the liver. Primarily excreted in urine. Not removed by hemodialysis. **Half-life:** 9–12 hr (increased in impaired renal function).

USES

Management of hypertension, alone or in combination with diuretics, other medications. **OFF-LABEL:** Angina pectoris, premature ventricular contractions, supraventricular arrhythmias.

PRECAUTIONS

CONTRAINDICATIONS: Cardiogenic shock, marked sinus bradycardia, overt cardiac failure, second- or third-degree heart block. **CAUTIONS:** Renal or hepatic impairment, peripheral vascular disease, hyperthyroidism, diabetes, inadequate cardiac function, bronchospastic disease.

 LIFESPAN CONSIDERATIONS: Pregnancy/Lactation: Readily crosses placenta; distributed in breast milk. Avoid use during first trimester. May produce bradycardia, apnea, hypoglycemia, hypothermia during delivery, low birth-weight infants. **Pregnancy Category C (D if used in second or third trimester). Children:** Safety and efficacy not established. **Elderly:** Age-related peripheral vascular disease may increase risk of decreased peripheral circulation.

INTERACTIONS

DRUG: Cimetidine: May increase bisoprolol blood concentration. **Diuretics, other antihypertensives:** May increase the hypotensive effect of bisoprolol. **Insulin, oral hypoglycemics:** May mask symptoms of hypoglycemia and prolong the hypoglycemic effect of these drugs. **NSAIDs:** May decrease antihypertensive effect. **Sympathomimetics, xanthines:** May mutually inhibit effects. **HERBAL:** None known. **FOOD:** None known. **LAB VALUES:** May increase ANA titer and BUN, serum lipoprotein, creatinine, potassium, uric acid, and triglyceride levels.

AVAILABILITY (Rx)

TABLETS: 5 mg, 10 mg.

ADMINISTRATION/HANDLING

PO
• Give without regard to food. • Scored tablet may be crushed.

INDICATIONS/ROUTES/DOSAGE

HYPERTENSION
PO: ADULTS: Initially, 2.5–5 mg/day. May increase up to 20 mg/day. ELDERLY: Initially, 2.5 mg/day. May increase by 2.5–5 mg/day. **Maximum:** 20 mg/day.

DOSAGE IN HEPATIC IMPAIRMENT
For adults and elderly patients with cirrhosis or hepatitis whose creatinine clearance is less than 40 ml/minute, initially give 2.5 mg.

SIDE EFFECTS

FREQUENT: Hypotension manifested as dizziness, nausea, diaphoresis, headache, cold extremities, fatigue, constipation or diarrhea. **OCCASIONAL:** Insomnia, flatulence, urinary frequency, impotence or decreased libido. **RARE:** Rash, arthralgia, myalgia, confusion (especially in the elderly), altered taste.

ADVERSE REACTIONS/ TOXIC EFFECTS

Overdose may produce profound bradycardia and hypotension. Abrupt withdrawal may result in diaphoresis, palpitations, headache, and tremulousness. Bisoprolol administration may precipitate CHF and MI in patients with heart disease, thyroid storm in those with thyrotoxicosis, and peripheral ischemia in those with existing peripheral vascular disease. Hypoglycemia may occur in patients with previously controlled diabetes. Thrombocytopenia, including unusual bruising and bleeding, occurs rarely.

NURSING CONSIDERATIONS

BASELINE ASSESSMENT

Assess baseline renal and liver function tests. Assess BP, apical pulse immediately before drug is administered (if pulse is 60/min or less or systolic BP is less than 90 mm Hg, withhold medications, contact physician).

INTERVENTION/EVALUATION

Assess pulse for quality, irregular rate, bradycardia. Assist with ambulation if dizziness occurs. Assess for peripheral edema (usually, first area of lower extremity swelling is behind medial malleolus in ambulatory, sacral area in bedridden). Monitor stool frequency, consistency.

PATIENT/FAMILY TEACHING

• Do not abruptly discontinue medication. • Compliance with therapy regimen is essential to control hypertension. • If dizziness occurs, sit or lie down immediately. • Avoid tasks that require alertness, motor skills until response to drug is established. • Teach patients how to take pulse properly before each dose and to report excessively slow pulse rate (less than 60 beats/min), peripheral numbness, dizziness. • Do not use nasal decongestants, OTC cold preparations (stimulants) without physician approval. • Restrict salt, alcohol intake.

---

bivalirudin

bye-**vail**-ih-rhu-din

(Angiomax)

◆ CLASSIFICATION

PHARMACOTHERAPEUTIC: Thrombin inhibitor. **CLINICAL:** Anticoagulant.

ACTION

An anticoagulant that specifically and reversibly inhibits thrombin by binding to its receptor sites. **Therapeutic Effect:** Decreases acute ischemic complications in patients with unstable angina pectoris.

PHARMACOKINETICS

Route	Onset	Peak	Duration
IV	Immediate	N/A	1 hr

Primarily eliminated by kidneys. Twenty-five percent removed by hemodialysis. **Half-life:** 25 min (increased in moderate to severe renal impairment).

USES

Anticoagulant in patients with unstable angina undergoing percutaneous transluminal coronary angioplasty (PTCA) in conjunction with aspirin. Patients with heparin induced thrombocytopenia (HIT) and thrombosis syndrome (HITTS) while undergoing percutaneous coronary intervention.

PRECAUTIONS

CONTRAINDICATIONS: Active major bleeding. **CAUTIONS:** Conditions associated with increased risk of bleeding (e.g., bacterial endocarditis, recent major bleeding, cerebrovascular accident [CVA], stroke, intracerebral surgery, hemorrhagic diathesis, severe hypertension, severe renal or hepatic impairment, recent major surgery).

⌛ **LIFESPAN CONSIDERATIONS: Pregnancy/Lactation:** Unknown if drug is distributed in breast milk or crosses placenta. **Pregnancy Category B. Children:** Safety and efficacy not established. **Elderly:** Age-related renal impairment may require dosage adjustment.

INTERACTIONS

DRUG: Platelet aggregation inhibitors other than aspirin, thrombolytics warfarin: May increase the risk of bleeding complications. **HERBAL: Ginkgo biloba:** May increase the risk of bleeding. **FOOD:** None known. **LAB VALUES:** Prolongs aPTT and PT.

AVAILABILITY (Rx)

INJECTION, POWDER FOR RECONSTITUTION: 250 mg.

ADMINISTRATION/HANDLING

IV

Reconstitution • To each 250-mg vial add 5 ml sterile water for injection. • Gently swirl until all material is dissolved. • Further dilute each vial in 50 ml D_5W or 0.9% NaCl to yield final concentration of 5 mg/ml (1 vial in 50 ml, 2 vials in 100 ml, 5 vials in 250 ml). • If low-rate infusion is used after the initial infusion, reconstitute the 250-mg vial with added 5 ml sterile water for injection. • Gently swirl until all material is dissolved. • Further dilute each vial in 500 ml D_5W or 0.9% NaCl to yield final concentration of 0.5 mg/ml. • Produces a clear, colorless solution (do not use if cloudy or contains a precipitate).

Rate of administration • Adjust IV infusion based on aPTT or patient's body weight.

Storage • Store unreconstituted vials at room temperature. • Reconstituted solution may be refrigerated for 24 hr or less. • Diluted drug with a concentration of 0.5–5 mg/ml is stable at room temperature for 24 hr or less.

IV INCOMPATIBILITIES

Do not mix with other medications.

INDICATIONS/ROUTES/DOSAGE

ANTICOAGULANT IN PATIENTS WITH UNSTABLE ANGINA, HITS, OR HITTS WHO ARE UNDERGOING PTCA IN CONJUNCTION WITH ASPIRIN

IV: ADULTS, ELDERLY: 0.75 mg/kg as IV bolus followed by IV infusion at rate of 1.75 mg/kg/hr for duration of procedure. After initial 4-hr infusion is completed, may give additional IV infusion at rate of 0.2 mg/ kg/hr for 20 hr or less, if necessary.

DOSAGE IN RENAL IMPAIRMENT

GFR	Dosage Reduced by
30–59 ml/min	20%
10–29 ml/min	60%
Dialysis	90%

SIDE EFFECTS

FREQUENT (42%): Back pain. **OCCASIONAL (15%–12%):** Nausea, headache, hypotension, generalized pain. **RARE (8%–4%):** Injection site pain, insomnia, hypertension, anxiety, vomiting, pelvic or abdominal pain, bradycardia, nervousness, dyspepsia, fever, urine retention.

ADVERSE REACTIONS/ TOXIC EFFECTS

A hemorrhagic event occurs rarely and is characterized by a fall in BP or Hct.

NURSING CONSIDERATIONS

BASELINE ASSESSMENT

Assess CBC, bleeding time, renal function. Determine initial BP.

INTERVENTION/EVALUATION

Monitor aPTT, Hct, urine and stool culture for occult blood, renal function studies. Assess for decrease in BP, increase in pulse rate. Question for increase in amount of discharge during menses. Assess urine for hematuria.

black cohosh

(Black Cohosh Softgel, Remifemin)

Also known as baneberry, bugbane, bugwort, fairy candles.

◆CLASSIFICATION

HERBAL: See Appendix G.

ACTION

Mechanism of action unknown. A phyto-estrogen that may have estrogen-like effects. **Effect:** Reduces symptoms of menopause (e.g., hot flashes).

USES

Treatment of symptoms of menopause, induction of labor in pregnant women. May reduce lipids and/or blood pressure (especially when combined with prescription medications). Mild sedative action.

PRECAUTIONS

CONTRAINDICATIONS: Preterm pregnancy (has menstrual and uterine stimulant effects that may increase risk of miscarriage). Not to be taken for longer than 6 mo. **CAUTIONS:** Patients with breast, uterine, ovarian cancer; endometriosis; uterine fibroids.

⌛ **LIFESPAN CONSIDERATIONS: Pregnancy/Lactation:** Contraindicated. **Children:** Safety and efficacy not established. **Elderly:** No age-related precautions noted.

INTERACTIONS

DRUG: Antihypertensives: May increase action of these drugs. **Tamoxifen:** May have additive antiproliferative effect with this drug. **HERBAL:** None known. **FOOD:** None known. **LAB VALUES:** May decrease serum luteinizing hormone (LH) concentration.

AVAILABILITY

CAPSULES (SOFT GELATIN): 40 mg. **TABLETS:** 20 mg.

INDICATIONS/ROUTES/DOSAGE

MENOPAUSE, INDUCING LABOR, LIPIDS AND/OR BP, SEDATIVE
PO: ADULTS, ELDERLY: 20–80 mg twice a day.

SIDE EFFECTS

Nausea, headache, dizziness, weight gain, visual changes, migraines.

ADVERSE REACTIONS/ TOXIC EFFECTS

Overdosage may cause nausea/vomiting, decreased heart rate, diaphoresis. May produce hepatotoxicity.

NURSING CONSIDERATIONS

BASELINE ASSESSMENT

Assess if patient is pregnant or breast-feeding (contraindicated).

INTERVENTION/EVALUATION

Monitor BP, lipid levels.

PATIENT/FAMILY TEACHING

• Inform physician if pregnancy occurs or planning to become pregnant, breast-feeding. • Do not take for longer than 6 mo.

---

bleomycin sulfate

blee-oh-**my**-sin
(Blenoxane)

◆ CLASSIFICATION

PHARMACOTHERAPEUTIC: Glycopeptide antibiotic. **CLINICAL:** Antineoplastic, sclerosing agent (see p. 72C).

ACTION

A glycopeptide antibiotic whose mechanism of action is unknown. Is most effective in the G_2 phase of cell division. **Therapeutic Effect:** Appears to inhibit DNA synthesis and, to a lesser extent, RNA and protein synthesis.

PHARMACOKINETICS

Protein binding: Low (1%). Metabolism varies. Excreted in urine as unchanged drug. **Half-life:** 115 min.

USES
Treatment of Hodgkin's and non-Hodgkin's lymphoma, malignant pleural effusions, squamous cell carcinoma (e.g., head, neck, penis, cervix, vulva), testicular carcinoma. **OFF-LABEL:** Treatment of mycosis fungoides, osteosarcoma, ovarian tumors, renal carcinoma, soft-tissue sarcoma.

PRECAUTIONS
CONTRAINDICATIONS: Previous allergic reaction. **CAUTIONS:** Severe renal or pulmonary impairment.

LIFESPAN CONSIDERATIONS: Pregnancy/Lactation: May cause fetal harm. Avoid breast-feeding. **Pregnancy Category D. Children:** Safety and efficacy not established. **Elderly:** Increased risk of pulmonary toxicity.

INTERACTIONS
DRUG: Cisplatin: May decrease bleomycin clearance and increase the risk of bleomycin toxicity (from cisplatin-induced renal impairment). **Live-virus vaccines:** May potentiate virus replication, increase vaccine side effects, and decrease the patient's antibody response to the vaccine. **Other antineoplastics:** May increase the risk of bleomycin toxicity. **HERBAL:** None known. **FOOD:** None known. **LAB VALUES:** None known.

AVAILABILITY (Rx)
POWDER FOR INJECTION (BLENOXANE): 15 units, 30 units.

ADMINISTRATION/HANDLING
◄ **ALERT** ► May be carcinogenic, mutagenic, or teratogenic. Handle with extreme care during preparation/administration.

IV

Reconstitution • Reconstitute 15-unit vial with at least 5 ml (30-unit vial with at least 10 ml) 0.9% NaCl to provide a concentration not greater than 3 units/ml.

Rate of administration • Administer over at least 10 min for IV injection.

Storage • Refrigerate powder. • After reconstitution with 0.9% NaCl, solution is stable for 24 hr at room temperature.

IM, SUBCUTANEOUS
Rate of administration • Reconstitute 15-unit vial with 1–5 ml (30-unit vial with 2–10 ml) sterile water for injection, 0.9% NaCl injection, or bacteriostatic water for injection to provide concentration of 3–15 units/ml. Do not use D_5W.

Storage • Refrigerate powder. • After reconstitution with 0.9% NaCl, solution is stable for 24 hr at room temperature.

IV INCOMPATIBILITIES
None known by Y-site administration.

IV COMPATIBILITIES
Cefepime (Maxipime), dacarbazine (DTIC), dexamethasone (Decadron), diphenhydramine (Benadryl), fludarabine (Fludara), gemcitabine (Gemzar), ondansetron (Zofran), paclitaxel (Taxol), piperacillin and tazobactam (Zosyn), vinblastine (Velban), vinorelbine (Navelbine).

INDICATIONS/ROUTES/DOSAGE
AS MONOTHERAPY FOR TREATMENT OF HODGKIN'S AND NON-HODGKIN'S LYMPHOMA, MALIGNANT PLEURAL EFFUSIONS, SQUAMOUS CELL CARCINOMA (E.G., HEAD, NECK, PENIS, CERVIX, VULVA), TESTICULAR CARCINOMA
IV, IM, SUBCUTANEOUS: ADULTS, ELDERLY: 10–20 units/m² (0.25–0.5 units/kg) 1–2 times a wk.
IV (CONTINUOUS): ADULTS, ELDERLY: 15 units/m² over 24 hr for 4 days.

IN COMBINATION THERAPY FOR TREATMENT OF HODGKIN'S AND

NON-HODGKIN'S LYMPHOMA, MALIGNANT PLEURAL EFFUSIONS, SQUAMOUS CELL CARCINOMA (E.G., HEAD, NECK, PENIS, CERVIX, VULVA), TESTICULAR CARCINOMA

IV, IM: ADULTS, ELDERLY: 3–4 units/m^2.

AS A SCLEROSING AGENT TO TREAT MALIGNANT PLEURAL EFFUSIONS AND PREVENT RECURRENT PLEURAL EFFUSIONS.

INTRAPLEURAL: ADULTS, ELDERLY: 60–240 units as a single injection.

DOSAGE IN RENAL IMPAIRMENT

Creatinine Clearance	Dosage
10–50 ml/min	75% of normal dosage
Less than 10 ml/min	50% of normal dosage

SIDE EFFECTS

FREQUENT: Anorexia, weight loss, erythematous skin swelling, urticaria, rash, striae, vesiculation, hyperpigmentation (particularly at areas of pressure, skin folds, cuticles, IM injection sites, and scars), stomatitis (usually evident 1–3 wk after initial therapy); may also be accompanied by decreased skin sensitivity followed by skin hypersensitivity, nausea, vomiting, alopecia, and-with parenteral form-fever or chills (typically occurring a few hours after large single dose and lasting 4–12 hr).

ADVERSE REACTIONS/ TOXIC EFFECTS

Interstitial pneumonitis occurs in 10% of patients and occasionally progresses to pulmonary fibrosis. This condition appears to be dose- or age-related, occurring more often in patients receiving a total dose greater than 400 units and those older than 70 yr. Nephrotoxicity and hepatotoxicity occur infrequently.

NURSING CONSIDERATIONS

BASELINE ASSESSMENT
Obtain chest x-rays q1–2wk.

INTERVENTION/EVALUATION
Monitor breath sounds for pulmonary toxicity (rales, rhonchi). Observe for dyspnea. Monitor hematologic, pulmonary function, liver, renal function tests. Assess skin daily for cutaneous toxicity. Monitor for stomatitis (burning or erythema of oral mucosa at inner margin of lips), hematologic toxicity (fever, sore throat, signs of local infection, unusual bruising or bleeding), symptoms of anemia (excessive fatigue, weakness).

PATIENT/FAMILY TEACHING
• Fever or chills reaction occurs less frequently with continued therapy.
• Improvement of Hodgkin's disease, testicular tumors noted within 2 wk, squamous cell carcinoma within 3 wk.
• Do not have immunizations without doctor's approval (drug lowers body's resistance). • Avoid contact with those who have recently taken live virus vaccine or have a cold.

---

bortezomib

bor-**teh**-zoe-mib
(Velcade)

•CLASSIFICATION
PHARMACOTHERAPEUTIC: Proteasome inhibitor. **CLINICAL:** Antineoplastic.

ACTION
A proteasome inhibitor, antineoplastic agent that degrades conjugated proteins required for cell-cycle progression and mitosis, disrupting cell proliferation.

Therapeutic Effect: Produces antitumor and chemosensitizing activity and cell death.

PHARMACOKINETICS

Distributed to tissues and organs, with highest level in the GI tract and liver. Protein binding: 83%. Primarily metabolized by enzymatic action. Rapidly cleared from the circulation. Significant biliary excretion, with lesser amount excreted in the urine. Half-life: 9–15 hr.

USES

Treatment of multiple myeloma in patients who have had one prior treatment and disease progression during that therapy.

PRECAUTIONS

CONTRAINDICATIONS: Hypersensitivity to boron or mannitol. CAUTIONS: History of syncope, patients receiving medication known to be associated with hypotension, dehydrated patients, renal or hepatic impairment.

⌛ LIFESPAN CONSIDERATIONS: Pregnancy/Lactation: May induce degenerative effects in the ovary, degenerative changes in the testes. May affect male and female fertility. Breast-feeding not recommended. Pregnancy Category D. Children: Safety and efficacy not established. Elderly: Increased incidence of grades 3 and 4 thrombocytopenia.

INTERACTIONS

DRUG: Oral antidiabetics: May alter the response of these drugs. FOOD: None known. HERBAL: None known. LAB VALUES: May significantly decrease blood Hgb and Hct levels and neutrophil, platelet, and WBC counts.

AVAILABILITY (Rx)

POWDER FOR INJECTION: 3.5 mg.

ADMINISTRATION/HANDLING

 IV

Reconstitution • Reconstitute vial with 3.5 ml 0.9% NaCl.

Rate of administration • Give as a bolus IV injection.

Storage • Store unopened vials at room temperature. Once reconstituted, solution may be stored at room temperature up to 8 hr after preparation.

INDICATIONS/ROUTES/DOSAGE

MULTIPLE MYELOMA

IV: ADULTS, ELDERLY: Treatment cycle consists of 1.3 mg/m² twice weekly on days 1, 4, 8, and 11 for 2 wk followed by a 10-day rest period on days 12 to 21. Consecutive doses separated by at least 72 hr.

DOSAGE ADJUSTMENT GUIDELINES

Therapy is withheld at onset of grade 3 nonhematological or grade 4 hematological toxicities, excluding neuropathy. When symptoms resolve, therapy is restarted at a 25% reduced dosage.

NEUROPATHIC PAIN, PERIPHERAL SENSORY NEUROPATHY

IV: ADULTS, ELDERLY: For grade 1 with pain or grade 2 (interfering with function but not activities of daily living [ADL]), 1 mg/m². For grade 2 with pain or grade 3 (interfering with ADL), withhold drug until toxicity is resolved, then reinitiate with 0.7 mg/m². For grade 4 (permanent sensory loss that interferes with function), discontinue bortezomib.

SIDE EFFECTS

EXPECTED (65%–36%): Fatigue, malaise, asthenia, nausea, diarrhea, anorexia, constipation, fever, vomiting. FREQUENT (28%–21%): Headache, insomnia, arthralgia, limb pain, edema, paresthesia, dizziness, rash. OCCASIONAL (18%–11%): Dehydration, cough, anxiety, bone pain, muscle cramps, myalgia, back pain, abdominal pain, taste alteration, dyspepsia, pruritus, hypotension (including orthostatic hypotension), rigors, blurred vision.

ADVERSE REACTIONS/ TOXIC EFFECTS

Thrombocytopenia occurs in 40% of patients. Platelet count peaks at day 11 and returns to baseline by day 21. GI and intracerebral hemorrhage are associated with drug-induced thrombocytopenia. Anemia occurs in 32% of patients. New onset or worsening neuropathy occurs in 37% of patients. Symptoms may improve in some patients when bortezomib is discontinued. Pneumonia occurs occasionally.

NURSING CONSIDERATIONS

BASELINE ASSESSMENT

Obtain baseline CBC; monitor CBC, especially platelet count, throughout treatment. Antiemetics, antidiarrheals may be effective in preventing, treating nausea, vomiting, diarrhea.

INTERVENTION/EVALUATION

Routinely assess BP; monitor patient for orthostatic hypotension. Maintain strict I&O. Encourage adequate fluid intake to prevent dehydration. Monitor temperature and be alert to high potential for fever. Monitor for peripheral neuropathy (burning sensation, neuropathic pain, paresthesia, hyperesthesia). Avoid IM injections, rectal temperatures, other traumas that may induce bleeding.

PATIENT/FAMILY TEACHING

• Discuss importance of pregnancy testing, avoidance of pregnancy, measures to prevent pregnancy. • Increase fluid intake. • Avoid tasks requiring mental alertness, motor skills until response to drug is established.

bosentan

bo-sen-tan
(Tracleer)
Do not confuse Tracleer with Tricor.

CLASSIFICATION

PHARMACOTHERAPEUTIC: Endothelin receptor antagonist. **CLINICAL:** Vasodilator, neurohormonal blocker.

ACTION

An endothelin receptor antagonist that blocks endothelin-1, the neurohormone that constricts pulmonary arteries. **Therapeutic Effect:** Improves exercise ability and slows clinical worsening of pulmonary arterial hypertension (PAH).

PHARMACOKINETICS

Highly bound to plasma proteins, mainly albumin. Metabolized in the liver. Eliminated by biliary excretion. **Half-life:** Approximately 5 hr.

USES

Treatment of PAH in those with class III or IV symptoms (World Health Organization). **OFF-LABEL:** CHF, pulmonary hypertension secondary to scleroderma.

PRECAUTIONS

CONTRAINDICATIONS: Administration with cyclosporine or glyburide, pregnancy. **EXTREME CAUTION:** Moderate to severe hepatic impairment. **CAUTIONS:** Mild hepatic impairment.

⌛ **LIFESPAN CONSIDERATIONS: Pregnancy/Lactation:** May induce male infertility, atrophy of seminiferous

---

tubules of the testes; reduce sperm count. Expected to cause fetal harm, teratogenic effects, including malformations of head, mouth, face, large vessels. Breast-feeding not recommended. **Pregnancy Category X. Children:** Safety and efficacy not established. **Elderly:** Use caution in dosage due to higher frequency of decreased hepatic, renal, cardiac function.

INTERACTIONS

DRUG: Atorvastatin, glyburide, hormonal contraceptives (including oral, injectable, and implantable), lovastatin, simvastatin, warfarin: May decrease the plasma concentrations of these drugs. **Cyclosporine, ketoconazole:** May increase plasma concentration of bosentan. **HERBAL:** None known. **FOOD:** None known. **LAB VALUES:** May increase serum bilirubin, AST, and ALT levels. May decrease blood Hgb and Hct levels.

AVAILABILITY (Rx)

TABLETS: 62.5 mg, 125 mg.

ADMINISTRATION/HANDLING

• Give in the morning and evening, with or without food. • Do not crush or chew film-coated tablets.

INDICATIONS/ROUTES/DOSAGE

PAH IN THOSE WITH WORLD HEALTH ORGANIZATION CLASS III OR IV SYMPTOMS
PO: ADULTS, ELDERLY: 62.5 mg twice a day for 4 wk; then increase to maintenance dosage of 125 mg twice a day. CHILDREN WEIGHING LESS THAN 40 KG: 62.5 mg twice a day.
◀ **ALERT** ▶ When discontinuing adult/elderly dosage, reduce dosage to 62.5 mg twice a day for 3–7 days to avoid clinical deterioration.

DOSAGE BASED ON TRANSAMINASE ELEVATIONS
Any elevation accompanied by symptoms of liver injury or serum bilirubin 2 or more times upper limit of normal, stop treatment. AST/ALT greater than 3 or less than 6 times upper limit of normal, reduce dose or interrupt treatment. AST/ALT greater than 5 or less than 9 times upper limit of normal, stop treatment. AST/ALT greater than 8 times upper limit of normal, stop treatment.

SIDE EFFECTS

OCCASIONAL: Headache, nasopharyngitis, flushing. **RARE:** Dyspepsia (heartburn, epigastric distress), fatigue, pruritus, hypotension.

ADVERSE REACTIONS/ TOXIC EFFECTS

Abnormal hepatic function, lower extremity edema, and palpitations occur rarely.

BASELINE ASSESSMENT
Pregnancy must be excluded before the start of treatment and prevented thereafter. A negative result from a urine or serum pregnancy test performed during the first 5 days of a normal menstrual period and at least 11 days after the last act of sexual intercourse must be obtained. Monthly follow-up pregnancy tests must be maintained.

INTERVENTION/EVALUATION
Assess hepatic enzyme levels (aminotransferase) before initiating therapy and then monthly thereafter. If elevation in hepatic enzymes is noted, changes in monitoring and treatment must be initiated. If clinical symptoms of hepatic injury (nausea, vomiting, fever, abdominal pain, fatigue, jaundice) occur or if serum bilirubin level increases, stop treatment. Monitor Hgb levels at 1 and 3 mo of treatment, then q3mo. Monitor Hgb, Hct levels for decrease.

PATIENT/FAMILY TEACHING
• Discuss importance of pregnancy testing, avoidance of pregnancy, measures to prevent pregnancy.

botulinum toxin type A

botch-you-lin-em **tocks**-in **tipe A**
(Botox, Botox Cosmetic ✦)

◆CLASSIFICATION
PHARMACOTHERAPEUTIC: Neurotoxin. **CLINICAL:** Neuromuscular conduction blocker.

ACTION
A neurotoxin that blocks neuromuscular conduction by binding to receptor sites on motor nerve endings, and inhibiting the release of acetylcholine, resulting in muscle denervation. **Therapeutic Effect:** Reduces muscle activity.

PHARMACOKINETICS
In the treatment of blepharospasm, each treatment lasts approximately 3 mo. In the treatment of strabismus, the paralysis lasts for 2–6 wk and gradually resolves over an additional 2–6 wk. In the treatment of hemifacial spasm, treatment may last 6 mo.

USES
Treatment of strabismus, blepharospasm associated with dystonia; cervical dystonia. Temporary improvement of brow furrow lines in those 65 yr and younger. **OFF-LABEL:** Treatment of dynamic muscle contracture in children with cerebral palsy, focal task-specific dystonia, head and neck tremor unresponsive to drug therapy, hemifacial spasms, laryngeal dystonia, oromandibular dystonia, spasmoditic torticollis, writer's cramp.

PRECAUTIONS
CONTRAINDICATIONS: Infection at proposed injection sites. **CAUTIONS:** Patients with neuromuscular junctional disorders (amyotrophic lateral sclerosis, motor neuropathy, myasthenia gravis, Lambert-Eaton syndrome) may experience significant systemic effects (severe dysphagia, respiratory compromise).

⌛ LIFESPAN CONSIDERATIONS: **Pregnancy/Lactation:** Unknown if drug crosses placenta or is distributed is breast milk. **Pregnancy Category C. Children:** Safety and efficacy not established. **Elderly:** No age-related precautions noted.

INTERACTIONS
DRUG: Aminoglycoside antibiotics, other drugs that interfere with neuromuscular transmission (such as curare-like compounds): May potentiate the effects of botulinum toxin type A. **HERBAL:** None known. **FOOD:** None known. **LAB VALUES:** None known.

AVAILABILITY (Rx)
INJECTION: 100 units/vial.

ADMINISTRATION/HANDLING
IM

Reconstitution • 0.9% NaCl is recommended diluent. • For resulting dose of units/0.1 ml, draw up 1 ml diluent to provide 10 units, 2 ml to provide 5 units, 4 ml to provide 2.5 units, or 8 ml to provide 1.25 units. • Slowly, gently inject diluent into the vial, avoid bubbles, rotate vial gently to mix.

Rate of administration • Administer within 4 hr after reconstitution. • To be injected into affected muscle using 25-, 27-, or 30-gauge needle for superficial muscles and a 22-gauge needle for deeper musculature.

Storage • Store in freezer. • Administer within 4 hr after removal from freezer and reconstituted. • May store reconstituted solution in refrigerator for up to 4 hr. • Appears as a clear, colorless solution (discard if particulate matter is present).

INDICATIONS/ROUTES/DOSAGE

CERVICAL DYSTONIA IN PATIENTS WHO HAVE PREVIOUSLY TOLERATED BOTULINUM TOXIN TYPE A

IM: ADULTS, ELDERLY: Mean dose of 236 units (range: 198–300 units) divided among the affected muscles, based on patient's head and neck position, localization of pain, muscle hypertrophy, patient response, and adverse reaction history.

CERVICAL DYSTONIA IN PATIENTS WHO HAVE NOT PREVIOUSLY BEEN TREATED WITH BOTULINUM TOXIN TYPE A

IM: ADULTS, ELDERLY: Administer at lower dosage than for patients who have previously tolerated the drug.

STRABISMUS

IM: ADULTS, CHILDREN OLDER THAN 12 YR: 1.25–2.5 units into any one muscle. CHILDREN 2 MO–12 YR: 1–2.5 units into any one muscle.

BLEPHAROSPASM

IM: ADULTS, CHILDREN 12 YR AND OLDER: Initially, 1.25–2.5 units. May increase up to 2.5–5.0 units at repeat treatments. **Maximum:** 5 units per injection or cumulative dose of 200 units over a 30 day period.

CEREBRAL PALSY SPASTICITY

IM: CHILDREN OLDER THAN 18 MO: 1–6 units/ kg. **Maximum:** 50 units per injection site. No more than 400 units per visit or during a 3 mo period.

IMPROVEMENT OF BROW FURROW

IM: ADULTS 65 YR AND YOUNGER: Individualized.

SIDE EFFECTS

◄ **ALERT** ► Side effects usually occur within the first week after injection. **FREQUENT (15%–11%):** Localized pain, tenderness, or bruising at injection site; localized weakness in injected muscle; upper respiratory tract infection; neck pain; headache. **OCCASIONAL (10%–2%):** Increased cough, flu-like symptoms, back pain, rhinitis, dizziness, hypertonia, soreness at injection site, asthenia, dry mouth, nausea, somnolence. **RARE:** Stiffness, numbness, diplopia, ptosis.

ADVERSE REACTIONS/ TOXIC EFFECTS

Mild to moderate dysphagia occurs in approximately 20% of patients. Arrhythmias and severe dysphagia (manifested as aspiration, pneumonia, and dyspnea) occur rarely. Overdose produces systemic weakness and muscle paralysis.

NURSING CONSIDERATIONS

BASELINE ASSESSMENT

Assess onset, type, location, duration of dystonia.

INTERVENTION/EVALUATION

Clinical improvement begins within first 2 wk after injection. Maximum benefit appears at approximately 6 wk after injection.

PATIENT/FAMILY TEACHING

• Resume activity slowly and carefully. • Seek medical attention immediately if swallowing, speech, respiratory difficulties appear.

botulinum toxin type B

botch-you-lin-em **tocks**-in **tipe B** (Myobloc)

◆CLASSIFICATION

PHARMACOTHERAPEUTIC: Neurotoxin. **CLINICAL:** Neuromuscular conduction blocker.

ACTION

A neurotoxin that inhibits acetylcholine release at the neuromuscular junction. **Therapeutic Effect:** Produces flaccid paralysis.

PHARMACOKINETICS

The duration of effect is 12–16 wk at doses of 5,000 or 10,000 units.

USES

Treatment of cervical dystonia (CD) to reduce severity of abnormal head position, neck pain associated with CD.

PRECAUTIONS

CONTRAINDICATIONS: None known. **CAUTIONS:** Patients with neuromuscular junctional disorders (amyotrophic lateral sclerosis, motor neuropathy, myasthenia gravis, Lambert-Eaton syndrome) may experience significant systemic effects (severe dysphagia, respiratory compromise).

⏳ **LIFESPAN CONSIDERATIONS: Pregnancy/Lactation:** Unknown if drug crosses placenta or is distributed in breast milk. **Pregnancy Category C. Children:** Safety and efficacy not established. **Elderly:** No age-related precautions noted.

INTERACTIONS

DRUG: Aminoglycoside antibiotics, other drugs that interfere with neuromuscular transmission (such as curare-like compounds): May potentiate the effects of botulinum toxin type B. **HERBAL:** None known. **FOOD:** None known. **LAB VALUES:** None known.

AVAILABILITY (Rx)

INJECTION: 2,500 units, 5,000 units, 10,000 units.

ADMINISTRATION/HANDLING

IM

Reconstitution • 0.9% NaCl is recommended diluent. • Slowly, gently inject diluent into the vial; avoid bubbles, rotate vial gently to mix.

Rate of administration • Administer within 4 hr after reconstitution. • To be injected into affected muscle using 25-, 27-, or 30-gauge needle for superficial muscles and a 22-gauge needle for deeper musculature.

Storage • May be refrigerated for up to 21 mo. Do not freeze. • Administer within 4 hr after removal from refrigerator and reconstituted. • May store reconstituted solution in refrigerator for up to 4 hr. • Appears as a clear, colorless solution (discard if particulate matter is present).

INDICATIONS/ROUTES/DOSAGE

TO REDUCE THE SEVERITY OF SYMPTOMS IN PATIENTS WITH CERVICAL DYSTONIA WHO HAVE PREVIOUSLY TOLERATED BOTULINUM TOXIN TYPE B
IM: ADULTS, ELDERLY: 2,500–5,000 units divided among the affected muscles.

TO REDUCE THE SEVERITY OF SYMPTOMS IN PATIENTS WITH CERVICAL DYSTONIA WHO HAVE NOT PREVIOUSLY BEEN TREATED WITH BOTULINUM TOXIN TYPE B
IM: ADULTS, ELDERLY: Administer at lower dosage than for patients who have previously tolerated the drug.

SIDE EFFECTS

◀ **ALERT** ▶ Side effects usually occur within the first week after the injection. **FREQUENT (19%–12%):** Infection, neck pain, headache, injection site pain, dry mouth. **OCCASIONAL (10%–4%):** Flu-like symptoms, generalized pain, increased cough, back pain, myasthenia. **RARE:** Dizziness, nausea, rhinitis, headache, vomiting, edema, allergic reaction.

ADVERSE REACTIONS/ TOXIC EFFECTS

Mild to moderate dysphagia occurs in approximately 10% of patients. Arrhythmias and severe dysphagia (manifested as aspiration, pneumonia, and dyspnea) occur rarely. Overdose produces systemic weakness and muscle paralysis.

NURSING CONSIDERATIONS

BASELINE ASSESSMENT
Assess onset, type, location, duration of dystonia.

INTERVENTION/EVALUATION
Duration of effect lasts between 12–16 wk at doses of 5,000 units or 10,000 units.

PATIENT/FAMILY TEACHING
• Resume activity slowly and carefully.
• Seek medical attention immediately if swallowing, speech, respiratory difficulties appear.

Brethine, *see terbutaline*

---

bretylium tosylate

bre-**till**-ee-um
(Bretylate ✤, Bretylol)
See Antiarrhythmics

Brevibloc, *see esmolol*

---

brimonidine

(Alphagan)
See Antiglaucoma agents (p. 47C)

---

brinzolamide

(Azopt)
See Antiglaucoma agents (p. 48C)

---

bromocriptine mesylate

broe-moe-**krip**-teen
(Apo-Bromocriptine ✤, Parlodel)
Do not confuse bromocriptine with benztropine, or Parlodel with pindolol.

◆CLASSIFICATION

PHARMACOTHERAPEUTIC: Dopamine agonist. **CLINICAL:** Infertility therapy adjunct, antihyperprolactinemic, lactation inhibitor, antidyskinetic, growth hormone suppressant.

ACTION

A dopamine agonist that directly stimulates dopamine receptors in the corpus striatum and inhibits prolactin secretion. Also suppresses secretion of growth hormone. **Therapeutic Effect:** Improves symptoms of parkinsonism, suppresses galactorrhea, and reduces serum growth hormone concentrations in acromegaly.

PHARMACOKINETICS

Indication	Onset	Peak	Duration
Prolactin lowering	2 hr	8 hr	24 hr
Antiparkinson	0.5–1.5 hr	2 hr	N/A
Growth hormone suppressant	1–2 hr	4–8 wk	4–8 hr

Minimally absorbed from the GI tract. Protein binding: 90%–96%. Metabolized in the liver. Excreted in feces by biliary secretion. **Half-life:** 15 hr.

USES

Treatment of pituitary prolactinomas, conditions associated with hyperprolactinemia (amenorrhea, galactorrhea, hypogonadism, infertility), parkinsonism. OFF-LABEL: Treatment of cocaine addiction, hyperprolactinemia associated with pituitary adenomas, neuroleptic malignant syndrome.

PRECAUTIONS

CONTRAINDICATIONS: Hypersensitivity to ergot alkaloids, peripheral vascular disease, pregnancy, severe ischemic heart disease, uncontrolled hypertension. **CAUTIONS:** Impaired hepatic or cardiac function, hypertension, psychiatric disorders.

⧗ LIFESPAN CONSIDERATIONS: **Pregnancy/Lactation:** Not recommended during pregnancy or while breastfeeding. **Pregnancy Category C. Children:** Safety and efficacy not established. **Elderly:** CNS effects may occur more frequently.

INTERACTIONS

DRUG: Alcohol: May produce a disulfiram-like reaction (chest pain, confusion, flushed face, nausea, vomiting). **Erythromycin, ritonavir:** May increase bromocriptine blood concentration and risk of toxicity. **Estrogens, progestins:** May decrease the effects of bromocriptine. **Haloperidol, MAOIs, phenothiazines, risperidone:** May decrease bromocriptine's prolactin-lowering effect. **Hypotension-producing medications:** May increase hypotension. **Levodopa:** May increase the effects of bromocriptine. HERBAL: None known. FOOD: None known. LAB VALUES: May increase plasma growth hormone concentration.

AVAILABILITY (Rx)

CAPSULES: 5 mg. TABLETS: 2.5 mg.

ADMINISTRATION/HANDLING

PO
• Patient should be lying down before administering first dose. • Give after food intake (decreases incidence of nausea).

INDICATIONS/ROUTES/DOSAGE

HYPERPROLACTINEMIA
PO: ADULTS, ELDERLY: Initially, 1.25–2.5 mg at bedtime. May increase by 2.5 mg q3–7days up to 5–7.5 mg/day in divided doses. Maintenance: 2.5 mg 2–3 times a day.

PITUITARY PROLACTINOMAS
PO: ADULTS, ELDERLY: Initially, 1.25 mg 2–3 times a day. May gradually increase over several weeks to 10–20 mg/day in divided doses. Maintenance: 2.5–20 mg/day in divided doses.

PARKINSONISM
PO: ADULTS, ELDERLY: Initially, 1.25 mg 1–2 times a day. May take single doses at bedtime. May increase by 2.5 mg/day at 14–28 day intervals. Maintenance: 2.5–40 mg/day in divided doses. **Maximum:** 100 mg/day.

ACROMEGALY
PO: ADULTS, ELDERLY: Initially, 1.25–2.5 mg at bedtime. May increase by

1.25–2.5 mg q3–7days up to 30 mg/day in divided doses. Maintenance: 10–30 mg/day in divided doses. **Maximum:** 100 mg/day.

SIDE EFFECTS

FREQUENT: Nausea (49%), headache (19%), dizziness (17%). **OCCASIONAL (7%–3%):** Fatigue, lightheadedness, vomiting, abdominal cramps, diarrhea, constipation, nasal congestion, somnolence, dry mouth. **RARE:** Muscle cramps, urinary hesitancy.

ADVERSE REACTIONS/ TOXIC EFFECTS

Visual or auditory hallucinations have been noted in patients with Parkinson's disease. Long-term, high-dose therapy may produce continuing rhinorrhea, syncope, GI hemorrhage, peptic ulcer, and severe abdominal pain.

NURSING CONSIDERATIONS

BASELINE ASSESSMENT

Evaluation of pituitary (rule out tumor) should be done before treatment for hyperprolactinemia with amenorrhea or galactorrhea, infertility. Obtain pregnancy test.

INTERVENTION/EVALUATION

Assist with ambulation if dizziness is noted after administration. Assess for therapeutic response (decrease in engorgement, parkinsonism symptoms). Monitor for constipation.

PATIENT/FAMILY TEACHING

• To reduce lightheadedness, rise slowly from lying to sitting position, permit legs to dangle momentarily before standing. Avoid sudden posture changes. • Avoid tasks that require alertness, motor skills until response to drug is established. • Must use contraceptive measures (other than oral) during treatment. • Report any watery nasal discharge to physician.

brompheniramine

(Brovex, Brovex CT)
See Antihistamines (p. 49C)

budesonide

byew-**des**-oh-nyd

(Entocort EC, Pulmicort Respules, Pulmicort Turbuhaler, Rhinocort, Rhinocort Aqua)

◆CLASSIFICATION

PHARMACOTHERAPEUTIC: Glucocorticosteroid. **CLINICAL:** Antiinflammatory, antiallergy (see pp. 67C, 83C).

ACTION

A glucocorticoid that inhibits the accumulation of inflammatory cells and decreases and prevents tissues from responding to the inflammatory process. **Therapeutic Effect:** Relieves symptoms of allergic rhinitis or Crohn's disease.

PHARMACOKINETICS

Minimally absorbed from nasal tissue; moderately absorbed from inhalation. Protein binding: 88%. Primarily metabolized in the liver. **Half-life:** 2–3 hr.

USES

Nasal: Management of seasonal or perennial allergic rhinitis, nonallergic rhinitis. **Inhalation:** Maintenance or prophylaxis therapy for bronchial asthma. **Oral:** Treatment of mild to moderate active Crohn's disease. Maintenance of clinical remission of mild to moderate Crohn's disease. **OFF-LABEL:** Treatment of vasomotor, rhinitis.

PRECAUTIONS

CONTRAINDICATIONS: Hypersensitivity to any corticosteroid or its components, persistently positive sputum cultures for *Candida albicans*, primary treatment of status asthmaticus, systemic fungal infections, untreated localized infection involving nasal mucosa. **CAUTIONS:** Adrenal insufficiency, cirrhosis, glaucoma, hypothyroidism, untreated infection, osteoporosis, tuberculosis.

⧗ **LIFESPAN CONSIDERATIONS: Pregnancy/Lactation:** Unknown if drug crosses placenta or is distributed in breast milk. **Pregnancy Category B. Children:** Prolonged treatment or high dosages may decrease short-term growth rate, cortisol secretion. **Elderly:** No age-related precautions noted.

INTERACTIONS

DRUG: Bupropion: May lower the seizure threshold. **Itraconazole, ketoconazole:** May increase the plasma concentration of budesonide. **HERBAL:** None known. **FOOD: Grapefruit, grapefruit juice:** May increase the systemic exposure of budesonide. **LAB VALUES:** None known.

AVAILABILITY (Rx)

CAPSULES (ENTOCORT EC): 3 mg. **POWDER FOR ORAL INHALATION (PULMICORT TURBUHALER):** 200 mcg per inhalation. **SUSPENSION FOR ORAL INHALATION (PULMICORT RESPULES):** 0.25 mg/2 ml; 0.5 mg/2 mg. **NASAL SPRAY (RHINOCORT AQUA):** 32 mcg/spray.

ADMINISTRATION/HANDLING

INHALATION
• Shake container well. Instruct patient to exhale completely, place mouthpiece between lips, inhale, hold breath as long as possible before exhaling. • Allow at least 1 min between inhalations. • Rinse mouth after each use to decrease dry mouth, hoarseness.

INTRANASAL
• Instruct patient to clear nasal passages before use. • Tilt head slightly forward. • Insert spray tip into nostril, pointing toward nasal passages, away from nasal septum. • Spray into 1 nostril while holding other nostril closed, instruct patient to concurrently inspire through nostril to allow medication as high into nasal passages as possible.

INDICATIONS/ROUTES/DOSAGE

RHINITIS
INTRANASAL (RHINOCORT AQUA):
ADULTS, ELDERLY, CHILDREN 6 YR AND OLDER: 1 spray in each nostril once a day. **Maximum:** 8 sprays/day for adults and children 12 yr and older; 4 sprays/day for children younger than 12 yr.

BRONCHIAL ASTHMA
NEBULIZATION: CHILDREN 6 MO–8 YR: 0.25–1 mg/day titrated to lowest effective dosage.
INHALATION: ADULTS, ELDERLY, CHILDREN 6 YR AND OLDER: Initially, 200–400 mcg twice a day. **Maximum:** Adults: 800 mcg twice a day. Children: 400 mcg twice a day.

CROHN'S DISEASE
PO: ADULTS, ELDERLY: 9 mg once a day for up to 8 wk.

SIDE EFFECTS

FREQUENT (greater than 3%): Nasal: Mild nasopharyngeal irritation, burning, stinging, or dryness; headache; cough. **Inhalation:** Flu-like symptoms, headache, pharyngitis. **OCCASIONAL (3%–1%): Nasal:** Dry mouth, dyspepsia, rebound congestion, rhinorrhea, loss of taste. **Inhalation:** Back pain, vomiting, altered taste, voice changes, abdominal pain, nausea, dyspepsia.

ADVERSE REACTIONS/ TOXIC EFFECTS

An acute hypersensitivity reaction marked by urticaria, angioedema, and severe bronchospasm, occurs rarely.

NURSING CONSIDERATIONS

BASELINE ASSESSMENT
Question for hypersensitivity to any corticosteroids, components.

INTERVENTION/EVALUATION
Monitor for relief of symptoms.

PATIENT/FAMILY TEACHING
• Improvement noted in 24 hr, but full effect may take 3–7 days. • Contact physician if no improvement in symptoms, sneezing, nasal irritation occurs.

bumetanide

byew-**met**-ah-nide
(Bumex, Burinex ✦)

◆ CLASSIFICATION
PHARMACOTHERAPEUTIC: Loop.
CLINICAL: Diuretic (see p. 89C).

ACTION

A loop diuretic that enhances excretion of sodium, chloride, and to lesser degree, potassium, by direct action at the ascending limb of the loop of Henle and in the proximal tubule. Therapeutic Effect: Produces diuresis.

PHARMACOKINETICS

Route	Onset	Peak	Duration
PO	30–60 min	60–120 min	4–6 hr
IV	Rapid	15–30 min	2–3 hr
IM	40 min	60–120 min	4–6 hr

Completely absorbed from the GI tract (absorption decreased in CHF and nephrotic syndrome). Protein binding: 94%–96%. Partially metabolized in the liver. Primarily excreted in urine. Not removed by hemodialysis. Half-life: 1–1.5 hr.

USES

Treatment of edema associated with CHF, chronic renal failure (including nephrotic syndrome), hepatic cirrhosis with ascites, treatment of acute pulmonary edema. OFF-LABEL: Treatment of hypercalcemia, hypertension.

PRECAUTIONS

CONTRAINDICATIONS: Anuria, hepatic coma, severe electrolyte depletion. CAUTIONS: Hypersensitivity to sulfonamides, renal/hepatic impairment, diabetes mellitus, elderly/debilitated.

⧖ LIFESPAN CONSIDERATIONS: Pregnancy/Lactation: Unknown if drug is distributed in breast milk. Pregnancy Category C (D if used in pregnancy-induced hypertension). Children: Safety and efficacy not established. Elderly: May be more sensitive to hypotension/electrolyte effects. Increased risk for circulatory collapse or thrombolytic episode. Age-related renal impairment may require reduced or extended dosage interval.

INTERACTIONS

DRUG: Amphotericin B, nephrotoxic and ototoxic medications: May increase the risk of nephrotoxicity and ototoxicity. Anticoagulants, heparin: May decrease the effects of these drugs. Lithium: May increase the risk of lithium toxicity. Other hypokalemia-causing medications: May increase the risk of hypokalemia. HERBAL: None known. FOOD: None known. LAB VALUES: May increase blood glucose, BUN, serum uric acid, and urinary phosphate levels. May decrease serum calcium, chloride, magnesium, potassium, and sodium levels.

AVAILABILITY (Rx)

TABLETS: 0.5 mg, 1 mg, 2 mg.
INJECTION: 0.25 mg/ml.

ADMINISTRATION/HANDLING

IV

Rate of administration • May give undiluted but is compatible with D₅W, 0.9% NaCl, or lactated Ringer's solution. • Administer IV push over 1–2 min. • May give through Y tube or 3-way stopcock. • May give as continuous infusion.

Storage • Store at room temperature. • Stable for 24 hr if diluted.

PO
• Give with food to avoid GI upset, preferably with breakfast (may prevent nocturia).

IV INCOMPATIBILITY

Midazolam (Versed).

IV COMPATIBILITIES

Aztreonam (Azactam), cefepime (Maxipime), diltiazem (Cardizem), dobutamine (Dobutrex), furosemide (Lasix), lorazepam (Ativan), milrinone (Primacor), morphine, piperacillin and tazobactam (Zosyn), propofol (Diprivan).

INDICATIONS/ROUTES/DOSAGE

EDEMA

PO: ADULTS, CHILDREN OLDER THAN 18 YR: 0.5–2 mg as a single dose in the morning. May repeat at q4–5h. ELDERLY: 0.5 mg/day, increased as needed.
IV, IM: ADULTS, ELDERLY: 0.5–2 mg/dose; may repeat in 2–3 hr. Or 0.5–1 mg/hr by continuous IV infusion.

HYPERTENSION

PO: ADULTS, ELDERLY: Initially, 0.5 mg/day.

Range: 1–4 mg/day. **Maximum:** 5 mg/day. Larger doses may be given 2–3 doses/day.

USUAL PEDIATRIC DOSAGE

IV, IM, PO: CHILDREN: 0.015–0.1 mg/kg/dose q6–24h. **Maximum:** 10 mg/day.

SIDE EFFECTS

EXPECTED: Increased urinary frequency and urine volume. **FREQUENT:** Orthostatic hypotension, dizziness. **OCCASIONAL:** Blurred vision, diarrhea, headache, anorexia, premature ejaculation, impotence, dyspepsia. **RARE:** Rash, urticaria, pruritus, asthenia, muscle cramps, nipple tenderness.

ADVERSE REACTIONS/TOXIC EFFECTS

Vigorous diuresis may lead to profound water and electrolyte depletion, resulting in hypokalemia, hyponatremia, dehydration, coma, and circulatory collapse. Ototoxicity—manifested as deafness, vertigo, or tinnitus—may occur, especially in patients with severe renal impairment and those taking other ototoxic drugs. Blood dyscrasias and acute hypotensive episodes have been reported.

NURSING CONSIDERATIONS

BASELINE ASSESSMENT

Check vital signs, especially BP for hypotension, before administration. Assess baseline electrolytes; particularly check for low serum potassium. Assess edema, skin turgor, mucous membranes for hydration status. Initiate I&O.

INTERVENTION/EVALUATION

Continue to monitor BP, vital signs, electrolytes, I&O, weight. Note extent of diuresis. Watch for changes from initial assessment (hypokalemia may result in muscle strength changes, tremor, muscle cramps, altered mental status, cardiac arrhythmias; hyponatremia may result in confusion, thirst, cold/clammy skin).

• Expect increased frequency and volume of urination. • Report hearing abnormalities (e.g., sense of fullness in ears, tinnitus) to physician. • Eat foods high in potassium such as whole grains (cereals), legumes, meat, bananas, apricots, orange juice, potatoes (white, sweet), raisins. • Get up slowly from sitting/lying position.

Bumex, *see bumetanide*

Buminate, *see albumin*

---

bupivacaine

(Marcaine, Sensorcaine)
See Anesthetics: local (p. 4C)

---

buprenorphine

(Buprenex)
See Opioid analgesics

---

*buPROPion

byew-**pro**-peon
(Wellbutrin, <u>Wellbutrin SR</u>, Wellbutrin XL, Zyban SR, Zyban SR Refill)
Do not confuse bupropion with buspirone, Wellbutrin with Wellcovorin or Wellferon, or Zyban with Zagam.

•CLASSIFICATION

PHARMACOTHERAPEUTIC: Aminoketone. **CLINICAL:** Antidepressant, smoking cessation aid (see p. 38C).

ACTION

An aminoketone that blocks the reuptake of neurotransmitters, including serotonin and norepinephrine at CNS presynaptic membranes, increasing their availability at postsynaptic receptor sites. Also reduces the firing rate of noradrenergic neurons. **Therapeutic Effect:** Relieves depression and nicotine withdrawal symptoms.

PHARMACOKINETICS

Rapidly absorbed from the GI tract. Protein binding: 84%. Crosses the blood-brain barrier. Undergoes extensive first-pass metabolism in the liver to active metabolite. Primarily excreted in urine. **Half-life:** 14 hr.

USES

Treatment of depression, particularly endogenous depression, exhibited as persistent and prominent dysphoria (occurring nearly every day for at least 2 wk) manifested by 4 of 8 symptoms: change in appetite, change in sleep pattern, increased fatigue, impaired concentration, feelings of guilt or worthlessness, loss of interest in usual activities, psychomotor agitation or retardation, or suicidal tendencies. Also used to assist in smoking cessation. **OFF-LABEL:** Treatment of attention deficit hyperactivity disorder in adults and children.

PRECAUTIONS

CONTRAINDICATIONS: Current or prior diagnosis of anorexia nervosa or bulimia, seizure disorder, use within 14 days of

---

MAOIs, concomitant use of other bupropion products. **CAUTIONS:** History of seizure, cranial trauma; those currently taking antipsychotics, antidepressants; impaired renal, hepatic function.

⧖ **LIFESPAN CONSIDERATIONS: Pregnancy/Lactation:** Unknown if drug crosses placenta or is distributed in breast milk. **Pregnancy Category B. Children:** More sensitive to increased dosage, toxicity, increased risk of suicidal ideation, worsening of depression. Safety and efficacy not established in those younger than 18 yr. **Elderly:** More sensitive to anticholinergic, sedative, cardiovascular effects. Age-related renal impairment may require dosage adjustment.

INTERACTIONS

DRUG: Alcohol, lithium, ritonavir, steroids, trazodone, tricyclic antidepressants: May increase the risk of seizures. **Fosphenytoin, phenytoin, phenobarbital:** May decrease the effectiveness of bupropion. **Haloperidol:** May increase plasma levels of haloperidol. **Levodopa:** May increase the risk of adverse effects including nausea, vomiting, excitation, restlessness, and postural tremor. **MAOIs:** May increase the risk of neuroleptic malignant syndrome and acute bupropion toxicity. **HERBAL:** None known. **FOOD:** None known. **LAB VALUES:** May decrease serum WBC count.

AVAILABILITY (Rx)

TABLETS (WELLBUTRIN): 75 mg, 100 mg. **TABLETS (EXTENDED-RELEASE [WELLBUTRIN XL]):** 150 mg, 300 mg. **TABLETS (SUSTAINED-RELEASE [WELLBUTRIN SR]):** 100 mg, 150 mg, 200 mg. **TABLETS (SUSTAINED-RELEASE [ZYBAN SR, ZYBAN SR REFILL]):** 150 mg.

ADMINISTRATION/HANDLING

PO

• Give with or without food (give with food to reduce GI irritation). • Give at least 4-hr interval for immediate onset and 8-hr interval for sustained-release tablet to avoid seizures. • Avoid bedtime dosage (decreases risk of insomnia). • Do not crush sustained-release preparations.

INDICATIONS/ROUTES/DOSAGE

DEPRESSION

PO (IMMEDIATE RELEASE): ADULTS: Initially, 100 mg twice a day. May increase to 100 mg 3 times a day no sooner than 3 days after beginning therapy. **Maximum:** 450 mg/day. ELDERLY: 37.5 mg twice a day. May increase by 37.5 mg q3–4days. Maintenance: Lowest effective dosage.

PO (SUSTAINED-RELEASE): ADULTS: Initially, 150 mg/day as a single dose in the morning. May increase to 150 mg twice a day as early as day 4 after beginning therapy. **Maximum:** 400 mg/day. ELDERLY: Initially, 50–100 mg/day. May increase by 50–100 mg/day q3–4 days. Maintenance: Lowest effective dosage.

PO (EXTENDED-RELEASE): ADULTS: 150 mg once a day. May increase to 300 mg once a day. **Maximum:** 450 mg a day.

SMOKING CESSATION

PO: ADULTS: Initially, 150 mg a day for 3 days; then 150 mg twice a day for 7–12 wk.

DOSAGE IN LIVER IMPAIRMENT

Mild-moderate: use caution, reduce dosage. **Severe:** use extreme caution, maximum dose. Wellbutrin: 75 mg/day. Wellbutrin SR: 100 mg/day or 150 mg every other day. Wellbutrin XL: 150 mg every other day. Zyban: 150 mg every other day.

SIDE EFFECTS

FREQUENT **(32%–18%):** Constipation, weight gain or loss, nausea, vomiting, anorexia, dry mouth, headache, diaphoresis, tremor, sedation, insomnia, dizziness, agitation. **OCCASIONAL (10%–5%):** Diarrhea, akinesia, blurred vision, tachycardia, confusion, hostility, fatigue.

ADVERSE REACTIONS/ TOXIC EFFECTS

The risk of seizures increases in patients taking more than 150 mg/dose of bupropion, in patients with a history of bulimia or seizure disorders and in patients discontinuing drugs that may lower the seizure threshold.

NURSING CONSIDERATIONS

BASELINE ASSESSMENT

For those on long-term therapy, liver and renal function tests should be performed periodically.

INTERVENTION/EVALUATION

Closely supervise suicidal-risk patient during early therapy (as depression lessens, energy level improves, increasing suicide potential). Assess appearance, behavior, speech pattern, level of interest, mood.

PATIENT/FAMILY TEACHING

• Full therapeutic effect may be noted in 4 wk. • Avoid tasks that require alertness, motor skills until response to drug is established.

*busPIRone hydrochloride

byew-spear-own

(BuSpar, BuSpar Dividose, Buspirex ✦, Bustab ✦)

Do not confuse buspirone with bupropion.

CLASSIFICATION

PHARMACOTHERAPEUTIC: Nonbarbiturate. **CLINICAL:** Antianxiety (see p. 12C).

ACTION

Although its exact mechanism of action is unknown, this nonbarbiturate is thought to bind to serotonin and dopamine receptors in the CNS. The drug may also increase norepinephrine metabolism in the locus ceruleus. **Therapeutic Effect:** Produces anxiolytic effect.

PHARMACOKINETICS

Rapidly and completely absorbed from the GI tract. Protein binding: 95%. Undergoes extensive first-pass metabolism. Metabolized in the liver to active metabolite. Primarily excreted in urine. Not removed by hemodialysis. **Half-life:** 2–3 hr.

USES

Short-term management (up to 4 wk) of anxiety disorders. **OFF-LABEL:** Augmenting medication for antidepressants; management of aggression in mental retardation and secondary mental disorders, major depression, panic attack; premenstrual syndrome (aches, pain, fatigue, irritability).

PRECAUTIONS

CONTRAINDICATIONS: Concurrent use of MAOIs, severe hepatic or renal impairment. **CAUTIONS:** Renal or hepatic impairment.

⧖ **LIFESPAN CONSIDERATIONS: Pregnancy/Lactation:** Unknown if drug crosses placenta or is distributed in breast milk. **Pregnancy Category B. Children:** Safety and efficacy not established. **Elderly:** No age-related precautions noted.

INTERACTIONS

DRUG: Alcohol, other CNS depressants: Potentiates effects of buspirone and may increase sedation. **Erythromycin, itraconazole:** May increase buspirone blood concentration and risk of toxicity. **MAOIs:** May increase BP. **HERBAL: Gingko biloba, St. John's wort:** May cause changes in mental status. **Kava kava:** May increase sedation. **FOOD: Grapefruit, grapefruit juice:** May increase buspirone blood concentration and risk of toxicity. **LAB VALUES:** None known.

AVAILABILITY (Rx)

TABLETS: 5 mg (BuSpar), 7.5 mg, 10 mg (BuSpar), 15 mg (BuSpar, BuSpar Dividose), 30 mg (BuSpar Dividose).

ADMINISTRATION/HANDLING

PO
• Give without regard to food. • Tablets may be crushed.

INDICATIONS/ROUTES/DOSAGE

SHORT-TERM MANAGEMENT (UP TO 4 WK) OF ANXIETY DISORDERS
PO: ADULTS: 5 mg 2–3 times a day or 7.5 mg twice a day. May increase by 5 mg/day every 2–4 days. Maintenance: 15–30 mg/day in 2–3 divided doses. **Maximum:** 60 mg/day. **ELDERLY:** Initially, 5 mg twice a day. May increase by 5 mg/day every 2–3 days. **Maximum:** 60 mg/day. **CHILDREN:** Initially, 5 mg/day. May increase by 5 mg/day at weekly intervals. **Maximum:** 60 mg/day.

SIDE EFFECTS

FREQUENT (12%–6%): Dizziness, somnolence, nausea, headache. **OCCASIONAL (5%–2%):** Nervousness, fatigue, insomnia, dry mouth, lightheadedness, mood swings, blurred vision, poor concentration, diarrhea, paraesthesia. **RARE:** Muscle pain and stiffness, nightmares, chest pain, involuntary movements.

ADVERSE REACTIONS/ TOXIC EFFECTS

Buspirone does not appear to cause drug tolerance, psychological or physical dependence, or withdrawal syndrome. Overdose may produce severe nausea, vomiting, dizziness, drowsiness, abdominal distention, and excessive pupil contraction.

NURSING CONSIDERATIONS

BASELINE ASSESSMENT

Offer emotional support to anxious patient. Assess motor responses (agitation, trembling, tension), autonomic responses (cold, clammy hands; diaphoresis).

INTERVENTION/EVALUATION

For those on long-term therapy, liver and renal function tests, blood counts should be performed periodically. Assist with ambulation if drowsiness, lightheadedness occur. Evaluate for therapeutic response: calm, facial expression, decreased restlessness, insomnia.

PATIENT/FAMILY TEACHING

• Improvement may be noted in 7–10 days, but optimum therapeutic effect generally takes 3–4 wk. • Drowsiness usually disappears during continued therapy. • If dizziness occurs, change position slowly from recumbent to sitting position before standing. • Avoid tasks that require alertness, motor skills until response to drug is established.

busulfan

bew-**sull**-fan
(Busulfex, Myleran)
Do not confuse Myleran with Alkeran, Leukeran, or Mylicon.

◆CLASSIFICATION

PHARMACOTHERAPEUTIC: Alkylating agent. **CLINICAL:** Antineoplastic (see p. 72C).

ACTION

An alkylating agent that interferes with DNA replication and RNA synthesis. Cell cycle-phase nonspecific. **Therapeutic Effect:** Disrupts nucleic acid function and causes myelosuppression.

PHARMACOKINETICS

Completely absorbed from the GI tract. Protein binding: 33%. Metabolized in the liver. Primarily excreted in urine. Minimally removed by hemodialysis. **Half-life:** 2.5 hr.

USES

Treatment of chronic myelogenous leukemia (CML). **OFF-LABEL:** Treatment of acute myelocytic leukemia.

PRECAUTIONS

CONTRAINDICATIONS: Disease resistance to previous therapy with this drug. **EXTREME CAUTION:** Compromised bone marrow reserve. **CAUTIONS:** Chickenpox, herpes zoster, infection, history of gout. ⌛ **LIFESPAN CONSIDERATIONS: Pregnancy/Lactation:** If possible, avoid use during pregnancy, especially first trimester. May cause fetal harm. Unknown if distributed in breast milk. Breast-feeding not recommended. **Pregnancy Category D. Children/ Elderly:** No age-related precautions noted.

INTERACTIONS

DRUG: Antigout medications: May decrease the effects of these drugs. **Bone marrow depressants:** May increase the risk of myelosuppression. **Fosphenytoin, phenytoin:** May decrease plasma concentrations of busulfan. **Live-virus vaccines:** May potentiate virus replication, increase vaccine side effects, and decrease the patient's antibody response to the vaccine. **HERBAL:** None known. **FOOD:** None known. **LAB VALUES:** May decrease serum magnesium, potassium, phosphates, and sodium levels. May increase blood glucose, BUN, and serum calcium, alkaline phosphatase, bilirubin, creatinine, and ALT levels.

AVAILABILITY (Rx)

TABLETS (MYLERAN): 2 mg. **INJECTION SOLUTION (BUSULFAN):** 60-mg ampule.

ADMINISTRATION/HANDLING

◀ **ALERT** ▶ May be carcinogenic, mutagenic, or teratogenic. Handle with extreme care during administration. Use of gloves recommended. If contact occurs with skin/mucosa, wash thoroughly with water.

 IV

Reconstitution • Dilute with 0.9% NaCl or D₅W only. The diluent quantity must be 10 times the volume of busulfan (e.g., 9.3 ml busulfan must be diluted with 93 ml diluent). • Use filter to withdraw busulfan from ampule. • Add busulfan to calculated diluent. • Use infusion pump to administer busulfan.

Rate of administration • Infuse over 2 hr. • Before and after infusion, flush catheter line with 5 ml 0.9% NaCl or D₅W.

Storage • Refrigerate ampules. • Following dilution, stable for 8 hr at room temperature, 12 hr if refrigerated when diluted with 0.9% NaCl.

PO
• Give at same time each day. • Give on empty stomach if nausea/vomiting occur.

▦ IV INCOMPATIBILITIES

Don't mix busulfan with any other medications.

INDICATIONS/ROUTES/DOSAGE

REMISSION INDUCTION IN CML

PO: ADULTS, ELDERLY: 4–8 mg/day up to 12 mg/day. Maintenance: 1–4 mg/day to 2 mg/wk. Continue until WBC count is 10,000–20,000/mm^3, resume when WBC count reaches 50,000/mm^3. CHILDREN: 0.06–0.12 mg/kg/day. Maintenance: Titrate to maintain leukocyte count above 40,000/mm^3, reduce dose by 50% if count is 30,000–40,000/mm^3, and discontinue if the count is 20,000/mm^3 or less.

MARROW ABLATIVE CONDITIONING FOR BONE MARROW TRANSPLANTATION

IV: ADULTS, ELDERLY, CHILDREN WEIGHING MORE THAN 12 KG: 0.8 mg/kg/dose q6h for total of 16 doses. (Use IBW or ABW, whichever is lower). CHILDREN WEIGHING 12 KG OR LESS: 1.1 mg/kg/dose (IBW) q6h for 16 doses.
PO: ADULTS, ELDERLY, CHILDREN: 1 mg/kg/dose (IBW) q6h for 16 doses.

SIDE EFFECTS

EXPECTED (98%–72%): Nausea, stomatitis, vomiting, anorexia, insomnia, diarrhea, fever, abdominal pain, anxiety. **FREQUENT (69%–44%):** Headache, rash, asthenia, infection, chills, tachycardia, dyspepsia. **OCCASIONAL (38%–16%):** Constipation, dizziness, edema, pruritus, cough, dry mouth, depression, abdominal enlargement, pharyngitis, hiccups, back pain, alopecia, myalgia. **RARE (13%–5%):** Injection site pain, arthralgia, confusion, hypotension, lethargy.

ADVERSE REACTIONS/ TOXIC EFFECTS

Busulfan's major adverse effect is myelosuppression resulting in hematologic toxicity, as evidenced by anemia, severe leukopenia, and severe thrombocytopenia. Very high busulfan dosages may produce blurred vision, muscle twitching, and tonic-clonic seizures. Long-term therapy (more than 4 yr) may produce pulmonary syndrome ("busulfan lung"), characterized by persistent cough, congestion, crackles, and dyspnea. Hyperuricemia may produce uric acid nephropathy, renal calculi, and acute renal failure.

NURSING CONSIDERATIONS

BASELINE ASSESSMENT

CBC with differential, liver/renal function studies should be performed weekly (dosage based on hematologic values).

INTERVENTION/EVALUATION

Monitor lab values diligently for evidence of bone marrow depression. Assess mouth for onset of stomatitis (redness/ulceration of oral mucous membranes, gum inflammation, difficulty swallowing). Initiate antiemetics to prevent nausea/vomiting. Monitor daily bowel activity, stool consistency.

PATIENT/FAMILY TEACHING

• Maintain adequate daily fluid intake (may protect against renal impairment). • Report consistent cough, congestion, difficulty breathing. • Promptly report fever, sore throat, signs of local infection, unusual bruising/bleeding from any site. • Do not have immunizations without physician's approval (drug lowers body's resistance). • Avoid contact with those who have recently taken live virus vaccine. • Take at same time each day. • Contraception is recommended during therapy.

butenafine

(Mentax)
See Antifungals: topical (p. 44C)

butorphanol tartrate ▷

byew-**tore**-phen-awl
(Stadol, Stadol NS)

Do not confuse butorphanol with butabarbital or Stadol with Haldol.

◆CLASSIFICATION

PHARMACOTHERAPEUTIC: Opioid (**Schedule IV**). **CLINICAL:** Analgesic, anesthesia adjunct (see p. 127C).

ACTION

An opioid that binds to opiate receptor sites in the CNS. Reduces intensity of pain stimuli incoming from sensory nerve endings. Therapeutic Effect: Alters pain perception and emotional response to pain.

PHARMACOKINETICS

Route	Onset	Peak	Duration
IM	10–30 min	30–60 min	3–4 hr
IV	Less than 1 min	30 min	2–4 hr
Nasal	15 min	1–2 hr	4–5 hr

Rapidly absorbed after IM injection. Protein binding: 80%. Extensively metabolized in the liver. Primarily excreted in urine. Half-life: 2.5–4 hr.

USES

Management of pain (including postoperative pain). **Nasal:** Migraine headache pain. **Parenteral:** Preoperative, preanesthetic medication, supplement balanced anesthesia, relief of pain during labor.

PRECAUTIONS

CONTRAINDICATIONS: CNS disease that affects respirations, hypersensitivity to the preservative benzethonium chloride, physical dependence on other opioid analgesics, preexisting respiratory depression, pulmonary disease. **CAUTIONS:** Hepatic/renal impairment, elderly, debilitated, head injury, hypertension, use before biliary tract surgery (produces spasm of sphincter of Oddi), MI, narcotic dependence.

⧖ LIFESPAN CONSIDERATIONS: **Pregnancy/Lactation:** Readily crosses placenta. Distributed in breast milk. Breast-feeding not recommended. **Pregnancy Category C, D if used for prolonged time, high dose at term. Children:** Safety and efficacy not known in those younger than 18 yr. **Elderly:** May be more sensitive to effects; adjust dose and interval.

INTERACTIONS

DRUG: **Alcohol, CNS depressants:** May increase CNS or respiratory depression and hypotension. **Buprenorphine:** Effects may be decreased with buprenorphine. **MAOIs:** May produce severe, fatal reaction unless dose is reduced by ¼. HERBAL: None known. FOOD: None known. LAB VALUES: None known.

AVAILABILITY (Rx)

INJECTION (STADOL): 1 mg/ml, 2 mg/ml. **NASAL SPRAY (STADOL NS):** 10 mg/ml.

ADMINISTRATION/HANDLING

INTRANASAL

• Instruct patient to blow nose to clear nasal passages as much as possible. • Tilt head slightly forward, insert spray tip into nostril, pointing toward nasal passages, away from nasal septum. • Spray into nostril while holding other nostril closed, concurrently inspire through nose to permit medication as high into nasal passages as possible.

✱ IV INCOMPATIBILITIES

Amphotericin B complex (Abelcet, AmBisome, Amphotec).

IV COMPATIBILITIES

Atropine, diphenhydramine (Benadryl), droperidol (Inapsine), hydroxyzine (Vistaril), morphine, promethazine (Phenergan), propofol (Diprivan).

INDICATIONS/ROUTES/DOSAGE

ANALGESIA

IV: ADULTS: 0.5–2 mg q3–4h as needed. ELDERLY: 1 mg q4–6h as needed.
IM: ADULTS: 1–4 mg q3–4h as needed. ELDERLY: 1 mg q4–6h as needed.

MIGRAINE

NASAL: ADULTS: 1 mg or 1 spray in one nostril. May repeat in 60–90 min. May repeat 2-dose sequence q3–4h as needed. Alternatively, 2 mg or 1 spray each nostril if patient remains recumbent, may repeat in 3–4 hr.

SIDE EFFECTS

FREQUENT: Parenteral: Somnolence (43%), dizziness (19%). **Nasal:** Nasal congestion (13%), insomnia (11%). **OCCASIONAL: Parenteral (9%–3%):** Confusion, diaphoresis, clammy skin, lethargy, headache, nausea, vomiting, dry mouth. **Nasal (9%–3%):** Vasodilation, constipation, unpleasant taste, dyspnea, epistaxis, nasal irritation, upper respiratory tract infection, tinnitus. **RARE: Parenteral:** Hypotension, pruritus, blurred vision, sensation of heat, CNS stimulation, insomnia. **Nasal:** Hypertension, tremor, ear pain, paresthesia, depression, sinusitis.

ADVERSE REACTIONS/ TOXIC EFFECTS

Abrupt withdrawal after prolonged use may produce symptoms of narcotic withdrawal, such as abdominal cramping, rhinorrhea, lacrimation, anxiety, increased temperature, and piloerection or goose bumps. Overdose results in severe respiratory depression, skeletal muscle flaccidity, cyanosis, and extreme somnolence progressing to seizures, stupor, and coma. Tolerance to analgesic effect and physical dependence may occur with chronic use.

NURSING CONSIDERATIONS

BASELINE ASSESSMENT

Obtain vital signs before giving medication. If respirations are 12/min or less (20/min or less in children), withhold medication, contact physician. Assess onset, type, location, duration of pain. Effect of medication is reduced if full pain recurs before next dose. Protect from falls. During labor, assess fetal heart tones, uterine contractions.

INTERVENTION/EVALUATION

Monitor for change in respirations, BP, rate/quality of pulse. Initiate deep breathing, coughing exercises, particularly in those with impaired pulmonary function. Change patient's position q2–4h. Assess for clinical improvement, record onset of relief of pain.

PATIENT/FAMILY TEACHING

• Change positions slowly to avoid dizziness. • Avoid tasks that require alertness, motor skills until response to drug is established. • Instruct patient on proper use of nasal spray. • Avoid use of alcohol, CNS depressants.

Byetta, *see exenatide*

---

cabergoline

cab-**err**-go-leen
(Dostinex)

•CLASSIFICATION
CLINICAL: Antihyperprolactinemic.

ACTION
Agonist at dopamine D_2 receptors suppressing prolactin secretion. **Therapeutic Effect:** Shrinks prolactinomas, restores gonadal function.

PHARMACOKINETICS
Extensive tissue distribution. Protein binding: 40%–42%. Hydrolyzed to inactive metabolite. Excreted primarily in feces. **Half-life:** 63–69 hr.

USES
Treatment of hyperprolactinemic disorders, either idiopathic or due to pituitary adenomas.

PRECAUTIONS
CONTRAINDICATIONS: Uncontrolled hypertension, hypersensitivity to ergot alkaloids. **CAUTIONS:** Hepatic impairment.

⧗ **LIFESPAN CONSIDERATIONS: Pregnancy/Lactation:** Adequate studies not done. Unknown if distributed in breast milk. Not recommended during pregnancy. **Pregnancy Category B. Children/Elderly:** Safety and efficacy not established.

INTERACTIONS
DRUG: Other antihypertensives: May increase hypotensive effect if given concurrently. **HERBAL:** None known. **FOOD:** None known. **LAB VALUES:** None known.

AVAILABILITY (Rx)
TABLETS: 0.5 mg.

INDICATIONS/ROUTES/DOSAGE
HYPERPROLACTINEMIA
PO: ADULTS, ELDERLY: Initially, 0.25 mg twice a wk. May increase by 0.25 mg a wk at 4-wk intervals up to a maximum of 1 mg twice a wk according to patient's serum prolactin level.

SIDE EFFECTS
FREQUENT (29%): Nausea. **OCCASIONAL (20%–5%):** Headache, vertigo, dizziness, dyspepsia, postural hypotension, constipation. **RARE (4%–2%):** Vomiting, dry mouth, diarrhea, flatulence.

ADVERSE REACTIONS/ TOXIC EFFECTS
Overdosage may produce nasal congestion, syncope, hallucinations.

NURSING CONSIDERATIONS

BASELINE ASSESSMENT
Obtain baseline hepatic function tests.

INTERVENTION/EVALUATION
Monitor prolactin levels monthly until prolactin levels equalize.

PATIENT/FAMILY TEACHING
• To reduce hypotensive effect, rise slowly from lying to sitting position, permit legs to dangle momentarily before rising.

caffeine citrate

(Cafcit)

ACTION
Stimulates medullary respiratory center. Appears to increase sensitivity of respiratory center to stimulatory effects of CO_2. **Therapeutic Effect:** Increases alveolar ventilation, reducing severity, frequency of apneic episodes.

USES
Short-term treatment of apnea in premature infants from 28 wk to younger than 33 wk gestational age.

PRECAUTIONS
Pregnancy Category B.

AVAILABILITY (Rx)
INJECTION: 20 mg/ml. **ORAL SOLUTION:** 20 mg/ml.

INDICATIONS/ROUTES/DOSAGE
APNEA
PO, IV: Loading dose: 10–20 mg/kg as caffeine citrate (5–10 mg/kg as caffeine base). If theophylline given within previous 72 hr, a modified dose (50%–75%) may be given. Maintenance: 5 mg/kg/day as caffeine citrate (2.5 mg/kg/day as caffeine base). Dosage adjusted based on patient response.

SIDE EFFECTS
FREQUENT (10%–5%): Feeding intolerance, rash.

ADVERSE REACTIONS/ TOXIC EFFECTS
Sepsis, necrotizing enterocolitis may be noted.

NURSING CONSIDERATIONS

INTERVENTION/EVALUATION
Monitor respirations diligently. Assess skin for rash.

calcitonin

kal-sih-**toe**-nin

(Calcimar, Caltine ❁, Cibacalcin, Fortical, Miacalcin, Miacalcin Nasal)

Do not confuse calcitonin with calcitriol.

◆CLASSIFICATION
PHARMACOTHERAPEUTIC: Synthetic hormone. **CLINICAL:** Calcium regulator, bone resorption inhibitor, osteoporosis therapy.

ACTION
A synthetic hormone that decreases osteoclast activity in bones, decreases tubular reabsorption of sodium and calcium in the kidneys, and increases absorption of calcium in the GI tract. Therapeutic Effect: Regulates serum calcium concentrations.

PHARMACOKINETICS
Injection form rapidly metabolized (primarily in kidneys); primarily excreted in urine. Nasal form rapidly absorbed. Half-life: 70–90 min (injection); 43 min (nasal).

USES
Parenteral: Treatment of Paget's disease, hypercalcemia, postmenopausal osteoporosis, osteogenesis imperfecta. **Intranasal:** Postmenopausal osteoporosis. OFF-LABEL: Treatment of secondary osteoporosis due to drug therapy or hormone disturbance.

PRECAUTIONS
CONTRAINDICATIONS: Hypersensitivity to gelatin desserts or salmon protein. **CAUTIONS:** History of allergy, renal dysfunction.
⧖ LIFESPAN CONSIDERATIONS: **Pregnancy/Lactation:** Drug does not cross placenta; unknown if distributed in breast milk. Safe usage during lactation not established (inhibits lactation in animals). **Pregnancy Category C. Children:** Safety and efficacy not established. **Elderly:** No age-related precautions noted.

INTERACTIONS
DRUG: None known. **HERBAL:** None known. **FOOD:** None known. **LAB VALUES:** None known.

AVAILABILITY (Rx)

INJECTION (MIACALCIN): 200 international units/ml (calcitonin-salmon), 500 mg (calcitonin-human). **NASAL SPRAY (FORTICAL, MIACALCIN NASAL):** 200 international units/activation (calcitonin-salmon).

ADMINISTRATION/HANDLING

IM, SUBCUTANEOUS
• May be administered subcutaneously or IM. No more than 2-ml dose should be given IM. • Skin test should be performed before therapy in patients suspected of sensitivity to calcitonin. • Bedtime administration may reduce nausea, flushing.

INTRANASAL
• Refrigerate unopened nasal spray. Store at room temperature after initial use. • Instruct patient to clear nasal passages as much as possible. • Tilt head slightly forward, insert spray tip into nostril, pointing toward nasal passages, away from nasal septum. • Spray into nostril while patient holds other nostril closed and concurrently inspires through nose to permit medication as high into nasal passage as possible.

INDICATIONS/ROUTES/DOSAGE

SKIN TESTING BEFORE TREATMENT IN PATIENTS WITH SUSPECTED SENSITIVITY TO CALCITONIN-SALMON
INTRACUTANEOUS: ADULTS, ELDERLY: Prepare a 10-international units/ml dilution; withdraw 0.05 ml from a 200-international units/ml vial in a tuberculin syringe; fill up to 1 ml with 0.9% NaCl. Take 0.1 ml and inject intracutaneously on inner aspect of forearm. Observe after 15 min; a positive response is the appearance of more than mild erythema or wheal.

PAGET'S DISEASE
IM, SUBCUTANEOUS: ADULTS, ELDERLY: Initially, 100 international units/day. Maintenance: 50 international units/day or 50–100 international units every 1–3 days.
INTRANASAL: ADULTS, ELDERLY: 200–400 international units/day.

OSTEOPOROSIS IMPERFECTA
IM, SUBCUTANEOUS: ADULTS: 2 international units/kg 3 times a week.

POSTMENOPAUSAL OSTEOPOROSIS
IM, SUBCUTANEOUS: ADULTS, ELDERLY: 100 international units/day with adequate calcium and vitamin D intake.
INTRANASAL: ADULTS, ELDERLY: 200 international units/day as a single spray, alternating nostrils daily.

HYPERCALCEMIA
IM, SUBCUTANEOUS: ADULTS, ELDERLY: Initially, 4 international units/kg q12h; may increase to 8 international units/kg q12h if no response in 2 days; may further increase to 8 international units/kg q6h if no response in another 2 days.

SIDE EFFECTS

FREQUENT: IM, Subcutaneous (10%): Nausea (may occur 30 min after injection, usually diminishes with continued therapy), inflammation at injection site. **Nasal (12%–10%):** Rhinitis, nasal irritation, redness, sores. **OCCASIONAL: IM, Subcutaneous (5%–2%):** Flushing of face or hands. **Nasal (5%–3%):** Back pain, arthralgia, epistaxis, headache. **RARE: IM, Subcutaneous:** Epigastric discomfort, dry mouth, diarrhea, flatulence. **Nasal:** Itching of earlobes, pedal edema, rash, diaphoresis.

ADVERSE REACTIONS/ TOXIC EFFECTS

Patients with a protein allergy may develop a hypersensitivity reaction.

NURSING CONSIDERATIONS

BASELINE ASSESSMENT
Establish baseline electrolytes.

C

INTERVENTION/EVALUATION
Ensure rotation of injection sites; check for inflammation. Assess vertebral bone mass (document stabilization/improvement). Assess for allergic response: rash, urticaria, swelling, shortness of breath, tachycardia, hypotension.

PATIENT/FAMILY TEACHING
• Instruct patient and family on aseptic technique, proper injection of medication, including rotation of sites. • Nausea is transient and usually decreases with continued therapy. • Notify physician immediately if rash, itching, shortness of breath, significant nasal irritation occur. • Explain to the patient and family that improvement in biochemical abnormalities and bone pain usually occurs in the first few months of treatment. • Explain to patients with neurologic lesions, improvement may take more than a year.

---

calcium acetate
(PhosLo)
calcium carbonate
(Apo-Cal 🍁, Calsan 🍁, Caltrate, Caltrate 600 🍁, Dicarbosil, Maalox Quick Dissolve, OsCal 🍁, Os-Cal 500, Titralac, Tums)
calcium chloride
calcium citrate
(Citracal, Citracal Prenatal Rx, Cal-Citrate)
calcium glubionate
(Calcione, Calciquid)
calcium gluconate

kal-see-um

Do not confuse OsCal with Asacol, Citracal with Citrucel, or PhosLo with PhosChol.

◆CLASSIFICATION
PHARMACOTHERAPEUTIC: Electrolyte replenisher. **CLINICAL:** Antacid, antihypocalcemic, antihyperkalemic, antihypermagnesemic, antihyperphosphatemic (see p. 10C).

ACTION
An electrolyte that is essential for the function and integrity of the nervous, muscular, and skeletal systems. Calcium plays an important role in normal cardiac and renal function, respiration, blood coagulation, and cell membrane and capillary permeability. It helps regulate the release and storage of neurotransmitters and hormones, and it neutralizes or reduces gastric acid (increase pH). Calcium acetate combines with dietary phosphate to form insoluble calcium phosphate. **Therapeutic Effect:** Replaces calcium in deficiency states; controls hyperphosphatemia in end-stage renal disease.

PHARMACOKINETICS
Moderately absorbed from the small intestine (absorption depends on presence of vitamin D metabolites and patient's pH). Primarily eliminated in feces.

USES
Parenteral: Acute hypocalcemia (e.g., neonatal hypocalcemic tetany, alkalosis), electrolyte depletion, cardiac arrest (strengthens myocardial contractions), hyperkalemia (reverses cardiac depression), hypermagnesemia (aids in reversing CNS depression). **Calcium Carbonate:** Antacid, treatment and prevention of calcium deficiency or hyperphosphatemia. **Calcium Citrate:** Antacid, treatment and prevention of calcium deficiency or hyperphosphatemia. **Calcium Acetate:** Controls hyperphosphatemia in end-stage renal disease.

PRECAUTIONS

CONTRAINDICATIONS: Calcium renal calculi, digoxin toxicity, hypercalcemia, hypercalciuria, sarcoidosis, ventricular fibrillation. **Calcium Acetate:** Decreased renal function, hypoparathyroidism. **CAUTIONS:** Dehydration, history of renal calculi, chronic renal impairment, decreased cardiac function, ventricular fibrillation during cardiac resuscitation.

 LIFESPAN CONSIDERATIONS: Pregnancy/Lactation: Distributed in breast milk. Unknown whether calcium chloride or gluconate is distributed in breast milk. **Pregnancy Category C. Children:** Extreme irritation, possible tissue necrosis or sloughing with IV. Restrict IV use due to small vasculature. **Elderly:** Oral absorption may be decreased.

INTERACTIONS

DRUG: Digoxin: May increase the risk of arrhythmias. **Etidronate, gallium:** May antagonize the effects of these drugs. **Ketoconazole, phenytoin, tetracyclines:** May decrease the absorption of these drugs. **Magnesium (parenteral), methenamine:** May decrease the effects of these drugs. **HERBAL:** None known. **FOOD:** None known. **LAB VALUES:** May increase blood pH, and serum gastrin and calcium levels. May decrease serum phosphate and potassium levels.

AVAILABILITY

CALCIUM ACETATE
GELCAP (PHOSLO): 667 mg (equivalent to 169 mg elemental calcium). **TABLET (PHOSLO):** 667 mg (equivalent to 169 mg elemental calcium).
CALCIUM CARBONATE
TABLETS: equivalent to 500 mg elemental calcium (Os-Cal 500), equivalent to 600 mg elemental calcium (Caltrate 600). **TABLETS (CHEWABLE):** equivalent to 200 mg elemental calcium (Tums), equivalent to 500 mg elemental calcium

(Os-Cal 500), 600 mg (Maalox Quick Dissolve).
CALCIUM CHLORIDE
INJECTION: 10% (100 mg/ml) equivalent to 27.2 mg elemental calcium per ml.
CALCIUM CITRATE
TABLETS: 125 mg (Citracal Prenatal Rx), 250 mg (equivalent to 53 mg elemental calcium) (Cal-Citrate), 950 mg (equivalent to 200 mg elemental calcium) (Citracal).
CALCIUM GLUBIONATE
SYRUP: 1.8 g/5 ml (equivalent to 115 mg of elemental calcium per 5 ml).
CALCIUM GLUCONATE
INJECTION: 10% (equivalent to 9 mg elemental calcium per ml).

ADMINISTRATION/HANDLING

IV

DILUTION

Calcium chloride • May give undiluted or may dilute with equal amount 0.9% NaCl or sterile water for injection.

Calcium gluconate • May give undiluted or may dilute in up to 1,000 ml NaCl.

Rate of administration

Calcium chloride • Give by slow IV push: 0.5–1 ml/min (rapid administration may produce bradycardia, metallic or chalky taste, drop in BP, sensation of heat, peripheral vasodilation).

Calcium gluconate • Give by IV push: 0.5–1 ml/min (rapid administration may produce vasodilation, drop in BP, arrhythmias, syncope, cardiac arrest). • Maximum rate for intermittent IV infusion is 200 mg/min (e.g., 10 ml/min when 1 g diluted with 50 ml diluent).

Storage • Store at room temperature.
PO
• Take tablets with full glass of water 0.5–1 hr after meals. Give syrup before meals (increases absorption), diluted in juice, water. • Chew chewable tablets well before swallowing.

C

⊞ IV INCOMPATIBILITIES

Calcium chloride: Amphotericin B complex (Abelcet, AmBisone, Amphotec), propofol (Diprivan), sodium bicarbonate. **Calcium gluconate:** Amphotericin B complex (Abelcet, AmBisome, Amphotec), fluconazole (Diflucan).

IV COMPATIBILITIES

Calcium chloride: Amikacin (Amikin), dobutamine (Dobutrex), lidocaine, milrinone (Primacor), morphine, norepinephrine (Levophed). **Calcium gluconate:** Ampicillin, aztreonam (Azactam), cefazolin (Ancef), cefepime (Maxipime), ciprofloxacin (Cipro), dobutamine (Dobutrex), enalapril (Vasotec), famotidine (Pepcid), furosemide (Lasix), heparin, lidocaine, magnesium sulfate, meropenem (Merrem IV), midazolam (Versed), milrinone (Primacor), norepinephrine (Levophed), piperacillin and tazobactam (Zosyn), potassium chloride, propofol (Diprivan).

INDICATIONS/ROUTES/DOSAGE

HYPERPHOSPHATEMIA

PO (CALCIUM ACETATE): ADULTS, ELDERLY: 2 tablets 3 times a day with meals. May increase gradually to bring serum phosphate level to less than 6 mg/dl as long as hypercalcemia does not develop.

HYPOCALCEMIA

PO (CALCIUM CARBONATE): ADULTS, ELDERLY: 1–2 g/day in 3–4 divided doses. CHILDREN: 45–65 mg/kg/day in 3–4 divided doses.

PO (CALCIUM GLUBIONATE): ADULTS, ELDERLY: 6–18 g/day in 4–6 divided doses. CHILDREN, INFANTS: 0.6–2 g/kg/day in 4 divided doses. NEONATES: 1.2 g/kg/day in 4–6 divided doses.

IV (CALCIUM CHLORIDE): ADULTS, ELDERLY: 0.5–1 g repeated q4–6h as needed. CHILDREN: 2.5–5 mg/kg/dose in q4–6h.

IV (CALCIUM GLUCONATE): ADULTS, ELDERLY: 2–15 g/24 hr. CHILDREN: 200–500 mg/kg/day.

ANTACID

PO (CALCIUM CARBONATE): ADULTS, ELDERLY: 1–2 tabs (5–10 ml) in q2h as needed.

OSTEOPOROSIS

PO (CALCIUM CARBONATE): ADULTS, ELDERLY: 1,200 mg/day.

CARDIAC ARREST

IV (CALCIUM CHLORIDE): ADULTS, ELDERLY: 2–4 mg/kg. May repeat q10 min. CHILDREN: 20 mg/kg. May repeat in 10 min.

HYPOCALCEMIA TETANY

IV (CALCIUM CHLORIDE): ADULTS, ELDERLY: 1 g may repeat in 6 hr. CHILDREN: 10 mg/kg over 5–10 min. May repeat in q6–8h.

IV (CALCIUM GLUCONATE): ADULTS, ELDERLY: 1–3 g until therapeutic response achieved. CHILDREN: 100–200 mg/kg/dose in 6–8 hr.

SUPPLEMENT

PO (CALCIUM CITRATE): ADULTS, ELDERLY: 0.5–2 g 2–4 times a day.

SIDE EFFECTS

FREQUENT: PO: Chalky taste. **Parenteral:** Hypotension; flushing; feeling of warmth; nausea; vomiting; pain, rash, redness, or burning at injection site; diaphoresis. **OCCASIONAL: PO:** Mild constipation, fecal impaction, peripheral edema, metabolic alkalosis (muscle pain, restlessness, slow breathing, altered taste). **Calcium Carbonate:** Milk-alkali syndrome (headache, decreased appetite, nausea, vomiting, unusual tiredness). **RARE:** Difficult or painful urination.

ADVERSE REACTIONS/ TOXIC EFFECTS

Hypercalcemia is a serious adverse effect of calcium acetate use. Early signs include constipation, headache, dry mouth, increased thirst, irritability, decreased appetite, metallic taste, fatigue, weakness, and depression. Later signs include confusion, somnolence, hypertension, photosensitivity, arrhythmias, nausea, vomiting, and increased painful urination.

NURSING CONSIDERATIONS

BASELINE ASSESSMENT
Assess BP, EKG and cardiac rhythm, renal function, serum magnesium, phosphate, potassium concentrations.

INTERVENTION/EVALUATION
Monitor BP, EKG, cardiac rhythm, serum magnesium, phosphate, potassium, renal function. Monitor serum, urine calcium concentrations. Monitor for signs of hypercalcemia.

PATIENT/FAMILY TEACHING
• Stress importance of diet. • Take tablets with full glass of water, $\frac{1}{2}$–1 hr after meals. • Give liquid before meals. • Do not take within 1–2 hr of other oral medications, fiber-containing foods. • Avoid excessive alcohol, tobacco, caffeine.

calfactant

cal-**fac**-tant
(Infasurf)

CLASSIFICATION
PHARMACOTHERAPEUTIC: Natural lung extract. **CLINICAL:** Pulmonary surfactant.

ACTION
A natural lung extract that reduces alveolar surface tension, stabilizing the alveoli. **Therapeutic Effect:** Restores surface activity to infant lungs, improves lung compliance and respiratory gas exchange.

PHARMACOKINETICS
No studies have been performed.

USES
Prevention of respiratory distress syndrome (RDS) in premature infants younger than 29 wk of gestational age; treatment of premature infants younger than 72 hr of age who develop RDS and require endotracheal intubation.

PRECAUTIONS
CONTRAINDICATIONS: None known. **CAUTIONS:** Hypersensitivity to calfactant.

⧗ **LIFESPAN CONSIDERATIONS: Pregnancy/Lactation, Elderly:** Not indicated in these patient populations. **Pregnancy Category: This drug is not indicated for use in pregnant women. Children:** Used only in neonates. No age-related precautions noted.

INTERACTIONS
DRUG: None known. **HERBAL:** None known. **FOOD:** None known. **LAB VALUES:** None known.

AVAILABILITY (Rx)
INTRATRACHEAL SUSPENSION: 35-mg/ml vials.

ADMINISTRATION/HANDLING
INTRATRACHEAL
• Refrigerate. • Unopened, unused vials may be returned to refrigerator only once after having been warmed to room temperature. • Do not shake. • Enter vial only once, discard unused suspension.

INDICATIONS/ROUTES/DOSAGE
RDS
INTRATRACHEAL: NEONATES: 3 ml/kg of birth weight administered as soon as possible after birth in 2 doses of

C

1.5 ml/kg. Repeat 3-ml/kg doses, up to a total of 3 doses given 12 hr apart.

SIDE EFFECTS

FREQUENT: Cyanosis (65%), airway obstruction (39%), bradycardia (34%), reflux of surfactant into endotracheal tube (21%), need for manual ventilation (16%). **OCCASIONAL:** Need for reintubation (3%).

ADVERSE REACTIONS/ TOXIC EFFECTS

None known.

NURSING CONSIDERATIONS

BASELINE ASSESSMENT

Drug must be administered in highly supervised setting. Clinicians in charge of care of neonate must be experienced with intubation, ventilator management. Offer emotional support to parents.

INTERVENTION/EVALUATION

Monitor infant with arterial or transcutaneous measurement of systemic O_2, CO_2. Assess lung sounds for rales, moist breath sounds.

Camptosar, *see* irinotecan

Cancidas, *see caspofungin*

---

candesartan cilexetil

kan-de-**sar**-tan sill-**ex**-eh-til (Atacand)

FIXED-COMBINATION(S)

Atacand HCT: candesartan/hydrochlorothiazide (a diuretic): 16 mg/12.5 mg; 32 mg/12.5 mg.

◆CLASSIFICATION

PHARMACOTHERAPEUTIC: Angiotensin II receptor antagonist. **CLINICAL:** Antihypertensive (see p. 8C).

ACTION

An angiotensin II receptor, type AT_1, antagonist that blocks the vasoconstrictor and aldosterone-secreting effects of angiotensin II, inhibiting the binding of angiotensin II to the AT_1 receptors. Therapeutic Effect: Causes vasodilation, decreases peripheral resistance, and decreases BP.

PHARMACOKINETICS

Route	Onset	Peak	Duration
PO	2–3 hr	6–8 hr	Greater than 24 hr

Rapidly, completely absorbed. Protein binding: greater than 99%. Undergoes minor hepatic metabolism to inactive metabolite. Excreted unchanged in urine and in the feces through the biliary system. Not removed by hemodialysis. Half-life: 9 hr.

USES

Treatment of hypertension alone or in combination with other antihypertensives, heart failure (reduces risk of death from cardiovascular causes, reduce hospitalization for heart failure).

PRECAUTIONS

CONTRAINDICATIONS: Hypersensitivity to candesartan. **CAUTIONS:** Severe CHF, dehydration (increased risk for hypotension), renal/hepatic impairment, renal artery stenosis.

✐ see color pill atlas   ✒ herb   <u>underlined</u> – top prescribed drug

⧗ **LIFESPAN CONSIDERATIONS: Pregnancy/Lactation:** Unknown if distributed in breast milk. May cause fetal/neonatal morbidity/mortality. **Pregnancy Category C (D if used in second or third trimester). Children:** Safety and efficacy not established. **Elderly:** No age-related precautions noted.

INTERACTIONS

DRUG: Lithium: May increase the risk of lithium toxicity. **HERBAL: Ma huang, yohimbe:** May reduce the effectiveness of candesartan. **FOOD:** None known. **LAB VALUES:** May increase BUN, serum alkaline phosphatase, serum bilirubin, serum creatinine, AST, and ALT levels. May decrease blood Hgb and Hct levels.

AVAILABILITY (Rx)

TABLETS: 4 mg, 8 mg, 16 mg, 32 mg.

ADMINISTRATION/HANDLING

PO
• Give without regard to food.

INDICATIONS/ROUTES/DOSAGE

HYPERTENSION ALONE OR IN COMBINATION WITH OTHER ANTIHYPERTENSIVES
PO: ADULTS, ELDERLY, PATIENTS WITH MILDLY IMPAIRED LIVER OR KIDNEY FUNCTION: Initially, 16 mg once a day in those who are not volume depleted. Can be given once or twice a day with total daily doses of 8–32 mg. Give lower dosage in those treated with diuretics or with severely impaired renal function.

HEART FAILURE
PO: ADULTS, ELDERLY: Initially, 4 mg once daily. May double dose at approximately 2-wk intervals up to a target dose of 32 mg/day.

SIDE EFFECTS

OCCASIONAL (6%–3%): Upper respiratory tract infection, dizziness, back and leg pain. **RARE (2%–1%):** Pharyngitis, rhinitis, headache, fatigue, diarrhea, nausea, dry cough, peripheral edema.

ADVERSE REACTIONS/ TOXIC EFFECTS

Overdosage may manifest as hypotension and tachycardia. Bradycardia occurs less often. Institute supportive measures.

NURSING CONSIDERATIONS

BASELINE ASSESSMENT

Obtain BP, apical pulse immediately before each dose, in addition to regular monitoring (be alert to fluctuations). If excessive reduction in BP occurs, place patient in supine position, feet slightly elevated. Question possibility of pregnancy (see Pregnancy Category). Assess medication history (especially diuretic). Question for history of hepatic/renal impairment, renal artery stenosis. Obtain BUN, serum creatinine, AST, ALT, alkaline phosphatase, bilirubin, Hgb, Hct.

INTERVENTION/EVALUATION

Maintain hydration (offer fluids frequently). Assess for evidence of upper respiratory infection. Assist with ambulation if dizziness occurs. Monitor all serum levels. Assess BP for hypertension/hypotension.

PATIENT/FAMILY TEACHING

• Inform female patient regarding consequences of second- and third-trimester exposure to candesartan. • Report pregnancy to physician as soon as possible. • Avoid tasks that require alertness, motor skills until response to drug is established. • Report any sign of infection (sore throat, fever). • Do not stop taking medication. • Explain need for lifelong control. • Caution against exercising during hot weather (risk of dehydration, hypotension).

capecitabine

cap-eh-**site**-ah-bean

(Xeloda)

Do not confuse Xeloda with Xenical.

◆ CLASSIFICATION

PHARMACOTHERAPEUTIC: Antimetabolite. **CLINICAL:** Antineoplastic (see p. 72C).

ACTION

An antimetabolite that is enzymatically converted to 5-fluorouracil (5-FU). Inhibits enzymes necessary for synthesis of essential cellular components. Therapeutic Effect: Interferes with DNA synthesis, RNA processing, and protein synthesis.

PHARMACOKINETICS

Readily absorbed from the GI tract. Protein binding: less than 60%. Metabolized in the liver. Primarily excreted in urine. Half-life: 45 min.

USES

Treatment of metastatic breast cancer resistant to other therapy, colon cancer. Adjuvant (post-surgery) treatment of Dukes' C colon cancer.

PRECAUTIONS

CONTRAINDICATIONS: Severe renal impairment, dihydropyrimidine dehydrogenase (DPD) deficiency, hypersensitivity to 5-FU. **CAUTIONS:** Existing bone marrow depression, chickenpox, herpes zoster, hepatic impairment, moderate renal impairment, previous cytotoxic therapy/radiation therapy.

LIFESPAN CONSIDERATIONS: Pregnancy/Lactation: May be harmful to fetus. Unknown if distributed in breast milk. **Pregnancy Category D.**

Children: Safety and efficacy in those younger than 18 yr not established. **Elderly:** May be more sensitive to GI side effects.

INTERACTIONS

DRUG: **Phenytoin:** May increase phenytoin levels and associated phenytoin toxicity. **Warfarin:** May alter the effects of warfarin. HERBAL: None known. FOOD: None known. LAB VALUES: May increase serum alkaline phosphatase, bilirubin, AST, and ALT levels. May decrease blood Hct, Hgb level, and WBC count.

AVAILABILITY (Rx)

TABLETS: 150 mg, 500 mg.

ADMINISTRATION/HANDLING

• Give within 30 min of a meal.

INDICATIONS/ROUTES/DOSAGE

METASTATIC BREAST CANCER, COLON CANCER, ADJUVANT (POST-SURGERY) TREATMENT OF DUKES' C COLON CANCER

PO: ADULTS, ELDERLY: Initially, 2,500 mg/m^2/day in 2 equally divided doses approximately q12h for 2 wk. Follow with a 1-wk rest period; given in 3-wk cycles. Administer 950 mg/m^2 twice a day in patients with creatinine clearance of 30–50 ml/min (not recommended in patients with creatinine clearance less than 30 ml/min).

DOSAGE IN RENAL IMPAIRMENT
Creatinine clearance 50–80 ml/min: No adjustment. **Creatinine clearance 30–49 ml/min:** 75% of normal dose. **Creatinine clearance less than 30 ml/min:** Not recommended.

SIDE EFFECTS

FREQUENT (greater than 5%): Diarrhea (sometimes severe), nausea, vomiting, stomatitis, hand-and-foot syndrome (painful palmar-plantar swelling with paresthesia, erythema, and blistering), fatigue, anorexia, dermatitis. **OCCASIONAL (less than 5%):** Constipation, dyspepsia, nail disorder, headache, dizziness, insomnia, edema, myalgia.

ADVERSE REACTIONS/ TOXIC EFFECTS

Serious reactions may include myelosuppression (evidenced by neutropenia, thrombocytopenia, and anemia), cardiovascular toxicity (marked by angina, cardiomyopathy, and deep vein thrombosis), respiratory toxicity (marked by dyspnea, epistaxis, and pneumonia), and lymphedema.

NURSING CONSIDERATIONS

BASELINE ASSESSMENT

Assess sensitivity to capecitabine or 5-fluorouracil. Obtain baseline Hgb, Hct, serum chemistries.

INTERVENTION/EVALUATION

Monitor for severe diarrhea; if dehydration occurs, fluid and electrolyte replacement therapy should be ordered. Assess hands/feet for erythema (chemotherapy induced). Monitor CBC for evidence of bone marrow depression. Monitor for blood dyscrasias (fever, sore throat, signs of local infection, unusual bruising/bleeding from any site), symptoms of anemia (excessive fatigue, weakness).

PATIENT/FAMILY TEACHING

• Inform patient of potential for, and need to notify physician if, nausea, vomiting, possibly severe diarrhea, hand-and-foot syndrome, stomatitis occur. • Do not have immunizations without physician's approval (drug lowers body's resistance). • Avoid contact with those who have recently received live virus vaccine. • Promptly report fever higher than 100.5°F, sore throat, signs of local infection, unusual bruising/bleeding from any site.

Capoten, *see captopril*

C

capsaicin

cap-**say**-sin

(ArthriCare, Axsain, Capzasin-P, Zostrix)

Do not confuse Zostrix with Zestril or Zovirax.

◆CLASSIFICATION

PHARMACOTHERAPEUTIC: Counterirritant. **CLINICAL:** Topical analgesic.

ACTION

Depletes/prevents reaccumulation of the chemomediator of pain impulses (substance P) from peripheral sensory neurons to CNS. **Therapeutic Effect:** Relieves pain.

USES

Treatment of neuralgia (e.g., pain with herpes zoster, painful diabetic neuropathy), osteoarthritis, rheumatoid arthritis. **OFF-LABEL:** Treatment of neurogenic pain, pruritis associated with hemodialysis and exposure to water.

PRECAUTIONS

CONTRAINDICATIONS: None known. **CAUTIONS:** For external use only. **Pregnancy Category C.**

INTERACTIONS

DRUG: None known. **HERBAL:** None known. **FOOD:** None known. **LAB VALUES:** None known.

AVAILABILITY (Rx)

CREAM: ARTHRICARE, AXSAIN, CAPZASIN-P, ZOSTRIX: 0.025%; **CAPZASIN-HP,**

C

ZOSTRIX HP: 0.075%. **LOTION: ARTHRI-CARE:** 0.025%. **STICK: ZOSTRIX:** 0.025%; **ZOSTRIX HP:** 0.075%.

INDICATIONS/ROUTES/DOSAGE
USUAL TOPICAL DOSAGE
TOPICAL: ADULTS, ELDERLY, CHILDREN 2 YR AND OLDER: Apply directly to affected area 3–4 times a day. Continue for 14–28 days for optimal clinical response.

SIDE EFFECTS
FREQUENT (greater than 30%): Burning, stinging, erythema at application site.

ADVERSE REACTIONS/ TOXIC EFFECTS
None known.

NURSING CONSIDERATIONS

PATIENT/FAMILY TEACHING
• Avoid contact with eyes, broken or irritated skin. • Transient burning may occur on application; usually disappears after 72 hr. • Wash hands immediately after application. • If there is no improvement or condition deteriorates after 28 days, discontinue use and consult physician.

captopril

cap-toe-pril
(Capoten, Novo-Captoril ✦)
Do not confuse captopril with Capitrol.

FIXED-COMBINATION(S)
Capozide: captopril/hydrochlorothiazide (a diuretic): 25 mg/15 mg; 25 mg/25 mg; 50 mg/15 mg; 50 mg/25 mg.

◆CLASSIFICATION
PHARMACOTHERAPEUTIC: Angiotensin-converting enzyme (ACE) inhibitor. **CLINICAL:** Antihypertensive, vasodilator (see p. 7C).

ACTION
An ACE inhibitor that suppresses the renin-angiotensin-aldosterone system and prevents conversion of angiotensin I to angiotensin II, a potent vasoconstrictor; may also inhibit angiotensin II at local vascular and renal sites. Decreases plasma angiotensin II, increases plasma renin activity, and decreases aldosterone secretion. **Therapeutic Effect:** Reduces peripheral arterial resistance, pulmonary capillary wedge pressure; improves cardiac output and exercise tolerance.

PHARMACOKINETICS

Route	Onset	Peak	Duration
PO	0.25 hr	0.5–1.5 hr	Dose-related

Rapidly, well absorbed from the GI tract (absorption is decreased in the presence of food). Protein binding: 25%–30%. Metabolized in the liver. Primarily excreted in urine. Removed by hemodialysis. **Half-life:** less than 3 hr (increased in those with impaired renal function).

USES
Treatment of hypertension, CHF, diabetic nephropathy, post-MI for prevention of ventricular failure. **OFF-LABEL:** Diagnosis of anatomic renal artery stenosis, hypertensive crisis, rheumatoid arthritis.

PRECAUTIONS
CONTRAINDICATIONS: History of angioedema from previous treatment with ACE inhibitors. **CAUTIONS:** Renal

impairment, those with sodium depletion or on diuretic therapy, dialysis, hypovolemia, coronary/cerebrovascular insufficiency.

⧗ **LIFESPAN CONSIDERATIONS: Pregnancy/Lactation:** Crosses placenta; distributed in breast milk. May cause fetal/neonatal mortality/morbidity. **Pregnancy Category C (D if used in second or third trimester). Children:** Safety and efficacy not established. **Elderly:** May be more sensitive to hypotensive effects; caution recommended.

INTERACTIONS

DRUG: Alcohol, antihypertensives, diuretics: May increase the effects of captopril. **Lithium:** May increase lithium blood concentration and risk of lithium toxicity. **NSAIDs:** May decrease the effects of captopril. **Potassium-sparing diuretics, potassium supplements:** May cause hyperkalemia. **HERBAL:** None known. **FOOD: All food:** Food significantly reduces drug absorption by 30%–40%. **LAB VALUES:** May increase BUN, serum alkaline phosphatase, serum bilirubin, serum creatinine, serum potassium, AST, and ALT levels. May decrease serum sodium levels. May cause positive antinuclear antibody titer.

AVAILABILITY (Rx)

TABLETS: 12.5 mg, 25 mg, 50 mg, 100 mg.

ADMINISTRATION/HANDLING
PO
• Best taken 1 hr before meals for maximum absorption (food significantly decreases drug absorption). • Tablets may be crushed.

INDICATIONS/ROUTES/DOSAGE
HYPERTENSION
PO: ADULTS, ELDERLY: Initially, 12.5–25 mg 2–3 times a day. After 1–2 wk, may increase to 50 mg 2–3 times a day. Diuretic may be added if no response in additional 1–2 wk. If taken in combination with diuretic, may increase to 100–150 mg 2–3 times a day after 1–2 wk. Maintenance: 25–150 mg 2–3 times a day. **Maximum:** 450 mg/day.

CHF
PO: ADULTS, ELDERLY: Initially, 6.25–25 mg 3 times a day. Increase to 50 mg 3 times a day. After at least 2 wk, may increase to 50–100 mg 3 times a day. **Maximum:** 450 mg/day.

POST-MYOCARDIAL INFARCTION, IMPAIRED LIVER FUNCTION
PO: ADULTS, ELDERLY: 6.25 mg a day, then 12.5 mg 3 times a day. Increase to 25 mg 3 times a day over several days up to 50 mg 3 times a day over several weeks.

DIABETIC NEPHROPATHY PREVENTION OF KIDNEY FAILURE
PO: ADULTS, ELDERLY: 25 mg 3 times a day. CHILDREN: Initially 0.3–0.5 mg/kg/dose titrated up to a maximum of 6 mg/kg/day in 2–4 divided doses. NEONATES: Initially, 0.05–0.1 mg/kg/dose q8–24h titrated up to 0.5 mg/kg/dose given q6–24h.

DOSAGE IN RENAL IMPAIRMENT
Creatinine clearance 10–50 ml/min: 75% of normal dosage. **Creatinine clearance less than 10 ml/min:** 50% of normal dosage.

SIDE EFFECTS
FREQUENT (7%–4%): Rash. **OCCASIONAL (4%–2%):** Pruritus, dysgeusia (altered taste). **RARE (less than 2%–0.5%):** Headache, cough, insomnia, dizziness, fatigue, paraesthesia, malaise, nausea, diarrhea or constipation, dry mouth, tachycardia.

ADVERSE REACTIONS/ TOXIC EFFECTS
Excessive hypotension ("first-dose syncope") may occur in patients with CHF and in those who are severely salt

and volume depleted. Angioedema (swelling of face and lips) and hyperkalemia occur rarely. Agranulocytosis and neutropenia may be noted in those with collagen vascular disease, including scleroderma and systemic lupus erythematosus, and impaired renal function. Nephrotic syndrome may be noted in those with history of renal disease.

NURSING CONSIDERATIONS

BASELINE ASSESSMENT

Obtain BP immediately before each dose, in addition to regular monitoring (be alert to fluctuations). If excessive reduction in BP occurs, place patient in supine position with legs elevated. In patients with prior renal disease or receiving dosages greater than 150 mg/day, urine test for protein by dipstick method should be made with first urine of day before therapy begins and periodically thereafter. In patients with renal impairment, autoimmune disease, or taking drugs that affect leukocytes or immune response, CBC should be performed before beginning therapy, q2wk for 3 mo, then periodically thereafter.

INTERVENTION/EVALUATION

Assess skin for rash, pruritus. Assist with ambulation if dizziness occurs. Monitor urinalysis for proteinuria. Assess for anorexia secondary to altered taste perception. Monitor serum potassium levels in those on concurrent diuretic therapy.

PATIENT/FAMILY TEACHING

• Several weeks may be needed for full therapeutic effect of BP reduction. • Skipping doses or voluntarily discontinuing drug may produce severe, rebound hypertension. • Avoid alcohol.

carbachol

(Isopto-Carbachol)

See Antiglaucoma agents (p. 46C)

carbamazepine

car-bah-**may**-zeh-peon

(Apo-Carbamazepine ✦, Carbatrol, Epitol, Equetro, Tegretol, Tegretol XR)

Do not confuse Tegretol with Cartrol, Topamax, Toprol XL, Toradol, or Trental.

CLASSIFICATION

PHARMACOTHERAPEUTIC: Iminostilbene derivative. **CLINICAL:** Anticonvulsant, antineuralgic, antimanic, antipsychotic (see p. 33C).

ACTION

An iminostilbene derivative that decreases sodium and calcium ion influx into neuronal membranes, reducing posttetanic potentiation at synapses. **Therapeutic Effect:** Reduces seizure activity.

PHARMACOKINETICS

Slowly and completely absorbed from the GI tract. Protein binding: 75%. Metabolized in the liver to active metabolite. Primarily excreted in urine. Not removed by hemodialysis. **Half-life:** 25–65 hr (decreased with chronic use).

USES

Partial seizures with complex symptomatology, generalized tonic-clonic seizures, mixed seizure patterns, pain relief of trigeminal neuralgia, diabetic neuropathy. **OFF-LABEL:** Treatment of alcohol withdrawal, diabetes insipidus, neurogenic pain, psychotic disorders.

PRECAUTIONS

CONTRAINDICATIONS: Concomitant use of MAOIs, history of myelosuppression,

---

hypersensitivity to tricyclic antidepressants. **CAUTIONS:** Mental illness, increased intraocular pressure (IOP), history of atypical absence seizures, cardiac, hepatic, renal impairment.

⧗ **LIFESPAN CONSIDERATIONS: Pregnancy/Lactation:** Crosses placenta; distributed in breast milk. Accumulates in fetal tissue. **Pregnancy Category D. Children:** Behavioral changes more likely to occur. **Elderly:** More susceptible to confusion, agitation, AV block, bradycardia, syndrome of inappropriate antidiuretic hormone (SIADH).

INTERACTIONS

DRUG: Anticoagulants, clarithromycin, diltiazem, erythromycin, estrogens, propoxyphene, quinidine, steroids: May decrease the effects of these drugs. **Antipsychotics, haloperidol, tricyclic antidepressants:** May increase CNS depressant effects. **Cimetidine:** May increase carbamazepine blood concentration and risk of toxicity. **Isoniazid:** May increase metabolism of isoniazid; may increase carbamazepine blood concentration and risk of toxicity. **MAOIs:** May cause seizures and hypertensive crisis. **Other anticonvulsants, barbiturates, benzodiazepines, valproic acid:** May increase the metabolism of these drugs. **Verapamil:** May increase the toxicity of carbamazepine. **HERBAL:** None known. **FOOD: Grapefruit, grapefruit juice:** May increase the absorption and blood concentration of carbamazepine. **LAB VALUES:** May increase BUN and blood glucose levels and serum alkaline phosphatase, bilirubin, AST, ALT, protein, cholesterol, HDL, and triglyceride levels. May decrease serum calcium and thyroid hormone (T_3, T_4, T_4 index) levels. Therapeutic serum level is 4–12 mcg/ml; toxic serum level is greater than 12 mcg/ml.

AVAILABILITY (Rx)

CAPSULES (EXTENDED-RELEASE): 100 mg (Carbatrol, Equetro), 200 mg (Carbatrol, Equetro), 300 mg (Carbatrol, Equetro), 400 mg (Carbatrol). **SUSPENSION (TEGRETOL):** 100 mg/5 ml. **TABLETS (EPITOL, TEGRETOL):** 200 mg. **TABLETS (CHEWABLE [TEGRETOL]):** 100 mg. **TABLETS (EXTENDED-RELEASE [TEGRETOL XR]):** 100 mg, 200 mg, 400 mg.

ADMINISTRATION/HANDLING
PO
• Store oral suspension, tablets at room temperature. • Give with meals to reduce risk of GI distress. • Shake oral suspension well. Do not administer simultaneously with other liquid medicine. • Do not crush extended-release tablets.

INDICATIONS/ROUTES/DOSAGE
SEIZURE CONTROL
PO: ADULTS, CHILDREN OLDER THAN 12 YR: Initially, 200 mg twice a day. May increase dosage by 200 mg/day at weekly intervals. Range: 400–1,200 mg/day in 2–4 divided doses. **Maximum:** 1.6–2.4 g/day. CHILDREN 6–12 YR: Initially, 100 mg twice a day. May increase by 100 mg/day at weekly intervals. Range: 400–800 mg/day. **Maximum:** 1,000 mg/day. CHILDREN YOUNGER THAN 6 YR: Initially 5 mg/kg/day. May increase at weekly intervals to 20 mg/kg/day up to 20 mg/kg/day. **Maximum:** 35 mg/kg/day. ELDERLY: Initially 100 mg 1–2 times a day. May increase by 100 mg/day at weekly intervals. Usual dose 400–1,000 mg/day.

TRIGEMINAL NEURALGIA, DIABETIC NEUROPATHY
PO: ADULTS: Initially, 100 mg twice a day. May increase by 100 mg twice a day up to 400–800 mg/day. **Maximum:** 1200 mg/day. ELDERLY: Initially 100 mg 1–2 times a day. May increase by 100 mg/day at weekly intervals. Usual dose 400–1,000 mg/day.

BIPOLAR DISORDER

PO: ADULTS, ELDERLY: Initially, 400 mg/day in 2 divided doses. May adjust dose in 200 mg increments. **Maximum:** 1,600 mg/day in divided doses.

SIDE EFFECTS

FREQUENT: Drowsiness, dizziness, nausea, vomiting. **OCCASIONAL:** Visual abnormalities (spots before eyes, difficulty focusing, blurred vision), dry mouth or pharynx, tongue irritation, headache, fluid retention, diaphoresis, constipation or diarrhea, behavioral changes in children.

ADVERSE REACTIONS/ TOXIC EFFECTS

Toxic reactions may include blood dyscrasias (such as aplastic anemia, agranulocytosis, thrombocytopenia, leukopenia, leukocytosis, and eosinophilia), cardiovascular disturbances (such as CHF, hypotension or hypertension, thrombophlebitis and arrhythmias), and dermatologic effects (such as rash, urticaria, pruritus, and photosensitivity). Abrupt withdrawal may precipitate status epilepticus.

NURSING CONSIDERATIONS

BASELINE ASSESSMENT

Seizures: Review history of seizure disorder (intensity, frequency, duration, level of consciousness [LOC]). Provide safety precautions, quiet, dark environment. CBC, serum iron determination, urinalysis, BUN should be performed before therapy begins and periodically during therapy.

INTERVENTION/EVALUATION

Seizures: Observe frequently for recurrence of seizure activity. Monitor for therapeutic serum levels. Assess for clinical improvement (decrease in intensity, frequency of seizures). Assess for clinical evidence of early toxic signs

(fever, sore throat, mouth ulcerations, unusual bruising or bleeding, joint pain). **Neuralgia:** Avoid triggering tic douloureux (draft, talking, washing face, jarring bed, hot, warm, cold food or liquids). Therapeutic serum level: 4–12 mcg/ml; toxic serum level: greater than 12 mcg/ml.

PATIENT/FAMILY TEACHING

• Do not abruptly withdraw medication after long-term use (may precipitate seizures). • Strict maintenance of drug therapy is essential for seizure control. • Drowsiness usually disappears during continued therapy. • Avoid tasks that require alertness, motor skills until response to drug is established. • Report visual disturbances. • Blood tests should be repeated frequently during first 3 mo of therapy and at monthly intervals thereafter for 2–3 yr. • Do not take oral suspension simultaneously with other liquid medicine. • Do not take with grapefruit juice.

carbenicillin

(Geocillin)

See Antibiotic: penicillins (p. 28C)

carbidopa/levodopa

car-bih-dope-ah/**lev**-oh-dope-ah

(Atamet, Apo-Levocarb ✦, Parcopa, Sinemet, Sinemet CR)

FIXED-COMBINATION(S)

Stalevo: carbidopa/levodopa/ entacapone (antiparkinson agent): 12.5 mg/50 mg/200 mg, 25 mg/ 100 mg/200 mg, 37.5 mg/150 mg/ 200 mg.

✐ see color pill atlas   ◢ herb   underlined – top prescribed drug

◆**CLASSIFICATION**

PHARMACOTHERAPEUTIC: Dopamine precursor. **CLINICAL:** Antiparkinson agent.

ACTION

Levodopa is converted to dopamine in the basal ganglia, thus increasing dopamine concentration in brain and inhibiting hyperactive cholinergic activity. Carbidopa prevents peripheral breakdown of levodopa, allowing more levodopa to be available for transport into the brain. Therapeutic Effect: Reduces tremor.

PHARMACOKINETICS

Carbidopa is rapidly and completely absorbed from the GI tract. Widely distributed. Excreted primarily in urine. Levodopa is converted to dopamine. Excreted primarily in urine. Half-life: 1–2 hr (carbidopa); 1–3 hr (levodopa).

USES

Treatment of idiopathic Parkinson's disease (paralysis agitans), postencephalitic parkinsonism, symptomatic parkinsonism following CNS injury by CO_2 poisoning, manganese intoxication.

PRECAUTIONS

CONTRAINDICATIONS: Angle-closure glaucoma, use within 14 days of MAOIs, skin lesions (Sinemet CR), history of melanoma (Sinemet CR). **CAUTIONS:** History of MI, bronchial asthma (tartrazine sensitivity), emphysema; severe cardiac, pulmonary, renal, hepatic, endocrine disease; active peptic ulcer; treated open-angle glaucoma.

⧗ LIFESPAN CONSIDERATIONS: Pregnancy/Lactation: Unknown if drug crosses placenta or is distributed in breast milk. May inhibit lactation. Do not breast-feed. **Pregnancy Category C.** Children: Safety and efficacy not established in those younger than 18 yr.

Elderly: More sensitive to effects of levodopa. Anxiety, confusion, nervousness more common when receiving anticholinergics.

INTERACTIONS

DRUG: **Anticonvulsants, benzodiazepines, haloperidol, phenothiazines:** May decrease the effects of carbidopa and levodopa. **MAOIs:** May increase the risk of hypertensive crisis. **Selegiline:** May increase levodopa-induced dyskinesias, nausea, orthostatic hypotension, confusion, and hallucinations. HERBAL: None known. FOOD: None known. LAB VALUES: May increase BUN level and serum LDH, alkaline phosphatase, bilirubin, AST, and ALT levels.

AVAILABILITY (Rx)

TABLETS (ATAMET, SINEMET): 10 mg carbidopa/100 mg levodopa, 25 mg carbidopa/100 mg levodopa, 25 mg carbidopa/250 mg levodopa. **TABLETS (ORAL-DISINTEGRATING [PARCOPA]):** 10 mg carbidopa/100 mg levodopa, 25 mg carbidopa/100 mg levodopa, 25 mg carbidopa/250 mg levodopa. **TABLETS (EXTENDED-RELEASE [SINEMET CR]):** 25 mg carbidopa/100 mg levodopa, 50 mg carbidopa/200 mg levodopa.

ADMINISTRATION/HANDLING

PO
• Scored tablets may be crushed. • Give without regard to food. • Do not crush sustained-release tablet; may cut in half.

PO (PARCOPA)
• Place oral disintegrating tablet on top of tongue. Tablet will dissolve in seconds, patient to swallow with saliva. It is not necessary to administer with liquid.

INDICATIONS/ROUTES/DOSAGE

PARKINSONISM
PO: ADULTS: Initially, 25/100 mg 2–4 times a day. May increase up 200/2,000 mg daily. ELDERLY: Initially, 25/100 mg

---

twice a day. May increase as necessary. When converting a patient from Sinemet to Sinemet CR (50 mg/200 mg), dosage is based on the total daily dose of levodopa, as follows:

Sinemet	Sinemet CR
300–400 mg	1 tablet twice a day
500–600 mg	1.5 tablet twice a day or 1 tab 3 times a day
700–800 mg	4 tablets in 3 or more divided doses
900–1,000 mg	5 tablets in 3 or more divided doses

Intervals between doses of Sinemet CR should be 4–8 hr while awake.

SIDE EFFECTS

FREQUENT: Uncontrolled movements of face, tongue, arms, or upper body; nausea and vomiting (80%); anorexia (50%). **OCCASIONAL:** Depression, anxiety, confusion, nervousness, urine retention, palpitations, dizziness, light-headedness, decreased appetite, blurred vision, constipation, dry mouth, flushed skin, headache, insomnia, diarrhea, unusual fatigue, darkening of urine and sweat. **RARE:** Hypertension, ulcer, hemolytic anemia (marked by fatigue).

ADVERSE REACTIONS/ TOXIC EFFECTS

Patients on long-term therapy have a high incidence of involuntary choreiform, dystonic, and dyskinetic movements. Numerous mild to severe CNS and psychiatric disturbances may occur, including reduced attention span, anxiety, nightmares, daytime somnolence, euphoria, fatigue, paranoia, psychotic episodes, depression, and hallucinations.

NURSING CONSIDERATIONS

BASELINE ASSESSMENT

Instruct patient to void before giving medication (reduces risk of urinary retention).

INTERVENTION/EVALUATION

Be alert to neurologic effects: headache, lethargy, mental confusion, agitation. Monitor for evidence of dyskinesia (difficulty with movement). Assess for clinical reversal of symptoms (improvement of tremor of head and hands at rest, mask-like facial expression, shuffling gait, muscular rigidity).

PATIENT/FAMILY TEACHING

• Avoid tasks that require alertness, motor skills until response to drug is established. • Avoid alcoholic beverages during therapy. • Sugarless gum, sips of tepid water may relieve dry mouth. • Take with food to minimize GI upset. • Effects may be delayed from several weeks to months. • May cause darkening of urine or sweat (not harmful). • Instruct patient taking oral disintegrating tablet to report any uncontrolled movement of face, eyelids, mouth, tongue, arms, hands, legs; mental changes; palpitations; severe or persistent nausea/vomiting; difficulty urinating.

carboplatin

car-bow-**play**-tin

(<u>Paraplatin</u>, Paraplatin-AQ ❧)

Do not confuse carboplatin with Cisplatin or Platinol.

◆ CLASSIFICATION

PHARMACOTHERAPEUTIC: Platinum coordination complex. **CLINICAL:** Antineoplastic (see p. 72C).

ACTION

A platinum coordination complex that inhibits DNA synthesis by cross-linking with DNA strands, preventing cell division. Cell cycle-phase nonspecific. **Therapeutic Effect:** Interferes with DNA function.

PHARMACOKINETICS

Protein binding: Low. Hydrolyzed in solution to active form. Primarily excreted in urine. Half-life: 2.6–5.9 hr.

USES

Treatment of ovarian carcinoma. OFF-LABEL: Brain tumors, Hodgkin's and non-Hodgkin's lymphomas, malignant melanoma, retinoblastoma, treatment of breast, bladder, endometrial, esophageal, small cell lung, non-small cell lung, head and neck, and testicular carcinomas.

PRECAUTIONS

CONTRAINDICATIONS: History of severe allergic reaction to cisplatin, platinum compounds, or mannitol; severe bleeding, severe myelosuppression. CAUTIONS: Chickenpox, herpes zoster, renal impairment.

LIFESPAN CONSIDERATIONS: Pregnancy/Lactation: If possible, avoid use during pregnancy, especially first trimester. May cause fetal harm. Unknown if distributed in breast milk. Breast-feeding not recommended. Pregnancy Category D. Children: Safety and efficacy not established. Elderly: Peripheral neurotoxicity increased, myelotoxicity may be more severe. Age-related renal impairment may require decreased dosage, more careful monitoring of blood counts.

INTERACTIONS

DRUG: Bone marrow depressants: May increase myelosuppression. Live-virus vaccines: May potentiate virus replication, increase vaccine side effects, and decrease the patient's antibody response to the vaccine. Nephrotoxic, ototoxic medications: May increase the risk of nephrotoxicity. HERBAL: None known. FOOD: None known. LAB VALUES: May decrease serum electrolyte levels, including calcium, magnesium, potassium, and sodium. High dosages (more than 4 times the recommended dosage) may elevate BUN and serum alkaline phosphatase, bilirubin, creatinine, and AST levels.

AVAILABILITY (Rx)

POWDER FOR INJECTION: 50 mg, 150 mg, 450 mg. INJECTION SOLUTION: 10 mg/ml.

ADMINISTRATION/HANDLING

‹ ALERT › May be carcinogenic, mutagenic, or teratogenic. Handle with extreme care during preparation/administration.

 IV

Reconstitution • Reconstitute immediately before use. • Do not use aluminum needles or administration sets that come in contact with drug (may produce black precipitate, loss of potency). • Reconstitute each 50 mg with 5 ml sterile water for injection, D₅W, or 0.9% NaCl to provide concentration of 10 mg/ml. • May be further diluted with D₅W or 0.9% NaCl to provide concentration as low as 0.5 mg/ml.

Rate of administration • Infuse over 15–60 min. • Rarely, anaphylactic reaction occurs minutes after administration. Use of epinephrine, corticosteroids alleviates symptoms.

Storage • Store vials at room temperature. • After reconstitution, solution is stable for 8 hr. Discard unused portion after 8 hr.

IV INCOMPATIBILITIES

Amphotericin B complex (Abelcet, AmBisome, Amphotec).

IV COMPATIBILITIES

Etoposide (VePesid), granisetron (Kytril), ondansetron (Zofran), paclitaxel (Taxol).

INDICATIONS/ROUTES/DOSAGE

OVARIAN CARCINOMA (MONOTHERAPY)

IV: ADULTS: 360 mg/m² on day 1, every 4 wk. Don't repeat dose until neutrophil and platelet counts are within acceptable levels. Adjust drug dosage in previously treated patients based on lowest post-treatment platelet or neutrophil count. Increase dosage only once to no more than 125% of starting dose.

OVARIAN CARCINOMA (COMBINATION THERAPY)

IV: ADULTS: 300 mg/m² (with cyclophosphamide) on day 1, every 4 wk. Don't repeat dose until neutrophil and platelet counts are within acceptable levels. CHILDREN: 300–600 mg/m² every 4 wk for solid tumor, or 175 mg/m² every 4 wk for brain tumor.

DOSAGE IN RENAL IMPAIRMENT

Initial dosage is based on creatinine clearance; subsequent dosages are based on the patient's tolerance and degree of myelosuppression.

Creatinine Clearance	Dosage Day 1
60 ml/min or greater	360 mg/m²
41–59 ml/min	250 mg/m²
16–40 ml/min	200 mg/m²

SIDE EFFECTS

FREQUENT: Nausea (75%–80%), vomiting (65%). **OCCASIONAL:** Generalized pain (17%), diarrhea or constipation (6%), peripheral neuropathy (4%). **RARE (3%–2%):** Alopecia, asthenia, hypersensitivity reaction (erythema, pruritus, rash, urticaria).

ADVERSE REACTIONS/ TOXIC EFFECTS

Myelosuppression may be severe, resulting in anemia, infection, (sepsis, pneumonia), and bleeding. Prolonged treatment may result in peripheral neurotoxicity.

NURSING CONSIDERATIONS

BASELINE ASSESSMENT

Offer emotional support. Do not repeat treatment until WBC recovers from previous therapy. Transfusions may be needed in those receiving prolonged therapy (myelosuppression increased in those with previous therapy, renal impairment).

INTERVENTION/EVALUATION

Monitor hematologic status, pulmonary function studies, liver and renal function tests. Monitor for fever, sore throat, signs of local infection, unusual bruising or bleeding from any site, symptoms of anemia (excessive fatigue, weakness).

PATIENT/FAMILY TEACHING

• Nausea, vomiting generally abate in less than 24 hr. • Do not have immunizations without physician's approval (drug lowers body's resistance). • Avoid contact with those who have recently received live virus vaccine.

Cardizem, *see diltiazem*

---

carisoprodol

(Soma)

See Skeletal muscle relaxants

---

carmustine

car-**muss**-teen

(BiCNU, Gliadel Wafer)

◆ CLASSIFICATION

PHARMACOTHERAPEUTIC: Alkylating agent, nitrosourea. **CLINICAL:** Antineoplastic (see p. 72C).

ACTION

An alkylating agent and nitrosourea that inhibits DNA and RNA synthesis by cross-linking with DNA and RNA strands, preventing cell division. Cell cycle-phase nonspecific. **Therapeutic Effect:** Interferes with DNA and RNA function.

PHARMACOKINETICS

Crosses blood-brain barrier. Metabolized in liver. Excreted in urine. **Half-life:** 1.4 min (first phase); 17.8 min (second phase).

USES

Treatment of brain tumors, Hodgkin's lymphomas, non-Hodgkin's lymphomas, multiple myeloma. **Gliadel Wafer:** Adjunct to surgery to prolong survival in recurrent glioblastoma multiforme. **OFF-LABEL:** Treatment of colorectal, hepatic, or GI carcinoma, malignant melanoma, mycosis fungoides.

PRECAUTIONS

CONTRAINDICATIONS: None known. **CAUTIONS:** Patients with decreased platelet, leukocyte, erythrocyte counts.

LIFESPAN CONSIDERATIONS: Pregnancy/Lactation: Avoid during pregnancy, particularly first trimester; may cause fetal harm. Unknown if distributed in breast milk; do not breastfeed. **Pregnancy Category D. Children:** Safety and efficacy not established in children. **Elderly:** No age-related precautions noted.

INTERACTIONS

DRUG: Bone marrow depressants, cimetidine: May enhance carmustine's myelosuppressive effect. **Hepatotoxic, nephrotoxic medications:** May increase the risk of hepatotoxicity or nephrotoxicity. **Live-virus vaccines:** May potentiate virus replication, increase vaccine side effects, and decrease the patient's antibody response to the vaccine. **HERBAL:** None known. **FOOD:** None known. **LAB VALUES:** May increase BUN, and serum alkaline phosphatase, bilirubin, AST, and ALT levels.

AVAILABILITY (Rx)

POWDER FOR INJECTION (BICNU): 100 mg. **IM PLANT DEVICE (GLIADEL WAFER):** 7.7 mg.

ADMINISTRATION/HANDLING

◀ **ALERT** ▶ May be carcinogenic, mutagenic, or teratogenic. Wear protective gloves during preparation of drug; may cause transient burning, brown staining of skin.

 IV

Reconstitution • Reconstitute 100-mg vial with 3 ml sterile dehydrated (absolute) alcohol, followed by 27 ml sterile water for injection to provide concentration of 3.3 mg/ml. • Further dilute with 50–250 ml D$_5$W or 0.9% NaCl.

Rate of administration • Infuse over 1–2 hr (shorter duration may produce intense burning pain at injection site, intense flushing of skin, conjunctiva). • Flush IV line with 5–10 ml 0.9% NaCl or D$_5$W before and after administration to prevent irritation at injection site.

Storage • Refrigerate unopened vials of dry powder. • Reconstituted vials are stable for 8 hr at room temperature or 24 hr if refrigerated. • Solutions further diluted to 0.2 mg/ml with D$_5$W or 0.9% NaCl are stable for 48 hr if refrigerated or an additional 8 hr at room temperature. • Solutions appear clear, colorless to yellow. • Discard if precipitate forms, color change occurs, or oily film develops on bottom of vial.

IV INCOMPATIBILITY

Allopurinol (Aloprim).

INDICATIONS/ROUTES/DOSAGE

DISSEMINATED HODGKIN'S DISEASE, NON-HODGKIN'S LYMPHOMA, MULTIPLE MYELOMA, AND PRIMARY AND METASTATIC BRAIN TUMORS IN PREVIOUSLY UNTREATED PATIENTS (MONOTHERAPY)

IV (BiCNU): ADULTS, ELDERLY: 150–200 mg/m^2 as a single dose q6–8wk or 75–100 mg/m^2 on 2 successive days q6–8wk. CHILDREN: 200–250 mg/m^2 q4–6wk as a single dose.

◀ ALERT ▶ Next dosage is based on clinical and hematologic response to previous dose (platelets greater than 100,000/mm^3 and leukocytes greater than 4,000/mm^3).

IMPLANTATION: (GLIADEL WAFER): ADULTS, ELDERLY, CHILDREN: Up to 8 wafers (62.6 mg) may be placed in resection cavity.

SIDE EFFECTS

FREQUENT: Nausea and vomiting within minutes to 2 hr after administration (may last up to 6 hr). OCCASIONAL: Diarrhea, esophagitis, anorexia, dysphagia. RARE: Thrombophlebitis.

ADVERSE REACTIONS/ TOXIC EFFECTS

Hematologic toxicity due to myelosuppression occurs frequently. Thrombocytopenia occurs about 4 wk after carmustine treatment begins and lasts 1–2 wk. Leukopenia is evident 5–6 wk after treatment begins and lasts 1–2 wk. Anemia occurs less frequently and is less severe. Mild, reversible hepatotoxicity also occurs frequently. Prolonged high-dose carmustine therapy may produce impaired renal function and pulmonary toxicity (pulmonary infiltrate or fibrosis).

NURSING CONSIDERATIONS

BASELINE ASSESSMENT

Perform CBC, renal/liver function studies before beginning therapy and periodically thereafter. Perform blood counts weekly during and for at least 6 wk after therapy ends.

INTERVENTION/EVALUATION

Monitor CBC, BUN, serum transaminase, alkaline phosphatase, bilirubin; pulmonary, renal/liver function tests. Monitor for hematologic toxicity (fever, sore throat, signs of local infection, unusual bruising or bleeding from any site) or symptoms of anemia (excessive fatigue, weakness). Monitor lung sounds for pulmonary toxicity (dyspnea, fine lung rales).

PATIENT/FAMILY TEACHING

• Maintain adequate daily fluid intake (may protect against renal impairment). • Do not have immunizations without doctor's approval (drug lowers body's resistance). • Avoid contact with those who have recently received live virus vaccine. • Contact physician if nausea/vomiting continues at home.

---

carteolol

(Cartrol, Ocupress)
See Beta-adrenergic blockers (pp. 47C, 64C)

---

carvedilol

car-**veh**-dih-lol
(Coreg)
Do not confuse carvedilol with carteolol.

◆CLASSIFICATION

PHARMACOTHERAPEUTIC: Beta-adrenergic blocker. CLINICAL: Antihypertensive (see p. 64C).

ACTION

An antihypertensive that possesses non-selective beta-blocking and alpha-adrenergic blocking activity. Causes vasodilation. **Therapeutic Effect:** Reduces cardiac output, exercise-induced tachycardia, and reflex ortho-static tachycardia; reduces peripheral vascular resistance.

PHARMACOKINETICS

Route	Onset	Peak	Duration
PO	30 min	1–2 hr	24 hr

Rapidly and extensively absorbed from the GI tract. Protein binding: 98%. Metabolized in the liver. Excreted primarily via bile into feces. Minimally removed by hemodialysis. **Half-life:** 7–10 hr. Food delays rate of absorption.

USES

Treatment of mild to severe heart failure, left ventricular dysfunction following MI, hypertension. Reduces risk of second MI in patients with damaged heart or heart failure. **OFF-LABEL:** Treatment of angina pectoris, idiopathic cardiomyopathy.

PRECAUTIONS

CONTRAINDICATIONS: Bronchial asthma or related bronchospastic conditions, cardiogenic shock, pulmonary edema, second- or third-degree AV block, severe bradycardia. **CAUTIONS:** CHF controlled with digitalis, diuretics, angiotensin-converting enzyme (ACE) inhibitor; peripheral vascular disease; anesthesia; diabetes mellitus; hypoglycemia; thyrotoxicosis; hepatic impairment.

⌛ **LIFESPAN CONSIDERATIONS: Pregnancy/Lactation:** Unknown if drug crosses placenta or is distributed in breast milk. May produce bradycardia, apnea, hypoglycemia, hypothermia during delivery, low birth-weight infants. **Pregnancy Category C (D if used in the**

second or third trimester). **Children:** Safety and efficacy not established. **Elderly:** Incidence of dizziness may be increased.

INTERACTIONS

DRUG: Calcium blockers: Increase risk of conduction disturbances. **Catapres:** May potentiate BP effects. **Cimetidine:** May increase carvedilol blood concentration. **Digoxin:** Increases concentrations of this drug. **Diuretics, other antihypertensives:** May increase hypotensive effect. **Insulin, oral hypoglycemics:** May mask symptoms of hypoglycemia and prolong hypoglycemic effect of these drugs. **Rifampin:** Decreases carvedilol blood concentration. **HERBAL:** None known. **FOOD:** None known. **LAB VALUE:** None known.

AVAILABILITY (Rx)

TABLETS: 3.125 mg, 6.25 mg, 12.5 mg, 25 mg.

ADMINISTRATION/HANDLING

PO
• Give with food (slows rate of absorption, reduces risk of orthostatic effects).
• Take standing systolic BP 1 hr after dosing as guide for tolerance.

INDICATIONS/ROUTES/DOSAGE

HYPERTENSION
PO: ADULTS, ELDERLY: Initially, 6.25 mg twice a day. May double at 7- to 14-day intervals to highest tolerated dosage. **Maximum:** 50 mg/day.

CHF
PO: ADULTS, ELDERLY: Initially, 3.125 mg twice a day. May double at 2-wk intervals to highest tolerated dosage. **Maximum:** For patients weighing more than 85 kg, give 50 mg twice a day, for those weighing 85 kg or less, give 25 mg twice a day.

LEFT VENTRICULAR DYSFUNCTION
PO: ADULTS, ELDERLY: Initially, 3.125–6.25 mg twice a day. May increase at intervals of 3–10 days up to 25 mg twice a day.

SIDE EFFECTS

Carvedilol is generally well tolerated, with mild and transient side effects. **FREQUENT (6%–4%):** Fatigue, dizziness. **OCCASIONAL (2%):** Diarrhea, bradycardia, rhinitis, back pain. **RARE (less than 2%):** Orthostatic hypotension, somnolence, UTI, viral infection.

ADVERSE REACTIONS/ TOXIC EFFECTS

Overdose may produce profound bradycardia, hypotension, bronchospasm, cardiac insufficiency, cardiogenic shock, and cardiac arrest. Abrupt withdrawal may result in diaphoresis, palpitations, headache, and tremors. Carvedilol administration may precipitate CHF and MI in patients with heart disease; thyroid storm in those with thyrotoxicosis; and peripheral ischemia in those with existing peripheral vascular disease. Hypoglycemia may occur in patients with previously controlled diabetes.

NURSING CONSIDERATIONS

BASELINE ASSESSMENT

Assess BP, apical pulse immediately before drug is administered (if pulse is 60/min or less or systolic BP is less than 90 mm Hg, withhold medication, contact physician).

INTERVENTION/EVALUATION

Monitor BP for hypotension, respiration for dyspnea. Assess pulse for quality, irregular rate, bradycardia. Monitor EKG for cardiac arrhythmias. Assist with ambulation if dizziness occurs. Assess for evidence of CHF: dyspnea (particularly on exertion or lying down), night cough, peripheral edema, distended neck veins. Monitor I&O (increase in weight, decrease in urine output may indicate CHF).

PATIENT/FAMILY TEACHING

• Full antihypertensive effect noted in 1–2 wk. • Contact lens wearers may experience decreased lacrimation. • Take with food. • Do not abruptly discontinue medication. Compliance with therapy regimen is essential to control hypertension. • Avoid tasks that require alertness, motor skills until response to drug is established. • Report excessive fatigue, prolonged dizziness. • Do not use nasal decongestants, OTC cold preparations (stimulants) without physician approval. • Monitor BP, pulse before taking medication. • Restrict salt, alcohol intake.

cascara sagrada

cass-**care**-ah sah-**graud**-ah (Cascara Sagrada)

FIXED-COMBINATION(S)

With milk of magnesia, a saline laxative.

CLASSIFICATION

PHARMACOTHERAPEUTIC: GI stimulant. **CLINICAL:** Laxative (see p. 110C).

ACTION

A GI stimulant that has a direct effect on colonic smooth musculature, by stimulating intramural nerve plexi. **Therapeutic Effect:** Promotes fluid and ion accumulation in the colon, increasing peristalsis and promoting a laxative effect.

PHARMACOKINETICS

Poorly absorbed following PO administration. Metabolized in the intestinal wall. Excreted in urine and bile. **Half life:** Unknown.

USES

Temporary relief of constipation, sometimes used with milk of magnesia.

PRECAUTIONS

CONTRAINDICATIONS: Abdominal pain, appendicitis, intestinal obstruction, nausea, vomiting. **CAUTIONS:** None known.

⧗ **LIFESPAN CONSIDERATIONS: Pregnancy/Lactation:** May be distributed in breast milk. **Pregnancy Category C. Children:** Safety and efficacy not established in children younger than 6 yr. **Elderly:** No age-related precautions noted.

INTERACTIONS

DRUG: Oral medications: May decrease transit time of concurrently administered oral medications, decreasing the absorption of cascara sagrada. **HERBAL:** None known. **FOOD:** None known. **LAB VALUES:** May increase blood glucose level. May decrease serum calcium and potassium levels.

AVAILABILITY (Rx)

LIQUID: (18% alcohol) 1 g/ml. **TABLETS:** 150 mg, 325 mg.

INDICATIONS/ROUTES/DOSAGE

TREATMENT OF CONSTIPATION
PO: ADULTS, ELDERLY: 5 ml or 1–2 tablets at bedtime. CHILDREN 2–11 yr: 2.5 ml, 1–3 ml as a single dose. INFANT: 1.25 ml, 0.5–2 ml as a single dose.

SIDE EFFECTS

FREQUENT: Pink-red, red-violet, red-brown, or yellow-brown discoloration of urine. **OCCASIONAL:** Some degree of abdominal discomfort, nausea, mild cramps, faintness.

ADVERSE REACTIONS/ TOXIC EFFECTS

Long-term use may result in laxative dependence, chronic constipation, and loss of normal bowel function. Prolonged use or overdose may result in electrolyte or metabolic disturbances (such as hypokalemia, hypocalcemia, and metabolic acidosis or alkalosis), as well as persistent diarrhea, vomiting, muscle weakness, malabsorption, and weight loss.

NURSING CONSIDERATIONS

INTERVENTION/EVALUATION
Encourage adequate fluid intake. Assess bowel sounds for peristalsis. Monitor daily bowel activity/stool consistency; record time of evacuation. Assess for abdominal disturbances. Monitor serum electrolytes in those exposed to prolonged/frequent/excessive use of medication.

PATIENT/FAMILY TEACHING
• Urine may turn pink-red, red-violet, red-brown, yellow-brown (only temporary, not harmful). • Institute measures to promote defecation: increase fluid intake, exercise, high-fiber diet. • Laxative effect generally occurs in 6–12 hr but may take 24 hr. • Do not use in presence of nausea, vomiting, abdominal pain longer than 1 wk. • Do not take other oral medication within 1 hr of taking this medicine (decreased effectiveness due to increased peristalsis).

Casodex, see bicalutamide

caspofungin acetate

cas-poe-**fun**-gin
(Cancidas)

◆CLASSIFICATION
CLINICAL: Antifungal.

ACTION

An antifungal that inhibits the synthesis of glucan, a vital component of fungal cell formation, thereby damaging the fungal cell membrane. **Therapeutic Effect:** Fungistatic.

PHARMACOKINETICS

Distributed in tissue. Extensively bound to albumin. Protein binding: 97%. Slowly metabolized in liver to active metabolite. Excreted primarily in urine and to a lesser extent in feces. Not removed by hemodialysis. **Half-life:** 40–50 hr.

USES

Treatment of invasive aspergillosis, candidemia, intra-abdominal abscess, peritonitis, esophageal candidiasis. Empiric therapy for presumed fungal infections in febrile neutropenia.

PRECAUTIONS

CONTRAINDICATIONS: None known. **CAUTIONS:** Myelosuppression, renal insufficiency, hepatic impairment.

⧖ **LIFESPAN CONSIDERATIONS: Pregnancy/Lactation:** May be embryotoxic. Crosses placental barrier. Distributed in breast milk. **Pregnancy Category C. Children:** Safety and efficacy not established. **Elderly:** Age-related moderate renal impairment may require dosage adjustment.

INTERACTIONS

DRUG: Carbamazepine, cyclosporine, dexamethasone, efavirenz, nelfinavir, nevirapine, phenytoin, rifampin: May increase blood concentration of caspofungin. **Tacrolimus:** May decrease the effect of tacrolimus. **HERBAL:** None known. **FOOD:** None known. **LAB VALUES:** May increase PT as well as serum alkaline phosphatase, serum bilirubin, serum creatinine, LDH, AST, ALT, serum uric acid, urine pH, urine protein, urine RBC, and urine WBC levels. May decrease Hgb, Hct, platelet count, and serum albumin, serum bicarbonate, serum protein, and serum potassium levels.

AVAILABILITY (Rx)

POWDER FOR INJECTION: 50-mg, 70-mg vials.

ADMINISTRATION/HANDLING

 IV

Reconstitution • For a 70-mg dose, add 10.5 ml of 0.9% NaCl to the 70-mg vial. Transfer 10 ml of reconstituted solution to 250 ml 0.9% NaCl. • For a 50-mg dose, add 10.5 ml of 0.9% NaCl to the 50-mg vial. Transfer 10 ml of the reconstituted solution to 100 ml or 250 ml 0.9% NaCl. • For a 35-mg dose, add 10.5 ml of 0.9% NaCl to the 50-mg vial. Transfer 7 ml of the reconstituted solution to 100 ml or 250 ml 0.9% NaCl.

Rate of administration • Infuse over 60 min.

Storage • Refrigerate but warm to room temperature before preparing with diluent. • Reconstituted solution, prior to preparation of patient infusion solution, may be stored at room temperature for 1 hr before infusion. • Final infusion solution can be stored at room temperature for 24 hr. • Discard if solution contains particulate or is discolored.

▦ IV INCOMPATIBILITIES

Don't mix caspofungin with any other medication or use dextrose as a diluent.

INDICATIONS/ROUTES/DOSAGE

ASPERGILLOSIS

IV: ADULTS, ELDERLY, CHILDREN OLDER THAN 12 YR: Give single 70-mg loading dose on day 1, followed by 50 mg/day thereafter. For patients with moderate hepatic insufficiency, daily dose reduced to 35 mg.

INVASIVE CANDIDIASIS

IV: ADULTS, ELDERLY: Initially, 70 mg followed by 50 mg daily.

ESOPHAGEAL CANDIDIASIS

IV: ADULTS, ELDERLY: 50 mg a day.

EMPIRIC THERAPY

IV: ADULTS, ELDERLY: Initially, 70 mg then 50 mg/day. May increase to 70 mg/day.

SIDE EFFECTS

FREQUENT (26%): Fever. **OCCASIONAL (11%–4%):** Headache, nausea, phlebitis. **RARE (3% or less):** Paresthesia, vomiting, diarrhea, abdominal pain, myalgia, chills, tremor, insomnia.

ADVERSE REACTIONS/ TOXIC EFFECTS

Hypersensitivity reactions (characterized by rash, facial swelling, pruritus, and a sensation of warmth) may occur.

NURSING CONSIDERATIONS

BASELINE ASSESSMENT

Determine baseline temperature, liver function tests. Assess allergies.

INTERVENTION/EVALUATION

Assess for signs and symptoms of hepatic dysfunction. Monitor hepatic enzyme test results in patients with preexisting hepatic dysfunction.

Catapres, *see clonidine*

Catapres TTS, *see clonidine*

---

cefaclor

sef-a-klor

(Apo-Cefaclor ✤, Ceclor, Ceclor CD, Ceclor Pulvules)

◆CLASSIFICATION

PHARMACOTHERAPEUTIC: Second-generation cephalosporin. **CLINICAL:** Antibiotic (see p. 21C).

ACTION

A second-generation cephalosporin that binds to bacterial cell membranes and inhibits cell wall synthesis. **Therapeutic Effect:** Bactericidal.

PHARMACOKINETICS

Well absorbed from the GI tract. Protein binding: 25%. Widely distributed. Primarily excreted unchanged in urine. Moderately removed by hemodialysis. **Half-life:** 0.6–0.9 hr (increased in impaired renal function).

USES

Treatment of susceptible infections due to *S. pneumoniae, S. pyogenes, S. aureus, H. influenzae, E. coli, M. catarrhalis,* Klebsiella species, *P. mirabilis* including acute otitis media, bronchitis, pharyngitis/tonsillitis, respiratory tract, skin/skin structure and urinary tract infections.

PRECAUTIONS

CONTRAINDICATIONS: History of anaphylactic reaction to penicillins or hypersensitivity to cephalosporins. **CAUTIONS:** Renal impairment, history of GI disease (especially ulcerative colitis, antibiotic-associated colitis), concurrent use of nephrotoxic medications.

⏳ **LIFESPAN CONSIDERATIONS: Pregnancy/Lactation:** Readily crosses placenta. Distributed in breast milk. **Pregnancy Category B. Children:** No age-related precautions noted in those older than 1 mo. **Elderly:** Age-related renal impairment may require dosage adjustment.

INTERACTIONS

DRUG: Probenecid: May increase cefaclor blood concentration. **HERBAL:** None known. **FOOD:** None known. **LAB VALUES:** May increase BUN level and serum alkaline phosphatase, bilirubin, creatinine, LDH, AST, and ALT levels. May cause a positive direct or indirect Coombs' test.

AVAILABILITY (Rx)

CAPSULES (CECLOR PULVULES): 250 mg, 500 mg. **ORAL SUSPENSION (CECLOR):** 125 mg/5 ml, 187 mg/5 ml, 250 mg/5 ml, 375 mg/5 ml. **TABLETS (EXTENDED-RELEASE [CECLOR CD]):** 375 mg, 500 mg. **TABLETS (CHEWABLE [RANICLOR]):** 125 mg, 187 mg, 250 mg, 375 mg.

ADMINISTRATION/HANDLING

PO

• After reconstitution, oral solution is stable for 14 days if refrigerated. • Shake oral suspension well before using. • Give without regard to food; if GI upset occurs, give with food or milk. • Do not cut, crush, or chew extended-release tablets.

INDICATIONS/ROUTES/DOSAGE

BRONCHITIS

PO (EXTENDED-RELEASE): ADULTS, ELDERLY: 500 mg q12h for 7 days.

LOWER RESPIRATORY TRACT INFECTIONS

PO: ADULTS, ELDERLY: 250–500 mg q8h.

OTITIS MEDIA

PO: CHILDREN: 20–40 mg/kg/day in 2–3 divided doses. **Maximum:** 1 g/day.

PHARYNGITIS, SKIN/SKIN STRUCTURE INFECTIONS, TONSILLITIS

PO (EXTENDED-RELEASE): ADULTS, ELDERLY: 375 mg q12h.
PO (REGULAR-RELEASE): ADULTS, ELDERLY: 250–500 mg q8h. CHILDREN: 20–40 mg/kg/day in 2–3 divided doses. **Maximum:** 1 g/day.

URINARY TRACT INFECTIONS

PO: ADULTS, ELDERLY: 250–500 mg q8h. CHILDREN: 20–40 mg/kg/day in 2–3 divided doses q8h. **Maximum:** 1 g/day.
PO (EXTENDED-RELEASE): ADULTS, CHILDREN OLDER THAN 16 YR: 375–500 mg q12h.

DOSAGE IN RENAL IMPAIRMENT

Decreased dosage may be necessary in patients with creatinine clearance less than 40 ml/min.

SIDE EFFECTS

FREQUENT: Oral candidiasis, mild diarrhea, mild abdominal cramping, vaginal candidiasis. **OCCASIONAL:** Nausea, serum sickness-like reaction (marked by fever and joint pain; usually occurs after the second course of therapy and resolves after the drug is discontinued). **RARE:** Allergic reaction (pruritus, rash, and urticaria).

ADVERSE REACTIONS/TOXIC EFFECTS

Antibiotic-associated colitis and other superinfections may result from altered bacterial balance. Nephrotoxicity may occur, especially in patients with pre-existing renal disease. Patients with a history of allergies, especially to penicillin, are at increased risk for developing a severe hypersensitivity reaction, marked by severe pruritus, angioedema, bronchospasm, and anaphylaxis.

NURSING CONSIDERATIONS

BASELINE ASSESSMENT

Question for history of allergies, particularly cephalosporins, penicillins.

INTERVENTION/EVALUATION

Assess oral cavity for white patches on mucous membranes, tongue (thrush). Monitor bowel activity and stool consistency carefully; mild GI effects may be tolerable, but increasing severity may indicate onset of antibiotic-associated colitis. Monitor I&O, renal function test results for nephrotoxicity. Be alert for superinfection: severe genital/anal pruritus, abdominal pain, severe mouth soreness, moderate to severe diarrhea.

PATIENT/FAMILY TEACHING

• Continue therapy for full length of treatment. • Doses should be evenly spaced. • May cause GI upset (may take with food or milk). • Refrigerate oral suspension.

---

cefadroxil

sef-a-**drox**-ill
(Duricef)

♦ CLASSIFICATION

PHARMACOTHERAPEUTIC: First-generation cephalosporin. **CLINICAL:** Antibiotic (see p. 21C).

ACTION

A first-generation cephalosporin that binds to bacterial cell membranes and inhibits cell wall synthesis. **Therapeutic Effect:** Bactericidal.

PHARMACOKINETICS

Well absorbed from the GI tract. Protein binding: 15%–20%. Widely distributed. Primarily excreted unchanged in urine. Removed by hemodialysis. **Half-life:** 1.2–1.5 hr (increased in impaired renal function).

USES

Treatment of susceptible infections due to group A *streptooccci, staphylococci, S. pneumoniae, H. influenzae,* Klebsiella species, *E. coli, P. mirabilis* including impetigo, pharyngitis/tonsillitis, skin/skin structure and urinary tract infections.

PRECAUTIONS

CONTRAINDICATIONS: History of anaphylactic reaction to penicillins or hypersensitivity to cephalosporins. **CAUTIONS:** Renal impairment, history of GI disease (especially ulcerative colitis, antibiotic-associated colitis), concurrent use of nephrotoxic medications.

⌛ **LIFESPAN CONSIDERATIONS: Pregnancy/Lactation:** Readily crosses placenta. Distributed in breast milk. **Pregnancy Category B. Children:** No age-related precautions noted. **Elderly:** Age-related renal impairment may require dosage adjustment.

INTERACTIONS

DRUG: Probenecid: Increases cefadroxil blood concentration. **HERBAL:** None known. **FOOD:** None known. **LAB VALUES:** May increase BUN level and serum alkaline phosphatase, bilirubin, creatinine, LDH, AST, and ALT levels. May cause a positive direct or indirect Coombs' test.

AVAILABILITY (Rx)

CAPSULES: 500 mg. **ORAL SUSPENSION:** 125 mg/5 ml, 250 mg/5 ml, 500 mg/5 ml. **TABLETS:** 1 g.

ADMINISTRATION/HANDLING

PO
• After reconstitution, oral solution is stable for 14 days if refrigerated. • Shake oral suspension well before using. • Give without regard to meals; if GI upset occurs, give with food or milk.

INDICATIONS/ROUTES/DOSAGE

UTIs
PO: ADULTS, ELDERLY: 1–2 g/day as a single dose or in 2 divided doses. CHILDREN: 30 mg/kg/day in 2 divided doses. **Maximum:** 2 g/day.

SKIN AND SKIN-STRUCTURE INFECTIONS, GROUP A BETA-HEMOLYTIC STREPTOCOCCAL PHARYNGITIS, TONSILLITIS
PO: ADULTS, ELDERLY: 1–2 g in 2 divided doses. CHILDREN: 30 mg/kg/day in 2 divided doses. **Maximum:** 2 g/day.

IMPETIGO
PO: CHILDREN: 30 mg/kg/day as a single or in 2 divided doses. **Maximum:** 2 g/day.

DOSAGE IN RENAL IMPAIRMENT
After an initial 1-g dose, dosage and frequency are modified based on creatinine clearance and the severity of the infection.

C

Creatinine Clearance	Dosage Interval
25–50 ml/min	500 mg q12h
10–25 ml/min	500 mg q24h
0–10 ml/min	500 mg q36h

SIDE EFFECTS

FREQUENT: Oral candidiasis, mild diarrhea, mild abdominal cramping, vaginal candidiasis. **OCCASIONAL:** Nausea, unusual bruising or bleeding, serum sickness-like reaction (marked by fever and joint pain; usually occurs after the second course of therapy and resolves after the drug is discontinued). **RARE:** Allergic reaction (rash, pruritus, urticaria), thrombophlebitis (pain, redness, swelling at injection site).

ADVERSE REACTIONS/ TOXIC EFFECTS

Antibiotic-associated colitis and other superinfections may result from altered bacterial balance. Nephrotoxicity may occur, especially in patients with pre-existing renal disease. Patients with a history of allergies, especially to penicillin, are at increased risk for developing a severe hypersensitivity reaction, marked by severe pruritus, angioedema, bronchospasm, and anaphylaxis.

NURSING CONSIDERATIONS

BASELINE ASSESSMENT

Question for history of allergies, particularly cephalosporins, penicillins.

INTERVENTION/EVALUATION

Assess oral cavity for white patches on mucous membranes, tongue. Monitor bowel activity and stool consistency carefully; mild GI effects may be tolerable, but increasing severity may indicate onset of antibiotic-associated colitis. Monitor I&O, renal function test results for nephrotoxicity. Be alert for superinfection: genital/anal pruritus, moniliasis, abdominal pain, sore mouth/tongue, moderate to severe diarrhea.

PATIENT/FAMILY TEACHING

• Continue therapy for full length of treatment. • Doses should be evenly spaced. • May cause GI upset (may take with food or milk). • Refrigerate oral suspension.

cefazolin sodium

cef-ah-**zoe**-lin

(Ancef, Kefzol)

Do not confuse cefazolin with cefprozil or Cefzil.

CLASSIFICATION

PHARMACOTHERAPEUTIC: First-generation cephalosporin. **CLINICAL:** Antibiotic (see p. 21C).

ACTION

A first-generation cephalosporin that binds to bacterial cell membranes and inhibits cell wall synthesis. **Therapeutic Effect:** Bactericidal.

PHARMACOKINETICS

Widely distributed. Protein binding: 85%. Primarily excreted unchanged in urine. Moderately removed by hemodialysis. **Half-life:** 1.4–1.8 hr (increased in impaired renal function).

USES

Treatment of susceptible infections due to *S. aureus, S. epidermidis,* Group A *beta-hemolytic streptococci, S. pneumoniae, E. coli, P. mirabilis,* Klebsiella species, *H. influenzae* including biliary tract, bone and joint, genital, respiratory tract, skin and skin structure and urinary tract infections, endocarditis, peri-operative prophylaxis, septicemia.

PRECAUTIONS

CONTRAINDICATIONS: History of anaphylactic reaction to penicillins or hypersensitivity to cephalosporins. **CAUTIONS:** Renal impairment, history of GI disease (especially ulcerative colitis, antibiotic-associated colitis), concurrent use of nephrotoxic medications.

⌛ **LIFESPAN CONSIDERATIONS: Pregnancy/Lactation:** Readily crosses placenta; distributed in breast milk. **Pregnancy Category B. Children:** No age-related precautions noted. **Elderly:** Age-related renal impairment may require reduced dosage.

INTERACTIONS

DRUG: Probenecid: Increases cefazolin blood concentration. **HERBAL:** None known. **FOOD:** None known. **LAB VALUES:** May increase BUN level and serum alkaline phosphatase, bilirubin, creatinine, LDH, AST, and ALT levels. May cause a positive direct or indirect Coombs' test.

AVAILABILITY (Rx)

POWDER FOR INJECTION (ANCEF, KEFZOL): 500 mg, 1 g, 5 g, 10 g. **READY-TO-HANG INFUSION (ANCEF):** 500 mg/50 ml, 1 g/50 ml.

ADMINISTRATION/HANDLING

 IV

Reconstitution • Reconstitute each 1 g with at least 10 ml sterile water for injection. • May further dilute in 50–100 ml D₅W or 0.9% NaCl (decreases incidence of thrombophlebitis).

Rate of administration • For IV push, administer over 3–5 min. • For intermittent IV infusion (piggyback), infuse over 20–30 min.

Storage • Solution appears light yellow to yellow. • IV infusion (piggyback) stable for 24 hr at room temperature, 96 hr if refrigerated. • Discard if precipitate forms.

IM

• To minimize discomfort, inject deep IM slowly. • Less painful if injected into gluteus maximus rather than lateral aspect of thigh.

▨ IV INCOMPATIBILITIES

Amikacin (Amikin), amiodarone (Cordarone), hydromorphone (Dilaudid).

IV COMPATIBILITIES

Calcium gluconate, diltiazem (Cardizem), famotidine (Pepcid), heparin, insulin (regular), lidocaine, magnesium sulfate, midazolam (Versed), morphine, multivitamins, potassium chloride, propofol (Diprivan), total parenteral nutrition (TPN), vecuronium (Norcuron).

INDICATIONS/ROUTES/DOSAGE

UNCOMPLICATED UTIs
IV, IM: ADULTS, ELDERLY: 1 g q12h.

MILD TO MODERATE INFECTIONS
IV, IM: ADULTS, ELDERLY: 250–500 mg q8–12h.

SEVERE INFECTIONS
IV, IM: ADULTS, ELDERLY: 0.5–1 g q6–8h.

LIFE-THREATENING INFECTIONS
IV, IM: ADULTS, ELDERLY: 1–1.5 g q6h. **Maximum:** 12 g/day.

PERIOPERATIVE PROPHYLAXIS
IV, IM: ADULTS, ELDERLY: 1 g 30–60 min before surgery, 0.5–1 g during surgery, and q6–8h for up to 24 hr postoperatively.

USUAL PEDIATRIC DOSAGE
CHILDREN: 50–100 mg/kg/day in divided doses q8h. **Maximum:** 6 g/day. NEONATES OLDER THAN 7 DAYS: 40–60 mg/kg/day in divided doses q8–12h. NEONATES 7 DAYS AND YOUNGER: 40 mg/kg/day in divided doses q12h.

DOSAGE IN RENAL IMPAIRMENT
Dosing frequency is modified based on creatinine clearance.

Creatinine Clearance	Dosage Interval
10–30 ml/min	Usual dose q12h
Less than 10 ml/min	Usual dose q24h

SIDE EFFECTS

FREQUENT: Discomfort with IM administration, oral candidiasis, mild diarrhea, mild abdominal cramping, vaginal candidiasis. **OCCASIONAL:** Nausea, serum sickness-like reaction (marked by fever and joint pain; usually occurs after the second course of therapy and resolves after the drug is discontinued). **RARE:** Allergic reaction (rash, pruritus, urticaria), thrombophlebitis (pain, redness, swelling at injection site).

ADVERSE REACTIONS/ TOXIC EFFECTS

Antibiotic-associated colitis and other superinfections may result from altered bacterial balance. Nephrotoxicity may occur, especially in patients with preexisting renal disease. Patients with a history of allergies, especially to penicillin, are at increased risk for developing a severe hypersensitivity reaction, marked by severe pruritus, angioedema, bronchospasm, and anaphylaxis.

NURSING CONSIDERATIONS

BASELINE ASSESSMENT

Question for history of allergies, particularly cephalosporins, penicillins.

INTERVENTION/EVALUATION

Evaluate IM site for induration and tenderness. Assess oral cavity for white patches on mucous membranes, tongue. Monitor bowel activity and stool consistency carefully; mild GI effects may be tolerable, but increasing severity may indicate onset of antibiotic-associated colitis. Monitor I&O, renal function reports for nephrotoxicity. Be alert for superinfection: severe genital/anal pruritus, abdominal pain, severe mouth soreness, moderate to severe diarrhea.

PATIENT/FAMILY TEACHING

• Discomfort may occur with IM injection.

cefdinir

sef-di-neer
(Omnicef)

CLASSIFICATION

PHARMACOTHERAPEUTIC: Third-generation cephalosporin. **CLINICAL:** Antibiotics (see p. 22C).

ACTION

A third-generation cephalosporin that binds to bacterial cell membranes and inhibits cell wall synthesis. **Therapeutic Effect:** Bactericidal.

PHARMACOKINETICS

Moderately absorbed from the GI tract. Protein binding: 60%–70%. Widely distributed. Not appreciably metabolized. Primarily excreted unchanged in urine. Minimally removed by hemodialysis. **Half-life:** 1–2 hr (increased in impaired renal function).

USES

Treatment of susceptible infections due to *S. pyogenes, S. pneumoniae, H. influenzae, H. parainfluenzae, M. catarrhalis* including community-acquired pneumonia, acute exacerbation of chronic bronchitis, acute maxillary sinusitis, pharyngitis, tonsillitis, uncomplicated skin/skin structure infections, otitis media.

PRECAUTIONS

CONTRAINDICATIONS: History of anaphylactic reaction to penicillins or hypersensitivity to cephalosporins. **CAUTIONS:** Hypersensitivity to penicillins or other drugs; history of GI disease (e.g., colitis); renal impairment, hepatic impairment.

⌛ **LIFESPAN CONSIDERATIONS: Pregnancy/Lactation:** Crosses placenta. Not detected in breast milk. **Pregnancy Category B. Children:** Newborns, infants

may have lower renal clearance. **Elderly:** Age-related renal impairment may require decreased dosage or increased dosing interval.

INTERACTIONS

DRUG: Aminoglycosides: May increase the risk of nephrotoxicity. **Antacids:** Decrease cefdinir blood concentration. **Probenecid:** Increases cefdinir blood concentration. **HERBAL:** None known. **FOOD:** None known. **LAB VALUES:** May increase serum alkaline phosphatase, bilirubin, LDH, AST, and ALT levels. May produce a false-positive reaction for ketones in urine.

AVAILABILITY (Rx)

CAPSULES: 300 mg. **ORAL SUSPENSION:** 125 mg/5 ml, 250 mg/5 ml.

ADMINISTRATION/HANDLING

PO
• Give without regard to food. • To reconstitute oral suspension, for the 60-ml bottle, add 39 ml water; for the 120-ml bottle, add 65 ml water. • Shake oral suspension well before administering. • Store mixed suspension at room temperature. Discard unused portion after 10 days.

INDICATIONS/ROUTES/DOSAGE

COMMUNITY-ACQUIRED PNEUMONIA
PO: ADULTS, ELDERLY, CHILDREN 13 YR AND OLDER: 300 mg q12h for 10 days.

ACUTE EXACERBATION OF CHRONIC BRONCHITIS
PO: ADULTS, ELDERLY: 300 mg q12h for 5–10 days.

ACUTE MAXILLARY SINUSITIS
PO: ADULTS, ELDERLY, CHILDREN 13 YR AND OLDER: 300 mg q12h or 600 mg q24h for 10 days. CHILDREN 6 MO–12 YR: 7 mg/kg q12h or 14 mg/kg q24h for 10 days.

PHARYNGITIS OR TONSILLITIS
PO: ADULTS, ELDERLY, CHILDREN 13 YR AND OLDER: 300 mg q12h for 5–10 days or 600 mg q24h for 10 days. CHILDREN 6 MO–12 YR: 7 mg/kg q12h for 5–10 days or 14 mg/kg q24h for 10 days.

UNCOMPLICATED SKIN OR SKIN-STRUCTURE INFECTIONS
PO: ADULTS, ELDERLY, CHILDREN 13 YR AND OLDER: 300 mg q12h for 10 days. CHILDREN 6 MO–12 YR: 7 mg/kg q12h for 10 days.

ACUTE BACTERIAL OTITIS MEDIA
PO (CAPSULES): CHILDREN: 6 MO–12 YR. 7 mg/kg q12h or 14 mg/kg q24h for 10 days.

USUAL PEDIATRIC DOSAGE FOR ORAL SUSPENSION
CHILDREN WEIGHING 81–95 LB (37–43 KG): 12.5 ml (2.5 tsp) q12h or 25 ml (5 tsp) q24h. CHILDREN WEIGHING 61–80 LB (28–36 KG): 10 ml (2 tsp) q12h or 20 ml (4 tsp) q24h. CHILDREN WEIGHING 41–60 LB (19–27 KG): 7.5 ml (1 tsp) q12h or 15 ml (3 tsp) q24h. CHILDREN WEIGHING 20–40 LB (9–18 KG): 5 ml (1 tsp) q12h or 10 ml (2 tsp) q24h. INFANTS WEIGHING LESS THAN 20 LB (LESS THAN 9 KG): 2.5 ml (½ tsp) q12h or 5 ml (1 tsp) q24h.

DOSAGE IN RENAL IMPAIRMENT
For patients with creatinine clearance less than 30 ml/min, dosage is 300 mg/day as single daily dose. For hemodialysis patients, dosage is 300 mg or 7 mg/kg/dose every other day.

SIDE EFFECTS

FREQUENT: Oral candidiasis, mild diarrhea, mild abdominal cramping, vaginal candidiasis. **OCCASIONAL:** Nausea, serum sickness-like reaction (marked by fever and joint pain; usually occurs after the second course of therapy and resolves after the drug is discontinued). **RARE:** Allergic reaction (rash, pruritus, urticaria).

ADVERSE REACTIONS/ TOXIC EFFECTS

Antibiotic-associated colitis and other superinfections may result from altered bacterial balance. Nephrotoxicity may occur, especially in patients with preexisting renal disease. Patients with a history of allergies, especially to penicillin, are at increased risk for developing a severe hypersensitivity reaction, marked by severe pruritus, angioedema, bronchospasm, and anaphylaxis.

NURSING CONSIDERATIONS

BASELINE ASSESSMENT

Question for hypersensitivity to cefdinir or other cephalosporins, penicillins.

INTERVENTION/EVALUATION

Monitor bowel activity and stool consistency carefully; mild GI effects may be tolerable, but increasing severity may indicate onset of antibiotic-associated colitis. Be alert for superinfection (e.g., genital/anal pruritus, ulceration or changes in oral mucosa, moderate to severe diarrhea, new/increased fever). Monitor hematology reports.

PATIENT/FAMILY TEACHING

• Take antacids 2 hr before or following medication. • Continue medication for full length of treatment; do not skip doses. • Doses should be evenly spaced. • Report persistent diarrhea to nurse/physician.

cefditoren

sef-dih-**toe**-rin

(Spectracef)

◆CLASSIFICATION

PHARMACOTHERAPEUTIC: Third-generation cephalosporin. **CLINICAL:** Antibiotic.

ACTION

A third-generation cephalosporin that binds to bacterial cell membranes and inhibits cell wall synthesis. **Therapeutic Effect:** Bactericidal.

PHARMACOKINETICS

Moderately absorbed from the GI tract. Protein binding: 88%. Not metabolized. Excreted in the urine. Minimally removed by hemodialysis. **Half-life:** 1.6 hr (half-life increased with impaired renal function).

USES

Treatment of susceptible infections due to *S. pneumoniae, S. pyogenes, S. aureus, H. influenzae, M. catarrhalis* including acute bacterial exacerbations of chronic bronchitis, pharyngitis or tonsillitis, uncomplicated skin and skin-structure infections, community-acquired pneumonia.

PRECAUTIONS

CONTRAINDICATIONS: Carnitine deficiency, inborn errors of metabolism, known allergy to cephalosporins, hypersensitivity to milk protein. **CAUTIONS:** Hypersensitivity to penicillins or other drugs; allergies; history of GI disease (e.g., colitis); renal impairment.

⧖ **LIFESPAN CONSIDERATIONS: Pregnancy/Lactation:** Unknown if distributed in breast milk. **Pregnancy Category B. Children:** Safety and efficacy not established in those younger than 12 yr. **Elderly:** Age-related renal impairment may require reduced dosage adjustment.

INTERACTIONS

DRUG: **Antacids containing magnesium or aluminum, H_2 receptor antagonists:** May decrease the absorption of cefditoren. **Probenecid:** May increase the absorption of cefditoren. **HERBAL:** None known. **FOOD:** **High-fat meals:** Increase the cefditoren plasma concentration. **LAB VALUES:** May cause a positive direct or indirect Coombs' test and a false-positive reaction to glycosuria.

AVAILABILITY (Rx)
TABLETS: 200 mg.

ADMINISTRATION/HANDLING
PO
• Give with food (enhances absorption).

INDICATIONS/ROUTES/DOSAGE
PHARYNGITIS, TONSILLITIS, SKIN INFECTIONS
PO: ADULTS, ELDERLY, CHILDREN OLDER THAN 12 YR: 200 mg twice a day for 10 days.

ACUTE EXACERBATION OF CHRONIC BRONCHITIS
PO: ADULTS, ELDERLY, CHILDREN OLDER THAN 12 YR: 400 mg twice a day for 10 days.

COMMUNITY-ACQUIRED PNEUMONIA
PO: ADULTS, ELDERLY, CHILDREN OLDER THAN 12 YR: 400 mg 2 twice a day for 14 days.

DOSAGE IN RENAL IMPAIRMENT
Dosage and frequency are modified based on creatinine clearance.

Creatinine Clearance	Dosage
50–80 ml/min	No adjustment necessary.
30–49 ml/min	200 mg twice a day
Less than 30 ml/min	200 mg once a day

SIDE EFFECTS
OCCASIONAL (11%): Diarrhea. **RARE (4%–1%):** Nausea, headache, abdominal pain, vaginal candidiasis, dyspepsia, vomiting.

ADVERSE REACTIONS/ TOXIC EFFECTS
Antibiotic-associated colitis and other superinfections may occur. Patients with a history of allergies, especially to penicillin, are at increased risk for developing a severe hypersensitivity reaction, marked by severe pruritus, angioedema, bronchospasm, and anaphylaxis.

NURSING CONSIDERATIONS

BASELINE ASSESSMENT
Question for history of allergies, particularly cephalosporins, penicillins.

INTERVENTION/EVALUATION
Monitor pattern of bowel activity and stool consistency; mild GI effects may be tolerable, but increasing severity may indicate onset of antibiotic-associated colitis. Be alert for superinfection: severe genital or anal pruritus, abdominal pain, stomatitis, moderate to severe diarrhea. Monitor carnitine deficiency (muscle damage, hypoglycemia, fatigue, confusion).

PATIENT/FAMILY TEACHING
• Continue medication for full length of treatment; do not skip doses. • Doses should be evenly spaced. • May cause GI upset (may take with food).

cefepime
sef-eh-**peem**
(Maxipime)
Do not confuse cefepime with ceftidine.

CLASSIFICATION
PHARMACOTHERAPEUTIC: Fourth-generation cephalosporin. **CLINICAL:** Antibiotic (see p. 23C).

ACTION
A fourth-generation cephalosporin that binds to bacterial cell membranes and inhibits cell wall synthesis. **Therapeutic Effect:** Bactericidal.

PHARMACOKINETICS
Well absorbed after IM administration. Protein binding: 20%. Widely distributed. Primarily excreted unchanged in urine. Removed by hemodialysis.

Half-life: 2–2.3 hr (increased in impaired renal function, and in the elderly).

USES

Susceptible infections due to aerobic gram negative organisms including *P. aeruginosa,* gram positive organisms including *S. aureus.* Treatment of empiric febrile neutropenia, intra-abdominal, skin and skin-structure, urinary tract infections, pneumonia.

PRECAUTIONS

CONTRAINDICATIONS: History of anaphylactic reaction to penicillins or hypersensitivity to cephalosporins. **CAUTIONS:** Renal impairment.

⏳ **LIFESPAN CONSIDERATIONS:** **Pregnancy/Lactation:** Unknown if distributed in breast milk. **Pregnancy Category B. Children:** No age-related precautions noted in those older than 2 mo. **Elderly:** Age-related renal impairment may require reduced dosage or increased dosing interval.

INTERACTIONS

DRUG: Aminoglycosides: May increase the risk of nephrotoxicity and ototoxicity. **Probenecid:** May increase cefepime blood concentration. **HERBAL:** None known. **FOOD:** None known. **LAB VALUES:** May increase serum alkaline phosphatase, bilirubin, LDH, AST, and ALT levels. May cause a positive direct or indirect Coombs' test.

AVAILABILITY (Rx)

POWDER FOR INJECTION: 500 mg, 1 g, 2 g.

ADMINISTRATION/HANDLING

💧 IV

Reconstitution • Add 5 ml to 500-mg vial (10 ml for 1-g and 2-g vials). • Further dilute with 50–100 ml 0.9% NaCl, or D_5W.

Rate of administration • For IV push, administer over 3–5 min. • For intermittent IV infusion (piggyback), infuse over 30 min.

Storage • Solution is stable for 24 hr at room temperature, 7 days if refrigerated.

IM

• Add 1.3 ml sterile water for injection, 0.9% NaCl, or D_5W to 500-mg vial. (2.4 ml for 1-g and 2-g vials). • Inject into a large muscle mass (e.g., upper gluteus maximus).

▨ IV INCOMPATIBILITIES

Acyclovir (Zovirax), amphotericin (Fungizone), cimetidine (Tagamet), ciprofloxacin (Cipro), cisplatin (Platinol), dacarbazine (DTIC), daunorubicin (Cerubidine), diazepam (Valium), diphenhydramine (Benadryl), dobutamine (Dobutrex), dopamine (Intropin), doxorubicin (Adriamycin), droperidol (Inapsine), famotidine (Pepcid), ganciclovir (Cytovene), haloperidol (Haldol), magnesium, magnesium sulfate, mannitol, meperidine (Demerol), metoclopramide (Reglan), morphine, ofloxacin (Floxin), ondansetron (Zofran), vancomycin (Vancocin).

IV COMPATIBILITIES

Bumetanide (Bumex), calcium gluconate, furosemide (Lasix), hydromorphone (Dilaudid), lorazepam (Ativan), propofol (Diprivan).

INDICATIONS/ROUTES/DOSAGE

PNEUMONIA

IV: ADULTS, ELDERLY: 1–2 g q12h for 7–10 days. CHILDREN 2 MO AND OLDER: 50 mg/kg q12h. **Maximum:** 2 g/dose.

INTRA-ABDOMINAL INFECTIONS

IV: ADULTS, ELDERLY: 2 g q12h for 10 days.

SKIN AND SKIN STRUCTURE INFECTIONS

IV: ADULTS, ELDERLY: 2 g q12h for 10 days. CHILDREN 2 MO AND OLDER: 50 mg/kg q12h. **Maximum:** 2 g/dose.

✐ see color pill atlas   🌿 herb   underlined – top prescribed drug

UTI₃

IV: ADULTS, ELDERLY: 0.5–2 g q12h for 7–10 days. CHILDREN 2 MO AND OLDER: 50 mg/kg q12h. **Maximum:** 2 g/dose.

FEBRILE NEUTROPENIA

IV: ADULTS, ELDERLY: 2 g q8h. CHILDREN 2 MO AND OLDER: 50 mg/kg q8h. **Maximum:** 2 g/dose.

DOSAGE IN RENAL IMPAIRMENT

Dosage and frequency are modified based on creatinine clearance and the severity of the infection.

Creatinine Clearance	Dose Range
30–60 ml/min	0.5 g q24h–2 g q12h
11–29 ml/min	0.5–2 g q24h
10 ml/min or less	0.25–1 g q24h

SIDE EFFECTS

FREQUENT: Discomfort with IM administration, oral candidiasis, mild diarrhea, mild abdominal cramping, vaginal candidiasis. **OCCASIONAL:** Nausea, serum sickness-like reaction (marked by fever and joint pain; usually occurs after the second course of therapy and resolves after the drug is discontinued). **RARE:** Allergic reaction (rash, pruritus, urticaria), thrombophlebitis (pain, redness, swelling at injection site).

ADVERSE REACTIONS/ TOXIC EFFECTS

Antibiotic-associated colitis manifested and other superinfections may result from altered bacterial balance. Nephrotoxicity may occur, especially in patients with preexisting renal disease. Patients with a history of allergies, especially to penicillin, are at increased risk for developing a severe hypersensitivity reaction, marked by severe pruritus, angioedema, bronchospasm, and anaphylaxis.

NURSING CONSIDERATIONS

BASELINE ASSESSMENT

Question for history of allergies, particularly cephalosporins, penicillins.

INTERVENTION/EVALUATION

Evaluate IM site for induration and tenderness. Assess oral cavity for white patches on mucous membranes, tongue. Monitor pattern of bowel activity and stool consistency carefully; mild GI effects may be tolerable, but increasing severity may indicate onset of antibiotic-associated colitis. Monitor I&O, renal function reports for nephrotoxicity. Be alert for superinfection: severe genital or anal pruritus, abdominal pain, severe mouth soreness, moderate to severe diarrhea.

PATIENT/FAMILY TEACHING

• Discomfort may occur with IM injection. • Continue therapy for full length of treatment. • Doses should be evenly spaced.

cefixime

sef-ih-zeem
(Suprax)
Do not confuse Suprax with Sporanox, Surbex, or Surfak.

CLASSIFICATION

PHARMACOTHERAPEUTIC: Third-generation cephalosporin. **CLINICAL:** Antibiotic.

ACTION

A third-generation cephalosporin that binds to bacterial cell membranes and inhibits cell wall synthesis. **Therapeutic Effect:** Bactericidal.

PHARMACOKINETICS

Moderately absorbed from the GI tract. Protein binding: 65%–70%. Widely distributed. Primarily excreted unchanged in urine. Minimally removed by hemodialysis. **Half-life:** 3–4 hr (increased in renal impairment).

C

USES

Treatment of susceptible infections due to *S. pneumoniae, S. pyogenes, M. catarrhalis, H. influenzae, N. gonorrhoeae, E. coli, P. mirabilis* including otitis media, acute bronchitis, acute exacerbations of chronic bronchitis, pharyngitis, tonsillitis, uncomplicated UTI, uncomplicated gonorrhea.

PRECAUTIONS

CONTRAINDICATIONS: History of anaphylactic reaction to penicillins, hypersensitivity to cephalosporins.   **CAUTIONS:** Hypersensitivity to penicillins or other drugs; allergies; history of GI disease (e.g., colitis); renal impairment.

⌛ **LIFESPAN CONSIDERATIONS: Pregnancy/Lactation:** Not recommended during labor and delivery. Unknown if distributed in breast milk. **Pregnancy Category B. Children:** Safety and efficacy not established in those younger than 6 mo. **Elderly:** Age-related renal impairment may require dosage adjustment.

INTERACTIONS

DRUG: Probenecid: Increases serum concentration of cefixime. **HERBAL:** None known. **FOOD:** None known. **LAB VALUES:** May increase BUN and serum alkaline phosphatase, bilirubin, creatinine, AST, and ALT levels. May increase LDH level. May cause a positive direct or indirect Coombs' test.

AVAILABILITY (Rx)

ORAL SUSPENSION: 100 mg/5 ml. **TABLETS:** 200 mg, 400 mg.

ADMINISTRATION/HANDLING
PO
• Give without regard to food. • After reconstitution, oral suspension is stable for 14 days at room temperature. • Do not refrigerate. • Shake oral suspension well before administering.

INDICATIONS/ROUTES/DOSAGE
OTITIS MEDIA, ACUTE BRONCHITIS, ACUTE EXACERBATIONS OF CHRONIC BRONCHITIS, PHARYNGITIS, TONSILLITIS, AND UNCOMPLICATED UTIs
PO: ADULTS, ELDERLY, CHILDREN WEIGHING MORE THAN 50 KG: 400 mg/day as a single dose or in 2 divided doses. CHILDREN 6 MO–12 YR WEIGHING LESS THAN 50 KG: 8 mg/kg/day as a single dose or in 2 divided doses. **Maximum:** 400 mg.

UNCOMPLICATED GONORRHEA
PO: ADULTS: 400 mg as a single dose.

DOSAGE IN RENAL IMPAIRMENT
Dosage is modified based on creatinine clearance.

Creatinine Clearance	% of Usual Dose
21–60 ml/min	75%
20 ml/min or less	50%

SIDE EFFECTS
FREQUENT: Oral candidiasis, mild diarrhea, mild abdominal cramping, vaginal candidiasis.   **OCCASIONAL:** Nausea, serum sickness-like reaction (marked by arthralgia and fever; usually occurs after second course of therapy and resolves after drug is discontinued). **RARE:** Allergic reaction (rash, pruritus, urticaria).

ADVERSE REACTIONS/ TOXIC EFFECTS

Antibiotic-associated colitis and other superinfections may result from altered bacterial balance. Nephrotoxicity may occur, especially in patients with preexisting renal disease. Patients with a history of allergies, especially to penicillin, are at increased risk for developing a severe hypersensitivity reaction, marked by severe pruritus, angioedema, bronchospasm, and anaphylaxis.

NURSING CONSIDERATIONS

BASELINE ASSESSMENT

Question for hypersensitivity to cefixime or other cephalosporins, penicillins, other drugs.

INTERVENTION/EVALUATION

Assess oral cavity for white patches on mucous membranes, tongue. Monitor bowel activity and stool consistency; mild GI effects may be tolerable, but increasing severity may indicate onset of antibiotic-associated colitis. Monitor renal function reports for evidence of nephrotoxicity. Be alert for superinfection: severe genital/anal pruritus, abdominal pain, stomatitis, moderate to severe diarrhea.

PATIENT/FAMILY TEACHING

• Continue medication for full length of treatment; do not skip doses. • Doses should be evenly spaced. • May cause GI upset (may take with food or milk).

Cefotan, *see cefotetan*

---

cefotaxime sodium

sef-oh-**taks**-eem

(Claforan)

Do not confuse cefotaxime with cefoxitin, ceftizoxime, or cefuroxime, or Claforan with Claritin.

◆CLASSIFICATION

PHARMACOTHERAPEUTIC: Third-generation cephalosporin. **CLINICAL:** Antibiotic (see p. 22C).

ACTION

A third-generation cephalosporin that binds to bacterial cell membranes and inhibits cell wall synthesis. **Therapeutic Effect:** Bactericidal.

PHARMACOKINETICS

Widely distributed, including to CSF. Protein binding: 30%–50%. Partially metabolized in the liver to active metabolite. Primarily excreted in urine. Moderately removed by hemodialysis. **Half-life:** 1 hr (increased in impaired renal function).

USES

Treatment of susceptible infections due to gram-negative organisms including bone and joint, GU, gynecologic, intra-abdominal, lower respiratory tract, and skin/skin structure infections, septicemia, meningitis, preoperative prophylaxis. **OFF-LABEL:** Treatment of Lyme disease.

PRECAUTIONS

CONTRAINDICATIONS: History of anaphylactic reaction to penicillins or hypersensitivity to cephalosporins. **CAUTIONS:** Concurrent use of nephrotoxic medications, history of GI disease (especially ulcerative colitis, antibiotic-associated colitis), renal impairment with creatinine clearance less than 20 ml/min.

⧗ **LIFESPAN CONSIDERATIONS: Pregnancy/Lactation:** Readily crosses placenta. Distributed in breast milk. **Pregnancy Category B. Children:** No age-related precautions noted. **Elderly:** Age-related renal impairment may require dosage adjustment.

INTERACTIONS

DRUG: Probenecid: May increase cefotaxime blood concentration. **HERBAL:** None known. **FOOD:** None known. **LAB VALUES:** May increase liver function test results and produce a positive direct or indirect Coombs' test.

AVAILABILITY (Rx)

POWDER FOR INJECTION: 500 mg, 1 g, 2 g, 10 g. **INTRAVENOUS SOLUTIONS:** 1 g/50 ml, 2 g/50 ml.

ADMINISTRATION/HANDLING
IV

Reconstitution • Reconstitute with 10 ml sterile water for injection to provide a concentration of 50 mg, 95 mg, or 180 mg/ml for 500-mg, 1-g, or 2-g vials, respectively. • May further dilute with 50–100 ml 0.9% NaCl or D₅W.

Rate of administration • For IV push, administer over 3–5 min. • For intermittent IV infusion (piggyback), infuse over 20–30 min.

Storage • Solution appears light yellow to amber. IV infusion (piggyback) may darken in color (does not indicate loss of potency). • IV infusion (piggyback) is stable for 24 hr at room temperature, 5 days if refrigerated. • Discard if precipitate forms.

IM

• Reconstitute with sterile water for injection or bacteriostatic water for injection. • Add 2, 3, or 5 ml to 500-mg, 1-g, or 2-g vial, respectively, providing a concentration of 230 mg, 300 mg, or 330 mg/ml, respectively. • To minimize discomfort, inject deep IM slowly. Less painful if injected into gluteus maximus than lateral aspect of thigh. For 2-g IM dose, give at 2 separate sites.

IV INCOMPATIBILITIES

Allopurinol (Aloprim), filgrastim (Neupogen), fluconazole (Diflucan), hetastarch (Hespan), pentamidine (Pentam IV), vancomycin (Vancocin).

IV COMPATIBILITIES

Diltiazem (Cardizem), famotidine (Pepcid), hydromorphone (Dilaudid), lorazepam (Ativan), magnesium sulfate, midazolam (Versed), morphine, propofol (Diprivan), total parenteral nutrition (TPN).

INDICATIONS/ROUTES/DOSAGE

UNCOMPLICATED INFECTIONS
IV, IM: ADULTS, ELDERLY: 1 g q12h.

MILD TO MODERATE INFECTIONS
IV, IM: ADULTS, ELDERLY: 1–2 g q8h.

SEVERE INFECTIONS
IV, IM: ADULTS, ELDERLY: 2 g q6–8h.

LIFE-THREATENING INFECTIONS
IV, IM: ADULTS, ELDERLY: 2 g q4h. CHILDREN: 2 g q4h. **Maximum:** 12 g/day.

GONORRHEA
IM: ADULTS: (**Male**): 1 g as a single dose. (**Female**): 0.5 g as a single dose.

PERIOPERATIVE PROPHYLAXIS
IV, IM: ADULTS, ELDERLY: 1 g 30–90 min before surgery.

CESAREAN SECTION
IV: ADULTS: 1 g as soon as umbilical cord is clamped, then 1 g 6 and 12 hr after first dose.

USUAL PEDIATRIC DOSAGE
CHILDREN WEIGHING 50 KG OR MORE: 1–2 g q6–8h. CHILDREN 1 MO–12 YR WEIGHING LESS THAN 50 KG: 100–200 mg/kg/day in divided doses q6–8h.

DOSAGE IN RENAL IMPAIRMENT
For patients with creatinine clearance less than 20 ml/min give half of dose at usual dosing intervals.

SIDE EFFECTS

FREQUENT: Discomfort with IM administration, oral candidiasis, mild diarrhea, mild abdominal cramping, vaginal candidiasis. **OCCASIONAL:** Nausea, serum sickness-like reaction (marked by fever and joint pain; usually occurs after the second course of therapy and resolves after the drug is discontinued). **RARE:** Allergic reaction (rash, pruritus, urticaria), thrombophlebitis (pain, redness, swelling at injection site).

ADVERSE REACTIONS/ TOXIC EFFECTS

Antibiotic-associated colitis and other superinfections may result from altered bacterial balance. Nephrotoxicity may occur, especially in patients with pre-existing renal disease. Patients with a history of allergies, especially to penicillin, are at increased risk for developing a severe hypersensitivity reaction, marked by severe pruritus, angioedema, bronchospasm, and anaphylaxis.

NURSING CONSIDERATIONS

BASELINE ASSESSMENT

Question for history of allergies, particularly cephalosporins, penicillins.

INTERVENTION/EVALUATION

Check IM injection sites for induration, tenderness. Assess oral cavity for white patches on mucous membranes, tongue. Monitor bowel activity and stool consistency carefully; mild GI effects may be tolerable, but increasing severity may indicate onset of antibiotic-associated colitis. Monitor I&O, renal function reports for nephrotoxicity. Be alert for superinfection: severe genital/anal pruritus, abdominal pain, severe mouth soreness, moderate to severe diarrhea.

PATIENT/FAMILY TEACHING

- Discomfort may occur with IM injection. • Doses should be evenly spaced. • Continue antibiotic therapy for full length of treatment.

cefotetan disodium

seh-fo-**teh**-tan

(Cefotan)

Do not confuse cefotetan with cefoxitin or Ceftin.

◆CLASSIFICATION

PHARMACOTHERAPEUTIC: Second-generation cephalosporin. **CLINICAL:** Antibiotic (see p. 21C).

ACTION

A second-generation cephalosporin that binds to bacterial cell membranes and inhibits cell wall synthesis. **Therapeutic Effect:** Bactericidal.

PHARMACOKINETICS

Protein binding: 78%–91%. Primarily excreted unchanged in urine. Minimally removed by hemodialysis. **Half-life:** 3–4.6 hr (increased in impaired renal function).

USES

Treatment of susceptible infections due to *S. pneumoniae*, *S. aureus*, gram-negative enteric bacilli, anaerobes (e.g., Bacteroides species) including bone and joint, gynecologic, intra-abdominal, lower respiratory, skin/skin structure and urinary tract infections, perioperative prophylaxis.

PRECAUTIONS

CONTRAINDICATIONS: History of anaphylactic reaction to penicillins or hypersensitivity to cephalosporins. **CAUTIONS:** Renal impairment, history of GI disease (especially ulcerative colitis, antibiotic-associated colitis), concurrent use of nephrotoxic medications.

🔲 LIFESPAN CONSIDERATIONS: **Pregnancy/Lactation:** Readily crosses placenta. Distributed in breast milk. **Pregnancy Category B. Children:** Safety and efficacy not established. **Elderly:** Age-related renal impairment may require dosage adjustment.

INTERACTIONS

DRUG: Alcohol: May produce a disulfiram-like reaction (facial flushing, headache, nausea, pruritus, tachycardia).

Heparin, other anticoagulants: May increase the risk of bleeding. **HERBAL:** None known. **FOOD:** None known. **LAB VALUES:** May increase BUN level and serum alkaline phosphatase, creatinine, AST, and ALT levels. May prolong prothrombin time and produce a positive direct or indirect Coombs' test. Interferes with crossmatching procedures and hematologic tests.

AVAILABILITY (Rx)

POWDER FOR INJECTION: 1 g, 2 g, 10 g. **INTRAVENOUS SOLUTION:** 1 g/50 ml, 2 g/50 ml.

ADMINISTRATION/HANDLING

◀ **ALERT** ▶ Give by IM injection, IV push, intermittent IV infusion (piggyback).

 IV

Reconstitution • Reconstitute each 1 g with 10 ml sterile water for injection to provide a concentration of 95 mg/ml. • May further dilute with 50–100 ml 0.9% NaCl or D_5W.

Rate of administration • For IV push, administer over 3–5 min. • For intermittent IV infusion (piggyback), infuse over 20–30 min.

Storage • Solution appears colorless to light yellow. • Color change to deep yellow does not indicate loss of potency. • IV infusion (piggyback) is stable for 24 hr at room temperature, 96 hr if refrigerated. • Discard if precipitate forms.

IM
• Add 2 or 3 ml sterile water for injection or other appropriate diluent to 1 g or 2 g providing a concentration of 400 mg/ml or 500 mg/ml, respectively. • Less painful if injected deep IM slowly into gluteus maximus rather than lateral aspect of thigh.

▓ IV INCOMPATIBILITY

Vancomycin (Vancocin).

IV COMPATIBILITIES

Diltiazem (Cardizem), famotidine (Pepcid), heparin, insulin (regular), morphine, propofol (Diprivan).

INDICATIONS/ROUTES/DOSAGE

UTIs
IV, IM: ADULTS, ELDERLY: 1–2 g in divided doses q12–24h.

MILD TO MODERATE INFECTIONS
IV, IM: ADULTS, ELDERLY: 1–2 g q12h.

SEVERE INFECTIONS
IV, IM: ADULTS, ELDERLY: 2 g q12h.

LIFE-THREATENING INFECTIONS
IV, IM: ADULTS, ELDERLY: 3 g q12h.

PERIOPERATIVE PROPHYLAXIS
IV: ADULTS, ELDERLY: 1–2 g 30–60 min before surgery.

CESAREAN SECTION
IV: ADULTS: 1–2 g as soon as umbilical cord is clamped.

USUAL PEDIATRIC DOSAGE
CHILDREN: 40–80 mg/kg/day in divided doses q12h. **Maximum:** 6 g/day.

DOSAGE IN RENAL IMPAIRMENT
Dosing frequency is modified based on creatinine clearance and the severity of the infection.

Creatinine Clearance	Dosage Interval
10–30 ml/min	Usual dose q24h
Less than 10 ml/min	Usual dose q48h

SIDE EFFECTS

FREQUENT: Discomfort with IM administration, oral candidiasis, mild diarrhea, mild abdominal cramping, vaginal candidiasis. **OCCASIONAL:** Nausea, unusual bleeding or bruising, serum sickness-like reaction (marked by fever and joint pain; usually occurs after the second course of therapy and resolves after the drug is discontinued). **RARE:** Allergic reaction (rash, pruritus, urticaria), thrombophlebitis (pain, redness, swelling at injection site).

ADVERSE REACTIONS/ TOXIC EFFECTS

Antibiotic-associated colitis and other superinfections may result from altered bacterial balance. Nephrotoxicity may occur, especially in patients with pre-existing renal disease. Patients with a history of allergies, especially to penicillin, are at increased risk for developing a severe hypersensitivity reaction, marked by severe pruritus, angioedema, bronchospasm, and anaphylaxis.

NURSING CONSIDERATIONS

BASELINE ASSESSMENT

Question for history of allergies, particularly cephalosporins, penicillins.

INTERVENTION/EVALUATION

Evaluate IV site for phlebitis (heat, pain, red streaking over vein). Check IM injection sites for induration, tenderness. Assess oral cavity for white patches on mucous membranes, tongue. Monitor bowel activity and stool consistency carefully; mild GI effects may be tolerable, but increasing severity may indicate onset of antibiotic-associated colitis. Monitor I&O, renal function reports for nephrotoxicity. Be alert for superinfection: severe genital/anal pruritus, abdominal pain, severe mouth soreness, moderate to severe diarrhea.

PATIENT/FAMILY TEACHING

• Discomfort may occur with IM injection. • Doses should be evenly spaced. • Continue antibiotic therapy for full length of treatment. • Avoid alcohol/alcohol-containing preparations (e.g., cough syrups, cold medicines) during and for 72 hr after last dose of cefotetan.

---

cefoxitin sodium

se-**fox**-i-tin
(Mefoxin)

Do not confuse cefoxitin with cefotaxime, cefotetan, or Cytoxan.

CLASSIFICATION

PHARMACOTHERAPEUTIC: Second-generation cephalosporin. **CLINICAL:** Antibiotic (see p. 21C).

ACTION

A second-generation cephalosporin that binds to bacterial cell membranes and inhibits cell wall synthesis. **Therapeutic Effect:** Bactericidal.

PHARMACOKINETICS

Well distributed. Protein binding: 41%–75%. Primarily excreted in urine. Removed by hemodialysis. **Half-life:** 0.8–1 hr.

USES

Treatment of susceptible infections due to *S. pneumoniae, S. aureus,* gram-negative enteric bacilli, anaerobes (e.g., bacteroides species) including bone and joint, gynecologic, intra-abdominal, lower respiratory, skin and skin-structure and urinary tract infections, perioperative prophylaxis.

PRECAUTIONS

CONTRAINDICATIONS: History of anaphylactic reaction to penicillins or hypersensitivity to cephalosporins. **CAUTIONS:** Renal impairment, history of GI disease (especially ulcerative colitis, antibiotic-associated colitis), concurrent use of nephrotoxic medications.

⧗ LIFESPAN CONSIDERATIONS: **Pregnancy/Lactation:** Readily crosses placenta; distributed in breast milk. **Pregnancy Category B. Children:** No age-related precautions noted. **Elderly:** Age-related renal impairment may require dosage adjustment.

INTERACTIONS

DRUG: Probenecid: Increases serum concentration of cefoxitin. **HERBAL:** None known. **FOOD:** None known. **LAB VALUES:** May increase BUN level and serum alkaline phosphatase, creatinine, AST, and ALT levels. May produce a positive direct or indirect Coombs' test. Interferes with crossmatching procedures and hematologic tests.

AVAILABILITY (Rx)

POWDER FOR INJECTION: 1 g, 2 g, 10 g. **INTRAVENOUS SOLUTION:** 1 g/50 ml, 2 g/50 ml.

ADMINISTRATION/HANDLING

◀ **ALERT** ▶ Give IM, IV push, intermittent IV infusion (piggyback).

 IV

Reconstitution • Reconstitute each 1 g with 10 ml sterile water for injection to provide concentration of 95 mg/ml. • May further dilute with 50–100 ml 0.9% sterile water for injection, NaCl, or D_5W.

Rate of administration • For IV push, administer over 3–5 min. • For intermittent IV infusion (piggyback), infuse over 15–30 min.

Storage • Solution appears colorless to light amber but may darken (does not indicate loss of potency). • IV infusion (piggyback) is stable for 24 hr at room temperature, 48 hr if refrigerated. • Discard if precipitate forms.

IM
• Reconstitute each 1 g with 2 ml sterile water for injection or lidocaine to provide concentration of 400 mg/ml. • To minimize discomfort, inject deep IM slowly. Less painful if injected into gluteus maximus than lateral aspect of thigh.

▓ IV INCOMPATIBILITIES

Filgrastim (Neupogen), pentamidine (Pentam IV), vancomycin (Vancocin).

IV COMPATIBILITIES

Diltiazem (Cardizem), famotidine (Pepcid), heparin, hydromorphone (Dilaudid), magnesium sulfate, morphine, multivitamins, propofol (Diprivan).

INDICATIONS/ROUTES/DOSAGE

MILD TO MODERATE INFECTIONS
IV, IM: ADULTS, ELDERLY: 1–2 g q6–8h.

SEVERE INFECTIONS
IV, IM: ADULTS, ELDERLY: 1 g q4h or 2 g q6–8h up to 2 g q4h.

PERIOPERATIVE PROPHYLAXIS
IV, IM: ADULTS, ELDERLY: 2 g 30–60 min before surgery, then q6h for up to 24 hr after surgery. CHILDREN OLDER THAN 3 MO: 30–40 mg/kg 30–60 min before surgery, then q6h for up to 24 hr after surgery.

CESAREAN SECTION
IV: ADULTS: 2 g as soon as umbilical cord is clamped, then 2 g 4 and 8 hr after first dose, then q6h for up to 24 hr.

USUAL PEDIATRIC DOSAGE
CHILDREN OLDER THAN 3 MO: 80–160 mg/kg/day in 4–6 divided doses. **Maximum:** 12 g/day. NEONATES: 90–100 mg/kg/day in divided doses q6–8h.

DOSAGE IN RENAL IMPAIRMENT
After a loading dose of 1–2 g, dosage and frequency are modified based on creatinine clearance and the severity of the infection.

Creatinine Clearance	Dosage
30–50 ml/min	1–2 g q8–12h
10–29 ml/min	1–2 g q12–24h
5–9 ml/min	500 mg–1 g q12–24h
Less than 5 ml/min	500 mg–1 g q24–48h

SIDE EFFECTS

FREQUENT: Discomfort with IM administration, oral candidiasis, mild diarrhea, mild abdominal cramping, vaginal candidiasis. **OCCASIONAL:** Nausea, serum sickness-like reaction (marked by fever and joint pain; usually occurs after the second course of therapy and resolves after the drug is discontinued). **RARE:** Allergic reaction (pruritus, rash, urticaria), thrombophlebitis (pain, redness, swelling at injection site).

ADVERSE REACTIONS/ TOXIC EFFECTS

Antibiotic-associated colitis and other superinfections may result from altered bacterial balance. Nephrotoxicity may occur, especially in patients with pre-existing renal disease. Patients with a history of allergies, especially to penicillin, are at increased risk for developing a severe hypersensitivity reaction, marked by severe pruritus, angioedema, bronchospasm, and anaphylaxis.

NURSING CONSIDERATIONS

BASELINE ASSESSMENT

Question for history of allergies, particularly cephalosporins, penicillins.

INTERVENTION/EVALUATION

Evaluate IV site for phlebitis (heat, pain, red streaking over vein). Assess IM injection sites for induration, tenderness. Assess oral cavity for white patches on mucous membranes, tongue. Monitor bowel activity and stool consistency carefully; mild GI effects may be tolerable, but increasing severity may indicate onset of antibiotic-associated colitis. Monitor I&O, renal function reports for nephrotoxicity. Be alert for superinfection: severe genital or anal pruritus, abdominal pain, severe mouth soreness, moderate to severe diarrhea.

PATIENT/FAMILY TEACHING

• Discomfort may occur with IM injection. • Doses should be evenly spaced. • Continue antibiotic therapy for full length of treatment.

cefpodoxime proxetil

sef-poe-**docks**-em
(Vantin)

Do not confuse Vantin with Ventolin.

CLASSIFICATION

PHARMACOTHERAPEUTIC: Third-generation cephalosporin. **CLINICAL:** Antibiotic (see p. 21C).

ACTION

A third-generation cephalosporin that binds to bacterial cell membranes and inhibits cell wall synthesis. Therapeutic Effect: Bactericidal.

PHARMACOKINETICS

Well absorbed from the GI tract (food increases absorption). Protein binding: 21%–40%. Widely distributed. Primarily excreted unchanged in urine. Partially removed by hemodialysis. Half-life: 2.3 hr (increased in impaired renal function and elderly patients).

USES

Treatment of susceptible infections due to *S. pneumoniae, S pyogenes, S. aureus, H. influenzae, M. catarrhalis, E. coli,* Proteus, Klebsiella including acute maxillary sinusitis, chronic bronchitis, community acquired pneumonia, gonorrhea, otitis media, pharyngitis or tonsillitis, skin and skin-structure and urinary tract infections.

PRECAUTIONS

CONTRAINDICATIONS: History of anaphylactic reaction to penicillins or hypersensitivity to cephalosporins. **CAUTIONS:** Renal impairment, history of allergies or GI disease (especially ulcerative colitis, antibiotic-associated colitis), concurrent use of nephrotoxic medications.

⊠ LIFESPAN CONSIDERATIONS: **Pregnancy/Lactation:** Readily crosses placenta. Distributed in breast milk. **Pregnancy Category B. Children:** Safety and efficacy not established in those younger than 6 mo.   **Elderly:** Age-related renal impairment may require dosage adjustment.

INTERACTIONS

DRUG: Antacids, H$_2$ antagonists: May decrease cefpodoxime absorption. **Probenecid:** May increase cefpodoxime blood concentration. **HERBAL:** None known. **FOOD:** None known. **LAB VALUES:** May increase BUN level and serum alkaline phosphatase, bilirubin, creatinine, LDH, AST, and ALT levels. May produce a positive direct or indirect Coombs' test.

AVAILABILITY (Rx)

ORAL SUSPENSION: 50 mg/5 ml, 100 mg/5 ml. **TABLETS:** 100 mg, 200 mg.

ADMINISTRATION/HANDLING
PO
• Administer with food to enhance absorption. • After reconstitution, oral suspension is stable for 14 days if refrigerated.

INDICATIONS/ROUTES/DOSAGE
CHRONIC BRONCHITIS, PNEUMONIA
PO: ADULTS, ELDERLY, CHILDREN OLDER THAN 13 YR: 200 mg q12h for 10–14 days.

GONORRHEA, RECTAL GONOCOCCAL INFECTION (FEMALE PATIENTS ONLY)
PO: ADULTS, CHILDREN OLDER THAN 13 YR: 200 mg as a single dose.

SKIN AND SKIN-STRUCTURE INFECTIONS
PO: ADULTS, ELDERLY, CHILDREN OLDER THAN 13 YR: 400 mg q12h for 7–14 days.

PHARYNGITIS, TONSILLITIS
PO: ADULTS, ELDERLY, CHILDREN OLDER THAN 13 YR: 100 mg q12h for 5–10 days. CHILDREN 6 MO–13 YR: 5 mg/kg q12h for 5–10 days. **Maximum:** 100 mg/dose.

ACUTE MAXILLARY SINUSITIS
PO: ADULTS, CHILDREN OLDER THAN 13 YR: 200 mg twice a day for 10 days. CHILDREN 2 MO–13 YR: 5 mg/kg q12h for 10 days. **Maximum:** 200 mg/dose.

UTIs
PO: ADULTS, ELDERLY, CHILDREN OLDER THAN 13 YR: 100 mg q12h for 7 days.

ACUTE OTITIS MEDIA
PO: CHILDREN 6 MO–13 YR: 5 mg/kg q12h for 5 days. **Maximum:** 400 mg/dose.

DOSAGE IN RENAL IMPAIRMENT
For patients with creatinine clearance less than 30 ml/min, usual dose is given q24h. For patients on hemodialysis, usual dose is given 3 times/wk after dialysis.

SIDE EFFECTS

FREQUENT: Oral candidiasis, mild diarrhea, mild abdominal cramping, vaginal candidiasis. **OCCASIONAL:** Nausea, serum sickness-like reaction (marked by fever and joint pain; usually occurs after the second course of therapy and resolves after the drug is discontinued). **RARE:** Allergic reaction (pruritus, rash, urticaria).

ADVERSE REACTIONS/TOXIC EFFECTS

Antibiotic-associated colitis and other superinfections may result from altered bacterial balance. Nephrotoxicity may occur, especially in patients with preexisting renal disease. Patients with a history of allergies, especially to penicillin, are at increased risk for developing a severe hypersensitivity reaction, marked by severe pruritus, angioedema, bronchospasm, and anaphylaxis.

NURSING CONSIDERATIONS

BASELINE ASSESSMENT
Question for history of allergies, particularly cephalosporins, penicillins.

INTERVENTION/EVALUATION

Assess oral cavity for white patches on mucous membranes, tongue. Monitor pattern of bowel activity and stool consistency carefully; mild GI effects may be tolerable, but increasing severity may indicate onset of antibiotic-associated colitis. Monitor I&O, renal function reports for nephrotoxicity. Be alert for superinfection: severe genital or anal pruritus, abdominal pain, severe mouth soreness, moderate to severe diarrhea.

PATIENT/FAMILY TEACHING

• Doses should be evenly spaced. • Shake oral suspension well before using. • Continue antibiotic therapy for full length of treatment. • Take with food. • Refrigerate oral suspension.

cefprozil

sef-**proz**-ill
(Cefzil)
Do not confuse cefprozil with Cefazolin or Cefzil with Cefol, Ceftin, or Kefzol.

CLASSIFICATION

PHARMACOTHERAPEUTIC: Second-generation cephalosporin. **CLINICAL:** Antibiotic (see p. 21C).

ACTION

A second-generation cephalosporin that binds to bacterial cell membranes and inhibits cell wall synthesis. **Therapeutic Effect:** Bactericidal.

PHARMACOKINETICS

Well absorbed from the GI tract. Protein binding: 36%–45%. Widely distributed. Primarily excreted unchanged in urine. Moderately removed by hemodialysis. **Half-life:** 1.3 hr (increased in impaired renal function).

USES

Treatment of susceptible infections due to *S. pneumoniae, S pyogenes, S. aureus, H. influenzae, M. catarrhalis* including pharyngitis or tonsillitis, otitis media, secondary bacterial infection of acute bronchitis, acute bacterial exacerbation of chronic bronchitis, uncomplicated skin and skin-structure infections, acute sinusitis.

PRECAUTIONS

CONTRAINDICATIONS: History of anaphylactic reaction to penicillins or hypersensitivity to cephalosporins. **CAUTIONS:** Renal impairment, history of GI disease (especially ulcerative colitis, antibiotic-associated colitis), concurrent use of nephrotoxic medications.

⌛ **LIFESPAN CONSIDERATIONS: Pregnancy/Lactation:** Readily crosses placenta. Distributed in breast milk. **Pregnancy Category B. Children:** Safety and efficacy not established in those younger than 6 mo. **Elderly:** Age-related renal impairment may require dosage adjustment.

INTERACTIONS

DRUG: Probenecid: Increases serum concentration of cefprozil. **HERBAL:** None known. **FOOD:** None known. **LAB VALUES:** May increase liver function test results. May produce a positive direct or indirect Coombs' test. Interferes with crossmatching procedures and hematologic tests.

AVAILABILITY (Rx)

ORAL SUSPENSION: 125 mg/5 ml, 250 mg/5 ml. **TABLETS:** 250 mg, 500 mg.

ADMINISTRATION/HANDLING

PO
• After reconstitution, oral suspension is stable for 14 days if refrigerated. • Shake oral suspension well before using. • Give without regard to food; if GI upset occurs, give with food or milk.

INDICATIONS/ROUTES/DOSAGE

PHARYNGITIS, TONSILLITIS
PO: ADULTS, ELDERLY: 500 mg q24h for 10 days. CHILDREN 2–12 YR: 7.5 mg/kg q12h for 10 days. **Maximum:** 1 g/day.

ACUTE BACTERIAL EXACERBATION OF CHRONIC BRONCHITIS, SECONDARY BACTERIAL INFECTION OF ACUTE BRONCHITIS
PO: ADULTS, ELDERLY: 500 mg q12h for 10 days.

SKIN AND SKIN-STRUCTURE INFECTIONS
PO: ADULTS, ELDERLY, CHILDREN OLDER THAN 12 YR: 250–500 mg q12h for 10 days. CHILDREN 2–12 YR: 20 mg/kg q24h for 10 days. **Maximum:** 1 g/day.

ACUTE SINUSITIS
PO: ADULTS, ELDERLY: 250–500 mg q12h for 10 days. CHILDREN 6 MO–12 YR: 7.5–15 mg/kg q12h for 10 days.

OTITIS MEDIA
PO: CHILDREN 6 MO–12 YR: 15 mg/kg q12h for 10 days. **Maximum:** 1 g/day.

DOSAGE IN RENAL IMPAIRMENT
Patients with creatinine clearance less than 30 ml/min receive 50% of usual dose at usual interval.

SIDE EFFECTS

FREQUENT: Oral candidiasis, mild diarrhea, mild abdominal cramping, vaginal candidiasis. **OCCASIONAL:** Nausea, serum sickness reaction (marked by fever and joint pain; usually occurs after the second course of therapy and resolves after the drug is discontinued). **RARE:** Allergic reaction (pruritus, rash, urticaria).

ADVERSE REACTIONS/ TOXIC EFFECTS

Antibiotic-associated colitis and other superinfections may result from altered bacterial balance. Nephrotoxicity may occur, especially in patients with pre-existing renal disease. Patients with a history of allergies, especially to penicillin, are at increased risk for developing a severe hypersensitivity reaction, marked by severe pruritus, angioedema, bronchospasm, and anaphylaxis.

NURSING CONSIDERATIONS

BASELINE ASSESSMENT
Question for history of allergies, particularly cephalosporins, penicillins.

INTERVENTION/EVALUATION
Assess oral cavity for evidence of stomatitis. Monitor pattern of bowel activity and stool consistency carefully; mild GI effects may be tolerable, but increasing severity may indicate onset of antibiotic-associated colitis. Monitor I&O, renal function reports for nephrotoxicity. Be alert for superinfection: severe genital or anal pruritus, abdominal pain, severe mouth soreness, moderate to severe diarrhea.

PATIENT/FAMILY TEACHING
• Doses should be evenly spaced. • Continue antibiotic therapy for full length of treatment. • May cause GI upset (may take with food or milk).

ceftazidime

sef-**taz**-ih-deem

(Ceptaz, <u>Fortaz</u>, Tazicef, Tazidime)
Do not confuse ceftazidime with ceftizoxime.

◆CLASSIFICATION
PHARMACOTHERAPEUTIC: Third-generation cephalosporin. **CLINICAL:** Antibiotic (see p. 22C).

ACTION

A third-generation cephalosporin that binds to bacterial cell membranes and inhibits cell wall synthesis. **Therapeutic Effect:** Bactericidal.

PHARMACOKINETICS

Widely distributed (including to cerebrospinal fluid [CSF]). Protein binding: 5%–17%. Primarily excreted unchanged in urine. Removed by hemodialysis. Half-life: 2 hr (increased in impaired renal function).

USES

Treatment of susceptible infections due to gram negative organisms including Pseudomonas and Enterobacteraceae including bone and joint, CNS (including meningitis), gynecologic, intra-abdominal, lower respiratory tract, skin and skin-structure, and urinary tract infections, septicemia.

PRECAUTIONS

CONTRAINDICATIONS: History of anaphylactic reaction to penicillins or hypersensitivity to cephalosporins. **CAUTIONS:** Renal impairment, history of GI disease (especially ulcerative colitis, antibiotic-associated colitis), concurrent use of nephrotoxic medications.

⏳ **LIFESPAN CONSIDERATIONS: Pregnancy/Lactation:** Readily crosses placenta. Distributed in breast milk. **Pregnancy Category B. Children:** No age-related precautions noted. **Elderly:** Age-related renal impairment may require dosage adjustment.

INTERACTIONS

DRUG: Aminoglycosides, diuretics (e.g., furosemide): May increase the risk of nephrotoxicity. **HERBAL:** None known. **FOOD:** None known. **LAB VALUES:** May increase BUN level and serum alkaline phosphatase, creatinine, LDH, AST, and ALT levels. May produce a positive direct or indirect Coombs' test. Interferes with crossmatching procedures and hematologic tests.

AVAILABILITY (Rx)

POWDER FOR INJECTION (FORTAZ, TAZICEF, TAZIDIME): 500 mg, 1 g, 2 g.

ADMINISTRATION/HANDLING

◀ **ALERT** ▶ Give by IM injection, direct IV injection, or intermittent IV infusion (piggyback).

 IV

Reconstitution • Add 10 ml sterile water for injection to each 1 g to provide concentration of 90 mg/ml. • May further dilute with 50–100 ml 0.9% NaCl, D_5W, or other compatible diluent.

Rate of administration • For IV push, administer over 3–5 min. • For intermittent IV infusion (piggyback), infuse over 15–30 min.

Storage • Solution appears light yellow to amber, tends to darken (color change does not indicate loss of potency). • IV infusion (piggyback) stable for 18 hr at room temperature, 7 days if refrigerated. • Discard if precipitate forms.

IM

• For reconstitution, add 1.5 ml sterile water for injection or lidocaine 1% to 500 mg or 3 ml to 1-g vial to provide a concentration of 280 mg/ml. • To minimize discomfort, inject deep IM slowly. Less painful if injected into gluteus maximus than lateral aspect of thigh.

▦ IV INCOMPATIBILITIES

Amphotericin B complex (Abelcet, AmBisome, Amphotec), doxorubicin liposomal (Doxil), fluconazole (Diflucan), idarubicin (Idamycin), midazolam (Versed), pentamidine (Pentam IV), vancomycin (Vancocin), total parenteral nutrition (TPN).

IV COMPATIBILITIES

Diltiazem (Cardizem), famotidine (Pepcid), heparin, hydromorphone (Dilaudid), morphine, propofol (Diprivan).

INDICATIONS/ROUTES/DOSAGE

UTIs
IV, IM: ADULTS: 250–500 mg q8–12h.

MILD TO MODERATE INFECTIONS
IV, IM: ADULTS: 1 g q8–12h.

UNCOMPLICATED PNEUMONIA, SKIN AND SKIN-STRUCTURE INFECTIONS
IV, IM: ADULTS: 0.5–1 g q8h.

BONE AND JOINT INFECTIONS
IV, IM: ADULTS: 2 g q12h.

MENINGITIS, SERIOUS GYNECOLOGIC AND INTRA-ABDOMINAL INFECTIONS
IV, IM: ADULTS: 2 g q8h.

PSEUDOMONAL PULMONARY INFECTIONS IN PATIENTS WITH CYSTIC FIBROSIS
IV: ADULTS: 30–50 mg/kg q8h. **Maximum:** 6 g/day.

USUAL ELDERLY DOSAGE
ELDERLY (NORMAL RENAL FUNCTION): 500 mg–1 g q12h.

USUAL PEDIATRIC DOSAGE
CHILDREN 1 MO–12 YR: 100–150 mg/kg/day in divided doses q8h. **Maximum:** 6 g/day. NEONATES 0–4 WK: 100–150 mg/kg/day in divided doses q8–12h.

DOSAGE IN RENAL IMPAIRMENT
After an initial 1-g dose, dosage and frequency are modified based on creatinine clearance and the severity of the infection.

Creatinine Clearance	Dosage
31–50 ml/min	1 g q12h
16–30 ml/min	1 g q24h
6–15 ml/min	500 mg q24h
Less than 5 ml/min	500 mg q48h

SIDE EFFECTS

FREQUENT: Discomfort with IM administration, oral candidiasis, mild diarrhea, mild abdominal cramping, vaginal candidiasis. **OCCASIONAL:** Nausea, serum sickness-like reaction (marked by fever and joint pain; usually occurs after the second course of therapy and resolves after the drug is discontinued). **RARE:** Allergic reaction (pruritus, rash, urticaria), thrombophlebitis (pain, redness, swelling at injection site).

ADVERSE REACTIONS/ TOXIC EFFECTS

Antibiotic-associated colitis and other superinfections may result from altered bacterial balance. Nephrotoxicity may occur, especially in patients with preexisting renal disease. Patients with a history of allergies, especially to penicillin, are at increased risk for developing a severe hypersensitivity reaction, marked by severe pruritus, angioedema, bronchospasm, and anaphylaxis.

NURSING CONSIDERATIONS

BASELINE ASSESSMENT
Question for history of allergies, particularly cephalosporins, penicillins.

INTERVENTION/EVALUATION
Evaluate IV site for phlebitis (heat, pain, red streaking over vein). Assess IM injection sites for induration, tenderness. Check oral cavity for white patches on mucous membranes, tongue. Monitor pattern of bowel activity and stool consistency carefully; mild GI effects may be tolerable, but increasing severity may indicate onset of antibiotic-associated colitis. Monitor I&O, renal function reports for nephrotoxicity. Be alert for superinfection: severe genital/anal pruritus, abdominal pain, severe mouth soreness, moderate to severe diarrhea.

PATIENT/FAMILY TEACHING
• Discomfort may occur with IM injection. • Doses should be evenly spaced. • Continue antibiotic therapy for full length of treatment.

ceftibuten

sef-tih-**byew**-ten
(Cedax)

CLASSIFICATION

PHARMACOTHERAPEUTIC: Third-generation cephalosporin. **CLINICAL:** Antibiotic (see p. 23C).

ACTION

A third-generation cephalosporin that binds to bacterial cell membranes and inhibits cell wall synthesis. **Therapeutic Effect:** Bactericidal.

PHARMACOKINETICS

Rapidly absorbed from the GI tract. Protein binding: 65%–77%. Excreted primarily in urine. **Half-life:** 2–3 hr.

USES

Treatment of susceptible infections due to *S. pneumoniae, S pyogenes, H. influenzae, M. catarrhalis* including chronic bronchitis, acute bacterial otitis media, pharyngitis, tonsillitis.

PRECAUTIONS

CONTRAINDICATIONS: History of anaphylactic reaction to penicillins or hypersensitivity to cephalosporins. **CAUTIONS:** Hypersensitivity to penicillins or other drugs, history of GI disease (e.g., colitis), renal impairment.

⧗ **LIFESPAN CONSIDERATIONS: Pregnancy/Lactation:** Unknown if drug crosses placenta or is distributed in breast milk. **Pregnancy Category B. Children:** Safety and efficacy not established in children younger than 6 mo. **Elderly:** Age-related renal impairment may require dosage adjustment.

INTERACTIONS

DRUG: Aminoglycosides: Increased risk of nephrotoxicity. **Probenecid:** Increases serum ceftibuten level. **HERBAL:** None known. **FOOD:** None known. **LAB VALUES:** May increase BUN level and serum alkaline phosphatase, bilirubin, creatinine, LDH, AST, and ALT levels. May produce a positive direct or indirect Coombs' test.

AVAILABILITY (Rx)

CAPSULES: 400 mg. **ORAL SUSPENSION:** 90 mg/5 ml.

INDICATIONS/ROUTES/DOSAGE

CHRONIC BRONCHITIS

PO: ADULTS, ELDERLY: 400 mg/day once a day for 10 days.

PHARYNGITIS, TONSILLITIS

PO: ADULTS, ELDERLY: 400 mg once a day for 10 days. CHILDREN OLDER THAN 6 MO: 9 mg/kg once a day for 10 days. **Maximum:** 400 mg/day.

OTITIS MEDIA

PO: CHILDREN OLDER THAN 6 MO: 9 mg/kg once a day for 10 days. **Maximum:** 400 mg/day.

DOSAGE IN RENAL IMPAIRMENT

Dosage is modified based on creatinine clearance.

Creatinine Clearance	Dosage
50 ml/min and higher	400 mg or 9 mg/kg q24h
30–49 ml/min	200 mg or 4.5 mg/kg q24h
Less than 30 ml/min	100 mg or 2.25 mg/kg q24h

SIDE EFFECTS

FREQUENT: Oral candidiasis, mild diarrhea (discharge, itching). **OCCASIONAL:** Nausea, serum sickness-like reaction (marked by fever and joint pain; usually occurs after the second course of therapy and resolves after the drug is discontinued). **RARE:** Allergic reaction (rash, pruritus, urticaria).

ADVERSE REACTIONS/ TOXIC EFFECTS

Antibiotic-associated colitis and other superinfections may result from altered bacterial balance. Nephrotoxicity may occur, especially in patients with pre-existing renal disease. Patients with a history of allergies, especially to penicillin, are at increased risk for developing a severe hypersensitivity reaction, marked by severe pruritus, angioedema, bronchospasm, and anaphylaxis.

NURSING CONSIDERATIONS

BASELINE ASSESSMENT

Question for history of allergies, particularly cephalosporins, penicillins.

INTERVENTION/EVALUATION

Assess oral cavity for white patches on mucous membranes, tongue. Monitor pattern of bowel activity and stool consistency carefully; mild GI effects may be tolerable, but increasing severity may indicate onset of antibiotic-associated colitis. Monitor I&O, serum renal function reports for nephrotoxicity. Be alert for superinfection: severe genital or anal pruritus, abdominal pain, severe mouth soreness, moderate to severe diarrhea.

PATIENT/FAMILY TEACHING

• Continue medication for full length of treatment; do not skip doses. • Doses should be evenly spaced. • May cause GI upset (may take with food or milk).

Ceftin, *see cefuroxime*

---

ceftizoxime sodium

sef-ti-**zox**-eem
(Cefizox)

Do not confuse ceftizoxime with cefotaxime or ceftazidime.

◆CLASSIFICATION

PHARMACOTHERAPEUTIC: Third-generation cephalosporin. **CLINICAL:** Antibiotic (see p. 23C).

ACTION

A third-generation cephalosporin that binds to bacterial cell membranes and inhibits cell wall synthesis. **Therapeutic Effect:** Bactericidal.

PHARMACOKINETICS

Widely distributed (including to CSF). Protein binding: 30%. Primarily excreted unchanged in urine. Moderately removed by hemodialysis. **Half-life:** 1.7 hr (increased in impaired renal function).

USES

Treatment of intra-abdominal, biliary tract, respiratory tract, GU tract, skin, bone infections; gonorrhea; meningitis; septicemia; pelvic inflammatory disease (PID).

PRECAUTIONS

CONTRAINDICATIONS: History of anaphylactic reaction to penicillins or hypersensitivity to cephalosporins. **CAUTIONS:** History of GI disease (especially ulcerative colitis, antibiotic-associated colitis), hepatic/renal impairment.

⏳ **LIFESPAN CONSIDERATIONS: Pregnancy/Lactation:** Readily crosses placenta. Distributed in breast milk. **Pregnancy Category B. Children:** Associated with transient elevations of eosinophils, serum AST, ALT, creatine kinase. **Elderly:** Age-related renal impairment may require dosage adjustment.

INTERACTIONS

DRUG: Probenecid: Increases serum concentration of ceftizoxime. **HERBAL:** None known. **FOOD:** None known. **LAB VALUES:** May increase BUN level and serum alkaline phosphatase, creatinine, AST, and ALT levels. May produce a positive direct or indirect Coombs' test.

AVAILABILITY (Rx)

INTRAVENOUS SOLUTION: 1 g/50 ml, 2 g/50 ml. **POWDER FOR INJECTION:** 500 mg, 1 g, 2 g, 10 g.

ADMINISTRATION/HANDLING
 IV

Reconstitution • Add 5 ml sterile water for injection to each 0.5 g to provide concentration of 95 mg/ml. • May further dilute with 50–100 ml 0.9% NaCl, D_5W, or other compatible fluid.

Rate of administration • For IV push, administer over 3–5 min. • For intermittent IV infusion (piggyback), infuse over 15–30 min.

Storage • Solution appears clear to pale yellow. Color change from yellow to amber does not indicate loss of potency. • IV infusion (piggyback) is stable for 24 hr at room temperature, 96 hr if refrigerated. • Discard if precipitate forms.

IM
• Add 1.5 ml sterile water for injection to each 0.5 g to provide concentration of 270 mg/ml. • Inject deep IM slowly to minimize discomfort. • When giving 2-g dose, divide dose and give in different large muscle masses.

🔲 IV INCOMPATIBILITY
Filgrastim (Neupogen).

IV COMPATIBILITIES
Hydromorphone (Dilaudid), morphine, propofol (Diprivan).

INDICATIONS/ROUTES/DOSAGE
UNCOMPLICATED UTIs
IV, IM: ADULTS, ELDERLY: 500 mg q12h.

MILD, MODERATE, OR SEVERE INFECTIONS OF THE BILIARY, RESPIRATORY, AND GU TRACTS; SKIN, BONE, AND INTRA-ABDOMINAL INFECTIONS; MENINGITIS; AND SEPTICEMIA
IV, IM: ADULTS, ELDERLY: 1–2 g q8–12h.

LIFE-THREATENING INFECTIONS OF THE BILIARY, RESPIRATORY, AND GU TRACTS; SKIN, BONE AND INTRA-ABDOMINAL INFECTIONS; MENINGITIS; AND SEPTICEMIA
IV: ADULTS, ELDERLY: 3–4 g q8h, up to 2 g q4h.

PELVIC INFLAMMATORY DISEASE (PID)
IV: ADULTS: 2 g q4–8h.

UNCOMPLICATED GONORRHEA
IM: ADULTS: 1 g one time.

USUAL PEDIATRIC DOSAGE
IV, IM: CHILDREN: OLDER THAN 6 MO: 50 mg/kg q6–8h. **Maximum:** 12 g/day.

DOSAGE IN RENAL IMPAIRMENT
After a loading dose of 0.5–1 g, dosage and frequency are modified based creatinine clearance and the severity of the infection.

Creatinine Clearance	Dosage
50–79 ml/min	0.5 g–1.5 g q8h
5–49 ml/min	0.25 g–1 g q12h
Less than 5 ml/min	0.25–0.5 g q24h or 0.5 g–1 g q48h

SIDE EFFECTS
FREQUENT: Discomfort with IM administration, oral candidiasis, mild diarrhea, mild abdominal cramping, vaginal candidiasis. **OCCASIONAL:** Nausea, serum sickness-like reaction (fever, joint pain; usually occurs after the second course of therapy and resolves after the drug is discontinued). **RARE:** Allergic reaction (rash, pruritus, urticaria), thrombophlebitis (pain, redness, swelling at injection site).

ADVERSE REACTIONS/ TOXIC EFFECTS
Antibiotic-associated colitis manifested and other superinfections may result from altered bacterial balance. Nephrotoxicity may occur, especially in patients with preexisting renal disease. Patients with a history of allergies, especially to penicillin, are at increased risk for developing a severe hypersensitivity reaction, marked by severe pruritus, angioedema, bronchospasm, and anaphylaxis.

NURSING CONSIDERATIONS

BASELINE ASSESSMENT

Question for history of allergies, particularly cephalosporins, penicillins.

INTERVENTION/EVALUATION

Assess oral cavity for white patches on mucous membranes, tongue. Monitor bowel activity and stool consistency carefully; mild GI effects may be tolerable, but increasing severity may indicate onset of antibiotic-associated colitis. Monitor I&O, renal function reports for nephrotoxicity. Be alert for superinfection: severe genital or anal pruritus, abdominal pain, severe mouth soreness, moderate to severe diarrhea.

PATIENT/FAMILY TEACHING

• Doses should be evenly spaced.
• Continue therapy for full length of treatment. • Discomfort may occur with IM injection.

---

ceftriaxone sodium

sef-try-**ax**-zone

(Rocephin, Rocephin IM Convenience Kit)

CLASSIFICATION

PHARMACOTHERAPEUTIC: Third-generation cephalosporin. **CLINICAL:** Antibiotic (see p. 23C).

ACTION

A third-generation cephalosporin that binds to bacterial cell membranes and inhibits cell wall synthesis. **Therapeutic Effect:** Bactericidal.

PHARMACOKINETICS

Widely distributed (including to CSF). Protein binding: 83%–96%. Primarily excreted unchanged in urine. Not removed by hemodialysis. **Half-life:** 4.3–4.6 hr IV; 5.8–8.7 hr IM (increased in impaired renal function).

USES

Treatment of susceptible infections due to gram-negative aerobic organisms, some gram positive organisms including respiratory tract, GU tract, skin, bone, intra-abdominal, biliary tract infections; septicemia; meningitis; gonorrhea; Lyme disease; acute bacterial otitis media.

PRECAUTIONS

CONTRAINDICATIONS: History of anaphylactic reaction to penicillins or hypersensitivity to cephalosporins. **CAUTIONS:** Renal/hepatic impairment, history of GI disease (especially ulcerative colitis, antibiotic-associated colitis), concurrent administration of nephrotoxic medications.

⧖ **LIFESPAN CONSIDERATIONS: Pregnancy/Lactation:** Readily crosses placenta. Distributed in breast milk. **Pregnancy Category B. Children:** May displace bilirubin from serum albumin. Caution in hyperbilirubinemic neonates. **Elderly:** Age-related renal impairment may require dosage adjustment.

INTERACTIONS

DRUG: None known. **HERBAL:** None known. **FOOD:** None known. **LAB VALUES:** May increase BUN level and serum alkaline phosphatase, bilirubin, creatinine, AST, and ALT levels. May produce a positive direct or indirect Coombs' test. Interferes with cross-matching procedures and hematologic tests.

AVAILABILITY (Rx)

KIT (INTRAMUSCULAR [ROCEPHIN IM CONVENIENCE KIT]): 500 mg, 1 g. **INTRAVENOUS SOLUTION (ROCEPHIN):** 1 g/50 ml, 2 g/50 ml. **POWDER FOR INJECTION (ROCEPHIN):** 250 mg, 500 mg, 1 g, 2 g, 10 g.

✐ see color pill atlas   🌿 herb   underlined – top prescribed drug

ADMINISTRATION/HANDLING

 IV

Reconstitution • Add 2.4 ml sterile water for injection to each 250 mg to provide concentration of 100 mg/ml. • May further dilute with 50–100 ml 0.9% NaCl, D₅W.

Rate of administration • For intermittent IV infusion (piggyback), infuse over 15–30 min for adults, 10–30 min in children, neonates. • Alternating IV sites, use large veins to reduce potential for phlebitis.

Storage • Solution appears light yellow to amber. • IV infusion (piggyback) is stable for 3 days at room temperature, 10 days if refrigerated. • Discard if precipitate forms.

IM
• Add 0.9 ml sterile water for injection, 0.9% NaCl, D₅W, bacteriostatic water and 0.9% benzyl alcohol or lidocaine to each 250 mg to provide concentration of 250 mg/ml. (ml/min) • To minimize discomfort, inject deep IM slowly. Less painful if injected into gluteus maximus than lateral aspect of thigh.

🔲 IV INCOMPATIBILITIES

Aminophylline, amphotericin B complex (Abelcet, AmBisome, Amphotec), filgrastim (Neupogen), fluconazole (Diflucan), labetalol (Normodyne), pentamidine (Pentam IV), vancomycin (Vancocin).

IV COMPATIBILITIES

Diltiazem (Cardizem), heparin, lidocaine, morphine, propofol (Diprivan), total parenteral nutrition (TPN).

INDICATIONS/ROUTES/DOSAGE

MILD TO MODERATE INFECTIONS
IV, IM: ADULTS, ELDERLY: 1–2 g as a single dose or in 2 divided doses.

SERIOUS INFECTIONS
IV, IM: ADULTS, ELDERLY: Up to 4 g/day in 2 divided doses. CHILDREN: 50–75 mg/kg/day in divided doses q12h. **Maximum:** 2 g/day.

SKIN AND SKIN-STRUCTURE INFECTIONS
IV, IM: CHILDREN: 50–75 mg/kg/day as a single dose or in 2 divided doses. **Maximum:** 2 g/day.

MENINGITIS
IV: CHILDREN: Initially, 75 mg/kg, then 100 mg/kg/day as a single dose or in divided doses q12h. **Maximum:** 4 g/day.

LYME DISEASE
IV: ADULTS, ELDERLY: 2–4 g a day for 10–14 days.

ACUTE BACTERIAL OTITIS MEDIA
IM: CHILDREN: 50 mg/kg once a day for 3 days. **Maximum:** 1 g/day.

PERIOPERATIVE PROPHYLAXIS
IV, IM: ADULTS, ELDERLY: 1 g 0.5–2 hr before surgery.

UNCOMPLICATED GONORRHEA
IM: ADULTS: 250 mg plus doxycycline one time.

DOSAGE IN RENAL IMPAIRMENT
Dosage modification is usually unnecessary but liver and renal function test results should be monitored in those with both renal and liver impairment or severe renal impairment.

SIDE EFFECTS

FREQUENT: Discomfort with IM administration, oral candidiasis, mild diarrhea, mild abdominal cramping, vaginal candidiasis. **OCCASIONAL:** Nausea, serum sickness-like reaction (marked by fever and joint pain; usually occurs after the second course of therapy and resolves after the drug is discontinued). **RARE:** Allergic reaction (rash, pruritus, urticaria), thrombophlebitis (pain, redness, swelling at injection site).

ADVERSE REACTIONS/ TOXIC EFFECTS

Antibiotic-associated colitis and other superinfections may result from altered bacterial balance. Nephrotoxicity may occur, especially in patients with preexisting renal disease. Patients with a history of allergies, especially to penicillin, are at increased risk for developing a severe hypersensitivity reaction, marked by severe pruritus, angioedema, bronchospasm, and anaphylaxis.

NURSING CONSIDERATIONS

BASELINE ASSESSMENT

Question for history of allergies, particularly cephalosporins, penicillins.

INTERVENTION/EVALUATION

Assess oral cavity for white patches on mucous membranes, tongue. Monitor bowel activity and stool consistency carefully; mild GI effects may be tolerable, but increasing severity may indicate onset of antibiotic-associated colitis. Monitor I&O, renal function reports for nephrotoxicity. Be alert for superinfection: severe genital or anal pruritus, abdominal pain, severe mouth soreness, moderate to severe diarrhea.

PATIENT/FAMILY TEACHING

• Discomfort may occur with IM injection. • Doses should be evenly spaced. • Continue antibiotic therapy for full length of treatment.

cefuroxime axetil

(Ceftin)

sef-yur-**ox**-ime

Do not confuse cefuroxime with cefotaxime or deferoxamine or Ceftin with Cefzil.

cefuroxime sodium

(Kefurox, Zinacef)

◆CLASSIFICATION

PHARMACOTHERAPEUTIC: Second-generation cephalosporin. **CLINICAL:** Antibiotic (see p. 22C).

ACTION

A second-generation cephalosporin that binds to bacterial cell membranes and inhibits cell wall synthesis. **Therapeutic Effect:** Bactericidal.

PHARMACOKINETICS

Rapidly absorbed from the GI tract. Protein binding: 33%–50%. Widely distributed (including to CSF). Primarily excreted unchanged in urine. Moderately removed by hemodialysis. **Half-life:** 1.3 hr (increased in impaired renal function).

USES

Treatment of susceptible infections due to group B *streptococci,* pneumococci, staphylococci, *H. influenzae, E. coli,* Enterobacter, Klebsiella including acute/chronic bronchitis, gonorrhea, impetigo, early Lyme disease, otitis media, pharyngitis/tonsillitis, sinusitis, skin and skin-structure and urinary tract infections.

PRECAUTIONS

CONTRAINDICATIONS: History of anaphylactic reaction to penicillins or hypersensitivity to cephalosporins. **CAUTIONS:** Renal impairment, history of GI disease (especially ulcerative colitis, antibiotic-associated colitis), concurrent use of nephrotoxic medications.

⌛ **LIFESPAN CONSIDERATIONS: Pregnancy/Lactation:** Readily crosses placenta. Distributed in breast milk. **Pregnancy Category B. Children:** No age-related precautions noted. **Elderly:** Age-related renal impairment may require dosage adjustment.

INTERACTIONS

DRUG: Probenecid: Increases serum concentration of cefuroxime. **HERBAL:** None known. **FOOD:** None known. **LAB VALUES:** May increase serum alkaline phosphatase, bilirubin, LDH, AST and ALT levels. May produce a positive direct or indirect Coombs' test. Interferes with

---

crossmatching procedures, hematologic tests.

AVAILABILITY (Rx)

ORAL SUSPENSION (AXETIL): 125 mg/5 ml, 250 mg/5 ml. **TABLETS (CEFTIN):** 125 mg, 250 mg, 500 mg. **POWDER FOR INJECTION (ZINACEF):** 750 mg, 1.5 g, 7.5 g. **POWDER FOR INJECTION (ADDVANTAGE VIAL [ZINACEF]):** 750 mg, 1.5 g. **POWDER FOR INJECTION (INFUSION PACK [ZINACEF]):** 750 mg, 1.5 g. **INTRAVENOUS SOLUTION (ZINACEF):** 750 mg/50 ml, 1.5 g/50 ml.

ADMINISTRATION/HANDLING

🖊 IV

Reconstitution • Reconstitute 750 mg in 8 ml (1.5 g in 14 ml) sterile water for injection to provide a concentration of 100 mg/ml. • For intermittent IV infusion (piggyback), further dilute with 50–100 ml 0.9% NaCl or D_5W.

Rate of administration • For IV push, administer over 3–5 min. • For intermittent IV infusion (piggyback), infuse over 15–60 min.

Storage • Solution appears light yellow to amber; may darken, but color change does not indicate loss of potency. • IV infusion (piggyback) is stable for 24 hr at room temperature, 7 days if refrigerated. • Discard if precipitate forms.

IM
• To minimize discomfort, inject deep IM slowly. Less painful if injected into gluteus maximus than lateral aspect of thigh.

PO
• Give tablets without regard to food. If GI upset occurs, give with food or milk. • Avoid crushing tablets due to bitter taste. • Suspension must be given with food.

🔲 IV INCOMPATIBILITIES

Filgrastim (Neupogen), fluconazole (Diflucan), midazolam (Versed), vancomycin (Vancocin).

IV COMPATIBILITIES

Diltiazem (Cardizem), hydromorphone (Dilaudid), morphine, propofol (Diprivan), total parenteral nutrition (TPN).

INDICATIONS/ROUTES/DOSAGE

AMPICILLIN-RESISTANT INFLUENZA; BACTERIAL MENINGITIS; EARLY LYME DISEASE; GU TRACT, GYNECOLOGIC, SKIN, AND BONE INFECTIONS; SEPTICEMIA; GONORRHEA, AND OTHER GONOCOCCAL INFECTIONS

IV, IM: ADULTS, ELDERLY: 750 mg–1.5 g q8h. CHILDREN: 75–100 mg/kg/day divided q8h. **Maximum:** 8 g/day. NEONATES: 50–100 mg/kg/day divided q12h.
PO: ADULTS, ELDERLY: 125–500 mg twice a day, depending on the infection.

PHARYNGITIS, TONSILLITIS
PO: CHILDREN 3 MO–12 YR: 125 mg (tablets) q12h or 20 mg/kg/day (suspension) in 2 divided doses.

ACUTE OTITIS MEDIA, ACUTE BACTERIAL MAXILLARY SINUSITIS, IMPETIGO
PO: CHILDREN 3 MO–12 YR: 250 mg (tablets) q12h or 30 mg/kg/day (suspension) in 2 divided doses.

BACTERIAL MENINGITIS
IV: CHILDREN 3 MO–12 YR: 200–240 mg/kg/day in divided doses q6–8h.

PERIOPERATIVE PROPHYLAXIS
IV: ADULTS, ELDERLY: 1.5 g 30–60 min before surgery and 750 mg q8h after surgery.

USUAL NEONATAL DOSAGE
IV, IM: NEONATES: 20–100 mg/kg/day in divided doses q12h.

DOSAGE IN RENAL IMPAIRMENT
Adult dosage and frequency are modified based on creatinine clearance and the severity of the infection.

Creatinine Clearance	Dosage
Greater than 20 ml/min	750 mg–1 g q8h
10–20 ml/min	750 mg q12h
Less than 10 ml/min	750 mg q24h

SIDE EFFECTS

FREQUENT: Discomfort with IM administration, oral candidiasis, mild diarrhea, mild abdominal cramping, vaginal candidiasis. **OCCASIONAL:** Nausea, serum sickness-like reaction (marked by fever and joint pain; usually occurs after the second course of therapy and resolves after the drug is discontinued). **RARE:** Allergic reaction (rash, pruritus, urticaria), thrombophlebitis (pain, redness, swelling at injection site).

ADVERSE REACTIONS/ TOXIC EFFECTS

Antibiotic-associated colitis and other superinfections may result from altered bacterial balance. Nephrotoxicity may occur, especially in patients with pre-existing renal disease. Patients with a history of allergies, especially to penicillin, are at increased risk for developing a severe hypersensitivity reaction, marked by severe pruritus, angioedema, bronchospasm, and anaphylaxis.

NURSING CONSIDERATIONS

BASELINE ASSESSMENT

Question for history of allergies, particularly cephalosporins, penicillins.

INTERVENTION/EVALUATION

Assess oral cavity for white patches on mucous membranes, tongue. Monitor bowel activity and stool consistency carefully; mild GI effects may be tolerable, but increasing severity may indicate onset of antibiotic-associated colitis. Monitor I&O, renal function reports for nephrotoxicity. Be alert for superinfection: severe genital/anal pruritus, abdominal pain, severe mouth soreness, moderate to severe diarrhea.

PATIENT/FAMILY TEACHING

• Discomfort may occur with IM injection. • Doses should be evenly spaced. • Continue antibiotic therapy for full length of treatment. • May cause GI upset (may take with food or milk).

Cefzil, *see cefprozil*

Celebrex, *see celecoxib*

---

celecoxib

sell-eh-**cox**-ib

(<u>Celebrex</u>)

Do not confuse Celebrex with Cerebyx or Celexa.

◆CLASSIFICATION

PHARMACOTHERAPEUTIC: Nonsteroidal anti-inflammatory. **CLINICAL:** Anti-inflammatory (see p. 116C).

ACTION

An NSAID that inhibits cyclo-oxygenase-2, the enzyme responsible for prostaglandin synthesis. Mechanism of action in treating familial adenomatous polyposis is unknown. **Therapeutic Effect:** Reduces inflammation and relieves pain.

PHARMACOKINETICS

Widely distributed. Protein binding: 97%. Metabolized in the liver. Primarily eliminated in feces. **Half-life:** 11.2 hr.

USES

Relief of signs/symptoms of osteoarthritis, rheumatoid arthritis in adults. Treatment of acute pain, menstrual

---

◆ see color pill atlas   *◆ herb*   <u>underlined</u> – top prescribed drug

C

pain. Used to reduce number of adenomatous colorectal polyps in familial adenomatous polyposis (FAP). Relief of signs/symptoms associated with ankylosing spondylitis.

PRECAUTIONS

◄ **ALERT** ► May increase cardiovascular risk when high doses given to prevent colon cancer.
CONTRAINDICATIONS: Hypersensitivity to aspirin, NSAIDs, or sulfonamides. **CAUTIONS:** Past history of peptic ulcer, older than 60 yr, those receiving anticoagulant therapy, steroids, alcohol consumption, smoking.

⌛ **LIFESPAN CONSIDERATIONS: Pregnancy/Lactation:** Unknown if drug crosses placenta or is distributed in breast milk. Avoid use during third trimester (may adversely affect fetal cardiovascular system: premature closure of ductus arteriosus). **Pregnancy Category C (D if used in third trimester or near delivery). Children:** Safety and efficacy not established in those younger than 18 yr. **Elderly:** No age-related precautions noted.

INTERACTIONS

DRUG: Fluconazole: May increase celecoxib blood level. **Lithium:** May increase lithium blood levels. **Warfarin:** May increase the risk of bleeding. **HERBAL:** None known. **FOOD:** None known. **LAB VALUES:** May increase AST and ALT levels.

AVAILABILITY (Rx)

CAPSULES: 100 mg, 200 mg, 400 mg.

ADMINISTRATION/HANDLING

PO
• Give without regard to food. • Do not crush or break capsules.

INDICATIONS/ROUTES/DOSAGE

OSTEOARTHRITIS
PO: ADULTS, ELDERLY: 200 mg/day as a single dose or 100 mg twice a day.

RHEUMATOID ARTHRITIS
PO: ADULTS, ELDERLY: 100–200 mg twice a day.

ACUTE PAIN
PO: ADULTS, ELDERLY: Initially, 400 mg with additional 200 mg on day 1, if needed. Maintenance: 200 mg twice a day as needed.

FAMILIAL ADENOMATOUS POLYPOSIS
PO: ADULTS, ELDERLY: 400 mg twice daily (with food).

PRIMARY DYSMENORRHEA
PO: ADULTS: 200 mg twice a day as needed (with food).

ANKYLOSING SPONDYLITIS
PO: ADULTS, ELDERLY: 200 mg/day as a single dose or in 2 divided doses. May increase to 400 mg/day if no effect is seen after 6 wk.

SIDE EFFECTS

FREQUENT (greater than 5%): Diarrhea, dyspepsia, headache, upper respiratory tract infection. **OCCASIONAL (5%–1%):** Abdominal pain, flatulence, nausea, back pain, peripheral edema, dizziness, rash.

ADVERSE REACTIONS/ TOXIC EFFECTS

There is an increased risk of cardiovascular events, including MI and cerebrovascular accident, and serious, potentially life-threatening, GI bleeding.

NURSING CONSIDERATIONS

BASELINE ASSESSMENT

Assess onset, type, location, duration of pain/inflammation. Inspect appearance of affected joints for immobility, deformity, skin condition.

INTERVENTION/EVALUATION

Evaluate for therapeutic response: pain relief, decreased stiffness, swelling, increased joint mobility, decreased tenderness, improved grip strength.

C

PATIENT/FAMILY TEACHING
• If GI upset occurs, take with food.
• Avoid aspirin, alcohol (increases risk of GI bleeding).

Celexa, *see citalopram*

CellCept, *see mycophenolate*

Cenestin, *see conjugated estrogens*

---

cephalexin

cef-ah-**lex**-in
(Apo-Cephalex ✦, Biocef, Keflex, Keftab, Novolexin ✦)

• CLASSIFICATION
PHARMACOTHERAPEUTIC: First-generation cephalosporin. **CLINICAL:** Antibiotic (see p. 21C).

ACTION
A first-generation cephalosporin that binds to bacterial cell membranes and inhibits cell wall synthesis. **Therapeutic Effect:** Bactericidal.

PHARMACOKINETICS
Rapidly absorbed from the GI tract. Protein binding: 10%–15%. Widely distributed. Primarily excreted unchanged in urine. Moderately removed by hemodialysis. **Half-life:** 0.9–1.2 hr (increased in impaired renal function).

USES
Treatment of susceptible infections due to Staphylococci, group A *Streptococcus, K. pneumoniae, E. coli, P. mirabilis, H. influenzae, M. catarrhalis* including respiratory tract, GU tract, skin, soft tissue, bone infections; otitis media; rheumatic fever prophylaxis; follow-up to parenteral therapy.

PRECAUTIONS
CONTRAINDICATIONS: History of anaphylactic reaction to penicillins or hypersensitivity to cephalosporins. **CAUTIONS:** Renal impairment, history of GI disease (especially ulcerative colitis, antibiotic-associated colitis), concurrent use of nephrotoxic medications.

⌛ **LIFESPAN CONSIDERATIONS: Pregnancy/Lactation:** Readily crosses placenta. Distributed in breast milk. **Pregnancy Category B. Children:** No age-related precautions noted. **Elderly:** Age-related renal impairment may require dosage adjustment.

INTERACTIONS
DRUG: Probenecid: Increases serum concentration of cephalexin. **HERBAL:** None known. **FOOD:** None known. **LAB VALUES:** May increase serum alkaline phosphatase, AST, and ALT levels. May produce a positive direct or indirect Coombs' test. Interferes with crossmatching procedures and hematologic tests.

AVAILABILITY (Rx)
CAPSULES: 250 mg (Keflex), 500 mg (Biocef, Keflex). **POWDER FOR ORAL SUSPENSION (BIOCEF, KEFLEX):** 125 mg/5 ml, 250 mg/5 ml. **TABLETS:** 250 mg, 500 mg.

ADMINISTRATION/HANDLING
PO
• After reconstitution, oral suspension is stable for 14 days if refrigerated.
• Shake oral suspension well before using. • Give without regard to food. If GI upset occurs, give with food or milk.

INDICATIONS/ROUTES/DOSAGE

BONE INFECTIONS, PROPHYLAXIS OF RHEUMATIC FEVER, FOLLOW-UP TO PARENTERAL THERAPY
PO: ADULTS, ELDERLY: 250–500 mg q6h up to 4 g/day.

STREPTOCOCCAL PHARYNGITIS, SKIN AND SKIN-STRUCTURE INFECTIONS, UNCOMPLICATED CYSTITIS
PO: ADULTS, ELDERLY: 500 mg q12h.

USUAL PEDIATRIC DOSAGE
CHILDREN: 25–100 mg/kg/day in 2–4 divided doses.

OTITIS MEDIA
PO: CHILDREN: 75–100 mg/kg/day in 4 divided doses.

DOSAGE IN RENAL IMPAIRMENT
After usual initial dose, dosing frequency is modified based on creatinine clearance and the severity of the infection.

Creatinine Clearance	Dosage Interval
10–40 ml/min	Usual dose q8–12h
Less than 10 ml/min	Usual dose q12–24h

SIDE EFFECTS

FREQUENT: Oral candidiasis, mild diarrhea, mild abdominal cramping, vaginal candidiasis. **OCCASIONAL:** Nausea, serum sickness-like reaction (marked by fever and joint pain; usually occurs after the second course of therapy and resolves after the drug is discontinued). **RARE:** Allergic reaction (rash, pruritus, urticaria).

ADVERSE REACTIONS/ TOXIC EFFECTS

Antibiotic-associated colitis and other superinfections may result from altered bacterial balance. Nephrotoxicity may occur, especially in patients with preexisting renal disease. Patients with a history of allergies, especially to penicillin, are at increased risk for developing a severe hypersensitivity reaction, marked by severe pruritus, angioedema, bronchospasm, and anaphylaxis.

NURSING CONSIDERATIONS

BASELINE ASSESSMENT
Question for history of allergies, particularly cephalosporins, penicillins.

INTERVENTION/EVALUATION
Assess oral cavity for white patches on mucous membranes, tongue. Monitor bowel activity and stool consistency carefully; mild GI effects may be tolerable, but increasing severity may indicate onset of antibiotic-associated colitis. Monitor I&O, renal function reports for nephrotoxicity. Be alert for superinfection: severe genital or anal pruritus, abdominal pain, severe mouth soreness, moderate to severe diarrhea.

PATIENT/FAMILY TEACHING
• Doses should be evenly spaced.
• Continue therapy for full length of treatment. • May cause GI upset (may take with food or milk). • Refrigerate oral suspension.

Cerebyx, *see fosphenytoin*

Cervidil, *see dinoprostone*

---

cetirizine

sih-**tier**-eh-zeen
(Reactine ✤, Zyrtec)
Do not confuse Zyrtec with Zantac or Zyprexa.

FIXED-COMBINATION(S)

Zyrtec D 12 hour Tablets: cetirizine/pseudoephedrine: 5 mg/120 mg.

◆ CLASSIFICATION

PHARMACOTHERAPEUTIC: Second-generation piperazine. **CLINICAL:** Antihistamine (see p. 49C).

ACTION

A second-generation piperazine that competes with histamine for H_1-receptor sites on effector cells in the GI tract, blood vessels, and respiratory tract. **Therapeutic Effect:** Prevents allergic response, produces mild bronchodilation, blocks histamine-induced bronchitis.

PHARMACOKINETICS

Route	Onset	Peak	Duration
PO	Less than 1 hr	4–8 hr	Less than 24 hr

Rapidly and almost completely absorbed from the GI tract (absorption not affected by food). Protein binding: 93%. Undergoes low first-pass metabolism; not extensively metabolized. Primarily excreted in urine (more than 80% as unchanged drug). **Half-life:** 6.5–10 hr.

USES

Relief of symptoms (sneezing, rhinorrhea, postnasal discharge, nasal pruritus, ocular pruritus, tearing) of seasonal and perennial allergic rhinitis (hay fever). Treatment of chronic urticaria (hives). **OFF-LABEL:** Treatment of bronchial asthma.

PRECAUTIONS

CONTRAINDICATIONS: Hypersensitivity to cetirizine or hydroxyzine. **CAUTIONS:** Impaired hepatic or renal function.

May cause drowsiness at dosage greater than 10 mg/day.

⧗ **LIFESPAN CONSIDERATIONS: Pregnancy/Lactation:** Not recommended during early months of pregnancy. Unknown if excreted in breast milk (breast-feeding not recommended). **Pregnancy Category B. Children:** Less likely to cause anticholinergic effects. **Elderly:** More sensitive to anticholinergic effects (e.g., dry mouth, urinary retention). Dizziness, sedation, confusion more likely to occur.

INTERACTIONS

DRUG: Alcohol, other CNS depressants: May increase CNS depression. **HERBAL:** None known. **FOOD:** None known. **LAB VALUES:** May suppress wheal and flare reactions to antigen skin testing, unless drug is discontinued 4 days before testing.

AVAILABILITY (Rx)

SYRUP: 5 mg/5 ml. **TABLETS:** 5 mg, 10 mg. **TABLETS (CHEWABLE):** 5 mg, 10 mg.

ADMINISTRATION/HANDLING

PO
- Give without regard to food.

INDICATIONS/ROUTES/DOSAGE

ALLERGIC RHINITIS, URTICARIA

PO: ADULTS, ELDERLY, CHILDREN OLDER THAN 5 YR: Initially, 5–10 mg/day as a single or in 2 divided doses. CHILDREN 2–5 YR: 2.5 mg/day. May increase up to 5 mg/day as a single or in 2 divided doses. CHILDREN 12–23 MO: Initially, 2.5 mg/day. May increase up to 5 mg/day in 2 divided doses. CHILDREN 6–11 MO: 2.5 mg once a day.

DOSAGE IN RENAL OR HEPATIC IMPAIRMENT

For adult and elderly patients with renal impairment (creatinine clearance of 11–31 ml/min), those receiving hemodialysis (creatinine clearance of less than 7 ml/min), and those with

---

✐ see color pill atlas   ◣ herb   underlined – top prescribed drug

C

hepatic impairment, dosage is decreased to 5 mg once a day.

SIDE EFFECTS

OCCASIONAL (10%–2%): Pharyngitis; dry mucous membranes, nose, or throat; nausea and vomiting; abdominal pain; headache; dizziness; fatigue; thickening of mucus; somnolence; photosensitivity; urine retention.

ADVERSE REACTIONS/ TOXIC EFFECTS

Children may experience paradoxical reactions, including restlessness, insomnia, euphoria, nervousness, and tremor. Dizziness, sedation, and confusion are more likely to occur in elderly patients.

NURSING CONSIDERATIONS

BASELINE ASSESSMENT

Assess lung sounds. Assess severity of rhinitis, urticaria, other symptoms. Obtain baseline liver function tests.

INTERVENTION/EVALUATION

For upper respiratory allergies, increase fluids to maintain thin secretions and offset thirst. Monitor symptoms for therapeutic response.

PATIENT/FAMILY TEACHING

• Avoid tasks that require alertness, motor skills until response to drug is established (may cause drowsiness). • Avoid alcohol during antihistamine therapy. • Avoid prolonged exposure to sunlight.

---

cetrorelix

(Cetrotide)
See Fertility agents (p. 91C)

---

cetuximab ▷

ceh-**tux**-ih-mab
(Erbitux)

◆**CLASSIFICATION**

PHARMACOTHERAPEUTIC: Monoclonal antibody. **CLINICAL:** Antineoplastic.

ACTION

A monoclonal antibody that binds to the epidermal growth factor receptor (EGFR), a glycoprotein on normal and tumor cells, thus inhibiting cell growth and inducing apoptosis. Therapeutic Effect: Inhibits the growth and survival of tumor cells that overexpress EGFR.

PHARMACOKINETICS

Reaches steady state levels by the third weekly infusion. Clearance decreases as dose increases. Half-life: 114 hr (Range: 75–188 hr).

USES

As a single agent or in combination with irinotecan for treatment of EGFR-expressing, metastatic colorectal carcinoma in patients who are refractory or intolerant to irinotecan-based chemotherapy. Treatment of advanced squamous cell cancer of head and neck (with radiation). Treatment of head and neck cancer that metastasized (as monotherapy). OFF-LABEL: Breast cancer, tumors over-expressing EGFR.

PRECAUTIONS

CONTRAINDICATIONS: None known. **CAUTIONS:** Hypersensitivity to murine proteins.

⧗ LIFESPAN CONSIDERATIONS: **Pregnancy/Lactation:** Crosses placental barrier; has potential to cause fetal harm, abortifacient. Do not breast-feed. **Pregnancy Category C. Children:** Safety

---

C

and efficacy not established. **Elderly:** No age-related precautions noted.

INTERACTIONS

DRUG: None known. **HERBAL:** None known. **FOOD:** None known. **LAB VALUES:** May decrease WBC count, Hct, and Hgb level.

AVAILABILITY (Rx)

INJECTION: 2 mg/ml.

ADMINISTRATION/HANDLING

IV

‹ **ALERT** › Do not give by IV push or bolus.

Reconstitution • Solution should appear clear, colorless; may contain a small amount of visible, white particulates. • Do not shake or dilute. • Infuse with a low protein-binding 0.22 micron in-line filter.

Rate of administration • First dose should be given as a 120-min IV infusion. • Maintenance infusion should be infused over 60 min. • Maximum infusion rate should not exceed 5 ml/min.

Storage • Refrigerate vials. • Preparations in infusion containers are stable for up to 12 hr if refrigerated, up to 8 hr at room temperature. • Discard any unused portion.

IV COMPATIBILITY

Irinotecan (Camptosar).

INDICATIONS/ROUTES/DOSAGE

HEAD AND NECK CANCER, METASTATIC COLORECTAL CARCINOMA
IV: ADULTS, ELDERLY: Initially, 400 mg/m^2 as a loading dose. Maintenance: 250 mg/m^2 infused over 60 min weekly.

SIDE EFFECTS

FREQUENT (90%–25%): Acneiform rash, malaise, fever, nausea, diarrhea, constipation, headache, abdominal pain, anorexia, vomiting. **OCCASIONAL (16%–10%):** Nail disorder, back pain, stomatitis, peripheral edema, pruritus, cough, insomnia. **RARE (9%–5%):** Weight loss, depression, dyspepsia, conjunctivitis, alopecia.

ADVERSE REACTIONS/ TOXIC EFFECTS

Anemia occurs in 10% of patients. A severe infusion reaction, characterized by rapid onset of airway obstruction, a precipitous drop in BP, and severe urticaria, occurs rarely. Dermatologic toxicity, pulmonary embolus, leukopenia, and renal failure occur rarely.

NURSING CONSIDERATIONS

BASELINE ASSESSMENT

Monitor Hgb, Hct. Assess signs and symptoms for evidence of anemia. Question patient regarding possibility of pregnancy. Advise patient to avoid pregnancy due to potential to cause fetal harm.

INTERVENTION/EVALUATION

Diligently monitor patient for evidence of infusion reaction characterized by rapid onset of bronchospasm, stridor, hoarseness, urticaria, and/or hypotension. Be aware that the patient may experience first severe infusion reaction during later infusions. Assess skin for evidence of dermatologic toxicity manifested by development of inflammatory sequelae, dry skin, exfoliative dermatitis, or rash.

PATIENT/FAMILY TEACHING

• Do not have immunizations without physician's approval (lowers body's resistance). • Avoid contact with anyone who recently received a live virus vaccine. • Avoid crowds, those with infection. • Instruct patient to wear sunscreen and limit sun exposure during therapy (sunlight can exacerbate skin reactions).

---

chamomile

ka-mow-meal

Also known as German chamomile, pinheads (Blossom 120/jar, 45/jar, 30/jar).

CLASSIFICATION

HERBAL: See Appendix G.

ACTION

Antiallergic, anti-inflammatory action due to inhibiting release of histamine. Possesses antiallergic, antiflatulent, antispasmodic, mild sedative, anti-inflammatory action.

USES

Treatment of symptoms of flatulence, travel sickness, diarrhea, insomnia, GI spasms.

PRECAUTIONS

CONTRAINDICATIONS: Pregnancy. **CAUTIONS:** Patients with asthma (may exacerbate condition) and those allergic to ragweed, aster, daisies, chrysanthemums.

⏳ **LIFESPAN CONSIDERATIONS: Pregnancy/Lactation:** Contraindicated. A teratogen, affects menstrual cycle, has uterine stimulant effects. **Children:** Safety and efficacy not established. **Elderly:** No age-related precautions noted.

INTERACTIONS

DRUG: **Aspirin, clopidrogel, dalteparin, enoxaparin, heparin, warfarin:** May increase the risk of bleeding, anticoagulation, when taken with chamomile. **Benzodiazepines:** May have additive effects. HERBAL: **Ginsing, kava kava, St. John's wort, valerian:** Sedation effects may increase when taken with chamomile. **Feverfew, garlic, ginger, ginkgo, licorice:** May increase the risk of bleeding. FOOD: None known. LAB VALUES: None known.

AVAILABILITY

WHOLE FLOWERS: 30 g/jar, 45 g/jar, 120 g/jar.

INDICATIONS/ROUTES/DOSAGE

FLATULENCE, TRAVEL SICKNESS, DIARRHEA, INSOMNIA, GI SPASMS
PO: ADULTS, ELDERLY: 2–8 g of dried flower heads 3 times a day or 1 cup of tea 3–4 times a day.

SIDE EFFECTS

Allergic reaction (e.g., contact dermatitis, severe hypersensitivity reaction, anaphylactic reaction), eye irritation.

ADVERSE REACTIONS/TOXIC EFFECTS

Anaphylactic reaction (bronchospasm, severe pruritus, angioedema).

NURSING CONSIDERATIONS

BASELINE ASSESSMENT

Assess if patient is pregnant, breastfeeding, or asthmatic. Assess if patient is taking other medications, especially those that increase risk of bleeding or have sedative properties. Assess for allergies to ragweed, aster, daisies, chrysanthemums.

INTERVENTION/EVALUATION

Monitor for signs of allergic reaction.

PATIENT/FAMILY TEACHING

• Inform physician if pregnancy occurs or if planning to become pregnant or breast-feed. • May cause mild sedation. • Avoid tasks that require alertness, motor skills until response to herbal is established. • Avoid use with other sedatives, alcohol, anticoagulants.

chloral hydrate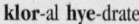

klor-al hye-drate

(Aquachloral Supprettes, Novochlor-hydrate ✤, PMS-Chloral Hydrate ✤, Somnote)

◆CLASSIFICATION

PHARMACOTHERAPEUTIC: Nonbarbiturate chloral derivative. **CLINICAL:** Sedative, hypnotic.

ACTION

A nonbarbiturate chloral derivative that produces CNS depression. Therapeutic Effect: Induces quiet, deep sleep, with only a slight decrease in respiratory rate and BP.

PHARMACOKINETICS

Readily absorbed from the GI tract following PO administration. Well absorbed following rectal administration. Protein binding: 70%–80%. Metabolized in liver and erythrocytes to the active metabolite, trichloroethanol, which may be further metabolized to inactive metabolites. Excreted in urine. Half-life: 7–10 hr (trichloroethanol).

USES

Sedative/hypnotic for dental or diagnostic procedures, sedative before EEG evaluations.

PRECAUTIONS

CONTRAINDICATIONS: Gastritis, marked hepatic or renal impairment, severe cardiac disease. **CAUTIONS:** History of drug abuse, clinical depression.

⧖ LIFESPAN CONSIDERATIONS: **Pregnancy/Lactation:** Crosses placenta; distributed in breast milk. **Pregnancy Category C. Children:** Safety and efficacy not established. **Elderly:** No age-related precautions noted.

INTERACTIONS

DRUG: **Alcohol, other CNS depressants:** May increase the effects of chloral hydrate. **Furosemide (IV):** May alter BP and cause diaphoresis if given within 24 hr after chloral hydrate. **Warfarin:** May increase the effect of warfarin. HERBAL: None known. FOOD: None known. LAB VALUES: May interfere with copper sulfate test for glycosuria, fluorometric tests for urine catecholamines, urinary 17-hydroxycorticosteroid determinations.

AVAILABILITY (Rx)

CAPSULES (SOMNOTE): 500 mg. **SYRUP:** 500 mg/5 ml. **SUPPOSITORIES (AQUA-CHLORAL SUPPRETTES):** 324 mg, 648 mg.

ADMINISTRATION/HANDLING

PO
• Give capsules with a full glass of water or fruit juice. Swallow capsules whole; do not chew. • Dilute the dose of syrup in water to minimize gastric irritation.

RECTAL
• Store suppositories at room temperature; don't refrigerate.

INDICATIONS/ROUTES/DOSAGE

PREMEDICATION FOR DENTAL OR MEDICAL PROCEDURES
PO, RECTAL: ADULTS: 0.5–1 g. CHILDREN: 75 mg/kg up to 1 g total.

PREMEDICATION FOR EEG
PO, RECTAL: ADULTS: 0.5–1.5 g. CHILDREN: 25–50 mg/kg/dose 30–60 min prior to EEG. May repeat in 30 min. **Maximum:** 1 g for infants, 2 g for children.

SIDE EFFECTS

OCCASIONAL: Gastric irritation (nausea, vomiting, flatulence, diarrhea), rash, sleepwalking. **RARE:** Headache, paradoxical CNS hyperactivity or nervousness in children, excitement or restlessness in the elderly (particularly in patients with pain).

ADVERSE REACTIONS/ TOXIC EFFECTS

Overdose may produce somnolence, confusion, slurred speech, severe incoordination, respiratory depression, and coma. Allergic-type reaction may occur in those with tartrazine sensitivity.

NURSING CONSIDERATIONS

BASELINE ASSESSMENT

Assess BP, pulse, respirations immediately before administration. Provide safety measures, e.g., raise bedrails. Provide environment conducive to sleep (back rub, quiet environment, low lighting).

INTERVENTION/EVALUATION

Monitor mental status, vital signs. Gastric irritation decreased by diluting dose in water. Assess sleep pattern. Assess elderly and children for paradoxical reaction. Evaluate for therapeutic response to insomnia: decrease in number of nocturnal awakenings, increase in length of sleep.

PATIENT/FAMILY TEACHING

• Take capsule with a full glass of water or fruit juice. • Swallow capsules whole; do not chew. • If taking at home before procedure, do not drive. • Do not abruptly withdraw medication after long-term use. • Tolerance, dependence may occur with prolonged use.

---

chlorambucil

klor-**am**-bew-sill

(Leukeran)

Do not confuse Leukeran with Alkeran, Chloromycetin, Leukine, or Mylleran.

•CLASSIFICATION

PHARMACOTHERAPEUTIC: Alkylating agent, nitrogen mustard. **CLINICAL:** Antineoplastic (see p. 72C).

ACTION

An alkylating agent and nitrogen mustard that inhibits DNA and RNA synthesis by cross-linking with DNA and RNA strands. Cell cycle–phase nonspecific. **Therapeutic Effect:** Interferes with nucleic acid function.

PHARMACOKINETICS

Rapidly and completely absorbed from the GI tract. Protein binding: 99%. Rapidly metabolized in the liver to active metabolite. Not removed by hemodialysis. **Half-life:** 1.5 hr; metabolite 2.5 hr.

USES

Treatment of chronic lymphocytic leukemia, Hodgkin's and non-Hodgkin's lymphomas. **OFF-LABEL:** Treatment of cutaneous T-cell lymphomas, epithelial carcinoma, hairy cell leukemia, nephrotic syndrome, ovarian or testicular carcinoma, polycythemia vera, trophoblastic gestational tumors.

PRECAUTIONS

CONTRAINDICATIONS: Previous allergic reaction or disease resistance to drug. **EXTREME CAUTIONS:** Within 4 wk after full-course radiation therapy or myelosuppressive drug regimen.

LIFESPAN CONSIDERATIONS: Pregnancy/Lactation: If possible, avoid use during pregnancy, especially first trimester. Breast-feeding not recommended. **Pregnancy Category D. Children:** No age-related precautions. When taken for nephritic syndrome, may increase seizures. **Elderly:** No age-related precautions noted.

INTERACTIONS

DRUG: **Antigout medications:** May decrease the effect of these drugs. **Bone marrow depressants:** May increase bone myelosuppression. **Live-virus vaccines:** May potentiate virus replication, increase vaccine side effects and decrease the patient's antibody response to the vaccine. **Other immunosuppressants (including steroids):** May increase the risk of infection or development of neoplasms. HERBAL: None known. FOOD: None known. LAB VALUES: May increase serum alkaline phosphatase, serum uric acid, and AST levels.

AVAILABILITY (Rx)

TABLETS: 2 mg.

ADMINISTRATION/HANDLING

PO
• Give without regard to food.

INDICATIONS/ROUTES/DOSAGE

PALLIATIVE TREATMENT OF ADVANCED HODGKIN'S DISEASE, ADVANCED MALIGNANT (NON-HODGKIN'S) LYMPHOMA (INCLUDING GIANT FOLLICULAR LYMPHOMA AND LYMPHOSARCOMA), CHRONIC LYMPHOCYTIC LEUKEMIA

PO: ADULTS, ELDERLY, CHILDREN: For initial or short-course therapy, 0.1–0.2 mg/kg/day as a single or in divided doses for 3–6 wk (average dose, 4–10 mg/day). Alternatively, 0.4 mg/kg initially as a single daily dose every 2 wk and increased by 0.1 mg/kg every 2 wk until response and myelosuppression occur. Maintenance: 0.03–0.1 mg/kg/day (average dose, 2–4 mg/day).

SIDE EFFECTS

EXPECTED: GI effects such as nausea, vomiting, anorexia, diarrhea, and abdominal distress (generally mild, last less than 24 hr and occur only if single dose exceeds 20 mg). OCCASIONAL: Rash or dermatitis, pruritus, cold sores. RARE: Alopecia, urticaria, erythema, hyperuricemia.

ADVERSE REACTIONS/TOXIC EFFECTS

Hematologic toxicity due to severe myelosuppression occurs frequently and may include neutropenia, leukopenia, progressive lymphopenia, anemia and thrombocytopenia. After discontinuation of short-course therapy, thrombocytopenia and leukopenia usually last for 1–2 wk but may persist for 3–4 wk. The neutrophil count may continue to decrease for up to 10 days after the last dose. Hematologic toxicity appears to be less severe with intermittent rather than continuous drug administration. Overdosage may produce seizures in children. Excessive serum uric acid level and hepatotoxicity occur rarely.

NURSING CONSIDERATIONS

BASELINE ASSESSMENT

CBC should be performed before therapy and each week during therapy, WBC count performed 3–4 days following each weekly CBC during first 3–6 wk of therapy (4–6 wk if patient on intermittent dosing schedule).

INTERVENTION/EVALUATION

Monitor for hematologic toxicity (fever, sore throat, signs of local infection, unusual bruising or bleeding from any site), symptoms of anemia (excessive fatigue, weakness). Assess skin for rash, pruritus, urticaria.

PATIENT/FAMILY TEACHING

• Increase fluid intake (may protect against hyperuricemia). • Do not have immunizations without doctor's approval (drug lowers body's resistance). • Avoid contact with those who have recently received live virus vaccine. • Promptly report fever, sore throat, signs of local infection, unusual bruising or bleeding from any site.

chlordiazepoxide ℮

klor-dye-az-e-**pox**-ide
(Apo-Chlordiazepoxide ✤, Libritabs, Librium, Novopoxide ✤)
Do not confuse Librium with Librax.

FIXED-COMBINATION(S)

Limbitrol: amitriptyline/chlordiazepoxide: 5 mg/12.5 mg; 10 mg/25 mg. **Librax:** chlordiazepoxide-clidinium: 5 mg/2.5 mg.

◆CLASSIFICATION

PHARMACOTHERAPEUTIC: Benzodiazepine. **CLINICAL:** Antianxiety (see p. 11C).

ACTION

A benzodiazepine that enhances the action of the inhibitory neurotransmitter gamma-aminobutyric acid in the CNS. **Therapeutic Effect:** Produces anxiolytic effect.

USES

Management of anxiety disorders, acute alcohol withdrawal symptoms; short-term relief of symptoms of anxiety, preop anxiety, tension. **OFF-LABEL:** Treatment of panic disorder, tension headache, tremors.

PRECAUTIONS

CONTRAINDICATIONS: Acute alcohol intoxication, acute angle-closure glaucoma. **CAUTIONS:** Impaired renal/hepatic function.

⌛ **LIFESPAN CONSIDERATIONS: Pregnancy/Lactation:** Crosses placenta; distributed in breast milk. **Pregnancy Category D. Children/Elderly:** Reduce initial dose, increase dosage gradually (prevents excessive sedation).

INTERACTIONS

DRUG: Alcohol, other CNS depressants: May increase CNS depression. **Azole antifungals:** May increase the serum concentrations of chlordiazepoxide and increase the risk of toxicity. **HERBAL: Kava kava, valerian:** May increase CNS depression. **St. John's wort:** May decrease the effectiveness of chlordiazepoxide. **FOOD:** None known. **LAB VALUES:** Therapeutic serum drug level is 1–3 mcg/ml; toxic serum drug level is greater than 5 mcg/ml.

AVAILABILITY (Rx)

CAPSULES: 5 mg (Librium), 10 mg (Libritabs, Librium), 25 mg (Librium). **INJECTION POWDER FOR RECONSTITUTION (LIBRIUM):** 100 mg.

ADMINISTRATION/HANDLING

◀ **ALERT** ▶ Expect to use the smallest effective chlordiazepoxide dose in elderly or debilitated patients and patients with hepatic disease or a low serum albumin level.
• Keep the patient recumbent for up to 3 hr after parenteral administration to reduce the drug's hypotensive effect.

INDICATIONS/ROUTES/DOSAGE
ALCOHOL WITHDRAWAL SYMPTOMS
PO: ADULTS, ELDERLY: 50–100 mg. May repeat q2–4h. **Maximum:** 300 mg/24 hr.

ANXIETY
PO: ADULTS: 15–100 mg/day in 3–4 divided doses. ELDERLY: 5 mg 2–4 times a day.
IV, IM: ADULTS: Initially, 50–100 mg, then 25–50 mg 3–4 times a day as needed.

PRE-OPERATIVE ANXIETY
IM: ADULTS, ELDERLY: 50–100 mg once.

SIDE EFFECTS

FREQUENT: Pain at IM injection site; somnolence, ataxia, dizziness, confusion with oral dose (particularly in elderly or debilitated patients). **OCCASIONAL:** Rash,

---

✤ Canadian trade name   ℮ see **evolve**   ☞ High Alert drug

peripheral edema, GI disturbances. **RARE:** Paradoxical CNS reactions, such as hyperactivity or nervousness in children and excitement or restlessness in the elderly (generally noted during first 2 wk of therapy, particularly in presence of uncontrolled pain).

ADVERSE REACTIONS/ TOXIC EFFECTS

IV administration may produce pain, swelling, thrombophlebitis, and carpal tunnel syndrome. Abrupt or too-rapid withdrawal may result in pronounced restlessness, irritability, insomnia, hand tremors, abdominal or muscle cramps, diaphoresis, vomiting, and seizures. Overdose results in somnolence, confusion, diminished reflexes, and coma.

NURSING CONSIDERATIONS

BASELINE ASSESSMENT

Assess BP, pulse, respirations immediately before administration. Patient must remain recumbent for up to 3 hr (individualized) after parenteral administration to reduce hypotensive effect.

INTERVENTION/EVALUATION

Assess motor responses (agitation, tremors, tension), autonomic responses (cold or clammy hands, diaphoresis). Assess children, elderly for paradoxical reaction, particularly during early therapy. Assist with ambulation if drowsiness, ataxia occur. Therapeutic serum level: 1–3 mcg/ml; toxic serum level: greater than 5 mcg/ml.

PATIENT/FAMILY TEACHING

• Discomfort may occur with IM injection. • Drowsiness usually disappears during continued therapy. • If dizziness occurs, change positions slowly from recumbent to sitting before standing. • Smoking reduces drug effectiveness. • Do not abruptly withdraw medication after long-term therapy.

chloroprocaine

(Nesacaine)

See Anesthetics: local (p. 4C)

chloroquine

klor-oh-kwin

(Aralen)

◆ CLASSIFICATION

PHARMACOTHERAPEUTIC: Amebicide. **CLINICAL:** Antimalarial.

ACTION

Concentrates in parasite acid vesicles. May interfere with parasite protein synthesis. **Therapeutic Effect:** Increases pH (inhibits parasite growth).

USES

Suppression/chemoprophylaxis of malaria in chloroquine-sensitive areas. Treatment of uncomplicated or mild to moderate malaria, extraintestinal amebiasis. **OFF-LABEL:** Treatment of sarcoid-associated hypercalcemia, juvenile arthritis, rheumatoid arthritis, systemic lupus erythematosus, solar urticaria, chronic cutaneous vasculitis.

PRECAUTIONS

CONTRAINDICATIONS: Hypersensitivity to 4-aminoquinolones, retinal or visual field changes, psoriasis, porphyria. **CAUTIONS:** Alcoholism, severe hematologic disorders, hepatic disease, neurologic disorders, G6PD deficiency. Children are especially susceptible to chloroquine fatalities. **Pregnancy Category C.**

INTERACTIONS

DRUG: Penicillamine: May increase concentration of this drug; concurrent use may increase risk of hematologic/renal or severe skin reaction. **HERBAL:** None known. **FOOD:** None known. **LAB VALUES:** Acute decrease in Hct, Hgb, RBC count may occur.

AVAILABILITY (Rx)
TABLETS: 250 mg, 500 mg.

INDICATIONS/ROUTES/DOSAGE
◀ **ALERT** ▶ Chloroquine PO$_4$ 500 mg = 300 mg base; chloroquine HCl 50 mg = 40 mg base.

CHLOROQUINE PHOSPHATE
TREATMENT OF MALARIA
(acute attack): Dose (mg base)

Dose	Time	Adults	Children
Initial	Day 1	600 mg	10 mg/kg
Second	6 hr later	300 mg	5 mg/kg
Third	Day 2	300 mg	5 mg/kg
Fourth	Day 3	300 mg	5 mg/kg

SUPPRESSION OF MALARIA
PO: ADULTS: 500 mg (300 mg base)/wk on same day each week beginning 2 wk before exposure; continue for 6–8 wk after leaving endemic area. CHILDREN: 5 mg base/kg/wk. If therapy is not begun before exposure, then.
PO: ADULTS: 600 mg base initially given in 2 divided doses 6 hr apart. CHILDREN: 10 mg base/kg.

AMEBIASIS
PO: ADULTS: 1 g (600 mg base) a day for 2 days; then, 500 mg (300 mg base) a day for at least 2–3 wk. CHILDREN: 10 mg base/kg once daily for 2–3 wk. **Maximum:** 300 mg base a day.

SIDE EFFECTS
FREQUENT: Mild transient headache, anorexia, nausea/vomiting. **OCCASIONAL:** Visual disturbances (blurring, difficulty focusing) anxiety, fatigue, pruritus (especially of palms, soles, scalp), bleaching of hair, irritability, personality changes, diarrhea, skin eruptions. **RARE:** Stomatitis (redness/burning of oral mucosa, gingivitis, glossitis), exfoliative dermatitis.

ADVERSE REACTIONS/ TOXIC EFFECTS
Ocular toxicity (tinnitus), ototoxicity (reduced hearing). Prolonged therapy: peripheral neuritis and neuromyopathy, hypotension, EKG changes, agranulocytosis, aplastic anemia, thrombocytopenia, seizures, psychosis. Overdosage: headache, vomiting, visual disturbance, drowsiness, seizures, hypokalemia followed by cardiovascular collapse, death.

NURSING CONSIDERATIONS
INTERVENTION/EVALUATION
Check for, promptly report any visual disturbances. Evaluate for GI distress. Monitor liver function tests, assess for fatigue, jaundice, other signs of hepatic effects. Assess skin/buccal mucosa, inquire about pruritus. Check vital signs, be alert to signs/symptoms of overdosage (especially with parenteral administration, children). Notify physician of tinnitus, reduced hearing. With prolonged therapy, test for muscle weakness.

PATIENT/FAMILY TEACHING
• IM administration may cause local discomfort. • Continue drug for full length of treatment. • Notify physician of **any** new symptom, visual difficulties, decreased hearing, tinnitus immediately. • Periodic lab, visual tests are important part of therapy.

chlorothiazide
(Diuril)
See Diuretics (p. 88C)

chlorpheniramine
(Chlor-Trimeton, Teldrin)
See Antihistamines (p. 50C)

*chlorproMAZINE ℮

klor-**proe**-ma-zeen
(Chlorpromanyl ♣, Largactil ♣, Thorazine)

Do not confuse chlorpromazine with chlorpropamide, clomipramine, or prochlorperazine, or Thorazine with thiamide or thioridazine.

CLASSIFICATION

PHARMACOTHERAPEUTIC: Phenothiazine. **CLINICAL:** Antipsychotic, antiemetic, antianxiety, antineuralgia adjunct (see p. 58C).

ACTION

A phenothiazine that blocks dopamine neurotransmission at postsynaptic dopamine receptor sites. Possesses strong anticholinergic, sedative, and antiemetic effects; moderate extrapyramidal effects; and slight antihistamine action. **Therapeutic Effect:** Relieves nausea and vomiting; improves psychotic conditions; controls intractable hiccups and porphyria.

USES

Management of psychotic disorders, manic phase of manic-depressive illness, severe nausea/vomiting, severe behavioral disturbances in children. Relief of intractable hiccups, acute intermittent porphyria. OFF-LABEL: Treatment of choreiform movement of Huntington's disease.

PRECAUTIONS

CONTRAINDICATIONS: Comatose states, myelosuppression, severe cardiovascular disease, severe CNS depression, subcortical brain damage. **CAUTIONS:** Impaired respiratory/hepatic/renal/cardiac function, alcohol withdrawal, history of seizures, urinary retention, glaucoma, prostatic hypertrophy, hypocalcemia (increases susceptibility to dystonias).

⌛ **LIFESPAN CONSIDERATIONS: Pregnancy/Lactation:** Crosses placenta; distributed in breast milk. **Pregnancy Category C. Children:** Those with acute illnesses (chickenpox, measles, gastroenteritis, CNS infection) are at risk of developing neuromuscular, extrapyramidal symptoms (EPS), particularly dystonias. **Elderly:** Susceptible to anticholinergic, neuromuscular, EPS.

INTERACTIONS

DRUG: **Alcohol, other CNS depressants:** May increase respiratory depression and the hypotensive effects of chlorpromazine. **Antithyroid agents:** May increase the risk of agranulocytosis. **Extrapyramidal symptom-producing medications:** Increased risk of extrapyramidal symptoms. **Hypotensives:** May increase hypotension. **Levodopa:** May decrease the effects of levodopa. **Lithium:** May decrease the absorption of chlorpromazine and produce adverse neurologic effects. **MAOIs, tricyclic antidepressants:** May increase the anticholinergic and sedative effects of chlorpromazine. HERBAL: None known. FOOD: None known. LAB VALUES: May produce false-positive pregnancy and phenylketonuria (PKU) test results. May cause EKG changes, including Q- and T-wave disturbances. Therapeutic serum level is 50–300 mcg/ml; toxic serum level is greater than 750 mcg/ml.

AVAILABILITY (Rx)

ORAL CONCENTRATE: 30 mg/ml, 100 mg/ml. **SYRUP:** 10 mg/5 ml. **TABLETS:** 10 mg, 25 mg, 50 mg, 100 mg, 200 mg. **CAPSULES (SUSTAINED-RELEASE):** 30 mg, 75 mg, 150 mg. **INJECTION:** 25 mg/ml. **SUPPOSITORIES:** 25 mg, 100 mg.

---

* "Tall Man" lettering   ℘ see color pill atlas   ♪ herb   underlined – top prescribed drug

ADMINISTRATION/HANDLING

IM

◄ **ALERT** ► Do not give chlorpromazine by the subcutaneous route (risk for severe tissue necrosis). • Dilute the injection solution as prescribed, with sodium chloride for injection or 2% procaine to reduce injection site irritation. • Slowly inject the drug deep into a large muscle, such as the gluteus maximus rather than the lateral aspect of the thigh, to minimize discomfort.

PO

• Avoid skin contact with the oral concentrate and syrup to prevent contact dermatitis. • A slight yellow color in the oral concentrate or syrup won't affect the drug's potency; discard if markedly discolored or if it contains precipitate. • Dilute each dose of oral concentrate immediately before administration with 60 ml or more of water, coffee, tea, milk, carbonated beverage, tomato or fruit juice, simple syrup, orange syrup, soup, or pudding. Use immediately and discard any remaining mixture.

RECTAL

• Wash hands with soap and water before using suppository. • Remove the foil or wrapper from the suppository before inserting it. • Lie patient on left side with left leg straight or slightly bent, and right knee bent upward. Gently push the pointed end of the suppository into the rectum about 1 inch. • Have patient remain lying down for about 15 min to keep the suppository from coming out before it melts. • Wash hands after inserting the suppository.

INDICATIONS/ROUTES/DOSAGE

SEVERE NAUSEA OR VOMITING

PO: ADULTS, ELDERLY: 10–25 mg q4–6h. CHILDREN: 0.5–1 mg/kg q4–6h.

IV, IM: ADULTS, ELDERLY: 25–50 mg q4–6h. CHILDREN: 0.5–1 mg/kg q6–8h.

RECTAL: ADULTS, ELDERLY: 50–100 mg q6–8h. CHILDREN: 1 mg/kg q6–8h.

PSYCHOTIC DISORDERS

PO: ADULTS, ELDERLY: 30–800 mg/day in 1–4 divided doses. CHILDREN OLDER THAN 6 MO: 0.5–1 mg/kg q4–6h.

IV, IM: ADULTS, ELDERLY: Initially, 25 mg; may repeat in 1–4 hr. May gradually increase to 400 mg q4–6h. Usual dose: 300–800 mg/day. CHILDREN OLDER THAN 6 MO: 0.5–1 mg/kg q6–8h. **Maximum:** 75 mg/day for children 5–12 yr; 40 mg/day for children younger than 5 yr.

INTRACTABLE HICCUPS

PO, IV, IM: ADULTS: 25–50 mg 3 times a day.

PORPHYRIA

PO: ADULTS: 25–50 mg 3–4 times a day.

IM: ADULTS, ELDERLY: 25 mg 3–4 times a day.

SIDE EFFECTS

FREQUENT: Somnolence, blurred vision, hypotension, color vision or night vision disturbances, dizziness, decreased sweating, constipation, dry mouth, nasal congestion. **OCCASIONAL:** Urinary retention, photosensitivity, rash, decreased sexual function, swelling or pain in breasts, weight gain, nausea, vomiting, abdominal pain, tremors.

ADVERSE REACTIONS/ TOXIC EFFECTS

EPS appear to be dose related and are divided into three categories: akathisia (including inability to sit still, tapping of feet), parkinsonian symptoms (such as mask-like face, tremors, shuffling gait, hypersalivation), and acute dystonias (including torticollis, opisthotonos, and oculogyric crisis). A dystonic reaction may also produce diaphoresis and pallor. Tardive dyskinesia, including tongue protrusion, puffing of the cheeks, and puckering of the mouth is a rare reaction that may be irreversible. Abrupt discontinuation after long-term therapy may precipitate nausea, vomiting, gastritis, dizziness, and tremors. Blood dyscrasias, particularly agranulocytosis and mild leukopenia, may occur. Chlorpromazine may lower the seizure threshold.

NURSING CONSIDERATIONS

BASELINE ASSESSMENT

Avoid skin contact with solution (contact dermatitis). **Antiemetic:** Assess for dehydration (poor skin turgor, dry mucous membranes, longitudinal furrows in tongue). **Antipsychotic:** Assess behavior, appearance, emotional status, response to environment, speech pattern, thought content.

INTERVENTION/EVALUATION

Monitor BP for hypotension. Assess for EPS. Monitor WBC, differential count for blood dyscrasias, fine tongue movement (may be early sign of tardive dyskinesia). Supervise suicidal-risk patient closely during early therapy (as depression lessens, energy level improves, increasing suicide potential). Assess for therapeutic response (interest in surroundings, improvement in self-care, increased ability to concentrate, relaxed facial expression). Therapeutic serum level: 50–300 mcg/ml; toxic serum level: greater than 750 mcg/ml.

PATIENT/FAMILY TEACHING

• Full therapeutic response may take up to 6 wk. • Urine may darken. • Do not abruptly withdraw from long-term drug therapy. • Report visual disturbances. • Drowsiness generally subsides during continued therapy. • Avoid tasks that require alertness, motor skills until response to drug is established. • Avoid alcohol, exposure to sunlight.

*chlorproPAMIDE

(Diabinese)
See Antidiabetics (p. 41C)

chlorzoxazone

(Paraflex, Parafon Forte DSC)
See Skeletal muscle relaxants (p. 137C)

cholestyramine resin

coal-es-**tie**-rah-meen
(Novo-Cholamine ✦, Prevalite, Questran, Questran Lite)
Do not confuse Questran with Quarzan.

◆CLASSIFICATION

PHARMACOTHERAPEUTIC: Bile acid sequestrant. **CLINICAL:** Antihyperlipoproteinemic (see p. 52C).

ACTION

An antihyperlipoproteinemic that binds with bile acids in the intestine, forming an insoluble complex. Binding results in partial removal of bile acid from enterohepatic circulation. **Therapeutic Effect:** Removes LDL cholesterol from plasma.

PHARMACOKINETICS

Not absorbed from the GI tract. Decreases in serum LDL apparent in 5–7 days and in serum cholesterol in 1 mo. Serum cholesterol returns to baseline levels about 1 mo after drug is discontinued.

USES

Adjunct to dietary therapy to decrease elevated serum cholesterol levels in patients with primary hypercholesterolemia. Relief of pruritus associated with partial biliary obstruction. **OFF-LABEL:** Treatment of diarrhea (due to bile acids), hyperoxaluria.

PRECAUTIONS

CONTRAINDICATIONS: Complete biliary obstruction, hypersensitivity to cholestyramine or tartrazine (frequently seen in aspirin hypersensitivity). **CAUTIONS:** GI dysfunction (especially constipation), hemorrhoids, hematologic disorders, osteoporosis.

⧗ **LIFESPAN CONSIDERATIONS: Pregnancy/Lactation:** Not systemically absorbed. May interfere with maternal absorption of fat-soluble vitamins. **Pregnancy Category B. Children:** No age-related precautions noted. Limited experience in those younger than 10 yr. **Elderly:** Increased risk of GI side effects, adverse nutritional effects.

INTERACTIONS

DRUG: Anticoagulants: May increase effects of these drugs by decreasing level of vitamin K. **Digoxin, folic acid, penicillins, propranolol, tetracyclines, thiazides, thyroid hormones, other medications:** May bind and decrease absorption of these drugs. **Mycophenolate mofetil:** May reduce mycophenolic acid exposure. **Oral vancomycin:** Binds and decreases the effects of oral vancomycin. **Warfarin:** May decrease warfarin absorption. **HERBAL:** None known. **FOOD:** None known. **LAB VALUES:** May increase serum alkaline phosphatase, serum magnesium, AST, and ALT levels. May decrease serum calcium, potassium, and sodium levels. May prolong PT.

AVAILABILITY (Rx)

POWDER FOR ORAL SUSPENSION: 4 g/5 g (Questran Light), 4 g/9 g (Prevalite, Questran).

ADMINISTRATION/HANDLING

PO

• Give other drugs at least 1 hr before or 4–6 hr following cholestyramine (capable of binding drugs in GI tract).
• Do not give in dry form (highly irritating). Mix with 3–6 oz water, milk, fruit juice, soup. • Place powder on surface for 1–2 min (prevents lumping), then mix thoroughly. • Excessive foaming with carbonated beverages; use extra large glass and stir slowly. • Administer before meals.

INDICATIONS/ROUTES/DOSAGE

HYPERCHOLESTEROLEMIA

PO: ADULTS, ELDERLY: Initially, 4 g 1–2 times a day. Maintenance: 8–16 g/day in divided doses. **Maximum:** 24 g/day. **CHILDREN:** 80 mg/kg 3 times a day.

PRURITIS

PO: ADULTS, ELDERLY: Initially, 4 g 1–2 times a day. Maintenance: 8–16 g/day in divided doses. **Maximum:** 24 g/day.

SIDE EFFECTS

FREQUENT: Constipation (may lead to fecal impaction), nausea, vomiting, abdominal pain, indigestion. **OCCASIONAL:** Diarrhea, belching, bloating, headache, dizziness. **RARE:** Gallstones, peptic ulcer disease, malabsorption syndrome.

ADVERSE REACTIONS/ TOXIC EFFECTS

GI tract obstruction, hyperchloremic acidosis, and osteoporosis secondary to calcium excretion may occur. High dosage may interfere with fat absorption, resulting in steatorrhea.

NURSING CONSIDERATIONS

BASELINE ASSESSMENT

Question for history of hypersensitivity to cholestyramine, tartrazine, aspirin. Obtain baseline serum cholesterol, triglycerides, electrolytes, hepatic enzyme level.

INTERVENTION/EVALUATION

Determine pattern of bowel activity and stool consistency. Evaluate food tolerance, abdominal discomfort, flatulence. Monitor blood chemistries.

Encourage several glasses of water between meals.

PATIENT/FAMILY TEACHING
• Complete full course of therapy; do not omit or change doses. • Take other drugs at least 1 hr before or 4–6 hr after cholestyramine. • Never take in dry form; mix with 3–6 oz water, milk, fruit juice, soup (place powder on surface for 1–2 min to prevent lumping, then mix well). • Use extra large glass, stir slowly when mixing with carbonated beverages due to foaming. • Take before meals, drink several glasses of water between meals. • Eat high-fiber foods (whole grain cereals, fruits, vegetables) to reduce potential for constipation.

chorionic gonadotropin, hCG

kore-ee-**on**-ik goe-**nad**-oh-troe-pin
(APL, Humegon 🍂, Novarel, Pregnyl, Profasi HP 🍂)

CLASSIFICATION
PHARMACOTHERAPEUTIC: Gonadotropin. **CLINICAL:** Infertility therapy adjunct, diagnostic aid (hypogonadism).

ACTION
Stimulates production of gonadal steroid hormones by stimulating interstitial cells (Leydig cells) of the testes to produce androgen and the corpus luteum of the ovary to produce progesterone. **Therapeutic Effect:** Androgen stimulation in the male causes production of secondary sex characteristics and may stimulate descent of testes when no anatomic impediment exists. In women of childbearing age with normally functioning ovaries, causes maturation of corpus luteum and triggers ovulation.

USES
Treatment of hypogonadotropic hypogonadism, prepubertal cryptorchidism. Induces ovulation. **OFF-LABEL:** Diagnosis of male hypogonadism, treatment of corpus luteum dysfunction.

PRECAUTIONS
CONTRAINDICATIONS: Precocious puberty, carcinoma of the prostate, other androgen-dependent neoplasia. Undiagnosed abnormal vaginal bleeding, fibroid tumors of uterus, ovarian cyst or enlargement not associated with polycystic ovarian disease. Active thrombophlebitis. **CAUTIONS:** Prepubertal males, conditions aggravated by fluid retention (cardiac/renal disease, epilepsy, migraine, asthma), polycystic ovarian disease. **Pregnancy Category C.**

INTERACTIONS
DRUG: None known. **HERBAL:** None known. **FOOD:** None known. **LAB VALUES:** None known.

AVAILABILITY (Rx)
INJECTION (POWDER FOR RECONSTITUTION): 10,000 units.

ADMINISTRATION/HANDLING
IM USE ONLY
• Following reconstitution, stable for 30–90 days when stored at 2°–15°C.

INDICATIONS/ROUTES/DOSAGE
PREPUBERTAL CRYPTORCHIDISM, HYPOGONADOTROPIC HYPOGONADISM
IM: CHILDREN: Dosage is individualized based on indication, age, weight of patient, and physician preference.
INDUCTION OF OVULATION AND PREGNANCY
IM: ADULTS (AFTER PRETREATMENT WITH MENOTROPINS): 5,000–10,000 international

---

units 1 day after last dose of menotropins.

SIDE EFFECTS

FREQUENT: Pain at injection site. **Induction of ovulation:** Ovarian cysts, uncomplicated ovarian enlargement. **OCCASIONAL**: Enlarged breasts, headache, irritability, fatigue, depression. **Induction of ovulation:** Severe ovarian hyperstimulation, peripheral edema. **Cryptorchidism:** Precocious puberty (acne, deepening voice, penile growth, pubic/axillary hair).

ADVERSE REACTIONS/TOXIC EFFECTS

When used with menotropins: increased risk of arterial thromboembolism, ovarian hyperstimulation with high incidence (20%) of multiple births (premature deliveries and neonatal prematurity), ruptured ovarian cysts.

NURSING CONSIDERATIONS

BASELINE ASSESSMENT

Obtain baseline weight, BP.

INTERVENTION/EVALUATION

Assess for edema: weigh every 2–3 days, report weight gain greater than 5 lb/wk; monitor BP periodically during treatment; check for decreased urinary output, peripheral edema.

PATIENT/FAMILY TEACHING

• Promptly report abdominal pain, vaginal bleeding, signs of precocious puberty in males (deepening of voice; axillary, facial, pubic hair; acne; penile growth), signs of edema. • In anovulation treatment, begin recording daily basal temperature; initiate intercourse daily beginning the day preceding human chorionic gonadotropin (hCG) treatment. • Possibility of multiple births.

ciclopirox

(Loprox, Penlac)
See Antifungals: topical (p. 44C)

cidofovir

ci-**dah**-fo-veer
(Vistide)

◆ CLASSIFICATION

PHARMACOTHERAPEUTIC: Anti-infective. **CLINICAL**: Antiviral (see p. 60C).

ACTION

An anti-infective that inhibits viral DNA synthesis by incorporating itself into the growing viral DNA chain. **Therapeutic Effect:** Suppresses replication of cytomegalovirus (CMV).

PHARMACOKINETICS

Protein binding: less than 6%. Excreted primarily unchanged in urine. Effect of hemodialysis unknown. **Elimination half-life:** 1.4–3.8 hr.

USES

Treatment of CMV retinitis in those with acquired immunodeficiency syndrome (AIDS). **OFF-LABEL:** Treatment of acyclovir-resistant herpes simplex virus, adenovirus, foscarnet-resistant CMV, ganciclovir-resistant CMV, varicella-zoster virus.

PRECAUTIONS

CONTRAINDICATIONS: Direct intraocular injection, history of clinically severe hypersensitivity to probenecid or other sulfa-containing drugs, renal function impairment (serum creatinine level greater than 1.5 mg/dl, creatinine clearance of 55 ml/min or less, or urine protein level greater than 100 mg/dl). **CAUTION:** Preexisting diabetes.

⏳ **LIFESPAN CONSIDERATIONS: Pregnancy/Lactation:** Embryotoxic (reduced fetal body weight) in animals. Unknown if excreted in breast milk. Do not administer to breast-feeding women. HIV-infected women should not breast-feed. **Pregnancy Category C. Children:** Safety and efficacy not established. **Elderly:** Age-related renal impairment may require dosage adjustment.

INTERACTIONS

DRUG: Nephrotoxic medications (such as aminoglycosides, amphotericin B, foscarnet, IV pentamidine): Increase the risk of nephrotoxicity. **HERBAL:** None known. **FOOD:** None known. **LAB VALUES:** May decrease neutrophil count and serum bicarbonate, phosphate, and uric acid levels. May elevate serum creatinine levels.

AVAILABILITY (Rx)

INJECTION: 75 mg/ml (5-ml ampule).

ADMINISTRATION/HANDLING

◀ **ALERT** ▶ Do not exceed recommended dosage, frequency, infusion rate.

 IV

Reconstitution • Dilute in 100 ml 0.9% NaCl.

Rate of administration • Infuse over 1 hr. • IV hydration with 0.9% NaCl and probenecid therapy must be used with each cidofovir infusion (minimizes risk of nephrotoxicity). • Ingestion of food before each dose of probenecid may reduce nausea and vomiting. An antiemetic may reduce potential for nausea.

Storage • Store at controlled room temperature (68°–77°F). • Admixtures may be refrigerated for no more than 24 hr. • Allow refrigerated admixtures to warm to room temperature before use.

🖫 IV INCOMPATIBILITIES

No information available for Y-site administration.

INDICATIONS/ROUTES/DOSAGE

CMV RETINITIS IN PATIENTS WITH AIDS (IN COMBINATION WITH PROBENECID)

IV INFUSION: ADULTS: **Induction:** Usual dosage, 5 mg/kg at constant rate over 1 hr once weekly for 2 consecutive wk. Give 2 g of PO probenecid 3 hr before cidofovir dose, and then give 1 g 2 hr and 8 hr after completion of the 1-hr cidofovir infusion (total of 4 g). In addition, give 1 L of 0.9% NaCl over 1–2 hr immediately before the cidofovir infusion. If tolerated, a second liter may be infused over 1–3 hr at the start of the infusion or immediately afterward. **Maintenance:** 5 mg/kg cidofovir at constant rate over 1 hr once every 2 wk.

DOSAGE IN RENAL IMPAIRMENT

Changes During Therapy: If creatinine increases by 0.3–0.4 mg/dl, reduce dose to 3 mg/kg; if creatinine increases by 0.5 mg/dl or greater or development of 3+ or greater proteinuria, discontinue therapy.

Preexisting Renal Impairment: Do not use with serum creatinine greater than 1.5 mg/dl, creatinine clearance less than 55 ml/min or urine protein 100 mg/dl or greater (2+ or greater proteinuria).

SIDE EFFECTS

FREQUENT: Nausea, vomiting (65%), fever (57%), asthenia (46%), rash (30%), diarrhea (27%), headache (27%), alopecia (25%), chills (24%), anorexia (22%), dyspnea (22%), abdominal pain (17%).

ADVERSE REACTIONS/ TOXIC EFFECTS

Serious adverse reactions may include proteinuria (80%), nephrotoxicity (53%), neutropenia (31%), elevated serum creatinine levels (29%), infection

---

(24%), anemia (20%), ocular hypotony (a decrease in intraocular pressure 12%), and pneumonia (9%). Concurrent use of probenecid may produce a hypersensitivity reaction characterized by a rash, fever, chills, and anaphylaxis. Acute renal failure occurs rarely.

NURSING CONSIDERATIONS

BASELINE ASSESSMENT
For those taking zidovudine, temporarily discontinue zidovudine administration or decrease zidovudine dose by 50% on days of infusion (probenecid reduces metabolic clearance of zidovudine). Closely monitor renal function (urinalysis, serum creatinine) during therapy.

INTERVENTION/EVALUATION
Monitor serum creatinine, urine protein, WBC count before each dose. Monitor for proteinuria (may be early indicator of dose-dependent nephrotoxicity). Periodically monitor visual acuity, ocular symptoms.

PATIENT/FAMILY TEACHING
• Obtain regular follow-up ophthalmologic exams. • Those of childbearing age should use effective contraception during and for 1 mo after treatment. • Men should practice barrier contraceptive methods during and for 3 mo after treatment. • Do not breast-feed. • Must complete full course of probenecid with each cidofovir dose.

---

cilostazol

sill-oh-**stay**-zole

(Pletal)

Do not confuse Pletal with Plendil.

•CLASSIFICATION

PHARMACOTHERAPEUTIC: Phosphodiesterase III inhibitor. **CLINICAL:** Antiplatelet.

ACTION
A phosphodiesterase III inhibitor that inhibits platelet aggregation. Dilates vascular beds with greatest dilation in femoral beds. **Therapeutic Effect:** Improves walking distance in patients with intermittent claudication.

PHARMACOKINETICS
Moderately absorbed from the GI tract. Protein binding: 95%–98%. Extensively metabolized in the liver. Excreted primarily in the urine and, to a lesser extent, in the feces. Not removed by hemodialysis. **Half-life:** 11–13 hr. Therapeutic effect is usually noted in 2–4 wk but may take as long as 12 wk.

USES
Reduction of symptoms of intermittent claudication indicated by increased walking distance without leg pain.

PRECAUTIONS
CONTRAINDICATIONS: CHF of any severity; hemostatic disorders or active pathologic bleeding, such as bleeding peptic ulcer and intracranial bleeding. **CAUTIONS:** None known.

⧗ **LIFESPAN CONSIDERATIONS: Pregnancy/Lactation:** Unknown if drug crosses placenta or is distributed in breast milk. **Pregnancy Category C. Children:** Safety and efficacy not established. **Elderly:** No age-related precautions noted.

INTERACTIONS
DRUG: Aspirin: May potentiate inhibition of platelet aggregation. **Clarithromycin, diltiazem, erythromycin, fluconazole, fluoxetine, omeprazole, sertraline:** May increase concentration of cilostazol. **HERBAL:** None known. **FOOD: Grapefruit, grapefruit juice:** May increase blood concentration and risk of toxicity of cilostazol. **LAB VALUES:** May increase BUN and serum creatinine levels. May decrease Hgb and Hct.

AVAILABILITY (Rx)

TABLETS: 50 mg, 100 mg.

ADMINISTRATION/HANDLING

PO
• Give at least 30 min before or 2 hr after meals. • Do not take with grapefruit juice.

INDICATIONS/ROUTES/DOSAGE

INTERMITTENT CLAUDICATION

PO: ADULTS, ELDERLY: 100 mg twice a day at least 30 min before or 2 hr after meals. 50 mg twice a day during concurrent therapy with clarithromycin, diltiazem, erythromycin, fluconazole, fluoxetine, omeprazole, or sertraline.

SIDE EFFECTS

FREQUENT (34%–10%): Headache, diarrhea, palpitations, dizziness, pharyngitis. **OCCASIONAL (7%–3%):** Nausea, rhinitis, back pain, peripheral edema, dyspepsia, abdominal pain, tachycardia, cough, flatulence, myalgia. **RARE (2%–1%):** Leg cramps, paresthesia, rash, vomiting.

ADVERSE REACTIONS/ TOXIC EFFECTS

Signs and symptoms of overdose are noted by severe headache, diarrhea, hypotension, and cardiac arrhythmias.

NURSING CONSIDERATIONS

BASELINE ASSESSMENT

Assess platelet count, Hgb, Hct before treatment and periodically during treatment.

PATIENT/FAMILY TEACHING

• Take on an empty stomach (at least 30 min before or 2 hr after meals). • Do not take with grapefruit juice.

Ciloxan, see *ciprofloxacin*

---

cimetidine

sih-**met**-ih-deen
(Apo-Cimetidine ✤, Novocimetine ✤, Peptol ✤, Tagamet, Tagamet HB)
Do not confuse cimetidine with simethicone.

◆CLASSIFICATION

PHARMACOTHERAPEUTIC: H_2 receptor antagonist. **CLINICAL:** Antiulcer, gastric acid secretion inhibitor (see p. 95C).

ACTION

An antiulcer agent and gastric acid secretion inhibitor that inhibits histamine action at histamine 2 receptor sites of parietal cells. **Therapeutic Effect:** Inhibits gastric acid secretion during fasting, at night, or when stimulated by food, caffeine, or insulin.

PHARMACOKINETICS

Well absorbed from the GI tract. Protein binding: 15%–20%. Widely distributed. Metabolized in the liver. Primarily excreted in urine. Not removed by hemodialysis. **Half-life:** 2 hr; increased with impaired renal function.

USES

Short-term treatment of active duodenal ulcer. Prevention of duodenal ulcer recurrence, upper GI bleeding in critically ill patients. Treatment of active benign gastric ulcer, pathologic GI hypersecretory conditions, gastroesophageal reflux disease (GERD). **OTC use:** Heartburn, acid indigestion, sour stomach. **OFF-LABEL:** Prevention of aspiration pneumonia; treatment of acute urticaria, chronic warts, upper GI bleeding.

PRECAUTIONS

CONTRAINDICATIONS: Hypersensitivity to other H_2-antagonists.

✎ see color pill atlas   ✒ herb   <u>underlined</u> – top prescribed drug

CAUTIONS: Impaired renal/hepatic function, elderly. Cimetidine may interfere with skin tests.

 LIFESPAN CONSIDERATIONS: Pregnancy/Lactation: Crosses placenta. Distributed in breast milk. In infants, may suppress gastric acidity, inhibit drug metabolism, produce CNS stimulation. **Pregnancy Category B. Children:** Long-term use may induce cerebral toxicity, affect hormonal system. **Elderly:** More likely to experience confusion, especially in patients with renal impairment.

INTERACTIONS

DRUG: Antacids: May decrease the absorption of cimetidine. **Calcium channel blockers, cyclosporine, lidocaine, metoprolol, metronidazole, oral anticoagulants, oral antidiabetics, phenytoin, propranolol, theophylline, tricyclic antidepressants:** May decrease the metabolism and increase the blood concentrations of these drugs. **Ketoconazole:** May decrease the absorption of ketoconazole. **HERBAL:** None known. **FOOD:** None known. **LAB VALUES:** Interferes with skin tests using allergen extracts. May increase prolactin, serum creatinine, and transaminase levels. May decrease parathyroid hormone concentration.

AVAILABILITY (Rx)

TABLETS (TAGAMET HB): 100 mg (OTC), 200 mg. **TABLETS (TAGAMET):** 200 mg, 300 mg, 400 mg, 800 mg. **LIQUID (TAGAMET):** 300 mg/5 ml. **LIQUID (TAGAMET HB):** 200 mg/20 ml. **INJECTION (TAGAMET):** 150 mg/ml.

ADMINISTRATION/HANDLING

IV

Dilution • Dilute each 300 mg (2 ml) with 18 ml 0.9% NaCl, 0.45% NaCl, 0.2% NaCl, D_5W, $D_{10}W$, Ringer's solution, or lactated Ringer's solution to a total volume of 20 ml.

Rate of administration • For IV push, administer over not less than 2 min (prevents arrhythmias, hypotension). • For intermittent IV (piggyback) administration, infuse over 15–20 min. • For IV infusion, dilute with 100–1,000 ml 0.9% NaCl, D_5W, or other compatible solution (see Dilution) and infuse over 24 hr.

Storage • Store at room temperature. • Reconstituted drug is stable for 48 hr at room temperature.

IM

• Administer undiluted. • Inject deep into large muscle mass.

PO

• Give without regard to food. Best given with meals and at bedtime. • Do not administer within 1 hr of antacids.

IV INCOMPATIBILITIES

Allopurinol (Aloprim), amphotericin B complex (Abelcet, AmBisome, Amphotec), cefepime (Maxipime).

IV COMPATIBILITIES

Aminophylline, diltiazem (Cardizem), furosemide (Lasix), heparin, hydromorphone (Dilaudid), insulin (regular), lidocaine, lorazepam (Ativan), midazolam (Versed), morphine, potassium chloride, propofol (Diprivan).

INDICATIONS/ROUTES/DOSAGE

ACTIVE ULCER

PO: ADULTS, ELDERLY: 300 mg 4 times a day or 400 mg twice a day or 800 mg at bedtime.
IV, IM: ADULTS, ELDERLY: 300 mg q6h or 150 mg as single dose followed by 37.5 mg/hr continuous infusion.

PREVENTION OF DUODENAL ULCER

PO: ADULTS, ELDERLY: 400–800 mg at bedtime.

GASTRIC HYPERSECRETORY SECRETIONS

PO, IV, IM: ADULTS, ELDERLY: 300–600 mg q6h. **Maximum:** 2,400 mg/day. CHILDREN: 20–40 mg/kg/day in divided doses q6h.

INFANTS: 10–20 mg/kg/day in divided doses q6–12h. NEONATES: 5–10 mg/kg/day in divided doses q8–12h.

GASTROINTESTINAL REFLUX DISEASE

PO: ADULTS, ELDERLY: 800 mg twice a day or 400 mg 4 times a day for 12 wk.

OTC USE

PO: ADULTS, ELDERLY: 100 mg up to 30 min before meals. **Maximum:** 2 doses/day.

PREVENTION OF UPPER GI BLEEDING

IV INFUSION: ADULTS, ELDERLY: 50 mg/hr.

DOSAGE IN RENAL IMPAIRMENT

Dosage is based on a 300-mg dose in adults. Dosage interval is modified based on creatinine clearance.

Creatinine Clearance	Dosage Interval
Greater than 40 ml/min	q6h
20–40 ml/min	q8h or decrease dose by 25%
Less than 20 ml/min	q12h or decrease dose by 50%

Give after hemodialysis and q12h between dialysis sessions.

SIDE EFFECTS

OCCASIONAL (4%–2%): Headache. **Elderly and severely ill patients, patients with impaired renal function:** Confusion, agitation, psychosis, depression, anxiety, disorientation, hallucinations. Effects reverse 3–4 days after discontinuance. **RARE (less than 2%):** Diarrhea, dizziness, somnolence, nausea, vomiting, gynecomastia, rash, impotence.

ADVERSE REACTIONS/ TOXIC EFFECTS

Rapid IV administration may produce cardiac arrhythmias and hypotension.

NURSING CONSIDERATIONS

BASELINE ASSESSMENT

Do not administer antacids concurrently (separate by 1 hr).

INTERVENTION/EVALUATION

Monitor BP for hypotension during IV infusion. Assess for GI bleeding: hematemesis, blood in stool. Check mental status in elderly, severely ill, those with renal impairment.

PATIENT/FAMILY TEACHING

• May produce transient discomfort at IM injection site. • Do not take antacids within 1 hr of cimetidine administration. • Avoid tasks that require alertness, motor skills until drug response is established. • Avoid smoking. • Report any blood in vomitus/stool, or dark, tarry stool.

---

cinacalcet

sin-ah-**kal**-set
(Sensipar)

◆CLASSIFICATION

PHARMACOTHERAPEUTIC: Calcium receptor agonist. **CLINICAL:** Calcimimetic.

ACTION

A calcium receptor agonist that increases the sensitivity of the calcium-sensing receptor on the parathyroid gland to extracellular calcium, thus lowering the parathyroid hormone (PTH) levels. **Therapeutic Effect:** Decreases serum calcium and PTH levels.

PHARMACOKINETICS

Extensively distributed after PO administration. Protein binding: 93%–97%. Rapidly and extensively metabolized by multiple enzymes. Primarily eliminated in urine with a lesser amount excreted in feces. **Half-life:** 30–40 hr.

USES

Treatment of hypercalcemia in patients with parathyroid carcinoma. Treatment of secondary hyperparathyroidism in patients on dialysis with chronic renal disease. **OFF-LABEL:** Primary hyperthyroidism.

PRECAUTIONS

CONTRAINDICATIONS: None known. **CAUTIONS:** Hepatic function impairment.

⌛ **LIFESPAN CONSIDERATIONS: Pregnancy/Lactation:** May cross placental barrier; unknown if distributed in breast milk. Safe usage during lactation not established (potential adverse reaction in infants). **Pregnancy Category C. Children:** Safety and efficacy not established. **Elderly:** No age-related precautions noted.

INTERACTIONS

DRUG: Amitriptyline: Increases amitriptyline plasma concentration. **Erythromycin, itraconazole, ketoconazole:** Increase cinacalcet plasma concentration. **Flecainide, thioridazine, tricyclic antidepressants, vinblastine:** May require dosage adjustment of these drugs. **HERBAL:** None known. **FOOD: High-fat meals:** Increase cinacalcet plasma concentration. **LAB VALUES:** Reduces serum calcium level.

AVAILABILITY (Rx)

TABLETS: 30 mg, 60 mg, 90 mg.

ADMINISTRATION/HANDLING

PO
• Store at room temperature. • Do not break or crush film-coated tablets. • Administer with food or shortly after a meal.

INDICATIONS/ROUTES/DOSAGE

HYPERCALCEMIA IN PARATHYROID CARCINOMA
PO: ADULTS, ELDERLY: Initially, 30 mg twice a day. Titrate dosage sequentially (60 mg twice a day, 90 mg twice a day, and 90 mg 3–4 times a day) every 2–4 wk as needed to normalize serum calcium levels.

SECONDARY HYPERPARATHYROIDISM IN PATIENTS ON DIALYSIS
PO: ADULTS, ELDERLY: Initially, 30 mg once a day. Titrate dosage sequentially (60, 90, 120, and 180 mg once a day) every 2–4 wk.

SIDE EFFECTS

FREQUENT (31%–21%): Nausea, vomiting, diarrhea. **OCCASIONAL (15%–10%):** Myalgia, dizziness. **RARE (7%–5%):** Asthenia, hypertension, anorexia, non-cardiac chest pain.

ADVERSE REACTIONS/ TOXIC EFFECTS

Overdose may lead to hypocalcemia.

NURSING CONSIDERATIONS

BASELINE ASSESSMENT
Establish baseline serum electrolyte levels.

INTERVENTION/EVALUATION
Monitor serum calcium level. Assess pattern of bowel activity and stool consistency. Obtain order for antidiarrheal, antiemetic medication to prevent serum electrolyte imbalance. Assess for evidence of dizziness and institute fall risk precautions.

PATIENT/FAMILY TEACHING
• Instruct patient to take cinacalcet with food or shortly after a meal. • Notify physician or nurse immediately if vomiting, diarrhea occurs.

Cipro, *see ciprofloxacin*

Cipro IV, *see ciprofloxacin*

---

ciprofloxacin hydrochloride

sip-row-**flocks**-ah-sin

(<u>Ciloxan</u>, <u>Cipro</u>, <u>Cipro I.V.</u>, Cipro XR, Proquin XR)

Do not confuse ciprofloxacin or Ciproxin with Ciloxan, cinoxacin, or Cytoxan.

FIXED-COMBINATION(S)

Cipro HC Otic: ciprofloxacin/hydrocortisone (a steroid): 0.2%/1%. **CiproDex Otic:** ciprofloxacin/dexamethasone (a corticosteroid): 0.3%/0.1%.

◆CLASSIFICATION

PHARMACOTHERAPEUTIC: Fluoroquinolone. **CLINICAL:** Anti-infective (see p. 24C).

ACTION

A fluoroquinolone that inhibits the enzyme DNA gyrase in susceptible bacteria, interfering with bacterial cell replication. **Therapeutic Effect:** Bactericidal.

PHARMACOKINETICS

Well absorbed from the GI tract (food delays absorption). Protein binding: 20%–40%. Widely distributed (including to CSF). Metabolized in the liver to active metabolite. Primarily excreted in urine. Minimal removal by hemodialysis. **Half-life:** 4–6 hr (increased in impaired renal function and the elderly).

USES

Treatment of susceptible infections due to *E. coli, K. pneumoniae, E. cloacae, P. mirabilis, P. vulgaris, P. aeruginosa, H. influenzae, M. catarrhalis, S. pneumoniae, S. aureus* (methicillin susceptible), *S. epidermidis, S. pyogenes, C. jejuni,* Shigella species, *S. typhi* including intra-abdominal, bone and joint, lower respiratory tract, skin and skin-structure, and urinary tract infections, infectious diarrhea, prostatitis, sinusitis, typhoid fever, febrile neutropenia. **OFF-LABEL:** Treatment of chancroid.

PRECAUTIONS

CONTRAINDICATIONS: Hypersensitivity to ciprofloxacin or other quinolones; for ophthalmic administration: vaccinia, varicella, epithelial herpes simplex, keratitis, mycobacterial infection, fungal disease of ocular structure, use after uncomplicated removal of a foreign body. **CAUTIONS:** Renal impairment, CNS disorders, seizures, those taking theophylline, caffeine. Suspension not for use in an NG tube.

⏳ **LIFESPAN CONSIDERATIONS: Pregnancy/Lactation:** Unknown if distributed in breast milk. If possible, do not use during pregnancy/lactation (risk of arthropathy to fetus/infant). **Pregnancy Category C. Children:** Safety and efficacy not established in those younger than 18 yr. **Elderly:** Age-related renal impairment may require dosage adjustment.

INTERACTIONS

DRUG: Antacids, iron preparations, sucralfate: May decrease ciprofloxacin absorption. **Antidiabetic agents:** May produce changes in blood glucose and increase the risk of hypoglycemia or hyperglycemia. **Caffeine, oral anticoagulants:** May increase the effects of these drugs. **Corticosteroids:** May increase the risk for tendon rupture. **Fosphenytoin, phenytoin:** May increase or decrease fosphenytoin or phenytoin levels. **Probenecid:** May increase the serum levels of ciprofloxacin. **Theophylline:** Decreases clearance and may increase blood concentration and risk of toxicity of theophylline. **HERBAL: Fennel:** May decrease the bioavailability of ciprofloxacin and cause possible treatment failure. **Guar gum:** May cause changes in blood glucose and increase the risk of hypoglycemia or hyperglycemia. FOOD: **Dairy:** May decrease ciprofloxacin concentrations. LAB VALUES: May increase BUN and serum alkaline phosphatase, bilirubin, creatinine, LDH, AST, and ALT levels.

AVAILABILITY (Rx)

TABLETS (CIPRO): 100 mg, 250 mg, 500 mg, 750 mg. **TABLETS (EXTENDED-RELEASE [CIPRO XR]):** 500 mg, 1,000 mg. **TABLETS (EXTENDED-RELEASE [PROQUIN XR]):** 500 mg. **INFUSION (CIPRO I.V.):** 200 mg/100 ml, 400 mg/200 ml. **INTRAVENOUS SOLUTION (CIPRO I.V.):** 10 mg/ml. **OPHTHALMIC OINTMENT (CILOXAN):** 0.3%. **OPHTHALMIC SUSPENSION (CILOXAN):** 0.3%. **ORAL SUSPENSION, POWDER FOR RECONSTITUTION (CIPRO):** 250 mg/5 ml, 500 mg/5 ml.

ADMINISTRATION/HANDLING

 IV

Reconstitution • Available prediluted in infusion container ready for use.

Rate of administration • Infuse over 60 min.

Storage • Store at room temperature. • Solution appears clear, colorless to slightly yellow.

PO
• May be given without regard to food (preferred dosing time: 2 hr after meals). • Do not administer antacids (aluminum, magnesium) within 2 hr of ciprofloxacin. • Encourage cranberry juice, citrus fruits (acidifies urine). • Suspension may be stored for 14 days at room temperature.

OPHTHALMIC
• Tilt patient's head back; place solution in conjunctival sac. • Have patient close eyes; press gently on lacrimal sac for 1 min. • Do not use ophthalmic solutions for injection. • Unless infection is very superficial, systemic administration generally accompanies ophthalmic use.

▦ IV INCOMPATIBILITIES

Aminophylline, ampicillin and sulbactam (Unasyn), cefepime (Maxipime), dexamethasone (Decadron), furosemide (Lasix), heparin, hydrocortisone (Solu-Cortef), methylprednisolone (Solu-Medrol), phenytoin (Dilantin), sodium bicarbonate, total parenteral nutrition (TPN).

IV COMPATIBILITIES

Calcium gluconate, diltiazem (Cardizem), dobutamine (Dobutrex), dopamine (Intropin), lidocaine, lorazepam (Ativan), magnesium, midazolam (Versed), potassium chloride.

INDICATIONS/ROUTES/DOSAGE

BONE, JOINT INFECTIONS
IV: ADULTS, ELDERLY: 400 mg q12h for 4–6 wk.
PO: ADULTS, ELDERLY: 500 mg q12h for 4–6 wk.

CONJUNCTIVITIS
OPHTHALMIC: ADULTS, ELDERLY: 1–2 drops q2h for 2 days, then 2 drops q4h for next 5 days.

CORNEAL ULCER
OPHTHALMIC: ADULTS, ELDERLY: 2 drops q15min for 6 hr, then 2 drops q30min for the remainder of first day, 2 drops q1h on second day, and 2 drops q4h on days 3–14.

CYSTIC FIBROSIS
IV: CHILDREN: 30 mg/kg/day in 2–3 divided doses. **Maximum:** 1.2 g/day.
PO: CHILDREN: 40 mg/kg/day. **Maximum:** 2 g/day.

FEBRILE NEUTROPENIA
IV: ADULTS, ELDERLY: 400 mg q8h for 7–14 days (in combination).

GONORRHEA
PO: ADULTS, ELDERLY: 250 mg as a single dose.

INFECTIOUS DIARRHEA
PO: ADULTS, ELDERLY: 500 mg q12h for 5–7 days.

INTRA-ABDOMINAL INFECTIONS (WITH METRONIDAZOLE)
IV: ADULTS, ELDERLY: 400 mg q12h for 7–14 days.
PO: ADULTS, ELDERLY: 500 mg q12h for 7–14 days.

LOWER RESPIRATORY TRACT INFECTIONS
IV: ADULTS, ELDERLY: 400 mg q12h for 7–14 days.
PO: ADULTS, ELDERLY: 500 mg q12h for 7–14 days (750 mg q12h for 7–14 days for severe or complicated infections).

NOSOCOMIAL PNEUMONIA
IV: ADULTS, ELDERLY: 400 mg q8h for 10–14 days.

PROSTATITIS
IV: ADULTS, ELDERLY: 400 mg q12h for 28 days.
PO: ADULTS, ELDERLY: 500 mg q12h for 28 days.

SINUSITIS
IV: ADULTS, ELDERLY: 400 mg q12h for 10 days.
PO: ADULTS, ELDERLY: 500 mg q12h for 10 days.

SKIN AND SKIN STRUCTURE INFECTIONS
IV: ADULTS, ELDERLY: 400 mg q12h for 7–14 days.
PO: ADULTS, ELDERLY: 500 mg q12h for 7–14 days (750 mg q12h for severe or complicated infections).

SUSCEPTIBLE INFECTIONS
IV: ADULTS, ELDERLY: 400 mg q8–12h.
PO: ADULTS, ELDERLY: 500–750 mg q12h.

TYPHOID FEVER
PO: ADULTS, ELDERLY: 500 mg q12h for 10 days.

UTIs
IV: ADULTS, ELDERLY: 200 mg q12h for 7–14 days (400 mg q12h for severe or complicated infections).
PO: ADULTS, ELDERLY: 100–250 mg q12h for 3 days for acute uncomplicated infections; 250 mg q12h for 7–14 days for mild to moderate infections; 500 mg q12h for 7–14 days for severe or complicated infections.

DOSAGE IN RENAL IMPAIRMENT
Dosage and frequency are modified based on creatinine clearance and the severity of the infection.

Creatinine Clearance	Dosage Interval
Less than 30 ml/min	Usual dose q18–24h

HEMODIALYSIS
ADULTS, ELDERLY: 250–500 mg q24h (after dialysis).

PERITONEAL DIALYSIS
ADULTS, ELDERLY: 250–500 mg q24h (after dialysis).

SIDE EFFECTS
FREQUENT (5%–2%): Nausea, diarrhea, dyspepsia, vomiting, constipation, flatulence, confusion, crystalluria. **Ophthalmic:** Burning, crusting in corner of eye. **OCCASIONAL (less than 2%):** Abdominal pain or discomfort, headache, rash. **Ophthalmic:** Bad taste, sensation of something in eye, eyelid redness or itching. **RARE (less than 1%):** Dizziness, confusion, tremors, hallucinations, hypersensitivity reaction, insomnia, dry mouth, paresthesia.

ADVERSE REACTIONS/ TOXIC EFFECTS
Superinfection (especially enterococcal or fungal), nephropathy, cardiopulmonary arrest, chest pain, and cerebral thrombosis may occur. Hypersensitivity reactions, including photosensitivity (as evidenced by rash, pruritus, blisters, edema, and burning skin), have occurred in patients receiving fluoroquinolones. Arthropathy may occur if the drug is given to children younger than 18 years. Sensitization to the ophthalmic form of the drug may contraindicate later systemic use of ciprofloxacin.

NURSING CONSIDERATIONS

BASELINE ASSESSMENT
Question for history of hypersensitivity to ciprofloxacin, quinolones.

INTERVENTION/EVALUATION
Evaluate food tolerance. Determine pattern of bowel activity. Monitor for dizziness, headache, visual changes, tremors. Assess for chest, joint pain. **Ophthalmic:** Observe therapeutic response.

PATIENT/FAMILY TEACHING
• Do not skip doses; take full course of therapy. • Take with 8 oz water; drink several glasses of water between meals. • Eat and drink high sources of ascorbic acid (cranberry juice, citrus fruits) to prevent crystalluria. • Do not take antacids (reduces/destroys effectiveness). • Shake suspension well before using; do not chew microcapsules in suspension. • Sugarless gum or hard candy may relieve bad taste. • **Ophthalmic:** Explain possibility of crystal precipitate forming, usual resolution in 1–7 days.

---

cisatracurium

(Nimbex)
See Neuromuscular blockers (p. 111C)

---

cisplatin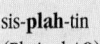

sis-**plah**-tin
(Platinol-AQ)
Do not confuse cisplatin with carboplatin, or Platinol with Paraplatin or Patanol.

◆CLASSIFICATION
PHARMACOTHERAPEUTIC: Platinum coordination complex. **CLINICAL:** Antineoplastic (see p. 72C).

ACTION
A platinum coordination complex that inhibits DNA and, to a lesser extent, RNA, protein synthesis by cross-linking with DNA strands, preventing cell division. Cell cycle–phase nonspecific. **Therapeutic Effect:** Interferes with DNA function.

PHARMACOKINETICS
Widely distributed. Protein binding: greater than 90%. Undergoes rapid nonenzymatic conversion to inactive metabolite. Excreted in urine. Removed by hemodialysis. **Half-life:** 58–73 hr (increased with impaired renal function).

USES
Treatment of metastatic testicular tumors, metastatic ovarian tumors, advanced bladder carcinoma. **OFF-LABEL:** Adrenocortical, anal, biliary tract, breast, cervical, endometrial, esophageal, gastric, head and neck, lung (small cell, non–small cell), primary hepatocellular, prostatic skin, thyroid, vulvar carcinomas; germ cell, gestational trophoblastic, and ovarian germ cell tumors; Hodgkin's and non-Hodgkin's lymphomas; Kaposi's sarcoma, malignant melanoma, neuroblastoma, osteosarcoma, soft tissue sarcoma, Wilm's tumor.

PRECAUTIONS
CONTRAINDICATIONS: Hearing impairment, myelosuppression, preexisting renal impairment. **CAUTIONS:** Previous therapy with other antineoplastic agents, radiation.

⧖ **LIFESPAN CONSIDERATIONS: Pregnancy/Lactation:** If possible, avoid use during pregnancy, especially first trimester. Breast-feeding not recommended.

Pregnancy Category D. Children: Ototoxic effects may be more severe. Elderly: Age-related renal impairment may require dosage adjustment.

INTERACTIONS

DRUG: **Antigout medications:** May decrease the effects of these drugs. **Bone marrow depressants:** May increase myelosuppression. **Fosphenytoin, phenytoin:** May decrease phenytoin plasma concentrations. **Live-virus vaccines:** May potentiate virus replication, increase vaccine side effects, and decrease the patient's antibody response to the vaccine. **Nephrotoxic, ototoxic medications:** May increase the risk of nephrotoxicity or ototoxicity. HERBAL: None known. FOOD: None known. LAB VALUES: May increase BUN and serum creatinine, uric acid, and AST levels. May decrease creatinine clearance and serum calcium, magnesium, phosphate, potassium, and sodium levels. May cause a positive Coombs' test result.

AVAILABILITY (Rx)

INTRAVENOUS SOLUTION: 1 mg/ml.

ADMINISTRATION/HANDLING

◀ ALERT ▶ Wear protective gloves during handling of cisplatin. May be carcinogenic, mutagenic, or teratogenic. Handle with extreme care during preparation/administration.

 IV

Reconstitution • For IV infusion, dilute desired dose in up to 1,000 ml D_5W, 0.33% or 0.45% NaCl containing 12.5–50 g mannitol/L.

Rate of administration • Infuse over 2–24 hr. • Avoid rapid infusion (increases risk of nephrotoxicity, ototoxicity). • Monitor for anaphylactic reaction during first few minutes of IV infusion.

Storage • Protect from sunlight; do not refrigerate (may precipitate). Discard if precipitate forms.

▦ IV INCOMPATIBILITIES

Amifostine (Ethyol), amphotericin B complex (Abelcet, AmBisome, Amphotec), cefepime (Maxipime), piperacillin and tazobactam (Zosyn), sodium bicarbonate, thiotepa.

IV COMPATIBILITIES

Etoposide (VePesid), granisetron (Kytril), heparin, hydromorphone (Dilaudid), lorazepam (Ativan), magnesium sulfate, mannitol, morphine, ondansetron (Zofran).

INDICATIONS/ROUTES/DOSAGE

BLADDER CARCINOMA

IV: ADULTS, ELDERLY: (Single agent): 50–70 mg/m^2 q3–4wk.

OVARIAN TUMORS

IV: ADULTS, ELDERLY: (Single Agent): 100 mg/m^2 q4wk. (Combination): 75–100 mg/m^2 q4wk in combination with cyclophosphamide.

TESTICULAR TUMORS

IV: ADULTS, ELDERLY: 20 mg/m^2 daily for 5 days in combination.

DOSAGE IN RENAL IMPAIRMENT

Dosage is modified based on creatinine clearance.

Creatinine Clearance	% of Dose
10–50 ml/min	75%
Less than 10 ml/min	50%

SIDE EFFECTS

FREQUENT: Nausea, vomiting (generally beginning 1–4 hr after administration and lasting up to 24 hr); myelosuppression (affecting 25%–30% of patients with recovery generally occurring in 18–23 days). **OCCASIONAL:** Peripheral neuropathy (with prolonged therapy [4–7 mo]). Pain or redness at injection site, loss of taste or appetite. **RARE:** Hemolytic anemia, blurred vision, stomatitis.

ADVERSE REACTIONS/ TOXIC EFFECTS

An anaphylactic reaction manifested as angioedema, wheezing, tachycardia, and hypotension, may occur in the first few minutes of IV administration in patients previously exposed to cisplatin. Nephrotoxicity occurs in 28%–36% of patients treated with a single dose of cisplatin, usually during the second week of therapy. Ototoxicity, including tinnitus and hearing loss, occurs in 31% of patients treated with a single dose of cisplatin. It may be more severe in children and may become more frequent or severe with repeated doses.

NURSING CONSIDERATIONS

BASELINE ASSESSMENT

Patients should be well hydrated before and 24 hr after medication to ensure good urinary output, decrease risk of nephrotoxicity.

INTERVENTION/EVALUATION

Measure all vomitus (general guideline requiring immediate notification of physician: 750 ml/8 hr, urinary output less than 100 ml/hr). Monitor I&O q1–2h beginning with pretreatment hydration, continue for 48 hr after cisplatin therapy. Assess vital signs q1–2h during infusion. Monitor urinalysis, renal function reports for nephrotoxicity.

PATIENT/FAMILY TEACHING

• Report signs of ototoxicity (tinnitus, hearing loss). • Do not have immunizations without physician's approval (lowers body's resistance). • Avoid contact with those who have recently taken oral polio vaccine. • Contact physician if nausea or vomiting continues at home. • Teach signs of peripheral neuropathy.

citalopram hydrobromide

sigh-**tail**-oh-pram high-dro-**broh**-mide

(Celexa)

Do not confuse Celexa with Celebrex, Zyprexa, or Cerebyx.

CLASSIFICATION

PHARMACOTHERAPEUTIC: Serotonin reuptake inhibitor. **CLINICAL:** Antidepressant (see p. 37C).

ACTION

A selective serotonin reuptake inhibitor that blocks the uptake of the neurotransmitter serotonin at CNS presynaptic neuronal membranes, increasing its availability at postsynaptic receptor sites. Therapeutic Effect: Relieves depression.

PHARMACOKINETICS

Well absorbed after PO administration. Protein binding: 80%. Primarily metabolized in the liver. Primarily excreted in feces with a lesser amount eliminated in urine. Half-life: 35 hr.

USES

Treatment of depression. OFF-LABEL: Treatment of alcohol abuse, dementia, diabetic neuropathy, obsessive-compulsive disorder, panic disorder, smoking cessation.

PRECAUTIONS

CONTRAINDICATIONS: Sensitivity to citalopram, use within 14 days of MAOIs. **CAUTIONS:** Hepatic/renal impairment, history of seizures, mania, hypomania. ⌛ LIFESPAN CONSIDERATIONS: **Pregnancy/Lactation:** Distributed in breast milk. **Pregnancy Category C. Children:** May cause increased anticholinergic effects, hyperexcitability.

C

Elderly: More sensitive to anticholinergic effects (e.g., dry mouth), more likely to experience dizziness, sedation, confusion, hypotension, hyperexcitability.

INTERACTIONS

DRUG: **Antifungals, cimetidine, macrolide antibiotics:** May increase the citalopram plasma level. **Carbamazepine:** May decrease the citalopram plasma level. **Lithium:** May increase lithium concentration and/or increase the risk of serotonin syndrome. **MAOIs:** May cause serotonin syndrome, marked by autonomic hyperactivity, coma, diaphoresis, excitement, hyperthermia, and rigidity, and neuroleptic malignant syndrome. **Metoprolol:** Increases the metoprolol plasma level. HERBAL: **Ginkgo biloba, St. John's wort:** May increase the risk of serotonin syndrome. FOOD: None known. LAB VALUES: May reduce serum sodium level.

AVAILABILITY (Rx)

ORAL SOLUTION: 10 mg/5 ml. **TABLETS:** 10 mg, 20 mg, 40 mg. **TABLETS (ORALLY DISINTEGRATING):** 10 mg, 20 mg, 40 mg.

ADMINISTRATION/HANDLING

PO
. Give without regard to food. . Scored tablets may be crushed.

PO (ORALLY DISINTEGRATING)
. Place tablet on tongue, allow to dissolve. . Swallow with saliva.

INDICATIONS/ROUTES/DOSAGE

DEPRESSION
PO: ADULTS: Initially, 20 mg once a day in the morning or evening. May increase in 20-mg increments at intervals of no less than 1 wk. **Maximum:** 60 mg/day. ELDERLY, PATIENTS WITH HEPATIC IMPAIRMENT: 20 mg/day. May titrate to 40 mg/day only for nonresponding patients.

SIDE EFFECTS

FREQUENT (21%–11%): Nausea, dry mouth, somnolence, insomnia, diaphoresis. **OCCASIONAL (8%–4%):** Tremor, diarrhea, abnormal ejaculation, dyspepsia, fatigue, anxiety, vomiting, anorexia. **RARE (3%–2%):** Sinusitis, sexual dysfunction, menstrual disorder, abdominal pain, agitation, decreased libido.

ADVERSE REACTIONS/ TOXIC EFFECTS

Overdose is manifested as dizziness, drowsiness, tachycardia, somnolence, confusion, and seizures.

NURSING CONSIDERATIONS

BASELINE ASSESSMENT
Liver/renal function tests, blood counts should be performed periodically for patients on long-term therapy. Observe and record behavior. Assess psychological status, thought content, sleep pattern, appearance, interest in environment.

INTERVENTION/EVALUATION
Closely supervise suicidal-risk patient during early therapy (as energy level improves, suicide potential increases). Assess appearance, behavior, speech pattern, level of interest, mood.

PATIENT/FAMILY TEACHING
. Do not stop taking medication or increase dosage. . Avoid alcohol. . Avoid tasks that require alertness, motor skills until response to drug is established.

citrates

sih-traits

(Bicitra, Citrolith, Oracit, Polycitra, Polycitra-K, Polycitra-LC, Urocit-K)

CLASSIFICATION
CLINICAL: Alkalinizer.

ACTION

These alkalinizers increase the solubility of cystine in urine and the ionization of

C

uric acid to urate ion. The increase in urinary pH and urinary citrate level decreases calcium ion activity and the saturation of calcium oxalate. Citrates also increase the plasma bicarbonate and buffer excess hydrogen ion concentration. **Therapeutic Effect:** Increase blood and urinary pH and reverse metabolic acidosis.

USES

Treatment of metabolic acidosis.

PRECAUTIONS

CONTRAINDICATIONS: Acute dehydration, anuria, azotemia, heat cramps, hypersensitivity to citrates, severe myocardial damage, severe renal impairment, sodium-restricted diet, untreated Addison's disease. **Urocit-K:** Concurrent use of anticholinergics, delayed gastric emptying, intestinal obstruction or stricture, severe peptic ulcer disease. **CAUTIONS:** Those with CHF, hypertension, pulmonary edema. May increase risk of urolithiasis.

⌛ **LIFESPAN CONSIDERATIONS: Pregnancy/Lactation:** Unknown if drug crosses placenta or is distributed in breast milk. **Pregnancy Category C (potassium citrate); other forms not expected to cause fetal harm. Children:** Safety and efficacy not established. **Elderly:** No age-related precautions noted.

INTERACTIONS

DRUG: Angiotensin-converting enzyme (ACE) inhibitors, NSAIDs, potassium-containing medications, potassium-sparing diuretics: May increase the risk of hyperkalemia. **Antacids:** May increase the risk of systemic alkalosis. **Methenamine:** May decrease the effects of methenamine. **Quinidine:** May increase the excretion of quinidine. **HERBAL:** None known. **FOOD:** None known. **LAB VALUES:** None known.

AVAILABILITY (Rx)

TABLETS: 5 mEq, 10 mEq. **TABLETS (CITROLITH):** 50 mg potassium citrate and 950 mg sodium citrate. **SYRUP (POLYCITRA):** 550 mg potassium citrate, plus 500 mg sodium citrate, plus 334 mg citric acid per 5 ml. **ORAL SOLUTION:** 490 mg sodium citrate and 640 mg citric acid per 5 ml (Oracit), 500 mg sodium citrate and 334 mg citric acid per 5 ml (Bicitra), 550 mg potassium citrate, 500 mg sodium citrate, and 334 mg citric acid per 5 ml (Polycitra-LC), 1,100 mg potassium citrate and 334 mg citric acid per 5 ml (Polycitra-K).

ADMINISTRATION/HANDLING

• Give after meals and at bedtime.

INDICATIONS/ROUTES/DOSAGE

METABOLIC ACIDOSIS

PO: ADULTS, ELDERLY: 15–30 ml after meals and at bedtime or 30–60 mEq/day in 3–4 divided doses. CHILDREN: 5–15 ml after meals and at bedtime or 2–3 mEq/kg/day in 3–4 divided doses.

SIDE EFFECTS

OCCASIONAL: Diarrhea, mild abdominal pain, nausea, vomiting.

ADVERSE REACTIONS/ TOXIC EFFECTS

Metabolic alkalosis, bowel obstruction or perforation, hyperkalemia, and hypernatremia occur rarely.

NURSING CONSIDERATIONS

INTERVENTION/EVALUATION

Assess urinary pH, EKG in patients with cardiac disease, serum acid-base balance, CBC, Hgb, Hct, serum creatinine.

PATIENT/FAMILY TEACHING

• Take after meals. • Mix in water or juice; follow with additional liquid if desired.

cladribine ⚑

clad-rih-bean

(Leustatin)

Do not confuse Leustatin with lovastatin.

◆ CLASSIFICATION

PHARMACOTHERAPEUTIC: Antimetabolite. **CLINICAL:** Antineoplastic (see p. 72C).

ACTION

Disrupts cellular metabolism by incorporating into DNA of dividing cells. Cytotoxic to both actively dividing and quiescent lymphocytes, monocytes. **Therapeutic Effect:** Prevents DNA synthesis.

PHARMACOKINETICS

Primarily excreted in urine. **Half-life:** 5.4 hr.

USES

Treatment for active hairy cell leukemia defined by clinically significant anemia, neutropenia, thrombocytopenia. **OFF-LABEL:** Chronic lymphocytic leukemia, non-Hodgkin's lymphoma, acute myeloid leukemia, autoimmune hemolytic anemia.

PRECAUTIONS

CONTRAINDICATIONS: None known. **CAUTIONS:** Renal/hepatic impairment, bone marrow suppression.

⧖ **LIFESPAN CONSIDERATIONS: Pregnancy/Lactation:** May produce fetal harm; may be embryotoxic and fetotoxic; potential for serious reactions in breastfed infants. **Pregnancy Category D. Children:** Safety and efficacy not established. **Elderly:** No age-related precautions noted.

INTERACTIONS

DRUG: Bone marrow depressants: May increase bone marrow depression. **Cyclophosphamide:** High dosages of cladribine with this drug and total body irradiation may cause severe, irreversible neurologic toxicity, acute renal dysfunction. **Nephrotoxic, neurotoxic medications:** May increase toxicity. **Live virus vaccines:** May potentiate virus replication, increase vaccine side effects, decrease patient's antibody response to vaccine. **HERBAL:** None known. **FOOD:** None known. **LAB VALUES:** None known.

AVAILABILITY (Rx)

INJECTION (SOLUTION): 1 mg/ml.

ADMINISTRATION/HANDLING

💧 IV

Reconstitution • Must dilute before administration. • Wear gloves, protective clothing during handling; if contact with skin, rinse with copious amounts of water. • Add calculated dose (0.09 mg/kg) to 500 ml 0.9% NaCl. Avoid D$_5$W (increases degradation of medication).

Rate of administration • Monitor vital signs during infusion, especially during first hour. Observe for hypotension, bradycardia (usually both do not occur during same course). • Immediately discontinue administration if severe hypersensitivity reaction occurs.

Storage • Refrigerate unopened vials. • May refrigerate dilution solution for no more than 8 hr before administration. • Solution is stable for at least 24 hr at room temperature. • Discard unused portion.

▦ IV INCOMPATIBILITIES

Do not mix with other IV drugs/additives or infuse concurrently via a common IV line.

INDICATIONS/ROUTES/DOSAGE

HAIRY CELL LEUKEMIA

IV INFUSION: ADULTS, CHILDREN: 0.09 mg/kg/day as continuous infusion for 7 days.

CHRONIC LYMPHOCYTIC LEUKEMIA

IV INFUSION: ADULTS, ELDERLY: 0.1 mg/kg/day days 1–7.

CHRONIC MYELOGENOUS LEUKEMIA

IV INFUSION: ADULTS, ELDERLY: 15 mg/m^2/day days 1–5. Give as a 1-hr infusion.

USUAL PEDIATRIC DOSAGE

IV: 0.09–0.1 mg/kg/day for 7 days. May repeat q28–35days.

SIDE EFFECTS

FREQUENT: Fever (69%), fatigue (45%), nausea (28%), rash (27%), headache (22%), injection site reactions (19%), anorexia (17%), vomiting (13%). **OCCASIONAL (10%–5%):** Diarrhea, cough, purpura, chills, diaphoresis, constipation, dizziness, petechiae, myalgia, shortness of breath, malaise, pruritus, erythema, insomnia, edema, tachycardia, abdominal/trunk pain, epistaxis, arthralgia.

ADVERSE REACTIONS/TOXIC EFFECTS

Myelosuppression characterized as severe neutropenia (less than 500 cells/mm^3); severe anemia (Hgb less than 8.5 g/dl), thrombocytopenia occur commonly. High-dose treatment may produce acute nephrotoxicity (increased BUN, serum creatinine levels) and/or neurotoxicity (irreversible motor weakness of upper or lower extremities).

NURSING CONSIDERATIONS

BASELINE ASSESSMENT

Offer emotional support to patient, family. Perform neurologic function tests before chemotherapy. Use strict asepsis; protect patient from infection.

INTERVENTION/EVALUATION

Monitor temperature, report fever promptly. Assess for signs of infection. Assess skin for evidence of rash, purpura, petechiae. Monitor Hgb, Hct, BUN, serum creatinine, platelet count, WBC, potassium, sodium.

PATIENT/FAMILY TEACHING

• Narrow margin between therapeutic and toxic response. • Avoid crowds, persons with known infections; report signs of infection at once (fever, flu-like symptoms). • Do not have immunizations without physician's approval (drug lowers body's resistance). • Avoid contact with those who have recently received live virus vaccine. • Women of childbearing potential should not become pregnant during treatment.

Clarinex, *see desloratadine*

clarithromycin

clair-**rith**-row-my-sin
(Biaxin, Biaxin XL, Biaxin XL-Pak)

◆CLASSIFICATION

PHARMACOTHERAPEUTIC: Macrolide. **CLINICAL:** Antibiotic (see p. 25C).

ACTION

A macrolide that binds to ribosomal receptor sites of susceptible organisms, inhibiting protein synthesis of the bacterial cell wall. **Therapeutic Effect:** Bacteriostatic; may be bactericidal with high dosages or very susceptible microorganisms.

PHARMACOKINETICS

Well absorbed from the GI tract. Protein binding: 65%–75%. Widely distributed.

C

Metabolized in the liver to active metabolite. Primarily excreted in urine. Not removed by hemodialysis. **Half-life:** 3–7 hr; metabolite 5–7 hr (increased in impaired renal function).

USES

Treatment of susceptible infections due to *C. pneumoniae, H. influenzae, H. parainfluenzae, H. pylori, M. catarrhalis, M. avium, M. pneumoniae, S. aureus, S pneumoniae, S. pyogenes.* including bacterial exacerbation of bronchitis, otitis media, acute maxillary sinusitis, *Mycobacterium avium* complex (MAC), pharyngitis, tonsillitis, *H. pylori* duodenal ulcer, bacterial pneumonia, skin and soft tissue infections. Prevention of MAC disease. **Biaxin XL:** Treatment of community-acquired pneumonia.

PRECAUTIONS

CONTRAINDICATIONS: Hypersensitivity to other macrolide antibiotics. **CAUTIONS:** Hepatic or renal dysfunction, elderly with severe renal impairment.

⧗ **LIFESPAN CONSIDERATIONS: Pregnancy/Lactation:** Unknown if distributed in breast milk. **Pregnancy Category C. Children:** Safety and efficacy not established in those younger than 6 mo. **Elderly:** Age-related renal impairment may require dosage adjustment.

INTERACTIONS

DRUG: Carbamazepine, digoxin, theophylline: May increase blood concentration and toxicity of these drugs. **Rifampin:** May decrease clarithromycin blood concentration. **Warfarin:** May increase warfarin effects. **Zidovudine:** May decrease blood concentration of zidovudine. **HERBAL:** None known. **FOOD:** None known. **LAB VALUES:** May (rarely) increase BUN, AST, and ALT levels.

AVAILABILITY (Rx)

ORAL SUSPENSION (BIAXIN): 125 mg/5 ml, 250 mg/5 ml. **TABLETS (BIAXIN):** 250 mg, 500 mg. **TABLETS (EXTENDED-RELEASE [BIAXIN XL, BIAXIN XL PAK]):** 500 mg.

ADMINISTRATION/HANDLING

PO
• Give without regard to food. • Do not crush or break tablets.

INDICATIONS/ROUTES/DOSAGE

BRONCHITIS
PO: ADULTS, ELDERLY: 250–500 mg q12h for 7–14 days.
PO (EXTENDED-RELEASE): ADULTS, ELDERLY: 1 g once daily for 7 days.

SKIN, SOFT TISSUE INFECTIONS
PO: ADULTS, ELDERLY: 250 mg q12h for 7–14 days. CHILDREN: 7.5 mg/kg q12h for 10 days. **Maximum:** 1 g/day.

MAC PROPHYLAXIS
PO: ADULTS, ELDERLY: 500 mg twice a day. CHILDREN: 7.5 mg/kg q12h. **Maximum:** 500 mg twice a day.

MAC TREATMENT
PO: ADULTS, ELDERLY: 500 mg twice a day in combination. CHILDREN: 7.5 mg/kg q12h in combination. **Maximum:** 500 mg twice a day.

PHARYNGITIS, TONSILLITIS
PO: ADULTS, ELDERLY: 250 mg q12h for 10 days. CHILDREN: 7.5 mg/kg q12h for 10 days. **Maximum:** 1 g/day.

PNEUMONIA
PO: ADULTS, ELDERLY: 250 mg q12h for 7–14 days. CHILDREN: 7.5 mg/kg q12h.
PO (EXTENDED-RELEASE): ADULTS, ELDERLY: 1 g/day.

MAXILLARY SINUSITIS
PO: ADULTS, ELDERLY: 500 mg q12h or 1,000 mg (2 × 500 mg extended-release) once daily for 14 days. CHILDREN: 7.5 mg/kg q12h. **Maximum:** 500 mg twice a day.

✑ see color pill atlas   ✑ herb   underlined – top prescribed drug

H. PYLORI
PO: ADULTS, ELDERLY: 500 mg q8–12h for 10–14 days in combination.

ACUTE OTITIS MEDIA
PO: CHILDREN: 7.5 mg/kg q12h for 10 days.

DOSAGE IN RENAL IMPAIRMENT
For patients with creatinine clearance less than 30 ml/min, reduce dose by 50% and administer once or twice a day.

SIDE EFFECTS

OCCASIONAL (6%–3%): Diarrhea, nausea, altered taste, abdominal pain. **RARE (2%–1%):** Headache, dyspepsia.

ADVERSE REACTIONS/ TOXIC EFFECTS

Antibiotic-associated colitis and other superinfections may result from altered bacterial balance. Hepatotoxicity and thrombocytopenia occur rarely.

NURSING CONSIDERATIONS

BASELINE ASSESSMENT
Question patient for history of hepatitis, allergies to clarithromycin, erythromycins.

INTERVENTION/EVALUATION
Monitor pattern of bowel activity and stool consistency carefully; mild GI effects may be tolerable, but increasing severity may indicate onset of antibiotic-associated colitis. Be alert for superinfection: genital or anal pruritus, abdominal pain, mouth soreness, moderate to severe diarrhea.

PATIENT/FAMILY TEACHING
• Continue therapy for full length of treatment. • Doses should be evenly spaced. • Take medication with 8 oz water without regard to food.

Claritin, *see loratadine*

clemastine fumarate

kleh-**mass**-teen
(Contac 12 Hour Allergy, Dayhistol Allergy, Tavist Allergy)

◆CLASSIFICATION

PHARMACOTHERAPEUTIC: Ethanolamine. **CLINICAL:** Antihistamine (see p. 50C).

ACTION

An ethanolamine that competes with histamine on effector cells in the GI tract, blood vessels, and respiratory tract. **Therapeutic Effect:** Relieves allergy symptoms, including urticaria, rhinitis, and pruritus.

PHARMACOKINETICS

Route	Onset	Peak	Duration
PO	15–60 min	5–7 hr	10–12 hr

Well absorbed from the GI tract. Metabolized in the liver. Excreted primarily in urine. **Half-life:** 21 hr.

USES

Perennial and seasonal allergic rhinitis, allergic symptoms (e.g., urticaria).

PRECAUTIONS

CONTRAINDICATIONS: Angle-closure glaucoma, hypersensitivity to clemastine, use within 14 days of MAOIs. **CAUTIONS:** Peptic ulcer, GI/GU obstruction, asthma, prostatic hypertrophy.

⧗ **LIFESPAN CONSIDERATIONS: Pregnancy/Lactation:** Excreted in breast milk. **Pregnancy Category B. Children:** Safety and efficacy not established in those younger than 6 yr. **Elderly:** Age-related renal impairment may require dosage adjustment.

INTERACTIONS

DRUG: Alcohol, other CNS depressants: May increase CNS depression.

MAOIs: May increase the anticholinergic and CNS depressant effects of clemastine. HERBAL: None known. FOOD: None known. LAB VALUES: May suppress wheal and flare reactions to antigen skin testing unless drug is discontinued 4 days before testing.

AVAILABILITY (Rx)

SYRUP (TAVIST): 0.67 mg/5 ml. **TABLETS:** 1.34 mg (Contac 12 Hour Allergy), 2.68 mg (Tavist).

ADMINISTRATION/HANDLING
PO
• Give without regard to food. • Scored tablets may be crushed. Do not crush extended-release or film-coated forms.

INDICATIONS/ROUTES/DOSAGE
ALLERGIC RHINITIS, URTICARIA
PO: ADULTS, CHILDREN OLDER THAN 11 YR: 1.34 mg twice a day up to 2.68 mg 3 times a day. **Maximum:** 8.04 mg/day. CHILDREN 6–11 YR: 0.67–1.34 mg twice a day. **Maximum:** 4.02 mg/day. CHILDREN YOUNGER THAN 6 YR: 0.05 mg/kg/day divided into 2–3 doses per day. **Maximum:** 1.34 mg/day. ELDERLY: 1.34 mg 1–2 times a day.

SIDE EFFECTS
FREQUENT: Somnolence, dizziness, urine retention, thickening of bronchial secretions, dry mouth, nose, or throat; in elderly, sedation, dizziness, hypotension. **OCCASIONAL:** Epigastric distress, flushing, blurred vision, tinnitus, paresthesia, diaphoresis, chills.

ADVERSE REACTIONS/TOXIC EFFECTS
A hypersensitivity reaction, marked by eczema, pruritus, rash, cardiac disturbances, angioedema, and photosensitivity, may occur. Overdose symptoms may vary from CNS depression, including sedation, apnea, cardiovascular collapse, and death to severe paradoxical reaction, such as hallucinations, tremor, and seizures. Children may experience paradoxical reactions, such as restlessness, insomnia, euphoria, nervousness, and tremors. Overdose in children may result in hallucinations, seizures, and death.

NURSING CONSIDERATIONS
BASELINE ASSESSMENT
If patient is experiencing allergic reaction, obtain history of recently ingested foods, drugs, environmental exposure, recent emotional stress. Monitor rate, depth, rhythm, type of respiration; quality and rate of pulse. Assess lung sounds for rhonchi, wheezing, rales.

INTERVENTION/EVALUATION
Monitor BP, especially in elderly (increased risk of hypotension). Monitor children closely for paradoxical reaction.

PATIENT/FAMILY TEACHING
• Tolerance to antihistaminic effect generally does not occur; tolerance to sedative effect may occur. • Avoid tasks that require alertness, motor skills until response to drug is established. • Dry mouth, drowsiness, dizziness may be an expected response of drug. • Avoid alcoholic beverages during antihistamine therapy. • Coffee, tea may help reduce drowsiness.

Climara, see estradiol

clindamycin
klin-da-**mye**-sin

(Cleocin HCl, Cleocin Ovules, Cleocin Pediatric, Cleocin Phosphate, Cleocin T, Cleocin Vaginal, Clinda-Derm, Clindagel, Clindamax, Clindesse, Clindets Pledget, Dalacin ✥, Dalacin C ✥)

CLASSIFICATION
PHARMACOTHERAPEUTIC: Lincosamide. **CLINICAL:** Antibiotic.

ACTION
A lincosamide antibiotic that inhibits protein synthesis of the bacterial cell wall by binding to bacterial ribosomal receptor sites. Topically, it decreases fatty acid concentration on the skin. **Therapeutic Effect:** Bacteriostatic. Prevents outbreaks of acne vulgaris.

PHARMACOKINETICS
Rapidly absorbed from the GI tract. Protein binding: 92%–94%. Widely distributed. Metabolized in the liver to some active metabolites. Primarily excreted in urine. Not removed by hemodialysis. **Half-life:** 2.4–3 hr (increased in impaired renal function and premature infants).

USES
Treatment of bone and joint, pelvic, intra-abdominal, pneumonia, septicemia, skin and soft tissue infections. **OFF-LABEL:** Treatment of actinomycosis, babesiosis, erysipelas, malaria, otitis media, *Pneumocystis carinii* pneumonia, sinusitis, toxoplasmosis.

PRECAUTIONS
CONTRAINDICATIONS: History of antibiotic-associated colitis, regional enteritis, or ulcerative colitis; hypersensitivity to clindamycin or lincomycin; known allergy to tartrazine dye. **CAUTIONS:** Severe renal or hepatic dysfunction, concomitant use of neuromuscular blocking agents, neonates. Topical preparations should not be applied to abraded areas or near eyes.

⏳ **LIFESPAN CONSIDERATIONS:** **Pregnancy/Lactation:** Readily crosses placenta. Distributed in breast milk. **Topical/vaginal:** Unknown if distributed in breast milk. **Pregnancy Category B.**

Children: Caution in those younger than 1 mo. **Elderly:** No age-related precautions noted.

INTERACTIONS
DRUG: Adsorbent antidiarrheals: May delay absorption of clindamycin. **Chloramphenicol, erythromycin:** May antagonize the effects of clindamycin. **Neuromuscular blockers:** May increase the effects of these drugs. **HERBAL:** None known. **FOOD:** None known. **LAB VALUES:** May increase serum alkaline phosphatase, AST, and ALT levels.

AVAILABILITY (Rx)
CAPSULES (CLEOCIN HCl): 75 mg, 150 mg, 300 mg. **POWDER FOR RECONSTITUTION (CLEOCIN PEDIATRIC):** 75 mg/5 ml. **INTRAVENOUS SOLUTION (CLEOCIN PHOSPHATE):** 150 mg/ml, 300 mg-5%/50 ml, 600 mg-5%/50 ml, 900 mg-5%/50 ml. **TOPICAL GEL (CLEOCIN T, CLINDAGEL, CLINDAMAX):** 1%. **TOPICAL LOTION (CLEOCIN T):** 1%. **TOPICAL SOLUTION (CLEOCIN T, CLINDADERM):** 1%. **TOPICAL SWAB (CLEOCIN T, CLINDETS PLEDGET):** 1%. **VAGINAL CREAM (CLEOCIN VAGINAl):** 2%. **VAGINAL SUPPOSITORY (CLEOCIN OVULES):** 100 mg.

ADMINISTRATION/HANDLING
 IV

Reconstitution • Dilute 300–600 mg with 50 ml D_5W or 0.9% NaCl (900–1,200 mg with 100 ml). • Never exceed concentration of 18 mg/ml.

Rate of administration • 50 ml (300–600 mg) piggyback is infused over 10–20 min; 100 ml (900 mg–1.2 g) piggyback is infused over 30–40 min. Severe hypotension or cardiac arrest can occur with too rapid administration. • No more than 1.2 g should be given in a single infusion.

Storage • IV infusion (piggyback) is stable for 16 days at room temperature.
IM
• Do not exceed 600 mg/dose.
• Administer deep IM.
PO
• Store capsules at room temperature.
• After reconstitution, oral solution is stable for 2 wk at room temperature.
• Do not refrigerate oral solution (avoids thickening). • Give with 8 oz water. Give without regard to food.
TOPICAL
• Wash skin and allow to dry completely before giving drug. • Shake the topical lotion well before each use. • Apply the liquid, solution, or gel in a thin film to affected area. • Avoid contact with eyes or abraded areas.
VAGINAL, CREAM OR SUPPOSITORY
• Use one applicatorful or suppository at bedtime. • Fill the applicator that comes with cream or suppository to indicated level. • Instruct the patient to lie on the back with knees drawn upward and spread apart. • Insert applicator into vagina and push plunger to release the medication. • Withdraw and wash applicator with soap and warm water. • Wash hands promptly to avoid spreading infection.

▧ IV INCOMPATIBILITIES

Allopurinol (Aloprim), filgrastim (Neupogen), fluconazole (Diflucan), idarubicin (Idamycin).

IV COMPATIBILITIES

Amiodarone (Cordarone), diltiazem (Cardizem), heparin, hydromorphone (Dilaudid), magnesium sulfate, midazolam (Versed), morphine, multivitamins, propofol (Diprivan), total parenteral nutrition (TPN).

INDICATIONS/ROUTES/DOSAGE
SUSCEPTIBLE INFECTIONS
IV, IM: ADULTS, ELDERLY: 600–2,700 mg/ day in 2–4 divided doses. CHILDREN

1 MO–16 YR: 20–40 mg/kg/day in 2–4 divided doses. **Maximum:** 4.8 g/day. CHILDREN YOUNGER THAN 1 MO: 15–20 mg/kg/ day in 2–3 divided doses.
PO: ADULTS, ELDERLY: 150–450 mg q6h. CHILDREN: 8–20 mg/kg/day in 3–4 divided doses.

BACTERIAL VAGINOSIS
PO: ADULTS, ELDERLY: 300 mg twice a day for 7 days.
INTRAVAGINAL: ADULTS: One applicatorful at bedtime for 3–7 days or 1 suppository at bedtime for 3 days.
INTRAVAGINAL (CLINDESSE CREAM): ADULTS: One applicatorful once at any time of the day.

ACNE VULGARIS
TOPICAL: ADULTS: Apply thin layer to affected area twice a day.

SIDE EFFECTS

FREQUENT: Systemic: Abdominal pain, nausea, vomiting, diarrhea. **Topical:** Dry scaly skin. **Vaginal:** Vaginitis, pruritus. **OCCASIONAL: Systemic:** Phlebitis or thrombophlebitis with IV administration, pain and induration at IM injection site, allergic reaction, urticaria, pruritus. **Topical:** Contact dermatitis, abdominal pain, mild diarrhea, burning or stinging. **Vaginal:** Headache, dizziness, nausea, vomiting, abdominal pain. **RARE: Vaginal:** Hypersensitivity reaction.

ADVERSE REACTIONS/ TOXIC EFFECTS

Antibiotic-associated colitis and other superinfections may occur during and several weeks after clindamycin therapy (including the topical form). Blood dyscrasias (leukopenia, thrombocytopenia) and nephrotoxicity (proteinuria, azotemia, oliguria) occur rarely.

NURSING CONSIDERATIONS

BASELINE ASSESSMENT
Question patient for history of allergies, particularly to clindamycin, lincomycin,

aspirin. Avoid, if possible, concurrent use of neuromuscular blocking agents.

INTERVENTION/EVALUATION

Monitor patterns of bowel activity and stool consistency; report diarrhea promptly due to potential for serious colitis (even with topical or vaginal). Assess skin for rash (dryness, irritation) with topical application. With all routes of administration, assess for superinfection: severe diarrhea, genital or anal pruritus, increased fever, change of oral mucosa.

PATIENT/FAMILY TEACHING

• Continue therapy for full length of treatment. • Doses should be evenly spaced. • Take oral doses with 8 oz water. • Caution should be used when applying topical clindamycin concurrently with peeling or abrasive acne agents, soaps, alcohol-containing cosmetics to avoid cumulative effect. • Do not apply topical preparations near eyes, abraded areas. • Notify the physician if severe persistent diarrhea, cramps, or bloody stool occur. • **Vaginal:** In event of accidental contact with eyes, rinse with copious amounts of cool tap water. • Do not engage in sexual intercourse during treatment. • Advise the patient to wear a sanitary napkin to protect clothes against stains. Tampons should not be used.

---

clobetasol

(Temovate)

See Corticosteroids: topical (p. 86C)

---

clofarabine

klo-**fare**-ah-been
(Clolar)

◆ CLASSIFICATION

PHARMACOTHERAPEUTIC: Antimetabolite. **CLINICAL:** Antineoplastic.

ACTION

Metabolized intracellularly to ribonucleotide reductase. Alters mitochondrial membrane necessary in DNA synthesis. **Therapeutic Effect:** Decreases cell replication and affects cell repair. Produces cell death.

PHARMACOKINETICS

Protein binding: 47%, primarily to albumin. Metabolized intracellularly. Partially excreted unchanged in urine. **Half-Life:** 5.2 hr.

USES

Treatment of relapsed or refractory acute lymphoblastic leukemia (ALL) in pediatric patients (1–21 yr) whose disease relapsed after or was refractory to at least 2 prior regimens.

PRECAUTIONS

CONTRAINDICATIONS: None known. **CAUTIONS:** Renal/hepatic impairment, dehydration, hypotension.

⏳ **LIFESPAN CONSIDERATIONS: Pregnancy/Lactation:** May cause fetal harm. Breast-feeding not recommended. **Pregnancy Category D. Children:** Safety and efficacy not established. **Elderly:** No age-related precautions noted.

INTERACTIONS

DRUG: None known. **HERBAL:** None known. **FOOD:** None known. **LAB VALUES:** May increase serum creatinine, uric acid, AST, ALT, bilirubin. May decrease WBCs, Hgb, Hct, thrombocytes.

AVAILABILITY (Rx)

INJECTION, SOLUTION: 20 mg/20 ml.

C

ADMINISTRATION/HANDLING
 IV

Reconstitution • Filter clofarabine through a sterile, 0.2 micrometer syringe filter prior to further dilution with D_5W or 0.9% NaCl.

Rate of administration • Administer drug over 2 hr. • Continuously infuse IV fluids to decrease risk of tumor lysis syndrome, other adverse events.

Storage • Store undiluted and diluted solution at room temperature. • Use diluted solution within 24 hr.

▨ IV INCOMPATIBILITIES
Do not administer any other medication through the same IV line.

INDICATIONS/ROUTES/DOSAGE
ALL
IV: CHILDREN 1–21 YR: 52 mg/m^2 over 2 hr once daily for 5 consecutive days; repeat q2–6wk following recovery or return to baseline organ function.

SIDE EFFECTS
FREQUENT: Vomiting (83%); nausea (75%); diarrhea (53%); pruritus (47%); headache (46%); fever, dermatitis (41%); rigors (38%); abdominal pain, fatigue (36%); tachycardia (34%); epistaxis (31%); anorexia (30%); petechiae, limb pain, hypotension (29%); anxiety (22%); constipation (21%); edema (20%). **OCCASIONAL:** Cough (19%); mucosal inflammation, erythema, flushing (18%); hematuria (17%); dizziness (16%); gingival bleeding (15%); injection site pain, respiratory distress, pharyngitis (14%); back pain, palmar-plantar erythrodysesthesia syndrome (13%); myalgia, oral candidiasis (13%); hypertension (11%); depression, irritability, arthralgia, anorexia (11%). **RARE (10%):** Tremor, weight gain, somnolence.

ADVERSE REACTIONS/ TOXIC EFFECTS
Neutropenia occurs in 57% of patients; pericardial effusion in 35%; left ventricular systolic dysfunction in 27%; hepatomegaly, jaundice in 15%; pleural effusion, pneumonia, bacteremia, in 10%; capillary leak syndrome in less than 10%.

NURSING CONSIDERATIONS

BASELINE ASSESSMENT
Monitor Hgb, Hct; assess for signs and symptoms of anemia. Question patient regarding possibility of pregnancy. Assess AST, ALT, bilirubin, creatinine clearance, BUN, and creatinine levels prior to therapy.

INTERVENTION/EVALUATION
Monitor BP, hepatic and renal function tests. Monitor daily bowel activity, stool consistency. Assess for GI disturbances. Assess skin for pruritus, dermatitis, petechiae, erythema on palms of hands and soles of feet. Assess for fever, sore throat; obtain blood cultures to detect evidence of infection.

PATIENT/FAMILY TEACHING
• Do not have immunizations without physician's approval (drug lowers body's resistance). • Avoid contact with anyone who recently received a live virus vaccine. • Avoid crowds, those with infection. • Avoid pregnancy due to risk of fetal harm; advise patients of childbearing potential to use effective contraception. • Maintain fastidious oral hygiene and frequent handwashing. • Notify physician if fever, respiratory distress, or prolonged nausea, vomiting, or diarrhea occurs.

*clomiPRAMINE hydrochloride

klow-**mih**-prah-meen

(Anafranil, Apo-Clomipramine ✤, Novo-Clopamine ✤)

Do not confuse clomipramine with chlorpromazine, clomiphene, or imipramine, or Anafranil with alfentanil, enalapril, or nafarelin.

✦CLASSIFICATION

PHARMACOTHERAPEUTIC: Tricyclic. **CLINICAL:** Antidepressant (see p. 36C).

ACTION

A tricyclic antidepressant that blocks the reuptake of neurotransmitters, such as norepinephrine and serotonin, at CNS presynaptic membranes, increasing their availability at postsynaptic receptor sites. Therapeutic Effect: Reduces obsessive-compulsive behavior.

USES

Treatment of obsessive-compulsive disorder manifested as repetitive tasks producing marked distress, time-consuming, or significant interference with social or occupational behavior. OFF-LABEL: Treatment of bulimia nervosa, cataplexy associated with narcolepsy, mental depression, neurogenic pain, panic disorder, ejaculatory disorders, pervasive developmental disorder.

PRECAUTIONS

CONTRAINDICATIONS: Acute recovery period after MI, use within 14 days of MAOIs. **CAUTIONS:** Prostatic hypertrophy, history of urinary retention/obstruction, glaucoma, diabetes mellitus, seizures, hyperthyroidism, cardiac/hepatic/renal disease, schizophrenia, increased intraocular pressure, hiatal hernia. **Pregnancy Category C.**

INTERACTIONS

DRUG: Alcohol, other CNS depressants: May increase CNS and respiratory depression and the hypotensive effects of clomipramine. **Antithyroid agents:** May increase the risk of agranulocytosis. **Cimetidine:** May increase clomipramine blood concentration and risk of toxicity. **Clonidine, guanadrel:** May decrease the effects of these drugs. **MAOIs:** May increase the risk of neuroleptic malignant syndrome, seizures, hyperpyresis, and hypertensive crisis. **Phenothiazines:** May increase the anticholinergic and sedative effects of clomipramine. **Sympathomimetics:** May increase the risk of cardiac effects. **HERBAL: St. John's wort:** May increase the risk of serotonin syndrome. **FOOD:** None known. **LAB VALUES:** May alter the blood glucose level and EKG readings.

AVAILABILITY (Rx)

CAPSULES: 25 mg, 50 mg, 75 mg.

INDICATIONS/ROUTES/DOSAGE

OBSESSIVE-COMPULSIVE DISORDER
PO: ADULTS, ELDERLY: Initially, 25 mg/day. May gradually increase to 100 mg/day in the first 2 wk. **Maximum:** 250 mg/day. CHILDREN 10 YR AND OLDER: Initially, 25 mg/day. May gradually increase up to maximum of 200 mg/day.

SIDE EFFECTS

FREQUENT: Somnolence, fatigue, dry mouth, blurred vision, constipation, sexual dysfunction (42%), ejaculatory failure (20%), impotence, weight gain (18%), delayed micturition, orthostatic hypotension, diaphoresis, impaired concentration, increased appetite, urine retention. **OCCASIONAL:** GI disturbances (such as nausea, GI distress, and metallic taste), asthenia, aggressiveness, muscle weakness. **RARE:** Paradoxical reactions (agitation, restlessness, nightmares, insomnia), extrapyramidal symptoms, (particularly fine hand tremor), laryngitis, seizures.

ADVERSE REACTIONS/TOXIC EFFECTS

Overdose may produce seizures; cardiovascular effects, such as severe orthostatic hypotension, dizziness, tachycardia, palpitations, and arrhythmias; and altered temperature regulation, including hyperpyrexia or hypothermia. Abrupt discontinuation after prolonged therapy may produce headache, malaise, nausea, vomiting, and vivid dreams. Anemia and agranulocytosis have been noted.

NURSING CONSIDERATIONS

INTERVENTION/EVALUATION

Closely supervise suicidal-risk patient during early therapy (as depression lessens, energy level improves, increasing suicide potential). Assess appearance, behavior, speech pattern, level of interest, mood.

PATIENT/FAMILY TEACHING

• May cause dry mouth, constipation, blurred vision. • Tolerance to postural hypotension, sedative, anticholinergic effects usually develop during early therapy. • Maximum therapeutic effect may be noted in 2–4 wk. • Do not abruptly discontinue medication. • Avoid tasks that require alertness, motor skills until response to drug is established. • Avoid alcohol.

clonazepam

klon-**nah**-zih-pam

(Clonapam 🍁, Klonopin, Klonopin Wafer, Rivotril 🍁)

Do not confuse clonazepam with clonidine or lorazepam.

CLASSIFICATION

PHARMACOTHERAPEUTIC: Benzodiazepine. **CLINICAL:** Anticonvulsant, antianxiety (see p. 33C).

ACTION

A benzodiazepine that depresses all levels of the CNS; inhibits nerve impulse transmission in the motor cortex and suppresses abnormal discharge in petit mal seizures. **Therapeutic Effect:** Produces anxiolytic and anticonvulsant effects.

PHARMACOKINETICS

Well absorbed from the GI tract. Protein binding: 85%. Metabolized in the liver. Excreted in urine. Not removed by hemodialysis. **Half-life:** 18–50 hr.

USES

Adjunct in treatment of Lennox-Gastaut syndrome (petit mal variant epilepsy); akinetic, myoclonic seizures; absence seizures (petit mal). Treatment of panic disorder. **OFF-LABEL:** Adjunctive treatment of seizures; treatment of simple, complex partial, and tonic-clonic seizures.

PRECAUTIONS

CONTRAINDICATIONS: Narrow-angle glaucoma, significant hepatic disease, hypersensitivity to benzodiazepines. **CAUTIONS:** Impaired renal/hepatic function, chronic respiratory disease.

⌛ **LIFESPAN CONSIDERATIONS: Pregnancy/Lactation:** Crosses placenta. May be distributed in breast milk. Chronic ingestion during pregnancy may produce withdrawal symptoms, CNS depression in neonates. **Pregnancy Category D. Children:** Long-term use may adversely affect physical or mental development. **Elderly:** Usually more sensitive to CNS effects (e.g., ataxia, dizziness, oversedation). Use low dosage, increase gradually.

INTERACTIONS

DRUG: Alcohol, other CNS depressants: May increase CNS depressant effect. **Azole antifungals:** May increase serum concentrations and the potential for clonazepam toxicity. **HERBAL: Kava kava:** May increase sedation. **St. John's wort:** May decrease clonazepam effectiveness. **FOOD:** None known. **LAB VALUES:** None known.

AVAILABILITY (Rx)

TABLETS (KLONOPIN): 0.5 mg, 1 mg, 2 mg. **TABLETS (DISINTEGRATING [KLONOPIN WAFER]):** 0.125 mg, 0.25 mg, 0.5 mg, 1 mg, 2 mg.

ADMINISTRATION/HANDLING

PO
• Give without regard to food. • Tablets may be crushed.

INDICATIONS/ROUTES/DOSAGE

ADJUNCTIVE TREATMENT OF LENNOX-GASTAUT SYNDROME (PETIT MAL VARIANT) AND AKINETIC, MYOCLONIC, AND ABSENCE (PETIT MAL) SEIZURES
PO: ADULTS, ELDERLY, CHILDREN 10 YR AND OLDER: 1.5 mg/day; may be increased in 0.5- to 1-mg increments every 3 days until seizures are controlled. Don't exceed maintenance dosage of 20 mg/day. INFANTS, CHILDREN YOUNGER THAN 10 YR OR WEIGHING LESS THAN 30 KG: 0.01–0.03 mg/kg/day in 2–3 divided doses; may be increased by up to 0.5 mg every 3 days until seizures are controlled. Don't exceed maintenance dosage of 0.2 mg/kg/day.

PANIC DISORDER
PO: ADULTS, ELDERLY: Initially, 0.25 mg twice a day; increased in increments of 0.125–0.25 mg twice a day every 3 days. **Maximum:** 4 mg/day.

SIDE EFFECTS

FREQUENT: Mild, transient drowsiness; ataxia; behavioral disturbances (aggression, irritability, agitation), especially in children. **OCCASIONAL:** Rash, ankle or facial edema, nocturia, dysuria, change in appetite or weight, dry mouth, sore gums, nausea, blurred vision. **RARE:** Paradoxical CNS reactions, including hyperactivity or nervousness in children and excitement or restlessness in the elderly (particularly in the presence of uncontrolled pain).

ADVERSE REACTIONS/TOXIC EFFECTS

Abrupt withdrawal may result in pronounced restlessness, irritability, insomnia, hand tremors, abdominal or muscle cramps, diaphoresis, vomiting, and status epilepticus. Overdose results in somnolence, confusion, diminished reflexes, and coma.

NURSING CONSIDERATIONS

BASELINE ASSESSMENT

Review history of seizure disorder (frequency, duration, intensity, level of consciousness [LOC]). For panic attack, assess motor responses (agitation, trembling, tension), autonomic responses (cold/clammy hands, diaphoresis).

INTERVENTION/EVALUATION

Assess children, elderly for paradoxical reaction, particularly during early therapy. Implement safety measures and observe frequently for recurrence of seizure activity. Assist with ambulation if drowsiness, ataxia occur. For those on long-term therapy, liver/renal function tests, blood counts should be performed periodically. Evaluate for therapeutic response: decreased intensity and frequency of seizures or, if used in panic attack, calm facial expression, decreased restlessness.

PATIENT/FAMILY TEACHING

• Drowsiness usually diminishes with continued therapy. • Avoid tasks that require alertness, motor skills until response to drug is established. • Smoking reduces drug effectiveness. • Do not abruptly withdraw medication after long-term therapy. • Strict maintenance of drug therapy is essential for seizure control. • Avoid alcohol.

---

clonidine

klon-ih-deen

(Catapres, <u>Catapres-TTS-1</u>, <u>Catapres-TTS-2</u>, <u>Catapres-TTS-3</u>, Clonidine TTS-1, Clonidine TTS-2, Clonidine TTS-3, Dixarit 🍁, Duraclon)

Do not confuse clonidine with clomiphene, Klonopin, or quinidine, or Catapres with Cetapred.

FIXED-COMBINATION(S)

Combipres: clonidine/chlorthalidone (a diuretic): 0.1 mg/15 mg, 0.2 mg/15 mg, 0.3 mg/15 mg.

◆CLASSIFICATION

PHARMACOTHERAPEUTIC: Antiadrenergic, sympatholytic. **CLINICAL:** Antihypertensive (see p. 54C).

ACTION

An antiadrenergic, sympatholytic agent that prevents pain signal transmission to the brain and produces analgesia at pre- and post-alpha-adrenergic receptors in the spinal cord. **Therapeutic Effect:** Reduces peripheral resistance; decreases BP and heart rate.

PHARMACOKINETICS

Route	Onset	Peak	Duration
PO	0.5–1 hr	2–4 hr	Up to 8 hr

Well absorbed from the GI tract. Transdermal best absorbed from the chest and upper arm; least absorbed from the thigh. Protein binding: 20%–40%. Metabolized in the liver. Primarily excreted in urine. Minimally removed by hemodialysis. **Half-life:** 12–16 hr (increased with impaired renal function).

USES

Treatment of hypertension alone or in combination with other antihypertensive agents. Treatment of severe pain in cancer patients. **Epidural:** Combined with opiates for relief of severe pain. **OFF-LABEL:** ADHD, diagnosis of pheochromocytoma, opioid withdrawal, prevention of migraine headaches, treatment of diarrhea in diabetes mellitus, treatment of dysmenorrhea, menopausal flushing.

PRECAUTIONS

CONTRAINDICATIONS: Epidural contraindicated in those patients with bleeding diathesis or infection at the injection site, those receiving anticoagulation therapy. **CAUTIONS:** Severe coronary insufficiency, recent MI, cerebrovascular disease, chronic renal failure, Raynaud's disease, thromboangiitis obliterans.

⌛ LIFESPAN CONSIDERATIONS: **Pregnancy/Lactation:** Crosses placenta. Distributed in breast milk. **Pregnancy Category C. Children:** More sensitive to effects, use caution. **Elderly:** May be more sensitive to hypotensive effect. Age-related renal impairment may require dosage adjustment.

INTERACTIONS

DRUG: Beta blockers: Discontinuing these drugs may increase risk

---

of clonidine-withdrawal hypertensive crisis. **Tricyclic antidepressants:** May decrease effect of clonidine. HERBAL: **Yohimbe:** May decrease the effectiveness of clonidine. FOOD: None known. LAB VALUES: None known.

AVAILABILITY (Rx)

TABLETS (CATAPRES): 0.1 mg, 0.2 mg, 0.3 mg. **TRANSDERMAL PATCH:** 2.5 mg (release at 0.1 mg/24 hr) (Catapres-TTS-1, Clonidine TTS-1), 5 mg (release at 0.2 mg/24 hr) (Catapres-TTS-2, Clonidine TTS-2), 7.5 mg (release at 0.3 mg/24 hr) (Catapres-TTS-3, Clonidine TTS-3). **INJECTION (DURACLON):** 100 mcg/ml, 500 mcg/ml.

ADMINISTRATION/HANDLING

PO
• Give without regard to food. • Tablets may be crushed. • Give last oral dose just before retiring.

TRANSDERMAL
• Apply transdermal system to dry, hairless area of intact skin on upper arm or chest. • Rotate sites (prevents skin irritation). • Do not trim patch to adjust dose.

▨ IV INCOMPATIBILITIES
None known.

IV COMPATIBILITIES

Bupivacaine (Marcaine, Sensorcaine), fentanyl (Sublimaze), heparin, ketamine (Ketalar), lidocaine, lorazepam (Ativan).

INDICATIONS/ROUTES/DOSAGE

HYPERTENSION
PO: ADULTS: Initially, 0.1 mg twice a day. Increase by 0.1–0.2 mg q2–4days. Maintenance: 0.2–1.2 mg/day in 2–4 divided doses up to maximum of 2.4 mg/day. ELDERLY: Initially, 0.1 mg at bedtime. May increase gradually. CHILDREN: Initially, 5–10 mcg/kg/day in divided doses q8–12h. Increase at 5- to 7-day intervals up to 25 mcg/kg/

day in divided doses q6h. **Maximum:** 0.9 mg/day.
TRANSDERMAL: ADULTS, ELDERLY: System delivering 0.1 mg/24 hr up to 0.6 mg/24 hr q7days.

ATTENTION DEFICIT HYPERACTIVITY DISORDER (ADHD)
PO: CHILDREN: Initially 0.05 mg/day. May increase by 0.05 mg/day q3–7days up to 3–5 mcg/kg/day in divided doses 3–4 times a day. **Maximum:** 0.3–0.4 mg/day.

SEVERE PAIN
EPIDURAL: ADULTS, ELDERLY: 30–40 mcg/hr. CHILDREN: Initially, 0.5 mcg/kg/hr, not to exceed adult dose.

SIDE EFFECTS

FREQUENT: Dry mouth (40%), somnolence (33%), dizziness (16%), sedation, constipation (10%). **OCCASIONAL (5%– 1%): Tablets, Injection:** Depression, swelling of feet, loss of appetite, decreased sexual ability, itching eyes, dizziness, nausea, vomiting, nervousness. **Transdermal:** Itching, reddening or darkening of skin. **RARE (less than 1%):** Nightmares, vivid dreams, cold feeling in fingers and toes.

ADVERSE REACTIONS/ TOXIC EFFECTS

Overdose produces profound hypotension, irritability, bradycardia, respiratory depression, hypothermia, miosis (pupillary constriction), arrhythmias, and apnea. Abrupt withdrawal may result in rebound hypertension associated with nervousness, agitation, anxiety, insomnia, hand tingling, tremor, flushing, and diaphoresis.

NURSING CONSIDERATIONS

BASELINE ASSESSMENT
Obtain BP immediately before each dose is administered, in addition to regular monitoring (be alert to BP fluctuations).

INTERVENTION/EVALUATION

Monitor pattern of daily bowel activity and stool consistency. If clonidine is to be withdrawn, discontinue concurrent beta-blocker therapy several days before discontinuing clonidine (prevents clonidine withdrawal hypertensive crisis). Slowly reduce clonidine dosage over 2–4 days.

PATIENT/FAMILY TEACHING

• Sugarless gum, sips of tepid water may relieve dry mouth. • To reduce hypotensive effect, rise slowly from lying to sitting position, permit legs to dangle momentarily before standing. • Skipping doses or voluntarily discontinuing drug may produce severe, rebound hypertension. • Side effects tend to diminish during therapy.

---

clopidogrel 🏳

klow-**pih**-duh-grel

(Plavix)

Do not confuse Plavix with Paxil.

◆CLASSIFICATION

PHARMACOTHERAPEUTIC: Thienopyridine derivative. **CLINICAL:** Antiplatelet (see p. 31C).

ACTION

A thienopyridine derivative that inhibits binding of the enzyme adenosine phosphate (ADP) to its platelet receptor and subsequent ADP-mediated activation of a glycoprotein complex. **Therapeutic Effect:** Inhibits platelet aggregation.

PHARMACOKINETICS

Route	Onset	Peak	Duration
PO	1 hr	2 hr	N/A

Rapidly absorbed. Protein binding: 98%. Extensively metabolized by the liver. Eliminated equally in the urine and feces. **Half-life:** 8 hr.

USES

Reduction of MI, stroke, vascular death in patients with documented atherosclerosis. Treatment of acute coronary syndrome. **OFF-LABEL:** Graft patency (saphenous vein), mitral regurgitation, mitral stenosis, noncardioembolic stroke, percutaneous coronary intervention.

PRECAUTIONS

CONTRAINDICATIONS: Active bleeding, coagulation disorders, severe hepatic disease. **CAUTIONS:** Hypertension, hepatic or renal impairment, history of bleeding, hematologic disorders, preoperative patients.

⌛ **LIFESPAN CONSIDERATIONS: Pregnancy/Lactation:** Unknown if drug crosses placenta or is distributed in breast milk. **Pregnancy Category B. Children:** Safety and efficacy not established. **Elderly:** No age-related precautions noted.

INTERACTIONS

DRUG: Fluvastatin, other NSAIDs, phenytoin, tamoxifen, tolbutamide, torsemide, warfarin: May interfere with metabolism of these drugs. **HERBAL: Ginger, ginkgo biloba:** May increase the risk of bleeding. **FOOD:** None known. **LAB VALUES:** Prolongs bleeding time.

AVAILABILITY (Rx)

TABLETS: 75 mg.

ADMINISTRATION/HANDLING

PO

• Give without regard to food. • Do not crush coated tablets.

INDICATIONS/ROUTES/DOSAGE

MI, STROKE REDUCTION
PO: ADULTS, ELDERLY: 75 mg once a day.

ACUTE CORONARY SYNDROME
PO: ADULTS, ELDERLY: Initially, 300 mg loading dose, then 75 mg once a day (in combination with aspirin).

SIDE EFFECTS

FREQUENT (15%): Skin disorders. **OCCASIONAL (8%–6%):** Upper respiratory tract infection, chest pain, flu-like symptoms, headache, dizziness, arthralgia. **RARE (5%–3%):** Fatigue, edema, hypertension, abdominal pain, dyspepsia, diarrhea, nausea, epistaxis, dyspnea, rhinitis.

ADVERSE REACTIONS/ TOXIC EFFECTS

Agranulocytosis, aplastic anemia/ pancytopenia, and thrombotic thrombocytopenic purpura (TTP) occur rarely. Cases of bleeding with fatal outcome (especially intracranial, GI, and retroperitoneal hemorrhage) have been reported. Hepatitis, hypersensitivity reactions, anaphylactoid reactions, and angioedema have also been reported.

NURSING CONSIDERATIONS

BASELINE ASSESSMENT
Perform platelet counts before drug therapy, q2days during the first week of treatment, and weekly thereafter until therapeutic maintenance dose is reached. Abrupt discontinuation of drug therapy produces an elevation of platelet count within 5 days.

INTERVENTION/EVALUATION
Monitor platelet count for evidence of thrombocytopenia. Assess BUN, serum creatinine, bilirubin, AST, ALT, WBC, Hgb, signs and symptoms of hepatic insufficiency during therapy.

PATIENT/FAMILY TEACHING
• Inform patient that it may take longer to stop bleeding during drug therapy. • Report any unusual bleeding. • All physicians and dentists must be informed if clopidogrel is being taken, especially before surgery is scheduled or before taking any new drug.

clorazepate dipotassium   ⓔ

klor-**az**-e-pate

(Novo-Clopate ✽, Tranxene SD, Tranxene SD Half-Strength, Tranxene T-Tab)

Do not confuse clorazepate with clofibrate.

CLASSIFICATION

PHARMACOTHERAPEUTIC: Benzodiazepine. **CLINICAL:** Antianxiety, anticonvulsant (see p. 11C).

ACTION

A benzodiazepine that depresses all levels of the CNS, including limbic and reticular formation, by binding to benzodiazepine receptor sites on the gamma-aminobutyric acid (GABA) receptor complex. Modulates GABA, a major inhibitory neurotransmitter in the brain. **Therapeutic Effect:** Produces anxiolytic effect, suppresses seizure activity.

USES

Management of anxiety disorders, short-term relief of anxiety symptoms, partial seizures, acute alcohol withdrawal symptoms.

PRECAUTIONS

CONTRAINDICATIONS: Acute narrow-angle glaucoma. **CAUTIONS:** Impaired renal/hepatic function, acute alcohol intoxication.

⧗ **LIFESPAN CONSIDERATIONS:** Pregnancy/Lactation: Crosses placenta; distributed in breast milk. **Pregnancy Category D. Children:** May experience paradoxical excitement. **Elderly:** Increased risk of dizziness, sedation, confusion, hypotension, hyperexcitability.

INTERACTIONS

DRUG: Alcohol, other CNS depressants: May increase CNS depressant effects. **Azole antifungals:** May increase the serum concentration of clorazepate and the potential for clorazepate toxicity. **HERBAL: Kava kava, valerian:** May increase CNS depression. **St. John's wort:** May decrease clorazepate effectiveness. **FOOD:** None known. **LAB VALUES:** Therapeutic serum drug level is 0.12–1.5 mcg/ml; toxic serum drug level is greater than 5 mcg/ml.

AVAILABILITY (Rx)

TABLETS (TRANXENE T-TAB): 3.75 mg, 7.5 mg, 15 mg. **TABLETS (SUSTAINED-RELEASE):** 11.25 mg (Tranxene SD Half-Strength), 22.5 mg (Tranxene SD).

ADMINISTRATION/HANDLING

◄ **ALERT** ► If the patient must change to another anticonvulsant, plan to decrease clorazepate dosage gradually as low-dose therapy begins with the replacement drug.

INDICATIONS/ROUTES/DOSAGE

ANXIETY

PO (REGULAR-RELEASE): ADULTS, ELDERLY: 7.5–15 mg 2–4 times a day.

PO (SUSTAINED-RELEASE): ADULTS, ELDERLY: 11.25 mg or 22.5 mg once a day at bedtime.

ANTICONVULSANT

PO: ADULTS, ELDERLY, CHILDREN OLDER THAN 12 YR: Initially, 7.5 mg 2–3 times a day. May increase by 7.5 mg at weekly intervals. **Maximum:** 90 mg/day. CHILDREN 9–12 YR: Initially, 3.75–7.5 mg twice a day. May increase by 2.75 mg at weekly intervals. **Maximum:** 60 mg/day in 2–3 divided doses.

ALCOHOL WITHDRAWAL

PO: ADULTS, ELDERLY: Initially, 30 mg, then 15 mg 2–4 times a day on first day. Gradually decrease dosage over subsequent days. **Maximum:** 90 mg/day.

SIDE EFFECTS

FREQUENT: Somnolence. **OCCASIONAL:** Dizziness, GI disturbances, nervousness, blurred vision, dry mouth, headache, confusion, ataxia, rash, irritability, slurred speech. **RARE:** Paradoxical CNS reactions, such as hyperactivity or nervousness in children and excitement or restlessness in the elderly or debilitated (generally noted during first 2 wk of therapy, particularly in presence of uncontrolled pain).

ADVERSE REACTIONS/ TOXIC EFFECTS

Abrupt or too-rapid withdrawal may result in pronounced restlessness, irritability, insomnia, hand tremors, abdominal or muscle cramps, diaphoresis, vomiting, and seizures. Overdose results in somnolence, confusion, diminished reflexes, and coma.

NURSING CONSIDERATIONS

BASELINE ASSESSMENT

Anxiety: Assess autonomic response (cold or clammy hands, diaphoresis), motor response (agitation, trembling, tension). Offer emotional support to anxious patient. **Seizures:** Review history of seizure disorder (intensity, frequency, duration, level of consciousness [LOC]). Observe frequently for recurrence of seizure activity. Initiate seizure precautions.

INTERVENTION/EVALUATION

Assess for paradoxical reaction, particularly during early therapy. Assist with ambulation if drowsiness, dizziness occur. Evaluate for therapeutic response: **Anxiety:** Calm facial expression; decreased restlessness. **Seizures:** Decrease in intensity/frequency of seizures. Therapeutic serum level: Peak: 0.12–1.5 mcg/ml; toxic serum level: greater than 5 mcg/ml.

PATIENT/FAMILY TEACHING

• Do not abruptly withdraw medication after long-term use (may precipitate seizures). • Strict maintenance of drug therapy is essential for seizure control. • Drowsiness usually disappears during continued therapy. • Avoid tasks that require alertness, motor skills until response to drug is established. • If dizziness occurs, change positions slowly from recumbent to sitting position before standing. • Smoking reduces drug effectiveness. • Avoid alcohol.

---

clotrimazole

kloe-**try**-mah-zole
(Canesten ✤, Clotrimaderm ✤, Cruex, Gyne-Lotrimin, Lotrimin, Mycelex, Mycelex-G)

Do not confuse clotrimazole with cotrimoxazole, or Lotrimin with Lotrisone, or Mycelex, Mycelex-G with Myoflex.

FIXED-COMBINATION(S)

Lotrisone: clotrimazole/betamethasone (a corticosteroid): 1%/0.05%.

◆CLASSIFICATION

PHARMACOTHERAPEUTIC: Antiinfective. **CLINICAL:** Antifungal (see p. 44C).

ACTION

Binds with phospholipids in fungal cell membrane. **Therapeutic Effect:** Altered cell membrane permeability inhibits yeast growth.

USES

Oral Lozenges: Treatment/prophylaxis of oropharyngeal candidiasis due to *Candida* sp. **Topical:** Treatment of tinea pedis, tinea cruris, tinea corporis, tinea versicolor, cutaneous candidiasis (moniliasis) due to *Candida albicans.* **Intravaginal:** Treatment of vulvovaginal candidiasis (moniliasis) due to *Candida* sp. OFF-LABEL: **Topical:** Treatment of paronychia, tinea barbae, tinea capitis.

PRECAUTIONS

CONTRAINDICATIONS: Hypersensitivity to clotrimazole or any ingredient in preparation, children younger than 3 yr. **CAUTIONS:** Hepatic disorder with oral therapy.

⧗ LIFESPAN CONSIDERATIONS: **Pregnancy/Lactation: Oral:** Unknown if distributed in breast milk. **Pregnancy Category C. Topical:** Unknown if distributed in breast milk. No adverse effects noted in fetus when given in 2nd or 3rd trimesters. **Pregnancy Category B. Vaginal:** Unknown if distributed in breast milk. **Pregnancy Category B. Children: Oral:** No specific problems noted in children 3 yr and older. Not recommended in children younger than 3 yr. **Topical:** No age-related precautions noted. **Vaginal:** Safety and efficacy not established in children up to 12 yr of age. **Elderly: Oral/Topical/Vaginal:** No age-related precautions noted.

INTERACTIONS

DRUG: None known. HERBAL: None known. FOOD: None known. LAB VALUES: May increase serum AST levels.

AVAILABILITY (Rx)

TOPICAL CREAM (Cruex, Lotrimin): 1%. **TOPICAL SOLUTION (Lotrimin):** 1%. **VAGINAL CREAM (Mycelex):** 1%, 2%. **VAGINAL TABLET (Gyne-Lotrimin):** 200 mg. **TROCHE (Mycelex):** 10 mg.

✤ Canadian trade name ⓔ see *evolve* ☛ High Alert drug

C

ADMINISTRATION/HANDLING

PO
• Lozenges must be dissolved in mouth longer than 15–30 min for oropharyngeal therapy. • Swallow saliva.

TOPICAL
• Rub well into affected, surrounding areas. • Do not apply occlusive covering or other preparations to affected area.

VAGINAL
• Use vaginal applicator; insert high into vagina.

INDICATIONS/ROUTES/DOSAGE

ORAL-LOCAL/OROPHARYNGEAL
PO: ADULTS, ELDERLY, CHILDREN 3 YR AND OLDER: 10 mg 5 times a day for 14 days.

PROPHYLAXIS VS. OROPHARYNGEAL CANDIDIASIS
PO: ADULTS, ELDERLY: 10 mg 3 times a day.

USUAL TOPICAL DOSAGE
TOPICAL: ADULTS, ELDERLY, CHILDREN 3 YR AND OLDER: Twice a day. Therapeutic effect may take up to 8 wk.

VULVOVAGINAL CANDIDIASIS
VAGINAL (TABLETS): ADULTS, ELDERLY, CHILDREN 12 YR AND OLDER: 1 tablet (100 mg) at bedtime for 7 days; 2 tablets (200 mg) at bedtime for 3 days; or 500-mg tablet one time.
VAGINAL (CREAM): ADULTS, ELDERLY, CHILDREN 12 YR AND OLDER: (1%): One applicator at bedtime for 7 days. (2%): One applicator at bedtime for 3 days.

SIDE EFFECTS

FREQUENT: PO: Nausea, vomiting, diarrhea, abdominal pain. OCCASIONAL: Topical: Itching, burning, stinging, erythema, urticaria. Vaginal: Mild burning (tablets/cream); irritation, cystitis (cream). RARE: Vaginal: Itching, rash, lower abdominal cramping, headache.

ADVERSE REACTIONS/ TOXIC EFFECTS

None known.

NURSING CONSIDERATIONS

BASELINE ASSESSMENT
Assess patient's ability to understand and follow directions regarding use of oral lozenges.

INTERVENTION/EVALUATION
With oral therapy, assess for nausea, vomiting. With topical therapy, check skin for erythema, urticaria, blistering; inquire about itching, burning, stinging. With vaginal therapy, evaluate for vulvovaginal irritation, abdominal cramping, urinary frequency, discomfort.

PATIENT/FAMILY TEACHING
• Continue for full length of therapy. • Inform physician of increased irritation. • Avoid contact with eyes. • Topical: Keep areas clean, dry; wear light clothing to promote ventilation. • Separate personal items, linens. • Vaginal: Continue use during menses. • Refrain from sexual intercourse or advise partner to use condom during therapy.

cloxacillin

(Tegopen)
See Antibiotic: penicillins (p. 27C)

clozapine   ⓔ

klo-za-peen
(Clozaril, FazaClo)
Do not confuse clozapine with Cloxapen or clofazimine, or Clozaril with Clinoril or Colazal.

◆CLASSIFICATION
PHARMACOTHERAPEUTIC: Dibenzodiazepine derivative. CLINICAL: Antipsychotic (see p. 58C).

🖋 see color pill atlas   🌿 herb   underlined – top prescribed drug

ACTION

A dibenzodiazepine derivative that interferes with the binding of dopamine at dopamine receptor sites; binds primarily at nondopamine receptor sites. **Therapeutic Effect:** Diminishes schizophrenic behavior.

USES

Management of severely ill schizophrenic patients who fail to respond to other antipsychotic therapy. Recurrent suicidal behavior.

PRECAUTIONS

CONTRAINDICATIONS: Coma, concurrent use of other drugs that may suppress bone marrow function, history of clozapine-induced agranulocytosis or severe granulocytopenia, myeloproliferative disorders, paralytic ileus, severe CNS depression. **CAUTIONS:** History of seizures, cardiovascular disease, myocarditis; impaired respiratory, hepatic, renal function; alcohol withdrawal; urinary retention; glaucoma; prostatic hypertrophy. **Pregnancy Category B.**

INTERACTIONS

DRUG: **Alcohol, other CNS depressants:** May increase CNS depressant effects. **Bone marrow depressants:** May increase myelosuppression. **Citalopram:** May increase concentration. **Lithium:** May increase the risk of confusion, dyskinesia, and seizures. **Phenobarbital:** Decreases clozapine blood concentration. HERBAL: None known. FOOD: None known. LAB VALUES: May increase serum glucose cholesterol and triglycerides.

AVAILABILITY (Rx)

TABLETS (CLOZARIL): 12.5 mg, 25 mg, 100 mg, 200 mg. **TABLETS (ORALLY-DISINTEGRATING [FAZACLO]):** 25 mg, 100 mg.

ADMINISTRATION/HANDLING

PO
• Give without regard to food.

INDICATIONS/ROUTES/DOSAGE

SCHIZOPHRENIC DISORDERS, REDUCE SUICIDAL BEHAVIOR
◀ **ALERT** ▶ For initiation of therapy, must have WBC equal to or greater than 3,500 mm^3 and ANC equal to or greater than 2,000 mm^3.
PO: ADULTS: Initially, 25 mg once or twice a day. May increase by 25–50 mg/day over 2 wk until dosage of 300–450 mg/day is achieved. May further increase by 50–100 mg/day no more than once or twice a week, Range: 200–600 mg/day. **Maximum:** 900 mg/day. ELDERLY: Initially, 25 mg/day. May increase by 25 mg/day. **Maximum:** 450 mg/day.

SIDE EFFECTS

FREQUENT: Somnolence (39%), salivation (31%), tachycardia (25%), dizziness (19%), constipation (14%). **OCCASIONAL:** Hypotension (9%); headache (7%); tremor, syncope, diaphoresis, dry mouth (6%); nausea, visual disturbances (5%); nightmares, restlessness, akinesia, agitation, hypertension, abdominal discomfort or heartburn, weight gain (4%). **RARE:** Rigidity, confusion, fatigue, insomnia, diarrhea, rash.

ADVERSE REACTIONS/ TOXIC EFFECTS

◀ **ALERT** ▶ Blood dyscrasias, particularly agranulocytosis and mild leukopenia, may occur.
Seizures occur in about 3% of patients. Overdose produces CNS depression (including sedation, coma, and delirium), respiratory depression, and hypersalivation.

NURSING CONSIDERATIONS

BASELINE ASSESSMENT

Obtain baseline WBC and absolute neutrophil count (ANC) before initiating treatment and monitor WBC and ANC count every week for first 6 mo of continuous therapy, then biweekly for

C

6 mo. If CBC and ANC are normal after 12 mo, then monthly monitoring of CBC and ANC is recommended. Assess behavior, appearance, emotional status, response to environment, speech pattern, thought content.

INTERVENTION/EVALUATION

Monitor BP for hypertension/hypotension. Assess pulse for tachycardia (common side effect). Monitor CBC for blood dyscrasias. Supervise suicidal-risk patient closely during early therapy (as depression lessens, energy level improves, increasing suicide potential). Assess for therapeutic response (interest in surroundings, improvement in self-care, increased ability to concentrate, relaxed facial expression).

PATIENT/FAMILY TEACHING

• Do not abruptly withdraw from long-term drug therapy. • Drowsiness generally subsides during continued therapy. • Avoid tasks that require alertness, motor skills until response to drug is established. • Avoid alcohol.

---

cocaine

koe-**kane**

FIXED-COMBINATION(S)

AC Gel: cocaine/epinephrine (a sympathomimetic): 11.8%/1:1,000. **TAC:** tetracaine/epinephrine/cocaine: 0.5%/1:2,000/11.8%.

◆CLASSIFICATION

PHARMACOTHERAPEUTIC: Amide. **CLINICAL:** Topical anesthetic.

ACTION

Decreases membrane permeability; increases norepinephrine at postsynaptic receptor sites, producing intense vasoconstriction. **Therapeutic Effect:** Blocks conduction of nerve impulses.

USES

Topical anesthesia for mucous membranes of orolaryngeal, nasal areas; minor, uncomplicated facial lacerations.

PRECAUTIONS

CONTRAINDICATIONS: Hypersensitivity to cocaine, local anesthetics; systemic or ophthalmic use. **CAUTIONS:** Hypertension, severe cardiovascular disease, thyrotoxicosis, infants, those with severely traumatized mucosa in area of intended application. **Pregnancy Category C (X if nonmedical use).**

INTERACTIONS

DRUG: Beta-blockers: Effects of these drugs may be decreased. **Cholinesterase inhibitors:** May increase effects, risk of toxicity. **CNS stimulation-producing agents:** May increase CNS effects. **Sympathomimetics:** Increase CNS stimulation, risk of cardiovascular effects. **Tricyclic antidepressants, digoxin, methyldopa:** May increase arrhythmias. **HERBAL:** None known. **FOOD:** None known. **LAB VALUES:** None known.

AVAILABILITY (Rx)

TOPICAL SOLUTION: 4%, 10%.

INDICATIONS/ROUTES/DOSAGE

USUAL TOPICAL DOSAGE
TOPICAL: ADULTS, ELDERLY: 1%–10% solution. **Maximum single dose:** 1 mg/kg.

SIDE EFFECTS

FREQUENT: Loss of sense of smell/taste.

ADVERSE REACTIONS/TOXIC EFFECTS

Repeated nasal application may produce stuffy nose, chronic rhinitis. Early signs of overdosage may include increased BP, increased pulse, palpitations, chills/fever, agitation, anxiety, confusion, inability to remain still, nausea, vomiting, abdominal pain, diaphoresis, tachypnea, dilated pupils. Advanced signs of overdosage may include arrhythmias, CNS

---

hemorrhage, CHF, seizures, delirium, hyperreflexia, loss of bladder/bowel control, respiratory weakness. Late signs of overdosage may include loss of reflexes, muscle paralysis, dilated pupils, diminished level of consciousness (LOC), cyanosis, pulmonary edema, cardiac/respiratory failure.

NURSING CONSIDERATIONS

INTERVENTION/EVALUATION

Monitor for anesthetic response. Be alert to CNS stimulation. Assess for euphoria; restlessness; increased BP, pulse, respirations. Be prepared to provide ventilatory support and emergency medications in event of progression of CNS response.

PATIENT/FAMILY TEACHING

• Do not eat or chew gum until sensation returns when used for throat anesthesia. • One time or infrequent use for procedures will not cause dependence. • Report feelings of euphoria, restlessness, tachycardia if these develop during procedure.

---

codeine phosphate ▷

koe-deen
(Codeine Phosphate Injection)

codeine sulfate

(Contin ✤)

Do not confuse codeine with Cardene or Lodine.

FIXED-COMBINATION(S)

Capital with Codeine, Tylenol with Codeine: acetaminophen/codeine: 120 mg/12 mg per 5 ml. **Tylenol with Codeine:** acetaminophen/codeine: 300 mg/15 mg, 300 mg/30 mg, 300 mg/60 mg.

◆CLASSIFICATION

PHARMACOTHERAPEUTIC: Opioid agonist. **CLINICAL:** Analgesic: **Schedule II;** fixed-combination form: **Schedule III** (see p. 127C).

ACTION

An opioid agonist that binds to opioid receptors at many cites in the CNS, particularly in the medulla. This action inhibits the ascending pain pathways. Therapeutic Effect: Alters the perception of and emotional response to pain, suppresses cough reflex.

PHARMACOKINETICS

Well absorbed following PO administration. Protein binding: Very low. Metabolized in liver. Excreted in urine. Half-life: 2.5–3.5 hr.

USES

Relief of mild to moderate pain and/or nonproductive cough. OFF-LABEL: Treatment of diarrhea.

PRECAUTIONS

CONTRAINDICATIONS: Premature infants. **EXTREME CAUTION:** CNS depression, anoxia, hypercapnia, respiratory depression, seizures, acute alcoholism, shock, untreated myxedema, respiratory dysfunction. **CAUTIONS:** Increased intracranial pressure (ICP), hepatic impairment, acute abdominal conditions, hypothyroidism, prostatic hypertrophy, Addison's disease, urethral stricture, chronic obstructive pulmoney disease (COPD). **Pregnancy Category C (D if used for prolonged periods or at high dosages at term).**

INTERACTIONS

DRUG: **Alcohol, other CNS depressants:** May increase CNS or respiratory depression, and hypotension. **MAOIs:** May produce a severe, sometimes fatal reaction; plan to administer a test dose,

---

which is $\frac{1}{4}$ of usual codeine dose. HERBAL: None known. FOOD: None known. LAB VALUES: May increase serum amylase and lipase levels.

AVAILABILITY (Rx)

TABLETS (PHOSPHATE): 30 mg, 60 mg.
TABLETS (SULFATE): 15 mg, 30 mg, 60 mg.
ORAL SOLUTION: 15 mg/5 ml. INJECTION: 15 mg/ml, 30 mg/ml, 60 mg/ml.

ADMINISTRATION/HANDLING

◀ ALERT ▶ Be aware that ambulatory patients and patients not in severe pain may be more prone to dizziness, hypotension, nausea, and vomiting than patients in the supine position and those in severe pain.

◀ ALERT ▶ Expect to reduce the initial dosage in elderly and debilitated patients; those with hypothyroidism, Addison's disease, or renal insufficiency; and those using other CNS depressants concurrently.

IM, SUBCUTANEOUS
• Inspect drug for cloudiness or precipitate. If present, discard drug.

PO
• Give codeine with food or milk to minimize adverse GI effects.

INDICATIONS/ROUTES/DOSAGE

ANALGESIA
PO, IM, SUBCUTANEOUS: ADULTS, ELDERLY: 30 mg q4–6h. Range: 15–60 mg. CHILDREN: 0.5–1 mg/kg q4–6h. **Maximum: 60 mg/dose.**

COUGH
PO: ADULTS, ELDERLY, CHILDREN 12 YR AND OLDER: 10–20 mg q4–6h. CHILDREN 6–11 YR: 5–10 mg q4–6h. CHILDREN 2–5 YR: 2.5–5 mg q4–6h.

DOSAGE IN RENAL IMPAIRMENT
Dosage is modified based on creatinine clearance.

Creatinine Clearance	Dosage
10–50 ml/min	75% of usual dose
Less than 10 ml/min	50% of usual dose

SIDE EFFECTS

FREQUENT: Constipation, somnolence, nausea, vomiting. OCCASIONAL: Paradoxical excitement, confusion, palpitations, facial flushing, decreased urination, blurred vision, dizziness, dry mouth, headache, hypotension (including orthostatic hypotension), decreased appetite, injection site redness, burning, or pain. RARE: Hallucinations, depression, abdominal pain, insomnia.

ADVERSE REACTIONS/ TOXIC EFFECTS

Too-frequent use may result in paralytic ileus. Overdose may produce cold and clammy skin, confusion, seizures, decreased BP, restlessness, pinpoint pupils, bradycardia, respiratory depression, decreased LOC, and severe weakness. The patient who uses codeine repeatedly may develop a tolerance to the drug's analgesic effect as well as physical dependence.

NURSING CONSIDERATIONS

BASELINE ASSESSMENT
Analgesic: Assess onset, type, location, duration of pain. Effect of medication is reduced if full pain response recurs before next dose. **Antitussive:** Assess type, severity, frequency of cough, sputum production.

INTERVENTION/EVALUATION
Monitor daily bowel activity and stool consistency. Increase fluid intake, environmental humidity to improve viscosity of lung secretions. Initiate deep breathing, coughing exercises. Assess for clinical improvement; record onset of relief of pain, cough.

PATIENT/FAMILY TEACHING
• Change positions slowly to avoid orthostatic hypotension. • Avoid tasks that require alertness, motor skills until response to drug is established. • Tolerance or dependence may occur

with prolonged use of high dosages.
• Avoid alcohol.

colchicine

kol-chi-seen
(Colchicine)

✦CLASSIFICATION
PHARMACOTHERAPEUTIC: Alkaloid.
CLINICAL: Antigout.

ACTION
An alkaloid that decreases leukocyte motility, phagocytosis, and lactic acid production. **Therapeutic Effect:** Decreases urate crystal deposits and reduces inflammatory process.

PHARMACOKINETICS
Rapidly absorbed from the GI tract. Highest concentration is in the liver, spleen, and kidney. Protein binding: 30%–50%. Reenters the intestinal tract by biliary secretion and is reabsorbed from the intestines. Partially metabolized in the liver. Eliminated primarily in feces.

USES
Treatment of acute gouty arthritis, prophylaxis of recurrent gouty arthritis. **OFF-LABEL:** To reduce frequency of recurrence of familial Mediterranean fever; treatment of acute calcium pyrophosphate deposition, amyloidosis, biliary cirrhosis, recurrent pericarditis, sarcoid arthritis.

PRECAUTIONS
CONTRAINDICATIONS: Blood dyscrasias; severe cardiac, GI, hepatic, or renal disorders. **CAUTIONS:** Hepatic impairment, elderly, debilitated.

⧗ **LIFESPAN CONSIDERATIONS:** Pregnancy/Lactation: Unknown if drug crosses placenta or is distributed in breast milk. **Pregnancy Category D.**

Children: Safety and efficacy not established. **Elderly:** May be more susceptible to cumulative toxicity. Age-related renal impairment may increase risk of myopathy.

INTERACTIONS
DRUG: Bone marrow depressants: May increase the risk of blood dyscrasias. **Clarithromycin, erythromycin:** May increase plasma levels of colchicine and increase the risk of toxicity. **NSAIDs:** May increase the risk of bone marrow depression, neutropenia, and thrombocytopenia. **HERBAL:** None known. **FOOD:** None known. **LAB VALUES:** May increase serum alkaline phosphatase and AST levels. May decrease platelet count.

AVAILABILITY (Rx)
TABLETS: 0.5 mg, 0.6 mg. **INJECTION:** 0.5 mg/ml.

ADMINISTRATION/HANDLING
 IV

◀ **ALERT ▶** Subcutaneous or IM administration produce severe local reaction. Use via IV route only. Avoid concurrent IV and oral administration.

Reconstitution • May dilute with 0.9% NaCl or sterile water for injection. • Do not dilute with D_5W.

Rate of administration • Administer over 2–5 min.

Storage • Store at room temperature.
PO
• Give without regard to food.

▦ IV INCOMPATIBILITIES
No information available via Y-site administration.

INDICATIONS/ROUTES/DOSAGE
ACUTE GOUTY ARTHRITIS
PO: ADULTS, ELDERLY: Initially, 0.6–1.2 mg;

then 0.6 mg q1–2h until pain is relieved or nausea, vomiting, or diarrhea occurs. Total dose: 6 mg.
IV: ADULTS, ELDERLY: Initially, 1–2 mg; then 0.5 mg q6h until satisfactory response. **Maximum:** 4 mg/wk or 4 mg/one course of treatment. If pain recurs, may give 1–2 mg/day for several days but no sooner than 7 days after a full course of IV therapy (total of 4 mg).

CHRONIC GOUTY ARTHRITIS
PO: ADULTS, ELDERLY: 0.6 mg every other day up to 3 times a day.

SIDE EFFECTS

FREQUENT: PO: Nausea, vomiting, abdominal discomfort. **OCCASIONAL: PO:** Anorexia. **RARE:** Hypersensitivity reaction, including angioedema. **Parenteral:** Nausea, vomiting, diarrhea, abdominal discomfort, pain or redness at injection site, neuritis in injected arm.

ADVERSE REACTIONS/ TOXIC EFFECTS

Bone marrow depression, including aplastic anemia, agranulocytosis, and thrombocytopenia, may occur with long-term therapy. Overdose initially causes a burning feeling in the skin or throat, severe diarrhea, and abdominal pain. The patient then experiences fever, seizures, delirium, and renal impairment, marked by hematuria and oliguria. The third stage of overdose causes hair loss, leukocytosis, and stomatitis.

NURSING CONSIDERATIONS

BASELINE ASSESSMENT
Instruct patient to drink 8–10 glasses (8 oz) of fluid daily while taking medication. Medication should be discontinued if any GI symptoms occur.

INTERVENTION/EVALUATION
Discontinue medication immediately if GI symptoms occur. Encourage high

fluid intake (3,000 ml a day). Monitor I&O (output should be at least 2,000 ml a day). Assess serum uric acid levels. Assess for therapeutic response (reduced joint tenderness, swelling, redness, limitation of motion).

PATIENT/FAMILY TEACHING
• Encourage low-purine food intake, drink 8–10 glasses (8 oz) of fluid daily while taking medication. • Report skin rash, sore throat, fever, unusual bruising/bleeding, weakness, fatigue, numbness. • Stop medication as soon as gout pain is relieved or at first sign of nausea, vomiting, diarrhea.

colesevelam

koh-le-**sev**-e-lam
(Welchol)

CLASSIFICATION
PHARMACOTHERAPEUTIC: Bile acid sequestrant. **CLINICAL:** Antihyperlipidemic agent (see p. 52C).

ACTION
A bile acid sequestrant and nonsystemic polymer that binds with bile acids in the intestines, preventing their reabsorption and removing them from the body. **Therapeutic Effect:** Decreases LDL cholesterol.

USES
Adjunctive therapy to diet, exercise used either alone or in combination with an hydroxamethylglutaryl CoA reductase inhibitor (e.g., simvastatin) to decrease elevated LDL cholesterol in patients with primary hypercholesterolemia (Fredrickson type IIa).

PRECAUTIONS
CONTRAINDICATIONS: Complete biliary

obstruction. **CAUTIONS:** Dysphagia, swallowing disorders, severe GI motility disorders, major GI tract surgery, those susceptible to fat-soluble vitamin deficiency. **Pregnancy Category B.**

INTERACTIONS

DRUG: **Aspirin, clindamycin, digoxin, furosemide, glipizide, hydrocortisone, imipramine, NSAIDs, phenytoin, propranolol, tetracyclines, thiazide diuretics, vitamins A, D, E, K:** May decrease the absorption of these drugs. **HERBAL:** None known. **FOOD:** None known. **LAB VALUES:** None known.

AVAILABILITY (Rx)

TABLETS: 625 mg.

INDICATIONS/ROUTES/DOSAGE

TO DECREASE LDL CHOLESTEROL LEVEL IN PRIMARY HYPERCHOLESTEROLEMIA (FREDRICKSON TYPE IIA)
PO: ADULTS, ELDERLY: 3 tablets with meals twice a day or 6 tablets once a day with a meal. May increase daily dose to 7 tablets a day.

SIDE EFFECTS

FREQUENT: (12%–8%) Flatulence, constipation, infection, dyspepsia (heartburn, epigastric distress).

ADVERSE REACTIONS/ TOXIC EFFECTS

GI tract obstruction may occur.

NURSING CONSIDERATIONS

BASELINE ASSESSMENT
Assess baseline lab results: cholesterol, triglycerides, liver function tests.

INTERVENTION/EVALUATION
Monitor cholesterol, triglyceride lab results for therapeutic response. Assess pattern of bowel activity and stool consistency.

PATIENT/FAMILY TEACHING
• Follow special diet (important part of treatment). • Periodic lab tests are essential part of therapy. • Do not take other medications without physician's knowledge.

colestipol
(Colestid)
See Antihyperlipidemics

Combivent, see
albuterol and ipratropium

Combivir, see lamivudine and zidovudine

Concerta, see
methylphenidate

conjugated estrogens

ess-troe-jenz
(Cenestin, C.E.S. 🍁, Congest 🍁, Enjuvia, Premarin, Premarin Intravenous, Premarin Vaginal)
Do not confuse Premarin with Primaxin or Remeron.

FIXED-COMBINATION(S)
Premphase, Prempro: estrogen/ methyltestosterone (an androgen): 0.3 mg/1.5 mg; 0.45 mg/1.5 mg; 0.625 mg/2.5 mg; 0.625 mg/5 mg.

C

◆CLASSIFICATION

PHARMACOTHERAPEUTIC: Estrogen.
CLINICAL: Hormone.

ACTION

An estrogen that increases synthesis of DNA, RNA, and various proteins in target tissues; reduces release of gonadotropin-releasing hormone from the hypothalamus; and reduces follicle-stimulating hormone (FSH) and leuteinizing hormone (LH) release from the pituitary gland. **Therapeutic Effect:** Promotes normal growth, promotes development of female sex organs, and maintains GU function and vasomotor stability. Prevents accelerated bone loss by inhibiting bone resorption, restoring balance of bone resorption and formation. Inhibits LH and decreases serum concentration of testosterone.

PHARMACOKINETICS

Well absorbed from the GI tract. Widely distributed. Protein binding: 50%–80%. Metabolized in the liver. Primarily excreted in urine.

USES

Management of moderate to severe vasomotor symptoms associated with menopause. Treatment of atrophic vaginitis, kraurosis vulvae, female hypogonadism and castration, primary ovarian failure. Retardation of osteoporosis in post-menopausal women. Palliative treatment of inoperable, progressive cancer of the prostate in men and of the breast in postmenopausal women. **OFF-LABEL:** Prevention of estrogen deficiency–induced premenopausal osteoporosis. **Cream:** Prevention of nosebleeds.

PRECAUTIONS

CONTRAINDICATIONS: Breast cancer with some exceptions, hepatic disease, thrombophlebitis, undiagnosed vaginal bleeding. **CAUTIONS:** Asthma, epilepsy, migraine headaches, diabetes, cardiac or renal dysfunction.

⧗ **LIFESPAN CONSIDERATIONS: Pregnancy/Lactation:** Distributed in breast milk. May be harmful to fetus. Not for use during lactation. **Pregnancy Category X. Children:** Safety and efficacy not established. **Elderly:** No age-related precautions noted.

INTERACTIONS

DRUG: Bromocriptine: May interfere with the effects of bromocriptine. **Cyclosporine:** May increase blood cyclosporine concentration and the risk of hepatotoxicity and nephrotoxicity. **Hepatotoxic medications:** May increase the risk of hepatotoxicity. **HERBAL:** None known. **FOOD:** None known. **LAB VALUES:** May increase blood glucose, HDL, serum calcium, and triglyceride levels. May decrease serum cholesterol levels and LDH concentrations. May affect serum metapyrone testing and thyroid function tests.

AVAILABILITY (Rx)

TABLETS: 0.3 mg (Cenestin, Premarin), 0.45 mg (Cenestin, Premarin), 0.625 mg (Cenestin, Enjuvia, Premarin), 0.9 mg (Cenestin, Premarin), 1.25 mg (Cenestin, Enjuvia, Premarin), 2.5 mg (Cenestin, Premarin). **INJECTION (PREMARIN INTRAVENOUS):** 25 mg. **VAGINAL CREAM (PREMARIN VAGINAL):** 0.625 mg/g.

ADMINISTRATION/HANDLING

💧 **IV**

Reconstitution • Reconstitute with 5 ml sterile water for injection containing benzyl alcohol (diluent provided). • Slowly add diluent, shaking gently. Avoid vigorous shaking.

Rate of administration • Give slowly to prevent flushing reaction.

Storage • Refrigerate vials for IV use. • Reconstituted solution stable for 60 days if refrigerated. • Do not use if solution darkens or precipitate forms.

PO
• Administer at the same time each day. • Give with milk or food if nausea occurs.

▓ IV INCOMPATIBILITIES

No information available via Y-site administration.

INDICATIONS/ROUTES/DOSAGE

VASOMOTOR SYMPTOMS ASSOCIATED WITH MENOPAUSE, ATROPHIC VAGINITIS, KRAUROSIS VULVAE
PO: ADULTS, ELDERLY: 0.3–0.625 mg/day cyclically (21 days on, 7 days off) or continuously.
INTRAVAGINAL: ADULTS, ELDERLY: 0.5–2 g/day cyclically, such as 21 days on and 7 days off.

FEMALE HYPOGONADISM
PO: ADULTS: 0.3–0.625 mg/day in divided doses for 20 days; then a rest period of 10 days.

FEMALE CASTRATION, PRIMARY OVARIAN FAILURE
PO: ADULTS: Initially, 1.25 mg/day cyclically. Adjust dosage, upward or downward, according to severity of symptoms and patient response. For maintenance, adjust dosage to lowest level that will provide effective control.

OSTEOPOROSIS
PO: ADULTS, ELDERLY: 0.3–0.625 mg/day, cyclically, such as 25 days on and 5 days off.

BREAST CANCER
PO: ADULTS, ELDERLY: 10 mg 3 times a day for at least 3 mo.

PROSTATE CANCER
PO: ADULTS, ELDERLY: 1.25–2.5 mg 3 times a day.

ABNORMAL UTERINE BLEEDING
PO: ADULTS: 1.25 mg q4h for 24 hr, then 1.25 mg/day for 7–10 days.

IV, IM: ADULTS: 25 mg; may repeat once in 6–12 hr.

SIDE EFFECTS

FREQUENT: Vaginal bleeding, such as spotting or breakthrough bleeding; breast pain or tenderness; gynecomastia. **OCCASIONAL:** Headache, hypertension, intolerance to contact lenses. **High-doses:** Anorexia, nausea. **RARE:** Loss of scalp hair, depression.

ADVERSE REACTIONS/ TOXIC EFFECTS

Prolonged administration may increase the risk of breast, cervical, endometrial, hepatic, and vaginal carcinoma; cerebrovascular disease, coronary heart disease, gallbladder disease, and hypercalcemia.

NURSING CONSIDERATIONS

BASELINE ASSESSMENT
Question for hypersensitivity to estrogen, previous jaundice, thromboembolic disorders associated with pregnancy, estrogen therapy.

INTERVENTION/EVALUATION
Assess BP periodically. Check for edema; weigh daily. Promptly report signs or symptoms of thromboembolic, thrombotic disorders: sudden severe headache, shortness of breath, vision/speech disturbance, weakness or numbness of an extremity, loss of coordination, pain in chest, groin, or leg.

PATIENT/FAMILY TEACHING
• Avoid smoking due to increased risk of heart attack and blood clots. • Explain importance of diet and exercise when taken to retard osteoporosis. • Teach how to perform Homans' test, signs and symptoms of blood clots (report these to physician immediately). • Notify physician of abnormal vaginal bleeding, depression. • Teach female patients to perform

C

breast self-exam. • Report weight gain of more than 5 lb a wk. • Stop taking medication and contact physician if pregnancy is suspected.

Copaxone, *see glatiramer*

Cordarone, *see amiodarone*

Coreg, *see carvedilol*

Corlopam, *see fenoldopam*

---

cortisone acetate

kor-ti-sone
(Cortone)

Do not confuse cortisone with Cort-Dome.

◆**CLASSIFICATION**

PHARMACOTHERAPEUTIC: Adrenocortical steroid. **CLINICAL:** Glucocorticoid (see p. 83C).

ACTION

An adrenocortical steroid that inhibits the accumulation of inflammatory cells at inflammation sites, phagocytosis, lysosomal enzyme release and synthesis, and release of mediators of inflammation. **Therapeutic Effect:** Prevents or suppresses cell-mediated immune reactions. Decreases or prevents tissue response to inflammatory process.

USES

Treatment of adrenocortical insufficiency, conditions treated by immunosuppression, inflammatory conditions.

PRECAUTIONS

CONTRAINDICATIONS: Hypersensitivity to corticosteroids, administration of live virus vaccine, peptic ulcers (except in life-threatening situations), systemic fungal infection. **CAUTIONS:** Thromboembolic disorders, history of tuberculosis (may reactivate disease), hypothyroidism, cirrhosis, nonspecific ulcerative colitis, CHF, hypertension, psychosis, renal insufficiency, seizure disorders. Prolonged therapy should be discontinued slowly.

⌛ **LIFESPAN CONSIDERATIONS: Pregnancy/Lactation:** Crosses placenta; distributed in breast milk. **Pregnancy Category C (D if used in the first trimester). Children:** Monitor growth, developments of children, infants on prolonged steroid therapy. **Elderly:** Higher risk for hypertension, osteoporosis.

INTERACTIONS

DRUG: Amphotericin: May increase hypokalemia. **Bupropion:** May lower the seizure threshold. **Digoxin:** May increase digoxin toxicity caused by hypokalemia. **Diuretics, insulin, oral hypoglycemics, potassium supplements:** May decrease the effects of these drugs. **Fluoroquinolones:** May increase the risk for tendon rupture. **Hepatic enzyme inducers:** May decrease the effects of cortisone. **Live-virus vaccines:** May decrease the patient's antibody response to vaccine, increase vaccine side effects, and potentiate virus replication. **HERBAL: Echinacea, Ma huang:** May decrease corticosteroid effectiveness. **FOOD:** None known. **LAB VALUES:** May increase blood glucose and serum lipid, amylase, and sodium levels. May

---

decrease serum calcium, potassium, and thyroxine levels.

AVAILABILITY (Rx)

TABLETS: 5 mg, 10 mg, 25 mg. **INJECTABLE SUSPENSION:** 25 mg/ml, 50 mg/ml.

INDICATIONS/ROUTES/DOSAGE

Dosage is dependent on the condition being treated and patient response.

ADRENOCORTICAL INSUFFICIENCY

PO: ADULTS, ELDERLY: 12–15 mg/m^2 divided as $\frac{2}{3}$ in the morning and $\frac{1}{3}$ in the afternoon. CHILDREN: 0.5–0.75 mg/kg/day in 3 divided doses.

IM: CHILDREN: 0.25–0.35 mg/kg/day.

INFLAMMATORY CONDITIONS

PO: ADULTS, ELDERLY: 25–300 mg/day. CHILDREN: 2.5–10 mg/kg/day in 3–4 divided doses.

IM: ADULTS, ELDERLY: 25–300 mg/day. CHILDREN: 1–5 mg/kg/day in 1–2 doses/day.

SIDE EFFECTS

FREQUENT: Insomnia, heartburn, anxiety, abdominal distention, increased diaphoresis, acne, mood swings, increased appetite, facial flushing, delayed wound healing, increased susceptibility to infection, diarrhea or constipation. **OCCASIONAL:** Headache, edema, change in skin color, frequent urination. **RARE:** Tachycardia, allergic reaction (such as rash and hives), psychological changes, hallucinations, depression.

ADVERSE REACTIONS/ TOXIC EFFECTS

Long-term therapy may cause hypocalcemia, hypokalemia, muscle wasting in arms and legs, osteoporosis, spontaneous fractures, amenorrhea, cataracts, glaucoma, peptic ulcer disease, and CHF. Abrupt withdrawal following long-term therapy may cause anorexia, nausea, fever, headache, joint pain, rebound inflammation, fatigue, weakness, lethargy, dizziness, and orthostatic hypotension.

NURSING CONSIDERATIONS

BASELINE ASSESSMENT

Question for hypersensitivity to any of the corticosteroids. Obtain baseline values for weight, BP, serum glucose, cholesterol, electrolytes.

INTERVENTION/EVALUATION

Be alert to infection (reduced immune response): sore throat, fever, vague symptoms. For patients on long-term therapy, monitor for hypocalcemia (muscle twitching, cramps, positive Trousseau's or Chvostek's signs), hypokalemia (weakness or muscle cramps, numbness or tingling [especially lower extremities], nausea/vomiting, irritability, EKG changes). Assess emotional status, ability to sleep.

PATIENT/FAMILY TEACHING

• Do not change dose or schedule or stop taking drug; **must** taper off under medical supervision. • Notify physician of fever, sore throat, muscle aches, sudden weight gain/swelling. • Inform dentist or other physicians of cortisone therapy now or within past 12 mo.

cosyntropin

koe-syn-**troe**-pin

(Cortrosyn)

Do not confuse Cortrosyn with Cotazym.

◆CLASSIFICATION

PHARMACOTHERAPEUTIC: Adrenocortical steroid. **CLINICAL:** Glucocorticoid.

ACTION

Stimulates initial reaction in synthesis of adrenal steroids from cholesterol.

Therapeutic Effect: Increases endogenous corticoid synthesis.

USES

Diagnostic testing of adrenocortical function.

PRECAUTIONS

CONTRAINDICATIONS: Hypersensitivity to cosyntropin or corticotropin. **CAUTIONS:** None known. **Pregnancy Category C.**

INTERACTIONS

DRUG: None known. **HERBAL:** None known. **FOOD:** None known. **LAB VALUES:** None known.

AVAILABILITY (Rx)

POWDER FOR INJECTION: 0.25 mg.

INDICATIONS/ROUTES/DOSAGE

ADRENOCORTICAL INSUFFICIENCY

IM, IV: ADULTS, ELDERLY, CHILDREN OLDER THAN 2 YR: 0.25–0.75 mg. CHILDREN 2 YR AND YOUNGER: 0.125 mg. NEONATES: 0.015 mg/kg/dose.
IV INFUSION: ADULTS, ELDERLY, CHILDREN OLDER THAN 2 YR: 0.25 mg over 4–8 hr at 0.04 mg/hr.

SIDE EFFECTS

OCCASIONAL: Nausea, vomiting. **RARE:** Hypersensitivity reaction (fever, pruritus).

ADVERSE REACTIONS/ TOXIC EFFECTS

None known.

NURSING CONSIDERATIONS

BASELINE ASSESSMENT

Hold cortisone, hydrocortisone, spironolactone on the test day. Ensure that baseline plasma cortisol concentration has been drawn before start of test or 24-hr urine for 17-KS or 17-OHCS is initiated.

INTERVENTION/EVALUATION

Adhere to time frame for blood draws; monitor urine collection if indicated.

PATIENT/FAMILY TEACHING

• Explain procedure, purpose of the test.

---

co-trimoxazole (sulfamethoxazole-trimethoprim)

koe-try-**mox**-oh-zole

(Apo-Sulfatrim ✸, Bactrim, Bactrim DS, Bactrim Pediatric, Bethaprim, Bethaprim Pediatric, Novotrimel ✸, Septra, Septra DS, Sulfatrim Pediatric, Sulfatrim Suspension, Uroplus, Uroplus DS)

Do not confuse Bactrim with bacitracin, co-trimoxazole with clotrimazole, or Septra with Sectral or Septa.

FIXED-COMBINATION(S)

Zotrim: co-trimoxazole/phenazopyridine. **Bactrim, Septra** (sulfa-methoxazole/trimethoprim): 5:1 ratio remains constant in all dosage forms (e.g., 400 mg/ 80 mg).

◆CLASSIFICATION

PHARMACOTHERAPEUTIC: Sulfonamide/folate antagonist. **CLINICAL:** Antibiotic.

ACTION

A sulfonamide and folate antagonist that blocks bacterial synthesis of essential nucleic acids. **Therapeutic Effect:** Bactericidal in susceptible microorganisms.

PHARMACOKINETICS

Rapidly and well absorbed from the GI tract. Protein binding: 45%–60%. Widely distributed. Metabolized in the liver. Excreted in urine. Minimally removed by hemodialysis. Half-life: sulfamethoxazole 6–12 hr, trimethoprim 8–10 hr (increased in impaired renal function).

USES

Treatment of susceptible infecitons due to *S. pneumoniae, H. influenzae, E. coli,* Klebsiella species, Enterobacter species, *M. morganii, P. mirabilis, P. vulgaris, S. flexneri, Pneumocystis carinii* including acute or complicated and recurrent or chronic UTI, *Pneumocystis carinii* pneumonia (PCP), shigellosis, enteritis, otitis media, chronic bronchitis, traveler's diarrhea. Prophylaxis of PCP. OFF-LABEL: Treatment of bacterial endocarditis; gonorrhea; meningitis; septicemia; sinusitis; and biliary tract, bone, joint, chancroid, chlamydial, intra-abdominal, skin and soft-tissue infections.

PRECAUTIONS

CONTRAINDICATIONS: Hypersensitivity to trimethoprim or any sulfonamides, infants younger than 2 mo, megaloblastic anemia due to folate deficiency. **CAUTIONS:** Those with G6PD deficiency, renal or hepatic impairment.

⌛ **LIFESPAN CONSIDERATIONS: Pregnancy/Lactation:** Contraindicated during pregnancy at term and during lactation. Readily crosses placenta. Distributed in breast milk. May produce kernicterus in newborns. **Pregnancy Category C. Children:** Contraindicated in those younger than 2 mo, may increase risk of kernicterus in newborn. **Elderly:** Increased risk for severe skin reaction, bone marrow depression, decreased platelet count.

INTERACTIONS

DRUG: **Hemolytics:** May increase the risk of toxicity. **Hepatotoxic medications:** May increase the risk of hepatotoxicity. **Hydantoin anticonvulsants, oral antidiabetics, warfarin:** May increase or prolong the effects of these drugs and increase their risk of toxicity. **Methenamine:** May form a precipitate. **Methotrexate:** May increase the effects of methotrexate. HERBAL: None known. FOOD: None known. LAB VALUES: May increase BUN and serum alkaline phosphatase, creatinine, potassium, AST, and ALT levels.

AVAILABILITY (Rx)

◀ ALERT ▶ All dosage forms have same 5:1 ratio of sulfamethoxazole (SMX) to trimethoprim (TMP).

ORAL SUSPENSION (BACTRIM PEDIATRIC, BETHAPRIM PEDIATRIC, SEPTRA, SULFATRIM, SULFATRIM PEDIATRIC): SMX 200 mg and TMP 40 mg per 5 ml. **TABLETS (BACTRIM, SEPTRA, UROPLUS):** SMX 400 mg and TMP 80 mg. **TABLETS (DOUBLE STRENGTH [BACTRIM DS, SEPTRA DS, UROPLUS DS]):** SMX 800 mg and TMP 160 mg. **INJECTION:** SMX 80 mg and TMP 16 mg per ml.

ADMINISTRATION/HANDLING

💉 IV

Reconstitution • For IV infusion (piggyback), dilute each 5 ml with 75–125 l D_5W. • Do not mix with other drugs or solutions.

Rate of administration • Infuse over 60–90 min. Must avoid bolus or rapid infusion. • Do not give IM. • Ensure adequate hydration.

Storage • IV infusion (piggyback) stable for 2–6 hr (use immediately). • Discard if cloudy or precipitate forms.

PO
• Store tablets, suspension at room temperature. • Administer on empty

stomach with 8 oz water. • Give several extra glasses of water/day.

▒ IV INCOMPATIBILITIES

Fluconazole (Diflucan), foscarnet (Foscavir), midazolam (Versed), vinorelbine (Navelbine), total parenteral nutrition (TPN).

IV COMPATIBILITIES

Diltiazem (Cardizem), heparin, hydromorphone (Dilaudid), lorazepam (Ativan), magnesium sulfate, morphine.

INDICATIONS/ROUTES/DOSAGE

CHRONIC BRONCHITIS

PO: ADULTS, ELDERLY: 1 double-strength or 2 single-strength tablets or 20 ml suspension q12h for 14 days.

PCP

PO: ADULTS, ELDERLY: 1 double-strength tablet daily or 3 times a week or 1 single-strength tablet daily. CHILDREN 1 MO AND OLDER: 150 mg/m^2 as trimethoprim each day in 2 divided doses 3 times a week on consecutive days.

PCP TREATMENT

PO, IV: ADULTS, ELDERLY, CHILDREN 2 MO AND OLDER: 15–20 mg/kg as trimethoprim a day in 4 divided doses for 14–21 days.

SHIGELLOSIS

PO: ADULTS, ELDERLY: 1 double-strength tablet or 2 single-strength tablets or 20 ml suspension q12h for 5 days.
IV: CHILDREN: 8–10 mg/kg as trimethoprim a day in 2–4 divided doses for up to 5 days.

OTITIS MEDIA

PO: CHILDREN 2 MO AND OLDER: 8 mg/kg trimethoprim a day q12h for 10 days.

UTIs

PO: ADULTS, ELDERLY: 1 double-strength or 2 single-strength tablets or 20 ml suspension q12h for 10–14 days. CHILDREN 2 MO AND OLDER: 8 mg/kg as trimethoprim a day in 2 divided doses for 10 days.

TRAVELERS' DIARRHEA

PO: ADULTS, ELDERLY: 1 double-strength or 2 single-strength tablets or 20 ml suspension q12h for 5 days.

DOSAGE IN RENAL IMPAIRMENT

Dosage and frequency are modified based on creatinine clearance, the severity of the infection and the serum concentration of the drug. For those with creatinine clearance of 15–30 ml/min, a 50% dosage reduction is recommended.

SIDE EFFECTS

FREQUENT: Anorexia, nausea, vomiting, rash (generally 7–14 days after therapy begins), urticaria. OCCASIONAL: Diarrhea, abdominal pain, pain or irritation at the IV infusion site. RARE: Headache, vertigo, insomnia, seizures, hallucinations, depression.

ADVERSE REACTIONS/ TOXIC EFFECTS

Rash, fever, sore throat, pallor, purpura, cough, and shortness of breath may be early signs of serious adverse reactions. Fatalities have occasionally occurred after Stevens-Johnson syndrome, toxic epidermal necrolysis, fulminant hepatic necrosis, agranulocytosis, aplastic anemia, and other blood dyscrasias in patients taking sulfonamides. Myelosuppression, decreased platelet count and severe dermatologic reactions may occur, especially in the elderly.

NURSING CONSIDERATIONS

BASELINE ASSESSMENT

Obtain history for hypersensitivity to trimethoprim or any sulfonamide, sulfite sensitivity, bronchial asthma. Determine renal, hepatic, hematologic baselines.

INTERVENTION/EVALUATION

Determine pattern of bowel activity. Assess skin for rash, pallor, purpura.

Check IV site, flow rate. Monitor renal, hepatic, hematology reports. Assess I&O. Check for CNS symptoms: headache, vertigo, insomnia, hallucinations. Monitor vital signs at least twice a day. Monitor for cough, shortness of breath. Assess for overt bleeding, ecchymosis, swelling.

PATIENT/FAMILY TEACHING

• Continue medication for full length of therapy. • Space doses evenly around the clock. • Take oral doses with 8 oz water and drink several extra glasses of water daily. • Notify physician of new symptoms immediately, especially rash, other skin changes, bleeding/bruising, fever, sore throat.

Coumadin, *see warfarin*

Cozaar, *see losartan*

Crestor, *see rosuvastatin*

Crixivan, *see indinavir*

---

cromolyn sodium

kroe-moe-lin

(Apo-Cromolyn ✤, Crolom, Gastrocom, Intal, Nasalcrom, Nalcrom ✤, Novo-Cromolyn ✤)

◆CLASSIFICATION

PHARMACOTHERAPEUTIC: Mast cell stabilizer. **CLINICAL:** Antiasthmatic, antiallergic (see p. 67C).

ACTION

An antiasthmatic and antiallergic agent that prevents mast cell release of histamine, leukotrienes, and slow-reacting substances of anaphylaxis by inhibiting degranulation after contact with antigens. **Therapeutic Effect:** Helps prevent symptoms of asthma, allergic rhinitis, mastocytosis, and exercise-induced bronchospasm.

PHARMACOKINETICS

Minimal absorption after PO, inhalation, or nasal administration. Absorbed portion excreted in urine or by biliary system. **Half-life:** 80–90 min.

USES

Oral inhalation, nebulization: Prophylactic management of severe bronchial asthma, exercise-induced bronchospasm. **Intranasal:** Perennial or seasonal allergic rhinitis. **Systemic:** Symptomatic treatment of systemic mastocytosis, food allergy, treatment of inflammatory bowel disease (IBD). **Ophthalmic:** Conjunctivitis.

PRECAUTIONS

CONTRAINDICATIONS: Status asthmaticus. **CAUTIONS:** Coronary artery disease, arrhythmias, tapering dose or discontinuing (symptoms may recur).

⧗ LIFESPAN CONSIDERATIONS: **Pregnancy/Lactation:** Unknown if drug crosses placenta or is distributed in breast milk. **Pregnancy Category B. Children:** No age-related precautions noted. **Elderly:** Age-related renal/hepatic impairment may require dosage adjustment.

INTERACTIONS

DRUG: None known. **HERBAL:** None known. **FOOD:** None known. **LAB VALUES:** None known.

AVAILABILITY (Rx)

ORAL CONCENTRATE (GASTROCROM): 100 mg/5 ml. **ORAL CAPSULES (GASTRO-CROM):** 100 mg. **NASAL SPRAY (NASAL-CROM):** 40 mg/ml. **SOLUTION FOR NEBULIZATION (INTAL):** 10 mg/ml. **SOLUTION FOR ORAL INHALATION (INTAL):** 800 mcg/inhalation. **OPHTHAL-MIC SOLUTION (CROLOM, OPTICROM):** 4%.

ADMINISTRATION/HANDLING

PO
• Give at least 30 min before meals.
• Pour contents of capsule in hot water, stirring until completely dissolved; add equal amount cold water while stirring. • Do not mix with fruit juice, milk, food.

INHALATION
• Shake container well; exhale completely; place mouthpiece fully into mouth, inhale deeply and slowly while depressing the canister; hold breath as long as possible before exhaling. • Wait 1–10 min before inhaling second dose (allows for deeper bronchial penetration). • Rinse mouth with water immediately after inhalation (prevents mouth and throat dryness). **Nebulization, inhalation capsules:** Inhalation capsules are not to be swallowed; instruct patient on use of Spinhaler.

NASAL
• Nasal passages should be clear (may require nasal decongestant). • Inhale through nose.

OPHTHALMIC
• Place finger on lower eyelid; pull down until pocket is formed between eye and lower lid. • Hold dropper above pocket; place prescribed number of drops in pocket. • Instruct patient to close eyes gently so that medication will not be squeezed out of sac. • Apply gentle finger pressure to the lacrimal sac at inner canthus for 1 min after installation (lessens risk of systemic absorption).

INDICATIONS/ROUTES/DOSAGE

ASTHMA
INHALATION   (NEBULIZATION):
ADULTS, ELDERLY, CHILDREN OLDER THAN 2 YR: 20 mg 3–4 times a day.
AEROSOL SPRAY: ADULTS, ELDERLY, CHILDREN 12 YR AND OLDER: Initially, 2 sprays 4 times a day. Maintenance: 2–4 sprays 3–4 times a day. CHILDREN 5–11 YR: Initially, 2 sprays 4 times a day, then 1–2 sprays 3–4 times a day.

PREVENTION OF BRONCHOSPASM
INHALATION   (NEBULIZATION):
ADULTS, ELDERLY, CHILDREN OLDER THAN 2 YR: 20 mg within 1 hr before exercise or exposure to allergens.
AEROSOL SPRAY: ADULTS, ELDERLY, CHILDREN OLDER THAN 5 YR: 2 sprays within 1 hr before exercise or exposure to allergens.

FOOD ALLERGY, INFLAMMATORY BOWEL DISEASE
PO: ADULTS, ELDERLY, CHILDREN OLDER THAN 12 YR: 200–400 mg 4 times a day. CHILDREN 2–12 YR: 100–200 mg 4 times a day. **Maximum:** 40 mg/kg/day.

ALLERGIC RHINITIS
INTRANASAL: ADULTS, ELDERLY, CHILDREN OLDER THAN 6 YR: 1 spray each nostril 3–4 times a day. May increase up to 6 times a day.

SYSTEMIC MASTOCYTOSIS
PO: ADULTS, ELDERLY, CHILDREN OLDER THAN 12 YR: 200 mg 4 times a day. CHILDREN 2–12 YR: 100 mg 4 times a day. **Maximum:** 40 mg/kg/day. CHILDREN YOUNGER THAN 2 YR: 20 mg/kg/day in 4 divided doses. **Maximum:** 30 mg/kg/day (children 6 mo–2 yr).

CONJUNCTIVITIS
OPHTHALMIC: ADULTS, ELDERLY, CHILDREN OLDER THAN 4 YR: 1–2 drops in both eyes 4–6 times a day.

SIDE EFFECTS

FREQUENT: PO: Headache, diarrhea.

Inhalation: Cough, dry mouth and throat, stuffy nose, throat irritation, unpleasant taste. **Nasal:** Nasal burning, stinging, or irritation; increased sneezing. **Ophthalmic:** Eye burning or stinging. **OCCASIONAL: PO:** Rash, abdominal pain, arthralgia, nausea, insomnia. **Inhalation:** Bronchospasm, hoarseness, lacrimation. **Nasal:** Cough, headache, unpleasant taste, postnasal drip. **Ophthalmic:** Lacrimation and itching of eye. **RARE: Inhalation:** Dizziness, painful urination, arthralgia, myalgia, rash. **Nasal:** Epistaxis, rash. **Ophthalmic:** Chemosis or edema of conjunctiva, eye irritation.

ADVERSE REACTIONS/ TOXIC EFFECTS

Anaphylaxis occurs rarely when cromolyn is given by the inhalation, nasal, or oral route.

NURSING CONSIDERATIONS

INTERVENTION/EVALUATION

Monitor rate, depth, rhythm, type of respiration; quality and rate of pulse. Assess lung sounds for rhonchi, wheezing, rales. Observe for cyanosis (lips, fingernails for blue or dusky color in light-skinned patients; gray in dark-skinned patients).

PATIENT/FAMILY TEACHING

• Increase fluid intake (decreases lung secretion viscosity). • Rinsing mouth with water immediately after inhalation may prevent mouth/throat dryness. • Effect of therapy dependent on administration at regular intervals.

cyanocobalamin (vitamin B$_{12}$)

sye-an-oh-koe-**bal**-a-min
(Bedoz ✤, Nascobal)

◆ CLASSIFICATION

PHARMACOTHERAPEUTIC: Coenzyme. **CLINICAL:** Vitamin, antianemic (see p. 145C).

ACTION

Acts as a coenzyme for various metabolic functions, including fat and carbohydrate metabolism and protein synthesis. **Therapeutic Effect:** Necessary for cell growth and replication, hematopoiesis, and myelin synthesis.

PHARMACOKINETICS

In the presence of calcium, absorbed systemically in lower half of ileum. Initially, bound to intrinsic factor; this complex passes down intestine, binding to receptor sites on ileal mucosa. Protein binding: High. Metabolized in the liver. Primarily eliminated unchanged in urine. **Half-life:** 6 days.

USES

Prophylaxis, treatment of pernicious anemia, vitamin B$_{12}$ deficiency. Deficiency generally occurs concurrently with other B-vitamin deficiencies.

PRECAUTIONS

CONTRAINDICATIONS: Folic acid deficiency anemia, hereditary optic nerve atrophy, history of allergy to cobalamins. **CAUTIONS:** None known.

⌛ **LIFESPAN CONSIDERATIONS: Pregnancy/Lactation:** Crosses placenta. Excreted in breast milk. **Pregnancy Category A (C if used in doses above recommended daily allowance). Children/Elderly:** No age-related precautions noted.

INTERACTIONS

DRUG: Alcohol, colchicines: May decrease the absorption of cyanocobalamin. **Ascorbic acid:** May destroy cyanocobalamin. **Folic acid**

(large doses): May decrease cyanocobalamin blood concentration. **HERBAL:** None known. **FOOD:** None known. **LAB VALUES:** None known.

AVAILABILITY (Rx)

TABLETS 50 mcg, 100 mcg, 250 mcg, 500 mcg, 1,000 mcg, 5,000 mcg. **TABLETS (EXTENDED-RELEASE):** 1,500 mcg. **INJECTION:** 1,000 mcg/ml. **NASAL GEL (NASCOBAL):** 500 mcg/0.1 ml.

ADMINISTRATION/HANDLING

IM, SUBCUTANEOUS
• Avoid the IV route because cyanocobalamin is rapidly eliminated.

PO
• Give with food (increases absorption).

INTRANASAL
• Clear both nostrils. • Pull the clear cover off the top of the pump. • Press down firmly and quickly on the pump's finger grips until a droplet of gel appears at the top of the pump. Then press down on the finger grips two more times. • Place the tip of the pump about halfway into the patient's nostril, pointing the tip toward the back of the nose. • Press down firmly and quickly on the finger grips to release medication into one nostril while pressing the other nostril closed. • Massage the medicated nostril for a few seconds. • Administer the nasal preparation at least 1 hr before or 1 hr after the patient consumes hot foods or liquids.

INDICATIONS/ROUTES/DOSAGE

PERNICIOUS ANEMIA
IM, SUBCUTANEOUS: ADULTS, ELDERLY: 100 mcg/day for 7 days, then every other day for 7 days, then every 3–4 days for 2–3 wk. Maintenance: 100 mcg/mo (oral 1,000–2,000 mcg/day). CHILDREN: 30–50 mcg/day for 2 or more wk. Maintenance: 100 mcg/mo. NEONATES: 1,000 mcg/day for 2 or more wk. Maintenance: 50 mcg/mo.

INTRANASAL: ADULTS, ELDERLY: 500 mcg once a wk.

UNCOMPLICATED VITAMIN B₁₂ DEFICIENCY
PO: ADULTS, ELDERLY: 1,000–2,000 mcg/day.
IM, SUBCUTANEOUS: ADULTS, ELDERLY: 100 mcg/day for 5–10 days, followed by 100–200 mcg/mo.

COMPLICATED VITAMIN B₁₂ DEFICIENCY
IM, SUBCUTANEOUS: ADULTS, ELDERLY: 1,000 mcg (with IM or IV folic acid 15 mg) as a single dose, then 1,000 mcg/day plus oral folic acid 5 mg/day for 7 days.

SIDE EFFECTS

OCCASIONAL: Diarrhea, pruritus.

ADVERSE REACTIONS/ TOXIC EFFECTS

Impurities in preparation may cause a rare allergic reaction. Peripheral vascular thrombosis, pulmonary edema, hypokalemia, and CHF may occur.

NURSING CONSIDERATIONS

BASELINE ASSESSMENT
Before and during therapy, assess for signs and symptoms of vitamin B₁₂ deficiency (anorexia, ataxia, fatigue, hyporeflexia, insomnia, irritability, loss of positional sense, pallor, palpitations on exertion).

INTERVENTION/EVALUATION
Assess for CHF, pulmonary edema, hypokalemia in cardiac patients receiving subcutaneous/IM therapy. Monitor serum potassium levels (3.5–5 mEq/L), serum B₁₂ (200–800 mcg/ml), rise in reticulocyte count (peaks in 5–8 days). Assess for reversal of deficiency symptoms: hyporeflexia, loss of positional sense, ataxia, fatigue, irritability, insomnia, anorexia, pallor, palpitation on exertion. Therapeutic response to treatment usually dramatic within 48 hr.

PATIENT/FAMILY TEACHING

• Lifetime treatment may be necessary with pernicious anemia. • Report symptoms of infection. • Foods rich in vitamin B_{12} include organ meats, clams, oysters, herring, red snapper, muscle meats, fermented cheese, dairy products, egg yolks. • Use nasal preparation at least 1 hr before or 1 hr after consuming hot foods or liquids.

---

cyclobenzaprine hydrochloride 🖊

sye-kloe-**ben**-za-preen
(Flexeril, Flexitec ✤, Novo-Cyclo-prine ✤)

Do not confuse cyclobenzaprine with cycloserine or cyproheptadine, or Flexeril with Floxin.

◆ CLASSIFICATION

CLINICAL: Skeletal muscle relaxant.

ACTION

A centrally acting skeletal muscle relaxant that reduces tonic somatic muscle activity at the level of the brainstem. Therapeutic Effect: Relieves local skeletal muscle spasm.

PHARMACOKINETICS

Route	Onset	Peak	Duration
PO	1 hr	3–4 hr	12–24 hr

Well but slowly absorbed from the GI tract. Protein binding: 93%. Metabolized in the GI tract and the liver. Primarily excreted in urine. Half-life: 1–3 days.

USES

Treatment of muscle spasm associated with acute painful musculoskeletal conditions. OFF-LABEL: Treatment of fibromyalgia.

PRECAUTIONS

CONTRAINDICATIONS: Acute recovery phase of MI, arrhythmias, CHF, heart block, conduction disturbances, hyperthyroidism, use within 14 days of MAOIs. **CAUTIONS:** Renal/hepatic impairment, history of urinary retention, angle-closure glaucoma, increased intraocular pressure (IOP).

⏳ LIFESPAN CONSIDERATIONS: **Pregnancy/Lactation:** Unknown if drug crosses placenta or is distributed in breast milk. **Pregnancy Category B. Children:** Safety and efficacy not established. **Elderly:** Increased sensitivity to anticholinergic effects (e.g., confusion, urinary retention).

INTERACTIONS

DRUG: **Alcohol, other CNS depression-producing medications (such as tricyclic antidepressants):** May increase CNS depression. **MAOIs:** May increase the risk of hypertensive crisis and severe seizures. **Tramadol:** May increase the risk of seizures. HERBAL: None known. FOOD: None known. LAB VALUES: None known.

AVAILABILITY (Rx)

TABLETS: 5 mg, 10 mg.

ADMINISTRATION/HANDLING

PO
• Give without regard to food.

INDICATIONS/ROUTES/DOSAGE

ACUTE, PAINFUL MUSCULOSKELETAL CONDITIONS
PO: ADULTS: Initially, 5 mg 3 times a day. May increase to 10 mg 3 times a day. ELDERLY: 5 mg 3 times a day.

DOSAGE IN HEPATIC IMPAIRMENT
MILD: 5 mg 3 times a day. MODERATE AND SEVERE: Not recommended.

SIDE EFFECTS

FREQUENT: Somnolence (39%), dry mouth (27%), dizziness (11%). **RARE (3%–1%):** Fatigue, asthenia, blurred vision, headache, nervousness, confusion, nausea, constipation, dyspepsia, unpleasant taste.

ADVERSE REACTIONS/ TOXIC EFFECTS

Overdose may result in visual hallucinations, hyperactive reflexes, muscle rigidity, vomiting, and hyperpyrexia.

NURSING CONSIDERATIONS

BASELINE ASSESSMENT

Record onset, type, location, duration of muscular spasm. Check for immobility, stiffness, swelling.

INTERVENTION/EVALUATION

Assist with ambulation at all times. Evaluate for therapeutic response: decreased intensity of skeletal muscle pain/tenderness, improved mobility, decrease in stiffness.

PATIENT/FAMILY TEACHING

• Drowsiness usually diminishes with continued therapy. • Avoid tasks that require alertness, motor skills until response to drug is established. • Avoid alcohol, other depressants while taking medication. • Avoid sudden changes in posture. • Sugarless gum, sips of water may relieve dry mouth.

---

cyclophos- ⚑
phamide

sye-kloe-**foss**-fa-mide

(Cytoxan, Cytoxan Lyophilized, Neosar, Procytox ✦)

Do not confuse Cytoxan with cefoxitin, Ciloxan, cyclosporine, or Cytotec.

CLASSIFICATION

PHARMACOTHERAPEUTIC: Alkylating agent. **CLINICAL:** Antineoplastic (see p. 73C).

ACTION

An alkylating agent that inhibits DNA and RNA protein synthesis by cross-linking with DNA and RNA strands, preventing cell growth. Cell cycle–phase nonspecific. Therapeutic Effect: Potent immunosuppressant.

PHARMACOKINETICS

Well absorbed from the GI tract. Protein binding: Low. Crosses the blood-brain barrier. Metabolized in the liver to active metabolites. Primarily excreted in urine. Removed by hemodialysis. Half-life: 3–12 hr.

USES

Treatment of acute lymphocytic, acute nonlymphocytic, chronic myelocytic, chronic lymphocytic leukemias; ovarian, breast carcinomas; neuroblastoma, retinoblastoma, Hodgkin's, non-Hodgkin's lymphomas; multiple myeloma, mycosis fungoides, nephrotic syndrome. OFF-LABEL: Adrenocortical, bladder, cervical, endometrial, prostatic, testicular carcinomas; Ewing's sarcoma; multiple sclerosis: non–small cell, small cell lung cancer; organ transplant rejection; osteosarcoma; ovarian germ cell, primary brain, trophoblastic tumors; rheumatoid arthritis; soft-tissue sarcomas; systemic dermatomyositis, systemic lupus erythematosus, Wilms' tumor.

PRECAUTIONS

CONTRAINDICATIONS: Severe bone marrow suppression. **CAUTIONS:** Severe leukopenia, thrombocytopenia, tumor infiltration of bone marrow, previous therapy with other antineoplastic agents, radiation.

C

LIFESPAN CONSIDERATIONS: Pregnancy/Lactation: If possible, avoid use during pregnancy. May cause fetal malformations (limb abnormalities, cardiac anomalies, hernias). Distributed in breast milk. Breast-feeding not recommended. **Pregnancy Category D.** **Children:** No age-related precautions noted. **Elderly:** Age-related renal impairment may require dosage adjustment.

INTERACTIONS

DRUG: Allopurinol, bone marrow depressants: May increase myelosuppression. **Antigout medications:** May decrease the effects of these drugs. **Cytarabine:** May increase the risk of cardiomyopathy. **Immunosuppressants:** May increase the risk of infection and development of neoplasms. **Live-virus vaccines:** May potentiate virus replication, increase vaccine side effects, and decrease the patient's antibody response to the vaccine. **HERBAL:** None known. **FOOD:** None known. **LAB VALUES:** May increase serum uric acid levels.

AVAILABILITY (Rx)

TABLETS (CYTOXAN): 25 mg, 50 mg. **POWDER FOR INJECTION (NEOSAR):** 100 mg, 200 mg, 500 mg, 1 g, 2 g. **POWDER FOR INJECTION (LYOPHILIZED [CYTOXAN LYOPHILIZED]):** 100 mg, 200 mg, 500 mg, 1 g, 2 g.

ADMINISTRATION/HANDLING

◀ ALERT ▶ May be carcinogenic, mutagenic, or teratogenic. Handle with extreme care during preparation/ administration.

 IV

Reconstitution • For IV push, reconstitute each 100 mg with 5 ml sterile water for injection or bacteriostatic water for injection to provide concentration of 20 mg/ml. • Shake to dissolve. Allow to stand until clear.

Rate of administration • May give by IV push or further dilute with 250 ml D₅W, 0.9% NaCl, 0.45% NaCl, lactated Ringer's (LR) solution or D₅W/LR. • Infuse each 100 mg or fraction thereof over 15 min or longer. • IV route may produce faintness, facial flushing, diaphoresis, oropharyngeal sensation.

Storage • Reconstituted solution is stable for 24 hr at room temperature or up to 6 days if refrigerated.

PO
• Give on an empty stomach. If GI upset occurs, give with food.

IV INCOMPATIBILITIES
Amphotericin B complex (Abelcet, AmBisome, Amphotec).

IV COMPATIBILITIES

Granisetron (Kytril), heparin, hydromorphone (Dilaudid), lorazepam (Ativan), morphine, ondansetron (Zofran), propofol (Diprivan).

INDICATIONS/ROUTES/DOSAGE

OVARIAN ADENOCARCINOMA, BREAST CARCINOMA, HODGKIN'S DISEASE, NON-HODGKIN'S LYMPHOMA, MULTIPLE MYELOMA, LEUKEMIA (ACUTE LYMPHOBLASTIC, ACUTE MYELOGENOUS, ACUTE MONOCYTIC, CHRONIC GRANULOCYTIC, CHRONIC LYMPHOCYTIC), MYCOSIS FUNGOIDES, DISSEMINATED NEUROBLASTOMA, RETINOBLASTOMA
PO: ADULTS: 1–5 mg/kg/day. CHILDREN: Initially, 2–8 mg/kg/day. Maintenance: 2–5 mg/kg twice a week.
IV: ADULTS: 40–50 mg/kg in divided doses over 2–5 days; or 10–15 mg/kg every 7–10 days or 3–5 mg/kg twice a week. CHILDREN: 2–8 mg/kg/day for 6 days or total dose for 7 days once a week.

BIOPSY-PROVEN MINIMAL-CHANGE NEPHROTIC SYNDROME

PO: ADULTS, CHILDREN: 2.5–3 mg/kg/day for 60–90 days.

SIDE EFFECTS

EXPECTED: Marked leukopenia 8–15 days after initial therapy. **FREQUENT:** Nausea, vomiting (beginning about 6 hr after administration and lasting about 4 hr); alopecia (33%). **OCCASIONAL:** Diarrhea, darkening of skin and fingernails, stomatitis, headache, diaphoresis. **RARE:** Pain or redness at injection site.

ADVERSE REACTIONS/ TOXIC EFFECTS

Cyclophosphamide's major toxic effect is myelosuppression resulting in blood dyscrasias, such as leukopenia, anemia, thrombocytopenia, and hypoprothrombinemia. Expect leukopenia to resolve in 17–28 days. Anemia generally occurs after large doses or prolonged therapy. Thrombocytopenia may occur 10–15 days after drug initiation. Hemorrhagic cystitis occurs commonly in long-term therapy, especially in pediatric patients. Pulmonary fibrosis and cardiotoxicity have been noted with high doses. Amenorrhea, azoospermia, and hyperkalemia may also occur.

NURSING CONSIDERATIONS

BASELINE ASSESSMENT

Obtain WBC count weekly during therapy or until maintenance dose is established, then at 2- to 3-wk intervals.

INTERVENTION/EVALUATION

Monitor CBC, serum uric acid concentration, blood chemistries. Monitor WBC closely during initial therapy. Monitor for hematologic toxicity (fever, sore throat, signs of local infection, unusual bruising or bleeding from any site),

symptoms of anemia (excessive fatigue, weakness). Recovery from marked leukopenia due to bone marrow depression can be expected in 17–28 days.

PATIENT/FAMILY TEACHING

• Encourage copious fluid intake, frequent voiding (assists in preventing cystitis) at least 24 hr before, during, after therapy. • Do not have immunizations without physician's approval (drug lowers body's resistance). • Avoid contact with those who have recently received live virus vaccine. • Promptly report fever, sore throat, signs of local infection, unusual bruising or bleeding from any site. • Alopecia is reversible, but new hair growth may have different color or texture.

*cycloSPORINE

sye-kloe-**spor**-in
(Gengraf, Neoral, Restasis, Sandimmune)

Do not confuse cyclosporine with cycloserine, cyclophosphamide, or Cyklokapron.

CLASSIFICATION

PHARMACOTHERAPEUTIC: Cyclic polypeptide. **CLINICAL:** Immunosuppressant (see p. 106C).

ACTION

A cyclic polypeptide that inhibits both cellular and humoral immune responses by inhibiting interleukin-2, a proliferative factor needed for T-cell activity. Therapeutic Effect: Prevents organ rejection and relieves symptoms of psoriasis and arthritis.

PHARMACOKINETICS

Variably absorbed from the GI tract. Protein binding: 90%. Widely distributed. Metabolized in the liver. Eliminated primarily by biliary or fecal excretion. Not removed by hemodialysis. **Half-life:** Adults, 10–27 hr; children, 7–19 hr.

USES

Prevents organ rejection of kidney, liver, heart in combination with steroid therapy. Treatment of chronic allograft rejection in those previously treated with other immunosuppressives. **Capsules/Solution:** Treatment of severe, active rheumatoid arthritis, psoriasis. **Ophthalmic:** Chronic dry eyes. OFF-LABEL: Treatment of alopecia areata, aplastic anemia, atopic dermatitis, Behçet's disease, biliary cirrhosis, prevention of corneal transplant rejection.

PRECAUTIONS

CONTRAINDICATIONS: History of hypersensitivity to cyclosporine or polyoxyethylated castor oil. **CAUTIONS:** Hepatic, renal, cardiac impairment; malabsorption syndrome; pregnancy; chickenpox; herpes zoster infection; hypokalemia. **Ophthalmic:** Active eye infection.

⏳ LIFESPAN CONSIDERATIONS: **Pregnancy/Lactation:** Readily crosses placenta. Distributed in breast milk. Avoid breast-feeding. **Pregnancy Category C. Children:** No age-related precautions noted in transplant patients. **Elderly:** Increased risk of hypertension, increased serum creatinine.

INTERACTIONS

DRUG: **ACE inhibitors, potassium-sparing diuretics, potassium supplements:** May cause hyperkalemia. **Cimetidine, danazol, diltiazem, erythromycin, ketoconazole:** May increase cyclosporine concentration and risk of hepatotoxicity and nephrotoxicity. **Immunosuppressants:** May increase risk of infection and lymphoproliferative disorders. **Live-virus vaccines:** May increase vaccine side effects, potentiate virus replication, and decrease the patient's antibody response to the vaccine. **Lovastatin:** May increase the risk of acute renal failure and rhabdomyolysis. HERBAL: **St. John's wort:** May alter cyclosporine absorption. FOOD: **Grapefruit, grapefruit juice:** May increase the absorption and risk of toxicity of cyclosporine. LAB VALUES: May increase BUN and serum alkaline phosphatase, amylase, bilirubin, creatinine, potassium, uric acid, AST, and ALT levels. May decrease serum magnesium level. Therapeutic peak serum level is 50–300 ng/ml; toxic serum level is greater than 400 ng/ml.

AVAILABILITY (Rx)

CAPSULES (SOFTGEL [GENGRAF, NEORAL, SANDIMMUNE]): 25 mg, 100 mg. **ORAL SOLUTION (SANDIMMUNE):** 50-ml bottle with calibrated liquid measuring device. **INJECTION (SANDIMMUNE):** 50 mg/ml. **OPHTHALMIC EMULSION (RESTASIS):** 0.05%.

ADMINISTRATION/HANDLING

◀ ALERT ▶ Oral solution available in bottle form with calibrated liquid measuring device. Oral form should replace IV administration as soon as possible.

 IV

Reconstitution • Dilute each ml concentrate with 20–100 ml 0.9% NaCl or D_5W.

Rate of administration • Infuse over 2–6 hr. • Monitor patient continuously for first 30 min after instituting infusion and frequently thereafter for hypersensitivity reaction (facial flushing, dyspnea).

Storage • Store parenteral form at room temperature. • Protect IV solution from light. • After diluted, stable for 24 hr.

C

PO
- Oral solution may be mixed in glass container with milk, chocolate milk, orange juice (preferably at room temperature). Stir well. Drink immediately. • Add more diluent to glass container. Mix with remaining solution to ensure total amount is given. • Dry outside of calibrated liquid measuring device before replacing in cover. Do not rinse with water. • Avoid refrigeration of oral solution (separation of solution may occur). Discard oral solution after 2 mo once bottle is opened.

OPHTHALMIC
- Invert vial several times to obtain a uniform suspension. • Instruct the patient to remove contacts before administration (may reinsert 15 min after administration). • May use with artificial tears.

▨ IV INCOMPATIBILITIES
Amphotericin B complex (Abelcet, AmBisome, Amphotec), magnesium.

IV COMPATIBILITY
Propofol (Diprivan).

INDICATIONS/ROUTES/DOSAGE

TRANSPLANTATION, PREVENTION OF ORGAN REJECTION
PO: ADULTS, ELDERLY, CHILDREN: 10–18 mg/kg/dose given 4–12 hr prior to organ transplantation. Maintenance: 5–15 mg/kg/day in divided doses then tapered to 3–10 mg/kg/day.
IV: ADULTS, ELDERLY, CHILDREN: Initially, 5–6 mg/kg/dose given 4–12 hr prior to organ transplantation. Maintenance: 2–10 mg/kg/day in divided doses.

RHEUMATOID ARTHRITIS
PO: ADULTS, ELDERLY: Initially, 2.5 mg/kg a day in 2 divided doses. May increase by 0.5–0.75 mg/kg/day. **Maximum:** 4 mg/kg/day.

PSORIASIS
PO: ADULTS, ELDERLY: Initially, 2.5 mg/kg/day in 2 divided doses. May increase by 0.5 mg/kg/day. **Maximum:** 4 mg/kg/day.

DRY EYE
OPHTHALMIC: ADULTS, ELDERLY: Instill 1 drop in each affected eye q12h.

SIDE EFFECTS

FREQUENT: Mild to moderate hypertension (26%), hirsutism (21%), tremor (12%). **OCCASIONAL (4%–2%):** Acne, leg cramps, gingival hyperplasia (marked by red, bleeding, and tender gums), paresthesia, diarrhea, nausea, vomiting, headache. **RARE (less than 1%):** Hypersensitivity reaction, abdominal discomfort, gynecomastia, sinusitis.

ADVERSE REACTIONS/ TOXIC EFFECTS

Mild nephrotoxicity occurs in 25% of renal transplant patients, 38% of cardiac transplant patients, and 37% of liver transplant patients, generally 2–3 mo after transplantation (more severe toxicity is generally occurs soon after transplantation). Hepatotoxicity occurs in 4% of renal transplant patients, 7% of cardiac transplant patients, and 4% of liver transplant patients, generally within the first month after transplantation. Both toxicities usually respond to dosage reduction. Severe hyperkalemia and hyperuricemia occur occasionally.

NURSING CONSIDERATIONS

BASELINE ASSESSMENT
If nephrotoxicity occurs, mild toxicity is generally noted 2–3 mo after transplantation; more severe toxicity noted early after transplantation; hepatotoxicity may be noted during first month after transplantation.

INTERVENTION/EVALUATION

Diligently monitor BUN, serum creatinine, bilirubin, AST, ALT, LDH serum levels for evidence of hepatotoxicity, nephrotoxicity (mild toxicity noted by slow rise in serum levels; more overt toxicity noted by rapid rise in levels; hematuria also noted in nephrotoxicity). Monitor serum potassium level for evidence of hyperkalemia. Encourage diligent oral hygiene (gum hyperplasia). Monitor BP for evidence of hypertension. Therapeutic serum level: Peak: 50–300 ng/ml; toxic serum level: greater than 400 ng/ml.

PATIENT/FAMILY TEACHING

• Essential to repeat blood testing on a routine basis while receiving medication. • Headache, tremor may occur as a response to medication. • Avoid grapefruit, grapefruit juice (increases concentration, side effects).

---

cyproheptadine hydrochloride @

sigh-pro-**hep**-tah-deen
(Periactin)

Do not confuse cyproheptadine with cyclobenzaprine, or Periactin with Persantine.

CLASSIFICATION

PHARMACOTHERAPEUTIC: Phenothiazine. **CLINICAL:** Antihistamine (see p. 50C).

ACTION

Competes with histamine for H_1-receptor sites on effector cells in the GI tract, blood vessels, and respiratory tract. **Therapeutic Effect:** Relieves allergic conditions (urticaria, pruritus).

USES

Relief of nasal allergies, allergic dermatitis, urticaria, hypersensitivity reactions. **OFF-LABEL:** Stimulates appetite in underweight patients, those with anorexia nervosa. Treatment of vascular cluster headaches.

PRECAUTIONS

CONTRAINDICATIONS: Exacerbation of asthma, patients receiving MAOIs. **CAUTIONS:** Narrow-angle glaucoma, peptic ulcer, prostatic hypertrophy, pyloroduodenal or bladder neck obstruction, asthma, chronic obstructive pulmonary disease (COPD), increased intraocular pressure (IOP), cardiovascular disease, hyperthyroidism, hypertension, seizure disorders. **Pregnancy Category B.**

INTERACTIONS

DRUG: Alcohol, CNS depressants: May increase CNS depressant effects. **MAOIs:** May increase anticholinergic, CNS depressant effects. **HERBAL:** None known. **FOOD:** None known. **LAB VALUES:** May suppress wheal, flare reactions to antigen skin testing unless antihistamines discontinued 4 days before testing.

AVAILABILITY (Rx)

TABLETS: 4 mg. **SYRUP:** 2 mg/5 ml.

ADMINISTRATION/HANDLING

PO
• Give without regard to food. • Scored tablets may be crushed.

INDICATIONS/ROUTES/DOSAGE

ALLERGIC CONDITION

PO: ADULTS, CHILDREN 15 YR AND OLDER: 4 mg 3 times a day. May increase dosage but do not exceed 0.5 mg/kg/day or 36 mg a day. CHILDREN 7–14 YR: 4 mg 2–3 times a day, or 0.25 mg/kg

---

a day in divided doses. **Maximum:** 16 mg a day.   CHILDREN 2–6 YR: 2 mg 2–3 times a day, or 0.25 mg/kg a day in divided doses. **Maximum:** 12 mg a day.

USUAL ELDERLY DOSAGE

PO: Initially, 4 mg twice a day.

◄ **ALERT** ► Reduce dosage in patients with severe hepatic impairment.

SIDE EFFECTS

FREQUENT: Drowsiness, dizziness, muscular weakness, dry mucous membranes, urinary retention, thickening of bronchial secretions. Sedation, dizziness, hypotension more likely noted in elderly. **OCCASIONAL:** Epigastric distress, flushing of skin, visual disturbances, hearing disturbances, paresthesia, diaphoresis, chills.

ADVERSE REACTIONS/ TOXIC EFFECTS

Children may experience dominant paradoxical reaction (restlessness, insomnia, euphoria, anxiety, tremors). Overdosage in children may result in hallucinations, seizures, death. Hypersensitivity reaction (eczema, pruritus, rash, cardiac arrhythmias, angioedema, photosensitivity) may occur. Overdosage may vary from CNS depression (sedation, apnea, cardiovascular collapse, death) to severe paradoxical reaction (hallucinations, tremor, seizures).

NURSING CONSIDERATIONS

BASELINE ASSESSMENT

If patient is experiencing allergic reaction, obtain history of recently ingested foods, drugs, environmental exposure, recent emotional stress.

INTERVENTION/EVALUATION

Monitor BP, especially in elderly (increased risk of hypotension). Monitor children closely for paradoxical reaction.

PATIENT/FAMILY TEACHING

• Tolerance to antihistaminic effect generally does not occur; tolerance to sedative effect may occur. • Avoid tasks that require alertness, motor skills until response to drug is established. • Dry mouth, drowsiness, dizziness may be an expected response of drug. • Avoid alcoholic beverages during antihistamine therapy.

---

cytarabine

sigh-**tar**-ah-bean

(Ara-C, Cytosar ♣ , Cytosar-U)

Do not confuse cytarabine with Cytadren, Cytovene, or vidarabine.

◆CLASSIFICATION

PHARMACOTHERAPEUTIC: Antimetabolite. **CLINICAL:** Antineoplastic (see p. 73C).

ACTION

An antimetabolite that is converted intracellularly to a nucleotide. Cell cycle–specific for S phase of cell division. Therapeutic Effect: May inhibit DNA synthesis. Potent immunosuppressive activity.

PHARMACOKINETICS

Widely distributed; moderate amount crosses the blood-brain barrier. Protein binding: 15%. Primarily excreted in urine. Half-life: 1–3 hr.

USES

Treatment of acute lymphocytic, acute non-lymphocytic, chronic myelocytic, meningeal leukemias. OFF-LABEL: Carcinomatous meningitis, Hodgkin's and non-Hodgkin's lymphomas, myelodysplastic syndrome.

C

PRECAUTIONS

CONTRAINDICATIONS: None known. **CAUTIONS:** Hepatic impairment.

⧖ **LIFESPAN CONSIDERATIONS: Pregnancy/Lactation:** If possible, avoid use during pregnancy. May cause fetal malformations. Unknown if distributed in breast milk. Breast-feeding not recommended. **Pregnancy Category D. Children:** No age-related precautions noted. **Elderly:** Age-related renal impairment may require dosage adjustment.

INTERACTIONS

DRUG: Antigout medications: May decrease the effects of these drugs. **Bone marrow depressants:** May increase myelosuppression. **Cyclophosphamide:** May increase the risk of cardiomyopathy. **Live-virus vaccines:** May potentiate virus replication, increase vaccine side effects, and decrease the patient's antibody response to the vaccine. **HERBAL:** None known. **FOOD:** None known. **LAB VALUES:** May increase serum alkaline phosphatase, bilirubin, uric acid, and AST levels.

AVAILABILITY (Rx)

INJECTION POWDER: 100 mg, 500 mg, 1 g, 2 g. **INJECTION SOLUTION:** 20 mg/ml, 50 mg/ml, 100 mg/ml.

ADMINISTRATION/HANDLING

◄ **ALERT** ► May give by subcutaneous, IV push, IV infusion, or intrathecal routes. May be carcinogenic, mutagenic, or teratogenic (embryonic deformity). Handle with extreme care during preparation/administration.

IV, SUBCUTANEOUS, INTRATHECAL

IV

Reconstitution • Reconstitute 100-mg vial with 5 ml bacteriostatic water for injection with benzyl alcohol (10 ml for 500 mg vial) to provide concentration of 20 mg/ml and 50 mg/ml, respectively. • Dose may be further diluted with up to 1,000 ml D_5W or 0.9% NaCl for IV infusion. • For intrathecal use, reconstitute vial with preservative-free 0.9% NaCl or patient's spinal fluid. Dose usually administered in 5–15 ml of solution, after equivalent volume of cerebrospinal fluid (CSF) removed.

Rate of administration • For IV push, give over 1–3 min. • For IV infusion, give over 30 min–24 hr.

Storage • Reconstituted solution is stable for 48 hr at room temperature. • IV infusion solutions at concentration up to 0.5 mg/ml is stable for 7 days at room temperature. • Discard if slight haze develops.

▩ IV INCOMPATIBILITIES

Amphotericin B complex (Abelcet, AmBisome, Amphotec), ganciclovir (Cytovene), heparin, insulin (regular).

IV COMPATIBILITIES

Dexamethasone (Decadron), diphenhydramine (Benadryl), filgrastim (Neupogen), granisetron (Kytril), hydromorphone (Dilaudid), lorazepam (Ativan), morphine, ondansetron (Zofran), potassium chloride, propofol (Diprivan), total parenteral nutrition (TPN).

INDICATIONS/ROUTES/DOSAGE

TO INDUCE REMISSION IN ACUTE LYMPHOCYTIC LEUKEMIA, ACUTE AND CHRONIC MYELOCYTIC LEUKEMIA, MENINGEAL LEUKEMIA, OR NON-HODGKIN'S LYMPHOMA IN CHILDREN

IV: ADULTS, ELDERLY, CHILDREN: 200 mg/m²/day for 5 days q2wk as monotherapy or 100–200 mg/m²/day for 5- to 10-day course of therapy every q2–4wk in combination therapy.

INTRATHECAL: ADULTS, ELDERLY, CHILDREN: 5–7.5 mg/m^2 every 2–7 days.

TO MAINTAIN REMISSION IN ACUTE LYMPHOCYTIC LEUKEMIA, ACUTE AND CHRONIC MYELOCYTIC LEUKEMIA, MENINGEAL LEUKEMIA, OR NON-HODGKIN'S LYMPHOMA IN CHILDREN

IV: ADULTS, ELDERLY, CHILDREN: 70–200 mg/m^2/day for 2–5 days every month.
IM, SUBCUTANEOUS: ADULTS, ELDERLY, CHILDREN: 1–1.5 mg/m^2 as single dose q1–4wk.
INTRATHECAL: ADULTS, ELDERLY, CHILDREN: 5–7.5 mg/m^2 every 2–7 days.

SIDE EFFECTS

FREQUENT: IV, Subcutaneous (33%–16%): Asthenia, fever, pain, altered taste and smell, nausea, vomiting (risk greater with IV push than with continuous IV infusion). **Intrathecal (28%–11%):** Headache, asthenia, altered taste and smell, confusion, somnolence, nausea, vomiting. **OCCASIONAL: IV, Subcutaneous (11%–7%):** Abnormal gait, somnolence, constipation, back pain, urinary incontinence, peripheral edema, headache, confusion. **Intrathecal (7%–3%):** Peripheral edema, back pain, constipation, abnormal gait, urinary incontinence.

ADVERSE REACTIONS/ TOXIC EFFECTS

Myelosuppression may result in blood dyscrasias, such as leukopenia, anemia, thrombocytopenia, megaloblastosis, and reticulocytopenia, after a single IV dose. Leukopenia, anemia, and thrombocytopenia should be expected with daily or continuous IV therapy. Cytarabine syndrome, (as evidenced by fever, myalgia, rash, conjunctivitis, malaise, and chest pain) and hyperuricemia may occur. High-dose cytarabine therapy may produce severe CNS, GI, and pulmonary toxicity.

NURSING CONSIDERATIONS

BASELINE ASSESSMENT

Leukocyte count decreases within 24 hr after initial dose, continues to decrease for 7–9 days followed by brief rise at 12 days, decreases again at 15–24 days, then rises rapidly for next 10 days. Platelet count decreases 5 days after drug initiation to its lowest count at 12–15 days, then rises rapidly for next 10 days.

INTERVENTION/EVALUATION

Monitor CBC for evidence of bone marrow depression. Monitor for blood dyscrasias (fever, sore throat, signs of local infection, unusual bruising or bleeding from any site), symptoms of anemia (excessive fatigue, weakness). Monitor for signs of neuropathy (gait disturbances, handwriting difficulties, numbness).

PATIENT/FAMILY TEACHING

• Increase fluid intake (may protect against hyperuricemia). • Do not have immunizations without physician's approval (drug lowers body's resistance). • Avoid contact with those who have recently received live virus vaccine. • Promptly report fever, sore throat, signs of local infection, unusual bruising or bleeding from any site.

dacarbazine

day-**car**-bah-zeen
(DTIC ♦, DTIC-Dome)

Do not confuse dacarbazine with Dicarbosil or procarbazine.

◆CLASSIFICATION

PHARMACOTHERAPEUTIC: Alkylating agent. **CLINICAL:** Antineoplastic (see p. 73C).

ACTION

An alkylating antineoplastic agent that forms methyldiazonium ions, which attack nucleophilic groups in DNA. Cross-links DNA strands. Therapeutic Effect: Inhibits DNA, RNA, and protein synthesis.

PHARMACOKINETICS

Minimally crosses the blood-brain barrier. Protein binding: 5%. Metabolized in the liver. Excreted in urine. Half-life: 5 hr (increased in impaired renal function).

USES

Treatment of metastatic malignant melanoma, second-line therapy of Hodgkin's disease. OFF-LABEL: Treatment of islet cell carcinoma, neuroblastoma, soft-tissue sarcoma.

PRECAUTIONS

CONTRAINDICATIONS: Demonstrated hypersensitivity to dacarbazine. **CAUTIONS:** Hepatic impairment.

⌛ LIFESPAN CONSIDERATIONS: **Pregnancy/Lactation:** If possible, avoid use during pregnancy, especially first trimester. Breast-feeding not recommended. **Pregnancy Category C. Children:** Safety and efficacy not established. **Elderly:** Age-related renal impairment may require dosage adjustment.

INTERACTIONS

DRUG: **Bone marrow depressants:** May enhance myelosuppression. **Live-virus vaccines:** May potentiate virus replication, increase vaccine side effects, and decrease the patient's antibody response to the vaccine. HERBAL: None known. FOOD: None known. LAB VALUES: May increase BUN, serum alkaline phosphatase, AST, and ALT levels.

AVAILABILITY (Rx)

POWDER FOR INJECTION: 100-mg vials, 200-mg vials, 500-mg vials.

ADMINISTRATION/HANDLING

◄ ALERT ► May give by IV push or IV infusion. May be carcinogenic, mutagenic, or teratogenic. Handle with extreme care during preparation/administration.

 IV

Reconstitution • Reconstitute 100-mg vial with 9.9 ml sterile water for injection (19.7 ml for 200-mg vial) to provide concentration of 10 mg/ml.

Rate of administration • Give IV push over 2–3 min. • For IV infusion, further dilute with up to 250 ml D₅W or 0.9% NaCl. Infuse over 15–30 min. • Apply hot packs if local pain, burning sensation, irritation at injection site occurs. • Avoid extravasation (stinging, swelling, coolness, slight or no blood return at injection site).

Storage • Protect from light; refrigerate vials. • Color change from ivory to pink indicates decomposition; discard. • Solution containing 10 mg/ml is stable for 8 hr at room temperature or 72 hr if refrigerated. • Solution diluted with up to 500 ml D₅W or 0.9% NaCl is stable for at least 8 hr at room temperature or 24 hr if refrigerated.

🔲 IV INCOMPATIBILITIES

Allopurinol (Aloprim), cefepime (Maxipime), heparin, piperacillin and tazobactam (Zosyn).

IV COMPATIBILITIES

Etoposide (VePesid), granisetron (Kytril), ondansetron (Zofran), paclitaxel (Taxol).

INDICATIONS/ROUTES/DOSAGE

MALIGNANT MELANOMA

IV: ADULTS, ELDERLY: 2–4.5 mg/kg/day for 10 days, repeated q4wk; or 250 mg/m² a day for 5 days, repeated q3wk.

HODGKIN'S DISEASE

IV: ADULTS, ELDERLY: 150 mg/m²/day for 5 days, repeated q4wk; or 375 mg/m² once, repeated every 15 days (as combination therapy). CHILDREN: 375 mg/m² on days 1 and 15; repeated every 28 days (as combination therapy).

SOLID TUMORS

IV: CHILDREN: 200–470 mg/m²/day over 5 days every 21–28 days.

NEUROBLASTOMA

IV: CHILDREN: 800–900 mg/m² as single dose on day 1 of therapy, repeated q3–4wk (as combination therapy).

SIDE EFFECTS

FREQUENT (90%): Nausea, vomiting, anorexia (occurs within 1 hr of initial dose, may last up to 12 hr). **OCCASIONAL:** Facial flushing, paresthesia, alopecia, flu-like symptoms (fever, myalgia, malaise), dermatologic reactions, confusion, blurred vision, headache, lethargy. **RARE:** Diarrhea, stomatitis, photosensitivity.

ADVERSE REACTIONS/ TOXIC EFFECTS

Myelosuppression may result in blood dyscrasias, such as leukopenia and thrombocytopenia, generally 2–4 wk after the last dacarbazine dose. Hepatotoxicity occurs rarely.

NURSING CONSIDERATIONS

BASELINE ASSESSMENT

Some clinicians recommend food and fluids be restricted 4–6 hr before treatment; other clinicians believe good hydration to within 1 hr of treatment will avoid dehydration due to vomiting. Conflicting reports of effectiveness of administering antiemetics for nausea, vomiting.

INTERVENTION/EVALUATION

Monitor leukocyte, erythrocyte, platelet counts for evidence of bone marrow depression. Monitor for hematologic toxicity (fever, sore throat, signs of local infection, unusual bleeding or bruising from any site).

PATIENT/FAMILY TEACHING

• Tolerance to GI effects occurs rapidly (generally after 1–2 days of treatment). • Do not have immunizations without physician's approval (drug lowers body's resistance). • Avoid contact with those who have recently received live virus vaccine. • Promptly report fever, sore throat, signs of local infection, unusual bleeding or bruising from any site. • Notify physician for persistent nausea, vomiting.

daclizumab

day-**cly**-zu-mab
(Zenapax)

◆CLASSIFICATION

PHARMACOTHERAPEUTIC: Monoclonal antibody. **CLINICAL:** Immunosuppressive (see p. 106C).

ACTION

A monoclonal antibody that binds to the interleukin-2 (IL-2) receptor complex, inhibiting the IL-2–mediated activation of T lymphocytes, a critical pathway in the cellular immune response involved in allograft rejection. **Therapeutic Effect:** Prevents organ rejection.

PHARMACOKINETICS

Half-life: **Adults:** 20 days. **Children:** 13 days.

USES

Prophylaxis of acute organ rejection in patients receiving renal transplants (in combination with an immunosuppressive regimen). OFF-LABEL: Treatment of aplastic anemia, graft vs. host disease.

PRECAUTIONS

CONTRAINDICATIONS: None known. **CAUTIONS:** Infection, history of malignancy.

⧗ LIFESPAN CONSIDERATIONS: **Pregnancy/Lactation:** Unknown if drug crosses placenta or is distributed in breast milk. **Pregnancy Category C. Children/Elderly:** No age-related precautions noted.

INTERACTIONS

DRUG: None known. HERBAL: None known. FOOD: None known. LAB VALUES: None known.

AVAILABILITY (Rx)

INJECTION: 5 mg/ml.

ADMINISTRATION/HANDLING

 IV

Reconstitution • Dilute in 50 ml 0.9% NaCl. • Invert gently. • Avoid shaking.

Rate of administration • Infuse over 15 min.

Storage • Protect from light; refrigerate vials. • Once reconstituted, stable for 4 hr at room temperature, 24 hr if refrigerated.

▓ IV INCOMPATIBILITIES

Don't mix daclizumab with any other drugs.

INDICATIONS/ROUTES/DOSAGE

PREVENTION OF ACUTE RENAL TRANSPLANT REJECTION (IN

COMBINATION WITH AN IMMUNOSUPPRESSIVE)

IV: ADULTS, CHILDREN: 1 mg/kg over 15 min q14days for 5 doses, beginning no more than 24 hr before transplantation. **Maximum:** 100 mg.

SIDE EFFECTS

OCCASIONAL (greater than 2%): Constipation, nausea, diarrhea, vomiting, abdominal pain, edema, headache, dizziness, fever, pain, fatigue, insomnia, weakness, arthralgia, myalgia, diaphoresis.

ADVERSE REACTIONS/ TOXIC EFFECTS

Hypersensitivity reaction, which occurs rarely, is characterized by dyspnea, tachycardia, dysphagia, peripheral edema, rash, and pruritus.

NURSING CONSIDERATIONS

BASELINE ASSESSMENT

Obtain baseline serum levels, vital signs, particularly BP, pulse.

INTERVENTION/EVALUATION

Diligently monitor all serum levels, CBC. Assess BP for hypertension or hypotension; pulse for evidence of tachycardia. Question for GI disturbances, urinary changes. Monitor for presence of wound infection, signs of systemic infection (fever, sore throat), unusual bleeding or bruising.

PATIENT/FAMILY TEACHING

• Report difficulty in breathing or swallowing, tachycardia, rash, itching, swelling of lower extremities, weakness. • Avoid pregnancy.

Dalmane, *see flurazepam*

---

dalteparin sodium ⚑

dawl-teh-pear-in
(Fragmin)

⋆CLASSIFICATION

PHARMACOTHERAPEUTIC: Low molecular weight heparin. **CLINICAL:** Anticoagulant (see p. 29C).

ACTION

An antithrombin that inhibits factor Xa and thrombin in the presence of low-molecular-weight heparin. Only slightly influences platelet aggregation, PT, and aPTT. Therapeutic Effect: Produces anticoagulation.

PHARMACOKINETICS

Route	Onset	Peak	Duration
Subcutaneous	N/A	4 hr	N/A

Protein binding: less than 10%. Half-life: 3–5 hr.

USES

Treatment of unstable angina and non–Q-wave MI to prevent ischemic events. Prevention of deep vein thrombosis (DVT) in patients undergoing hip replacement or abdominal surgery who are at risk of thromboembolic complications. Those at risk are 40 yr and older, obese, undergoing surgery under general anesthesia lasting longer than 30 min, malignancy or history of DVT or pulmonary embolism. Prevention of DVT or pulmonary embolism in acutely ill patients with severely restricted mobility.

PRECAUTIONS

CONTRAINDICATIONS: Active major bleeding; concurrent heparin therapy; hypersensitivity to dalteparin, heparin, or pork products; thrombocytopenia associated with positive in vitro test for antiplatelet antibody. **CAUTIONS:** Conditions with increased risk of hemorrhage, bacterial endocarditis, history of heparin-induced thrombocytopenia, renal or hepatic impairment, uncontrolled hypertension, history of recent GI ulceration or hemorrhage, hypertensive or diabetic retinopathy. When neuraxial anesthesia (epidural or spinal anesthesia) or spinal puncture is employed, patients anticoagulated or scheduled to be anticoagulated with dalteparin for prevention of thromboembolic complications are at risk of developing an epidural or spinal hematoma which can result in long-term or permanent paralysis.

⌛ LIFESPAN CONSIDERATIONS: **Pregnancy/Lactation:** Use with caution, particularly during last trimester, immediate postpartum period (increased risk of maternal hemorrhage). Unknown if distributed in breast milk. **Pregnancy Category B. Children:** Safety and efficacy not established. **Elderly:** No age-related precautions noted.

INTERACTIONS

DRUG: **Anticoagulants, platelet inhibitors:** May increase risk of bleeding. HERBAL: None known. FOOD: None known. LAB VALUES: Increases (reversible) LDH, serum alkaline phosphatase, AST, and ALT levels.

AVAILABILITY (Rx)

SYRINGE: 2,500 international units/0.2 ml, 5,000 international units/0.2 ml, 7,500 international units/0.3 ml, 10,000 international units/ml. **VIAL:** 10,000 international units/ml, 25,000 international units/ml.

ADMINISTRATION/HANDLING

SUBCUTANEOUS

• Store at room temperature. • Instruct patient to sit/lie down before administering by deep subcutaneous injection. • Inject in U-shaped area around the navel, upper outer side of thigh, upper outer quadrangle of buttock. • Use a fine needle (25–26 gauge) to minimize tissue trauma. • Introduce entire length of needle (½ inch) into skin fold held between thumb and forefinger, holding needle during injection at a 45°–90° angle. • Do not rub injection site after administration (prevents bruising). • Alternate the administration site with each injection.

INDICATIONS/ROUTES/DOSAGE

LOW- TO MODERATE-RISK ABDOMINAL SURGERY

SUBCUTANEOUS: ADULTS, ELDERLY: 2,500 international units 1–2 hr before surgery, then daily for 5–10 days.

HIGH-RISK ABDOMINAL SURGERY

SUBCUTANEOUS: ADULTS, ELDERLY: 5,000 international units 1–2 hr before surgery, then daily for 5–10 days.

TOTAL HIP SURGERY

SUBCUTANEOUS: ADULTS, ELDERLY: 2,500 international units 1–2 hr before surgery, then 2,500 units 6 hrs after surgery, then 5,000 units/day for 7–10 days.

UNSTABLE ANGINA, NON–Q-WAVE MI

SUBCUTANEOUS: ADULTS, ELDERLY: 120 international units/kg q12h (**Maximum:** 10,000 international units/dose) given with aspirin until clinically stable.

PREVENTION OF DVT OR PULMONARY EDEMA IN THE ACUTELY ILL PATIENT

SUBCUTANEOUS: ADULTS, ELDERLY: 5,000 international units once a day.

SIDE EFFECTS

OCCASIONAL (7%–3%): Hematoma at injection site. **RARE (less than 1%):** Hypersensitivity reaction (chills, fever, pruritus, urticaria, asthma, rhinitis, lacrimation, headache); mild, local skin irritation.

ADVERSE REACTIONS/ TOXIC EFFECTS

Overdose may lead to bleeding complications ranging from local ecchymoses to major hemorrhage. Thrombocytopenia occurs rarely.

NURSING CONSIDERATIONS

BASELINE ASSESSMENT

Assess CBC, especially platelet count. Determine initial BP.

INTERVENTION/EVALUATION

Periodically monitor CBC, platelet count, stool for occult blood (no need for daily monitoring in patients with normal presurgical coagulation parameters). Assess for any sign of bleeding: bleeding at surgical site, hematuria, blood in stool, bleeding from gums, petechiae, bruising or bleeding at injection sites.

PATIENT/FAMILY TEACHING

• Usual length of therapy is 5–10 days. • Do not take any OTC medication (especially aspirin) without consulting physician. • Report bleeding, bruising, dizziness or lightheadedness, rash, itching, fever, swelling, breathing difficulty. • Rotate injection sites daily. • Teach proper injection technique. • Excessive bruising at injection site may be lessened by ice massage before injection.

---

danazol   ℮

dan-ah-zole

(Cyclomen �֍, Danocrine)

Do not confuse Danocrine with Dantrium.

◆CLASSIFICATION

PHARMACOTHERAPEUTIC: Testosterone derivative. **CLINICAL:** Androgen, hormone.

ACTION

Suppresses the pituitary-ovarian axis by inhibiting the output of pituitary gonadotropins. In endometriosis, causes atrophy of both normal and ectopic endometrial tissue. For fibrocystic breast disease, follicle stimulating hormone (FSH) and luteinizing hormone (LH) are depressed. Inhibits steroid synthesis and binding of steroids to their receptors in breast tissue. Increases serum levels of esterase inhibitor. **Therapeutic Effect:** Produces anovulation, amenorrhea. Reduces production of estrogen. Corrects biochemical deficiency as seen in hereditary angioedema.

USES

Palliative treatment of endometriosis, fibrocystic breast disease; prophylactic treatment of hereditary angioedema. **OFF-LABEL:** Treatment of gynecomastia, menorrhagia, precocious puberty.

PRECAUTIONS

CONTRAINDICATIONS: Severe cardiac/hepatic/renal function impairment. Active or history of thromboembolic disease, androgen tumor, abnormal vaginal bleeding. **CAUTIONS:** Renal impairment, cardiac impairment, epilepsy, migraine headaches, diabetes. **Pregnancy Category X.**

INTERACTIONS

DRUG: Anticoagulants: The effects of these drugs may be enhanced. **Cyclosporine, tacrolimus:** May increase nephrotoxicity with these drugs. **HERBAL:** None known. **FOOD:** None known. **LAB VALUES:** May increase hepatic function values.

AVAILABILITY (Rx)

CAPSULES: 50 mg, 100 mg, 200 mg.

INDICATIONS/ROUTES/DOSAGE

◀ **ALERT** ▶ Initiate therapy during menstruation or when patient is not pregnant.

ENDOMETRIOSIS

PO: ADULTS: 200–800 mg a day in 2 divided doses for 3–9 mo.

FIBROCYSTIC BREAST DISEASE

PO: ADULTS: 100–400 mg a day in 2 divided doses.

HEREDITARY ANGIOEDEMA

PO: ADULTS: Initially, 200 mg 2–3 times a day. Decrease dosage by 50% or less at 1- to 3-mo intervals. If attack occurs, increase dosage by up to 200 mg a day.

SIDE EFFECTS

FREQUENT: Females: Amenorrhea, breakthrough bleeding/spotting, decreased breast size, weight gain, irregular menstrual period. **OCCASIONAL: Males/Females:** Edema, rhabdomyolysis (muscle cramps, unusual fatigue), virilism (acne, oily skin), flushed skin, altered moods. **RARE: Males/Females:** Hematuria, gingivitis, carpal tunnel syndrome, cataracts, severe headache, vomiting, rash, photosensitivity. **Females:** Enlarged clitoris, hoarseness, deepening voice, hair growth, monilial vaginitis. **Males:** Decreased testicle size.

ADVERSE REACTIONS/ TOXIC EFFECTS

Jaundice may occur in those receiving 400 mg or more per day. Hepatic dysfunction, eosinophilia, thrombocytopenia, pancreatitis occur rarely.

NURSING CONSIDERATIONS

BASELINE ASSESSMENT

Inquire about menstrual cycle: Therapy should begin during menstruation. Establish baseline weight, BP.

INTERVENTION/EVALUATION

Weigh 2–3 times a wk; report 5 lb or more/wk gain or swelling of fingers/feet. Monitor BP periodically. Check for jaundice (yellow sclera/skin, dark urine, clay-colored stools).

• Patient should use nonhormonal contraceptive during therapy. • Do not take drug, notify physician if pregnancy suspected (risk to fetus). • Stress importance of full length of therapy, regular visits to physician's office (liver function tests, CBC, serum amylase, lipase). • Notify physician promptly of masculinizing effects (may not be reversible), weight gain, muscle cramps, fatigue. • Spotting/bleeding may occur in first months of therapy for endometriosis (does not mean lack of efficacy). • In fibrocystic breast disease, irregular menstrual periods and amenorrhea may occur with or without ovulation.

dantrolene sodium

dan-troe-leen

(Dantrium, Dantrium Intravenous)

Do not confuse Dantrium with Daraprim.

CLASSIFICATION

CLINICAL: Skeletal muscle relaxant.

ACTION

A skeletal muscle relaxant that reduces muscle contraction by interfering with release of calcium ion. Reduces calcium ion concentration. Therapeutic Effect: Dissociates excitation-contraction coupling. Interferes with catabolic process associated with malignant hyperthermic crisis.

PHARMACOKINETICS

Poorly absorbed from the GI tract. Protein binding: High. Metabolized in the liver. Primarily excreted in urine. Half-life: IV: 4–8 hr; PO: 8.7 hr.

USES

PO: Relief of symptoms of spasticity due to spinal cord injuries, stroke, cerebral palsy, multiple sclerosis, especially flexor spasms, concomitant pain, clonus, muscular rigidity. **Parenteral:** Management of fulminant hypermetabolism of skeletal muscle due to malignant hyperthermia crisis. OFF-LABEL: Relief of exercise-induced pain in patients with muscular dystrophy, treatment of flexor spasms and neuroleptic malignant syndrome.

PRECAUTIONS

CONTRAINDICATIONS: Active hepatic disease. CAUTIONS: Cardiac/pulmonary impairment, history of previous hepatic disease.

⧖ LIFESPAN CONSIDERATIONS: **Pregnancy/Lactation:** Readily crosses placenta. Do not use in breast-feeding mothers. **Pregnancy Category C. Children:** No age-related precautions noted in those 5 yr and older. **Elderly:** No information available.

INTERACTIONS

DRUG: **Central nervous system (CNS) depressants:** May increase CNS depression with short-term use. **Liver toxic medications:** May increase the risk of liver toxicity with chronic use. HERBAL: None known. FOOD: None known. LAB VALUES: May alter liver function test results.

AVAILABILITY (Rx)

CAPSULES (DANTRIUM): 25 mg, 50 mg, 100 mg. POWDER FOR INJECTION (DANTRIUM INTRAVENOUS): 20-mg vial.

ADMINISTRATION/HANDLING

IV

Reconstitution • Reconstitute 20-mg vial with 60 ml sterile water for injection to provide concentration of 0.33 mg/ml.

Rate of administration • For IV infusion, administer over 1 hr. • Diligently monitor for extravasation (high pH of

IV preparation). May produce severe complications.

Storage • Store at room temperature. • Use within 6 hr after reconstitution. Solution is clear, colorless. Discard if cloudy, precipitate formed.

PO
• Give without regard to food.

▦ IV INCOMPATIBILITY
None known.

INDICATIONS/ROUTES/DOSAGE
SPASTICITY
PO: ADULTS, ELDERLY: Initially, 25 mg/day. Increase to 25 mg 2–4 times a day, then by 25-mg increments up to 100 mg 2–4 times a day. CHILDREN: Initially, 0.5 mg/kg twice a day. Increase to 0.5 mg/kg 3–4 times a day, then in increments of 0.5 mg/kg/day up to 3 mg/kg 2–4 times a day. **Maximum:** 400 mg/day.

PREVENTION OF MALIGNANT HYPERTHERMIC CRISIS
PO: ADULTS, ELDERLY, CHILDREN: 4–8 mg/kg/day in 3–4 divided doses 1–2 days before surgery; give last dose 3–4 hr before surgery.
IV: ADULTS, ELDERLY, CHILDREN: 2.5 mg/kg about 1.25 hr before surgery.

MANAGEMENT OF MALIGNANT HYPERTHERMIC CRISIS
IV: ADULTS, ELDERLY, CHILDREN: Initially a minimum of 1 mg/kg rapid IV; may repeat up to total cumulative dose of 10 mg/kg. May follow with 4–8 mg/kg/day PO in 4 divided doses up to 3 days after crisis.

SIDE EFFECTS
FREQUENT: Drowsiness, dizziness, weakness, general malaise, diarrhea (mild). **OCCASIONAL:** Confusion, diarrhea (may be severe), headache, insomnia, constipation, urinary frequency. **RARE:** Paradoxical CNS excitement or restlessness, paresthesia, tinnitus, slurred speech, tremor, blurred vision, dry mouth, nocturia, impotence, rash, pruritus.

ADVERSE REACTIONS/TOXIC EFFECTS
There is a risk of hepatotoxicity, most notably in females, those 35 yr of age and older, and those taking other medications concurrently. Overt hepatitis noted most frequently between 3rd and 12th mo of therapy. Overdosage results in vomiting, muscular hypotonia, muscle twitching, respiratory depression, and seizures.

NURSING CONSIDERATIONS
BASELINE ASSESSMENT
Obtain baseline liver function tests (AST, ALT, alkaline phosphatase, total bilirubin). Record onset, type, location, duration of muscular spasm. Check for immobility, stiffness, swelling.

INTERVENTION/EVALUATION
Assist with ambulation. For those on long-term therapy, liver/renal function tests, CBC should be performed periodically. Evaluate for therapeutic response: decreased intensity of skeletal muscle pain, spasm.

PATIENT/FAMILY TEACHING
• Drowsiness usually diminishes with continued therapy. • Avoid tasks that require alertness, motor skills until response to drug is established. • Avoid alcohol/other depressants while taking medication. • Report continued weakness, fatigue, nausea, diarrhea, skin rash, itching, bloody or tarry stools.

daptomycin
dap-toe-my-sin
(Cubicin)

◆CLASSIFICATION

PHARMACOTHERAPEUTIC: Lipopeptide antibacterial agent. **CLINICAL:** Antibiotic.

ACTION

A lipopeptide antibacterial agent that binds to bacterial membranes and causes a rapid depolarization of the membrane potential. The loss of membrane potential leads to inhibition of protein, DNA, and RNA synthesis. **Therapeutic Effect:** Bactericidal.

PHARMACOKINETICS

Widely distributed. Protein binding: 90%. Primarily excreted unchanged in urine. Moderately removed by hemodialysis. **Half-life:** 7–8 hr (increased in impaired renal function).

USES

Treatment of complicated skin and skin-structure infections caused by susceptible strains of gram-positive pathogens, including penicillin-resistant *Streptococcus pneumoniae*, methicillin-resistant *Staphyloccus aureus*, vancomycin-resistant enterococci.

PRECAUTIONS

CONTRAINDICATIONS: None known. **CAUTIONS:** Renal impairment, history of or current musculoskeletal disorders (risk of exacerbation), pregnancy.

⧗ **LIFESPAN CONSIDERATIONS: Pregnancy/Lactation:** Unknown if drug is distributed in breast milk. **Pregnancy Category B. Children:** Safety and efficacy not established in those younger than 18 yr. **Elderly:** No age-related precautions noted.

INTERACTIONS

DRUG: Hydroxamethylglutaryl-CoA (HMG-CoA) reductase inhibitors: May cause myopathy. **Tobramycin:**

Increases the serum concentration of daptomycin. **HERBAL:** None known. **FOOD:** None known. **LAB VALUES:** May increase serum CPK levels. May alter liver function test results.

AVAILABILITY (Rx)

POWDER FOR INJECTION: 250 mg/vial, 500 mg/vial.

ADMINISTRATION/HANDLING

 IV

Reconstitution • Reconstitute 250-mg vial with 5 ml 0.9% NaCl; reconstitute 500-mg vial with 10 ml 0.9% NaCl. Further dilute in 50 ml 0.9% NaCl.

Rate of administration • For intermittent IV infusion (piggyback), infuse over 30 min.

Storage • Refrigerate. • Appears as pale yellow to light brown lyophilized cake. • Reconstituted solution is stable for 12 hr at room temperature or up to 48 hr if refrigerated. • Inspect for particulate matter.

▨ IV INCOMPATIBILITIES

Diluents containing dextrose. If the same IV line is used to administer different drugs, the line should be flushed with 0.9% NaCl.

INDICATIONS/ROUTES/DOSAGE

COMPLICATED SKIN AND SKIN-STRUCTURE INFECTIONS
IV: ADULTS, ELDERLY: 4 mg/kg every 24 hr for 7–14 days.

DOSAGE IN RENAL IMPAIRMENT
For patients with creatinine clearance of less than 30 ml/min, dosage is 4 mg/kg q48h for 7–14 days.

SIDE EFFECTS

FREQUENT (6%–5%): Constipation, nausea, peripheral injection site reactions, headache, diarrhea. **OCCASIONAL (4%–3%):** Insomnia, rash, vomiting. **RARE (less than 3%):** Pruritus, dizziness, hypotension.

ADVERSE REACTIONS/ TOXIC EFFECTS

Skeletal muscle myopathy, characterized by muscle pain and weakness, particularly of the distal extremities, occurs rarely. Antibiotic-associated colitis and other superinfections may result from altered bacterial balance.

NURSING CONSIDERATIONS

BASELINE ASSESSMENT

Obtain culture and sensitivity test before first dose (therapy may begin before results are known).

INTERVENTION/EVALUATION

Assess oral cavity for white patches on mucous membranes, tongue. Monitor pattern of bowel activity and stool consistency carefully; mild GI effects may be tolerable, but increasing severity may indicate onset of antibiotic-associated colitis. Be alert for superinfection: severe genital or anal pruritus, abdominal pain, severe mouth soreness, moderate to severe diarrhea. Monitor for dizziness, institute appropriate measures.

PATIENT/FAMILY TEACHING

• Report rash, headache, nausea, any new symptom.

---

darbepoetin alfa

dar-bee-eh-poe-**ee**-tin

(Aranesp)

Do not confuse Aranesp with Aricept.

◆CLASSIFICATION

PHARMACOTHERAPEUTIC: Glycoprotein. **CLINICAL:** Hematopoietic.

ACTION

A glycoprotein that stimulates formation of RBCs in bone marrow; increases serum half-life of epoetin. Therapeutic Effect: Induces erythropoiesis and release of reticulocytes from bone marrow.

PHARMACOKINETICS

Well absorbed after subcutaneous administration. Half-life: 48.5 hr.

USES

Treatment of anemia associated with chronic renal failure, chemotherapy-induced anemia.

PRECAUTIONS

CONTRAINDICATIONS: History of sensitivity to mammalian cell-derived products or human albumin, uncontrolled hypertension. **CAUTIONS:** Patients with known porphyria (impairment of erythrocyte formation in bone marrow or responsible for hepatic impairment), hemolytic anemia, sickle cell anemia, thalassemia, history of seizures.

⌛ LIFESPAN CONSIDERATIONS: Pregnancy/Lactation: Unknown if drug crosses placenta or is distributed in breast milk. **Pregnancy Category C. Children:** Safety and efficacy not established. **Elderly:** Age-related renal impairment may require dosage adjustment.

INTERACTIONS

DRUG: None known. HERBAL: None known. FOOD: None known. LAB VALUES: May increase BUN, serum phosphorus, potassium, serum creatinine, serum uric acid, and sodium levels. May decrease bleeding time, serum iron concentration, and serum ferritin.

AVAILABILITY (Rx)

INJECTION: 25 mcg/ml, 40 mcg/ml, 60 mcg/ml, 100 mcg/ml, 150 mcg/ml, 200 mcg/ml, 300 mcg/ml. **PREFILLED SYRINGE:** 25 mcg/0.42 ml, 40 mcg/ 0.4 ml, 60 mcg/0.3 ml, 100 mcg/0.5 ml, 200 mcg/0.4 ml, 300 mcg/0.6 ml, 500 mcg/ml.

ADMINISTRATION/HANDLING

◄ **ALERT** ► Avoid excessive agitation of vial; do not shake (will cause foaming).

 IV

Reconstitution • No reconstitution necessary.

Rate of administration • May be given as an IV bolus.

Storage • Refrigerate vials. Vigorous shaking may denature medication, rendering it inactive.

SUBCUTANEOUS

• Use 1 dose per vial; do not reenter vial. Discard unused portion. May be mixed in a syringe with bacteriostatic 0.9% NaCl with benzyl alcohol 0.9% (bacteriostatic saline) at a 1:1 ratio (benzyl alcohol acts as a local anesthetic; may reduce injection site discomfort).

▨ IV INCOMPATIBILITIES

Do not mix with other medications.

INDICATIONS/ROUTES/DOSAGE

ANEMIA IN CHRONIC RENAL FAILURE
IV BOLUS, SUBCUTANEOUS: ADULTS, ELDERLY: Initially, 0.45 mcg/kg once weekly. Adjust dosage to achieve and maintain a target Hgb not to exceed 12 g/dl. Do not increase dosage more frequently than once monthly. Limit increases in Hgb by less than 1 g/dl over any 2-wk period.

ANEMIA ASSOCIATED WITH CHEMOTHERAPY
IV, SUBCUTANEOUS: ADULTS, ELDERLY: 2.25 mcg/kg/dose once a wk or 500 mcg every 3 wk. May increase up to 4.5 mcg/kg/dose once a week.

SIDE EFFECTS

FREQUENT: Myalgia, hypertension or hypotension, headache, diarrhea.
OCCASIONAL: Fatigue, edema, vomiting, reaction at administration site, asthenia, dizziness.

ADVERSE REACTIONS/ TOXIC EFFECTS

Vascular access thrombosis, CHF, sepsis, arrhythmias, and anaphylactic reaction occur rarely.

NURSING CONSIDERATIONS

BASELINE ASSESSMENT
Assess BP before drug administration (80% of patients with chronic renal failure have history of hypertension). BP often rises during early therapy in those with history of hypertension. Assess serum iron (transferrin saturation should be greater than 20%) and serum ferritin (greater than 100 ng/ml) before and during therapy. Consider that all patients will eventually need supplemental iron therapy. Establish baseline CBC (especially note Hct).

INTERVENTION/EVALUATION
Monitor Hct level diligently (if level increases greater than 4 points in 2 wk, dosage should be reduced). Monitor Hgb, serum ferritin, CBC with differential, serum creatinine, BUN, potassium, phosphorus, reticulocyte count. Monitor BP aggressively for increase (25% of patients taking medication require antihypertension therapy, dietary restrictions).

PATIENT/FAMILY TEACHING
• Frequent blood tests needed to determine correct dose. • Inform physician if severe headache develops. • Avoid tasks requiring alertness, motor skills until response to drug is established.

---

darifenacin hydrochloride

dare-ih-**fen**-ah-sin
(Enablex)

D

◆CLASSIFICATION

PHARMACOTHERAPEUTIC: Muscarinic receptor antagonist. **CLINICAL:** Urinary antispasmodic.

ACTION

Acts as a direct antagonist at muscarinic receptor sites in cholinergically innervated organs. Receptor blockade limits bladder contractions. **Therapeutic Effect:** Reduces symptoms of bladder irritability/overactivity (urge incontinence, urinary urgency and frequency), improves bladder capacity.

PHARMACOKINETICS

Well absorbed from GI tract. Protein binding: 98%. Extensively metabolized in liver. Primarily excreted in urine; a lesser amount eliminated in feces. **Half-life:** 24–29 hr.

USES

Management of symptoms of bladder overactivity (urge incontinence, urinary urgency and frequency).

PRECAUTIONS

CONTRAINDICATIONS: Uncontrolled narrow-angle glaucoma, paralytic ileus, GI/GU obstruction, urine retention, severe hepatic impairment. **CAUTIONS:** Bladder outflow obstruction, non-obstructive prostatic hyperplasia, urine retention, GI obstructive disorders, decreased GI motility, constipation, hiatal hernia, reflux esophagitis, ulcerative colitis, controlled narrow-angle glaucoma, myasthenia gravis.

⧖ **LIFESPAN CONSIDERATIONS:** Pregnancy/Lactation: Unknown if drug crosses placenta or is distributed in breast milk. **Pregnancy Category C.**

Children: Safety and efficacy not established. **Elderly:** No age-related precautions noted.

INTERACTIONS

DRUG: Anticholinergic drugs: Darifenacin may increase anticholinergic adverse effects. **Clarithromycin, itraconazole, ketoconazole, nefazodone, nelfinavir, ritonavir:** May increase levels of darifenacin, daily dose should not exceed 7.5 mg/day. **Digoxin:** Darifenacin may increase digoxin levels. **Flecainide, imipramine, thioridazine, tricyclic antidepressants:** Caution should be taken with concurrent administration of darifenacin. **HERBAL:** None known. **FOOD:** None known. **LAB VALUES:** None known.

AVAILABILITY (Rx)

TABLETS (EXTENDED-RELEASE): 7.5 mg, 15 mg.

ADMINISTRATION/HANDLING

PO

• Give without regard to food. • Do not crush extended-release tablets; swallow them whole.

INDICATIONS/ROUTES/DOSAGE

OVERACTIVE BLADDER

PO: ADULTS, ELDERLY: Initially, 7.5 mg once daily. If response is not adequate after at least 2 wk, may increase to 15 mg once daily. Do not exceed 7.5 mg once daily in moderate hepatic impairment.

SIDE EFFECTS

FREQUENT (35%–21%): Dry mouth, constipation. **OCCASIONAL (8%–4%):** Dyspepsia, headache, nausea, abdominal pain. **RARE (3%–2%):** Asthenia, diarrhea, dizziness, ocular dryness.

ADVERSE REACTIONS/ TOXIC EFFECTS

Urinary tract infection occurs occasionally.

NURSING CONSIDERATIONS

BASELINE ASSESSMENT

Monitor voiding pattern and assess signs and symptoms of overactive bladder prior to therapy as baseline.

INTERVENTION/EVALUATION

Monitor I&O. Palpate bladder for urine retention. Monitor bowel activity, stool consistency for evidence of constipation. Relieve dry mouth with sips of tepid water. Assess for relief of symptoms of overactive bladder (urge incontinence, urinary frequency and urgency).

PATIENT/FAMILY TEACHING

• Swallow tablet whole; do not crush, divide, or chew. • Increase fluid intake to reduce risk of constipation. • Avoid tasks that require alertness or motor skills until response to drug is established.

Darvocet-N, *see*
propoxyphene

DAUNOrubicin ⚑

dawn-oh-**rue**-bih-sin
(Cerubidine, DaunoXome)
Do not confuse daunorubicin with dactinomycin or doxorubicin.

CLASSIFICATION

PHARMACOTHERAPEUTIC: Anthracycline antibiotic. **CLINICAL:** Antineoplastic (see p. 73C).

ACTION

An anthracycline antibiotic that inhibits DNA and DNA-dependent RNA synthesis by binding with DNA strands. Liposomal encapsulation increases uptake by tumors, prolongs drug action, and may decrease toxicity. **Therapeutic Effect:** Prevents cell division.

PHARMACOKINETICS

Widely distributed. Protein binding: High. Does not cross the blood-brain barrier. Metabolized in the liver to active metabolite. Excreted in urine; eliminated by biliary excretion. **Half-life:** 18.5 hr; metabolite: 26.7 hr.

USES

Cerubidine: Treatment of leukemias (acute lymphocytic [ALL] and acute non-lymphocytic [ANLL]) in combination with other agents. **DaunoXome:** Advanced HIV-related Kaposi's sarcoma. **OFF-LABEL:** Treatment of chronic myelocytic leukemia, Ewing's sarcoma, neuroblastoma, non-Hodgkin's lymphoma, Wilms' tumor.

PRECAUTIONS

CONTRAINDICATIONS: Arrhythmias, CHF, left ventricular ejection fraction less than 40%, preexisting myelosuppression. **CAUTIONS:** Those with hepatic, biliary, renal impairment.

⌛ **LIFESPAN CONSIDERATIONS: Pregnancy/Lactation:** If possible, avoid use during pregnancy, especially first trimester. May cause fetal harm. Breastfeeding not recommended. **Pregnancy Category D. Children:** Safety and efficacy not established. **Elderly:** Cardiotoxicity may be more frequent; reduced bone marrow reserves requires caution. Age-related renal impairment may require dosage adjustment.

INTERACTIONS

DRUG: Antigout medications: May decrease the effects of these drugs.

Bone marrow depressants: May enhance myelosuppression. **Live-virus vaccines:** May potentiate virus replication, increase vaccine side effects, and decrease the patient's antibody response to the vaccine. HERBAL: None known. FOOD: None known. LAB VALUES: May increase serum alkaline phosphatase, bilirubin, uric acid, and AST levels.

AVAILABILITY (Rx)

POWDER FOR INJECTION (CERUBIDINE): 20 mg. **SOLUTION FOR INJECTION (CERUBIDINE):** 5 mg/ml. **INJECTION (DAUNOXOME):** 2 mg/ml.

ADMINISTRATION/HANDLING

IV

◄ ALERT ► Give by IV push or IV infusion. IV infusion not recommended due to vein irritation, risk of thrombophlebitis. Avoid small veins, swollen or edematous extremities, areas overlying joints and tendons. May be carcinogenic, mutagenic, or teratogenic. Handle with extreme care during preparation/administration.

Reconstitution

Cerubidine • Reconstitute each 20-mg vial with 4 ml sterile water for injection to provide concentration of 5 mg/ml. • Gently agitate vial until completely dissolved.

Daunoxome • Must dilute with equal part D$_5$W to provide concentration of 1 mg/ml. • Do not use any other diluent.

Rate of administration

Cerubidine • For IV push, withdraw desired dose into syringe containing 10–15 ml 0.9% NaCl. Inject over 2–3 min into tubing of running IV solution of D$_5$W or 0.9% NaCl. • For IV infusion, further dilute with 100 ml D$_5$W or 0.9% NaCl. Infuse over 30–45 min. • Extravasation produces immediate pain,

severe local tissue damage. Aspirate as much infiltrated drug as possible, then infiltrate area with hydrocortisone sodium succinate injection (50–100 mg hydrocortisone) and/or isotonic sodium thiosulfate injection or ascorbic acid injection (1 ml of 5% injection). Apply cold compresses.

Daunoxome • Infuse over 60 min.

Storage

Cerubidine • Reconstituted solution is stable for 24 hr at room temperature or 48 hr if refrigerated. • Color change from red to blue-purple indicates decomposition; discard.

Daunoxome • Refrigerate unopened vials • Reconstituted solution is stable for 6 hr if refrigerated. • Do not use if opaque.

IV INCOMPATIBILITIES

Allopurinol (Aloprim), aztreonam (Azactam), cefepime (Maxipime), fludarabine (Fludara), piperacillin and tazobactam (Zosyn). **DaunoXome:** Don't mix with any other solution, especially NaCl or bacteriostatic agents (such as benzyl alcohol).

IV COMPATIBILITIES

Cytarabine (Cytosar), etoposide (VePesid), filgrastim (Neupogen), granisetron (Kytril), ondansetron (Zofran).

INDICATIONS/ROUTES/DOSAGE

ALL

IV (CERUBIDINE): ADULTS, ELDERLY: 45 mg/m^2 on days 1, 2, and 3 of induction course. CHILDREN 2 YR AND OLDER: 25 mg/m^2 on day 1 of every wk. CHILDREN YOUNGER THAN 2 YR BODY SURFACE AREA LESS THAN 0.5: 1 mg/kg/dose.

ANLL

IV (CERUBIDINE): ADULTS YOUNGER THAN 60 YR: 45 mg/m^2 on days 1, 2, and 3 of induction course then on days 1 and 2 of subsequent courses. ADULTS 60 YR AND OLDER: 30 mg/m² on days 1, 2, and 3 of induction course, then on days 1 and 2 of subsequent courses.

KAPOSI'S SARCOMA

IV (DAUNOXOME): ADULTS: 20–40 mg/m² over 1 hr repeated q2wk; or 100 mg/m² q3wk.

DOSAGE IN RENAL IMPAIRMENT

ALL, ANLL: CREATININE CLEARANCE LESS THAN 10 ML/MIN: 75% of normal dose. SERUM CREATININE GREATER THAN 3 MG/DL: 50% of normal dose.

KAPOSI'S SARCOMA: SERUM CREATININE GREATER THAN 3 MG/DL: 50% of normal dose.

DOSAGE IN HEPATIC IMPAIRMENT

ALL, ANLL: BILIRUBIN 1.2–3 MG/DL: 75% of normal dose. BILIRUBIN 3.1–5 MG/DL: 50% of normal dose. BILIRUBIN GREATER THAN 5 MG/DL: Daunorubicin is not recommended for use in this patient population.

KAPOSI'S SARCOMA: BILIRUBIN 1.2–3 MG/DL: 75% of normal dose. BILIRUBIN GREATER THAN 3 MG/DL: 50% of normal dose.

SIDE EFFECTS

FREQUENT: Complete alopecia (scalp, axillary, pubic), nausea, vomiting (beginning a few hr after administration and lasting 24–48 hr. **DaunoXome:** Mild to moderate nausea, fatigue, fever. **OCCASIONAL:** Diarrhea, abdominal pain, esophagitis, stomatitis, transverse pigmentation of fingernails and toenails. **RARE:** Transient fever, chills.

ADVERSE REACTIONS/ TOXIC EFFECTS

Myelosuppression may cause hematologic toxicity, manifested as severe leukopenia, anemia, and thrombocytopenia. Platelet and WBC counts typically decrease in 10–14 days and return to normal levels by the third week of daunorubicin treatment. The risk of cardiotoxicity (either acute, manifested as transient EKG abnormalities, or chronic, manifested as CHF) increases when the total cumulative dose exceeds 550 mg/m² in adults, 300 mg/m² in children older than 2 yr, or 10 mg/kg in children younger than 2 yr.

NURSING CONSIDERATIONS

BASELINE ASSESSMENT

Obtain WBC, platelet, erythrocyte counts before and at frequent intervals during therapy. EKG should be obtained before therapy. Antiemetics may be effective in preventing, treating nausea.

INTERVENTION/EVALUATION

Monitor for stomatitis (burning, erythema of oral mucosa). May lead to ulceration within 2–3 days. Assess skin, nailbeds for hyperpigmentation. Monitor hematologic status, renal/liver function studies, serum uric acid level. Assess pattern of daily bowel activity/stool consistency. Monitor for hematologic toxicity (fever, sore throat, signs of local infection, unusual bruising or bleeding from any site), symptoms of anemia (excessive fatigue, weakness).

PATIENT/FAMILY TEACHING

• Urine may turn reddish color for 1–2 days after beginning therapy. • Alopecia is reversible, but new hair growth may have different color or texture. • New hair growth resumes about 5 wk after last therapy dose. • Maintain fastidious oral hygiene. • Do not have immunizations without physician's approval (drug lowers body's resistance). • Avoid contact with those who have recently received live virus vaccine. • Promptly report fever, sore throat, signs of local infection, unusual bruising/bleeding from any site. • Increase fluid intake (may protect against hyperuricemia). • Contact physician for persistent nausea or vomiting.

---

* "Tall Man" lettering   🍁 Canadian trade name   ⓔ see **evolve**   ▶ High Alert drug

DDAVP, *see desmopressin*

Decadron, *see*
dexamethasone

deferasirox

daeh-fur-**ah**-sir-ox
(Exjade)

• **CLASSIFICATION**

PHARMACOTHERAPEUTIC: Iron chelating agent. **CLINICAL:** Iron reduction.

ACTION

Selective for iron. Binds iron with a high affinity in a 2:1 ratio. **Therapeutic Effect:** Induces iron excretion.

PHARMACOKINETICS

Well absorbed following oral administration. Protein binding: 99%. Minimally metabolized. Primarily excreted in feces with a lesser amount eliminated in urine. **Half-life:** 8–16 hr.

USES

Treatment of chronic iron overload due to blood transfusions (transfusional hemosiderosis) in patients 2 yr and older.

PRECAUTIONS

CONTRAINDICATIONS: None known. **CAUTIONS:** Renal impairment, hepatic impairment, preexisting hearing loss, vision disturbances.

⌛ **LIFESPAN CONSIDERATIONS: Pregnancy/Lactation:** Unknown if drug crosses placenta or is distributed in breast milk. **Pregnancy Category B.**

Children: Not recommended for children younger than 2 yr. **Elderly:** No age-related precautions noted.

INTERACTIONS

DRUG: Aluminum-containing antacids: May decrease effects of deferasirox. Separate by 1 hr. **Other iron-chelating agents:** Increase risk of toxic effects. **HERBAL:** None known. **FOOD: Food:** Bioavailability is variably increased if deferasirox is taken with food. **LAB VALUES:** Decreases serum ferritin. May increase serum creatinine, transaminase, AST, ALT, urine protein.

AVAILABILITY (Rx)

TABLETS: 125 mg, 250 mg, 500 mg (Exjade).

ADMINISTRATION/HANDLING
PO

• Give on an empty stomach 30 min before food. • Tablets should not be chewed or swallowed whole. • Disperse tablet by stirring in water, apple juice or orange juice until a fine suspension is achieved. • Dosage less than 1 gram should be dispersed in 2.5 ounces of liquid, dosage more than 1 gram should be dispersed in 7 ounces of liquid. If any residue remains in glass, resuspend with a small amount of liquid.

INDICATIONS/ROUTES/DOSAGE
IRON OVERLOAD
PO: ADULTS, ELDERLY, CHILDREN 2 YR AND OLDER: Initially, 20 mg/kg once daily. Adjust dosage of 5 or 10 mg/kg every 3–6 mo based on serum ferritin levels. **Maximum:** 30 mg/kg once daily.

SIDE EFFECTS

FREQUENT (19%–10%): Fever, headache, abdominal pain, cough, nasopharyngitis, diarrhea, nausea, vomiting. **OCCASIONAL (9%–4%):** Rash, arthralgia, fatigue, back pain, urticaria. **RARE (1%):** Edema, sleep disorder, dizziness, anxiety.

✐ see color pill atlas   🌿 herb   underlined – top prescribed drug

ADVERSE REACTIONS/ TOXIC EFFECTS

Bronchitis, pharyngitis, acute tonsillitis, ear infection occur occasionally. Hepatitis, auditory disturbances, ocular abnormalities occur rarely.

NURSING CONSIDERATIONS

BASELINE ASSESSMENT

Obtain baseline serum creatinine, ALT, AST, serum transaminase and monthly thereafter. Auditory and ophthalmic testing should be obtained before therapy and annually therafter. Monitor serum ferritin monthly.

INTERVENTION/EVALUATION

Treatment should be interrupted if serum ferritin levels are consistently less than 500 mcg/L. Suspend treatment if severe rash occurs.

PATIENT/FAMILY TEACHING

• Take on an empty stomach 30 min before food. • Do not chew or swallow tablet whole; disperse tablet completely in water, apple juice or orange juice; drink resulting suspension immediately. • Do not take aluminum-containing antacids concurrently.

---

deferoxamine mesylate

deaf-er-**ox**-ah-meen

(Desferal)

Do not confuse deferoxamine with cefuroxime, or Desferal with Desyrel or Disophrol.

◆ CLASSIFICATION

CLINICAL: Antidote.

ACTION

Binds with iron to form complex. **Therapeutic Effect:** Promotes urine excretion of iron.

USES

Treatment of acute iron toxicity, chronic iron toxicity secondary to multiple transfusions associated with some chronic anemias (e.g., thalassemia). **OFF-LABEL:** Treatment/diagnosis of aluminum toxicity.

PRECAUTIONS

CONTRAINDICATIONS: Severe renal disease, anuria, primary hemochromatosis. **CAUTIONS:** Renal impairment. **Pregnancy Category C.**

INTERACTIONS

DRUG: Vitamin C: May increase effect. **HERBAL:** None known. **FOOD:** None known. **LAB VALUES:** May cause a falsely high total iron-binding capacity (TIBC).

AVAILABILITY (Rx)

INJECTION: 500 mg, 2 g.

ADMINISTRATION/HANDLING

◀ **ALERT** ▶ Reconstitute each 500-mg vial with 2 ml sterile water for injection to provide a concentration of 250 mg/ml.

IV

• For IV infusion, further dilute with 0.9% NaCl, D$_5$W, and administer at no more than 15 mg/kg/hr. • A too rapid IV administration may produce skin flushing, urticaria, hypotension, shock.

IM

• Inject deeply into upper outer quadrant of buttock; may give undiluted.

SUBCUTANEOUS

• Administer subcutaneous very slowly; may give undiluted.

IV INCOMPATIBILITY

Do not mix with any other IV medications.

INDICATIONS/ROUTES/DOSAGE

ACUTE IRON INTOXICATION

IM: ADULTS: Initially, 1 g, then 0.5 g q4h for 2 doses; may give additional doses of

---

0.5 g q4–12h. CHILDREN: 50 mg/kg/dose
q6h. **Maximum:** 6 g/day.
IV: ADULTS: 15 mg/kg/hr. CHILDREN: 15 mg/
kg/hr. **Maximum:** 6 g/day.

CHRONIC IRON OVERLOAD

SUBCUTANEOUS: ADULTS: 1–2 g/day
over 8–24 hr. CHILDREN: 20–50 mg/kg/day
over 8–12 hr. **Maximum:** 2 g/day.
IM: ADULTS: 0.5–1 g/day. Also, 2 g with
each unit blood.
IV: ADULTS, CHILDREN: 2 g after each
unit blood at 15 mg/kg/hr. **Maximum:**
12 g/day.

SIDE EFFECTS

FREQUENT: Pain, induration at injection
site, urine color change (to orange-
rose). **OCCASIONAL:** Abdominal discomfort, diarrhea, leg cramps, impaired
vision.

ADVERSE REACTIONS/ TOXIC EFFECTS

High-frequency hearing loss, tinnitus has
been noted.

NURSING CONSIDERATIONS

BASELINE ASSESSMENT

Assess serum iron levels, total iron-
binding capacity before and during
therapy.

INTERVENTION/EVALUATION

Question for evidence of hearing loss
(neurotoxicity). Periodic slit-lamp ophthalmic exams should be obtained in
those treated for chronic iron overload.
For IV administration, monitor serum
ferritin, iron, TIBC, body weight, growth,
BP. If using subcutaneous technique,
monitor for pruritus, erythema, skin
irritation, edema.

PATIENT/FAMILY TEACHING

• Inform patient medication may
produce discomfort at IM or subcutaneous injection site. • Urine will appear
reddish.

delavirdine mesylate

deh-la-**ver**-deen
(Rescriptor)
**Do not confuse Rescriptor with
Retrovin or Ritonavir.**

◆CLASSIFICATION

PHARMACOTHERAPEUTIC: Non-
nucleoside reverse transcriptase
inhibitor. **CLINICAL:** Antiretroviral
(see pp. 60C, 104C).

ACTION

A nonnucleoside reverse transcriptase
inhibitor that binds directly to HIV-1
reverse transcriptase and blocks RNA-
and DNA-dependent DNA polymerase
activities. Therapeutic Effect: Interrupts HIV replication, slowing the
progression of HIV infection.

PHARMACOKINETICS

Rapidly absorbed after PO administration. Protein binding: 98%. Primarily
distributed in plasma. Metabolized in
the liver. Eliminated in feces and urine.
Half-life: 2–11 hr.

USES

Treatment of HIV infection (in combination with other antivirals).

PRECAUTIONS

CONTRAINDICATIONS: None   known.
CAUTIONS: Hepatic impairment.
⌛ LIFESPAN CONSIDERATIONS: **Preg-
nancy/Lactation:** Unknown if drug
crosses placenta or is distributed in
breast milk. **Pregnancy Category C.
Children:** Safety and efficacy not established in those younger than 16 yr.
Elderly: Safety   and   efficacy   not
established.

INTERACTIONS

DRUG: **Benzodiazepines, calcium channel blockers:** May cause life-threatening adverse reactions. **Carbamazepine, phenobarbital, phenytoin:** May decrease delavirdine blood concentration. **H$_2$ blockers:** May decrease delavirdine absorption. **Rifampin:** May decrease delavirdine blood concentrations. HERBAL: None known. FOOD: None known. LAB VALUES: May increase AST and ALT levels. May decrease neutrophil count.

AVAILABILITY (Rx)

TABLETS: 100 mg, 200 mg.

ADMINISTRATION/HANDLING

PO
• May disperse in water before consumption. • Give without regard to food. • Patients with achlorhydria should take with orange juice, cranberry juice.

INDICATIONS/ROUTES/DOSAGE

HIV INFECTION (IN COMBINATION WITH OTHER ANTIRETROVIRALS)
PO: ADULTS: 400 mg 3 times a day.

SIDE EFFECTS

FREQUENT (18%): Rash, pruritus. OCCASIONAL (greater than 2%): Headache, nausea, diarrhea, fatigue, anorexia.

ADVERSE REACTIONS/ TOXIC EFFECTS

Hepatic failure, severe rash, hemolytic anemia, rhabdomyolysis, erythema multiforme, Stevens-Johnson syndrome and acute kidney failure have been reported.

NURSING CONSIDERATIONS

BASELINE ASSESSMENT

Obtain baseline laboratory testing, especially liver function tests, before initiation of therapy and at periodic intervals during therapy. Offer emotional support.

INTERVENTION/EVALUATION

Assess skin for rash. Question if nausea is noted. Assess pattern of bowel activity and stool consistency. Assess eating pattern; monitor for weight loss. Monitor lab values carefully, particularly liver function.

PATIENT/FAMILY TEACHING

• Do not take any medications, including OTC drugs, without consulting physician. • Small, frequent meals may offset anorexia, nausea. • Delavirdine is not a cure for HIV infection, nor does it reduce risk of transmission to others.

demecarium

(Humorsol)
See Antiglaucoma agents

demeclocycline hydrochloride

deh-meh-clo-**sigh**-clean
(Declomycin)

◆**CLASSIFICATION**

PHARMACOTHERAPEUTIC: Tetracycline. CLINICAL: Antibiotic.

ACTION

A tetracycline antibiotic that inhibits bacterial protein synthesis by binding to ribosomal receptor sites; also inhibits ADH-induced water reabsorption. Therapeutic Effect: Bacteriostatic; also produces water diuresis.

PHARMACOKINETICS

Food and dairy products interfere with absorption. Protein binding: 41%–91%. Metabolized in liver. Excreted in urine.

Removed by hemodialysis. Half-life: 10–15 hr.

USES

Treatment of acne, gonorrhea, pertussis, chronic bronchitis, UTIs, syndrome of inappropriate ADH secretion (SIADH).

PRECAUTIONS

CONTRAINDICATIONS: Children 8 yr and younger, last half of pregnancy. **CAUTIONS:** Renal impairment, sun/ultraviolet exposure (severe photosensitivity reaction).

⌛ **LIFESPAN CONSIDERATIONS: Pregnancy/Lactation:** Crosses placenta; distributed in breast milk. May inhibit skeletal growth of fetus; avoid use in last half of pregnancy. **Pregnancy Category D. Children:** Not recommended in those 8 yr and younger; may cause permanent discoloration of teeth, enamel hypoplasia; may inhibit skeletal growth. **Elderly:** No age-related precautions noted.

INTERACTIONS

DRUG: Antacids containing aluminum, calcium, or magnesium; laxatives containing magnesium; oral iron preparations: Impair the absorption of demeclocycline. **Cholestyramine, colestipol:** May decrease demeclocycline absorption. **Oral contraceptives:** May decrease the effects of oral contraceptives. **HERBAL:** None known. **FOOD: Dairy products:** May decrease demeclocycline absorption. **LAB VALUES:** May increase BUN and serum alkaline phosphatase, amylase, bilirubin, AST, and ALT levels.

AVAILABILITY (Rx)

TABLETS: 150 mg, 300 mg.

ADMINISTRATION/HANDLING

PO
• Give antacids containing aluminum, calcium, or magnesium; laxatives containing magnesium; or oral iron preparations 1–2 hr before or after demeclocycline because they may impair the drug's absorption.

INDICATIONS/ROUTES/DOSAGE

MILD TO MODERATE INFECTIONS, INCLUDING ACNE, PERTUSSIS, CHRONIC BRONCHITIS, AND UTIs
PO: ADULTS, ELDERLY: 150 mg 4 times a day or 300 mg 2 times a day. CHILDREN OLDER THAN 8 YR: 8–12 mg/kg/day in 2–4 divided doses.

UNCOMPLICATED GONORRHEA
PO: ADULTS: Initially, 600 mg, then 300 mg q12h for 4 days for total of 3 g.

SIADH
PO: ADULTS, ELDERLY: Initially, 900–1,200 mg/day in 3–4 divided doses, then decrease dose to 600–900 mg/day in divided doses.

SIDE EFFECTS

FREQUENT: Anorexia, nausea, vomiting, diarrhea, dysphagia, possibly severe photosensitivity, (with moderate to high demeclocycline dosage). **OCCASIONAL:** Urticaria, rash; diabetes insipidus syndrome, marked by polydipsia, polyuria, and weakness (with long-term therapy).

ADVERSE REACTIONS/TOXIC EFFECTS

Superinfection (especially fungal), anaphylaxis, and benign intracranial hypertension occur rarely. Bulging fontanelles occur rarely in infants.

NURSING CONSIDERATIONS

BASELINE ASSESSMENT
Question for history of allergies, especially to tetracyclines.

INTERVENTION/EVALUATION
Determine pattern of bowel activity and stool consistency. Assess food intake, tolerance. Monitor I&O, renal function test results. Assess for rash. Be alert

to superinfection: diarrhea, ulceration or changes of oral mucosa, tongue, anal/genital pruritus. Monitor BP, level of consciousness (LOC) (potential for increased intracranial pressure [ICP]).

PATIENT/FAMILY TEACHING

• Continue antibiotic for full length of treatment. • Space doses evenly. • Take oral doses on empty stomach with full glass of water. • Avoid sun/ultraviolet light exposure.

Demedex, *see torsemide*

Demerol, *see meperidine*

---

denileukin diftitox

den-ee-**lew**-kin
(Ontak)

CLASSIFICATION

PHARMACOTHERAPEUTIC: Biologic response modifier. **CLINICAL:** Antineoplastic (see p. 73C).

ACTION

A cytotoxic fusion protein that targets cells expressing interleukin-2 (IL-2) receptors. After binding to IL-2 receptor, directs cytocidal action to malignant cutaneous T-cell lymphoma (CTCL) cells. Therapeutic Effect: Causes inhibition of protein synthesis and cell death.

USES

Treatment of persistent/recurrent T-cell lymphoma whose malignant cells express the CD25 component of the IL-2 receptor.

PRECAUTIONS

CONTRAINDICATIONS: None known. **CAUTIONS:** Preexisting cardiovascular disease, hypoalbuminemia. **Pregnancy Category C.**

INTERACTIONS

DRUG: None known. HERBAL: None known. FOOD: None known. LAB VALUES: May decrease serum albumin, calcium, potassium, WBC count, Hgb, Hct. Increases serum transaminase level.

AVAILABILITY (Rx)

SOLUTION FOR INJECTION: 150 mcg/ml.

ADMINISTRATION/HANDLING

IV

Reconstitution • Thaw in refrigerator for up to 24 hr or at room temperature for 1–2 hr. • Inject calculated dose into empty infusion bag. No more than 9 ml 0.9% NaCl to be added to each ml denileukin.

Rate of administration • Infuse over 15 min.

Storage • Store frozen. • Solutions for IV infusion stable for 6 hr.

IV INCOMPATIBILITIES

Do not mix with any other IV medications.

INDICATIONS/ROUTES/DOSAGE

CTCL
IV INFUSION: ADULTS: 9 or 18 mcg/kg/day for 5 consecutive days q21days. Infuse over at least 15 min.

SIDE EFFECTS

FREQUENT: Two distinct syndromes occur commonly: A hypersensitivity reaction (69%), consisting of 2 or more of the following: hypotension, back pain, dyspnea, vasodilation,

---

vascular leak syndrome characterized by hypotension, edema, hypoalbuminemia, rash, chest tightness, tachycardia, dysphagia, syncope. Also, a flu-like symptom complex (91%), consisting of 2 or more of the following: fever, chills, nausea, vomiting, diarrhea, myalgia, arthralgia. **OCCASIONAL (25%–10%):** Dizziness, chest pain, vasodilation, decreased weight, rhinitis, pruritus.

ADVERSE REACTIONS/ TOXIC EFFECTS

Pancreatitis, acute renal insufficiency, hematuria, hypothyroidism or hyperthyroidism occur rarely.

NURSING CONSIDERATIONS

BASELINE ASSESSMENT

CBC, blood chemistries (including renal/liver function tests), chest x-ray should be performed before therapy and weekly thereafter. Assess serum albumin level before initiation of each treatment (should be equal to or greater than 3 g/dl).

INTERVENTION/EVALUATION

Monitor serum albumin for hypoalbuminemia (generally occurs 1–2 wk after administration). Monitor for evidence of infection (lowered immune response: sore throat, fever, other vague symptoms).

PATIENT/FAMILY TEACHING

• At home, increase fluid intake (protects against renal impairment). • Do not have immunizations without physician's approval (drug lowers body resistance); avoid contact with those who have recently taken live virus vaccine.

Depacon, see *valproic acid*

Depakene, see *valproic acid*

Depakote, see *valproic acid*

Depakote ER, see *valproic acid*

Depo-Medrol, see *methylprednisolone*

Depo-Provera, see *medroxyprogesterone*

---

desipramine hydrochloride

deh-**sip**-rah-meen

(Apo-Desipramine ✦, Norpramin, Novo-Desipramine ✦)

Do not confuse desipramine with clomipramine, disopyramide, imipramine, or nortriptyline.

◆CLASSIFICATION

PHARMACOTHERAPEUTIC: Tricyclic. **CLINICAL:** Antidepressant (see p. 36C).

ACTION

A tricyclic antidepressant that blocks the reuptake of neurotransmitters, such

---

as norepinephrine and serotonin, at presynaptic membranes, increasing their availability at postsynaptic receptor sites. Also has strong anticholinergic activity. **Therapeutic Effect:** Relieves depression.

PHARMACOKINETICS

Rapidly and well absorbed from the GI tract. Protein binding: 90%. Metabolized in the liver. Primarily excreted in urine. Minimally removed by hemodialysis. **Half-life:** 12–27 hr.

USES

Treatment of various forms of depression, often in conjunction with psychotherapy. **OFF-LABEL:** Treatment of attention deficit hyperactivity disorder, bulimia nervosa, cataplexy associated with narcolepsy, cocaine withdrawal, neurogenic pain, panic disorder.

PRECAUTIONS

CONTRAINDICATIONS: Angle-closure glaucoma, use within 14 days of MAOIs. **CAUTIONS:** Cardiovascular disease, cardiac conduction disturbances, urinary retention, seizure disorders, hyperthyroidism, those taking thyroid replacement therapy.

🔲 LIFESPAN CONSIDERATIONS: **Pregnancy/Lactation:** Crosses placenta. Minimally distributed in breast milk. **Pregnancy Category C. Children:** Not recommended in those 6 yr and younger. Children and adolescents with major depressive disorder (MDD) and other psychiatric disorders are at an increased risk of suicidal thinking and behavior while taking desipramine, especially during the first few months of treatment. **Elderly:** Use lower dosages (higher dosages not tolerated, increases risk of toxicity).

INTERACTIONS

DRUG: **Alcohol, other CNS depressants:** May increase CNS and respiratory depression and the hypotensive effects of desipramine. **Antithyroid agents:** May increase the risk of agranulocytosis. **Cimetidine:** May increase desipramine blood concentration and risk of toxicity. **Clonidine, guanadrel:** May decrease the effects of these drugs. **MAOIs:** May increase the risk of neuroleptic malignant syndrome, hyperpyrexia, hypertensive crisis, and seizures. **Phenothiazines:** May increase the anticholinergic and sedative effects of desipramine. **Phenytoin:** May decrease the desipramine blood concentration. **Sympathomimetics:** May increase the risk of cardiac effects. **HERBAL: St. John's wort:** May increase desipramine's pharmacologic effects and risk of toxicity. **FOOD:** None known. **LAB VALUES:** May alter blood glucose level and EKG readings. Therapeutic serum drug level is 115–300 ng/ml; toxic serum drug level is greater than 400 ng/ml.

AVAILABILITY (Rx)

TABLETS: 10 mg, 25 mg, 50 mg, 75 mg, 100 mg, 150 mg.

ADMINISTRATION/HANDLING

PO
◀ **ALERT** ▶ Make sure at least 14 days elapse between the use of MAOIs and desipramine.
• Give with food or milk if GI distress occurs.

INDICATIONS/ROUTES/DOSAGE

DEPRESSION

PO: ADULTS: 75 mg/day. May gradually increase to 150–200 mg/day. **Maximum:** 300 mg/day. ELDERLY: Initially, 10–25 mg/day. May gradually increase to 75–100 mg/day. **Maximum:** 300 mg/day. CHILDREN OLDER THAN 12 YR: Initially, 25–50 mg/day. May gradually increase to 100 mg/day. **Maximum:** 150 mg/day. CHILDREN 6–12 YR: 1–3 mg/kg/day. **Maximum:** 5 mg/kg/day.

SIDE EFFECTS

FREQUENT: Somnolence, fatigue, dry mouth, blurred vision, constipation, delayed micturition, orthostatic hypotension, diaphoresis, impaired concentration, increased appetite, urine retention. **OCCASIONAL:** GI disturbances (such as nausea, GI distress, metallic taste). **RARE:** Paradoxical reactions (agitation, restlessness, nightmares, insomnia), extrapyramidal symptoms (particularly fine hand tremor).

ADVERSE REACTIONS/ TOXIC EFFECTS

Overdose may produce confusion, seizures, somnolence, arrhythmias, fever, hallucinations, dyspnea, vomiting, and unusual fatigue or weakness. Abrupt discontinuation after prolonged therapy may produce severe headache, malaise, nausea, vomiting, and vivid dreams.

NURSING CONSIDERATIONS

BASELINE ASSESSMENT

For those on long-term therapy, liver/renal function tests, blood counts should be performed periodically. For those at risk for arrhythmias, perform a baseline EKG.

INTERVENTION/EVALUATION

Supervise suicidal-risk patient closely during early therapy (as depression lessens, energy level improves, increasing suicide potential). Assess appearance, behavior, speech pattern, level of interest, mood. Therapeutic serum level: 115–300 ng/ml; toxic serum level: greater than 400 ng/ml. Monitor EKG if patient has history of arrhythmias.

PATIENT/FAMILY TEACHING

• Change positions slowly to avoid hypotensive effect. • Tolerance to postural hypotension, sedative, anticholinergic effects usually develops during early therapy. • Maximum therapeutic effect may be noted in 2–4 wk. • Do not abruptly discontinue medication.

desloratadine

des-low-**rah**-tah-deen

(Aerius ❧, Clarinex, Clarinex Redi-Tabs)

Do not confuse Clarinex with Claritin.

FIXED-COMBINATION(S)

Clarinex-D 24 Hour: desloratadine/pseudoephedrine, (a sympathomimetic): 5 mg/240 mg. **Clarinex-D 12 Hour:** desloratadine/pseudoephedrine: 2.5 mg/ 120 mg.

CLASSIFICATION

PHARMACOTHERAPEUTIC: H_1 antagonist. **CLINICAL:** Nonsedating antihistamine.

ACTION

A nonsedating antihistamine that exhibits selective peripheral histamine H_1 receptor blocking action. Competes with histamine at receptor sites. Therapeutic Effect: Prevents allergic responses mediated by histamine, such as rhinitis and urticaria.

PHARMACOKINETICS

Rapidly and almost completely absorbed from the GI tract. Distributed mainly in liver, lungs, GI tract, and bile. Metabolized in the liver to active metabolite and undergoes extensive first-pass metabolism. Eliminated in urine and feces. Half-life: 27 hr (increased in the elderly and in renal or hepatic impairment).

USES

Relief of nasal symptoms of rhinitis (sneezing, rhinorrhea, itching or tearing of eyes, stuffiness), chronic idiopathic urticaria (hives).

PRECAUTIONS

CONTRAINDICATIONS: None known. **CAUTIONS:** Hepatic impairment. Safety in children younger than 6 yr unknown.

LIFESPAN CONSIDERATIONS: Pregnancy/Lactation: Excreted in breast milk. **Pregnancy Category C. Children/Elderly:** More sensitive to anticholinergic effects (e.g., dry mouth, nose, throat). Safety in children younger than 6 yr unknown.

INTERACTIONS

DRUG: Erythromycin, ketoconazole: May increase desloratadine blood concentration. **HERBAL:** None known. **FOOD:** None known. **LAB VALUES:** May suppress wheal and flare reactions to antigen skin testing unless the drug is discontinued 4 days before testing.

AVAILABILITY (Rx)

TABLETS (CLARINEX): 5 mg. **TABLETS (ORALLY DISINTEGRATING [CLARINEX REDITABS]):** 2.5 mg, 5 mg. **SYRUP (CLARINEX):** 2.5 mg/5 ml.

ADMINISTRATION/HANDLING

PO
• Do not crush or break film-coated tablets.

INDICATIONS/ROUTES/DOSAGE

ALLERGIC RHINITIS, URTICARIA
PO: ADULTS, ELDERLY, CHILDREN OLDER THAN 12 YR: 5 mg once a day. CHILDREN 6–12 YR: 2.5 mg once a day. CHILDREN 1–5 YR: 1.25 mg once a day. CHILDREN 6–11 MO: 1 mg once a day.

DOSAGE IN HEPATIC OR RENAL IMPAIRMENT
Dosage is decreased to 5 mg every other day.

SIDE EFFECTS

FREQUENT (12%): Headache. **OCCASIONAL (3%):** Dry mouth, somnolence. **RARE (less than 3%):** Fatigue, dizziness, diarrhea, nausea.

ADVERSE REACTIONS/TOXIC EFFECTS

None known.

NURSING CONSIDERATIONS

BASELINE ASSESSMENT
Assess lung sounds for wheezing; skin for urticaria, hives.

INTERVENTION/EVALUATION
For upper respiratory allergies, increase fluids to decrease viscosity of secretions, offset thirst, replace loss of fluids from diaphoresis. Monitor symptoms for therapeutic response.

PATIENT/FAMILY TEACHING
• Does not cause drowsiness; however, if blurred vision or eye pain occurs, do not drive or perform activities requiring visual acuity. • Avoid alcohol.

desmopressin

des-moe-**press**-in
(DDAVP, DDAVP Nasal, DDAVP Rhinal Tube, Minirin, Octostim , Stimate)

CLASSIFICATION

PHARMACOTHERAPEUTIC: Synthetic pituitary hormone. **CLINICAL:** Antidiuretic.

ACTION

A synthetic pituitary hormone that increases reabsorption of water by increasing permeability of collecting ducts of the kidneys. Also serves as a plasminogen activator. **Therapeutic Effect:** Increases plasma factor VIII (antihemophilic factor). Decreases urinary output.

PHARMACOKINETICS

Route	Onset	Peak	Duration
PO	1 hr	2–7 hr	6–8 hr
IV	15–30 min	1.5–3 hr	N/A
Intranasal	15 min–1 hr	1–5 hr	5–21 hr

Poorly absorbed after oral or nasal administration. Metabolism: Unknown. **Half-life:** **Oral:** 1.5–2.5 hr. **Intranasal:** 3.3–3.5 hr. **IV:** 0.4–4 hr.

USES

DDAVP Intranasal: Primary nocturnal enuresis, central cranial diabetes insipidus. **Parenteral:** Central cranial diabetes insipidus, hemophilia A, von Willebrand's disease (type I). **Stimate intranasal:** Hemophilia A, von Willebrand's disease (type I). **PO:** Central cranial diabetes insipidus. OFF-LABEL: Prophylaxis and treatment of central diabetes insipidus, treatment of hemophilia A, primary nocturnal enuresis, von Willebrand's disease.

PRECAUTIONS

CONTRAINDICATIONS: Hemophilia A with factor VIII levels less than 5%; hemophilia B; severe type I, type IIB, or platelet-type von Willebrand's disease. **CAUTIONS:** Predisposition to thrombus formation, conditions with fluid or electrolyte imbalance, coronary artery disease, hypertensive cardiovascular disease.

⌛ LIFESPAN CONSIDERATIONS: **Pregnancy Category B. Children:** Caution in neonates, those younger than 3 mo (increased risk of fluid balance problems). Careful fluid restrictions recommended in infants. **Elderly:** Increased risk of hyponatremia, water intoxication.

INTERACTIONS

DRUG: **Carbamazepine, chlorpropamide, clofibrate:** May increase the effects of desmopressin. **Demeclocycline, lithium, norepinephrine:** May decrease effects of desmopressin. HERBAL: None known. FOOD: None known. LAB VALUES: None known.

AVAILABILITY (Rx)

TABLETS (DDAVP): 0.1 mg, 0.2 mg. **INJECTION (DDAVP):** 4 mcg/ml. **NASAL**

SOLUTION (DDAVP): 100 mcg/ml. **NASAL SPRAY:** 1.5 mg/ml (150 mcg/spray) (Stimate), 100 mcg/ml (10 mcg/spray) (DDAVP).

ADMINISTRATION/HANDLING

 IV

Reconstitution • For IV infusion, dilute in 10–50 ml 0.9% NaCl.

Rate of administration • Infuse over 15–30 min. • For preop use, administer 30 min before procedure. • Monitor BP, pulse during IV infusion. • IV dose = $\frac{1}{10}$ intranasal dose.

Storage • Refrigerate. Stable for 2 wk at room temperature.

SUBCUTANEOUS

• Estimate response by adequate sleep duration. • Morning and evening doses should be adjusted separately.

INTRANASAL

• Refrigerate DDAVP nasal solution and Stimate nasal spray. Nasal solution and Stimate nasal spray are stable for 3 wk at room temperature if unopened. • DDAVP nasal spray is stable at room temperature. • A calibrated catheter (rhinyle) is used to draw up a measured quantity of desmopressin; with one end inserted in the nose, patient blows on the other end to deposit the solution deep in the nasal cavity. • For infants, young children, obtunded patients, an air-filled syringe may be attached to the catheter to deposit the solution.

INDICATIONS/ROUTES/DOSAGE

PRIMARY NOCTURNAL ENURESIS

PO: CHILDREN 12 YR AND OLDER: 0.2–0.6 mg once before bedtime.

INTRANASAL: CHILDREN 6 YR AND OLDER: Initially, 20 mcg (0.2 ml) at bedtime; use ½ dose in each nostril. Adjust to maximum of 40 mcg/day. Range: 10–40 mcg.

CENTRAL CRANIAL DIABETES INSIPIDUS

PO: ADULTS, ELDERLY, CHILDREN 12 YR AND

OLDER: Initially, 0.05 mg twice a day. Range: 0.1–1.2 mg/day in 2–3 divided doses. CHILDREN YOUNGER THAN 12 YR: Initially, 0.05 mg; then twice a day. Range: 0.1–0.8 mg daily.

IV, SUBCUTANEOUS: ADULTS, ELDERLY, CHILDREN 12 YR AND OLDER: 2–4 mcg/day in 2 divided doses or $\frac{1}{10}$ of maintenance intranasal dose.

INTRANASAL (USE 100 MCG/ML CONCENTRATION): ADULTS, ELDERLY, CHILDREN OLDER THAN 12 YR: 5–40 mcg (0.05–0.4 ml) in 1–3 doses/day. CHILDREN 3 MO–12 YR: Initially, 5 mcg (0.05 ml)/day. Range: 5–30 mcg (0.05–0.3 ml)/day.

HEMOPHILIA A, VON WILLEBRAND'S DISEASE (TYPE I)

IV INFUSION: ADULTS, ELDERLY, CHILDREN WEIGHING MORE THAN 10 KG.: 0.3 mcg/kg diluted in 50 ml 0.9% NaCl. CHILDREN WEIGHING 10 KG AND LESS: 0.3 mcg/kg diluted in 10 ml 0.9% NaCl.

INTRANASAL (USE 1.5 MG/ML CONCENTRATION PROVIDING 150 MCG/ SPRAY): ADULTS, ELDERLY, CHILDREN 12 YR AND OLDER WEIGHING MORE THAN 50 KG: 300 mcg; use 1 spray in each nostril. ADULTS, ELDERLY, CHILDREN 12 YR AND OLDER WEIGHING 50 KG OR LESS: 150 mcg as a single spray.

SIDE EFFECTS

OCCASIONAL: IV: Pain, redness, or swelling at injection site; headache; abdominal cramps; vulval pain; flushed skin; mild BP elevation; nausea with high dosages. **Nasal:** Rhinorrhea, nasal congestion, slight BP elevation.

ADVERSE REACTIONS/ TOXIC EFFECTS

Water intoxication or hyponatremia, marked by headache, somnolence, confusion, decreased urination, rapid weight gain, seizures, and coma, may occur in overhydration. Children, elderly patients, and infants are especially at risk.

NURSING CONSIDERATIONS

BASELINE ASSESSMENT

Establish baselines for BP, pulse, weight, serum electrolytes, urine specific gravity. Check lab values for factor VIII coagulant concentration for hemophilia A, von Willebrand's disease; bleeding times.

INTERVENTION/EVALUATION

Check BP, pulse with IV infusion. Monitor patient weight, fluid intake, urine volume, urine specific gravity, osmolality, serum electrolytes for diabetes insipidus. Assess factor VIII antigen levels, aPTT, factor VIII activity level for hemophilia.

PATIENT/FAMILY TEACHING

• Avoid overhydration. • Teach proper technique for intranasal administration. • Inform physician if headache, shortness of breath, heartburn, nausea, abdominal cramps occur.

---

desonide

(Otic Tridesilon, Tridesilon)
See Corticosteroids: topical (p. 86C)

---

desoximetasone

(Topicort)
See Corticosteroids: topical (p. 86C)

Desyrel, *see trazodone*

Detrol, *see tolterodine*

D

Detrol LA, *see tolterodine*

dexamethasone

dex-a-**meth**-a-sone

(Adrenocot, Cortastat, Cortastat 10, Cortastat LA, Dalalone, Dalalone D.P., Dalalone L.A., Decadron, Decadron 5-12 Pak, Decadron Phosphate Injectable, Decaject, De-Sone LA, Dexacen-4, Dexamethasone Intensol, Dexasone, Dexasone LA, Dexpak Taperpak, Diodex ✦, Hexadrol, Hexadrol Phosphate, Maxidex, Solurex, Solurex LA)

Do not confuse dexamethasone with desoximetasone or dextramethophan, or Maxidex with Maxzide.

FIXED-COMBINATION(S)

Ciprodex Otic: dextramethasone/ ciprofloxacin (antibiotic): 0.1%/ 0.3%. **Dexacidin, Maxitrol:** dexamethasone/neomycin/polymyxin (anti-infectives): 0.1%/3.5 mg/ 10,000 units per g or ml.

✦ CLASSIFICATION

PHARMACOTHERAPEUTIC: Long-acting glucocorticoid. **CLINICAL:** Corticosteroid (see pp. 83C, 86C).

ACTION

A long-acting glucocorticoid that inhibits accumulation of inflammatory cells at inflammation sites, phagocytosis, lysosomal enzyme release and synthesis, and release of mediators of inflammation. Therapeutic Effect: Prevents and suppresses cell and tissue immune reactions and inflammatory process.

PHARMACOKINETICS

Rapidly, completely absorbed from the GI tract after oral administration. Widely distributed. Protein binding: High. Metabolized in the liver. Primarily excreted in urine. Minimally removed by hemodialysis. Half-life: 3–4.5 hr.

USES

Acute exacerbations of chronic allergic disorders, cerebral edema, conditions treated by immunosupression, inflammatory conditions, ototis externa, ophthalmic conditions including corneal injury, inflammatory conditions, infective conjunctivitis. OFF-LABEL: Antiemetic, croup.

PRECAUTIONS

CONTRAINDICATIONS: Active untreated infections, fungal, tuberculosis, or viral diseases of the eye. **CAUTIONS:** Respiratory tuberculosis, untreated systemic infections, ocular herpes simplex, hyperthyroidism, cirrhosis, ulcerative colitis, hypertension, osteoporosis patients at high thromboembolic risk, CHF, seizure disorders, peptic ulcer, diabetes. Prolonged use may result in cataracts, glaucoma.

⧖ LIFESPAN CONSIDERATIONS: **Pregnancy/Lactation:** Crosses placenta. Distributed in breast milk. **Pregnancy Category C (D if used in the first trimester). Children:** Prolonged treatment with high-dose therapy may decrease short-term growth rate, cortisol secretion. **Elderly:** Higher risk for developing hypertension, osteoporosis.

INTERACTIONS

DRUG: **Amphotericin:** May increase hypokalemia. **Digoxin:** May increase digoxin toxicity caused by hypokalemia. **Diuretics, insulin, oral hypoglycemics, potassium supplements:** May decrease the effects of these drugs. **Hepatic enzyme inducers:** May decrease the effects of dexamethasone. **Live-virus vaccines:** May decrease the patient's antibody response to vaccine, increase vaccine side effects, and potentiate virus replication. **HERBAL:** None known. **FOOD:** None known. **LAB VALUES:** May increase blood glucose and serum lipid, amylase, and sodium levels. May decrease serum calcium, potassium, and thyroxine levels.

AVAILABILITY (Rx)

NASAL AEROSOL: 100 mcg. **OPHTHALMIC OINTMENT (DECADRON, MAXIDEX):** 0.05%. **OPHTHALMIC SOLUTION (DECADRON):** 0.1%. **OPHTHALMIC SUSPENSION (MAXIDEX):** 0.1%. **ORAL CONCENTRATE (DEXAMETHASONE INTENSOL):** 1 mg/ml. **ORAL SOLUTION:** 0.5 mg/5 ml, 1 mg/ml. **TABLETS:** 0.25 mg, 0.5 mg (Decadron), 0.75 mg (Decadron, Decadron 5–12 Pak), 1 mg, 1.5 mg (Dexpak Taperpak), 2 mg, 4 mg (Decadron, Hexadrol), 6 mg. **TOPICAL AEROSOL:** 0.01%, 0.04%. **TOPICAL CREAM (DECADRON):** 0.1%. **TOPICAL GEL:** 0.1%. **INJECTABLE SOLUTION:** 4 mg/ml (Adrenocot, Cortastat, Dalalone, Decadron Phosphate Injectable, Decaject, Dexacen-4, Dexasone, Hexadrol Phosphate, Solurex), 10 mg/ml (Cortastat 10, Dexasone, Hexadrol Phosphate). **INJECTABLE SUSPENSION:** 8 mg/ml (Cortastat LA, Dalalone LA, De-Sone LA, Dexasone LA, Solurex LA), 16 mg/ml (Dalalone D.P.).

ADMINISTRATION/HANDLING

 IV

◄ **ALERT** ► Dexamethasone sodium phosphate may be given by IV push or IV infusion.

• For IV push, give over 1–4 min. • For IV infusion, mix with 0.9% NaCl or D_5W and infuse over 15–30 min. • For neonate, solution must be preservative free. • IV solution must be used within 24 hr.

IM

• Give deep IM, preferably in gluteus maximus.

PO

• Give with milk or food.

OPHTHALMIC

• Place finger on lower eyelid and pull out until a pocket is formed between eye and lower lid. • Hold dropper above pocket and place correct number of drops (¼–½ inch ointment) into pocket. • Close eye gently.

Solution: Apply digital pressure to lacrimal sac for 1–2 min (minimizes drainage into nose and throat, reducing risk of systemic effects).

Ointment: Close eye for 1–2 min. Instruct patient to roll eyeball (increases contact area of drug to eye). Remove excess solution or ointment around eye with tissue. • Ointment may be used at night to reduce frequency of solution administration. • As with other corticosteroids, taper dosage slowly when discontinuing.

TOPICAL

• Gently cleanse area before application. • Use occlusive dressings only as ordered. • Apply sparingly and rub into area thoroughly.

⊞ IV INCOMPATIBILITIES

Ciprofloxacin (Cipro), daunorubicin (Cerubidine), idarubicin (Idamycin), midazolam (Versed).

IV COMPATIBILITIES

Aminophylline, cimetidine (Tagamet), cisplatin (Platinol), cyclophosphamide (Cytoxan), cytarabine (Cytosar), docetaxel (Taxotere), doxorubicin (Adriamycin), etoposide (VePesid), granisetron (Kytril), heparin, hydromorphone (Dilaudid), lorazepam (Ativan), morphine, ondansetron (Zofran), paclitaxel (Taxol), potassium chloride, propofol (Diprivan), total parenteral nutrition (TPN).

INDICATIONS/ROUTES/DOSAGE

ANTI-INFLAMMATORY

PO, IV, IM: ADULTS, ELDERLY: 0.75–9 mg/day in divided doses q6–12h. CHILDREN: 0.08–0.3 mg/kg/day in divided doses q6–12h.

CEREBRAL EDEMA

IV: ADULTS, ELDERLY: Initially, 10 mg, then 4 mg (IV or IM) q6h.

PO, IV, IM: CHILDREN: Loading dose of 1–2 mg/kg, then 1–1.5 mg/kg/day in divided doses q4–6h.

NAUSEA AND VOMITING IN CHEMOTHERAPY PATIENTS

IV: ADULTS, ELDERLY: 8–20 mg once, then 4 mg (PO) q4–6h or 8 mg q8h. CHILDREN: 10 mg/m^2/dose (**Maximum:** 20 mg), then 5 mg/m^2/dose q6h.

USUAL TOPICAL DOSAGE

TOPICAL: ADULTS, ELDERLY, CHILDREN: Apply to affected area 3–4 times a day.

PHYSIOLOGIC REPLACEMENT

PO, IV, IM: CHILDREN: 0.03–0.15 mg/kg/day in divided doses q6–12h.

USUAL OPHTHALMIC DOSAGE, OCULAR INFLAMMATORY CONDITIONS

OINTMENT: ADULTS, ELDERLY, CHILDREN: Thin coating 3–4 times/day.

SUSPENSION: ADULTS, ELDERLY, CHILDREN: Initially, 2 drops q1h while awake and q2h at night for 1 day, then reduce to 3–4 times/day.

SIDE EFFECTS

FREQUENT: Inhalation: Cough, dry mouth, hoarseness, throat irritation. **Intranasal:** Burning, mucosal dryness. **Ophthalmic:** Blurred vision. **Systemic:** Insomnia, facial swelling or cushingoid appearance, moderate abdominal distention, indigestion, increased appetite, nervousness, facial flushing, diaphoresis. **OCCASIONAL: Inhalation:** Localized fungal infection, such as thrush. **Intranasal:** Crusting inside nose, nosebleed, sore throat, ulceration of nasal mucosa. **Ophthalmic:** Decreased vision, watering of eyes, eye pain, burning, stinging, redness of eyes, nausea, vomiting. **Systemic:** Dizziness, decreased or blurred vision. **Topical:** Allergic contact dermatitis, purpura or blood-containing blisters, thinning of skin with easy bruising, telangiectasis or raised dark red spots on skin.

RARE: Inhalation: Increased bronchospasm, esophageal candidiasis. **Intranasal:** Nasal and pharyngeal candidiasis, eye pain. **Systemic:** General allergic reaction (such as rash and hives); pain, redness, or swelling at injection site; psychological changes; false sense of well-being; hallucinations; depression.

ADVERSE REACTIONS/ TOXIC EFFECTS

Long-term therapy may cause muscle wasting (especially in the arms and legs), osteoporosis, spontaneous fractures, amenorrhea, cataracts, glaucoma, peptic ulcer disease, and CHF. The ophthalmic form may cause glaucoma, ocular hypertension, and cataracts. Abrupt withdrawal following long-term therapy may cause severe joint pain, severe headache, anorexia, nausea, fever, rebound inflammation, fatigue, weakness, lethargy, dizziness, and orthostatic hypotension.

NURSING CONSIDERATIONS

BASELINE ASSESSMENT

Question for hypersensitivity to any of the corticosteroids. Obtain baselines for height, weight, BP, serum glucose, electrolytes.

INTERVENTION/EVALUATION

Monitor I&O, daily weight. Assess for edema. Evaluate food tolerance and bowel activity. Report hyperacidity promptly. Check vital signs at least twice a day. Be alert to infection: sore throat, fever, vague symptoms. Monitor serum electrolytes. Monitor for hypercalcemia (muscle twitching, cramps), hypokalemia (weakness, muscle cramps, numbness or tingling, especially lower extremities, nausea or vomiting, irritability). Assess emotional status, ability to sleep.

PATIENT/FAMILY TEACHING

• Do not change dose/schedule or stop taking drug. • **Must** taper off gradually under medical supervision. • Notify physician of fever, sore throat, muscle aches, sudden weight gain or edema. • Severe stress (serious infection, surgery, trauma) may require increased dosage. • Inform dentist, other physicians of dexamethasone therapy now or within past 12 mo. • **Topical:** Apply after shower/bath for best absorption.

dexmedetomidine hydrochloride

decks-meh-deh-**tome**-ih-deen
(Precedex)
Do not confuse Precedex with Peridex or Percocet.

•CLASSIFICATION

PHARMACOTHERAPEUTIC: Alpha$_2$-agonist. **CLINICAL:** Nonbarbiturate sedative, hypnotic.

ACTION

A selective alpha$_2$-adrenergic agonist. Therapeutic Effect: Produces analgesic, hypnotic, and sedative effects.

USES

Sedation of initially intubated and mechanically ventilated adults during treatment in intensive care setting. OFF-LABEL: Pain relief, treatment of shivering.

PRECAUTIONS

CONTRAINDICATIONS: None known. **CAUTIONS:** Advanced heart block, severe CHF, impaired hepatic or renal function, hypovolemia. **Pregnancy Category C.**

INTERACTIONS

DRUG: **Anesthetics, opioids, other sedative-hypnotics:** May enhance the effects of dexmedetomidine.

HERBAL: None known. FOOD: None known. LAB VALUES: May increase serum potassium, alkaline phosphatase, AST, and ALT levels.

AVAILABILITY (Rx)

INJECTION: 100 mcg/ml.

ADMINISTRATION/HANDLING

 IV

Reconstitution • Dilute 2 ml of dexmedetomidine with 48 ml 0.9 NaCl.

Rate of administration • Give as maintenance infusion.

Storage • Store at room temperature.

▧ IV INCOMPATIBILITIES

Do not mix dexmedetomidine with any other medications.

INDICATIONS/ROUTES/DOSAGE

SEDATION BEFORE, DURING, AND AFTER INTUBATION AND MECHANICAL VENTILATION WHILE IN ICU
IV: ADULTS: Loading dose of 1 mcg/kg over 10 min followed by maintenance infusion of 0.2–0.7 mcg/kg/hr. ELDERLY: May require decreased dosage. No guidelines available.

SIDE EFFECTS

FREQUENT: Hypotension (30%), nausea (11%). **OCCASIONAL (3%–2%):** Pain, fever, oliguria, thirst.

ADVERSE REACTIONS/ TOXIC EFFECTS

Bradycardia, atrial fibrillation, hypoxia, anemia, pain, and pleural effusion may occur with too-rapid IV infusion.

NURSING CONSIDERATIONS

INTERVENTION/EVALUATION
Monitor EKG for atrial fibrillation, pulse for bradycardia, BP for hypotension, level of sedation. Assess respiratory rate, rhythm. Monitor ventilator settings.

dexmethylphenidate hydrochloride

dex-meth-ill-**fen**-i-date
(Focalin, Focalin XR)

CLASSIFICATION

CLINICAL: CNS stimulant (**Schedule II**).

ACTION

A CNS stimulant that blocks the reuptake of norepinephrine and dopamine into presynaptic neurons, increasing the release of these neurotransmitters into the synaptic cleft. **Therapeutic Effect:** Decreases motor restlessness and fatigue; increases motor activity, mental alertness, and attention span; elevates mood.

PHARMACOKINETICS

Route	Onset	Peak	Duration
PO	N/A	N/A	4–5 hr

Readily absorbed from the GI tract. Plasma concentrations increase rapidly. Metabolized in the liver. Excreted unchanged in urine. **Half-life:** 2.2 hr.

USES

Adjunct in the treatment of attention deficit hyperactivity disorder (ADHD) with moderate to severe distractability, short attention spans, hyperactivity, emotional impulsivity in children 6 yr and older.

PRECAUTIONS

CONTRAINDICATIONS: Diagnosis or family history of Tourette syndrome; glaucoma; history of marked agitation, anxiety, or tension; motor tics; use within 14 days of MAOIs. **CAUTIONS:** Cardiovascular disease, seizure disorder, psychosis. Avoid use in those with a history of substance abuse.

⧗ **LIFESPAN CONSIDERATIONS: Pregnancy/Lactation:** Unknown if excreted in breast milk. **Pregnancy Category C. Children:** May be more susceptible to developing anorexia, insomnia, abdominal pain, weight loss. Chronic use may inhibit growth. In psychotic children, may exacerbate symptoms of behavior disturbance, thought disorder. **Elderly:** No age-related precautions noted.

INTERACTIONS

DRUG: Amitriptyline, phenobarbital, phenytoin, primidone: Dosage of these drugs may need to be decreased. **MAOIs:** May increase the effects of dexmethylphenidate. **Other CNS stimulants:** May have an additive effect. **Warfarin:** May inhibit the metabolism of warfarin. **HERBAL:** None known. **FOOD:** None known. **LAB VALUES:** None known.

AVAILABILITY (Rx)

TABLETS (FOCALIN): 2.5 mg, 5 mg, 10 mg. **CAPSULES (EXTENDED-RELEASE [FOCALIN XR]):** 5 mg, 10 mg, 20 mg.

ADMINISTRATION/HANDLING

PO

• Do not give drug in afternoon or evening (causes insomnia). • Tablets may be crushed. • Give without regard to food. • Swallow extended-release capsules whole; do not chew, crush, or divide tablets. • May sprinkle contents of extended-release capsules on a small amount of applesauce. • Give extended-release capsules once each day in the morning, before breakfast.

INDICATIONS/ROUTES/DOSAGE

ADHD

PO (PATIENTS NEW TO DEXMETHYLPHENIDATE OR METHYLPHENIDATE): ADULTS, ELDERLY: 2.5 mg twice a day (5 mg/day). May adjust dosage

---

in 2.5- to 5-mg increments. **Maximum:** 20 mg/day.

PO (PATIENTS CURRENTLY TAKING METHYLPHENIDATE): ADULTS, ELDERLY: Half the methylphenidate dosage. **Maximum:** 20 mg/day.

PO [EXTENDED-RELEASE (PATIENTS NEW TO DEXMETHYLPHENIDATE OR METHYLPHENIDATE)]: ADULTS, ELDERLY: Initially, 10 mg/day. CHILDREN: Initially, 5 mg/day. May increase dosage at weekly intervals. **Maximum:** 20 mg/day.

PO [EXTENDED-RELEASE (PATIENTS CURRENTLY TAKING METHYLPHENIDATE)]: ADULTS, ELDERLY: Half the methylphenidate dosage. **Maximum:** 20 mg/day. Patients using Focalin may be switched to the same daily dose for Focalin XR.

SIDE EFFECTS

FREQUENT: Abdominal pain, nausea, anorexia, fever. **OCCASIONAL:** Tachycardia, arrhythmias, palpitations, insomnia, twitching. **RARE:** Blurred vision, rash, arthralgia.

ADVERSE REACTIONS/ TOXIC EFFECTS

Withdrawal after prolonged therapy may unmask symptoms of the underlying disorder. Dexmethylphenidate may lower the seizure threshold in those with a history of seizures. Overdose produces excessive sympathomimetic effects, including vomiting, tremor, hyperreflexia, seizures, confusion, hallucinations, and diaphoresis. Prolonged administration to children may delay growth. Neuroleptic malignant syndrome occurs rarely.

NURSING CONSIDERATIONS

INTERVENTION/EVALUATION

CBC, differential, platelet count should be performed routinely during therapy. If paradoxical return of attention deficit occurs, dosage should be reduced or discontinued. Weigh pediatric patient regularly to detect delayed growth.

PATIENT/FAMILY TEACHING

• Avoid tasks that require alertness, motor skills until response to drug is established. • Report any increase in seizures. • The last dose should be given several hours before bedtime to prevent insomnia. • Report anxiety, fever.

dexrazoxane

dex-ray-**zoks**-ane
(Zinecard)

CLASSIFICATION

PHARMACOTHERAPEUTIC: Cytoprotective agent. **CLINICAL:** Antineoplastic.

ACTION

An antineoplastic adjunct and cytoprotective agent that binds to intracellular iron in myocardial cell membranes preventing the generation of free radicals by anthracyclines such as doxorubicin. Therapeutic Effect: Protects against anthracycline-induced cardiomyopathy.

PHARMACOKINETICS

Rapidly distributed after IV administration. Not bound to plasma proteins. Primarily excreted in urine. Removed by peritoneal dialysis. Half-life: 2.1–2.5 hr.

USES

Reduction of incidence, severity of cardiomyopathy associated with doxorubicin therapy in women with metastatic breast cancer. Not recommended with initiation of doxorubicin therapy.

PRECAUTIONS

CONTRAINDICATIONS: Hypersensitivity to nonanthracycline chemotherapy regimens. **CAUTIONS:** Chemotherapeutic agents that are additive to myelosuppression, concurrent fluorouracil, adriamycin, cyclophosphamide (FAC) therapy.

⏳ **LIFESPAN CONSIDERATIONS: Pregnancy/Lactation:** May be embryotoxic, teratogenic. Unknown if distributed in breast milk. Breast-feeding not recommended. **Pregnancy Category C. Children:** Safety and efficacy not established. **Elderly:** Information not available.

INTERACTIONS

DRUG: Concurrent FAC (5-fluorouracil, adriamycin, cyclophosphamide) therapy: May produce severe blood dyscrasias. **HERBAL:** None known. **FOOD:** None known. **LAB VALUES:** Concurrent FAC therapy may produce abnormal liver or renal function test results.

AVAILABILITY (Rx)

POWDER FOR INJECTION: 250 mg (10 mg/ml reconstituted in 25-ml single-use vial), 500 mg (10 mg/ml reconstituted in 50-ml single-use vial).

ADMINISTRATION/HANDLING

◀ **ALERT** ▶ Do not mix with other drugs. Use caution in handling and preparation of reconstituted solution (glove use recommended).

 IV

Reconstitution • Reconstitute with 0.167 molar (M/6) sodium lactate injection to give concentration of 10 mg dexrazoxane for each ml of sodium lactate. • May further dilute with 0.9% NaCl or D_5W. Concentration should range from 1.3–5 mg/ml.

Rate of administration • Give reconstituted solution by slow IV push or IV infusion over 15–30 min. • After infusion is completed, and before a total elapsed time of 30 min from beginning of dexrazoxane infusion, give IV injection of doxorubicin.

Storage • Store vials at room temperature. • Reconstituted solution is stable for 6 hr at room temperature or if refrigerated. Discard unused solution.

🎞 IV INCOMPATIBILITIES

Don't mix dexrazoxane with other medications.

INDICATIONS/ROUTES/DOSAGE

REDUCTION OF INCIDENCE AND SEVERITY OF CARDIOMYOPATHY ASSOCIATED WITH DOXORUBICIN THERAPY IN WOMEN WITH METASTATIC BREAST CANCER
IV: ADULTS, CHILDREN: Recommended dosage ratio is 10 parts dexrazoxane to 1 part doxorubicin (for example, 500 mg/m² dexrazoxane for every 50 mg/m² doxorubicin).

SIDE EFFECTS

FREQUENT: Alopecia, nausea, vomiting, fatigue, malaise, anorexia, stomatitis, fever, infection, diarrhea. **OCCASIONAL:** Pain at injection site, neurotoxicity, phlebitis, dysphagia, streaking or erythema at injection site. **RARE:** Urticaria, skin reaction.

ADVERSE REACTIONS/ TOXIC EFFECTS

Patients receiving FAC therapy concurrently with dexrazoxane are at increased risk for severe leukopenia, granulocytopenia, and thrombocytopenia. In case of overdose, excess dexrazoxane can be removed with peritoneal dialysis or hemodialysis.

NURSING CONSIDERATIONS

BASELINE ASSESSMENT

Use gloves when preparing solution. If powder/solution comes in contact with skin, wash immediately with soap and water. Antiemetics may be effective in preventing, treating nausea.

INTERVENTION/EVALUATION

Frequently monitor CBC with differential for evidence of blood dyscrasias. Assess for stomatitis (burning/erythema of oral mucosa at inner margin of lips, sore throat, difficulty swallowing). Monitor hematologic status, renal/hepatic function studies, cardiac function. Assess pattern of daily bowel activity/stool consistency. Monitor for hematologic toxicity (fever, signs of local infection, unusual bruising/bleeding from any site).

PATIENT/FAMILY TEACHING

• Alopecia is reversible, but new hair growth may have different color/texture. • New hair growth resumes 2–3 mo after last therapy dose. • Maintain fastidious oral hygiene. • Promptly report fever, sore throat, signs of local infection. • Contact physician if persistent nausea/vomiting continues at home.

dextran, low molecular weight (dextran 40)

dex-tran
(Gentran LMD, Rheomacrodex ✦)

dextran, high molecular weight (dextran 75)

(Gentran, Macrodex)

Do not confuse Gentran with Genprine.

◆CLASSIFICATION

PHARMACOTHERAPEUTIC: Branched polysaccharide. **CLINICAL:** Plasma volume expander.

ACTION

A branched polysaccharide that produces plasma volume expansion due to high colloidal osmotic effect. Draws interstitial fluid into the intravascular space. May also increase blood flow in microcirculation. **Therapeutic Effect:** Increases central venous pressure, cardiac output, stroke volume, BP, urine output, capillary perfusion, and pulse pressure. Decreases heart rate, peripheral resistance, and blood viscosity. Corrects hypovolemia.

USES

Fluid replacement, blood volume expander in treatment of hypovolemia, shock, impending shock.

PRECAUTIONS

CONTRAINDICATIONS: Hypervolemia, renal failure, severe bleeding disorders, severe CHF, severe thrombocytopenia. **CAUTIONS:** Those with extreme dehydration, chronic hepatic disease.

⧗ LIFESPAN CONSIDERATIONS: **Pregnancy/Lactation:** Crosses placenta; unknown if distributed in breast milk. **Pregnancy Category C. Children:** No age-related precautions noted. **Elderly:** No age-related precautions noted.

INTERACTIONS

DRUG: None known. **HERBAL:** None known. **FOOD:** None known. **LAB VALUES:** Prolongs bleeding time and depresses platelet count. Decreases clotting factors V, VIII, and IX.

AVAILABILITY (Rx)

INJECTION (HIGH MOLECULAR WEIGHT [GENTRAN]): 6% dextran 70 in 500 ml 0.9% NaCl. **INJECTION (LOW MOLECULAR WEIGHT [GENTRAN LMD]):** 10% dextran 40 in 500 ml D₅W, 10% dextran 40 in 500 ml 0.9% NaCl.

ADMINISTRATION/HANDLING
 IV

Rate of administration • Give by IV infusion only. • Monitor patient closely during first 15 min of infusion for anaphylactoid reaction. Monitor vital signs q5min. • Monitor urine flow rates during administration (if oliguria/anuria occurs, dextran 40 should be discontinued and osmotic diuretic given [minimizes vascular overloading]). • Monitor central venous pressure (CVP) when given by rapid infusion. If there is a precipitous rise in CVP, immediately discontinue drug (overexpansion of blood volume). • Monitor BP diligently during infusion; if marked hypotension occurs, stop infusion immediately (imminent anaphylactic reaction). • If evidence of blood volume overexpansion occurs, discontinue drug until blood volume adjusts via diuresis.

Storage • Store at room temperature. • Use only clear solutions. • Discard partially used containers.

⊞ IV INCOMPATIBILITIES
Do not add medications to dextran solution.

INDICATIONS/ROUTES/DOSAGE
VOLUME EXPANSION, SHOCK
IV: ADULTS, ELDERLY: 500–1,000 ml at a rate of 20–40 ml/min. **Maximum:** 20 ml/kg for first 24 hr, and 10 ml/kg thereafter. CHILDREN: Total dose not to exceed 20 ml/kg on day 1 and 10 ml/kg/day thereafter.

SIDE EFFECTS
OCCASIONAL: Mild hypersensitivity reaction, including urticaria, nasal congestion, wheezing.

ADVERSE REACTIONS/TOXIC EFFECTS
Severe or fatal anaphylaxis, manifested by marked hypotension and cardiac or respiratory arrest, may occur early during IV infusion, generally in those not previously exposed to IV dextran.

INTERVENTION/EVALUATION
Monitor urine output closely (increased output generally occurs in oliguric patients after dextran administration). If no increase is observed after 500 ml dextran is infused, discontinue drug until diuresis occurs. Monitor for fluid overload (peripheral and/or pulmonary edema, impending CHF symptoms). Assess lung sounds for rales. Monitor CVP (detects overexpansion of blood volume). Monitor vital signs and observe closely for allergic reaction. Assess for bleeding, especially following surgery or in those on anticoagulant therapy (overt bleeding, especially at surgical site, bruising, petechiae development).

dextroamphetamine sulfate

dex-troe-am-**fet**-a-meen

(Dexedrine, Dexedrine Spansule, Dextrostat)

Do not confuse dextroamphetamine with dextromethorphan, or Dexedrine with Dextran or Excedrin.

•CLASSIFICATION
PHARMACOTHERAPEUTIC: Amphetamine (**Schedule II**). **CLINICAL:** CNS stimulant.

ACTION
An amphetamine that enhances the action of dopamine and norepinephrine by blocking their reuptake from synapses; also inhibits monoamine oxidase and facilitates the release of catecholamines. **Therapeutic Effect:** Increases motor activity and mental alertness; decreases motor restlessness, drowsiness, and fatigue; suppresses appetite.

PHARMACOKINETICS

Well absorbed following PO administration. Metabolized in liver. Excreted in urine. Removed by hemodialysis. Half-life: 7–34 hr.

USES

Treatment of narcolepsy; treatment of attention deficit disorder (ADD) in hyperactive children; short-term treatment to assist caloric restriction in exogenous obesity.

PRECAUTIONS

CONTRAINDICATIONS: Advanced arteriosclerosis, agitated states, glaucoma, history of drug abuse, hypersensitivity to sympathomimetic amines, hyperthyroidism, moderate to severe hypertension, symptomatic cardiovascular disease, use within 14 days of MAOIs. **CAUTIONS:** Elderly, debilitated, tartrazine-sensitive patients.

⌛ LIFESPAN CONSIDERATIONS: **Pregnancy/Lactation:** Distributed in breast milk. **Pregnancy Category C. Children:** - Safety and efficacy not established in children younger than 3 yr. **Elderly:** Age-related cardiovascular, cerebrovascular disease, and hepatic or renal impairment may increase risk of side effects.

INTERACTIONS

DRUG: **Beta blockers:** May increase the risk of bradycardia, heart block, and hypertension. **Digoxin:** May increase the risk of arrhythmias. **MAOIs:** May prolong and intensify the effects of dextroamphetamine. **Meperidine:** May increase the risk of hypotension, respiratory depression, seizures, and vascular collapse. **Other CNS stimulants:** May increase the effects of dextroamphetamine. **Thyroid hormones:** May increase the effects of either drug. **Tricyclic antidepressants:** May increase cardiovascular effects. HERBAL: None known. FOOD: None known. LAB VALUES: May increase plasma corticosteroid concentration.

AVAILABILITY (Rx)

CAPSULES (SUSTAINED-RELEASE [DEXEDRINE SPANSULE]): 5 mg, 10 mg, 15 mg. **TABLETS:** 5 mg (Dexedrine), 10 mg (Dexedrine, Dextrostat).

INDICATIONS/ROUTES/DOSAGE
NARCOLEPSY

PO: ADULTS, CHILDREN OLDER THAN 12 YR: Initially, 10 mg/day. Increase by 10 mg/day at weekly intervals until therapeutic response is achieved. CHILDREN 6–12 YR: Initially, 5 mg/day. Increase by 5 mg/day at weekly intervals until therapeutic response is achieved. **Maximum:** 60 mg/day.

ATTENTION DEFICIT HYPERACTIVITY DISORDER (ADHD)

PO: CHILDREN 6 YR AND OLDER: Initially, 5 mg once or twice a day. Increase by 5 mg/day at weekly intervals until therapeutic response is achieved. CHILDREN 3–5 YR: Initially, 2.5 mg/day. Increase by 2.5 mg/day at weekly intervals until therapeutic response is achieved. Range: 0.1–0.5 mg/kg/dose. **Maximum:** 40 mg/day.

APPETITE SUPPRESSANT

PO: ADULTS: 5–30 mg daily in divided doses of 5–10 mg each, given 30–60 min before meals; or 1 extended-release capsule in the morning.

SIDE EFFECTS

FREQUENT: Irregular pulse, increased motor activity, talkativeness, nervousness, mild euphoria, insomnia. **OCCASIONAL:** Headache, chills, dry mouth, GI distress, worsening depression in patients who are clinically depressed, tachycardia, palpitations, chest pain, dizziness, decreased appetite.

ADVERSE REACTIONS/ TOXIC EFFECTS

Overdose may produce skin pallor or flushing, arrhythmias, and psychosis. Abrupt withdrawal after prolonged use of high doses may produce lethargy lasting for weeks. Prolonged administration to children with ADHD may inhibit growth.

NURSING CONSIDERATIONS

INTERVENTION/EVALUATION

Monitor for CNS overstimulation, increase in BP, weight loss.

PATIENT/FAMILY TEACHING

• Normal dosage levels may produce tolerance to drug's anorexic mood-elevating effects within a few weeks. • Avoid tasks that require alertness, motor skills until response to drug is established. • Dry mouth may be relieved with sugarless gum, sips of tepid water. • Take early in day. • May mask extreme fatigue. • Report pronounced anxiety, dizziness, decreased appetite, dry mouth.

DHEA

Also known as prasterone.

◆ CLASSIFICATION

HERBAL: See Appendix G.

ACTION

Produced in adrenal glands and liver, metabolized to androstenedione, major precursor to androgens and estrogens. Also produced in the CNS and concentrated in the limbic regions; may function as an excitatory neuroregulator. **Effect:** Androgen or estrogen-like hormonal effects may be responsible for DHEA benefits.

USES

Used for increasing strength, energy, muscle mass; stimulation of immune system; improving cognitive function and memory; improving depressed mood/fatigue in HIV patients. Treatment of atherosclerosis, hyperglycemia, cancer; prevention of osteoporosis; increase bone mineral density.

PRECAUTIONS

CONTRAINDICATIONS: None known. **CAUTIONS:** May increase risk of prostate, breast, hormone-sensitive cancers. Avoid use in those with breast, uterine, ovarian cancer; endometriosis; uterine fibroids; diabetes (can increase insulin resistance/sensitivity); depression (may increase risk of adverse psychiatric effects).

⧖ **LIFESPAN CONSIDERATIONS: Pregnancy/Lactation:** May adversely affect pregnancy by increasing androgen levels; avoid use. **Children:** Safety and efficacy not established. **Elderly:** Age-related hepatic impairment may require dosage adjustment.

INTERACTIONS

DRUG: Estrogen/androgen therapy: DHEA use may interfere with estrogen/androgen therapy. **Triazolam:** Concentration may increase. **HERBAL:** None known. **FOOD:** None known. **LAB VALUES:** None known.

AVAILABILITY (OTC)

CAPSULES: 25 mg. **TABLETS:** 25 mg.

INDICATIONS/ROUTES/DOSAGE

DEPRESSION
PO: ADULTS, ELDERLY: 30–90 mg/day.

USUAL ADULT DOSAGE
PO: ADULTS, ELDERLY: 25–50 mg/day.

SIDE EFFECTS

Acne, hair loss, hirsutism, voice deepening, insulin resistance, altered menstrual cycle, hypertension, abdominal pain, fatigue, headache, nasal congestion.

ADVERSE REACTIONS/ TOXIC EFFECTS

None known.

NURSING CONSIDERATIONS

BASELINE ASSESSMENT

Assess for hormone-sensitive tumors (may stimulate growth). Avoid use of hormone replacement therapy.

INTERVENTION/EVALUATION

Assess changes in mood, sleep pattern. Monitor changes in aggressiveness, irritability, restlessness.

PATIENT/FAMILY TEACHING

• Avoid use in pregnancy/lactation; concurrent hormone replacement therapy. • Lower dosage if acne develops.

Diabeta, *see glyburide*

---

diazepam

dye-**az**-e-pam

(Apo-Diazepam ✤, Diastat, Diastat Pediatric, Diazemuls ✤, Dizac, Valium, Vivol ✤)

Do not confuse diazepam with diazoxide or Ditropan, or Valium with Valcyte.

CLASSIFICATION

PHARMACOTHERAPEUTIC: Benzodiazepine (**Schedule IV**). **CLINICAL:** Antianxiety, skeletal muscle relaxant, anticonvulsant (see pp. 11C, 34C, 138C).

ACTION

A benzodiazepine that depresses all levels of the CNS by enhancing the action of gamma-aminobutyric acid, a major inhibitory neurotransmitter in the brain. Therapeutic Effect: Produces anxiolytic effect, elevates the seizure threshold, produces skeletal muscle relaxation.

PHARMACOKINETICS

Route	Onset	Peak	Duration
PO	30 min	1–2 hr	2–3 hr
IV	1–5 min	15 min	15–60 min
IM	15 min	30–90 min	30–90 min

Well absorbed from the GI tract. Widely distributed. Protein binding: 98%. Metabolized in the liver to active metabolite. Excreted in urine. Minimally removed by hemodialysis. Half-life: 20–70 hr (increased in hepatic dysfunction and the elderly).

USES

Short-term relief of anxiety symptoms, preanesthetic medication, relief of acute alcohol withdrawal. Adjunct for relief of acute musculoskeletal conditions, treatment of seizures (IV route used for termination of status epilepticus). **Gel:** Control of increased seizure activity in refractory epilepsy in those on stable regimens. OFF-LABEL: Treatment of panic disorder, tension headache, tremors.

PRECAUTIONS

CONTRAINDICATIONS: Angle-closure glaucoma, coma, preexisting CNS depression, respiratory depression, severe, uncontrolled pain. **CAUTIONS:** Those receiving other CNS depressants, renal or hepatic impairment, hypoalbuminemia.

⌛ LIFESPAN CONSIDERATIONS: **Pregnancy/Lactation:** Crosses placenta. Distributed in breast milk. May increase risk of fetal abnormalities if administered during first trimester of pregnancy. Chronic ingestion during pregnancy may produce withdrawal symptoms, CNS depression in neonates. **Pregnancy Category D. Children/Elderly:** Use small initial doses with gradual increases to avoid ataxia, excessive sedation.

INTERACTIONS

DRUG: **Alcohol, other CNS depressants:** May increase CNS depression. HERBAL: **Kava kava, valerian:** May increase CNS depression. FOOD: None known. LAB VALUES: May elevate serum LDH, alkaline phosphatase, bilirubin, AST, and ALT levels. May produce abnormal renal function test results. Therapeutic serum drug level is 0.5–2 mcg/ml; toxic serum drug level is greater than 3 mcg/ml.

AVAILABILITY (Rx)

ORAL CONCENTRATE (DIAZEPAM INTENSOL): 5 mg/ml. **ORAL SOLUTION:** 5 mg/5 ml. **TABLETS (VALIUM):** 2 mg, 5 mg, 10 mg. **INJECTION:** 5 mg/ml. **RECTAL GEL (DIASTAT):** 5 mg/ml.

ADMINISTRATION/HANDLING

 IV

Rate of administration • Give by IV push into tubing of a flowing IV solution as close to the vein insertion point as possible. • Administer directly into a large vein (reduces risk of thrombosis and phlebitis). Do not use small veins (e.g., wrist or dorsum of hand). • Administer IV at rate not exceeding 5 mg/min. For children, give over a 3-min period (a too rapid IV may result in hypotension, respiratory depression). • Monitor respirations q5–15min for 2 hr.

Storage • Store at room temperature.

IM
• Injection may be painful. Inject deeply into deltoid muscle.

PO
• Give without regard to meals. • Dilute oral concentrate with water, juice, carbonated beverages; may also be mixed in semisolid food (applesauce, pudding). • Tablets may be crushed. • Do not crush or break capsule.

⬛ IV INCOMPATIBILITIES

Amphotericin B complex (Abelcet, AmBisome, Amphotec), cefepime (Maxipime), diltiazem (Cardizem), fluconazole (Diflucan), foscarnet (Foscavir), heparin, hydrocortisone (Solu-Cortef), hydromorphone (Dilaudid), meropenem (Merrem IV), potassium chloride, propofol (Diprivan), vitamins.

IV COMPATIBILITIES

Dobutamine (Dobutrex), fentanyl, morphine.

INDICATIONS/ROUTES/DOSAGE

ANXIETY, SKELETAL MUSCLE RELAXATION

PO: ADULTS: 2–10 mg 2–4 times a day. ELDERLY: 2–5 mg 2–4 times a day. CHILDREN: 0.12–0.8 mg/kg/day in divided doses q6–8h.

IV, IM: ADULTS: 2–10 mg repeated in 3–4 hr. CHILDREN: 0.04–0.3 mg/kg/dose q2–4h. **Maximum:** 0.6 mg/kg in an 8-hr period.

PREANESTHESIA

IV: ADULTS, ELDERLY: 5–15 mg 5–10 min before procedure. CHILDREN: 0.2–0.3 mg/kg. **Maximum:** 10 mg.

ALCOHOL WITHDRAWAL

PO: ADULTS, ELDERLY: 10 mg 3–4 times during first 24 hr, then reduced to 5–10 mg 3–4 times a day as needed. IV, IM: ADULTS, ELDERLY: Initially, 10 mg, followed by 5–10 mg q3–4h.

STATUS EPILEPTICUS

IV: ADULTS, ELDERLY: 5–10 mg q10–15min up to 30 mg/8 hr. CHILDREN 5 YR AND OLDER: 0.05–0.3 mg/kg/dose q15–30min. **Maximum:** 10 mg/dose. CHILDREN 1 MO TO YOUNGER THAN 5 YR: 0.05–0.3 mg/kg/dose q15–30min. **Maximum:** 5 mg/dose.

CONTROL OF INCREASED SEIZURE ACTIVITY IN PATIENTS WITH REFRACTORY EPILEPSY WHO ARE ON STABLE REGIMENS OF ANTICONVULSANTS

RECTAL GEL: ADULTS, CHILDREN 12 YR AND OLDER: 0.2 mg/kg; may be repeated

---

✒ see color pill atlas   ✒ herb   underlined – top prescribed drug

in 4–12 hr. CHILDREN 6–11 YR: 0.3 mg/kg; may be repeated in 4–12 hr. CHILDREN 2–5 YR: 0.5 mg/kg; may be repeated in 4–12 hr.

SIDE EFFECTS

FREQUENT: Pain with IM injection, somnolence, fatigue, ataxia. **OCCASIONAL:** Slurred speech, orthostatic hypotension, headache, hypoactivity, constipation, nausea, blurred vision. **RARE:** Paradoxical CNS reactions, such as hyperactivity or nervousness in children and excitement or restlessness in the elderly or debilitated (generally noted during first 2 wk of therapy, particularly in presence of uncontrolled pain).

ADVERSE REACTIONS/ TOXIC EFFECTS

IV administration may produce pain, swelling, thrombophlebitis, and carpal tunnel syndrome. Abrupt or too-rapid withdrawal may result in pronounced restlessness, irritability, insomnia, hand tremor, abdominal or muscle cramps, diaphoresis, vomiting, and seizures. Abrupt withdrawal in patients with epilepsy may produce an increase in the frequency or severity of seizures. Overdose results in somnolence, confusion, diminished reflexes, and coma.

NURSING CONSIDERATIONS

BASELINE ASSESSMENT

Assess BP, pulse, respirations immediately before administration. Patient must remain recumbent for up to 3 hr (individualized) after parenteral administration to reduce hypotensive effect. **Anxiety:** Assess autonomic response (cold, clammy hands, diaphoresis), motor response (agitation, trembling, tension). **Musculoskeletal spasm:** Record onset, type, location, duration of pain. Check for immobility, stiffness, swelling. **Seizures:** Review history of seizure disorder (length, intensity, frequency, duration, level of consciousness

[LOC]). Observe frequently for recurrence of seizure activity. Initiate seizure precautions.

INTERVENTION/EVALUATION

Monitor heart rate, respiratory rate, BP. Assess children, elderly for paradoxical reaction, particularly during early therapy. Evaluate for therapeutic response: decrease in intensity and frequency of seizures; calm, facial expression, decreased restlessness; decreased intensity of skeletal muscle pain. Therapeutic serum level: 0.5–2 mcg/ml; toxic serum level: greater than 3 mcg/ml.

PATIENT/FAMILY TEACHING

• Avoid alcohol. • Limit caffeine. • May cause drowsiness, impair ability to perform activities requiring mental alertness (e.g., driving). • May be habit forming. • Avoid abrupt discontinuation after prolonged use.

dibucaine

(Nupercainal)
See Anesthetics: local

diclofenac

dye-**klo**-feh-nak
(Cataflam, Diclotec ❧, Novo-Difenac ❧, Solaraze, Voltaren, Voltaren Ophthalmic, Voltaren XR)
Do not confuse diclofenac with Diflucan or Duphalac, or Voltaren with Verelan.

FIXED-COMBINATION(S)

Arthrotec: diclofenac/misoprostol (an antisecretory gastric protectant): 50 mg/200 mcg; 75 mg/200 mcg.

◆CLASSIFICATION

PHARMACOTHERAPEUTIC: Nonsteroidal anti-inflammatory. **CLINICAL:** Analgesic, anti-inflammatory (see p. 116C).

ACTION

An NSAID that inhibits prostaglandin synthesis, reducing the intensity of pain. Also constricts the iris sphincter. May inhibit angiogenesis (the formation of blood vessels) by inhibiting substance P or blocking the angiogenic effects of prostaglandin E. **Therapeutic Effect:** Produces analgesic and anti-inflammatory effects. Prevents miosis during cataract surgery. May reduce angiogenesis in inflamed tissue.

PHARMACOKINETICS

Route	Onset	Peak	Duration
PO	30 min	2–3 hr	Up to 8 hr

Completely absorbed from the GI tract; penetrates cornea after ophthalmic administration (may be systemically absorbed). Protein binding: greater than 99%. Widely distributed. Metabolized in the liver. Primarily excreted in urine. Minimally removed by hemodialysis. **Half-life:** 1.2–2 hr.

USES

Oral: (Immediate-release): Treatment of rheumatoid arthritis, osteoarthritis, ankylosing spondylitis, primary dysmenorrhea. (Delayed-release): Treatment of rheumatoid arthritis, osteoarthritis, ankylosing spondylitis. (Extended-release): Treatment of rheumatoid arthritis, osteoarthritis. **Ophthalmic:** Treatment of photophobia and pain in patients undergoing corneal refractive surgery. **Topical:** Treatment of actinic keratoses. **OFF-LABEL:** Treatment of vascular headaches (oral); to reduce the occurrence and severity of cystoid macular edema after cataract surgery (ophthalmic form).

PRECAUTIONS

CONTRAINDICATIONS: Hypersensitivity to aspirin, diclofenac, and other NSAIDs; porphyria. **CAUTIONS:** CHF, hypertension, renal/hepatic impairment, history of GI disease. Avoid topical gel to open skin wounds, infections, exfoliative dermatitis, eyes, neonates, infants, children.

⧗ **LIFESPAN CONSIDERATIONS: Pregnancy/Lactation:** Crosses placenta. Unknown if distributed in breast milk. Avoid use during last trimester (may adversely affect fetal cardiovascular system: premature closure of ductus arteriosus). **Pregnancy Category B (D if used in third trimester or near delivery; C for ophthalmic solution). Children:** Safety and efficacy not established. **Elderly:** GI bleeding or ulceration more likely to cause serious adverse effects. Age-related renal impairment may increase risk of hepatic or renal toxicity; reduced dosage recommended.

INTERACTIONS

DRUG: Acetylcholine, carbachol: May decrease the effects of these drugs (with ophthalmic diclofenac). **Antihypertensives, diuretics:** May decrease the effects of these drugs. **Aspirin, other salicylates:** May increase the risk of GI side effects such as bleeding. **Bone marrow depressants:** May increase the risk of hematologic reactions. **Epinephrine, other antiglaucoma medications:** May decrease the antiglaucoma effect of these drugs. **Heparin, oral anticoagulants, thrombolytics:** May increase the effects of these drugs. **Lithium:** May increase the blood concentration and risk of toxicity of lithium. **Methotrexate:** May increase the risk of methotrexate toxicity. **Probenecid:** May increase diclofenac blood concentration.

HERBAL: Ginkgo biloba: May increase the risk of bleeding. **FOOD:** None known. **LAB VALUES:** May increase BUN level; urine protein level; and serum LDH, potassium, alkaline phosphatase, creatinine, AST, and ALT levels. May decrease serum uric acid level.

AVAILABILITY (Rx)

TOPICAL GEL (SOLARAZE): 3%. **TABLETS (IMMEDIATE-RELEASE [CATAFLAM]):** 50 mg. **TABLETS (DELAYED-RELEASE [VOLTAREN]):** 25 mg, 50 mg, 75 mg. **TABLETS (EXTENDED-RELEASE [VOLTAREN XR]):** 100 mg. **OPHTHALMIC SOLUTION (VOLTAREN OPHTHALMIC):** 0.1%.

ADMINISTRATION/HANDLING

PO
• Do not crush or break enteric-coated form. • May give with food, milk, or antacids if GI distress occurs.

OPHTHALMIC
• Place finger on lower eyelid and pull out until pocket is formed between eye and lower lid. Hold dropper above pocket and place prescribed number of drops in pocket. • Close eye gently. Apply digital pressure to lacrimal sac for 1–2 min (minimized drainage into nose and throat, reducing risk of systemic effects). • Remove excess solution with tissue.

INDICATIONS/ROUTES/DOSAGE

OSTEOARTHRITIS
PO (CATAFLAM, VOLTAREN): ADULTS, ELDERLY: 50 mg 2–3 times a day.
PO (VOLTAREN XR): ADULTS, ELDERLY: 100–200 mg/day as a single dose.

RHEUMATOID ARTHRITIS
PO (CATAFLAM, VOLTAREN): ADULTS, ELDERLY: 50 mg 2–4 times a day. **Maximum:** 225 mg/day.
PO (VOLTAREN XR): ADULTS, ELDERLY: 100 mg once a day. **Maximum:** 100 mg twice a day.

ANKYLOSING SPONDYLITIS
PO (VOLTAREN): ADULTS, ELDERLY: 100–125 mg/day in 4–5 divided doses.

ANALGESIA, PRIMARY DYSMENORRHEA
PO (CATAFLAM): ADULTS, ELDERLY: 50 mg 3 times a day.

USUAL PEDIATRIC DOSAGE
CHILDREN: 2–3 mg/kg/day in 2–4 divided doses.

ACTINIC KERATOSES
TOPICAL: ADULTS, ADOLESCENTS: Apply twice a day to lesion for 60–90 days.

CATARACT SURGERY
OPHTHALMIC: ADULTS, ELDERLY: Apply 1 drop to eye 4 times a day commencing 24 hr after cataract surgery. Continue for 2 wk afterward.

PAIN, RELIEF OF PHOTOPHOBIA IN PATIENTS UNDERGOING CORNEAL REFRACTIVE SURGERY
OPHTHALMIC: ADULTS, ELDERLY: Apply 1–2 drops to affected eye 1 hr before surgery, within 15 min after surgery, then 4 times a day for up to 3 days.

SIDE EFFECTS

FREQUENT (9%–4%): PO: Headache, abdominal cramps, constipation, diarrhea, nausea, dyspepsia. **Ophthalmic:** Burning or stinging on instillation, ocular discomfort. **OCCASIONAL (3%–1%): PO:** Flatulence, dizziness, epigastric pain. **Ophthalmic:** Ocular itching or tearing. **RARE (less than 1%): PO:** Rash, peripheral edema or fluid retention, visual disturbances, vomiting, drowsiness.

ADVERSE REACTIONS/ TOXIC EFFECTS

Overdose may result in acute renal failure. Rare reactions with long-term use include peptic ulcer disease, GI bleeding, gastritis, a severe hepatic reaction (jaundice), nephrotoxicity (hematuria, dysuria, proteinuria), and a severe hypersensitivity reaction (bronchospasm or angioedema).

NURSING CONSIDERATIONS

BASELINE ASSESSMENT

Anti-inflammatory: Assess onset, type, location, duration of pain and inflammation. Inspect appearance of affected joints for immobility, deformities, skin condition.

INTERVENTION/EVALUATION

Monitor for headache, dyspepsia. Monitor pattern of daily bowel activity and stool consistency. Evaluate for therapeutic response: relief of pain, stiffness, swelling; increase in joint mobility; reduced joint tenderness; improved grip strength.

PATIENT/FAMILY TEACHING

• Swallow tablet whole; do not crush or chew. • Avoid aspirin, alcohol during therapy (increases risk of GI bleeding). • If GI upset occurs, take with food, milk. • Report skin rash, itching, weight gain, changes in vision, black stools, persistent headache. • **Ophthalmic:** Do not use hydrogel soft contact lenses. • **Topical:** Avoid exposure to sunlight or sun lamps. • Inform physician if rash occurs.

---

dicloxacillin sodium

(Dycill, Dynapen, Pathocil)

See Antibiotic: penicillins (p. 27C)

---

dicyclomine hydrochloride

dye-**sye**-kloe-meen

(Bentyl, Bentylol ✤, Dicyclocot, Formulex ✤, Lomine ✤)

Do not confuse dicyclomine with doxycycline or dyclonime, or Bentyl with Aventyl or Benadryl.

✦CLASSIFICATION

CLINICAL: GI antispasmodic, anticholinergic.

ACTION

A GI antispasmodic and anticholinergic agent that directly acts as a relaxant on smooth muscle. **Therapeutic Effect:** Reduces tone and motility of GI tract.

PHARMACOKINETICS

Route	Onset	Peak	Duration
PO	1–2 hr	N/A	4 hr

Readily absorbed from the GI tract. Widely distributed. Metabolized in the liver. **Half-life:** 9–10 hr.

USES

Treatment of functional disturbances of GI motility (e.g., irritable bowel syndrome).

PRECAUTIONS

CONTRAINDICATIONS: Bladder neck obstruction due to prostatic hyperplasia, coronary vasospasm, intestinal atony, myasthenia gravis in patients not treated with neostigmine, narrow-angle glaucoma, obstructive disease of the GI tract, paralytic ileus, severe ulcerative colitis, tachycardia secondary to cardiac insufficiency or thyrotoxicosis, toxic megacolon, unstable cardiovascular status in acute hemorrhage. **EXTREME CAUTION:** Autonomic neuropathy, known or suspected GI infections, diarrhea, mild to moderate ulcerative colitis. **CAUTIONS:** Hyperthyroidism, hepatic or renal disease, hypertension, tachyarrhythmias, CHF, coronary artery disease, gastric ulcer, esophageal reflux or hiatal hernia associated with reflux esophagitis, infants, elderly, chronic obstructive pulmonary disease (COPD).

⧗ LIFESPAN CONSIDERATIONS: **Pregnancy/Lactation:** Unknown if drug crosses placenta or is distributed in breast milk. **Pregnancy Category B. Children:** Infants, young children more susceptible to toxic effects. **Elderly:** May cause excitement, agitation, drowsiness, confusion.

INTERACTIONS

DRUG: **Antacids, antidiarrheals:** May decrease the absorption of dicyclomine. **Ketoconazole:** May decrease the absorption of ketoconazole. **Other anticholinergics:** May increase the effects of dicyclomine. **Potassium chloride:** May increase the severity of GI lesions with the wax matrix formulation of potassium chloride. HERBAL: None known. FOOD: None known. LAB VALUES: None known.

AVAILABILITY (Rx)

CAPSULES (BENTYL): 10 mg. **TABLETS (BENTYL):** 20 mg. **SYRUP (BENTYL):** 10 mg/5 ml. **INJECTION (BENTYL, DICYCLOCOT):** 10 mg/ml.

ADMINISTRATION/HANDLING
- Store capsules, tablets, syrup, parenteral form at room temperature.

IM
- Injection should appear colorless.
- Do not administer IV or subcutaneous. • Inject deep into large muscle mass. • Do not give for longer than 2 days.

PO
- Dilute oral solution with equal volume of water just before administration.
- May give without regard to meals (food may slightly decrease absorption).

INDICATIONS/ROUTES/DOSAGE

FUNCTIONAL DISTURBANCES OF GI MOTILITY

PO: ADULTS: 10–20 mg 3–4 times a day up to 40 mg 4 times/day. CHILDREN OLDER THAN 2 YR: 10 mg 3–4 times a day. CHILDREN 6 MO–2 YR: 5 mg 3–4 times a day. ELDERLY: 10–20 mg 4 times a day. May increase to 160 mg/day.
IM: ADULTS: 20 mg q4–6h.

SIDE EFFECTS

FREQUENT: Dry mouth (sometimes severe), constipation, diminished sweating ability. **OCCASIONAL:** Blurred vision; photophobia; urinary hesitancy; somnolence (with high dosage); agitation, excitement, confusion, or somnolence noted in elderly (even with low dosages); transient light-headedness (with IM route), irritation at injection site (with IM route). **RARE:** Confusion, hypersensitivity reaction, increased intraocular pressure, nausea, vomiting, unusual fatigue.

ADVERSE REACTIONS/ TOXIC EFFECTS

Overdose may produce temporary paralysis of ciliary muscle; pupillary dilation; tachycardia; palpitations; hot, dry, or flushed skin; absence of bowel sounds; hyperthermia; increased respiratory rate; EKG abnormalities; nausea; vomiting; rash over face or upper trunk; CNS stimulation; and psychosis (marked by agitation, restlessness, rambling speech, visual hallucinations, paranoid behavior, and delusions, followed by depression).

NURSING CONSIDERATIONS

BASELINE ASSESSMENT
Before giving medication, instruct patient to void (reduces risk of urinary retention).

INTERVENTION/EVALUATION
Monitor daily bowel activity and stool consistency. Assess for urinary retention. Monitor changes in BP, temperature. Be alert for fever (increased risk of hyperthermia). Assess skin turgor, mucous membranes to evaluate hydration status (encourage adequate fluid intake), bowel sounds for peristalsis.

PATIENT/FAMILY TEACHING

• Do not become overheated during exercise in hot weather (may result in heat stroke). • Avoid hot baths, saunas. • Avoid tasks that require alertness, motor skills until response to drug is established. • Do not take antacids or antidiarrheals within 1 hr of taking this medication (decreased effectiveness).

didanosine

dye-**dan**-o-seen
(Videx, Videx-EC)

CLASSIFICATION

PHARMACOTHERAPEUTIC: Purine nucleoside analogue. **CLINICAL:** Antiviral (see pp. 60C, 102C).

ACTION

A purine nucleoside analogue that is intracellularly converted into a triphosphate, which interferes with RNA-directed DNA polymerase (reverse transcriptase). **Therapeutic Effect:** Inhibits replication of retroviruses, including HIV.

PHARMACOKINETICS

Variably absorbed from the GI tract. Protein binding: less than 5%. Rapidly metabolized intracellularly to active form. Primarily excreted in urine. Partially (20%) removed by hemodialysis. **Half-life:** 1.5 hr; metabolite: 8–24 hr.

USES

Treatment of HIV infection in combination with other antiretroviral agents.

PRECAUTIONS

CONTRAINDICATIONS: Hypersensitivity to didanosine or any of its components. **CAUTIONS:** Renal or hepatic impairment, alcoholism, elevated triglycerides, T-cell counts less than 100 cells/mm^3; extreme caution with history of pancreatitis. Phenylketonuria and sodium-restricted diets due to phenylalanine, sodium content of preparations.

⌛ **LIFESPAN CONSIDERATIONS: Pregnancy/Lactation:** Use during pregnancy only if clearly needed. Discontinue breast-feeding during didanosine therapy. **Pregnancy Category B. Children:** Well tolerated in children older than 3 mo. **Elderly:** Age-related renal impairment may require dosage adjustment.

INTERACTIONS

DRUG: Dapsone, flouroquinolones, itraconazole, ketoconazole, tetracyclines: May decrease absorption of these drugs. **Medications producing pancreatitis or peripheral neuropathy:** May increase the risk of pancreatitis or peripheral neuropathy. **Stavudine:** May increase the risk of fatal lactic acidosis in pregnancy. **HERBAL:** None known. **FOOD: All foods:** Decreases absorption of didanosine. **LAB VALUES:** May increase serum alkaline phosphatase, amylase, bilirubin, lipase, triglyceride, AST, ALT, and uric acid levels. May decrease serum potassium levels.

AVAILABILITY (Rx)

CAPSULES (DELAYED-RELEASE): 125 mg (Videx), 200 mg (Videx-EC), 250 mg (Videx-EC), 400 mg (Videx-EC). **PEDIATRIC POWDER FOR ORAL SOLUTION (VIDEX):** 10 mg/ml. **POWDER FOR ORAL SOLUTION (VIDEX):** 100 mg, 167 mg, 250 mg. **TABLETS (CHEWABLE [VIDEX]):** 25 mg, 50 mg, 100 mg, 150 mg, 200 mg.

ADMINISTRATION/HANDLING
PO

• Store at room temperature. • Tablets dispersed in water are stable for 1 hr at room temperature; after reconstitution of buffered powder, oral solution is

---

stable for 4 hr at room temperature. • Pediatric powder for oral solution following reconstitution as directed, stable for 30 days refrigerated. • Give 1 hr before or 2 hr after meals (food decreases rate and extent of absorption). • **Chewable tablets:** Thoroughly crush and disperse in at least 30 ml water before swallowing. Mixture should be stirred well (2–3 min) and swallowed immediately. • **Buffered powder for oral solution:** Reconstitute before administration by pouring contents of packet into 4 oz water; stir until completely dissolved (up to 2–3 min). Do not mix with fruit juice or other acidic liquid (didanosine is unstable at acidic pH). • **Unbuffered pediatric powder:** Add 100–200 ml water to 2 or 4 g, respectively, to provide concentration of 20 mg/ml. Immediately mix with equal amount of antacid to provide concentration of 10 mg/ml. Shake thoroughly before removing each dose. • **Enteric-coated capsules:** Swallow whole, take on empty stomach.

INDICATIONS/ROUTES/DOSAGE

HIV INFECTION (IN COMBINATION WITH OTHER ANTIRETROVIRALS)

PO (CHEWABLE TABLETS): ADULTS, CHILDREN 13 YR AND OLDER, WEIGHING 60 KG AND MORE: 200 mg q12h or 400 mg once a day. ADULTS, CHILDREN 13 YR AND OLDER, WEIGHING LESS THAN 60 KG: 125 mg q12h or 250 mg once a day. CHILDREN 3 MO–12 YR: 180–300 mg/m^2/day in divided doses q12h. CHILDREN YOUNGER THAN 3 MO: 50 mg/ m^2/day in divided doses q12h.

PO (DELAYED-RELEASE CAP-SULES): ADULTS, CHILDREN 13 YR AND OLDER, WEIGHING 60 KG AND MORE: 400 mg once a day. ADULTS, CHILDREN 13 YR AND OLDER, WEIGHING LESS THAN 60 KG: 250 mg once a day.

PO (ORAL SOLUTION): ADULTS, CHIL-DREN 13 YR AND OLDER WEIGHING 60 KG AND MORE: 250 mg q12h. ADULTS, CHILDREN 13 YR AND OLDER WEIGHING LESS THAN 60 KG: 167 mg q12h.

PO (PEDIATRIC POWDER FOR ORAL SOLUTION): CHILDREN 3 MO–12 YR: 180–300 mg/m^2/day in divided doses q12h. CHILDREN YOUNGER THAN 3 MO: 50 mg/ m^2/day in divided doses q12h.

DOSAGE IN RENAL IMPAIRMENT
Patients weighing less than 60 kg:

CrCl	Tablets	Oral Solution	Delayed-Release Capsules
30–59 ml/min	75 mg twice a day	100 mg twice a day	125 mg once a day
10–29 ml/min	100 mg once a day	100 mg once a day	125 mg once a day
Less than 10 ml/min	75 mg once a day	100 mg once a day	N/A

CrCl = creatinine clearance

Patients weighing 60 kg or more:

CrCl	Tablets	Oral Solution	Delayed-Release Capsules
30–59 ml/ min	100 mg twice a day	100 mg twice a day	200 mg once a day
10–29 ml/ min	150 mg once a day	167 mg once a day	125 mg once a day
Less than 10 ml/ min	100 mg once a day	100 mg once a day	125 mg once a day

CrCl = creatinine clearance

SIDE EFFECTS

FREQUENT: Adults (greater than 10%): Diarrhea, neuropathy, chills and fever. **Children (greater than 25%):** Chills, fever, decreased appetite, pain, malaise, nausea, vomiting, diarrhea, abdominal pain, headache, nervousness, cough, rhinitis, dyspnea, asthenia, rash, pruritus. **OCCASIONAL: Adults (9%–2%):** Rash, pruritus, headache, abdominal pain, nausea, vomiting, pneumonia, myopathy, decreased appetite, dry mouth, dyspnea. **Children**

(25%–10%): Failure to thrive, weight loss, stomatitis, oral thrush, ecchymosis, arthritis, myalgia, insomnia, epistaxis, pharyngitis.

ADVERSE REACTIONS/ TOXIC EFFECTS

Pneumonia and opportunistic infections occur occasionally. Peripheral neuropathy, potentially fatal pancreatitis, retinal changes, and optic neuritis are the major toxic effects.

NURSING CONSIDERATIONS

BASELINE ASSESSMENT

Obtain baseline values for CBC, serum renal and liver function tests, vital signs, weight.

INTERVENTION/EVALUATION

In event of abdominal pain, nausea or vomiting, elevated serum amylase, triglycerides, contact physician before administering medication (potential for pancreatitis). Be alert to sensation of burning feet, "restless leg syndrome" (unable to find comfortable position for legs or feet), lack of coordination or other signs of peripheral neuropathy. Monitor pattern of bowel activity and stool consistency. Check skin for rash, eruptions. Monitor blood chemistry, CBC. Assess for opportunistic infections: onset of fever, oral mucosa changes, cough, other respiratory symptoms. Check weight at least twice per wk. Assess for visual or auditory difficulty; provide protection from light if photophobia develops.

PATIENT/FAMILY TEACHING

• Avoid alcohol. • Inform physician if numbness, tingling, persistent severe abdominal pain, nausea or vomiting occur. • Shake oral suspension well before use, keep refrigerated. • Discard solution after 30 days and obtain new supply.

Diflucan, *see fluconazole*

---

diflunisal

dye-**flew**-neh-sol

(Apo-Diflunisal 🍁, Dolobid, Novo-Diflunisal 🍁)

Do not confuse diflunisal with Dicarbosil or Dolobid with Slo-bid.

◆CLASSIFICATION

PHARMACOTHERAPEUTIC: Nonsteroidal anti-inflammatory. **CLINICAL:** Antirheumatic, analgesic, vascular headache suppressant (see p. 116C).

ACTION

A nonsteroidal anti-inflammatory that inhibits prostaglandin synthesis, reducing inflammatory response and intensity of pain stimulus reaching sensory nerve endings. Therapeutic Effect: Produces analgesic and anti-inflammatory effect.

PHARMACOKINETICS

Route	Onset	Peak	Duration
PO	1 hr	2–3 hr	8–12 hr

Completely absorbed from the GI tract. Widely distributed. Protein binding: greater than 99%. Metabolized in liver. Primarily excreted in urine. Not removed by hemodialysis. Half-life: 8–12 hr.

USES

Treatment of mild to moderate pain, rheumatoid arthritis, osteoarthritis. OFF-LABEL: Treatment of psoriatic arthritis, vascular headache.

PRECAUTIONS

CONTRAINDICATIONS: Active GI bleeding, factor VII or factor IX deficiencies, hypersensitivity to aspirin or NSAIDs.

CAUTIONS: Renal or hepatic impairment, edema, elevated hepatic function tests, platelet or bleeding disorders, peptic ulcer disease, erosive gastritis, vitamin K deficiency.

⧗ **LIFESPAN CONSIDERATIONS: Pregnancy/Lactation:** Crosses placenta. Distributed in breast milk. Avoid use during last trimester (may adversely affect fetal cardiovascular system: premature closure of ductus arteriosus). **Pregnancy Category C (D if used in third trimester or near delivery). Children:** Safety and efficacy not established. **Elderly:** GI bleeding or ulceration more likely to cause serious adverse effects. Age-related renal impairment may increase risk of hepatic or renal toxicity; decreased dosage recommended.

INTERACTIONS

DRUG: Antihypertensives, diuretics: May decrease the effects of these drugs. **Aspirin, salicylates:** May increase the risk of GI bleeding and side effects. **Bone marrow depressants:** May increase the risk of hematologic reactions. **Heparin, oral anticoagulants, thrombolytics:** May increase the effects of these drugs. **Lithium:** May increase the blood concentration and risk of toxicity of lithium. **Methotrexate:** May increase the risk of toxicity of methotrexate. **Probenecid:** May increase diflunisal blood concentration. **HERBAL: Ginkgo biloba:** May increase the risk of bleeding. **FOOD:** None known. **LAB VALUES:** May increase serum AST and ALT levels. May decrease serum uric acid levels.

AVAILABILITY (Rx)

TABLETS: 250 mg, 500 mg.

ADMINISTRATION/HANDLING

PO
• May give with water, milk, or meals.
• Do not crush or break film-coated tablets.

INDICATIONS/ROUTES/DOSAGE

MILD TO MODERATE PAIN
PO: ADULTS, ELDERLY: Initially, 0.5–1 g, then 250–500 mg q8–12h. **Maximum:** 1.5 g/day.

OSTEOARTHRITIS
PO: ADULTS, ELDERLY: 500–750 mg/day in divided doses.

RHEUMATOID ARTHRITIS
PO: ADULTS, ELDERLY: 0.5–1 g/day in 2 divided doses. **Maximum:** 1.5 g/day.

SIDE EFFECTS

Side effects are less common with short-term treatment.
OCCASIONAL (9%–3%): Nausea, dyspepsia (heartburn, indigestion, epigastric pain), diarrhea, headache, rash. **RARE (3%–1%):** Vomiting, constipation, flatulence, dizziness, somnolence, insomnia, fatigue, tinnitus.

ADVERSE REACTIONS/ TOXIC EFFECTS

Overdosage may produce drowsiness, vomiting, nausea, diarrhea, hyperventilation, tachycardia, diaphoresis, stupor, and coma. Peptic ulcer, GI bleeding, gastritis, and severe hepatic reaction, including cholestasis, jaundice occur rarely. Nephrotoxicity, including dysuria, hematuria, proteinuria, and nephrotic syndrome, and severe hypersensitivity reaction, marked by bronchospasm and angioedema, occur rarely.

NURSING CONSIDERATIONS

BASELINE ASSESSMENT
Assess onset, type, location, duration of pain and inflammation. Inspect appearance of affected joints for immobility, deformities, skin condition.

INTERVENTION/EVALUATION
Monitor for nausea, dyspepsia. Assess skin for evidence of rash. Monitor pattern of daily bowel activity and stool consistency. Evaluate for therapeutic

response: relief of pain, stiffness, swelling; increase in joint mobility; reduced joint tenderness; improved grip strength.

PATIENT/FAMILY TEACHING

• Swallow tablet whole; do not crush or chew. • If GI upset occurs, take with food, milk. • Report GI distress, headache, rash.

Digitek, *see digoxin*

---

digoxin ⚑

di-**jox**-in

(Digitek, Lanoxicaps, Lanoxin)

Do not confuse digoxin with Desoxyn or doxepin, or Lanoxin with Levsinex or Lonox.

⬩CLASSIFICATION

PHARMACOTHERAPEUTIC: Cardiac glycoside. **CLINICAL:** Antiarrhythmic, cardiotonic (see p. 80C).

ACTION

A cardiac glycoside that increases the influx of calcium from extracellular to intracellular cytoplasm. Therapeutic Effect: Potentiates the activity of the contractile cardiac muscle fibers and increases the force of myocardial contraction. Slows the heart rate by decreasing conduction through the SA and AV nodes.

PHARMACOKINETICS

Route	Onset	Peak	Duration
PO	0.5–2 hr	28 hr	3–4 days
IV	5–30 min	1–4 hr	3–4 days

Readily absorbed from the GI tract. Widely distributed. Protein binding: 30%.

Partially metabolized in the liver. Primarily excreted in urine. Minimally removed by hemodialysis. Half-life: 36–48 hr (increased with impaired renal function and in the elderly).

USES

Prophylactic management and treatment of CHF, control of ventricular rate in patients with atrial fibrillation. Treatment and prevention of recurrent paroxysmal atrial tachycardia.

PRECAUTIONS

CONTRAINDICATIONS: Ventricular fibrillation, ventricular tachycardia unrelated to CHF. **CAUTIONS:** Renal/hepatic impairment, hypokalemia, advanced cardiac disease, acute MI, incomplete AV block, cor pulmonale, hyperthyroidism, hypothyroidism, pulmonary disease, severe bradycardia, sick sinus syndrome, ventricular tachycardia, Wolff-Parkinson-White syndrome.

⌛ LIFESPAN CONSIDERATIONS: Pregnancy/Lactation: Crosses placenta. Distributed in breast milk. Pregnancy Category C. Children: Premature infants more susceptible to toxicity. Elderly: Age-related hepatic or renal impairment may require dosage adjustment. Increased risk of loss of appetite.

INTERACTIONS

◀ ALERT ▶ Digoxin and regular human insulin are physically compatible for 3 hr in 0.9% sodium chloride. In dextrose 5% and water, a slight haze develops within 1 hr. Do not allow digoxin and insulin to come in contact with each other in an IV for over 15 min.
DRUG: **Amiodarone:** May increase digoxin blood concentration and risk of toxicity; may have an additive effect on the SA and AV nodes. **Amphotericin, glucocorticoids, potassium-depleting diuretics:** May increase risk of toxicity due to hypokalemia. **Antiarrhythmics, parenteral calcium, sympathomimetics:** May increase

---

risk of arrhythmias. **Antidiarrheals, cholestyramine, colestipol, sucralfate:** May decrease absorption of digoxin. **Diltiazem, fluoxetine, quinidine, verapamil:** May increase digoxin blood concentration. **Parenteral magnesium:** May cause cardiac conduction changes and heart block. **HERBAL: Siberian ginseng:** May increase serum digoxin levels. **St. John's wort:** May reduce digoxin efficacy. **FOOD: All food:** May decrease peak digoxin concentrations. **LAB VALUES:** None known.

AVAILABILITY (Rx)

CAPSULES (LANOXICAPS): 50 mcg, 100 mcg, 200 mcg. **ELIXIR (LANOXIN):** 50 mcg/ml. **TABLETS (DIGITEK, LANOXIN):** 125 mcg, 250 mcg. **INJECTION (LANOXIN):** 100 mcg/ml, 250 mcg/ml.

ADMINISTRATION/HANDLING

◀ **ALERT** ▶ IM rarely used (produces severe local irritation, erratic absorption). If no other route possible, give deep into muscle followed by massage. Give no more than 2 ml at any one site.

 IV

• May give undiluted or dilute with at least a 4-fold volume of sterile water for injection, or D_5W (less than this may cause a precipitate). Use immediately.
• Give IV slowly over at least 5 min.

PO

• May give without regard to meals.
• Tablets may be crushed.

🏵 IV INCOMPATIBILITIES

Amphotericin B complex (Abelcet, AmBisome, Amphotec), fluconazole (Diflucan), foscarnet (Foscavir), propofol (Diprivan).

IV COMPATIBILITIES

Cimetidine (Tagamet), diltiazem (Cardizem), furosemide (Lasix), heparin, insulin regular (physically compatible for 3 hr in 0.9% NaCl. In D_5W, a slight haze

develops within 1 hr.), lidocaine, midazolam (Versed), milrinone (Primacor), morphine, potassium chloride.

INDICATIONS/ROUTES/DOSAGE

RAPID LOADING DOSE FOR THE MANAGEMENT AND TREATMENT OF CHF; CONTROL OF VENTRICULAR RATE IN PATIENTS WITH ATRIAL FIBRILLATION; TREATMENT AND PREVENTION OF RECURRENT PAROXYSMAL ATRIAL TACHYCARDIA

PO: ADULTS, ELDERLY: Initially, 0.5–0.75 mg, additional doses of 0.125–0.375 mg at 6- to 8-hr intervals. Range: 0.75–1.25 mg. CHILDREN 10 YR AND OLDER: 10–15 mcg/kg. CHILDREN 5–9 YR: 20–35 mcg/kg. CHILDREN 2–4 YR: 30–40 mcg/kg. CHILDREN 1–23 MO: 35–60 mcg/kg. NEONATE, FULL-TERM: 25–35 mcg/kg. NEONATE, PREMATURE: 20–30 mcg/kg.

IV: ADULTS, ELDERLY: 0.6–1 mg. CHILDREN 10 YR AND OLDER: 8–12 mcg/kg. CHILDREN 5–9 YR: 15–30 mcg/kg. CHILDREN 2–4 YR: 25–35 mcg/kg. CHILDREN 1–23 MO: 30–50 mcg/kg. NEONATES, FULL-TERM: 20–30 mcg/kg. NEONATES, PREMATURE: 15–25 mcg/kg.

MAINTENANCE DOSAGE FOR CHF; CONTROL OF VENTRICULAR RATE IN PATIENTS WITH ATRIAL FIBRILLATION; TREATMENT AND PREVENTION OF RECURRENT PAROXYSMAL ATRIAL TACHYCARDIA

PO, IV: ADULTS, ELDERLY: 0.125–0.375 mg/day. CHILDREN: 25%–35% loading dose (20%–30% for premature neonates).

DOSAGE IN RENAL IMPAIRMENT
Dosage adjustment is based on creatinine clearance. Total digitalizing dose: decrease by 50% in end-stage renal disease.

Creatinine Clearance	Dosage
10–50 ml/min	25%–75% usual
Less than 10 ml/min	10%–25% usual

SIDE EFFECTS

None known. However, there is a very narrow margin of safety between a therapeutic and toxic result. Long-term therapy may produce mammary gland enlargement in women but is reversible when drug is withdrawn.

ADVERSE REACTIONS/ TOXIC EFFECTS

The most common early manifestations of digoxin toxicity are GI disturbances (anorexia, nausea, vomiting) and neurologic abnormalities (fatigue, headache, depression, weakness, drowsiness, confusion, nightmares). Facial pain, personality change, and ocular disturbances (photophobia, light flashes, halos around bright objects, yellow or green color perception) may be noted.

NURSING CONSIDERATIONS

BASELINE ASSESSMENT

Assess apical pulse for 60 sec (30 sec if on maintenance therapy). If pulse is 60 or less/min (70 or less/min for children), withhold drug, contact physician. Blood samples are best taken 6–8 hr after dose or just before next dose.

INTERVENTION/EVALUATION

Monitor pulse for bradycardia, EKG for arrhythmias for 1–2 hr after administration (excessive slowing of pulse may be a first clinical sign of toxicity). Assess for GI disturbances, neurologic abnormalities (signs of toxicity) q2–4h during loading dose (daily during maintenance). Monitor serum potassium, magnesium levels. Therapeutic serum level: 0.8–2 ng/ml; toxic serum level: greater than 2 ng/ml.

PATIENT/FAMILY TEACHING

• Stress importance of follow-up visits, blood tests. • Teach patient to take apical pulse correctly and to report pulse 60 or less/min (or as indicated by physician). • Ensure patient understands signs of toxicity and need to notify physician if any occur. • Wear/ carry identification of digoxin therapy and inform dentist, other physician of taking digoxin. • Do not increase or skip doses. • Do not take OTC medications without consulting physician. • Inform physician of decreased appetite, nausea/vomiting, diarrhea, visual changes.

digoxin immune FAB

di-**jox**-in

(Digibind, DigiFab)

Do not confuse digoxin immune FAB with Desoxyn or doxepin.

CLASSIFICATION

CLINICAL: Antidote.

ACTION

An antidote that binds molecularly to digoxin in the extracellular space. **Therapeutic Effect:** Makes digoxin unavailable for binding at its site of action on cells in the body.

PHARMACOKINETICS

Route	Onset	Peak	Duration
IV	30 min	N/A	3–4 days

Widely distributed into extracellular space. Excreted in urine. **Half-life:** 15–20 hr.

USES

Treatment of potentially life-threatening digoxin toxicity including acute digoxin ingestion of greater than 10 mg in adults or greater than 4 mg in children, chronic ingestion leading to digoxin concentrations greater than 6 ng/ml in adults or greater than 4 ng/ml in children, or clinical signs of digoxin toxicity (e.g., life-threatening ventricular arrhythmias, progressive bradycardia, 2nd or

3rd degree heart block not responsive to atropine).

PRECAUTIONS

CONTRAINDICATIONS: None known. **CAUTIONS:** Cardiac, renal impairment. ⌛ LIFESPAN CONSIDERATIONS: **Pregnancy/Lactation:** Unknown if drug crosses placenta or is distributed in breast milk. **Pregnancy Category C. Children:** No age-related precautions noted. **Elderly:** Age-related renal impairment may require dosage adjustment.

INTERACTIONS

DRUG: None known. HERBAL: None known. FOOD: None known. LAB VALUES: May alter serum potassium level. Serum digoxin concentration may increase precipitously and persist for up to 1 wk until FAB/digoxin complex is eliminated from the body.

AVAILABILITY (Rx)

POWDER FOR INJECTION: 38-mg vial (Digibind), 40-mg vial (DigiFab).

ADMINISTRATION/HANDLING

 IV

Reconstitution • Reconstitute each 38-mg vial with 4 ml sterile water for injection to provide a concentration of 9.5 mg/ml. • Further dilute with 50 ml 0.9% NaCl.

Rate of administration • Infuse over 30 min (recommended that solution be infused through a 0.22-micron filter). • If cardiac arrest imminent, may give IV push.

Storage • Refrigerate vials. • After reconstitution, is stable for 4 hr if refrigerated. • Use immediately after reconstitution.

⬛ IV INCOMPATIBILITY

None known.

INDICATIONS/ROUTES/DOSAGE

POTENTIALLY LIFE-THREATENING DIGOXIN OVERDOSE

IV: ADULTS, ELDERLY, CHILDREN: Dosage varies according to amount of digoxin to be neutralized. Refer to manufacturer's dosing guidelines.

SIDE EFFECTS

RARE: Allergic reaction.

ADVERSE REACTIONS/ TOXIC EFFECTS

Hyperkalemia may occur as a result of digitalis toxicity. Signs and symptoms of hyperkalemia include diarrhea, paresthesia of extremities, heaviness of legs, decreased BP, cold skin, grayish pallor, hypotension, mental confusion, irritability, flaccid paralysis, tented T waves, widening QRS interval, and ST depression. Hypokalemia may develop rapidly when the effect of digitalis is reversed. Signs and symptoms of hypokalemia include muscle cramping, nausea, vomiting, hypoactive bowel sounds, abdominal distention, difficulty breathing, and orthostatic hypotension. Low cardiac output and CHF may occur rarely.

NURSING CONSIDERATIONS

BASELINE ASSESSMENT

Obtain serum digoxin level before administering drug. If drawn less than 6 hr before last digoxin dose, serum digoxin level may be unreliable. Those with renal impairment may require more than 1 wk before serum digoxin assay is reliable. Assess muscle strength, mental status.

INTERVENTION/EVALUATION

Closely monitor temperature, BP, EKG, serum potassium level during and after drug is administered. Watch for changes from initial assessment (hypokalemia may result in muscle strength changes, tremor, muscle cramps, change in mental status, cardiac arrhythmias;

hyponatremia may result in confusion, thirst, cold or clammy skin).

dihydroergotamine

See ergotamine

dihydrotachysterol

See vitamin D

Dilacor XR, see diltiazem

Dilantin, see phenytoin

Dilaudid, see hydromorphone

diltiazem hydrochloride

dil-**tye**-a-zem

(Apo-Diltiaz ✶, Cardizem, Cardizem CD, Cardizem LA, Cardizem SR, Cartia XT, Dilacor XR, Diltia XT, Diltiazem Hydrochloride XT, Novo-Diltiazem ✶, Taztia XT, Tiazac)

Do not confuse Cardizem with Cardene or Cardene SR, or Tiazac with Ziac.

FIXED-COMBINATION(S)

Teczem: diltiazem/enalapril (angiotensin-converting enzyme [ACE] inhibitor): 180 mg/5 mg.

♦ CLASSIFICATION

PHARMACOTHERAPEUTIC: Calcium channel blocker. **CLINICAL:** Antianginal, antihypertensive, antiarrhythmic (see pp. 16C, 69C).

ACTION

An antianginal, antihypertensive, and antiarrhythmic agent that inhibits calcium movement across cardiac and vascular smooth-muscle cell membranes. This action causes the dilation of coronary arteries, peripheral arteries, and arterioles. Therapeutic Effect: Decreases heart rate and myocardial contractility, slows SA and AV conduction and decreases total peripheral vascular resistance by vasodilation.

PHARMACOKINETICS

Route	Onset	Peak	Duration
PO	0.5–1 hr	N/A	N/A
PO (extended-release)	2–3 hr	N/A	N/A
IV	3 min	N/A	N/A

Well absorbed from the GI tract. Protein binding: 70%–80%. Undergoes first-pass metabolism in the liver to active metabolite. Primarily excreted in urine. Not removed by hemodialysis. Half-life: 3–8 hr.

USES

PO: Treatment of angina due to coronary artery spasm (Prinzmetal's variant angina), chronic stable angina (effort-associated angina). **Extended-Release:** Treatment of essential hypertension, angina. **Cardizem LA:** Treatment of chronic stable angina. **Parenteral:** Temporary control of rapid ventricular rate in atrial fibrillation/flutter. Rapid conversion of paroxysmal supraventricular tachycardia (PSVT) to normal sinus rhythm.

PRECAUTIONS

CONTRAINDICATIONS: Acute MI, pulmonary congestion, hypersensitivity to diltiazem or other calcium channel blockers, second- or third-degree AV block (except in the presence of a pacemaker), severe hypotension (less than 90 mm Hg, systolic), sick sinus syndrome. **CAUTIONS:** Renal or hepatic impairment, CHF.

⧗ LIFESPAN CONSIDERATIONS: **Pregnancy/Lactation:** Distributed in breast milk. **Pregnancy Category C. Children:** No age-related precautions noted. **Elderly:** Age-related renal impairment may require dosage adjustment.

INTERACTIONS

DRUG: **Beta blockers:** May have additive effect. **Carbamazepine, quinidine, theophylline:** May increase diltiazem blood concentration and risk of toxicity. **Digoxin:** May increase serum digoxin concentration. **Procainamide, quinidine:** May increase risk of QT-interval prolongation. HERBAL: None known. FOOD: None known. LAB VALUES: PR interval may be increased.

AVAILABILITY (Rx)

CAPSULES (SUSTAINED-RELEASE [CARDIZEM SR]): 60 mg, 90 mg, 120 mg. **CAPSULES (EXTENDED-RELEASE [CARDIZEM CD]):** 120 mg (Cardizem CD, Cartia XT, Dilacor XR, Diltia XT, Taztia XT, Tiazac), 180 mg (Cardizem CD, Cartia XT, Dilacor XR, Diltia XT, Taztia XT, Tiazac), 240 mg (Cardizem CD, Cartia XT, Dilacor XR, Diltia XT, Taztia XT, Tiazac), 300 mg (Cardizem CD, Cartia XT, Taztia XT, Tiazac), 360 mg (Cardizem CD, Taztia XT, Tiazac), 420 mg (Tiazac). **TABLETS (CARDIZEM):** 30 mg, 60 mg, 90 mg, 120 mg. **TABLETS (EXTENDED-RELEASE [CARDIZEM LA]):** 120 mg, 180 mg, 240 mg, 300 mg, 360 mg, 420 mg. **INJECTION (READY-TO-HANG INFUSION):** 1 mg/ml.

ADMINISTRATION/HANDLING

▣ IV

Reconstitution • Add 125 mg to 100 ml D$_5$W, 0.9% NaCl to provide a concentration of 1 mg/ml. Add 250 mg to 250 or 500 ml diluent to provide a concentration of 0.83 mg/ml or 0.45 mg/ml, respectively. Maximum concentration: 1.25 g/250 ml (5 mg/ml).

Rate of administration • Infuse per dilution/rate chart provided by manufacturer.

Storage • Refrigerate vials. • After dilution, stable for 24 hr.

PO
• Give before meals and at bedtime. • Tablets may be crushed. • Do not crush sustained-release capsules.

▦ IV INCOMPATIBILITIES

Acetazolamide (Diamox), acyclovir (Zovirax), aminophylline, ampicillin, ampicillin/sulbactam (Unasyn), cefoperazone (Cefobid), diazepam (Valium), furosemide (Lasix), heparin, insulin, nafcillin, phenytoin (Dilantin), rifampin (Rifadin), sodium bicarbonate.

IV COMPATIBILITIES

Albumin, aztreonam (Azactam), bumetanide (Bumex), cefazolin (Ancef), cefotaxime (Claforan), ceftazidime (Fortaz), ceftriaxone (Rocephin), cefuroxime (Zinacef), cimetidine (Tagamet), ciprofloxacin (Cipro), clindamycin (Cleocin), digoxin (Lanoxin), dobutamine (Dobutrex), dopamine (Intropin), gentamicin (Garamycin), hydromorphone (Dilaudid), lidocaine, lorazepam (Ativan), metoclopramide (Reglan), metronidazole (Flagyl), midazolam (Versed), morphine, multivitamins, nitroglycerin, norepinephrine (Levophed), potassium chloride, potassium phosphate, tobramycin (Nebcin), vancomycin (Vancocin).

INDICATIONS/ROUTES/DOSAGE

ANGINA

PO (CARDIZEM): ADULTS, ELDERLY: Initially, 30 mg 4 times a day. Range: 180–360 mg/day.

PO (CARDIZEM CD, CARTIA XT, DILACOR XR, DILTIA XT, TIAZAC): ADULTS, ELDERLY: Initially, 120–180 mg/day. **Maximum:** 480 mg/day.

PO (CARDIZEM LA): ADULTS, ELDERLY: Initially, 180 mg/day. May increase at intervals of 7–14-day intervals. **Maximum:** 360 mg/day.

HYPERTENSION

PO (CARDIZEM CD, CARTIA XT, DILACOR XR, DILTIA XT, TIAZAC): ADULTS, ELDERLY: Initially, 180–240 mg/day. Range: 180–420 mg/day, **Tiazac:** 120–540 mg/day.

PO (CARDIZEM SR): ADULTS, ELDERLY: Initially, 60–120 mg twice a day. May increase at 14-day intervals. Maintenance: 240–360 mg/day.

PO (CARDIZEM LA): ADULTS, ELDERLY: Initially, 180–240 mg/day. May increase at 14-day intervals. Range: 120–540 mg/day.

TEMPORARY CONTROL OF RAPID VENTRICULAR RATE IN ATRIAL FIBRILLATION OR FLUTTER, RAPID CONVERSION OF PAROXYSMAL SUPRAVENTRICULAR TACHYCARDIA TO NORMAL SINUS RHYTHM.

IV PUSH: ADULTS, ELDERLY: Initially, 0.25 mg/kg actual body weight over 2 min. May repeat in 15 min at dose of 0.35 mg/kg actual body weight. Subsequent doses individualized.

IV INFUSION: ADULTS, ELDERLY: After initial bolus injection, may begin infusion at 5–10 mg/hr; may increase by 5 mg/hr up to a maximum of 15 mg/hr. Infusion duration should not exceed 24 hr.

SIDE EFFECTS

FREQUENT (10%–5%): Peripheral edema, dizziness, light-headedness, headache, bradycardia, asthenia (loss of strength, weakness). **OCCASIONAL (5%–2%):** Nausea, constipation, flushing, EKG changes. **RARE (less than 2%):** Rash, micturition disorder (polyuria, nocturia, dysuria, frequency of urination), abdominal discomfort, somnolence.

ADVERSE REACTIONS/ TOXIC EFFECTS

Abrupt withdrawal may increase frequency or duration of angina. CHF and second- and third-degree AV block occur rarely. Overdose produces nausea, somnolence, confusion, slurred speech, and profound bradycardia.

NURSING CONSIDERATIONS

BASELINE ASSESSMENT

Concurrent therapy of sublingual nitroglycerin may be used for relief of anginal pain. Record onset, type (sharp, dull, squeezing), radiation, location, intensity, duration of anginal pain, and precipitating factors (exertion, emotional stress). Assess baseline renal and liver function tests. Assess BP, apical pulse immediately before drug is administered.

INTERVENTION/EVALUATION

Assist with ambulation if dizziness occurs. Assess for peripheral edema behind medial malleolus (sacral area in bedridden patients). Monitor pulse rate for bradycardia. With IV therapy, assess BP, renal and liver function tests, EKG. Question for asthenia, headache.

PATIENT/FAMILY TEACHING

• Do not abruptly discontinue medication. • Compliance with therapy regimen is essential to control anginal pain. • To avoid hypotensive effect, rise slowly from lying to sitting position, wait momentarily before standing. • Avoid tasks that require alertness, motor skills until response to drug is established. • Contact physician or nurse if palpitations, shortness of breath, pronounced dizziness, nausea, or constipation occurs.

*dimenhyDRINATE

(Dramamine)
See Antihistamines (p. 50C)

dinoprostone

dye-noe-**pros**-tone
(Cervidil, Prepidil, Prostin E$_2$)
Do not confuse Cervidil or Prepidil with bepridil or Prostin with Prostigmin.

◆ CLASSIFICATION

PHARMACOTHERAPEUTIC: Prostaglandin. **CLINICAL:** Oxytocic, abortifacient, antihemorrhagic.

ACTION

A prostaglandin that directly acts on the myometrium, causing softening and dilation effect of the cervix. Therapeutic Effect: Stimulates myometrial contractions in gravid uterus.

PHARMACOKINETICS

Undergoes rapid enzymatic deactivation primarily in maternal lungs. Protein binding: 73%. Primarily excreted in urine. Half-life: Less than 5 min.

USES

Suppository: To induce abortion from the 12th wk of pregnancy through the second trimester; to evacuate uterine contents in missed abortion or intrauterine fetal death up to 28 wk gestational age (as calculated from the first day of the last normal menstrual period), benign hydatidiform mole. Treatment of postpartum or postabortion hemorrhage, induction of labor at or near term. **Gel:** Ripening unfavorable cervix in pregnant women at or near term with medical or obstetric need for labor induction. Induction of labor at or near term. **Vaginal insert:** Initiation and/or cervical ripening in patients having medical indication for induction of labor.

PRECAUTIONS

CONTRAINDICATIONS: Gel: Active cardiac, hepatic, pulmonary or renal disease; acute pelvic inflammatory disease (PID); fetal malpresentation; grand multiparae with 6 or more previous term pregnancy cases with nonvertex presentation; history of cesarean section or major uterine surgery; history of difficult labor and /or traumatic delivery; hypersensitivity to other prostaglandins; placenta previa or unexplained vaginal bleeding during this pregnancy; patients for whom vaginal delivery is not indicated, such as vasa previa or active herpes genitalia; significant cephalopelvic disproportion. **Vaginal suppository:** Active cardiac, hepatic, pulmonary, or renal disease; acute PID. **CAUTIONS:** Cervicitis, infected endocervical lesions or acute vaginitis, history of asthma, hypotension or hypertension, anemia, jaundice, diabetes, epilepsy, uterine fibroids, compromised (scarred) uterus, history of cardiovascular, renal, or hepatic disease.

⌛ LIFESPAN CONSIDERATIONS: **Pregnancy/Lactation: Suppository:** Teratogenic, therefore abortion must be complete. **Gel:** Sustained uterine hyperstimulation may affect fetus (e.g., abnormal heart rate). **Pregnancy Category C. Children/Elderly:** Not used in these patient populations.

INTERACTIONS

DRUG: **Oxytocics:** May cause uterine hypertonus, possibly resulting in uterine rupture or cervical laceration. HERBAL: None known. FOOD: None known. LAB VALUES: None known.

AVAILABILITY (Rx)

VAGINAL GEL (PREPIDIL): 0.5 mg. **VAGINAL INSERTS (CERVIDIL):** 10 mg.

VAGINAL SUPPOSITORIES (PROSTIN E$_2$ VAGINAL CREAM): 20 mg.

ADMINISTRATION/HANDLING

GEL
• Refrigerate. • Use caution in handling, prevent skin contact. Wash hands thoroughly with soap and water following administration. • Bring to room temperature just before use (avoid forcing the warming process). • Assemble dosing apparatus as described in manufacturer insert. • Place patient in dorsal position with cervix visualized using a speculum. • Introduce gel into cervical canal just below level of internal os. • Have patient remain in supine position at least 15–30 min (minimizes leakage from cervical canal).

SUPPOSITORY
• Keep frozen (less than 4ºF); bring to room temperature just before use. • Administer only in hospital setting with emergency equipment available. • Warm suppository to room temperature before removing foil wrapper. • Avoid skin contact due to risk of absorption. • Insert high in vagina. • Patient should remain supine for 10 min after administration.

INDICATIONS/ROUTES/DOSAGE

ABORTIFACIENT
INTRAVAGINAL: ADULTS: 20 mg (or one suppository) high into vagina. May repeat at 3- to 5-hr intervals until abortion occurs. Do not administer for longer than 2 days. **Maximum:** 240 mg.

RIPENING OF UNFAVORABLE CERVIX
INTRACERVICAL (PREPIDIL): ADULTS: Initially, 0.5 mg (2.5 ml); if no cervical or uterine response, may repeat 0.5-mg dose in 6 hr. **Maximum:** 1.5 mg (7.5 ml) for a 24-hr period.
INTRACERVICAL (CERVIDIL): ADULTS: 10 mg over 12-hr period; remove upon onset of active labor or 12 hr after insertion.

SIDE EFFECTS

FREQUENT: Vomiting (66%), diarrhea (40%), nausea (33%). **OCCASIONAL:** Headache (10%), chills or shivering (10%), hives, bradycardia, increased uterine pain accompanying abortion, peripheral vasoconstriction. **RARE:** Flushing, vulvae edema.

ADVERSE REACTIONS/ TOXIC EFFECTS

Overdose may cause uterine hypertonicity with spasm and tetanic contraction, leading to cervical laceration or perforation, and uterine rupture or hemorrhage.

NURSING CONSIDERATIONS

BASELINE ASSESSMENT
Offer emotional support. **Suppository:** Obtain orders for antiemetics, antidiarrheals, meperidine, other pain medication for abdominal cramps. Assess any uterine activity, vaginal bleeding. **Gel:** Assess Bishop score. Assess degree of effacement (determines size of shielded endocervical catheter).

INTERVENTION/EVALUATION
Suppository: Check strength, duration, frequency of contractions and monitor vital signs q15min until stable, then hourly until abortion complete. Check resting uterine tone. Administer medications for relief of GI effects if indicated or for abdominal cramps. **Gel:** Monitor uterine activity (onset of uterine contractions), fetal status (heart rate), character of cervix (dilation, effacement). Have patient remain recumbent 12 hr after application with continuous electronic monitoring of fetal heart rate and uterine activity. Record maternal vital signs at least hourly in presence of uterine activity. Reassess Bishop score.

PATIENT/FAMILY TEACHING
• **Suppository:** Report fever, chills, foul-smelling/increased vaginal discharge, uterine cramps or pain promptly.

Diovan, *see valsartan*

Diovan HCT, *see* *hydrochlorothiazide and valsartan*

*diphenhydrAMINE hydrochloride

dye-fen-**hye**-dra-meen

(Allerdry ✦, Banophen, Benadryl, Diphen, Diphenhist, Genahist, Nytol ✦)

Do not confuse diphenhydr-amine with dimenhydrinate, or Benadryl with benazepril, Bentyl, or Benylin, or Banophen with baclofen.

FIXED-COMBINATION(S)

Advil PM: diphenhydramine/ ibuprofen (NSAID): 38 mg/200 mg. With calamine, an astringent, and camphor, a counterirritant **(Caladryl).**

*CLASSIFICATION

PHARMACOTHERAPEUTIC: Ethanol-amine. **CLINICAL:** Antihistamine, anticholinergic, antipruritic, anti-tussive, antiemetic, antidyskinetic (see p. 50C).

ACTION

An ethanolamine that competitively blocks the effects of histamine at periph-eral H_1 receptor sites. Therapeutic Effect: Produces anticholinergic, anti-pruritic, antitussive, antiemetic, antidys-kinetic, and sedative effects.

PHARMACOKINETICS

Route	Onset	Peak	Duration
PO	15–30 min	1–4 hr	4–6 hr
IV, IM	Less than 15 min	1–4 hr	4–6 hr

Well absorbed after PO or parenteral administration. Protein binding: 98%–99%. Widely distributed. Metabolized in the liver. Primarily excreted in urine. Half-life: 1–4 hr.

USES

Treatment of allergic reactions, parkin-sonism; prevention and treatment of nausea, vomiting, vertigo due to motion sickness; antitussive; short-term manage-ment of insomnia. Topical form used for relief of pruritus, insect bites, skin irritations.

PRECAUTIONS

CONTRAINDICATIONS: Acute exacerba-tion of asthma, use within 14 days of MAOIs. **CAUTIONS:** Narrow-angle glau-coma, peptic ulcer, prostatic hyper-trophy, pyloroduodenal or bladder neck obstruction, asthma, chronic obstructive pulmonary disease (COPD), increased intraocular pressure (IOP), cardiovascular disease, hyperthyroidism, hypertension, seizure disorders.

⊠ LIFESPAN CONSIDERATIONS: **Preg-nancy/Lactation:** Crosses placenta. Detected in breast milk (may produce irritability in breast-fed infants). Increased risk of seizures in neonates, premature infants if used during third trimester of pregnancy. May prohibit lactation. **Pregnancy Category B. Children:** Not recommended in new-borns or premature infants (increased risk of paradoxical reaction). **Elderly:** Increased risk for dizziness, sedation, confusion, hypotension, hyperexcit-ability.

INTERACTIONS

DRUG: Alcohol, other CNS depressants: May increase CNS depressant effects. **Anticholinergics:** May increase anticholinergic effects. **MAOIs:** May increase the anticholinergic and CNS depressant effects of diphenhydramine. **HERBAL:** None known. **FOOD:** None known. **LAB VALUES:** May suppress wheal and flare reactions to antigen skin testing unless the drug is discontinued 4 days before testing.

AVAILABILITY (OTC)

CAPSULES: 25 mg (Banophen, Diphen, Genahist), 50 mg (Nytol). **SYRUP (DIPHEN, DIPHENHIST):** 12.5 mg/5 ml. **TABLETS (BANOPHEN, BENADRYL, GENAHIST, NYTOL):** 25 mg, 50 mg. **INJECTION (BENADRYL):** 50 mg/ml. **CREAM (BENADRYL):** 1%, 2%. **SPRAY (BENADRYL):** 1%, 2%.

ADMINISTRATION/HANDLING

 IV

• May be given undiluted. • Give IV injection over at least 1 min.

IM

• Give deep IM into large muscle mass.

PO

• Give without regard to meals. • Scored tablets may be crushed. • Do not crush capsules or film-coated tablets.

▨ IV INCOMPATIBILITIES

Allopurinol (Aloprim), amphotericin B complex (Abelcet, AmBisome, Amphotec), cefepime (Maxipime), dexamethasone (Decadron), foscarnet (Foscavir).

IV COMPATIBILITIES

Atropine, cisplatin (Platinol), cyclophosphamide (Cytoxan), cytarabine (Ara-C), droperidol (Inapsine), fentanyl, glycopyrrolate (Robinul), heparin, hydrocortisone (Solu-Cortef), hydromorphone (Dilaudid), hydroxyzine (Vistaril), lidocaine, metoclopramide (Reglan), ondansetron (Zofran), promethazine (Phenergan), potassium chloride, propofol (Diprivan).

INDICATIONS/ROUTES/DOSAGE
MODERATE TO SEVERE ALLERGIC REACTION
PO, IV, IM: ADULTS, ELDERLY: 25–50 mg q4h. **Maximum:** 400 mg/day. CHILDREN: 5 mg/kg/day in divided doses q6–8h. **Maximum:** 300 mg/day.

MOTION SICKNESS
PO: ADULTS, ELDERLY, CHILDREN 12 YR AND OLDER: 25–50 mg q4–6h. **Maximum:** 300 mg/day. CHILDREN 6–11 YR: 12.5–25 mg q4–6h. **Maximum:** 150 mg/day. CHILDREN 2–5 YR: 6.25 mg q4–6h. **Maximum:** 37.5 mg/day.

PARKINSON'S DISEASE
PO: ADULTS, ELDERLY: 25–50 mg 3–4 times a day.

ANTITUSSIVE
PO: ADULTS, ELDERLY, CHILDREN 12 YR AND OLDER: 25 mg q4h. **Maximum:** 150 mg/day. CHILDREN 6–11 YR: 12.5 mg q4h. **Maximum:** 75 mg/day. CHILDREN 2–5 YR: 6.25 mg q4h. **Maximum:** 37.5 mg/day.

NIGHTTIME SLEEP AID
PO: ADULTS, ELDERLY, CHILDREN 12 YR AND OLDER: 50 mg at bedtime. CHILDREN 2–11 YR: 1 mg/kg/dose. **Maximum:** 50 mg.

PRURITUS
TOPICAL: ADULTS, ELDERLY, CHILDREN 12 YR AND OLDER: Apply 1% or 2% cream or spray 3–4 times a day. CHILDREN 2–11 YR: Apply 1% cream or spray 3–4 times a day.

SIDE EFFECTS

FREQUENT: Somnolence, dizziness, muscle weakness, hypotension, urine retention, thickening of bronchial secretions, dry mouth, nose, throat, or lips; in elderly, sedation, dizziness, hypotension. **OCCASIONAL:** Epigastric distress, flushing, visual or hearing disturbances, paresthesia, diaphoresis, chills.

ADVERSE REACTIONS/ TOXIC EFFECTS

Hypersensitivity reactions, such as eczema, pruritus, rash, cardiac disturbances, and photosensitivity, may occur. Overdose symptoms may vary from CNS depression, including sedation, apnea, hypotension, cardiovascular collapse, and death, to severe paradoxical reactions, such as hallucinations, tremor, and seizures. Children and neonates may experience paradoxical reactions, including restlessness, insomnia, euphoria, nervousness, and tremors. Overdosage in children may result in hallucinations, seizures, and death.

NURSING CONSIDERATIONS

BASELINE ASSESSMENT

If patient is having acute allergic reaction, obtain history of recently ingested foods, drugs, environmental exposure, emotional stress. Monitor rate, depth, rhythm, type of respiration, quality and rate of pulse. Assess lung sounds for rhonchi, wheezing, rales.

INTERVENTION/EVALUATION

Monitor BP, especially in elderly (increased risk of hypotension). Monitor children closely for paradoxical reaction.

PATIENT/FAMILY TEACHING

• Tolerance to antihistaminic effect generally does not occur; tolerance to sedative effect may occur. • Avoid tasks that require alertness, motor skills until response to drug is established. • Dry mouth, drowsiness, dizziness may be an expected response of drug. • Avoid alcohol.

diphenoxylate hydrochloride with atropine sulfate

dye-fen-**ox**-i-late

(Lomocot, Lomotil, Lonox, Vi-Atro)

Do not confuse Lomotil with Lamictal or Lonox with Lanoxin, Loprox, or Lovenox.

FIXED-COMBINATION(S)

Lomotil: diphenoxylate/atropine (anticholinergic, antispasmodic): 2.5 mg/0.025 mg.

CLASSIFICATION

PHARMACOTHERAPEUTIC: Meperidine derivative. **CLINICAL:** Antidiarrheal (see p. 43C).

ACTION

A meperidine derivative that acts locally and centrally on gastric mucosa. Therapeutic Effect: Reduces intestinal motility.

PHARMACOKINETICS

Well absorbed from the GI tract. Metabolized in the liver to active metabolite. Primarily eliminated in feces. Half-life: 2.5 hr; metabolite, 12–24 hr.

USES

Adjunctive treatment of acute, chronic diarrhea.

PRECAUTIONS

CONTRAINDICATIONS: Children younger than 2 yr, dehydration, jaundice, narrow-angle glaucoma, severe hepatic disease. **CAUTIONS:** Cirrhosis, renal/hepatic disease, renal impairment, acute ulcerative colitis.

⌛ LIFESPAN CONSIDERATIONS: **Pregnancy/Lactation:** Unknown if drug crosses placenta or is distributed

---

* "Tall Man" lettering   ❧ Canadian trade name   ⓔ see **evolve**   ⮞ High Alert drug

in breast milk. **Pregnancy Category C. Children:** Not recommended (increased susceptibility to toxicity, including respiratory depression). **Elderly:** More susceptible to anticholinergic effects, confusion, respiratory depression.

INTERACTIONS

DRUG: **Alcohol, other CNS depressants:** May increase CNS depressant effects. **Anticholinergics:** May increase the effects of atropine. **Digoxin:** May increase serum digoxin levels. **MAOIs:** May precipitate hypertensive crisis. HERBAL: None known. FOOD: None known. LAB VALUES: May increase serum amylase level.

AVAILABILITY (Rx)

TABLETS (LOMOTIL, LONOX): 2.5 mg diphenoxylate/0.025 mg atropine. **LIQUID (LOMOTIL):** 2.5 mg/5 ml.

ADMINISTRATION/HANDLING

PO
• Give without regard to meals. If GI irritation occurs, give with food. • Use liquid for children 2–12 yr (use graduated dropper for administration of liquid medication).

INDICATIONS/ROUTES/DOSAGE

DIARRHEA
PO: ADULTS, ELDERLY: Initially, 15–20 mg/day in 3–4 divided doses; then 5–15 mg/day in 2–3 divided doses. CHILDREN 9–12 YR: 2 mg 5 times a day. CHILDREN 6–8 YR: 2 mg 4 times a day. CHILDREN 2–5 YR: 2 mg 3 times a day.

SIDE EFFECTS

FREQUENT: Somnolence, light-headedness, dizziness, nausea. **OCCASIONAL:** Headache, dry mouth. **RARE:** Flushing, tachycardia, urine retention, constipation, paradoxical reaction (marked by restlessness and agitation), blurred vision.

ADVERSE REACTIONS/TOXIC EFFECTS

Dehydration may predispose to diphenoxylate toxicity. Paralytic ileus and toxic megacolon (marked by constipation, decreased appetite, and stomach pain with nausea or vomiting) occur rarely. Severe anticholinergic reaction, manifested by severe lethargy, hypotonic reflexes, and hyperthermia, may result in severe respiratory depression and coma.

NURSING CONSIDERATIONS

BASELINE ASSESSMENT
Check baseline hydration status: skin turgor, mucous membranes for dryness, urinary status.

INTERVENTION/EVALUATION
Encourage adequate fluid intake. Assess bowel sounds for peristalsis. Monitor daily bowel activity, stool consistency; record time of evacuation. Assess for abdominal disturbances. Discontinue medication if abdominal distention occurs.

PATIENT/FAMILY TEACHING
• Avoid tasks that require alertness, motor skills until response to drug is established. • Avoid alcohol, barbiturates. • Contact physician if fever, palpitations occur or diarrhea persists. • Report abdominal distention.

dipivefrin

(Propine)
See Antiglaucoma agents (p. 47C)

Diprivan, *see propofol*

---

dipyridamole

dye-pie-**rid**-ah-mole

(Apo-Dipyridamole ❦, Apo-Dipyridamole FC ❦, Novodipirado l ❦, Persantine)

Do not confuse Aggrenox with Aggrastat, or dipyridamole with disopyramide, or Persantin with Periactin.

FIXED-COMBINATION(S)

Aggrenox: dipyridamole/aspirin (antiplatelet): 200 mg/25 mg.

CLASSIFICATION

PHARMACOTHERAPEUTIC: Blood modifier, platelet aggregation inhibitor. **CLINICAL:** Antiplatelet, antianginal, diagnostic agent (see p. 31C).

ACTION

A blood modifier and platelet aggregation inhibitor that inhibits the activity of adenosine deaminase and phosphodiesterase, enzymes causing accumulation of adenosine and cyclic adenosine monophosphate. Therapeutic Effect: Inhibits platelet aggregation; may cause coronary vasodilation.

PHARMACOKINETICS

Slowly, variably absorbed from the GI tract. Widely distributed. Protein binding: 91%–99%. Metabolized in the liver. Primarily eliminated via biliary excretion. Half-life: 10–15 hr.

USES

Adjunct to warfarin (Coumadin) anticoagulant therapy in prevention of postop thromboembolic complications of cardiac valve replacement. **IV:** Alternative to exercise in thallium myocardial perfusion imaging for evaluation of coronary artery disease. OFF-LABEL: Reduces risk of reinfarction in patients recovering from MI, treatment of transient ischemic attacks (TIAs).

PRECAUTIONS

CONTRAINDICATIONS: None known. **CAUTIONS:** Hypotension.

⧗ LIFESPAN CONSIDERATIONS: **Pregnancy/Lactation:** Distributed in breast milk. **Pregnancy Category C. Children:** Safety and efficacy not established. **Elderly:** No age-related precautions noted.

INTERACTIONS

DRUG: **Anticoagulants, aspirin, heparin, salicylates, thrombolytics:** May increase the risk of bleeding with these drugs. HERBAL: **Ginkgo biloba:** May increase the risk of bleeding. FOOD: None known. LAB VALUES: None known.

AVAILABILITY (Rx)

TABLETS: 25 mg, 50 mg, 75 mg. **INJECTION:** 5 mg/ml.

ADMINISTRATION/HANDLING

🖫 IV

• Dilute to at least 1:2 ratio with 0.9% NaCl or D_5W for total volume of 20–50 ml (undiluted may cause irritation). • Infuse over 4 min. • Inject thallium within 5 min after dipyridamole infusion.

PO
• Best taken on empty stomach with full glass of water.

🞉 IV INCOMPATIBILITIES

No information available via Y-site administration.

INDICATIONS/ROUTES/DOSAGE

PREVENTION OF THROMBOEMBOLIC DISORDERS

PO: ADULTS, ELDERLY: 75–100 mg 4 times a day in combination with other medications. CHILDREN: 3–6 mg/kg/day in 3 divided doses.

D

DIAGNOSTIC AID

IV: ADULTS, ELDERLY (BASED ON WEIGHT): 0.142 mg/kg/min infused over 4 min; although a maximum hasn't been determined, doses greater than 60 mg have been determined to be unnecessary for any patient.

SIDE EFFECTS

FREQUENT (14%): Dizziness. **OCCASIONAL (6%–2%):** Abdominal distress, headache, rash. **RARE (less than 2%):** Diarrhea, vomiting, flushing, pruritus.

ADVERSE REACTIONS/ TOXIC EFFECTS

Overdose produces peripheral vasodilation, resulting in hypotension.

NURSING CONSIDERATIONS

BASELINE ASSESSMENT

Assess for presence of chest pain. Obtain baseline BP, pulse. When used as antiplatelet, check hematologic status.

INTERVENTION/EVALUATION

Assist with ambulation if dizziness occurs. Assess BP for hypotension. Assess skin for flushing, rash.

PATIENT/FAMILY TEACHING

• Avoid alcohol. • If nausea occurs, cola, unsalted crackers, dry toast may relieve effect. • Therapeutic response may not be achieved before 2–3 mo of continuous therapy. • Use caution when getting up suddenly from lying or sitting position.

dirithromycin

die-**rith**-ro-my-sin

(Dynabac, Dynabac D5-Pak)

Do not confuse Dynabac with Dynacin or DynaCirc.

◆ CLASSIFICATION

PHARMACOTHERAPEUTIC: Macrolide. **CLINICAL:** Antibiotic (see p. 25C).

ACTION

A macrolide that binds to ribosomal receptor sites of susceptible organisms, inhibiting bacterial protein synthesis. Therapeutic Effect: Bactericidal or bacteriostatic, depending on drug dosage.

PHARMACOKINETICS

Rapidly absorbed from the GI tract. Protein binding: 15%–30%. Widely distributed into tissues and within cells. Eliminated primarily unchanged by biliary excretion. Not removed by hemodialysis. Half-life: 30–44 hr.

USES

Treatment of susceptible infections due to *H. influenzae, Legionella pneumophila, M. catarrhalis, M. pneumoniae, S. pneumoniae, S. pyogenes* including acute bacterial exacerbation of acute or chronic bronchitis, pharyngitis or tonsillitis, community-acquired pneumonia, uncomplicated skin and skin-structure infections.

PRECAUTIONS

CONTRAINDICATIONS: Hypersensitivity to other macrolide antibiotics. **CAUTIONS:** Hepatic or renal impairment.

⧗ LIFESPAN CONSIDERATIONS: **Pregnancy/Lactation:** Unknown if distributed in breast milk. **Pregnancy Category C. Children:** Safety and efficacy not established in those younger than 12 yr. **Elderly:** No age-related precautions noted.

INTERACTIONS

DRUG: **Aluminum- and magnesium-containing antacids:** May decrease dirithromycin blood concentration. **Carbamazepine, cyclosporine, theophylline, warfarin:** Serum concentrations of these drugs may increase when taken with dirithromycin. **H₂ antagonists:** Increase dirithromycin absorption. HERBAL: None known. FOOD: None known. LAB VALUES: May increase serum creatine kinase (CK) and potassium levels as well as blood eosinophil, neutrophil and platelet counts.

AVAILABILITY (Rx)

TABLETS (ENTERIC-COATED [DYNABAC, DYNABAC D5-PAK]): 250 mg.

ADMINISTRATION/HANDLING

PO
• Administer with food or within 1 hr of meal (food increases absorption).
• Swallow whole (do not cut, crush, or chew tablets).

INDICATIONS/ROUTES/DOSAGE

PHARYNGITIS, TONSILLITIS
PO: ADULTS, ELDERLY, CHILDREN 12 YR AND OLDER: 500 mg once a day for 10 days.

ACUTE OR CHRONIC BRONCHITIS, SKIN AND SKIN-STRUCTURE INFECTIONS
PO: ADULTS, ELDERLY, CHILDREN 12 YR AND OLDER: 500 mg once a day for 7 days.

COMMUNITY-ACQUIRED PNEUMONIA
PO: ADULTS, ELDERLY, CHILDREN 12 YR AND OLDER: 500 mg once a day for 14 days.

SIDE EFFECTS

FREQUENT (10%–8%): Abdominal pain, headache, nausea, diarrhea. **OCCASIONAL (3%–2%):** Vomiting, dyspepsia, dizziness, nonspecific pain, asthenia. **RARE (less than 2%):** Increased cough, flatulence, rash, dyspnea, pruritus and urticaria, insomnia.

ADVERSE REACTIONS/ TOXIC EFFECTS

Antibiotic-associated colitis and other superinfections may result from altered bacterial balance.

NURSING CONSIDERATIONS

BASELINE ASSESSMENT
Question for history of allergies to dirithromycin, erythromycins.

INTERVENTION/EVALUATION
Monitor for improvement in signs and symptoms of infection, WBC. Check for GI discomfort, nausea, headache, diarrhea. Determine pattern of bowel activity and stool consistency. Evaluate for superinfection: genital or anal pruritus, sore mouth or tongue, moderate to severe diarrhea.

PATIENT/FAMILY TEACHING
• Continue therapy for full length of treatment. • Take medication with food or within 1 hr of meal. • Do not take with aluminum or magnesium-containing antacids.

disopyramide phosphate

dye-soe-**peer**-a-mide
(Norpace, Norpace CR, Rythmodan ✦, Rythmodan LA ✦)
Do not confuse disopyramide with desipramine, dipyridamole, or Rythmol.

◆CLASSIFICATION

CLINICAL: Antiarrhythmic (see p. 13C).

ACTION

An antiarrhythmic that prolongs the refractory period of the cardiac cell by direct effect, decreasing myocardial excitability and conduction velocity. Therapeutic Effect: Depresses myocardial contractility. Has anticholinergic and negative inotropic effects.

D

PHARMACOKINETICS

Rapidly and almost completely absorbed from the GI tract. Protein binding: 50%–65%. Metabolized in liver. Excreted in urine. Removed by hemodialysis. Half-life: 4–10 hr.

USES

Suppression and prevention of ventricular ectopy (unifocal/multifocal premature ventricular contractions, episodes of ventricular tachycardia). OFF-LABEL: Prophylaxis and treatment of supraventricular tachycardia.

PRECAUTIONS

CONTRAINDICATIONS: Cardiogenic shock, congenital QT prolongation, narrow-angle glaucoma (unless patient is undergoing cholinergic therapy), preexisting second- or third-degree AV block, preexisting urinary retention. CAUTIONS: CHF, myasthenia gravis, prostatic hypertrophy, sick sinus syndrome (bradycardia/tachycardia), Wolff-Parkinson-White syndrome, bundle-branch block, renal or hepatic impairment.

⏳ LIFESPAN CONSIDERATIONS: Pregnancy/Lactation: Distributed in breast milk. Pregnancy Category C. Children: Safety and efficacy not established in children. Elderly: Increased sensitivity to anticholinergic effects.

INTERACTIONS

DRUG: Other antiarrhythmics, including diltiazem, propranolol, verapamil: May prolong cardiac conduction, decrease cardiac output. Pimozide: May increase cardiac arrhythmias. HERBAL: None known. FOOD: None known. LAB VALUES: May decrease blood glucose levels. May cause EKG changes. May increase serum cholesterol and triglyceride levels. Therapeutic serum level is 2–8 mcg/ml and the toxic serum level is greater than 8 mcg/ml.

AVAILABILITY (Rx)

CAPSULES (NORPACE): 100 mg, 150 mg. CAPSULES (EXTENDED-RELEASE [NORPACE CR]): 100 mg, 150 mg.

ADMINISTRATION/HANDLING

PO
• Administer immediate-release capsules in divided doses. • Swallow extended-release capsules whole.

INDICATIONS/ROUTES/DOSAGE

SUPPRESSION AND PREVENTION OF VENTRICULAR ECTOPY, UNIFOCAL OR MULTIFOCAL PREMATURE VENTRICULAR CONTRACTIONS, PAIRED VENTRICULAR CONTRACTIONS (COUPLETS), AND EPISODES OF VENTRICULAR TACHYCARDIA

PO: ADULTS, ELDERLY WEIGHING 50 KG AND MORE: 150 mg q6h (300 mg q12h with extended-release). ADULTS, ELDERLY WEIGHING LESS THAN 50 KG: 100 mg q6h (200 mg q12h with extended-release).

USUAL PEDIATRIC DOSAGE

PO (IMMEDIATE-RELEASE CAPSULES): CHILDREN 12–18 YR: 6–15 mg/kg/day in divided doses q6h. CHILDREN 5–11 YR: 10–15 mg/kg/day in divided doses q6h. CHILDREN 1–4 YR: 10–20 mg/kg/day in divided doses q6h. CHILDREN YOUNGER THAN 1 YR: 10–30 mg/kg/day in divided doses q6h.

DOSAGE IN RENAL IMPAIRMENT

With or without loading dose of 150 mg:

Creatinine Clearance	Dosage
40 ml/min and higher	100 mg q6h (extended-release 200 mg q12h)
30–39 ml/min	100 mg q8h
15–29 ml/min	100 mg q12h
Less than 15 ml/min	100 mg q24h

DOSAGE IN LIVER IMPAIRMENT

ADULTS, ELDERLY WEIGHING 50 KG AND MORE: 100 mg q6h (200 mg q12h with extended-release).

✐ see color pill atlas   ✐ herb   underlined – top prescribed drug

DOSAGE IN CARDIOMYOPATHY, CARDIAC DECOMPENSATION

ADULTS, ELDERLY WEIGHING 50 KG AND MORE: No loading dose; 100 mg q6–8h with gradual dosage adjustments.

SIDE EFFECTS

FREQUENT (greater than 9%): Dry mouth (32%), urinary hesitancy, constipation. **OCCASIONAL (9%–3%):** Blurred vision, dry eyes, nose, or throat, urinary retention, headache, dizziness, fatigue, nausea. **RARE (less than 1%):** Impotence, hypotension, edema, weight gain, shortness of breath, syncope, chest pain, nervousness, diarrhea, vomiting, decreased appetite, rash, itching.

ADVERSE REACTIONS/ TOXIC EFFECTS

May produce or aggravate CHF. May produce severe hypotension, shortness of breath, chest pain, syncope (especially in patients with primary cardiomyopathy or CHF). Hepatotoxicity occurs rarely.

NURSING CONSIDERATIONS

BASELINE ASSESSMENT

Before giving medication, instruct patient to void (reduces risk of urinary retention).

INTERVENTION/EVALUATION

Monitor EKG for cardiac changes, particularly widening of QRS complex, prolongation of PR and QT intervals. Monitor BP, EKG, serum potassium, glucose, hepatic enzymes. Monitor I&O (be alert to urinary retention). Assess for evidence of CHF (cough, dyspnea [particularly on exertion], rales at base of lungs, fatigue). Assist with ambulation if dizziness occurs. Therapeutic serum level: 2–8 mcg/ml; toxic serum level: greater than 8 mcg/ml.

PATIENT/FAMILY TEACHING

• Report shortness of breath, productive cough. • Do not use nasal decongestants, OTC cold preparations (stimulants) without physician approval. • Restrict salt, alcohol intake.

Ditropan, *see oxybutynin*

Ditropan XL, *see oxybutynin*

---

*DOBUTamine hydrochloride

doe-**byoo**-ta-meen

(Dobutrex)

Do not confuse dobutamine with dopamine.

CLASSIFICATION

PHARMACOTHERAPEUTIC: Sympathomimetic. **CLINICAL:** Cardiac stimulant (see p. 142C).

ACTION

A direct-acting inotropic agent acting primarily on beta$_1$-adrenergic receptors. **Therapeutic Effect:** Decreases preload and afterload, and enhances myocardial contractility, stroke volume, and cardiac output. Improves renal blood flow and urine output.

PHARMACOKINETICS

Route	Onset	Peak	Duration
IV	1–2 min	10 min	Length of infusion

Metabolized in the liver. Primarily excreted in urine. Not removed by hemodialysis. Half-life: 2 min.

D

USES

Short-term management of cardiac decompensation.

PRECAUTIONS

CONTRAINDICATIONS: Hypovolemia patients, idiopathic hypertrophic subaortic stenosis, sulfite sensitivity. **CAUTIONS:** Atrial fibrillation, hypertension, hypovolemia, severe coronary artery disease, MI.

⌛ **LIFESPAN CONSIDERATIONS: Pregnancy/Lactation:** Unknown if drug crosses placenta or is distributed in breast milk. Has not been administered to pregnant women. **Pregnancy Category B. Children/Elderly:** No age-related precautions noted.

INTERACTIONS

DRUG: Beta blockers: May antagonize the effects of dobutamine. **Digoxin:** May increase the risk of arrhythmias and enhance the inotropic effect of both drugs. **Entacapone:** May increase the risk of arrhythmias, hypertension, and tachycardias. **MAOIs, oxytocics, tricyclic antidepressants:** May increase the adverse effects of dobutamine, such as arrhythmias and hypertension. **HERBAL:** None known. **FOOD:** None known. **LAB VALUES:** Decreases serum potassium level.

AVAILABILITY (Rx)

INFUSION (READY-TO-USE): 1 mg/ml, 2 mg/ml, 4 mg/ml. **INJECTION:** 12.5-mg/ml vial.

ADMINISTRATION/HANDLING

◂ **ALERT** ▸ Correct hypovolemia with volume expanders before dobutamine infusion. Those with atrial fibrillation should be digitalized before infusion. Administer by IV infusion only.

▢ IV

Reconstitution • Dilute 250-mg ampule with 10 ml sterile water for injection or D₅W for injection. Resulting solution: 25 mg/ml. Add additional 10 ml of diluent if not completely dissolved (resulting solution: 12.5 mg/ml). • Further dilute 250-mg vial with D₅W or 0.9% NaCl. Maximum concentration: 3.125 g/250 ml (12.5 mg/ml).

Rate of administration • Use infusion pump to control flow rate. • Titrate dosage to individual response. • Infiltration causes local inflammatory changes. • Extravasation may cause dermal necrosis.

Storage • Store at room temperature. Freezing produces crystallization. • Pink discoloration of solution (due to oxidation) does not indicate loss of potency if used within recommended time period. • Further diluted solution for infusion must be used within 24 hr.

▨ IV INCOMPATIBILITIES

Acyclovir (Zovirax), alteplase (Activase), amphotericin B complex (Abelcet, AmBisome, Amphotec), bumetanide (Bumex), cefepime (Maxipime), foscarnet (Foscavir), furosemide (Lasix), heparin, piperacillin/tazobactam (Zosyn).

IV COMPATIBILITIES

Amiodarone (Cordarone), calcium chloride, calcium gluconate, diltiazem (Cardizem), dopamine (Intropin), enalapril (Vasotec), famotidine (Pepcid), hydromorphone(Dilaudid),insulin(regular), lidocaine, lorazepam (Ativan), magnesium sulfate, midazolam (Versed), milrinone (Primacor), morphine, nitroglycerin, norepinephrine (Levophed), potassium chloride, propofol (Diprivan), total parenteral nutrition (TPN).

INDICATIONS/ROUTES/DOSAGE

SHORT-TERM MANAGEMENT OF CARDIAC DECOMPENSATION
IV INFUSION: ADULTS, ELDERLY, CHILDREN: 2.5–20 mcg/kg/min. Rarely, drug can be infused at a rate of up to 40 mcg/kg/

min to increase cardiac output. NEONATES: 2–15 mcg/kg/min.

SIDE EFFECTS

FREQUENT (greater than 5%): Increased heart rate, increased BP. **OCCASIONAL (5%–3%):** Pain at injection site. **RARE (3%–1%):** Nausea, headache, anginal pain, shortness of breath, fever.

ADVERSE REACTIONS/ TOXIC EFFECTS

Overdose may produce a marked increase in heart rate (by 30 beats/min or higher) marked increase in BP (by 50 mm Hg or higher), anginal pain, and premature ventricular contractions (PVCs).

NURSING CONSIDERATIONS

BASELINE ASSESSMENT

Patient must be on continuous cardiac monitoring. Determine weight (for dosage calculation). Obtain initial BP, heart rate, respirations. Correct hypovolemia before drug therapy.

INTERVENTION/EVALUATION

Continuously monitor for cardiac rate, arrhythmias. With physician, establish parameters for adjusting rate or stopping infusion. Maintain accurate I&O; measure urine output frequently. Assess serum potassium levels and dobutamine plasma level (therapeutic range: 40–190 ng/ml). Monitor BP continuously (hypertension greater risk in patients with preexisting hypertension). Check cardiac output and pulmonary wedge pressure or central venous pressure (CVP) frequently. Immediately notify physician of decreased urine output, cardiac arrhythmias, significant increase in BP, heart rate, or less commonly hypotension.

Dobutrex, *see dobutamine*

---

docetaxel ⚑

dox-eh-**tax**-el
(Taxotere)
Do not confuse docetaxel with Taxol.

CLASSIFICATION

PHARMACOTHERAPEUTIC: Antimitotic agent, taxoid. **CLINICAL:** Antineoplastic (see p. 73C).

ACTION

An antimitotic agent belonging to the taxoid family that disrupts the microtubular cell network, which is essential for cellular function. Therapeutic Effect: Inhibits cellular mitosis.

PHARMACOKINETICS

Distributed into peripheral compartments. Protein binding: 94%. Extensively metabolized. Excreted primarily in feces, with lesser amount in urine. Half-life: 11.1 hr.

USES

Treatment of locally advanced or metastatic breast carcinoma after the failure of any prior chemotherapy. Treatment of metastatic non–small cell lung cancer. Treatment of metastatic prostate cancer (with prednisone). Treatment of stomach cancer. OFF-LABEL: Bladder, esophageal, gastric, head and neck, ovarian, small cell lung carcinoma.

PRECAUTIONS

CONTRAINDICATIONS: History of severe hypersensitivity to drugs formulated with polysorbate 80, neutrophil count less than 1,500 cells/mm³. **CAUTIONS:** Hepatic impairment, bone marrow depression, herpes zoster, chickenpox, preexisting pleural effusion, infection, chemotherapy or radiation.

⌛ LIFESPAN CONSIDERATIONS: Pregnancy/Lactation: May cause fetal

---

harm. Unknown if distributed in breast milk; do not breast-feed. **Pregnancy Category D. Children:** Safety and efficacy not established in those younger than 16 yr. **Elderly:** No age-related precautions noted.

INTERACTIONS

DRUG: **Bone marrow depressants:** May increase myelosuppression. **Cyclosporine, erythromycin, ketoconazole:** May significantly inhibit docetaxel metabolism. **Live virus vaccines:** May potentiate replication, increase vaccine side effects, and decrease the patient's antibody response to the vaccine. HERBAL: None known. FOOD: None known. LAB VALUES: May significantly increase BUN level and serum alkaline phosphatase, bilirubin, creatinine, AST, and ALT levels. Reduces blood neutrophil, thrombocyte, and WBC counts.

AVAILABILITY (Rx)

INJECTION: 20 mg/0.5 ml with diluent, 80 mg/2 ml with diluent.

ADMINISTRATION/HANDLING

◂ ALERT ▸ Because docetaxel may be carcinogenic, mutagenic, or teratogenic, handle the drug with extreme care during preparation and administration.

◂ ALERT ▸ Dilution is required before administration. Patient should be premedicated with oral corticosteroids (e.g., dexamethasone 16 mg/day for 5 days beginning day 1 before docetaxel therapy; reduces severity of fluid retention, hypersensitivity reaction).

 IV

Reconstitution • Withdraw contents of diluent (provided by manufacturer) and add to vial of docetaxel. • Gently rotate to ensure thorough mixing to provide a solution of 10 mg/ml. • Withdraw dose and add to 250 ml 0.9% NaCl or D₅W in glass or polyolefin

container to provide a final concentration of 0.3–0.9 mg/ml.

Rate of administration • Administer as a 1-hr infusion. • Monitor closely for hypersensitivity reaction (i.e., flushing, localized skin reaction, bronchospasm [may occur within a few min after beginning infusion]).

Storage • Refrigerate vial. Freezing does not adversely affect drug. • Protect from bright light. • Stand vial at room temperature for 5 min before administering (do not store in PVC bags). • Remixed solution is stable for 8 hr either at room temperature or if refrigerated.

🏵 IV INCOMPATIBILITIES

Amphotericin B (Fungizone), doxorubicin liposomal (DaunoXome), methylprednisolone (Solu-Medrol), nalbuphine (Nubain).

IV COMPATIBILITIES

Bumetanide (Bumex), calcium gluconate, dexamethasone (Decadron), diphenhydramine (Benadryl), dobutamine (Dobutrex), dopamine (Inotropin), furosemide (Lasix), granisetron (Kytril), heparin, hydromorphone (Dilaudid), lorazepam (Ativan), magnesium sulfate, mannitol, morphine, ondansetron (Zofran), potassium chloride.

INDICATIONS/ROUTES/DOSAGE
BREAST CARCINOMA

IV: ADULTS: $60–100$ mg/m² given over 1 hr q3wk. If patient develops febrile neutropenia, a neutrophil count less than 500 cells/mm³ for longer than 1 wk, severe or cumulative cutaneous reactions, or severe peripheral neuropathy with initial dose of 100 mg/m², dosage should be decreased to 75 mg/m². If reaction continues, dosage should be further reduced to 55 mg/m² or therapy should be discontinued. Patients who don't experience the above symptoms at a dose of 60 mg/m² may tolerate an increased docetaxel dose.

NON–SMALL CELL LUNG CARCINOMA
IV: ADULTS: 75 mg/m² q3wk. Adjust dosage if toxicity occurs.

PROSTATE CANCER
IV: ADULTS, ELDERLY: 75 mg/m² q3wk with concurrent administration of prednisone 5 mg twice a day.

SIDE EFFECTS

FREQUENT: Alopecia (80%), asthenia (62%), hypersensitivity reaction such as dermatitis (59% decreases to 16% in those pretreated with oral corticosteroids), fluid retention (49%), stomatitis (43%), nausea and diarrhea (40%), fever (30%), nail changes (28%), vomiting (24%), myalgia (19%). **OCCASIONAL:** Hypotension, edema, anorexia, headache, weight gain, infection (urinary tract, injection site, indwelling catheter tip), dizziness. **RARE:** Dry skin, sensory disorders (vision, speech, taste), arthralgia, weight loss, conjunctivitis, hematuria, proteinuria.

ADVERSE REACTIONS/ TOXIC EFFECTS

In patients with normal liver function tests, neutropenia (neutrophil count less than 2,000 cells/mm³) and leukopenia (WBC count less than 4,000 cells/mm³) occur in 96% of patients; anemia (hemoglobin level less than 11 g/dl) occurs in 90% of patients; thrombocytopenia (platelet count less than 100,000 cells/mm³) occur in 8% of patients; and infection occurs in 28% of patients. Neurosensory and neuromotor effects, such as distal paresthesias and weakness, occur in 54% and 13% of patients, respectively.

NURSING CONSIDERATIONS

BASELINE ASSESSMENT
Offer emotional support to patient and family. Antiemetics may be effective in preventing, treating nausea, vomiting. Patient should be pretreated with corticosteroids before therapy to reduce fluid retention, hypersensitivity reaction.

INTERVENTION/EVALUATION
Frequent monitoring of blood counts is essential, particularly neutrophil count (less than 1,500 cells/mm³ requires discontinuation of therapy). Monitor renal and liver function tests; serum uric acid levels. Observe for cutaneous reactions characterized by rash with eruptions, mainly on hands or feet. Assess for extravascular fluid accumulation: rales in lungs, dependent edema, dyspnea at rest, pronounced abdominal distention (due to ascites).

PATIENT/FAMILY TEACHING
• Alopecia is reversible, but new hair growth may have different color or texture. • New hair growth resumes 2–3 mo after last therapy dose. • Maintain fastidious oral hygiene. • Do not have immunizations without physician approval (drug lowers body's resistance). • Avoid those who have recently taken live virus vaccine.

docusate

dok-yoo-sate

(Apo-Docusate ✽, Colace, Colax-C ✽, Diocto, Docusoft-S, Novo-Ducosate ✽, PMS-Docusate ✽, Pro-Cal-Sof, Regulex ✽, Selax ✽, Soflax ✽, Surfak)

CLASSIFICATION

PHARMACOTHERAPEUTIC: Bulk-producing laxative. **CLINICAL:** Stool softener (see p. 109C).

ACTION

A bulk-producing laxative that decreases surface film tension by mixing liquid and bowel contents. **Therapeutic**

Effect: Increases infiltration of liquid to form a softer stool.

PHARMACOKINETICS

Minimal absorption from the GI tract. Acts in small and large intestines. Results usually occur 1–2 days after first dose, but may take 3–5 days.

USES

Stool softener for those who need to avoid straining during defecation; constipation associated with hard, dry stools.

PRECAUTIONS

CONTRAINDICATIONS: Acute abdominal pain, concomitant use of mineral oil, intestinal obstruction, nausea, vomiting. **CAUTIONS:** Do not use for longer than 1 wk.

⌛ **LIFESPAN CONSIDERATIONS: Pregnancy/Lactation:** Unknown if drug is distributed in breast milk. **Pregnancy Category C. Children:** Not recommended in children younger than 6 yr. **Elderly:** No age-related precautions noted.

INTERACTIONS

DRUG: Danthron, mineral oil: May increase the absorption of danthron or mineral oil. **HERBAL:** None known. **FOOD:** None known. **LAB VALUES:** None known.

AVAILABILITY (OTC)

CAPSULES: 50 mg (Colace), 100 mg (Colace, Ducosoft-S), 240 mg (Surfak). **LIQUID (COLACE):** 50 mg/5 ml (sodium). **SYRUP (COLACE, DIOCTO):** 60 mg/15 ml.

ADMINISTRATION/HANDLING

• Drink 6–8 glasses of water a day (aids stool softening). • Give each dose with full glass of water or fruit juice. • Administer docusate liquid with milk, fruit juice, or infant formula (masks bitter taste).

INDICATIONS/ROUTES/DOSAGE
STOOL SOFTENER

PO: ADULTS, ELDERLY, CHILDREN 12 YR AND OLDER: 50–500 mg/day in 1–4 divided doses. CHILDREN 6–11 YR: 40–150 mg/day in 1–4 divided doses. CHILDREN 3–5 YR: 20–60 mg/day in 1–4 divided doses. CHILDREN YOUNGER THAN 3 YR: 10–40 mg in 1–4 divided doses.

SIDE EFFECTS

OCCASIONAL: Mild GI cramping, throat irritation (with liquid preparation). **RARE:** Rash.

ADVERSE REACTIONS/ TOXIC EFFECTS

None known.

NURSING CONSIDERATIONS

INTERVENTION/EVALUATION

Encourage adequate fluid intake. Assess bowel sounds for peristalsis. Monitor daily bowel activity/stool consistency, record time of evacuation.

PATIENT/FAMILY TEACHING

• Institute measures to promote defecation: increase fluid intake, exercise, high-fiber diet. • Do not use for longer than 1 wk.

dolasetron

dole-**ah**-seh-tron

(<u>Anzemet</u>)

Do not confuse Anzemet with Aldomet.

◆ **CLASSIFICATION**

PHARMACOTHERAPEUTIC: Selective receptor antagonist. **CLINICAL:** Antiemetic.

ACTION

A 5-HT$_3$ receptor antagonist that acts centrally in the chemoreceptor trigger zone and peripherally at the vagal nerve terminals. **Therapeutic Effect:** Prevents nausea and vomiting.

PHARMACOKINETICS

Readily absorbed from the GI tract after PO administration. Protein binding: 69%–77%. Metabolized in the liver. Primarily excreted in urine. Unknown if removed by hemodialysis. **Half-life:** 5–10 hr.

USES

Oral: Prevention of nausea or vomiting associated with cancer chemotherapy, including high-dose cisplatin; prevention of postop nausea or vomiting. **Injection:** Treatment of postop nausea or vomiting. **OFF-LABEL:** Radiation therapy induced nausea and vomiting.

PRECAUTIONS

CONTRAINDICATIONS: None known. **CAUTIONS:** Those who have or may have prolongation of cardiac conduction intervals, hypokalemia, hypomagnesemia, those taking diuretics with potential for inducing electrolyte disturbances, congenital long QT syndrome, those taking antiarrhythmics that may lead to QT prolongation and cumulative high-dose anthracycline therapy.

⧖ **LIFESPAN CONSIDERATIONS: Pregnancy/Lactation:** Unknown if drug is distributed in breast milk. **Pregnancy Category B. Children:** Safety and efficacy not established in those younger than 2 yr. **Elderly:** No age-related precautions noted.

INTERACTIONS

DRUG: None known. **HERBAL:** None known. **FOOD:** None known. **LAB VALUES:** May transiently increase AST and ALT levels.

AVAILABILITY (Rx)

TABLETS: 50 mg, 100 mg. **INJECTION:** 20 mg/ml in single use 0.625 ml amps,

0.625 ml fill in 2 ml Carpuject and 5 ml vials.

ADMINISTRATION/HANDLING

 IV

Reconstitution • May dilute in 0.9% NaCl, D_5W, D_5W with 0.45% NaCl, D_5W with lactated Ringer's, lactated Ringer's, or 10% mannitol injection to 50 ml.

Rate of administration • Can be given as IV push as rapidly as 100 mg/30 sec. • Intermittent IV infusion (piggyback) may be infused over 15 min.

Storage • Store vials at room temperature. • After dilution, solution is stable for 24 hr at room temperature or 48 hr if refrigerated.

PO
• Do not cut, break, or chew film-coated tablets. • For children 2–16 yr, injection form may be mixed in apple or apple-grape juice for oral dosing at 1.8 mg/kg up to a maximum of 100 mg.

⊞ IV INCOMPATIBILITIES

No information available for Y-site administration.

INDICATIONS/ROUTES/DOSAGE

PREVENTION OF CHEMOTHERAPY-INDUCED NAUSEA AND VOMITING
PO: ADULTS: 100 mg within 1 hr of chemotherapy. CHILDREN 2–16 YR: 1.8 mg/kg within 1 hr of chemotherapy. **Maximum:** 100 mg.
IV: ADULTS, CHILDREN 1–16 YR: 1.8 mg/kg as a single dose 30 min before chemotherapy. **Maximum:** 100 mg.

TREATMENT OR PREVENTION OF POSTOPERATIVE NAUSEA OR VOMITING
PO: ADULTS: 100 mg within 2 hr of surgery. CHILDREN 2–16 YR: 1.2 mg/kg within 2 hr of surgery. **Maximum:** 100 mg.
IV: ADULTS: 12.5 mg 15 min before cessation of anesthesia or as soon as nausea occurs. CHILDREN 2–16 YR: 0.35

D

mg/kg 15 min before cessation of anesthesia or as soon as nausea occurs. **Maximum:** 12.5 mg.

SIDE EFFECTS

FREQUENT (10%–5%): Headache, diarrhea, fatigue. **OCCASIONAL (5%–1%):** Fever, dizziness, tachycardia, dyspepsia.

ADVERSE REACTIONS/ TOXIC EFFECTS

Overdose may produce a combination of CNS stimulant and depressant effects.

NURSING CONSIDERATIONS

BASELINE ASSESSMENT

Assess for dehydration if excessive vomiting occurs (poor skin turgor, dry mucous membranes, longitudinal furrows in tongue). Provide emotional support.

INTERVENTION/EVALUATION

Monitor for therapeutic relief from nausea or vomiting, EKG in high-risk patients. Maintain quiet, supportive atmosphere.

Dolobid, *see diflunisal*

Dolophine, *see* *methadone*

---

donepezil hydrochloride

doh-**neh**-peh-zil

(Aricept, Aricept ODT)

Do not confuse Aricept with Aciphex or Ascriptin.

◆ CLASSIFICATION

PHARMACOTHERAPEUTIC: Cholinesterase inhibitor. **CLINICAL:** Cholinergic.

ACTION

A cholinesterase inhibitor that inhibits the enzyme acetylcholinesterase, thus increasing the concentration of acetylcholine at cholinergic synapses and enhancing cholinergic function in the CNS. **Therapeutic Effect:** Slows the progression of Alzheimer's disease.

PHARMACOKINETICS

Well absorbed after PO administration. Protein binding: 96%. Extensively metabolized. Eliminated in urine and feces. **Half-life:** 70 hr.

USES

Treatment of mild to moderate dementia of Alzheimer's disease. **OFF-LABEL:** Treatment of attention deficit hyperactivity disorder, autism, behavioral syndromes in dementia.

PRECAUTIONS

CONTRAINDICATIONS: History of hypersensitivity to piperidine derivatives. **CAUTIONS:** Asthma, chronic obstructive pulmonary disease (COPD), bladder outflow obstruction, history of ulcer disease, those on concurrent NSAIDs, "sick sinus syndrome" or other supraventricular cardiac conduction conditions, seizures.

⧖ **LIFESPAN CONSIDERATIONS: Pregnancy/Lactation:** Unknown if drug is distributed in breast milk. **Pregnancy Category C. Children:** Safety and efficacy not established. **Elderly:** No age-related precautions noted.

INTERACTIONS

DRUG: Anticholinergics: May decrease the effect of anticholinergics.

Cholinergic agonists, neuromuscular blockers, succinylcholine: May increase the synergistic effects of these drugs. **Ketoconazole, quinidine:** May inhibit the metabolism of donepezil. **NSAIDs:** May increase gastric acid secretion of NSAIDs. **Paroxetine:** May decrease the metabolism and increase the blood concentration of donepezil. HERBAL: None known. FOOD: None known. LAB VALUES: May increase blood glucose and serum creatine kinase and LDH concentrations. May decrease the serum potassium level.

AVAILABILITY (Rx)

TABLETS (ARICEPT): 5 mg, 10 mg.
TABLETS (ORALLY-DISINTEGRATING [ARICEPT ODT]): 5 mg, 10 mg.

ADMINISTRATION/HANDLING

PO
• May be given without regard to meals or time of administration, although it is suggested dose be given in the evening, just before bedtime.

INDICATIONS/ROUTES/DOSAGE

ALZHEIMER'S DISEASE
PO: ADULTS, ELDERLY: Initially, 5 mg/day at bedtime. May increase at 4–6 wk interval to 10 mg/day at bedtime.

SIDE EFFECTS

FREQUENT (11%–8%): Nausea, diarrhea, headache, insomnia, nonspecific pain, dizziness. **OCCASIONAL (6%–3%):** Mild muscle cramps, fatigue, vomiting, anorexia, ecchymosis. **RARE (3%–2%):** Depression, abnormal dreams, weight loss, arthritis, somnolence, syncope, frequent urination.

ADVERSE REACTIONS/ TOXIC EFFECTS

Overdose may result in cholinergic crisis, characterized by severe nausea, increased salivation, diaphoresis, bradycardia, hypotension, flushed skin, abdominal pain, respiratory depression, seizures, and cardiorespiratory collapse. Increasing muscle weakness may result in death if respiratory muscles are involved. The antidote is 1–2 mg IV atropine sulfate with subsequent doses based on therapeutic response.

NURSING CONSIDERATIONS

BASELINE ASSESSMENT
Obtain baseline vital signs. Assess history for peptic ulcer, urinary obstruction, asthma, COPD, seizure disorder, cardiac conduction disturbances.

INTERVENTION/EVALUATION
Monitor for cholinergic reaction: GI discomfort or cramping, feeling of facial warmth, excessive salivation and diaphoresis, lacrimation, pallor, urinary urgency, dizziness. Monitor for nausea, diarrhea, headache, insomnia.

PATIENT/FAMILY TEACHING
• Report nausea, vomiting, diarrhea, diaphoresis, increased salivary secretions, severe abdominal pain, dizziness.
• May take without regard to food.
• Not a cure for Alzheimer's disease but may slow the progression of symptoms.

dong quai

Also known as **Chinese angelica, dang gui, tang kuei, toki.**

CLASSIFICATION
HERBAL: See Appendix G.

ACTION
Competitively inhibits estradiol binding to estrogen receptors. Has vasodilation, antispasmodic, CNS stimulant activity. Effect: Reduces symptoms of menopause.

USES
Gynecologic ailments, including menstrual cramps, menopause symptoms;

uterine stimulant. Also used to control hypertension and as anti-inflammatory, vasodilator, immunosuppressant, analgesic, antipyretic.

PRECAUTIONS

CONTRAINDICATIONS: Pregnancy due to uterine stimulant effect, bleeding disorders, excessive menstrual flow. **CAUTIONS:** Lactation; breast, ovarian, uterine cancer.

⧗ **LIFESPAN CONSIDERATIONS: Pregnancy/Lactation:** Contraindicated. **Children:** Safety and efficacy not established. **Elderly:** No age-related precautions noted.

INTERACTIONS

DRUG: Warfarin: Anticoagulant effect and risk of bleeding is increased. **HERBAL: Feverfew, garlic, ginger, ginkgo, ginseng:** May increase risk of bleeding. **FOOD:** None known. **LAB VALUES:** May increase PT/INR.

AVAILABILITY (Rx)

DONG QUAI SOFTGEL: 200 mg, 530 mg, 565 mg.

INDICATIONS/ROUTES/DOSAGE

GYNECOLOGIC AILMENTS, OTHER PURPORTED USES
PO: ADULTS, ELDERLY: 3–4 g a day in divided doses with meals.

SIDE EFFECTS

Diarrhea, photosensitivity, nausea, vomiting, anorexia, increased menstrual flow.

ADVERSE REACTIONS/ TOXIC EFFECTS

None known.

NURSING CONSIDERATIONS

BASELINE ASSESSMENT

Assess if patient is pregnant or breast-feeding, taking other medications, especially those that increase risk of bleeding.

INTERVENTION/EVALUATION

Assess for hypersensitivity reaction.

PATIENT/FAMILY TEACHING

• Inform physician if pregnant or planning to become pregnant. • Do not breast-feed. • May cause photosensitivity reaction; sunscreen or protective clothing should be worn.

*DOPamine hydrochloride ⚑

dope-a-meen
(Intropin)

Do not confuse dopamine with dobutamine or Dopram, or Inotropin with Isoptin.

◆ CLASSIFICATION

PHARMACOTHERAPEUTIC: Sympathomimetic (adrenergic agonist). **CLINICAL:** Cardiac stimulant, vasopressor (see p. 142C).

ACTION

A sympathomimetic (adrenergic agonist) that stimulates adrenergic receptors. Effects are dose dependent. Low dosages (less than 5 mcg/kg/min) stimulate dopaminergic receptors, causing renal vasodilation. Low to moderate dosages (10 mcg/kg/min or less) have a positive inotropic effect by direct action and release of norepinephrine. High dosages (greater than 10 mcg/kg/min) stimulate alpha-receptors. **Therapeutic Effect:** With low dosages, increases renal blood flow, urine flow, and sodium excretion. With low to moderate dosages, increases myocardial contractility, stroke volume, and cardiac output. With high dosages, increases peripheral resistance, renal vasoconstriction, and systolic and diastolic BP.

PHARMACOKINETICS

Route	Onset	Peak	Duration
IV	1–2 min	N/A	Less than 10 min

Widely distributed. Does not cross blood-brain barrier. Metabolized in the liver, kidney, and plasma. Primarily excreted in urine. Not removed by hemodialysis. Half-life: 2 min.

USES

Prophylaxis and treatment of acute hypotension, shock (associated with MI, trauma, renal failure, cardiac decompensation, open heart surgery), treatment of low cardiac output, CHF.

PRECAUTIONS

CONTRAINDICATIONS: Pheochromocytoma, sulfite sensitivity, uncorrected tachyarrhythmias, ventricular fibrillation. **CAUTIONS:** Ischemic heart disease, occlusive vascular disease, hypovolemia, recent use of MAOIs, or ventricular arrhythmias.

LIFESPAN CONSIDERATIONS: **Pregnancy/Lactation:** Unknown if drug crosses placenta or is distributed in breast milk. **Pregnancy Category C. Children:** Recommended close hemodynamic monitoring (gangrene due to extravasation reported). **Elderly:** No age-related precautions noted.

INTERACTIONS

DRUG: **Beta blockers:** May decrease the effects of dopamine. **Digoxin:** May increase the risk of arrhythmias. **Ergot alkaloids:** May increase vasoconstriction. **MAOIs:** May increase cardiac stimulation and vasopressor effects. **Tricyclic antidepressants:** May increase cardiovascular effects. HERBAL: None known. FOOD: None known. LAB VALUES: None known.

AVAILABILITY (Rx)

INJECTION: 40 mg/ml, 80 mg/ml, 160 mg/ml. **INJECTION (PREMIX WITH DEXTROSE):** 80 mg/100 ml, 160 mg/100 ml, 320 mg/100 ml.

ADMINISTRATION/HANDLING

◀ ALERT ▶ Blood volume depletion must be corrected before administering dopamine (may be used concurrently with fluid replacement).

 IV

Reconstitution • Available prediluted in 250 or 500 ml D₅W or dilute each 5-ml (200-mg) ampule in 250–500 ml 0.9% NaCl, D₅W/0.45 NaCl, D₅W/0.45 NaCl, D₅W/lactated Ringer's or lactated Ringer's (concentration is dependent on dosage and fluid requirement of patient); 250 ml solution yields 800 mcg/ml; 500 ml solution yields 400 mcg/ml. Maximum concentration: 3.2 g/250 ml (12.8 mg/ml).

Rate of administration • Administer into large vein (antecubital fossa or central line) to prevent extravasation. • Use infusion pump to control rate of flow. • Titrate each patient to the desired hemodynamic or renal response (optimum urine flow determines dosage).

Storage • Do not use solutions darker than slightly yellow or discolored to yellow, brown, or pink to purple (indicates decomposition of drug). • Stable for 24 hr after dilution.

IV INCOMPATIBILITIES

Acyclovir (Zovirax), amphotericin B complex (Abelcet, AmBisome, Amphotec), cefepime (Maxipime), furosemide (Lasix), insulin, sodium bicarbonate.

IV COMPATIBILITIES

Amiodarone (Cordarone), calcium chloride, diltiazem (Cardizem), dobutamine (Dobutrex), enalapril (Vasotec), heparin, hydromorphone (Dilaudid), labetalol (Trandate), levofloxacin (Levaquin), lidocaine, lorazepam (Ativan), methylprednisolone (Solu-Medrol), midazolam (Versed), milrinone (Primacor), morphine, nicardipine (Cardene), nitroglycerin, norepinephrine (Levophed), piperacillin/tazobactam (Zosyn), potassium chloride, propofol (Diprivan), total parenteral nutrition (TPN).

INDICATIONS/ROUTES/DOSAGE

TREATMENT AND PREVENTION OF ACUTE HYPOTENSION; SHOCK (ASSOCIATED WITH CARDIAC DECOMPENSATION, MI, OPEN HEART SURGERY, RENAL FAILURE, OR TRAUMA), TREATMENT OF LOW CARDIAC OUTPUT, TREATMENT OF CHF
IV: ADULTS, ELDERLY: 1 mcg/kg/min up to 50 mcg/kg/min titrated to desired response. CHILDREN: 1–20 mcg/kg/min. **Maximum:** 50 mcg/kg/min. NEONATES: 1–20 mcg/kg/min.

SIDE EFFECTS

FREQUENT: Headache, ectopic beats, tachycardia, anginal pain, palpitations, vasoconstriction, hypotension, nausea, vomiting, dyspnea. **OCCASIONAL:** Piloerection or goose bumps, bradycardia, widening of QRS complex.

ADVERSE REACTIONS/ TOXIC EFFECTS

High doses may produce ventricular arrhythmias. Patients with occlusive vascular disease are at high-risk for further compromise of circulation to the extremities, which may result in gangrene. Tissue necrosis with sloughing may occur with extravasation of IV solution.

NURSING CONSIDERATIONS

BASELINE ASSESSMENT

Check for MAOI therapy within last 2–3 wk (requires dosage reduction). Patient must be on continuous cardiac monitoring. Determine weight (for dosage calculation). Obtain initial BP, heart rate, respirations.

INTERVENTION/EVALUATION

Continuously monitor for cardiac arrhythmias. Measure urine output frequently. If extravasation occurs, immediately infiltrate the affected tissue with 10–15 ml 0.9% NaCl solution containing 5–10 mg phentolamine mesylate. Monitor BP, heart rate, respirations q15min during administration (or more often if indicated). Assess cardiac output, pulmonary wedge pressure, or central venous pressure (CVP) frequently. Assess peripheral circulation (palpate pulses, note color/temperature of extremities). Immediately notify physician of decreased urine output, cardiac arrhythmias, significant changes in BP or heart rate (or failure to respond to increase or decrease in infusion rate), decreased peripheral circulation (cold, pale, or mottled extremities). Taper dosage before discontinuing because abrupt cessation of therapy may result in marked hypotension. Be alert to excessive vasoconstriction (as evidenced by decreased urine output, increased heart rate or arrhythmias, a disproportionate increase in diastolic BP, decrease in pulse pressure); slow or temporarily stop the infusion, notify physician.

dorzolamide

(Trusopt)
See Antiglaucoma agents (p. 48C)

doxacurium chloride

(Nuromax)
See Neuromuscular blockers (p. 111C)

---

* "Tall Man" lettering   see color pill atlas   herb   underlined – top prescribed drug

doxazosin mesylate

dox-ay-**zoe**-sin

(Apo-Doxazosin ♣, Cardura)

Do not confuse doxazosin with doxapram, doxepin, or doxorubicin, or Cardura with Cardene, Cordarone, Coumadin, K-Dur, or Ridaura.

CLASSIFICATION

PHARMACOTHERAPEUTIC: Alpha-adrenergic blocker. **CLINICAL:** Antihypertensive (see p. 55C).

ACTION

An antihypertensive that selectively blocks alpha₁-adrenergic receptors, decreasing peripheral vascular resistance. Therapeutic Effect: Causes peripheral vasodilation and lowers of BP. Also relaxes smooth muscle of bladder and prostate.

PHARMACOKINETICS

Route	Onset	Peak	Duration
PO	N/A	2–6 hr	24 hr

Well absorbed from the GI tract. Protein binding: 98%–99%. Metabolized in the liver. Primarily eliminated in feces. Not removed by hemodialysis. Half-life: 19–22 hr.

USES

Treatment of mild to moderate hypertension. Used alone or in combination with other antihypertensives. Treatment of benign prostatic hyperplasia alone or in combination with finasteride (Proscar).

PRECAUTIONS

CONTRAINDICATIONS: Hypersensitivity to other quinazolines. **CAUTIONS:** Carcinoma of the prostate, chronic renal failure, hepatic impairment, recent cerebrovascular accident (CVA).

🕸 LIFESPAN CONSIDERATIONS: **Pregnancy/Lactation:** Unknown if drug crosses placenta or is distributed in breast milk. **Pregnancy Category C. Children:** Safety and efficacy not established. **Elderly:** May be more sensitive to hypotensive effects.

INTERACTIONS

DRUG: **Estrogen, NSAIDs:** May decrease the effect of doxazosin. **Hypotension-producing medications, such as antihypertensives and diuretics:** May increase the effect of doxazosin. **Sildenafil, tadalafil, vardenafil:** May potentiate hypotensive effects. HERBAL: None known. FOOD: None known. LAB VALUES: None known.

AVAILABILITY (Rx)

TABLETS: 1 mg, 2 mg, 4 mg, 8 mg.

ADMINISTRATION/HANDLING

PO
• Give without regard to food.

INDICATIONS/ROUTES/DOSAGE

MILD TO MODERATE HYPERTENSION
PO: ADULTS: Initially, 1 mg once a day. May increase to a maximum of 16 mg/day. ELDERLY: Initially, 0.5 mg once a day.

BENIGN PROSTATIC HYPERPLASIA, ALONE OR IN COMBINATION WITH FINASTERIDE (PROSCAR)
PO: ADULTS, ELDERLY: Initially, 1 mg/day. May increase q1–2wk. **Maximum:** 8 mg/day.

SIDE EFFECTS

FREQUENT (20%–10%): Dizziness, asthenia, headache, edema. **OCCASIONAL (9%–3%):** Nausea, pharyngitis, rhinitis, pain in extremities, somnolence. **RARE (3%–1%):** Palpitations, diarrhea, constipation, dyspnea, myalgia, altered vision, dizziness, nervousness.

♣ Canadian trade name   🅮 see **evolve**   ▸ High Alert drug

ADVERSE REACTIONS/ TOXIC EFFECTS

First-dose syncope (hypotension with sudden loss of consciousness) may occur 30–90 min following initial dose of 2 mg or greater, a too-rapid increase in dosage, or addition of another antihypertensive agent to therapy. First-dose syncope may be preceded by tachycardia (pulse rate of 120–160 beats/min).

NURSING CONSIDERATIONS

BASELINE ASSESSMENT

Give first dose at bedtime. If initial dose is given during daytime, patient must remain recumbent for 3–4 hr. Assess BP, pulse immediately before each dose, and q15–30min until BP is stabilized (be alert to fluctuations).

INTERVENTION/EVALUATION

Monitor pulse diligently (first-dose syncope may be preceded by tachycardia). Assess for edema, headache. Assist with ambulation if dizziness, light-headedness occurs.

PATIENT/FAMILY TEACHING

• Full therapeutic effect may not occur for 3–4 wk. • May cause syncope (fainting). • Avoid tasks that require alertness, motor skills until response to drug is established.

doxepin hydrochloride

dox-eh-pin

(Apo-Doxepin ✤, Novo-Doxepin ✤, Prudoxin, Sinequan, Zonalon)

Do not confuse doxepin with doxapram, doxazosin, or Doxidan, or Sinequan with saquinavir.

CLASSIFICATION

PHARMACOTHERAPEUTIC: Tricyclic. **CLINICAL:** Antidepressant, antianxiety, antineuralgic, antiulcer, antipruritic (see p. 37C).

ACTION

A tricyclic antidepressant, antianxiety agent, antineuralgic agent, antipruritic, and antiulcer agent that increases synaptic concentrations of norepinephrine and serotonin. Therapeutic Effect: Produces antidepressant and anxiolytic effects.

PHARMACOKINETICS

Rapidly and well absorbed from the GI tract. Protein binding: 80%–85%. Metabolized in the liver to active metabolite. Primarily excreted in urine. Not removed by hemodialysis. Half-life: 6–8 hr. **Topical:** Absorbed through the skin. Distributed to body tissues. Metabolized to active metabolite. Excreted in urine.

USES

Treatment of various forms of depression, often in conjunction with psychotherapy. Treatment of anxiety. **Topical:** Treatment of pruritus associated with eczema. OFF-LABEL: Treatment of neurogenic pain, panic disorder; prevention of vascular headache, pruritus in idiopathic urticaria.

PRECAUTIONS

CONTRAINDICATIONS: Angle-closure glaucoma, hypersensitivity to other tricyclic antidepressants, urine retention. **CAUTIONS:** Bipolar disorder, cardiac/hepatic/renal disease, diabetes mellitus, glaucoma, history of seizures, history of urinary retention/obstruction, hyperthyroidism, prostatic hypertrophy.

⏳ LIFESPAN CONSIDERATIONS: **Pregnancy/Lactation:** Unknown if doxepin crosses placenta or is distributed in breast milk. **Pregnancy Category C (B for topical form). Children:** Safety and efficacy not established in children younger than 12 yr. Be aware that children with major depressive disorder (MDD) may be at an increased risk of suicidal thinking and behavior. **Elderly:** Increased risk of excessive sedation (lower dosages recommended).

INTERACTIONS

DRUG: Alcohol, other CNS depressants: May increase CNS and respiratory depression and the hypotensive effects of doxepin. **Antithyroid agents:** May increase the risk of agranulocytosis. **Cimetidine:** May increase doxepin blood concentration and risk of toxicity. **Clonidine, guanadrel:** May decrease the effects of these drugs. **MAOIs:** May increase the risk of seizures, hyperpyrexia, and hypertensive crisis. **Phenothiazines:** May increase the anticholinergic and sedative effects of doxepin. **Sympathomimetics:** May increase cardiac effects. **HERBAL: St. John's wort:** May increase the risk of serotonin syndrome. **FOOD:** None known. **LAB VALUES:** May alter blood glucose levels and EKG readings. Therapeutic serum drug level is 110–250 ng/ml; toxic serum drug level is greater than 300 ng/ml.

AVAILABILITY (Rx)

CAPSULES (SINEQUAN): 10 mg, 25 mg, 50 mg, 75 mg, 100 mg, 150 mg. **ORAL CONCENTRATE (SINEQUAN):** 10 mg/ml. **CREAM (PRUDOXIN, ZONALON):** 5%.

ADMINISTRATION/HANDLING

PO

• Give with food or milk if GI distress occurs. • Dilute concentrate in 4-oz glass of water, milk, orange, grapefruit, tomato, prune, pineapple juice. Incompatible with carbonated drinks. • Give the larger portion of the daily dose at bedtime.

TOPICAL

• Apply thin film of cream on affected areas of the skin. • Don't use for more than 8 days. • Don't use occlusive dressings.

INDICATIONS/ROUTES/DOSAGE

DEPRESSION, ANXIETY

PO: ADULTS: 30–150 mg/day at bedtime or in 2–3 divided doses. May increase to 300 mg/day. ELDERLY: Initially, 10–25 mg at bedtime. May increase by 10–25 mg/day every 3–7 days. **Maximum:** 75 mg/day. ADOLESCENTS: Initially, 25–50 mg/day as a single dose or in divided doses. May increase to 100 mg/day. CHILDREN 12 YR AND YOUNGER: 1–3 mg/kg/day.

PRURITUS ASSOCIATED WITH ECZEMA

TOPICAL: ADULTS, ELDERLY: Apply thin film 4 times a day.

SIDE EFFECTS

FREQUENT: Oral: Orthostatic hypotension, somnolence, dry mouth, headache, increased appetite, weight gain, nausea, unusual fatigue, unpleasant taste. **Topical:** Edema; increased pruritus and eczema; burning, tingling, or stinging at application site; altered taste; dizziness; drowsiness; dry skin; dry mouth; fatigue; headache; thirst. **OCCASIONAL: Oral:** Blurred vision, confusion, constipation, hallucinations, difficult urination, eye pain, irregular heartbeat, fine muscle tremors, nervousness, impaired sexual function, diarrhea, diaphoresis, heartburn, insomnia. **Topical:** Anxiety, skin irritation or cracking, nausea. **RARE: Oral:** Allergic reaction, alopecia, tinnitus, breast enlargement. **Topical:** Fever, photosensitivity.

ADVERSE REACTIONS/TOXIC EFFECTS

Abrupt or too-rapid withdrawal may result in headache, malaise, nausea, vomiting, and vivid dreams. Overdose may produce seizures, dizziness, and cardiovascular effects, such as severe orthostatic hypotension, tachycardia, palpitations, and arrhythmias.

NURSING CONSIDERATIONS

BASELINE ASSESSMENT

Assess BP, pulse, EKG (those with history of cardiovascular disease). Peform CBC and blood chemistry tests before long-term therapy. Assess patient's appearance, behavior, level of interest, mood, sleep pattern.

INTERVENTION/EVALUATION

Monitor BP, pulse, weight. Perform CBC, blood chemistry tests periodically to assess renal/hepatic function. Supervise suicidal-risk patient closely during early therapy (as depression lessens, energy level improves, increasing suicide potential). Assess appearance, behavior, speech pattern, level of interest, mood. Therapeutic serum level: 110–250 ng/ml; toxic serum level: greater than 300 ng/ml.

PATIENT/FAMILY TEACHING

• Do not discontinue abruptly. • Change positions slowly to avoid dizziness. • Avoid tasks that require alertness, motor skills until response to drug is established. • Do not cover affected area with occlusive dressing after applying cream. • May cause dry mouth. • Avoid alcohol, limit caffeine. • May increase appetite. • Avoid exposure to sunlight/artificial light source. • Therapeutic effect may be noted within 2–5 days, maximum effect within 2–3 wk.

doxercalciferol

(Hectorol)
See vitamin D

Doxil, *see doxorubicin*

DOXOrubicin

dox-o-**roo**-bi-sin
(Adriamycin, Adriamycin PFS, Adriamycin RDF, Caelyx, <u>Doxil</u>, Rubex)
Do not confuse doxorubicin with daunorubicin, or Adriamycin with idamycin or idarubicin.

CLASSIFICATION

PHARMACOTHERAPEUTIC: Anthracycline antibiotic. **CLINICAL:** Antineoplastic (see p. 73C).

ACTION

An anthracycline antibiotic that inhibits DNA and DNA-dependent RNA synthesis by binding with DNA strands. Liposomal encapsulation increases uptake by tumors, prolongs drug action, and may decrease toxicity. Therapeutic Effect: Prevents cell division.

PHARMACOKINETICS

Widely distributed. Protein binding: 74%–76%. Does not cross the blood-brain barrier. Metabolized rapidly in the liver to active metabolite. Primarily eliminated by biliary system. Not removed by hemodialysis. Half-life: 16 hr; metabolite, 32 hr.

USES

Adriamycin, Rubex: Treatment of acute lymphocytic, non-lymphocytic leukemia, breast, gastric, small cell lung, ovarian, epithelial, thyroid, bladder carcinomas, neuroblastoma, Wilms' tumor, Hodgkin's, non-Hodgkin's lymphoma, osteosarcoma, soft tissue sarcoma. **Doxil:** Treatment of AIDS-related Kaposi's sarcoma, metastatic ovarian cancer. OFF-LABEL: Carcinoid

---

tumors; Ewing's sarcoma; germ cell, gestational trophoblastic, and prostatic tumors; multiple myeloma; retinoblastoma; treatment of cervical, endometrial, esophageal, head or neck, non–small cell lung, pancreatic carcinoma.

PRECAUTIONS

CONTRAINDICATIONS: Cardiomyopathy; preexisting myelosuppression; previous or concomitant treatment with cyclophosphamide, idarubicin, mitoxantrone, or irradiation of the cardiac region; severe CHF. **CAUTIONS:** Bone marrow suppression, CHF, hepatic impairment. life-threatening arrhythmias.

LIFESPAN CONSIDERATIONS: Pregnancy/Lactation: If possible, avoid use during pregnancy, especially first trimester. Breast-feeding not recommended. **Pregnancy Category D. Children/Elderly:** Cardiotoxicity may be more frequent in those younger than 2 yr or older than 70 yr.

INTERACTIONS

DRUG: Antigout medications: May decrease the effects of these drugs. **Bone marrow depressants:** May increase myelosuppression. **Daunorubicin:** May increase the risk of cardiotoxicity. **Live-virus vaccines:** May potentiate virus replication, increase vaccine side effects, and decrease the patient's antibody response to the vaccine. **HERBAL:** None known. **FOOD:** None known. **LAB VALUES:** May cause EKG changes and increase serum uric acid level. Doxil may reduce neutrophil and RBC counts.

AVAILABILITY (Rx)

INJECTION, POWDER FOR RECONSTITUTION: 10 mg (Adriamycin RDF), 20 mg (Adriamycin RDF), 50 mg (Adriamycin RDF, Rubex), 100 mg (Rubex), 150 mg (Adriamycin RDF). **INJECTION SOLUTION**

(ADRIAMYCIN PFS): 2 mg/ml. **LIPID COMPLEX (DOXIL):** 2 mg/ml.

ADMINISTRATION/HANDLING

◀ **ALERT** ▶ Wear gloves. If powder or solution comes in contact with skin, wash thoroughly. Avoid small veins; swollen or edematous extremities; areas overlying joints, tendons. **Doxil:** Do not use with in-line filter or mix with any diluent except D_5W. May be carcinogenic, mutagenic, or teratogenic. Handle with extreme care during preparation/administration.

 IV

Reconstitution • Reconstitute each 10-mg vial with 5 ml preservative-free 0.9% NaCl (10 ml for 20 mg; 25 ml for 50 mg) to provide concentration of 2 mg/ml. • Shake vial; allow contents to dissolve. • Withdraw appropriate volume of air from vial during reconstitution (avoids excessive pressure buildup). • May be further diluted with 50 ml D_5W or 0.9% NaCl and give as a continuous infusion through a central venous line.

Rate of administration • For IV push, administer into tubing of freely running IV infusion of D_5W or 0.9% NaCl, preferably via butterfly needle over 3–5 min (avoids local erythematous streaking along vein and facial flushing). • Must test for flashback q30sec to be certain needle remains in vein during injection. • Extravasation produces immediate pain, severe local tissue damage. Terminate administration immediately; withdraw as much medication as possible, obtain extravasation kit, follow protocol.

Storage • Store at room temperature. • Reconstituted solution is stable for 24 hr at room temperature or 48 hr if refrigerated. • Protect from prolonged exposure to sunlight; discard unused solution.

DOXIL

Reconstitution • Dilute each dose in 250 ml D_5W.

Rate of administration • Give as infusion over 30 min. Do not use in-line filters.

Storage • Refrigerate unopened vials. • After solution is diluted, use within 24 hr.

🔅 IV INCOMPATIBILITIES

Doxorubicin: Allopurinol (Aloprim), amphotericin B complex (Abelcet, AmBisome, Amphotec), cefepime (Maxipime), furosemide (Lasix), ganciclovir (Cytovene), heparin, piperacillin and tazobactam (Zosyn), propofol (Diprivan). **Doxil:** Don't mix with any other medications.

IV COMPATIBILITIES

Dexamethasone (Decadron), diphenhydramine (Benadryl), etoposide (VePesid), granisetron (Kytril), hydromorphone (Dilaudid), lorazepam (Ativan), morphine, ondansetron (Zofran), paclitaxel (Taxol).

INDICATIONS/ROUTES/DOSAGE

TO PRODUCE REGRESSION IN ACUTE LYMPHOBLASTIC AND MYELOBLASTIC LEUKEMIA; BREAST, BRONCHOGENIC, GASTRIC, OVARIAN, THYROID, AND TRANSITIONAL CELL BLADDER CARCINOMAS; HODGKIN'S DISEASE; NON-HODGKIN'S LYMPHOMAS; NEUROBLASTOMA; PRIMARY LIVER CANCER; SOFT-TISSUE AND BONE SARCOMAS; AND WILMS' TUMOR

IV: ADULTS: $60–75$ mg/m² as a single dose every 21 days, 20 mg/m² once weekly, or $25–30$ mg/m²/day on $2–3$ successive days q4wk. Because of the risk of cardiotoxicity, don't exceed a cumulative dose of 550 mg/m² ($400–450$ mg/m² for those previously treated with related compounds or irradiation of cardiac region). CHILDREN: $35–75$ mg/m² as a

single dose q3wk or $20–30$ mg/m² weekly, or $60–90$ mg/m² as continuous infusion over 96 hr q3–4wk.

KAPOSI'S SARCOMA

IV (DOXIL): ADULTS: 20 mg/m² q3wk infused over 30 min.

OVARIAN CANCER

IV (DOXIL): ADULTS: 50 mg/m² q4wk.

DOSAGE IN HEPATIC IMPAIRMENT

Dosage is modified based on serum bilirubin level.

Serum Bilirubin Concentration	% of Normal Dose
1.2–3 mg/dl	50%
Greater than 3 mg/dl	25%

SIDE EFFECTS

FREQUENT: Complete alopecia (scalp, axillary, pubic hair), nausea, vomiting, stomatitis, esophagitis (especially if drug is given on several successive days), reddish urine. **Doxil:** Nausea. **OCCASIONAL:** Anorexia, diarrhea; hyperpigmentation of skin, nailbeds, and phalangeal and dermal creases. **RARE:** Fever, chills, conjunctivitis, lacrimation.

ADVERSE REACTIONS/ TOXIC EFFECTS

Myelosuppression may cause hematologic toxicity (manifested principally as leukopenia and, to lesser extent, anemia and thrombocytopenia), usually within 10–15 days of starting therapy. Blood counts typically return to normal levels by the third week. Cardiotoxicity (either acute, manifested as transient EKG abnormalities, or chronic, manifested as CHF) may occur.

NURSING CONSIDERATIONS

BASELINE ASSESSMENT

Obtain WBC, platelet, erythrocyte counts before and at frequent intervals during therapy. Obtain EKG before therapy,

---

liver function studies before each dose. Antiemetics may be effective in preventing, treating nausea.

INTERVENTION/EVALUATION

Monitor for stomatitis (burning or erythema of oral mucosa at inner margin of lips, difficulty swallowing). May lead to ulceration of mucous membranes within 2–3 days. Assess skin, nailbeds for hyperpigmentation. Monitor hematologic status, renal and liver function studies, serum uric acid levels. Assess pattern of daily bowel activity and stool consistency. Monitor for hematologic toxicity (fever, sore throat, signs of local infection, unusual bruising or bleeding from any site), symptoms of anemia (excessive fatigue, weakness).

PATIENT/FAMILY TEACHING

• Alopecia is reversible, but new hair growth may have different color, texture. New hair growth resumes 2–3 mo after last therapy dose. • Maintain fastidious oral hygiene. • Do not have immunizations without physician's approval (drug lowers body's resistance). • Avoid contact with those who have recently received live virus vaccine. • Promptly report fever, sore throat, signs of local infection, unusual bruising or bleeding from any site. • Contact physician for persistent nausea or vomiting. • Avoid alcohol (may cause GI irritation, a common side effect with liposomal doxorubicin).

doxycycline

dox-i-**sye**-kleen

(Adoxa, Apo-Doxy ✦, Atridox, Doryx, Doxy-100, Doxy-Caps, Doxycin ✦, Monodox, Periostat, Vibramycin, Vibramycin Calcium, Vibramycin Hyclate, Vibramycin Monohydrate, Vibra-Tabs).

> **Do not confuse doxycycline with Dicyclomine or doxylamine, or Monodox with Monopril.**

◆CLASSIFICATION

PHARMACOTHERAPEUTIC: Tetracycline. **CLINICAL:** Antibiotic.

ACTION

A tetracycline antibiotic that inhibits bacterial protein synthesis by binding to ribosomes. Therapeutic Effect: Bacteriostatic.

PHARMACOKINETICS

Rapidly and almost completely absorbed after PO administration. Protein binding: greater than 90%. Metabolized in liver. Partially excreted in urine; partially eliminated in bile. Half-life: 15–24 hr.

USES

Treatment of susceptible infections due to *H. ducreyi, Pasteurella pestis, tularnsis,* Bacteroides species, *V. cholerae,* Brucella species, *Rickettsiae, Y. pestis, Francisella tularesis, M. pneumoniae* including brucellosis, chlamydia, cholera, granuloma inguinale, lymphogranuloma venereum, malaria prophylaxis, nongonococcal urethritis, pelvic inflammatory disease, plague, psittacosis, relapsing fever, rickettsia infections, primary and secondary syphilis, tularemia. OFF-LABEL: Treatment of atypical mycobacterial infections, gonorrhea, malaria, rheumatoid arthritis; prevention of Lyme disease; prevention or treatment of traveler's diarrhea.

PRECAUTIONS

CONTRAINDICATIONS: Children 8 yr and younger, hypersensitivity to tetracyclines or sulfites, last half of pregnancy, severe hepatic dysfunction. **CAUTIONS:** Sun or ultraviolet light exposure (severe photosensitivity reaction).

⌛ **LIFESPAN CONSIDERATIONS: Pregnancy/Lactation:** Crosses placenta; distributed in breast milk. **Pregnancy Category D. Children:** May cause permanent discoloration of teeth, enamel hypoplasia. **Elderly:** No age-related precautions noted.

INTERACTIONS

DRUG: Antacids containing aluminum, calcium, or magnesium; laxatives containing magnesium: Decrease doxycycline absorption. **Barbiturates, carbamazepine, phenytoin:** May decrease doxycycline blood concentrations. **Cholestyramine, colestipol:** May decrease doxycycline absorption. **Oral contraceptives:** May decrease the effects of oral contraceptives. **Oral iron preparations:** Impair absorption of doxycycline. **HERBAL:** None known. **FOOD:** None known. **LAB VALUES:** May increase serum alkaline phosphatase, amylase, bilirubin, AST, and ALT levels. May alter CBC.

AVAILABILITY (Rx)

CAPSULES: 50 mg (Monodox), 75 mg (Doryx), 100 mg (Doryx, Monodox, Vibramycin). **ORAL SUSPENSION (VIBRAMYCIN):** 25 mg/5 ml. **SYRUP (VIBRAMYCIN):** 50 mg/5 ml. **TABLETS:** 20 mg (Periostat), 50 mg (Adoxa), 75 mg (Adoxa), 100 mg (Adoxa, Vibra-Tabs). **INJECTION, POWDER FOR RECONSTITUTION (DOXY-100):** 100 mg.

ADMINISTRATION/HANDLING

◄ **ALERT** ▶ Do not administer IM or subcutaneous. Space doses evenly around clock.

💉 **IV**

Reconstitution • Reconstitute each 100-mg vial with 10 ml sterile water for injection for concentration of 10 mg/ml. • Further dilute each 100 mg with at least 100 ml D₅W, 0.9% NaCl, lactated Ringer's.

Rate of administration • Give by intermittent IV infusion (piggyback). • Infuse over 1–4 hr.

Storage • After reconstitution, IV infusion (piggyback) is stable for 12 hr at room temperature or 72 hr if refrigerated. • Protect from direct sunlight. Discard if precipitate forms.

PO

• Store capsules, tablets at room temperature. • Oral suspension is stable for 2 wk at room temperature. • Give with full glass of fluid. • May take with food or milk.

▦ IV INCOMPATIBILITIES

Allopurinol (Aloprim), heparin, piperacillin and tazobactam (Zosyn).

IV COMPATIBILITIES

Amiodarone (Cordarone), diltiazem (Cardizem), hydromorphone (Dilaudid), magnesium sulfate, morphine, propofol (Diprivan), total parenteral nutrition (TPN).

INDICATIONS/ROUTES/DOSAGE

RESPIRATORY, SKIN, AND SOFT-TISSUE INFECTIONS; UTIs; PELVIC INFLAMMATORY DISEASE (PID); BRUCELLOSIS; TRACHOMA; ROCKY MOUNTAIN SPOTTED FEVER; TYPHUS; Q FEVER; RICKETTSIA; SEVERE ACNE (ADOXA); SMALLPOX; PSITTACOSIS; ORNITHOSIS; GRANULOMA INGUINALE; LYMPHOGRANULOMA VENEREUM; INTESTINAL AMEBIASIS (ADJUNCTIVE TREATMENT); PREVENTION OF RHEUMATIC FEVER
PO: ADULTS, ELDERLY: Initially, 100 mg q12h, then 100 mg/day as single dose or 50 mg q12h for severe infections. CHILDREN 8 YR AND OLDER AND WEIGHING MORE THAN 45 KG: 2–4 mg/kg/day divided q12–24h. **Maximum:** 200 mg/day.
IV: ADULTS, ELDERLY: Initially, 200 mg as 1–2 infusions; then 100–200 mg/day in 1–2 divided doses. CHILDREN 8 YR AND OLDER: 2–4 mg/kg/day divided q12–24h.

Maximum: 200 mg/day.

ACUTE GONOCOCCAL INFECTIONS
PO: ADULTS: Initially, 200 mg, then 100 mg at bedtime on first day; then 100 mg twice a day for 14 days.

SYPHILIS
PO, IV: ADULTS: 200 mg/day in divided doses for 14–28 days.

TRAVELER'S DIARRHEA
PO: ADULTS, ELDERLY: 100 mg/day during a period of risk (up to 14 days) and for 2 days after returning home.

PERIODONTITIS
PO: ADULTS: 20 mg twice a day.

SIDE EFFECTS

FREQUENT: Anorexia, nausea, vomiting, diarrhea, dysphagia, possibly severe photosensitivity. **OCCASIONAL:** Rash, urticaria.

ADVERSE REACTIONS/ TOXIC EFFECTS

Superinfection (especially fungal) and benign intracranial hypertension (headache, visual changes) may occur. Hepatoxicity, fatty degeneration of the liver, and pancreatitis occur rarely.

NURSING CONSIDERATIONS

BASELINE ASSESSMENT
Question for history of allergies, especially to tetracyclines, sulfites.

INTERVENTION/EVALUATION
Determine pattern of bowel activity and stool consistency. Assess skin for rash. Monitor level of consciousness (LOC) due to potential for increased intracranial pressure (ICP). Be alert for superinfection: diarrhea, ulceration or changes of oral mucosa, anal/genital pruritus.

PATIENT/FAMILY TEACHING
• Avoid unnecessary exposure to sunlight. • Do not take with antacids, iron products, dairy products. • Complete

full course of therapy. • After application of dental gel, avoid brushing teeth, flossing the treated areas for 7 days.

D

dronabinol

droe-**nab**-i-nol
(Marinol)
Do not confuse dronabinol with droperidol.

CLASSIFICATION

PHARMACOTHERAPEUTIC: Controlled substance (**Schedule III**). **CLINICAL:** Antinausea, antiemetic, appetite stimulant.

ACTION

An antiemetic and appetite stimulant that may act by inhibiting vomiting control mechanisms in the medulla oblongata. **Therapeutic Effect:** Inhibits vomiting and stimulates appetite.

PHARMACOKINETICS

Well absorbed after PO administration. Protein binding: 97%. Undergoes first-pass metabolism. Is highly lipid soluble. Primarily excreted in feces. **Half-life:** 4 hr.

USES

Prevention, treatment of nausea, vomiting due to cancer chemotherapy; appetite stimulant in AIDS, cancer patients. **OFF-LABEL:** Postoperative nausea and vomiting.

PRECAUTIONS

CONTRAINDICATIONS: Treatment of nausea and vomiting not caused by chemotherapy, hypersensitivity to sesame oil or tetrahydrocannabinol products. **CAUTIONS:** Cardiac disorders, history of psychiatric illness, history of substance abuse, hypertension. Not recommended in children.

⏳ LIFESPAN CONSIDERATIONS: Pregnancy/Lactation: Unknown if drug crosses placenta. Distributed in breast milk. **Pregnancy Category C. Children:** Not recommended. **Elderly:** Monitor carefully during therapy.

INTERACTIONS

DRUG: **Alcohol, other CNS suppressants:** May increase CNS depression. HERBAL: None known. FOOD: None known. LAB VALUES: None known.

AVAILABILITY (Rx)

CAPSULES (GELATIN [MARINOL]): 2.5 mg, 5 mg, 10 mg.

ADMINISTRATION/HANDLING

PO

• Refrigerate capsules. • Give before meals.

INDICATIONS/ROUTES/DOSAGE

PREVENTION OF CHEMOTHERAPY-INDUCED NAUSEA AND VOMITING

PO: ADULTS, CHILDREN: Initially, 5 mg/m^2 1–3 hr before chemotherapy, then q2–4h after chemotherapy for total of 4–6 doses a day. May increase by 2.5 mg/m^2 up to 15 mg/m^2 per dose.

APPETITE STIMULANT

PO: ADULTS: Initially, 2.5 mg twice a day (before lunch and dinner). Range: 2.5–20 mg/day.

SIDE EFFECTS

FREQUENT (24%–3%): Euphoria, dizziness, paranoid reaction, somnolence. **OCCASIONAL (less than 3%–1%):** Asthenia, ataxia, confusion, abnormal thinking, depersonalization. **RARE (less than 1%):** Diarrhea, depression, nightmares, speech difficulties, headache, anxiety, tinnitus, flushed skin.

ADVERSE REACTIONS/ TOXIC EFFECTS

Mild intoxication may produce increased sensory awareness (including taste, smell, and sound), altered time perception, reddened conjunctiva, dry mouth, and tachycardia. Moderate intoxication may produce memory impairment and urine retention. Severe intoxication may produce lethargy, decreased motor coordination, slurred speech, and orthostatic hypotension.

NURSING CONSIDERATIONS

BASELINE ASSESSMENT

Assess dehydration status if excessive vomiting occurs (skin turgor, mucous membranes, urine output).

INTERVENTION/EVALUATION

Supervise closely for serious mood, behavior responses, especially in patients with a history of psychiatric illness. Monitor BP, heart rate.

PATIENT/FAMILY TEACHING

• Change positions slowly to avoid dizziness. • Relief from nausea/vomiting generally occurs within 15 min of drug administration. • Don't take any other medications, including OTC, without physician approval. • Avoid alcohol, barbiturates. • Avoid tasks that require alertness, motor skills until response to drug is established. • For appetite stimulation, take before lunch and dinner.

droperidol

droe-**pear**-ih-dall
(Inapsine)

◆CLASSIFICATION

PHARMACOTHERAPEUTIC: General anesthetic. **CLINICAL:** Anesthesia adjunct, antiemetic.

ACTION

Antagonizes dopamine neurotransmission at synapses by blocking postsynaptic dopamine receptor sites; partially blocks adrenergic receptor binding sites. **Therapeutic Effect:** Produces tranquilization, antiemetic effect.

PHARMACOKINETICS

Onset	Peak	Duration
IM		
3–10 min	30 min	2–4 hr
IV		
3–10 min	30 min	2–4 hr

Well absorbed after IM administration. Crosses blood-brain barrier. Metabolized in liver. Primarily excreted in urine. **Half-life:** 2.3 hr.

USES

Treatment of nausea/vomiting associated with surgical and diagnostic procedures. **OFF-LABEL:** Adjunct in induction and maintenance of general and regional anesthesia, produces sedation for diagnostic procedures, treatment of acute psychotic episodes.

PRECAUTIONS

CONTRAINDICATIONS: Known or suspected QT interval prolongation, congenital long QT syndrome. **CAUTIONS:** Hepatic/renal/cardiac impairment (may cause cardiac arrhythmias during administration).

LIFESPAN CONSIDERATIONS: Pregnancy/Lactation: Crosses placenta. Unknown if drug is distributed in breast milk. **Pregnancy Category C.** **Children:** Dystonias more likely. **Elderly:** May be more sensitive to sedative, hypotensive effects.

INTERACTIONS

DRUG: Anti-hypertensives: May increase hypotension. **CNS depressants:** May increase CNS depressant effect. **HERBAL:** None known. **FOOD:** None known. **LAB VALUES:** None known.

AVAILABILITY (Rx)

INJECTION: 2.5 mg/ml.

ADMINISTRATION/HANDLING

◀ **ALERT** ▶ Patient must remain recumbent for 30–60 min in head-low position with legs raised, to minimize hypotensive effect.

Storage • Store parenteral form at room temperature.

 IV

• May give undiluted as IV push over 2–5 min. • Dose for high-risk patients should be added to D$_5$W or lactated Ringer's injection to a concentration of 1 mg/50 ml and given as an IV infusion.

IM

• Inject slowly, deep IM into upper outer quadrant of gluteus maximus.

▦ IV INCOMPATIBILITIES

Allopurinol (Aloprim), amphotericin B complex (Abelcet, AmBisome, Amphotic), cefepime (Maxipime), foscarnet (Foscavir), heparin, methotrexate, piperacillin/tazobactam (Zosyn).

IV COMPATIBILITIES

Atropine, diphenhydramine (Benadryl), glycopyrrolate (Robinul), metoclopramide (Reglan), midazolam (Versed), morphine, potassium chloride, promethazine (Phenergan).

INDICATIONS/ROUTES/DOSAGE

NAUSEA, VOMITING

IM, IV: ADULTS, ELDERLY: Initially, 2.5 mg. Additional doses of 1.25 mg may be given to achieve desired effect. CHILDREN 2–12 YR: 0.05–0.06 mg/kg (maximum initial dose of 0.1 mg/kg). Additional dose may be given to achieve desired effect.

SIDE EFFECTS

FREQUENT: Mild to moderate hypotension. **OCCASIONAL:** Tachycardia, postop drowsiness, dizziness, chills, shivering.

RARE: Postop nightmares, facial sweating, bronchospasm.

ADVERSE REACTIONS/ TOXIC EFFECTS

May produce cardiac arrhythmias. Extrapyramidal symptoms (EPS) may appear as akathisia (motor restlessness), dystonias: torticollis (neck muscle spasm), opisthotonos (rigidity of back muscles), oculogyric crisis (rolling back of eyes).

NURSING CONSIDERATIONS

BASELINE ASSESSMENT

Assess vital signs. Have patient void. Raise side rails. Instruct patient to remain recumbent.

INTERVENTION/EVALUATION

Monitor BP, pulse diligently for hypotensive reaction during and after procedure. Assess pulse for tachycardia. Monitor for EPS. Evaluate for therapeutic response from anxiety: a calm facial expression, decreased restlessness. Monitor for decreased nausea, vomiting.

---

drotrecogin alfa

dro-trae-**coe**-gin-**al**-fa
(Xigris)

◆**CLASSIFICATION**

PHARMACOTHERAPEUTIC: Activated protein C. **CLINICAL:** Antisepsis agent.

ACTION

A recombinant form of human-activated protein C that exerts an antithrombotic effect by inhibiting Factors Va and VIIIa and may exert an indirect profibrinolytic effect by inhibiting plasminogen activator inhibitor-1 and limiting the generation of activated thrombin-activatable-fibrinolysis-inhibitor. The drug may also exert an anti-inflammatory effect by inhibiting tumor necrosis factor (TNF) production by monocytes, by blocking leukocyte adhesion to selectins, and by limiting thrombin-induced inflammatory responses. **Therapeutic Effect:** Produces anti-inflammatory, antithrombotic, and profibrinolytic effects.

PHARMACOKINETICS

Inactivated by endogenous plasma protease inhibitors. Clearance occurs within 2 hr of initiating infusion. **Half-life:** 1.6 hr.

USES

Treatment of severe sepsis or septic shock with evidence of organ dysfunction in patients at high risk for death.

PRECAUTIONS

CONTRAINDICATIONS: Active internal bleeding, evidence of cerebral herniation, intracranial neoplasm or mass lesion, presence of an epidural catheter, recent (within the past 3 mo) hemorrhagic stroke, recent (within the past 2 mo) intracranial or intraspinal surgery or severe head trauma, trauma with an increased risk of life-threatening bleeding. **CAUTIONS:** Concurrent use of heparin, platelet count less than 30,000/mm^3, prolonged PT, recent (6 wk or less) GI bleeding, recent (3 days or less) thrombolytic therapy, recent (7 days or less) anticoagulant or aspirin therapy, intracranial aneurysm, chronic severe hepatic disease.

⧗ **LIFESPAN CONSIDERATIONS: Pregnancy/Lactation:** Unknown if the drug can cause fetal harm. Unknown if excreted in breast milk. **Pregnancy Category C. Children/Elderly:** Safety and efficacy not established.

INTERACTIONS

DRUG: None known. **HERBAL:** None known. **FOOD:** None known. **LAB VALUES:** May prolong aPTT.

D

AVAILABILITY (Rx)
POWDER FOR INFUSION: 5 mg, 20 mg.

ADMINISTRATION/HANDLING
 IV

Reconstitution • Reconstitute 5-mg vials with 2.5 ml sterile water for injection and 20-mg vials with 10 ml sterile water for injection. Resulting concentration is 2 mg/ml. • Slowly add the sterile water for injection by swirling; do not shake or invert vial. • Further dilute with 0.9% NaCl. • Withdraw amount from vial and add to infusion bag containing 0.9% NaCl for a final concentration of between 100 and 200 mcg/ml; direct the stream to the side of the bag (minimizes agitation). • Invert infusion bag to mix solution.

Rate of administration • Administer via a dedicated IV line or a dedicated lumen of a multilumen central venous line (CVL). • Administer infusion rate of 24 mcg/kg/hr for 96 hr. • If infusion is interrupted, restart drug at 24 mcg/kg/hr.

Storage • Store unreconstituted vials at room temperature. • Start infusion within 3 hr after reconstitution.

▨ IV INCOMPATIBILITIES
Don't mix drotrecogin alfa with other medications.

IV COMPATIBILITIES
Lactated Ringer's solution, 0.9% NaCl and dextrose are the only solutions that can be administered through the same line.

INDICATIONS/ROUTES/DOSAGE
SEVERE SEPSIS
IV INFUSION: ADULTS, ELDERLY: 24 mcg/kg/hr for 96 hr. Immediately stop infusion if clinically significant bleeding is identified.

SIDE EFFECTS
None known.

ADVERSE REACTIONS/TOXIC EFFECTS
Bleeding (intrathoracic, retroperitoneal, GI, GU, intra-abdominal, intracranial) occurs in about 2% of patients.

NURSING CONSIDERATIONS
BASELINE ASSESSMENT
Criteria that must be met before initiating drug therapy: age older than 18 yr, no pregnancy or breast-feeding, actual body weight less than 135 kg, 3 or more systemic inflammatory response criteria (fever, heart rate over 90 beats/min, respiratory rate over 20 breaths/min, increased WBC count), and at least one sepsis-induced organ or system failure (cardiovascular, renal, respiratory, hematologic, or unexplained metabolic acidosis).

INTERVENTION/EVALUATION
Monitor closely for hemorrhagic complication.

Dulcolax, *see bisacodyl*

---

duloxetine
dew-**lox**-ah-teen
(Cymbalta)

◆CLASSIFICATION
CLINICAL: Antidepressant.

ACTION
An antidepressant that appears to inhibit serotonin and norepinephrine reuptake at CNS neuronal presynaptic membranes;

---

is a less potent inhibitor of dopamine reuptake. **Therapeutic Effect:** Relieves depression.

PHARMACOKINETICS

Well absorbed from the GI tract. Protein binding: greater than 90%. Extensively metabolized to active metabolites. Excreted primarily in urine and, to a lesser extent, in feces. **Half-life:** 8–17 hr.

USES

Treatment of major depression exhibited as persistent, prominent dysphoria (occurring nearly every day for at least 2 wk) manifested by 4 of 8 symptoms: change in appetite, change in sleep pattern, increased fatigue, impaired concentration, feelings of guilt or worthlessness, loss of interest in usual activities, psycho-motor agitation or retardation, or suicidal tendencies. **OFF-LABEL:** Treatment of chronic pain syndromes, fibromyalgia, stress incontinence, urinary incontinence.

PRECAUTIONS

CONTRAINDICATIONS: End-stage renal disease (creatinine clearance less than 30 ml/min), severe hepatic impairment, uncontrolled angle-closure glaucoma, use within 14 days of MAOIs. **CAUTIONS:** Renal impairment, history of alcoholism, chronic liver disease, hepatic insufficiency, history of seizures, history of mania, conditions that may slow gastric emptying, those with suicidal ideation and behavior.

⧖ **LIFESPAN CONSIDERATIONS: Pregnancy/Lactation:** May produce neonatal adverse reactions (constant crying, feeding difficulty, hyperreflexia, irritability). Unknown if distributed in breast milk; do not breast-feed. **Pregnancy Category C. Children:** Safety and efficacy not established. **Elderly:** Caution required when increasing dosage.

INTERACTIONS

DRUG: Alcohol: Increases the risk of hepatic injury. **Fluoxetine, fluvoxamine, paroxetine, quinidine, quinolone antimicrobials:** May increase duloxetine plasma concentration. **MAOIs:** May cause serotonin syndrome, characterized by autonomic hyperactivity, coma, diaphoresis, excitement, hyperthermia, and rigidity. **Tricyclic antidepressants (TCAs):** May increase tricyclic antidepressant serum concentrations and potential toxicity. **Thioridazine:** May produce ventricular arrhythmias. **Warfarin:** May increase the warfarin plasma concentration. **HERBAL: St John's wort:** May increase adverse effects. **FOOD:** None known. **LAB VALUES:** May increase serum bilirubin, AST, and ALT levels.

AVAILABILITY (Rx)

CAPSULES: 20 mg, 30 mg, 60 mg.

ADMINISTRATION/HANDLING

◀ **ALERT** ▶ Allow at least 14 days to elapse between the use of MAOIs and duloxetine.

PO
• Give without regard to meals. Give with food or milk if GI distress occur. • Do not crush or chew enteric-coated capsules. • Do not sprinkle capsule contents on food or mix with liquids.

INDICATIONS/ROUTES/DOSAGE

MAJOR DEPRESSIVE DISORDER
PO: ADULTS: 20 mg twice a day, increased up to 60 mg/day as a single dose or in 2 divided doses.

DIABETIC NEUROPATHY PAIN
PO: ADULTS: 60 mg once a day.

SIDE EFFECTS

FREQUENT (20%–11%): Nausea, dry mouth, constipation, insomnia.

✒ see color pill atlas   ✒ herb   underlined – top prescribed drug

OCCASIONAL (9%–5%): Dizziness, fatigue, diarrhea, somnolence, anorexia, diaphoresis, vomiting. RARE (4%–2%): Blurred vision, erectile dysfunction, delayed or failed ejaculation, anorgasmia, anxiety, decreased libido, hot flashes.

ADVERSE REACTIONS/ TOXIC EFFECTS

Duloxetine use may slightly increase the patient's heart rate. Colitis, dysphagia, gastritis, and irritable bowel syndrome occur rarely.

NURSING CONSIDERATIONS

BASELINE ASSESSMENT
Assess appearance, behavior, speech pattern, level of interest, mood, sleep pattern.

INTERVENTION/EVALUATION
For those on long-term therapy, serum chemistry profile to assess hepatic function should be performed periodically. Supervise suicidal risk patient closely during early therapy (as depression lessens, energy level improves, increasing suicide potential).

PATIENT/FAMILY TEACHING
• Therapeutic effect may be noted within 1–4 wk. • Do not abruptly discontinue medication. • Avoid tasks that require alertness, motor skills until response to drug is established. • Inform physician if intention of pregnancy or if pregnancy occurs. • Inform physician if anxiety, agitation, panic attacks, worsening of depression occurs. • Avoid heavy alcohol intake (associated with severe hepatic injury).

DuoNeb, see albuterol and ipratropium

Duragesic, see fentanyl

Duramorph, see morphine

dutasteride

do-tah-**stir**-eyed
(Avodart)

CLASSIFICATION
PHARMACOTHERAPEUTIC: Androgen hormone inhibitor. CLINICAL: Benign prostatic hyperplasia agent.

ACTION

An androgen hormone inhibitor that inhibits 5-alpha reductase, an intracellular enzyme that converts testosterone into dihydrotestosterone (DHT) in the prostate gland, reducing the serum DHT level. Therapeutic Effect: Reduces size of the prostate gland.

PHARMACOKINETICS

Route	Onset	Peak	Duration
PO	24 hr	N/A	3–8 wk

Moderately absorbed after PO administration. Widely distributed. Protein binding: 99%. Metabolized in the liver. Primarily excreted in feces. Half-life: Up to 5 wk.

USES

Treatment of benign prostatic hyperplasia (BPH). OFF-LABEL: Treatment of hair loss.

PRECAUTIONS

CONTRAINDICATIONS: Females, physical handling of tablets by those who are or may be pregnant. **CAUTIONS:** Hepatic disease or impairment, obstructive uropathy, preexisting sexual dysfunction (e.g., reduced male libido, impotence). **Pregnancy Category X.**

INTERACTIONS

DRUG: Cimetidine, ciprofloxacin, diltiazem, ketoconazole, ritonavir, verapamil: May increase dutasteride plasma concentrations. **HERBAL:** None known. **FOOD:** None known. **LAB VALUES:** Decreases the serum prostate-specific antigen (PSA) level.

AVAILABILITY (Rx)

CAPSULE: 0.5 mg.

ADMINISTRATION/HANDLING

PO
• Do not open or break capsules. • Give without regard to meals.

INDICATIONS/ROUTES/DOSAGE

BENIGN PROSTATIC HYPERPLASIA (BPH)
PO: ADULTS, ELDERLY (MEN ONLY): 0.5 mg once a day.

SIDE EFFECTS

OCCASIONAL: Gynecomastia, sexual dysfunction (decreased libido, impotence, and decreased volume of ejaculate).

ADVERSE REACTIONS/
TOXIC EFFECTS

Toxicity may be manifested as rash, diarrhea, and abdominal pain. Allergic reaction characterized as rash, pruritus, urticaria, and localized edema, occurs rarely.

NURSING CONSIDERATIONS

BASELINE ASSESSMENT

Serum PSA determination should be performed in patients with BPH before beginning therapy and periodically thereafter.

INTERVENTION/EVALUATION

Diligently monitor I&O. Assess for signs/symptoms of BPH (hesitancy, reduced force of urinary stream, postvoid dribbling, sensation of incomplete bladder emptying).

PATIENT/FAMILY TEACHING

• Discuss potential for impotence; volume of ejaculate may be decreased during treatment. • May not notice improved urinary flow for up to 6 mo after treatment. • Women who may be or are pregnant should not handle capsules (risk of fetal anomaly to male fetus).

Dyazide, *see hydrochlorothiazide and triamterene*

DynaCirc, *see isradipine*

---

echinacea

Also known as black susans, comb flower, red sunflower, scurvy root.

◆CLASSIFICATION

HERBAL: See Appendix G.

ACTION

Stimulates immune system. Possesses antiviral/immune stimulatory effects. Increases phagocytosis, lymphocyte activity (possibly by releasing tumor necrosis factor (TNF), interleukin-1, interferon). **Effect:** Prevents/reduces symptoms associated with upper respiratory infections.

USES

Immune system stimulant used for treatment/prevention of the common cold and other upper respiratory infections. Also used for UTIs, vaginal candidiasis.

PRECAUTIONS

CONTRAINDICATIONS: Pregnancy/lactation, children 2 yr and younger, those with autoimmune disease (e.g., multiple sclerosis, systemic lupus erythematosus [SLE], HIV/AIDS), tuberculosis, history of allergic conditions. **CAUTIONS:** Diabetes (may alter control of blood sugar). Do not use for more than 8 wk (may decrease effectiveness).

⧗ **LIFESPAN CONSIDERATIONS: Pregnancy/Lactation:** Contraindicated. **Pregnancy Category C. Children:** Safety and efficacy not established in those younger than 2 yr. **Elderly:** No age-related precautions noted.

INTERACTIONS

DRUG: Immunosuppressant therapy (e.g., corticosteroids, cyclosporine, mycophenolate): May be interfered with during echinacea use. **Topical econazole:** May reduce recurring vaginal candida infections. **HERBAL:** None known. **FOOD:** None known. **LAB VALUES:** None known.

AVAILABILITY (OTC)

CAPSULES: 200 mg, 380 mg, 400 mg, 500 mg. **POWDER:** 25 g, 100 g, 500 g. **TINCTURE:** 475 mg/ml.

INDICATIONS/ROUTES/DOSAGE

USUAL ADULT DOSAGE
PO: ADULTS, ELDERLY: 6–9 ml herbal juice for a maximum of 8 wk.
◀ **ALERT** ▶ A variety of doses have been used depending on the preparation.

SIDE EFFECTS

Well tolerated. May cause allergic reaction (urticaria, acute asthma/dyspnea, angioedema), fever, nausea, vomiting, diarrhea, unpleasant taste, abdominal pain, dizziness.

ADVERSE REACTIONS/ TOXIC EFFECTS

None known.

NURSING CONSIDERATIONS

BASELINE ASSESSMENT

Assess if patient is pregnant or breastfeeding, history of autoimmune disease, receiving immunosuppressant therapy.

INTERVENTION/EVALUATION

Assess for hypersensitivity reaction, improvement in infection.

PATIENT/FAMILY TEACHING

• Do not use during pregnancy or lactation, children younger than 2 yr.
• Do not use for more than 8 wk without at least 1-wk rest.

echothiophate

(Phospholine Iodide)

See Antiglaucoma agents (p. 46C)

Ecotrin, *see aspirin*

edetate calcium

See Appendix L

EES, *see erythromycin*

efalizumab

ef-ah-**liz**-ewe-mab

(Raptiva)

◆ CLASSIFICATION

PHARMACOTHERAPEUTIC: Monoclonal antibody. **CLINICAL:** Immunosuppressive.

ACTION

A monoclonal antibody that interferes with lymphocyte activation by binding to the lymphocyte antigen, inhibiting the adhesion of leukocytes to other cell types. Therapeutic Effect: Prevents the release of cytokines and the growth and migration of circulating total lymphocytes, predominant in psoriatic lesions.

PHARMACOKINETICS

Clearance is affected by body weight, not by gender or race, after subcutaneous injection. Serum concentration reaches steady state at 4 wk. Mean time to elimination: 25 days.

USES

Treatment of adults 18 yr and older with chronic moderate to severe plaque psoriasis who are candidates for systemic therapy or phototherapy.

PRECAUTIONS

CONTRAINDICATIONS: Concurrent use of immunosuppressive agents, hypersensitivity to any murine or humanized monoclonal antibody preparation. **CAUTIONS:** History of malignancy, chronic infection, history of recurrent infection, asthma, history of allergic reaction.

⧗ **LIFESPAN CONSIDERATIONS: Pregnancy/Lactation:** Unknown if drug is distributed in breast milk. **Pregnancy Category C. Children:** Not indicated for use in pediatric patients. **Elderly:** Age-related increased incidence of infection requires cautious use in the elderly.

INTERACTIONS

DRUG: Immunosuppressive agents: Increase the risk of infection. **Live-virus vaccines:** Decrease the immune response. **HERBAL:** None known. **FOOD:** None known. **LAB VALUES:** May increase the lymphocyte count.

AVAILABILITY (Rx)

POWDER FOR INJECTION: 150 mg, designed to deliver 125 mg/1.25 ml.

ADMINISTRATION/HANDLING
SUBCUTANEOUS

Reconstitution • Slowly inject 1.3 ml sterile water for injection provided into the efalizumab vial, using the provided prefilled diluent syringe. • Swirl vial gently to dissolve; do not shake (shaking causes foaming). • Dissolution takes less than 5 min.

Rate of administration • Administer into thigh, abdomen, buttocks, or upper arm.

Storage • Refrigerate unopened vial. • Reconstituted solution may be stored at room temperature for up to 8 hr.

INDICATIONS/ROUTES/DOSAGE
PSORIASIS

SUBCUTANEOUS: ADULTS, ELDERLY: Initially, 0.7 mg/kg followed by weekly doses of 1 mg/kg. **Maximum:** 200 mg (single dose).

SIDE EFFECTS

FREQUENT (32%–10%): Headache, chills, nausea, injection site pain. **OCCASIONAL (8%–7%):** Myalgia, flu-like symptoms, fever. **RARE (4%):** Back pain, acne.

ADVERSE REACTIONS/ TOXIC EFFECTS

Hypersensitivity reaction, malignancies, serious infections (abscess, cellulitis, postoperative wound infection, pneumonia), thrombocytopenia, and worsening of psoriasis occur rarely.

NURSING CONSIDERATIONS

BASELINE ASSESSMENT

Inform patient of treatment duration and required monitoring procedures. Obtain CBC to assess platelet count, lymphocyte before therapy and periodically thereafter. Inform patient of increased risk of developing an infection while undergoing treatment. Assess skin before therapy and document extent and location of psoriasis lesions.

INTERVENTION/EVALUATION

Assess skin throughout therapy for evidence of improvement of psoriasis lesions. Monitor for worsening of lesions. Offer patient teaching to assure accurate and sterile preparation and self-injection of medication.

PATIENT/FAMILY TEACHING

• If appropriate, patients may self-inject after proper training in the preparation and injection technique. • Inform physician or nurse if bleeding from the gums, bruising or petechiae of the skin, or onset of signs of infection occurs. • If new diagnosis of malignancy occurs, inform physician of current treatment with efalizumab. • Advise patients not to undergo phototherapy treatments.

efavirenz

eh-fah-**vir**-enz

(Sustiva)

Do not confuse Sustiva with Survanta.

CLASSIFICATION

PHARMACOTHERAPEUTIC: Nonnucleoside reverse transcriptase inhibitor. **CLINICAL:** Antiretroviral (see pp. 61C, 104C).

ACTION

A nonnucleoside reverse transcriptase inhibitor that inhibits the activity of HIV reverse transcriptase of HIV-1 and the transcription of HIV-1 RNA to DNA. **Therapeutic Effect:** Interrupts HIV replication, slowing the progression of HIV infection.

PHARMACOKINETICS

Rapidly absorbed after PO administration. Protein binding: 99%. Metabolized to major isoenzymes in the liver. Eliminated in urine and feces. **Half-life:** 40–55 hr.

USES

Treatment of HIV infection in combination with other appropriate antiretroviral agents.

PRECAUTIONS

CONTRAINDICATIONS: Concurrent use with ergot derivatives, midazolam, or triazolam; efavirenz as monotherapy. **CAUTIONS:** History of mental illness, substance abuse, hepatic impairment.

⏳ **LIFESPAN CONSIDERATIONS: Pregnancy/Lactation:** Breast-feeding not recommended. **Pregnancy Category D. Children:** Safety and efficacy not established in those younger than 3 yr; may have increased incidence of rash. **Elderly:** No age-related precautions noted.

INTERACTIONS

DRUG: Alcohol, psychoactive drugs: May produce additive CNS effects. **Clarithromycin:** Decreases clarithromycin plasma levels. **Ergot derivatives, midazolam, triazolam:** May cause serious or life-threatening reactions, such as arrhythmias, prolonged sedation, or respiratory depression. **Indinavir, saquinavir:** Decreases the plasma concentrations of these drugs. **Nelfinavir, ritonavir:** Increases the plasma concentrations of these drugs. **Phenobarbital, rifabutin, rifampin:** Lowers efavirenz plasma concentration. **Warfarin:** Alters warfarin plasma concentration. **HERBAL:** None known. **FOOD: High-fat meals:** May increase drug absorption. **LAB VALUES:** May produce false-positive urine test results for cannabinoid and increase total cholesterol, AST, ALT, and serum triglyceride levels.

AVAILABILITY (Rx)

CAPSULES: 50 mg, 100 mg, 200 mg.
TABLETS: 600 mg.

ADMINISTRATION/HANDLING
PO
• Give without regard to meals. • Avoid high-fat meal (may increase absorption).

INDICATIONS/ROUTES/DOSAGE

HIV INFECTION (IN COMBINATION WITH OTHER ANTIRETROVIRALS)
PO: ADULTS, ELDERLY, CHILDREN 3 YR AND OLDER WEIGHING 40 KG OR MORE: 600 mg once a day at bedtime. CHILDREN 3 YR AND OLDER WEIGHING 32.5 KG–LESS THAN 40 KG: 400 mg once a day. CHILDREN 3 YR AND OLDER WEIGHING 25 KG–LESS THAN 32.5 KG: 350 mg once a day. CHILDREN 3 YR AND OLDER WEIGHING 20 KG–LESS THAN 25 KG: 300 mg once a day. CHILDREN 3 YR AND OLDER WEIGHING 15 KG–LESS THAN 20 KG: 250 mg once a day. CHILDREN 3 YR AND OLDER WEIGHING 10 KG–LESS THAN 15 KG: 200 mg once a day.

SIDE EFFECTS

FREQUENT (52%): Mild to severe: Dizziness, vivid dreams, insomnia, confusion, impaired concentration, amnesia, agitation, depersonalization, hallucinations, euphoria, somnolence (mild symptoms don't interfere with daily activities; severe symptoms interrupt daily activities). **OCCASIONAL: Mild to moderate:** Maculopapular rash (27%); nausea, fatigue, headache, diarrhea, fever, cough (less than 26%) (moderate symptoms may interfere with daily activities).

ADVERSE REACTIONS/TOXIC EFFECTS

Serious psychiatric adverse experiences (aggressive reactions, agitation, delusions, emotional lability, mania, neurosis, paranoia, psychosis, suicide) have been reported.

NURSING CONSIDERATIONS

BASELINE ASSESSMENT
Offer emotional support to patient and family. Obtain baseline AST, ALT in patients with history of hepatitis B or C; serum cholesterol or triglycerides before initiating therapy and at intervals during therapy. Obtain history of all prescription and OTC medication (high level of drug interaction).

INTERVENTION/EVALUATION
Monitor for CNS, psychological symptoms: severe acute depression, including suicidal ideation or attempts, dizziness, impaired concentration, somnolence, abnormal dreams, insomnia (begins during first or second day of therapy, generally resolves in 2–4 wk). Assess for evidence of rash (common side effect). Monitor hepatic enzyme studies for abnormalities. Assess for headache, nausea, diarrhea.

PATIENT/FAMILY TEACHING
• Avoid high-fat meals during therapy.
• If rash appears, contact physician

immediately. • CNS, psychological symptoms occur in more than half the patients and may manifest as dizziness, impaired concentration, delusions, depression. • Take medication every day as prescribed. • Do not alter dose or discontinue medication without informing physician. • Avoid tasks that require alertness, motor skills until response to drug is established. • Drug is not a cure for HIV infection, nor does it reduce risk of transmission to others.

Effexor, *see venlafaxine*

Effexor CR, *see venlafaxine*

Effexor XR, *see venlafaxine*

Efudex, *see fluorouracil*

Elavil, *see amitriptyline*

eletriptan

el-eh-**trip**-tan
(Relpax)

E

CLASSIFICATION

PHARMACOTHERAPEUTIC: Serotonin receptor agonist. **CLINICAL:** Antimigraine.

ACTION

A serotonin receptor agonist that binds selectively to vascular receptors, producing a vasoconstrictive effect on cranial blood vessels. **Therapeutic Effect:** Relieves migraine headache.

PHARMACOKINETICS

Well absorbed after PO administration. Metabolized by the liver to inactive metabolite. Eliminated in urine. **Half-life:** 4.4 hr (increased in hepatic impairment and the elderly (older than 65 yr).

USES

Treatment of acute migraine headache with or without aura.

PRECAUTIONS

CONTRAINDICATIONS: Arrhythmias associated with conduction disorders, cerebrovascular syndrome including strokes and transient ischemic attacks (TIAs), coronary artery disease, hemiplegic or basilar migraine, ischemic heart disease, peripheral vascular disease including ischemic bowel disease, severe hepatic impairment, uncontrolled hypertension, use within 24 hr of treatment with another 5-HT1 agonist, an ergotamine-containing or ergot-type medication such as dihydroergotamine (DHE) or methysergide. **CAUTIONS:** Mild to moderate renal or hepatic impairment, controlled hypertension, history of cerebrovascular accident (CVA).

⧗ LIFESPAN CONSIDERATIONS: **Pregnancy/Lactation:** May decrease possibility of ovulation. Distributed in breast milk. **Pregnancy Category C. Children:** Safety and efficacy not established in patients younger than 18 yr.

Elderly: Increased risk of hypertension in patients older than 65 yr.

INTERACTIONS

DRUG: Clarithromycin, itraconazole, ketoconazole, nefazodone, nelfinavir, ritonavir: May decrease eletriptan metabolism. **Ergotamine-containing medications:** May produce a vasospastic reaction. **Sibutramine:** May produce serotonin syndrome (marked by altered level of consciousness [LOC], CNS irritability, motor weakness, myoclonus, and shivering). **HERBAL:** None known. **FOOD:** None known. **LAB VALUES:** None known.

AVAILABILITY (Rx)

TABLETS: 20 mg, 40 mg.

ADMINISTRATION/HANDLING

PO

• Do not crush or break film-coated tablets.

INDICATIONS/ROUTES/DOSAGE

ACUTE MIGRAINE HEADACHE

PO: ADULTS, ELDERLY: 20–40 mg. If headache improves but then returns, dose may be repeated after 2 hr. **Maximum:** 80 mg/day.

SIDE EFFECTS

OCCASIONAL (6%–5%): Dizziness, somnolence, asthenia, nausea. **RARE (3%–2%):** Paresthesia, headache, dry mouth, warm or hot sensation, dyspepsia, dysphagia.

ADVERSE REACTIONS/ TOXIC EFFECTS

Cardiac reactions (including ischemia, coronary artery vasospasm, and MI) and noncardiac vasospasm-related reactions (such as hemorrhage and CVA) occur rarely, particularly in patients with hypertension, diabetes, or a strong family history of coronary artery disease; obese patients; smokers; males older than 40 yr; and postmenopausal women.

NURSING CONSIDERATIONS

BASELINE ASSESSMENT

Question patient regarding onset, location, duration of migraine, possible precipitating symptoms. Obtain baseline BP for evidence of uncontrolled hypertension (contraindication).

INTERVENTION/EVALUATION

Assess for relief of migraine headache, potential for photophobia, phonophobia (sound sensitivity, nausea, vomiting).

PATIENT/FAMILY TEACHING

• Take a single dose as soon as symptoms of an actual migraine attack appear. • Medication is intended to relieve migraine headaches, not to prevent or reduce number of attacks. • Avoid tasks that require alertness, motor skills until response to drug is established. • If palpitations, pain or tightness in chest or throat, sudden or severe abdominal pain, pain or weakness of extremities occur, contact physician immediately.

Elidel, *see pimecrolimus*

Eloxatin, *see oxaliplatin*

emtricitabine

em-trih-**sit**-ah-bean
(Emtriva)

FIXED-COMBINATION(S)

Truvada: emtricitabine/tenofovir (an antiretroviral): 200 mg/300 mg.

CLASSIFICATION

PHARMACOTHERAPEUTIC: Nucleoside reverse transcriptase inhibitor. **CLINICAL:** Antiretroviral agent.

ACTION

An antiretroviral that inhibits HIV-1 reverse transcriptase by incorporating itself into viral DNA, resulting in chain termination. **Therapeutic Effect:** Interrupts HIV replication, slowing the progression of HIV infection.

PHARMACOKINETICS

Rapidly and extensively absorbed from the GI tract. Excreted primarily in urine (86%) and, to a lesser extent, in feces (14%); 30% removed by hemodialysis. Unknown if removed by peritoneal dialysis. **Half-life:** 10 hr.

USES

Used in combination with other antiretroviral agents for treatment of HIV-1 infection in adults.

PRECAUTIONS

CONTRAINDICATIONS: None known. **CAUTIONS:** Hepatic or renal impairment.

⌛ **LIFESPAN CONSIDERATIONS: Pregnancy/Lactation:** Breast-feeding not recommended. **Pregnancy Category B. Children:** Safety and effectiveness not established. **Elderly:** Age-related renal impairment may require dosage adjustment.

INTERACTIONS

DRUG: None known. **HERBAL:** None known. **FOOD:** None known. **LAB VALUES:** May elevate serum amylase, lipase, ALT, AST, and triglyceride levels. May alter blood glucose levels.

AVAILABILITY (Rx)

CAPSULES: 200 mg. **ORAL SOLUTION:** 10 mg/ml.

ADMINISTRATION/HANDLING

PO
• Give without regard to food.

INDICATIONS/ROUTES/DOSAGE

HIV INFECTION (IN COMBINATION WITH OTHER ANTIRETROVIRALS)
PO: ADULTS, ELDERLY: 200 mg once a day.

DOSAGE IN RENAL IMPAIRMENT
Dosage and frequency are modified based on creatinine clearance.

Creatinine Clearance	Dosage
30–49 ml/min	200 mg q48h
15–29 ml/min	200 mg q72h
Less than 15 ml/min, hemodialysis patients	200 mg q96h

SIDE EFFECTS

FREQUENT (23%–13%): Headache, rhinitis, rash, diarrhea, nausea. **OCCASIONAL (14%–4%):** Cough, vomiting, abdominal pain, insomnia, depression, paresthesia, dizziness, peripheral neuropathy, dyspepsia, myalgia. **RARE (3%–2%):** Arthralgia, abnormal dreams.

ADVERSE REACTIONS/ TOXIC EFFECTS

Lactic acidosis and hepatomegaly with steatosis occur rarely and may be severe.

NURSING CONSIDERATIONS

BASELINE ASSESSMENT

Obtain baseline laboratory testing, especially serum liver function tests, triglycerides before beginning and at periodic intervals during emtricitabine therapy. Offer emotional support.

INTERVENTION/EVALUATION

Monitor pattern of bowel activity and stool. Question for evidence of nausea, pruritus (itching). Assess skin for rash, urticaria (hives). Monitor serum chemistry tests for marked lab abnormalities.

E

PATIENT/FAMILY TEACHING
PATIENT/FAMILY TEACHING
• May cause redistribution of body fat.
• Continue therapy for full length of treatment. • Emtricitabine is not a cure for HIV infection, nor does it reduce risk of transmission to others.
• Patients may continue to acquire illnesses associated with advanced HIV infection.

enalapril maleate ✐

en-**al**-ah-pril

(AApo-Enalapril ✦, <u>Vasotec</u>)

Do not confuse enalapril with Anafranil, Eldepryl, or ramipril.

FIXED-COMBINATION(S)

Lexxel: enalapril/felodipine (calcium channel blocker): 5 mg/2.5 mg; 5 mg/5 mg. **Teczem:** enalapril/diltiazem (calcium channel blocker): 5 mg/180 mg. **Vaseretic:** enalapril/hydrochlorothiazide (diuretic): 5 mg/12.5 mg; 10 mg/25 mg.

◦CLASSIFICATION

PHARMACOTHERAPEUTIC: Angiotensin-converting enzyme (ACE) inhibitor. **CLINICAL:** Antihypertensive, vasodilator (see p. 7C).

ACTION

This ACE inhibitor suppresses the renin-angiotensin-aldosterone system, and prevents conversion of angiotensin I to angiotensin II, a potent vasoconstrictor; may inhibit angiotensin II at local vascular, renal sites. Decreases plasma angiotensin II, increases plasma renin activity, decreases aldosterone secretion. **Therapeutic Effect:** In hypertension, reduces peripheral arterial resistance. In congestive heart failure (CHF), increases cardiac output; decreases peripheral vascular resistance, BP, pulmonary capillary wedge pressure, heart size.

PHARMACOKINETICS

Route	Onset	Peak	Duration
PO	1 hr	4–6 hr	24 hr
IV	15 min	1–4 hr	6 hr

Readily absorbed from the GI tract (not affected by food). Protein binding: 50%–60%. Converted to active metabolite. Primarily excreted in urine. Removed by hemodialysis. **Half-life:** 11 hr (half-life is increased in those with impaired renal function).

USES

Treatment of hypertension alone or in combination with other antihypertensives. Adjunctive therapy for CHF. **OFF-LABEL:** Diabetic nephropathy, hypertension due to scleroderma renal crisis, hypertensive crisis, idiopathic edema, renal artery stenosis, rheumatoid arthritis, post MI for prevention of ventricular failure.

PRECAUTIONS

CONTRAINDICATIONS: History of angioedema from previous treatment with ACE inhibitors. **CAUTIONS:** Renal impairment, those with sodium depletion or on diuretic therapy, dialysis, hypovolemia, coronary/cerebrovascular insufficiency.

⧗ **LIFESPAN CONSIDERATIONS: Pregnancy/Lactation:** Crosses placenta. Distributed in breast milk. May cause fetal/neonatal mortality, morbidity. **Pregnancy Category D (C if used in first trimester). Children:** Safety and efficacy not established. **Elderly:** May be more susceptible to hypotensive effects.

INTERACTIONS

DRUG: Alcohol, antihypertensives, diuretics: May increase the effects of enalapril. **HERBAL:** None known.

✐ see color pill atlas   ✦ herb   <u>underlined</u> – top prescribed drug

FOOD: None known. **LAB VALUES:** May increase BUN and serum alkaline phosphatase, serum bilirubin, serum creatinine, serum potassium, AST, and ALT levels. May decrease serum sodium levels. May cause positive ANA titer.

AVAILABILITY (Rx)

TABLETS: 2.5 mg, 5 mg, 10 mg, 20 mg.
INJECTION: 1.25 mg/ml.

ADMINISTRATION/HANDLING

 IV

Reconstitution • May give undiluted or dilute with D_5W or 0.9% NaCl.

Rate of administration • For IV push, give undiluted over 5 min. • For IV piggyback, infuse over 10–15 min.

Storage • Store parenteral form at room temperature. • Use only clear, colorless solution. • Diluted IV solution is stable for 24 hr at room temperature.

PO
• Give without regard to food. • Tablets may be crushed.

⊞ IV INCOMPATIBILITIES

Amphotericin B (Fungizone), amphotericin B complex (Abelcet, AmBisome, Amphotec), cefepime (Maxipime), phenytoin (Dilantin).

IV COMPATIBILITIES

Calcium gluconate, dobutamine (Dobutrex), dopamine (Inotropin), fentanyl (Sublimaze), heparin, lidocaine, magnesium sulfate, morphine, nitroglycerin, potassium chloride, potassium phosphate, propofol (Diprivan).

INDICATIONS/ROUTES/DOSAGE

HYPERTENSION ALONE OR IN COMBINATION WITH OTHER ANTIHYPERTENSIVES
PO: ADULTS, ELDERLY: Initially, 2.5–5 mg / day. May increase at 1–2 wk intervals. Range: 10–40 mg/day in 1–2 divided doses. CHILDREN: 0.1 mg/kg/day in 1–2

divided doses. **Maximum:** 0.5 mg/kg/day. NEONATES: 0.1 mg/kg/day q24h.
IV: ADULTS, ELDERLY: 0.625–1.25 mg q6h up to 5 mg q6h. CHILDREN, NEONATES: 5–10 mcg/kg/dose q8–24h.

ADJUNCTIVE THERAPY FOR CHF
PO: ADULTS, ELDERLY: Initially, 2.5–5 mg / day. Range: 5–20 mg/day in 2 divided doses.

DOSAGE IN RENAL IMPAIRMENT
Dosage is modified based on creatinine clearance.

Creatinine Clearance	% Usual Dose
10–50 ml/min	75–100
Less than 10 ml/min	50

SIDE EFFECTS

FREQUENT (7%–5%): Headache, dizziness. **OCCASIONAL (3%–2%):** Orthostatic hypotension, fatigue, diarrhea, cough, syncope. **RARE (less than 2%):** Angina, abdominal pain, vomiting, nausea, rash, asthenia (loss of strength, energy).

ADVERSE REACTIONS/TOXIC EFFECTS

Excessive hypotension ("first-dose syncope") may occur in patients with CHF and in those who are severely salt or volume depleted. Angioedema (swelling of face, lips) and hyperkalemia occur rarely. Agranulocytosis and neutropenia may be noted in patients with collagen vascular diseases, including scleroderma and systemic lupus erythematosus, and impaired renal function. Nephrotic syndrome may be noted in those with history of renal disease.

NURSING CONSIDERATIONS

BASELINE ASSESSMENT
Obtain BP immediately before each dose (be alert to fluctuations). In patients with renal impairment, autoimmune disease, or taking drugs that affect leukocytes/immune response, CBC should be performed before beginning

---

therapy, q2wk for 3 mo, then periodically thereafter.

INTERVENTION/EVALUATION

Assist with ambulation if dizziness occurs. Monitor serum potassium, BUN, serum creatinine levels, BP. Monitor pattern of daily bowel activity and stool consistency.

PATIENT/FAMILY TEACHING

• To reduce hypotensive effect, rise slowly from lying to sitting position, permit legs to dangle from bed momentarily before standing. • Several weeks may be needed for full therapeutic effect of BP reduction. • Skipping doses or voluntarily discontinuing drug may produce severe, rebound hypertension. • Limit alcohol intake. • Inform physician if vomiting, diarrhea, excessive perspiration, swelling of face, lips, tongue, difficulty in breathing occurs.

Enbrel, *see etanercept*

---

enfuvirtide

en-**few**-vir-tide

(Fuzeon)

Do not confuse Fuzeon with Furoxone.

◆ CLASSIFICATION

PHARMACOTHERAPEUTIC: Fusion inhibitor. **CLINICAL:** Antiretroviral agent.

ACTION

A fusion inhibitor that interferes with the entry of HIV-1 into CD4+ cells by inhibiting the fusion of viral and cellular membranes. **Therapeutic Effect:** Impairs HIV replication, slowing the progression of HIV infection.

PHARMACOKINETICS

Comparable absorption when injected into subcutaneous tissue of abdomen, arm, or thigh. Protein binding: 92%. Undergoes catabolism to amino acids. Half-life: 3.8 hr.

USES

Used in combination with other antiretroviral agents for treatment of HIV-1 infection in treatment-experienced patients with evidence of HIV-1 replication.

PRECAUTIONS

CONTRAINDICATIONS: None known. **CAUTIONS:** None known.

⌛ **LIFESPAN CONSIDERATIONS: Pregnancy/Lactation:** Breast-feeding not recommended. **Pregnancy Category B. Children:** Safety and effectiveness not established in children 6 yr and younger. **Elderly:** No age-related precautions noted.

INTERACTIONS

DRUG: None known. **HERBAL:** None known. **FOOD:** None known. **LAB VALUES:** May elevate blood glucose and serum amylase, creatine kinase (CK), lipase, triglyceride, AST, and ALT levels. May decrease blood hemoglobin levels and WBC count.

AVAILABILITY (Rx)

POWDER FOR INJECTION: 108-mg (approximately 90 mg/ml when reconstituted) vials.

ADMINISTRATION/HANDLING

SUBCUTANEOUS

Reconstitution • Reconstitute with 1.1 ml sterile water for injection. • Visually inspect vial for particulate matter. Solution should appear clear, colorless. • Discard unused portion.

Rate of administration • Administer into the upper arm, anterior thigh, abdomen. Rotate injection sites.

✐ see color pill atlas   ✑ herb   underlined – top prescribed drug

Storage • Store at room temperature. • Refrigerate reconstituted solution; use within 24 hr. • Bring reconstituted solution to room temperature before injection.

INDICATIONS/ROUTES/DOSAGE

HIV INFECTION (IN COMBINATION WITH OTHER ANTIRETROVIRALS)

SUBCUTANEOUS: ADULTS, ELDERLY: 90 mg (1 ml) twice a day. CHILDREN 6–16 YR: 2 mg/kg twice a day. **Maximum:** 90 mg twice a day.

Pediatric dosing guidelines

Weight: kg (lb)	Dose: mg (ml)
11–15.5 (24–34)	27 (0.3)
15.6–20 (35–44)	36 (0.4)
20.1–24.5 (45–54)	45 (0.5)
24.6–29 (55–64)	54 (0.6)
29.1–33.5 (65–74)	63 (0.7)
33.6–38 (75–84)	72 (0.8)
38.1–42.5 (85–94)	81 (0.9)
Greater than 42.5 (greater than 94)	90 (1)

SIDE EFFECTS

EXPECTED (98%): Local injection site reactions (pain, discomfort, induration, erythema, nodules, cysts, pruritus, ecchymosis). **FREQUENT (26%–16%):** Diarrhea, nausea, fatigue. **OCCASIONAL (11%–4%):** Insomnia, peripheral neuropathy, depression, cough, decreased appetite or weight loss, sinusitis, anxiety, asthenia, myalgia, cold sores. **RARE (3%–2%):** Constipation, influenza, upper abdominal pain, anorexia, conjunctivitis.

ADVERSE REACTIONS/ TOXIC EFFECTS

Enfuvirtide use may potentiate bacterial pneumonia. Hypersensitivity (rash, fever, chills, rigors, hypotension), thrombocytopenia, neutropenia, and renal insufficiency or failure may occur rarely.

NURSING CONSIDERATIONS

BASELINE ASSESSMENT

Obtain baseline laboratory testing, especially serum liver function tests, triglycerides before beginning enfuvirtide therapy and at periodic intervals during therapy. Offer emotional support.

INTERVENTION/EVALUATION

Assess skin for local injection site hypersensitivity reaction. Question for evidence of nausea, fatigue. Assess sleep pattern. Monitor for insomnia, signs and symptoms of depression. Monitor serum chemistry tests for marked laboratory abnormalities.

PATIENT/FAMILY TEACHING

• Advise patient that an increased rate of bacterial pneumonia has occurred with enfuvirtide therapy and to seek medical attention if cough with fever, rapid, difficult breathing occurs. • Continue therapy for full length of treatment. • Enfuvirtide is not a cure for HIV infection, nor does it reduce risk of transmission to others; patient must continue practices to prevent HIV transmission.

enoxacin

(Penetrex)

See Antibiotic: fluoroquinolones (p. 24C)

enoxaparin sodium

en-**ox**-ah-pear-in

(Klexane ✤, Lovenox)

Do not confuse Lovenox with Lotronex.

◆ CLASSIFICATION

PHARMACOTHERAPEUTIC: Low-molecular-weight heparin. **CLINICAL:** Anticoagulant (see p. 30C).

E

ACTION

A low-molecular-weight heparin that potentiates the action of antithrombin III and inactivates coagulation factor Xa. **Therapeutic Effect:** Produces anticoagulation. Does not significantly influence bleeding time, PT, or aPTT.

PHARMACOKINETICS

Route	Onset	Peak	Duration
Subcutaneous	N/A	3–5 hr	12 hr

Well absorbed after subcutaneous administration. Eliminated primarily in urine. Not removed by hemodialysis. **Half-life:** 4.5 hr.

USES

Prevention of postop deep vein thrombosis (DVT) following hip or knee replacement surgery, abdominal surgery. Long-term DVT prevention following hip replacement surgery, nonsurgical acute illness. Treatment of unstable angina, non–Q-wave MI, acute DVT (with warfarin). OFF-LABEL: Prevention of DVT following general surgical procedures.

PRECAUTIONS

CONTRAINDICATIONS: Active major bleeding, concurrent heparin therapy, hypersensitivity to heparin or pork products, thrombocytopenia associated with positive in vitro test for antiplatelet antibodies. **CAUTIONS:** Conditions with increased risk of hemorrhage, history of heparin-induced thrombocytopenia, renal impairment, elderly, uncontrolled arterial hypertension, history of recent GI ulceration or hemorrhage. When neuraxial anesthesia (epidural or spinal anesthesia) or spinal puncture is employed, patients anticoagulated or scheduled to be anticoagulated with enoxaparin for prevention of thromboembolic complications are at risk of developing an epidural or spinal hematoma which can result in long-term or permanent paralysis.

⏳ **LIFESPAN CONSIDERATIONS: Pregnancy/Lactation:** Use with caution, particularly during last trimester, immediate postpartum period (increased risk of maternal hemorrhage). Unknown if excreted in breast milk. **Pregnancy Category B. Children:** Safety and efficacy not established. **Elderly:** May be more susceptible to bleeding.

INTERACTIONS

DRUG: Anticoagulants, platelet inhibitors: May increase bleeding. **HERBAL:** None known. **FOOD:** None known. **LAB VALUES:** Increases (reversible) LDH, serum alkaline phosphatase, AST, and ALT levels.

AVAILABILITY (Rx)

INJECTION: 30 mg/0.3 ml, 40 mg/0.4 ml, 60 mg/0.6 ml, 80 mg/0.8 ml, 100 mg/ml, 120 mg/0.8 ml, 150 mg/ml in prefilled syringes.

ADMINISTRATION/HANDLING

◀ **ALERT** ▶ Do not mix with other injections or infusions. Do not give IM.

SUBCUTANEOUS
• Parenteral form appears clear and colorless to pale yellow. • Store at room temperature. • Instruct patient to lie down before administering by deep subcutaneous injection. • Inject between left and right anterolateral and left and right posterolateral abdominal wall. • Introduce entire length of needle (½ inch) into skin fold held between thumb and forefinger, holding skin fold during injection.

INDICATIONS/ROUTES/DOSAGE

PREVENTION OF DVT AFTER HIP AND KNEE SURGERY
SUBCUTANEOUS: ADULTS, ELDERLY: 30 mg twice a day, generally for 7–10 days.

E

PREVENTION OF DVT AFTER ABDOMINAL SURGERY

SUBCUTANEOUS: ADULTS, ELDERLY: 40 mg a day for 7–10 days.

PREVENTION OF LONG-TERM DVT IN NONSURGICAL ACUTE ILLNESS

SUBCUTANEOUS: ADULTS, ELDERLY: 40 mg once a day for 3 wk.

PREVENTION OF ISCHEMIC COMPLICATIONS OF UNSTABLE ANGINA AND NON–Q-WAVE MI (WITH ORAL ASPIRIN THERAPY)

SUBCUTANEOUS: ADULTS, ELDERLY: 1 mg/kg q12h.

ACUTE DVT

SUBCUTANEOUS: ADULTS, ELDERLY: 1 mg/kg q12h or 1.5 mg/kg once daily.

USUAL PEDIATRIC DOSAGE

SUBCUTANEOUS: CHILDREN: 0.5 mg/kg q12h (prophylaxis); 1 mg/kg q12h (treatment).

DOSAGE IN RENAL IMPAIRMENT

Clearance of enoxaparin is decreased when creatinine clearance is less than 30 ml/min. Monitor patient and adjust dosage as necessary. When enoxaparin is used in abdominal, hip, or knee surgery or acute illness, the dosage in renal impairment is 30 mg once a day. When enoxaparin is used to treat DVT, angina, or MI the dosage in renal impairment is 1 mg/kg once a day.

SIDE EFFECTS

OCCASIONAL (4%–1%): Injection site hematoma, nausea, peripheral edema.

ADVERSE REACTIONS/ TOXIC EFFECTS

Overdose may lead to bleeding complications ranging from local ecchymoses to major hemorrhage. Antidote: Protamine sulfate (1% solution) equal to the dose of enoxaparin injected. One mg protamine sulfate neutralizes 1 mg enoxaparin. A second dose of 0.5 mg protamine sulfate per 1 mg enoxaparin may be given if aPTT tested 2–4 hr after first injection remains prolonged.

NURSING CONSIDERATIONS

BASELINE ASSESSMENT

Assess CBC, including platelet count.

INTERVENTION/EVALUATION

Periodically monitor CBC, platelet count, stool for occult blood (no need for daily monitoring in patients with normal presurgical coagulation parameters). Assess for any sign of bleeding: bleeding at surgical site, hematuria, blood in stool, bleeding from gums, petechiae, bruising, bleeding from injection sites.

PATIENT/FAMILY TEACHING

- Usual length of therapy is 7–10 days.
- Do not take any OTC medication (especially aspirin) without consulting physician.

entacapone

en-**tah**-cah-pone
(Comtan)

FIXED-COMBINATION(S)

Stalevo: entacapone/carbidopa-levodopa (an antiparkinson agent) 200 mg/12.5 mg/50 mg; 200 mg/ 25 mg/100 mg; 200 mg/37.5 mg/ 150 mg.

CLASSIFICATION

PHARMACOTHERAPEUTIC: Enzyme inhibitor. **CLINICAL:** Antiparkinson agent.

ACTION

An antiparkinson agent that inhibits the enzyme, catechol-*O*-methyltransferase (COMT), potentiating dopamine activity and increasing the duration of action of levodopa. **Therapeutic Effect:** Decreases signs and symptoms of Parkinson's disease.

✤ Canadian trade name   Ⓔ see **evolve**   ▶ High Alert drug

PHARMACOKINETICS

Rapidly absorbed after PO administration. Protein binding: 98%. Metabolized in the liver. Primarily eliminated by biliary excretion. Not removed by hemodialysis. Half-life: 2.4 hr.

USES

In conjunction with levodopa/carbidopa, improves quality of life in patients with Parkinson's disease.

PRECAUTIONS

CONTRAINDICATIONS: Hypersensitivity, use within 14 days of MAOIs. **CAUTIONS:** Renal or hepatic impairment. May increase risk of orthostatic hypotension and syncope, exacerbate dyskinesias.

⧗ LIFESPAN CONSIDERATIONS: **Pregnancy/Lactation:** Unknown if distributed in breast milk. **Pregnancy Category C. Children:** Not used in children. **Elderly:** No age-related precautions noted.

INTERACTIONS

DRUG: **Ampicillin, cholestyramine, erythromycin, probenecid:** May decrease the excretion of entacapone. **Bitolterol, dobutamine, dopamine, epinephrine, isoetharine, isoproterenol, epinephrine, methyldopa, norepinephrine:** May increase the risk of arrhythmias and changes in BP. **Nonselective MAOIs (including phenelzine):** May inhibit catecholamine metabolism. **Other CNS depressants:** May increase CNS depression. HERBAL: None known. FOOD: None known. LAB VALUES: None known.

AVAILABILITY (Rx)

TABLETS: 200 mg.

ADMINISTRATION/HANDLING

PO

• Give without regard to food.

INDICATIONS/ROUTES/DOSAGE

ADJUNCTIVE TREATMENT OF PARKINSON'S DISEASE

PO: ADULTS, ELDERLY: 200 mg concomitantly with each dose of carbidopa and levodopa up to a maximum of 8 times a day (1,600 mg).

SIDE EFFECTS

FREQUENT (greater than 10%): Dyskinesia, nausea, dark yellow or orange urine and sweat, diarrhea. OCCASIONAL (9%–3%): Abdominal pain, vomiting, constipation, dry mouth, fatigue, back pain. RARE (less than 2%): Anxiety, somnolence, agitation, dyspepsia, flatulence, diaphoresis, asthenia, dyspnea.

ADVERSE REACTIONS/ TOXIC EFFECTS

Hallucinations have been reported.

NURSING CONSIDERATIONS

INTERVENTION/EVALUATION

Monitor for evidence of dyskinesia (difficulty with movement). Assess for clinical reversal of symptoms (improvement of tremor of head and hands at rest, mask-like facial expression, shuffling gait, muscular rigidity). Monitor BP. Assess for orthostatic hypotension, diarrhea.

PATIENT/FAMILY TEACHING

• Avoid tasks that require alertness, motor skills until response to drug is established. • May cause color change in urine or sweat (dark yellow, orange). • Report any uncontrolled movement of face, eyelids, mouth, tongue, arms, hands, legs.

entecavir

en-**tech**-ah-veer
(Baraclude)

CLASSIFICATION

PHARMACOTHERAPEUTIC: Reverse transcriptase inhibitor. **CLINICAL:** Antiretroviral.

ACTION

A nucleoside analogue that inhibits hepatitis B viral polymerase, an enzyme blocking reverse transcriptase activity. **Therapeutic Effect:** Interferes with viral DNA synthesis.

PHARMACOKINETICS

Poorly absorbed from the GI tract. Protein binding: 13%. Extensively distributed into tissues. Partially metabolized in liver. Eliminated mainly in urine. **Half-life:** 5–6 days (half-life increased in renal impairment).

USES

Treatment of chronic hepatitis B infection with evidence of active viral replication and either evidence of persistent transaminase elevations or histologically-active disease.

PRECAUTIONS

CONTRAINDICATIONS: None known. **CAUTIONS:** Renal impairment, patients receiving concurrent therapy which may reduce renal function, hepatic transplant patients receiving concurrent therapy of cyclosporine or tacrolimus.

LIFESPAN CONSIDERATIONS: Pregnancy/Lactation: Unknown if drug crosses placenta or is distributed in breast milk. **Pregnancy Category C. Children:** Safety and efficacy not established in children younger than 16 yr. **Elderly:** Age-related renal impairment may require dosage adjustment.

INTERACTIONS

DRUG: Drugs that reduce renal function: May increase serum concentrations of either entecavir or the coadministered drug. **HERBAL:** None known. **FOOD: Food:** Delays absorption, decreases concentration. **LAB VALUES:** May increase amylase, lipase, bilirubin, ALT, AST, creatinine, glucose. May decrease albumin, platelets.

AVAILABILITY (Rx)

FILM-COATED TABLETS: 0.5 mg, 1 mg. **ORAL SOLUTION:** 0.05 mg/ml.

ADMINISTRATION/HANDLING

PO
• Administer tablets on an empty stomach (at least 2 hr after a meal and 2 hr before the next meal). • Do not dilute or mix oral solution with water or any other solvent or liquid. • Each bottle of the oral solution is accompanied by a dosing spoon. Before administering, hold the spoon in a vertical position and fill it gradually to the mark corresponding to the prescribed dose.

Storage • Store both tablets and oral solution at room temperature.

INDICATIONS/ROUTES/DOSAGE

CHRONIC HEPATITIS B, NO PREVIOUS NUCLEOSIDE TREATMENT
PO: ADULTS, ELDERLY, CHILDREN 16 YR AND OLDER: 0.5 mg once daily.

CHRONIC HEPATITIS B, RECEIVING LAMIVUDINE OR KNOWN LAMIVUDINE RESISTANCE
PO: ADULTS, ELDERLY, CHILDREN 16 YR AND OLDER: 1 mg once daily.

DOSAGE IN RENAL IMPAIRMENT

Creatinine clearance	Dosage
50 ml/min and greater	0.5 mg once daily
30–49 ml/min	0.25 mg once daily
10–29 ml/min	0.15 mg once daily
9 ml/min and less	0.05 mg once daily

SIDE EFFECTS

OCCASIONAL (4%–3%): Headache, fatigue. **RARE (less than 1%):** Diarrhea, dyspepsia, nausea, vomiting, dizziness, insomnia.

ADVERSE REACTIONS/ TOXIC EFFECTS

Lactic acidosis, severe hepatomegaly with steatosis have been reported. Severe, acute exacerbations of hepatitis B have been reported in patients who have discontinued therapy; reinitiation of antihepatitis B therapy may be required. Hematuria occurs occasionally.

NURSING CONSIDERATIONS

BASELINE ASSESSMENT

Obtain baseline laboratory testing, especially hepatic function tests, before beginning therapy and at periodic intervals during therapy. Offer emotional support. Obtain medication history.

INTERVENTION/EVALUATION

Hepatic function should be monitored closely with both clinical and laboratory follow-up for at least several months in patients who discontinue anti-hepatitis B therapy. For patients on therapy, closely monitor amylase, lipase, bilirubin, ALT, AST, creatinine, glucose, albumin, platelet count. Assess for evidence of GI discomfort.

PATIENT/FAMILY TEACHING

• Take medication at least 2 hr after a meal and 2 hr before the next meal.
• Avoid transmission of Hepatitis B infection to others through sexual contact or blood contamination.
• Notify physician immediately if unusual muscle pain, abdominal pain with nausea and vomiting, cold feeling in the arms and legs, and dizziness occur (signs and symptoms signaling onset of lactic acidosis).

epinephrine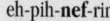

eh-pih-**nef**-rin

(Adrenalin, EpiPen, EpiPen 2-Pak, EpiPen Auto Injector, EpiPen Jr. Auto-Injector, Primatene, Sus-Phrine Injection)

Do not confuse epinephrine with ephedrine.

FIXED-COMBINATION(S)

LidoSite: epinephrine/lidocaine (anesthetic): 0.1%/10%.

CLASSIFICATION

PHARMACOTHERAPEUTIC: Sympathomimetic (adrenergic agonist). **CLINICAL:** Antiglaucoma, bronchodilator, cardiac stimulant, antiallergic, antihemorrhagic, priapism reversal agent (see pp. 47C, 142C).

ACTION

A sympathomimetic, adrenergic agonist that stimulates alpha-adrenergic receptors causing vasoconstriction and pressor effects, beta$_1$-adrenergic receptors, resulting in cardiac stimulation, and beta$_2$-adrenergic receptors, resulting in bronchial dilation and vasodilation. With ophthalmic form, increases outflow of aqueous humor from anterior eye chamber. Therapeutic Effect: Relaxes smooth muscle of the bronchial tree, produces cardiac stimulation, and dilates skeletal muscle vasculature. The ophthalmic form dilates pupils and constricts conjunctival blood vessels.

PHARMACOKINETICS

Route	Onset	Peak	Duration
IM	5–10 min	20 min	1–4 hr
Subcutaneous	5–10 min	20 min	1–4 hr
Inhalation	3–5 min	20 min	1–3 hr
Ophthalmic	1 hr	4–8 hr	12–24 hr

Well absorbed after parenteral administration; minimally absorbed after inhalation. Metabolized in the liver, other tissues, and sympathetic nerve endings. Excreted in urine. The ophthalmic form may be systemically absorbed as a result of drainage into nasal pharyngeal passages. Mydriasis occurs within several min and persists several hr; vasoconstriction occurs within 5 min, and lasts less than 1 hr.

USES

Systemic: Treatment of asthma (acute exacerbation, reversible bronchospasm), anaphylaxis, cardiac arrest. **Ophthalmic:** Management of chronic open-angle glaucoma. OFF-LABEL: **Systemic:** Treatment of gingival or pulpal hemorrhage, priapism. **Ophthalmic:** Treatment of conjunctival congestion during surgery, secondary glaucoma.

PRECAUTIONS

CONTRAINDICATIONS: Cardiac arrhythmias, cerebrovascular insufficiency, hypertension, hyperthyroidism, ischemic heart disease, narrow-angle glaucoma, shock. **CAUTIONS:** Elderly, diabetes mellitus, angina pectoris, tachycardia, MI, severe renal or hepatic impairment, psychoneurotic disorders, hypoxia.

⏳ LIFESPAN CONSIDERATIONS: **Pregnancy/Lactation:** Crosses placenta. Distributed in breast milk. **Pregnancy Category C. Children/Elderly:** No age-related precautions noted.

INTERACTIONS

DRUG: **Beta blockers:** May decrease the effects of beta blockers. **Digoxin, sympathomimetics:** May increase risk of arrhythmias. **Ergonovine, methergine, oxytocin:** May increase vasoconstriction. **MAOIs, tricyclic antidepressants:** May increase cardiovascular effects. HERBAL: None known. FOOD: None known. LAB VALUES: May decrease serum potassium level.

AVAILABILITY (Rx)

INJECTION (ADRENALIN): 0.1 mg/ml, 1 mg/ml. **INJECTION:** 0.3 mg/0.3 ml (EpiPen Auto Injector), 0.15 mg/0.3 ml (EpiPen Jr Auto-Injector, EpiPen 2-Pak). **INHALATION (AEROSOL [PRIMATENE MIST]):** 0.2 mg/inhalation. **INHALATION SOLUTION:** 1%, 2.25%. **OPHTHALMIC SOLUTION (EPIFRIN):** 0.5%, 1%, 2%. **SUBCUTANEOUS SUSPENSION (SUS-PHRINE INJECTION):** 5 mg/ml. **TOPICAL SOLUTION (ADRENALIN, TOPICAL):** 1:100.

ADMINISTRATION/HANDLING

 IV

Reconstitution • For injection, dilute each 1 mg of 1;1,000 solution with 10 ml 0.9 NaCl to provide 1;10,000 solution and inject each 1 mg or fraction thereof 1 min or more. • For infusion, further dilute with 250–500 D₅W. Maximum concentration: 64 mg/250 ml.

Rate of administration • For IV infusion, give at 1–10 mcg/min (titrate to desired response).

Storage • Store parenteral forms at room temperature. • Do not use if solution appears discolored or contains a precipitate.

SUBCUTANEOUS
• Shake ampule thoroughly. • Use tuberculin syringe for injection into lateral deltoid region. • Massage rejection site (minimizes vasoconstriction effect).

INHALANT
• Shake container well. • Have the patient exhale completely as possible. • Place the mouthpiece fully into the patient's mouth, then while holding the inhaler upright, have the patient inhale deeply and slowly while pressuring the top of the canister. • Instruct the patient to hold his or her breath as long as possible before exhaling, then exhale slowly. • Wait 1 min between inhalations when multiple inhalations are ordered to allow for deeper bronchial penetration.

• Have the patient rinse his or her mouth with water immediately after inhalation to prevent mouth and throat dryness.

NEBULIZER
• Approximately 10 drops (not more) of Adrenalin Chloride solution 1:100 should be placed in the reservoir of the nebulizer, the nozzle of which is placed just inside the partially opened mouth. • As the bulb is squeezed once or twice instruct the patient to inhale deeply, drawing the vaporized solution into the lungs. • Have the patient rinse his or her mouth with water immediately after inhalation to prevent mouth and throat dryness. • When the nebulizer is not in use, it should be stoppered and kept in an upright position.

OPHTHALMIC
• Place a finger on the lower eyelid and pull it out until a pocket is formed between the eye and lower lid. • Hold the dropper above the pocket and place the prescribed number of drops into pocket. • Close eye gently so the medication will not be squeezed out of the sac. • Apply gentle digital pressure to the lacrimal sac at the inner canthus for 1 min after installation to lessen the risk of systemic absorption.

✷ IV INCOMPATIBILITY
Ampicillin (Omnipen, Polycillin).

IV COMPATIBILITIES
Calcium chloride, calcium gluconate, diltiazem (Cardizem), dobutamine (Dobutrex), dopamine (Intropin), fentanyl (Sublimaze), heparin, hydromorphone (Dilaudid), lorazepam (Ativan), midazolam (Versed), milrinone (Primacor), morphine, nitroglycerin, norepinephrine (Levophed), potassium chloride, propofol (Diprivan).

INDICATIONS/ROUTES/DOSAGE
ANAPHYLAXIS
IM: ADULTS, ELDERLY: 0.3 mg (0.3 ml of 1:1,000 solution). May repeat if anaphylaxis persists. CHILDREN: 0.15–0.3 mg or 0.01 mg/kg for patients weighing less than 30 kg. May repeat if anaphylaxis persists.

ASTHMA
SUBCUTANEOUS: ADULTS, ELDERLY: 0.2–0.5 mg (0.2–0.5 ml of 1:1,000 solution) q2h as needed. In severe attacks, may repeat q20min times 3 doses. CHILDREN: 0.01 ml/kg/dose (1:1,000 solution). **Maximum:** 0.4–0.5 ml/dose. May repeat q15–20min for 3–4 doses or q4h as needed.
INHALATION: ADULTS, ELDERLY, CHILDREN 4 YR AND OLDER: 1 inhalation, wait at least 1 min. May repeat once. Do not use again for at least 3 hr.

CARDIAC ARREST
IV: ADULTS, ELDERLY: Initially, 1 mg. May repeat q3–5min as needed. CHILDREN: Initially, 0.01 mg/kg (0.1 ml/kg of a 1:10,000 solution). May repeat q3–5min as needed.
ENDOTRACHEAL: CHILDREN: 0.1 mg/kg (0.1 ml/kg of a 1:1,000 solution). May repeat q3–5min as needed.

HYPERSENSITIVITY REACTION
IM, SUBCUTANEOUS: ADULTS, ELDERLY: 0.3–0.5 mg q15–20min.
SUBCUTANEOUS: CHILDREN: 0.01 mg/kg q15min for 2 doses, then q4h. **Maximum single dose:** 0.5 mg.
INHALATION: ADULTS, ELDERLY, CHILDREN 4 YR AND OLDER: 1 inhalation, may repeat in at least 1 min. Give subsequent doses no sooner than 3 hr.
NEBULIZER: ADULTS, ELDERLY, CHILDREN 4 YR AND OLDER: 1–3 deep inhalations. Give subsequent doses no sooner than 3 hr.

GLAUCOMA
OPHTHALMIC: ADULTS, ELDERLY: 1–2 drops 1–2 times a day.

SIDE EFFECTS
FREQUENT: Systemic: Tachycardia, palpitations, nervousness. **Ophthalmic:** Headache, eye irritation, watering of eyes. **OCCASIONAL: Systemic:** Dizziness, light-headedness, facial flushing,

headache, diaphoresis, increased BP, nausea, trembling, insomnia, vomiting, fatigue. **Ophthalmic:** Blurred or decreased vision, eye pain. **RARE: Systemic:** Chest discomfort or pain, arrhythmias, bronchospasm, dry mouth or throat.

ADVERSE REACTIONS/ TOXIC EFFECTS

Excessive doses may cause acute hypertension or arrhythmias. Prolonged or excessive use may result in metabolic acidosis due to increased serum lactic acid concentrations. Metabolic acidosis may cause disorientation, fatigue, hyperventilation, headache, nausea, vomiting, and diarrhea.

NURSING CONSIDERATIONS

INTERVENTION/EVALUATION

Monitor for vital sign changes. Assess lung sounds for rhonchi, wheezing, rales. Monitor ABGs. In cardiac arrest, monitor EKG, patient condition.

PATIENT/FAMILY TEACHING

• Avoid excessive use of caffeine derivatives (chocolate, coffee, tea, cola, cocoa). • **Ophthalmic:** Slight burning, stinging may occur on initial instillation. • Report any new symptoms (tachycardia, shortness of breath, dizziness) immediately: may be systemic effects.

epirubicin ⚑

eh-pea-**rew**-bih-sin

(Ellence, Pharmorubicin ✢, Pharmorubicin PFS ✢, Pharmorubicin RDS ✢)

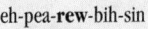

◆CLASSIFICATION

PHARMACOTHERAPEUTIC: Anthracycline antibiotic. **CLINICAL:** Antineoplastic (see p. 73C).

ACTION

An anthracycline antibiotic whose exact mechanism is unknown but may include formation of a complex with DNA and subsequent inhibition of DNA, RNA, and protein synthesis. Also inhibits DNA helicase activity, preventing enzymatic separation of double-stranded DNA and interfering with replication and transcription. Therapeutic Effect: Produces antiproliferative and cytotoxic activity.

PHARMACOKINETICS

Widely distributed into tissues. Protein binding: 77%. Metabolized in the liver and RBCs. Primarily eliminated through biliary excretion. Not removed by hemodialysis. Half-life: 33 hr.

USES

Component of adjuvant therapy in patients with evidence of axillary node tumor involvement following resection of primary breast cancer. OFF-LABEL: Esophageal, gastric, small cell lung, non–small cell lung, ovarian carcinomas; Hodgkin's, non-Hodgkin's lymphomas; soft tissue sarcoma; neoplasms of bladder.

PRECAUTIONS

CONTRAINDICATIONS: Baseline neutrophil count less than 1,500/mm^3, hypersensitivity to epirubicin, previous treatment with anthracyclines up to maximum cumulative dose, recent MI, severe hepatic impairment, severe myocardial insufficiency. **CAUTIONS:** Renal or hepatic impairment.

⚖ LIFESPAN CONSIDERATIONS: Pregnancy/Lactation: May cause fetal harm. Unknown if distributed in breast milk. Pregnancy Category D. Children: Safety and efficacy not established. Elderly: No age-related precautions noted but monitor for toxicity.

INTERACTIONS

DRUG: Blood dyscrasia-causing medications: May increase the

E

patient's risk of developing leukopenia or thrombocytopenia. **Bone marrow depressants:** May cause additive bone marrow suppression. **Calcium channel blockers:** May increase the patient's risk of developing heart failure. **Cimetidine:** May increase epirubicin serum concentration and toxicity. **Hepatotoxic medications:** May increase the risk of hepatotoxicity. **Live-virus vaccines:** May potentiate virus replication, increase vaccine side effects, and decrease the patient's antibody response to the vaccine. HERBAL: None known. FOOD: None known. LAB VALUES: None known.

AVAILABILITY (Rx)

INJECTION: 2-mg/ml single-use vials.

ADMINISTRATION/HANDLING

◄ ALERT ▶ Exclude pregnant staff from working with epirubicin; wear protective clothing. If accidental contact with skin or eyes occurs, flush area immediately with copious amounts of water.

 IV

Reconstitution • Ready-to-use vials require no reconstitution.

Rate of administration • Infuse medication into tubing of free-flowing IV of 0.9% NaCl or D_5W over 3–5 min.

Storage • Refrigerate vial. • Protect from light. • Use within 24 hr of first penetration of rubber stopper. • Discard unused portion.

✺ IV INCOMPATIBILITIES

Heparin, fluorouracil (5-FU). Don't mix epirubicin in same syringe with other medications.

INDICATIONS/ROUTES/DOSAGE

BREAST CANCER

IV: ADULTS: Initially, 100–120 mg/m² in repeated cycles of 3–4 wk, in combination with 5-FU and Cytoxan. Total dose may be given on day 1 of each cycle or in equally divided doses on days 1 and 8 of each cycle.

SIDE EFFECTS

FREQUENT (83%–70%): Nausea, vomiting alopecia, amenorrhea. OCCASIONAL (9%–5%): Stomatitis, diarrhea, hot flashes. RARE (2%–1%): Rash, pruritus, fever, lethargy, conjunctivitis.

ADVERSE REACTIONS/ TOXIC EFFECTS

The risk of cardiotoxicity (either acute, manifested as transient EKG abnormalities, or chronic, manifested as CHF) increases when the total cumulative dose exceeds 900 mg/m². Extravasation during administration may result in severe local tissue necrosis. Myelosuppression may cause hematologic toxicity, manifested principally as leukopenia and, to lesser extent, anemia and thrombocytopenia.

NURSING CONSIDERATIONS

BASELINE ASSESSMENT

Obtain WBC, platelet, erythrocyte counts before and at frequent intervals during therapy. Obtain EKG before therapy, serum liver function studies before each dose. Antiemetics may be effective in preventing, treating nausea.

INTERVENTION/EVALUATION

Monitor for stomatitis (may lead to ulceration of mucous membranes within 2–3 days). Monitor blood counts for evidence of myelosuppression, renal and liver function studies, cardiac function. Assess pattern of daily bowel activity and stool consistency. Monitor for hematologic toxicity (fever, sore throat, signs of local infection, unusual bruising or bleeding from any site), symptoms of anemia (excessive fatigue, weakness).

PATIENT/FAMILY TEACHING

• Alopecia is reversible, but new hair growth may have different color, texture.

New hair growth resumes 2–3 mo after last therapy dose. • Maintain fastidious oral hygiene. • Do not have immunizations without physician's approval (drug lowers body's resistance). • Avoid contact with those who have recently received live virus vaccine. • Promptly report fever, sore throat, signs of local infection, easy unusual bruising or bleeding from any site.

Epivir, *see lamivudine*

eplerenone

eh-**pleh**-reh-known
(Inspra)

•CLASSIFICATION
PHARMACOTHERAPEUTIC: Aldosterone receptor antagonist. **CLINICAL:** Antihypertensive.

ACTION
An aldosterone receptor antagonist that binds to the mineralocorticoid receptors in the kidney, heart, blood vessels, and brain, blocking the binding of aldosterone. **Therapeutic Effect:** Reduces BP.

PHARMACOKINETICS
Absorption unaffected by food. Protein binding: 50%. No active metabolites. Excreted in the urine with a lesser amount eliminated in the feces. Not removed by hemodialysis. **Half-life:** 4–6 hr.

USES
Treatment of hypertension alone or in combination with other antihypertensive agents. Treatment of CHF following acute myocardial infarction (AMI).

PRECAUTIONS
CONTRAINDICATIONS: Concurrent use of potassium supplements or potassium-sparing diuretics (such as amiloride, spironolactone, and triamterene), or strong inhibitors of the cytochrome P450 3A4 enzyme system (including ketoconazole and itraconazole), creatinine clearance less than 50 ml/min, serum creatinine level greater than 2 mg/dl in males or 1.8 mg/dl in females, serum potassium level greater than 5.5 mEq/L, type 2 diabetes mellitus with microalbuminuria. **CAUTIONS:** Hepatic function impairment, hyperkalemia.

LIFESPAN CONSIDERATIONS: Pregnancy/Lactation: Unknown if drug crosses placenta or is distributed in breast milk. **Pregnancy Category B. Children:** Safety and efficacy not established. **Elderly:** No age-related precautions noted.

INTERACTIONS
DRUG: Angiotensin-converting enzyme (ACE) inhibitors, angiotensin II antagonists, erythromycin, fluconazole, saquinavir, verapamil: Increase risk of hyperkalemia. **HERBAL: St. John's wort:** Decreases eplerenone effectiveness. **FOOD: Grapefruit, grapefruit juice:** Produces small increase in serum potassium level. **LAB VALUES:** May increase serum potassium level. May decrease serum sodium level.

AVAILABILITY (Rx)
TABLETS: 25 mg, 50 mg.

ADMINISTRATION/HANDLING
• Do not break, crush, or chew film-coated tablets.

INDICATIONS/ROUTES/DOSAGE
HYPERTENSION
PO: ADULTS, ELDERLY: 50 mg once a day. If 50 mg once a day produces an inadequate BP response, may increase

dosage to 50 mg twice a day. If patient is concurrently receiving erythromycin, saquinavir, verapamil, or fluconazole, reduce initial dose to 25 mg once a day.

CHF FOLLOWING MI

PO: ADULTS, ELDERLY: Initially, 25 mg once a day. If tolerated, titrate up to 50 mg once a day within 4 wk.

SIDE EFFECTS

RARE (3%–1%): Dizziness, diarrhea, cough, fatigue, flu-like symptoms, abdominal pain.

ADVERSE REACTIONS/ TOXIC EFFECTS

Hyperkalemia may occur, particularly in patients with type 2 diabetes mellitus and microalbuminuria.

NURSING CONSIDERATIONS

BASELINE ASSESSMENT

Obtain BP, apical pulse immediately before each dose, in addition to regular monitoring (be alert to fluctuations). If excessive reduction in BP occurs, place patient in supine position, feet slightly elevated.

INTERVENTION/EVALUATION

Assist with ambulation if dizziness occurs. Monitor serum potassium levels. Assess BP for hypertension and hypotension. Monitor pattern of daily bowel activity and stool consistency. Assess for evidence of flu-like symptoms.

PATIENT/FAMILY TEACHING

• Avoid tasks that require alertness, motor skills until response to drug is established (possible dizziness effect). • Discuss need for lifelong control. • Caution against exercising during hot weather (risk of dehydration, hypotension).

epoetin alfa

eh-po-**ee**-tin-**al**-fa

(Epogen, Eprex 🍁, Procrit)

Do not confuse Epogen with Neupogen.

◆CLASSIFICATION

PHARMACOTHERAPEUTIC: Glycoprotein. **CLINICAL:** Erythropoietin.

ACTION

A glycoprotein that stimulates division and differentiation of erythroid progenitor cells in bone marrow. **Therapeutic Effect:** Induces erythropoiesis and releases reticulocytes from bone marrow.

PHARMACOKINETICS

Well absorbed after subcutaneous administration. Following administration, an increase in reticulocyte count occurs within 10 days, and increases in Hgb, Hct, and RBC count are seen within 2–6 wk. **Half-life:** 4–13 hr.

USES

Treatment of anemia in patients receiving or who have received chemotherapy, those with chronic renal failure, HIV-infected patients on zidovudine (AZT) therapy, those scheduled for elective nonvascular surgery, reducing need for allogenic blood transfusions. **OFF-LABEL:** Anemia associated with frequent blood donations, anemia in critically ill patients, malignancy, management of hepatitis C, myelodysplastic syndromes.

PRECAUTIONS

CONTRAINDICATIONS: History of sensitivity to mammalian cell-derived products or human albumin, uncontrolled hypertension. **CAUTIONS:** Patients with known porphyria (impairment of erythrocyte formation in bone marrow); history of seizures.

⊠ **LIFESPAN CONSIDERATIONS: Pregnancy/Lactation:** Unknown if drug crosses placenta or is distributed in breast milk. **Pregnancy Category C. Children:** Safety and efficacy not established in those 12 yr and younger. **Elderly:** No age-related precautions noted.

INTERACTIONS

DRUG: Heparin: An increase in RBC volume may enhance blood clotting. Heparin dosage may need to be increased. **HERBAL:** None known. **FOOD:** None known. **LAB VALUES:** May increase BUN, serum phosphorus, serum potassium, serum creatinine, serum uric acid, and sodium levels. May decrease bleeding time, iron concentration, and serum ferritin levels.

AVAILABILITY (Rx)

INJECTION (EPOGEN, PROCRIT): 2,000 units/ml, 3,000 units/ml, 4,000 units/ml, 10,000 units/ml, 20,000 units/ml, 40,000 units/ml.

ADMINISTRATION/HANDLING

◀ **ALERT** ▶ Avoid excessive agitation of vial; do not shake (foaming).

 IV

Reconstitution • No reconstitution necessary.

Rate of administration • May be given as an IV bolus.

Storage • Refrigerate. • Vigorous shaking may denature medication, rendering it inactive.

SUBCUTANEOUS
• Use 1 dose per vial; do not reenter vial. Discard unused portion. May be mixed in a syringe with bacteriostatic 0.9% NaCl with benzyl alcohol 0.9% (bacteriostatic saline) at a 1:1 ratio (benzyl alcohol acts as a local anesthetic; may reduce injection site discomfort).

IV INCOMPATIBILITIES
Do not mix with other medications.

INDICATIONS/ROUTES/DOSAGE
TREATMENT OF ANEMIA IN CHEMOTHERAPY PATIENTS
IV, SUBCUTANEOUS: ADULTS, ELDERLY, CHILDREN: 150 units/kg/dose 3 times a wk. **Maximum:** 1,200 units/kg/wk.

REDUCTION OF ALLOGENIC BLOOD TRANSFUSIONS IN ELECTIVE SURGERY
SUBCUTANEOUS: ADULTS, ELDERLY: 300 units/kg/day 10 days before day of, and 4 days after surgery.

CHRONIC RENAL FAILURE
IV BOLUS, SUBCUTANEOUS: ADULTS, ELDERLY: Initially, 50–100 units/kg 3 times a wk. Target Hct range: 30%–36%. Adjust dosage no earlier than 1-mo intervals unless prescribed. Decrease dosage if Hct is increasing and approaching 36%. Plan to temporarily withhold doses if Hct continues to rise and to reinstate lower dosage when Hct begins to decrease. If Hct increases by more than 4 points in 2 wk, monitor Hct twice a wk for 2–6 wk. Increase dose if Hct does not increase 5–6 points after 8 wk (with adequate iron stores) and if Hct is below target range. Maintenance: *For patients on dialysis:* 75 units/kg 3 times a wk. Range: 12.5–525 units/kg. *For patients not on dialysis:* 75–150 units/kg/wk.

HIV INFECTION IN PATIENTS TREATED WITH AZT
IV, SUBCUTANEOUS: ADULTS: Initially, 100 units/kg 3 times a wk for 8 wk; may increase by 50–100 units/kg 3 times a wk. Evaluate response q4–8wk thereafter. Adjust dosage by 50–100 units/kg 3 times a wk. If dosages larger than 300 units/kg 3 times a wk are not eliciting response, it is unlikely patient will respond. Maintenance: Titrate to maintain desired Hct.

E

E

SIDE EFFECTS

PATIENTS RECEIVING CHEMOTHERAPY
FREQUENT (20%–17%): Fever, diarrhea, nausea, vomiting, edema. **OCCASIONAL (13%–11%):** Asthenia, shortness of breath, paresthesia. **RARE (5%–3%):** Dizziness, trunk pain.

PATIENTS WITH CHRONIC RENAL FAILURE
FREQUENT (24%–11%): Hypertension, headache, nausea, arthralgia. **OCCASIONAL (9%–7%):** Fatigue, edema, diarrhea, vomiting, chest pain, skin reactions at administration site, asthenia, dizziness.

PATIENTS WITH HIV INFECTION TREATED WITH AZT
FREQUENT (38%–15%): Fever, fatigue, headache, cough, diarrhea, rash, nausea. **OCCASIONAL (14%–9%):** Shortness of breath, asthenia, skin reaction at injection site, dizziness.

ADVERSE REACTIONS/ TOXIC EFFECTS

Hypertensive encephalopathy, thrombosis, cerebrovascular accident, MI, and seizures have occurred rarely. Hyperkalemia occurs occasionally in patients with chronic renal failure, usually in those who do not conform to medication regimen, dietary guidelines, and frequency of dialysis regimen.

NURSING CONSIDERATIONS

BASELINE ASSESSMENT
Assess BP before drug initiation (80% of patients with chronic renal failure have history of hypertension). BP often rises during early therapy in patients with history of hypertension. Consider that all patients eventually need supplemental iron therapy. Assess serum iron (should be greater than 20%) and serum ferritin (should be greater than 100 ng/ml) before and during therapy. Establish baseline CBC (especially note Hct). Monitor aggressively for increased BP (25% of patients on medication require antihypertensive therapy, dietary restrictions).

INTERVENTION/EVALUATION
Monitor Hct level diligently (if level increases greater than 4 points in 2 wk, dosage should be reduced); assess CBC routinely. Monitor temperature, especially in cancer patients on chemotherapy and zidovudine-treated HIV patients. Monitor BUN, serum uric acid, creatinine, phosphorus, potassium, especially in chronic renal failure patients.

PATIENT/FAMILY TEACHING
• Frequent blood tests needed to determine correct dosage. • Inform physician if severe headache develops. • Avoid potentially hazardous activity during first 90 days of therapy (increased risk of seizures in renal patients during first 90 days).

Epogen, see epoetin alfa

epoprostenol sodium, PG₂, PGX, prostacyclin

e-poe-**pros**-ten-ol
(Flolan)

◆ CLASSIFICATION
PHARMACOTHERAPEUTIC: Vasodilator. **CLINICAL:** Antihypertensive.

ACTION

An antihypertensive that directly dilates pulmonary and systemic arterial vascular beds and inhibits platelet aggregation.

Therapeutic Effect: Reduces right and left ventricular afterload; increases cardiac output and stroke volume.

USES

Long-term treatment of primary pulmonary hypertension in class III and IV patients (New York Heart Association). OFF-LABEL: Cardiopulmonary bypass surgery; hemodialysis; pulmonary hypertension associated with acute respiratory distress syndrome, systemic lupus erythematosus, or congenital heart disease; neonatal pulmonary hypertension; refractory CHF; severe community-acquired pneumonia.

PRECAUTIONS

CONTRAINDICATIONS: Long-term use in patients with CHF (severe ventricular systolic dysfunction). **CAUTIONS:** Elderly. LIFESPAN CONSIDERATIONS: **Pregnancy/Lactation:** Unknown if drug crosses placenta or is distributed in breast milk. **Pregnancy Category B. Children:** Safety and efficacy not established. **Elderly:** No age-related precautions noted.

INTERACTIONS

DRUG: **Acetate in dialysis fluids, other vasodilators:** May increase hypotensive effect. **Anticoagulants, antiplatelets:** May increase the risk of bleeding. **Vasoconstrictors:** May decrease effects of epoprostenol. HERBAL: None known. FOOD: None known. LAB VALUES: None known.

AVAILABILITY (Rx)

INJECTION, POWDER FOR RECONSTITUTION: 0.5 mg, 1.5 mg.

ADMINISTRATION/HANDLING
IV

Reconstitution • Must use diluent provided by manufacturer. • Follow instructions of manufacturer for dilution to specific concentrations.

Rate of administration • Give as a pump infusion only.

Storage • Store unopened vial at room temperature. • Do not freeze. • Reconstituted solutions may be refrigerated within 48 hr.

IV INCOMPATIBILITIES

Don't mix epoprostenol with other medications.

INDICATIONS/ROUTES/DOSAGE

LONG-TERM TREATMENT OF NEW YORK HEART ASSOCIATION CLASS III AND IV PRIMARY PULMONARY HYPERTENSION

IV INFUSION: ADULTS, ELDERLY: Procedure to determine dose range: Initially, 2 ng/kg/min, increased in increments of 2 ng/kg/min q15min until dose-limiting adverse effects occur. Chronic infusion: Start at 4 ng/kg/min less than the maximum dose rate tolerated during acute dose ranging (or $\frac{1}{2}$ of the maximum rate if rate was less than 5 ng/kg/min).

SIDE EFFECTS

FREQUENT: Acute Phase: Flushing (58%), headache (49%), nausea (32%), vomiting (32%), hypotension (16%), anxiety (11%), chest pain (11%), dizziness (8%). **Chronic Phase (greater than 20%):** Dyspnea, asthenia, dizziness, headache, chest pain, nausea, vomiting, palpitations, edema, jaw pain, tachycardia, flushing, myalgia, nonspecific muscle pain, paresthesia, diarrhea, anxiety, chills, fever, or flu-like symptoms. **OCCASIONAL: Acute Phase (5%–2%):** Bradycardia, abdominal pain, muscle pain, dyspnea, back pain. **Chronic Phase (20%–10%):** Rash, depression, hypotension, pallor, syncope, bradycardia, ascites. **RARE (less than 2%): Acute Phase:** Paresthesia. **Chronic Phase (less than 2%):** Diaphoresis, dyspepsia, tachycardia.

E

ADVERSE REACTIONS/ TOXIC EFFECTS

Overdose may cause hyperglycemia or ketoacidosis manifested as increased urination, thirst, and fruitlike breath odor. Angina, MI, and thrombocytopenia occur rarely. Abrupt withdrawal, including a large reduction in dosage or interruption in drug delivery, may produce rebound pulmonary hypertension as evidenced by dyspnea, dizziness, and asthenia.

NURSING CONSIDERATIONS

INTERVENTION/EVALUATION

Monitor standing and supine BP for several hours after any dosage adjustment. Assess for therapeutic response: improvement in pulmonary function, decreased dyspnea on exertion (DOE), fatigue, syncope, chest pain, pulmonary vascular resistance, pulmonary arterial pressure.

PATIENT/FAMILY TEACHING

• Instruct patient about drug reconstitution, drug administration, care of the permanent central venous catheter. • Brief interruptions in drug delivery may result in rapid, deteriorating symptoms. • Drug therapy will be necessary for a prolonged period, possibly years.

eprosartan

eh-pro-**sar**-tan

(Teveten)

FIXED COMBINATION(S)

Teveten HCT: eprosartan/hydrochlorothiazide (a diuretic) 400 mg/12.5 mg.

CLASSIFICATION

PHARMACOTHERAPEUTIC: Angiotensin II receptor antagonist. **CLINICAL:** Antihypertensive (see p. 8C).

ACTION

An angiotensin II receptor antagonist that blocks the vasoconstrictor and aldosterone-secreting effects of angiotensin II, inhibiting the binding of angiotensin II to the AT_1 receptors. **Therapeutic Effect:** Causes vasodilation, decreases peripheral resistance, and decreases BP.

PHARMACOKINETICS

Rapidly absorbed after PO administration. Protein binding: 98%. Undergoes first-pass metabolism in the liver to active metabolites. Excreted in urine and biliary system. Minimally removed by hemodialysis. **Half-life:** 5–9 hr.

USES

Treatment of hypertension.

PRECAUTIONS

CONTRAINDICATIONS: Bilateral renal artery stenosis, hyperaldosteronism. **CAUTIONS:** Unilateral renal artery stenosis, preexisting renal insufficiency, significant aortic or mitral stenosis.

⧗ **LIFESPAN CONSIDERATIONS: Pregnancy/Lactation:** Has caused fetal and neonatal morbidity and mortality. Potential for adverse effects on breastfeeding infant. Do not breast-feed. **Pregnancy Category C (D if used in second or third trimester). Children:** Safety and efficacy not established. **Elderly:** No age-related precautions noted.

INTERACTIONS

DRUG: None known. **HERBAL:** None known. **FOOD:** None known. **LAB VALUES:** May increase BUN, serum alkaline phosphatase, serum bilirubin, serum creatinine, AST, and ALT levels. May decrease blood Hgb and Hgb levels.

AVAILABILITY (Rx)

TABLETS: 400 mg, 600 mg.

ADMINISTRATION/HANDLING

PO

• Give without regard to food. • Do not crush or break tablets.

INDICATIONS/ROUTES/DOSAGE

HYPERTENSION

PO: ADULTS, ELDERLY: Initially, 600 mg/day. Range: 400–800 mg/day.

SIDE EFFECTS

OCCASIONAL (5%–2%): Headache, cough, dizziness. **RARE (less than 2%):** Muscle pain, fatigue, diarrhea, upper respiratory tract infection, dyspepsia.

ADVERSE REACTIONS/ TOXIC EFFECTS

Overdosage may manifest as hypotension and tachycardia. Bradycardia occurs less often.

NURSING CONSIDERATIONS

BASELINE ASSESSMENT

Obtain BP, apical pulse immediately before each dose, in addition to regular monitoring (be alert to fluctuations). Question for possibility of pregnancy (see Pregnancy Category), history of hepatic or renal impairment, renal artery stenosis. Assess medication history (especially diuretic).

INTERVENTION/EVALUATION

Monitor BP, electrolytes, serum creatinine, BUN, urinalysis, pulse for tachycardia.

PATIENT/FAMILY TEACHING

• Inform female patient regarding consequences of second and third trimester exposure to medication. • Avoid tasks that require alertness, motor skills until response to drug is established (possible dizziness effect). • Restrict sodium, alcohol intake. • Follow diet, control weight. • Do not stop taking medication. Discuss need for lifelong control. • Caution against exercising during hot weather (risk of dehydration, hypotension). • Check BP regularly.

---

eptifibatide

ep-tih-**fye**-bah-tide
(Integrilin)

◆CLASSIFICATION

PHARMACOTHERAPEUTIC: Glycoprotein IIb/IIIa inhibitor. **CLINICAL:** Antiplatelet, antithrombotic (see p. 31C).

ACTION

A glycoprotein IIb/IIIa inhibitor that rapidly inhibits platelet aggregation by preventing binding of fibrinogen to receptor sites on platelets. **Therapeutic Effect:** Prevents closure of treated coronary arteries. Also prevents acute cardiac ischemic complications.

USES

Treatment of patients with acute coronary syndrome (ACS), including those managed medically and those undergoing percutaneous coronary intervention (PCI).

PRECAUTIONS

CONTRAINDICATIONS: Active internal bleeding, AV malformation or aneurysm, history of cerebrovascular accident (CVA) within 2 yr or CVA with residual neurologic defect, history of vasculitis, intracranial neoplasm, oral anticoagulant use within last 7 days unless PT is less than 1.22 times the control, recent (6 wk or less) GI or GU bleeding, recent (6 wk or less) surgery or trauma, prior IV dextran use before or during percutaneous transluminal coronary angioplasty (PTCA), severe uncontrolled hypertension, thrombocytopenia (less than 100,000 cells/mcL).

CAUTIONS: Patients who weigh less than 75 kg; those 65 yr and older; history of GI disease; patients receiving thrombolytics, heparin, aspirin, PTCA less than 12 hr of onset of symptoms for acute MI, prolonged PTCA (greater than 70 min), failed PTCA. **Pregnancy Category B.**

INTERACTIONS

DRUG: Anticoagulants, heparin: May increase the risk of hemorrhage. **Dextran, other platelet aggregation inhibitors (such as aspirin), thrombolytic agents:** May increase the risk of bleeding. **HERBAL:** None known. **FOOD:** None known. **LAB VALUES:** Increases aPTT, PT, and clotting time. Decreases platelet count.

AVAILABILITY (Rx)

INJECTION SOLUTION: 0.75 mg/ml, 2 mg/ml.

ADMINISTRATION/HANDLING

IV

Reconstitution • Withdraw bolus dose from 10-ml vial (2 mg/ml); for IV infusion withdraw from 100-ml vial (0.75 mg/ml). IV push and infusion administration may be given undiluted.

Rate of administration • Give bolus dose IV push over 1–2 min.

Storage • Store vials in refrigerator. Solution appears clear, colorless. Do not shake. Discard any unused portion left in vial or if preparation contains *any* opaque particles.

IV INCOMPATIBILITIES

Administer in separate line; do not add other medications to infusion solution.

INDICATIONS/ROUTES/DOSAGE

ADJUNCT TO PERCUTANEOUS CORONARY INTERVENTION (PCI)
IV BOLUS, IV INFUSION: ADULTS, ELDERLY: 180 mcg/kg before PCI

initiation; then continuous drip of 2 mcg/kg/min and a second 180 mcg/kg bolus 10 min after the first. **Maximum:** 15 mg/h. Continue until hospital discharge or for up to 18–24 hr. Minimum 12 hr is recommended. Concurrent aspirin and heparin therapy is recommended.

ACUTE CORONARY SYNDROME
IV BOLUS, IV INFUSION: ADULTS, ELDERLY: 180 mcg/kg bolus then 2 mcg/kg/min until discharge or coronary artery bypass graft, up to 72 hr. **Maximum:** 15 mg/h. Concurrent aspirin and heparin therapy is recommended.

DOSAGE IN RENAL IMPAIRMENT
Creatinine clearance less than 50 ml/min: Use 180 mcg/kg bolus (**Maximum:** 22.6 mg) and 1 mcg/kg/min infusion (**Maximum:** 7.5 mg/h).

SIDE EFFECTS

OCCASIONAL (7%): Hypotension.

ADVERSE REACTIONS/ TOXIC EFFECTS

Minor to major bleeding complications may occur, most commonly at arterial access site for cardiac catheterization.

NURSING CONSIDERATIONS

BASELINE ASSESSMENT

Assess platelet count, Hgb, Hct before treatment. If platelet count less than 90,000/mm^3, additional platelet counts should be obtained routinely to avoid thrombocytopenia.

INTERVENTION/EVALUATION

Diligently monitor for potential bleeding, particularly at other arterial, venous puncture sites. If possible, urinary catheters, nasogastric tubes should be avoided.

Erbitux, *see cetuximab*

ergoloid mesylates

ur-go-loyd mess-**ah**-lates

◆CLASSIFICATION
PHARMACOTHERAPEUTIC: Ergot alkaloid. **CLINICAL:** Psychotherapeutic.

ACTION
Central action decreases vascular tone, slows heart rate. Peripheral action blocks alpha-adrenergic receptors. **Therapeutic Effect:** Improves O_2 uptake, improves cerebral metabolism.

USES
Treatment of age-related (those older than 60 yr) decline in mental capacity (cognitive/interpersonal skills, mood, self-care, apparent motivation).

PRECAUTIONS
CONTRAINDICATIONS: Acute or chronic psychosis, regardless of etiology. **CAUTIONS:** Bradycardia, hypotension. **Pregnancy Category C.**

INTERACTIONS
DRUG: None known. **HERBAL:** None known. **FOOD:** None known. **LAB VALUES:** None known.

AVAILABILITY (Rx)
TABLETS (SUBLINGUAL): 1 mg. **TABLETS (ORAL):** 1 mg.

INDICATIONS/ROUTES/DOSAGE
AGE-RELATED DECLINE IN MENTAL CAPACITY
PO, SUBLINGUAL: ADULTS, ELDERLY: Initially, 1 mg 3 times a day. Range: 1.5–12 mg a day.

SIDE EFFECTS
OCCASIONAL: GI distress, transient nausea, sublingual irritation.

ADVERSE REACTIONS/ TOXIC EFFECTS
Overdose may produce blurred vision, dizziness, syncope, headache, flushed face, nausea, vomiting, decreased appetite, stomach cramps, stuffy nose.

E

NURSING CONSIDERATIONS

BASELINE ASSESSMENT
Exclude possibility that patient's signs/symptoms arise from a possibly reversible, treatable condition secondary to systemic disease, neurologic disease, primary disturbance of mood prior to administering medication.

INTERVENTION/EVALUATION
Monitor BP, pulse, peripheral circulation. Assess for relief of symptoms.

PATIENT/FAMILY TEACHING
• Elimination of symptoms appears gradually: results may not be noted for 3–4 wk. • May cause nausea, GI upset. • Allow sublingual tablets to dissolve completely under tongue.

ergotamine tartrate

er-**got**-a-meen
(Cafergot ♣, Ergomar, Ergostat, Gynergen, Medihaler Ergotamine ♣)

dihydroergotamine

(D.H.E. 45, Dihydroergotamine Sandoz ♣, Migranal)

FIXED-COMBINATION(S)
Bellergal-S: ergotamine/belladonna (anticholinergic)/phenobarbital (sedative-hypnotic): 0.6 mg/0.2 mg/

---

40 mg. **Cafergot, Wigraine:** ergotamine/caffeine (stimulant): 1 mg/100 mg; 2 mg/100 mg.

CLASSIFICATION

PHARMACOTHERAPEUTIC: Ergotamine derivative. **CLINICAL:** Antimigraine.

ACTION

An ergotamine derivative and alpha-adrenergic blocker that directly stimulates vascular smooth muscle, resulting in peripheral and cerebral vasoconstriction. May also have antagonist effects on serotonin. **Therapeutic Effect:** Suppresses vascular headaches.

PHARMACOKINETICS

Slowly and incompletely absorbed from the GI tract; rapidly and extensively absorbed after rectal administration. Protein binding: greater than 90%. Undergoes extensive first-pass metabolism in the liver to active metabolite. Eliminated in feces by the biliary system. **Half-life:** 21 hr.

USES

Ergotamine: Prevents or aborts vascular headaches (e.g., migraine, cluster headaches). **Dihydroergotamine:** Treatment of migraine headache with or without aura. Injection used to treat cluster headache. **OFF-LABEL:** Prevention of deep venous thrombosis, prevention and treatment of orthostatic hypotension, pulmonary thromboembolism.

PRECAUTIONS

CONTRAINDICATIONS: Coronary artery disease, hypertension, impaired hepatic or renal function, malnutrition, peripheral vascular diseases (such as thromboangiitis obliterans, syphilitic arteritis, severe arteriosclerosis, thrombophlebitis, and Raynaud's disease), sepsis, severe pruritus. **CAUTIONS:** None known.

LIFESPAN CONSIDERATIONS: Pregnancy/Lactation: Contraindicated in pregnancy (produces uterine stimulant action, resulting in possible fetal death or retarded fetal growth); increases vasoconstriction of placental vascular bed. Drug distributed in breast milk. May produce diarrhea, vomiting in neonate. May prohibit lactation. **Pregnancy Category X. Children:** No precautions in those 6 yr and older, but use only when unresponsive to other medication. **Elderly:** Age-related occlusive peripheral vascular disease increases risk of peripheral vasoconstriction. Age-related renal impairment may require dosage adjustment.

INTERACTIONS

DRUG: Beta blockers, erythromycin: May increase the risk of vasospasm. **Ergot alkaloids, systemic vasoconstrictors:** May increase pressor effect. **Nitroglycerin:** May decrease the effects of nitroglycerin. **HERBAL:** None known. **FOOD:** None known. **LAB VALUES:** None known.

AVAILABILITY (Rx)

TABLETS (SUBLINGUAL [ERGOMAR]): 2 mg. **INJECTION (DHE 45):** 1 mg/ml. **NASAL SPRAY (MIGRANAL):** 0.5 mg/spray. **SUPPOSITORIES (ERGOTAMINE AND CAFFEINE):** 2 mg, with 100 mg caffeine.

ADMINISTRATION/HANDLING

SUBLINGUAL
• Place under tongue; do not swallow.

INDICATIONS/ROUTES/DOSAGE

VASCULAR HEADACHES
PO (CAFERGOT [FIXED-COMBINATION OF ERGOTAMINE AND CAFFEINE]): ADULTS, ELDERLY: 2 mg at onset of headache, then 1–2 mg q30min. **Maximum:** 6 mg/episode; 10 mg/wk.
PO, SUBLINGUAL: CHILDREN: 1 mg at onset of headache, then 1 mg q30min. **Maximum:** 3 mg/episode.

IV: ADULTS, ELDERLY: 1 mg at onset of headache; may repeat hourly. **Maximum:** 2 mg/day; 6 mg/wk.

SUBLINGUAL: ADULTS, ELDERLY: 1 tablet at onset of headache, then 1 tablet q30min. **Maximum:** 3 tablets/24 hr; 5 tablets/wk.

IM, SUBCUTANEOUS (DIHYDRO-ERGOTAMINE): ADULTS, ELDERLY: 1 mg at onset of headache; may repeat hourly. **Maximum:** 3 mg/day; 6 mg/wk.

INTRANASAL: ADULTS, ELDERLY: 1 spray (0.5 mg) into each nostril; may repeat in 15 min. **Maximum:** 4 sprays/day; 8 sprays/wk.

RECTAL: ADULTS, ELDERLY: 1 suppository at onset of headache; may repeat dose in 1 hr. **Maximum:** 2 suppositories/episode; 5 suppositories/wk.

SIDE EFFECTS

OCCASIONAL (5%–2%): Cough, dizziness. **RARE (less than 2%):** Myalgia, fatigue, diarrhea, upper respiratory tract infection, dyspepsia.

ADVERSE REACTIONS/TOXIC EFFECTS

Prolonged administration or excessive dosage may produce ergotamine poisoning, manifested as nausea and vomiting; paresthesia, muscle pain or weakness; precordial pain; tachycardia or bradycardia; and hypertension or hypotension. Vasoconstriction of peripheral arteries and arterioles may result in localized edema and pruritus. Muscle pain will occur when walking and later, even at rest. Other rare effects include confusion, depression, drowsiness, seizures, and gangrene.

NURSING CONSIDERATIONS

BASELINE ASSESSMENT

Question for history of peripheral vascular disease, renal or hepatic impairment, possibility of pregnancy. Question regarding onset, location, duration of migraine, possible precipitating symptoms.

INTERVENTION/EVALUATION

Monitor closely for evidence of ergotamine overdosage as result of prolonged administration or excessive dosage.

PATIENT/FAMILY TEACHING

• Initiate therapy at first sign of migraine headache. • Report if there is need to progressively increase dose to relieve vascular headaches or if palpitations, nausea, vomiting, numbness or tingling of fingers or toes, pain or weakness of extremities is noted. • Discuss contraception with physician; report suspected pregnancy immediately (Pregnancy Category X).

erlotinib

er-**low**-tih-nib
(Tarceva)

CLASSIFICATION

PHARMACOTHERAPEUTIC: Human epidermal growth factor. **CLINICAL:** Antineoplastic.

ACTION

A human epidermal growth factor that inhibits tyrosine kinases (TK) associated with transmembrane cell surface receptors found on both normal and cancer cells. One such receptor is epidermal growth factor receptor (EGFR). **Therapeutic Effect:** TK activity appears to be vitally important to cell proliferation and survival.

PHARMACOKINETICS

About 60% is absorbed after PO administration; bioavailability is increased by food to almost 100%. Protein binding: 93%. Extensively metabolized in liver. Primarily eliminated in feces; minimal excretion in urine. **Half-life:** 36 hr.

USES

Treatment of locally advanced or metastatic non–small cell lung cancer after failure of at least one prior chemotherapy regimen. Treatment of locally advanced, unresectable, or metastatic pancreatic cancer (in combination with gemcitabine). OFF-LABEL: Salvage therapy of advanced or metastatic breast, colorectal, and head and neck tumors.

PRECAUTIONS

CONTRAINDICATIONS: Pregnancy. **CAUTIONS:** Severe hepatic or renal impairment.

⏳ LIFESPAN CONSIDERATIONS: **Pregnancy/Lactation:** Unknown if drug crosses the placenta or is distributed in breast milk. **Pregnancy Category D. Children:** Safety and efficacy not established. **Elderly:** No age-related precautions noted.

INTERACTIONS

DRUG: **Atanzavir, clarithromycin, indinavir, itraconazole, ketoconazole, nefazodone, nelfinavir, ritonavir, saquinavir, telithromycin:** May increase the level and effects of erlotinib. **Carbamazepine, phenobarbital, phenytoin, rifampin:** May decrease the levels and effects of erlotinib. **Warfarin:** May increase risk of bleeding with erlotinib. HERBAL: **St. John's wort:** May decrease the level and effects of erlotinib. FOOD: None known. LAB VALUES: May increase ALT, AST, bilirubin levels.

AVAILABILITY (Rx)

TABLETS: 25 mg, 100 mg, 150 mg.

ADMINISTRATION/HANDLING

PO
• Give at least 1 hr before or 2 hr after ingestion of food.

INDICATIONS/ROUTES/DOSAGE

LUNG CANCER
PO: ADULTS, ELDERLY: 150 mg/day until disease progression or unacceptable toxicity occurs.

PANCREATIC CANCER
PO: ADULTS, ELDERLY: 100 mg/day in combination with gemcitabine until disease progression or unacceptable toxicity occurs.

SIDE EFFECTS

FREQUENT (greater than 10%): Fatigue, anxiety, headache, depression, insomnia, rash, pruritus, dry skin, erythema, diarrhea, anorexia, nausea, vomiting, mucositis, xerostomia, pain, constipation, dyspepsia, weight loss, abnormal taste, abdominal pain, arthralgia, dyspnea, cough, infection. **OCCASIONAL (10%–1%):** Keratitis, pneumonitis. **RARE (less than 1%):** Corneal ulceration, gastrointestinal bleeding, interstitial lung disease.

ADVERSE REACTIONS/ TOXIC EFFECTS

GI bleeding and increased hepatic enzymes have been reported.

NURSING CONSIDERATIONS

BASELINE ASSESSMENT
Obtain hepatic enzyme levels and CBC before beginning therapy.

INTERVENTION/EVALUATION
Assess hepatic enzyme levels and CBC periodically.

PATIENT/FAMILY TEACHING
• Take drug on an empy stomach.
• Notify physician if rash, blood in stool, diarrhea, irritated eyes, and fever occur.

---

ertapenem

er-tah-**pen**-em
(Invanz)

◆ **CLASSIFICATION**
PHARMACOTHERAPEUTIC: Carbapenem. **CLINICAL:** Antibiotic.

ACTION

A carbapenem that penetrates the bacterial cell wall of microorganisms and binds to penicillin-binding proteins, inhibiting cell wall synthesis. Therapeutic Effect: Produces bacterial cell death.

PHARMACOKINETICS

Almost completely absorbed after IM administration. Protein binding: 85%–95%. Widely distributed. Primarily excreted in urine with smaller amount eliminated in feces. Removed by hemodialysis. Half-life: 4 hr.

USES

Treatment of susceptible infections due to *S. aureus* (methicillin suceptible only), *S. agalactiae*, *S. pneumoniae* (penicillin susceptible only), *S. pyogenes*, *E. coli*, *H. influenzae* (beta-lactamase negative strains only), *K. pneumoniae*, *M. catarrhalis*, *Bacteroides* species, *C. clostridioforme*, *Peptostreptococcus* species, including moderate to severe intra-abdominal, skin and skin-structure infections; community-acquired pneumonia; complicated UTI; acute pelvic infection; adult diabetic foot infections without osteomyelitis.

PRECAUTIONS

CONTRAINDICATIONS: History of hypersensitivity to beta-lactams (imipenem and cilastin, meropenem), hypersensitivity to amide-type local anesthetics (IM). **CAUTIONS:** Hypersensitivity to penicillins, cephalosporins, other allergens; impaired renal function; CNS disorders, especially brain lesions or history of seizures.

⌛ **LIFESPAN CONSIDERATIONS: Pregnancy/Lactation:** Distributed in breast milk. **Pregnancy Category B. Children:** Safety and efficacy not established in those younger than 18 yr.

Elderly: Advanced or end-stage renal insufficiency may require dosage adjustment.

INTERACTIONS

DRUG: **Probenecid:** Reduces renal excretion of ertapenem. HERBAL: None known. FOOD: None known. LAB VALUES: May increase serum alkaline phosphatase, AST and ALT levels. May decrease platelet count, blood Hct and Hgb levels, and serum potassium level.

AVAILABILITY (Rx)

INJECTION POWDER FOR RECONSTITUTION: 1-g.

ADMINISTRATION/HANDLING

 IV

Reconstitution • Dilute 1-g vial with 10 ml 0.9% NaCl or bacteriostatic water for injection. • Shake well to dissolve. • Further dilute with 50 ml 0.9% NaCl.

Rate of administration • Give by intermittent IV infusion (piggyback). Do not give IV push. • Infuse over 20–30 min.

Storage • Solution appears colorless to yellow (variation in color does not affect potency). • Discard if solution contains precipitate. • Reconstituted solution is stable for 6 hr at room temperature or 24 hr if refrigerated.

IM
• Reconstitute with 3.2 ml 1% lidocaine HCl injection (without epinephrine). • Shake vial thoroughly. • Inject deep in large muscle mass (gluteal or lateral part of thigh). • Administer suspension within 1 hr after preparation.

▨ IV INCOMPATIBILITIES

Do not mix or infuse ertapenem with any other medications. Do not use diluents or IV solutions containing dextrose.

IV COMPATIBILITIES

Sterile water for injection, 0.9% NaCl.

E

INDICATIONS/ROUTES/DOSAGE

INTRA-ABDOMINAL INFECTION
IV, IM: ADULTS, ELDERLY: 1 g/day for 5–14 days.

SKIN AND SKIN STRUCTURE INFECTION
IV, IM: ADULTS, ELDERLY: 1 g/day for 7–14 days.

PNEUMONIA, UTI
IV, IM: ADULTS, ELDERLY: 1 g/day for 10–14 days.

PELVIC INFECTION
IV, IM: ADULTS, ELDERLY: 1 g/day for 3–10 days.

DIABETIC FOOT INFECTION
IV, IM: ADULTS, ELDERLY: 1 g/day for 7–14 days.

DOSAGE IN RENAL IMPAIRMENT
For adults and elderly patients with creatinine clearance less than 30 ml/min: dosage is 500 mg once a day.

SIDE EFFECTS

FREQUENT (10%–6%): Diarrhea, nausea, headache. **OCCASIONAL (5%–2%):** Altered mental status, insomnia, rash, abdominal pain, constipation, vomiting, edema, fever. **RARE (less than 2%):** Dizziness, cough, oral candidiasis, anxiety, tachycardia, phlebitis at IV site.

ADVERSE REACTIONS/ TOXIC EFFECTS

Antibiotic-associated colitis and other superinfections may occur. Anaphylactic reactions have been reported. Seizures may occur in those with CNS disorders (including patients with brain lesions or a history of seizures), bacterial meningitis, or severe renal impairment.

NURSING CONSIDERATIONS

BASELINE ASSESSMENT
Question for history of allergies, particularly to beta-lactams, penicillins, cephalosporins. Inquire about history of seizures.

INTERVENTION/EVALUATION
Monitor pattern of daily bowel activity and stool consistency. Monitor for nausea, vomiting. Evaluate hydration status. Evaluate for inflammation at IV injection site. Assess skin for rash. Observe mental status; be alert to tremors, possible seizures. Assess sleep pattern for evidence of insomnia.

PATIENT/FAMILY TEACHING
• Notify physician in event of tremors, seizures, rash, diarrhea, other new symptoms.

Eryc, *see erythromycin*

Erythrocin, *see erythromycin*

erythromycin

er-rith-row-**my**-sin

(A/T/S, Akne-Mycin, Apo-Erythro Base ♣, EES, Emgel, E-Mycin, Erybid ♣, Eryc, Eryc-125 ♣, Eryc-250 ♣, Erycette, EryDerm, Erygel, EryPed, Erymax, Ery-Tab, Erythra-Derm, Erythrocin, Erythromid ♣, PCE Dispertab, Romycin, Roymicin, Staticin, Theramycin, Theramycin Z, T-Stat)

Do not confuse erythromycin with azithromycin or Ethmozine, or Eryc with Emct.

FIXED-COMBINATION(S)

Eryzole, Pediazole: erythromycin/sulfisoxazole (sulfonamide): 200 mg/600 mg per 5 ml.

◆ CLASSIFICATION

PHARMACOTHERAPEUTIC: Macrolide. **CLINICAL:** Antibiotic, antiacne (see p. 26C).

ACTION

A macrolide that reversibly binds to bacterial ribosomes, inhibiting bacterial protein synthesis. **Therapeutic Effect:** Bacteriostatic.

PHARMACOKINETICS

Variably absorbed from the GI tract (depending on dosage form used). Protein binding: 70%–90%. Widely distributed. Metabolized in the liver. Primarily eliminated in feces by bile. Not removed by hemodialysis. **Half-life:** 1.4–2 hr (increased in impaired renal function).

USES

Treatment of susceptible infections due to *S. pyogenes*, *S. pneumoniae*, *S. aureus*, *M. pneumoniae*, *Legionella*, diphtheria, pertussis, chancroid, *Chlamydia*, *N. gonorrheae*, *E. histolytica*, syphilis, nongonococcal urethritis, *Campylobacter* gastroenteritis including. **Topical:** Treatment of acne vulgaris. **Ophthalmic:** Prevention of gonococcal ophthalmia neonatorum. **OFF-LABEL: Systemic:** Treatment of acne vulgaris, chancroid, *Campylobacter* enteritis, gastroparesis, Lyme disease. **Topical:** Treatment of minor bacterial skin infections. **Ophthalmic:** Treatment of blepharitis, conjunctivitis, keratitis, chlamydial trachoma.

PRECAUTIONS

CONTRAINDICATIONS: Administration of fixed-combination product, Pediazole, to infants younger than 2 mo; history of hepatitis due to macrolides; hypersensitivity to macrolides; preexisting hepatic disease. **CAUTIONS:** Hepatic dysfunction. If combination therapy is used (Pediazole), consider precautions of sulfonamides. IV route may cause tachycardia, prolonged QT interval.

LIFESPAN CONSIDERATIONS: Pregnancy/Lactation: Crosses placenta. Distributed in breast milk. Erythromycin estolate may increase hepatic enzymes in pregnant women. **Pregnancy Category B. Children/Elderly:** No age-related precautions noted. High dosage in those with decreased hepatic or renal function increases risk of hearing loss.

INTERACTIONS

DRUG: Buspirone, cyclosporine, felodipine, lovastatin, simvastatin: May increase the blood concentration and toxicity of these drugs. **Carbamazepine:** May inhibit the metabolism of carbamazepine. **Chloramphenicol, clindamycin:** May decrease the effects of these drugs. **Hepatotoxic medications:** May increase the risk of hepatotoxicity. **Theophylline:** May increase the risk of theophylline toxicity. **Warfarin:** May increase warfarin's effects. **HERBAL:** None known. **FOOD:** None known. **LAB VALUES:** May increase serum alkaline phosphatase, bilirubin, AST, and ALT levels.

AVAILABILITY (Rx)

TOPICAL GEL (A/T/S, EMGEL, ERYGEL): 2%. **INJECTION POWDER FOR RECONSTITUTION (ERYTHROCIN):** 500 mg, 1 g. **OPHTHALMIC OINTMENT (ROYMICIN):** 0.5%. **ORAL SUSPENSION (ERYPED, EES):** 200 mg/5 ml, 400 mg/5 ml. **TOPICAL OINTMENT (AKNE-MYCIN):** 2%. **TOPICAL SOLUTION:** 1.5% (Staticin), 2% (A/T/S, Erymax, EryDerm, Erythra-Derm, Romycin, Theramycin Z, T-Stat). **TOPICAL SWAB (ERYCETTE, T-STAT):** 2%. **TABLETS (CHEWABLE [ERY-PED]):** 200 mg. **TABLETS:** 250 mg (E-Mycin, Ery-Tab, Erythrocin), 333 mg (Ery-Tab, E-Mycin, PCE Dispertab), 400 mg (EES), 500 mg (E-Mycin, Ery-Tab, Erythrocin, PCE Dispertab). **CAPSULES (ENTERIC-COATED [ERYC]):** 250 mg.

ADMINISTRATION/HANDLING

IV

Reconstitution • Reconstitute each 500 mg with 10 ml sterile water for injection without preservative to provide a concentration of 50 mg/ml. • Further dilute with 100–250 ml D₅W or 0.9% NaCl.

Rate of administration • For intermittent IV infusion (piggyback), infuse over 20–60 min. • For continuous infusion, infuse over 6–24 hr.

Storage • Store parenteral form at room temperature. • Initial reconstituted solution in vial is stable for 2 wk refrigerated or 24 hr at room temperature. • Diluted IV solutions stable for 8 hr at room temperature or 24 hr if refrigerated. • Discard if precipitate forms.

PO
• Store capsules, tablets at room temperature. • Oral suspension is stable for 14 days at room temperature. • Administer erythromycin base, stearate 1 hr before or 2 hr following food. Erythromycin estolate, ethylsuccinate may be given without regard to meals, but optimal absorption occurs when given on empty stomach. • Give with 8 oz water. • If swallowing difficulties exist, sprinkle capsule contents on teaspoon of applesauce, follow with water. • Do not swallow chewable tablets whole.

OPHTHALMIC
• Place finger on lower eyelid, pull out until a pocket is formed between eye and lower lid. Place ¼–½ inch layer of ointment into pocket. • Have patient close eye gently for 1–2 min, rolling eyeball (increases contact area of drug to eye). • Remove excess ointment around eye with tissue.

⊞ IV INCOMPATIBILITY
Fluconazole (Diflucan).

IV COMPATIBILITIES
Aminophylline, amiodarone (Cordarone), diltiazem (Cardizem), heparin, hydromorphone (Dilaudid), lidocaine, lorazepam (Ativan), magnesium sulfate, midazolam (Versed), morphine, multivitamins, potassium chloride, total parenteral nutrition (TPN).

INDICATIONS/ROUTES/DOSAGE
MILD TO MODERATE INFECTIONS OF THE UPPER AND LOWER RESPIRATORY TRACT, PHARYNGITIS, SKIN INFECTIONS
PO: ADULTS, ELDERLY: 250 mg q6h, 500 mg q12h, or 333 mg q8h. **Maximum:** 4 g/day. CHILDREN: 30–50 mg/kg/day in divided doses up to 60–100 mg/kg/day for severe infections. NEONATES: 20–40 mg/kg/day in divided doses q6–12h.
IV: ADULTS, ELDERLY, CHILDREN: 15–20 mg/kg/day in divided doses. **Maximum:** 4 g/day.

PREOPERATIVE INTESTINAL ANTISEPSIS
PO: ADULTS, ELDERLY: 1 g at 1 PM, 2 PM, and 11 PM on day before surgery (with neomycin). CHILDREN: 20 mg/kg at 1 PM, 2 PM, and 11 PM on day before surgery (with neomycin).

ACNE VULGARIS
TOPICAL: ADULTS: Apply thin layer to affected area twice a day.

GONOCOCCAL OPHTHALMIA NEONATORUM
OPHTHALMIC: NEONATES: 0.5–2 cm no later than 1 hr after delivery.

SIDE EFFECTS
FREQUENT: IV: Abdominal cramping or discomfort, phlebitis or thrombophlebitis. **Topical:** Dry skin (50%). **OCCASIONAL:** Nausea, vomiting, diarrhea, rash, urticaria. **RARE: Ophthalmic:** Sensitivity reaction with increased irritation, burning, itching, and inflammation. **Topical:** Urticaria.

ADVERSE REACTIONS/ TOXIC EFFECTS
Antibiotic-associated colitis and other superinfections may occur. High dosages in patients with renal impairment may lead to reversible hearing loss. Anaphylaxis and hepatotoxicity occur rarely.

Ventricular arrhythmias and prolonged QT interval occur rarely with the IV drug form.

NURSING CONSIDERATIONS

BASELINE ASSESSMENT

Question for history of allergies (particularly erythromycins), hepatitis.

INTERVENTION/EVALUATION

Determine pattern of bowel activity and stool consistency. Assess skin for rash. Assess for hepatotoxicity: malaise, fever, abdominal pain, GI disturbances. Evaluate for superinfection. Check for phlebitis (heat, pain, red streaking over vein). Monitor for high-dose hearing loss.

PATIENT/FAMILY TEACHING

• Continue therapy for full length of treatment. • Doses should be evenly spaced. • Do *not* swallow chewable tablets whole. • Take medication with 8 oz water 1 hr before or 2 hr following food or beverage. • **Ophthalmic:** Report burning, itching, inflammation. • **Topical:** Report excessive skin dryness, itching, burning. • Improvement of acne may not occur for 1–2 mo; maximum benefit may take 3 mo; therapy may last months or years. • Use caution if using other topical acne preparations containing peeling or abrasive agents, medicated or abrasive soaps, cosmetics containing alcohol (e.g., astringents, aftershave lotion).

---

escitalopram

es-sih-**tail**-oh-pram
(Lexapro)

◆CLASSIFICATION

PHARMACOTHERAPEUTIC: Serotonin reuptake inhibitor. **CLINICAL:** Antidepressant (see p. 37C).

ACTION

A selective serotonin reuptake inhibitor that blocks the uptake of the neurotransmitter serotonin at neuronal presynaptic membranes, increasing its availability at postsynaptic receptor sites. **Therapeutic Effect:** Relieves depression.

PHARMACOKINETICS

Well absorbed after PO administration. Primarily metabolized in the liver. Primarily excreted in feces with a lesser amount eliminated in urine. **Half-life:** 35 hr.

USES

Treatment of major depressive disorder exhibited as persistent, prominent dysphoria (occurring nearly every day for at least 2 wk) manifested by 4 of 8 symptoms: appetite change, sleep pattern change, increased fatigue, impaired concentration, feelings of guilt or worthlessness, loss of interest in usual activities, psychomotor agitation or retardation, suicidal tendencies. Treatment of generalized anxiety disorder (GAD). **OFF-LABEL:** Mixed anxiety and depressive disorder.

PRECAUTIONS

CONTRAINDICATIONS: Breast-feeding, use within 14 days of MAOIs. **CAUTIONS:** Hepatic/renal impairment; history of seizures, mania, hypomania; concurrent use of CNS depressants.

⏳ LIFESPAN CONSIDERATIONS: **Pregnancy/Lactation:** Distributed in breast milk. **Pregnancy Category C. Children:** May cause increased anticholinergic effects or hyperexcitability. **Elderly:** More sensitive to anticholinergic effects (e.g., dry mouth), more likely to experience dizziness, sedation, confusion, hypotension, hyperexcitability.

INTERACTIONS

DRUG: Alcohol, other CNS suppressants: May increase CNS depression.

Antifungals, cimetidine, macrolide antibiotics: May increase plasma level of escitalopram. **Carbamazepine:** May decrease plasma level of escitalopram. **Lithium:** May increase lithium concentration and increase the risk of serotonin syndrome. **MAOIs:** May cause serotonin syndrome, marked by autonomic hyperactivity, coma, diaphoresis, excitement, hyperthermia, and rigidity, and neuroleptic malignant syndrome. **Metoprolol:** Increases plasma level of metoprolol. **HERBAL: Ginkgo biloba, St. John's wort:** May increase the risk of serotonin syndrome. **FOOD:** None known. **LAB VALUES:** May reduce serum sodium level.

AVAILABILITY (Rx)

ORAL SOLUTION: 5 mg/5 ml. **TABLETS:** 5 mg, 10 mg, 20 mg.

ADMINISTRATION/HANDLING
PO

• Give without regard to food. • Do not crush film-coated tablets.

INDICATIONS/ROUTES/DOSAGE

DEPRESSION, GENERAL ANXIETY DISORDER (GAD)
PO: ADULTS: Initially, 10 mg once a day in the morning or evening. May increase to 20 mg after a minimum of 1 wk. ELDERLY, PATIENTS WITH HEPATIC IMPAIRMENT: 10 mg/day.

SIDE EFFECTS

FREQUENT (21%–11%): Nausea, dry mouth, somnolence, insomnia, diaphoresis. **OCCASIONAL (8%–4%):** Tremor, diarrhea, abnormal ejaculation, dyspepsia, fatigue, anxiety, vomiting, anorexia. **RARE (3%–2%):** Sinusitis, sexual dysfunction, menstrual disorder, abdominal pain, agitation, decreased libido.

ADVERSE REACTIONS/ TOXIC EFFECTS

Overdose is manifested as dizziness, drowsiness, tachycardia, somnolence, confusion, and seizures.

NURSING CONSIDERATIONS
BASELINE ASSESSMENT

For patients on long-term therapy, liver/renal function tests, blood counts should be performed periodically. Observe/record behavior. Assess psychological status, thought content, sleep pattern, appearance, interest in environment.

INTERVENTION/EVALUATION

Supervise suicidal-risk patient closely during early therapy (as energy level improves, suicide potential increases). Assess appearance, behavior, speech pattern, level of interest, mood.

PATIENT/FAMILY TEACHING

• Do not stop taking medication or increase dosage. • Avoid use of alcohol. • Avoid tasks that require alertness, motor skills until response to drug is established.

Eskalith, see lithium carbonate

esmolol hydrochloride 🏳

ess-moe-lol
(Brevibloc)

◆ CLASSIFICATION

PHARMACOTHERAPEUTIC: Beta$_1$ adrenergic blocker. **CLINICAL:** Antiarrhythmic (see pp. 15C, 64C).

ACTION

An antiarrhythmic that selectively blocks beta$_1$-adrenergic receptors. **Therapeutic Effect:** Slows sinus heart rate, decreases cardiac output, reducing BP.

PHARMACOKINETICS

Rapidly metabolized primarily by esterase in the cytosol of red blood cells. Protein binding: 55%. Less than 1%–2% excreted in urine. Half-life: 9 min.

USES

Treatment of supraventricular tachycardia and atrial fibrillation or flutter, treatment of tachycardia and/or hypertension especially intraoperative or postop.

PRECAUTIONS

CONTRAINDICATIONS: Cardiogenic shock, overt cardiac failure, second- and third-degree heart block, sinus bradycardia. **CAUTIONS:** History of allergy, bronchial asthma, emphysema, bronchitis, CHF, diabetes, renal impairment.

LIFESPAN CONSIDERATIONS: Pregnancy/Lactation: Crosses placenta; distributed in breast milk. **Pregnancy Category C. Children:** Safety and efficacy not established. **Elderly:** No age-related precautions noted.

INTERACTIONS

DRUG: Insulin, oral hypoglycemics: May mask symptoms of hypoglycemia and prolong hypoglycemic effect of these drugs. **MAOIs:** May cause significant hypertension. **Sympathomimetics, xanthines:** May mutually inhibit effects. **HERBAL:** None known. **FOOD:** None known. **LAB VALUES:** None known.

AVAILABILITY (Rx)

INJECTION: 10 mg/ml, 20 mg/ml, 250 mg/ml.

ADMINISTRATION/HANDLING

◀ **ALERT** ▶ Give by IV infusion. Avoid butterfly needles, very small veins.

 IV

Reconstitution • The 250 mg/ml ampule is not for direct IV injection but must be diluted to a final concentration not to exceed 10 mg/ml (prevents vein irritation). • For IV infusion, remove 20 ml from 500-ml container of D₅W, Ringer's, D₅W/Ringer's, D₅W/lactated D₅W/0.9% NaCl, D₅W/0.45% NaCl, 0.9% NaCl, lactated Ringer's or 0.45% NaCl and dilute 250 mg/ml concentration esmolol to remaining 480 ml of solution to provide concentration of 10 mg/ml. Maximum concentration: 10 g/250 ml (40 mg/ml).

Rate of administration • Administer by controlled infusion device; titrate to tolerance and response. • Infuse IV loading dose over 1–2 min. • Hypotension (systolic BP less than 90 mm Hg) is greatest during first 30 min of IV infusion.

Storage • Use only clear and colorless to light yellow solution. • After dilution, solution is stable for 24 hr. • Discard solution if it is discolored or if precipitate forms.

🔹 IV INCOMPATIBILITIES

Amphotericin B complex (Abelcet, AmBisome, Amphotec), furosemide (Lasix).

IV COMPATIBILITIES

Amiodarone (Cordarone), diltiazem (Cardizem), dopamine (Intropin), heparin, magnesium, midazolam (Versed), potassium chloride, propofol (Diprivan).

INDICATIONS/ROUTES/DOSAGE

ARRHYTHMIAS

IV: ADULTS, ELDERLY: Initially, loading dose of 500 mcg/kg/min for 1 min, followed by 50 mcg/kg/min for 4 min. If optimum response is not attained in 5 min, give second loading dose of 500 mcg/kg/min for 1 min, followed by infusion of 100 mcg/kg/min for 4 min. Additional loading doses can be given and infusion increased by 50 mcg/kg/min, up to 200 mcg/kg/min, for 4 min. Once desired response is attained, cease loading dose and increase infusion by no more than 25 mcg/kg/min. Interval between doses may be increased to 10 min. Infusion usually administered over 24–48 hr in most patients. Range: 50–200 mcg/kg/min, with average dose of 100 mcg/kg/min.

INTRA-OPERATIVE TACHYCARDIA OR HYPERTENSION (IMMEDIATE CONTROL)
IV: ADULTS, ELDERLY: Initially, 80 mg over 30 sec, then 150 mcg/kg/min infusion up to 300 mcg/kg/min.

SIDE EFFECTS

Esmolol is generally well tolerated, with transient and mild side effects. **FREQUENT:** Hypotension (systolic BP less than 90 mm Hg) manifested as dizziness, nausea, diaphoresis, headache, cold extremities, fatigue. **OCCASIONAL:** Anxiety, drowsiness, flushed skin, vomiting, confusion, inflammation at injection site, fever.

ADVERSE REACTIONS/ TOXIC EFFECTS

Overdose may produce profound hypotension, bradycardia, dizziness, syncope, drowsiness, breathing difficulty, bluish fingernails or palms of hands, and seizures. Esmolol administration may potentiate insulin-induced hypoglycemia in diabetic patients.

NURSING CONSIDERATIONS

BASELINE ASSESSMENT

Assess BP, apical pulse immediately before drug is administered (if pulse is 60 or less/min or systolic BP is 90 mm Hg or less, withhold medication, contact physician).

INTERVENTION/EVALUATION

Monitor BP for hypotension, EKG, heart rate, respiratory rate, development of diaphoresis, dizziness (usually first sign of impending hypotension). Assess pulse for quality, irregular rate, bradycardia, extremities for coldness. Assist with ambulation if dizziness occurs. Assess for nausea, diaphoresis, headache, fatigue.

esomeprazole

es-oh-**mep**-rah-zole
(Nexium, Nexium IV)

CLASSIFICATION

PHARMACOTHERAPEUTIC: Proton pump inhibitor. **CLINICAL:** Gastric acid inhibitor (see p. 134C).

ACTION

A proton pump inhibitor that is converted to active metabolites that irreversibly bind to and inhibit hydrogen-potassium adenosine triphosphates, an enzyme on the surface of gastric parietal cells. Inhibits hydrogen ion transport into gastric lumen. **Therapeutic Effect:** Increases gastric pH, reducing gastric acid production.

PHARMACOKINETICS

Well absorbed after oral administration. Protein binding: 97%. Extensively metabolized by the liver. Primarily excreted in urine. **Half-life:** 1–1.5 hr.

USES

Short-term treatment (4–8 wk) of erosive esophagitis (diagnosed by endoscopy); symptomatic gastroesophageal reflux disease (GERD). Used in triple therapy with amoxicillin and clarithromycin for treatment of *H. pylori* infection in patients with duodenal ulcer. Reduce risk of NSAID gastric ulcer.

PRECAUTIONS

CONTRAINDICATIONS: Hypersensitivity to benzimidazoles. **CAUTIONS:** None known.

⧗ **LIFESPAN CONSIDERATIONS: Pregnancy/Lactation:** Unknown if drug crosses placenta or is distributed in breast milk. **Pregnancy Category B. Children:** Safety and efficacy not established. **Elderly:** No age-related precautions noted.

INTERACTIONS

DRUG: **Digoxin, iron, ketoconazole:** May decrease the concentration of digoxin, iron, and ketoconazole. HERBAL: None known. FOOD: None known. LAB VALUES: None known.

AVAILABILITY (Rx)

CAPSULES (DELAYED-RELEASE, MAGNESIUM [NEXIUM]): 20 mg, 40 mg. POWDER FOR SOLUTION (SODIUM [NEXIUM IV]): 20 mg, 40 mg.

ADMINISTRATION/HANDLING

 IV

Reconstitution • Reconstitution for IV push, add 5 mL of 0.9% NaCl to the vial with esomeprazole. • When administering a 20 mg dose, use only half of the reconstituted solution. • Discard any unused solution.

Infusion • Dissolve the content of one vial with esomeprazole in up to 100 ml 0.9% sodium chloride for IV use.

Rate of administration • For IV push, administer over not less than 3 min. For intermittent infusion (piggyback) infuse over 15–30 min. • Flush line with 0.9% NaCl injection, lactated Ringer's, or D₅W, both before and after administration.

Storage • Use only clear and colorless to very slightly yellow solution. • Discard solution if particulate matter is present.

PO
• Give more than 1 hr before eating. • Do not crush or chew capsule; swallow whole. For those with difficulty swallowing capsules, open capsule and mix pellets with 1 tbsp applesauce. Swallow spoonful without chewing.

IV INCOMPATIBILITIES

Don't mix esomeprazole with any other medications through the same IV line or tubing.

INDICATIONS/ROUTES/DOSAGE

EROSIVE ESOPHAGITIS
PO: ADULTS, ELDERLY: 20–40 mg once daily for 4–8 wk.
IV: ADULTS, ELDERLY: 20 or 40 mg once daily by IV injection over at least 3 min or IV infusion over 10–30 min.

TO MAINTAIN HEALING OF EROSIVE ESOPHAGITIS
PO: ADULTS, ELDERLY: 20 mg/day.

GASTROESOPHAGEAL REFLUX DISEASE, TO REDUCE THE RISK OF NSAID-INDUCED GASTRIC ULCER
PO: ADULTS, ELDERLY: 20 mg once a day for 4 wk.

DUODENAL ULCER CAUSED BY *HELICOBACTER PYLORI*
PO: ADULTS, ELDERLY: 40 mg (esomeprazole) once a day, with amoxicillin 1,000 mg and clarithromycin 500 mg twice a day for 10 days.

SIDE EFFECTS

FREQUENT (7%): Headache. OCCASIONAL (3%–2%): Diarrhea, abdominal pain, nausea. RARE (less than 2%): Dizziness, asthenia or loss of strength, vomiting, constipation, rash, cough.

ADVERSE REACTIONS/ TOXIC EFFECTS

None known.

INTERVENTION/EVALUATION

Evaluate for therapeutic response (i.e., relief of GI symptoms). Question if GI discomfort, nausea, diarrhea occur.

PATIENT/FAMILY TEACHING

• Report headache. • Take more than 1 hr before eating. • For patients with difficulty swallowing capsules, open capsule and mix pellets with 1 tbsp applesauce. Swallow spoonful without chewing.

Estrace, *see estradiol*

Estraderm, *see estradiol*

estradiol

ess-tra-**dye**-ole

(Alora, <u>Climara</u>, Delestrogen, Depo-Estradiol, Esclim, Estrace, Estraderm, Estradot ❧, Estrasorb, Estrogel, Estring, Femring, Menostar, Oesclim ❧, Vagifem, Vivelle, <u>Vivelle Dot</u>)

Do not confuse Estraderm with Testoderm.

FIXED-COMBINATION(S)

Activella: estradiol/norethindrone (hormone): 1 mg/0.5 mg. **Climara PRO:** estradiol/levonorgestrel (progestin): 0.045 mg/24 hr/0.015 mg/ 24 hr. **Combi-patch:** estradiol/ norethindrone (hormone): 0.05 mg/0.14 mg; 0.05 mg/0.25 mg. **Femhrt:** estradiol/norethindrone (hormone): 5 mcg/1 mg. **Lunelle:** estradiol/medroxy-progesterone (progestin): 5 mg/25 mg per 0.5 ml.

CLASSIFICATION

PHARMACOTHERAPEUTIC: Estrogen. **CLINICAL:** Estrogen, antineoplastic.

ACTION

An estrogen that increases synthesis of DNA, RNA, and proteins in target tissues; reduces release of gonadotropin-releasing hormone from the hypothalamus; and reduces follicle-stimulating hormone and luteinizing hormone (LH) release from the pituitary. **Therapeutic Effect:** Promotes normal growth, promotes development of female sex organs, and maintains GU function and vasomotor stability. Prevents accelerated bone loss by inhibiting bone resorption, restoring balance of bone resorption and formation. Inhibits LH and decreases serum testosterone concentration.

PHARMACOKINETICS

Well absorbed from the GI tract. Widely distributed. Protein binding: 50%–80%. Metabolized in the liver. Primarily excreted in urine. **Half-life:** Unknown.

USES

Treatment of moderate to severe vasomotor symptoms associated with menopause, hypoestrogenism (due to hypogonadism, primary ovarian failure), breast cancer, prostate cancer, prevention of osteoporosis, vaginal atrophy, atrophic vaginitis. **OFF-LABEL:** Treatment of Turner's syndrome.

PRECAUTIONS

CONTRAINDICATIONS: Abnormal vaginal bleeding, active arterial thrombosis, blood dyscrasias, estrogen-dependent cancer, known or suspected breast cancer, pregnancy, thrombophlebitis or thromboembolic disorders, thyroid dysfunction. **CAUTIONS:** Renal/hepatic insufficiency, diseases that may be exacerbated by fluid retention, diabetes mellitus, endometriosis, hypercalcemia, hyperlipidemias, hypertension, hypocalcemia, hypothyroidism, history of jaundice during pregnancy, or vaginal infection, children in whom bone growth is not complete.

⧖ **LIFESPAN CONSIDERATIONS: Pregnancy/Lactation:** Distributed in breast milk. May be harmful to infant. Not for use during breast-feeding. **Pregnancy Category X. Children:** Caution in those whom bone growth is not complete (may accelerate epiphyseal closure). **Elderly:** No age-related precautions noted.

✐ see color pill atlas   ❧ herb   <u>underlined</u> – top prescribed drug

INTERACTIONS

DRUG: Bromocriptine: May interfere with the effects of bromocriptine. **Cyclosporine:** May increase blood cyclosporine concentration and the risk of hepatotoxicity and nephrotoxicity. **Hepatotoxic medications:** May increase the risk of hepatotoxicity. **HERBAL: Saw palmetto:** Increases the effects of saw palmetto. **St. John's wort:** May decrease plasma concentrations and effectiveness of estrogens. **FOOD:** None known. **LAB VALUES:** May increase blood glucose, HDL, serum calcium, and triglyceride levels. May decrease serum cholesterol levels and LDH concentrations. May affect metapyrone testing and thyroid function tests.

AVAILABILITY (Rx)

TABLETS (ESTRACE): 0.5 mg, 1 mg, 2 mg. **EMULSION (TOPICAL [ESTRASORB]):** 2.5 mg/g. **INJECTION (CYPIONATE [DEPO-ESTRADIOL]):** 5 mg/ml. **INJECTION (VALERATE [DELESTROGEN]):** 10 mg/ml. **TOPICAL GEL (ESTROGEL):** 1.25 g. **TRANSDERMAL SYSTEM (ALORA):** twice weekly: 0.025 mg, 0.05 mg, 0.075 mg, 0.1 mg. **TRANSDERMAL SYSTEM (CLIMARA):** once weekly: 0.025 mg, 0.0375 mg, 0.05 mg, 0.06 mg, 0.075 mg, 0.1 mg. **TRANSDERMAL SYSTEM (ESCLIM):** twice weekly: 0.025 mg, 0.0375 mg, 0.05 mg, 0.075 mg, 0.1 mg. **TRANSDERMAL SYSTEM (ESTRADERM):** twice weekly: 0.05 mg, 0.1 mg. **TRANSDERMAL SYSTEM (MENOSTAR):** once a week: 1 mg. **TRANSDERMAL SYSTEM (VIVELLE):** twice weekly: 0.025 mg, 0.0375 mg, 0.05 mg, 0.075 mg, 0.1 mg. **TRANSDERAMAL SYSTEM (VIVELLE DOT):** twice weekly: 0.0375 mg, 0.05 mg, 0.075 mg, 0.1 mg. **VAGINAL CREAM (ESTRACE):** 0.1 mg/g. **VAGINAL RING (ESTRING):** 2 mg. **VAGINAL RING (FEMRING):** 0.05 mg. **VAGINAL TABLET (VAGIFEM):** 25 mcg.

ADMINISTRATION/HANDLING

IM
• Rotate vial to disperse drug in solution. • Inject deep IM in large muscle mass.

PO
• Administer at the same time each day.

TRANSDERMAL
◀ **ALERT** ▶ Transdermal Climara is administered once weekly; other transdermal forms of estradiol are applied twice weekly. • Remove old patch; select new site (buttocks are alternative application site). • Peel off protective strip to expose adhesive surface. • Apply to clean, dry, intact skin on the trunk of the body (area with as little hair as possible). • Press in place for at least 10 sec (do not apply to the breasts or waistline).

VAGINAL
• Apply at bedtime for best absorption. • Insert end of filled applicator into vagina, directed slightly toward sacrum; push plunger down completely. • Avoid skin contact with cream (prevents skin absorption).

INDICATIONS/ROUTES/DOSAGE

PROSTATE CANCER
IM (ESTRADIOL VALERATE): ADULTS, ELDERLY: 30 mg or more q1–2wk.
PO: ADULTS, ELDERLY: 10 mg 3 times a day for at least 3 mo.

BREAST CANCER
PO: ADULTS, ELDERLY: 10 mg 3 times a day for at least 3 mo.

OSTEOPOROSIS PROPHYLAXIS IN POST-MENOPAUSAL FEMALES
PO: ADULTS, ELDERLY: 0.5 mg/day cyclically (3 wk on, 1 wk off).
TRANSDERMAL (CLIMARA): ADULTS, ELDERLY: Initially, 0.025 mg weekly, adjust dose as needed.
TRANSDERMAL (ALORA, VIVELLE, VIVELLE-DOT): ADULTS, ELDERLY: Initially, 0.025 mg patch twice weekly, adjust dose as needed.
TRANSDERMAL (ESTRADERM): ADULTS, ELDERLY: 0.05 mg twice weekly.
TRANSDERMAL (MENOSTAR): ADULTS, ELDERLY: 1 mg weekly.

E

FEMALE HYPOESTROGENISM
PO: ADULTS, ELDERLY: 1–2 mg/day, adjust dose as needed.
IM (CYPIONATE): ADULTS, ELDERLY: 1.5–2 mg monthly.
IM (ESTRADIOL VALERATE): ADULTS, ELDERLY: 10–20 mg q4wk.

VASOMOTOR SYMPTOMS ASSOCIATED WITH MENOPAUSE
PO: ADULTS, ELDERLY: 1–2 mg/day cyclically (3 wk on, 1 wk off), adjust dose as needed.
IM (ESTRADIOL CYPIONATE): ADULTS, ELDERLY: 1–5 mg q3–4wk.
IM (ESTRADIOL VALERATE): ADULTS, ELDERLY: 10–20 mg q4wk.
TOPICAL EMULSION (ESTRASORB): ADULTS, ELDERLY: 3.84 g once a day in the morning.
TOPICAL GEL (ESTROGEL): ADULTS, ELDERLY: 1.25 g/day.
TRANSDERMAL (CLIMARA): ADULTS, ELDERLY: 0.025 mg weekly. Adjust dose as needed.
TRANSDERMAL (ALORA, ESCLIM, ESTRADER, VIVELLE-DOT): ADULTS, ELDERLY: 0.05 mg twice a wk.
TRANSDERMAL (VIVELLE): ADULTS, ELDERLY: 0.0375 mg twice a wk.
VAGINAL RING (FEMRING): ADULTS, ELDERLY: 0.05 mg. May increase to 0.1 mg if needed.

VAGINAL ATROPHY
VAGINAL RING (ESTRING): ADULTS, ELDERLY: 2 mg.

ATROPHIC VAGINITIS
VAGINAL TABLET (VAGIFEM): ADULTS, ELDERLY: Initially, 1 tablet/day for 2 wk. Maintenance: 1 tablet twice a week.

SIDE EFFECTS

FREQUENT: Anorexia, nausea, swelling of breasts, peripheral edema marked by swollen ankles and feet. **Transdermal:** Skin irritation, redness. **OCCASIONAL:** Vomiting, especially with high doses; headache that may be severe; intolerance to contact lenses; hypertension; glucose intolerance; brown spots on exposed skin. **Vaginal:** Local irritation, vaginal discharge, changes in vaginal bleeding, including spotting, and breakthrough or prolonged bleeding. **RARE:** Chorea or involuntary movements, hirsutism or abnormal hairiness, loss of scalp hair, depression.

ADVERSE REACTIONS/ TOXIC EFFECTS

Estrogen therapy may increase the risk of developing coronary heart disease, hypercalcemia, gallbladder disease, cerebrovascular disease, and breast cancer. Prolonged administration increases the risk of gallbladder disease, thromboembolic disease, and breast, cervical, vaginal, endometrial, and hepatic carcinoma. Cholestatic jaundice occurs rarely.

NURSING CONSIDERATIONS

BASELINE ASSESSMENT
Question for hypersensitivity to estrogen, previous jaundice, thromboembolic disorders associated with pregnancy, estrogen therapy. Question for possibility of pregnancy (Pregnancy Category X).

INTERVENTION/EVALUATION
Monitor BP, weight, serum calcium, glucose, hepatic enzymes.

PATIENT/FAMILY TEACHING
• Limit alcohol, caffeine. • Inform physician if sudden headache, vomiting, disturbance of vision/speech, numbness/weakness of extremities, chest pain, calf pain, shortness of breath, severe abdominal pain, mental depression, unusual bleeding occurs.

---

estramustine ⚑ phosphate sodium

es-trah-**mew**-steen
(Emcyt)

Do not confuse Emcyt with Eryc.

CLASSIFICATION
PHARMACOTHERAPEUTIC: Alkylating agent, estrogen/nitrogen mustard. **CLINICAL:** Antineoplastic (see p. 74C).

ACTION
An alkylating agent, estrogen and nitrogen mustard that binds to microtubule-associated proteins, causing their disassembly. **Therapeutic Effect:** Reduces serum testosterone concentration.

PHARMACOKINETICS
Well absorbed from the GI tract. Highly localized in prostatic tissue. Rapidly dephosphorylated during absorption into peripheral circulation. Metabolized in the liver. Primarily eliminated in feces by biliary system. **Half-life:** 20 hr.

USES
Treatment of metastatic or progressive carcinoma of prostate gland.

PRECAUTIONS
CONTRAINDICATIONS: Active thrombophlebitis or thromboembolic disorders (unless the tumor is the cause of the thromboembolic disorder and the benefits outweigh the risk), hypersensitivity to estradiol or nitrogen mustard. **CAUTIONS:** History of thrombophlebitis, thrombosis, thromboembolic disorders; cerebrovascular, coronary artery disease; hepatic impairment; metabolic bone disease in those with hypercalcemia, renal insufficiency.

⌛ **LIFESPAN CONSIDERATIONS: Pregnancy/Lactation, Pregnancy Category C. Children:** Not used in this population. **Elderly:** Age-related renal impairment and/or peripheral vascular disease may require dosage adjustment.

INTERACTIONS
DRUG: Calcium-containing antacids: May impair estramustine absorption. **Hepatotoxic medications:** May increase the risk of hepatotoxicity. **HERBAL:** None known. **FOOD: Milk, dairy products, and other calcium-rich foods:** May impair estramustine absorption. **LAB VALUES:** May increase blood glucose level and serum bilirubin, cortisol, LDH, phospholipid, prolactin, AST, sodium, and triglyceride levels. May decrease urine pregnanediol level and serum antithrombin III, folate, and phosphate levels. May alter thyroid function test results.

AVAILABILITY (Rx)
CAPSULES: 140 mg.

ADMINISTRATION/HANDLING
PO
• Refrigerate capsules (may remain at room temperature for 24–48 hr without loss of potency). • Give with water 1 hr before or 2 hr after meals.

INDICATIONS/ROUTES/DOSAGE
PROSTATIC CARCINOMA
PO: ADULTS, ELDERLY: 10–16 mg/kg/day or 140 mg 4 times a day.

SIDE EFFECTS
FREQUENT: Peripheral edema of lower extremities, breast tenderness or enlargement, diarrhea, flatulence, nausea. **OCCASIONAL:** Increase in BP, thirst, dry skin, ecchymosis, flushing, alopecia, night sweats. **RARE:** Headache, rash, fatigue, insomnia, vomiting.

ADVERSE REACTIONS/ TOXIC EFFECTS
Estramustine use may exacerbate CHF and increase the risk of pulmonary emboli, thrombophlebitis, and cerebrovascular accident.

E

🍁 Canadian trade name   ℮ see **evolve**   ▶ High Alert drug

NURSING CONSIDERATIONS

INTERVENTION/EVALUATION
Monitor BP periodically.

PATIENT/FAMILY TEACHING
• Do not take with milk, milk products, calcium-rich food, calcium-containing antacids. • Use contraceptive measures during therapy. • If headache (migraine or severe), vomiting, disturbed speech or vision, dizziness, numbness, shortness of breath, calf pain, chest pain or pressure, unexplained cough occurs, contact physician.

estropipate

ess-troe-**pie**-pate
(Ogen, Ortho-Est)

CLASSIFICATION
PHARMACOTHERAPEUTIC: Estrogen.
CLINICAL: Hormone.

ACTION
An estrogen that increases synthesis of DNA, RNA, and proteins in target tissues; reduces release of gonadotropin-releasing hormone from the hypothalamus; and reduces follicle-stimulating hormone (FSH) and luteinizing hormone (LH) from the pituitary. **Therapeutic Effect:** Promotes normal growth, promotes development of female sex organs, and maintains GU function and vasomotor stability. Prevents accelerated bone loss by inhibiting bone resorption, restoring balance of bone resorption and formation. Inhibits LH and decreases serum testosterone concentration.

USES
Treatment of vasomotor symptoms associated with menopause, vulvar and vaginal atrophy, hypoestrogenism, osteoporosis prophylaxis.

PRECAUTIONS
CONTRAINDICATIONS: Abnormal vaginal bleeding, active arterial thrombosis, blood dyscrasias, estrogen-dependent cancer, known or suspected breast cancer, pregnancy, thrombophlebitis or thromboembolic disorders, thyroid dysfunction. **CAUTIONS:** Renal or hepatic insufficiency, diseases that may be exacerbated by fluid retention. **Pregnancy Category X.**

INTERACTIONS
DRUG: Bromocriptine: May interfere with the effects of bromocriptine. **Cyclosporine:** May increase blood cyclosporine concentration and the risk of hepatotoxicity and nephrotoxicity. **Hepatotoxic medications:** May increase the risk of hepatotoxicity. **HERBAL: Saw palmetto:** Increases the effects of saw palmetto. **FOOD:** None known. **LAB VALUES:** May increase blood glucose, HDL, serum calcium, and triglyceride levels. May decrease serum cholesterol and LDH concentrations. May affect metapyrone testing and thyroid function tests.

AVAILABILITY (Rx)
TABLETS (OGEN, ORTHO-EST): 0.625 mg (0.75 mg estropipate), 1.25 mg (1.5 mg estropipate), 2.5 mg (3 mg estropipate). **VAGINAL CREAM (OGEN):** 1.5 mg/g.

ADMINISTRATION/HANDLING
• Administer estropipate at the same time each day. • Store in a tightly-closed container.

INDICATIONS/ROUTES/DOSAGE
VASOMOTOR SYMPTOMS, ATROPHIC VAGINITIS, KRAUROSIS VULVAE
PO: ADULTS, ELDERLY: 0.625–5 mg/day cyclically.

ATROPHIC VAGINITIS, KRAUROSIS VULVAE
INTRAVAGINAL: ADULTS, ELDERLY: 2–4 g/day cyclically.

FEMALE HYPOGONADISM, CASTRATION, PRIMARY OVARIAN FAILURE
PO: ADULTS, ELDERLY: 1.25–7.5 mg/day for 21 days; then off for 8–10 days. Repeat if bleeding does not occur by end of off cycle.

PREVENTION OF OSTEOPOROSIS
PO: ADULTS, ELDERLY: 0.625 mg/day (25 days of 31-day cycle/mo).

SIDE EFFECTS

FREQUENT: Anorexia, nausea, swelling of breasts, peripheral edema marked by swollen ankles and feet. **OCCASIONAL:** Vomiting, especially with high doses; headache that may be severe; intolerance to contact lenses; hypertension; glucose intolerance; brown spots on exposed skin. **Vaginal:** Local irritation, vaginal discharge, changes in vaginal bleeding, including spotting, and breakthrough or prolonged bleeding. **RARE:** Chorea or involuntary movements, hirsutism or abnormal hairiness, loss of scalp hair, depression.

ADVERSE REACTIONS/ TOXIC EFFECTS

Prolonged administration may increase the risk of breast, cervical, endometrial, hepatic, and vaginal carcinoma; cerebrovascular disease, coronary heart disease, gallbladder disease, and hypercalcemia. Cholestatic jaundice occurs rarely.

NURSING CONSIDERATIONS

BASELINE ASSESSMENT
Question for hypersensitivity to estrogen, previous jaundice, thromboembolic disorders associated with pregnancy, estrogen therapy. Question for possibility of pregnancy (Pregnancy Category X).

INTERVENTION/EVALUATION
Promptly report signs or symptoms of thromboembolic or thrombotic disorders: sudden severe headache, shortness of breath, vision or speech disturbance, numbness of an extremity.

PATIENT/FAMILY TEACHING
• Avoid smoking due to increased risk of heart attack and blood clots. • Notify physician of abnormal vaginal bleeding, depression. • With vaginal application, remain recumbent at least 30 min after application; do not use tampons. • Stop taking the medication and contact physician at once if pregnancy is suspected.

eszopiclone

es-zoe-**pick**-lone
(Lunesta)

CLASSIFICATION
PHARMACOTHERAPEUTIC: Non-benzodiazepine. **CLINICAL:** Hypnotic Schedule IV.

ACTION

May interact with GABA-receptor complexes at binding domains located close to or allosterically coupled to benzodiazepine receptors. **Therapeutic Effect:** Prevents insomnia and/or difficulty maintaining sleep during the night.

PHARMACOKINETICS

Rapidly absorbed following PO administration. Weakly bound to plasma proteins. Metabolized in the liver. Excreted in urine. **Half-life:** 5–6 hr.

USES

Long-term treatment of insomnia in patients who experience difficulty falling asleep as well as treatment of patients who are unable to sleep through the night (sleep maintenance difficulty).

PRECAUTIONS

CONTRAINDICATIONS: None known. **CAUTIONS:** Hepatic impairment compromised respiratory function, clinical depression.

⧗ **LIFESPAN CONSIDERATIONS: Pregnancy/Lactation:** Unknown if drug crosses placenta or is distributed in breast milk. **Pregnancy Category C. Children:** Safety and efficacy not established. **Elderly:** Those with impaired motor or cognitive performance may require dosage adjustment.

INTERACTIONS

DRUG: Alcohol: Concurrent use has additive effect: decreased psychomotor function. **Aminoglutethimide, carbamazepine, nafcillin, nevirapine, phenobarbital, phenytoin, rifampicin:** May decrease the levels or effects of eszopiclone. **CYP3A4 inhibitors (clarithromycin, itraconazole, ketoconazole, nefazodone, nelfinavir, ritonavir, troleandomycin):** May increase the serum levels, effects of eszopiclone. **Olanzapine:** Concurrent use may lead to decreased psychomotor function. **HERBAL: Gotu kola, kava kava, St. John's wort, valerian:** May increase CNS depression. **FOOD: Heavy meals:** Onset of action may be reduced if taken with or immediately after a heavy meal. **LAB VALUES:** None known.

AVAILABILITY (Rx)

TABLETS, FILM-COATED: 1 mg, 2 mg, 3 mg (Lunesta).

ADMINISTRATION/HANDLING

PO
• Should be administered immediately before bedtime. • Do not give with or immediately following a high-fat meal. • Do not crush or break tablet.

INDICATIONS/ROUTES/DOSAGE

INSOMNIA
PO: ADULTS: 2 mg before bedtime. **Maximum:** 3 mg. **Concurrent use with CYP3A4 INHIBITORS:** 1 mg before bedtime; if needed, dose may

be increased to 2 mg. ELDERLY: Initially, 1 mg before bedtime. **Maximum:** 2 mg.

SLEEP MAINTENANCE DIFFICULTY
PO: ADULTS: 2 mg before bedtime.

SIDE EFFECTS

FREQUENT (34%–21%): Unpleasant taste, headache. **OCCASIONAL (10%–4%):** Somnolence, dry mouth, dyspepsia, dizziness, nervousness, nausea, rash, pruritus, depression, diarrhea. **RARE (3%–2%):** Hallucinations, anxiety, confusion, abnormal dreams, decreased libido, neuralgia.

ADVERSE REACTIONS/TOXIC EFFECTS

Chest pain, peripheral edema occurs occasionally.

NURSING CONSIDERATIONS

BASELINE ASSESSMENT

Assess BP, pulse, respirations. Raise bed rails, provide call light. Provide environment conducive to sleep (quiet environment, low or no lighting, TV off).

INTERVENTION/EVALUATION

Assess sleep pattern of patient. Evaluate for therapeutic response: decrease in number of nocturnal awakenings, increase in length of sleep.

PATIENT/FAMILY TEACHING

• Do not abruptly withdraw medication following long-term use. • Avoid alcohol. • At least 8 hr must be devoted for sleep time before daily activity begins. • Advise the patient to take eszopiclone immediately before bedtime.

etanercept

ee-tan-er-cept
(Enbrel)

CLASSIFICATION

PHARMACOTHERAPEUTIC: Protein.
CLINICAL: Antiarthritic.

ACTION

A protein that binds to tumor necrosis factor (TNF), blocking its interaction with cell surface receptors. Elevated levels of TNF, which is involved in inflammatory and immune responses, are found in the synovial fluid of rheumatoid arthritis patients. Therapeutic Effect: Relieves symptoms of rheumatoid arthritis.

PHARMACOKINETICS

Well absorbed after subcutaneous administration. Half-life: 115 hr.

USES

Reduces signs and symptoms of moderately to severely active rheumatoid arthritis (RA). Treatment of active juvenile RA, ankylosing spondylitis, psoriatic arthritis. Treatment of chronic moderate to severe plaque psoriasis. Improvement of physical function in patients with psoriatic arthritis. OFF-LABEL: Treatment of Crohn's disease, reactive arthritis.

PRECAUTIONS

CONTRAINDICATIONS: Serious active infection or sepsis. **CAUTIONS:** History of recurrent infections, illnesses that predispose to infection (e.g., diabetes). LIFESPAN CONSIDERATIONS: Pregnancy/Lactation: Unknown if drug is excreted in breast milk. Pregnancy Category B. Children: No age-related precautions noted in those 4 yr and older. Elderly: No age-related precautions noted.

INTERACTIONS

DRUG: None known. HERBAL: None known. FOOD: None known. LAB VALUES: None known.

AVAILABILITY (Rx)

POWDER FOR INJECTION: 25 mg.
PREFILLED SYRINGE: 50 mg.

ADMINISTRATION/HANDLING

◂ ALERT ▸ Do not add other medications to solution. Do not use filter during reconstitution or administration.

SUBCUTANEOUS
• Reconstitute with 1 ml of bacteriostatic water for injection (0.9% benzyl alcohol). Do not reconstitute with other diluents. • Slowly inject the diluent into the vial. Some foaming will occur. To avoid excessive foaming, slowly swirl contents until powder is dissolved (less than 5 min). • Visually inspect solution for particles, discoloration. Reconstituted solution should appear clear, colorless. If discolored, cloudy, or particles remain, discard solution; do not use. • Withdraw all the solution into syringe. Final volume should be approx. 1 ml. • Inject into thigh, abdomen, upper arm. Rotate injection sites. • Give new injection at least 1 inch from an old site and never into area where skin is tender, bruised, red, hard. • Refrigerate. • Once reconstituted, may be stored up to 6 hr if refrigerated.

INDICATIONS/ROUTES/DOSAGE

RHEUMATOID ARTHRITIS, PSORIATIC ARTHRITIS, ANKYLOSING SPONDYLITIS
SUBCUTANEOUS: ADULTS, ELDERLY: 25 mg twice weekly given 72–96 hr apart. Alternative weekly dosing: 0.8 mg/kg/dose once a wk. **Maximum:** 50 mg/wk. **Maximum:** 25 mg/dose.

JUVENILE RHEUMATOID ARTHRITIS
SUBCUTANEOUS: CHILDREN 4–17 YR: 0.4 mg/kg (**Maximum:** 25 mg dose) twice weekly given 72–96 hr apart. Alternative weekly dosing: 50 mg once weekly. **Maximum:** 25 mg/dose.

PLAQUE PSORIASIS
SUBCUTANEOUS: ADULTS, ELDERLY: 50 mg twice a wk (give 3–4 days apart) for 3 mo. Maintenance: 50 mg once a wk.

E

SIDE EFFECTS

FREQUENT (37%): Injection site erythema, pruritus, pain, and swelling; abdominal pain, vomiting (more common in children than adults). **OCCASIONAL (16%–4%):** Headache, rhinitis, dizziness, pharyngitis, cough, asthenia, abdominal pain, dyspepsia. **RARE (less than 3%):** Sinusitis, allergic reaction.

ADVERSE REACTIONS/ TOXIC EFFECTS

Infections (such as pyelonephritis, cellulitis, osteomyelitis, wound infection, leg ulcer, septic arthritis, diarrhea, bronchitis, and pneumonia), occur in 38%–29% of patients. Rare adverse effects include heart failure, hypertension, hypotension, pancreatitis, GI hemorrhage, and dyspnea. The patient also may develop autoimmune antibodies.

NURSING CONSIDERATIONS

BASELINE ASSESSMENT

Assess onset, type, location, duration of pain or inflammation. If a significant exposure to varicella virus has occurred during treatment, therapy should be temporarily discontinued and treatment with varicella-zoster immune globulin considered.

INTERVENTION/EVALUATION

Assess for joint swelling, pain, tenderness. Monitor erythrocyte sedimentation rate (ESR) or C-reactive protein level, CBC with differential, platelet count.

PATIENT/FAMILY TEACHING

• Instruct in subcutaneous injection technique, including areas of the body acceptable as injection sites. • Injection site reaction generally occurs in first month of treatment and decreases in frequency during continued therapy. • Do not receive live vaccines during treatment. • Inform physician if persistent fever, bruising, bleeding, pallor occurs.

ethambutol

eth-**am**-byoo-tol
(Etibi ✽, Myambutol)

Do not confuse ethambutol or Myambutol with Nembutal.

CLASSIFICATION

PHARMACOTHERAPEUTIC: Isonicotinic acid derivative. **CLINICAL:** Antitubercular.

ACTION

An isonicotinic acid derivative that interferes with RNA synthesis. **Therapeutic Effect:** Suppresses the multiplication of mycobacteria.

PHARMACOKINETICS

Rapidly and well absorbed from the GI tract. Protein binding: 20%–30%. Widely distributed. Metabolized in the liver. Primarily excreted in urine. Removed by hemodialysis. **Half-life:** 3–4 hr (increased in impaired renal function).

USES

In conjunction with at least one other antitubercular agent for initial treatment and retreatment of clinical tuberculosis. **OFF-LABEL:** Treatment of atypical mycobacterial infections such as *Mycobacterium avium* complex (MAC).

PRECAUTIONS

CONTRAINDICATIONS: Optic neuritis. **CAUTIONS:** Renal dysfunction, gout, ocular defects: diabetic retinopathy, cataracts, recurrent ocular inflammatory conditions. Not recommended for children 13 yr and younger.

⧗ **LIFESPAN CONSIDERATIONS: Pregnancy/Lactation:** Crosses placenta. Excreted in breast milk. **Pregnancy Category B. Children:** Safety and efficacy

---

not established in those younger than 13 yr. **Elderly:** Age-related renal impairment may require dosage adjustment.

INTERACTIONS

DRUG: Neurotoxic medications: May increase the risk of neurotoxicity. **HERBAL:** None known. **FOOD:** None known. **LAB VALUES:** May increase serum uric acid levels.

AVAILABILITY (Rx)

TABLETS: 100 mg, 400 mg.

ADMINISTRATION/HANDLING

PO
• Give with food (decreases GI upset).

INDICATIONS/ROUTES/DOSAGE

TUBERCULOSIS, OTHER MYOBACTERIAL DISEASES
PO: ADULTS, ELDERLY: 15–25 mg/kg/day. **Maximum:** 1.6 g/dose. CHILDREN: 15–20 mg/kg/day. **Maximum:** 1 g/day.

DOSAGE IN RENAL IMPAIRMENT
Dosage interval is modified based on creatinine clearance.

Creatinine Clearance	Dosage Interval
10–50 ml/min	q24–36h
Less than 10 ml/min	q48h

SIDE EFFECTS

OCCASIONAL: Acute gouty arthritis (chills, pain, swelling of joints with hot skin), confusion, abdominal pain, nausea, vomiting, anorexia, headache. **RARE:** Rash, fever, blurred vision, eye pain, red-green color blindness.

ADVERSE REACTIONS/ TOXIC EFFECTS

Optic neuritis (more common with high-dosage or long-term ethambutol therapy), peripheral neuritis, thrombocytopenia, and an anaphylactoid reaction occur rarely.

NURSING CONSIDERATIONS

BASELINE ASSESSMENT
Evaluate initial CBC, renal and liver test results.

INTERVENTION/EVALUATION
Assess for vision changes (altered color perception, decreased visual acuity may be first signs): discontinue drug and notify physician immediately. Give with food if GI distress occurs. Monitor serum uric acid. Assess for hot, painful, or swollen joints, especially big toe, ankle, knee (gout). Report numbness, tingling, burning of extremities (peripheral neuritis).

PATIENT/FAMILY TEACHING
• Do not skip doses; take for full length of therapy (may take months or years).
• Notify physician immediately of any visual problem (visual effects generally reversible with discontinuation of ethambutol but in rare cases may take up to 1 yr to disappear or may be permanent); promptly report swelling or pain of joints, numbness or tingling/burning of extremities.

ethosuximide

(Zarontin)
See Anticonvulsants

etidronate disodium

eh-**tye**-droe-nate
(Didronel, Didronel I.V.)
Do not confuse etidronate with etidocaine or etomidate.

◆CLASSIFICATION
PHARMACOTHERAPEUTIC: Bisphosphonate. **CLINICAL:** Calcium regulator.

ACTION

A bisphosphonate that decreases mineral release and matrix in bone and inhibits osteocytic osteolysis. **Therapeutic Effect:** Decreases bone resorption.

PHARMACOKINETICS

Variable absorption following PO administration. Not metabolized. Approximately 50% of drug is excreted in urine. Unabsorbed drug is excreted intact in feces. **Half-life:** 1–6 hr (oral); 6 hr (IV).

USES

PO: Treatment of symptomatic Paget's disease of the bone, prevention and treatment of heterotopic ossification following hip replacement or due to spinal injury. **IV:** Treatment of hypercalcemia associated with malignant neoplasms inadequately managed by dietary modification, oral hydration; treatment of hypercalcemia of malignancy persisting after adequate hydration has been restored.

PRECAUTIONS

CONTRAINDICATIONS: Clinically overt osteomalacia. **CAUTIONS:** Those with restricted calcium, vitamin D intake, renal impairment, hyperphosphatemia.

⧗ **LIFESPAN CONSIDERATIONS: Pregnancy/Lactation:** Unknown if drug is distributed in breast milk. **Pregnancy Category C** (parenteral), **B** (oral). **Children:** Safety and efficacy not established. **Elderly:** Prone to overhydration when treated with parenteral etidronate in conjunction with hydration therapy.

INTERACTIONS

DRUG: Antacids containing aluminum, calcium, magnesium mineral supplements: May decrease the absorption of etidronate. **HERBAL:** None

known. **FOOD: Foods with calcium:** May decrease the absorption of etidronate. **LAB VALUES:** None known.

AVAILABILITY (Rx)

TABLETS (DIDRONEL): 200 mg, 400 mg. **INJECTION (DIDRONEL I.V.):** 300-mg ampule (50 mg/ml).

ADMINISTRATION/HANDLING

💧 IV

Reconstitution • Must dilute with at least 250 ml 0.9% NaCl or D_5W.

Rate of administration • Infuse over at least 2 hr.

Storage • Store at room temperature.

▦ IV INCOMPATIBILITIES

Do not mix with other medications.

INDICATIONS/ROUTES/DOSAGE

PAGET'S DISEASE

PO: ADULTS, ELDERLY: Initially, 5–10 mg/kg/day not to exceed 6 mo, or 11–20 mg/kg/day not to exceed 3 mo. Repeat only after drug-free period of at least 90 days.

HETEROTOPIC OSSIFICATION CAUSED BY SPINAL CORD INJURY

PO: ADULT, ELDERLY: 20 mg/kg/day for 2 wk; then 10 mg/kg/day for 10 wk.

HETEROTOPIC OSSIFICATION COMPLICATING TOTAL HIP REPLACEMENT

PO: ADULTS, ELDERLY: 20 mg/kg/day for 1 mo before surgery; then 20 mg/kg/day for 3 mo after surgery.

HYPERCALCEMIA ASSOCIATED WITH MALIGNANCY

IV: ADULTS, ELDERLY: 7.5 mg/kg/day for 3 days. For retreatment, allow 7 days between treatment courses. Follow with oral therapy on day after last infusion. Begin with 20 mg/kg/day for 30 days; may extend up to 90 days.

✑ see color pill atlas   ◣ herb   underlined – top prescribed drug

SIDE EFFECTS

FREQUENT: Nausea; diarrhea; continuing or more frequent bone pain in patients with Paget's disease. **OCCASIONAL:** Bone fractures, especially of the femur. **Parenteral:** Metallic, altered taste. **RARE:** Hypersensitivity reaction.

ADVERSE REACTIONS/ TOXIC EFFECTS

Nephrotoxicity, including hematuria, dysuria, and proteinuria, has occurred with parenteral route.

NURSING CONSIDERATIONS

BASELINE ASSESSMENT

Obtain baseline laboratory tests, especially serum electrolytes, renal function.

INTERVENTION/EVALUATION

Assess for diarrhea. Monitor electrolytes. Check I&O, BUN, serum creatinine in patients with renal impairment. Evaluate pain in patients with Paget's disease.

PATIENT/FAMILY TEACHING

• May take up to 3 mo for therapeutic response. • Ensure milk, dairy products in diet for calcium, vitamin D. • Take medication on empty stomach, 2 hr after food, vitamins, antacids.

etodolac

eh-**toe**-doe-lack

(Apo-Etodolac ✹, Lodine, Lodine XL, Ultradol ✹)

Do not confuse Lodine with codeine or iodine.

◆CLASSIFICATION

PHARMACOTHERAPEUTIC: NSAID. **CLINICAL:** Nonsteroidal anti-inflammatory, analgesic (see p. 116C).

ACTION

An NSAID that produces analgesic and anti-inflammatory effects by inhibiting prostaglandin synthesis. **Therapeutic Effect:** Reduces the inflammatory response and intensity of pain.

PHARMACOKINETICS

Route	Onset	Peak	Duration
PO (analgesic)	30 min	N/A	4–12 hr

Completely absorbed from the GI tract. Protein binding: greater than 99%. Widely distributed. Metabolized in the liver. Primarily excreted in urine. Not removed by hemodialysis. **Half-life:** 6–7 hr.

USES

Acute and long-term treatment of osteoarthritis, management of pain, treatment of rheumatoid arthritis. **OFF-LABEL:** Treatment of acute gouty arthritis, vascular headache.

PRECAUTIONS

◀ **ALERT** ▶ There is an increased risk of cardiovascular events (including MI and cerebrovascular accident [CVA]) and serious and potentially life-threatening GI bleeding associated with the use of etodolac.

CONTRAINDICATIONS: Active peptic ulcer disease, chronic inflammation of GI tract, GI bleeding or ulceration, history of hypersensitivity to aspirin or NSAIDs. **CAUTIONS:** Renal/hepatic impairment, history of GI tract disease, predisposition to fluid retention.

⧗ **LIFESPAN CONSIDERATIONS: Pregnancy/Lactation:** Unknown if drug crosses placenta or is distributed in breast milk. Avoid use during last trimester (may adversely affect fetal cardiovascular system: premature closure of ductus arteriosus). **Pregnancy**

E

Category C (D if used in third trimester or near delivery). **Children:** Safety and efficacy not established. **Elderly:** GI bleeding, ulceration more likely to cause serious adverse effects. Age-related renal impairment may increase risk of hepatic/renal toxicity; decreased dosage recommended.

INTERACTIONS

DRUG: Antihypertensives, diuretics: May decrease the effects of these drugs. **Aspirin, other salicylates:** May increase the risk of GI side effects such as bleeding. **Bone marrow depressants:** May increase the risk of hematologic reactions. **Heparin, oral anticoagulants, thrombolytics:** May increase the effects of these drugs. **Lithium:** May increase the blood concentration and risk of toxicity of lithium. **Methotrexate:** May increase the risk of methotrexate toxicity. **Probenecid:** May increase etodolac blood concentration. **HERBAL: Feverfew, ginkgo biloba:** May increase the risk of bleeding. **FOOD:** None known. **LAB VALUES:** May increase bleeding time, liver function test results, and serum creatinine level. May decrease serum uric acid level.

AVAILABILITY (Rx)

CAPSULES (LODINE): 200 mg, 300 mg. **TABLETS (LODINE):** 400 mg, 500 mg. **TABLETS (EXTENDED-RELEASE [LODINE XL]):** 400 mg, 500 mg, 600 mg.

ADMINISTRATION/HANDLING

PO
• Do not crush or break capsules, extended-releases. • May give with food, milk, antacids if GI distress occurs.

INDICATIONS/ROUTES/DOSAGE

OSTEOARTHRITIS, RHEUMATOID ARTHRITIS
PO (IMMEDIATE-RELEASE): ADULTS, ELDERLY: Initially, 300 mg 2–3 times

a day or 400–500 mg twice a day. Maintenance: 600–1,000 mg/day in 2–4 divided doses.
PO (EXTENDED-RELEASE): ADULTS, ELDERLY: 400–1,000 mg once daily. **Maximum:** 1,200 mg/day.

JUVENILE RHEUMATOID ARTHRITIS
PO (EXTENDED-RELEASE): CHILDREN 6–16 YR: 1,000 mg in children weighing more than 60 kg, 800 mg once daily in children weighing 46–60 kg, 600 mg once daily in children weighing 31–45 kg, 400 mg once daily in children weighing 20–30 kg.

ANALGESIA
PO: ADULTS, ELDERLY: 200–400 mg q6–8h as needed. **Maximum:** 1,200 mg/day.

SIDE EFFECTS

OCCASIONAL (9%–4%): Dizziness, headache, abdominal pain or cramps, bloated feeling, diarrhea, nausea, indigestion. **RARE (3%–1%):** Constipation, rash, pruritus, visual disturbances, tinnitus.

ADVERSE REACTIONS/ TOXIC EFFECTS

Overdose may result in acute renal failure. There is an increased risk of cardiovascular events (including MI and CVA) and serious and potentially life-threatening GI bleeding. Rare reactions with long-term use include peptic ulcer disease, GI bleeding, gastritis, severe hepatic reactions (jaundice), nephrotoxicity (hematuria, dysuria, proteinuria), and a severe hypersensitivity reaction (bronchospasm, angioedema).

NURSING CONSIDERATIONS

BASELINE ASSESSMENT
Assess onset, type, location, duration of pain/inflammation. Inspect appearance of affected joints for immobility, deformities, skin condition.

INTERVENTION/EVALUATION

Monitor CBC, hepatic/renal function. Observe for bleeding/ecchymosis. Evaluate for therapeutic response: relief of pain, stiffness, swelling; increase in joint mobility; reduced joint tenderness; improved grip strength.

PATIENT/FAMILY TEACHING

• Swallow capsule whole; do not crush or chew. • Avoid aspirin, alcohol during therapy (increases risk of GI bleeding). • Report GI distress, visual disturbances, rash, edema, headache. • Report any signs of bleeding. • Take with food, milk, antacid if GI distress occurs. • Avoid tasks that require alertness, motor skills until response to drug is established (dizziness).

---

etoposide, VP-16 ▷

eh-**toe**-poe-side

(Etopophos, Toposar, VePesid)

Do not confuse VePesid with Pepcid or Versed.

◆CLASSIFICATION

PHARMACOTHERAPEUTIC: Epipodophyllotoxin. **CLINICAL:** Antineoplastic (see p. 74C).

ACTION

An epipodophyllotoxin that induces single- and double-stranded breaks in DNA. Cell cycle-dependent and phase-specific; most effective in the S and G_2 phases of cell division. **Therapeutic Effect:** Inhibits or alters DNA synthesis.

PHARMACOKINETICS

Variably absorbed from the GI tract. Rapidly distributed, low concentrations in CSF. Protein binding: 97%. Metabolized in the liver. Primarily

excreted in urine. Not removed by hemodialysis. **Half-life:** 3–12 hr.

USES

Treatment of testicular tumors, small cell lung carcinoma. **OFF-LABEL:** Acute lymphocytic, acute nonlymphocytic leukemias; Ewing's and Kaposi's sarcoma; Hodgkin's and non-Hodgkin's lymphomas; endometrial, gastric, non–small cell lung carcinomas; multiple myeloma, myelodysplastic syndromes, neuroblastoma, osteosarcoma, ovarian germ cell tumors; primary brain, gestational trophoblastic tumors; soft tissue sarcomas, Wilms' tumor.

PRECAUTIONS

CONTRAINDICATIONS: Pregnancy. **CAUTIONS:** Hepatic/renal impairment, bone marrow suppression.

⧖ **LIFESPAN CONSIDERATIONS: Pregnancy/Lactation:** If possible, avoid use during pregnancy, especially first trimester. May cause fetal harm. Breastfeeding not recommended. **Pregnancy Category D. Children:** Safety and efficacy not established. **Elderly:** Age-related renal impairment may require dosage adjustment.

INTERACTIONS

DRUG: Bone marrow depressants: May increase myelosuppression. **Live-virus vaccines:** May potentiate virus replication, increase vaccine side effects, and decrease the patient's antibody response to the vaccine. **HERBAL:** None known. **FOOD:** None known. **LAB VALUES:** None known.

AVAILABILITY (Rx)

CAPSULES (VEPESID): 50 mg. **INJECTION (TOPOSAR, VEPESID):** 20 mg/ml. **INJECTION (WATER-SOLUBLE [ETOPOPHOS]):** 100 mg/ml.

ADMINISTRATION/HANDLING

◀ **ALERT** ▶ Administer by slow IV infusion. Wear gloves when preparing

---

E

solution. If powder or solution comes in contact with skin, wash immediately and thoroughly with soap, water. May be carcinogenic, mutagenic, teratogenic. Handle with extreme care during preparation and administration.

IV

Reconstitution

VEPESID • Dilute each 100 mg (5 ml) with at least 250 ml D₅W or 0.9% NaCl to provide concentration of 0.4 mg/ml (500 ml for concentration of 0.2 mg/ml).

ETOPOPHOS • Reconstitute each 100 mg with 5–10 ml sterile water for injection, D₅W, or 0.9% NaCl to provide concentration of 20 mg/ml or 10 mg/ml, respectively. • May give without further dilution or further dilute to concentration as low as 0.1 mg/ml with 0.9% NaCl or D₅W.

Rate of administration

VEPESID • Infuse slowly, over 30–60 min (rapid IV may produce marked hypotension). • Monitor for anaphylactic reaction during infusion (chills, fever, dyspnea, diaphoresis, lacrimation, sneezing, throat, back, or chest pain).

ETOPOPHOS • May give over as little as 5 min up to 210 min.

Storage

VEPESID • Store injection at room temperature before dilution. • Concentrate for injection is clear, yellow. • Diluted solution is stable at room temperature for 96 hr at 0.2 mg/ml, 48 hr at 0.4 mg/ml. • Discard if crystallization occurs.

ETOPOPHOS • Refrigerate vials. • Stable for 24 hr after reconstitution.

PO

Storage • Refrigerate gelatin capsules.

▧ IV INCOMPATIBILITIES

VePesid: Cefepime (Maxipime), filgrastim (Neupogen), idarubicin (Idamycin). **Etopophos:** Amphotericin B (Fungizone), cefepime (Maxipime), chlorpromazine (Thorazine), methylprednisolone (Solu-Medrol), prochlorperazine (Compazine).

IV COMPATIBILITIES

VePesid: Carboplatin (Paraplatin), cisplatin (Platinol), cytarabine (Cytosar), daunorubicin (Cerubidine), doxorubicin (Adriamycin), granisetron (Kytril), mitoxantrone (Novantrone), ondansetron (Zofran). **Etopophos:** Carboplatin (Paraplatin), cisplatin (Platinol), cytarabine (Cytosar), dacarbazine (DTIC-Dome), daunorubicin (Cerubidine), dexamethasone (Decadron), diphenhydramine (Benadryl), doxorubicin (Adriamycin), granisetron (Kytril), magnesium sulfate, mannitol, mitoxantrone (Novantrone), ondansetron (Zofran), potassium chloride.

INDICATIONS/ROUTES/DOSAGE

REFRACTORY TESTICULAR TUMORS

IV: ADULTS: 50–100 mg/m²/day on days 1–5, or 100 mg/m²/day on days 1, 3, 5 (as combination therapy).

ACUTE MYELOCYTIC LEUKEMIA

IV: CHILDREN: 150 mg/m²/day for 2–3 days and 2–3 cycles.

BRAIN TUMOR

IV: CHILDREN: 150 mg/m²/day on days 2 and 3 of treatment course.

NEUROBLASTOMA

IV: CHILDREN: 100 mg/m²/day on days 1–5 of treatment course; repeated q4wk.

SMALL-CELL LUNG CARCINOMA

PO: ADULTS: Twice the IV dose rounded to nearest 50 mg. Give once a day for doses 400 mg or less, in divided doses for dosages greater than 400 mg.

IV: ADULTS: 35 mg/m²/day for 4 consecutive days up to 50 mg/m²/day for 5 consecutive days (as combination therapy).

LEUKEMIA, RHABDOMYOSARCOMA
CHILDREN: 60–150 mg/m²/day for 2–5 days q3–6wk.

DOSAGE IN RENAL IMPAIRMENT
Creatinine clearance 10–50 ml/min: 75% of normal dose. **Creatinine clearance less than 10 ml/min:** 50% of normal dose.

SIDE EFFECTS

FREQUENT (66%–43%): Mild to moderate nausea and vomiting, alopecia. **OCCASIONAL (13%–6%):** Diarrhea, anorexia, stomatitis. **RARE (2% or less):** Hypotension, peripheral neuropathy.

ADVERSE REACTIONS/ TOXIC EFFECTS

Myelosuppression may result in hematologic toxicity, manifested as anemia, leukopenia (occurring 7–14 days after drug administration), thrombocytopenia (occurring 9–16 days after administration) and, to lesser extent, pancytopenia. Bone marrow recovery occurs by day 20. Hepatotoxicity occurs occasionally.

NURSING CONSIDERATIONS

BASELINE ASSESSMENT
Obtain hematology tests before and at frequent intervals during therapy. Antiemetics readily control nausea, vomiting.

INTERVENTION/EVALUATION
Monitor Hgb, Hct, WBC, platelet count. Assess pattern of daily bowel activity and stool consistency. Monitor for hematologic toxicity (fever, sore throat, signs of local infection, unusual ecchymosis or bleeding from any site), symptoms of anemia (excessive fatigue, weakness).

Assess for paresthesias (peripheral neuropathy). Monitor for stomatitis.

PATIENT/FAMILY TEACHING
• Alopecia is reversible, but new hair growth may have different color, texture. • Do not have immunizations without physician's approval (drug lowers body's resistance). • Avoid contact with those who have recently received live virus vaccine. • Promptly report fever, sore throat, signs of local infection, unusual bruising or bleeding from any site.

Eulexin, *see flutamide*

Evista, *see raloxifene*

Exelon, *see rivastigmine*

exemestane

x-eh-**mess**-tane
(Aromasin)

CLASSIFICATION
PHARMACOTHERAPEUTIC: Hormone. **CLINICAL:** Antineoplastic (see p. 74C).

ACTION

Inactivates aromatase, the principal enzyme that converts androgens to estrogens in both premenopausal and postmenopausal women, thereby lowering the circulating estrogen level. **Therapeutic Effect:** Inhibits the growth of breast cancers that are stimulated by estrogens.

PHARMACOKINETICS

Rapidly absorbed after PO administration. Protein binding: 90%. Distributed extensively into tissues. Metabolized in the liver; eliminated in urine and feces. **Half-life:** 24 hr.

USES

Treatment of advanced breast cancer in postmenopausal women whose disease has progressed following tamoxifen therapy. Adjuvant treatment of postmenopausal women with estrogen-receptor positive early breast cancer after 2–3 yr of tamoxifen therapy for completion of 5 consecutive years of adjuvant hormonal therapy. **OFF-LABEL:** Prevention of prostate cancer.

PRECAUTIONS

CONTRAINDICATIONS: Pregnancy. **CAUTIONS:** Do not give to premenopausal women.

⌛ **LIFESPAN CONSIDERATIONS: Pregnancy/Lactation:** Indicated for postmenopausal women. **Pregnancy Category D. Children:** Not indicated in children. **Elderly:** No age-related precautions noted.

INTERACTIONS

DRUG: None known. **HERBAL:** None known. **FOOD:** None known. **LAB VALUES:** May increase serum alkaline phosphatase, AST, and ALT levels.

AVAILABILITY (Rx)

TABLETS: 25 mg.

ADMINISTRATION/HANDLING

PO
• Give after a meal.

INDICATIONS/ROUTES/DOSAGE

BREAST CANCER
PO: ADULTS, ELDERLY: 25 mg once a day after a meal. 50 mg/day when used

concurrently with potent CYP3A4 inducers (e.g., rifampin, phenytoin).

SIDE EFFECTS

FREQUENT (22%–10%): Fatigue, nausea, depression, hot flashes, pain, insomnia, anxiety, dyspnea. **OCCASIONAL (8%–5%):** Headache, dizziness, vomiting, peripheral edema, abdominal pain, anorexia, flu-like symptoms, diaphoresis, constipation, hypertension. **RARE (4%):** Diarrhea.

ADVERSE REACTIONS/TOXIC EFFECTS

MI has been reported.

NURSING CONSIDERATIONS

INTERVENTION/EVALUATION

Monitor for onset of depression. Assess sleep pattern. Monitor for and assist with ambulation if dizziness occurs. Assess for headache. Offer antiemetic for nausea and vomiting.

PATIENT/FAMILY TEACHING

• Notify physician if nausea, hot flashes become unmanageable. • Avoid tasks that require alertness, motor skills until response to drug is established. • Best taken after meals and at the same time each day.

---

exenatide

ex-**nah**-tide
(Byetta)

♦ CLASSIFICATION

PHARMACOTHERAPEUTIC: Antihyperglycemic. **CLINICAL:** Antidiabetic.

ACTION

Stimulates release of insulin from beta cells of the pancreas, mimics enhancement of glucose-dependent insulin secretion, suppresses elevated glucagon secretion, slows gastric emptying. **Therapeutic Effect:** Improves glycemic control by reducing fasting and postprandial glucose concentrations in patients with type 2 diabetes mellitus.

PHARMACOKINETICS

Minimal systemic metabolism. Eliminated by glomerular filtration with subsequent proteolytic degradation. **Half-life:** 2.4 hr.

USES

Adjunct to diet and exercise to improve glycemic control in patients with type 2 diabetes mellitus who are taking metformin (Glucophage) and a sulfonylurea.

PRECAUTIONS

CONTRAINDICATIONS: Diabetic ketoacidosis, type 1 diabetes mellitus. Not recommended in severe renal impairment, severe GI disease. **CAUTIONS:** Mild-to-moderate renal function impairment.

⧖ **LIFESPAN CONSIDERATIONS:** Pregnancy/Lactation: Unknown if distributed in breast milk. **Pregnancy Category C. Children:** Safety and efficacy not established. **Elderly:** No age-related precautions noted.

INTERACTIONS

DRUG: Antibiotics, acetaminophen, digoxin, lisinopril, lovastatin, oral contraceptives: Reduce or delay optimal drug absorption and peak levels of these drugs if administered within 1 hr of exenatide dose. **Ethanol:** Increases the risk of hypoglycemia. **HERBAL:** None known. **FOOD:** None known. **LAB VALUES:** Decreases glucose serum levels.

AVAILABILITY (Rx)

SUBCUTANEOUS (PREFILLED PEN): 5 mcg/dose in 1.2 ml, 10 mcg/dose in 2.4 ml (Byetta).

ADMINISTRATION/HANDLING

SUBCUTANEOUS
• May be given in thigh, abdomen, or upper arm. • Rotation of injection sites is essential; maintain careful record. • Give at any time within 60 min before morning and evening meal.

Storage • Refrigerate prefilled pens. • Discard if freezing occurs. • Discard pen 30 days after initial use.

INDICATIONS/ROUTE/DOSAGE

DIABETES MELLITUS
SUBCUTANEOUS: ADULTS, ELDERLY: 5 mcg per dose given twice a day at any time with the 60 min period before the morning and evening meal. Dose may be increased to 10 mcg twice a day after 1 mo of therapy.

SIDE EFFECTS

FREQUENT (44%): Nausea. **OCCASIONAL (13%–6%):** Diarrhea, vomiting, dizziness, jitteriness, dyspepsia. **RARE (less than 6%):** Weakness, decreased appetite.

ADVERSE REACTIONS/ TOXIC EFFECTS

With concurrent sulfonylurea, hypoglycemia occurs in 36% when given a 10 mcg dose exenatide, 16% when given a 5 mcg dose.

NURSING CONSIDERATIONS

BASELINE ASSESSMENT
Check blood glucose concentration before administration. Discuss lifestyle to determine extent of learning, emotional needs. Assure follow-up instruction if patient or family does not

thoroughly understand diabetes management or glucose-testing technique. At least 1 mo should elapse to assess response to drug before new dose adjustment is made.

INTERVENTION/EVALUATION

Monitor blood glucose and food intake. Assess for hypoglycemia (cool wet skin, tremors, dizziness, anxiety, headache, tachycardia, numbness in mouth, hunger, diplopia) or hyperglycemia (polyuria, polyphagia, polydipsia, nausea, vomiting, dim vision, fatigue, deep rapid breathing). Be alert to conditions that alter glucose requirements: fever, increased activity or stress, surgical procedures.

PATIENT/FAMILY TEACHING

• Diabetes mellitus requires lifelong control. • Prescribed diet and exercise is principal part of treatment; do not skip or delay meals. • Continue to adhere to dietary instructions, a regular exercise program, and regular testing of blood glucose. • When taking combination drug therapy with a sulfonylurea, have a source of glucose available to treat symptoms of low blood sugar.

Exjade, *see deferasirox*

---

ezetimibe

eh-**zeh**-tih-myb
(Zetia)
Do not confuse Zetia with Zestril.

FIXED-COMBINATION(S)

Vytorin: ezetimibe/simvastatin (Hydroxamethyglutaryl CoA [HMG-CoA] reductase inhibitor): 10 mg/10 mg, 10 mg/20 mg, 10 mg/40 mg, 10 mg/80 mg.

◆CLASSIFICATION

PHARMACOTHERAPEUTIC: Antihyperlipidemic. **CLINICAL:** Anticholesterol agent.

ACTION

An antihyperlipidemic that inhibits cholesterol absorption in the small intestine, leading to a decrease in the delivery of intestinal cholesterol to the liver. **Therapeutic Effect:** Reduces total serum cholesterol, LDL cholesterol, and triglyceride levels; and increases HDL cholesterol concentration.

PHARMACOKINETICS

Well absorbed following oral administration. Protein binding: greater than 90%. Metabolized in the small intestine and liver. Excreted by the kidneys and bile. **Half-life:** 22 hr.

USES

Adjunct to diet for treatment of primary hypercholesterolemia (monotherapy or in combination with HMG-CoA reductase inhibitors), homozygous sitosterolemia, homozygous familial hypercholesterolemia (combined with atrovastatin or simvastatin).

PRECAUTIONS

CONTRAINDICATIONS: Concurrent use of an hydroxamethylglutaryl-CoA (HMG-CoA) reductase inhibitor (atorvastatin, fluvastatin, lovastatin, pravastatin, or simvastatin) in patients with

---

active hepatic disease or unexplained persistent elevations in serum transaminase levels, moderate or severe hepatic insufficiency. **CAUTIONS:** Diabetes, hypothyroidism, obstructive liver disease, chronic renal failure, hepatic impairment.

⧖ **LIFESPAN CONSIDERATIONS: Pregnancy/Lactation:** Unknown if drug crosses placenta or is distributed in breast milk. **Pregnancy Category C.** **Children:** Safety and efficacy not established in patients 10 yr and younger. **Elderly:** Age-related mild hepatic impairment may require dosage adjustment. Not recommended in patients with moderate or severe hepatic impairment.

INTERACTIONS

DRUG: **Aluminum and magnesium-containing antacids, cyclosporine, fenofibrate, gemfibrozil:** Increase ezetimibe plasma concentration. **Cholestyramine resin:** Decreases drug effectiveness. **HERBAL:** None known. **FOOD:** None known. **LAB VALUES:** May increase serum alkaline phosphatase, serum bilirubin, AST, and ALT levels.

AVAILABILITY (Rx)

TABLETS: 10 mg.

ADMINISTRATION/HANDLING

• Give without regard to food.

INDICATIONS/ROUTES/DOSAGE

HYPERCHOLESTEROLEMIA
PO: ADULTS, ELDERLY: Initially, 10 mg once a day, given with or without food. If the patient is also receiving a bile acid sequestrant, give ezetimibe at least 2 hr before or at least 4 hr after the bile acid sequestrant.

SITOSTEROLEMIA
PO: ADULTS, ELDERLY: 10 mg/day.

SIDE EFFECTS

OCCASIONAL (4%–3%): Back pain, diarrhea, arthralgia, sinusitis, abdominal pain. **RARE (2%):** Cough, pharyngitis, fatigue.

ADVERSE REACTIONS/ TOXIC EFFECTS

Hepatitis, hypersensitivity reactions, myopathy, and rhabdomyolysis occur rarely.

NURSING CONSIDERATIONS

BASELINE ASSESSMENT
Obtain serum cholesterol, triglycerides, liver function tests, blood counts during initial therapy and periodically during treatment. Treatment should be discontinued if hepatic enzyme levels persist more than 3 times normal limit.

INTERVENTION/EVALUATION
Monitor pattern of daily bowel activity and stool consistency. Question patient for signs and symptoms of back pain, abdominal disturbances. Monitor serum cholesterol, triglyceride concentrations for therapeutic response.

PATIENT/FAMILY TEACHING
• Periodic laboratory tests are essential part of therapy. • Do not stop medication without consulting physician.

E

---

famciclovir

fam-**sigh**-klo-veer

(Famvir)

Do not confuse Famvir with Femhrt.

◆ CLASSIFICATION

PHARMACOTHERAPEUTIC: Synthetic nucleoside. **CLINICAL:** Antiviral (see p. 61C).

ACTION

A synthetic nucleoside that inhibits viral DNA synthesis. **Therapeutic Effect:** Suppresses replication of herpes simplex virus and varicella-zoster virus.

PHARMACOKINETICS

Rapidly and extensively absorbed after PO administration. Protein binding: 20%–25%. Rapidly metabolized to penciclovir by enzymes in the GI wall, liver, and plasma. Eliminated unchanged in urine. Removed by hemodialysis. **Half-life:** 2 hr.

USES

Management of acute herpes zoster (shingles), treatment and suppression of recurrent genital herpes, treatment of recurrent mucocutaneous herpes simplex in HIV patients.

PRECAUTIONS

CONTRAINDICATIONS: Hypersensitivity to penciclovir cream. **CAUTIONS:** Renal or hepatic impairment.

⧖ **LIFESPAN CONSIDERATIONS: Pregnancy/Lactation:** Increased mammary adenocarcinoma in animals. Unknown if excreted in breast milk. **Pregnancy Category B. Children:** Safety and efficacy not established. **Elderly:** Age-related renal impairment may require dosage adjustment.

INTERACTIONS

DRUG: Probenecid: May increase the famciclovir plasma concentration. **HERBAL:** None known. **FOOD:** None known. **LAB VALUES:** None known.

AVAILABILITY (Rx)

TABLETS: 125 mg, 250 mg, 500 mg.

ADMINISTRATION/HANDLING

PO

- Give without regard to meals.

INDICATIONS/ROUTES/DOSAGE

HERPES ZOSTER

PO: ADULTS: 500 mg q8h for 7 days.

GENITAL HERPES, FIRST EPISODE

PO: ADULTS, ELDERLY: 250 mg 3 times a day for 7–10 days.

RECURRENT GENITAL HERPES

PO: ADULTS: 125 mg twice a day for 5 days.

SUPPRESSION OF RECURRENT GENITAL HERPES

PO: ADULTS: 250 mg twice a day for up to 1 yr.

RECURRENT HERPES SIMPLEX

PO: ADULTS: 500 mg twice a day for 7 days.

DOSAGE IN RENAL IMPAIRMENT

Dosage and frequency are modified based on creatinine clearance.

Creatinine Clearance	Herpes Zoster	Genital Herpes
40–59 ml/min	500 mg q12h	125 mg q12h
20–39 ml/min	500 mg q24h	125 mg q24h
Less than 20 ml/min	250 mg q24h	125 mg q24h

DOSAGE IN HEMODIALYSIS PATIENTS

For adults with herpes zoster, give 250 mg after each dialysis treatment; for adults with genital herpes, give 125 mg after each dialysis treatment.

✐ see color pill atlas   ⬗ herb   underlined – top prescribed drug

F

SIDE EFFECTS

FREQUENT: Headache (23%), nausea (12%). **OCCASIONAL (10%–2%):** Dizziness, somnolence, numbness of feet, diarrhea, vomiting, constipation, decreased appetite, fatigue, fever, pharyngitis, sinusitis, pruritus. **RARE (less than 2%):** Insomnia, abdominal pain, dyspepsia, flatulence, back pain, arthralgia.

ADVERSE REACTIONS/ TOXIC EFFECTS

Urticaria, hallucinations, and confusion (including delirium, disorientation, confusional state, occurring predominantly in the elderly) have been reported.

NURSING CONSIDERATIONS

INTERVENTION/EVALUATION

Evaluate cutaneous lesions. Be alert to neurologic effects: headache, dizziness. Provide analgesics, comfort measures; especially exhausting in elderly.

PATIENT/FAMILY TEACHING

• Drink adequate fluids. • Fingernails should be kept short, hands clean. • Do not touch lesions with fingers to avoid spreading infection to new site. • **Genital herpes:** Continue therapy for full length of treatment. • Space doses evenly. • Avoid contact with lesions during duration of outbreak to prevent cross-contamination. • Notify physician if lesions recur or do not improve.

famotidine

fah-**mow**-tih-deen

(Novo-Famotidine ♣ Pepcid, Pepcid AC, Ulcidine ♣)

FIXED-COMBINATION(S)

Pepcid Complete: famotidine/calcium chloride/magnesium hydroxide (antacids): 10 mg/800 mg/ 165 mg.

◆CLASSIFICATION

PHARMACOTHERAPEUTIC: H_2 receptor antagonist. **CLINICAL:** Antiulcer, gastric acid secretion inhibitor (see p. 96C).

ACTION

An antiulcer agent and gastric acid secretion inhibitor that inhibits histamine action at histamine 2 receptors of parietal cells. **Therapeutic Effect:** Inhibits gastric acid secretion when fasting, at night, or when stimulated by food, caffeine, or insulin.

PHARMACOKINETICS

Route	Onset	Peak	Duration
PO	1 hr	1–4 hr	10–12 hr
IV	1 hr	0.5–3 hr	10–12 hr

Rapidly, incompletely absorbed from the GI tract. Protein binding: 15%–20%. Partially metabolized in the liver. Primarily excreted in urine. Not removed by hemodialysis. **Half-life:** 2.5–3.5 hr (increased with impaired renal function).

USES

Short-term treatment of active duodenal ulcer. Prevention, maintenance of duodenal ulcer recurrence. Treatment of active benign gastric ulcer, pathologic GI hypersecretory conditions. Short-term treatment of gastroesophageal reflux disease (GERD), including erosive esophagitis. OTC formulation for relief of heartburn, acid indigestion, sour stomach. **OFF-LABEL.** Autism, prevention of aspiration pneumonitis, *H. pylori* eradication

PRECAUTIONS

CONTRAINDICATIONS: None known. **CAUTIONS:** Renal or hepatic impairment.

♣ Canadian trade name   ℮ see **evolve**   ☛ High Alert drug

⧗ **LIFESPAN CONSIDERATIONS: Pregnancy/Lactation:** Unknown if drug crosses placenta or is distributed in breast milk. **Pregnancy Category B. Children:** No age-related precautions noted. **Elderly:** Confusion more likely to occur, especially in those with renal or hepatic impairment.

INTERACTIONS

DRUG: Antacids: May decrease the absorption of famotidine. **Ketoconazole:** May decrease the absorption of ketoconazole. **HERBAL:** None known. **FOOD:** None known. **LAB VALUES:** Interferes with skin tests using allergen extracts. May increase liver enzyme levels.

AVAILABILITY (Rx)

ORAL SUSPENSION (PEPCID): 40 mg/5 ml. **TABLETS:** 10 mg (Pepcid AC [OTC]), 20 mg (Pepcid, Pepcid AC), 40 mg (Pepcid). **TABLETS (CHEWABLE [PEPCID AC]):** 10 mg (OTC). **CAPSULES (PEPCID AC):** 10 mg. **INJECTION (PEPCID):** 10 mg/ml.

ADMINISTRATION/HANDLING
 IV

Reconstitution • For IV push, dilute 20 mg with 5–10 ml 0.9% NaCl, D₅W, D₁₀W, lactated Ringer's, or 5% sodium bicarbonate. • For intermittent infusion (piggyback), dilute with 50–100 ml D₅W, or 0.9% NaCl.

Rate of administration • IV push given over at least 2 min. • Infuse piggyback over 15–30 min.

Storage • Refrigerate unreconstituted vials. • IV solution appears clear, colorless. • After dilution, IV solution is stable for 48 hr at room temperature.

PO
• Store tablets, suspension at room temperature. • Following reconstitution, oral suspension is stable for 30 days at room temperature. • Give without regard to meals. Best given after meals and/or at bedtime. • Shake suspension well before use.

▦ IV INCOMPATIBILITIES
Amphotericin B complex (Abelcet, AmBisome, Amphotec), cefepime (Maxipime), furosemide (Lasix), piperacillin/tazobactam (Zosyn).

IV COMPATIBILITIES

Calcium gluconate, dobutamine (Dobutrex), dopamine (Intropin), heparin, hydromorphone (Dilaudid), insulin (regular), lidocaine, lorazepam (Ativan), magnesium sulfate, midazolam (Versed), morphine, nitroglycerin, norepinephrine (Levophed), potassium chloride, potassium phosphate, propofol (Diprivan), total parenteral nutrition (TPN).

INDICATIONS/ROUTES/DOSAGE
ACUTE TREATMENT OF DUODENAL AND GASTRIC ULCERS
PO: ADULTS, ELDERLY, CHILDREN 12 YR AND OLDER: 40 mg/day at bedtime. CHILDREN 1–11 YR: 0.5 mg/kg/day at bedtime. **Maximum:** 40 mg/day.

DUODENAL ULCER MAINTENANCE
PO: ADULTS, ELDERLY: 20 mg/day at bedtime.

GASTROESOPHAGEAL REFLUX DISEASE
PO: ADULTS, ELDERLY, CHILDREN 12 YR AND OLDER: 20 mg twice a day. CHILDREN 1–11 YR: 1 mg/kg/day in 2 divided doses. CHILDREN 3 MO–11 MO: 0.5 mg/kg/dose twice a day. CHILDREN YOUNGER THAN 3 MO: 0.5 mg/kg/dose once a day.

ESOPHAGITIS
PO: ADULTS, ELDERLY, CHILDREN 12 YR AND OLDER: 2–40 mg twice a day.

HYPERSECRETORY CONDITIONS
PO: ADULTS, ELDERLY, CHILDREN 12 YR AND OLDER: Initially, 20 mg q6h. May increase up to 160 mg q6h.

ACID INDIGESTION, HEARTBURN (OVER-THE-COUNTER)
PO: ADULTS, ELDERLY, CHILDREN 12 YR AND OLDER: 10–20 mg 15–60 min before eating. **Maximum:** 2 doses per day.

USUAL PARENTERAL DOSAGE

IV: ADULTS, ELDERLY, CHILDREN 12 YR AND OLDER: 20 mg q12h.

DOSAGE IN RENAL IMPAIRMENT

Dosing frequency is modified based on creatinine clearance.

Creatinine Clearance	Dosing Frequency
10–50 ml/min	q24h
Less than 10 ml/min	q36–48h

SIDE EFFECTS

OCCASIONAL (5%): Headache. **RARE (2% or less):** Constipation, diarrhea, dizziness.

ADVERSE REACTIONS/ TOXIC EFFECTS

None known.

NURSING CONSIDERATIONS

INTERVENTION/EVALUATION

Assess pattern of daily bowel activity and stool consistency. Monitor for diarrhea and constipation, headache.

PATIENT/FAMILY TEACHING

• May take without regard to meals or antacids. • Report headache. • Avoid excessive amounts of coffee, aspirin. • If symptoms of heartburn, acid indigestion, sour stomach persist with medication, consult physician.

Famvir, *see famciclovir*

Faslodex, *see fulvestrant*

---

felodipine

feh-**low**-dih-peen
(Plendil, Renedil ♣)

Do not confuse Plendil with Pletal, or Renedil with Prinivil.

FIXED-COMBINATION(S)

Lexxel: felodipine/enalapril (angiotensin-converting enzyme [ACE] inhibitor): 2.5 mg/5 mg; 5 mg/5 mg.

✦CLASSIFICATION

PHARMACOTHERAPEUTIC: Calcium channel blocker. **CLINICAL:** Antihypertensive, antianginal (see p. 69C).

ACTION

An antihypertensive and antianginal agent that inhibits calcium movement across cardiac and vascular smooth-muscle cell membranes. Potent peripheral vasodilator (does not depress SA or AV nodes). **Therapeutic Effect:** Increases myocardial contractility, heart rate, and cardiac output; decreases peripheral vascular resistance and BP.

PHARMACOKINETICS

Route	Onset	Peak	Duration
PO	2–5 hr	N/A	N/A

Rapidly, completely absorbed from the GI tract. Protein binding: greater than 99%. Undergoes first-pass metabolism in the liver. Primarily excreted in urine. Not removed by hemodialysis. **Half-life:** 11–16 hr.

USES

Management of hypertension. May be used alone or with other antihypertensives. **OFF-LABEL:** Treatment of CHF, chronic angina pectoris, Raynaud's phenomenon.

PRECAUTIONS

CONTRAINDICATIONS: None known. **CAUTIONS:** Severe left ventricular dysfunction, CHF, hepatic or renal impairment, hypertrophic cardiomyopathy, edema, concomitant administration with beta-blockers/digoxin.

⧗ **LIFESPAN CONSIDERATIONS: Pregnancy/Lactation:** Unknown if drug crosses placenta or is distributed in breast milk. **Pregnancy Category C. Children:** Safety and efficacy not established. **Elderly:** May experience greater hypotension response. Constipation may be more problematic.

INTERACTIONS

DRUG: Beta blockers: May have additive effect. **Digoxin:** May increase digoxin blood concentration. **Erythromycin:** May increase felodipine blood concentration and risk of toxicity. **Hypokalemia-producing agents (such as furosemide and certain other diuretics):** May increase risk of arrhythmias. **Procainamide, quinidine:** May increase risk of QT-interval prolongation. **HERBAL: DHEA:** May increase felodipine blood concentration. **FOOD: Grapefruit, grapefruit juice:** May increase the absorption and blood concentration of felodipine. **LAB VALUES:** None known.

AVAILABILITY (Rx)

TABLETS (EXTENDED-RELEASE): 2.5 mg, 5 mg, 10 mg.

ADMINISTRATION/HANDLING

PO
• Give without regard to food. • Do not crush or break tablets.

INDICATIONS/ROUTES/DOSAGE

HYPERTENSION

PO: ADULTS: Initially, 5 mg/day as single dose. ELDERLY, PATIENTS WITH IMPAIRED HEPATIC FUNCTION: Initially, 2.5 mg/day. Adjust dosage at no less than 2-wk intervals. Maintenance: 2.5–10 mg/day. Range: 2.5–20 mg/day.

SIDE EFFECTS

FREQUENT (22%–18%): Headache, peripheral edema. **OCCASIONAL (6%–4%):** Flushing, respiratory infection, dizziness, light-headedness, asthenia (loss of strength, weakness). **RARE (less than 3%):** Paresthesia, abdominal discomfort, nervousness, muscle cramping, cough, diarrhea, constipation.

ADVERSE REACTIONS/TOXIC EFFECTS

Overdose produces nausea, somnolence, confusion, slurred speech, hypotension, and bradycardia.

NURSING CONSIDERATIONS

BASELINE ASSESSMENT

Assess BP, apical pulse immediately before drug administration (if pulse is 60 or less/min or systolic BP is less than 90 mm Hg, withhold medication, contact physician).

INTERVENTION/EVALUATION

Assist with ambulation if lightheadedness, dizziness occur. Assess for peripheral edema behind media malleolus (sacral area in bedridden patients). Monitor pulse rate for bradycardia. Assess skin for flushing. Monitor hepatic enzyme tests. Question for headache, asthenia.

PATIENT/FAMILY TEACHING

• Do not abruptly discontinue medication. • Compliance with therapy regimen is essential to control hypertension. • To avoid hypotensive effect, rise slowly from lying to sitting position. Wait momentarily before standing. • Avoid tasks that require alertness, motor skills until response to drug is established. • Contact physician or nurse if palpitations, shortness of breath, pronounced dizziness, nausea occurs. • Swallow tablet whole; do not crush or chew. • Avoid grapefruit juice.

fenofibrate

fen-oh-**figh**-brate

(Antara, Apo-Fenofibrate ✤, Lipidil Supra, Lipofen, Lofibra, <u>Tricor</u>, Triglide)

Do not confuse Tricor with Tracleer.

◆CLASSIFICATION

CLINICAL: Antihyperlipidemic (see p. 53C).

ACTION

An antihyperlipidemic that enhances synthesis of lipoprotein lipase and reduces triglyceride-rich lipoproteins and VLDLs. **Therapeutic Effect:** Increases VLDL catabolism and reduces total plasma triglyceride levels.

PHARMACOKINETICS

Well absorbed from the GI tract. Absorption increased when given with food. Protein binding: 99%. Rapidly metabolized in the liver to active metabolite. Excreted primarily in urine; lesser amount in feces. Not removed by hemodialysis. **Half-life:** 20 hr.

USES

Adjunct to diet in treatment of hypertriglyceride levels at risk of pancreatitis. Reduction of low density lipoprotein cholesterol (LDL-C), total cholesterol, triglycerides and apo-lipoprotein B in patients with primary hypercholesterolemia or mixed dyslipidemia.

PRECAUTIONS

CONTRAINDICATIONS: Gallbladder disease, severe renal or hepatic dysfunction (including primary biliary cirrhosis, unexplained persistent liver function abnormality). **CAUTIONS:** Anticoagulant therapy, history of hepatic disease, substantial alcohol consumption.

⧖ **LIFESPAN CONSIDERATIONS: Pregnancy/Lactation:** Safety in pregnancy not established. Avoid use in breastfeeding mothers. **Pregnancy Category C. Children:** Safety and efficacy not established. **Elderly:** No age-related precautions noted.

INTERACTIONS

DRUG: Anticoagulants: Potentiates effects of these drugs. **Bile acid sequestrants:** May impede fenofibrate absorption. **Cyclosporine:** Increases risk of nephrotoxicity. **HMG-CoA reductase inhibitors:** Increases risk of severe myopathy, rhabdomyolysis, and acute renal failure. **HERBAL:** None known. **FOOD: All foods:** Increase absorption of fenofibrate. **LAB VALUES:** May increase BUN and serum creatine kinase (CK), AST, and ALT, levels. May decrease blood Hgb and Hct levels, serum uric acid level, and WBC count.

AVAILABILITY (Rx)

CAPSULES: 43 mg (Antara), 50 mg (Lipofen), 67 mg (Lofibra), 87 mg (Antara), 100 mg (Lipofen), 130 mg (Antara), 134 mg (Lofibra), 150 mg (Lipofen), 200 mg (Lipidil Supra, Lofibra). **TABLETS:** 48 mg (Tricor), 50 mg (Triglide), 54 mg (Lofibra), 145 mg (Tricor), 160 mg (Lofibra, Triglide).

ADMINISTRATION/HANDLING

PO

• Give Lofibra with meals. • Antara, Tricor, and Triglide may be given without regard to food. • Administer fenofibrate preparations 1 hr before or 4–6 hr after giving bile acid sequestrant.

INDICATIONS/ROUTES/DOSAGE

HYPERTRIGLYCERIDEMIA

PO (ANTARA): ADULTS, ELDERLY: 43–130 mg/day.

PO (LOFIBRA): ADULTS, ELDERLY: 67–200 mg/day with meals.
PO (TRICOR): ADULTS, ELDERLY: 48–145 mg/day.
PO (TRIGLIDE): ADULTS, ELDERLY: 50–160 mg/day.

HYPERCHOLESTEROLEMIA
PO (ANTARA): ADULTS, ELDERLY: 130 mg/day.
PO (LOFIBRA): ADULTS, ELDERLY: 200 mg/day with meals.
PO (TRICOR): ADULTS, ELDERLY: 145 mg/day.
PO (TRIGLIDE): ADULTS, ELDERLY: 160 mg/day.

SIDE EFFECTS

FREQUENT (8%–4%): Pain, rash, headache, asthenia or fatigue, flu symptoms, dyspepsia, nausea and vomiting, rhinitis. **OCCASIONAL (3%–2%):** Diarrhea, abdominal pain, constipation, flatulence, arthralgia, decreased libido, dizziness, pruritus. **RARE (less than 2%):** Increased appetite, insomnia, polyuria, cough, blurred vision, eye floaters, earache.

ADVERSE REACTIONS/ TOXIC EFFECTS

Fenofibrate may increase excretion of cholesterol into bile, leading to cholelithiasis. Pancreatitis, hepatitis, thrombocytopenia, and agranulocytosis occur rarely.

NURSING CONSIDERATIONS

BASELINE ASSESSMENT
Obtain serum cholesterol, triglycerides, liver function tests (including ALT), blood counts during initial therapy and periodically during treatment. Treatment should be discontinued if hepatic enzyme levels persist greater than 3 times normal limit.

INTERVENTION/EVALUATION
For patients on concurrent therapy with hydroxamethylglutaryl-CoA (HMG-CoA)

reductase inhibitors, monitor for complaints of myopathy (muscle pain, weakness). Monitor serum CK levels. Monitor serum cholesterol, triglyceride concentrations for therapeutic response.

PATIENT/FAMILY TEACHING
• Take with food. • Inform physician if diarrhea, constipation, nausea becomes severe. • Report skin rash or irritation, insomnia, muscle pain, tremors or dizziness.

fenoldopam

phen-**ole**-doe-pam
(Corlopam)

◆ **CLASSIFICATION**
PHARMACOTHERAPEUTIC: Vasodilator (dopamine receptor agonist). **CLINICAL:** Antihypertensive.

ACTION

A rapid-acting vasodilator. An agonist for D_1-like dopamine receptors; also produces vasodilation in coronary, renal, mesenteric, and peripheral arteries. **Therapeutic Effect:** Reduces systolic and diastolic BP and increases heart rate.

PHARMACOKINETICS

After IV administration, metabolized in the liver. Primarily excreted in urine. Unknown if removed by hemodialysis. **Half-life:** Approximately 5 min.

USES

Short-term (48 hr or less) management of severe hypertension when rapid, but quickly reversible, emergency reduction of BP is clinically indicated, including malignant hypertension with deteriorating end-organ function.

OFF-LABEL: Prevention of contrast media-induced nephrotoxicity.

PRECAUTIONS

CONTRAINDICATIONS: Sensitivity to sulfites. **CAUTIONS:** Glaucoma, intraocular hypertension, tachycardia, hypotension, hypokalemia, sulfite sensitivity.

 LIFESPAN CONSIDERATIONS: Pregnancy/Lactation: Unknown if distributed in breast milk. **Pregnancy Category B. Children:** Safety and efficacy not established. **Elderly:** No age-related precautions noted.

INTERACTIONS

DRUG: Beta blockers: May produce excessive hypotension. **HERBAL:** None known. **FOOD:** None known. **LAB VALUES:** May elevate BUN, blood glucose, serum LDH, and serum transaminase levels. May decrease serum potassium levels.

AVAILABILITY (Rx)

INJECTION: 10 mg/ml.

ADMINISTRATION/HANDLING

◄ **ALERT** ► Must give by continuous IV infusion, not as a bolus injection.

IV

Reconstitution • Each 10 mg (1 ml) must be diluted with 250 ml 0.9% NaCl or D_5W to provide a concentration of 40 mcg/ml.

Rate of administration • Administer as IV infusion at initial rate of 0.1 mcg/kg/min. • Use infusion pump.

Storage • Store ampules at room temperature. • Diluted solution is stable for 24 hr. Discard any solution not used within 24 hr.

▦ IV INCOMPATIBILITIES

Do not mix fenoldopam with other medications. Specific IV incompatibilities are not available.

INDICATIONS/ROUTES/DOSAGE

SHORT-TERM MANAGEMENT OF SEVERE HYPERTENSION WHEN RAPID, BUT QUICKLY REVERSIBLE EMERGENCY REDUCTION OF BP IS CLINICALLY INDICATED, INCLUDING MALIGNANT HYPERTENSION WITH DETERIORATING END-ORGAN FUNCTION

IV INFUSION (CONTINUOUS): ADULTS, ELDERLY: Initially, 0.1 mcg/kg/min. May increase in increments of 0.05–0.1 mcg/kg/min until target BP is achieved. Usual length of treatment is 1–6 hr with tapering of dose q15–30min. Average rate: 0.25–0.5 mcg/kg/min. **Maximum rate:** 1.6 mcg/kg/min. CHILDREN: Initially, 0.2 mcg/kg/min. May increase increments of 0.3–0.5 mcg/kg/min q20–30min. Dosage greater than 0.8 mcg/kg/min have resulted in tachycardia with no additional benefit.

SIDE EFFECTS

EXPECTED: Beta blockers may cause unforeseen hypotension. **OCCASIONAL:** Headache (7%), flushing (3%), nausea (4%), hypotension (2%). **RARE (2% or less):** Nervousness or anxiety, vomiting, constipation, nasal congestion, diaphoresis, back pain.

ADVERSE REACTIONS/ TOXIC EFFECTS

Excessive hypotension occurs occasionally. Substantial tachycardia may lead to ischemic cardiac events or worsened heart failure. Allergic-type reactions, including anaphylaxis and life-threatening asthmatic exacerbation, may occur in patients with sulfite sensitivity.

NURSING CONSIDERATIONS

BASELINE ASSESSMENT

Determine initial BP, apical pulse. It is essential to diligently monitor BP, EKG during infusion to avoid hypotension and too rapid decrease of BP. Assess medication history (especially beta-blockers). Obtain baseline serum electrolytes, particularly potassium, and periodically thereafter during infusion. Question asthmatic patients for history of sulfite sensitivity. Check with physician for desired BP range parameters.

INTERVENTION/EVALUATION

Monitor rate of infusion frequently. Monitor EKG for tachycardia (may lead to ischemic heart disease, MI, angina, extrasystoles, worsening heart failure). Monitor closely for symptomatic hypotension.

---

fenoprofen calcium

fen-oh-**proe**-fen
(Nalfon)

Do not confuse Nalfon with Naldecon.

◆CLASSIFICATION

PHARMACOTHERAPEUTIC: NSAID. **CLINICAL:** Nonsteroidal anti-inflammatory, analgesic, antigout, vascular headache prophylactic/suppressant (see p. 116C).

ACTION

An NSAID that produces analgesic and anti-inflammatory effects by inhibiting prostaglandin synthesis. Therapeutic Effect: Reduces the inflammatory response and intensity of pain.

PHARMACOKINETICS

Rapidly absorbed following PO administration. Protein binding: 99%. Metabolized in liver. Primarily excreted in urine; small amount excreted in feces. Half-life: 3 hr.

USES

Treatment of acute or long-term mild to moderate pain, symptomatic treatment of acute and/or chronic rheumatoid arthritis, osteoarthritis.

OFF-LABEL: Treatment of ankylosing spondylitis, psoriatic arthritis, vascular headaches.

PRECAUTIONS

CONTRAINDICATIONS: Active peptic ulcer disease, chronic inflammation of GI tract, GI bleeding or ulceration, history of hypersensitivity to aspirin or NSAIDs, significant renal impairment. **CAUTIONS:** Renal or hepatic impairment, history of GI tract diseases, predisposition to fluid retention.

⧗ **LIFESPAN CONSIDERATIONS: Pregnancy/Lactation:** Crosses placenta; distributed in breast milk. **Pregnancy Category B (D if used in third trimester or near delivery). Children:** Safety and efficacy not established. **Elderly:** Age-related renal, hepatic impairment may increase risk of hepatotoxicity, renal toxicity.

INTERACTIONS

DRUG: Antihypertensives, diuretics: May decrease the effects of these drugs. **Aspirin, other salicylates:** May increase the risk of GI side effects such as bleeding. **Bone marrow depressants:** May increase the risk of hematologic reactions. **Heparin, oral anticoagulants, thrombolytics:** May increase the effects of these drugs. **Lithium:** May increase the blood concentration and risk of toxicity of lithium. **Methotrexate:** May increase the risk of methotrexate toxicity. **Probenecid:** May increase fenoprofen blood concentration. **HERBAL:** None known. **FOOD:** None known. **LAB VALUES:** May increase bleeding time, BUN and blood glucose levels, and serum protein, alkaline phosphatase, LDH, creatinine, AST, and ALT levels.

AVAILABILITY (Rx)

CAPSULES: 200 mg, 300 mg. **TABLETS:** 600 mg.

✎ see color pill atlas   ⬥ herb   <u>underlined</u> – top prescribed drug

ADMINISTRATION/HANDLING

PO
◄ **ALERT** ▶ Don't exceed a fenoprofen dosage of 3.2 g a day, as prescribed. Do not crush, open, or break capsules.

INDICATIONS/ROUTES/DOSAGE

MILD TO MODERATE PAIN
PO: ADULTS, ELDERLY: 200 mg q4–6h as needed.

RHEUMATOID ARTHRITIS, OSTEOARTHRITIS
PO: ADULTS, ELDERLY: 300–600 mg 3–4 times a day.

SIDE EFFECTS

FREQUENT (9%–3%): Headache, somnolence, dyspepsia, nausea, vomiting, constipation. **OCCASIONAL (2%–1%):** Dizziness, pruritus, nervousness, asthenia, diarrhea, abdominal cramps, flatulence, tinnitus, blurred vision, peripheral edema and fluid retention.

ADVERSE REACTIONS/ TOXIC EFFECTS

Overdose may result in acute hypotension and tachycardia. Rare reactions with long-term use include peptic ulcer disease, GI bleeding, gastritis, severe hepatic reaction (jaundice), nephrotoxicity (hematuria, dysuria, proteinuria), and a severe hypersensitivity reaction (bronchospasm, angioedema).

NURSING CONSIDERATIONS

BASELINE ASSESSMENT
Assess onset, type, location, duration of pain or inflammation. Inspect appearance of affected joints for immobility, deformities, skin condition.

INTERVENTION/EVALUATION
Assist with ambulation if somnolence, drowsiness or dizziness occurs. Monitor for evidence of dyspepsia. Monitor pattern of daily bowel activity and stool consistency. Check behind medial malleolus for fluid retention (usually first area noted). Evaluate for therapeutic response: relief of pain, stiffness, swelling; increased joint mobility; reduced joint tenderness; improved grip strength.

PATIENT/FAMILY TEACHING
• Swallow capsule whole; do not crush or chew. • Avoid tasks that require alertness, motor skills until response to drug is established. • If GI upset occurs, take with food, milk. • Avoid aspirin, alcohol during therapy (increases risk of GI bleeding).

---

fentanyl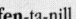

fen-ta-nill

(Actiq, <u>Duragesic</u>, Sublimaze)

Do not confuse fentanyl with alfentanil.

✦CLASSIFICATION

PHARMACOTHERAPEUTIC: Opioid, narcotic agonist **(Schedule II)**. **CLINICAL:** Analgesic (see p. 128C).

ACTION

An opioid agonist that binds to opioid receptors in the CNS, reducing stimuli from sensory nerve endings and inhibiting ascending pain pathways. **Therapeutic Effect:** Alters pain reception and increases the pain threshold.

PHARMACOKINETICS

Route	Onset	Peak	Duration
IV	1–2 min	3–5 min	0.5–1 hr
IM	7–15 min	20–30 min	1–2 hr
Transdermal	6–8 hr	24 hr	72 hr
Transmucosal	5–15 min	20–30 min	1–2 hr

Well absorbed after IM or topical administration. Transmucosal form absorbed through the buccal mucosa and GI

---

tract. Protein binding: 80%–85%. Metabolized in the liver. Primarily eliminated by biliary system. **Half-life:** 2–4 hr IV; 17 hr transdermal; 6.6 hr transmucosal.

USES

For sedation, pain relief, preop medication; adjunct to general or regional anesthesia. Management of chronic pain *(transdermal)*. **Actiq:** Treatment breakthrough for pain in chronic cancer or AIDS-related pain.

PRECAUTIONS

CONTRAINDICATIONS: Increased intracranial pressure, severe hepatic or renal impairment, severe respiratory depression. **CAUTIONS:** Bradycardia; renal, hepatic, respiratory disease; head injuries; altered level of consciousness (LOC); use of MAOI within 14 days; transdermal not recommended in those younger than 12 yr or younger than 18 yr and weighing less than 50 kg.

⚖ **LIFESPAN CONSIDERATIONS: Pregnancy/Lactation:** Readily crosses placenta. Unknown if distributed in breast milk. May prolong labor if administered in latent phase of first stage of labor or before cervical dilation of 4–5 cm has occurred. Respiratory depression may occur in neonate if mother received opiates during labor. **Pregnancy Category C (D if used for prolonged periods or at high dosages at term). Children:** PATCH: Safety and efficacy not established in those younger than 12 yr. Neonates more susceptible to respiratory depressant effects. **Elderly:** May be more susceptible to respiratory depressant effects. Age-related renal impairment may require dosage adjustment.

INTERACTIONS

DRUG: Benzodiazepines, CNS depressants: May increase the risk of hypotension and respiratory depression.

Buprenorphine: May decrease the effects of fentanyl. **HERBAL:** None known. **FOOD:** None known. **LAB VALUES:** May increase serum amylase and lipase concentrations.

AVAILABILITY (Rx)

INJECTION (SUBLIMAZE): 50 mcg/ml. **TRANSDERMAL PATCH (DURAGESIC):** 12 mcg/hr, 25 mcg/hr, 50 mcg/hr, 75 mcg/hr, 100 mcg/hr. **TRANSMUCOSAL LOZENGES (ACTIQ):** 200 mcg, 400 mcg, 600 mcg, 800 mcg, 1,200 mcg, 1,600 mcg.

ADMINISTRATION/HANDLING

 IV

Rate of administration • For initial anesthesia induction dosage, give small amount, via tuberculin syringe. • Give by slow IV injection (over 1–2 min). • Too rapid IV increases risk of severe adverse reactions (skeletal, thoracic muscle rigidity resulting in apnea, laryngospasm, bronchospasm, peripheral circulatory collapse, anaphylactoid effects, cardiac arrest). • Opiate antagonist (naloxone) should be readily available.

TRANSDERMAL

• Apply to nonhairy area of intact skin of upper torso. • Use flat, nonirritated site. • Firmly press evenly for 10–20 sec, ensuring adhesion is in full contact with skin and edges are completely sealed. • Use only water to cleanse site before application (soaps, oils, etc., may irritate skin). • Rotate sites of application. • Carefully fold used patches so that system adheres to itself; discard in toilet.

TRANSMUCOSAL

• Suck lozenge vigorously.

Storage • Store parenteral form at room temperature.

⚜ **IV INCOMPATIBILITY**
Phenytoin (Dilantin).

IV COMPATIBILITIES

Atropine, bupivacaine (Marcaine, Sensorcaine), clonidine (Duraclon), diltiazem (Cardizem), diphenhydramine (Benadryl), dobutamine (Dobutrex), dopamine (Intropin), droperidol (Inapsine), heparin, hydromorphone (Dilaudid), ketorolac (Toradol), lorazepam (Ativan), metoclopramide (Reglan), midazolam (Versed), milrinone (Primacor), morphine, nitroglycerin, norepinephrine (Levophed), ondansetron (Zofran), potassium chloride, propofol (Diprivan).

INDICATIONS/ROUTES/DOSAGE

SEDATION IN MINOR PROCEDURES, ANALGESIA

IV, IM: ADULTS, ELDERLY, CHILDREN 12 YR AND OLDER: 0.5–1 mcg/kg/dose; may repeat in 30–60 min. CHILDREN 1–11 YR: 1–2 mcg/kg/dose. CHILDREN YOUNGER THAN 1 YR: 1–4 mcg/kg/dose.

PREOPERATIVE SEDATION, POSTOPERATIVE PAIN, ADJUNCT TO REGIONAL ANESTHESIA

IV, IM: ADULTS, ELDERLY, CHILDREN 12 YR AND OLDER: 50–100 mcg/dose.

ADJUNCT TO GENERAL ANESTHESIA

IV: ADULTS, ELDERLY, CHILDREN 12 YR AND OLDER: 2–50 mcg/kg.

USUAL TRANSDERMAL DOSE

ADULTS, ELDERLY, CHILDREN 12 YR AND OLDER: Initially, 25 mcg/hr. May increase after 3 days.

USUAL TRANSMUCOSAL DOSE

ADULTS, CHILDREN: 200–400 mcg for breakthrough cancer pain.

USUAL EPIDURAL DOSE

ADULTS, ELDERLY: Bolus dose of 100 mcg, followed by continuous infusion of 10 mcg/ml concentration at 4–12 ml/hr.

CONTINUOUS ANALGESIA

IV: ADULTS, ELDERLY, CHILDREN 1–12 YR: Bolus dose of 1–2 mcg/kg, followed by continuous infusion of 1 mcg/kg/hr. Range: 1–5 mcg/kg/hr. CHILDREN YOUNGER THAN 1 YR: Bolus dose of 1–2 mcg/kg, followed by continuous infusion of 0.5–1 mcg/kg/hr.

DOSAGE IN RENAL IMPAIRMENT

Dosage is modified based on creatinine clearance.

Creatinine Clearance	Dosage
10–50 ml/min	75% of usual dose
Less than 10 ml/min	50% of usual dose

SIDE EFFECTS

FREQUENT: IV: Postoperative drowsiness, nausea, vomiting. **Transdermal (10%–3%):** Headache, pruritus, nausea, vomiting, diaphoresis, dyspnea, confusion, dizziness, somnolence, diarrhea, constipation, decreased appetite. **OCCASIONAL: IV:** Postoperative confusion, blurred vision, chills, orthostatic hypotension, constipation, difficulty urinating. **Transdermal (3%–1%):** Chest pain, arrhythmias, erythema, pruritus, swelling of skin, syncope, agitation, tingling or burning of skin.

ADVERSE REACTIONS/ TOXIC EFFECTS

Overdose or too rapid IV administration may produce severe respiratory depression and skeletal and thoracic muscle rigidity (which may lead to apnea), laryngospasm, bronchospasm, cold and clammy skin, cyanosis, and coma. The patient who uses fentanyl repeatedly may develop a tolerance to the drug's analgesic effect.

NURSING CONSIDERATIONS

BASELINE ASSESSMENT

Resuscitative equipment, opiate antagonist (naloxone 0.5 mcg/kg) must be available. Establish baseline BP, respirations. Assess type, location, intensity, duration of pain.

INTERVENTION/EVALUATION

Assist with ambulation. Encourage patient to turn, cough, deep breathe q2h. Monitor respiratory rate, BP, heart rate, oxygen saturation. Assess for relief of pain.

PATIENT/FAMILY TEACHING

• Avoid alcohol; do not take other medications without consulting physician. • Do not perform activities requiring alertness, coordination. • Teach patient proper transdermal application. • Use as directed to avoid overdosage; potential for physical dependence with prolonged use. • After long-term use, must be discontinued slowly.

Feosol, *see ferrous sulfate*

Fergon, *see ferrous gluconate*

Fer-In-Sol, *see ferrous sulfate*

Ferrlicit, *see sodium ferric gluconate complex*

---

ferrous fumarate

fair-us **fume**-ah-rate
(Femiron, Feostat, Ferro-Sequels, Nephro-Fer, Palafer ✤)

ferrous gluconate

fair-us **glue**-kuh-nate
(Apo-Ferrous Gluconate ✤, Fergon)

ferrous sulfate

fair-us **sul**-fate
(Apo-Ferrous Sulfate ✤, Fer-In-Sol, Fer-Iron, Slow-Fe)

FIXED-COMBINATION(S)

Ferro-Sequels: ferrous fumarate/docusate (stool softener): 150 mg/100 mg.

CLASSIFICATION

PHARMACOTHERAPEUTIC: Enzymatic mineral. **CLINICAL:** Iron preparation (see p. 97C).

ACTION

An enzymatic mineral that is as an essential component in the formation of Hgb, myoglobin, and enzymes. Promotes effective erythropoiesis and transport and utilization of oxygen (O_2). **Therapeutic Effect:** Prevents iron deficiency.

PHARMACOKINETICS

Absorbed in the duodenum and upper jejunum. Ten percent absorbed in patients with normal iron stores; increased to 20%–30% in those with inadequate iron stores. Primarily bound to serum transferrin. Excreted in urine, sweat, and sloughing of intestinal mucosa and by menses. **Half-life:** 6 hr.

USES

Prevention and treatment of iron deficiency anemia due to inadequate diet, malabsorption, pregnancy, blood loss.

PRECAUTIONS

CONTRAINDICATIONS: Hemochromatosis, hemosiderosis, hemolytic anemias, peptic ulcer disease, regional enteritis, ulcerative colitis. **CAUTIONS:** Bronchial asthma, iron hypersensitivity, alcoholism, intestinal tract inflammation, hepatic or renal impairment.

⧖ **LIFESPAN CONSIDERATIONS: Pregnancy/Lactation:** Crosses placenta. Excreted in breast milk. **Pregnancy Category A. Children/Elderly:** No age-related precautions noted.

INTERACTIONS

DRUG: Antacids, calcium supplements, pancreatin, pancrelipase: May decrease the absorption of ferrous fumarate, ferrous gluconate, and ferrous sulfate. **Etidronate, quinolones, tetracyclines:** May decrease the absorption of etidronate, quinolones, and tetracyclines. **HERBAL:** None known. **FOOD: Eggs, milk:** Inhibit ferrous fumarate absorption. **LAB VALUES:** May increase serum bilirubin and iron levels. May decrease serum calcium level. May obscure occult blood in stools.

AVAILABILITY (OTC)

FERROUS FUMARATE
TABLETS: 63 mg (20 mg elemental iron) (Femiron), 350 mg (115 mg elemental iron) (Nephro-Fer). **TABLETS (CHEWABLE [FEOSTAT]):** 100 mg (33 mg elemental iron). **TABLETS (TIME-RELEASE [FERRO-SEQUELS]):** 150 mg (50 mg elemental iron).
FERROUS GLUCONATE
TABLETS: 240 mg (27 mg elemental iron) (Fergon), 325 mg (36 mg elemental iron).
FERROUS SULFATE
TABLETS: 325 mg (65 mg elemental iron). **TABLETS (TIMED-RELEASE [SLOW-FE]):** 160 mg (50 mg elemental iron). **ELIXIR:** 220 mg/5 ml (44 mg elemental iron per 5 ml). **ORAL DROPS (FER-IN-SOL, FER-IRON):** 75 mg/0.6 ml.

ADMINISTRATION/HANDLING
PO
• Store all forms (tablets, capsules, suspension, drops) at room temperature. • Ideally, give between meals with water but may give with meals if GI discomfort occurs. • Transient staining of mucous membranes, teeth occurs with liquid iron preparation. To avoid this, place liquid on back of tongue with dropper or straw. • Avoid simultaneous administration of antacids or tetracycline. • Do not crush sustained-release preparations.

INDICATIONS/ROUTES/DOSAGE
IRON DEFICIENCY ANEMIA
Dosage is expressed in terms of milligrams of elemental iron, degree of anemia, patient weight, and presence of any bleeding. Expect to use periodic hematologic determinations as guide to therapy.
PO (FERROUS FUMARATE): ADULTS, ELDERLY: 60–100 mg twice a day. CHILDREN: 3–6 mg/kg/day in 2–3 divided doses.
PO (FERROUS GLUCONATE): ADULTS, ELDERLY: 60 mg 2–4 times a day. CHILDREN: 3–6 mg/kg/day in 2–3 divided doses.
PO (FERROUS SULFATE): ADULTS, ELDERLY: 325 mg 2–4 times a day. CHILDREN: 3–6 mg/kg/day in 2–3 divided doses.

PREVENTION OF IRON DEFICIENCY
PO (FERROUS FUMARATE): ADULTS, ELDERLY: 60–100 mg/day. CHILDREN: 1–2 mg/kg/day.
PO (FERROUS GLUCONATE): ADULTS, ELDERLY: 60 mg/day. CHILDREN: 1–2 mg/kg/day.
PO (FERROUS SULFATE): ADULTS, ELDERLY: 325 mg/day. CHILDREN: 1–2 mg/kg/day.

SIDE EFFECTS
OCCASIONAL: Mild, transient nausea. **RARE:** Heartburn, anorexia, constipation, diarrhea.

ADVERSE REACTIONS/ TOXIC EFFECTS
Large doses may aggravate existing GI tract disease, such as peptic ulcer disease, regional enteritis, and ulcerative colitis. Severe iron poisoning occurs

F

most often in children and is manifested as vomiting, severe abdominal pain, diarrhea, and dehydration, followed by hyperventilation, pallor or cyanosis, and cardiovascular collapse.

NURSING CONSIDERATIONS

BASELINE ASSESSMENT

To prevent mucous membrane and teeth staining with liquid preparation, use dropper or straw and allow solution to drop on back of tongue. Eggs, milk inhibit absorption.

INTERVENTION/EVALUATION

Monitor serum iron, total iron-binding capacity, reticulocyte count, Hgb, ferritin. Monitor daily pattern of bowel activity and stool consistency. Assess for clinical improvement, record relief of iron deficiency symptoms (fatigue, irritability, pallor, paresthesia of extremities, headache).

PATIENT/FAMILY TEACHING

• Expect stool color to darken. • If GI discomfort occurs, take after meals or with food. • Do not take within 2 hr of antacids (prevents absorption).

---

feverfew

Also known as bachelor's button, featherfew, midsummer daisy, Santa maria.

◆CLASSIFICATION

HERBAL: See Appendix G.

ACTION

Exact mechanism unknown. May inhibit platelet aggregation, serotonin release from platelets, leukocytes. Also inhibits/blocks prostaglandin synthesis. **Effect:** Reduces pain intensity, vomiting, noise sensitivity with severe migraine headaches.

USES

Fever, headache, prevention of migraine and menstrual irregularities, arthritis, psoriasis, allergies, asthma, vertigo.

PRECAUTIONS

CONTRAINDICATIONS: Pregnancy/lactation (may cause uterine contraction/abortion). Allergies to ragweed, chrysanthemums, marigolds, daisies. **CAUTIONS:** None known.

⧗ **LIFESPAN CONSIDERATIONS: Pregnancy/Lactation:** Contraindicated. **Children:** Safety and efficacy not established; avoid use. **Elderly:** No age-related precautions noted.

INTERACTIONS

DRUG: Anticoagulants, antiplatelets: May increase risk of bleeding. **NSAIDs:** May decrease effectiveness of feverfew. **HERBAL: Garlic, ginger, ginkgo:** May increase risk of bleeding. **FOOD:** None known. **LAB VALUES:** None known.

AVAILABILITY (Rx)

CAPSULES: 100 mg. **FEVERFEW LEAF:** 380 mg.

INDICATIONS/ROUTES/DOSAGE

MIGRAINE HEADACHE

PO: ADULTS, ELDERLY: 50–100 mg extract a day. **Leaf:** 50–125 mg a day.

SIDE EFFECTS

ORAL: Abdominal pain, muscle stiffness, pain, indigestion, diarrhea, flatulence, nausea, vomiting. **Chewing Leaf:** Mouth ulceration, inflammation of oral mucosa and tongue, swelling of lips, loss of taste.

ADVERSE REACTIONS/ TOXIC EFFECTS

Hypersensitivity reaction.

✐ see color pill atlas   ✐ herb   <u>underlined</u> – top prescribed drug

NURSING CONSIDERATIONS

BASELINE ASSESSMENT
Assess if patient is pregnant or breast-feeding (contraindicated).

INTERVENTION/EVALUATION
Assess for hypersensitivity reaction, mouth ulcers, muscle/joint pain.

PATIENT/FAMILY TEACHING
• Do not use during pregnancy or lactation. • Avoid use in children.

---

fexofenadine hydrochloride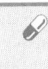

fex-**oh**-fen-eh-deen
(Allegra)

FIXED-COMBINATION(S)
Allegra D 12 Hour: fexofenadine/pseudoephedrine (sympathomimetic): 60 mg/120 mg. **Allegra-D 24 Hour:** 180 mg/240 mg.

◆CLASSIFICATION
PHARMACOTHERAPEUTIC: Piperidine. **CLINICAL:** Antihistamine (see p. 50C).

ACTION
A piperidine that competes with histamine for H_1-receptor sites on effector cells. **Therapeutic Effect:** Relieves allergic rhinitis symptoms.

PHARMACOKINETICS
Rapidly absorbed after PO administration. Protein binding: 60%–70%. Does not cross the blood-brain barrier. Minimally metabolized. Eliminated in feces and urine. Not removed by hemodialysis. **Half-life:** 14.4 hr (increased in renal impairment).

USES
Relief of seasonal allergic rhinitis, chronic idiopathic urticaria.

PRECAUTIONS
CONTRAINDICATIONS: None known. **CAUTIONS:** Severe renal impairment.
⧗ **LIFESPAN CONSIDERATIONS: Pregnancy/Lactation:** Unknown if drug crosses placenta or is distributed in breast milk. **Pregnancy Category C. Children:** Safety and efficacy not established in those younger than 12 yr. **Elderly:** No age-related precautions noted.

INTERACTIONS
DRUG: Antacids: May decrease fexofenadine absorption if given within 15 min of a fexofenadine dose. **HERBAL:** None known. **FOOD:** None known. **LAB VALUES:** May suppress wheal and flare reactions to antigen skin testing unless drug is discontinued at least 4 days before testing.

AVAILABILITY (Rx)
TABLETS: 30 mg, 60 mg, 180 mg.

ADMINISTRATION/HANDLING
PO
• Give without regard to food.

INDICATIONS/ROUTES/DOSAGE
ALLERGIC RHINITIS, URTICARIA
PO: ADULTS, ELDERLY, CHILDREN 12 YR AND OLDER: 60 mg twice a day or 180 mg once a day. CHILDREN 6–11 YR: 30 mg twice a day.

DOSAGE IN RENAL IMPAIRMENT
For adults, elderly, and children 12 yr and older, dosage is reduced to 60 mg once a day. For children 6–11 yr, dosage is reduced to 30 mg once a day.

SIDE EFFECTS
RARE (less than 2%): Somnolence, headache, fatigue, nausea, vomiting, abdominal distress, dysmenorrhea.

ADVERSE REACTIONS/ TOXIC EFFECTS

In rare cases, hypersensitivity reactions including rash, urticaria, pruritus, with manifestations characterized as angioedema, chest tightness, dyspnea, flushing, and systemic anaphylaxis have been reported.

NURSING CONSIDERATIONS

BASELINE ASSESSMENT

If patient is having an allergic reaction, obtain history of recently ingested foods, drugs, environmental exposure, emotional stress. Monitor rate, depth, rhythm, type of respiration; quality, rate of pulse. Assess lung sounds for rhonchi, wheezing, rales.

INTERVENTION/EVALUATION

Assess for therapeutic response; relief from allergy: itching, red, watery eyes, rhinorrhea, sneezing.

PATIENT/FAMILY TEACHING

• Avoid tasks that require alertness, motor skills until response to drug is established. • Avoid alcohol during antihistamine therapy. • Coffee, tea may help reduce drowsiness.

---

filgrastim

fill-**grass**-tim

(Neupogen)

Do not confuse Neupogen with Epogen or Nutramigen.

◆CLASSIFICATION

PHARMACOTHERAPEUTIC: Biologic modifier. **CLINICAL:** Granulocyte colony-stimulating factor (GCSF).

ACTION

A biologic modifier that stimulates production, maturation, and activation of neutrophils to increase their migration and cytotoxicity. **Therapeutic Effect:** Decreases incidence of infection.

PHARMACOKINETICS

Readily absorbed after subcutaneous administration. Not removed by hemodialysis. **Half-life:** 3.5 hr.

USES

Decrease infection incidence in patients with malignancies receiving myelosuppressive therapy associated with severe neutropenia, fever. Reduce neutropenia duration (and sequelae) in patient with nonmyeloid malignancies having myeloablative therapy followed by bone marrow transplant (BMT). Mobilization of hematopoietic progenitor cells into peripheral blood for collection by leukapheresis. Treatment of chronic, severe neutropenia. **OFF-LABEL:** Treatment of AIDS-related neutropenia, drug-induced neutropenia, myelodysplastic syndrome.

PRECAUTIONS

CONTRAINDICATIONS: Hypersensitivity to *Escherichia coli*–derived proteins, 24 hr before or after cytotoxic chemotherapy, concurrent use of other drugs that may result in lowered platelet count. **CAUTIONS:** Malignancy with myeloid characteristics due to a GCSF's potential to act as a growth factor; gout, psoriasis, preexisting cardiac conditions; those taking lithium.

⏳ **LIFESPAN CONSIDERATIONS: Pregnancy/Lactation:** Unknown if drug crosses placenta or is distributed in breast milk. **Pregnancy Category C. Children/Elderly:** No age-related precautions noted.

INTERACTIONS

DRUG: None known. **HERBAL:** None known. **FOOD:** None known. **LAB VALUES:** May increase LDH concentrations, leukocyte alkaline phosphatase

---

(LAP) scores, and serum alkaline phosphatase and uric acid levels.

AVAILABILITY (Rx)

INJECTION: 300 mcg/ml, 480 mcg/ 0.8 ml, 600 mcg/ml.

ADMINISTRATION/HANDLING

◀ **ALERT** ▶ May be given by subcutaneous injection, short IV infusion (15–30 min), or continuous IV infusion.

Reconstitution • Use single-dose vial, do not reenter vial. Do not shake. • Dilute with 10–50 ml D_5W to concentration of 15 mcg/ml or greater. For concentration from 5–14 mcg/ml, add 2 ml of 5% albumin to each 50 ml D_5W to provide a final concentration of 2 mg/ml. Do not dilute to a final concentration of less than 5 mcg/ml.

Rate of administration • For intermittent infusion (piggyback), infuse over 15–30 min. • For continuous infusion, give single dose over 4–24 hr. • In all situations, flush IV line with D_5W before and after administration.

Storage • Refrigerate vials. • Stable for up to 24 hr at room temperature (provided vial contents are clear and contain no particulate matter). Remains stable if accidentally exposed to freezing temperature.

SUBCUTANEOUS

Storage • Store in refrigerator, but remove before use and allow to warm to room temperature. • Aspirate syringe before injection (avoid intra-arterial administration).

▓ IV INCOMPATIBILITIES

Amphotericin (Fungizone), cefepime (Maxipime), cefotaxime (Claforan), cefoxitin (Mefoxin), ceftizoxime (Cefizox), ceftriaxone (Rocephin), cefuroxime (Zinacef), clindamycin (Cleocin), dactinomycin (Cosmegen), etoposide (VePesid), fluorouracil, furosemide (Lasix),

heparin, mannitol, methylprednisolone (Solu-Medrol), mitomycin (Mutamycin), prochlorperazine (Compazine), total parenteral nutrition (TPN).

IV COMPATIBILITIES

Bumetanide (Bumex), calcium gluconate, hydromorphone (Dilaudid), lorazepam (Ativan), morphine, potassium chloride.

INDICATIONS/ROUTES/DOSAGE

MYELOSUPPRESSION

IV OR SUBCUTANEOUS INFUSION, SUBCUTANEOUS INJECTION: ADULTS, ELDERLY: Initially, 5 mcg/ kg/day. May increase by 5 mcg/ kg for each chemotherapy cycle based on duration or severity of absolute neutrophil count nadir.

BONE MARROW TRANSPLANT

IV OR SUBCUTANEOUS INFUSION: ADULTS, ELDERLY, CHILDREN: 5–10 mcg/kg/ day. Adjust dosage daily during period of neutrophil recovery based on neutrophil response.

MOBILIZATION PROGENITOR CELLS

IV OR SUBCUTANEOUS INFUSION: ADULTS: 10 mcg/kg/day beginning at least 4 days before first leukapheresis and continuing until last leukapheresis.

CHRONIC NEUTROPENIA, CONGENITAL NEUTROPENIA

SUBCUTANEOUS: ADULTS, CHILDREN: 6 mcg/kg/dose twice a day.

IDIOPATHIC OR CYCLIC NEUTROPENIA

SUBCUTANEOUS: ADULTS, CHILDREN: 5 mcg/kg/dose once a day.

SIDE EFFECTS

FREQUENT: Nausea or vomiting (57%), mild to severe bone pain (22%) that occurs more frequently with high-dose IV form less frequently with low-dose subcutaneous form; alopecia (18%), diarrhea (14%), fever (12%), fatigue (11%). **OCCASIONAL (9%–5%):** Anorexia, dyspnea, headache, cough, rash.

RARE (less than 5%): Psoriasis, hematuria or proteinuria, osteoporosis.

ADVERSE REACTIONS/ TOXIC EFFECTS

Long-term administration occasionally produces chronic neutropenia and splenomegaly. Thrombocytopenia, MI, and arrhythmias occur rarely. Adult respiratory distress syndrome may occur in patients with sepsis.

NURSING CONSIDERATIONS

BASELINE ASSESSMENT

CBC, platelet count (differential) should be obtained before therapy initiation and twice weekly thereafter.

INTERVENTION/EVALUATION

In septic patients, be alert to adult respiratory distress syndrome. Closely monitor those with preexisting cardiac conditions. Monitor BP (transient decrease in BP may occur), temperature, CBC with differential, platelet count, Hct, serum uric acid, liver function tests.

PATIENT/FAMILY TEACHING

• Inform physician of fever, chills, severe bone pain, chest pain, palpitations.

---

finasteride

fin-**ah**-stir-eyd

(Propecia, <u>Proscar</u>)

Do not confuse Proscar with Posicor, ProSom, Prozac, or Psorcon.

◆CLASSIFICATION

PHARMACOTHERAPEUTIC: Androgen hormone inhibitor. **CLINICAL:** Benign prostatic hyperplasia agent.

ACTION

An androgen hormone inhibitor that inhibits 5-alpha reductase, an intracellular enzyme that converts testosterone into dihydrotestosterone (DHT) in the prostate gland, resulting in a decreased serum DHT level. **Therapeutic Effect:** Reduces size of the prostate gland.

PHARMACOKINETICS

Route	Onset	Peak	Duration
PO	24 hr	1–2 days	5–7 days

Rapidly absorbed from the GI tract. Protein binding: 90%. Widely distributed. Metabolized in the liver. **Half-life:** 6–8 hr. Onset of clinical effect: 3–6 mo of continued therapy.

USES

Proscar reduces risk of acute urinary retention, need for surgery in symptomatic benign prostatic hypertrophy (BPH alone or in combination with doxazosin [Cardura]). Most improvement noted in hesitancy, feeling of incomplete bladder emptying, interruption of urinary stream, difficulty initiating flow, dysuria, impaired size and force of urinary stream. **Propecia:** Treatment for hair loss. **OFF-LABEL:** Adjuvant monotherapy after radical prostatectomy in treatment of prostate cancer, female hirsutism.

PRECAUTIONS

CONTRAINDICATIONS: Exposure to the patient's semen or handling of finasteride tablets by those who are or may be pregnant. **CAUTIONS:** Hepatic function abnormalities.

⌛ **LIFESPAN CONSIDERATIONS: Pregnancy/Lactation:** Physical handling of tablet in those who may become or are pregnant. May produce abnormalities of external genitalia of male fetus. **Pregnancy Category X. Children:** Not indicated in children. **Elderly:** Efficacy not established.

INTERACTIONS

DRUG: None known. **HERBAL:** None known. **FOOD:** None known. **LAB VALUES:** Decreases the serum prostate-specific antigen (PSA) level, even in patients with prostate cancer.

AVAILABILITY (Rx)

TABLETS: 1 mg (Propecia), 5 mg (Proscar).

ADMINISTRATION/HANDLING

PO
• Do not break or crush film-coated tablets. • Give without regard to meals.

INDICATIONS/ROUTES/DOSAGE

BENIGN PROSTATIC HYPERPLASIA (BPH)
PO: ADULTS, ELDERLY: 5 mg once a day (for a minimum of 6 mo).

HAIR LOSS
PO: ADULTS: 1 mg/day.

SIDE EFFECTS

RARE (4%–2%): Gynecomastia, sexual dysfunction (impotence, decreased libido, decreased volume of ejaculate).

ADVERSE REACTIONS/ TOXIC EFFECTS

Hypersensitivity reactions, including rash, pruritus, urticaria, circumoral swelling, and testicular pain, have been reported.

NURSING CONSIDERATIONS

BASELINE ASSESSMENT
Digital rectal exam, serum PSA determination should be performed in those with BPH before initiating therapy and periodically thereafter.

INTERVENTION/EVALUATION
Diligent monitoring of I&O, especially in those with large residual urinary volume, severely diminished urinary flow for obstructive uropathy.

PATIENT/FAMILY TEACHING
• Patient should be aware of potential for impotence. • May not notice improved urinary flow even if prostate gland shrinks. • Need to take medication longer than 6 mo, and it is unknown if medication decreases need for surgery. • Because of potential risk to male fetus, women who are or may become pregnant should not handle tablets or be exposed to patient's semen. • Volume of ejaculate may be decreased during treatment.

Fioricet, see acetaminophen

Fiorinal, see aspirin

Flagyl, see metronidazole

flavocoxid

flay-**vox**-ah-sid
(Limbrel)

◆**CLASSIFICATION**
PHARMACOTHERAPEUTIC: Oral nutritional supplement. **CLINICAL:** Antiarthritis.

ACTION

An oral nutritional supplement that inhibits prostaglandin synthesis and arachidonic acid metabolism, reducing the production of leukotrienes. Also acts through an antioxidant mechanism.

Therapeutic Effect: Produces anti-inflammatory and analgesic effects and increases mobility.

PHARMACOKINETICS

Undergoes hydrolysis at the gut mucosal border. Food decreases absorption. Little hepatic metabolism.

USES

For clinical dietary management of mild to moderate osteoarthritis, including associated inflammation.

PRECAUTIONS

CONTRAINDICATIONS: History of peptic ulcer. **CAUTIONS:** History of stomach ulcers.

⧗ **LIFESPAN CONSIDERATIONS: Pregnancy/Lactation:** Unknown if drug crosses placenta or is distributed in breast milk. **Pregnancy Category not classified. Children:** Safety and efficacy not established in children younger than 18 yr. **Elderly:** No age-related precautions noted.

INTERACTIONS

DRUG: None known. **HERBAL:** None known. **FOOD: All foods:** Decrease the absorption of flavocoxid. **LAB VALUES:** None known.

AVAILABILITY (Rx)

CAPSULES: 250 mg.

ADMINISTRATION/HANDLING

PO
• Patient should not consume food 1 hr before or after taking flavocoxid (limits drug absorption).

INDICATIONS/ROUTES/DOSAGE

OSTEOARTHRITIS
PO: ADULTS 18 YR AND OLDER, ELDERLY: One 250-mg capsule q12h.

SIDE EFFECTS

RARE (2%): Increase in varicose veins, psoriasis, mild hypertension.

ADVERSE REACTIONS/TOXIC EFFECTS

GI bleeding, perforation, and ulceration occur rarely in patients currently or previously treated with NSAIDs or COX-2 inhibitors.

NURSING CONSIDERATIONS

BASELINE ASSESSMENT

Assess onset, type, location, duration of pain or inflammation. Inspect appearance of affected joint for immobility, deformities, skin condition.

INTERVENTION/EVALUATION

Assess for therapeutic response: relief of pain, stiffness, swelling; increased joint mobility, reduced joint tenderness, improved grip strength.

PATIENT/FAMILY TEACHING

• Food should not be consumed 1 hr before or after taking flavocoxid.

flavoxate

fla-**vox**-ate
(Urispas)

Do not confuse Urispas with Urised.

CLASSIFICATION

PHARMACOTHERAPEUTIC: Anticholinergic. **CLINICAL:** Antispasmodic.

ACTION

An anticholinergic that relaxes detrusor and other smooth muscle by cholinergic blockade, counteracting muscle spasm in the urinary tract. **Therapeutic Effect:** Produces anticholinergic, local anesthetic, and analgesic effects, relieving urinary symptoms.

PHARMACOKINETICS

Unknown absorption, distribution, metabolism. Protein binding: 50%–80%. Excreted in urine. **Half-life:** 10–20 hr.

USES

Symptomatic relief of dysuria, urgency, nocturia, frequency, incontinence associated with cystitis, prostatitis, urethritis, urethrocystitis, urethrotrigonitis.

PRECAUTIONS

CONTRAINDICATIONS: Duodenal or pyloric obstruction, GI hemorrhage or obstruction, ileus, lower urinary tract obstruction. **CAUTIONS:** Glaucoma.

⌛ **LIFESPAN CONSIDERATIONS: Pregnancy/Lactation:** Unknown if drug crosses placenta or is distributed in breast milk. **Pregnancy Category B. Children:** Safety and efficacy not established in children younger than 12 yr. **Elderly:** Higher risk of confusion.

INTERACTIONS

DRUG: None known. **HERBAL:** None known. **FOOD:** None known. **LAB VALUES:** None known.

AVAILABILITY (Rx)

TABLETS: 100 mg.

ADMINISTRATION/HANDLING

• Expect to reduce the dosage of flavoxate as symptoms improve.

INDICATIONS/ROUTES/DOSAGE

TO RELIEVE SYMPTOMS OF CYSTITIS, PROSTATITIS, URETHRITIS, URETHROCYSTITIS, OR URETHROTRIGONITIS
PO: ADULTS, ELDERLY, ADOLESCENTS: 100–200 mg 3–4 times a day.

SIDE EFFECTS

FREQUENT: Somnolence, dry mouth and throat. **OCCASIONAL:** Constipation, difficult urination, blurred vision, dizziness, headache, increased light sensitivity, nausea, vomiting, abdominal pain. **RARE:** Confusion (primarily in elderly), hypersensitivity, increased IOP, leukopenia.

ADVERSE REACTIONS/ TOXIC EFFECTS

Overdose may produce anticholinergic effects, including unsteadiness, severe dizziness, somnolence, fever, facial flushing, dyspnea, nervousness, and irritability.

NURSING CONSIDERATIONS

BASELINE ASSESSMENT

Assess for dysuria, urgency, frequency, incontinence, suprapubic pain.

INTERVENTION/EVALUATION

Monitor for symptomatic relief. Observe elderly, especially for mental confusion.

PATIENT/FAMILY TEACHING

• Avoid driving, other tasks requiring alertness, coordination, manual dexterity (blurred vision, drowsiness).

flecainide

(Tambocor)
See Antiarrhythmics (p. 15C)

Flexeril, *see cyclobenzaprine*

Flomax, *see tamsulosin*

Flonase, *see fluticasone*

Flovent, *see fluticasone*

Floxin Otic, *see ofloxacin*

F

fluconazole

flu-**con**-ah-zole
(Apo-Fluconazole ✥, <u>Diflucan</u>)
Do not confuse Diflucan with diclofenac.

◆CLASSIFICATION
CLINICAL: Antifungal.

ACTION

A fungistatic antifungal that interferes with cytochrome P-450, an enzyme necessary for ergosterol formation. **Therapeutic Effect:** Directly damages fungal membrane, altering its function.

PHARMACOKINETICS

Well absorbed from GI tract. Widely distributed, including to CSF. Protein binding: 11%. Partially metabolized in liver. Excreted unchanged primarily in urine. Partially removed by hemodialysis. **Half-life:** 20–30 hr (increased in impaired renal function).

USES

Prevention of candidiasis in patients undergoing bone marrow transplant receiving chemotherapy and/or radiation therapy, treatment of esophageal, oropharyngeal, disseminated, vulvovaginal, urinary tract candidiasis, treatment and suppression of cryptococcal meningitis. **OFF-LABEL:** Treatment of coccidioidomycosis, cryptococcosis, fungal pneumonia, onychomycosis, ringworm of the hand, septicemia.

PRECAUTIONS

CONTRAINDICATIONS: None known. **CAUTIONS:** Hepatic or renal impairment, hypersensitivity to other triazoles (e.g., itraconazole, terconazole), imidazoles (e.g., butoconazole, ketoconazole).

⧖ **LIFESPAN CONSIDERATIONS: Pregnancy/Lactation:** Unknown if excreted in breast milk. **Pregnancy Category C. Children:** No age-related precautions noted. **Elderly:** Age-related renal impairment may require dosage adjustment.

INTERACTIONS

DRUG: Cyclosporine: High fluconazole doses increase cyclosporine blood concentration. **Oral antidiabetics:** May increase blood concentration and effects of oral antidiabetics. **Phenytoin, warfarin:** May decrease the metabolism of these drugs. **Rifampin:** May increase fluconazole metabolism. **HERBAL:** None known. **FOOD:** None known. **LAB VALUES:** May increase serum alkaline phosphatase, serum bilirubin, AST, and ALT levels.

AVAILABILITY (Rx)

TABLETS: 50 mg, 100 mg, 150 mg, 200 mg. **POWDER FOR ORAL SUSPENSION:** 10 mg/ml, 40 mg/ml. **INJECTION:** 2 mg/ml (in 100- or 200-ml containers).

ADMINISTRATION/HANDLING
 IV

Rate of administration • Do not exceed maximum flow rate 200 mg/hr.

Storage • Store at room temperature. • Do not remove from outer wrap until ready to use. • Squeeze inner bag to check for leaks. • Do not use parenteral form if solution is cloudy, precipitate forms, seal is not intact, or it is discolored. • Do not add supplementary medication.

✐ see color pill atlas   ⬐ herb   <u>underlined</u> – top prescribed drug

PO

• Give without regard to meals. • PO and IV therapy equally effective; IV therapy for patient intolerant of the drug or unable to take orally.

IV INCOMPATIBILITIES

Amphotericin B (Fungizone), amphotericin B complex (Abelcet, Ambisome, Amphotec), ampicillin (Polycillin), calcium gluconate, cefotaxime (Claforan), ceftazidime (Fortaz), ceftriaxone (Rocephin), cefuroxime (Zinacef), chloramphenicol (Chloromycetin), clindamycin (Cleocin), co-trimoxazole (Bactrim), diazepam (Valium), digoxin (Lanoxin), erythromycin (Erythrocin), furosemide (Lasix), haloperidol (Haldol), hydroxyzine (Vistaril), imipenem and cilastatin (Primaxin), total parenteral nutrition (TPN).

IV COMPATIBILITIES

Diltiazem (Cardizem), dobutamine (Dobutrex), dopamine (Intropin), heparin, lorazepam (Ativan), midazolam (Versed), propofol (Diprivan).

INDICATIONS/ROUTES/DOSAGE

OROPHARYNGEAL CANDIDIASIS

PO, IV: ADULTS, ELDERLY: 200 mg once, then 100 mg/day for at least 14 days. CHILDREN: 6 mg/kg/day once, then 3 mg/kg/day.

ESOPHAGEAL CANDIDIASIS

PO, IV: ADULTS, ELDERLY: 200 mg once, then 100 mg/day (up to 400 mg/day) for 21 days and at least 14 days following resolution of symptoms. CHILDREN: 6 mg/kg/day once, then 3 mg/kg/day (up to 12 mg/kg/day) for 21 days at least 14 days following resolution of symptoms.

VAGINAL CANDIDIASIS

PO: ADULTS: 150 mg once.

PREVENTION OF CANDIDIASIS IN PATIENTS UNDERGOING BONE MARROW TRANSPLANTATION

PO: ADULTS: 400 mg/day.

SYSTEMIC CANDIDIASIS

PO, IV: ADULTS, ELDERLY: 400 mg once, then 200 mg/day (up to 400 mg/day) for at least 28 days and at least 14 days following resolution of symptoms. CHILDREN: 6–12 mg/kg/day.

URINARY CANDIDIASIS

PO, IV: ADULTS, ELDERLY: 50–200 mg/day.

CRYPTOCOCCAL MENINGITIS

PO, IV: ADULTS, ELDERLY: 400 mg once, then 200 mg/day (up to 800 mg/day) for 10–12 wk after CSF becomes negative (200 mg/day for suppression of relapse in patients with AIDS). CHILDREN: 12 mg/kg/day once, then 6–12 mg/kg/day (6 mg/kg/day for suppression of relapse in patients with AIDS).

ONYCHOMYCOSIS

PO: ADULTS: 150 mg/wk.

DOSAGE IN RENAL IMPAIRMENT

After a loading dose of 400 mg, the daily dosage is based on creatinine clearance.

Creatinine Clearance	% of Recommended Dose
Greater than 50 ml/min	100
21–50 ml/min	50
11–20 ml/min	25
Dialysis	Dose after dialysis

SIDE EFFECTS

OCCASIONAL (4%–1%): Hypersensitivity reaction (including chills, fever, pruritus, and rash), dizziness, drowsiness, headache, constipation, diarrhea, nausea, vomiting, abdominal pain.

ADVERSE REACTIONS/ TOXIC EFFECTS

Exfoliative skin disorders, serious hepatic effects, and blood dyscrasias (such as eosinophilia, thrombocytopenia, anemia, and leukopenia) have been reported rarely.

F

NURSING CONSIDERATIONS

BASELINE ASSESSMENT

Establish baselines for CBC, serum potassium, liver function studies.

INTERVENTION/EVALUATION

Assess for hypersensitivity reaction (chills, fever). Monitor serum liver and renal function tests, potassium, CBC, platelet count. Report rash, itching promptly. Monitor temperature at least daily. Determine pattern of bowel activity and stool consistency. Assess for dizziness; provide assistance as needed.

PATIENT/FAMILY TEACHING

• Avoid tasks that require alertness, motor skills until response to drug is established (dizziness, drowsiness). • Notify physician of dark urine, pale stool, jaundiced skin or sclera of eyes, rash with or without itching. • Patients with oropharyngeal infections should be taught appropriate oral hygiene. • Consult physician before taking any other medication.

fludarabine phosphate

flew-**dare**-ah-bean
(Fludara)
Do not confuse Fludara with FUDR.

◆ CLASSIFICATION

PHARMACOTHERAPEUTIC: Antimetabolite. **CLINICAL:** Antineoplastic (see p. 74C).

ACTION

An antimetabolite that inhibits DNA synthesis by interfering with DNA polymerase alpha, ribonucleotide reductase, and DNA primase. Therapeutic Effect: Induces cell death.

PHARMACOKINETICS

Rapidly dephosphorylated in serum, then phosphorylated intracellularly to active triphosphate. Primarily excreted in urine. Half-life: 7–20 hr.

USES

Treatment of chronic lymphocytic leukemia (CLL) in those who have not responded to or have not progressed with another standard alkylating agent.

PRECAUTIONS

CONTRAINDICATIONS: Concurrent use with pentostatin. **CAUTIONS:** Preexisting neurologic problems, renal insufficiency, bone marrow suppression.

⧖ LIFESPAN CONSIDERATIONS: **Pregnancy/Lactation:** If possible, avoid use during pregnancy, especially first trimester. May cause fetal harm. Not known whether distributed in breast milk. Breast-feeding not recommended. **Pregnancy Category D. Children:** Safety and efficacy not established. **Elderly:** Age-related renal impairment may require dosage adjustment.

INTERACTIONS

DRUG: **Antigout medications:** May decrease the effects of these drugs. **Bone marrow depressants:** May increase the risk of myelosuppression. **Live-virus vaccines:** May potentiate virus replication, increase vaccine side effects, and decrease the patient's antibody response to the vaccine. HERBAL: None known. FOOD: None known. LAB VALUES: May increase serum alkaline phosphatase, uric acid, and AST levels.

AVAILABILITY (Rx)

INJECTION POWDER FOR RECONSTITUTION: 50 mg.

ADMINISTRATION/HANDLING

‹ **ALERT** › Give by IV infusion. Do not add to other IV infusions. Avoid small veins; swollen, edematous extremities; areas overlying joints, tendons.

 IV

Reconstitution • Reconstitute 50-mg vial with 2 ml sterile water for injection to provide a concentration of 25 mg/ml. • Further dilute with 100–125 ml 0.9% NaCl or D_5W.

Rate of administration • Infuse over 30 min.

Storage • Store in refrigerator. • Handle with extreme care during preparation/administration. If contact with skin or mucous membranes occurs, wash thoroughly with soap and water; rinse eyes profusely with plain water. • After reconstitution, use within 8 hr; discard unused portion.

▨ IV INCOMPATIBILITIES

Acyclovir (Zovirax), amphotericin B (Fungizone), hydroxyzine (Vistaril), prochlorperazine (Compazine).

IV COMPATIBILITIES

Heparin, hydromorphone (Dilaudid), lorazepam (Ativan), magnesium sulfate, morphine, multivitamins, potassium chloride.

INDICATIONS/ROUTES/DOSAGE

CHRONIC LYMPHOCYTIC LEUKEMIA

IV: ADULTS: 25 mg/m^2 daily for 5 consecutive days. Continue for up to 3 additional cycles. Begin each course of treatment every 28 days.

NON-HODGKIN'S LYMPHOMA

IV: ADULTS, ELDERLY: Initially, 20 mg/m^2, then 30 mg/m^2/day for 48 hr.

DOSAGE IN RENAL IMPAIRMENT

Creatinine Clearance	Dosage
30–70 ml/min	Decrease dose by 20%
Less than 30 ml/min	not recommended

SIDE EFFECTS

FREQUENT: Fever (60%), nausea and vomiting (36%), chills (11%). **OCCASIONAL (20%–10%):** Fatigue, generalized pain, rash, diarrhea, cough, asthenia, stomatitis, dyspnea, peripheral edema. **RARE (7%–3%):** Anorexia, sinusitis, dysuria, hematuria, myalgia, paresthesia, headaches, visual disturbances.

ADVERSE REACTIONS/ TOXIC EFFECTS

Pneumonia occurs frequently. Severe hematologic toxicity (as evidenced by anemia, thrombocytopenia, and neutropenia) and GI bleeding may occur. Tumor lysis syndrome may start with flank pain and hematuria and may include hypercalcemia, hyperphosphatemia, hyperuricemia and renal failure. High-dosage therapy may produce acute leukemia, blindness, and coma.

NURSING CONSIDERATIONS

BASELINE ASSESSMENT

Assess baseline CBC, platelet, serum creatinine. Drug should be discontinued if intractable vomiting, diarrhea, stomatitis, GI bleeding occurs.

INTERVENTION/EVALUATION

Assess for fatigue, visual disturbances, peripheral edema. Assess for onset of pneumonia. Monitor for dyspnea, cough, rapidly falling WBC, intractable vomiting, diarrhea, GI bleeding (bright red or tarry stool). Assess oral mucosa for erythema, ulceration at inner margin of lips, sore throat, difficulty swallowing (stomatitis). Assess skin

F

for rash. Be alert to possible tumor lysis syndrome (onset of flank pain, hematuria).

PATIENT/FAMILY TEACHING

• Avoid crowds, exposure to infection. • Maintain fastidious oral hygiene. • Promptly report fever, sore throat, signs of local infection, unusual bruising or bleeding from any site. • Contact physician if nausea or vomiting continues.

fludrocortisone

floo-droe-**kor**-ti-sone

(Florinef)

Do not confuse Florinef with Fioricet or Florinal.

CLASSIFICATION

PHARMACOTHERAPEUTIC: Mineralocorticoid. **CLINICAL:** Glucocorticosteroid (see p. 83C).

ACTION

A mineralocorticoid that acts at distal tubules. Therapeutic Effect: Increases potassium and hydrogen ion excretion. Replaces sodium loss and raises blood pressure (with low dosages). Inhibits endogenous adrenal cortical secretion, thymic activity, and secretion of corticotropin by pituitary gland (with higher dosages).

PHARMACOKINETICS

Well absorbed from the GI tract. Protein binding: 42%. Widely distributed. Metabolized in the liver and kidney. Primarily excreted in urine. Half-life: 3.5 hr.

USES

Partial replacement therapy for primary and secondary adrenocortical insufficiency in Addison's disease. Adjunctive treatment of salt-losing forms of congenital adrenogenital syndrome. OFF-LABEL: Treatment of acidosis in renal tubular disorders, idiopathic orthostatic hypotension.

PRECAUTIONS

CONTRAINDICATIONS: CHF, systemic fungal infection. **CAUTIONS:** Hypertension, edema, renal impairment.

⧖ LIFESPAN CONSIDERATIONS: **Pregnancy/Lactation:** Unknown whether drug crosses placenta or is distributed in breast milk. **Pregnancy Category C. Children:** May cause growth suppression, inhibition of endogenous steroid production. **Elderly:** Studies not performed.

INTERACTIONS

DRUG: **Digoxin:** May increase the risk of digoxin toxicity caused by hypokalemia. **Hepatic enzyme inducers (such as phenytoin):** May increase the metabolism of fludrocortisone. **Hypokalemia-causing medications:** May increase the effects of fludrocortisone. **Sodium-containing medications:** May increase BP, incidence of edema, and serum sodium level. HERBAL: None known. FOOD: None known. LAB VALUES: May increase serum sodium level. May decrease Hct and serum potassium level.

AVAILABILITY (Rx)

TABLETS: 0.1 mg.

ADMINISTRATION/HANDLING

PO

• Give with food or milk.

INDICATIONS/ROUTES/DOSAGE

ADDISON'S DISEASE

PO: ADULTS, ELDERLY: 0.05–0.1 mg/day. Range: 0.1 mg 3 times a wk to 0.2 mg/day. Administration with cortisone or hydrocortisone preferred.

SALT-LOSING ADRENOGENITAL SYNDROME
PO: ADULTS, ELDERLY: 0.1–0.2 mg/day.
USUAL PEDIATRIC DOSAGE
CHILDREN: 0.05–0.1 mg/day.

SIDE EFFECTS

FREQUENT: Increased appetite, exaggerated sense of well-being, abdominal distention, weight gain, insomnia, mood swings. **High dosages, prolonged therapy, too rapid withdrawal:** Increased susceptibility to infection with masked signs and symptoms, delayed wound healing, hypokalemia, hypocalcemia, GI distress, diarrhea or constipation, hypertension. **OCCASIONAL:** Headache, dizziness, menstrual difficulty or amenorrhea, gastric ulcer development. **RARE:** Hypersensitivity reaction.

ADVERSE REACTIONS/ TOXIC EFFECTS

Long-term therapy may cause muscle wasting (especially in the arms and legs), osteoporosis, spontaneous fractures, amenorrhea, cataracts, glaucoma, peptic ulcer disease, and CHF. Abruptly withdrawing the drug after long-term therapy may cause anorexia, nausea, fever, headache, joint pain, rebound inflammation, fatigue, weakness, lethargy, dizziness, and orthostatic hypotension.

NURSING CONSIDERATIONS

BASELINE ASSESSMENT
Obtain baselines for weight, BP, blood glucose, serum electrolytes, chest x-ray, EKG.

INTERVENTION/EVALUATION
Monitor serum electrolytes, blood glucose, BP, serum renin. Taper dosage slowly if medication is to be discontinued.

PATIENT/FAMILY TEACHING
• Do not change dose or schedule or stop taking drug; must taper off gradually. • Report fever, sore throat, muscle aches, sudden weight gain or swelling, continuing headaches. • Maintain careful personal hygiene, avoid exposure to disease, trauma. • Severe stress (serious infection, surgery, trauma) may require increased dosage.

flumazenil

flew-**maz**-ah-nil
(Anexate ✤, Romazicon)

CLASSIFICATION

PHARMACOTHERAPEUTIC: Benzodiazepine receptor antagonist. **CLINICAL:** Antidote.

ACTION

An antidote that antagonizes the effect of benzodiazepines on the gamma-aminobutyric acid receptor complex in the CNS. **Therapeutic Effect:** Reverses sedative effect of benzodiazepines.

PHARMACOKINETICS

Route	Onset	Peak	Duration
IV	1–2 min	6–10 min	Less than 1 hr

Duration and degree of benzodiazepine reversal depend on dosage and plasma concentration. Protein binding: 50%. Metabolized by the liver; excreted in urine.

USES

Complete or partial reversal of sedative effects of benzodiazepines when general anesthesia has been induced and/or maintained with benzodiazepines, when sedation has been produced with benzodiazepines for diagnostic and therapeutic procedures, management of benzodiazepine overdosage.

PRECAUTIONS

CONTRAINDICATIONS: Anticholinergic signs (such as mydriasis, dry mucosa, and hypoperistalsis), arrhythmias, cardiovascular collapse, history of hypersensitivity to benzodiazepines, patients with signs of serious cyclic antidepressant overdose (such as motor abnormalities), patients who have been given a benzodiazepine for control of a potentially life-threatening condition (such as control of status epilepticus or increased intracranial pressure [ICP]). **CAUTIONS:** Head injury, hepatic impairment, alcoholism, drug dependency.

⌛ **LIFESPAN CONSIDERATIONS: Pregnancy/Lactation:** Unknown whether drug crosses placenta or is distributed in breast milk. Not recommended during labor, delivery. **Pregnancy Category C. Children:** No age-related precautions noted. **Elderly:** Benzodiazepine-induced sedation tends to be deeper, more prolonged, requiring careful monitoring.

INTERACTIONS

DRUG: Tricyclic antidepressants: May produces seizures and arrhythmias as flumazenil reverses the sedative effects of tricyclic antidepressants. **HERBAL:** None known. **FOOD:** None known. **LAB VALUES:** None known.

AVAILABILITY (Rx)

INJECTION: 0.1 mg/ml.

ADMINISTRATION/HANDLING

◄ **ALERT** ► Compatible with D_5W, lactated Ringer's, 0.9% NaCl.

Rate of administration • Reverse conscious sedation or general anesthesia: Give over 15 sec. • **Benzodiazepine overdose:** Give over 30 sec. • Administer through freely running IV infusion into large vein (local injection produces pain, inflammation at injection site).

Storage • Store parenteral form at room temperature. • Discard after 24 hr once medication is drawn into syringe, is mixed with any solutions, or if particulate/discoloration is noted. • Rinse spilled medication from skin with cool water.

▨ IV INCOMPATIBILITIES

No information available for Y-site administration.

IV COMPATIBILITIES

Aminophylline, cimetidine (Tagamet), dobutamine (Dobutrex), dopamine (Intropin), famotidine (Pepcid), heparin, lidocaine, procainamide (Pronestyl), ranitidine (Zantac).

INDICATIONS/ROUTES/DOSAGE

REVERSAL OF CONSCIOUS SEDATION OR GENERAL ANESTHESIA

IV: ADULTS, ELDERLY: Initially, 0.2 mg (2 ml) over 15 sec; may repeat dose in 45 sec; then at 60-sec intervals. **Maximum:** 1 mg (10-ml) total dose. CHILDREN, NEONATES: Initially, 0.01 mg/kg; may repeat in 45 sec, then at 60-sec intervals. **Maximum:** 0.2 mg single dose; 0.05 mg/kg or 1 mg cumulative dose.

BENZODIAZEPINE OVERDOSE

IV: ADULTS, ELDERLY: Initially, 0.2 mg (2 ml) over 30 sec; if desired level of consciousness (LOC) is not achieved after 30 sec, 0.3 mg (3 ml) may be given over 30 sec. Further doses of 0.5 mg (5 ml) may be administered over 30 sec at 60-sec intervals. **Maximum:** 3 mg (30 ml) total dose. CHILDREN, NEONATES: Initially, 0.01 mg/kg; may repeat in 45 sec, then at 60-sec intervals. **Maximum:** 0.2 mg single dose; 1 mg cumulative dose.

SIDE EFFECTS

FREQUENT (11%–4%): Agitation, anxiety, dry mouth, dyspnea, insomnia, palpitations, tremors, headache, blurred vision, dizziness, ataxia, nausea, vomiting, pain at injection site, diaphoresis. **OCCASIONAL (3%–1%):** Fatigue, flushing, auditory disturbances, thrombophlebitis, rash. **RARE (less than 1%):** Urticaria, pruritus, hallucinations.

ADVERSE REACTIONS/ TOXIC EFFECTS

Toxic effects, such as seizures and arrhythmias, of other drugs taken in overdose, especially tricyclic antidepressants, may emerge with reversal of sedative effect of benzodiazepines. Flumazenil may provoke a panic attack in those with a history of panic disorder.

NURSING CONSIDERATIONS

BASELINE ASSESSMENT

ABGs should be obtained before and at 30-min intervals during IV administration. Prepare to intervene in reestablishing airway, assisting ventilation (drug may not fully reverse ventilatory insufficiency induced by benzodiazepines). Note that effects of flumazenil may dissipate before effects of benzodiazepines.

INTERVENTION/EVALUATION

Properly manage airway, assist breathing, maintain circulatory access and support, perform internal decontamination by lavage and charcoal as required, provide adequate clinical evaluation. Monitor for reversal of benzodiazepine effect. Assess for possible resedation, respiratory depression, hypoventilation. Assess closely for return of unconsciousness (narcosis) for at least 1 hr after patient is fully alert.

PATIENT/FAMILY TEACHING

• Avoid ingestion of alcohol, tasks that require alertness, motor skills or taking nonprescription drugs until at least 18–24 hr after discharge.

flunisolide

floo-**niss**-oh-lide

(AeroBid, AeroBid-M, Aerospan, Bronalide ✤, Nasalide, Nasarel, Rhinalar ✤)

Do not confuse flunisolide with fluocinonide, or Nasalide with Nasalcrom.

◆CLASSIFICATION

PHARMACOTHERAPEUTIC: Adrenocorticosteroid. **CLINICAL:** Antiasthmatic, anti-inflammatory (see pp. 67C, 83C).

ACTION

An adrenocorticosteroid that controls the rate of protein synthesis, depresses migration of polymorphonuclear leukocytes, reverses capillary permeability, and stabilizes lysosomal membranes. **Therapeutic Effect:** Prevents or controls inflammation.

PHARMACOKINETICS

Rapidly absorbed from lungs and GI tract following inhalation. About 50% of dose is absorbed from the nasal mucosa following intranasal administration. Metabolized in liver. Partially excreted in urine and feces. **Half-life:** 1–2 hr.

USES

Inhalation: Long-term control of persistent bronchial asthma. Assists in reducing or discontinuing oral corticosteroid therapy. **Intranasal:** Relieves symptoms of seasonal or perennial rhinitis. **OFF-LABEL:** To prevent recurrence of nasal polyps after surgery.

PRECAUTIONS

CONTRAINDICATIONS: Hypersensitivity to any corticosteroid, persistently positive sputum cultures for *Candida albicans*, primary treatment of status asthmaticus, systemic fungal infections. **CAUTIONS:** Adrenal insufficiency.

⧗ **LIFESPAN CONSIDERATIONS: Pregnancy/Lactation:** Unknown if distributed in breast milk. **Pregnancy Category C. Children:** Safety and efficacy not established.   **Elderly:** No age-related cautions noted.

INTERACTIONS

DRUG: Bupropion: May lower the seizure threshold. **HERBAL:** None known. **FOOD:** None known. **LAB VALUES:** None known.

AVAILABILITY (Rx)

AEROSOL WITH ADAPTER (AEROBID): 250 mcg/activation. **AEROSOL (AEROBID-M):** 250 mcg/activation. **AEROSPAN:** 80 mcg/activation. **NASAL SPRAY (NAS-ALIDE, NASAREL):** 25 mcg/activation.

ADMINISTRATION/HANDLING

INHALATION

• Shake container well; instruct patient to exhale as completely as possible.
• Place mouthpiece fully into mouth; holding inhaler upright, instruct patient to inhale deeply, slowly while pressing the top of the canister and hold breath as long as possible before exhaling; then exhale slowly. • Wait 1 min between inhalations when multiple inhalations ordered (allows for deeper bronchial penetration). • Rinse mouth with water immediately after inhalation (prevents mouth and throat dryness).

INTRANASAL

• Clear nasal passages before use (topical nasal decongestants may be needed 5–15 min before use). • Instruct the patient to tilt head slightly forward. • Insert spray tip up in one nostril, pointing toward inflamed nasal turbinates, away from nasal septum. • Pump medication into one nostril while the patient holds other nostril closed and concurrently inspires through nose. • Discard opened nasal solution after 3 mo.

INDICATIONS/ROUTES/DOSAGE

LONG-TERM CONTROL OF BRONCHIAL ASTHMA, ASSISTS IN REDUCING OR DISCONTINUING ORAL CORTICOSTEROID THERAPY

INHALATION: ADULTS, ELDERLY: 2 inhalations twice a day, morning and evening. **Maximum:** 4 inhalations twice a day. CHILDREN 6–15 YR: 2 inhalations twice a day.

RELIEF OF SYMPTOMS OF PERENNIAL AND SEASONAL RHINITIS

INTRANASAL: ADULTS, ELDERLY: Initially, 2 sprays each nostril twice a day, may increase at 4–7 day intervals to 2 sprays 3 times a day. **Maximum:** 8 sprays in each nostril daily. CHILDREN 6–14 YR: Initially, 1 spray 3 times a day or 2 sprays twice a day. **Maximum:** 4 sprays in each nostril daily. Maintenance: 1 spray into each nostril each day.

SIDE EFFECTS

FREQUENT: Inhalation (25%–10%): Unpleasant taste, nausea, vomiting, sore throat, diarrhea, upset stomach, cold symptoms, nasal congestion. **OCCASIONAL: Inhalation (9%–3%):** Dizziness, irritability, nervousness, tremors, abdominal pain, heartburn, oropharynx candidiasis, edema. **Nasal:** Mild nasopharyngeal irritation or dryness, rebound congestion, bronchial asthma, rhinorrhea, altered taste.

ADVERSE REACTIONS/ TOXIC EFFECTS

An acute hypersensitivity reaction, marked by urticaria, angioedema, and severe bronchospasm, occurs rarely. A transfer from systemic to local steroid therapy may unmask previously suppressed bronchial asthma condition.

NURSING CONSIDERATIONS

BASELINE ASSESSMENT

Establish baseline assessment of asthma, rhinitis.

INTERVENTION/EVALUATION

Advise patients receiving bronchodilators by inhalation concomitantly with steroid inhalation therapy to use bronchodilator several minutes before corticosteroid aerosol (enhances penetration of steroid into bronchial tree). Monitor rate, depth, rhythm, type of respiration; quality and rate of pulse. Assess lung sounds for rhonchi, wheezing, rales. Monitor ABGs.

PATIENT/FAMILY TEACHING

• Do not change dose schedule or stop taking drug; must taper off gradually under medical supervision. • Maintain careful oral hygiene. • Rinse mouth with water immediately after inhalation (prevents mouth and throat dryness, fungal infection of mouth). • Increase fluid intake (decreases lung secretion viscosity). • **Intranasal:** Teach proper use of nasal spray. • Clear nasal passages before use. • Contact physician if no improvement in symptoms, sneezing or nasal irritation occurs. • Improvement usually noted in several days.

fluocinolone acetonide

(Flurosyn, Synalar, Synemol)

fluocinonide

(Lidex, Vanos, Vasoderm)
See Corticosteroids: topical (p. 86C)

fluorouracil, 5-FU ▷

phlur-oh-**your**-ah-sill
(Adrucil, Carac, Efudex, Fluoroplex)
Do not confuse Efudex with Efidac.

•CLASSIFICATION

PHARMACOTHERAPEUTIC: Antimetabolite. **CLINICAL:** Antineoplastic (see p. 74C).

ACTION

An antimetabolite that blocks formation of thymidylic acid. Cell cycle-specific for S phase of cell division. **Therapeutic Effect:** Inhibits DNA and RNA synthesis. Topical form destroys rapidly proliferating cells.

PHARMACOKINETICS

Widely distributed. Crosses the blood-brain barrier. Rapidly metabolized in tissues to active metabolite, which is localized intracellularly. Primarily excreted by lungs as carbon dioxide. Removed by hemodialysis. **Half-life:** 20 hr.

USES

Parenteral: Treatment of carcinoma of colon, rectum, breast, stomach, pancreas. Used in combination with levamisole after surgical resection in patients with Duke's stage C colon cancer. **Topical:** Treatment of multiple actinic, solar keratoses, superficial basal cell carcinomas. **OFF-LABEL: Parenteral:** Treatment of bladder, cervical, endometrial, head and neck, liver, lung, ovarian, or prostate carcinomas; pericardial, peritoneal, or pleural effusions. **Topical:** Treatment of actinic cheilitis, radiodermatitis.

PRECAUTIONS

CONTRAINDICATIONS: Major surgery within previous month, myelosuppression, poor nutritional status, potentially serious infections. **CAUTIONS:** History of high-dose pelvic irradiation, metastatic cell infiltration of bone marrow, hepatic or renal impairment.

▨ **LIFESPAN CONSIDERATIONS: Pregnancy/Lactation:** If possible, avoid use during pregnancy, especially first trimester. May cause fetal harm. Unknown whether distributed in breast milk. Breast-feeding not recommended. **Pregnancy Category D. Children:** No age-related precautions noted.

Elderly: Age-related renal impairment may require dosage adjustment.

INTERACTIONS

DRUG: Bone marrow depressants: May increase the risk of myelosuppression. **Live virus vaccines:** May potentiate virus replication, increase vaccine side effects, and decrease the patient's antibody response to the vaccine. **HERBAL:** None known. **FOOD:** None known. **LAB VALUES:** May decrease serum albumin level. May increase excretion of 5-hydroxyindoleacetic acid (5-HIAA) in urine. Topical form may cause eosinophilia, leukocytosis, thrombocytopenia, and toxic granulation.

AVAILABILITY (Rx)

INJECTION (ADRUCIL): 50 mg/ml. **TOPICAL CREAM:** 1% (Carac, Fluoroplex), 5% (Efudex). **TOPICAL SOLUTION:** 1% (Fluoroplex), 2% (Efudex).

ADMINISTRATION/HANDLING

◄ **ALERT** ▶ Give by IV injection or IV infusion. Do not add to other IV infusions. Avoid small veins, swollen or edematous extremities, areas overlying joints, tendons. May be carcinogenic, mutagenic, or teratogenic. Handle with extreme care during preparation/administration.

 IV

Reconstitution • IV push does not need to be diluted or reconstituted. • Inject through Y-tube or 3-way stopcock of free-flowing solution. • For IV infusion, further dilute with D_5W or 0.9% NaCl.

Rate of administration • Give IV push slowly over 1–2 min. • IV infusion is administered over 30 min–24 hr. • Extravasation produces immediate pain, severe local tissue damage. • Follow protocol.

Storage • Solution appears colorless to faint yellow. Slight discoloration does

not adversely affect potency or safety. • If precipitate forms, redissolve by heating, shaking vigorously; allow to cool to body temperature.

🔲 IV INCOMPATIBILITIES

Amphotericin B complex (Abelcet, AmBisome, Amphotec), droperidol (Inapsine), filgrastim (Neupogen), ondansetron (Zofran), vinorelbine (Navelbine).

IV COMPATIBILITIES

Granisetron (Kytril), heparin, hydromorphone (Dilaudid), leucovorin, morphine, potassium chloride, propofol (Diprivan), total parenteral nutrition (TPN).

INDICATIONS/ROUTES/DOSAGE

CARCINOMA OF BREAST, COLON, PANCREAS, RECTUM, AND STOMACH; IN COMBINATION WITH LEVAMISOLE AFTER SURGICAL RESECTION IN PATIENTS WITH DUKE'S STAGE C COLON CANCER

IV: ADULTS, ELDERLY, CHILDREN: Initially, 12 mg/kg/day for 4–5 days. **Maximum:** 800 mg/day. Maintenance: 6 mg/kg every other day for 4 doses repeated in 4 wk; or 15 mg/kg as a single bolus dose; or 5–15 mg/kg/wk as a single dose, not to exceed 1 g.

MULTIPLE ACTINIC OR SOLAR KERATOSES

TOPICAL (CARAC): ADULTS, ELDERLY: Apply once a day.
TOPICAL (EFUDEX, FLUOROPLEX): ADULTS, ELDERLY: Apply twice a day.

BASAL CELL CARCINOMA

TOPICAL (EFUDEX): ADULTS, ELDERLY: Apply twice a day for 3–6 wk up to 10–12 wk.

SIDE EFFECTS

OCCASIONAL: Parenteral: Anorexia, diarrhea, minimal alopecia, fever, dry skin, skin fissures, scaling, erythema. **Topical:** Pain, pruritus, hyperpigmentation, irritation, inflammation, and burning at application site; photosensitivity. **RARE:** Nausea, vomiting, anemia, esophagitis, proctitis, GI ulcer, confusion, headache, lacrimation, visual disturbances, angina, allergic reactions.

ADVERSE REACTIONS/ TOXIC EFFECTS

The earliest sign of toxicity, which may occur 4–8 days after beginning therapy, is stomatitis (as evidenced by dry mouth, burning sensation, mucosal erythema, and ulceration at inner margin of lips). Hematologic toxicity may be manifested as leukopenia (generally within 9–14 days after drug administration, but possibly as late as the 25th day), thrombocytopenia (within 7–17 days after administration), pancytopenia, or agranulocytosis. The most common dermatologic toxicity is a pruritic rash on the extremities or, less frequently, the trunk.

NURSING CONSIDERATIONS

BASELINE ASSESSMENT

Obtain CBC with differential, platelet count, serum renal and liver function tests.

INTERVENTION/EVALUATION

Monitor for rapidly falling WBC, intractable diarrhea, GI bleeding (bright red or tarry stool). Assess oral mucosa for stomatitis. Drug should be discontinued if intractable diarrhea, stomatitis, GI bleeding occurs. Assess skin for rash.

PATIENT/FAMILY TEACHING

• Maintain fastidious oral hygiene. • Inform physician of signs or symptoms of infection, unusual bruising or bleeding, visual changes, nausea, vomiting, diarrhea, chest pain, palpitations. • Avoid sunlight and artificial light sources; wear protective clothing, sunglasses, sunscreen. • **Topical:** Apply only to affected area. • Do not use occlusive coverings. • Be careful near eyes, nose, mouth. • Wash hands thoroughly after

application. • Treated areas may be unsightly for several weeks after therapy.

fluoxetine hydrochloride

floo-**ox**-e-teen

(Novo-Fluoxetine ❦, <u>Prozac</u>, Prozac Weekly, Rapiflux, Sarafem)

Do not confuse fluoxetine with fluvastatin, Prozac with Prilosec, Proscar, or ProSom; or Sarafem with Serophene.

FIXED-COMBINATION(S)

Symbyax: fluoxetine/olanzapine (an antipsychotic): 25 mg/6 mg, 50 mg/6 mg, 25 mg/12 mg, 50 mg/12 mg.

CLASSIFICATION

PHARMACOTHERAPEUTIC: Psychotherapeutic. **CLINICAL:** Antidepressant, antiobsessional agent, antibulimic (see p. 37C).

ACTION

A psychotherapeutic agent that selectively inhibits serotonin uptake in the CNS, enhancing serotonergic function. **Therapeutic Effect:** Relieves depression; reduces obsessive-compulsive and bulimic behavior.

PHARMACOKINETICS

Well absorbed from the GI tract. Crosses the blood-brain barrier. Protein binding: 94%. Metabolized in the liver to active metabolite. Primarily excreted in urine. Not removed by hemodialysis. **Half-life:** 2–3 days; metabolite 7–9 days.

USES

Treatment of clinical depression, obsessive-compulsive disorder (OCD), bulimia nervosa, premenstrual dysphoric disorder (PMDD), panic disorder.

OFF-LABEL: Treatment of body dysmorphic disorder, fibromyalgia, hot flashes, post-traumatic stress duisorder, Raynaud's phenomena.

PRECAUTIONS

CONTRAINDICATIONS: Use within 14 days of MAOIs. **CAUTIONS:** Seizure disorder, cardiac dysfunction, diabetes, those at high risk for suicide.

⧗ **LIFESPAN CONSIDERATIONS: Pregnancy/Lactation:** Unknown whether drug crosses placenta or is distributed in breast milk. **Pregnancy Category C. Children:** May be more sensitive to behavioral side effects (e.g., insomnia, restlessness). **Elderly:** No age-related precautions noted.

INTERACTIONS

DRUG: Alcohol, other CNS depressants: May increase CNS depression. **Highly protein-bound medications (including oral anticoagulants):** May increase adverse effects. **MAOIs:** May produce serotonin syndrome and neuroleptic malignant syndrome. **Phenytoin:** May increase phenytoin blood concentration and risk of toxicity. **HERBAL: St. John's wort:** May increase fluoxetine's pharmacologic effects and risk of toxicity. **FOOD:** None known. **LAB VALUES:** None known.

AVAILABILITY (Rx)

CAPSULES: 10 mg (Prozac, Sarafem), 20 mg (Prozac, Sarafem), 40 mg (Prozac). **CAPSULES (DELAYED-RELEASE [PROZAC WEEKLY]):** 90 mg. **ORAL SOLUTION (PROZAC):** 20 mg/5 ml. **TABLETS (PROZAC, RAPIFLUX):** 10 mg, 20 mg.

ADMINISTRATION/HANDLING

PO
• Give with food or milk if GI distress occurs.

INDICATIONS/ROUTES/DOSAGE

DEPRESSION
PO: ADULTS: Initially, 20 mg each morning. If therapeutic improvement does not occur after 2 wk, gradually increase to maximum of 80 mg/day in 2 equally divided doses in morning and at noon. Prozac Weekly: 90 mg/wk, begin 7 days after last dose of 20 mg. ELDERLY: Initially, 10 mg/day. May increase by 10–20 mg q2wk. CHILDREN 7–17 YR: Initially, 5–10 mg/day. Titrate upward as needed. Usual dosage is 20 mg/day.

PANIC DISORDER
PO: ADULTS, ELDERLY: Initially, 10 mg/day. May increase to 20 mg/day after 1 wk. **Maximum:** 60 mg/day.

BULIMIA NERVOSA
PO: ADULTS: 60 mg each morning.

OBSESSIVE-COMPULSIVE DISORDER (OCD)
PO: ADULTS, ELDERLY: 40–80 mg/day. CHILDREN 7–18 YR: Initially, 10 mg/day. May increase to 20 mg/day after 2 wk. Range: 10–80 mg/day.

PREMENSTRUAL DYSPHORIC DISORDER
PO: ADULTS: 20 mg/day.

SIDE EFFECTS

FREQUENT (more than 10%): Headache, asthenia, insomnia, anxiety, nervousness, somnolence, nausea, diarrhea, decreased appetite. **OCCASIONAL (9%–2%):** Dizziness, tremor, fatigue, vomiting, constipation, dry mouth, abdominal pain, nasal congestion, diaphoresis, rash. **RARE (less than 2%):** Flushed skin, light-headedness, impaired concentration.

ADVERSE REACTIONS/ TOXIC EFFECTS

Overdose may produce seizures, nausea, vomiting, agitation, and restlessness.

NURSING CONSIDERATIONS

BASELINE ASSESSMENT

For patients on long-term therapy, baseline liver and renal function tests, blood counts should be performed periodically thereafter.

INTERVENTION/EVALUATION
Supervise suicidal-risk patient closely during early therapy (as energy level improves, suicide potential increases). Assess appearance, behavior, speech pattern, level of interest, mood. Monitor pattern of daily bowel activity and stool consistency. Assess skin for appearance of rash. Monitor serum liver function tests, glucose, sodium, weight.

PATIENT/FAMILY TEACHING
• Maximum therapeutic response may require 4 or more wk of therapy. • Do not abruptly discontinue medication. • Avoid tasks that require alertness, motor skills until response to drug is established. • Avoid alcohol. • To avoid insomnia, take last dose of drug before 4 PM.

---

fluphenazine hydrochloride (oral)

fluphenazine decanoate (injection)

floo-**fen**-a-zeen
(Moditen ✽, Permitil, Prolixin, Prolixin Decanoate)
Do not confuse Moditen with Modane or Mobidin.

✦CLASSIFICATION
PHARMACOTHERAPEUTIC: Phenothiazine. **CLINICAL:** Antipsychotic (see p. 58C).

ACTION
A phenothiazine that antagonizes dopamine neurotransmission at synapses by blocking postsynaptic dopaminergic receptors in the brain. **Therapeutic Effect:** Decreases psychotic behavior. Also produces weak anticholinergic, sedative, and antiemetic effects and strong extrapyramidal effects.

PHARMACOKINETICS
Erratic absorption. Protein binding: greater than 90%. Metabolized in liver. Excreted in urine. **Half-life:** 33 hr.

USES
Management of psychotic disturbances (schizophrenia, delusions, hallucinations). **OFF-LABEL:** Treatment of neurogenic pain (adjunct to tricyclic antidepressants).

PRECAUTIONS
CONTRAINDICATIONS: Angle-closure glaucoma, myelosuppression, severe cardiac or hepatic disease, severe hypertension or hypotension, subcortical brain damage. **CAUTIONS:** Seizures, Parkinson's disease.

⌛ LIFESPAN CONSIDERATIONS: **Pregnancy/Lactation:** Crosses placenta; distributed in breast milk. **Pregnancy Category C. Children:** Those with acute illnesses (chickenpox, measles, gastroenteritis, CNS infection) are at risk of developing neuromuscular, extrapyramidal symptoms (EPS), particularly dystonias. **Elderly:** Susceptible to anticholinergic, effects.

INTERACTIONS
DRUG: **Alcohol, other CNS depressants:** May increase hypotensive and CNS and respiratory depressant effects. **Antithyroid agents:** May increase the risk of agranulocytosis. **EPS-producing medications:** May increase EPS. **Hypotension-producing medications:** May increase hypotension. **Levodopa:** May decrease the effects of this drug. **Lithium:** May decrease the absorption of fluphenazine and produce

---

adverse neurologic effects. **MAOIs, tricyclic antidepressants:** May increase anticholinergic and sedative effects. **HERBAL:** None known. **FOOD:** None known. **LAB VALUES:** May produce false-positive pregnancy and phenylketonuria test results. May cause EKG changes, including Q- and T-wave disturbances.

AVAILABILITY (Rx)

ELIXIR (PROLIXIN): 2.5 mg/5 ml. **ORAL CONCENTRATE (PERMITIL):** 5 mg/ml. **TABLETS (PROLIXIN):** 1 mg, 2.5 mg, 5 mg, 10 mg. **INJECTION:** 2.5 mg/ml (Prolixin), 25 mg/ml (Prolixin Decanoate).

ADMINISTRATION/HANDLING

• Avoid skin contact with the fluphenazine solution to prevent contact dermatitis.

INDICATIONS/ROUTES/DOSAGE

PSYCHOSIS

PO: ADULTS, ELDERLY: 0.5–10 mg/day in divided doses q6–8h.
IM: ADULTS, ELDERLY: 2.5–10 mg/day in divided doses q6–8h or 12.5 mg (decanoate) q2wk.

SIDE EFFECTS

FREQUENT: Hypotension, dizziness, and syncope (occur frequently after first injection, occasionally after subsequent injections, and rarely with oral doses). **OCCASIONAL:** Somnolence (during early therapy), dry mouth, blurred vision, lethargy, constipation or diarrhea, nasal congestion, peripheral edema, urine retention. **RARE:** Ocular changes, altered skin pigmentation (with prolonged use of high doses).

ADVERSE REACTIONS/ TOXIC EFFECTS

EPS appear to be related to high dosages and are divided into 3 categories: akathisia (inability to sit still, tapping of feet), parkinsonian symptoms (such as hypersalivation, masklike facial expression, shuffling gait, and tremors), and acute dystonias (such as torticollis, opisthotonos, and oculogyric crisis). Tardive dyskinesia, manifested as tongue protrusion, puffing of the cheeks, and chewing or puckering of the mouth occurs rarely but may be irreversible. Abrupt withdrawal after long-term therapy may precipitate dizziness, gastritis, nausea and vomiting, and tremors. Blood dyscrasias, particularly agranulocytosis and mild leukopenia, may occur. Fluphenzine use may lower the seizure threshold.

NURSING CONSIDERATIONS

BASELINE ASSESSMENT

Avoid skin contact with solution (contact dermatitis). Assess behavior, appearance, emotional status, response to environment, speech pattern, thought content.

INTERVENTION/EVALUATION

Monitor BP for hypotension. Monitor CBC for blood dyscrasias. Monitor for fine tongue movement (may be early sign of tardive dyskinesia). Supervise suicidal-risk patient closely during early therapy (as depression lessens, energy level improves, increasing suicide potential). Assess for therapeutic response (interest in surroundings, improvement in self-care, increased ability to concentrate, relaxed facial expression).

PATIENT/FAMILY TEACHING

• Full therapeutic effect may take up to 6 wk. • Urine may darken. • Do not abruptly withdraw from long-term drug therapy. • Drowsiness generally subsides during continued therapy. • Avoid tasks that require alertness, motor skills until response to drug is established.

---

see color pill atlas   *herb*   underlined – top prescribed drug

flurandrenolide

(Cordran)

**See Corticosteroids: topical
(p. 86C)**

flurazepam hydrochloride

flure-**az**-e-pam

(Apo-Flurazepam ✤, Dalmane)

Do not confuse Dalmane with Dialume.

⬥CLASSIFICATION

PHARMACOTHERAPEUTIC: Benzodiazepine (**Schedule IV**). **CLINICAL:** Sedative-hypnotic (see p. 136C).

ACTION

A benzodiazepine that enhances action of inhibitory neurotransmitter gamma-aminobutyric acid (GABA). **Therapeutic Effect:** Produces hypnotic effect due to CNS depression.

PHARMACOKINETICS

Route	Onset	Peak	Duration
PO	15–20 min	3–6 hr	7–8 hr

Well absorbed from the GI tract. Protein binding: 97%. Crosses the blood-brain barrier. Widely distributed. Metabolized in liver to active metabolite. Primarily excreted in urine. Not removed by hemodialysis. **Half-life:** 2.3 hr; metabolite: 40–114 hr.

USES

Short-term treatment of insomnia (4 wk or less). Reduces sleep-induction time, number of nocturnal awakenings; increases length of sleep.

PRECAUTIONS

CONTRAINDICATIONS: Acute alcohol intoxication, acute angle-closure glaucoma, hypersensitivity to other benzodiazepines, pregnancy or breast-feeding.
CAUTIONS: Renal or hepatic impairment.

⌛ **LIFESPAN CONSIDERATIONS: Pregnancy/Lactation:** Crosses placenta. May be distributed in breast milk. Chronic ingestion during pregnancy may produce withdrawal symptoms, CNS depression in neonates. **Pregnancy Category X. Children:** Safety and efficacy not established in those younger than 15 yr. **Elderly:** Use small initial doses with gradual dose increases to avoid ataxia, excessive sedation.

INTERACTIONS

DRUG: Alcohol, CNS depressants: May increase CNS depression. **Azole antifungals:** May increase flurazepam concentration and the potential for benzodiazepine toxicity. **HERBAL: Kava kava, valerian:** May increase CNS depression. **St. John's wort:** May reduce flurazepam effectiveness. **FOOD:** None known. **LAB VALUES:** None known.

AVAILABILITY (Rx)

CAPSULES: 15 mg, 30 mg.

ADMINISTRATION/HANDLING

PO
• Give without regard to meals.
• Capsules may be emptied and mixed with food.

INDICATIONS/ROUTES/DOSAGE

INSOMNIA
PO: ADULTS: 15–30 mg at bedtime. ELDERLY, DEBILITATED, LIVER DISEASE, LOW SERUM ALBUMIN, CHILDREN 15 YR AND OLDER: 15 mg at bedtime.

SIDE EFFECTS

FREQUENT: Drowsiness, dizziness, ataxia, sedation. Morning drowsiness may occur initially. **OCCASIONAL:** GI

✤ Canadian trade name   ⓔ see **evolve**   ☞ High Alert drug disturbances, nervousness, blurred vision, dry mouth, headache, confusion, skin rash, irritability, slurred speech. **RARE:** Paradoxical CNS excitement or restlessness, particularly noted in elderly or debilitated.

ADVERSE REACTIONS/ TOXIC EFFECTS

Abrupt or too-rapid withdrawal after long-term use may result in pronounced restlessness and irritability, insomnia, hand tremors, abdominal or muscle cramps, vomiting, diaphoresis, and seizures. Overdose results in somnolence, confusion, diminished reflexes, and coma.

NURSING CONSIDERATIONS

BASELINE ASSESSMENT

Assess BP, pulse, respirations immediately before administration. Raise bed rails. Provide environment conducive to sleep (back rub, quiet environment, low lighting).

INTERVENTION/EVALUATION

Assess for paradoxical reaction, particularly during early therapy. Evaluate for therapeutic response: decrease in number of nocturnal awakenings, increase in length of sleep duration.

PATIENT/FAMILY TEACHING

• Smoking reduces drug effectiveness. • Do not abruptly withdraw medication after long-term use. • May have disturbed sleep 1–2 nights after discontinuing. • Notify physician if pregnant or planning to become pregnant (Pregnancy Category X). • Avoid alcohol, other CNS depressants. • May be habit forming.

flurbiprofen

flure-bi-proe-fen

(Apo-Flurbiprofen ✲, Ansaid, Froben ✲, Froben SR ✲, Ocufen)

Do not confuse Ocufen with Ocuflox.

CLASSIFICATION

PHARMACOTHERAPEUTIC: Phenylalkanoic acid. **CLINICAL:** Nonsteroidal anti-inflammatory, antidysmenorrheal (see p. 116C).

ACTION

A phenylalkanoic acid that produces analgesic and anti-inflammatory effect by inhibiting prostaglandin synthesis. Also relaxes the iris sphincter. **Therapeutic Effect:** Reduces the inflammatory response and intensity of pain. Prevents or decreases miosis during cataract surgery.

PHARMACOKINETICS

Well absorbed from the GI tract; ophthalmic solution penetrates cornea after administration, and may be systemically absorbed. Protein binding: 99%. Widely distributed. Metabolized in the liver. Primarily excreted in urine. **Half-life:** 3–4 hr.

USES

Oral: Symptomatic treatment of acute and/or chronic rheumatoid arthritis, osteoarthritis, dysmenorrhea, pain. **Ophthalmic:** Inhibits intraoperative miosis. **OFF-LABEL: Oral:** Ankylosing spondylitis, dental pain, post-operative gynecologic pain.

PRECAUTIONS

CONTRAINDICATIONS: Active peptic ulcer, chronic inflammation of GI tract, GI bleeding or ulceration, history of hypersensitivity to aspirin or

NSAIDs. **CAUTIONS:** Renal or hepatic impairment, history of GI tract disease, predisposition to fluid retention, soft contact lens wearers, surgical patients with bleeding tendencies.

⌛ **LIFESPAN CONSIDERATIONS: Pregnancy/Lactation:** Crosses placenta. Unknown whether distributed in breast milk. Avoid use during last trimester (may adversely affect fetal cardiovascular system: premature closure of ductus arteriosus). **Pregnancy Category B (D if used in third trimester or near delivery; C for ophthalmic solution). Children:** Safety and efficacy not established. **Elderly:** GI bleeding or ulceration more likely to cause serious adverse effects. Age-related renal impairment may increase risk of hepatic or renal toxicity, decreased dosage recommended.

INTERACTIONS

DRUG: Acetylcholine, carbachol: May decrease the effects of these drugs (with ophthalmic flurbiprofen). **Antihypertensives, diuretics:** May decrease the effects of these drugs. **Aspirin, other salicylates:** May increase the risk of GI side effects such as bleeding. **Bone marrow depressants:** May increase the risk of hematologic reactions. **Epinephrine, other antiglaucoma medications:** May decrease the antiglaucoma effect of these drugs. **Heparin, oral anticoagulants, thrombolytics:** May increase the effects of these drugs. **Lithium:** May increase the blood concentration and risk of toxicity of lithium. **Methotrexate:** May increase the risk of methotrexate toxicity. **Probenecid:** May increase the flurbiprofen blood concentration. **HERBAL: Feverfew:** May decrease the effects of feverfew. **Ginkgo biloba:** May increase the risk of bleeding. **FOOD:** None known. **LAB VALUES:** May increase bleeding time and serum LDH, alkaline phosphatase, AST, and ALT levels.

AVAILABILITY (Rx)

TABLETS (ANSAID): 50 mg, 100 mg. **OPHTHALMIC SOLUTION (OCUFEN):** 0.03%.

ADMINISTRATION/HANDLING

PO
• Do not crush or break enteric-coated tablets. • May give with food, milk, antacids if GI distress occurs.

OPHTHALMIC
• Place finger on lower eyelid, pull out until pocket is formed between eye and lower lid. • Hold dropper above pocket, place prescribed number of drops into pocket. Close eye gently. • Apply digital pressure to lacrimal sac for 1–2 min (minimizes drainage into nose and throat, reducing risk of systemic effects). • Remove excess solution with tissue.

INDICATIONS/ROUTES/DOSAGE

RHEUMATOID ARTHRITIS, OSTEOARTHRITIS
PO: ADULTS, ELDERLY: 200–300 mg/day in 2–4 divided doses. **Maximum:** 100 mg/dose or 300 mg/day.

DYSMENORRHEA, PAIN
PO: ADULTS: 50 mg 4 times a day.

USUAL OPHTHALMIC DOSAGE
ADULTS, ELDERLY, CHILDREN: Apply 1 drop q30min starting 2 hr before surgery for total of 4 doses.

SIDE EFFECTS

OCCASIONAL: PO (9%–3%): Headache, abdominal pain, diarrhea, indigestion, nausea, fluid retention. **Ophthalmic:** Burning or stinging on instillation, keratitis, elevated intraocular pressure. **RARE (less than 3%): PO:** Blurred vision, flushed skin, dizziness, somnolence, nervousness, insomnia, unusual fatigue, constipation, decreased appetite, vomiting, confusion.

ADVERSE REACTIONS/ TOXIC EFFECTS

Overdose may result in acute renal failure. Rare reactions with long-term use include peptic ulcer disease, GI bleeding, gastritis, severe hepatic reaction (jaundice), nephrotoxicity (hematuria, dysuria, proteinuria), a severe hypersensitivity reaction (angioedema, bronchospasm) and cardiac arrhythmias.

NURSING CONSIDERATIONS

BASELINE ASSESSMENT

Anti-inflammatory: Assess onset, type, location, duration of pain or inflammation. Inspect appearance of affected joints for immobility, deformities, skin condition.

INTERVENTION/EVALUATION

Monitor for headache, dyspepsia, dizziness. Monitor pattern of daily bowel activity and stool consistency. **Systemic Use:** CBC, platelets, BUN, serum creatinine, liver function tests, occult blood loss. **Ocular:** Periodic eye exams. **Anti-inflammatory:** Evaluate for therapeutic response: relief of pain, stiffness, swelling; increased joint mobility; reduced joint tenderness; improved grip strength.

PATIENT/FAMILY TEACHING

• Swallow tablet whole; do not crush or chew. • Avoid aspirin, alcohol (increases risk of GI bleeding). • If GI upset occurs, take with food, milk. • Report GI distress, visual disturbances, rash, edema, headache. • **Ophthalmic:** Eye burning may occur with instillation.

---

flutamide ⚑

flew-tah-myd
(Euflex ✿, Eulexin, Novo-Flutamide ✿)

Do not confuse flutamide with Flumadine.

♦ CLASSIFICATION

PHARMACOTHERAPEUTIC: Anti-androgen, hormone. **CLINICAL:** Antineoplastic (see p. 74C).

ACTION

An antiandrogen hormone that inhibits androgen uptake and prevents androgen from binding to androgen receptors in target tissue. Used in conjunction with leuprolide to inhibit the stimulant effects of flutamide on serum testosterone levels. **Therapeutic Effect:** Suppresses testicular androgen production and decreases growth of prostate carcinoma.

PHARMACOKINETICS

Completely absorbed from the GI tract. Protein binding: 94%–96%. Metabolized in the liver to active metabolite. Primarily excreted in urine. Not removed by hemodialysis. **Half-life:** 6 hr (increased in elderly).

USES

Treatment of metastatic carcinoma of prostate (in combination with luteinizing hormone-releasing hormone [LHRH] analogues, e.g., leuprolide). Management of locally confined stages B_2-C, D_2 carcinoma. **OFF-LABEL:** Female hirsutism.

PRECAUTIONS

CONTRAINDICATIONS: Severe hepatic impairment. **CAUTIONS:** None known.

⌛ **LIFESPAN CONSIDERATIONS: Pregnancy/Lactation:** Not used in this patient population. **Pregnancy Category D. Children:** Not used in children. **Elderly:** No age-related precautions noted.

INTERACTIONS

DRUG: Warfarin: May increase the risk of bleeding. **HERBAL:** None known. **FOOD:** None known. **LAB VALUES:** May

---

✎ see color pill atlas   ✐ herb   <u>underlined</u> – top prescribed drug increase blood glucose level and serum estradiol, testosterone, bilirubin, creatinine, AST, and ALT levels.

AVAILABILITY (Rx)
CAPSULES: 125 mg.

ADMINISTRATION/HANDLING
PO
• Give without regard to food.

INDICATIONS/ROUTES/DOSAGE
PROSTATIC CARCINOMA
(IN COMBINATION WITH LEUPROLIDE)
PO: ADULTS, ELDERLY: 250 mg q8h.

SIDE EFFECTS
FREQUENT: Hot flashes (50%); decreased libido, diarrhea (24%); generalized pain (23%); asthenia (17%); constipation (12%); nausea, nocturia (11%). **OCCASIONAL (8%–6%):** Dizziness, paresthesia, insomnia, impotence, peripheral edema, gynecomastia. **RARE (5%–4%):** Rash, diaphoresis, hypertension, hematuria, vomiting, urinary incontinence, headache, flu-like syndromes, photosensitivity.

ADVERSE REACTIONS/ TOXIC EFFECTS
Hepatoxicity, including hepatic encephalopathy, and hemolytic anemia may be noted.

NURSING CONSIDERATIONS

INTERVENTION/EVALUATION
Periodically monitor liver function tests in long-term therapy.

PATIENT/FAMILY TEACHING
• Do not stop taking medication (both drugs must be continued). • Urine color may change to amber or yellow-green. • Avoid prolonged exposure to sun or tanning beds. Wear clothing to protect from ultraviolet exposure until tolerance is determined.

fluticasone propionate

flew-**tih**-cah-sewn

(Cutivate, <u>Flonase</u>, <u>Flovent</u>, Flovent Diskus, Flovent HFA)

FIXED-COMBINATION(S)
Advair: fluticasone/salmeterol (bronchodilator): 100 mcg/50 mcg; 250 mcg/50 mcg; 500 mcg/ 50 mcg.

CLASSIFICATION
PHARMACOTHERAPEUTIC: Corticosteroid. **CLINICAL:** Anti-inflammatory, antipruritic (see pp. 67C, 83C, 86C).

ACTION
A corticosteroid that controls the rate of protein synthesis, depresses migration of polymorphonuclear leukocytes, reverses capillary permeability, and stabilizes lysosomal membranes. **Therapeutic Effect:** Prevents or controls inflammation.

PHARMACOKINETICS
Inhalation/intranasal: Protein binding: 91%. Undergoes extensive first-pass metabolism in liver. Excreted in urine. **Half-life:** 3–7.8 hr. **Topical:** Amount absorbed depends on affected area and skin condition (absorption increased with fever, hydration, inflamed or denuded skin).

USES
Nasal: Relief of seasonal/perennial allergic rhinitis. **Topical:** Relief of inflammation/pruritus associated with steroid-responsive disorders (e.g., contact dermatitis, eczema). **Inhalation:** Long-term control of persistent bronchial asthma. Assists in reducing or discontinuing oral corticosteroid therapy.

PRECAUTIONS

CONTRAINDICATIONS: Primary treatment of status asthmaticus or other acute asthma episodes (inhalation); untreated localized infection of nasal mucosa. **CAUTIONS:** Active or quiescent tuberculosis, untreated fungal, bacterial, or systemic ocular herpes simplex viral infection.

⌛ **LIFESPAN CONSIDERATIONS: Pregnancy/Lactation:** Unknown if drug crosses placenta or is distributed in breast milk. **Pregnancy Category C. Children:** Safety and efficacy not established in those younger than 4 yr. Children 4 yr and older may experience growth suppression with prolonged or high doses. **Elderly:** No age-related precautions noted.

INTERACTIONS

DRUG: Bupropion: May lower the seizure threshold. **HERBAL:** None known. **FOOD:** None known. **LAB VALUES:** None known.

AVAILABILITY (Rx)

AEROSOL FOR ORAL INHALATION (FLOVENT, FLOVENT HFA): 44 mcg/inhalation, 110 mcg/inhalation, 220 mcg/inhalation. **POWDER FOR ORAL INHALATION (FLOVENT DISKUS):** 50 mcg, 100 mcg, 250 mcg. **INTRANASAL SPRAY (FLONASE):** 50 mcg/inhalation. **TOPICAL CREAM (CUTIVATE):** 0.05%. **TOPICAL OINTMENT (CUTIVATE):** 0.005%.

ADMINISTRATION/HANDLING

INHALATION

• Shake container well; instruct patient to exhale as completely as possible.
• Place mouthpiece fully into mouth; holding inhaler upright. Instruct patient to inhale deeply, slowly while pressing the top of the canister and to hold breath as long as possible before exhaling, then exhale slowly. • Wait 1 min between inhalations when multiple inhalations ordered (allows for deeper bronchial penetration). • Rinse mouth with water immediately after inhalation (prevents mouth/throat dryness).

INTRANASAL

• Clear nasal passages before use (topical nasal decongestants may be needed 5–15 min before use). • Tilt head slightly forward. • Insert spray tip up in 1 nostril, pointing toward inflamed nasal turbinates, away from nasal septum. • Pump medication into 1 nostril while holding other nostril closed, concurrently inspire through nose.

INDICATIONS/ROUTES/DOSAGE

ALLERGIC RHINITIS

INTRANASAL: ADULTS, ELDERLY: Initially, 200 mcg (2 sprays in each nostril once daily or 1 spray in each nostril q12h). Maintenance: 1 spray in each nostril once daily. **Maximum:** 200 mcg/day. CHILDREN 4 YR AND OLDER: Initially, 100 mcg (1 spray in each nostril once daily). **Maximum:** 200 mcg/day.

RELIEF OF INFLAMMATION AND PRURITUS ASSOCIATED WITH STEROID-RESPONSIVE DISORDERS, SUCH AS CONTACT DERMATITIS AND ECZEMA

TOPICAL: ADULTS, ELDERLY, CHILDREN 3 MO AND OLDER: Apply sparingly to affected area once or twice a day.

MAINTENANCE TREATMENT FOR ASTHMA FOR THOSE PREVIOUSLY TREATED WITH BRONCHODILATORS

INHALATION POWDER (FLOVENT DISKUS): ADULTS, ELDERLY, CHILDREN 12 YR AND OLDER: Initially, 100 mcg q12h. **Maximum:** 500 mcg/day.

INHALATION (ORAL [FLOVENT]): ADULTS, ELDERLY, CHILDREN 12 YR AND OLDER: 88 mcg twice a day. **Maximum:** 440 mcg twice a day.

MAINTENANCE TREATMENT FOR ASTHMA FOR THOSE PREVIOUSLY TREATED WITH INHALED STEROIDS

INHALATION POWDER (FLOVENT DISKUS): ADULTS, ELDERLY, CHILDREN

✏ see color pill atlas   🌿 herb   <u>underlined</u> – top prescribed drug

12 YR AND OLDER: Initially, 100–250 mcg q12h. **Maximum:** 500 mcg q12h.
INHALATION (ORAL [FLOVENT]): ADULTS, ELDERLY, CHILDREN 12 YR AND OLDER: 88–220 mcg twice a day. **Maximum:** 440 mcg twice a day.

MAINTENANCE TREATMENT FOR ASTHMA FOR THOSE PREVIOUSLY TREATED WITH ORAL STEROIDS INHALATION POWDER (FLOVENT DISKUS): ADULTS, ELDERLY, CHILDREN 12 YR AND OLDER: 500–1,000 mcg twice a day.
INHALATION (ORAL [FLOVENT]): ADULTS, ELDERLY, CHILDREN 12 YR AND OLDER: 880 mcg twice a day.

SIDE EFFECTS

FREQUENT: Inhalation: Throat irritation, hoarseness, dry mouth, cough, temporary wheezing, oropharyngeal candidiasis (particularly if mouth is not rinsed with water after each administration). **Intranasal:** Mild nasopharyngeal irritation; nasal burning, stinging, or dryness; rebound congestion; rhinorrhea; loss of taste. **OCCASIONAL: Inhalation:** Oral candidiasis. **Intranasal:** Nasal and pharyngeal candidiasis, headache. **Topical:** Skin burning, pruritus.

ADVERSE REACTIONS/ TOXIC EFFECTS

Deaths due to adrenal insufficiency have occurred in asthma patients during and after transfer from use of long-term systemic corticosteroids to less systemically available inhaled corticosteroids.

NURSING CONSIDERATIONS

BASELINE ASSESSMENT
Establish baseline history of skin disorder, asthma, rhinitis.

INTERVENTION/EVALUATION
Monitor rate, depth, rhythm, type of respiration; quality/rate of pulse. Assess lung sounds for rhonchi, wheezing, rales. Monitor ABGs. Assess oral

mucous membranes for evidence of candidiasis. Monitor growth in pediatric patients. **Topical:** Assess involved area for therapeutic response to irritation.

PATIENT/FAMILY TEACHING
• Advise patients receiving bronchodilators by inhalation concomitantly with steroid inhalation therapy to use bronchodilator several minutes before corticosteroid aerosol (enhances penetration of steroid into bronchial tree). • Do not change dose schedule or stop taking drug; must taper off gradually under medical supervision. • Maintain careful oral hygiene. • Rinse mouth with water immediately after inhalation (prevents mouth/throat dryness, fungal infection of mouth). • Increase fluid intake (decreases lung secretion viscosity). • **Intranasal:** Teach proper use of nasal spray. • Clear nasal passages before use. • Contact physician if no improvement in symptoms or sneezing/nasal irritation occurs. • Improvement noted in several days. • **Topical:** Rub thin film gently into affected area. • Use only for prescribed area and no longer than ordered. • Avoid contact with eyes.

fluvastatin

flu-vah-**stah**-tin
(Lescol, Lescol XL)

Do not confuse fluvastatin with fluoxetine.

CLASSIFICATION

PHARMACOTHERAPEUTIC: Hydroxamethylglutaryl-CoA (HMG-CoA) reductase inhibitor. **CLINICAL:** Antihyperlipidemic (see p. 52C).

ACTION
An antihyperlipidemic that inhibits HMG-CoA reductase, the enzyme that catalyzes

the early step in cholesterol synthesis. **Therapeutic Effect:** Decreases LDL cholesterol, VLDL, and plasma triglyceride levels. Slightly increases HDL cholesterol concentration.

PHARMACOKINETICS

Well absorbed from the GI tract and is unaffected by food. Does not cross the blood-brain barrier. Protein binding: greater than 98%. Primarily eliminated in feces. **Half-life:** 1.2 hr.

USES

Adjunct to diet therapy to decrease elevated total, LDL cholesterol concentrations in those with primary hypercholesterolemia (types IIa, IIb), those with combined hypercholesterolemia, hypertriglyceridemia. Treatment of elevated triglycerides, apolipoprotein, secondary prevention of coronary events.

PRECAUTIONS

CONTRAINDICATIONS: Active hepatic disease, lactation, pregnancy, unexplained increased serum transaminase levels. **CAUTIONS:** Anticoagulant therapy, history of hepatic disease, substantial alcohol consumption, major surgery; severe acute infection; trauma; hypotension; severe metabolic, endocrine, electrolyte disorders; uncontrolled seizures. Withholding or discontinuing fluvastatin may be necessary when patient is at risk for renal failure (secondary to rhabdomyolysis).

⏳ **LIFESPAN CONSIDERATIONS: Pregnancy/Lactation:** Contraindicated in pregnancy (suppression of cholesterol biosynthesis may cause fetal toxicity), lactation. Unknown whether drug is distributed in breast milk. **Pregnancy Category X. Children:** Safety and efficacy not established. **Elderly:** No age-related precautions noted.

INTERACTIONS

DRUG: Cyclosporine, **erythromycin, gemfibrozil, immunosuppressants,**

niacin: Increases the risk of acute renal failure and rhabdomyolysis with these drugs. **Cholestyramine:** May reduce the effectiveness of fluvastatin. **Phenytoin:** May increase the maximum plasma concentration of fluvastatin. **HERBAL: St. John's wort:** May reduce the effectiveness of fluvastatin. **FOOD:** None known. **LAB VALUES:** May increase serum creatine kinase (CK) and transaminase concentrations.

AVAILABILITY (Rx)

CAPSULES (LESCOL): 20 mg, 40 mg. **TABLETS (EXTENDED-RELEASE [LESCOL XL]):** 80 mg.

ADMINISTRATION/HANDLING
PO
• Give without regard to food.

INDICATIONS/ROUTES/DOSAGE
HYPERLIPOPROTEINEMIA
PO: ADULTS, ELDERLY: Initially, 20 mg/day (capsule) in the evening. May increase up to 40 mg/day. Maintenance: 20–40 mg/day in a single dose or divided doses. PATIENTS REQUIRING MORE THAN A 25% DECREASE IN LDL CHOLESTEROL: 40 mg (capsule) 1–2 times a day or 80 mg tablet once a day.

SIDE EFFECTS

FREQUENT (8%–5%): Headache, dyspepsia, back pain, myalgia, arthralgia, diarrhea, abdominal cramping, rhinitis. **OCCASIONAL (4%–2%):** Nausea, vomiting, insomnia, constipation, flatulence, rash, pruritus, fatigue, cough, dizziness.

ADVERSE REACTIONS/ TOXIC EFFECTS

Myositis (inflammation of voluntary muscle) with or without increased CK, and muscle weakness, occur rarely. These conditions may progress to frank rhabdomyolysis and renal impairment.

NURSING CONSIDERATIONS

BASELINE ASSESSMENT

Question for possibility of pregnancy before initiating therapy (Pregnancy Category X). Assess baseline lab results: serum cholesterol, triglycerides, liver function tests.

INTERVENTION/EVALUATION

Determine pattern of bowel activity. Check for headache, dizziness. Assess for rash, pruritus. Monitor serum cholesterol, triglyceride lab results for therapeutic response. Be alert for malaise, muscle cramping or weakness.

PATIENT/FAMILY TEACHING

• Follow special diet (important part of treatment). • Periodic lab tests are essential part of therapy. • Report promptly any muscle pain/weakness, especially if accompanied by fever, malaise.

fluvoxamine maleate

floo-**vox**-a-meen

(Luvox)

✦CLASSIFICATION

PHARMACOTHERAPEUTIC: Serotonin reuptake inhibitor. **CLINICAL:** Antidepressant, antiobsessive (see p. 37C).

ACTION

An antidepressant and antiobsessive agent that selectively inhibits neuronal reuptake of serotonin. **Therapeutic Effect:** Relieves depression and symptoms of obsessive-compulsive disorder (OCD).

PHARMACOKINETICS

Well absorbed following PO administration. Protein binding: 77%. Metabolized in liver. Excreted in urine. **Half-life:** 15.6 hr.

USES

Treatment of obsessive-compulsive disorder (OCD). **OFF-LABEL:** Treatment of anxiety disorders in children, depression, panic disorder.

PRECAUTIONS

CONTRAINDICATIONS: Use within 14 days of MAOIs, co-administration of thioridazine, terfenadine, astemizole, cisapride, or pimozide with fluvoxamine. **CAUTIONS:** Renal/hepatic impairment, elderly.

⧗ **LIFESPAN CONSIDERATIONS: Pregnancy/Lactation:** Unknown if drug crosses the placenta; distributed in breast milk. **Pregnancy Category C. Children:** Safety and efficacy not established **Elderly:** Potential for reduced serum clearance; maintain caution.

INTERACTIONS

DRUG: Benzodiazepines, carbamazepine, clozapine, theophylline: May increase the blood concentration and risk of toxicity of these drugs. **Cisapride:** May increase the risk of cardiotoxicity. **Lithium, tryptophan:** May enhance fluvoxamine's serotonergic effects. **MAOIs:** May produce serious reactions, including hyperthermia, rigidity, and myoclonus. **Tricyclic antidepressants:** May increase the fluvoxamine blood concentration. **Warfarin:** May increase the effects of warfarin. **HERBAL: St. John's wort:** May increase fluvoxamine's pharmacologic effects and risk of toxicity. **FOOD:** None known. **LAB VALUES:** May reduce sodium level.

AVAILABILITY (Rx)

TABLETS: 25 mg, 50 mg, 100 mg.

INDICATIONS/ROUTES/DOSAGE

OCD

PO: ADULTS: 50 mg at bedtime; may increase by 50 mg every 4–7 days. Dosages greater than 100 mg/day given in 2 divided doses. **Maximum:** 300 mg/day. CHILDREN 8–17 YR: 25 mg at bedtime; may increase by 25 mg every 4–7 days. Dosages greater than 50 mg/day given in 2 divided doses. **Maximum:** 200 mg/day.

SIDE EFFECTS

FREQUENT: Nausea (40%), headache, somnolence, insomnia (22%–21%). **OCCASIONAL (14%–8%):** Dizziness, diarrhea, dry mouth, asthenia, weakness, dyspepsia, constipation, abnormal ejaculation. **RARE (6%–3%):** Anorexia, anxiety, tremor, vomiting, flatulence, urinary frequency, sexual dysfunction, altered taste.

ADVERSE REACTIONS/ TOXIC EFFECTS

Overdose may produce seizures, nausea, vomiting, and extreme agitation and restlessness.

NURSING CONSIDERATIONS

INTERVENTION/EVALUATION

Supervise suicidal-risk patient closely during early therapy (as energy level improves, suicide potential increases). Assess appearance, behavior, speech pattern, level of interest, mood. Assist with ambulation if dizziness, somnolence occurs. Monitor pattern of bowel activity and stool consistency.

PATIENT/FAMILY TEACHING

• Maximum therapeutic response may require 4 wk or more of therapy. • Dry mouth may be relieved by sugarless gum, sips of tepid water. • Do not abruptly discontinue medication. • Avoid tasks that require alertness, motor skills until response to drug is established.

---

folic acid (vitamin B₉)

(Apo-Folic ✦, Folvite)

sodium folate

(Folvite-parenteral)

foe-lik

Do not confuse Folvite with Florvite.

CLASSIFICATION

PHARMACOTHERAPEUTIC: Coenzyme. **CLINICAL:** Nutritional supplement.

ACTION

A coenzyme that stimulates production of platelets, RBCs, and WBCs. **Therapeutic Effect:** Essential for nucleoprotein synthesis and maintenance of normal erythropoiesis.

PHARMACOKINETICS

PO form almost completely absorbed from the GI tract (upper duodenum). Protein binding: High. Metabolized in the liver and plasma to active form. Excreted in urine. Removed by hemodialysis.

USES

Treatment of megaloblastic, macrocytic anemia associated with pregnancy, infancy, childhood, inadequate dietary intake. **OFF-LABEL:** To decrease the risk of colon cancer.

PRECAUTIONS

CONTRAINDICATIONS: Anemias (aplastic, normocytic, pernicious, refractory). **CAUTIONS:** None known.

⧖ **LIFESPAN CONSIDERATIONS: Pregnancy/Lactation:** Distributed in breast milk. **Pregnancy Category A (C if used in doses above the recommended daily allowance). Children/**

Elderly: No age-related precautions noted.

INTERACTIONS

DRUG: Analgesics, carbamazepine, estrogens: May increase folic acid requirements. **Antacids, cholestyramine:** May decrease the absorption of folic acid. **Hydantoin anticonvulsants:** May decrease the effects of these drugs. **Methotrexate, triamterene, trimethoprim:** May antagonize the effects of folic acid. **HERBAL:** None known. **FOOD:** None known. **LAB VALUES:** May decrease vitamin B_{12} concentration.

AVAILABILITY (Rx)

TABLETS: 0.4 mg (OTC), 0.8 mg (OTC), 1 mg. **INJECTION:** 5 mg/ml.

ADMINISTRATION/HANDLING

◀ **ALERT** ▶ Parenteral form used in acutely ill, parenteral/enteral alimentation, those unresponsive to oral route in GI malabsorption syndrome. Dosage greater than 0.1 mg a day may conceal pernicious anemia.

INDICATIONS/ROUTES/DOSAGE

VITAMIN B_9 DEFICIENCY

PO, IV, IM, SUBCUTANEOUS: ADULTS, ELDERLY, CHILDREN 12 YR AND OLDER: Initially, 1 mg/day. Maintenance: 0.5 mg/day. CHILDREN 1–11 YR: Initially 1 mg/day. Maintenance: 0.1–0.4 mg/day. INFANTS: 50 mcg/day.

DIETARY SUPPLEMENT

PO, IV, IM, SUBCUTANEOUS: ADULTS, ELDERLY, CHILDREN 4 YR AND OLDER: 0.4 mg/day. CHILDREN 1–3 YR: 0.3 mg/day. CHILDREN YOUNGER THAN 1 YR: 0.1 mg/day. PREGNANT WOMEN: 0.6 mg/day.

SIDE EFFECTS

None known.

ADVERSE REACTIONS/TOXIC EFFECTS

Allergic hypersensitivity occurs rarely with parenteral form. Oral folic acid is nontoxic.

BASELINE ASSESSMENT

Pernicious anemia should be ruled out with Schilling test and vitamin B_{12} blood level before initiating therapy (may produce irreversible neurologic damage). Resistance to treatment may occur if decreased hematopoiesis, alcoholism, antimetabolic drugs, deficiency of vitamin B_6, B_{12}, C, E is evident.

INTERVENTION/EVALUATION

Assess for therapeutic improvement: improved sense of well-being, relief from iron deficiency symptoms (fatigue, shortness of breath, sore tongue, headache, pallor).

PATIENT/FAMILY TEACHING

• Eat foods rich in folic acid, including fruits, vegetables, organ meats.

follitropin alpha

(Gonal-F)
See Fertility agents (p. 92C)

fomepizole

(Antizol)
See Appendix L

fondaparinux sodium ▷

fond-dah-**pear**-in-ux
(Arixtra)

 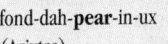

CLASSIFICATION

PHARMACOTHERAPEUTIC: Factor Xa inhibitor, pentasaccharide. **CLINICAL:** Antithrombotic.

ACTION

A factor Xa inhibitor and pentasaccharide that selectively binds to antithrombin, and increases its affinity for factor Xa, thereby inhibiting factor Xa and stopping the blood coagulation cascade. **Therapeutic Effect:** Indirectly prevents formation of thrombin and subsequently the fibrin clot.

PHARMACOKINETICS

Well absorbed after subcutaneous administration. Undergoes minimal, if any, metabolism. Highly bound to antithrombin III. Distributed mainly in blood and to a minor extent in extravascular fluid. Excreted unchanged in urine. Removed by hemodialysis. **Half-life:** 17–21 hr (prolonged in patients with impaired renal function).

USES

Prevention of venous thromboembolism in patients undergoing total hip replacement, hip fracture surgery, knee replacement surgery. Treatment of acute deep vein thrombosis (DVT), acute pulmonary embolism. Used concurrently with warfarin therapy. Prevention of DVT in patients undergoing abdominal surgery.

PRECAUTIONS

◀ **ALERT** ▶ When neuraxial anesthesia (epidural or spinal anesthesia) or spinal puncture is employed, patients anticoagulated or scheduled to be anticoagulated with fondaparinux sodium for prevention of thromboembolic complications are at risk of developing an epidural or spinal hematoma which can result in long-term or permanent paralysis. **CONTRAINDICATIONS:** Active major bleeding, bacterial endocarditis, body weight less than 50 kg, severe renal impairment (with creatinine clearance less than 30 ml/min), thrombocytopenia associated with antiplatelet antibody formation in the presence of fondaparinux. **CAUTIONS:** Conditions with increased risk of hemorrhage (GI ulceration, hemophilia, concurrent use of antiplatelet agents, severe uncontrolled hypertension, history of cerebrovascular accident [CVA]), history of heparin-induced thrombocytopenia, renal impairment, elderly, neuraxial anesthesia, indwelling epidural catheter use.

⏳ **LIFESPAN CONSIDERATIONS: Pregnancy/Lactation:** Use with caution, particularly during last trimester, immediate postpartum period (increased risk of maternal hemorrhage). Unknown if excreted in breast milk. **Pregnancy Category B. Children:** Safety and efficacy not established. **Elderly:** Age-related renal impairment may increase risk of bleeding.

INTERACTIONS

DRUG: Anticoagulants, platelet inhibitors: May increase bleeding. **HERBAL:** None known. **FOOD:** None known. **LAB VALUES:** Increases reversible serum creatinine, AST, and ALT levels. May decrease Hgb, Hct, and platelet count.

AVAILABILITY (Rx)

INJECTION: 2.5 mg/0.5 ml prefilled syringe.

ADMINISTRATION/HANDLING

SUBCUTANEOUS

• Parenteral form appears clear, colorless. Discard if discoloration or particulate matter is noted. • Store at room temperature. • Do not expel the air bubble from the prefilled syringe before injection. • Pinch a fold of skin at the injection site between thumb and forefinger. Introduce entire length of subcutaneous needle into skin fold during

---

injection. Inject into fatty tissue between left and right anterolateral or left and right posterolateral abdominal wall.
• Rotate injection sites.

INDICATIONS/ROUTES/DOSAGE
PREVENTION OF VENOUS THROMBOEMBOLISM
SUBCUTANEOUS: ADULTS: 2.5 mg once a day for 5–9 days after surgery. Initial dose should be given 6–8 hr after surgery. Dosage should be adjusted in the elderly and in those with renal impairment.

TREATMENT VENOUS THROMBOEMBOLISM, PULMONARY EMBOLISM
SUBCUTANEOUS: ADULTS, ELDERLY WEIGHING GREATER THAN 100 KG: 10 mg once daily. ADULTS, ELDERLY WEIGHING 50–100 KG: 7.5 mg once daily. ADULTS, ELDERLY WEIGHING LESS THAN 50 KG: 5 mg once daily.

SIDE EFFECTS
OCCASIONAL (14%): Fever. **RARE (4%–1%):** Injection site hematoma, nausea, peripheral edema.

ADVERSE REACTIONS/ TOXIC EFFECTS
Accidental overdose may lead to bleeding complications ranging from local ecchymoses to major hemorrhage. Thrombocytopenia occurs rarely.

NURSING CONSIDERATIONS
BASELINE ASSESSMENT
Assess CBC, including platelet count, baseline BUN, creatinine clearance.

INTERVENTION/EVALUATION
Periodically monitor CBC, platelet count, stool for occult blood (no need for daily monitoring in patients with normal presurgical coagulation parameters). Assess for any signs of bleeding: bleeding at surgical site, hematuria, blood in stool, bleeding from gums, petechiae, ecchymosis, bleeding from injection sites. Monitor BP and pulse; hypotension and tachycardia may indicate bleeding.

PATIENT/FAMILY TEACHING
• Usual length of therapy is 5–9 days.
• Do not take any OTC medication (especially aspirin, NSAIDs). • Consult physician if swelling in hands, feet is noted or unusual back pain, unusual bleeding or bruising, weakness, sudden or severe headache occurs.

formoterol fumarate
for-**moe**-ter-ol
(Foradil Aerolizer)

◆CLASSIFICATION
PHARMACOTHERAPEUTIC: Sympathomimetic (beta$_2$-adrenergic agonist). **CLINICAL:** Bronchodilator (see p. 66C).

ACTION
A long-acting bronchodilator that stimulates beta$_2$-adrenergic receptors in the lungs, resulting in relaxation of bronchial smooth muscle. Also inhibits release of mediators from various cells in the lungs, including mast cells, with little effect on heart rate. **Therapeutic Effect:** Relieves bronchospasm, reduces airway resistance. Improves bronchodilation, nighttime asthma control, and peak flow rates.

PHARMACOKINETICS

Route	Onset	Peak	Duration
Inhalation	1–3 min	0.5–1 hr	12 hr

Absorbed from bronchi after inhalation. Metabolized in the liver. Primarily excreted in urine. Unknown if removed by hemodialysis. **Half-life:** 10 hr.

USES

For long-term maintenance treatment of asthma, prevention of exercise-induced bronchospasm, treatment of broncho-constriction in patients with chronic obstructive pulmonary disease (COPD). Can be used concomitantly with short-acting beta-agonists, inhaled or systemic corticosteroids, theophylline therapy.

PRECAUTIONS

CONTRAINDICATIONS: None known. **CAUTIONS:** Hypertension, cardiovascular disease, convulsive disorder, thyrotoxicosis. May increase risk of severe asthma episodes.

⌛ **LIFESPAN CONSIDERATIONS: Pregnancy/Lactation:** Unknown if drug crosses placenta or is distributed in breast milk. **Pregnancy Category C. Children:** Safety and efficacy not established in children younger than 5 yr. **Elderly:** May be more sensitive to tremor or tachycardia due to age-related increased sympathetic sensitivity.

INTERACTIONS

DRUG: Beta blockers: May antagonize formoterol's bronchodilating effects. **Diuretics, steroids, xanthine derivatives:** May increase the risk of hypokalemia. **Drugs that can prolong QT interval (including erythromycin, quinidine, and thioridazine), MAOIs, tricyclic antidepressants:** May potentiate cardiovascular effects. **HERBAL:** None known. **FOOD:** None known. **LAB VALUES:** May decrease serum potassium level. May increase blood glucose level.

AVAILABILITY (Rx)

INHALATION POWDER IN CAPSULES: 12 mcg.

ADMINISTRATION/HANDLING

INHALATION

• Pull off Aerolizer Inhaler cover, twisting mouthpiece in direction of the arrow to open. • Place capsule in chamber. Capsule is pierced by pressing and releasing buttons on the side of the Aerolizer, once only. • Exhale completely; place mouthpiece into mouth, close lips. • Inhale quickly, deeply through mouth (this causes capsule to spin, dispensing the drug). Hold breath as long as possible before exhaling slowly. • Check capsule to make sure all the powder is gone. If not, inhale again to receive rest of the dose. Rinse mouth with water immediately after inhalation (prevents mouth/throat dryness).

Storage • Maintain capsules in individual blister pack until immediately before use. • Do not swallow capsules. • Do not use with a spacer.

INDICATIONS/ROUTES/DOSAGE

ASTHMA, COPD

INHALATION: ADULTS, ELDERLY, CHILDREN 5 YR AND OLDER: 12 mcg capsule q12h.

EXERCISE-INDUCED BRONCHOSPASM

INHALATION: ADULTS, ELDERLY, CHILDREN 5 YR AND OLDER: 12 mcg capsule at least 15 min before exercise. Do not repeat for another 12 hr.

SIDE EFFECTS

OCCASIONAL: Tremor, muscle cramps, tachycardia, insomnia, headache, irritability, irritation of mouth or throat.

ADVERSE REACTIONS/ TOXIC EFFECTS

Excessive sympathomimetic stimulation may produce palpitations, extrasystole, and chest pain.

NURSING CONSIDERATIONS

INTERVENTION/EVALUATION

Assess rate, depth, rhythm, type of respiration; quality and rate of pulse. Monitor EKG, serum potassium, ABG determinations. Assess lung sounds for wheezing (bronchoconstriction), rales.

PATIENT/FAMILY TEACHING
• Instruct patient in proper use of inhaler. • Increase fluid intake (decreases lung secretion viscosity). • Rinsing mouth with water immediately after inhalation may prevent mouth/throat irritation. • Avoid excessive use of caffeine derivatives (chocolate, coffee, tea, cola).

Fortaz, *see ceftazidime*

Fortovase, *see saquinavir*

Fosamax, *see alendronate*

---

fosamprenavir calcium

foss-am-**pren**-ah-vur
(Lexiva)

◆ **CLASSIFICATION**

PHARMACOTHERAPEUTIC: Antiretroviral. **CLINICAL:** Protease inhibitor.

ACTION

An antiretroviral that is rapidly converted to amprenavir, which inhibits HIV-1 protease by binding to the enzyme's active site, thus preventing the processing of viral precursors and resulting in the formation of immature, noninfectious viral particles. **Therapeutic Effect:** Impairs HIV replication and proliferation.

PHARMACOKINETICS

Rapidly absorbed after PO administration. Protein binding: 90%. Metabolized in the liver. Excreted in urine and feces. **Half-life:** 7.7 hr.

USES

Treatment of HIV infection in combination with other antiretroviral agents.

PRECAUTIONS

CONTRAINDICATIONS: Concurrent use of amprenavir, dihydroergotamine, ergonovine, ergotamine, flecainide, methylergonovine, midazolam, pimozide, propafenone, ritonavir, triazolam. **EXTREME CAUTION:** Hepatic impairment. **CAUTIONS:** Diabetes mellitus, elderly, renal impairment, known sulfonamide allergy.

⧖ **LIFESPAN CONSIDERATIONS: Pregnancy/Lactation:** Unknown if drug crosses placenta or is distributed in breast milk. **Pregnancy Category C. Children:** Safety and efficacy not established in children younger than 4 yr. **Elderly:** Age-related hepatic impairment may require decreased dosage.

INTERACTIONS

DRUG: Amiodarone, bepridil, ergotamine, lidocaine, midazolam, oral contraceptives, quinidine, triazolam, tricyclic antidepressants: May interfere with the metabolism of the these drugs. **Antacids, didanosine:** May decrease the absorption of fosamprenavir. **Carbamazepine, phenobarbital, phenytoin, rifampin:** May decrease fosamprenavir blood concentration. **Clozapine, hydroxamethylglutaryl-CoA (HMG-CoA) reductase inhibitors (statins), warfarin:** May increase the blood concentrations of these drugs. **HERBAL: St. John's wort:** May decrease fosamprenavir blood concentration. **FOOD:** None known. **LAB VALUES:** May increase serum lipase, triglyceride, AST, and ALT levels.

F

AVAILABILITY (Rx)

TABLETS: 700 mg (equivalent to 600 mg amprenavir).

ADMINISTRATION/HANDLING

PO

• Give without regard to meals. • Do not crush or break film-coated tablets.

INDICATIONS/ROUTES/DOSAGE

HIV INFECTION IN PATIENTS WHO HAVE NOT HAD PREVIOUS PROTEASE INHIBITOR THERAPY

PO: ADULTS, ELDERLY: 1,400 mg twice daily without ritonavir; or 1,400 mg once daily plus ritonavir 200 mg once daily; or 700 mg twice daily plus ritonavir 100 mg twice daily.

HIV INFECTION IN PATIENTS WHO HAVE HAD PREVIOUS PROTEASE INHIBITOR THERAPY

PO: ADULTS, ELDERLY: 700 mg twice daily plus ritonavir 100 mg twice daily.

CONCURRENT THERAPY WITH EFAVIRENZ

PO: ADULTS, ELDERLY: In patients receiving fosamprenavir plus once-daily ritonavir in combination with efavirenz, an additional 100 mg/day ritonavir (300 mg total/day) should be given.

SIDE EFFECTS

FREQUENT (39%–35%): Nausea, rash, diarrhea. **OCCASIONAL (19%–8%):** Headache, vomiting, fatigue, depression. **RARE (7%–2%):** Pruritus, abdominal pain, perioral paresthesia.

ADVERSE REACTIONS/ TOXIC EFFECTS

Severe and possibly life-threatening dermatologic reactions, including Stevens-Johnson syndrome, occur rarely. New onset or exacerbation of diabetes mellitus has been reported.

NURSING CONSIDERATIONS

BASELINE ASSESSMENT

Obtain baseline lab testing, especially liver function tests, before beginning therapy and at periodic intervals during therapy. Offer emotional support. Obtain medication history.

INTERVENTION/EVALUATION

Closely monitor for evidence of GI discomfort. Monitor pattern of bowel activity and stool consistency. Assess skin for evidence of rash. Monitor serum chemistry tests for marked laboratory abnormalities, particularly hepatic profile. Assess for opportunistic infections: onset of fever, oral mucosa changes, cough, or other respiratory symptoms.

PATIENT/FAMILY TEACHING

• Eat small, frequent meals to offset nausea, vomiting. • Continue therapy for full length of treatment. • Doses should be evenly spaced. • Medication is not a cure for HIV infection, nor does it reduce risk of transmission to others. • Patient may continue to experience illnesses, including opportunistic infections. • Diarrhea can be controlled with OTC medication.

foscarnet sodium

foss-**car**-net
(Foscavir)

CLASSIFICATION

CLINICAL: Antiviral (see p. 61C).

ACTION

An antiviral that selectively inhibits binding sites on virus-specific DNA polymerase and reverse transcriptase. **Therapeutic Effect:** Inhibits replication of herpes virus.

✎ see color pill atlas   🖛 herb   underlined – top prescribed drug

PHARMACOKINETICS

Sequestered into bone and cartilage. Protein binding: 14%–17%. Primarily excreted unchanged in urine. Removed by hemodialysis. **Half-life:** 3.3–6.8 hr (increased in impaired renal function).

USES

Treatment of herpes virus infections suspected to be caused by acyclovir-resistant or ganciclovir-resistant strains. Treatment of cytomegalovirus (CMV) retinitis.

PRECAUTIONS

CONTRAINDICATIONS: None known. **CAUTIONS:** Neurologic or cardiac abnormalities, history of renal impairment, altered calcium, other electrolyte levels.

⌛ **LIFESPAN CONSIDERATIONS: Pregnancy/Lactation:** Unknown if distributed in breast milk. **Pregnancy Category C. Children:** Safety and efficacy not established. **Elderly:** Age-related renal impairment may require dosage adjustment.

INTERACTIONS

DRUG: Nephrotoxic medications: May increase the risk of nephrotoxicity. **Pentamidine (IV):** May cause reversible hypocalcemia, hypomagnesemia, and nephrotoxicity. **Zidovudine (AZT):** May increase the risk of anemia. **HERBAL:** None known. **FOOD:** None known. **LAB VALUES:** May increase serum alkaline phosphatase, bilirubin, creatinine, AST, and ALT levels. May decrease serum magnesium and potassium levels. May alter serum calcium and phosphate concentrations.

AVAILABILITY (Rx)

INJECTION: 24 mg/ml.

ADMINISTRATION/HANDLING

 IV

Reconstitution • The standard 24 mg/ml solution may be used without dilution when central venous catheter is used for infusion; 24 mg/ml solution *must* be diluted to 12 mg/ml when peripheral vein catheter is being used. • Only D_5W or 0.9% NaCl solution for injection should be used for dilution.

Rate of administration • Because dosage is calculated on body weight, unneeded quantity may be removed before start of infusion to avoid overdosage. Aseptic technique must be used and solution administered within 24 hr of first entry into sealed bottle. • Do not give by IV injection or rapid infusion (increases toxicity). • Administer by IV infusion at a rate not faster than 1 hr for doses up to 60 mg/kg and 2 hr for doses greater than 60 mg/kg. • To minimize toxicity and phlebitis, use central venous lines or veins with adequate blood flow to permit rapid dilution, dissemination of foscarnet. • Use IV infusion pump to prevent accidental overdose.

Storage • Store parenteral vials at room temperature. • After dilution, stable for 24 hr at room temperature. • Do not use if solution is discolored or contains particulate material.

▨ IV INCOMPATIBILITIES

Acyclovir (Zovirax), amphotericin B (Fungizone), co-trimoxazole (Bactrim), diazepam (Valium), digoxin (Lanoxin), diphenhydramine (Benadryl), dobutamine (Dobutrex), droperidol (Inapsine), ganciclovir (Cytovene), haloperidol (Haldol), leucovorin, midazolam (Versed), pentamidine (Pentam IV), prochlorperazine (Compazine), vancomycin (Vancocin).

IV COMPATIBILITIES

Dopamine (Intropin), heparin, hydromorphone (Dilaudid), lorazepam (Ativan), morphine, potassium chloride, total parenteral nutrition (TPN).

INDICATIONS/ROUTES/DOSAGE

CYTOMEGALOVIRUS (CMV) RETINITIS

IV: ADULTS, ELDERLY: Initially, 60 mg/kg q8h or 100 mg/kg q12h for 2–3 wk. Maintenance: 90–120 mg/kg/day as a single IV infusion.

HERPES INFECTION

IV: ADULTS: 40 mg/kg q8–12h for 2–3 wk or until healed.

DOSAGE IN RENAL IMPAIRMENT

Dosages are individualized based on creatinine clearance. Refer to the dosing guide provided by the manufacturer.

SIDE EFFECTS

FREQUENT: Fever (65%); nausea (47%); vomiting, diarrhea (30%). **OCCASIONAL (5% or greater):** Anorexia, pain and inflammation at injection site, fever, rigors, malaise, headache, paresthesia, dizziness, rash, diaphoresis, abdominal pain. **RARE (5%–1%):** Back or chest pain, edema, flushing, pruritus, constipation, dry mouth.

ADVERSE REACTIONS/ TOXIC EFFECTS

Nephrotoxicity occurs to some extent in most patients. Seizures and serum mineral or electrolyte imbalances may be life-threatening.

NURSING CONSIDERATIONS

BASELINE ASSESSMENT

Obtain baseline serum mineral and electrolyte levels, vital signs, CBC values, renal function tests. Risk of renal impairment can be reduced by sufficient fluid intake to assure diuresis before and during therapy.

INTERVENTION/EVALUATION

Monitor serum creatinine, calcium, phosphorus, potassium, magnesium, Hgb, Hct. Obtain periodic ophthalmologic exams. Assess for signs of serum electrolyte imbalance, especially hypocalcemia (perioral tingling, numbness or paresthesia of extremities), hypokalemia (weakness, muscle cramps, numbness/tingling of extremities, irritability). Monitor renal function tests. Assess for tremors; provide safety measures for potential seizures. Assess for bleeding, anemia, developing superinfections.

PATIENT/FAMILY TEACHING

• Important to report perioral tingling, numbness in the extremities, paresthesias during or following infusion (may indicate electrolyte abnormalities).
• Tremors should be reported promptly due to potential for seizures.

fosfomycin tromethamine

foss-fo-**mye**-sin

(Monurol)

Do not confuse Monurol with Monopril.

◆CLASSIFICATION

PHARMACOTHERAPEUTIC: Antibiotic. **CLINICAL:** UTI agent.

ACTION

An antibiotic that prevents bacterial cell wall formation by inhibiting the synthesis of peptidoglycan. **Therapeutic Effect:** Bactericidal.

PHARMACOKINETICS

Rapidly absorbed following PO administration. Not bound to plasma proteins. Not metabolized. Partially excreted in urine; minimal elimination in feces. **Half-life:** 5.7 + 2.8 hr.

USES

Single-dose treatment for uncomplicated UTIs in women. **OFF-LABEL:** Serious UTI in men.

PRECAUTIONS

CONTRAINDICATIONS: None known. **CAUTIONS:** Renal impairment.

⌛ **LIFESPAN CONSIDERATIONS: Pregnancy/Lactation:** Unknown if drug crosses placenta or is distributed in breast milk. **Pregnancy Category B. Children:** Safety and efficacy not established in children younger than 12 yr. **Elderly:** Age-related renal impairment may require dosage adjustment.

INTERACTIONS

DRUG: Metoclopramide: Lowers serum concentration and urinary excretion of fosfomycin. **HERBAL:** None known. **FOOD:** None known. **LAB VALUES:** May increase blood eosinophil count and serum alkaline phosphatase, bilirubin, AST, and ALT levels. May alter platelet and WBC counts. May decrease blood Hct and Hgb levels.

AVAILABILITY (Rx)

POWDER FOR ORAL SOLUTION: 3 g.

ADMINISTRATION/HANDLING

• Give without regard to food.

INDICATIONS/ROUTES/DOSAGE

UTIs
PO (UNCOMPLICATED): FEMALES: 3 g mixed in 4 oz water as a single dose.
PO (COMPLICATED): MALES: 3 g/day q2–3days for 3 doses.

SIDE EFFECTS

OCCASIONAL (9%–3%): Diarrhea, nausea, headache, back pain. **RARE (less than 2%):** Dysmenorrhea, pharyngitis, abdominal pain, rash.

ADVERSE REACTIONS/ TOXIC EFFECTS

None known.

PATIENT/FAMILY TEACHING
• Symptoms should improve in 2–3 days. • Always mix medication with water before taking.

fosinopril

fo-**sin**-o-pril

(Monopril)

Do not confuse Monopril with Monurol.

CLASSIFICATION

PHARMACOTHERAPEUTIC: Angiotensin-converting enzyme (ACE) inhibitor. **CLINICAL:** Antihypertensive (see p. 7C).

ACTION

An ACE inhibitor that suppresses the renin-angiotensin-aldosterone system and prevents conversion of angiotensin I to angiotensin II, a potent vasoconstrictor; may also inhibit angiotensin II at local vascular and renal sites. Decreases plasma angiotensin II, increases plasma renin activity, and decreases aldosterone secretion. **Therapeutic Effect:** Reduces peripheral arterial resistance, pulmonary capillary wedge pressure; improves cardiac output, and exercise tolerance.

PHARMACOKINETICS

Route	Onset	Peak	Duration
PO	1 hr	2–6 hr	24 hr

Slowly absorbed from the GI tract. Protein binding: 97%–98%. Metabolized in the liver and GI mucosa to active metabolite. Primarily excreted in urine. Minimal removal by hemodialysis. **Half-life:** 11.5 hr.

F

USES

Treatment of hypertension. Used alone or in combination with other antihypertensives. Treatment of heart failure. OFF-LABEL: Treatment of diabetic and nondiabetic nephropathy, post-MI left ventricular dysfunction, renal crisis in scleroderma.

PRECAUTIONS

CONTRAINDICATIONS: History of angioedema from previous treatment with ACE inhibitors, pregnancy. **CAUTIONS:** Renal impairment, those with sodium depletion or on diuretic therapy, dialysis, hypovolemia, coronary or cerebrovascular insufficiency.

⧗ LIFESPAN CONSIDERATIONS: **Pregnancy/Lactation:** Crosses placenta. Distributed in breast milk. May cause fetal or neonatal mortality or morbidity. **Pregnancy Category C (D if used in second or third trimester). Children:** Safety and efficacy not established. Neonates, infants may be at increased risk for oliguria, neurologic abnormalities. **Elderly:** May be more sensitive to hypotensive effects.

INTERACTIONS

DRUG: **Alcohol, antihypertensives, diuretics:** May increase the effects of fosinopril. **Lithium:** May increase lithium blood concentration and risk of lithium toxicity. **NSAIDs:** May decrease the effects of fosinopril. **Potassium-sparing diuretics, potassium supplements:** May cause hyperkalemia. HERBAL: None known. FOOD: None known. LAB VALUES: May increase BUN, serum alkaline phosphatase, serum bilirubin, serum creatinine, serum potassium, AST, and ALT levels. May decrease serum sodium levels. May cause positive antinuclear antibody titer.

AVAILABILITY (Rx)

TABLETS: 10 mg, 20 mg, 40 mg.

ADMINISTRATION/HANDLING

PO

• Give without regard to food. • Tablets may be crushed.

INDICATIONS/ROUTES/DOSAGE

HYPERTENSION

PO: ADULTS, ELDERLY: Initially, 10 mg/day. Maintenance: 20–40 mg/day as a single or 2 divided doses. **Maximum:** 80 mg/day. CHILDREN 6–16 YR WEIGHING MORE THAN 50 KG: Initially, 5–10 mg/day.

HEART FAILURE

PO: ADULTS, ELDERLY: Initially, 10 mg/day. Maintenance: 20–40 mg/day. **Maximum:** 40 mg/day.

SIDE EFFECTS

FREQUENT (12%–9%): Dizziness, cough. **OCCASIONAL (4%–2%):** Hypotension, nausea, vomiting, upper respiratory tract infection.

ADVERSE REACTIONS/ TOXIC EFFECTS

Excessive hypotension ("first-dose syncope") may occur in patients with CHF and in those who are severely salt and volume depleted. Angioedema (swelling of face and lips) and hyperkalemia occur rarely. Agranulocytosis and neutropenia may be noted in those with collagen vascular disease, including scleroderma and systemic lupus erythematosus, and impaired renal function. Nephrotic syndrome may be noted in those with history of renal disease.

NURSING CONSIDERATIONS

BASELINE ASSESSMENT

Obtain BP immediately before each dose, in addition to regular monitoring (be alert to fluctuations). Renal function tests should be performed before beginning therapy. In patients with renal impairment, autoimmune disease, or taking drugs that affect leukocytes or immune response, CBC, differential count should be performed before therapy begins and q2wk for 3 mo, then periodically thereafter.

INTERVENTION/EVALUATION

If excessive reduction in BP occurs, place patient in supine position with legs elevated. Assist with ambulation if dizziness occurs. Assess for urinary frequency. Auscultate lung sounds for rales, wheezing in those with CHF. Monitor urinalysis for proteinuria. Monitor serum potassium levels in those on concurrent diuretic therapy.

PATIENT/FAMILY TEACHING

• Report any sign of infection (sore throat, fever). • Several weeks may be needed for full therapeutic effect of BP reduction. • Skipping doses or voluntarily discontinuing drug may produce severe, rebound hypertension. • To reduce hypotensive effect, rise slowly from lying to sitting position, permit legs to dangle from bed momentarily before standing. • Inform physician if vomiting, excessive perspiration, persistent cough develops.

fosphenytoin

fos-phen-ih-**toyn**
(Cerebyx)
Do not confuse Cerebyx with Celebrex or Celexa.

◆CLASSIFICATION

PHARMACOTHERAPEUTIC: Hydantoin. **CLINICAL:** Anticonvulsant (see p. 34C).

ACTION

A hydantoin anticonvulsant that stabilizes neuronal membranes by decreasing sodium and calcium ion influx into the neurons. Also decreases post-tetanic potentiation and repetitive discharge. **Therapeutic Effect:** Decreases seizure activity.

PHARMACOKINETICS

Completely absorbed after IM administration. Protein binding: 95%–99%. Rapidly and completely hydrolyzed to phenytoin after IM or IV administration. Time of complete conversion to phenytoin: 4 hr after IM injection; 2 hr after IV infusion. **Half-life:** 8–15 min (for conversion to phenytoin).

USES

Acute treatment, control of generalized convulsive status epilepticus; prevention, treatment of seizures occurring during neurosurgery; short-term substitution of oral phenytoin.

PRECAUTIONS

CONTRAINDICATIONS: Adams-Stokes syndrome; hypersensitivity to ethotoin, phenytoin, mephenytoin; second- or third-degree AV block; severe bradycardia; SA block. **CAUTIONS:** Porphyria, hypotension, severe myocardial insufficiency, renal or hepatic disease, hypoalbuminemia.

⧗ LIFESPAN CONSIDERATIONS: **Pregnancy/Lactation:** May increase frequency of seizures during pregnancy. Increased risk of congenital malformations. Unknown if excreted in breast milk. **Pregnancy Category D. Children:** Safety not established. **Elderly:** Lower dosage recommended.

INTERACTIONS

DRUG: **Alcohol, other CNS depressants:** May increase CNS depression. **Amiodarone, anticoagulants, cimetidine, disulfiram, fluoxetine, isoniazid, sulfonamides:** May increase fosphenytoin blood concentration, effects, and risk of toxicity. **Antacids:** May decrease fosphenytoin absorption. **Fluconazole, ketoconazole, miconazole:** May increase fosphenytoin blood

F

concentration. **Glucocorticoids:** May decrease the effects of glucocorticoids. **Lidocaine, propranolol:** May increase cardiac depressant effects. **Valproic acid:** May increase the blood concentration and decrease the metabolism of fosphenytoin. **Xanthines:** May increase the metabolism of xanthines. **HERBAL:** None known. **FOOD:** None known. **LAB VALUES:** May increase blood glucose, serum GGT, and serum alkaline phosphatase levels.

AVAILABILITY (Rx)

INJECTION: 75 mg/ml (equivalent to 50 mg/ml phenytoin).

ADMINISTRATION/HANDLING
 IV

Reconstitution • Dilute in D₅W or 0.9% NaCl to a concentration ranging from 1.5–25 mg PE/ml.

Rate of administration • Administer at rate of less than 150 mg PE/min (decreases risk of hypotension, arrhythmias).

Storage • Refrigerate. Do not store at room temperature for longer than 48 hr. • After dilution, solution is stable for 8 hr at room temperature or 24 hr if refrigerated.

IV INCOMPATIBILITY
Midazolam (Versed).

IV COMPATIBILITIES
Lorazepam (Ativan), phenobarbital, potassium chloride.

INDICATIONS/ROUTES/DOSAGE
STATUS EPILEPTICUS
IV: ADULTS: Loading dose: 15–20 mg phenytoin equivalent (PE)/kg infused at rate of 100–150 mg PE/min.

NONEMERGENT SEIZURES
IV, IM: ADULTS: Loading dose: 10–20 mg PE/kg. Maintenance: 4–6 mg PE/kg/day.

SHORT TERM SUBSTITUTION FOR ORAL PHENYTOIN
IV, IM: ADULTS: May substitute for oral phenytoin at same total daily dose.

SIDE EFFECTS
FREQUENT: Dizziness, paresthesia, tinnitus, pruritus, headache, somnolence. **OCCASIONAL:** Morbilliform rash.

ADVERSE REACTIONS/ TOXIC EFFECTS
An elevated fosphenytoin blood concentration may produce ataxia, nystagmus, diplopia, lethargy, slurred speech, nausea, vomiting, and hypotension. As the drug level increases, extreme lethargy may progress to coma.

NURSING CONSIDERATIONS

BASELINE ASSESSMENT
Review history of seizure disorder (intensity, frequency, duration, level of consciousness [LOC]). Initiate seizure precautions. Obtain vital signs, medication history (especially use of phenytoin, other anticonvulsants). Observe clinically.

INTERVENTION/EVALUATION
Measure cardiac function, EKG, respiratory function, BP during and immediately following infusion (10–20 min). Discontinue if skin rash appears. Interrupt or decrease rate if hypotension, arrhythmias are detected. Assess patient post-infusion (may feel dizzy, ataxic, drowsy). Assess blood levels of fosphenytoin (2 hr post IV infusion or 4 hr post IM injection).

PATIENT/FAMILY TEACHING
• Teach patients about their seizure condition and role in its management. • If noncompliance is an issue in causing acute seizures, discuss and address reasons for noncompliance. • Avoid tasks that require alertness, motor skills until response to drug is established.

 see color pill atlas   herb   underlined – top prescribed drug

Fragmin, *see dalteparin*

frovatriptan

fro-va-**trip**-tan

(Frova)

◆CLASSIFICATION

PHARMACOTHERAPEUTIC: Serotonin receptor agonist. **CLINICAL:** Antimigraine (see p. 56C).

ACTION

A serotonin receptor agonist that binds selectively to vascular receptors, producing a vasoconstrictive effect on cranial blood vessels. **Therapeutic Effect:** Relieves migraine headache.

PHARMACOKINETICS

Well absorbed after PO administration. Metabolized by the liver to inactive metabolite. Eliminated in urine. **Half-life:** 26 hr (increased in hepatic impairment).

USES

Treatment of acute migraine attack with or without aura in adults.

PRECAUTIONS

CONTRAINDICATIONS: Basilar or hemiplegic migraine, cerebrovascular or peripheral vascular disease, coronary artery disease, ischemic heart disease (including angina pectoris, history of MI, silent ischemia, and Prinzmetal's angina), severe hepatic impairment (Child-Pugh grade C), uncontrolled hypertension, use within 24 hr of ergotamine-containing preparations or another serotonin receptor agonist, use within 14 days of MAOIs. **CAUTIONS:** Mild to moderate hepatic impairment, patient profile suggesting cardiovascular risks.

⧗ **LIFESPAN CONSIDERATIONS: Pregnancy/Lactation:** Unknown if drug is excreted in breast milk. **Pregnancy Category C. Children:** Safety and efficacy not established. **Elderly:** Not recommended in the elderly.

INTERACTIONS

DRUG: Ergotamine-containing medications: May produce a vasospastic reaction. **Fluoxetine, fluvoxamine, paroxetine, sertraline:** May produce a vasospastic reaction. **Oral contraceptives:** Decrease frovatriptan clearance and volume of distribution. **Propranolol:** May dramatically increase frovatriptan plasma concentration. **HERBAL:** None known. **FOOD:** None known. **LAB VALUES:** None known.

AVAILABILITY (Rx)

TABLETS: 2.5 mg.

ADMINISTRATION/HANDLING

PO
• Do not crush or chew film-coated tablets.

INDICATIONS/ROUTES/DOSAGE

ACUTE MIGRAINE ATTACK

PO: ADULTS, ELDERLY: Initially 2.5 mg. If headache improves but then returns, dose may be repeated after 2 hr. **Maximum:** 7.5 mg/day.

SIDE EFFECTS

OCCASIONAL (8%–4%): Dizziness, paresthesia, fatigue, flushing. **RARE (3%–2%):** Hot or cold sensation, dry mouth, dyspepsia.

ADVERSE REACTIONS/ TOXIC EFFECTS

Cardiac reactions (including ischemia, coronary artery vasospasm, and MI), and noncardiac vasospasm-related reactions (such as cerebral hemorrhage and cerebrovascular accident [CVA]), occur rarely, particularly in patients with hypertension, diabetes, or a strong family history of coronary artery disease; obese patients; smokers; males older than 40 yr; and postmenopausal women.

NURSING CONSIDERATIONS

BASELINE ASSESSMENT
Question for history of peripheral vascular disease, renal or hepatic impairment, possibility of pregnancy. Question regarding onset, location, duration of migraine, possible precipitating symptoms.

INTERVENTION/EVALUATION
Assess for relief of migraine headache, potential for photophobia, phonophobia (sound sensitivity, nausea, vomiting).

PATIENT/FAMILY TEACHING
• Take a single dose as soon as symptoms of an actual migraine attack appear. • Medication is intended to relieve migraine headaches, not to prevent or reduce number of attacks. • Avoid tasks that require alertness, motor skills until response to drug is established. • If palpitations, pain, tightness in chest or throat, sudden or severe abdominal pain, pain or weakness of extremities occurs, contact physician immediately.

---

fulvestrant

full-**ves**-trant

(Faslodex)

Do not confuse Faslodex with Fosamax.

◆CLASSIFICATION
PHARMACOTHERAPEUTIC: Estrogen antagonist. **CLINICAL:** Antineoplastic (see p. 74C).

ACTION
An estrogen antagonist that competes with endogenous estrogen at estrogen receptor binding sites. **Therapeutic Effect:** Inhibits tumor growth.

PHARMACOKINETICS
Extensively and rapidly distributed after IM administration. Protein binding: 99%. Metabolized in the liver. Eliminated by hepatobiliary route; excreted in feces. **Half-life:** 40 days in postmenopausal women. Peak serum levels occur in 7–9 days.

USES
Treatment of hormone receptor–positive metastatic breast cancer in postmenopausal women with disease progression following antiestrogen therapy. **OFF-LABEL:** Endometriosis, uterine bleeding.

PRECAUTIONS
CONTRAINDICATIONS: Known or suspected pregnancy. **CAUTIONS:** Thrombocytopenia, bleeding diathesis, anticoagulant therapy, hepatic disease, reduced hepatic blood flow, estrogen receptor–negative breast cancer.

⧗ **LIFESPAN CONSIDERATIONS: Pregnancy/Lactation:** Do not administer to pregnant women. Unknown if excreted in breast milk. May cause fetal harm. **Pregnancy Category D. Children:** Not for use in children. **Elderly:** No age-related precautions noted.

INTERACTIONS
DRUG: None known. **HERBAL:** None known. **FOOD:** None known. **LAB VALUES:** None known.

AVAILABILITY (Rx)

PREFILLED SYRINGE: 50 mg/ml in 2.5-ml and 5-ml syringes.

ADMINISTRATION/HANDLING

IM

• Administer slowly into the buttock as a single 5-ml injection or 2 concurrent 2.5-ml injections.

INDICATIONS/ROUTES/DOSAGE

BREAST CANCER

IM: ADULTS, ELDERLY: 250 mg given once monthly.

SIDE EFFECTS

FREQUENT (26%–13%): Nausea, hot flashes, pharyngitis, asthenia, vomiting, vasodilatation, headache. **OCCASIONAL (12%–5%):** Injection site pain, constipation, diarrhea, abdominal pain, anorexia, dizziness, insomnia, paresthesia, bone or back pain, depression, anxiety, peripheral edema, rash, diaphoresis, fever. **RARE (2%–1%):** Vertigo, weight gain.

ADVERSE REACTIONS/ TOXIC EFFECTS

UTIs, vaginitis, anemia, thromboembolic phenomena, and leukopenia occur rarely.

NURSING CONSIDERATIONS

BASELINE ASSESSMENT

An estrogen receptor assay should be done before beginning therapy. Baseline CT should be performed initially and periodically thereafter for evidence of tumor regression.

INTERVENTION/EVALUATION

Monitor blood chemistry, plasma lipids. Be alert to increased bone pain, ensure adequate pain relief. Check for edema, especially of dependent areas. Monitor

for and assist with ambulation if asthenia or dizziness occurs. Assess for headache. Offer antiemetic for nausea and vomiting.

PATIENT/FAMILY TEACHING

• Notify physician if nausea, asthenia, hot flashes become unmanageable.

furosemide

feur-**oh**-sah-mide

(Apo-Furosemide ✤, Lasix)

Do not confuse Lasix with Lidex, Luvox, or Luxiq, or furosemide with Torsemide.

CLASSIFICATION

PHARMACOTHERAPEUTIC: Loop. **CLINICAL:** Diuretic (see p. 89C).

ACTION

A loop diuretic that enhances excretion of sodium, chloride, and potassium by direct action at the ascending limb of the loop of Henle. **Therapeutic Effect:** Produces diuresis and lowers BP.

PHARMACOKINETICS

Route	Onset	Peak	Duration
PO	30–60 min	1–2 hr	6–8 hr
IV	5 min	20–60 min	2 hr
IM	30 min	N/A	N/A

Well absorbed from the GI tract. Protein binding: 91%–97%. Partially metabolized in the liver. Primarily excreted in urine (nonrenal clearance increases in severe renal impairment). Not removed by hemodialysis. **Half-life:** 30–90 min (increased in renal or hepatic impairment, and in neonates).

USES

Treatment of edema associated with CHF, chronic renal failure (including nephrotic syndrome), hepatic cirrhosis, acute pulmonary edema. Treatment of hypertension, either alone or in combination with other antihypertensives. OFF-LABEL: Hypercalcemia.

PRECAUTIONS

CONTRAINDICATIONS: Anuria, hepatic coma, severe electrolyte depletion. **CAUTIONS:** Hepatic cirrhosis.

LIFESPAN CONSIDERATIONS: Pregnancy/Lactation: Crosses placenta. Distributed in breast milk. **Pregnancy Category C (D if used in pregnancy-induced hypertension). Children:** Half-life increased in neonates; may require increased dosage interval. **Elderly:** May be more sensitive to hypotensive, electrolyte effects, developing circulatory collapse, thromboembolic effect. Age-related renal impairment may require dosage adjustment.

INTERACTIONS

DRUG: **Amphotericin B, nephrotoxic and ototoxic medications:** May increase the risk of nephrotoxicity and ototoxicity. **Anticoagulants, heparin:** May decrease the effects of these drugs. **Lithium:** May increase the risk of lithium toxicity. **Other hypokalemia-causing medications:** May increase the risk of hypokalemia. **Probenecid:** May increase furosemide blood concentration. HERBAL: None known. FOOD: None known. LAB VALUES: May increase blood glucose, BUN, and serum uric acid levels. May decrease serum calcium, chloride, magnesium, potassium, and sodium levels.

AVAILABILITY (Rx)

ORAL SOLUTION: 10 mg/ml, 40 mg/5 ml. **TABLETS:** 20 mg, 40 mg, 80 mg. **INJECTION:** 10 mg/ml.

ADMINISTRATION/HANDLING

 IV

Rate of administration • May give undiluted but is compatible with D_5W, 0.9% NaCl, or lactated Ringer's solutions. • Administer each 40 mg or fraction by IV push over 1–2 min. Do not exceed administration rate of 4 mg/min in those with renal impairment.

Storage • Solution appears clear, colorless. • Discard yellow solutions.

IM
• Temporary pain at injection site may be noted.

PO
• Give with food to avoid GI upset, preferably with breakfast (may prevent nocturia).

🔲 IV INCOMPATIBILITIES

Ciprofloxacin (Cipro), diltiazem (Cardizem), dobutamine (Dobutrex), dopamine (Intropin), doxorubicin (Adriamycin), droperidol (Inapsine), esmolol (Brevibloc), famotidine (Pepcid), filgrastim (Neupogen), fluconazole (Diflucan), gemcitabine (Gemzar), gentamicin (Garamycin), idarubicin (Idamycin), labetalol (Trandate), meperidine (Demerol), metoclopramide (Reglan), midazolam (Versed), milrinone (Primacor), nicardipine (Cardene), ondansetron (Zofran), quinidine, thiopental (Pentothal), vecuronium (Norcuron), vinblastine (Velban), vincristine (Oncovin), vinorelbine (Navelbine).

IV COMPATIBILITIES

Aminophylline, amiodarone (Cordarone), bumetanide (Bumex), calcium gluconate, cimetidine (Tagamet), heparin, hydromorphone (Dilaudid), lidocaine, morphine, nitroglycerin, norepinephrine (Levophed), potassium chloride, propofol (Diprivan).

INDICATIONS/ROUTES/DOSAGE

EDEMA, HYPERTENSION

PO: ADULTS, ELDERLY: Initially, 20–80 mg/dose; may increase by 20–40 mg/dose q6–8h. May titrate up to 600 mg/day in severe edematous states. CHILDREN: 1–6 mg/kg/day in divided doses q6–12h. NEONATES: 1–4 mg/kg/dose 1–2 times a day.

IV, IM: ADULTS, ELDERLY: 20–40 mg/dose; may increase by 20 mg/dose q1–2h. CHILDREN: 1–2 mg/kg/dose q6–12h. NEONATES: 1–2 mg/kg/dose q12–24h.

IV INFUSION: ADULTS, ELDERLY: Bolus of 0.1 mg/kg, followed by infusion of 0.1 mg/kg/hr; may double q2h. **Maximum:** 0.4 mg/kg/hr. CHILDREN: 0.05 mg/kg/hr; titrate to desired effect.

SIDE EFFECTS

EXPECTED: Increased urinary frequency and urine volume. **FREQUENT:** Nausea, dyspepsia, abdominal cramps, diarrhea or constipation, electrolyte disturbances. **OCCASIONAL:** Dizziness, light-headedness, headache, blurred vision, paresthesia, photosensitivity, rash, fatigue, bladder spasm, restlessness, diaphoresis. **RARE:** Flank pain.

ADVERSE REACTIONS/ TOXIC EFFECTS

Vigorous diuresis may lead to profound water loss and electrolyte depletion, resulting in hypokalemia, hyponatremia, and dehydration. Sudden volume depletion may result in increased risk of thrombosis, circulatory collapse, and sudden death. Acute hypotensive episodes may occur, sometimes several days after beginning therapy. Ototoxicity—manifested as deafness, vertigo, or tinnitus—may occur, especially in patients with severe renal impairment. Furosemide use can exacerbate diabetes mellitus, systemic lupus erythematosus, gout, and pancreatitis. Blood dyscrasias have been reported.

NURSING CONSIDERATIONS

BASELINE ASSESSMENT

Check vital signs, especially BP for hypotension before administration. Assess baseline serum electrolytes, especially for hypokalemia. Assess skin turgor, mucous membranes for hydration status; observe for edema. Assess muscle strength, mental status. Note skin temperature, moisture. Obtain baseline weight. Initiate I&O monitoring.

INTERVENTION/EVALUATION

Monitor BP, vital signs, serum electrolytes, I&O, weight. Note extent of diuresis. Watch for changes from initial assessment (hypokalemia may result in changes in muscle strength, tremor, muscle cramps, change in mental status, cardiac arrhythmias). Hyponatremia may result in confusion, thirst, cold and clammy skin.

PATIENT/FAMILY TEACHING

• Expect increased frequency, volume of urination. • Report palpitations, signs of electrolyte imbalances (noted previously), hearing abnormalities (e.g., sense of fullness in ears, tinnitus). • Eat foods high in potassium such as whole grains (cereals), legumes, meat, bananas, apricots, orange juice, potatoes (white, sweet), raisins. • Avoid sun or sunlamps.

F

gabapentin

gah-bah-**pen**-tin

(Apo-Gabapentin ✱ , Gabarone, <u>Neurontin</u>, Novo-Gabapentin ✱)

Do not confuse Neurontin with Neoral, Noroxin.

CLASSIFICATION

CLINICAL: Anticonvulsant, antineuralgic (see p. 34C).

ACTION

An anticonvulsant and antineuralgic agent whose exact mechanism unknown. May increase the synthesis or accumulation of gamma-aminobutyric acid by binding to as-yet-undefined receptor sites in brain tissue. **Therapeutic Effect:** Reduces seizure activity and neuropathic pain.

PHARMACOKINETICS

Well absorbed from the GI tract (not affected by food). Protein binding: less than 5%. Widely distributed. Crosses the blood-brain barrier. Primarily excreted unchanged in urine. Removed by hemodialysis. **Half-life:** 5–7 hr (increased in impaired renal function and the elderly).

USES

Adjunct in treatment of partial seizures in children 12 yr and older and adults (with or without secondary generalized seizures, partial seizures in children 3–12 yr); adjunct in treatment of neuropathic pain, postherpetic neuralgia. **OFF-LABEL:** Treatment of bipolar disorder, chronic pain, diabetic peripheral neuropathy, essential tremor, hot flashes, hyperhidrosis, migraines, psychiatric disorders (social phobia).

PRECAUTIONS

CONTRAINDICATIONS: None known. **CAUTIONS:** Renal impairment.

LIFESPAN CONSIDERATIONS: Preg-
nancy/Lactation: Unknown whether it is distributed in breast milk. **Pregnancy Category C. Children:** Safety and efficacy not established in those 3 yr and younger. **Elderly:** Age-related renal impairment may require dosage adjustment.

INTERACTIONS

DRUG: Antacids (aluminum- and magnesium-containing): May decrease gabapentin's effectiveness. **HERBAL:** None known. **FOOD:** None known. **LAB VALUES:** May decrease serum WBC count.

AVAILABILITY (Rx)

CAPSULES (NEURONTIN): 100 mg, 300 mg, 400 mg. **ORAL SOLUTION (NEURONTIN):** 250 mg/5 ml. **TABLETS (NEURONTIN):** 100 mg, 300 mg, 400 mg, 600 mg, 800 mg.

ADMINISTRATION/HANDLING

PO
• Give without regard to meals; may give with food to avoid or reduce GI upset.
• If treatment is discontinued or anticonvulsant therapy is added, do so gradually over at least 1 wk (reduces risk of loss of seizure control).

INDICATIONS/ROUTES/DOSAGE

ADJUNCTIVE THERAPY FOR SEIZURE CONTROL
PO: ADULTS, ELDERLY, CHILDREN OLDER THAN 12 YR: Initially, 300 mg 3 times a day. May titrate dosage. Range: 900–1,800 mg/day in 3 divided doses. **Maximum:** 3,600 mg/day. CHILDREN 3–12 YR: Initially, 10–15 mg/kg/day in 3 divided doses. May titrate up to 25–35 mg/kg/day (for children 5–12 yr) and 40 mg/kg/day (for children 3–4 yr). **Maximum:** 50 mg/kg/day.

ADJUNCTIVE THERAPY FOR NEUROPATHIC PAIN
PO: ADULTS, ELDERLY: Initially, 100 mg 3 times a day; may increase by 300 mg/day

at weekly intervals. **Maximum:** 3,600 mg/day in 3 divided doses. CHILDREN: Initially, 5 mg/kg/dose at bedtime, followed by 5 mg/kg/dose for 2 doses on day 2, then 5 mg/kg/dose for 3 doses on day 3. Range: 8–35 mg/kg/day in 3 divided doses.

POSTHERPETIC NEURALGIA

PO: ADULTS, ELDERLY: 300 mg on day 1, 300 mg twice a day on day 2, and 300 mg 3 times a day on day 3. Titrate up to 1,800 mg/day.

DOSAGE IN RENAL IMPAIRMENT

Dosage and frequency are modified based on creatinine clearance:

Creatinine Clearance	Dosage
60 ml/min or higher	400 mg q8h
30–59 ml/min	300 mg q12h
16–29 ml/min	300 mg daily
Less than 16 ml/min	300 mg every other day
Hemodialysis	200–300 mg after each 4-hr hemodialysis session

SIDE EFFECTS

FREQUENT (19%–10%): Fatigue, somnolence, dizziness, ataxia. **OCCASIONAL (8%–3%):** Nystagmus, tremor, diplopia, rhinitis, weight gain. **RARE (less than 2%):** Nervousness, dysarthria, memory loss, dyspepsia, pharyngitis, myalgia.

ADVERSE REACTIONS/ TOXIC EFFECTS

Abrupt withdrawal may increase seizure frequency. Overdosage may result in diplopia, slurred speech, drowsiness, lethargy, and diarrhea.

NURSING CONSIDERATIONS

BASELINE ASSESSMENT

Review history of seizure disorder (type, onset, intensity, frequency, duration, level of consciousness [LOC]). Routine laboratory monitoring of serum levels unnecessary for safe use.

INTERVENTION/EVALUATION

Provide safety measures as needed. Monitor seizure frequency/duration, renal function, weight, behavior in children.

PATIENT/FAMILY TEACHING

• Take gabapentin only as prescribed; do not abruptly stop taking drug (may increase seizure frequency). • Avoid tasks that require alertness, motor skills until response to drug is established. • Avoid alcohol. • Carry identification card/bracelet to note seizure disorder/anticonvulsant therapy.

G

galantamine

gal-**an**-tah-mine

(Razadyne, Razadyne ER)
Do not confuse with Rozerem.

•CLASSIFICATION

PHARMACOTHERAPEUTIC: Cholinesterase inhibitor. **CLINICAL:** Antidementia.

ACTION

A cholinesterase inhibitor that inhibits the enzyme acetylcholinesterase, thus increasing the concentration of acetylcholine at cholinergic synapses and enhancing cholinergic function in the CNS. **Therapeutic Effect:** Slows the progression of Alzheimer's disease.

PHARMACOKINETICS

Rapidly absorbed from the GI tract. Protein binding: 18%. Distributed to blood cells; binds to plasma proteins, mainly albumin. Metabolized in the liver. Excreted in urine. **Half-life:** 7 hr.

USES

Treatment of mild to moderate dementia of Alzheimer's type.

PRECAUTIONS

CONTRAINDICATIONS: Severe hepatic or renal impairment. **CAUTIONS:** Moderate renal or hepatic impairment, history of ulcer disease, those on concurrent NSAIDs, asthma, chronic obstructive pulmonary disease (COPD), bladder outflow obstruction, supraventricular cardiac conduction conditions.

⌛ **LIFESPAN CONSIDERATIONS: Pregnancy/Lactation:** Unknown if drug crosses placenta or is distributed in breast milk. **Pregnancy Category B. Children:** Not prescribed for this patient population. **Elderly:** No age-related precautions noted, but use is not recommended in those with severe hepatic, renal impairment (creatinine clearance less than 9 ml/min).

INTERACTIONS

DRUG: Bethanechol, succinylcholine: May interfere with the effects of these drugs. **Cimetidine, erythromycin, ketoconazole, paroxetine:** May increase the galantamine blood concentration. **HERBAL:** None known. **FOOD:** None known. **LAB VALUES:** None known.

AVAILABILITY (Rx)

CAPSULES (EXTENDED-RELEASE [RAZADYNE ER]): 8 mg, 16 mg, 24 mg. **ORAL SOLUTION (RAZADYNE):** 4 mg/ml. **TABLETS (RAZADYNE):** 4 mg, 8 mg, 12 mg.

ADMINISTRATION/HANDLING

PO
• Give with morning and evening meals.

INDICATIONS/ROUTES/DOSAGE

ALZHEIMER'S DISEASE
PO: ADULTS, ELDERLY: Initially, 4 mg twice a day (8 mg/day). After a minimum of 4 wk (if well tolerated), may increase to 8 mg twice a day (16 mg/day). After another 4 wk, may increase to 12 mg twice daily (24 mg/day). Range: 16–24 mg/day in 2 divided doses.
PO (EXTENDED-RELEASE): ADULTS,

ELDERLY: 8–24 mg/day as a single daily dose.

DOSAGE IN RENAL IMPAIRMENT
For moderate impairment, maximum dosage is 16 mg/day. Drug is not recommended for patients with severe impairment.

SIDE EFFECTS

FREQUENT (17%–5%): Nausea, vomiting, diarrhea, anorexia, weight loss. **OCCASIONAL (9%–4%):** Abdominal pain, insomnia, depression, headache, dizziness, fatigue, rhinitis. **RARE (less than 3%):** Tremors, constipation, confusion, cough, anxiety, urinary incontinence.

ADVERSE REACTIONS/TOXIC EFFECTS

Overdose may cause cholinergic crisis, characterized by increased salivation, lacrimation, severe nausea and vomiting, bradycardia, respiratory depression, hypotension, and increased muscle weakness. Treatment usually consists of supportive measures and an anticholinergic such as atropine.

NURSING CONSIDERATIONS

BASELINE ASSESSMENT
Assess cognitive, behavioral, functional deficits of patient. Assess serum liver, renal function tests.

INTERVENTION/EVALUATION
Monitor cognitive, behavioral, functional status of patient. Evaluate EKG, periodic rhythm strips in patients with underlying arrhythmias. Assess for evidence of GI disturbances (nausea, vomiting, diarrhea, anorexia, weight loss).

PATIENT/FAMILY TEACHING
• Take with morning and evening meals (reduces risk of nausea). • Avoid tasks that require alertness, motor skills until response to drug is established. • Report persistent GI disturbances, excessive salivation, diaphoresis,

excessive tearing, excessive fatigue, insomnia, depression, dizziness, increased muscle weakness.

Gamimune N, *see immune globulin IV*

Gammagard S/D, *see immune globulin IV*

Gammar-P IV, *see immune globulin IV*

ganciclovir sodium

gan-**sy**-clo-ver
(Cytovene, Vitrasert)
Do not confuse Cytovene with Cytosar.

◆CLASSIFICATION
PHARMACOTHERAPEUTIC: Synthetic nucleoside. **CLINICAL:** Antiviral (see p. 61C).

ACTION
This synthetic nucleoside competes with viral DNA polymerase and is incorporated into growing viral DNA chains. **Therapeutic Effect:** Interferes with synthesis and replication of viral DNA.

PHARMACOKINETICS
Widely distributed. Protein binding: 1%–2%. Undergoes minimal metabolism. Excreted unchanged primarily in urine. Removed by hemodialysis. **Half-life:** 2.5–3.6 hr (increased in impaired renal function).

USES
Parenteral: Treatment of cytomegalovirus (CMV) retinitis in immunocompromised patients (e.g., HIV), prophylaxis of CMV infection in transplant patients. **Oral:** Maintenance treatment of CMV retinitis. **Implant:** Treatment of CMV retinitis. **OFF-LABEL:** Treatment of other CMV infections, such as gastroenteritis, hepatitis, and pneumonitis.

PRECAUTIONS
CONTRAINDICATIONS: Absolute neutrophil count less than 500/mm³, platelet count less than 25,000/mm³, hypersensitivity to acyclovir or ganciclovir, immunocompetent patients, patients with congenital or neonatal CMV disease. **CAUTIONS:** Patients with neutropenia, thrombocytopenia, renal impairment; children (long-term safety not determined due to potential for long-term carcinogenic and adverse reproductive effects).

⏳ **LIFESPAN CONSIDERATIONS: Pregnancy/Lactation:** Effective contraception should be used during therapy; ganciclovir should not be used during pregnancy. Breast-feeding should be discontinued; may be resumed no sooner than 72 hr after the last dose of ganciclovir. **Pregnancy Category C. Children:** Safety and efficacy not established in those younger than 12 yr. **Elderly:** Age-related renal impairment may require dosage adjustment.

INTERACTIONS
DRUG: Bone marrow depressants: May increase bone marrow depression. **Imipenem and cilastatin:** May increase the risk of seizures. **Zidovudine (AZT):** May increase the risk of hepatotoxicity. **HERBAL:** None known. **FOOD:** None known. **LAB VALUES:** May increase serum alkaline phosphatase, bilirubin,

AST, and ALT levels.

AVAILABILITY (Rx)

CAPSULES (CYTOVENE): 250 mg, 500 mg.
POWDER FOR INJECTION (CYTOVENE):
500 mg. **IMPLANT (VITRASERT):** 4.5 mg.

ADMINISTRATION/HANDLING
IV

Reconstitution • Reconstitute 500-mg vial with 10 ml sterile water for injection to provide a concentration of 50 mg/ml; do **not** use bacteriostatic water (contains parabens, which is incompatible with ganciclovir). • Further dilute with 100 ml D_5W, 0.9% NaCl, lactated Ringer's, or any combination thereof to provide a concentration of 5 mg/ml.

Rate of administration • Administer only by IV infusion over 1 hr. • Do not give by IV push or rapid IV infusion (increases risk of toxicity); protect from in filtration (high pH causes severe tissue irritation). • Use large veins to permit rapid dilution and dissemination of ganciclovir (minimizes phlebitis); central venous ports may reduce catheter-associated infection.

Storage • Store vials at room temperature. Do not refrigerate. • Reconstituted solution in vial is stable for 12 hr at room temperature. • After dilution, refrigerate, use within 24 hr. • Discard if precipitate forms, discoloration occurs. • Avoid exposure to skin, eyes, mucous membranes. • Latex gloves and safety glasses should be used during preparation/handling of solution. • Avoid inhalation. • If solution contacts skin or mucous membranes, wash thoroughly with soap and water; rinse eyes thoroughly with plain water.

PO
• Give with food.

⬚ IV INCOMPATIBILITIES
Aldesleukin (Proleukin), amifostine (Ethyol), aztreonam (Azactam), cefepime (Maxipime), cytarabine (ARA-C), doxorubicin (Adriamycin), fludarabine (Fludara), foscarnet (Foscavir), gemcitabine (Gemzar), ondansetron (Zofran), piperacillin and tazobactam (Zosyn), sargramostim (Leukine), total parenteral nutrition (TPN), vinorelbine (Navelbine).

IV COMPATIBILITIES
Amphotericin B, enalapril (Vasotec), filgrastim (Neupogen), fluconazole (Diflucan), propofol (Diprivan).

INDICATIONS/ROUTES/DOSAGE
CMV RETINITIS
IV: ADULTS, CHILDREN 3 MO AND OLDER: 10 mg/kg/day in divided doses q12h for 14–21 days, then 5 mg/kg/day as a single daily dose or 6 mg/kg 5 days a wk.

PREVENTION OF CMV DISEASE IN TRANSPLANT PATIENTS
IV: ADULTS, CHILDREN: 10 mg/kg/day in divided doses q12h for 7–14 days, then 5 mg/kg/day as a single daily dose.

OTHER CMV INFECTIONS
IV: ADULTS: Initially, 10 mg/kg/day in divided doses q12h for 14–21 days, then 5 mg/kg/day as a single daily dose. Maintenance: 1,000 mg 3 times a day or 500 mg q3h (6 times a day). CHILDREN: Initially, 10 mg/kg/day in divided doses q12h for 14–21 days, then 5 mg/kg/day as a single daily dose. Maintenance: 30 mg/kg/dose q8h.

INTRAVITREAL IMPLANT: ADULTS: 1 implant q6–9mo plus oral ganciclovir. CHILDREN 9 YR AND OLDER: 1 implant q6–9mo plus oral ganciclovir (30 mg/dose q8h).

ADULT DOSAGE IN RENAL IMPAIRMENT
Dosage and frequency are modified based on creatinine clearance.

CrCl	Induction Dosage	Maintenance Dosage	Oral
50–69 ml/min	2.5 mg/kg q12h	2.5 mg/kg q24h	1,500 mg/day

G

25–49 ml/min	2.5 mg/kg q24h	1.25 mg/kg q24h	1,000 mg/day
10–24 ml/min	1.25 mg/kg q24h	0.625 mg/kg q24h	500 mg/day
Less than 10 ml/min	1.25 mg/kg 3 times/wk	0.625 mg/kg 3 times/ wk	500 mg 3 times/ wk

CrCl = creatinine clearance

SIDE EFFECTS

FREQUENT: Diarrhea (41%), fever (40%), nausea (25%), abdominal pain (17%), vomiting (13%). **OCCASIONAL (11%–6%):** Diaphoresis, infection, paresthesia, flatulence, pruritus. **RARE (4%–2%):** Headache, stomatitis, dyspepsia, phlebitis.

ADVERSE REACTIONS/ TOXIC EFFECTS

Hematologic toxicity occurs commonly: leukopenia in 41%–29% of patients and anemia in 25%–19%. Intraocular insertion occasionally results in visual acuity loss, vitreous hemorrhage, and retinal detachment. GI hemorrhage occurs rarely.

NURSING CONSIDERATIONS

BASELINE ASSESSMENT

Evaluate hematologic baseline. Obtain specimens for support of differential diagnosis (urine, feces, blood, throat) because retinal infection is usually due to hematogenous dissemination.

INTERVENTION/EVALUATION

Monitor I&O, ensure adequate hydration (minimum 1,500 ml/24 hr). Diligently evaluate hematology reports for neutropenia, thrombocytopenia, decreased platelets. Question patient regarding vision, therapeutic improvement, complications. Assess for rash, pruritus.

PATIENT/FAMILY TEACHING

• Ganciclovir provides suppression, not cure, of CMV retinitis. • Frequent blood tests, eye exams are necessary during therapy because of toxic nature of drug. • Report any new symptom promptly. • May temporarily or permanently inhibit sperm production in men, suppress fertility in women. • Barrier contraception should be used during and for 90 days after therapy because of mutagenic potential.

ganirelix

(Antagon)
See Fertility agents (p. 93C)

garlic

Also known as ail, allium, nectar of the gods, poor man's treacle, stinking rose.

CLASSIFICATION

HERBAL: See Appendix G.

ACTION

Possesses antithrombotic properties, can increase fibrinolytic activity, decrease platelet aggregation, increase PT. Acts as an hydroxamethylglutaryl-CoA (HMG-CoA) reductase inhibitor (statins). **Effect:** Lowers serum cholesterol levels. Causes smooth muscle relaxation/vasodilation, reducing BP. Reduces oxidative stress and LDL oxidation, preventing age-related vascular changes, atherosclerosis. Prevents endothelial cell depletion, producing antioxidant effect.

USES

Treatment of hypertension, hyperlipidemia; prevention of coronary artery disease, age-related vascular changes, atherosclerosis.

PRECAUTIONS

CONTRAINDICATIONS: Patients with bleeding disorders. **CAUTIONS:** Diabetes (may decrease blood glucose levels), inflammatory GI conditions (may irritate the GI tract). Hypothyroidism (may reduce iodine uptake). May prolong bleeding time (discontinue 1–2 wk before surgery).

⏳ **LIFESPAN CONSIDERATIONS: Pregnancy/Lactation: Caution:** May stimulate labor and cause colic in infants. **Children:** Safety and efficacy not established (may be beneficial in children with hypercholesterolemia). **Elderly:** No age-related precautions noted.

INTERACTIONS

DRUG: Insulin, oral antidiabetic agents: May increase hypoglycemic effect. **Anticoagulants/antiplatelets (e.g., warfarin, aspirin, clopidogrel, enoxaparin):** Effects may be enhanced. **Cyclosporine, oral contraceptives:** May decrease effects of these drugs. **Saquinavir, other HIV antiretrovirals:** May decrease concentration/effect of garlic. **HERBAL: Feverfew, ginger, ginkgo, ginseng:** May increase risk of bleeding. **FOOD:** None known. **LAB VALUES:** May decrease blood glucose, serum cholesterol, increase INR.

AVAILABILITY (OTC)

CAPSULES: 100 mg, 300 mg, 500 mg, 1,000 mg, 1.5 g. **TABLETS:** 400 mg, 1,250 mg. **TEA. EXTRACT. OIL. POWDER.**

INDICATIONS/ROUTES/DOSAGE

HYPERLIPIDEMIA, HYPERTENSION
PO (CAPSULES, POWDER, TEA):
ADULTS, ELDERLY: 600–1,200 mg a day in divided doses 3 times a day.
◀ **ALERT** ▶ Appropriate doses for other conditions vary depending on the preparation used.

SIDE EFFECTS

Breath/body odor, oropharyngeal/ esophageal burning, heartburn, nausea, vomiting, diarrhea, allergic reactions (e.g., rhinitis, urticaria, angioedema).

ADVERSE REACTIONS/ TOXIC EFFECTS

None known.

NURSING CONSIDERATIONS

BASELINE ASSESSMENT

Assess serum lipid levels, determine whether patient is taking anticoagulants or antiplatelets. Assess if diabetic, taking insulin or oral hypoglycemic agents.

INTERVENTION/EVALUATION

Monitor CBC, coagulation studies, serum lipid levels, glucose levels. Assess for hypersensitivity reaction, contact dermatitis.

PATIENT/FAMILY TEACHING

• Avoid use in pregnancy or breastfeeding. • Inform all health care providers of garlic use. • Discontinue 1–2 wk before any procedure in which excessive bleeding may occur.

gatifloxacin

gat-ih-**flocks**-ah-sin
(<u>Tequin</u>, Tequin Teqpaq, Zymar)

◆**CLASSIFICATION**

PHARMACOTHERAPEUTIC: Fluoroquinolone. **CLINICAL:** Antibiotic (see p. 24C).

ACTION

A fluoroquinolone that inhibits two enzymes, topoisomerase II and IV, in susceptible microorganisms. **Therapeutic Effect:** Interferes with bacterial DNA replication. Prevents or delays resistance emergence. Bactericidal.

✐ see color pill atlas　　　✐ herb　　　<u>underlined</u> – top prescribed drug

PHARMACOKINETICS

Well absorbed from the GI tract after PO administration. Protein binding: 20%. Widely distributed. Metabolized in liver. Primarily excreted in urine. Half-life: 7–14 hr.

USES

Treatment of susceptible infections due to *S. pneumoniae, S. aureus, S. pyogenes, H. influenzae, M. catarrhalis, E. coli, M. pneumoniae, C. pneumoniae, Legionella pneumophila, P. mirabilis, N. gonorrhoeae* including infections due to acute bacterial exacerbation of chronic bronchitis, acute sinusitis, community-acquired pneumonia, uncomplicated skin and skin-structure infections, cystitis, complicated UTIs, pyelonephritis, urethral gonorrhea in men and women, endocervical and rectal gonorrhea in women. **Ophthalmic:** Topical treatment of bacterial conjunctivitis due to susceptible strains of bacteria.

PRECAUTIONS

CONTRAINDICATIONS: Hypersensitivity to quinolones diabetic patients. **CAUTIONS:** Renal or hepatic impairment, CNS disorders, cerebral atherosclerosis, seizures, those with prolonged QT interval,other medications known to prolong the QT interval (e.g., erythromycin, tricyclic antidepressants), uncorrected hypokalemia, those receiving quinidine, procainamide, amiodarone, sotalol.

⏳ **LIFESPAN CONSIDERATIONS: Pregnancy/Lactation:** Unknown if distributed in breast milk. **Pregnancy Category C. Children:** Safety and efficacy not established. **Elderly:** Age-related renal impairment may require dosage adjustment.

INTERACTIONS

DRUG: Antacids, digoxin, iron preparations: May decrease gatifloxacin plasma concentration and half-life.

Probenecid: May increase gatifloxacin plasma concentration and half-life. **HERBAL:** None known. **FOOD:** None known. **LAB VALUES:** None known.

AVAILABILITY (Rx)

TABLETS (TEQUIN, TEQUIN TEQPAQ): 200 mg, 400 mg. **INJECTION (TEQUIN):** 200-mg, 400-mg vials. **OPHTHALMIC SOLUTION (ZYMAR):** 0.3%.

ADMINISTRATION/HANDLING

 IV

Rate of administration • Infuse over 60 min. • Do not give by rapid or bolus IV.

Storage • Available prediluted and ready for use. • Also available in 20- and 40-ml vials, which must be diluted in 100–200 ml D_5W, 0.9% NaCl.

PO
• Give without regard to meals. • Oral gatifloxacin should be administered 4 hr before giving antacids, multivitamins, ferrous sulfate, buffered tablets or solutions.

OPHTHALMIC
• Tilt patient's head backward, have patient look up. • Gently pull lower eyelid down until pocket formed. • Hold dropper above pocket and without touching eyelid or conjunctival sac place drops into center of pocket. • Close eyes gently, apply gentle finger pressure to lacrimal sac at inner canthus. • Remove excess solution around eye with a tissue.

🔲 IV INCOMPATIBILITIES

Amphotericin (Fungizone), potassium phosphate.

IV COMPATIBILITIES

Aminophylline, calcium gluconate, hydromorphone (Dilaudid), lidocaine, lorazepam (Ativan), magnesium sulfate, methylprednisolone (Solu-Medrol), metoclopramide (Reglan), midazolam (Versed), morphine, nitroglycerin, potassium chloride, sodium phosphate.

INDICATIONS/ROUTES/DOSAGE

CHRONIC BRONCHITIS, COMPLICATED URINARY TRACT INFECTIONS, PYELONEPHRITIS, SKIN INFECTIONS
PO, IV: ADULTS, ELDERLY: 400 mg/day for 7–10 days (5 days for chronic bronchitis).

SINUSITIS
PO, IV: ADULTS, ELDERLY: 400 mg/day for 10 days.

PNEUMONIA
PO, IV: ADULTS, ELDERLY: 400 mg/day for 7–14 days.

CYSTITIS
PO, IV: ADULTS, ELDERLY: 400 mg as a single dose or 200 mg/day for 3 days.

URETHRAL GONORRHEA IN MEN AND WOMEN, ENDOCERVICAL AND RECTAL GONORRHEA IN WOMEN
PO, IV: ADULTS, ELDERLY: 400 mg as a single dose.

TOPICAL TREATMENT OF BACTERIAL CONJUNCTIVITIS DUE TO SUSCEPTIBLE STRAINS OF BACTERIA
OPHTHALMIC: ADULTS, ELDERLY, CHILDREN 1 YR AND OLDER: 1 drop q2h while awake for 2 days, then 1 drop up to 4 times/day for days 3–7.

DOSAGE IN RENAL IMPAIRMENT

Creatinine Clearance	Dosage
40 ml/min	400 mg/day
Less than 40 ml/min	Initially, 400 mg/day then 200 mg/day
Hemodialysis	Initially, 400 mg/day then 200 mg/day
Peritoneal dialysis	Initially, 400 mg/day then 200 mg/day

SIDE EFFECTS

OCCASIONAL (8%–3%): Nausea, vaginitis, diarrhea, headache, dizziness. **Ophthalmic:** conjunctival irritation, increased tearing, corneal inflammation. **RARE (3%–0.1%):** Abdominal pain, constipation, dyspepsia, stomatitis, edema, insomnia, abnormal dreams, diaphoresis, altered taste, rash. **Ophthalmic:** corneal swelling, dry eye, eye pain, eyelid swelling, headache, red eye, reduced visual acuity, altered taste.

ADVERSE REACTIONS/ TOXIC EFFECTS

Pseudomembranous colitis, as evidenced by severe abdominal pain and cramps, severe watery diarrhea, and fever, may occur. Superinfection, manifested as genital or anal pruritus, ulceration or changes in oral mucosa, and moderate to severe diarrhea, may occur.

NURSING CONSIDERATIONS

BASELINE ASSESSMENT
Determine hypersensitivity to gatifloxacin, quinolones before beginning drug therapy.

INTERVENTION/EVALUATION
Determine pattern of bowel activity and stool consistency. Assist with ambulation if dizziness occurs. Assess for headache, nausea, vaginitis. Monitor WBC, signs of infection, mental status.

PATIENT/FAMILY TEACHING
• Do not skip dose; take full course of therapy. • Take with 8 oz water; drink several glasses of water between meals. • Do not take antacids within 4 hr of medication (reduces or destroys effectiveness). • Avoid exposure to direct sunlight during therapy and for several days following treatment. • Avoid tasks that require alertness, motor skills until response to drug is established (potential for dizziness).

gefitinib ▷

geh-**fih**-tih-nib
(Iressa)

•CLASSIFICATION

PHARMACOTHERAPEUTIC: Epidermal growth factor receptor antibody. **CLINICAL:** Antineoplastic.

ACTION

Blocks the signaling pathway that binds to the epidermal growth factor receptor (EGFR) on the surface of normal and cancer cells. EGFR activates the enzyme tyrosine kinase, which sends signals instructing the cells to grow. **Therapeutic Effect:** Inhibits the growth of cancer cells.

PHARMACOKINETICS

Slowly absorbed and extensively distributed throughout the body. Protein binding: 90%. Undergoes extensive metabolism in the liver. Excreted in the feces. **Half-life:** 48 hr.

USES

Treatment in patients with locally advanced or metastatic non–small cell lung cancer after failure of platinum-based and docetaxel chemotherapies.

PRECAUTIONS

CONTRAINDICATIONS: None known. **CAUTIONS:** Severe renal impairment, hepatic impairment.

⧗ **LIFESPAN CONSIDERATIONS: Pregnancy/Lactation:** Has potential to cause fetal harm, potential abortifacient. Substitute formula feedings for breast-feedings. Those with child-bearing potential should use contraceptive methods during treatment and up to 12 mo following therapy. **Pregnancy Category D. Children:** Safety and efficacy not established. **Elderly:** No age-related precautions noted.

INTERACTIONS

DRUG: Cimetidine, phenytoin, ranitidine, rifampin, sodium bicarbonate: May decrease gefitinib blood concentration and effectiveness. **Itraconazole, ketoconazole:** Increases gefitinib blood concentration. **Metoprolol:** Increases the effect of metoprolol. **Warfarin:** Increases the risk of bleeding. **HERBAL:** None known. **FOOD:** None known. **LAB VALUES:** May increase serum alkaline phosphatase, bilirubin, AST, and ALT levels.

AVAILABILITY (Rx)

TABLETS: 250 mg.

ADMINISTRATION/HANDLING

• Give without regard to food. • Do not crush or break film-coated tablet.

INDICATIONS/ROUTES/DOSAGE

NON-SMALL CELL LUNG CANCER
PO: ADULTS, ELDERLY: 250 mg/day; may increase to 500 mg/day for patients receiving drugs that may decrease gefitinib blood concentrations, such as CYP3A4 inducers rifampin and phenytoin.

SIDE EFFECTS

FREQUENT (48%–25%): Diarrhea, rash, acne. **OCCASIONAL (13%–8%):** Dry skin, nausea, vomiting, pruritus. **RARE (7%–2%):** Anorexia, asthenia, weight loss, peripheral edema, eye pain.

ADVERSE REACTIONS/ TOXIC EFFECTS

Pancreatitis and ocular hemorrhage occur rarely. Hypersensitivity reaction produces angioedema and urticaria. Cases of interstitial lung disease have been reported.

NURSING CONSIDERATIONS

BASELINE ASSESSMENT

Antiemetics, antidiarrheals may be effective in preventing and treating nausea, vomiting, diarrhea. Patients with poorly

G

tolerated diarrhea may be helped by briefly interrupting drug therapy (up to 14 days).

INTERVENTION/EVALUATION

Encourage adequate fluid intake. Assess bowel sounds for hyperactivity. Monitor pattern of daily bowel activity and stool consistency. Assess skin for evidence of rash. Assess liver function test results.

PATIENT/FAMILY TEACHING

• Do not have immunizations without physician's approval (drug lowers body's resistance). • Avoid crowds, persons with known infections. • Report signs of infection at once (fever, flu-like symptoms). • Contact physician if severe or persistent diarrhea, nausea, vomiting, anorexia occurs. • Avoid pregnancy during therapy.

---

gemcitabine hydrochloride ▷

gem-**cih**-tah-bean
(Gemzar)

◆CLASSIFICATION

PHARMACOTHERAPEUTIC: Antimetabolite. **CLINICAL:** Antineoplastic (see p. 74C).

ACTION

An antimetabolite that inhibits ribonucleotide reductase, the enzyme necessary for catalyzing DNA synthesis. **Therapeutic Effect:** Produces death in cells undergoing DNA synthesis.

PHARMACOKINETICS

Not extensively distributed after IV infusion (increased with length of infusion). Protein binding: less than 10%. Excreted primarily in urine as metabolite. **Half-life:** 42–94 min (influenced by gender of patient and duration of infusion).

USES

Metastatic breast cancer in combination with paclitaxel. Treatment of locally advanced (stage II, III) or metastatic (stage IV) adenocarcinoma of pancreas. Indicated for patients previously treated with 5-fluorouracil. Monotherapy or in combination with cisplatin for treatment for locally advanced or metastatic non–small cell lung cancer. **OFF-LABEL:** Treatment of biliary tract carcinoma, gall bladder carcinoma, germ cell tumors (e.g., ovarian, testicular), Hodgkin's lymphoma, non-Hodgkin's lymphoma.

PRECAUTIONS

CONTRAINDICATIONS: None known. **CAUTIONS:** Renal or hepatic impairment. **⚠ LIFESPAN CONSIDERATIONS: Pregnancy/Lactation:** If possible, avoid use during pregnancy, especially first trimester. May cause fetal harm. Unknown if distributed in breast milk. Breastfeeding not recommended. **Pregnancy Category D. Children:** Safety and efficacy not established. **Elderly:** Increased risk of hematologic toxicity.

INTERACTIONS

DRUG: Bone marrow depressants: May increase the risk of myelosuppression. **Live virus vaccines:** May potentiate virus replication, increase vaccine side effects, and decrease the patient's antibody response to the vaccine. **HERBAL:** None known. **FOOD:** None known. **LAB VALUES:** May increase BUN level and serum alkaline phosphatase, bilirubin, creatinine, AST, and ALT levels.

AVAILABILITY (Rx)

POWDER FOR RECONSTITUTION: 200 mg, 1-g vials.

ADMINISTRATION/HANDLING

🖐 IV

Reconstitution • Use gloves when handling or preparing gemcitabine. • Reconstitute 200-mg or 1-g vial with

0.9% NaCl injection without preservative (5 ml or 25 ml, respectively) to provide a concentration of 40 mg/ml. • Shake to dissolve.

Rate of administration • May give without further dilution. • May be further diluted with 0.9% NaCl to a concentration as low as 0.1 mg/ml. • Infuse over 30 min.

Storage • Store at room temperature (refrigeration may cause crystallization). • Reconstituted solution is stable for 24 hr at room temperature.

IV INCOMPATIBILITIES

Acyclovir (Zovirax), amphotericin B (Fungizone), cefoperazone (Cefobid), furosemide (Lasix), ganciclovir (Cytovene), imipenem and cilastatin (Primaxin), irinotecan (Camptosar), methotrexate, methylprednisolone (Solu-Medrol), mitomycin (Mutamycin), piperacillin and tazobactam (Zosyn), prochlorperazine (Compazine).

IV COMPATIBILITIES

Bumetanide (Bumex), calcium gluconate, dexamethasone (Decadron), diphenhydramine (Benadryl), dobutamine (Dobutrex), dopamine (Intropin), granisetron (Kytril), heparin, hydrocortisone (Solu-Cortef), lorazepam (Ativan), ondansetron (Zofran), potassium.

INDICATIONS/ROUTES/DOSAGE

BREAST CANCER

IV INFUSION (IN COMBINATION WITH PACLITAXEL): ADULTS, ELDERLY: 1,250 mg/m^2 over 30 min on days 1 and 8 of each 21-day cycle.

NON SMALL-CELL LUNG CANCER
(IN COMBINATION WITH CISPLATIN)

IV: ADULTS, ELDERLY, CHILDREN: 1,000 mg/m^2 on days 1, 8, and 15, repeated every 28 days; or 1,250 mg/m^2 on days 1 and 8. Repeat every 21 days.

PANCREATIC CANCER

IV: ADULTS: 1,000 mg/m^2 once weekly for up to 7 wk or until toxicity

necessitates decreasing dosage or withholding the dose, followed by 1 wk of rest. Subsequent cycles should consist of once-weekly dose for 3 consecutive wk out of every 4 wk. For patients completing cycles at 1,000 mg/m^2, increase dose to 1,250 mg/m^2 as tolerated. Dose for next cycle may be increased to 1,500 mg/m^2.

DOSAGE REDUCTION GUIDELINES

Dosage adjustments should be based on granulocyte count and platelet count, as follows:

Absolute Granulocyte Counts (cells/mm^3)	Platelet Count (cells/mm^3)	% of Full Dose
1,000 and	100,000	100
500–999 or	50,000–99,000	75
Less than 500 or	Less than 50,000	Hold

SIDE EFFECTS

FREQUENT: Nausea and vomiting (69%); generalized pain (48%); fever (41%); mild to moderate pruritic rash (30%); mild to moderate dyspnea, constipation (23%); peripheral edema (20%). **OCCASIONAL (19%–10%):** Diarrhea, petechiae, alopecia, stomatitis, infection, somnolence, paresthesia. **RARE:** Diaphoresis, rhinitis, insomnia, malaise.

ADVERSE REACTIONS/ TOXIC EFFECTS

Severe myelosuppression, as evidenced by anemia, thrombocytopenia, and leukopenia, is a common reaction.

NURSING CONSIDERATIONS

BASELINE ASSESSMENT

CBC, renal and liver function tests should be performed beforestarting therapy and periodically thereafter. Drug should be suspended or dosage modified if bone marrow suppression is detected.

G

INTERVENTION/EVALUATION

Assess all lab results before giving each dose. Monitor for dyspnea, fever, pruritic rash, dehydration due to vomiting. Assess oral mucosa for erythema, ulceration at inner margin of lips, sore throat, difficulty swallowing (stomatitis). Assess skin for rash. Monitor for and report diarrhea. Provide antiemetics as needed.

PATIENT/FAMILY TEACHING

• Avoid crowds and exposure to infection. • Maintain fastidious oral hygiene. • Promptly report fever, sore throat, signs of local infection, easy bruising, rash. • Contact physician if nausea or vomiting continues at home.

---

gemfibrozil

gem-**fi**-broe-zil

(Apo-Gemfibrozil ✦, Lopid, Novo-Gemfibrozil ✦)

Do not confuse Lopid with Lorabid or Levbid.

⚫ CLASSIFICATION

PHARMACOTHERAPEUTIC: Fibric acid derivative. **CLINICAL:** Antihyperlipoproteinemic (see p. 53C).

ACTION

A fibric acid derivative that inhibits lipolysis of fat in adipose tissue; decreases liver uptake of free fatty acids and reduces hepatic triglyceride production. Inhibits synthesis of VLDL carrier apolipoprotein B. **Therapeutic Effect:** Lowers serum cholesterol and triglycerides (decreases VLDL, LDL; increases HDL).

PHARMACOKINETICS

Well absorbed from the GI tract. Protein binding: 99%. Metabolized in liver. Primarily excreted in urine. Not removed by hemodialysis. **Half-life:** 1.5 hr.

USES

Treatment of hyperlipidemia, decreases risk of coronary heart disease in patients with type IIB hyperlipidemia. Treatment of severe primary hyperlipidemia (types IV, V).

PRECAUTIONS

CONTRAINDICATIONS: Liver dysfunction (including primary biliary cirrhosis), preexisting gallbladder disease, severe renal dysfunction. **CAUTIONS:** Hypothyroidism, diabetes mellitus, estrogen or anticoagulant therapy.

⧗ **LIFESPAN CONSIDERATIONS: Pregnancy/Lactation:** Unknown if drug crosses placenta or is distributed in breast milk. Decision to discontinue nursing or drug should be based on potential for serious adverse effects. **Pregnancy Category C. Children:** Not recommended in those younger than 2 yr (cholesterol necessary for normal development). **Elderly:** Age-related renal impairment may require dosage adjustment.

INTERACTIONS

DRUG: Lovastatin: May cause rhabdomyolysis, leading to acute renal failure. **Pioglitazone, repaglinide, warfarin:** May increase the effect of these drugs. **HERBAL:** None known. **FOOD:** None known. **LAB VALUES:** May increase serum alkaline phosphatase, serum bilirubin, serum creatinine kinase, serum LDH concentrations, and AST and ALT levels. May decrease blood Hgb and Hct levels, leukocyte counts, and serum potassium levels.

AVAILABILITY (Rx)

TABLETS: 600 mg.

ADMINISTRATION/HANDLING

PO

• Give 30 min before morning and evening meals.

INDICATIONS/ROUTES/DOSAGE

HYPERLIPIDEMIA

PO: ADULTS, ELDERLY: 1,200 mg/day in 2 divided doses 30 min before breakfast and dinner.

SIDE EFFECTS

FREQUENT (20%): Dyspepsia. **OCCASIONAL (10%–2%):** Abdominal pain, diarrhea, nausea, vomiting, fatigue. **RARE (less than 2%):** Constipation, acute appendicitis, vertigo, headache, rash, pruritus, altered taste.

ADVERSE REACTIONS/ TOXIC EFFECTS

Cholelithiasis, cholecystitis, acute appendicitis, pancreatitis, and malignancy occur rarely.

NURSING CONSIDERATIONS

BASELINE ASSESSMENT

Assess baseline lab results: serum glucose, triglyceride, cholesterol levels; liver function tests; CBC.

INTERVENTION/EVALUATION

Determine pattern of bowel activity. Monitor LDL, VLDL, serum triglyceride, cholesterol lab results for therapeutic response. Assess for rash, pruritus. Check for headache, dizziness. Monitor liver function, hematology tests. Assess for pain, especially right upper quadrant or epigastric pain suggestive of adverse gallbladder effects. Monitor serum glucose for those receiving insulin, oral antihyperglycemics.

PATIENT/FAMILY TEACHING

• Follow special diet (important part of treatment). • Take before meals. • Periodic lab tests are essential part of therapy. • Notify physician if dizziness, blurred vision, abdominal pain, diarrhea, nausea, vomiting becomes pronounced.

gemifloxacin mesylate

gem-ih-**flocks**-ah-sin
(Factive)

CLASSIFICATION

PHARMACOTHERAPEUTIC: Fluoroquinolone. **CLINICAL:** Antibacterial.

ACTION

A fluoroquinolone that inhibits the enzyme DNA gyrase in susceptible microorganisms, interfering with bacterial cell replication and repair. Therapeutic Effect: Bactericidal.

PHARMACOKINETICS

Rapidly and well absorbed from the GI tract. Protein binding: 70%. Widely distributed. Penetrates well into lung tissue and fluid. Undergoes limited metabolism in the liver. Primarily excreted in feces; lesser amount eliminated in urine. Partially removed by hemodialysis. Half-life: 4–12 hr.

USES

Treatment of susceptible infections due to *S. pneumoniae, H. influenzae, H. parainfluenzae, M. catarrhalis, M. pneumoniae, C. pneumoniae, K. pneumoniae* including acute bacterial exacerbation of chronic bronchitis, community-acquired pneumonia of mild to moderate severity.

PRECAUTIONS

CONTRAINDICATIONS: Concurrent use of amiodarone, quinidine, procainamide, or sotalol; history of prolonged QTc interval; hypersensitivity to fluoroquinolones; uncorrected electrolyte disorders (such as hypokalemia and hypomagnesemia). **CAUTIONS:** Hepatic or renal impairment, clinically significant bradycardia, acute myocardial ischemia.

⌛ **LIFESPAN CONSIDERATIONS:** Pregnancy/Lactation: Has potential for teratogenic effects. Substitute formula feedings for breast-feedings. **Pregnancy Category C. Children:** Safety and efficacy not established in those 18 yr and younger. **Elderly:** Age-related renal impairment may require dosage adjustment.

INTERACTIONS

DRUG: Aluminum and magnesium-containing antacids, bismuth subsalicylate, didanosine, iron preparations and other metals, sucralfate, zinc preparations: May decrease the absorption of gemifloxacin. **Antipsychotics, class 1A and class III antiarrhythmics, erythromycin, tricyclic antidepressants:** May increase the risk of prolonged QTc interval and life-threatening arrhythmias. **Cyclosporine:** Increases the risk of nephrotoxicity. **Probenecid:** Increases gemifloxacin serum concentration. **HERBAL:** None known. **FOOD:** None known. **LAB VALUES:** May increase BUN and serum alkaline phosphatase, bilirubin, LDH, creatinine, AST, and ALT levels.

AVAILABILITY (Rx)

TABLETS: 320 mg.

ADMINISTRATION/HANDLING

PO
• Give without regard to meals. • Do not crush or break tablet. • Do not administer antacids with or within 2 hr of gemifloxacin.

INDICATIONS/ROUTES/DOSAGE

ACUTE BACTERIAL EXACERBATION OF CHRONIC BRONCHITIS
PO: ADULTS, ELDERLY: 320 mg once a day for 5 days.

COMMUNITY-ACQUIRED PNEUMONIA
PO: ADULTS, ELDERLY: 320 mg once a day for 7 days.

DOSAGE IN RENAL IMPAIRMENT

Dosage and frequency are modified based on creatinine clearance.

Creatinine Clearance	Dosage
Greater than 40 ml/min	320 mg once a day
40 ml/min or less	160 mg once a day

SIDE EFFECTS

OCCASIONAL (4%–2%): Diarrhea, rash, nausea. **RARE (1% or less):** Headache, abdominal pain, dizziness.

ADVERSE REACTIONS/ TOXIC EFFECTS

Antibiotic-associated colitis may result from altered bacterial balance. Hypersensitivity reactions, including photosensitivity (as evidenced by rash, pruritus, blisters, edema, and burning skin), have occurred. Tendonitis and rupture of the shoulder, hand, and Achilles tendons that required surgical repair or resulted in prolonged disability have been reported.

NURSING CONSIDERATIONS

BASELINE ASSESSMENT
Question for history of hypersensitivity to fluoroquinolone antibiotics.

INTERVENTION/EVALUATION
Monitor signs and symptoms of infection, WBC count, liver function tests. Encourage adequate fluid intake. Monitor pattern of daily bowel activity and stool consistency. Assess skin for evidence of rash. Be alert for superinfection (oral candidiasis, genital pruritus).

PATIENT/FAMILY TEACHING
• Take with 8 oz of water, without regard to food. • Drink several glasses of water between meals. • Complete full course of therapy. • Do not take

G

antacids with or within 2 hr of gemifloxacin dose (reduces or destroys effectiveness).

gemtuzumab ozogamicin ⚑

gem-**too**-zoo-mab
(Mylotarg)

◆CLASSIFICATION

PHARMACOTHERAPEUTIC: Monoclonal antibody. **CLINICAL:** Antineoplastic (see p. 74C).

ACTION

Binds to an antigen on the surface of leukemic blast cells, resulting in the formation of a complex that leads to the release of the antibiotic inside the myeloid cells. The antibiotic then binds to DNA, resulting in DNA double-strand breaks and cell death. **Therapeutic Effect:** Inhibits colony formation in cultures of adult leukemic bone marrow cells.

PHARMACOKINETICS

Elimination half-life: 45 hr after first infusion; 60 hr after second infusion.

USES

Treatment of patients with CD33 acute myloid leukemia (AML) in first relapse who are 60 yr and older and not considered candidates for cytotoxic chemotherapy.

PRECAUTIONS

CONTRAINDICATIONS: Hypersensitivity to any component of formulation, patients with anti-CD33 antibody (hP67.6), pregnancy. **CAUTIONS:** Hepatic impairment.

⌛ **LIFESPAN CONSIDERATIONS: Pregnancy/Lactation:** May cause fetal harm. Unknown if excreted in breast milk. **Pregnancy Category D. Children:** Safety and efficacy not established. **Elderly:** No age-related precautions noted.

INTERACTIONS

DRUG: None known. **HERBAL:** None known. **FOOD:** None known. **LAB VALUES:** May increase serum bilirubin, AST, and ALT levels. May decrease blood Hgb and Hct levels, platelet count, WBC count, and serum magnesium and potassium levels.

AVAILABILITY (Rx)

POWDER FOR INJECTION: 5 mg.

ADMINISTRATION/HANDLING

💧 IV

Reconstitution • Prepare in a biologic safety hood with fluorescent light off. • Allow vials to come to room temperature. • Reconstitute each vial with 5 ml sterile water for injection using sterile syringes to provide concentration of 1 mg/ml. • Gently swirl; inspect for particulate matter/discoloration. • Withdraw desired volume from each vial and inject into 100 ml 0.9% NaCl and place into a UV protectant bag.

Rate of administration • Do not give IV push or bolus. • Infuse over 2 hr. • Use separate line equipped with a low protein binding 1.2-micron filter. • May give through peripheral or central line.

Storage • Protect from direct and indirect sunlight and unshielded fluorescent light during preparation and administration. • Refrigerate, do not freeze. • Following reconstitution in vial, stable for 8 hr if refrigerated and protected from light. • Once diluted with 100 ml 0.9% NaCl, use immediately.

▦ IV INCOMPATIBILITIES

Don't mix gemtuzumab with any other medications.

INDICATIONS/ROUTES/DOSAGE

CD33 POSITIVE ACUTE MYELOID LEUKEMIA

IV: ADULTS 60 YR AND OLDER: 9 mg/m^2 infused over 2 hr repeated in 14 days for a total of 2 doses.

SIDE EFFECTS

◀ ALERT ▶ Most patients experience a postinfusion symptom complex of fever (85%), chills (73%), nausea (70%), and vomiting (63%) that resolves within 2–4 hr with supportive therapy. **FREQUENT (44%–31%):** Asthenia, diarrhea, abdominal pain, headache, stomatitis, dyspnea, epistaxis. **OCCASIONAL (25%–15%):** Constipation, neutropenic fever, nonspecific rash, herpes simplex infection, hypertension, hypotension, petechiae, peripheral edema, dizziness, insomnia, back pain. **RARE (14%–10%):** Pharyngitis, ecchymosis, dyspepsia, tachycardia, hematuria, rhinitis.

ADVERSE REACTIONS/TOXIC EFFECTS

Severe myelosuppression, characterized by neutropenia, anemia, and thrombocytopenia, occurs in 98% of all patients. Sepsis occurs in 25% of patients. Hepatotoxicity also may occur.

NURSING CONSIDERATIONS

BASELINE ASSESSMENT

Obtain baseline CBC, liver function studies, serum chemistry for comparison to expected myelosuppression. Use strict aseptic technique to protect patient from infection.

INTERVENTION/EVALUATION

Monitor CBC, blood chemistries, WBC, liver function studies. Monitor for myelosuppression (fever, sore throat, signs of local infection, unusual bruising or bleeding from any site), symptoms of anemia (excessive fatigue, weakness). Assess for impending stomatitis. Monitor BP for hypertension/hypotension.

PATIENT/FAMILY TEACHING

• Do not have immunizations without physician's approval (drug lowers body's resistance). • Avoid contact with those who have recently received live virus vaccine. • Promptly report fever, sore throat, signs of local infection, unusual bruising or bleeding from any site.

Gemzar, see gemcitabine

gentamicin sulfate

jen-ta-**mye**-sin

(Alcomicin ✦, Cidomycin ✦, Garamycin, Garamycin Ophthalmic, Garamycin Topical, Genoptic, Gentacidin, Gentak, Gentacidin, Ocu-Mycin)

◆CLASSIFICATION

PHARMACOTHERAPEUTIC: Aminoglycoside. **CLINICAL:** Antibiotic (see p. 19C).

ACTION

An aminoglycoside antibiotic that irreversibly binds to the protein of bacterial ribosomes. **Therapeutic Effect:** Interferes with protein synthesis of susceptible microorganisms. Bactericidal.

PHARMACOKINETICS

Rapid, complete absorption after IM administration. Protein binding: less than 30%. Widely distributed (doesn't cross the blood-brain barrier, low concentrations in CSF). Excreted unchanged in urine. Removed by hemodialysis. **Half-life:** 2–4 hr (increased in impaired renal function and neonates; decreased in cystic fibrosis and burn or febrile patients).

USES

Parenteral: Treatment of infections susceptible to Pseudomonas and other gram-negative organisms including skin and skin-structure, bone, joint, respiratory tract, intra-abdominal, complicated urinary tract, acute pelvic infections; postop; burns; septicemia; meningitis. **Ophthalmic:** Ointment or solution for superficial eye infections. **Topical:** Cream or ointment for superficial skin infections. Ophthalmic or topical applications may be combined with systemic administration for serious, extensive infections. OFF-LABEL: **Topical:** Prophylaxis of minor bacterial skin infections, treatment of dermal ulcer.

PRECAUTIONS

CONTRAINDICATIONS Hypersensitivity to other aminoglycosides (cross-sensitivity), or their components. Sulfite sensitivity may result in anaphylaxis, especially in asthmatic patients. **CAUTIONS:** Elderly, neonates because of renal insufficiency or immaturity; neuromuscular disorders (potential for respiratory depression), prior hearing loss, vertigo, renal impairment. Cumulative effects may occur with concurrent systemic administration and topical application to large areas.

⧖ LIFESPAN CONSIDERATIONS: **Pregnancy/Lactation:** Readily crosses placenta; unknown if distributed in breast milk. **Pregnancy Category C. Children:** Caution in neonates: Immature renal function increases half-life and toxicity. **Elderly:** Age-related renal impairment may require dosage adjustment.

INTERACTIONS

DRUG: Nephrotoxic mediations, other aminoglycosides, ototoxic medications: May increase the risk of nephrotoxicity or ototoxicity. **Neuromuscular blockers:** May increase neuromuscular blockade. **HERBAL:** None known. **FOOD:** None known.

LAB VALUES: May increase serum creatinine, serum bilirubin, BUN, serum LDH, AST, and ALT levels. May decrease serum calcium, magnesium, potassium, and sodium concentrations. Therapeutic peak serum level is 6–10 mcg/ml and trough is 0.5–2 mcg/ml. Toxic peak serum level is greater than 10 mcg/ml, and trough is greater than 2 mcg/ml.

AVAILABILITY (Rx)

INJECTION: 10 mg/ml, 40 mg/ml (Garamycin), 40 mg/50 ml-0.9%, 60 mg/50 ml-0.9%, 60 mg/100 ml-0.9%, 70 mg/50 ml-0.9%, 80 mg/50 ml-0.9%, 80 mg/100 ml-0.9%, 90 mg/100 ml-0.9%, 100 mg/50 ml-0.9%, 100 mg/ 100 ml-0.9%. **OPHTHALMIC SOLUTION (GARAMYCIN OPHTHALMIC, GENTACIDIN, GENOPTIC, GENTAK, OCU-MYCIN):** 0.3%. **OPHTHALMIC OINTMENT (GENTAK):** 0.3%. **CREAM (GARAMYCIN TOPICAL):** 0.1%. **OINTMENT:** 0.1%.

ADMINISTRATION/HANDLING

 IV

Reconstitution • Dilute with 50–200 ml D$_5$W or 0.9% NaCl. Amount of diluent for infants, children depends on individual needs.

Rate of administration • Infuse over 30–60 min for adults, older children; over 60–120 min for infants, young children.

Storage • Store vials at room temperature. • Solution appears clear or slightly yellow. • Intermittent IV infusion (piggyback) is stable for 24 hr at room temperature. • Discard if precipitate forms.

IM
• To minimize discomfort, give deep IM slowly. • Less painful if injected into gluteus maximus rather than lateral aspect of thigh.

INTRATHECAL
• Use only 2 mg/ml intrathecal preparation without preservative. • Mix with

G

10% estimated CSF volume or NaCl. • Use intrathecal forms immediately after preparation. Discard unused portion. • Give over 3–5 min.

OPHTHALMIC
• Place finger on lower eyelid, pull out until a pocket is formed between eye and lower lid. • Hold dropper above pocket, place correct number of drops (¼–½ inch ointment) into pocket. Close eye gently. • **Solution:** Apply digital pressure to lacrimal sac for 1–2 min (minimizes drainage into nose and throat, reducing risk of systemic effects). • **Ointment:** Close eye for 1–2 min, rolling eyeball (increases contact area of drug to eye). • Remove excess solution or ointment around eye with tissue.

TOPICAL
• Wash affected area with soap and water; allow to dry before applying. • Apply a small amount of gentamicin to the affected area and rub in gently.

▒ IV INCOMPATIBILITIES

Allopurinol (Aloprim), amphotericin B complex (Abelcet, AmBisome, Amphotec), furosemide (Lasix), heparin, hetastarch (Hespan), idarubicin (Idamycin), indomethacin (Indocin), propofol (Diprivan).

IV COMPATIBILITIES

Amiodarone (Cordarone), diltiazem (Cardizem), enalapril (Vasotec), filgrastim (Neupogen), hydromorphone (Dilaudid), insulin, lorazepam (Ativan), magnesium sulfate, midazolam (Versed), morphine, multivitamins, total parenteral nutrition (TPN).

INDICATIONS/ROUTES/DOSAGE

ACUTE PELVIC, BONE, INTRA-ABDOMINAL, JOINT, RESPIRATORY TRACT, BURN WOUND, POSTOP, AND SKIN OR SKIN-STRUCTURE INFECTIONS; COMPLICATED UTIs; SEPTICEMIA; MENINGITIS
IV, IM: ADULTS, ELDERLY: Usual dosage, 3–6 mg/kg/day in divided doses q8h or 4–6.6 mg/kg once a day. CHILDREN 5–12 YR: Usual dosage 2–2.5 mg/kg/dose q8h. CHILDREN YOUNGER THAN 5 YR: Usual dosage, 2.5 mg/kg/dose q8h. NEONATES: Usual dosage 2.5–3.5 mg/kg/dose q8–12h.

HEMODIALYSIS
IV, IM: ADULTS, ELDERLY: 0.5–0.7 mg/kg/dose after dialysis. CHILDREN: 1.25–1.75 mg/kg/dose after dialysis.
INTRATHECAL: ADULTS: 4–8 mg/day. CHILDREN 3 MO–12 YR: 1–2 mg/day. NEONATES: 1 mg/day.

SUPERFICIAL EYE INFECTIONS
OPHTHALMIC OINTMENT: ADULTS, ELDERLY: Usual dosage, apply thin strip to conjunctiva 2–3 times a day.
OPHTHALMIC SOLUTION: ADULTS, ELDERLY, CHILDREN: Usual dosage, 1–2 drops q2–4h up to 2 drops/hr.

SUPERFICIAL SKIN INFECTIONS
TOPICAL: ADULTS, ELDERLY: Usual dosage, apply 3–4 times/day.

DOSAGE IN RENAL IMPAIRMENT
Creatinine clearance greater than 41–60 ml/min: Dosage interval q12h. **Creatinine clearance 20–40 ml/min:** Dosage interval q24h. **Creatinine clearance less than 20 ml/min:** Monitor levels to determine dosage interval.

SIDE EFFECTS

OCCASIONAL: IM: Pain, induration. **IV:** Phlebitis, thrombophlebitis, hypersensitivity reactions (fever, pruritus, rash, urticaria). **Ophthalmic:** Burning, tearing, itching, blurred vision. **Topical:** Redness, itching. **RARE:** Alopecia, hypertension, weakness.

ADVERSE REACTIONS/ TOXIC EFFECTS

Nephrotoxicity (as evidenced by increased BUN and serum creatinine levels and decreased creatinine clearance) may be reversible if the drug is stopped at the first sign of symptoms. Irreversible ototoxicity (manifested as tinnitus, dizziness, ringing or roaring in the ears, and diminished hearing), and neurotoxicity (as evidenced by headache, dizziness, lethargy, tremor, and visual disturbances) occur occasionally. The risk of these effects increases with higher dosages or prolonged therapy and when the solution is applied directly to the mucosa. Superinfections, particularly with fungal infections, may result from bacterial imbalance no matter which administration route is used. Ophthalmic application may cause paresthesia of conjunctiva or mydriasis.

NURSING CONSIDERATIONS

BASELINE ASSESSMENT
Dehydration must be treated before beginning parenteral therapy. Establish baseline hearing acuity. Question for history of allergies, especially to aminoglycosides and sulfites (and parabens for topical/ophthalmic routes).

INTERVENTION/EVALUATION
Monitor I&O (maintain hydration), urinalysis (casts, RBCs, WBCs, decrease in specific gravity). Be alert to ototoxic, neurotoxic symptoms (see Adverse Reactions/Toxic Effects). Check IM injection site for induration. Evaluate IV site for phlebitis (heat, pain, red streaking over vein). Assess for rash (**ophthalmic:** redness, burning, itching, tearing; **topical:** redness, itching). Be alert for superinfection, particularly genital or anal pruritus, changes in oral mucosa, diarrhea. When treating patients with neuromuscular disorders, assess respiratory response carefully. Therapeutic serum level: Peak 6–10 mcg/ml; trough: 0.5–2 mcg/ml. Toxic serum level: Peak: greater than 10 mcg/ml; trough: greater than 2 mcg/ml.

PATIENT/FAMILY TEACHING
• Discomfort may occur with IM injection. • Blurred vision, tearing may occur briefly after each ophthalmic dose. • Notify physician in event of any hearing, visual, balance, urinary problems, even after therapy is completed. • **Ophthalmic:** Contact physician if tearing, redness, irritation continues. • **Topical:** Cleanse area gently before applying; notify physician if redness, itching occurs.

Geodon, *see ziprasidone*

ginger

Also known as black ginger, race ginger, zingiber.

CLASSIFICATION
HERBAL: See Appendix G.

ACTION
Possesses antipyretic, analgesic, antitussive, sedative properties. Increases GI motility; may act on serotonin receptors, primarily 5-HT$_3$. **Effect:** Reduces nausea/vomiting.

USES
Prevention of nausea/vomiting caused by motion sickness, early pregnancy, dyspepsia; treatment of rheumatoid arthritis.

PRECAUTIONS
CONTRAINDICATIONS: None known. **CAUTIONS:** Pregnancy; patients with bleeding conditions, diabetes (may cause hypoglycemia).

⧖ **LIFESPAN CONSIDERATIONS: Pregnancy/Lactation:** Use during pregnancy is controversial (large amounts act as an abortifacient). **Children:** Safety and efficacy not established. **Elderly:** No age-related precautions noted.

INTERACTIONS

DRUG: Anticoagulants, antiplatelets: Large amounts of ginger may increase risk of bleeding with these drugs. **HERBAL: Feverfew, garlic, ginkgo, ginseng:** May increase risk of bleeding. **FOOD:** None known. **LAB VALUES:** None known.

AVAILABILITY (Rx)

CAPSULES: 470 mg, 550 mg. **ROOT:** 470 mg, 550 mg. **EXTRACT. POWDER. TABLETS. TEA. TINCTURE.**

INDICATIONS/ROUTES/DOSAGE

MORNING SICKNESS

PO: ADULTS: 250 mg 4 times a day. **Maximum:** 4 g a day.

MOTION SICKNESS

PO: ADULTS: 1 g (dried powder root) 30 min before travel.

NAUSEA

PO: ADULTS: 550–1,100 mg 3 times a day.

ARTHRITIS

PO: ADULTS: 170 mg 3 times a day or 255 mg twice a day.

SIDE EFFECTS

Abdominal discomfort, heartburn, diarrhea, hypersensitivity reaction, nausea.

ADVERSE REACTIONS/ TOXIC EFFECTS

CNS depression, arrhythmias.

BASELINE ASSESSMENT

Assess for use of anticoagulants, antiplatelets (may increase risk of bleeding).

INTERVENTION/EVALUATION

Monitor for hypersensitivity reaction.

PATIENT/FAMILY TEACHING

• Use cautiously during pregnancy or breast-feeding.

---

ginkgo biloba

Also known as fossil tree, maidenhair tree, tanakan.

◆CLASSIFICATION

HERBAL: See Appendix G.

ACTION

Possesses antioxidant, free radical scavenging properties. **Effect:** Protects tissues from oxidative damage, prevents progression of tissue degeneration in patients with dementia. Inhibits platelet-activating factor bonding at numerous sites, decreasing platelet aggregation, smooth muscle contraction; may increase cardiac contractility and coronary blood flow. Decreases blood viscosity, improving circulation by relaxing vascular smooth muscle. Increases cerebral and peripheral blood flow, reduces vascular permeability. May influence neurotransmitter system (e.g., cholinergic).

USES

Dementia syndromes, including Alzheimer's. Improves cerebral, peripheral circulation. Improves conditions associated with cerebral vascular insufficiency (e.g., memory loss, difficulty concentrating, vertigo, tinnitus). Improves cognitive behavior and sleep patterns in patients with depression. Acts as an antioxidant.

PRECAUTIONS

CONTRAINDICATIONS: Pregnancy or lactation. **CAUTIONS:** Patients with bleeding disorders, diabetes; epileptic patients or those prone to seizures. Avoid use in couples having difficulty conceiving.

⧗ **LIFESPAN CONSIDERATIONS: Pregnancy/Lactation:** Contraindicated. **Children:** Safety and efficacy not established. Avoid use. **Elderly:** No age-related precautions noted.

INTERACTIONS

DRUG: Anticoagulants, antiplatelets (e.g., warfarin, aspirin, heparin, clopidogrel): May increase bleeding. **MAOIs:** Effects may be increased. **HERBAL: Feverfew, ginger, garlic, ginseng:** May increase risk of bleeding. **FOOD:** None known. **LAB VALUES:** May alter blood glucose levels.

AVAILABILITY (OTC)

CAPSULES: 40 mg, 60 mg. **TABLETS:** 40 mg, 60 mg. **FLUID EXTRACT. TINCTURE.**

INDICATIONS/ROUTES/DOSAGE

DEMENTIA
PO: ADULTS, ELDERLY: 120–240 mg a day (extract) in 2–3 doses.

VERTIGO, TINNITUS
PO: ADULTS, ELDERLY: 120–160 mg a day.

COGNITIVE FUNCTION
PO: ADULTS, ELDERLY: 120–600 mg a day.
‹ **ALERT** › Appropriate doses for other conditions vary; should be started at low doses, titrated to higher doses as needed.

SIDE EFFECTS

Headache, dizziness, palpitations, constipation, allergic skin reactions. Large doses may cause nausea, vomiting, diarrhea, fatigue, lack of muscle tone.

ADVERSE REACTIONS/ TOXIC EFFECTS

None known.

NURSING CONSIDERATIONS

BASELINE ASSESSMENT
Assess for use of anticoagulants or antiplatelets, MAOIs. Assess for history of bleeding disorders, diabetes, seizures.

INTERVENTION/EVALUATION
Monitor for hypersensitivity reaction, blood glucose levels.

PATIENT/FAMILY TEACHING
• Avoid use with anticoagulants or antiplatelets. • May take up to 6 mo before

effectiveness is noted. • Do not use during pregnancy or breast-feeding. • Avoid use in children.

ginseng

Also known as Asian ginseng, Chinese ginseng, red ginseng.

CLASSIFICATION

HERBAL: See Appendix G.

G

ACTION

Affects the hypothalamic-pituitary-adrenal axis. Appears to stimulate lymphocytic action. **Effect:** Reduces stress. Affects immune function.

USES

Increases resistance to stress. Boosts energy level. Enhances brain activity. Increases physical endurance. Aids in blood glucose control. Improves cognitive function, concentration, memory, work efficiency.

PRECAUTIONS

CONTRAINDICATIONS: Patients with bleeding tendencies, thrombosis. Avoid use during pregnancy or lactation. **CAUTIONS:** Patients with cardiac disorders, diabetes, hormone-sensitive cancers (e.g., breast, uterine, ovarian), endometriosis, uterine fibroids.

⌛ **LIFESPAN CONSIDERATIONS: Pregnancy/Lactation:** Insufficient information. Do not use. **Children:** Safety and efficacy not established. **Elderly:** No age-related precautions noted.

INTERACTIONS

DRUG: Anticoagulants, antiplatelets (e.g., aspirin, clopidogrel, enoxaparin, heparin, warfarin): May increase bleeding. **Oral antidiabetic agents, insulin:** May increase effects of these drugs. **Furosemide:** Effects may be decreased. **Immunosuppressants (e.g., cyclosporine, prednisone):** Effects may be interferred with when taken with ginseng. **HERBAL: Chamomile, feverfew, garlic, ginger, ginkgo:** May increase risk of bleeding. **FOOD: Coffee, tea:** May increase effect. **LAB VALUES:** May prolong aPTT, decrease serum glucose.

AVAILABILITY (OTC)

CAPSULES: 100 mg, 250 mg, 410 mg, 500 mg. **TABLETS:** 250 mg, 1,000 mg. **DRIED ROOT. EXTRACT. POWDER. TEA** (usually 1,500 mg/bag). **TINCTURE.**

INDICATIONS/ROUTES/DOSAGE

USUAL DOSAGE

PO: ADULTS, ELDERLY: **(Tablets/capsules):** 200–600 mg a day. **(Powder root):** 0.6–3 g 1–3 times a day. **(Tea— 1,500 mg):** 1–3 times a day.

SIDE EFFECTS

FREQUENT: Insomnia. **OCCASIONAL:** Vaginal bleeding, amenorrhea, palpitations, hypertension, diarrhea, headache, allergic reactions.

ADVERSE REACTIONS/ TOXIC EFFECTS

None known.

NURSING CONSIDERATIONS

BASELINE ASSESSMENT

Assess if patient is pregnant or breast-feeding. Assess if patient is diabetic, taking oral hypoglycemic agents, insulin. Assess for anticoagulant, immunosuppressant use. Determine baseline blood glucose.

INTERVENTION/EVALUATION

Monitor coagulation studies, serum glucose levels. Assess for hypersensitivity reaction, rash.

PATIENT/FAMILY TEACHING

• Avoid use in pregnancy or breast-feeding, children. • Avoid continuous use for longer than 3 mo.

glatiramer

glah-**tie**-rah-mir

(Copaxone)

Do not confuse Copaxone with Compazine.

CLASSIFICATION

PHARMACOTHERAPEUTIC: Immunosuppressive. **CLINICAL:** Neurologic agent.

ACTION

An immunosuppressive whose exact mechanism is unknown. May act by modifying immune processes thought to be responsible for the pathogenesis of multiple sclerosis (MS). **Therapeutic Effect:** Slows progression of MS.

PHARMACOKINETICS

Substantial fraction of glatiramer is hydrolyzed locally. Some fraction of injected material enters lymphatic circulation, reaching regional lymph nodes; some may enter systemic circulation intact.

USES

Treatment of relapsing, remitting multiple sclerosis.

PRECAUTIONS

CONTRAINDICATIONS: Hypersensitivity to mannitol. **CAUTIONS:** Immediate postinjection reaction (flushing, chest pain, palpitations, anxiety, dyspnea, urticaria).

⧗ **LIFESPAN CONSIDERATIONS: Pregnancy/Lactation:** Unknown if drug is distributed in breast milk. **Pregnancy Category B. Children:** Safety and efficacy not established. **Elderly:** Information not available.

INTERACTIONS

DRUG: None known. **HERBAL:** None known. **FOOD:** None known. **LAB VALUES:** None known.

AVAILABILITY (Rx)

INJECTION: 20 mg/ml in prefilled syringes.

ADMINISTRATION/HANDLING

SUBCUTANEOUS

• Refrigerate syringes. • Sites for self-injection include arms, abdomen, hips, and thighs. • The pre-filled syringe is suitable for single use only; unused portions should be discarded.

INDICATIONS/ROUTES/DOSAGE

MS

SUBCUTANEOUS: ADULTS, ELDERLY: 20 mg once a day.

SIDE EFFECTS

EXPECTED (73%–40%): Pain, erythema, inflammation, or pruritus at injection site; asthenia. **FREQUENT (27%–18%):** Arthralgia, vasodilation, anxiety, hypertonia, nausea, transient chest pain, dyspnea, flu-like symptoms, rash, pruritus. **OCCASIONAL (17%–10%):** Palpitations, back pain, diaphoresis, rhinitis, diarrhea, urinary urgency. **RARE (8%–6%):** Anorexia, fever, neck pain, peripheral edema, ear pain, facial edema, vertigo, vomiting.

ADVERSE REACTIONS/
TOXIC EFFECTS

Infection is a common effect. Lymphadenopathy occurs occasionally.

INTERVENTION/EVALUATION

Assess injection site for reaction. Monitor for fever, chills (evidence of infection).

PATIENT/FAMILY TEACHING

• Report difficulty in breathing or swallowing, rash, itching, swelling of lower extremities, fatigue. • Avoid pregnancy.

Gleevec, *see imatinib*

---

glimepiride

glim-**eh**-purr-eyd

(Amaryl)

Do not confuse glimepiride with glipizide or glyburide.

FIXED-COMBINATION(S)

Avandaryl: glimepiride, rosiglitazone (an antidiabetic): 1 mg/4 mg, 2 mg/4 mg, 4 mg/4 mg.

•CLASSIFICATION

PHARMACOTHERAPEUTIC: Second-generation sulfonylurea. **CLINICAL:** Hypoglycemic (see p. 41C).

ACTION

A second-generation sulfonylurea that promotes release of insulin from beta cells of the pancreas and increases insulin sensitivity at peripheral sites. **Therapeutic Effect:** Lowers blood glucose concentration.

PHARMACOKINETICS

Route	Onset	Peak	Duration
PO	N/A	2–3 hr	24 hr

Completely absorbed from the GI tract. Protein binding: greater than 99%. Metabolized in the liver. Excreted in urine and eliminated in feces. **Half-life:** 5–9.2 hr.

USES

Adjunct to diet, exercise in management of non–insulin dependent diabetes mellitus (type 2, NIDDM). Use in combination with insulin or metformin in patients whose diabetes is not controlled by diet, exercise in conjunction with oral hypoglycemic agent.

PRECAUTIONS

CONTRAINDICATIONS: Diabetic complications, such as ketosis, acidosis, and diabetic coma; monotherapy for type 1 diabetes mellitus; severe hepatic or renal impairment; stress situations, including severe infection, trauma, and surgery. **CAUTIONS:** Severe diarrhea, intestinal obstruction, prolonged vomiting, hepatic disease, hyperthyroidism (uncontrolled), impaired renal function, adrenal insufficiency, debilitation, malnutrition, pituitary insufficiency.

⧗ LIFESPAN CONSIDERATIONS: **Pregnancy/Lactation:** Not recommended for use during pregnancy. Unknown if distributed in breast milk. **Pregnancy Category C. Children:** Safety and efficacy not established. **Elderly:** Hypoglycemia may be difficult to recognize. Age-related renal impairment may increase sensitivity to glucose-lowering effect.

INTERACTIONS

DRUG: Beta blockers: May increase the hypoglycemic effect of glimepiride and mask signs of hypoglycemia. **Cimetidine, ciprofloxacin, fluconazole, MAOIs, quinidine, ranitidine, large doses of salicylates:** May increase the effects of glimepiride. **Corticosteroids, lithium, thiazide diuretics:** May decrease the effects of glimepiride. **Oral anticoagulants:** May increase the effects of oral anticoagulants. HERBAL: None known. FOOD: None known. LAB VALUES: May increase BUN and LDH concentrations and serum alkaline phosphatase, creatinine, and AST levels.

AVAILABILITY (Rx)

TABLETS: 1 mg, 2 mg, 4 mg.

ADMINISTRATION/HANDLING
PO
- Give with breakfast or first main meal.

INDICATIONS/ROUTES/DOSAGE
DIABETES MELLITUS

PO: ADULTS, ELDERLY: Initially, 1–2 mg once a day, with breakfast or first main meal. Maintenance: 1–4 mg once a day. After dose of 2 mg is reached, dosage should be increased in increments of up to 2 mg q1–2wk, based on blood glucose response. **Maximum:** 8 mg/day.

DOSAGE IN RENAL IMPAIRMENT
PO: ADULTS: 1 mg once/day.

SIDE EFFECTS

FREQUENT: Altered taste sensation, dizziness, somnolence, weight gain, constipation, diarrhea, heartburn, nausea, vomiting, stomach fullness, headache. **OCCASIONAL:** Increased sensitivity of skin to sunlight, peeling of skin, itching, rash.

ADVERSE REACTIONS/TOXIC EFFECTS

Overdose or insufficient food intake may produce hypoglycemia, especially with increased glucose demands. GI hemorrhage, cholestatic hepatic jaundice, leukopenia, thrombocytopenia, pancytopenia, agranulocytosis, and aplastic or hemolytic anemia occur rarely.

NURSING CONSIDERATIONS

BASELINE ASSESSMENT
Check blood glucose level. Discuss lifestyle to determine extent of learning, emotional needs. Ensure follow-up instruction if patient or family do not thoroughly understand diabetes management or blood glucose-testing technique.

INTERVENTION/EVALUATION

Monitor blood glucose level, food intake. Assess for hypoglycemia (cool, wet skin, tremors, dizziness, anxiety, headache, tachycardia, perioral numbness, hunger, diplopia), hyperglycemia (polyuria, polyphagia, polydipsia, nausea, vomiting, dim vision, fatigue, deep or rapid breathing). Be alert to conditions that alter glucose requirements: fever, increased activity or stress, surgical procedure.

PATIENT/FAMILY TEACHING

• Prescribed diet is principal part of treatment; do not skip or delay meals. • Carry candy, sugar packets, other sugar supplements for immediate response to hypoglycemia. • Wear medical alert identification. • Check with physician when glucose demands are altered (e.g., fever, infection, trauma, stress, heavy physical activity).

---

glipiZIDE

glip-ih-zide
(Glucotrol, Glucotrol XL)

Do not confuse glipizide with glimepiride or glyburide.

FIXED-COMBINATION(S)

Metaglip: glipizide/metformin (an antidiabetic): 2.5 mg/250 mg; 2.5 mg/500 mg; 5 mg/500 mg.

CLASSIFICATION

PHARMACOTHERAPEUTIC: Second-generation sulfonylurea. **CLINICAL:** Hypoglycemic (see p. 41C).

ACTION

A second-generation sulfonylurea that promotes the release of insulin from beta cells of the pancreas and increases insulin sensitivity at peripheral sites. **Therapeutic Effect:** Lowers blood glucose concentration.

PHARMACOKINETICS

Route	Onset	Peak	Duration
PO	15–30 min	2–3 hr	12–24 hr
Extended-release	2–3 hr	6–12 hr	24 hr

Well absorbed from the GI tract. Protein binding: 99%. Metabolized in the liver. Excreted in urine. Half-life: 2–4 hr.

USES

Adjunct to diet, exercise in management of stable, mild to moderately severe non–insulin dependent diabetes mellitus (type 2, NIDDM). May be used to supplement insulin in those with type 1 diabetes mellitus. May be used concomitantly with insulin or metformin to improve glycemic control.

PRECAUTIONS

CONTRAINDICATIONS: Diabetic ketoacidosis with or without coma, type 1 diabetes mellitus. **CAUTIONS:** Adrenal or pituitary insufficiency, hypoglycemic reactions, hepatic or renal impairment.

 LIFESPAN CONSIDERATIONS: Pregnancy/Lactation: Insulin is drug of choice during pregnancy; glipizide given within 1 mo of delivery may produce neonatal hypoglycemia. Drug crosses placenta. Distributed in breast milk. **Pregnancy Category C. Children:** Safety and efficacy not established. **Elderly:** Hypoglycemia may be difficult to recognize. Age-related renal impairment may increase sensitivity to glucose-lowering effect.

INTERACTIONS

DRUG: Beta blockers: May increase the hypoglycemic effect of glipizide and mask signs of hypoglycemia. **Cimetidine, ciprofloxacin, fluconazole, MAOIs, quinidine, ranitidine, large doses of salicylates:** May increase the effects of glipizide. **Corticosteroids, lithium, thiazide diuretics:** May decrease the effects of glipizide. **Oral anticoagulants:** May increase the effects of oral anticoagulants. HERBAL: None known. FOOD: None known. LAB VALUES: May increase BUN and LDH concentrations and serum alkaline phosphatase, creatinine, and AST levels.

AVAILABILITY (Rx)

TABLETS (GLUCOTROL): 5 mg, 10 mg.
TABLETS (EXTENDED-RELEASE [GLUCOTROL XL]): 2.5 mg, 5 mg, 10 mg.

ADMINISTRATION/HANDLING
PO
• May give with food (response better if taken 15–30 min before meals).
• Do not crush extended-release tablets.

INDICATIONS/ROUTES/DOSAGE
DIABETES MELLITUS
PO: ADULTS: Initially, 5 mg/day or 2.5 mg in the elderly or those with hepatic disease. Adjust dosage in 2.5- to 5-mg increments at intervals of several days. **Maximum single dose:** 15 mg. **Maximum dose/day:** 40 mg. Maintenance (extended-release tablet): 20 mg/day. ELDERLY: Initially, 2.5–5 mg/day. May increase by 2.5–5 mg/day q1–2wk.

SIDE EFFECTS
FREQUENT: Altered taste sensation, dizziness, somnolence, weight gain, constipation, diarrhea, heartburn, nausea, vomiting, stomach fullness, headache. **OCCASIONAL:** Increased sensitivity of skin to sunlight, peeling of skin, itching, rash.

ADVERSE REACTIONS/ TOXIC EFFECTS
Overdose or insufficient food intake may produce hypoglycemia, especially with increased glucose demands. GI hemorrhage, cholestatic hepatic jaundice, leukopenia, thrombocytopenia, pancytopenia, agranulocytosis, and aplastic or hemolytic anemia occurs rarely.

NURSING CONSIDERATIONS
BASELINE ASSESSMENT
Check blood glucose level. Discuss lifestyle to determine extent of learning, emotional needs. Ensure follow-up instruction if patient or family does not thoroughly understand diabetes management or blood glucose-testing technique.

INTERVENTION/EVALUATION
Monitor blood glucose level, food intake. Assess for hypoglycemia (cool, wet skin, tremors, dizziness, anxiety, headache, tachycardia, perioral numbness, hunger, diplopia), hyperglycemia (polyuria, polyphagia, polydipsia, nausea, vomiting, dim vision, fatigue, deep, rapid breathing). Be alert to conditions that alter glucose requirements: fever, increased activity or stress, surgical procedure.

PATIENT/FAMILY TEACHING
• Prescribed diet is principal part of treatment; do not skip or delay meals. • Carry candy, sugar packets, other sugar supplements for immediate response to hypoglycemia. • Wear medical alert identification. • Check with physician when glucose demands are altered (e.g., fever, infection, trauma, stress, heavy physical activity).

glucagon hydrochloride

glue-ka-gon
(GlucaGen, GlucaGen Diagnostic Kit, Glucagon, Glucagon Diagnostic Kit, Glucagon Emergency Kit)
Do not confuse glucagon with Glaucon.

◆CLASSIFICATION
PHARMACOTHERAPEUTIC: Glucose

elevating agent. **CLINICAL:** Antihypoglycemic, antispasmodic, antidote.

ACTION

A glucose elevating agent that promotes hepatic glycogenolysis, gluconeogenesis. Stimulates production of cyclic adenosine monophosphate (cAMP), which results in increased plasma glucose concentration, smooth muscle relaxation, and an inotropic myocardial effect. **Therapeutic Effect:** Increases plasma glucose level.

PHARMACOKINETICS

Onset of action occurs within 4–10 min following IM administration. Recovery occurs within 12–32 min. **Half-life:** 8–18 min.

USES

Treatment of severe hypoglycemia in diabetic patients. Not for use in chronic hypoglycemia or hypoglycemia due to starvation, adrenal insufficiency (hepatic glycogen unavailable). Diagnostic aid in radiographic examination of GI tract. **OFF-LABEL:** Treatment of esophageal obstruction due to foreign bodies, toxicity associated with beta blockers or calcium channel blockers.

PRECAUTIONS

CONTRAINDICATIONS: Hypersensitivity to glucagon or beef or pork proteins, known pheochromocytoma. **CAUTIONS:** History of insulinoma, pheochromocytoma.

⧗ **LIFESPAN CONSIDERATIONS: Pregnancy/Lactation:** Unknown if drug crosses placenta or is distributed in breast milk. **Pregnancy Category B. Children/Elderly:** No age-related precautions noted.

INTERACTIONS

DRUG: Anticoagulants: May increase the effects of these drugs. **HERBAL:** None known. **FOOD:** None known. **LAB VALUES:** May decrease serum potassium level.

AVAILABILITY (Rx)

POWDER FOR INJECTION (GLUCAGEN, GLUCAGEN DIAGNOSTIC KIT, GLUCAGON, GLUCAGON DIAGNOSTIC KIT, GLUCAGON EMERGENCY KIT): 1 mg.

ADMINISTRATION/HANDLING

◀ **ALERT** ▶ Place patient on side to prevent aspiration (glucagon, hypoglycemia may produce nausea/vomiting).

IV, IM, SUBCUTANEOUS

Reconstitution • Reconstitute powder with manufacturer's diluent when preparing doses of 2 mg or less. For doses greater than 2 mg, dilute with sterile water for injection. • To provide 1 mg glucagon/ml, use 1 ml diluent. For 1-mg vial of glucagon, use 10 ml diluent for 10-mg vial.

Rate of administration • Patient usually awakens in 5–20 min. Although 1–2 additional doses may be administered, concern for effects of continuing cerebral hypoglycemia requires consideration of parenteral glucose. • When patient awakens, give supplemental carbohydrate to restore hepatic glycogen and prevent secondary hypoglycemia. If patient fails to respond to glucagon, IV glucose is necessary.

Storage • Store vial at room temperature. • After reconstitution, is stable for 48 hr if refrigerated. If reconstituted with sterile water for injection, use immediately. Do not use glucagon solution unless clear.

▨ IV INCOMPATIBILITIES

Don't mix glucagon with any other medications.

INDICATIONS/ROUTES/DOSAGE

HYPOGLYCEMIA

IV, IM, SUBCUTANEOUS: ADULTS, ELDERLY, CHILDREN WEIGHING MORE THAN 20

G

KG: 0.5–1 mg. May give 1 or 2 additional doses if response is delayed. CHILDREN WEIGHING 20 KG OR LESS: 0.5 mg.

DIAGNOSTIC AID
IV, IM: ADULTS, ELDERLY: 0.25–2 mg 10 min prior to procedure.

SIDE EFFECTS

OCCASIONAL: Nausea, vomiting. **RARE:** Allergic reaction, such as urticaria, respiratory distress, and hypotension.

ADVERSE REACTIONS/ TOXIC EFFECTS

Overdose may produce persistent nausea and vomiting and hypokalemia, marked by severe weakness, decreased appetite, irregular heartbeat, and muscle cramps.

NURSING CONSIDERATIONS

BASELINE ASSESSMENT
Obtain immediate assessment, including history, clinical signs/symptoms. If hypoglycemic coma is established, give glucagon promptly.

INTERVENTION/EVALUATION
Monitor response time carefully. Have IV dextrose readily available in event patient does not awaken within 5–20 min. Assess for possible allergic reaction (urticaria, respiratory difficulty, hypotension). When patient is conscious, give carbohydrate.

PATIENT/FAMILY TEACHING
• Recognize significance of identifying symptoms of hypoglycemia: pale, cool skin; anxiety, difficulty concentrating, headache, hunger, nausea, shakiness, diaphoresis, unusual fatigue, unusual weakness, unconsciousness. • If symptoms of hypoglycemia develop, instruct patient, family, or friend to give sugar form first (orange juice, honey, hard candy, sugar cubes, table sugar dissolved in water or juice) followed by cheese and crackers, half a sandwich, or glass of milk.

Glucophage, *see* *metformin*

Glucophage XR, *see* *metformin*

glucosamine/ chondroitin

CLASSIFICATION
HERBAL: See Appendix G.

ACTION
Glucosamine: Necessary for synthesis of mucopolysaccharides, which comprise the body's tendons, ligaments, cartilage, synovial fluid. May decrease glucose-induced insulin secretion. **Effect:** Relieves symptoms of osteoarthritis. **Chondroitin:** Endogenously found in cartilage tissue, substrate for forming joint matrix structure. May have some anticoagulant properties. **Effect:** Relieves symptoms of osteoarthritis.

USES
Treatment of osteoarthritis.

PRECAUTIONS
CONTRAINDICATIONS: None known. **CAUTIONS: Glucosamine:** Diabetes (may increase insulin resistance). **Chondroitin:** None known.

INTERACTIONS
DRUG: Warfarin: Effects may increase. **Anticoagulant therapy:** Monitor.

Blood glucose may be increased with glucosamine. **HERBAL:** None known. **FOOD:** None known. **LAB VALUES:** Chondroitin may increase antifactor Xa level.

AVAILABILITY (OTC)

GLUCOSAMINE
CAPSULES: 500 mg. **TABLETS:** 500 mg.
CHONDROITIN
CAPSULES: 250 mg.
◀ **ALERT** ▶ Many combination products are available.

INDICATIONS/ROUTES/DOSAGE

OSTEOARTHRITIS

PO: ADULTS, ELDERLY: **(Glucosamine):** 500 mg 3 times a day or 1–2 g a day. **(Chondroitin):** 200–400 mg 2–3 times a day.

SIDE EFFECTS

GLUCOSAMINE: Mild GI symptoms (e.g., gas, bloating, cramps). **CHONDROITIN:** Well tolerated. May cause nausea, diarrhea, constipation, edema, alopecia, allergic reactions.

ADVERSE REACTIONS/ TOXIC EFFECTS

None known.

BASELINE ASSESSMENT

Determine whether patient is taking anticoagulants or antiplatelets, antidiabetic drugs. Assess if patient is pregnant or breast-feeding.

INTERVENTION/EVALUATION

Monitor effectiveness of therapy in relieving osteoarthritis symptoms. Monitor blood glucose levels.

PATIENT/FAMILY TEACHING

• Avoid use in pregnancy, breast-feeding, children. • May take several mo of therapy to be effective. • Glucosamine may alter blood glucose levels.

Glucotrol, *see glipizide*

Glucovance, *see glyburide and metformin*

---

*glyBURIDE

glye-byoo-ride

(Daonil ✤, DiaBeta, Euglucon ✤, Glycron, Glynase, Glynase Pres-Tab, Micronase)

Do not confuse glyburide with glimepiride or glipizide, or Micronase with Micro-K, Micronor.

FIXED-COMBINATION(S)

Glucovance: glyburide/metformin (an antidiabetic): 1.25 mg/250 mg; 2.5 mg/500 mg; 5 mg/500 mg.

CLASSIFICATION

PHARMACOTHERAPEUTIC: Second-generation sulfonylurea. **CLINICAL:** Hypoglycemic (see p. 41C).

ACTION

A second-generation sulfonylurea that promotes release of insulin from beta cells of the pancreas and increases insulin sensitivity at peripheral sites. **Therapeutic Effect:** Lowers blood glucose concentration.

PHARMACOKINETICS

Route	Onset	Peak	Duration
PO	0.25–1 hr	1–2 hr	12–24 hr

Well absorbed from the GI tract. Protein binding: 99%. Metabolized in the liver to weakly active metabolite. Primarily excreted in urine. Not removed by hemodialysis. Half-life: 1.4–1.8 hr.

USES

Adjunct to diet, exercise in management of stable, mild to moderately severe non–insulin dependent diabetes mellitus (type 2, NIDDM). May be used to supplement insulin in those with type 1 diabetes mellitus. May be used concomitantly with insulin or metformin to improve glycemic control.

PRECAUTIONS

CONTRAINDICATIONS: Diabetic ketoacidosis with or without coma, monotherapy for type 1 diabetes mellitus. **CAUTIONS:** Adrenal or pituitary insufficiency, hypoglycemic reactions, hepatic or renal impairment.

⌛ **LIFESPAN CONSIDERATIONS: Pregnancy/Lactation:** Crosses placenta. Distributed in breast milk. May produce neonatal hypoglycemia if given within 2 wk of delivery. **Pregnancy Category C. Children:** Safety and efficacy not established. **Elderly:** Hypoglycemia may be difficult to recognize. Age-related renal impairment may increase sensitivity to glucose-lowering effect.

INTERACTIONS

DRUG: Beta blockers: May increase the hypoglycemic effect of glyburide and mask signs of hypoglycemia. **Cimetidine, ciprofloxacin, fluconazole, MAOIs, quinidine, ranitidine, large doses of salicylates:** May increase the effects of glyburide. **Corticosteroids, lithium, thiazide diuretics:** May decrease the effects of glyburide. **Oral anticoagulants:** May increase the effects of oral anticoagulants. **HERBAL:** None known. **FOOD:** None known. **LAB VALUES:** May increase BUN and LDH concentrations and serum alkaline phosphatase, creatinine, and AST levels.

AVAILABILITY (Rx)

TABLETS (DIABETA, MICRONASE): 1.25 mg, 2.5 mg, 5 mg. **TABLETS (MICRONIZED [GLYCRON, GLYNASE]):** 1.5 mg, 3 mg, 4.5 mg, 6 mg.

ADMINISTRATION/HANDLING

PO
• May give with food (response better if taken 15–30 min before meals).

INDICATIONS/ROUTES/DOSAGE

DIABETES MELLITUS
PO: ADULTS: Initially 2.5–5 mg. May increase by 2.5 mg/day at weekly intervals. Maintenance: 1.25–20 mg/day. **Maximum:** 20 mg/day. ELDERLY: Initially, 1.25–2.5 mg/day. May increase by 1.25–2.5 mg/day at 1- to 3-wk intervals.
PO (MICRONIZED TABLETS): ADULTS, ELDERLY: Initially 0.75–3 mg/day. May increase by 1.5 mg/day at weekly intervals. Maintenance: 0.75–12 mg/day as a single dose or in divided doses.

DOSAGE IN RENAL IMPAIRMENT
Glyburide is not recommended in patients with creatinine clearance less than 50 ml/min.

SIDE EFFECTS

FREQUENT: Altered taste sensation, dizziness, somnolence, weight gain, constipation, diarrhea, heartburn, nausea, vomiting, stomach fullness, headache. **OCCASIONAL:** Increased sensitivity of skin to sunlight, peeling of skin, itching, rash.

---

* "Tall Man" lettering   ✐ see color pill atlas   ✐ herb   underlined – top prescribed drug

ADVERSE REACTIONS/ TOXIC EFFECTS

Overdose or insufficient food intake may produce hypoglycemia, especially in patients with increased glucose demands. Cholestatic jaundice, leukopenia, thrombocytopenia, pancytopenia, agranulocytosis, and aplastic or hemolytic anemia occur rarely.

NURSING CONSIDERATIONS

BASELINE ASSESSMENT

Check blood glucose level. Discuss lifestyle to determine extent of learning, emotional needs. Ensure follow-up instruction if patient or family does not thoroughly understand diabetes management or glucose-testing technique.

INTERVENTION/EVALUATION

Monitor blood glucose level, food intake. Assess for hypoglycemia (cool, wet skin; tremors, dizziness, anxiety, headache, tachycardia, perioral numbness, hunger, diplopia) hyperglycemia (polyuria, polyphagia, polydipsia, nausea, vomiting, dim vision, fatigue, deep, rapid breathing). Be alert to conditions that alter glucose requirements: fever, increased activity or stress, surgical procedure.

PATIENT/FAMILY TEACHING

• Prescribed diet is principal part of treatment; do not skip or delay meals. • Carry candy, sugar packets, other sugar supplements for immediate response to hypoglycemia. • Wear medical alert identification. • Check with physician when glucose demands are altered (e.g., fever, infection, trauma, stress, heavy physical activity).

glycopyrrolate

glye-koe-**pye**-roe-late

(Robinul, Robinul Forte)

Do not confuse Robinul with Reminyl.

◆CLASSIFICATION

PHARMACOTHERAPEUTIC: Quaternary anticholinergic. **CLINICAL:** Antimuscarinic, antiarrhythmic, cholinergic adjunct.

ACTION

A quaternary anticholinergic that inhibits action of acetylcholine at postganglionic parasympathetic sites in smooth muscle, secretory glands, and CNS. **Therapeutic Effect:** Reduces salivation and excessive secretions of respiratory tract; reduces gastric secretions and acidity.

USES

Inhibits salivation/excessive secretions of the respiratory tract. Reverses the muscarinic effects of cholinergic agents (e.g., neostigmine).

PRECAUTIONS

CONTRAINDICATIONS: Acute hemorrhage, myasthenia gravis, narrow-angle glaucoma, obstructive uropathy, paralytic ileus, tachycardia, ulcerative colitis. **CAUTIONS:** Those with fever, hyperthyroidism, hepatic/renal disease, hypertension, CHF, GI infections, diarrhea, reflux esophagitis. **Pregnancy Category B.**

INTERACTIONS

DRUG: Antacids, antidiarrheals: May decrease the absorption of glycopyrrolate. **Ketoconazole:** May decrease the absorption of ketoconazole. **Other anticholinergics:** May increase the effects of glycopyrrolate. **Potassium chloride:** May increase the severity of

G

GI lesions with the wax matrix formulation of potassium chloride. **HERBAL:** None known. **FOOD:** None known. **LAB VALUES:** May decrease serum uric acid levels.

AVAILABILITY (Rx)

INJECTION (ROBINUL): 0.2 mg/ml.

ADMINISTRATION/HANDLING

 IV

• Administer undiluted for direct injection through tubing of a free-flowing compatible IV solution.

IM

• Administer undiluted or diluted with D_5W, $D_{10}W$, or 0.9% NaCl.

⊞ IV INCOMPATIBILITY

None known.

IV COMPATIBILITIES

Diphenhydramine (Benadryl), droperidol (Inapsine), hydromorphone (Dilaudid), hydroxyzine (Vistaril), lidocaine, midazolam (Versed), morphine, promethazine (Phenergan).

INDICATIONS/ROUTES/DOSAGE

PREOPERATIVE INHIBITION OF SALIVATION AND EXCESSIVE RESPIRATORY TRACT SECRETIONS
IM: ADULTS, ELDERLY: 4 mcg/kg 30–60 min before procedure. CHILDREN 2 YR AND OLDER: 4 mcg/kg. CHILDREN YOUNGER THAN 2 YR: 4–9 mcg/kg.

TO BLOCK EFFECTS OF ANTICHOLINESTERASE AGENTS
IV: ADULTS, ELDERLY: 0.2 mg for each 1 mg neostigmine or 5 mg pyridostigmine.

SIDE EFFECTS

FREQUENT: Dry mouth, decreased sweating, constipation. **OCCASIONAL:** Blurred vision, gastric bloating, urinary hesitancy, somnolence (with high dosage), headache, intolerance to light, loss of taste, nervousness, flushing, insomnia, impotence, mental confusion or excitement (particularly in the elderly and children), temporary light-headedness (with parenteral form), local irritation (with parenteral form). **RARE:** Dizziness, faintness.

ADVERSE REACTIONS/ TOXIC EFFECTS

Overdose may produce temporary paralysis of ciliary muscle; pupillary dilation; tachycardia; palpitations; hot, dry, or flushed skin; absence of bowel sounds; hyperthermia; increased respiratory rate; EKG abnormalities; nausea; vomiting; rash over face or upper trunk; CNS stimulation; and psychosis (marked by agitation, restlessness, rambling speech, visual hallucinations, paranoid behavior, and delusions, followed by depression).

NURSING CONSIDERATIONS

BASELINE ASSESSMENT

Before giving medication, instruct patient to void (reduces risk of urinary retention).

INTERVENTION/EVALUATION

Monitor daily bowel activity/stool consistency. Palpate bladder for urinary retention. Monitor heart rate, changes in BP, temperature. Assess skin turgor, mucous membranes to evaluate hydration status (encourage adequate fluid intake), bowel sounds for peristalsis. Be alert for fever (increased risk of hyperthermia).

PATIENT/FAMILY TEACHING

• May cause dry mouth. • Take 30 min before meals (food decreases absorption of medication). • Use care not to become overheated during exercise in hot weather (may result in heat stroke). • Avoid hot baths, saunas. • Avoid tasks that require alertness, motor skills until response to drug is established. • Do not take antacids or medicine for diarrhea within 1 hr of taking this medication (decreased effectiveness).

gold sodium thiomalate

gold **soe**-dee-um thigh-oh-**mal**-ate
(Myochrysine)

CLASSIFICATION

PHARMACOTHERAPEUTIC: Gold compound. **CLINICAL:** Antirheumatic, anti-inflammatory.

ACTION

A gold compound whose mechanism of action is unknown. May decrease prostaglandin synthesis or alter cellular mechanisms by inhibiting sulfhydryl systems. **Therapeutic Effect:** Decreases synovial inflammation, retards cartilage and bone destruction, suppresses or prevents—but does not cure—arthritis and synovitis.

PHARMACOKINETICS

Completely bioavailable. Protein binding: Very high. Not broken down to elemental gold. 70% excreted in kidneys with 30% eliminated in feces. **Half-life:** Blood: 26 days, tissue 80 days.

USES

Treatment of progressive rheumatoid arthritis. **OFF-LABEL:** Treatment of psoriatic arthritis.

PRECAUTIONS

CONTRAINDICATIONS: Colitis; concurrent use of antimalarials, immunosuppressive agents, penicillamine, or phenylbutazone; CHF; exfoliative dermatitis; history of blood dyscrasias; severe hepatic or renal impairment; systemic lupus erythematosus; toxicity to gold or other heavy metals. **CAUTIONS:** None known.

LIFESPAN CONSIDERATIONS: Pregnancy/Lactation: Unknown if drug crosses placenta; distributed in breast milk. **Pregnancy Category C. Children:** No age-related precautions noted. **Elderly:** No age-related precautions noted.

INTERACTIONS

DRUG: Bone marrow depressants, hepatotoxic and nephrotoxic medications: May increase the risk of toxicity. **Penicillamine:** May increase the risk of adverse hematologic or renal effects. **HERBAL:** None known. **FOOD:** None known. **LAB VALUES:** May decrease Hgb level, Hct, and WBC and platelet counts. May increase urine protein level. May alter liver function test results.

AVAILABILITY (Rx)

INJECTION: 50 mg/ml.

ADMINISTRATION/HANDLING

Give gold sodium thiomalate as weekly injections, as prescribed.

◄ **ALERT** ► The possibility of toxic reactions should always be explained to the patient before therapy.

INDICATIONS/ROUTES/DOSAGE

RHEUMATOID ARTHRITIS
IM: ADULTS, ELDERLY: Initially, 10 mg, followed by 25 mg for second dose, then 25–50 mg/wk until improvement noted or total of 1 g has been administered. Maintenance: 25–50 mg q2wk for 2–20 wk; if stable, may increase intervals to q3–4wk. CHILDREN: Initially, 10 mg, then 1 mg/kg/wk up to a maximum single dose of 50 mg. Maintenance: 1 mg/kg/dose q2–4wk.

DOSAGE IN RENAL IMPAIRMENT
Dosage is modified based on creatinine clearance.

Creatinine Clearance	Dosage
50–80 ml/min	50% of usual dose
Less than 50 ml/min	Not recommended

SIDE EFFECTS

FREQUENT: Pruritic dermatitis, stomatitis, diarrhea, abdominal pain, nausea. **OCCASIONAL:** Vomiting, anorexia, flatulence, dyspepsia, conjunctivitis, photosensitivity. **RARE:** Constipation, urticaria, rash.

ADVERSE REACTIONS/ TOXIC EFFECTS

Signs and symptoms of gold toxicity include decreased Hgb level, decreased granulocyte count (less than 150,000/mm^3), proteinuria, hematuria, blood dyscrasias (anemia, leukopenia [WBC less than 4,000 mm^3], thrombocytopenia, and eosinophilia), glomerulonephritis, nephrotic syndrome, and cholestatic jaundice.

NURSING CONSIDERATIONS

BASELINE ASSESSMENT

Rule out pregnancy before beginning treatment; CBC, urinalysis, renal and liver function tests should be performed before therapy begins.

INTERVENTION/EVALUATION

Monitor pattern of daily bowel activity and stool consistency. Assess urine tests for proteinuria, hematuria. Monitor CBC, renal and liver function studies. Assess skin frequently for rash, purpura, ecchymoses. Assess oral mucous membranes, borders of tongue, palate, pharynx for ulceration, complaint of metallic taste sensation (signs of stomatitis). Evaluate for therapeutic response: relief of joint pain, stiffness, swelling; increased joint mobility; reduced joint tenderness; improved grip strength.

PATIENT/FAMILY TEACHING

• Therapeutic response may take 6 mo or longer. • Avoid exposure to sunlight (gray to blue pigment may appear). • Maintain diligent oral hygiene.

gonadorelin

go-nad-oh-**rell**-in

(Factrel, Lutrepulse)

Do not confuse gonadorelin with gonadotropin, Factrel with guanadrel or Sectral.

◆CLASSIFICATION

PHARMACOTHERAPEUTIC: Gonadotropin-releasing hormone. **CLINICAL:** Diagnostic agent.

ACTION

Stimulates release of luteinizing hormone (LH) from the anterior pituitary gland. **Therapeutic effect:** Stimulates release of gonadotropin-releasing hormone (GnRH) from hypothalamus.

PHARMACOKINETICS

	Onset	Peak	Duration
IV	NA	20 min	3–5 hr

Half-life: 4 min.

USES

Evaluation of hypothalamic pituitary gonadotropic function, evaluation of abnormal gonadotropin regulation as in precocious or delayed puberty, treatment of primary hypothalamic amenorrhea.

PRECAUTIONS

CONTRAINDICATIONS: None known. **CAUTIONS:** None known. **Pregnancy Category B.**

INTERACTIONS

DRUG: None known. **HERBAL:** None known. **FOOD:** None known. **LAB VALUES:** None known.

AVAILABILITY (Rx)

POWDER FOR INJECTION: 100 mcg (Factrel), 0.8 mg (Lutrepulse), 3.2 mg (Lutrepulse).

INDICATIONS/ROUTES/DOSAGE

◂ **ALERT** ▸ Test should be conducted in the absence of other drugs that affect pituitary secretion of gonadotropins.

GONADORELIN ACETATE

PRIMARY HYPOTHALAMIC AMENORRHEA

IV (LUTREPULSE) PUMP: ADULTS: 5 mcg q90min (range 1–20 mcg); treatment interval 21 days. Refer to manufacturer's manual for proper dilutions/settings on pump. Response usually occurs 2–3 wk after initiation. Continue additional 2 wk after ovulation occurs (maintains corpus luteum). **Note:** Pump will pulsate q90min for 7 days.

GONADORELIN HYDROCHLORIDE
DIAGNOSTIC AGENT

IV, SUBCUTANEOUS: ADULTS: 100 mcg. In females, perform test in early follicular phase of menstrual cycle.

SIDE EFFECTS

OCCASIONAL: Swelling, pain, itching at injection site with subcutaneous administration. Local or generalized skin rash with chronic subcutaneous administration. **RARE:** Headache, nausea, lightheadedness, abdominal discomfort, hypersensitivity reactions (bronchospasm, tachycardia, flushing, urticaria), induration at injection site.

ADVERSE REACTIONS/ TOXIC EFFECTS

Anaphylactic reaction occurs rarely.

NURSING CONSIDERATIONS

BASELINE ASSESSMENT
Ensure patient understands procedure before starting test. **Gonadorelin Acetate:** Patient instructions included with kit from manufacturer. **Gonadorelin Hydrochloride:** Draw venous blood sample (for LH) immediately before administration.

INTERVENTION/EVALUATION
Gonadorelin Acetate: With baseline pelvic ultrasound, perform follow-up studies. **Gonadorelin Hydrochloride:** Change cannula, IV site at 48-hr intervals. Ensure that protocol for test is maintained: usually venous blood samples (for LH) drawn after administration at intervals of 15, 30, 45, 60, 120 min.

G

---

goserelin acetate ▷

gos-**er**-ah-lin
(Zoladex, Zoladex LA ❀)

◆CLASSIFICATION
PHARMACOTHERAPEUTIC: Gonadotropin-releasing hormone analogue. **CLINICAL:** Antineoplastic (see pp. 75C, 93C).

ACTION
A gonadotropin-releasing hormone analogue and antineoplastic agent that stimulates the release of luteinizing hormone (LH) and follicle-stimulating hormone (FSH) from the anterior pituitary gland. In males, increases testosterone concentrations initially, then suppresses secretion of LH and FSH, resulting in decreased testosterone levels. **Therapeutic Effect:** In females, causes a reduction in ovarian size and function, reduction in uterine and mammary gland size, and regression of sex-hormone-responsive tumors.

In males, produces pharmacologic castration and decreases the growth of abnormal prostate tissue.

PHARMACOKINETICS

Protein binding: 27%. Metabolized in liver. Excreted in urine. **Half-life:** 4.2 hr (male); 2.3 hr (female).

USES

Treatment of advanced carcinoma of prostate as alternative when orchiectomy, estrogen therapy is either not indicated or unacceptable to patient. In combination with flutamide before and during radiation therapy for early stages of prostate cancer. Management of endometriosis. Treatment of advanced breast cancer in premenopausal and perimenopausal women. Endometrial thinning before ablation for dysfunctional uterine bleeding.

PRECAUTIONS

CONTRAINDICATIONS: Pregnancy. **CAUTIONS:** None known.

⧗ **LIFESPAN CONSIDERATIONS: Pregnancy/Lactation:** Crosses placenta; unknown if distributed in breast milk. **Pregnancy Category D (advanced breast cancer), X (endometriosis, endometrial thinning). Children:** Safety and efficacy not established. **Elderly:** No age-related precautions noted.

INTERACTIONS

DRUG: None known. **HERBAL:** None known. **FOOD:** None known. **LAB VALUES:** May increase serum prostatic acid phosphatase and testosterone levels.

AVAILABILITY (Rx)

IMPLANT (ZOLADEX): 3.6 mg, 10.8 mg.

ADMINISTRATION/HANDLING
IMPLANT

• Inspect the package for damage before opening. If the package is damaged, don't use the syringe. • Remove the sterile syringe from the package immediately before use. Examine the syringe for damage, and check that goserelin is visible in the translucent chamber. • Clean an area of skin on the upper abdominal wall with an alcohol swab. • Grasp the safety clip tab, pull it out and away from the needle, and discard it immediately. Then remove the needle cover. • Using aseptic technique, stretch or pinch the patient's skin with one hand, and grip the syringe barrel. Insert the needle into the subcutaneous tissue.

◀ **ALERT** ▶ The goserelin syringe should not be used for aspiration. If the needle penetrates a large vessel, you'll see blood instantly in the syringe chamber. If a vessel is penetrated, withdraw the needle and use a new syringe elsewhere.

• Direct the needle so that it parallels the abdominal wall. Push the needle in until the barrel hub touches the patient's skin. Withdraw the needle 1 cm to create a space to discharge goserelin. Fully depress the plunger to discharge the drug. • Withdraw the needle. Then bandage the site. Confirm the discharge of goserelin by ensuring that the tip of the plunger is visible within the tip of the needle. • Dispose of the used needle and syringe in a safe manner.

INDICATIONS/ROUTES/DOSAGE
PROSTATIC CARCINOMA

IMPLANT: ADULTS OLDER THAN 18 YR, ELDERLY: 3.6 mg every 28 days or 10.8 mg q12wk subcutaneously into upper abdominal wall.

BREAST CARCINOMA, ENDOMETRIOSIS

IMPLANT: ADULTS: 3.6 mg every 28 days subcutaneously into upper abdominal wall.

✎ see color pill atlas   ⬧ herb   underlined – top prescribed drug

ENDOMETRIAL THINNING
IMPLANT: ADULTS: 3.6 mg subcutaneously into upper abdominal wall as a single dose or in 2 doses 4 wk apart.

SIDE EFFECTS

FREQUENT: Headache (60%), hot flashes (55%), depression (54%), diaphoresis (45%), sexual dysfunction (21%), decreased erection (18%), lower urinary tract symptoms (13%). **OCCASIONAL (10%–5%):** Pain, lethargy, dizziness, insomnia, anorexia, nausea, rash, upper respiratory tract infection, hirsutism, abdominal pain. **RARE:** Pruritus.

ADVERSE REACTIONS/ TOXIC EFFECTS

Arrhythmias, CHF, and hypertension occur rarely. Ureteral obstruction and spinal cord compression have been observed. An immediate orchiectomy may be necessary if these conditions occur.

NURSING CONSIDERATIONS

INTERVENTION/EVALUATION

Monitor patient closely for worsening signs and symptoms of prostatic cancer, especially during first month of therapy.

PATIENT/FAMILY TEACHING

• Use contraceptive measures during therapy. • Inform physician if patient becomes pregnant or regular menstruation persists. • Breakthrough menstrual bleeding may occur if dose is missed. • Use nonhormonal methods of contraception.

granisetron

gran-**is**-eh-tron
(Kytril)

◆CLASSIFICATION

PHARMACOTHERAPEUTIC: Serotonin receptor antagonist. **CLINICAL:** Antiemetic.

G

ACTION

A 5-HT$_3$ receptor antagonist that acts centrally in the chemoreceptor trigger zone or peripherally at the vagal nerve terminals. **Therapeutic Effect:** Prevents nausea and vomiting.

PHARMACOKINETICS

Route	Onset	Peak	Duration
IV	1–3 min	N/A	24 hr

Rapidly and widely distributed to tissues. Protein binding: 65%. Metabolized in the liver to active metabolite. Eliminated in urine and feces. **Half-life:** 10–12 hr (increased in the elderly).

USES

Prevents nausea, vomiting associated with emetogenic cancer therapy (includes high-dose cisplatin). Prevention and treatment of postop nausea, vomiting. Prophylaxis of nausea and vomiting associated with cancer radiation therapy. **OFF-LABEL: PO:** Prophylaxis of nausea or vomiting associated with radiation therapy.

PRECAUTIONS

CONTRAINDICATIONS: None known. **CAUTIONS:** Safety in children younger than 2 yr not established. The use of granisetron following abdominal surgery or with chemotherapy-induced nausea and vomiting may mask a progressive ileus and/or gastric distention.

⧗ **LIFESPAN CONSIDERATIONS: Pregnancy/Lactation:** Unknown if drug is distributed in breast milk. **Pregnancy Category B. Children:** Safety and efficacy not established in patients younger than 2 yr. **Elderly:** No age-related precautions noted.

INTERACTIONS

DRUG: Hepatic enzyme inducers: May decrease the effects of granisetron. **HERBAL:** None known. **FOOD:** None known. **LAB VALUES:** May increase AST and ALT levels.

AVAILABILITY (Rx)

ORAL SOLUTION: 2 mg/10 ml. **TABLETS:** 1 mg. **INJECTION:** 0.1 mg/ml, 1 mg/ml.

ADMINISTRATION/HANDLING
▱ IV

Reconstitution • May be given undiluted or dilute with 20–50 ml 0.9% NaCl or D$_5$W. Do not mix with other medications.

Rate of administration • May give undiluted as IV push over 30 sec. • For IV piggyback, infuse over 5–20 min depending on volume of diluent used.

Storage • Appears as a clear, colorless solution. • Store at room temperature. • After dilution, is stable for at least 24 hr at room temperature. • Inspect for particulates, discoloration.

▨ IV INCOMPATIBILITY
Amphotericin B (Fungizone).

IV COMPATIBILITIES
Allopurinol (Aloprim), bumetanide (Bumex), calcium gluconate, carboplatin (Paraplatin), cisplatin (Platinol), cyclophosphamide (Cytoxan), cytarabine (Ara-C), dacarbazine (DTIC-Dome), dexamethasone (Decadron), diphenhydramine (Benadryl), docetaxel (Taxotere), doxorubicin (Adriamycin), etoposide (VePesid), gemcitabine (Gemzar), magnesium, mitoxantrone (Novantrone), paclitaxel (Taxol), potassium.

INDICATIONS/ROUTES/DOSAGE
PREVENTION OF CHEMOTHERAPY-INDUCED NAUSEA AND VOMITING
PO: ADULTS, ELDERLY: 2 mg 1 hr before chemotherapy or 1 mg 1 hr before and 12 hr after chemotherapy.
IV: ADULTS, ELDERLY, CHILDREN 2 YR AND OLDER: 10 mcg/kg/dose (or 1 mg/dose) within 30 min of chemotherapy.

PREVENTION OF RADIATION-INDUCED NAUSEA AND VOMITING
PO: ADULTS, ELDERLY: 2 mg once a day, given 1 hr before radiation therapy.

POSTOPERATIVE NAUSEA OR VOMITING
PO: ADULTS, ELDERLY, CHILDREN 4 YR AND OLDER: 20–40 mcg/kg as a single postoperative dose.
IV: ADULTS, ELDERLY: 1 mg as a single postoperative dose. CHILDREN OLDER THAN 4 YR: 20–40 mcg/kg. **Maximum:** 1 mg.

SIDE EFFECTS

FREQUENT **(21%–14%):** Headache, constipation, asthenia. **OCCASIONAL (8%–6%):** Diarrhea, abdominal pain. **RARE (less than 2%):** Altered taste, hypersensitivity reaction.

ADVERSE REACTIONS/TOXIC EFFECTS

Hypertension, hypotension, arrhythmias such as sinus bradycardia, atrial fibrillation, varying degrees of AV block, ventricular ectopy including non-sustained tachycardia, and EKG abnormalities have been observed. Rare cases of hypersensitivity reactions, sometimes severe (e.g., anaphylaxis, shortness of breath, hypotension, urticaria) have been reported.

✎ see color pill atlas   ⬤ herb   <u>underlined</u> – top prescribed drug

NURSING CONSIDERATIONS

BASELINE ASSESSMENT
Ensure that granisetron is given within 30 min of starting chemotherapy.

INTERVENTION/EVALUATION
Monitor for therapeutic effect. Assess for headache. Monitor frequency/consistency of stools.

PATIENT/FAMILY TEACHING
• Granisetron is effective shortly following administration; prevents nausea, vomiting. • Explain that transitory taste disorder may occur.

griseofulvin
griz-ee-oh-**full**-vin
(Fulvicin P/G, Fulvicin U/F, Grifulvin V, Grisactin 500, Griseofulicin, Gris-PEG)

♦CLASSIFICATION
CLINICAL: Antifungal.

ACTION
An antifungal that inhibits fungal cell mitosis by disrupting mitotic spindle structure. **Therapeutic Effect:** Fungistatic.

PHARMACOKINETICS
Ultramicrosize is almost completely absorbed. Absorption is significantly enhanced after a fatty meal. Extensively metabolized in liver. Minimal excretion in urine. **Half-life:** 24 hr.

USES
Treatment of susceptible tinea infections of the skin, hair, and nails including tinea (ringworm): t. capitis, t. corporis, t. cruris, t. pedis, t. unguium.

PRECAUTIONS
CONTRAINDICATIONS: Hepatocellular failure, porphyria. **CAUTIONS:** Exposure to sun or ultraviolet light (photosensitivity), hypersensitivity to penicillins.

⌛ LIFESPAN CONSIDERATIONS: **Pregnancy/Lactation:** Crosses placenta; unknown if distributed in breast milk. **Pregnancy Category C. Children:** Safety and efficacy not established in children younger than 2 yr. **Elderly:** No age-related precautions noted.

INTERACTIONS
DRUG: Oral contraceptives, warfarin: May decrease the effects of these drugs. **HERBAL:** None known. **FOOD:** None known. **LAB VALUES:** None known.

AVAILABILITY (Rx)
ORAL SUSPENSION (GRIFULVIN V): 125 mg/5 ml. **TABLETS (MICROSIZE [FULVICIN -U/F, GRISACTIN 500, GRIFULVIN V]):** 250 mg, 500 mg. **TABLETS (ULTRAMICROSIZE):** 125 mg (Fulvicin P/G, Gris-PEG), 165 mg (Fulvicin P/G), 250 mg (Fulvicin P/G, Gris-PEG), 330 mg (Fulvicin P/G, Griseofulicin).

INDICATIONS/ROUTES/DOSAGE
TINEA CAPITIS, TINEA CORPORIS, TINEA CRURIS, TINEA PEDIS, TINEA UNGUIUM
PO (MICROSIZE TABLETS, ORAL SUSPENSION): ADULTS: Usual dosage, 500–1,000 mg as a single dose or in divided doses. CHILDREN 2 YR AND OLDER: Usual dosage, 10–20 mg/kg/day.
PO (ULTRAMICROSIZE TABLETS): ADULTS: Usual dosage, 330–750 mg/day as a single dose or in divided doses. CHILDREN 2 YR AND OLDER: 5–10 mg/kg/day.

SIDE EFFECTS
OCCASIONAL: Hypersensitivity reaction (including pruritus, rash, and urticaria), headache, nausea, diarrhea, excessive thirst, flatulence, oral thrush, dizziness, insomnia. **RARE:** Paresthesia of hands

G

or feet, proteinuria, photosensitivity reaction.

ADVERSE REACTIONS/TOXIC EFFECTS

Granulocytopenia occurs rarely.

BASELINE ASSESSMENT

Question for history of allergies, especially to griseofulvin, penicillins.

INTERVENTION/EVALUATION

Assess skin for rash, response to therapy. Determine pattern of bowel activity and stool consistency. Question presence of headache: onset, location, type of discomfort. Assess for dizziness.

PATIENT/FAMILY TEACHING

• Prolonged therapy (weeks or months) usually is necessary. • Do not miss a dose; continue therapy as long as ordered. • Avoid alcohol (may produce tachycardia, flushing). • May cause photosensitivity reaction; avoid exposure to sunlight. • Maintain good hygiene (prevents superinfection). • Separate personal items in direct contact with affected areas. • Keep affected areas dry; wear light clothing for ventilation. • Take with foods high in fat such as milk, ice cream (reduces GI upset and assists absorption).

guaifenesin

gwye-**fen**-e-sin

(Allfen, Amibid LA, Balminil 🍁, Benylin E 🍁, Duratuss G, Fenesin, Ganidin NR, GG 200 NR, Guaibid-LA, Guaifenex G, Guaifenex LA, Gua-SR, Guiadrine G-1200, Guiatuss, Humavent LA, Humibid LA, Humibid Pediatric, Iofen, Iophen NR, Liquidbid, Liquidbid 1200, Liquidbid LA, Mucinex, Mucobid-L.A., Muco-Fen, Muco-Fen 1200, Muco-Fen 800, Organ-1 NR, Organidin NR, Pneumomist, Q-Bid LA, Respa-GF, Robitussin, Touro EX, Tussin)

Do not confuse guaifenesin with guanfacine.

FIXED-COMBINATION(S)

Mucinex D: guaifenesin/pseudoephedrine (a sympathomimetic): 600 mg/60 mg; 1,200 mg/120 mg. **Mucinex DM:** guaifenesin/dextromethorphan: 600 mg/30 mg; 1,200 mg/60 mg. **Robitussin AC:** guaifenesin/codeine (a narcotic analgesic): 100 mg/10 mg; 75 mg/2.5 mg per 5 ml. **Robitussin DM:** guaifenesin/dextromethorphan (a cough suppressant): 100 mg/10 mg per 5 ml.

CLASSIFICATION

CLINICAL: Expectorant.

ACTION

An expectorant that stimulates respiratory tract secretions by decreasing adhesiveness and viscosity of phlegm. **Therapeutic Effect:** Promotes removal of viscous mucus.

PHARMACOKINETICS

Well absorbed from the GI tract. Metabolized in the liver. Excreted in urine. **Half-life:** 1 hr.

USES

Expectorant for symptomatic treatment of coughs.

PRECAUTIONS

CONTRAINDICATIONS: None known. **CAUTIONS:** None known.

⌛ **LIFESPAN CONSIDERATIONS: Pregnancy/Lactation:** Unknown if drug crosses placenta or is distributed in breast milk. **Pregnancy Category C. Children:** Caution advised in patients younger than 2 yr with persistent cough. **Elderly:** No age-related precautions noted.

✎ see color pill atlas   🍁 herb   underlined – top prescribed drug

INTERACTIONS

DRUG: None known. **HERBAL:** None known. **FOOD:** None known. **LAB VALUES:** None known.

AVAILABILITY (OTC)

TABLETS (GG 200 NR, IOFEN, ORGAN-1 NR, ORGANIDIN NR): 200 mg. **TABLETS (EXTENDED-RELEASE):** 300 mg (Humibid Pediatric), 575 mg (Touro EX), 600 mg (Amibid LA, Fenesin, Guaibid-LA, Guaifenex LA, Gua-SR, Humavent LA, Humibid LA, Liquidbid, Liquidbid LA, Mucinex, Mucobid-L.A., Pneumomist, A-Bid LA, Respa-GF), 800 mg (Muco-Fen 800), 1,000 mg (Allfen, Muco-Fen), 1,200 mg (Duratuss G, Guaifenex G, Guiadrine G-1200, Liquidbid 1200, Muco-Fen 1200). **SYRUP (GANIDIN NR, GUIATUSS, IOPHEN NR, ROBITUSSIN, TUSSIN):** 100 mg/5 ml.

ADMINISTRATION/HANDLING

PO
• Store syrup, liquid, capsules at room temperature. • Give without regard to meals. • Do not crush or break extended-release capsule. May sprinkle contents on soft food, then swallow without crushing or chewing.

INDICATIONS/ROUTES/DOSAGE

EXPECTORANT
PO: ADULTS, ELDERLY, CHILDREN OLDER THAN 12 YR: 200–400 mg q4h. CHILDREN 6–12 YR: 100–200 mg q4h. **Maximum:** 1.2 g/day. CHILDREN 2–5 YR: 50–100 mg q4h. **Maximum:** 600 mg/day. CHILDREN YOUNGER THAN 2 YR: 12 mg/kg/day in 6 divided doses.
PO (EXTENDED-RELEASE): ADULTS, ELDERLY, CHILDREN OLDER THAN 12 YR: 600–1,200 mg q12h. **Maximum:** 2.4 g/day. CHILDREN 6–12 YR: 600 mg q12h. **Maximum:** 1.2 g/day.

SIDE EFFECTS

RARE: Dizziness, headache, rash, diarrhea, nausea, vomiting, abdominal pain.

ADVERSE REACTIONS/ TOXIC EFFECTS

Overdose may produce nausea and vomiting.

NURSING CONSIDERATIONS

BASELINE ASSESSMENT
Assess type, severity, frequency of cough. Increase fluid intake, environmental humidity to lower viscosity of lung secretions.

INTERVENTION/EVALUATION
Initiate deep breathing, coughing exercises, particularly in patients with pulmonary impairment. Assess for clinical improvement; record onset of relief of cough.

PATIENT/FAMILY TEACHING
• Avoid tasks that require alertness, motor skills until response to drug is established. • Do not take for chronic cough. • Inform physician if cough persists or if fever, rash, headache, sore throat is present with cough. • Maintain adequate hydration.

guanabenz
(Wytensin)
See Antihypertensives (p. 54C)

guanadrel
(Hylorel)
See Antihypertensives

guanfacine
(Tenex)
See Antihypertensives (p. 54C)

halcinonide

(Halog)
See Corticosteroids: topical

Haldol, *see haloperidol*

halobetasol

(Ultravate)
See Corticosteroids: topical (p. 87C)

haloperidol

hal-oh-**pear**-ih-dawl

(Apo-Haloperidol ✦, Haldol, Haldol Decanoate, Novoperidol ✦, Peridol ✦)

Do not confuse Haldol with Halcion, Halog, or Stadol.

◆ CLASSIFICATION

CLINICAL: Antipsychotic, antiemetic, antidyskinetic (see p. 58C).

ACTION

An antipsychotic, antiemetic, and antidyskinetic agent that competitively blocks postsynaptic dopamine receptors, interrupts nerve impulse movement, and increases turnover of dopamine in the brain. Has strong extrapyramidal and antiemetic effects; weak anticholinergic and sedative effects. **Therapeutic Effect:** Produces tranquilizing effect.

PHARMACOKINETICS

Readily absorbed from the GI tract. Protein binding: 92%. Extensively metabolized in the liver. Primarily excreted in urine. Not removed by hemodialysis. **Half-life:** 12–37 hr PO; 10–19 hr IV; 17–25 hr IM.

USES

Treatment of psychoses, Tourette's disorder, severe behavioral problems in children, emergency sedation of severely agitated/psychotic patients. **OFF-LABEL:** Treatment of Huntington's chorea, infantile autism, nausea or vomiting associated with cancer chemotherapy.

PRECAUTIONS

CONTRAINDICATIONS: Angle-closure glaucoma, CNS depression, myelosuppression, Parkinson's disease, severe cardiac or hepatic disease. **CAUTIONS:** Renal or hepatic impairment, cardiovascular disease, history of seizures.

⧖ **LIFESPAN CONSIDERATIONS: Pregnancy/Lactation:** Crosses placenta. Distributed in breast milk. **Pregnancy Category C. Children:** More susceptible to dystonias; not recommended in those younger than 3 yr. **Elderly:** More susceptible to orthostatic hypotension, anticholinergic effects and sedation, increased risk for extrapyramidal effects. Decreased dosage recommended.

INTERACTIONS

DRUG: Alcohol, other CNS depressants: May increase CNS depression. **Epinephrine:** May block alpha-adrenergic effects. **Extrapyramidal symptom-producing medications:** May increase extrapyramidal symptoms. **Lithium:** May increase neurologic toxicity. **HERBAL:** None known. **FOOD:** None known. **LAB VALUES:** None known. Therapeutic serum level is 0.2–1 mcg/ml; toxic serum level is greater than 1 mcg/ml.

AVAILABILITY (Rx)

ORAL CONCENTRATE: 1 mg/ml, 2 mg/ml. **TABLETS (HALDOL):** 0.5 mg, 1 mg, 2 mg, 5 mg, 10 mg, 20 mg. **INJECTION (LACTATE [HALDOL]):** 5 mg/ml. **INJECTION (DECANOATE [HALDOL DECANOATE]):** 50 mg/ml, 100 mg/ml.

ADMINISTRATION/HANDLING

 IV

‹ **ALERT** › Only haloperidol lactate is given IV.

Reconstitution • May give undiluted. • Flush with at least 2 ml 0.9% NaCl before and after administration. • May add to 30–50 ml most solutions (D_5W preferred).

Rate of administration • Give IV push at rate of 5 mg/min. • Infuse IV piggyback over 30 min. • For IV infusion, up to 25 mg/hr has been used (titrated to patient response).

Storage • Discard if precipitate forms, discoloration occurs. • Store at room temperature. • Protect from light, do not freeze.

IM

Parenteral administration: • Patient should remain recumbent for 30–60 min in head-low position with legs raised to minimize hypotensive effect. • Prepare Decanoate IM injection using 21-gauge needle. • Do not exceed maximum volume of 3 ml per IM injection site. • Inject slow, deep IM into upper outer quadrant of gluteus maximus.

PO

• Give without regard to meals. • Scored tablets may be crushed.

▦ IV INCOMPATIBILITIES

Allopurinol (Aloprim), amphotericin B complex (Abelcet, AmBisome, Amphotec), cefepime (Maxipime), fluconazole (Diflucan), foscarnet (Foscavir), heparin, nitroprusside (Nipride), piperacillin and tazobactam (Zosyn).

IV COMPATIBILITIES

Dobutamine (Dobutrex), dopamine (Intropin), fentanyl (Sublimaze), hydromorphone (Dilaudid), lidocaine, lorazepam (Ativan), midazolam (Versed), morphine, nitroglycerin, norepinephrine (Levophed), propofol (Diprivan).

INDICATIONS/ROUTES/DOSAGE

ACUTE PSYCHOSIS, DELIRIUM

IV: ADULTS, ELDERLY: 0.5–50 mg at a rate of 5 mg/min. May repeat as needed.

PSYCHOTIC DISORDER

PO: ADULTS, ELDERLY: Initially, 0.5–5 mg 2–3 times a day. **Maximum:** 100 mg/day.

SEVERE BEHAVIORAL PROBLEMS

PO: CHILDREN 3–12 YR, WEIGHING 15–40 KG: 0.05–0.075 mg/kg/day. Initially, 0.5 mg/day. May increase by 0.5 mg/day q5–7days divided into 2–3 doses a day.

TOURETTE'S DISORDER

PO: ADULTS, ELDERLY: 6–15 mg/day. May increase by 2 mg increments as needed. Maintenance: 9 mg/day. CHILDREN 3–12 YR, WEIGHING 15–40 KG: 0.05–0.075 mg/kg/day. Initially, 0.5 mg/day. May increase by 0.5 mg/day q5–7days divided into 2–3 doses a day.

SIDE EFFECTS

FREQUENT: Blurred vision, constipation, orthostatic hypotension, dry mouth, swelling or soreness of female breasts, peripheral edema. **OCCASIONAL:** Allergic reaction, difficulty urinating, decreased thirst, dizziness, decreased sexual function, drowsiness, nausea, vomiting, photosensitivity, lethargy.

ADVERSE REACTIONS/ TOXIC EFFECTS

Extrapyramidal symptoms appear to be dose-related and typically occur in the first few days of therapy. Marked drowsiness and lethargy, excessive salivation, and fixed stare occur frequently. Less common reactions include severe akathisia (motor restlessness) and acute dystonias (such as torticollis, opisthotonos, and oculogyric crisis). Tardive dyskinesia (tongue protrusion, puffing of the cheeks, chewing or puckering of the mouth) may occur during long-term therapy or after discontinuing the drug and may be irreversible. Elderly female patients have a greater risk of developing this reaction.

NURSING CONSIDERATIONS

BASELINE ASSESSMENT
Assess behavior, appearance, emotional status, response to environment, speech pattern, thought content.

INTERVENTION/EVALUATION
Supervise suicidal-risk patient closely during early therapy (as depression lessens, energy level improves, causing increased suicide potential). Monitor for rigidity, tremor, mask-like facial expression, fine tongue movement. Assess for therapeutic response (interest in surroundings, improvement in self-care, increased ability to concentrate, relaxed facial expression). Therapeutic serum level: 0.2–1 mcg/ml. Toxic serum level: greater than 1 mcg/ml.

PATIENT/FAMILY TEACHING
• Full therapeutic effect may take up to 6 wk. • Do not abruptly withdraw from long-term drug therapy. • Sugarless gum, sips of tepid water may relieve dry mouth. • Drowsiness generally subsides during continued therapy. • Avoid tasks that require alertness, motor skills until response to drug is established. • Avoid alcohol. • Report muscle stiffness. • Avoid exposure to sunlight, overheating, dehydration (increased risk of heat stroke).

haloprogin

(Halotex)
See Antifungals: topical

heparin sodium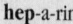

hep-a-rin

(Hep-Lock, Hep-Pak CVC, Hepalean ✷, Heparin Leo)

Do not confuse heparin with Hespan.

◆CLASSIFICATION
PHARMACOTHERAPEUTIC: Blood modifier. **CLINICAL:** Anticoagulant (see p. 30C).

ACTION
A blood modifier that interferes with blood coagulation by blocking conversion of prothrombin to thrombin and fibrinogen to fibrin. **Therapeutic Effect:** Prevents further extension of existing thrombi or new clot formation. Has no effect on existing clots.

PHARMACOKINETICS
Well absorbed following subcutaneous administration. Protein binding: Very high. Metabolized in the liver. Removed from the circulation via uptake by the reticuloendothelial system. Primarily excreted in urine. Not removed by hemodialysis. **Half-life:** 1–6 hr.

USES
Prophylaxis and/or treatment of thromboembolic disorders, including venous thrombosis, pulmonary embolism, peripheral arterial embolism, atrial fibrillation with embolism. Prevention of thromboembolus in cardiac and vascular surgery, dialysis procedures, blood transfusions, blood sampling for laboratory purposes. Adjunct in treatment of coronary occlusion with acute MI. Maintains patency of indwelling intravascular devices. Diagnosis, treatment of acute/chronic consumptive coagulation pathology (e.g., disseminated intravascular coagulation [DIC]). Prevents cerebral thrombosis in progressive strokes.

PRECAUTIONS

CONTRAINDICATIONS: Intracranial hemorrhage, severe hypotension, severe thrombocytopenia, subacute bacterial endocarditis, uncontrolled bleeding. **CAUTIONS:** IM injections, peptic ulcer disease, menstruation, recent surgery or invasive procedures, severe hepatic or renal disease.

⧗ **LIFESPAN CONSIDERATIONS: Pregnancy/Lactation:** Use with caution, particularly during last trimester, immediate postpartum period (increased risk of maternal hemorrhage). Does not cross placenta. Not distributed in breast milk. **Pregnancy Category C. Children:** No age-related precautions noted. Benzyl alcohol preservative may cause gasping syndrome in infants. **Elderly:** More susceptible to hemorrhage. Age-related renal impairment may increase risk of bleeding.

INTERACTIONS

DRUG: Antithyroid medications, cefoperazone, cefotetan, valproic acid: May cause hypoprothrombinemia. **Other anticoagulants, platelet aggregation inhibitors, thrombolytics:** May increase the risk of bleeding. **Probenecid:** May increase the effects of heparin. **HERBAL: Feverfew, ginkgo biloba:** May have additive effect. **FOOD:** None known. **LAB VALUES:** May increase free fatty acid, AST, and ALT levels. May decrease serum cholesterol and triglyceride levels.

AVAILABILITY (Rx)

INJECTION: 10 units/ml (Hep-Lock), 100 units/ml, 1,000 units/ml, 2,500 units/ml, 5,000 units/ml, 7,500 units/ml, 10,000 units/ml, 20,000 units/ml, 25,000 units/500 ml infusion. **INJECTABLE KIT (HEP-PAK CVC):** 20 units/ml, 100 units/ml.

ADMINISTRATION/HANDLING

◂ **ALERT** ▸ Do **not** give by IM injection (pain, hematoma, ulceration, erythema).

 IV

◂ **ALERT** ▸ Used in full-dose therapy. Intermittent IV produces higher incidence of bleeding abnormalities. Continuous IV route preferred.

Reconstitution • Dilute IV infusion in isotonic sterile saline, D₅W, or lactated Ringer's. • Invert container at least 6 times (ensures mixing, prevents pooling of medication).

Rate of administration • Use constant-rate IV infusion pump.

Storage • Store at room temperature.

SUBCUTANEOUS

◂ **ALERT** ▸ Used in low-dose therapy. • After withdrawal of heparin from vial, change needle before injection (prevents leakage along needle track). • Inject above iliac crest or in abdominal fat layer. Do not inject within 2 inches of umbilicus, or any scar tissue. • Withdraw needle rapidly, apply prolonged pressure at injection site. Do not massage. • Rotate injection sites.

▦ **IV INCOMPATIBILITIES**

Amiodarone (Cordarone), amphotericin B complex (Abelcet, AmBisome, Amphotec), ciprofloxacin (Cipro), dacarbazine (DTIC), diazepam (Valium), dobutamine (Dobutrex), doxorubicin (Adriamycin), droperidol (Inapsine), filgrastim (Neupogen), gentamicin (Garamycin), haloperidol (Haldol), idarubicin (Idamycin), labetalol (Trandate), nicardipine (Cardene), phenytoin (Dilantin), quinidine, tobramycin (Nebcin), vancomycin (Vancocin).

IV COMPATIBILITIES

Aminophylline, ampicillin/sulbactam (Unasyn), aztreonam (Azactam), calcium gluconate, cefazolin (Ancef), ceftazidime (Fortaz), ceftriaxone (Rocephin), digoxin (Lanoxin), diltiazem (Cardizem), dopamine (Intropin), enalapril (Vasotec), famotidine (Pepcid), fentanyl (Sublimaze), furosemide (Lasix), hydromorphone (Dilaudid), insulin, lidocaine, lorazepam (Ativan), magnesium sulfate, methylprednisolone (Solu-Medrol), midazolam (Versed), milrinone (Primacor), morphine, nitroglycerin, norepinephrine (Levophed), oxytocin (Pitocin), piperacillin/tazobactam (Zosyn), procainamide (Pronestyl), propofol (Diprivan), total parenteral nutrition (TPN).

INDICATIONS/ROUTES/DOSAGE

LINE FLUSHING

IV: ADULTS, ELDERLY, CHILDREN: 100 units q6–8h. INFANTS WEIGHING LESS THAN 10 KG: 10 units q6–8h.

TREATMENT OF VENOUS THROMBOSIS, PULMONARY EMBOLISM, PERIPHERAL ARTERIAL EMBOLISM, ATRIAL FIBRILLATION WITH EMBOLISM

INTERMITTENT IV: ADULTS, ELDERLY: Initially, 10,000 units, then 50–70 units/kg (5,000–10,000 units) q4–6h. CHILDREN 1 YR AND OLDER: Initially, 50–100 units/kg, then 50–100 units q4h.
IV INFUSION: ADULTS, ELDERLY: Loading dose: 80 units/kg, then 18 units/kg/hr, with adjustments based on aPTT. Range: 10–30 units/kg/hr. CHILDREN 1 YR AND OLDER: Loading dose: 75 units/kg, then 20 units/kg/hr with adjustments based on aPTT. CHILDREN YOUNGER THAN 1 YR: Loading dose: 75 units/kg, then 28 units/kg/hr.

PREVENTION OF VENOUS THROMBOSIS, PULMONARY EMBOLISM, PERIPHERAL ARTERIAL EMBOLISM, ATRIAL FIBRILLATION WITH EMBOLISM

SUBCUTANEOUS: ADULT, ELDERLY: 5,000 units q8–12h.

SIDE EFFECTS

OCCASIONAL: Itching, burning (particularly on soles of feet) caused by

vasospastic reaction. **RARE:** Pain, cyanosis of extremity 6–10 days after initial therapy lasting 4–6 hr; hypersensitivity reaction, including chills, fever, pruritus, urticaria, asthma, rhinitis, lacrimation, and headache.

ADVERSE REACTIONS/ TOXIC EFFECTS

Bleeding complications ranging from local ecchymoses to major hemorrhage occur more frequently in high-dose therapy, intermittent IV infusion, and in women 60 yr of age and older. Antidote: Protamine sulfate 1–1.5 mg, IV, for every 100 units heparin subcutaneous within 30 min of overdose, 0.5–0.75 mg for every 100 units heparin subcutaneous if within 30–60 min of overdose, 0.25–0.375 mg for every 100 units heparin subcutaneous if 2 hr have elapsed since overdose, 25–50 mg if heparin was given by IV infusion.

NURSING CONSIDERATIONS

BASELINE ASSESSMENT

Cross-check dose with co-worker. Determine aPTT before administration and 24 hr following initiation of therapy, then q24–48h for first week of therapy or until maintenance dose is established. Follow with aPTT determinations 1–2 times weekly for 3–4 wk. In long-term therapy, monitor 1–2 times a mo.

INTERVENTION/EVALUATION

Monitor aPTT (therapeutic dosage at 1.5–2.5 times normal) diligently. Assess Hct, platelet count, AST, ALT, urine and stool for occult blood, regardless of route of administration. Assess for decrease in BP, increase in pulse rate, complaint of abdominal/back pain, severe headache (may be evidence of hemorrhage). Question for increase in amount of discharge during menses. Assess peripheral pulses; skin for ecchymosis, petechiae. Check for excessive bleeding from minor cuts, scratches. Assess gums for erythema, gingival bleeding. Assess urine output for hematuria. Avoid IM injections of other medications due to potential for hematomas. When converting to Coumadin therapy, monitor PT results (will be 10%–20% higher while heparin is given concurrently).

PATIENT/FAMILY TEACHING

• Use electric razor, soft toothbrush to prevent bleeding. • Report any sign of red or dark urine, black or red stool, coffee-ground vomitus, blood-tinged mucus from cough. • Do not use any OTC medication without physician approval (may interfere with platelet aggregation). • Wear or carry identification that notes anticoagulant therapy. • Inform dentist, other physicians of heparin therapy.

Hepsera, *see adefovir*

Herceptin, *see*
trastuzumab

---

hetastarch

het-ah-starch
(Hespan, Hextend)

•CLASSIFICATION
CLINICAL: Plasma volume expander.

ACTION

A plasma volume expander that exerts osmotic pull on tissue fluids. **Therapeutic Effect:** Reduces hemoconcentration and blood viscosity; increases circulating blood volume.

PHARMACOKINETICS

Smaller molecules, less than 50,000 molecular weight, rapidly excreted by kidneys; larger molecules, 50,000 molecular weight and greater, slowly degraded to smaller-sized molecules, then excreted. **Half-life:** 17 days.

USES

Fluid replacement, plasma volume expansion in treatment of shock due to hemorrhage, burns, surgery, sepsis, trauma, leukapheresis.

PRECAUTIONS

CONTRAINDICATIONS: Anuria, oliguria, severe bleeding disorders, severe CHF. **CAUTIONS:** Thrombocytopenia, elderly or very young, pulmonary edema, CHF, renal impairment, hepatic disease, those on sodium restriction.

⏳ **LIFESPAN CONSIDERATIONS: Pregnancy/Lactation:** Unknown if drug crosses placenta or is distributed in breast milk. **Pregnancy Category C. Children:** Safety and efficacy not established. **Elderly:** Age-related renal impairment may require dosage adjustment.

INTERACTIONS

DRUG: None known. **HERBAL:** None known. **FOOD:** None known. **LAB VALUES:** May prolong bleeding, and clotting times, aPTT, and PT. May decrease Hct concentration.

AVAILABILITY (Rx)

INJECTION (HESPAN, HEXTEND): 6 g/ 100 ml 0.9% NaCl (500 ml infusion container).

ADMINISTRATION/HANDLING
💉 **IV**

Rate of administration • Administer only by IV infusion. • Do not add drugs or mix with other IV fluids. • In acute hemorrhagic shock, administer at rate approaching 1.2 g/kg (20 ml/kg) per

---

hour. Use slower rates for burns, septic shock. • Monitor central venous pressure (CVP) when given by rapid infusion. If there is a precipitous rise in CVP, immediately discontinue drug (overexpansion of blood volume).

Storage • Store solutions at room temperature. • Solution should appear clear, pale yellow to amber. Do not use if discolored (deep turbid brown) or if precipitate forms.

▨ IV INCOMPATIBILITIES

Amikacin (Amikin), ampicillin (Polycillin), cefazolin (Ancef, Kefzol), cefotaxime (Claforan), cefoxitin (Mefoxin), gentamicin (Garamycin), ranitidine (Zantac), tobramycin (Nebcin).

INDICATIONS/ROUTES/DOSAGE

PLASMA VOLUME EXPANDER

IV: ADULTS, ELDERLY: 500–1,000 ml (30–60 g) per dose. **Maximum total daily dose:** 1.2 g/kg or 1,500 ml (90 g). CHILDREN: 10 ml/kg/dose. **Maximum total daily dose:** 20 ml/kg.

LEUKAPHERESIS

IV: ADULTS, ELDERLY: 250–700 ml infused at a constant rate, usually 1:8 to venous whole blood.

SIDE EFFECTS

RARE: Allergic reaction resulting in vomiting, mild temperature elevation, chills, itching, submaxillary and parotid gland enlargement, peripheral edema of lower extremities, mild flu-like symptoms, headache, muscle aches.

ADVERSE REACTIONS/ TOXIC EFFECTS

Fluid overload may occur marked by increased BP and distended neck veins. Neurologic changes that may occur include headache, weakness, blurred vision, behavioral changes, incoordination, and isolated muscle twitching. Pulmonary edema may also occur, manifested by rapid breathing, crackles, wheezing, and coughing. Anaphylactic reaction, including periorbital edema, urticaria, and wheezing, may occur.

NURSING CONSIDERATIONS

INTERVENTION/EVALUATION

Monitor for fluid overload (peripheral and/or pulmonary edema, impending CHF symptoms). Assess lung sounds for wheezing, rales. During leukapheresis, monitor leukocyte and platelet counts, Hgb, Hct, PT, PTT, I&O. Monitor central venous BP (detects overexpansion of blood volume). Monitor urine output closely (increase in output generally occurs in oliguric patients following administration). Assess for periorbital edema, itching, wheezing, urticaria (allergic reaction). Monitor for oliguria, anuria, any change in output ratio. Monitor for bleeding from surgical/trauma sites.

Hivid, *see zalcitabine*

Humalog, *see insulin*

Humalog Mix 75 and 25 Pen, *see insulin*

Humira, *see adalimumab*

Humulin 70 and 30, *see insulin*

Humulin N, *see insulin*

Humulin R, *see insulin*

Hycamtin, *see topotecan*

*hydrALAZINE hydrochloride

hye-**dral**-a-zeen
(Apresoline, Novohylazin ✤)
Do not confuse hydralazine with hydroxyzine.

FIXED-COMBINATION(S)

Apresazide: hydralazine/hydrochlorothiazide (a diuretic): 25 mg/25 mg; 50 mg/50 mg; 100 mg/50 mg. **BiDil:** hydralazine/isosorbide (a nitrate): 37.5 mg/20 mg.

CLASSIFICATION

PHARMACOTHERAPEUTIC: Vasodilator. **CLINICAL:** Antihypertensive (see p. 55C).

ACTION

An antihypertensive with direct vasodilating effects on arterioles. **Therapeutic Effect:** Decreases BP and systemic resistance.

PHARMACOKINETICS

Route	Onset	Peak	Duration
PO	20–30 min	N/A	2–4 hr
IV	5–20 min	N/A	2–6 hr

Well absorbed from the GI tract. Widely distributed. Protein binding: 85%–90%. Metabolized in the liver to active metabolite. Primarily excreted in urine. Not removed by hemodialysis. **Half-life:** 3–7 hr (increased with impaired renal function).

USES

Management of moderate or severe hypertension. **OFF-LABEL:** Treatment of CHF, hypertension secondary to eclampsia and preeclampsia, primary pulmonary hypertension.

PRECAUTIONS

CONTRAINDICATIONS: Coronary artery disease, lupus erythematosus, rheumatic heart disease. **CAUTIONS:** Renal impairment, cerebrovascular disease.

⧗ **LIFESPAN CONSIDERATIONS: Pregnancy/Lactation:** Drug crosses placenta. Unknown if drug is distributed in breast milk. Thrombocytopenia, leukopenia, petechial bleeding, hematomas have occurred in newborns (resolved within 1–3 wk). **Pregnancy Category C. Children:** No age-related precautions noted. **Elderly:** More sensitive to hypotensive effects. Age-related renal impairment may require dosage adjustment.

INTERACTIONS

DRUG: Diuretics, other antihypertensives: May increase hypotensive effect. **HERBAL:** None known. **FOOD:** None known. **LAB VALUES:** May produce positive direct Coombs' test.

AVAILABILITY (Rx)

TABLETS: 10 mg, 25 mg, 50 mg, 100 mg. **INJECTION:** 20 mg/ml.

ADMINISTRATION/HANDLING

🏺 **IV**

Rate of administration • May give undiluted. • Give single dose over 1 min.

Storage • Store at room temperature.

PO
• Best given with food or regularly spaced meals. • Tablets may be crushed.

▦ IV INCOMPATIBILITIES

Aminophylline, ampicillin (Polycillin), furosemide (Lasix).

IV COMPATIBILITIES

Dobutamine (Dobutrex), heparin, hydrocortisone (Solu-Cortef), nitroglycerin, potassium.

INDICATIONS/ROUTES/DOSAGE

MODERATE TO SEVERE HYPERTENSION
PO: ADULTS: Initially, 10 mg 4 times a day. May increase by 10–25 mg/dose q2–5 days. **Maximum:** 300 mg/day. ELDERLY: Initially, 10 mg 2–3 times a day. May increase by 10–25 mg q2–3days. CHILDREN: Initially, 0.75–1 mg/kg/day in 2–4 divided doses, not to exceed 25 mg/dose. May increase over 3–4 wk. **Maximum:** 7.5 mg/kg/day (5 mg/kg/day in infants). **Maximum daily dose:** 200 mg.

IV, IM: ADULTS, ELDERLY: Initially, 10–20 mg/dose q4–6h. May increase to 40 mg/ dose. CHILDREN: Initially, 0.1–0.2 mg/kg/dose (**maximum:** 20 mg) q4–6h, as needed, up to 1.7–3.5 mg/kg/day in divided doses q4–6h.

DOSAGE IN RENAL IMPAIRMENT
Dosage interval is based on creatinine clearance.

Creatinine Clearance	Dosage Interval
10–50 ml/min	q8h
Less than 10 ml/min	q8–24h

SIDE EFFECTS

FREQUENT: Headache, palpitations, tachycardia (generally disappears in 7–10 days). **OCCASIONAL:** GI disturbance (nausea, vomiting, diarrhea), paraesthesia, fluid retention, peripheral edema, dizziness, flushed face, nasal congestion.

ADVERSE REACTIONS/ TOXIC EFFECTS

High dosage may produce lupus erythematosus–like reaction, including fever, facial rash, muscle and joint aches, and splenomegaly. Severe orthostatic hypotension, skin flushing, severe headache, myocardial ischemia, and cardiac arrhythmias may develop. Profound shock may occur with severe overdosage.

BASELINE ASSESSMENT
Obtain BP, pulse immediately before each dose, in addition to regular monitoring (be alert to fluctuations).

INTERVENTION/EVALUATION
Monitor for headache, palpitations, tachycardia. Assess for peripheral edema of hands, feet. Monitor pattern of daily bowel activity and stool consistency.

PATIENT/FAMILY TEACHING
• To reduce hypotensive effect, rise slowly from lying to sitting position, permit legs to dangle from bed momentarily before standing. • Unsalted crackers, dry toast may relieve nausea. • If taking high-dose therapy, report muscle/ joint aches, fever (lupus-like reaction).

hydro- chlorothiazide

high-drow-chlor-oh-**thigh**-ah-zide (Apo-Hydro ♣, Aquazide H, Esidrix, HydroDIURIL, Microzide, Oretic)

FIXED-COMBINATION(S)

Accuretic: hydrochlorothiazide/quinapril (an angiontensin-converting

---

enzyme [ACE] inhibitor): 12.5 mg/10 mg; 12.5 mg/20 mg; 25 mg/20 mg. **Aldactazide:** hydrochlorothiazide/spironolactone (a potassium-sparing diuretic): 25 mg/25 mg; 50 mg/50 mg. **Aldoril:** hydrochlorothiazide/methyldopa (an antihypertensive): 15 mg/250 mg; 25 mg/250 mg; 30 mg/500 mg; 50 mg/500 mg. **Apresazide:** hydrochlorothiazide/hydralazine (a vasodilator): 25 mg/25 mg; 50 mg/50 mg; 50 mg/100 mg. **Atacand HCT:** hydrochlorothiazide/candesartan (an angiotensin II receptor antagonist): 12.5 mg/16 mg; 12.5 mg/32 mg. **Avalide:** hydrochlorothiazide/irbesartan (an angiotensin II receptor antagonist): 12.5 mg/150 mg; 12.5 mg/300 mg; 25 mg/300 mg. **Benicar HCT:** hydrochlorothiazide/olmesartan (an angiotensin II receptor antagonist): 12.5 mg/20 mg; 12.5 mg/40 mg; 25 mg/40 mg. **Capozide:** hydrochlorothiazide/captopril (an ACE inhibitor): 15 mg/25 mg; 15 mg/50 mg; 25 mg/25 mg; 25 mg/50 mg. **Diovan HCT:** hydrochlorothiazide/valsartan (an angiotensin II receptor antagonist): 12.5 mg/80 mg; 12.5 mg/160 mg. **Dyazide/Maxide:** hydrochlorothiazide/triamterene (a potassium-sparing diuretic): 25 mg/37.5 mg; 25 mg/50 mg; 50 mg/75 mg. **Hyzaar:** hydrochlorothiazide/losartan (an angiotensin II receptor antagonist): 12.5 mg/50 mg; 12.5 mg/100 mg; 25 mg/100 mg. **Inderide:** hydrochlorothiazide/propranolol (a beta-blocker): 25 mg/40 mg; 25 mg/80 mg; 50 mg/80 mg; 50 mg/120 mg; 50 mg/160 mg. **Lopressor HCT:** hydrochlorothiazide/metoprolol (a beta-blocker): 25 mg/50 mg; 25 mg/100 mg; 50 mg/100 mg. **Lotensin HCT:** hydrochlorothiazide/bepridil (a calcium channel blocker): 6.25 mg/5 mg; 12.5 mg/10 mg; 12.5 mg/20 mg; 25 mg/20 mg. **Micardis HCT:**

hydrochlorothiazide/telmisartan (an angiotensin II receptor antagonist): 12.5 mg/40 mg; 12.5 mg/80 mg. **Moduretic:** hydrochlorothiazide/amiloride (a potassium-sparing diuretic): 50 mg/5 mg. **Normozide:** hydrochlorothiazide/labetalol (a beta-blocker): 25 mg/100 mg; 25 mg/300 mg. **Prinzide/Zestoretic:** hydrochlorothiazide/lisinopril (an ACE inhibitor): 12.5 mg/10 mg; 12.5 mg/20 mg; 25 mg/20 mg. **Teveten HCT:** hydrochlorothiazide/eprosartan (an angiotensin II receptor antagonist): 12.5 mg/600 mg; 25 mg/600 mg. **Timolide:** hydrochlorothiazide/timolol (a beta-blocker): 25 mg/10 mg. **Uniretic:** hydrochlorothiazide/moexipril (an ACE inhibitor): 12.5 mg/7.5 mg; 25 mg/15 mg. **Vaseretic:** hydrochlorothiazide/enalapril (an ACE inhibitor): 12.5 mg/5 mg; 25 mg/10 mg. **Ziac:** hydrochlorothiazide/bisoprolol (a beta-blocker): 6.25 mg/5 mg; 6.25 mg/10 mg.

CLASSIFICATION

PHARMACOTHERAPEUTIC: Sulfonamide derivative. **CLINICAL:** Thiazide diuretic, antihypertensive (see p. 88C).

ACTION

A sulfonamide derivative that acts as a thiazide diuretic and antihypertensive. As a diuretic blocks reabsorption of water, sodium, and potassium at the cortical diluting segment of the distal tubule. As an antihypertensive reduces plasma, extracellular fluid volume, and peripheral vascular resistance by direct effect on blood vessels. **Therapeutic Effect:** Promotes diuresis; reduces BP.

PHARMACOKINETICS

Route	Onset	Peak	Duration
PO (diuretic)	2 hr	4–6 hr	6–12 hr

Variably absorbed from the GI tract. Primarily excreted unchanged in urine. Not removed by hemodialysis. **Half-life:** 5.6–14.8 hr.

USES

Treatment of mild to moderate hypertension, edema in CHF, nephrotic syndrome. **OFF-LABEL:** Treatment of diabetes insipidus, prevention of calcium-containing renal calculi.

PRECAUTIONS

CONTRAINDICATIONS: Anuria, history of hypersensitivity to sulfonamides or thiazide diuretics, renal decompensation. **CAUTIONS:** Severe renal disease, hepatic impairment, diabetes mellitus, elderly or debilitated, thyroid disorders.

⌛ **LIFESPAN CONSIDERATIONS:** Pregnancy/Lactation: Crosses placenta. Small amount distributed in breast milk; breast-feeding not advised. **Pregnancy Category B (D if used in pregnancy-induced hypertension). Children:** No age-related precautions noted, except jaundiced infants may be at risk for hyperbilirubinemia. **Elderly:** May be more sensitive to hypotensive, electrolyte effects. Age-related renal impairment may require dosage adjustment.

INTERACTIONS

DRUG: **Cholestyramine, colestipol:** May decrease the absorption and effects of hydrochlorothiazide. **Digoxin:** May increase the risk of digoxin toxicity. associated with hydrochlorothiazide-induced hypokalemia. **Lithium:** May increase the risk of lithium toxicity. **HERBAL:** None known. **FOOD:** None known. **LAB VALUES:** May increase blood glucose and serum cholesterol, LDL, bilirubin, calcium, creatinine, uric acid, and triglyceride levels. May decrease urinary calcium, and serum magnesium, potassium, and sodium levels.

AVAILABILITY (Rx)

CAPSULES (MICROZIDE): 12.5 mg. **ORAL SOLUTION:** 50 mg/5 ml. **TABLETS (AQUAZIDE, ORETIC):** 25 mg, 50 mg, 100 mg.

ADMINISTRATION/HANDLING

PO

• May give with food or milk if GI upset occurs, preferably with breakfast (may prevent nocturia).

INDICATIONS/ROUTES/DOSAGE

EDEMA

PO: ADULTS, ELDERLY: 25–100 mg/day as a single or in divided doses. CHILDREN 2–12 YR: 1–2 mg/kg. **Maximum:** 100 mg/day. INFANTS YOUNGER THAN 2 YR: 1–2 mg/kg. **Maximum:** 37.5 mg/day.

HYPERTENSION

PO: ADULTS, ELDERLY: Initially, 12.5–25 mg once daily. May increase up to 50–100 mg/day as a single or in divided doses. CHILDREN 2–12 YR: 1–2 mg/kg. **Maximum:** 100 mg/day. INFANTS YOUNGER THAN 2 YR: 1–2 mg/kg. **Maximum:** 37.5 mg/day.

SIDE EFFECTS

EXPECTED: Increase in urinary frequency and urine volume. **FREQUENT:** Potassium depletion. **OCCASIONAL:** Orthostatic hypotension, headache, GI disturbances, photosensitivity.

ADVERSE REACTIONS/ TOXIC EFFECTS

Vigorous diuresis may lead to profound water and electrolyte depletion, resulting in hypokalemia, hyponatremia, and dehydration. Acute hypotensive episodes may occur. Hyperglycemia may occur during prolonged therapy. Pancreatitis, blood dyscrasias, pulmonary edema, allergic pneumonitis, and dermatologic reactions occur rarely. Overdose can lead to lethargy and coma without changes in electrolytes or hydration.

NURSING CONSIDERATIONS

BASELINE ASSESSMENT

Check vital signs, especially BP for hypotension before administration. Assess baseline electrolytes; particularly check for hypokalemia. Evaluate skin turgor, mucous membranes for hydration status. Evaluate for peripheral edema. Assess muscle strength, mental status. Note skin temperature, moisture. Obtain baseline weight. Initiate I&O.

INTERVENTION/EVALUATION

Continue to monitor BP, vital signs, electrolytes, I&O, daily weight. Note extent of diuresis. Watch for changes from initial assessment (hypokalemia may result in weakness, tremor, muscle cramps, nausea, vomiting, altered mental status, tachycardia; hyponatremia may result in confusion, thirst, cold and clammy skin). Be especially alert for potassium depletion in patients taking digoxin (cardiac arrhythmias). Potassium supplements are frequently ordered. Check for constipation (may occur with exercise diuresis).

PATIENT/FAMILY TEACHING

• Expect increased frequency and volume of urination. • To reduce hypotensive effect, rise slowly from lying to sitting position, permit legs to dangle momentarily before standing. • Eat foods high in potassium, such as whole grains (cereals), legumes, meat, bananas, apricots, orange juice, potatoes (white, sweet), raisins. • Protect skin from sun and ultraviolet rays (photosensitivity may occur).

hydrocodone bitartrate 🏳

high-drough-**koe**-doan
(Hycodan ❋, Robidone ❋)

FIXED-COMBINATION(S)

Anexsia: hydrocodone/acetaminophen (a non-narcotic analgesic): 5 mg/500 mg; 7.5 mg/650 mg; 10 mg/650 mg. **Duocet:** hydrocodone/acetaminophen: 5 mg/500 mg. **Hycet:** hydrocodone/acetaminophen: 7.5 mg/325 mg per 15 ml. **Hycodan:** hydrocodone/homatropine (an anticholinergic): 5 mg/1.5 mg. **Hycotuss, Vitussin:** hydrocodone/guaifenesin (an expectorant): 5 mg/100 mg. **Lorcet:** hydrocodone/acetaminophen: 7.5 mg/650 mg; 10 mg/650 mg. **Lortab Elixer:** hydrocodone/acetaminophen: 2.5 mg/167 mg per 5 ml. **Lortab with ASA:** hydrocodone/aspirin: 5 mg/500 mg. **Lortab:** hydrocodone/acetaminophen: 2.5 mg/500 mg; 5 mg/500 mg; 7.5 mg/500 mg; 10 mg/500 mg. **Norco:** hydrocodone/acetaminophen: 10 mg/325 mg. **Reprexain CIII:** hydrocodone/ibuprofen (an NSAID): 5 mg/200 mg. **Tussend:** hydrocodone/pseudoephedrine (a sympathomimetic)/guaifenesin (an expectorant): 2.5 mg/30 mg/100 mg per 5 ml. **Vicodin ES:** hydrocodone/acetaminophen: 7.5 mg/750 mg. **Vicodin HP:** hydrocodone/acetaminophen: 10 mg/650 mg. **Vicodin:** hydrocodone/acetaminophen: 5 mg/500 mg. **Vicoprofen:** hydrocodone/ibuprofen (an NSAID): 7.5 mg/200 mg. **Zydone:** hydrocodone/acetaminophen: 5 mg/400 mg; 7.5 mg/400 mg; 10 mg/400 mg.

◆CLASSIFICATION

PHARMACOTHERAPEUTIC: Opioid agonist (**Schedule III**). **CLINICAL:** Narcotic analgesic, antitussive (see p. 128C).

ACTION

A narcotic analgesic and antitussive that binds with opioid receptors in the

H

CNS. Therapeutic Effect: Alters the perception of and emotional response to pain; suppresses cough reflex.

PHARMACOKINETICS

Route	Onset	Peak	Duration
PO (analgesic)	10–20 min	30–60 min	4–6 hr
PO (antitussive)	N/A	N/A	4–6 hr

Well absorbed from the GI tract. Metabolized in the liver. Primarily excreted in urine. Half-life: 3.8 hr (increased in elderly).

USES

Relief of moderate to moderately severe pain, nonproductive cough.

PRECAUTIONS

CONTRAINDICATIONS: None known. **EXTREME CAUTION:** CNS depression, anoxia, hypercapnia, respiratory depression, seizures, acute alcoholism, shock, untreated myxedema, respiratory dysfunction. **CAUTIONS:** Increased intracranial pressure (ICP), hepatic impairment, acute abdominal conditions, hypothyroidism, prostatic hypertrophy, Addison's disease, urethral stricture, chronic obstructive pulmonary disease (COPD).

LIFESPAN CONSIDERATIONS: Pregnancy/Lactation: Readily crosses placenta. Distributed in breast milk. May prolong labor if administered in latent phase of first stage of labor, or before cervical dilation of 4–5 cm has occurred. Respiratory depression may occur in neonate if mother received opiates during labor. Regular use of opiates during pregnancy may produce withdrawal symptoms (irritability, excessive crying, tremors, hyperactive reflexes, fever, vomiting, diarrhea, yawning, sneezing, seizures) in the neonate. **Pregnancy Category C (D if used for prolonged periods or at high dosages at term). Children:** Those younger than 2 yr may be more susceptible to respiratory depression. **Elderly:** May be more susceptible to respiration depression, may cause paradoxical excitement. Age-related renal impairment, prostatic hypertrophy or obstruction may increase risk of urinary retention; dosage adjustment recommended.

INTERACTIONS

DRUG: Alcohol, other CNS depressants: May increase CNS or respiratory depression and hypotension. **MAOIs:** May produce a severe, sometimes fatal reaction; plan to administer ¼ of usual hydrocodone dose. **HERBAL:** None known. **FOOD:** None known. **LAB VALUES:** May increase serum amylase and lipase levels.

ADMINISTRATION/HANDLING

PO
• Give without regard to meals. • Tablets may be crushed.

INDICATIONS/ROUTES/DOSAGE

ANALGESIA
PO: ADULTS, CHILDREN OLDER THAN 12 YR: 5–15 mg q4–6h. ELDERLY: 2.5–10 mg q4–6h.

COUGH
PO: ADULTS, ELDERLY: 5–10 mg q4–6h as needed. **Maximum:** 15 mg/dose. CHILDREN: 0.6 mg/kg/day in 3–4 divided doses at intervals of at least 4 hr. **Maximum single dose:** 10 mg (children older than 12 yr), 5 mg (children 2–12 yr), 1.25 mg (children younger than 2 yr).
PO (EXTENDED-RELEASE): ADULTS: 10 mg q12h. CHILDREN 6–12 YR: 5 mg q12h.

SIDE EFFECTS

FREQUENT: Sedation, hypotension, diaphoresis, facial flushing, dizziness, somnolence. **OCCASIONAL:** Urine retention, blurred vision, constipation, dry mouth, headache, nausea, vomiting, difficult or painful urination, euphoria, dysphoria.

ADVERSE REACTIONS/ TOXIC EFFECTS

Overdose results in respiratory depression, skeletal muscle flaccidity, cold or clammy skin, cyanosis, and extreme somnolence progressing to seizures, stupor, and coma. The patient who uses hydrocodone repeatedly may develop a tolerance to the drug's analgesic effect as well as physical dependence. The drug may have a prolonged duration of action and cumulative effect in patients with hepatic or renal impairment.

NURSING CONSIDERATIONS

BASELINE ASSESSMENT

Obtain vital signs before giving medication. If respirations are 12/min or less (20/min or less in children), withhold medication, contact physician. **Analgesic:** Assess onset, type, location, duration of pain. Effect of medication is reduced if full pain recurs before next dose. **Antitussive:** Assess type, severity, frequency of cough.

INTERVENTION/EVALUATION

Palpate bladder for urinary retention. Monitor pattern of daily bowel activity and stool consistency. Initiate deep breathing and coughing exercises, particularly in patients with pulmonary impairment. Assess for clinical improvement; record onset of relief of pain or cough.

PATIENT/FAMILY TEACHING

• Change positions slowly to avoid orthostatic hypotension. • Avoid tasks that require alertness, motor skills until response to drug is established. • Tolerance or dependence may occur with prolonged use at high dosages. • Avoid alcohol. • Report nausea, vomiting, constipation, shortness of breath, difficulty breathing. • May take with food.

hydrocortisone

hye-dro-**kor**-ti-sone

(Acticort 100, Aeroseb-HC, A-HydroCort, Ala-Cort, Ala-Scalp HP, Anucort-HC, Anumed-HC, Anusol-HC, Anutone-HC, Caldecort, Cetacort, Colocort, Cortane, Cortaid, Cort-Dome High Potency, Cortef, Cortenema, Cortifoam, Cortizone-5, Cortizone-10, Emo-Cort ✤, Emcort, Gly-Cort, Hemorrhoidal HC, Hemril-30, Hemril-HC Uniserts, Hydrocortone, Hydrocortone Phosphate, Hytone, Instacort 10, Lacticare-HC, Locoid, Locoid Lipocream, Nupercainal Hydrocortisone Cream, Nutracort, Orabase HCA, Pandel, Penecort, Preparation H Hydrocortisone, Protocort, Proctocream-HC, Procto-Kit 1%, Procto-Kit 2.5%, Proctosert HC, Proctosol-HC, Proctozone HC, Rectasol-HC, Rederm, Scalp-Aid, Solu-Cortef, Texacort, WestCort).

FIXED-COMBINATION(S)

Cortisporin: hydrocortisone/neomycin/polymyxin (anti-infective): 5 mg/10,000 units/5 mg; 10 mg/10,000 units/5 mg.

♦CLASSIFICATION

PHARMACOTHERAPEUTIC: Adrenal corticosteroid. **CLINICAL:** Glucocorticoid (see pp. 83C, 87C).

ACTION

An adrenocortical steroid that inhibits accumulation of inflammatory cells at inflammation sites, phagocytosis, lysosomal enzyme release and synthesis and release of mediators of inflammation. **Therapeutic Effect:** Prevents or suppresses cell-mediated immune reactions. Decreases or prevents tissue response to inflammatory process.

PHARMACOKINETICS

Route	Onset	Peak	Duration
IV	N/A	4–6 hr	8–12 hr

Well absorbed after IM administration. Widely distributed. Metabolized in the liver. **Half-life:** Plasma, 1.5–2 hr; biologic, 8–12 hr.

USES

Management of adrenocortical insufficiency; relief of inflammation of corticosteroid-responsive dermatoses; adjunctive treatment of ulcerative colitis, status asthmaticus, shock.

PRECAUTIONS

CONTRAINDICATIONS: Fungal, tuberculosis, or viral skin lesions; serious infections. **CAUTIONS:** Hyperthyroidism, cirrhosis, ulcerative colitis, hypertension, osteoporosis, thromboembolic tendencies, CHF, seizure disorders, thrombophlebitis, peptic ulcer, diabetes.

⧗ **LIFESPAN CONSIDERATIONS: Pregnancy/Lactation:** Crosses placenta, distributed in breast milk. May produce left palate if used chronically during first trimester. Breast-feeding contraindicated. **Pregnancy Category C (D if used in first trimester). Children:** Prolonged treatment or high dosages may decrease short-term growth rate, cortisol secretion. **Elderly:** May be more susceptible to developing hypertension or osteoporosis.

INTERACTIONS

DRUG: Amphotericin: May increase hypokalemia. **Bupropion:** May lower the seizure threshold. **Digoxin:** May increase the risk of digoxin toxicity caused by hypokalemia. **Diuretics, insulin, oral hypoglycemics, potassium supplements:** May decrease the effects of these drugs. **Hepatic enzyme inducers:** May decrease the effects of

hydrocortisone. **Live virus vaccines:** May decrease the patient's antibody response to vaccine, increase vaccine side effects, and potentiate virus replication. **HERBAL:** None known. **FOOD:** None known. **LAB VALUES:** May increase blood glucose and serum lipid, amylase, and sodium levels. May decrease serum calcium, potassium, and thyroxine levels.

AVAILABILITY (Rx)

TABLETS (CORTEF): 5 mg, 10 mg, 20 mg. **ORAL SUSPENSION, CYPIONATE (CORTEF):** 10 mg/5 ml. **CREAM (RECTAL):** 1% (Nupercainal Hydrocortisone Cream, Cortizone-10, Preparation H Hydrocortisone, Proctocort, Procto-Kit 1%), 2.5% (Anusol-HC, Hemorrhoidal HC, Procto-Kit 2.5%, Proctosol-HC, Proctozone-HC). **CREAM, BUTYRATE (TOPICAL [LOCOID, LOCOID LIPOCREAM]):** 0.1%. **CREAM, PROBUTATE (TOPICAL [PANDEL]):** 0.1%. **CREAM, VALERATE (TOPICAL [WESTCORT]):** 0.2%. **CREAM (TOPICAL):** 0.5% (Cortizone-5 [OTC]), 1% (Ala-Cort, Caldecort, Cortizone-10, Hycort, Hytone, Penecort [OTC]), 2.5% (Hytone, Proctocream-HC). **FOAM (RECTAL [CORTIFOAM]):** 10%. **GEL (TOPICAL [INSTACORT 10]):** 1%. **LOTION:** 0.5% (Cetacort [OTC]), 1% (Ala-Cort, Cetacort, Cortone, Lacticare-HC, Nutracort [OTC]), 2.5% (Hytone, Lacticare-HC, Nutracort). **OINTMENT, BUTYRATE (TOPICAL [LOCOID]):** 0.1%. **OINTMENT, VALERATE (TOPICAL [WESTCORT]):** 0.2%. **OINTMENT (TOPICAL):** 0.5% (Cortizone-5 [OTC]), 1% (Anusol-HC, Cortaid, Cortizone-10, Hydrocortisone 1%, Hytone [OTC]), 2.5% (Hytone). **PASTE (TOPICAL [ORABASE HCA]):** 0.5%. **SOLUTION (TOPICAL):** 1% (Acticort 100, Gly-Cort, Penecort, Rederm, Scalp-Aid, Texacort), 2.5% (Texacort). **SOLUTION, BUTYRATE (TOPICAL [LOCOID]):** 0.1%. **SPRAY (TOPICAL [AEROSEB-HC]):** 0.5%. **SUPPOSITORIES:** 25 mg (Anucort-HC,

---

Anumed-HC, Anusol-HC, Anutone-HC, Cort-Dome High Potency, Hemorrhoidal HC, Hemril-HC, Proctosol-HC, Rectasol-HC), 30 mg (Emcort, Hemril-30, Protocort, Proctosert HC). **SUPPOSITORIES (RECTAL [COLOCORT, CORTENEMA]):** 100 mg/60 ml. **INJECTION (A-HYDRO-CORT, SOLU-CORTEF):** 100 mg, 250 mg, 500 mg, 1 g. **INJECTABLE SOLUTION, SODIUM PHOSPHATE (HYDROCORTONE PHOSPHATE):** 50 mg/ml. **INJECTABLE SUSPENSION, ACETATE:** 25 mg/ml, 50 mg/ml.

ADMINISTRATION/HANDLING

 IV

HYDROCORTISONE SODIUM SUCCINATE

• After reconstitution, use solution within 72 hr. Use immediately if further diluted with D_5W, 0.9% NaCl, or other compatible diluent. • Once reconstituted, solution is stable for 72 hr at room temperature.

Reconstitution • May further dilute with D_5W or 0.9% NaCl. For IV push, dilute to 50 mg/ml; for intermittent infusion, dilute to 1 mg/ml.

Rate of administration • Administer IV push over 3–5 min. Give intermittent infusion over 20–30 min.

Storage • Store at room temperature.

PO

• Give with food if GI distress occurs.

RECTAL

• Shake homogeneous suspension well.
• Instruct patient to lie on left side with left leg extended, right leg flexed.
• Gently insert applicator tip into rectum, pointed slightly toward navel (umbilicus). Slowly instill medication.

TOPICAL

• Gently cleanse area before application.
• Use occlusive dressings only as ordered. • Apply sparingly and rub into area thoroughly.

⚙ IV INCOMPATIBILITIES

Ciprofloxacin (Cipro), diazepam (Valium), idarubicin (Idamycin), midazolam (Versed), phenytoin (Dilantin).

IV COMPATIBILITIES

Aminophylline, amphotericin, calcium gluconate, cefepime (Maxipime), digoxin (Lanoxin), diltiazem (Cardizem), diphenhydramine (Benadryl), dopamine (Intropin), insulin, lidocaine, lorazepam (Ativan), magnesium sulfate, morphine, norepinephrine (Levophed), procainamide (Pronestyl), potassium chloride, propofol (Diprivan).

INDICATIONS/ROUTES/DOSAGE

ACUTE ADRENAL INSUFFICIENCY

IV: ADULTS, ELDERLY: 100 mg IV bolus; then 300 mg/day in divided doses q8h. CHILDREN: 1–2 mg/kg IV bolus; then 150–250 mg/day in divided doses q6–8h. INFANTS: 1–2 mg/kg/dose IV bolus; then 25–150 mg/day in divided doses q6–8h.

ANTI-INFLAMMATION, IMMUNOSUPPRESSION

IV, IM: ADULTS, ELDERLY: 15–240 mg q12h. CHILDREN: 1–5 mg/kg/day in divided doses q12h.
PO: ADULTS, ELDERLY: 15–240 mg q12h. CHILDREN: 2.5–10 mg/kg/day.

PHYSIOLOGIC REPLACEMENT

PO: CHILDREN: 0.5–0.75 mg/kg/day in divided doses q8h.
IM: CHILDREN: 0.25–0.35 mg/kg/day as a single dose.

STATUS ASTHMATICUS

IV: ADULTS, ELDERLY: 100–500 mg q6h. CHILDREN: 2 mg/kg/dose q6h.

SHOCK

IV: ADULTS, ELDERLY, CHILDREN 12 YR AND OLDER: 500 mg–2 g q2–6h. CHILDREN YOUNGER THAN 12 YR: 50 mg/kg. May repeat in 4 hr, then q24h as needed.

H

ADJUNCTIVE TREATMENT OF ULCERATIVE COLITIS

RECTAL: ADULTS, ELDERLY: 100 mg at bedtime for 21 nights or until clinical and proctologic remission occurs (may require 2–3 mo of therapy).

RECTAL (CORTIFOAM): ADULTS, ELDERLY: 1 applicator 1–2 times a day for 2–3 wk, then every second day until therapy ends.

TOPICAL: ADULTS, ELDERLY: Apply sparingly 2–4 times a day.

SIDE EFFECTS

FREQUENT: Insomnia, heartburn, nervousness, abdominal distention, diaphoresis, acne, mood swings, increased appetite, facial flushing, delayed wound healing, increased susceptibility to infection, diarrhea or constipation. **OCCASIONAL:** Headache, edema, change in skin color, frequent urination. **Topical:** Itching, redness, irritation. **RARE:** Tachycardia, allergic reaction (such as rash and hives), psychological changes, hallucinations, depression. **Topical:** Allergic contact dermatitis, purpura. **Systemic:** Absorption more likely with use of occlusive dressings or extensive application in young children.

ADVERSE REACTIONS/ TOXIC EFFECTS

Long-term therapy may cause hypocalcemia, hypokalemia, muscle wasting (especially in arms and legs), osteoporosis, spontaneous fractures, amenorrhea, cataracts, glaucoma, peptic ulcer disease, and CHF. Abruptly withdrawing the drug after long-term therapy may cause anorexia, nausea, fever, headache, sudden severe joint pain, rebound inflammation, fatigue, weakness, lethargy, dizziness, and orthostatic hypotension.

NURSING CONSIDERATIONS

BASELINE ASSESSMENT

Obtain baseline values for weight, BP, blood glucose, serum cholesterol, electrolytes. Check results of initial tests (e.g., tuberculosis [TB] skin test, x-rays, EKG).

INTERVENTION/EVALUATION

Assess for edema. Be alert to infection (reduced immune response): sore throat, fever, vague symptoms. Monitor pattern of bowel activity and stool consistency. Monitor electrolytes. Watch for hypocalcemia (muscle twitching, cramps), hypokalemia (weakness, numbness or tingling [especially lower extremities], nausea/vomiting, irritability, EKG changes). Assess emotional status, ability to sleep.

PATIENT/FAMILY TEACHING

• Notify physician of fever, sore throat, muscle aches, sudden weight gain or swelling. • Do not take aspirin or any other medication without consulting physician. • Limit caffeine, avoid alcohol. • Inform dentist, physicians of cortisone therapy now or within past 12 mo. • Caution against overuse of joints injected for symptomatic relief. • **Topical:** Apply after shower or bath for best absorption. • Do not cover unless physician orders; do not use tight diapers, plastic pants, coverings. • Avoid contact with eyes.

Hydrodiuril, see
hydrochlorothiazide

hydromorphone ⚑ *hydrochloride*

hye-droe-**mor**-fone

(Dilaudid, Dilaudid-5, Dilaudid HP, Hydromorph Contin ✿, Hydrostat IR)

Do not confuse with morphine or Dilantin.

❖ CLASSIFICATION

PHARMACOTHERAPEUTIC: Opioid agonist (**Schedule II**). **CLINICAL:** Narcotic analgesic, antitussive (see p. 128C).

ACTION

An opioid agonist that binds to opioid receptors in the CNS, reducing the intensity of pain stimuli from sensory nerve endings. Therapeutic Effect: Alters the perception of and emotional response to pain; suppresses cough reflex.

PHARMACOKINETICS

Route	Onset	Peak	Duration
PO	30 min	90–120 min	4 hr
IV	10–15 min	15–30 min	2–3 hr
IM	15 min	30–60 min	4–5 hr
Subcuta-neous	15 min	30–90 min	4 hr
Rectal	15–30 min	N/A	N/A

Well absorbed from the GI tract after IM administration. Widely distributed. Metabolized in the liver. Excreted in urine. Half-life: 1–3 hr.

USES

Relief of moderate to severe pain, persistent nonproductive cough.

PRECAUTIONS

CONTRAINDICATIONS: Obstetrical analgesia, respiratory depression in the absence of resuscitative equipment, status asthmaticus. **EXTREME CAUTION:** CNS depression, anoxia, hypercapnia, respiratory depression, seizures, acute alcoholism, shock, untreated myxedema, respiratory dysfunction. **CAUTIONS:** Increased intracranial pressure (ICP), hepatic impairment, acute abdominal conditions, hypothyroidism, prostatic hypertrophy, Addison's disease, urethral stricture, chronic obstructive pulmonary disease (COPD).

LIFESPAN CONSIDERATIONS: Pregnancy/Lactation: Readily crosses placenta. Unknown if distributed in breast milk. May prolong labor if administered in latent phase of first stage of labor or before cervical dilation of 4–5 cm has occurred. Respiratory depression may occur in neonate if mother receives opiates during labor. Regular use of opiates during pregnancy may produce withdrawal symptoms in the neonate (irritability, excessive crying, tremors, hyperactive reflexes, fever, vomiting, diarrhea, yawning, sneezing, seizures). **Pregnancy Category B (D if used for prolonged periods or at high dosages at term). Children:** Those younger than 2 yr may be more susceptible to respiratory depression. **Elderly:** May be more susceptible to respiratory depression, may cause paradoxical excitement. Age-related renal impairment, prostatic hypertrophy or obstruction may increase risk of urinary retention; dosage adjustment recommended.

INTERACTIONS

DRUG: Alcohol, other CNS depressants: May increase CNS or respiratory depression and hypotension. **MAOIs:** May produce a severe, sometimes fatal reaction; plan to administer ¼ of usual hydromorphone dose. **HERBAL: St. John's wort:** May increase sedation. **FOOD:** None known. **LAB VALUES:** May increase serum amylase and lipase concentrations.

AVAILABILITY (Rx)

LIQUID: 1 mg/ml (Dilaudid-5), 5 mg/5 ml (Dilaudid). **TABLETS:** 2 mg (Dilaudid, Hydrostat IR), 3 mg (Dilaudid, Hydrostat IR), 4 mg (Dilaudid), 8 mg (Dilaudid). **INJECTION:** 1 mg/ml (Dilaudid), 2 mg/ml (Dilaudid), 4 mg/ml (Dilaudid), 10 mg/ml (Dilaudid HP). **SUPPOSITORY (DILAUDID):** 3 mg.

ADMINISTRATION/HANDLING

 IV

◀ ALERT ▶ High concentration injection (10 mg/ml) should be used only in those tolerant to opiate agonists, currently receiving high doses of another opiate agonist for severe, chronic pain due to cancer.

Reconstitution • May give undiluted. • May further dilute with 5 ml sterile water for injection or 0.9% NaCl.

Rate of administration • Administer IV push very slowly (over 2–5 min). • Rapid IV increases risk of severe adverse reactions (chest wall rigidity, apnea, peripheral circulatory collapse, anaphylactoid effects, cardiac arrest).

Storage • Store at room temperature; protect from light. • Slight yellow discoloration of parenteral form does not indicate loss of potency.

IM, SUBCUTANEOUS
• Use short 25- to 30-gauge needle for subcutaneous injection. • Administer slowly; rotate injection sites. • Patients with circulatory impairment experience higher risk of overdosage because of delayed absorption of repeated administration.

PO
• Give without regard to meals. • Tablets may be crushed.

RECTAL
• Refrigerate suppositories. • Moisten suppository with cold water before inserting well up into rectum.

▓ IV INCOMPATIBILITIES
Amphotericin B complex (Abelcet, AmBisome, Amphotec), cefazolin (Ancef, Kefzol), diazepam (Valium), phenobarbital, phenytoin (Dilantin), total parenteral nutrition (TPN).

IV COMPATIBILITIES
Diltiazem (Cardizem), diphenhydramine (Benadryl), dobutamine (Dobutrex), dopamine (Intropin), fentanyl (Sublimaze), furosemide (Lasix), heparin, lorazepam (Ativan), magnesium sulfate, metoclopramide (Reglan), midazolam (Versed), milrinone (Primacor), morphine, propofol (Diprivan).

INDICATIONS/ROUTES/DOSAGE
ANALGESIA
PO: ADULTS, ELDERLY, CHILDREN WEIGHING 50 KG AND MORE: 2–4 mg q3–4h. Range: 2–8 mg/dose. CHILDREN OLDER THAN 6 MO AND WEIGHING LESS THAN 50 KG: 0.03–0.08 mg/kg/dose q3–4h.
IV: ADULTS, ELDERLY, CHILDREN WEIGHING MORE THAN 50 KG: 0.2–0.6 mg q2–3h. CHILDREN WEIGHING 50 KG OR LESS: 0.015 mg/kg/dose q3–6h as needed.
RECTAL: ADULTS, ELDERLY: 3 mg q4–8h.
PATIENT-CONTROLLED ANALGESIA (PCA)
IV: ADULTS, ELDERLY: 0.05–0.5 mg at 5–15 min lockout. **Maximum (4-hr):** 4–6 mg.
EPIDURAL: ADULTS, ELDERLY: Bolus dose of 1–1.5 mg at rate of 0.04–0.4 mg/hr. Demand dose of 0.15 mg at 30 min lockout.
COUGH
PO: ADULTS, ELDERLY, CHILDREN OLDER THAN 12 YR: 1 mg q3–4h. CHILDREN 6–12 YR: 0.5 mg q3–4h.

SIDE EFFECTS
FREQUENT: Somnolence, dizziness, hypotension (including orthostatic hypotension), decreased appetite. **OCCASIONAL:** Confusion, diaphoresis, facial flushing, urine retention, constipation, dry mouth, nausea, vomiting, headache, pain at injection site. **RARE:** Allergic reaction, depression.

ADVERSE REACTIONS/ TOXIC EFFECTS
Overdose results in respiratory depression, skeletal muscle flaccidity, cold

or clammy skin, cyanosis, and extreme somnolence progressing to seizures, stupor, and coma. The patient who uses hydromorphone repeatedly may develop a tolerance to the drug's analgesic effect as well as physical dependence. This drug may have a prolonged duration of action and cumulative effect in patients with hepatic or renal impairment.

NURSING CONSIDERATIONS

BASELINE ASSESSMENT

Obtain vital signs before giving medication. If respirations are 12/min or less (20/min or less in children), withhold medication, contact physician. **Analgesic:** Assess onset, type, location, duration of pain. Effect of medication is reduced if full pain recurs before next dose. **Antitussive:** Assess type, severity, frequency of cough.

INTERVENTION/EVALUATION

Monitor vital signs; assess for pain relief, cough. Assess breath sounds. Increase fluid intake, environmental humidity to decrease viscosity of lung secretions. To prevent pain cycles, instruct patient to request pain medication as soon as discomfort begins. Assess pattern of daily bowel activity and stool consistency. (especially in long-term use). Initiate deep breathing and coughing exercises, particularly in patients with pulmonary impairment. Assess for clinical improvement; record onset of relief of pain or cough.

PATIENT/FAMILY TEACHING

• Avoid alcohol, tasks that require alertness/motor skills until response to drug is established. • Tolerance or dependence may occur with prolonged use at high dosages. • Change positions slowly to avoid orthostatic hypotension.

hydroxychloroquine sulfate

hye-drox-ee-**klor**-oh-kwin

(Apo-Hydroxyquine ✤, Plaquenil)

Do not confuse hydroxychloroquine with hydrocortisone or hydroxyzine.

◆CLASSIFICATION

CLINICAL: Antimalarial, antirheumatic.

ACTION

An antimalarial and antirheumatic that concentrates in parasite acid vesicles, increasing the pH of the vesicles and interfering with parasite protein synthesis. Antirheumatic action may involve suppressing formation of antigens responsible for hypersensitivity reactions. Therapeutic Effect: Inhibits parasite growth.

PHARMACOKINETICS

Variable rate of absorption. Widely distributed in body tissues (eyes, kidneys, liver, lungs). Protein binding: 45%. Partially metabolized in liver. Partially excreted in urine. Half-life: 32 days (in plasma); 50 days (in blood).

USES

Treatment of falciparum malaria (terminates acute attacks, cures nonresistant strains); suppression of acute attacks and prolongation of interval between treatment/relapse in vivax, ovale, malariae malaria. Treatment of discoid or systematic lupus erythematosus, acute and chronic rheumatoid arthritis. OFF-LABEL: Treatment of juvenile arthritis, sarcoid-associated hypercalcemia.

H

PRECAUTIONS

CONTRAINDICATIONS: Long-term therapy for children, porphyria, psoriasis, retinal or visual field changes. **CAUTIONS:** Alcoholism, hepatic disease, G6PD deficiency. Children are especially susceptible to hydroxychloroquine fatalities.

⧗ **LIFESPAN CONSIDERATIONS: Pregnancy/Lactation:** Crosses placenta; distributed in breast milk. **Pregnancy Category C. Children:** Safety and efficacy not established. **Elderly:** No age-related precautions noted.

INTERACTIONS

DRUG: Aurothioglucose: May increase risk of blood dyscrasias. **Penicillamine:** May increase blood penicillamine concentration and the risk of hematologic, renal, or severe skin reactions. **HERBAL:** None known. **FOOD:** None known. **LAB VALUES:** None known.

AVAILABILITY (Rx)

TABLETS: 200 mg (155 mg base).

ADMINISTRATION/HANDLING

◀ **ALERT** ▶ Be aware that 200 mg hydroxychloroquine equals 155 mg base. Give the drug dose with food for treatment of malaria.

INDICATIONS/ROUTES/DOSAGE

TREATMENT OF ACUTE ATTACK OF MALARIA (DOSAGE IN MG BASE)

PO

Dose	Times	Adults	Children
Initial	Day 1	620 mg	10 mg/kg
Second	6 hr later	310 mg	5 mg/kg
Third	Day 2	310 mg	5 mg/kg
Fourth	Day 3	310 mg	5 mg/kg

SUPPRESSION OF MALARIA

PO: ADULTS: 310 mg base weekly on same day each wk, beginning 2 wk before entering an endemic area and continuing for 4–6 wk after leaving the area. CHILDREN: 5 mg base/kg/wk, beginning 2 wk before entering an endemic area and continuing for 4–6 wk after leaving the area. If therapy is not begun before exposure, administer a loading dose of 10 mg base/kg in 2 equally divided doses 6 hr apart, followed by the usual dosage regimen.

RHEUMATOID ARTHRITIS

PO: ADULTS: Initially, 400–600 mg (310–465 mg base) daily for 5–10 days, gradually increased to optimum response level. Maintenance (usually within 4–12 wk): Dosage decreased by 50% and then continued at maintenance dose of 200–400 mg/day. Maximum effect may not be seen for several mo.

LUPUS ERYTHEMATOSUS

PO: ADULTS: Initially, 400 mg once or twice a day for several wk or mo. Maintenance: 200–400 mg/day.

SIDE EFFECTS

FREQUENT: Mild, transient headache; anorexia; nausea; vomiting. **OCCASIONAL:** Visual disturbances, nervousness, fatigue, pruritus (especially of palms, soles, and scalp), irritability, personality changes, diarrhea. **RARE:** Stomatitis, dermatitis, impaired hearing.

ADVERSE REACTIONS/ TOXIC EFFECTS

Ocular toxicity, especially retinopathy, may occur and may progress even after drug is discontinued. Prolonged therapy may result in peripheral neuritis, neuromyopathy, hypotension, EKG changes, agranulocytosis, aplastic anemia, thrombocytopenia, seizures,

---

and psychosis. Overdosage may result in headache, vomiting, visual disturbances, drowsiness, seizures, and hypokalemia followed by cardiovascular collapse and death.

NURSING CONSIDERATIONS

BASELINE ASSESSMENT
Evaluate CBC, liver function.

INTERVENTION/EVALUATION
Monitor, report any visual disturbances promptly. Evaluate for GI distress. Give dose with food (for malaria). Monitor liver function tests. Assess skin/buccal mucosa; inquire about pruritus. Report impaired vision/hearing immediately.

PATIENT/FAMILY TEACHING
• Continue drug for full length of treatment. • In long-term therapy, therapeutic response may not be evident for up to 6 mo. • Immediately notify physician of **any** new symptom of visual difficulties, muscular weakness, impaired hearing, tinnitus.

---

hydroxyurea

high-**drocks**-ee-your-e-ah
(Droxia, Hydrea, Mylocel)

CLASSIFICATION
PHARMACOTHERAPEUTIC: Synthetic urea analogue. **CLINICAL:** Antineoplastic (see p. 75C).

ACTION
A synthetic urea analogue that inhibits DNA synthesis without interfering with RNA synthesis or protein. Therapeutic Effect: Interferes with the normal repair process of cancer cells damaged by irradiation.

PHARMACOKINETICS
Well absorbed from GI tract. Protein binding: 75%–80%. Metabolized in liver. Excreted in urine as urea and unchanged drug. Half-life: 3–4 hr.

USES
Treatment of melanoma; resistant chronic myelocytic leukemia; recurrent, metastatic, inoperable ovarian carcinoma. Also used in combination with radiation therapy for local control of primary squamous cell carcinoma of head or neck, excluding lip. Treatment of sickle cell anemia. OFF-LABEL: Treatment of cervical carcinoma, polycythemia vera; long-term suppression of HIV infection.

PRECAUTIONS
CONTRAINDICATIONS: WBC count less than $2,500/mm^3$ or platelet count less than $100,000/mm^3$. **CAUTIONS:** Previous irradiation therapy, other cytoxic drugs, renal or hepatic impairment.

LIFESPAN CONSIDERATIONS: **Pregnancy/Lactation:** Crosses placenta; distributed in breast milk. May be harmful to fetus. **Pregnancy Category D. Children:** Safety and efficacy not established. **Elderly:** More sensitive to hydroxyurea effects; may require lower dosage.

INTERACTIONS
DRUG: **Antigout medications:** May decrease the effects of these drugs. **Bone marrow depressants:** May increase myelosuppression. **Live-virus vaccines:** May potentiate virus replication, increase vaccine side effects, and decrease the patient's antibody response to the vaccine. HERBAL: None known.

FOOD: None known. **LAB VALUES:** May increase BUN and serum creatinine and uric acid levels.

AVAILABILITY (Rx)

CAPSULES: 200 mg (Droxia), 300 mg (Droxia), 400 mg (Droxia), 500 mg (Hydrea). **TABLETS (MYLOCEL):** 1,000 mg.

ADMINISTRATION/HANDLING

◄ **ALERT** ► Hydroxyurea dosage is individualized based on the patient's clinical response, tolerance of the drug's adverse effects, and actual or ideal body weight, whichever is less. When administering this drug in combination therapy, consult specific protocols for optimum dosage and sequence of drug administration.

◄ **ALERT** ► Expect therapy to be interrupted when platelet count falls below 100,000/mm^3 or WBC count falls below 2,500/mm^3 and to resume when counts return to normal.

INDICATIONS/ROUTES/DOSAGE

MELANOMA; RECURRENT, METASTATIC, OR INOPERABLE OVARIAN CARCINOMA

PO: ADULTS, ELDERLY: 80 mg/kg every 3 days or 20–30 mg/kg/day as a single dose.

CONTROL OF PRIMARY SQUAMOUS CELL CARCINOMA OF THE HEAD AND NECK, EXCLUDING LIPS (IN COMBINATION WITH RADIATION THERAPY)

PO: ADULTS, ELDERLY: 80 mg/kg every 3 days, beginning at least 7 days before starting radiation therapy.

RESISTANT CHRONIC MYELOCYTIC LEUKEMIA

PO: ADULTS, ELDERLY: 20–30 mg/kg once a day. CHILDREN: 10–20 mg/kg once a day.

HIV INFECTION

PO: ADULTS, ELDERLY: 500 mg twice a day with didanosine.

SICKLE CELL ANEMIA

PO: ADULTS, ELDERLY, CHILDREN: Initially, 15 mg/kg once a day. May increase by 5 mg/kg/day. **Maximum:** 35 mg/kg/day.

SIDE EFFECTS

FREQUENT: Nausea, vomiting, anorexia, constipation or diarrhea. **OCCASIONAL:** Mild, reversible rash; facial flushing; pruritus; fever; chills; malaise. **RARE:** Alopecia, headache, drowsiness, dizziness, disorientation.

ADVERSE REACTIONS/ TOXIC EFFECTS

Myelosuppression may cause hematologic toxicity (manifested as leukopenia and, to a lesser extent, thrombocytopenia and anemia).

NURSING CONSIDERATIONS

BASELINE ASSESSMENT

Obtain bone marrow studies, liver and renal function tests before therapy begins, periodically thereafter. Obtain Hgb, WBC, platelet count, serum uric acid at baseline, and weekly during therapy. Those with marked renal impairment may develop visual or auditory hallucinations, marked hematologic toxicity.

INTERVENTION/EVALUATION

Assess pattern of daily bowel activity and stool consistency. Monitor for hematologic toxicity (fever, sore throat, signs of local infection, unusual bleeding or bruising from any site), symptoms of anemia (excessive fatigue, weakness). Assess skin for rash, erythema. Monitor CBC with differential, platelet count, Hgb, renal and hepatic function, uric acid.

✐ see color pill atlas　　　✒ herb　　　underlined – top prescribed drug

PATIENT/FAMILY TEACHING

• Promptly report fever, sore throat, signs of local infection, unusual bleeding or bruising from any site.

*hydrOXYzine

high-**drox**-ih-zeen

(Apo-Hydroxyzine ♣, Atarax, Hyzine, Novohydroxyzin ♣, Vistacort, Vistaject-50, Vistaril, Vistaril IM)

Do not confuse hydroxyzine with hydralazine or hydroxyurea.

◆CLASSIFICATION

PHARMACOTHERAPEUTIC: Piperazine derivative. **CLINICAL:** Antihistamine, antianxiety, antispasmodic, antiemetic, antipruritic (see pp. 12C, 50C).

ACTION

A piperazine derivative that competes with histamine for receptor sites in the GI tract, blood vessels, and respiratory tract. May exert CNS depressant activity in subcortical areas. Diminishes vestibular stimulation and depresses labyrinthine function. **Therapeutic Effect:** Produces anxiolytic, anticholinergic, antihistaminic, and analgesic effects; relaxes skeletal muscle; controls nausea and vomiting.

PHARMACOKINETICS

Route	Onset	Peak	Duration
PO	15–30 min	N/A	4–6 hr

Well absorbed from the GI tract and after parenteral administration. Metabolized in the liver. Primarily excreted in urine. Not removed by hemodialysis.

Half-life: 20–25 hr (increased in the elderly).

PRECAUTIONS

CONTRAINDICATIONS: None known. **CAUTIONS:** Narrow-angle glaucoma, prostatic hypertrophy, bladder neck obstruction, asthma, COPD.

⧖ **LIFESPAN CONSIDERATIONS: Pregnancy/Lactation:** Unknown if drug crosses placenta or is distributed in breast milk. **Pregnancy Category C. Children:** Not recommended in newborns or premature infants (increased risk of anticholinergic effects). Paradoxical excitement may occur. **Elderly:** Increased risk of dizziness, sedation, confusion. Hypotension, hyperexcitability may occur.

INTERACTIONS

DRUG: Alcohol, other CNS depressants: May increase CNS depressant effects. **MAOIs:** May increase anticholinergic and CNS depressant effects. **HERBAL:** None known. **FOOD:** None known. **LAB VALUES:** May cause false-positive urine 17-hydroxycorticosteroid determinations.

AVAILABILITY (Rx)

CAPSULES (VISTARIL): 25 mg, 50 mg, 100 mg. **ORAL SUSPENSION (VISTARIL):** 25 mg/5 ml. **SYRUP (ATARAX):** 10 mg/5 ml. **TABLETS (ATARAX):** 110 mg, 25 mg, 50 mg, 100 mg. **INJECTION (HYZINE, VISTACORT, VISTAJECT-50, VISTARIL IM):** 25 mg/ml, 50 mg/ml.

ADMINISTRATION/HANDLING

IM

◄ **ALERT** ► Significant tissue damage, thrombosis, gangrene may occur if injection is given subcutaneous, intra-arterial, or by IV.

• IM may be given undiluted. • Use Z-track technique of injection to prevent

H

subcutaneous infiltration. • Inject deep IM into gluteus maximus or midlateral thigh in adults, midlateral thigh in children.

PO

• Shake oral suspension well. • Scored tablets may be crushed; do not crush or break capsule.

INDICATIONS/ROUTES/DOSAGE

ANXIETY
PO: ADULTS, ELDERLY: 25–100 mg 4 times a day. **Maximum:** 600 mg/day.

NAUSEA AND VOMITING
IM: ADULTS, ELDERLY: 25–100 mg/dose q4–6h.

PRURITUS
PO: ADULTS, ELDERLY: 25 mg 3–4 times a day.

PREOPERATIVE SEDATION
PO: ADULTS, ELDERLY: 50–100 mg.
IM: ADULTS, ELDERLY: 25–100 mg.

USUAL PEDIATRIC DOSAGE
PO: CHILDREN: 2 mg/kg/day in divided doses q6–8h.
IM: CHILDREN: 0.5–1 mg/kg/dose q4–6h.

SIDE EFFECTS

Side effects are generally mild and transient. **FREQUENT:** Somnolence, dry mouth, marked discomfort with IM injection. **OCCASIONAL:** Dizziness, ataxia, asthenia, slurred speech, headache, agitation, increased anxiety. **RARE:** Paradoxical CNS reactions, such as hyperactivity or nervousness in children and excitement or restlessness in elderly or debilitated patients (generally noted during first 2 wk of therapy, particularly in presence of uncontrolled pain).

ADVERSE REACTIONS/ TOXIC EFFECTS

A hypersensitivity reaction, including wheezing, dyspnea, and chest tightness, may occur.

NURSING CONSIDERATIONS

BASELINE ASSESSMENT
Anxiety: Offer emotional support to anxious patient. Assess motor responses (agitation, trembling, tension), autonomic responses (cold and clammy hands, diaphoresis). **Antiemetic:** Assess for dehydration (poor skin turgor, dry mucous membranes, longitudinal furrows in tongue).

INTERVENTION/EVALUATION
For those on long-term therapy, liver and renal function tests, blood counts should be performed periodically. Monitor lung sounds for signs of hypersensitivity reaction. Monitor serum electrolytes in patients with severe vomiting. Assess for paradoxical reaction, particularly during early therapy. Assist with ambulation if drowsiness, lightheadedness occurs.

PATIENT/FAMILY TEACHING
• Marked discomfort may occur with IM injection. • Sugarless gum, sips of tepid water may relieve dry mouth. • Drowsiness usually diminishes with continued therapy. • Avoid tasks that require alertness, motor skills until response to drug is established.

hyoscyamine

hye-oh-**sye**-a-meen
(Anaspaz, A-Spas S/L, Buscopan 🍁, Cystospaz, Cystospaz-M, Donnamar, Hyosine, IV-Stat, Levbid, Levsin, Levsin S/L, Levsinex, Neosol, NuLev, Spacol, Spacol T/S, Spasdel, Symax SL, Symax SR)

Do not confuse Anaspaz with Anaprox.

FIXED COMBINATIONS

Donnatal: hyoscyamine/atropine (anticholinergic)/phenobarbital (sedative)/scopolamine (anticholinergic): 0.1037 mg/0.0194 mg/16.2 mg/0.0065 mg.

CLASSIFICATION

PHARMACOTHERAPEUTIC: Anticholinergic. **CLINICAL:** Antimuscarinic, antispasmodic.

ACTION

A GI antispasmodic and anticholinergic agent that inhibits the action of acetylcholine at postganglionic (muscarinic) receptor sites. **Therapeutic Effect:** Decreases secretions (bronchial, salivary, sweat gland) and gastric juices and reduces motility of GI and urinary tract.

PHARMACOKINETICS

Completely absorbed following PO administration. Partially hydrolyzed. Majority of hyoscyamine dose is excreted unchanged in urine. Removed by hemodialysis. **Half-life:** 3.5 hr (immediate-release); 7 hr (sustained-release).

USES

Treatment of GI tract disorders caused by spasm. Adjunct for peptic ulcer, hypermotility disorders of lower urinary tract. Infant colic.

PRECAUTIONS

CONTRAINDICATIONS: GI or GU obstruction, myasthenia gravis, narrow-angle glaucoma, paralytic ileus, severe ulcerative colitis. **CAUTIONS:** Hyperthyroidism, CHF, cardiac arrhythmias, prostatic hypertrophy, neuropathy, chronic lung disease.

⧖ **LIFESPAN CONSIDERATIONS: Pregnancy/Lactation:** Crosses placenta; distributed in breast milk. **Pregnancy Category C. Children:** Safety and efficacy not established. **Elderly:** No age-related precautions noted.

INTERACTIONS

DRUG: Antacids, Antidiarrheals: May decrease the absorption of hyoscyamine. **Ketoconazole:** May decrease the absorption of this drug. **Other Anticholinergics:** May increase the effects of hyoscyamine. **Potassium Chloride:** May increase the severity of GI lesions with the matrix formulation of potassium chloride. **HERBAL:** None known. **FOOD:** None known. **LAB VALUES:** None known.

AVAILABILITY (Rx)

TABLETS (ANASPAZ, CYSTOSPAZ, LEVSIN, SPACOL): 0.125 mg. **TABLETS (ORAL-DISINTEGRATING [NULEV]):** 0.125 mg. **TABLETS (SUBLINGUAL [LEVSIN S/L, SYMAX SL]):** 0.125 mg. **TABLETS (EXTENDED-RELEASE [LEVBID, SPACOL T/S, SYMAX SR]):** 0.375 mg. **CAPSULES (EXTENDED-RELEASE [CYSTOSPAZ-M, LEVSINEX]):** 0.375 mg. **LIQUID (HYOSINE, SPACOL):** 0.125 mg/5 ml. **ORAL DROPS (HYOSINE, LEVSIN):** 0.125 mg/ml. **ORAL SOLUTION (HYOSINE, LEVSIN):** 0.125 mg/5 ml.

ADMINISTRATION/HANDLING

PO
• Give without regard to meals.
• Tablets may be crushed, chewed.
• Extended-release capsule should be swallowed whole.

PARENTERAL
• May give undiluted.

INDICATIONS/ROUTES/DOSAGE

GI TRACT DISORDERS

PO: ADULTS, ELDERLY, CHILDREN 12 YR AND OLDER: 0.125–0.25 mg q4h as needed. Extended-release: 0.375–0.75 mg q12h. **Maximum:** 1.5 mg/day. CHILDREN 2–11 YR: 0.0625–0.125 mg q4h as needed. Extended-release: 0.375 mg q12h. **Maximum:** 0.75 mg/day.

IV, IM: ADULTS, ELDERLY, CHILDREN 12 YR AND OLDER: 0.25–0.5 mg q4h for 1–4 doses.

HYPERMOTILITY OF LOWER URINARY TRACT

PO, SUBLINGUAL: ADULTS, ELDERLY: 0.15–0.3 mg 4 times a day; or extended-release 0.375 mg q12h.

INFANT COLIC

PO: INFANTS: Individualized drops dosed q4h as needed.

SIDE EFFECTS

FREQUENT: Dry mouth (sometimes severe), decreased sweating, constipation. **OCCASIONAL:** Blurred vision; bloated feeling; urinary hesitancy; somnolence (with high dosage); headache; intolerance to light; loss of taste; nervousness; flushing; insomnia; impotence; mental confusion or excitement (particularly in the elderly and children); temporary light-headedness (with parenteral form); local irritation (with parenteral form). **RARE:** Dizziness, faintness.

ADVERSE REACTIONS/ TOXIC EFFECTS

Overdose may produce temporary paralysis of ciliary muscle; pupillary dilation; tachycardia; palpitations; hot, dry, or flushed skin; absence of bowel sounds; hyperthermia; increased respiratory rate; EKG abnormalities; nausea; vomiting; rash over face or upper trunk; CNS stimulation; and psychosis (marked by agitation, restlessness, rambling speech, visual hallucinations, paranoid behavior, and delusions, followed by depression).

NURSING CONSIDERATIONS

BASELINE ASSESSMENT

Before giving medication, instruct patient to void (reduces risk of urinary retention).

INTERVENTION/EVALUATION

Monitor patterns of daily bowel activity and stool consistency. Palpate bladder for urinary retention. Monitor changes in BP, temperature. Assess skin turgor, mucous membranes to evaluate hydration status (encourage adequate fluid intake), bowel sounds for peristalsis. Be alert for fever (increased risk of hyperthermia).

PATIENT/FAMILY TEACHING

• May cause dry mouth; maintain good oral hygiene habits (lack of saliva may increase risk of cavities). • Inform physician of rash, eye pain, difficulty in urinating, constipation. • Avoid tasks that require alertness, motor skills until response to drug is established. • Avoid hot baths, saunas.

Hyzaar, *see hydrochlorothiazide and losartan*

---

ibandronate sodium

eye-**band**-droh-nate
(Boniva)

CLASSIFICATION
PHARMACOTHERAPEUTIC: Bisphosphonate. **CLINICAL:** Calcium regulator.

ACTION
A bisphosphonate that binds to bone hydroxyapatite (part of the mineral matrix of bone) and inhibits osteoclast activity. Therapeutic Effect: Reduces rate of bone turnover and bone resorption, resulting in a net gain in bone mass.

PHARMACOKINETICS
Absorbed in the upper GI tract. Extent of absorption impaired by food or beverages (other than plain water). Rapidly binds to bone. Unabsorbed portion is eliminated in urine. Protein binding: 90%. Half-life: 10–60 hr.

USES
Treatment/prevention of osteoporosis in postmenopausal women.

PRECAUTIONS
CONTRAINDICATIONS: Hypersensitivity to other bisphosphonates, including alendronate, etidronate, pamidronate, risedronate, and tiludronate; inability to stand or sit upright for at least 60 min; severe renal impairment with creatinine clearance less than 30 ml/min; uncorrected hypocalcemia. **CAUTIONS:** GI diseases (duodenitis, dysphagia, esophagitis, gastritis, ulcers [drug may exacerbate these conditions]), mild to moderate renal impairment.

⧗ LIFESPAN CONSIDERATIONS: **Pregnancy/Lactation:** Potential for teratogenic effects. Unknown if excreted in breast milk. Do not breast-feed. **Pregnancy Category C. Children:** Safety

and efficacy not established. **Elderly:** No age-related precautions noted.

INTERACTIONS
DRUG: **Antacids containing aluminum, calcium, magnesium; vitamin D:** Decrease the absorption of ibandronate. HERBAL: None known. FOOD: **Beverages other than plain water, dietary supplements, food:** Interfere with the absorption of ibandronate. LAB VALUES: May decrease serum alkaline phosphatase level. May increase blood cholesterol level.

AVAILABILITY (Rx)
TABLETS: 2.5 mg, 150 mg. **INJECTION:** 3 mg/3 ml syringe.

ADMINISTRATION/HANDLING
PO
• Give 60 min before first food, beverage of the day, on an empty stomach with 6–8 oz plain water (not mineral water) while the patient is standing or sitting in an upright position. • Patient cannot lie down for 60 min following drug administration. • Patient should not chew or suck the tablet (potential for oropharyngeal ulceration).

 IV
• Give over 15–20 sec.

INDICATIONS/ROUTES/DOSAGE
OSTEOPOROSIS
PO: ADULTS, ELDERLY: 2.5 mg daily. Alternatively, 150 mg once monthly.
IV: ADULTS, ELDERLY: 3 mg q3mo.

SIDE EFFECTS
FREQUENT (13%–6%): Back pain; dyspepsia, including epigastric distress and heartburn; peripheral discomfort; diarrhea; headache; myalgia. **IV:** Abdominal pain, dyspepsia, constipation, nausea, diarrhea. **OCCASIONAL (4%–3%):** Dizziness, arthralgia, asthenia. **RARE (2% or less):** Vomiting, hypersensitivity reaction.

ADVERSE REACTIONS/ TOXIC EFFECTS

Upper respiratory tract infection occurs occasionally. Overdose causes hypocalcemia, hypophosphatemia, and significant GI disturbances.

NURSING CONSIDERATIONS

BASELINE ASSESSMENT

Hypocalcemia, vitamin D deficiency must be corrected before beginning therapy. Obtain laboratory baselines, especially serum electrolytes, renal function. Obtain results of bone density study.

INTERVENTION/EVALUATION

Monitor electrolytes, especially serum calcium, alkaline phosphatase levels. Monitor renal and liver function tests.

PATIENT/FAMILY TEACHING

• Instruct patient that expected benefits occur only when medication is taken with full glass (6–8 oz) of plain water, first thing in the morning and at least 60 min before first food, beverage, medication of the day. Any other beverage (mineral water, orange juice, coffee) significantly reduces absorption of medication. • Do not lie down for at least 60 min after taking medication (potentiates delivery to stomach, reduces risk of esophageal irritation). • Consider weight-bearing exercises, modify behavioral factors (e.g., cigarette smoking, alcohol consumption).

---

ibritumomab tiuxetan 🚩

ih-brit-uh-**moe**-mab tea-**ux**-eh-an (Zevalin)

◆CLASSIFICATION

PHARMACOTHERAPEUTIC: Monoclonal antibody. **CLINICAL:** Antineoplastic (see p. 75C).

ACTION

Radioimmunotherapeutic agent that combines the targeting power of monoclonal antibodies (MAbs) with the cancer-killing ability of radiation. Ibritumomab tiuxetan is an immunoconjugate resulting from a bond between the monoclonal antibody ibritumomab with the chelator tiuxetan. This conjugate tightly binds yttrium-90 (Y-90) for radioimmunotherapy of B-cell non-Hodgkin's lymphoma and indium-111 for imaging in this protocol. **Therapeutic Effect:** Targets the CD antigen (present on B cells in greater than 90% of patients with B-cell non-Hodgkin's lymphoma), inducing cellular damage via formation of free radicals in the target and neighboring cells.

PHARMACOKINETICS

Tumor uptake is greater than normal tissue in non-Hodgkin's lymphoma. Most of dose is cleared by binding to tumor. Minimally excreted in urine. **Half-life:** 27–30 hr.

USES

Treatment of non-Hodgkin's lymphoma in combination with rituxumab in patients with relapsed or refractory low-grade, follicular, or CD20-positive transformed B-cell non-Hodgkin's lymphoma.

PRECAUTIONS

CONTRAINDICATIONS: Platelet count less than 100,000 cells/mm^3, neutrophil count less than 1,500 cells/mm^3, history of failed stem cell collection. **CAUTIONS:** Prior radio/immunotherapy with the rituzimab/ibritumomab tiuxetan regimen, mild thrombocytopenia, prior external beam radiation to 25% or greater of bone marrow, breast-feeding period, pregnancy, cardiovascular disease, hypertension/hypotension, history of hypersensitivity or anaphylaxis after use of other medications.

⧗ LIFESPAN CONSIDERATIONS: Pregnancy/Lactation: Has potential to cause fetal harm. Substitute formula feedings for breast-feedings. Those with childbearing potential should use contraceptive methods during treatment and up to 12 mo after therapy. **Pregnancy Category D. Children:** Safety and efficacy not established. **Elderly:** No age-related precautions noted.

INTERACTIONS

DRUG: Any medication that interferes with platelet function, anticoagulants: Increase potential for prolonged/severe thrombocytopenia. **Bone marrow depressants:** May increase bone marrow depression. **Live virus vaccines:** May potentiate virus replication, increase vaccine side effects, decrease patient's antibody response to vaccine. **HERBAL:** None known. **FOOD:** None known. **LAB VALUES:** Severe reduction of Hgb, Hct, platelet count, WBC count.

AVAILABILITY (Rx)

INJECTION: 3.2-mg vial of ibritumomab tiuxetan. (1.6 mg/ml).

ADMINISTRATION/HANDLING

• Indium-111 ibritumomab tiuxetan and Y-90 ibritumomab tiuxetan are radiopharmaceuticals and should be used only by physicians and other professionals trained and experienced in the safe use/handling of radionuclides.

Rate of administration • Administer IV push over 10 min (see Indications/Routes/Dosage).

▨ IV INCOMPATIBILITIES

Do not mix with any medications.

INDICATIONS/ROUTES/DOSAGE

NON-HODGKIN'S LYMPHOMA

IV: ADULTS, ELDERLY: Regimen consists of two steps: STEP 1: Single infusion of 250 mg/m^2 rituximab preceding (4 hr or less) a fixed dose of 5 mCi (1.6 mg total antibody dose) of indium-111 ibritumomab administered IV push over 10 min. STEP 2: Follows step 1 by 7–9 days and consists of a second infusion of 250 mg/m^2 rituximab preceding (4 hr or less) a fixed dose of 0.4 mCi/kg of Y-90 ibritumomab administered IV push over 10 min.

◄ ALERT ▸ Reduce dosage of ibritumomab to 0.3 mCi/kg in patients whose platelet count is 100,000–149,000 cells/mm^3.

SIDE EFFECTS

FREQUENT (43%–24%): Asthenia (loss of strength, energy), nausea, chills. **OCCASIONAL (17%–10%):** Fever, abdominal pain, dyspnea, headache, vomiting, dizziness, cough, oral candidiasis. **RARE (9%–5%):** Pruritus, diarrhea, back pain, peripheral edema, anorexia, rash, flushing, arthralgia, myalgia, ecchymosis, rhinitis, constipation, insomnia.

ADVERSE REACTIONS/ TOXIC EFFECTS

Thrombocytopenia (95%), neutropenia (77%), anemia (61%) may be severe and prolonged; may be followed by infection (29%). Hypersensitivity reaction produces hypotension, bronchospasm, angioedema. Severe cutaneouos or mucocutaneous reactions.

NURSING CONSIDERATIONS

BASELINE ASSESSMENT

Pretreatment with acetaminophen and diphenhydramine before each infusion may prevent infusion-related effects. Give emotional support to patient/family. Use strict asepsis; protect patient from infection. CBC, platelet count, blood chemistries should be obtained as a baseline before beginning therapy. ANC nadir is 62 days before recovery begins.

INTERVENTION/EVALUATION

Observe for a minimum of 1 hr following administration. Increase observation time if previous infusion reaction has occurred. Diligently monitor lab values for possibly severe/prolonged thrombocytopenia, neutropenia, anemia. Monitor for hematologic toxicity (fever, sore throat, signs of local infections, unusual bleeding/ecchymosis), symptoms of anemia (excessive fatigue, weakness). Assess for GI symptoms (nausea, vomiting, abdominal pain, diarrhea).

PATIENT/FAMILY TEACHING

• Do not have immunizations without physician's approval (drug lowers body's resistance). • Avoid crowds, persons with known infections. • Report signs of infection at once (fever, flu-like symptoms). • Contact physician if nausea/vomiting continues at home. • Avoid pregnancy during therapy.

---

ibuprofen

eye-**byoo**-pro-fen
(Advil, Advil Pediatric, Apo-Ibuprofen, Children's Advil, Children's Motrin, Ibu, Ibu-4, Ibu-6, Ibu-8, Ibu-Tab, Junior Advil, Junior Strength Motrin, Motrin, Novoprofen ♥, Pediacare Fever)

FIXED-COMBINATION(S)

Children's Advil Cold: ibuprofen/pseudoephedrine (a nasal decongestant): 100 mg/15 mg per 5 ml. **Combunox:** ibuprofen/oxycodone (a narcotic analgesic): 400 mg/5 mg. **Reprexain CIII:** ibuprofen/hydrocodone: 200 mg/5 mg. **Vicoprofen:** ibuprofen/hydrocodone (a narcotic analgesic): 200 mg/7.5 mg.

CLASSIFICATION

PHARMACOTHERAPEUTIC: Nonsteroidal anti-inflammatory. **CLINICAL:** Antirheumatic, analgesic, antipyretic, antidysmenorrheal, vascular headache suppressant (see p. 116C).

ACTION

An NSAID that inhibits prostaglandin synthesis. Also produces vasodilation by acting centrally on the heat-regulating center of the hypothalamus. **Therapeutic Effect:** Produces analgesic and anti-inflammatory effects and decreases fever.

PHARMACOKINETICS

Route	Onset	Peak	Duration
PO (analgesic)	0.5 hr	N/A	4–6 hr
PO (antirheumatic)	2 days	1–2 wk	N/A

Rapidly absorbed from the GI tract. Protein binding: greater than 90%. Metabolized in the liver. Primarily excreted in urine. Not removed by hemodialysis. **Half-life:** 2–4 hr.

USES

Treatment of inflammatory diseases, rheumatoid disorders (e.g., juvenile rheumatoid arthritis), mild to moderate pain, migraine pain, fever, dysmenorrhea, gouty arthritis. **OFF-LABEL:** Treatment of psoriatic arthritis, vascular headaches.

PRECAUTIONS

CONTRAINDICATIONS: Active peptic ulcer, chronic inflammation of GI tract, GI bleeding disorders or ulceration, history of hypersensitivity to aspirin or NSAIDs. **CAUTIONS:** CHF, hypertension, renal or hepatic impairment, dehydration, GI disease (e.g., bleeding, ulcers), concurrent anticoagulant use.

⧗ **LIFESPAN CONSIDERATIONS: Pregnancy/Lactation:** Unknown if drug crosses placenta or is distributed in breast milk. Avoid use during third trimester (may adversely affect fetal cardiovascular system: premature closure of ductus arteriosus). **Pregnancy Category B (D if used in third trimester or near delivery). Children:** Safety and efficacy not established in those younger than 6 mo. **Elderly:** GI bleeding and ulceration more likely to cause serious adverse effects. Age-related renal impairment may increase risk of hepatic or renal toxicity; reduced dosage recommended.

INTERACTIONS

DRUG: **Antihypertensives, diuretics:** May decrease the effects of these drugs. **Aspirin, other salicylates:** May increase the risk of GI side effects such as bleeding. **Bone marrow depressants:** May increase the risk of hematologic reactions. **Heparin, oral anticoagulants, thrombolytics:** May increase the effects of these drugs. **Lithium:** May increase the blood concentration and risk of toxicity of lithium. **Methotrexate:** May increase the risk of methotrexate toxicity. **Probenecid:** May increase the ibuprofen blood concentration. HERBAL: **Feverfew:** May decrease the effects of feverfew. **Ginkgo biloba:** May increase the risk of bleeding. FOOD: None known. LAB VALUES: May prolong bleeding time. May alter blood glucose level. May increase BUN level, and serum creatinine, potassium, AST, and ALT levels. May decrease blood Hgb and Hct.

AVAILABILITY (Rx)

CAPLETS (ADVIL, MENADOL, MOTRIN): 200 mg. **CAPSULES (ADVIL, ADVIL MIGRAINE):** 200 mg. **GELCAPS (ADVIL, MOTRIN IB):** 200 mg. **TABLETS:** 200 mg (Advil, Motrin IB [OTC]), 400 mg (Ibu, Ibu-4, Ibu-6, Ibu-8, Ibu-Tab, Motrin), 600 mg (Ibu, Ibu-4, Ibu-6, Ibu-8, Ibu-Tab, Motrin), 800 mg (Ibu, Ibu-4, Ibu-6, Ibu-8, Ibu-Tab, Motrin). **TABLETS (CHEWABLE):** 50 mg (Children's Advil, Children-Motrin), 100 mg (Junior Advil, Junior Strength Motrin). **ORAL SUSPENSION (ADVIL, CHILDREN'S ADVIL, CHILDREN'S MOTRIN):** 100 mg/ 5 ml (OTC). **ORAL DROPS (ADVIL PEDIATRIC, INFANT ADVIL, INFANT MOTRIN, CHILDREN'S MOTRIN, PEDIACARE FEVER):** 40 mg/ml.

ADMINISTRATION/HANDLING

PO

• Do not crush or break enteric-coated form. • Give with food, milk, antacids if GI distress occurs.

INDICATIONS/ROUTES/DOSAGE

ACUTE OR CHRONIC RHEUMATOID ARTHRITIS, OSTEOARTHRITIS, MIGRAINE PAIN, GOUTY ARTHRITIS
PO: ADULTS, ELDERLY: 400–800 mg 3–4 times a day. **Maximum:** 3.2 g/day.

MILD TO MODERATE PAIN, PRIMARY DYSMENORRHEA
PO: ADULTS, ELDERLY: 200–400 mg q4–6h as needed. **Maximum:** 1.6 g/day.

FEVER, MINOR ACHES OR PAIN
PO: ADULTS, ELDERLY: 200–400 mg q4–6h. **Maximum:** 1.6 g/day. CHILDREN: 5–10 mg/kg/dose q6–8h. **Maximum:** 40 mg/kg/day. OTC: 7.5 mg/kg/dose q6–8h. **Maximum:** 30 mg/kg/day.

JUVENILE ARTHRITIS
PO: CHILDREN: 30–70 mg/kg/day in 3–4 divided doses. **Maximum:** 400 mg/day in children weighing less than 20 kg, 600 mg/day in children weighing 20–30 kg, 800 mg/day in children weighing greater than 30–40 kg.

SIDE EFFECTS

OCCASIONAL (9%–3%): Nausea with or without vomiting, dyspepsia, dizziness, rash. **RARE (less than 3%):** Diarrhea or constipation, flatulence, abdominal cramps or pain, pruritus.

ADVERSE REACTIONS/ TOXIC EFFECTS

Acute overdose may result in metabolic acidosis. Rare reactions with long-term use include peptic ulcer disease, GI bleeding, gastritis, a severe hepatic reaction (cholestasis, jaundice), nephrotoxicity (dysuria, hematuria, proteinuria, nephrotic syndrome), and a severe hypersensitivity reaction (particularly in patients with systemic lupus erythematosus or other collagen diseases).

NURSING CONSIDERATIONS

BASELINE ASSESSMENT

Assess onset, type, location, duration of pain or inflammation. Inspect appearance of affected joints for immobility, deformities, skin condition. Assess temperature.

INTERVENTION/EVALUATION

Monitor for evidence of nausea, dyspepsia. Monitor CBC, liver and renal function tests. Monitor pattern of daily bowel activity and stool consistency. Assess skin for evidence of rash. Evaluate for therapeutic response: relief of pain, stiffness, swelling; increased joint mobility; reduced joint tenderness; improved grip strength. Monitor temperature for fever.

PATIENT/FAMILY TEACHING

• Avoid aspirin, alcohol during therapy (increases risk of GI bleeding). • If GI upset occurs, take with food, milk, antacids. • Do not crush or chew enteric-coated tablet. • May cause dizziness. • Avoid tasks that require alertness, motor skills until response to drug is established.

---

idarubicin hydrochloride ⚑

eye-dah-**roo**-bi-sin

(Idamycin PFS, Zavedos)

Do not confuse idarubicin with doxorubicin, or Idamycin with Adriamycin.

◆CLASSIFICATION

PHARMACOTHERAPEUTIC: Anthracycline antibiotic. **CLINICAL:** Antineoplastic (see p. 75C).

ACTION

An anthracycline antibiotic that inhibits nucleic acid synthesis by interacting with the enzyme topoisomerase II, which promotes DNA strand supercoiling. Therapeutic Effect: Causes death of rapidly dividing cells.

PHARMACOKINETICS

Widely distributed. Protein binding: 97%. Rapidly metabolized in the liver to active metabolite. Primarily eliminated by biliary excretion. Not removed by hemodialysis. Half-life: 4–46 hr; metabolite: 8–92 hr.

USES

Treatment of acute leukemias (AML, ANLL, ALL) accelerated phase or blast phase of chronic myelogenous leukemia (CML), breast cancer. OFF-LABEL: Autologous hematopoietic stem cell transplantation (in combination with busulfan).

PRECAUTIONS

CONTRAINDICATIONS: Preexisting arrhythmias, cardiomyopathy, myelosuppression, pregnancy, severe CHF. **CAUTIONS:** Renal or hepatic impairment, concurrent radiation therapy.

🖾 LIFESPAN CONSIDERATIONS: **Pregnancy/Lactation:** If possible, avoid use during pregnancy (may be embryotoxic). Unknown if drug is distributed in breast milk (advise to discontinue breast-feeding before drug initiation). **Pregnancy Category D. Children:** Safety and efficacy not established. **Elderly:** Cardiotoxicity may be more frequent. Caution in those with inadequate bone marrow reserves. Age-related renal impairment may require dosage adjustment.

INTERACTIONS

DRUG: **Antigout medications:** May decrease the effects of these drugs. **Bone marrow depressants:** May increase myelosuppression. **Live virus vaccines:** May potentiate virus replication, increase vaccine side effects, and decrease the patient's antibody response

---

to the vaccine. **HERBAL:** None known. **FOOD:** None known. **LAB VALUES:** May increase serum alkaline phosphatase, bilirubin, uric acid, AST, and ALT levels. May cause EKG changes.

AVAILABILITY (Rx)

INJECTION (IDAMYCIN PFS): 1 mg/ml in 5 ml, 10 ml vials.

ADMINISTRATION/HANDLING

◄ **ALERT** ▶ Give by free-flowing IV infusion (**never** subcutaneous or IM). Gloves, gowns, eye goggles recommended during preparation and administration of medication. If powder or solution comes in contact with skin, wash thoroughly. Avoid small veins, swollen or edematous extremities, areas overlying joints and tendons.

 IV

Reconstitution • Reconstitute each 10-mg vial with 10 ml 0.9% NaCl (5 ml/5-mg vial) to provide a concentration of 1 mg/ml.

Rate of administration • Administer into tubing of freely running IV infusion of D_5W or 0.9% NaCl, preferably via butterfly needle, **slowly** (longer than 10–15 min). • Extravasation produces immediate pain, severe local tissue damage. Terminate infusion immediately. Apply cold compresses for 30 min immediately, then q30min 4 times a day for 3 days. Keep extremity elevated.

Storage • Reconstituted solution is stable for 72 hr (3 days) at room temperature or 168 hr (7 days) if refrigerated. • Discard unused solution.

▩ IV INCOMPATIBILITIES

Acyclovir (Zovirax), allopurinol (Aloprim), ampicillin and sulbactam (Unasyn), cefazolin (Ancef, Kefzol), cefepime (Maxipime), ceftazidime (Fortaz), clindamycin (Cleocin), dexamethasone (Decadron), furosemide (Lasix),

hydrocortisone (Solu-Cortef), lorazepam (Ativan), meperidine (Demerol), methotrexate, piperacillin and tazobactam (Zosyn), sodium bicarbonate, teniposide (Vumon), vancomycin (Vancocin), vincristine (Oncovin).

IV COMPATIBILITIES

Diphenhydramine (Benadryl), granisetron (Kytril), magnesium, potassium.

INDICATIONS/ROUTES/DOSAGE

USUAL DOSAGE (AML, BREAST CANCER, ACCELERATED PHASE OR BLAST PHASE OF CML)
IV: ADULTS: 8–12 mg/m^2/day for 3 days in combination with Ara-C. CHILDREN (SOLID TUMOR): 5 mg/m^2 once a day for 3 days. CHILDREN (LEUKEMIA): 10–12 mg/m^2 once a day for 3 days.

DOSAGE IN HEPATIC OR RENAL IMPAIRMENT
Dosage is modified based on serum creatinine or bilirubin level.

Serum Level	Dose Reduction
Serum creatinine 2 mg/dl or more	25%
Serum bilirubin greater than 2.5 mg/dl	50%
Serum bilirubin greater than 5 mg/dl	Do not give

SIDE EFFECTS

FREQUENT: Nausea, vomiting (82%); complete alopecia (scalp, axillary, pubic hair) (77%); abdominal cramping, diarrhea (73%); mucositis (50%). **OCCASIONAL:** Hyperpigmentation of nailbeds, phalangeal and dermal creases (46%); fever (36%); headache (20%). **RARE:** Conjunctivitis, neuropathy.

ADVERSE REACTIONS/ TOXIC EFFECTS

Myelosuppression may cause hematologic toxicity (manifested principally as leukopenia and, to lesser extent, anemia and thrombocytopenia), usually within 10–15 days of starting therapy. Blood counts typically return to normal levels by the third week. Cardiotoxicity (either acute, manifested as transient EKG abnormalities, or chronic, manifested as CHF) may occur.

NURSING CONSIDERATIONS

BASELINE ASSESSMENT

Determine baseline renal and liver function, CBC results. Obtain EKG before therapy. Antiemetic before and during therapy may prevent or relieve nausea, vomiting. Inform patient of high potential for alopecia.

INTERVENTION/EVALUATION

Monitor CBC with differential, platelet count, EKG, renal and liver function tests. Monitor for hematologic toxicity (fever, sore throat, signs of local infection, unusual bleeding or ecchymosis from any site), symptoms of anemia (excessive fatigue, weakness). Avoid IM injections, rectal temperatures, other trauma that may precipitate bleeding. Check infusion site frequently for extravasation (causes severe local necrosis). Assess for potentially fatal CHF (dyspnea, rales, pulmonary edema), life-threatening arrhythmias.

PATIENT/FAMILY TEACHING

• Total body alopecia is frequent but reversible. • Assist with ways to cope with hair loss. • New hair growth resumes 2–3 mo after last therapy dose and may have different color, texture. • Maintain fastidious oral hygiene. • Avoid crowds, those with infections. • Teach patient and family the early signs of bleeding or infection. • Inform physician of fever, sore throat, bleeding, bruising. • Urine may turn pink or red. • Use contraceptive measures during therapy.

ifosfamide ⚑

eye-**fos**-fah-mide
(Ifex)

◆ CLASSIFICATION

PHARMACOTHERAPEUTIC: Alkylating agent. **CLINICAL:** Antineoplastic (see p. 75C).

ACTION

An alkylating agent that inhibits DNA and RNA protein synthesis by cross-linking with DNA and RNA strands, preventing cell growth. Cell cycle-phase nonspecific. **Therapeutic Effect:** Interferes with DNA and RNA function.

PHARMACOKINETICS

Metabolized in the liver to active metabolite. Crosses the blood-brain barrier (to a limited extent). Primarily excreted in urine. Removed by hemodialysis. **Half-life:** 15 hr.

USES

Chemotherapy of germ cell testicular carcinoma (used in combination with agents that protect against hemorrhagic cystitis). **OFF-LABEL:** Head and neck, breast, cervical, small cell lung, non-small cell lung, ovarian epithelial, bladder, or endometrial carcinomas, soft tissue sarcomas, Hodgkin's, non-Hodgkin's lymphomas, neuroblastoma, osteosarcoma, germ cell ovarian tumors, Wilm's tumor.

PRECAUTIONS

CONTRAINDICATIONS: Pregnancy, severe myelosuppression. **CAUTIONS:** Renal or hepatic impairment, compromised bone marrow function.

⌛ **LIFESPAN CONSIDERATIONS: Pregnancy/Lactation:** If possible, avoid use during pregnancy, especially first trimester. May cause fetal harm. Drug is distributed in breast milk. Breast-feeding not recommended. **Pregnancy Category D. Children:** Not intended for this patient population. **Elderly:** Age-related renal impairment may require dosage adjustment.

INTERACTIONS

DRUG: Bone marrow depressants: May increase myelosuppression. **Live-virus vaccines:** May potentiate virus replication, increase vaccine side effects, and decrease the patient's antibody response to the vaccine. **HERBAL:** None known. **FOOD:** None known. **LAB VALUES:** May increase BUN and serum bilirubin, creatinine, uric acid, AST, and ALT levels.

AVAILABILITY (Rx)

POWDER FOR INJECTION (IFEX): 1 g, 3 g.

ADMINISTRATION/HANDLING

◀ **ALERT** ▶ Hemorrhagic cystitis occurs if mesna is not given concurrently. Mesna should always be given with ifosfamide.

 IV

Reconstitution • Reconstitute 1-g vial with 20 ml sterile water for injection or bacteriostatic water for injection to provide a concentration of 50 mg/ml. Shake to dissolve. • Further dilute with D₅W or 0.9% NaCl to provide concentration of 0.6–20 mg/ml.

Rate of administration • Infuse over a minimum of 30 min. • Give with at least 2,000 ml PO or IV fluid (prevents bladder toxicity). • Give with a protectant against hemorrhagic cystitis (i.e., mesna).

Storage • Store vial at room temperature. • After reconstitution with bacteriostatic water for injection, solution is stable for 1 wk at room temperature, 3 wk if refrigerated (further diluted solution is stable for 6 wk if refrigerated). • Solution prepared with other diluents should be used within 6 hr.

IV INCOMPATIBILITIES

Cefepime (Maxipime), methotrexate.

IV COMPATIBILITIES

Granisetron (Kytril), ondansetron (Zofran).

INDICATIONS/ROUTES/DOSAGE

GERM CELL TESTICULAR CARCINOMA
IV: ADULTS: 700–2,000 mg/m²/day for 5 consecutive days. Repeat q3wk or after recovery from hematologic toxicity. Administer with mesna. CHILDREN: 1,200–1,800 mg/m²/day for 3–5 days q21–28 days.

SIDE EFFECTS

FREQUENT: Alopecia (83%); nausea, vomiting (58%). **OCCASIONAL (15%–5%):** Confusion, somnolence, hallucinations, infection. **RARE (less than 5%):** Dizziness, seizures, disorientation, fever, malaise, stomatitis.

ADVERSE REACTIONS/ TOXIC EFFECTS

Hemorrhagic cystitis with hematuria and dysuria occurs frequently if a protective agent (mesna) is not used. Myelosuppression, characterized by leukopenia and, to a lesser extent, thrombocytopenia occurs frequently. Pulmonary toxicity, hepatotoxicity, nephrotoxicity, cardiotoxicity, and CNS toxicity (manifested as confusion, hallucinations, somnolence, and coma) may require discontinuation of therapy.

NURSING CONSIDERATIONS

BASELINE ASSESSMENT

Obtain urinalysis before each dose. If hematuria occurs (greater than 10 RBCs per field), therapy should be withheld until resolution occurs. Obtain WBC, platelet count, Hgb before each dose.

INTERVENTION/EVALUATION

Monitor hematologic studies, urinalysis diligently. Assess for fever, sore throat, signs of local infection, unusual bleeding or ecchymosis from any site, symptoms of anemia (excessive fatigue, weakness).

PATIENT/FAMILY TEACHING

• Alopecia is reversible, but new hair growth may have a different color or texture. • Maintain copious daily fluid intake (protects against cystitis). • Do not have immunizations without physician's approval (drug lowers body's resistance). • Avoid contact with those who have recently received live virus vaccine. • Avoid crowds, those with infections. • Report unusual bleeding or bruising, fever, chills, sore throat, joint pain, sores in mouth or on lips, yellowing skin or eyes.

iloprost

eye-low-prost
(Ventavis)

•CLASSIFICATION

PHARMACOTHERAPEUTIC: Prostaglandin. **CLINICAL:** Vasodilator.

ACTION

A prostaglandin that dilates systemic and pulmonary arterial vascular beds, alters pulmonary vascular resistance, and suppresses vascular smooth muscle proliferation. **Therapeutic Effect:** Improves symptoms and exercise tolerance in patients with pulmonary hypertension; delays deterioration of condition.

PHARMACOKINETICS

Protein binding: 60%. Metabolized in liver. Primarily excreted in urine; minimal elimination in feces. **Half-life:** 20–30 min.

USES

Treatment of pulmonary arterial hypertension in patients with NYHA class III or IV symptoms. May be used in combination with bosentan for treatment of pulmonary arterial hypertension.

PRECAUTIONS

CONTRAINDICATIONS: None known. **CAUTIONS:** Hepatic impairment, concurrent conditions or medications that may increase risk of syncope.

⧗ **LIFESPAN CONSIDERATIONS: Pregnancy/Lactation:** Unknown if drug crosses placenta or is distributed is breast milk. **Pregnancy Category C. Children:** Safety and efficacy not established. **Elderly:** No age-related precautions noted.

INTERACTIONS

DRUG: Anticoagulants, antiplatelet agents: May increased the risk of bleeding. **Antihypertensives, other vasodilators:** May increase the hypotensive effects of iloprost. **HERBAL:** None known. **FOOD:** None known. **LAB VALUES:** May increase serum alkaline phosphatase and GGT levels.

AVAILABILITY (Rx)

SOLUTION FOR ORAL INHALATION: 10 mcg/ml (2-ml ampule).

ADMINISTRATION/HANDLING

ORAL INHALATION

• For inhalation only using Prodose ADD system. • Transfer entire contents of ampule into the medication chamber. • After use, discard remainder of medicine.

INDICATIONS/ROUTES/DOSAGE

PULMONARY HYPERTENSION IN PATIENTS WITH NYHA CLASS III OR IV SYMPTOMS
ORAL INHALATION: ADULTS: Initially, 2.5 mcg/dose; if tolerated, increased to 5 mcg/dose. Administer 6–9 times a day at intervals of 2 hr or longer while patient is awake. Maintenance: 5 mcg/dose. **Maximum daily dose:** 45 mcg.

SIDE EFFECTS

FREQUENT (39%–27%): Increased cough, headache, flushing. **OCCASIONAL (13%–11%):** Flu-like symptoms, nausea, lockjaw, jaw pain, hypotension. **RARE (8%–2%):** Insomnia, syncope, palpitations, vomiting, back pain, muscle cramps.

ADVERSE REACTIONS/ TOXIC EFFECTS

Hemoptysis and pneumonia occur occasionally. CHF, renal failure, dyspnea, and chest pain occur rarely.

NURSING CONSIDERATIONS

BASELINE ASSESSMENT
Assess BP and heart rate.

INTERVENTION/EVALUATION
Monitor the patient's heartbeat and BP during therapy. Assess for signs of pulmonary venous hypertension.

PATIENT/FAMILY TEACHING
• Instruct proper administration of the medication using the supplied inhalation system. • Advise the patient to discard any remaining solution in the medication chamber after each inhalation session.

---

imatinib mesylate ▷

ih-**mah**-tin-ib
(Gleevec)

CLASSIFICATION
PHARMACOTHERAPEUTIC: Protein tyrosine kinase inhibitor. **CLINICAL:** Antineoplastic (see p. 75C).

ACTION

Inhibits Bcr-Abl tyrosine kinase, an enzyme created by the Philadelphia chromosome abnormality found in patients with chronic myeloid leukemia (CML). **Therapeutic Effect:** Suppresses tumor growth during the three stages of CML; blast crisis, accelerated phase, and chronic phase.

PHARMACOKINETICS

Well absorbed after PO administration. Binds to plasma proteins, particularly albumin. Metabolized in the liver. Eliminated mainly in the feces as metabolites. **Half-life:** 18 hr.

USES

Treatment of CML in blast crisis, accelerated phase, or in chronic phase after failure of interferon-alpha therapy. Treatment of GI stromal tumors (GIST).

PRECAUTIONS

CONTRAINDICATIONS: Pregnancy. **CAUTIONS:** Hepatic or renal impairment.

⌛ **LIFESPAN CONSIDERATIONS: Pregnancy/Lactation:** Has potential for severe teratogenic effects. Avoid breastfeeding. **Pregnancy Category D. Children:** Safety and efficacy not established. **Elderly:** Increased frequency of fluid retention.

INTERACTIONS

DRUG: Carbamazepine, dexamethasone, phenobarbital, phenytoin, rifampicin: Decrease imatinib plasma concentration. **Clarithromycin, erythromycin, itraconazole, ketoconazole:** Increase imatinib plasma concentration. **Cyclosporine, pimozide:** May alter the therapeutic effects of these drugs. **Dihydropyridine calcium channel blockers, simvastatin, triazolo-benzodiazepines:** May increase the blood concentration of these drugs. **Live virus vaccines:** May potentiate viral replication, increase vaccine side effects, and decrease the patient's antibody response to the vaccine. **Warfarin:** Reduces the effect

---

of warfarin. HERBAL: **St. John's wort:** Decreases imatinib concentration. FOOD: None known. LAB VALUES: May increase serum bilirubin AST, and ALT levels. May decrease platelet count, WBC count, and serum potassium level.

AVAILABILITY (Rx)

TABLETS: 100 mg, 400 mg. **CAPSULES:** 100 mg.

ADMINISTRATION/HANDLING

PO
- Give with a meal and a large glass of water.

INDICATIONS/ROUTES/DOSAGE

CML
PO: ADULTS, ELDERLY: 400 mg/day for patients in chronic-phase CML; 600 mg/day for patients in accelerated phase or blast crisis. May increase dosage from 400 to 600 mg/day for patients in chronic phase or from 600 to 800 mg (given as 300–400 mg twice a day) for patients in accelerated phase or blast crisis in the absence of a severe drug reaction or severe neutropenia or thrombocytopenia in the following circumstances: progression of the disease, failure to achieve a satisfactory hematologic response after 3 mo or more of treatment, or loss of a previously achieved hematologic response. CHILDREN: 260 mg/m^2 a day as a single daily dose or in 2 divided doses.

GI STROMAL TUMORS
PO: ADULTS, ELDERLY: 400 or 600 mg once daily.

SIDE EFFECTS

FREQUENT (68%–24%): Nausea, diarrhea, vomiting, headache, fluid retention (periorbital, lower extremities), rash, musculoskeletal pain, muscle cramps, arthralgia. **OCCASIONAL (23%–10%):** Abdominal pain, cough, myalgia, fatigue, fever, anorexia, dyspepsia, constipation, night sweats, pruritus. **RARE (less than 10%):** Nasopharyngitis, petechiae, asthenia, epistaxis.

ADVERSE REACTIONS/TOXIC EFFECTS

Severe fluid retention (manifested as pleural effusion, pericardial effusion, pulmonary edema, and ascites) and hepatotoxicity occur rarely. Neutropenia and thrombocytopenia are expected responses to the drug. Respiratory toxicity, manifested as dyspnea and pneumonia, may occur.

NURSING CONSIDERATIONS

BASELINE ASSESSMENT

Obtain CBC weekly for first month, biweekly for second month, and periodically thereafter. Monitor liver function tests (serum transaminase, bilirubin, alkaline phosphatase) before beginning treatment and monthly thereafter.

INTERVENTION/EVALUATION

Assess periorbital area, lower extremities for early evidence of fluid retention. Monitor for unexpected rapid weight gain. Offer antiemetics to control nausea, vomiting. Monitor pattern of bowel activity and stool consistency. Monitor CBC for evidence of neutropenia, thrombocytopenia; assess liver function tests for hepatotoxicity. Duration of neutropenia or thrombocytopenia ranges from 2–4 wk.

PATIENT/FAMILY TEACHING

- Avoid crowds, those with known infection. - Avoid contact with anyone who recently received live virus vaccine; do not receive vaccinations. - Take with food and a full glass of water.

Imdur, see isosorbide

imipenem/cilastatin sodium

im-ih-**peh**-nem/sill-as-**tah**-tin
(<u>Primaxin IM</u>, <u>Primaxin IV</u>)

CLASSIFICATION

PHARMACOTHERAPEUTIC: Fixed-combination carbapenem. **CLINICAL:** Antibiotic.

ACTION

A fixed-combination carbapenem. Imipenem penetrates the bacterial cell membrane and binds to penicillin-binding proteins, inhibiting cell wall synthesis. Cilastatin competitively inhibits the enzyme dehydropeptidase, preventing renal metabolism of imipenem. Therapeutic Effect: Produces bacterial cell death.

PHARMACOKINETICS

Readily absorbed after IM administration. Protein binding: 13%–21%. Widely distributed. Metabolized in the kidneys. Primarily excreted in urine. Removed by hemodialysis. Half-life: 1 hr (increased in impaired renal function).

USES

Treatment of susceptible infections due to gram-negative, gram-positive and anaerobic organisms including respiratory tract, skin and skin-structure, gynecologic, bone or joint, intra-abdominal, complicated or uncomplicated urinary tract infections; endocarditis; polymicrobic infections; septicemia; serious nosocomial infections.

PRECAUTIONS

CONTRAINDICATIONS: IM: Severe shock or heart block, hypersensitivity to local anesthetics of the amide type. **IV:** Patients with meningitis. **CAUTIONS:** History of seizures, sensitivity to penicillins, renal impairment.

LIFESPAN CONSIDERATIONS: Pregnancy/Lactation: Crosses placenta. Distributed in cord blood, amniotic fluid, breast milk. **Pregnancy Category C. Children:** No precautions noted. **Elderly:** Age-related renal impairment may require dosage adjustment.

INTERACTIONS

DRUG: None known. **HERBAL:** None known. **FOOD:** None known. **LAB VALUES:** May increase BUN level and serum alkaline phosphatase, bilirubin, creatinine, LDH, AST and ALT levels. May decrease Hct and Hgb levels.

AVAILABILITY (Rx)

IV INJECTION (PRIMAXIN IV): 250 mg, 500 mg. **IM INJECTION (PRIMAXIN IM):** 500 mg, 750 mg.

ADMINISTRATION/HANDLING

 IV

Reconstitution • Dilute each 250- or 500-mg vial with 100 ml D_5W; 0.9% NaCl.

Rate of administration • Give by intermittent IV infusion (piggyback). Do not give IV push. • Infuse over 20–30 min (1-g dose over 40–60 min). • Observe patient during initial 30 min of first-time infusion for possible hypersensitivity reaction.

Storage • Solution appears colorless to yellow; discard if solution turns brown. • IV infusion (piggyback) is stable for 4 hr at room temperature, 24 hr if refrigerated. • Discard if precipitate forms.

IM
• Prepare with 1% lidocaine without epinephrine; 500-mg vial with 2 ml, 750-mg vial with 3 ml lidocaine HCl. • Administer suspension within 1 hr of preparation. • Do not mix with any other medications. • Inject deep in large muscle mass.

⊞ IV INCOMPATIBILITIES

Allopurinol (Aloprim), amphotericin B complex (Abelcet, AmBisome, Amphotec), fluconazole (Diflucan).

IV COMPATIBILITIES

Diltiazem (Cardizem), insulin, propofol (Diprivan), total parenteral nutrition (TPN).

INDICATIONS/ROUTES/DOSAGE

SERIOUS RESPIRATORY TRACT, SKIN AND SKIN-STRUCTURE, GYNECOLOGIC, BONE, JOINT, INTRA-ABDOMINAL, NOSOCOMIAL, AND POLYMICROBIC INFECTIONS; UTIs; ENDOCARDITIS; SEPTICEMIA

IV: ADULTS, ELDERLY: 2–4 g/day in divided doses q6h.

MILD TO MODERATE RESPIRATORY TRACT, SKIN AND SKIN-STRUCTURE, GYNECOLOGIC, BONE, JOINT, INTRA-ABDOMINAL, AND POLYMICROBIC INFECTIONS; UTIs; ENDOCARDITIS; SEPTICEMIA

IV: ADULTS, ELDERLY: 1–2 g/day in divided doses q6–8h. CHILDREN OLDER THAN 3 MO–12 YR: 60–100 mg/kg/day in divided doses q6h. **Maximum:** 4 g/day. CHILDREN 1–3 MO: 100 mg/kg/day in divided doses q6h. CHILDREN YOUNGER THAN 1 MO: 20–25 mg/kg/ dose q8–24h.

IM: ADULTS, ELDERLY: 500–750 mg q12h.

DOSAGE IN RENAL IMPAIRMENT

Dosage and frequency are modified based on creatinine clearance and the severity of the infection.

Creatinine Clearance	Dosage (IV)
31–70 ml/min	500 mg q8h
21–30 ml/min	500 mg q12h
5–20 ml/min	250 mg q12h

SIDE EFFECTS

OCCASIONAL (3%–2%): Diarrhea, nausea, vomiting. **RARE (2%–1%):** Rash.

ADVERSE REACTIONS/ TOXIC EFFECTS

Antibiotic-associated colitis and other superinfections may occur. Anaphylactic reactions have been reported.

NURSING CONSIDERATIONS

BASELINE ASSESSMENT

Question for history of allergies, particularly to beta-lactams, penicillins, cephalosporins. Inquire about history of seizures.

INTERVENTION/EVALUATION

Monitor renal, liver, hematologic function tests. Evaluate for phlebitis (heat, pain, red streaking over vein), pain at IV injection site. Assess for GI discomfort, nausea, vomiting. Determine pattern of bowel activity and stool consistency. Assess skin for rash. Be alert to tremors, possible seizures.

imipramine

ih-**mih**-prah-meen

(Apo-Imipramine ✦, Tofranil, Tofranil-PM)

Do not confuse imipramine with desipramine.

◆CLASSIFICATION

PHARMACOTHERAPEUTIC: Tricyclic. **CLINICAL:** Antidepressant, antineuritic, antipanic, antineuralgic, antinarcoleptic adjunct, anticataplectic, antibulimic (see p. 37C).

ACTION

A tricyclic antidepressant, antibulimic, anticataplectic, antinarcoleptic, antineuralgic, antineuritic, and antipanic agent that blocks the reuptake of neurotransmitters, such as norepinephrine and serotonin, at presynaptic membranes, increasing their concentration at post-synaptic receptor sites. **Therapeutic Effect:** Relieves depression and controls nocturnal enuresis.

USES

Treatment of various forms of depression, often in conjunction with psychotherapy. Treatment of nocturnal enuresis in children older than 6 yr. **OFF-LABEL:** Treatment of attention-deficit hyperactivity disorder, cataplexy associated with narcolepsy, neurogenic pain, panic disorder.

PRECAUTIONS

CONTRAINDICATIONS: Acute recovery period after MI, use within 14 days of MAOIs. **CAUTIONS:** Prostatic hypertrophy, history of urinary retention or obstruction, glaucoma, diabetes mellitus, history of seizures, hyperthyroidism, cardiac, hepatic or renal disease, schizophrenia, increased intraocular pressure, hiatal hernia. **Pregnancy Category D.**

INTERACTIONS

DRUG: Alcohol, other CNS depressants: May increase the hypotensive effects and CNS and respiratory depression caused by imipramine. **Antithyroid agents:** May increase the risk of agranulocytosis. **Cimetidine:** May increase imipramine blood concentration and risk of toxicity. **Clonidine, guanadrel:** May decrease the effects of these drugs. **MAOIs:** May increase the risk of neuroleptic malignant syndrome, hyperpyrexia, hypertensive crisis, and seizures. **Phenothiazines:** May increase the anticholinergic and sedative effects of imipramine. **Phenytoin:** May decrease the imipramine blood concentration. **Sympathomimetics:** May increase the risk of cardiac effects. **HERBAL: Ginkgo biloba:** May decrease seizure threshold. **St. John's wort:** May increase

imipramine's pharmacologic effects and risk of toxicity. **FOOD:** None known. **LAB VALUES:** May alter blood glucose levels and EKG readings. Therapeutic serum drug level is 225–300 ng/ml; toxic serum drug level is greater than 500 ng/ml.

AVAILABILITY (Rx)

TABLETS (TOFRANIL): 10 mg, 25 mg, 50 mg. **CAPSULES (TOFRANIL-PM):** 75 mg, 100 mg, 125 mg, 150 mg.

ADMINISTRATION/HANDLING

PO
• Give with food or milk if GI distress occurs. • Do not crush or break film-coated tablets.

INDICATIONS/ROUTES/DOSAGE

DEPRESSION
PO: ADULTS: Initially, 75–100 mg/day. May gradually increase to 300 mg/day then reduce dosage to effective maintenance level 50–150 mg/day. ELDERLY: Initially, 10–25 mg/day at bedtime. May increase by 10–25 mg every 3–7 days. Range: 50–150 mg/day. CHILDREN: 1.5 mg/kg/day. May increase by 1 mg/kg every 3–4 days. **Maximum:** 5 mg/kg/day.

ENURESIS
PO: CHILDREN OLDER THAN 6 YR: Initially, 10–25 mg at bedtime. May increase by 25 mg/day. **Maximum:** 50 mg for children older than 12 yr.

SIDE EFFECTS

FREQUENT: Somnolence, fatigue, dry mouth, blurred vision, constipation, delayed micturition, orthostatic hypotension, diaphoresis, impaired concentration, increased appetite, urine retention, photosensitivity. **OCCASIONAL:** GI disturbances (nausea, metallic taste). **RARE:** Paradoxical reactions, (agitation, restlessness, nightmares, insomnia), extrapyramidal symptoms (particularly fine hand tremor).

ADVERSE REACTIONS/ TOXIC EFFECTS

Overdose may produce seizures; cardio-vascular effects, such as severe ortho-static hypotension, dizziness, tachycardia, palpitations, and arrhythmias; and altered temperature regulation, including hyperpyrexia or hypothermia. Abrupt discontinuation after prolonged therapy may produce headache, malaise, nausea, vomiting, and vivid dreams.

NURSING CONSIDERATIONS

BASELINE ASSESSMENT

For patients on long-term therapy, liver and renal function tests, blood counts should be performed periodically.

INTERVENTION/EVALUATION

Supervise suicidal-risk patient closely during early therapy (as depression lessens, energy level improves, causing increased suicide potential). Assess appearance, behavior, speech pattern, level of interest, mood. Monitor pattern of daily bowel activity and stool consistency. Monitor BP, pulse for hypotension, arrhythmias. Assess for urinary retention by bladder palpation. Therapeutic serum level: 225–300 ng/ml; toxic serum level: greater than 500 ng/ml.

PATIENT/FAMILY TEACHING

• Change positions slowly to avoid hypotensive effect. • Tolerance to postural hypotension, sedative, anticholinergic effects usually develops during early therapy. • Therapeutic effect may be noted within 2–5 days, maximum effect within 2–3 wk. • Sugarless gum, sips of tepid water may relieve dry mouth. • Do not abruptly discontinue medication. • Avoid tasks that require alertness, motor skills until response to drug is established.

Imitrex, *see sumatriptan*

immune globulin IV (IGIV)

ih-**mewn glah**-byew-lin
(Carimune, Gamimune N 5%, Gamimune N 10%, Gammagard S/D, Gammar-P-IV, Gamunex, Iveegam EN, Octagam, Panglobulin, Polygam S/D, Sandoglobulin, Vivaglobin)
Do not confuse Sandoglobulin with Sandimmune or Sandostatin.

CLASSIFICATION
CLINICAL: Immune serum.

ACTION

An immune serum that increases antibody titer and antigen-antibody reaction. **Therapeutic Effect:** Provides passive immunity against infection; induces rapid increase in platelet count; produces anti-inflammatory effect.

PHARMACOKINETICS

Evenly distributed between intravascular and extravascular space. **Half-life:** 21–23 days.

USES

Treatment of patients with primary immunodeficiency syndromes, idiopathic thrombocytopenia purpura (ITP), Kawasaki disease; prevention of recurrent bacterial infections in patients with hypogammaglobulinemia associated with B-cell chronic lymphocytic leukemia (CLL). Treatment adjunct in bone marrow transplantation. **OFF-LABEL:** Control and prevention of infections in infants and children with immunosuppression due to AIDS or AIDS-related complex; prevention of acute infections in immunosuppressed patients; prevention and treatment of infections in high-risk, preterm, low-birth-weight neonates; treatment of chronic inflammatory demyelinating polyneuropathies and multiple sclerosis.

PRECAUTIONS

CONTRAINDICATIONS: Allergies to gamma globulin, thimerosal, or anti-IgA antibodies; isolated IgA deficiency. **CAUTIONS:** Cardiovascular disease, history of thrombosis, renal impairment, diabetes, volume depletion, sepsis, concomitant nephrotoxic drugs.

⌛ **LIFESPAN CONSIDERATIONS: Pregnancy/Lactation:** Unknown if drug crosses placenta or is distributed in breast milk. **Pregnancy Category C. Children/Elderly:** No age-related precautions noted.

INTERACTIONS

DRUG: Live virus vaccines: May increase vaccine side effects, potentiate virus replication, and decrease the patient's antibody response to the vaccine. **HERBAL:** None known. **FOOD:** None known. **LAB VALUES:** None known.

AVAILABILITY (Rx)

INJECTION SOLUTION: 5% (Gamimune N 5%, Octagam), 10% (Gammagard, Gamimune N 10%, Gamunex). **INJECTION POWDER FOR RECONSTITUTION:** 0.5 g (Iveegam EN), 1 g (Carimune, Gammar-P-IV, Iveegam EN, Panglobulin, Sandoglobulin), 2.5 g (Gammar-P-IV, Gammagard S/D, Iveegam EN, Polygam S/D, Sandoglobulin), 3 g (Carimune, Panglobulin, Sandoglobulin), 5 g (Gammar-P-IV, Gammagard S/D, Iveegam EN, Polygam S/D, Sandoglobulin), 6 g (Carimune, Panglobulin, Sandoglobulin), 10 g (Gammar-P-IV, Gammagard S/D, Polygam S/D, Sandoglobulin), 12 g (Carimune, Panglobulin, Sandoglobulin). **SUBCUTANEOUS FORMULATION:** (Vivaglobin) injection 160 mg/ml.

ADMINISTRATION/HANDLING

💉 IV

Reconstitution • Reconstitute only with diluent provided by manufacturer.

• Discard partially used or turbid preparations.

Rate of administration • Give by infusion only. • After reconstituted, administer via separate tubing. • Avoid mixing with other medication or IV infusion fluids. • Rate of infusion varies with product used. • Monitor vital signs, BP diligently during and immediately after IV administration (precipitous fall in BP may indicate anaphylactic reaction). Stop infusion immediately. Epinephrine should be readily available.

Storage • Refer to individual IV preparations for storage requirements, stability after reconstitution.

🔲 IV INCOMPATIBILITIES

Do not mix IGIV with any other medications.

INDICATIONS/ROUTES/DOSAGE

PRIMARY IMMUNODEFICIENCY SYNDROME

IV: ADULTS, ELDERLY, CHILDREN: 200–400 mg/kg once monthly.
SUBCUTANEOUS: ADULTS, ELDERLY: 100–200 mg/kg once weekly.

ITP

IV: ADULTS, ELDERLY, CHILDREN: 400–1,000 mg/kg/day for 2–5 days.

KAWASAKI DISEASE

IV: ADULTS, ELDERLY, CHILDREN: 2 g/kg as a single dose.

CLL

IV: ADULTS, ELDERLY, CHILDREN: 400 mg/kg q3–4wk.

BONE MARROW TRANSPLANT

IV: ADULTS, ELDERLY, CHILDREN: 400–500 mg/kg/dose every week for 12 wk, then every month.

SIDE EFFECTS

FREQUENT: Tachycardia, backache, headache, arthralgia, myalgia. **OCCASIONAL:** Fatigue, wheezing, injection site rash or pain, leg cramps, urticaria, bluish lips and nailbeds, lightheadedness.

ADVERSE REACTIONS/ TOXIC EFFECTS

Anaphylactic reactions are rare, but the incidence increases with repeated injections of IGIV. Keep epinephrine readily available. Overdose may produce chest tightness, chills, diaphoresis, dizziness, facial flushing, nausea, vomiting, fever, and hypotension. Hypersensitivity reaction, characterized by anxiety, arthralgia, dizziness, flushing, myalgia, palpitations, and pruritus, occurs rarely.

NURSING CONSIDERATIONS

BASELINE ASSESSMENT
Inquire about history of exposure to disease for both patient and family as appropriate. Have epinephrine readily available. Well hydrate patient before use.

INTERVENTION/EVALUATION
Control rate of IV infusion carefully; too-rapid infusion increases risk of precipitous fall in BP, signs of anaphylaxis (facial flushing, chest tightness, chills, fever, nausea, vomiting, diaphoresis). Assess patient closely during infusion, especially first hour; monitor vital signs continuously. Stop infusion temporarily if aforementioned signs noted. For treatment of ITP, monitor platelets.

PATIENT/FAMILY TEACHING
• Explain rationale for therapy. • Rapid response, lasts 1–3 mo. • Inform physician if sudden weight gain, fluid retention, edema, decreased urine output, shortness of breath occur.

Imodium A-D, see
loperamide

Increlex, *see mecasermin*

---

indapamide

in-**dap**-a-mide
(Lozide ✲, Lozol)
Do not confuse indapamide with iodamide or iopamidol.

◆CLASSIFICATION
PHARMACOTHERAPEUTIC: Thiazide.
CLINICAL: Diuretic, antihypertensive (see p. 88C).

ACTION
A thiazide-like diuretic that blocks reabsorption of water, sodium, and potassium at the cortical diluting segment of the distal tubule; also reduces plasma and extracellular fluid volume and peripheral vascular resistance by direct effect on blood vessels. **Therapeutic Effect:** Promotes diuresis and reduces BP.

PHARMACOKINETICS
Almost completely absorbed following PO administration. Protein binding: 71%–79%. Extensively metabolized in liver. Excreted in urine. **Half-life:** 14–15 hr.

USES
Management of hypertension. Treatment of edema associated with CHF, nephrotic syndrome.

PRECAUTIONS
CONTRAINDICATIONS: Anuria, hypersensitivity to sulfonamides. **CAUTIONS:** History of hypersensitivity to sulfonamides or thiazide diuretics, renal decompensation, anuria. Severe renal disease, hepatic impairment, diabetes mellitus, elderly or debilitated, thyroid disorders.

---

nancy/Lactation: Unknown if drug crosses placenta or is distributed in breast milk. **Pregnancy Category B (D if used in pregnancy-induced hypertension).** Children: Safety and efficacy not established. Elderly: May be more sensitive to hypotensive, electrolyte effects.

INTERACTIONS

DRUG: **Digoxin:** May increase the risk of digoxin toxicity associated with indapamide-induced hypokalemia. **Lithium:** May increase the risk of lithium toxicity. HERBAL: None known. FOOD: None known. LAB VALUES: May increase plasma renin activity. May decrease protein-bound iodine and serum calcium, potassium, and sodium levels.

AVAILABILITY (Rx)

TABLETS: 1.25 mg, 2.5 mg.

ADMINISTRATION/HANDLING

PO
• Give with food, milk if GI upset occurs, preferably with breakfast (may prevent nocturia). • Do not crush or break tablets.

INDICATIONS/ROUTES/DOSAGE

EDEMA
PO: ADULTS: Initially, 2.5 mg/day, may increase to 5 mg/day after 1 wk.

HYPERTENSION
PO: ADULTS, ELDERLY: Initially, 1.25 mg, may increase to 2.5 mg/day after 4 wk or 5 mg/day after additional 4 wk.

SIDE EFFECTS

FREQUENT (5% and greater): Fatigue, numbness of extremities, tension, irritability, agitation, headache, dizziness, light-headedness, insomnia, muscle cramps. OCCASIONAL (less than 5%): Tingling of extremities, urinary frequency, urticaria, rhinorrhea, flushing, weight loss, orthostatic hypotension, depression, blurred vision, nausea, vomiting, diarrhea or constipation, dry mouth, impotence, rash, pruritus.

ADVERSE REACTIONS/ TOXIC EFFECTS

Vigorous diuresis may lead to profound water and electrolyte depletion, resulting in hypokalemia, hyponatremia, and dehydration. Acute hypotensive episodes may occur. Hyperglycemia may occur during prolonged therapy. Pancreatitis, blood dyscrasias, pulmonary edema, allergic pneumonitis, and dermatologic reactions occur rarely. Overdose can lead to lethargy and coma without changes in electrolytes or hydration.

NURSING CONSIDERATIONS

BASELINE ASSESSMENT

Check vital signs, especially BP for hypotension, before administration. Assess baseline electrolytes, particularly check for hypokalemia. Observe for edema; assess skin turgor, mucous membranes for hydration status. Assess muscle strength, mental status. Note skin temperature, moisture. Obtain baseline weight. Initiate I&O.

INTERVENTION/EVALUATION

Continue to monitor BP, vital signs, electrolytes, I&O, weight. Note extent of diuresis. Watch for electrolyte disturbances (hypokalemia may result in weakness, tremor, muscle cramps, nausea, vomiting, altered mental status, tachycardia; hyponatremia may result in confusion, thirst, cold or clammy skin).

PATIENT/FAMILY TEACHING

• Expect increased frequency and volume of urination. • To reduce hypotensive effect, rise slowly from lying to sitting position, permit legs to dangle momentarily before standing. • Eat foods high in potassium such as whole grains (cereals), legumes, meat, bananas, apricots, orange juice, potatoes (white, sweet), raisins. • Take early in the day to avoid nocturia.

Inderal, *see propranolol*

Inderal LA, *see propranolol*

---

indinavir

in-**din**-oh-vir
(Crixivan)

Do not confuse indinavir with Denavir.

◆CLASSIFICATION

PHARMACOTHERAPEUTIC: Protease inhibitor. **CLINICAL:** Antiviral (see pp. 61C, 104C).

ACTION

A protease inhibitor that suppresses HIV protease, an enzyme necessary for splitting viral polyprotein precursors into mature and infectious viral particles. **Therapeutic Effect:** Interrupts HIV replication, slowing the progression of HIV infection.

PHARMACOKINETICS

Rapidly absorbed after PO administration. Protein binding: 60%. Metabolized in the liver. Primarily excreted in urine. Unknown if removed by hemodialysis. **Half-life:** 1.8 hr (increased in impaired hepatic function).

USES

Treatment of HIV infection as part of a multidrug regimen (at least 3 anti-retroviral agents). **OFF-LABEL:** Prophylaxis following occupational exposure to HIV.

PRECAUTIONS

CONTRAINDICATIONS: Concurrent use with terfenadine, cisapride, astemizole, triazolam, midazolam, pimozide, ergot derivatives; nephrolithiasis. **CAUTIONS:** Renal or hepatic impairment.

⧗ **LIFESPAN CONSIDERATIONS: Pregnancy/Lactation:** Unknown if excreted in breast milk. Breast-feeding not recommended in HIV-infected women. **Pregnancy Category C. Children:** Safety and efficacy not established. **Elderly:** Information not available.

INTERACTIONS

DRUG: Ergot derivatives: May increase the risk of ergotism. **Midazolam, triazolam:** Increases the risk of arrhythmias and prolonged sedation. **Pimozide:** May increase the risk of cardiotoxicity. **HERBAL: St. John's wort:** May decrease indinavir blood concentration and effect. **FOOD: Grapefruit, grapefruit juice:** May decrease indinavir blood concentration and effect. **High-fat, high-calorie, and high-protein meals:** May decrease indinavir blood concentration. **LAB VALUES:** May increase serum bilirubin (in 10% of patients), AST, and ALT levels.

AVAILABILITY (Rx)

CAPSULES: 100 mg, 200 mg, 333 mg, 400 mg.

ADMINISTRATION/HANDLING
PO
• Store at room temperature. • Protect from moisture (capsules sensitive to moisture; keep in original bottle). • Best given without food but with water only (optimal absorption) 1 hr before or 2 hr following a meal but may give with water, skim milk, juice, coffee, tea, light meal (e.g., dry toast with jelly).

• Do not give with meal high in fat, calories, protein. • If indinavir and didanosine re given concurrently, give at least 1 hr apart on an empty stomach.

INDICATIONS/ROUTES/DOSAGE

HIV INFECTION (IN COMBINATION WITH OTHER ANTIRETROVIRALS)

PO: ADULTS: 800 mg (two 400-mg capsules) q8h.
DOSAGE ADJUSTMENTS WHEN GIVEN CONCOMITANTLY: DELAVIRDINE, ITRACONAZOLE, KETOCONAZOLE: Reduce dose to 600 mg q8h. EFAVIRENZ: Increase dose to 1,000 mg q8h. LOPINAVIR/RITONAVIR: Reduce dose to 600 mg twice a day. NEVIRAPINE: Increase dose to 1,000 mg q8h. RIFABUTIN: Reduce rifabutin by ½ and increase indinavir to 1,000 mg q8h. RITONAVIR: 100–200 mg twice a day and indinavir 800 mg twice a day or ritonavir 400 mg twice a day and indinavir 400 mg twice a day.

HIV INFECTION IN PATIENTS WITH HEPATIC INSUFFICIENCY

PO: ADULTS: 600 mg q8h.

SIDE EFFECTS

FREQUENT: Nausea (12%), abdominal pain (9%), headache (6%), diarrhea (5%). **OCCASIONAL:** Vomiting, asthenia, fatigue (4%); insomnia; accumulation of fat in waist, abdomen, or back of neck. **RARE:** Abnormal taste sensation, heartburn, symptomatic urinary tract disease, transient renal dysfunction.

ADVERSE REACTIONS/ TOXIC EFFECTS

Nephrolithiasis (flank pain with or without hematuria) occurs in 4% of patients.

NURSING CONSIDERATIONS

BASELINE ASSESSMENT

Offer emotional support. Establish baseline lab values. Emphasize need for close monitoring of renal function (urinalysis, serum creatinine) during therapy.

INTERVENTION/EVALUATION

Encourage adequate hydration. Patient should drink 48 oz (1.5 L) of liquid for each 24 hr during therapy. Monitor for evidence of nephrolithiasis (flank pain, hematuria), contact physician if symptoms occur (therapy should be interrupted for 1–3 days). Monitor stool frequency and consistency. Assess for abdominal discomfort, headache. Monitor serum bilirubin, cholesterol, triglycerides, amylase, lipase, liver function tests, blood glucose, CD4 cell count, CBC.

PATIENT/FAMILY TEACHING

• Advise that indinavir is not a cure for HIV; condition may progress despite treatment. • If dose is missed, take next dose at regularly scheduled time (do **not** double the dose). • Best taken without food but water only (optimal absorption) 1 hr before or 2 hr following a meal but may take with water, skim milk, juice, coffee, tea, light carbohydrate meal. • Avoid the herb St. John's wort and grapefruits or grapefruit juice.

indomethacin

in-doe-**meth**-a-sin
(Apo-Indomethacin ✤, Indocid ✤, Indocin, Indocin-IV, Indocin-SR, Novomethacin ✤)

Do not confuse Indocin with Imodium or Vicodin.

◆ CLASSIFICATION

PHARMACOTHERAPEUTIC: Nonsteroidal anti-inflammatory. **CLINICAL:** Anti-inflammatory, analgesic (see p. 116C).

ACTION

An NSAID that produces analgesic and anti-inflammatory effects by inhibiting prostaglandin synthesis. Also increases the sensitivity of the premature ductus to the dilating effects of prostaglandins. **Therapeutic Effect:** Reduces the inflammatory response and intensity of pain. Closure of the patent ductus arteriosus.

PHARMACOKINETICS

Rectal absorption more rapid than oral administration. Protein binding: 99%. Metabolized in liver. Excreted in urine. Half-life: 4.5 hr.

USES

Treatment of active stages of rheumatoid arthritis, osteoarthritis, ankylosing spondylitis, acute gouty arthritis. Relieves acute bursitis and/or tendonitis. For closure of hemodynamically significant patent ductus arteriosus of premature infants weighing 500–1,750 g. OFF-LABEL: Treatment of fever due to malignancy, pericarditis, psoriatic arthritis, rheumatic complications associated with Paget's disease of bone, vascular headache.

PRECAUTIONS

CONTRAINDICATIONS: Active GI bleeding or ulcerations; hypersensitivity to aspirin, indomethacin, or other NSAIDs; renal impairment, thrombocytopenia. **CAUTIONS:** Cardiac dysfunction, hypertension, decreased renal or hepatic function, epilepsy, concurrent anticoagulant therapy.

☒ LIFESPAN CONSIDERATIONS: **Pregnancy/Lactation:** Crosses placenta; distributed in breast milk. **Pregnancy Category B (D if used after 34 wk gestation, close to delivery, or for longer than 48 hr). Children:** Safety and efficacy not established in those younger than 14 yr. **Elderly:** GI bleeding, ulceration increase risk of serious adverse effects.

INTERACTIONS

DRUG: **Aminoglycosides:** May increase the blood concentration of these drugs in neonates. **Antihypertensives, diuretics:** May decrease the effects of these drugs. **Aspirin, other salicylates:** May increase the risk of GI side effects such as bleeding. **Bone marrow depressants:** May increase the risk of hematologic reactions. **Heparin, oral anticoagulants, thrombolytics:** May increase the effects of these drugs. **Lithium:** May increase the blood concentration and risk of toxicity of lithium. **Methotrexate:** May increase the risk of methotrexate toxicity. **Probenecid:** May increase the indomethacin blood concentration. **Triamterene:** May potentiate acute renal failure. Don't give concurrently. HERBAL: **Feverfew:** May decrease the effects of feverfew. **Ginkgo biloba:** May increase the risk of bleeding. FOOD: None known. LAB VALUES: May prolong bleeding time. May alter blood glucose level. May increase BUN level, and serum creatinine, potassium, AST, and ALT levels. May decrease serum sodium level and platelet count.

AVAILABILITY (Rx)

CAPSULES (INDOCIN): 25 mg, 50 mg. **CAPSULES (SUSTAINED-RELEASE [INDOCIN SR]):** 75 mg. **ORAL SUSPENSION (INDOCIN):** 25 mg/5 ml. **POWDER FOR INJECTION (INDOCIN IV):** 1 mg. **SUPPOSITORIES:** 50 mg.

ADMINISTRATION/HANDLING

🖏 IV

Reconstitution • To 1-mg vial, add 1–2 ml preservative-free sterile water for injection or 0.9% NaCl to provide concentration of 1 mg or 0.5 mg/ml, respectively. • Do not further dilute.

Rate of administration • Administer over 5–10 sec. • Restrict fluid intake.

Storage • IV solutions made without preservatives should be used immediately. • Use IV immediately following reconstitution. • IV solution appears

---

clear; discard if cloudy or if precipitate form. • Discard unused portion.

PO
• Give after meals or with food or antacids. • Do not crush sustained-release capsules.

RECTAL
◄ **ALERT** ► IV injection preferred for patent ductus arteriosus in neonate (may give dose PO via NG tube or rectally).
• If suppository is too soft, chill for 30 min in refrigerator or run cold water over foil wrapper. • Moisten suppository with cold water before inserting well into rectum.

▒ IV INCOMPATIBILITIES
Amino acid injection, calcium gluconate, cimetidine (Tagamet), dobutamine (Dobutrex), dopamine (Intropin), gentamicin (Garamycin), tobramycin (Nebcin).

IV COMPATIBILITIES
Insulin, potassium.

INDICATIONS/ROUTES/DOSAGE
MODERATE TO SEVERE RHEUMATOID ARTHRITIS, OSTEOARTHRITIS, ANKYLOSING SPONDYLITIS
PO: ADULTS, ELDERLY: Initially, 25 mg 2–3 times a day; increased by 25–50 mg/wk up to 150–200 mg/day. Or 75 mg/day (extended-release) up to 75 mg twice a day. CHILDREN: 1–2 mg/kg/day. **Maximum:** 150–200 mg/day.

ACUTE GOUTY ARTHRITIS
PO: ADULTS, ELDERLY: Initially, 100 mg, then 50 mg 3 times a day.

ACUTE SHOULDER PAIN
PO: ADULTS, ELDERLY: 75–150 mg/day in 3–4 divided doses.

USUAL RECTAL DOSAGE
ADULTS, ELDERLY: 50 mg 4 times a day. CHILDREN: Initially, 1.5–2.5 mg/kg/day, increased up to 4 mg/kg/day. **Maximum:** 150–200 mg/day.

PATENT DUCTUS ARTERIOSUS
IV: NEONATES: Initially, 0.2 mg/kg. Subsequent doses are based on age, as follows: NEONATES OLDER THAN 7 DAYS: 0.25 mg/kg for 2nd and 3rd doses. NEONATES 2–7 DAYS: 0.2 mg/kg for 2nd and 3rd doses. NEONATES LESS THAN 48 HR: 0.1 mg/kg for 2nd and 3rd doses.

SIDE EFFECTS
FREQUENT (11%–3%): Headache, nausea, vomiting, dyspepsia, dizziness. **OCCASIONAL (less than 3%):** Depression, tinnitus, diaphoresis, somnolence, constipation, diarrhea, bleeding disturbances in patent ductus arteriosus. **RARE:** Hypertension, confusion, urticaria, pruritus, rash, blurred vision.

ADVERSE REACTIONS/ TOXIC EFFECTS
Paralytic ileus and ulceration of the esophagus, stomach, duodenum, or small intestine may occur. Patients with impaired renal function may develop hyperkalemia and worsening of renal impairment. Indomethacin use may aggravate epilepsy, parkinsonism, and depression or other psychiatric disturbances. Nephrotoxicity, including dysuria, hematuria, proteinuria, and nephrotic syndrome, occurs rarely. Metabolic acidosis or alkalosis, apnea, and bradycardia occur rarely in patients with patent ductus arteriosus.

NURSING CONSIDERATIONS

BASELINE ASSESSMENT
May mask signs of infection. Assess onset, type, location, duration of pain, fever, inflammation. Inspect appearance of affected joints for immobility, deformities, skin condition.

INTERVENTION/EVALUATION
Monitor for evidence of nausea, dyspepsia. Assist with ambulation if dizziness occurs. Evaluate for therapeutic response: relief of pain, stiffness, swelling;

increased joint mobility; reduced joint tenderness; improved grip strength. Monitor BUN, serum creatinine, potassium, hepatic function tests. In neonates, also monitor heart rate, heart sounds for murmur, BP, urine output, EKG, serum sodium, glucose, platelets.

PATIENT/FAMILY TEACHING

• Avoid aspirin, alcohol during therapy (increases risk of GI bleeding). • If GI upset occurs, take with food, milk. • Avoid tasks that require alertness, motor skills until response to drug is established. • Swallow capsule whole; do not crush or chew.

infliximab

in-**flicks**-ih-mab

(Remicade)

Do not confuse Remicade with Reminyl.

◆CLASSIFICATION

PHARMACOTHERAPEUTIC: Monoclonal antibody. **CLINICAL:** GI antiinflammatory.

ACTION

A monoclonal antibody that binds to tumor necrosis factor (TNF), inhibiting functional activity of TNF. Reduces infiltration of inflammatory cells. **Therapeutic Effect:** Decreases inflamed areas of the intestine.

PHARMACOKINETICS

Route	Onset	Peak	Duration
IV (Crohn's disease)	1–2 wk	N/A	8–48 wk
IV (Rheumatoid arthritis [RA])	3–7 days	N/A	6–12 wk

Absorbed into the GI tissue; primarily distributed in the vascular compartment. **Half-life:** 9.5 days.

USES

Treatment of moderate to severe Crohn's disease, treatment of patients with fistulizing Crohn's disease for reduction in number of draining enterocutaneous fistula(s), ankylosing spondylitis. First-line treatment of rheumatoid arthritis (with methotrexate). Reducing signs and symptoms, achieving clinical remission and mucosal healing, eliminating steroid use in patients with moderate to severe active ulcerative colitis. Treatment of ankylosing spondylitis, reducing signs and symptoms of active arthritis in patients with psoriatic arthritis. **OFF-LABEL:** CHF, juvenile arthritis, psoriasis, reactive arthritis, sciatica.

PRECAUTIONS

CONTRAINDICATIONS: Sensitivity to murine proteins, sepsis, serious active infection. **CAUTIONS:** History of recurrent infections.

⧗ **LIFESPAN CONSIDERATIONS: Pregnancy/Lactation:** Unknown if distributed in breast milk. **Pregnancy Category C. Children:** Safety and efficacy not established. **Elderly:** Use cautiously due to higher rate of infection.

INTERACTIONS

DRUG: Immunosuppressants: May reduce frequency of infusion reactions and antibodies to infliximab. **Live virus vaccines:** May decrease immune response. **HERBAL:** None known. **FOOD:** None known. **LAB VALUES:** None known.

AVAILABILITY (Rx)

POWDER FOR INJECTION: 100 mg.

ADMINISTRATION/HANDLING

⊡ **IV**

Reconstitution • Reconstitute each vial with 10 ml sterile water for injection, using 21-gauge or smaller needle. Direct the stream of sterile water to the glass wall of the vial. • Swirl the vial gently

to dissolve the contents. Do not shake.
• Allow the solution to stand for 5 min.
• Because infliximab is a protein, the solution may develop a few translucent particles; do not use if particles are opaque or foreign particles are present.
• Solution should appear colorless to light yellow and opalescent; do not use if discolored. • Withdraw and waste a volume of 0.9% NaCl from a 250-ml bag to equal the volume of reconstituted solution to be injected into the 250-ml bag (approximately 10 ml). Total dose to be infused should equal 250 ml.
• Slowly add the reconstituted infliximab solution to the 250-ml infusion bag. Gently mix. Infusion concentration should range between 0.4 and 4 mg/ml.
• Begin infusion within 3 hr after reconstitution.

Rate of administration • Administer IV infusion over 2 hr, using set with a low protein-binding filter.

Storage • Refrigerate vials.

░ IV INCOMPATIBILITIES
Do not infuse infliximab in the same IV line with other agents.

INDICATIONS/ROUTES/DOSAGE
CROHN'S DISEASE, MODERATE TO SEVERE, ULCERATIVE COLITIS, PSORIATIC ARTHRITIS
IV INFUSION: ADULTS, ELDERLY: Initially, 5 mg/kg at wk 0, 2, and 6. Maintenance: 5 mg/kg q8wk thereafter.

ANKYLOSING SPONDYLITIS
IV INFUSION: ADULTS, ELDERLY: Initially, 5 mg/kg at wk 0, 2, and 6. Maintenance: 5 mg/kg q6wk thereafter.

FISTULIZING CROHN'S DISEASE
IV INFUSION: ADULTS, ELDERLY: Initially, 5 mg/kg followed by additional 5-mg/kg doses at 2 and 6 wk after first infusion.

RHEUMATOID ARTHRITIS (RA)
IV INFUSION: ADULTS, ELDERLY: 3 mg/kg; followed by additional doses at 2 and 6 wk after first infusion. Then q8wk.

SIDE EFFECTS
FREQUENT (22%–10%): Headache, nausea, fatigue, fever. **OCCASIONAL (9%–5%):** Fever or chills during infusion, pharyngitis, vomiting, pain, dizziness, bronchitis, rash, rhinitis, cough, pruritus, sinusitis, myalgia, back pain. **RARE (4%–1%):** Hypotension or hypertension, paresthesia, anxiety, depression, insomnia, diarrhea, urinary tract infection.

ADVERSE REACTIONS/ TOXIC EFFECTS
Serious infections, including sepsis, occur rarely. Hypersensitivity reaction, lupus-like syndrome, and severe hepatic reactions may occur.

NURSING CONSIDERATIONS
BASELINE ASSESSMENT
Assess pattern of bowel activity and stool consistency. Check baseline hydration status: skin turgor for tenting mucous membranes, urinary status.

INTERVENTION/EVALUATION
Monitor urinalysis, erythrocyte sedimentation rate (ESR), BP. Monitor for signs of infection. **Crohn's Disease:** Monitor C-reactive protein, frequency of stools. Assess for abdominal pain. **Rheumatoid Arthritis:** Monitor C-reactive protein. Assess for decreased pain, swollen joints, stiffness.

insulin ⚑

in-sull-in
Rapid acting: INSULIN LISPRO: (Humalog), **INSULIN ASPART:** (Novolog), **INSULIN GLULISINE:** (Apidra), **INSULIN INHALED:** (Exubera), **REGULAR INSULIN:** (Humulin R, Novolin R)
Intermediate acting: NPH: (Humulin N, Novolin N, NPH Iletin II), **LENTE:** (Humulin L, Lente Iletin II, Novolin L)

Long acting: INSULIN DETEMIR: (Levemir), **INSULIN GLARGINE:** (Lantus Ultralente)

FIXED-COMBINATION(S)

Novolog Mix 70/30: aspart suspension 70% and aspart solution 30%. **Humalog Mix 75/25:** lispro suspension 75% and lispro solution 25%. **Humulin Mix 50/50:** NPH 50% and regular 50%. **Humulin 70/30, Novolin 70/30:** NPH 70% and rapid acting regular 30%.

CLASSIFICATION

PHARMACOTHERAPEUTIC: Exogenous insulin. **CLINICAL:** Antidiabetic (see p. 40C).

ACTION

An exogenous insulin that facilitates passage of glucose, potassium, and magnesium across the cellular membranes of skeletal and cardiac muscle and adipose tissue. Controls storage and metabolism of carbohydrates, protein, and fats. Promotes conversion of glucose to glycogen in the liver. **Therapeutic Effect:** Controls glucose levels in diabetic patients.

PHARMACOKINETICS

Drug Form	Onset (hr)	Peak (hr)	Duration (hr)
Glulisine	0.25	1	3–5
Lispro	0.25	0.5–1.5	4–5
Insulin aspart	1/6	1–3	3–5
Regular	0.5–1	2–4	5–7
Inhaled	0.5–1	2–4	5–7
NPH	1–2	6–14	24+
Lente	1–3	6–14	24+
Insulin glargine	N/A	N/A	24

USES

Treatment of insulin-dependent type 1 diabetes mellitus; non–insulin-dependent type 2 diabetes mellitus when diet and weight control therapy has failed to maintain satisfactory blood glucose levels or in event of pregnancy, surgery, trauma, infection, fever, severe renal, hepatic, or endocrine dysfunction. Regular insulin used for emergency treatment of ketoacidosis, to promote passage of glucose across cell membrane in hyperalimentation, to facilitate intracellular shift of potassium in hyperkalemia.

PRECAUTIONS

CONTRAINDICATIONS: Hypersensitivity or insulin resistance may require change of type or species source of insulin.

⌛ **LIFESPAN CONSIDERATIONS: Pregnancy/Lactation:** Insulin is drug of choice for diabetes in pregnancy; close medical supervision is needed. Following delivery, insulin needs may drop for 24–72 hr, then rise to pre-pregnancy levels. Not secreted in breast milk; lactation may decrease insulin requirements. **Pregnancy Category B. Children:** No age-related precautions noted. **Elderly:** Decreased vision, fine motor tremors may lead to inaccurate self-dosing.

INTERACTIONS

◀ **ALERT** ▶ Regular human insulin and digoxin are physically compatible for 3 hr in 0.9% sodium chloride. In dextrose 5% and water, a slight haze develops within 1 hr. Do not allow digoxin and insulin to come in contact with each other in an IV for over 15 min.
DRUG: Alcohol: May increase the effects of insulin. **Beta-adrenergic blockers:** May increase the risk of hyperglycemia or hypoglycemia; may mask signs and prolong periods of hypoglycemia. **Glucocorticoids, thiazide diuretics:** May increase blood glucose level. **HERBAL:** None known. **FOOD:** None known. **LAB VALUES:** May decrease serum magnesium, phosphate, and potassium concentrations.

AVAILABILITY

RAPID ACTING: Apidra, Exubera, Humulin R, Novolin R, Novolog, Humalog. **INTERMEDIATE ACTING:** Humulin L, Novolin L, Lente Iletin II, Humulin N, Novolin N, NPH IIletin II. **LONG ACTING:** Lantus Ultralente, Levemir. **INTERMEDIATE- AND SHORT-ACTING MIXTURES:** Humulin 50/50, Humulin 70/30, Humalog Mix 75/25, Humalog Mix 50/50, Novolin 70/30, Novolog Mix 70/30.

ADMINISTRATION/HANDLING

🖥 **IV (REGULAR)**

• Use only if solution is clear. • May give undiluted.

SUBCUTANEOUS

• Store currently used insulin at room temperature (avoid extreme temperatures, direct sunlight). Store extra vials in refrigerator. • Discard unused vials if not used for several weeks. • Give subcutaneously only. (Regular insulin is the **only** insulin that may be given IV, IM for ketoacidosis or in other specific situations. • Do not give cold insulin; warm to room temperature. • Rotate vial gently between hands; do not shake. Regular insulin should be clear; no insulin should have precipitate or discoloration. • Usually administered approximately 30 min before a meal (Insulin Lispro is given up to 15 min before meals). Check blood glucose concentration before administration; dosage highly individualized. • When insulin is mixed, regular insulin is always drawn up first. Mixtures must be administered at once (binding can occur within 5 min). Humalog may be mixed with Humulin N, Humulin L. • Subcutaneous injections may be given in thigh, abdomen, upper arm, buttocks, upper back if there is adequate adipose tissue. • Rotation of injection sites is essential; maintain careful record. • For home situations, prefilled syringes are stable for 1 wk if refrigerated (this includes mixtures once they have stabilized, e.g., 15 min for NPH/Regular, 24 hr for Lente/Regular). Prefilled syringes should be stored in vertical or oblique position to avoid plugging; plunger should be pulled back slightly and the syringe rocked to remix the solution before injection.

⚙ IV INCOMPATIBILITIES

Diltiazem (Cardizem), dopamine (Intropin), nafcillin (Nafcil).

IV COMPATIBILITIES

Amiodarone (Cordarone), ampicillin/sulbactam (Unasyn), cefazolin (Ancef), cimetidine (Tagamet), digoxin (Lanoxin): (physically compatible for 3 hr in 0.9% NaCl. In D₅W, water, a slight haze develops within 1 hr.), dobutamine (Dobutrex), famotidine (Pepcid), gentamicin, heparin, magnesium sulfate, metoclopramide (Reglan), midazolam (Versed), milrinone (Primacor), morphine, nitroglycerin, potassium chloride, propofol (Diprivan), vancomycin (Vancocin).

INDICATIONS/ROUTES/DOSAGE

TREATMENT OF INSULIN-DEPENDENT TYPE 1 DIABETES MELLITUS AND NON–INSULIN-DEPENDENT TYPE 2 DIABETES MELLITUS WHEN DIET OR WEIGHT CONTROL HAS FAILED TO MAINTAIN SATISFACTORY BLOOD GLUCOSE LEVELS OR IN EVENT OF FEVER, INFECTION, PREGNANCY, SURGERY, OR TRAUMA, OR SEVERE ENDOCRINE, HEPATIC OR RENAL DYSFUNCTION; EMERGENCY TREATMENT OF KETOACIDOSIS (REGULAR INSULIN); TO PROMOTE PASSAGE OF GLUCOSE ACROSS CELL MEMBRANE IN HYPERALIMENTATION (REGULAR INSULIN): TO FACILITATE INTRACELLULAR SHIFT OF POTASSIUM IN HYPERKALEMIA (REGULAR INSULIN)
SUBCUTANEOUS: ADULTS, ELDERLY, CHILDREN: 0.5–1 unit/kg/day. ADOLESCENTS (DURING GROWTH SPURT): 0.8–1.2 unit/kg/day.

INHALATION: ADULTS, ELDERLY: 0.05 mg/kg before meals.

SIDE EFFECTS

OCCASIONAL: Localized redness, swelling, and itching caused by improper injection technique or allergy to cleansing solution or insulin. **INFREQUENT:** Somogyi effect, including rebound hyperglycemia with chronically excessive insulin dosages: systemic allergic reaction, marked by rash, angioedema, and anaphylaxis; lipodystrophy or depression at injection site due to breakdown of adipose tissue; lipohypertrophy or accumulation of subcutaneous tissue at injection site due to inadequate site rotation. **RARE:** Insulin resistance.

ADVERSE REACTIONS/ TOXIC EFFECTS

Severe hypoglycemia caused by hyperinsulinism may occur with insulin overdose, decrease or delay of food intake, or excessive exercise and in those with brittle diabetes. Diabetic ketoacidosis may result from stress, illness, omission of insulin dose, or long-term poor insulin control.

NURSING CONSIDERATIONS

BASELINE ASSESSMENT

Check blood glucose level. Discuss lifestyle to determine extent of learning, emotional needs.

INTERVENTION/EVALUATION

Assess for hypoglycemia (refer to pharmacokinetics table for peak times and duration): cool, wet skin, tremors, dizziness, headache, anxiety, tachycardia, numbness in mouth, hunger, diplopia. Check sleeping patient for restlessness, diaphoresis. Check for hyperglycemia: polyuria (excessive urine output), polyphagia (excessive food intake), polydipsia (excessive thirst), nausea or vomiting, dim vision, fatigue, deep or rapid breathing (Kussmaul respirations). Be alert to conditions altering glucose requirements: fever, increased activity or stress, surgical procedure.

PATIENT/FAMILY TEACHING

• Prescribed diet is an essential part of treatment; do not skip or delay meals. • Carry candy, sugar packets, other sugar supplements for immediate response to hypoglycemia. • Wear or carry medical alert identification. • Check with physician when insulin demands are altered (e.g., fever, infection, trauma, stress, heavy physical activity). • Do not take other medication without consulting physician. • Weight control, exercise, hygiene (including foot care), and not smoking are integral parts of therapy. • Protect skin, limit sun exposure. • Inform dentist, physician, surgeon of medication before any treatment is given.

Integrillin, *see eptifibatide*

interferon alfa-2a ▷

inn-ter-**fear**-on
(Roferon-A)
Do not confuse interferon alfa-2a with interferon alfa-2b.

•CLASSIFICATION

PHARMACOTHERAPEUTIC: Biologic response modifier. **CLINICAL:** Antineoplastic (see p. 75C).

ACTION

A biological response modifier that inhibits viral replication in virus-infected cells, suppresses cell proliferation, increases phagocytic action of macrophage, and augments specific lymphocytic cell toxicity. **Therapeutic Effect:** Prevents rapid growth of malignant cells; inhibits hepatitis virus.

✐ see color pill atlas   ✒ herb   underlined – top prescribed drug

PHARMACOKINETICS

Well absorbed after IM and subcutaneous administration. Undergoes proteolytic degradation during reabsorption in kidneys. Half-life: 2 hr (IM); 3 hr (subcutaneous).

USES

Treatment of hairy cell leukemia, AIDS-related Kaposi's sarcoma, chronic myelogenous leukemia (CML), chronic hepatitis C. OFF-LABEL: Treatment of active, chronic hepatitis; bladder or renal carcinoma; malignant melanoma; multiple myeloma; mycosis fungoides; non-Hodgkin's lymphoma.

PRECAUTIONS

CONTRAINDICATIONS: Autoimmune hepatitis. CAUTIONS: Renal or hepatic impairment, seizure disorders, compromised CNS function, cardiac disease, history of cardiac abnormalities, myelosuppression.

LIFESPAN CONSIDERATIONS: Pregnancy/Lactation: If possible, avoid use during pregnancy. Breast-feeding not recommended. Pregnancy Category C. Children: Safety and efficacy not established. Elderly: Neurotoxicity, cardiotoxicity may occur more frequently. Age-related renal impairment may require dosage adjustment.

INTERACTIONS

DRUG: **Bone marrow depressants:** May have increase myelosuppression. HERBAL: None known. FOOD: None known. LAB VALUES: May increase serum LDH, alkaline phosphatase, AST, and ALT levels. May decrease Hct, blood Hgb level, and leukocyte and platelet counts.

AVAILABILITY (Rx)

INJECTION, VIAL: 6 million units/ml. INJECTION (PRE-FILLED SYRINGE): 3 million units/0.5 ml, 6 million units/0.5 ml, 9 million units/0.5 ml. INJECTION (SINGLE DOSE VIAL): 36 million units/ml.

ADMINISTRATION/HANDLING

◀ ALERT ▶ Subcutaneous route preferred for thrombocytopenic patients, those at risk for bleeding.

IM, SUBCUTANEOUS
• Refrigerate. • Do not shake vial. • Solution appears colorless. • Do not use if precipitate or discoloration occurs.

INDICATIONS/ROUTES/DOSAGE

HAIRY CELL LEUKEMIA
IM, SUBCUTANEOUS: ADULTS: Initially, 3 million units/day for 16–24 wk. Maintenance: 3 million units 3 times a wk. Do not use 36-million-unit vial.

CHRONIC MYELOGENOUS LEUKEMIA
IM, SUBCUTANEOUS: ADULTS: 9 million units/day. Continue treatment until worsening of disease.

MELANOMA
IM, SUBCUTANEOUS: ADULTS, ELDERLY: 12 million units/m^2 3 times a wk for 3 mo or 3 million units 3 times a wk .

AIDS-RELATED KAPOSI'S SARCOMA
IM, SUBCUTANEOUS: ADULTS: Initially, 36 million units/day for 10–12 wk, may give 3 million units on day 1, 9 million units on day 2, 18 million units on day 3, then 36 million units/day for remaining of 10–12 wk. Maintenance: 36 million units/day 3 times a wk.

CHRONIC HEPATITIS C
IM, SUBCUTANEOUS: ADULTS, ELDERLY: 6 million units 3 times a wk for 3 mo, then 3 million units 3 times a wk for 9 mo.

SIDE EFFECTS

FREQUENT (greater than 20%): Flu-like symptoms, nausea, vomiting, cough, dyspnea, hypotension, edema, chest pain, dizziness, diarrhea, weight loss, altered taste, abdominal discomfort, confusion, paresthesia, depression, visual and sleep disturbances, diaphoresis, lethargy.

OCCASIONAL (20%–5%): Alopecia (partial), rash, dry throat or skin, pruritus, flatulence, constipation, hypertension, palpitations, sinusitis. **RARE (less than 5%):** Hot flashes, hypermotility, Raynaud's syndrome, bronchospasm, earache, ecchymosis.

ADVERSE REACTIONS/ TOXIC EFFECTS

Arrhythmias, CVA, transient ischemic attacks, CHF, pulmonary edema, and MI occur rarely.

NURSING CONSIDERATIONS

BASELINE ASSESSMENT

CBC, platelet count, blood chemistries, urinalysis, renal or liver function tests should be performed before initial therapy and routinely thereafter.

INTERVENTION/EVALUATION

Offer emotional support. Monitor all levels of clinical function (numerous side effects). Encourage ample fluid intake, particularly during early therapy.

PATIENT/FAMILY TEACHING

• Clinical response may take 1–3 mo. • Flu-like symptoms tend to diminish with continued therapy. • Contact physician if nausea or vomiting continues at home. • Avoid alcohol while taking medication. • Avoid tasks that require alertness, motor skills until response to drug is established.

---

interferon alfa-2b ▷

inn-ter-**fear**-on

(Intron-A)

Do not confuse interferon alfa-2b with interferon alfa-2a.

FIXED-COMBINATION(S)

Rebetron: interferon alfa-2b/ribavirin (an antiviral): 3 million units/ 200 mg.

◆CLASSIFICATION

PHARMACOTHERAPEUTIC: Biologic response modifier. **CLINICAL:** Antineoplastic (see p. 75C).

ACTION

A biological response modifier that inhibits viral replication in virus-infected cells, suppresses cell proliferation, increases phagocytic action of macrophages, and augments specific cytotoxicity of lymphocytes for target cells. Therapeutic Effect: Prevents rapid growth of malignant cells; inhibits hepatitis virus.

PHARMACOKINETICS

Well absorbed after IM and subcutaneous administration. Undergoes proteolytic degradation during reabsorption in kidneys. Half-life: 2–3 hr.

USES

Treatment of hairy cell leukemia, condylomata acuminata (genital, venereal warts), AIDS-related Kaposi's sarcoma, chronic hepatitis (non-A, non-B/C), chronic hepatitis B (including children 1 yr and older), follicular lymphoma. OFF-LABEL: Treatment of bladder, cervical, or renal carcinoma; chronic myelocytic leukemia; laryngeal papillomatosis; multiple myeloma; mycosis fungoides.

PRECAUTIONS

CONTRAINDICATIONS: Autoimmune hepatitis, impaired hepatic function. **CAUTIONS:** Renal or hepatic impairment, seizure disorders, compromised CNS function, cardiac diseases, history of cardiac abnormalities, myelosuppression.

⧗ LIFESPAN CONSIDERATIONS: **Pregnancy/Lactation:** If possible, avoid use during pregnancy. Breast-feeding not recommended. **Pregnancy Category C. Children:** Safety and efficacy not established. **Elderly:** Neurotoxicity,

---

cardiotoxicity may occur more frequently. Age-related renal impairment may require dosage adjustment.

INTERACTIONS

DRUG: **Bone marrow depressants:** May increase myelosuppression. HERBAL: None known. FOOD: None known. LAB VALUES: May increase PT, aPTT, and serum LDH, alkaline phosphatase, AST, and ALT levels. May decrease blood Hgb level, Hct, and leukocyte and platelet counts.

AVAILABILITY (Rx)

INJECTION (MULTIDOSE VIAL): 6 million units/ml, 10 million units/ml. **INJECTION (SINGLE DOSE VIAL):** 3 million units/0.5 ml, 5 million units/0.5 ml, 10 million units/ml, 18 million units/ml, 25 million units/ml, 50 million units/ml. **INJECTION (PREFILLED SOLUTION):** 3 million units/ 0.2 ml, 5 million units/0.2 ml, 10 million units/0.2 ml.

ADMINISTRATION/HANDLING

🖉 IV

Reconstitution • Prepare immediately before use. • Reconstitute with diluent provided by manufacturer. • Withdraw desired dose and further dilute with 100 ml 0.9% NaCl to provide final concentration at least 10 million international units/100 ml.

Rate of administration • Administer over 20 min.

Storage • Refrigerate unopened vials (stable for 7 days at room temperature).

IM, SUBCUTANEOUS

• Do not give IM if platelets are less than 50,000/m³; give subcutaneous. • For hairy cell leukemia, reconstitute each 3 million international units vial with 1 ml bacteriostatic water for injection to provide concentration of 3 million international units/ml (1 ml to 5 million-international units vial; 2 ml to 10

million-international units vial; 5 ml to 25 million-international units vial provides concentration of 5 million international units/ml). • For condylomata acuminata, reconstitute each 10 million international units vial with 1 ml bacteriostatic water for injection to provide concentration of 10 million international units/ml. • For AIDS-related Kaposi's sarcoma, reconstitute 50 million international units vial with 1 ml bacteriostatic water for injection to provide concentration of 50 million international units/ml. • Agitate vial gently, withdraw with sterile syringe.

🖩 IV INCOMPATIBILITIES

Do not mix with other medications for Y-site administration.

INDICATIONS/ROUTES/DOSAGE

HAIRY CELL LEUKEMIA

IM, SUBCUTANEOUS: ADULTS: 2 million units/m² 3 times a week. If severe adverse reactions occur, modify dose or temporarily discontinue drug.

CONDYLOMA ACUMINATUM

INTRALESIONAL: ADULTS: 1 million units/lesion 3 times a week for 3 wk. Use only 10-million-unit vial, and reconstitute with no more than 1 ml diluent.

AIDS-RELATED KAPOSI'S SARCOMA

IM, SUBCUTANEOUS: ADULTS: 30 million units/m² 3 times a week. Use only 50-million-unit vials. If severe adverse reactions occur, modify dose or temporarily discontinue drug.

CHRONIC HEPATITIS C

IM, SUBCUTANEOUS: ADULTS: 3 million units 3 times a week for up to 6 mo. For patients who tolerate therapy and whose ALT level normalizes within 16 wk, therapy may be extended for up to 18–24 mo.

CHRONIC HEPATITIS B

IM, SUBCUTANEOUS: ADULTS: 30–35 million units weekly, either as 5 million units/day or 10 million units 3 times a week.

MALIGNANT MELANOMA

IV: ADULTS: Initially, 20 million units/m^2 5 times a week for 4 wk. Maintenance: 10 million units IM or subcutaneously 3 times a week for 48 wk.

FOLLICULAR LYMPHOMA

SUBCUTANEOUS: ADULTS: 5 million units 5 times a week for up to 18 mo.

SIDE EFFECTS

FREQUENT: Flu-like symptoms, rash (only in patients with hairy cell leukemia Kaposi's sarcoma). **Patients with Kaposi's sarcoma:** All previously mentioned side effects plus depression, dyspepsia, dry mouth or thirst, alopecia, rigors. **OCCASIONAL:** Dizziness, pruritus, dry skin, dermatitis, altered taste. **RARE:** Confusion, leg cramps, back pain, gingivitis, flushing, tremor, nervousness, eye pain.

ADVERSE REACTIONS/ TOXIC EFFECTS

Hypersensitivity reactions occur rarely. Severe flu-like symptoms may occur at higher doses.

NURSING CONSIDERATIONS

BASELINE ASSESSMENT

CBC, platelet count, blood chemistries, urinalysis, renal and liver function tests should be performed before initial therapy and routinely thereafter.

INTERVENTION/EVALUATION

Offer emotional support. Monitor all levels of clinical function (numerous side effects). Encourage ample fluid intake, particularly during early therapy.

PATIENT/FAMILY TEACHING

• Clinical response occurs in 1–3 mo. • Flu-like symptoms tend to diminish with continued therapy. • Some symptoms may be alleviated or minimized by bedtime doses. • Do not have immunizations without physician's approval (drug lowers body's resistance).

• Avoid contact with those who have recently received live virus vaccine. • Avoid tasks that require alertness, motor skills until response to drug is established. • Sips of tepid water may relieve dry mouth.

interferon beta-1a

inn-ter-**fear**-on

(Avonex, Avonex Prefilled Syringe, Rebif)

Do not confuse interferon beta-1a with interferon beta-1b or Avonex with Avelox.

CLASSIFICATION

PHARMACOTHERAPEUTIC: Biologic response modifier. **CLINICAL:** Multiple sclerosis agent.

ACTION

A biological response modifier that interacts with specific cell receptors found on the surface of human cells. **Therapeutic Effect:** Produces antiviral and immunoregulatory effects.

PHARMACOKINETICS

Peak serum levels attained 3–15 hr after IM administration. Biological markers increase within 12 hr and remain elevated for 4 days. **Half-life:** 10 hr (Avonex); 69 hr (Rebif).

USES

Treatment of relapsing multiple sclerosis to slow progression of physical disability, decrease frequency of clinical exacerbations. **OFF-LABEL:** Treatment of AIDS, AIDS-related Kaposi's sarcoma, condyloma acuminatum, malignant melanoma, renal cell carcinoma.

PRECAUTIONS

CONTRAINDICATIONS: Avonex: Hypersensitivity to natural or recombinant interferon beta, human albumin. **Rebif:** Hypersensitivity to natural or recombinant interferon, human albumin. **CAUTIONS:** Chronic progressive multiple sclerosis, children younger than 18 yr, depression.

⧗ **LIFESPAN CONSIDERATIONS: Pregnancy/Lactation:** Has abortifacient potential. Unknown if drug is distributed in breast milk. **Pregnancy Category C. Children:** Safety and efficacy not established. **Elderly:** No information available.

INTERACTIONS

DRUG: None known. **HERBAL:** None known. **FOOD:** None known. **LAB VALUES:** May increase blood glucose and BUN levels, and serum alkaline phosphatase, bilirubin, calcium, AST, and ALT levels. May decrease blood Hgb level and neutrophil, platelet, and WBC counts.

AVAILABILITY (Rx)

INJECTION POWDER FOR RECONSTITUTION (AVONEX): 30 mcg. **INJECTION SOLUTION (PREFILLED SYRINGE):** 22 mcg/ml (Rebif), 30 mcg/0.5 ml (Avonex Prefilled Syringe), 44 mcg/ml (Rebif). **TITRATION PACK (PREFILLED SYRINGE [REBIF]):** 8.8 mcg and 22 mcg.

ADMINISTRATION/HANDLING

IM (AVONEX) SYRINGE
• Refrigerate syringe. • Allow to warm to room temperature before use. • Use within 12 hr after removing from refrigerator.

IM (AVONEX) VIAL
• Refrigerate vials. • Following reconstitution, may refrigerate again but use within 6 hr if refrigerated. • Reconstitute 30 mcg *MicroPin* (6.6 million international units) vial with 1.1 ml diluent (supplied by manufacturer). • Gently swirl to dissolve medication; do not shake. • Discard if discolored, contains particulate matter. • Discard unused portion (contains no preservative).

SUBCUTANEOUS (REBIF)
• Refrigerate. May store at room temperature up to 30 days. Avoid heat, light. Administer at same time of day 3 days each wk. Doses to be separated by at least 48 hr.

INDICATIONS/ROUTES/DOSAGE

RELAPSING-REMITTING MULTIPLE SCLEROSIS

IM (AVONEX): ADULTS: 30 mcg once weekly.
SUBCUTANEOUS (REBIF): ADULTS: Initially 8.8 mcg 3 times a week, may increase to 44 mcg 3 times a week over 4–6 wk.

SIDE EFFECTS

FREQUENT: Headache (67%), flu-like symptoms (61%), myalgia (34%), upper respiratory tract infection (31%), depression with suicidal thoughts (25%), generalized pain (24%), asthenia, chills (21%), sinusitis (18%), infection (11%). **OCCASIONAL:** Abdominal pain, arthralgia (9%), chest pain, dyspnea (6%), malaise, syncope (4%). **RARE:** Injection site reaction, hypersensitivity reaction (3%).

ADVERSE REACTIONS/ TOXIC EFFECTS

Anemia occurs in 8% of patients. Severe hepatic injury, including hepatic failure, has been reported.

NURSING CONSIDERATIONS

BASELINE ASSESSMENT
Obtain Hgb, CBC, platelet count, blood chemistries including liver function tests. Assess home situation for support of therapy.

INTERVENTION/EVALUATION
Assess for headache, flu-like symptoms, myalgia. Periodically monitor lab results,

reevaluate injection technique. Assess for depression, suicidal ideation.

PATIENT/FAMILY TEACHING

• Do not change schedule or dosage without consultation with physician. • Instruct on correct reconstitution of product and administration, including aseptic technique. • Provide puncture-resistant container for used needles, syringes; explain proper disposal. • Explain that injection site reactions may occur. • These do not require discontinuation of therapy, but note type and extent carefully.

interferon beta-1b

inn-ter-**fear**-on
(Betaseron)
Do not confuse interferon beta-1b with interferon beta-1a.

◆ CLASSIFICATION

PHARMACOTHERAPEUTIC: Biologic response modifier. **CLINICAL:** Multiple sclerosis, cancer, AIDS agent.

ACTION

A biological response modifier that interacts with specific cell receptors found on the surface of human cells. **Therapeutic Effect:** Produces antiviral and immunoregulatory effects.

PHARMACOKINETICS

Because serum concentrations of interferon beta-1b are low or not detectable, pharmacokinetic information is not available. **Half-life:** 8 min–4.3 hr.

USES

Reduces frequency of clinical exacerbations in patients with relapsing-remitting multiple sclerosis (recurrent attacks of neurologic dysfunction).

OFF-LABEL: Treatment of acute non-A and non-B hepatitis, AIDS, AIDS-related Kaposi's sarcoma, malignant melanoma, renal cell carcinoma.

PRECAUTIONS

CONTRAINDICATIONS: Hypersensitivity to albumin or interferon. **CAUTIONS:** Chronic progressive multiple sclerosis, children younger than 18 yr.

⌛ **LIFESPAN CONSIDERATIONS: Pregnancy/Lactation:** Unknown if distributed in breast milk. **Pregnancy Category C. Children:** Safety and efficacy not established. **Elderly:** No information available.

INTERACTIONS

DRUG: None known. **HERBAL:** None known. **FOOD:** None known. **LAB VALUES:** May increase blood glucose and BUN levels, and serum alkaline phosphatase, bilirubin, calcium, AST, and ALT levels. May decrease blood Hgb level and neutrophil, platelet, and WBC counts.

AVAILABILITY (Rx)

POWDER FOR INJECTION: 0.3 mg (9.6 million units).

ADMINISTRATION/HANDLING

SUBCUTANEOUS

• Store vials at room temperature. • After reconstitution, stable for 3 hr if refrigerated. • Use within 3 hr of reconstitution. • Discard if discolored or contains a precipitate. • Reconstitute 0.3-mg (9.6 million international units) vial with 1.2 ml diluent (supplied by manufacturer) to provide concentration of 0.25 mg/ml (8 million units/ml). • Gently swirl to dissolve medication; do not shake. • Discard if discolored or contains particulate matter. • Withdraw 1 ml solution and inject subcutaneous into arms, abdomen, hips, or thighs using 27-gauge needle.

• Discard unused portion (contains no preservative).

INDICATIONS/ROUTES/DOSAGE
RELAPSING-REMITTING MULTIPLE SCLEROSIS
SUBCUTANEOUS: ADULTS: 0.25 mg (8 million units) every other day.

SIDE EFFECTS
FREQUENT: Injection site reaction (85%), headache (84%), flu-like symptoms (76%), fever (59%), asthenia (49%), myalgia (44%), sinusitis (36%), diarrhea, dizziness (35%), mental status changes (29%), constipation (24%), diaphoresis (23%), vomiting (21%). **OCCASIONAL:** Malaise (15%), somnolence (6%), alopecia (4%).

ADVERSE REACTIONS/ TOXIC EFFECTS
Seizures occur rarely.

NURSING CONSIDERATIONS

BASELINE ASSESSMENT
Obtain Hgb, CBC, platelet count, blood chemistries (including liver function tests). Assess home situation for support of therapy.

INTERVENTION/EVALUATION
Periodically monitor lab results, reevaluate injection technique. Assess for nausea (high incidence). Monitor sleep pattern. Monitor pattern of bowel activity and stool consistency. Assist with ambulation if dizziness occurs. Question for evidence of heartburn, epigastric discomfort. Monitor food intake. Assess for depression, suicidal ideation.

PATIENT/FAMILY TEACHING
• Inform physician of flu-like symptoms (occur commonly but decrease over time). • Wear sunscreens, protective clothing if exposed to sunlight or ultraviolet light until tolerance known.

interferon gamma-1b

inn-ter-**fear**-on
(Actimmune)

CLASSIFICATION
PHARMACOTHERAPEUTIC: Biologic response modifier. **CLINICAL:** Immunologic agent.

ACTION
A biological response modifier that induces activation of macrophages in blood monocytes to phagocytes, which is necessary in the body's cellular immune response to intracellular and extracellular pathogens. Enhances phagocytic function and antimicrobial activity of monocytes. **Therapeutic Effect:** Decreases signs and symptoms of serious infections in chronic granulomatous disease.

PHARMACOKINETICS
Slowly absorbed after subcutaneous administration. **Half-life:** 0.5–1 hr.

USES
Reduces frequency, severity of serious infections due to chronic granulomatous disease. Treatment of severe, malignant osteopetrosis.

PRECAUTIONS
CONTRAINDICATIONS: Hypersensitivity to *Escherichia coli*-derived products. **CAUTIONS:** Seizure disorders, compromised CNS function, preexisting cardiac disease (including ischemia, CHF, arrhythmias), myelosuppression.

⧗ **LIFESPAN CONSIDERATIONS: Pregnancy/Lactation:** Unknown if drug crosses placenta or is distributed in breast milk. **Pregnancy Category C. Children:** Safety and efficacy not established in those younger than 1 yr. Flu-like symptoms may occur more frequently. **Elderly:** No information available.

INTERACTIONS

DRUG: Bone marrow depressants: May increase myelosuppression. **HERBAL:** None known. **FOOD:** None known. **LAB VALUES:** None known.

AVAILABILITY (Rx)

INJECTION: 100 mcg (2 million units).

ADMINISTRATION/HANDLING

◄ **ALERT** ▶ Avoid excessive agitation of vial; do not shake.

SUBCUTANEOUS
• Refrigerate vials. Do not freeze. • Do not keep at room temperature for more than 12 hr; discard after 12 hr. • Vials are single dose; discard unused portion. • Solution is clear, colorless. Do not use if discolored, precipitate formed. • When given 3 times a wk, rotate injection sites.

INDICATIONS/ROUTES/DOSAGE

CHRONIC GRANULOMATOUS DISEASE; SEVERE, MALIGNANT OSTEOPETROSIS
SUBCUTANEOUS: ADULTS, CHILDREN OLDER THAN 1 YR: 50 mcg/m² (1.5 million units/m²) in patients with body surface area (BSA) greater than 0.5 m²; 1.5 mcg/kg/dose in patients with BSA 0.5 m² or less. Give 3 times a week.

SIDE EFFECTS

FREQUENT: Fever (52%); headache (33%); rash (17%); chills, fatigue, diarrhea (14%). **OCCASIONAL (13%–10%):** Vomiting, nausea. **RARE (6%–3%):** Weight loss, myalgia, anorexia.

ADVERSE REACTIONS/ TOXIC EFFECTS

Interferon gamma-1b may exacerbate preexisting CNS disturbances, including decreased mental status, gait disturbance, and dizziness, as well as cardiac disorders.

NURSING CONSIDERATIONS

BASELINE ASSESSMENT

CBC, platelet count, blood chemistries, urinalysis, renal and liver function tests should be performed before initial therapy and at 3-mo intervals during course of treatment.

INTERVENTION/EVALUATION

Monitor for flu-like symptoms (fever, chills, fatigue, myalgia). Assess skin for evidence of rash.

PATIENT/FAMILY TEACHING

• Flu-like symptoms (fever, chills, fatigue, muscle aches) are generally mild and tend to disappear as treatment continues. Symptoms may be minimized with bedtime administration. • Avoid tasks that require alertness, motor skills until response to drug is established. • If home use prescribed, instruct in proper technique of administration; care in proper disposal of needles, syringes. • Vials should remain refrigerated.

---

interleukin-2 (aldesleukin) ⚑

in-tur-**lew**-kin
(IL-2, <u>Proleukin</u>)
Do not confuse interleukin-2 with interferon 2.

• CLASSIFICATION

PHARMACOTHERAPEUTIC: Biologic response modifier. **CLINICAL:** Antineoplastic (see p. 70C).

ACTION

A biological response modifier that acts like human recombinant interleukin-2, promoting proliferation, differentiation, and recruitment of T and B cells, lymphokine-activated and natural cells, and thymocytes. Therapeutic Effect: Enhances cytolytic activity in lymphocytes.

PHARMACOKINETICS

Primarily distributed into plasma, lymphocytes, lungs, liver, kidney, and spleen. Metabolized to amino acids in the cells lining the kidneys. Half-life: 85 min.

USES

Treatment of metastatic renal cell carcinoma, metastatic melanoma. OFF-LABEL: Treatment of colorectal cancer, Kaposi's sarcoma, non-Hodgkin's lymphoma.

PRECAUTIONS

CONTRAINDICATIONS: Abnormal pulmonary function or thallium stress test results, bowel ischemia or perforation, coma or toxic psychosis lasting longer than 48 hr, GI bleeding requiring surgery, intubation lasting more than 72 hr, organ allografts, pericardial tamponade, renal dysfunction requiring dialysis for longer than 72 hr, repetitive or difficult-to-control seizures; retreatment in those who experience any of the following toxicities: angina, MI, recurrent chest pain with EKG changes, sustained ventricular tachycardia, uncontrolled or unresponsive cardiac rhythm disturbances. EXTREME CAUTION: Patients with normal thallium stress tests and pulmonary function tests who have history of prior cardiac or pulmonary disease. CAUTIONS: Patients with fixed requirements for large volumes of fluid (e.g., those with hypercalcemia), history of seizures.

LIFESPAN CONSIDERATIONS: Pregnancy/Lactation: Avoid use in those of either sex not practicing effective contraception. Pregnancy Category C. Children: Safety and efficacy not established. Elderly: Age-related renal impairment may require dosage adjustment; will not tolerate toxicity.

INTERACTIONS

DRUG: Antihypertensives: May increase hypotensive effect. Cardiotoxic, hepatotoxic, myelotoxic, or nephrotoxic medications: May increase the risk of toxicity. Glucocorticoids: May decrease the effects of interleukin-2. HERBAL: None known. FOOD: None known. LAB VALUES: May increase BUN and serum alkaline phosphatase, bilirubin, creatinine, AST, and ALT levels. May decrease serum calcium, magnesium, phosphorus, potassium, and sodium levels.

AVAILABILITY (Rx)

POWDER FOR INJECTION (PROLEUKIN): 22 million units (1.3 mg) (18 million units/ml when reconstituted).

ADMINISTRATION/HANDLING

◄ ALERT ► Hold administration in patients who develop moderate to severe lethargy or somnolence (continued administration may result in coma).

 IV

Reconstitution • Reconstitute 22 million units vial with 1.2 ml sterile water for injection to provide concentration of 18 million units/ml. Bacteriostatic water for injection or NaCl should not be used to reconstitute because of increased aggregation. • During reconstitution, direct the sterile water for injection at the side of vial. Swirl contents gently to avoid foaming. Do not shake.

Rate of administration • Further dilute dose in 50 ml D₅W and infuse over 15 min. Do not use an in-line filter.

• Solution should be warmed to room temperature before infusion. • Monitor diligently for drop in mean arterial BP (sign of capillary leak syndrome [CLS]). Continued treatment may result in significant hypotension (less than 90 mm Hg or a 20 mm Hg drop from baseline systolic pressure), edema, pleural effusion, altered mental status.

Storage • Refrigerate vials; do not freeze. • Reconstituted solution is stable for 48 hr refrigerated or at room temperature (refrigeration preferred).

⚙ IV INCOMPATIBILITIES

Ganciclovir (Cytovene), pentamidine (Pentam), prochlorperazine (Compazine), promethazine (Phenergan).

IV COMPATIBILITIES

Calcium gluconate, dopamine (Intropin), heparin, lorazepam (Ativan), magnesium, potassium.

INDICATIONS/ROUTES/DOSAGE

METASTATIC MELANOMA, METASTATIC RENAL CELL CARCINOMA
IV: ADULTS 18 YR AND OLDER: 600,000 units/kg q8h for 14 doses; followed by 9 days of rest, then another 14 doses for a total of 28 doses per course. Course may be repeated after rest period of at least 7 wk from date of hospital discharge.

SIDE EFFECTS

Side effects are generally self-limiting and reversible within 2–3 days after discontinuing therapy. **FREQUENT (89%–48%):** Fever, chills, nausea, vomiting, hypotension, diarrhea, oliguria or anuria, mental status changes, irritability, confusion, depression, sinus tachycardia, pain (abdominal, chest, back), fatigue, dyspnea, pruritus. **OCCASIONAL (47%–17%):** Edema, erythema, rash, stomatitis, anorexia, weight gain, infection (UTI, injection site, catheter tip), dizziness. **RARE (15%–4%):** Dry skin,

sensory disorders (vision, speech, taste), dermatitis, headache, arthralgia, myalgia, weight loss, hematuria, conjunctivitis, proteinuria.

ADVERSE REACTIONS/ TOXIC EFFECTS

Anemia, thrombocytopenia, and leukopenia occur commonly. GI bleeding and pulmonary edema occur occasionally. Capillary leak syndrome results in hypotension (systolic pressure less than 90 mm Hg or a 20-mm Hg drop from baseline systolic pressure), extravasation of plasma proteins and fluid into extravascular space, and loss of vascular tone. It may result in cardiac arrhythmias, angina, MI, and respiratory insufficiency. Other rare reactions include fatal malignant hyperthermia, cardiac arrest, cerebrovascular accident (CVA), pulmonary emboli, bowel perforation, gangrene, and severe depression leading to suicide.

NURSING CONSIDERATIONS

BASELINE ASSESSMENT

Patients with bacterial infection and with indwelling central lines should be treated with antibiotic therapy before treatment begins. All patients should be neurologically stable with a negative CT scan before treatment begins. CBC, blood chemistries (including electrolytes), renal and liver function tests, chest x-ray should be performed before therapy begins and daily thereafter.

INTERVENTION/EVALUATION

Monitor CBC with differential, platelets, electrolytes, renal and hepatic functions, weight, pulse oximetry. Determine serum amylase concentration frequently during therapy. Discontinue medication at first sign of hypotension and hold for moderate to severe lethargy (physician must decide whether therapy should continue). Assess altered mental status (irritability, confusion, depression), weight gain/loss. Maintain strict I&O. Assess for extravascular fluid accumulation (rales in lungs, edema in dependent areas).

PATIENT/FAMILY TEACHING

• Nausea may decrease during therapy. • At home, increase fluid intake (protects against renal impairment). • Do not have immunizations without physician's approval (drug lowers body resistance). • Avoid exposure to persons with infection. • Contact physician if fever, chills, lower back pain, difficulty with urination, unusual bleeding or bruising, black tarry stools, blood in urine, pinpoint red spots on skin occur. • Report symptoms of depression or suicidal ideation immediately.

ipecac syrup

ip-eh-kak
(PMS Ipecac Syrup ♣)

◆ **CLASSIFICATION**

PHARMACOTHERAPEUTIC: Antidote. **CLINICAL:** Antidote.

ACTION

Acts centrally by stimulating medullary chemoreceptor trigger zone and locally by irritating gastric mucosa. **Therapeutic Effect:** Produces emesis.

USES

Induces vomiting in early treatment of unabsorbed oral poisons, drug overdosage.

PRECAUTIONS

CONTRAINDICATIONS: Unconscious patients, those with absent gag reflex, seizures. Do not use for ingestion of strong bases or acids, corrosive substances, volatile oils, hydrocarbons with high potential for aspiration. **CAUTIONS:** Cardiovascular disease, bulimia. **Pregnancy Category C.**

INTERACTIONS

DRUG: **Antiemetics:** May decrease effect. HERBAL: None known. FOOD: **Carbonated beverages:** Cause stomach distention. **Milk, milk products:** Decrease effectiveness of ipecac. LAB VALUES: None known.

AVAILABILITY (OTC)

SYRUP: 70 mg/ml.

INDICATIONS/ROUTES/DOSAGE

◀ ALERT ▶ If vomiting has not occurred within 20 min after first dose, repeat dose (15 ml). If vomiting has not occurred within 30 min after last dose, initiate gastric lavage, activated charcoal.

EMETIC

PO: ADULTS, ELDERLY, CHILDREN OLDER THAN 12 YR: 15–30 ml; give with 3–4 glasses of water immediately following administration. CHILDREN 1–12 YR: 15 ml; follow with 1–2 glasses of water. CHILDREN 6 MO–YOUNGER THAN 1 YR: 5–10 ml; follow with 1 glass of water. If vomiting has not occurred within 30 min, repeat initial dosage.

SIDE EFFECTS

EXPECTED RESPONSE: Nausea, vomiting. After vomiting, diarrhea and CNS symptoms (drowsiness, mild CNS depression) commonly occur.

ADVERSE REACTIONS/ TOXIC EFFECTS

Cardiotoxicity may occur if ipecac syrup is not vomited (noted as hypotension, tachycardia/precordial chest pain, pulmonary congestion, dyspnea, ventricular tachycardia/fibrillation, cardiac arrest). Overdose may produce diarrhea, tachycardia, palpitations, nausea continuing over 30 min, abdominal pain, dyspnea, myalgia.

NURSING CONSIDERATIONS

BASELINE ASSESSMENT

Do not administer to semiconscious, unconscious, patient with active seizures. Gastric lavage, activated charcoal is necessary if vomiting does not occur within 30 min of second dose to avoid drug toxicity (bloody stools, vomiting, abdominal pain, hypotension, dyspnea, shock, cardiac disturbances, seizures, coma). Maintain patient in upright position to enhance emetic effect.

INTERVENTION/EVALUATION

Closely monitor vital signs, EKG during and following drug administration. Watch for changes from initial assessment. Check for reversal of poisoning or overdosage symptoms. Monitor daily bowel activity/stool consistency; record time of evacuation. Assess for dehydration if vomiting is excessive (poor skin turgor, dry mucous membranes, longitudinal furrows in tongue).

PATIENT/FAMILY TEACHING

• Avoid consuming carbonated beverages.

ipratropium bromide

ih-prah-**trow**-pea-um

(Apo-Ipravent ✹, Atrovent, Novo-Ipramide ✹, Nu-Ipratropium ✹, PMS-Ipratropium ✹)

Do not confuse Atrovent with Alupent.

FIXED-COMBINATION(S)

Combivent, Duoneb: ipratropime/albuterol (a bronchodilator): *Aerosol:* 18 mcg/103 mcg per actuation. *Solution:* 0.5 ml/2.5 ml per 3 ml.

✦ CLASSIFICATION

PHARMACOTHERAPEUTIC: Anticholinergic. **CLINICAL:** Bronchodilator.

ACTION

An anticholinergic that blocks the action of acetylcholine at parasympathetic sites in bronchial smooth muscle. **Therapeutic Effect:** Causes bronchodilation and inhibits nasal secretions.

PHARMACOKINETICS

Route	Onset	Peak	Duration
Inhalation	1–3 min	1–hr	4–6 hr

Minimal systemic absorption after inhalation. Metabolized in the liver (systemic absorption). Primarily eliminated in feces. **Half-life:** 1.5–4 hr.

USES

Inhalation: Maintenance treatment of bronchospasm due to chronic obstructive pulmonary disease (COPD), bronchitis, emphysema, asthma. Not to be used for immediate bronchospasm relief. **Nasal Spray:** Rhinorrhea (0.03% associated with perineal rhinitis, 0.06% associated with common cold), seasonal allergy.

PRECAUTIONS

CONTRAINDICATIONS: History of hypersensitivity to atropine, soya lecithin, or related food products such as soybean and peanut. **CAUTIONS:** Narrow-angle glaucoma, prostatic hypertrophy, bladder neck obstruction.

⧗ **LIFESPAN CONSIDERATIONS: Pregnancy/Lactation:** Unknown if distributed in breast milk. **Pregnancy Category B. Children/Elderly:** No age-related precautions noted.

INTERACTIONS

DRUG: Cromolyn inhalation solution: Avoid mixing these drugs because they form a precipitate. **HERBAL:** None known. **FOOD:** None known. **LAB VALUES:** None known.

AVAILABILITY (Rx)

ORAL INHALATION: 18 mcg/actuation. **AEROSOL SOLUTION FOR INHALATION:** 0.02%. **NASAL SPRAY:** 0.03%, 0.06%.

ADMINISTRATION/HANDLING

INHALATION

• Shake container well. • Exhale completely through mouth; place mouthpiece into mouth, close lips, holding inhaler upright. • Inhale deeply through mouth while fully depressing the top of canister. Hold breath as long as possible before exhaling slowly. • Wait 2 min before inhaling second dose (allows for deeper bronchial penetration). • Rinse mouth with water immediately after inhalation (prevents mouth/throat dryness).

NASAL

• Store at room temperature. • Initial pump priming requires 7 actuations of the pump. • If used regularly as recommended, no further priming is required. If not used for more than 24 hr, the pump will require 2 actuations, or if not used for more than 7 days, the pump will require 7 actuations to reprime.

INDICATIONS/ROUTES/DOSAGE

BRONCHOSPASM

INHALATION: ADULTS, ELDERLY: 2 inhalations 4 times a day. **Maximum:** 12 inhalations/day. CHILDREN 3-14 YR: 1–2 inhalations 3 times a day. **Maximum:** 6 inhalations/day.

NEBULIZATION: ADULTS, ELDERLY: 500 mcg 3–4 times a day. CHILDREN: 125–250 mcg 3 times a day.

RHINORRHEA (PERENNIAL ALLERGIC AND NON-ALLERGIC RHINITIS)

INTRANASAL (0.03%): ADULTS, ELDERLY, CHILDREN 6 YR AND OLDER: 2 sprays per nostril 2–3 times a day.

RHINORRHEA (COMMON COLD)

INTRANASAL (0.06%): ADULTS, ELDERLY: 2 sprays per nostril 3–4 times a day for up to 4 days. CHILDREN 5 YR AND OLDER: 2 sprays per nostril 3 times a day for up to 4 days.

RHINORRHEA (SEASONAL ALLERGY)

INTRANASAL (0.06%): ADULTS, ELDERLY, CHILDREN 5 YR AND OLDER: 2 sprays per nostril 4 times a day for up to 3 wk.

SIDE EFFECTS

FREQUENT: Inhalation (6%–3%): Cough, dry mouth, headache, nausea. **Nasal:** Dry nose and mouth, headache, nasal irritation. **OCCASIONAL: Inhalation (2%):** Dizziness, transient increased bronchospasm. **RARE (less than 1%): Inhalation:** Hypotension, insomnia, metallic or unpleasant taste, palpitations, urine retention. **Nasal:** Diarrhea or constipation, dry throat, abdominal pain, stuffy nose.

ADVERSE REACTIONS/ TOXIC EFFECTS

Worsening of angle-closure glaucoma, acute eye pain, and hypotension occur rarely.

NURSING CONSIDERATIONS

BASELINE ASSESSMENT

Offer emotional support (high incidence of anxiety due to difficulty in breathing, sympathomimetic response to drug).

INTERVENTION/EVALUATION

Monitor rate, depth, rhythm, type of respiration; quality, rate of pulse. Assess lung sounds for rhonchi, wheezing, rales. Monitor ABGs. Observe lips, fingernails for cyanosis (blue or dusky color in light-skinned patients; gray in dark-skinned patients). Observe for clavicular, sternal, intercostal retractions, hand tremor. Evaluate for clinical improvement (quieter, slower respirations, relaxed facial expression, cessation of retractions).

PATIENT/FAMILY TEACHING

• Increase fluid intake (decreases lung secretion viscosity). • Do not take more than 2 inhalations at any one time (excessive use may produce paradoxical bronchoconstriction or a decreased bronchodilating effect). • Rinsing mouth with water immediately after inhalation may prevent mouth and throat dryness. • Avoid excessive use of caffeine derivatives (chocolate, coffee, tea, cola, cocoa).

irbesartan

ir-beh-**sar**-tan

(Avapro)

FIXED-COMBINATION(S)

Avalide: irbesartan/hydrochlorothiazide (a diuretic): 150 mg/12.5 mg; 300 mg/12.5 mg, 300 mg/25 mg.

CLASSIFICATION

PHARMACOTHERAPEUTIC: Angiotensin II receptor antagonist. **CLINICAL:** Antihypertensive (see p. 8C).

ACTION

An angiotensin II receptor, type AT_1, antagonist that blocks the vasoconstrictor and aldosterone-secreting effects of angiotensin II, inhibiting the binding of angiotensin II to the AT_1 receptors. **Therapeutic Effect:** Causes vasodilation, decreases peripheral resistance, and decreases BP.

PHARMACOKINETICS

Rapidly and completely absorbed after PO administration. Protein binding: 90%. Undergoes hepatic metabolism to inactive metabolite. Recovered primarily in feces and, to a lesser extent, in urine. Not removed by hemodialysis. **Half-life:** 11–15 hr.

USES

Treatment of hypertension alone or in combination with other antihypertensives. Treatment of diabetic nephropathy. **OFF-LABEL:** Treatment of atrial fibrillation, CHF.

PRECAUTIONS

CONTRAINDICATIONS: Bilateral renal artery stenosis, biliary cirrhosis or obstruction, primary hyperaldosteronism, severe hepatic insufficiency. **CAUTIONS:** Mild to moderate hepatic dysfunction, sodium/water depletion, CHF, unilateral renal artery stenosis, coronary artery disease.

⧖ **LIFESPAN CONSIDERATIONS: Pregnancy/Lactation:** Unknown if drug is distributed in breast milk. May cause fetal or neonatal morbidity or mortality. **Pregnancy Category C (D if used in second or third trimester). Children:** Safety and efficacy not established. **Elderly:** No age-related precautions noted.

INTERACTIONS

DRUG: Diuretics: Produce additive hypotensive effects. **HERBAL:** None known. **FOOD:** None known. **LAB VALUES:** May slightly increase BUN and serum creatinine levels. May decrease blood Hgb level.

AVAILABILITY (Rx)

TABLETS: 75 mg, 150 mg, 300 mg.

ADMINISTRATION/HANDLING

PO

• Give without regard to meals.

INDICATIONS/ROUTES/DOSAGE

HYPERTENSION ALONE OR IN COMBINATION WITH OTHER ANTIHYPERTENSIVES

PO: ADULTS, ELDERLY, CHILDREN 13 YR AND OLDER: Initially, 75–150 mg/day. May increase to 300 mg/day. CHILDREN

6–12 YR: Initially, 75 mg/day. May increase to 150 mg/day.

NEPHROPATHY
PO: ADULTS, ELDERLY: Target dose of 300 mg/day.

SIDE EFFECTS

OCCASIONAL (9%–3%): Upper respiratory tract infection, fatigue, diarrhea, cough. **RARE (2%–1%):** Heartburn, dizziness, headache, nausea, rash.

ADVERSE REACTIONS/ TOXIC EFFECTS

Overdosage may manifest as hypotension and tachycardia. Bradycardia occurs less often.

BASELINE ASSESSMENT
Obtain BP, apical pulse immediately before each dose, in addition to regular monitoring (be alert to fluctuations). If excessive reduction in BP occurs, place patient in supine position, feet slightly elevated. Question possibility of pregnancy (see Pregnancy Category). Assess medication history (especially diuretic therapy).

INTERVENTION/EVALUATION
Maintain hydration (offer fluids frequently). Assess for evidence of upper respiratory infection. Assist with ambulation if dizziness occurs. Monitor electrolytes, renal and liver function tests, urinalysis, BP, pulse. Assess for hypotension.

PATIENT/FAMILY TEACHING
• Inform female patient regarding consequences of second- and third-trimester exposure to irbesartan. • Avoid tasks that require alertness, motor skills until response to drug is established (possible dizziness effect). • Report any sign of infection (sore throat, fever). • Caution against exercising during hot weather (risk of dehydration, hypotension).

irinotecan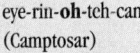

eye-rin-**oh**-tch-can
(Camptosar)

♦ CLASSIFICATION

PHARMACOTHERAPEUTIC: DNA topoisomerase inhibitor. **CLINICAL:** Antineoplastic (see p. 75C).

ACTION

A DNA topoisomerase inhibitor that inhibits the action of topoisomerase I, an enzyme that allows DNA replication by producing reversible single-strand breaks in DNA that relieve torsional strain. Irinotecan prevents religation of the DNA strand, resulting in damage to double-strand DNA and cell death. Therapeutic Effect: Kills cancer cells.

PHARMACOKINETICS

Metabolized to active metabolite in the liver after IV administration. Protein binding: 95% (metabolite). Excreted in urine and eliminated by biliary route. Half-life: 6 hr; metabolite, 10 hr.

USES

Treatment of metastatic carcinoma of colon or rectum in patients whose disease has recurred or progressed after 5-fluorouracil-based therapy. OFF-LABEL: Non–small cell lung cancer, refractory solid tumor configuration, untreated rhabdomyosarcoma.

PRECAUTIONS

CONTRAINDICATIONS: None known.
CAUTIONS: Patient previously receiving pelvic or abdominal irradiation (increased risk of myelosuppression), elderly older than 65 yr.

⚡ LIFESPAN CONSIDERATIONS: **Pregnancy/Lactation:** May cause fetal harm. Unknown if distributed in breast milk; discontinue breast-feeding. **Pregnancy Category C (first trimester), D (second and third trimester). Children:** Safety and efficacy not established. **Elderly:** Risk of diarrhea significantly increased.

INTERACTIONS

DRUG: **Diuretics:** May increase the risk of dehydration from vomiting and diarrhea. **Laxatives:** May increase the severity of diarrhea. **Live virus vaccines:** May potentiate virus replication, increase vaccine side effects, and decrease the patient's antibody response to the vaccine. **Other bone marrow depressants:** May increase the risk of myelosuppression. **Prochlorperazine:** May increase akathisia. HERBAL: **St. John's wort:** May decrease irinotecan effectiveness. FOOD: None known. LAB VALUES: May increase serum alkaline phosphatase and AST levels.

AVAILABILITY (Rx)

INJECTION: 20 mg/ml.

ADMINISTRATION/HANDLING

IV

Reconstitution • Dilute in D_5W (preferred) or 0.9% NaCl to concentration of 0.12 to 1.1 mg/ml.

Rate of administration • Administer all doses as IV infusion over 90 min. • Assess for extravasation (flush site with sterile water, apply ice if extravasation occurs).

Storage • Store vials at room temperature, protect from light. • Solution diluted in D_5W is stable for 48 hr if refrigerated. • Use within 24 hr if refrigerated or 6 hr if kept at room temperature. • Do not refrigerate solution if diluted with 0.9% NaCl.

IV INCOMPATIBILITY

Gemcitabine (Gemzar).

INDICATIONS/ROUTES/DOSAGE

CARCINOMA OF THE COLON OR RECTUM THAT HAS PROGRESSED OR RECURRED AFTER TREATMENT WITH 5-FLUOROURACIL

IV: ADULTS, ELDERLY: Initially, 125 mg/m^2 once weekly for 4 wk, followed by a rest period of 2 wk. Additional courses may be repeated q6wk. Dosage may be adjusted in 25–50 mg/m^2 increments to as high as 150 mg/m^2 or as low as 50 mg/m^2.

SIDE EFFECTS

EXPECTED: Nausea (64%), alopecia (49%), vomiting (45%), diarrhea (32%). **FREQUENT:** Constipation, fatigue (29%); fever (28%); asthenia (25%); skeletal pain (23%); abdominal pain, dyspnea (22%). **OCCASIONAL:** Anorexia (19%); headache, stomatitis (18%); rash (16%).

ADVERSE REACTIONS/TOXIC EFFECTS

Myelosuppression characterized as neutropenia occurs in 97% of patients; severe neutropenia—neutrophil count less than 50/mm^3—occurs in 78% of patients. Thrombocytopenia, anemia, and sepsis are common reactions.

NURSING CONSIDERATIONS

BASELINE ASSESSMENT

Offer emotional support to patient and family. Assess hydration status, electrolytes, CBC before each dose. Premedicate with antiemetics on day of treatment, starting at least 30 min before administration.

INTERVENTION/EVALUATION

Assess for early signs of diarrhea (preceded by complaints of diaphoresis, abdominal cramping). Monitor hydration status, I&O, electrolytes, CBC, Hgb, platelets. Monitor infusion site for signs of inflammation. Inform patient of possibility of alopecia. Assess skin for evidence of rash.

PATIENT/FAMILY TEACHING

• Inform patient of possible late diarrhea causing dehydration, electrolyte depletion. • Provide antiemetic and antidiarrheal regimen for subsequent use. • Do not have immunizations without physician's approval (drug lowers body's resistance). • Avoid contact with those who have recently received live virus vaccine. • Avoid crowds, those with infections.

iron dextran

iron **dex**-tran
(DexFerrum, Dexiron ♣, Infed, Infufer ♣)

◆ CLASSIFICATION

PHARMACOTHERAPEUTIC: Trace element. **CLINICAL:** Hematinic iron preparation.

ACTION

A trace element and essential component in the formation of Hgb. Necessary for effective erythropoiesis and transport and utilization of oxygen. Serves as cofactor of several essential enzymes. **Therapeutic Effect:** Replenishes Hgb and depleted iron stores.

PHARMACOKINETICS

Readily absorbed after IM administration. Most absorption occurs within 72 hr; remainder within 3–4 wk. Bound to protein to form hemosiderin, ferritin, or transferrin. No physiologic system of elimination. Small amounts lost daily in shedding of skin, hair, and nails and in feces, urine, and perspiration. **Half-life:** 5–20 hr.

USES

Treatment of established iron deficiency anemia. Use only when PO administration is not feasible or when rapid replenishment of iron is warranted.

PRECAUTIONS

CONTRAINDICATIONS: All anemias except iron deficiency anemia, including pernicious, aplastic, normocytic, and refractory. **EXTREME CAUTION:** Serious hepatic impairment. **CAUTIONS:** History of allergies, bronchial asthma, rheumatoid arthritis.

⌛ **LIFESPAN CONSIDERATIONS: Pregnancy/Lactation:** May cross placenta in some form (unknown). Trace distributed in breast milk. **Pregnancy Category C. Children/Elderly:** No age-related precautions noted.

INTERACTIONS

DRUG: None known. **HERBAL:** None known. **FOOD:** None known. **LAB VALUES:** None known.

AVAILABILITY (Rx)

INJECTION (DEXFERRUM, INFED): 50 mg/ml.

ADMINISTRATION/HANDLING

◀ **ALERT** ▶ Test dose is generally given before the full dosage; monitor patient for several minutes after injection due to potential for anaphylactic reaction.

 IV

Reconstitution • May give undiluted or dilute in 0.9% NaCl for infusion.

Rate of administration • Do not exceed IV administration rate of 50 mg/min (1 ml/min). A too rapid IV rate may produce flushing, chest pain, shock, hypotension, tachycardia. • Patient must remain recumbent 30–45 min after IV administration (minimizes postural hypotension).

Storage • Store at room temperature.

IM
• Draw up medication with one needle; use new needle for injection (minimizes

skin staining). • Administer deep IM in upper outer quadrant of buttock only. • Use Z-tract technique (displacement of subcutaneous tissue lateral to injection site before inserting needle) to minimize skin staining.

IV INCOMPATIBILITIES
No information available via Y-site administration.

INDICATIONS/ROUTES/DOSAGE
IRON DEFICIENCY ANEMIA (NO BLOOD LOSS)
Dosage is expressed in terms of milligrams of elemental iron, degree of anemia, patient weight, and presence of any bleeding. Expect to use periodic hematologic determinations as guide to therapy.
IV, IM: ADULTS, ELDERLY: Mg iron = 0.66 × weight (kg) × (100 − Hgb [g/dl])/14.8.

IRON REPLACEMENT SECONDARY TO BLOOD LOSS
IV, IM: ADULTS, ELDERLY: Replacement iron (mg) = blood loss (ml) times Hct.

MAXIMUM DAILY DOSAGES
ADULTS WEIGHING MORE THAN 50 KG: 100 mg.
CHILDREN WEIGHING 10–50 KG: 100 mg.
CHILDREN WEIGHING 5–LESS THAN 10 KG: 50 mg.
INFANTS WEIGHING LESS THAN 5 KG: 25 mg.

SIDE EFFECTS
FREQUENT: Allergic reaction (such as rash and itching), backache, myalgia, chills, dizziness, headache, fever, nausea, vomiting, flushed skin, pain or redness at injection site, brown discoloration of skin, metallic taste.

ADVERSE REACTIONS/TOXIC EFFECTS
Anaphylaxis has occurred during the first few minutes after injection, causing death rarely. Leukocytosis and lymphadenopathy occur rarely.

NURSING CONSIDERATIONS
BASELINE ASSESSMENT
Do not give concurrently with oral iron form (excessive iron may produce excessive iron storage [hemosiderosis]). Be alert to patients with rheumatoid arthritis or iron deficiency anemia (acute exacerbation of joint pain or swelling may occur). Inguinal lymphadenopathy may occur with IM injection. Assess for adequate muscle mass before injecting medication.

INTERVENTION/EVALUATION
Monitor IM site for abscess formation, necrosis, atrophy, swelling, brownish color to skin. Question patientt regarding soreness, pain, inflammation at or near IM injection site. Check IV site for phlebitis. Monitor serum ferritin levels.

PATIENT/FAMILY TEACHING
• Pain, brown staining may occur at injection site. • Oral iron should not be taken when receiving iron injections. • Stools often become black with iron therapy; this is harmless unless accompanied by red streaking, sticky consistency of stool, abdominal pain or cramping, which should be reported to physician. • Oral hygiene, hard candy, gum may reduce metallic taste. • Notify physician immediately if fever, back pain, headache occur.

iron sucrose
iron **sue**-crose
(Venofer)

CLASSIFICATION
PHARMACOTHERAPEUTIC: Trace element. **CLINICAL:** Hematinic iron preparation.

ACTION

A trace element that is an essential component in the formation of Hgb. It's necessary for effective erythropoiesis and oxygen transport capacity of blood, and transport and utilization of oxygen, and serves as cofactor of several essential enzymes. **Therapeutic Effect:** Replenishes body iron stores in patients who have iron deficiency anemia.

PHARMACOKINETICS

Distributed mainly in blood and to some extent in extravascular fluid. Iron sucrose is dissociated into iron and sucrose by the reticuloendothelial system. The sucrose component is eliminated mainly by urinary excretion. **Half-life:** 6 hr.

USES

Treatment of iron deficiency anemia in patients undergoing chronic hemodialysis or peritoneal dialysis who are receiving supplemental erythropoietin therapy. Treatment of iron deficiency anemia in patients with chronic kidney disease who are not undergoing dialysis. **OFF-LABEL:** Treatment of dystrophic epidermolysis bullosa.

PRECAUTIONS

CONTRAINDICATIONS: All anemias except iron deficiency anemia, including pernicious, aplastic, normocytic, and refractory anemia; evidence of iron overload. **CAUTIONS:** History of allergies, bronchial asthma; hepatic or renal or cardiac dysfunction.

LIFESPAN CONSIDERATIONS: Pregnancy/Lactation: Unknown if drug crosses placenta or is distributed in breast milk. **Pregnancy Category B. Children:** Safety and efficacy not established. **Elderly:** Age-related renal impairment may require dosage adjustment.

INTERACTIONS

DRUG: Oral iron preparations: May reduce the absorption of these preparations. **HERBAL:** None known. **FOOD:** None known. **LAB VALUES:** Increases Hgb and Hct, serum ferritin level, and serum transferrin saturation.

AVAILABILITY (Rx)

INJECTION: 20 mg/ml or 100 mg elemental iron in 5-ml single-dose vial.

ADMINISTRATION/HANDLING

◄ ALERT ► Administer directly into dialysis line during hemodialysis.

 IV

Reconstitution • May give undiluted as slow IV injection or IV infusion. For IV infusion, dilute each vial in maximum of 100 ml 0.9% NaCl immediately before infusion.

Rate of administration • For IV injection, administer into the dialysis line at a rate of 1 ml (20 mg iron) undiluted solution per min (5 min per vial). Do not exceed 1 vial per injection. **•** For IV infusion, administer into dialysis line (reduces risk of hypotensive episodes) at a rate of 100 mg iron over at least 15 min.

Storage • Store at room temperature.

IV INCOMPATIBILITIES

Do not mix with other medications or add to parenteral nutrition solution for IV infusion.

INDICATIONS/ROUTES/DOSAGE

IRON DEFICIENCY ANEMIA

Dosage is expressed in terms of milligrams of elemental iron.
IV: ADULTS, ELDERLY: 5 ml iron sucrose, or 100 mg elemental iron, delivered during dialysis; administer 1–3 times a wk to total dose of 1,000 mg in 10 doses. Give no more than 3 times a wk.

SIDE EFFECTS

FREQUENT (36%–23%): Hypotension, leg cramps, diarrhea.

ADVERSE REACTIONS/ TOXIC EFFECTS

Too rapid IV administration may produce severe hypotension, headache, vomiting, nausea, dizziness, paresthesia, abdominal and muscle pain, edema, and cardiovascular collapse. Hypersensitivity reaction occurs rarely.

NURSING CONSIDERATIONS

INTERVENTION/EVALUATION

Initially, monitor Hgb, Hct, serum ferritin, serum transferrin levels monthly then q2–3mo thereafter. Reliable serum iron values can be obtained 48 hr following administration.

isoetharine

(Bronkosol)
See Bronchodilators

isoflurophate

(Floropryl)
See Antiglaucoma agents

isoniazid

eye-**soe**-nye-a-zid
(INH, Isotamine ♣, Nydrazid, PMS Isoniazid ♣)

FIXED-COMBINATION(S)

Rifamate: isoniazid/rifampin (antitubercular): 150 mg/300 mg.
Rifater: isoniazid/pyrazinamide/rifampin (antitubercular): 50 mg/300 mg/120 mg.

◆CLASSIFICATION

PHARMACOTHERAPEUTIC: Isonicotinic acid derivative. **CLINICAL:** Antitubercular.

ACTION

An isonicotinic acid derivative that inhibits mycolic acid synthesis and causes disruption of the bacterial cell wall and loss of acid-fast properties in susceptible mycobacteria. Active only during bacterial cell division. **Therapeutic Effect:** Bactericidal against actively growing intracelleluar and extracellular susceptible mycobacteria.

PHARMACOKINETICS

Readily absorbed from the GI tract. Protein binding: 10%–15%. Widely distributed (including to CSF). Metabolized in the liver. Primarily excreted in urine. Removed by hemodialysis. **Half-life:** 0.5-5 hr.

USES

Treatment of susceptible mycobacterial infection due to *M. tuberculosis* and prophylactically due to exposure to tuberculosis.

PRECAUTIONS

CONTRAINDICATIONS: Acute hepatic disease, history of hypersensitivity reactions or hepatic injury with previous isoniazid therapy. **CAUTIONS:** Chronic hepatic disease, alcoholism, severe renal impairment. May be cross-sensitive with nicotinic acid, other chemically related medications.

⚠ LIFESPAN CONSIDERATIONS: **Pregnancy/Lactation:** Prophylaxis usually postponed until after delivery. Crosses placenta. Distributed in breast milk. **Pregnancy Category C. Children:** No age-related precautions noted. **Elderly:** More susceptible to developing hepatitis.

INTERACTIONS

DRUG: Alcohol: May increase isoniazid metabolism and the risk of hepatotoxicity. **Carbamazepine, Phenytoin:** May increase the toxicity of these drugs. **Disulfiram:** May increase CNS effects. **Hepatotoxic medications:** May increase the risk of hepatotoxicity. **Ketoconazole:** May decrease ketoconazole blood concentration. **HERBAL:** None known. **FOOD: Tyramine-containing foods:** May cause a hypertensive crisis. **LAB VALUES:** May increase serum bilirubin, AST, and ALT levels.

AVAILABILITY (Rx)

TABLETS: 100 mg, 300 mg. **SYRUP:** 50 mg/5 ml. **INJECTION (NYDRAZID):** 100 mg/ml.

ADMINISTRATION/HANDLING

PO
• Give 1 hr before or 2 hr following meals (may give with food to decrease GI upset, but will delay absorption).
• Administer at least 1 hr before antacids, especially those containing aluminum.

INDICATIONS/ROUTES/DOSAGE

TUBERCULOSIS (IN COMBINATION WITH ONE OR MORE ANTITUBERCULARS)
PO, IM: ADULTS, ELDERLY: 5 mg/kg/day as a single dose. **Maximum:** 300 mg/day. CHILDREN: 10–15 mg/kg/day as a single dose. **Maximum:** 300 mg/day.

PREVENTION OF TUBERCULOSIS
PO, IM: ADULTS, ELDERLY: 300 mg/day as a single dose. CHILDREN: 10 mg/kg/day as a single dose. **Maximum:** 300 mg/day.

SIDE EFFECTS

FREQUENT: Nausea, vomiting, diarrhea, abdominal pain. **RARE:** Pain at injection site, hypersensitivity reaction.

ADVERSE REACTIONS/ TOXIC EFFECTS

Rare reactions include neurotoxicity (as evidenced by ataxia and paraesthesia), optic neuritis, and hepatotoxicity.

NURSING CONSIDERATIONS

BASELINE ASSESSMENT
Question for history of hypersensitivity reactions, hepatic injury from isoniazid, sensitivity to nicotinic acid or chemically related medications. Ensure collection of specimens for culture, sensitivity. Evaluate initial hepatic function results.

INTERVENTION/EVALUATION
Monitor liver function test results and assess for hepatitis: anorexia, nausea, vomiting, weakness, fatigue, dark urine, jaundice (hold INH and inform physician promptly). Assess for paraesthesia of extremities (those especially at risk for neuropathy may be given pyridoxine prophylactically: malnourished, elderly, diabetics, patients with chronic hepatic disease [including alcoholics]). Be alert for fever, skin eruptions (hypersensitivity reaction).

PATIENT/FAMILY TEACHING
• Do not skip doses; continue taking isoniazid for full length of therapy (6–24 mo). • Take preferably 1 hr before or 2 hr following meals (with food if GI upset). • Avoid alcohol during treatment. • Do not take any other medications, including antacids, without consulting physician. • Must take isoniazid at least 1 hr before antacid. • Avoid tuna, sauerkraut, aged cheeses, smoked fish (provide list of tyramine-containing foods) that may cause reaction such as red or itching skin, palpitations, lightheadedness, hot or clammy feeling, headache; contact physician. • Notify physician of any new symptom, immediately for vision difficulties, nausea or vomiting, dark urine, yellowing of skin or eyes (jaundice), fatigue, paraesthesia of extremities.

isoproterenol

(Isuprel)

See Sympathomimetics

isosorbide dinitrate

eye-sew-**sore**-bide

(Apo-ISDN ✿, Cedocard ✿, Dilatrate, Dilatrate-SR, ISDN, Isochron, Isordil, Isordil Tembids, Isordil Titradose, Sorbitrate)

isosorbide mononitrate

(Imdur, ISMO, Monoket)

Do not confuse Isordil with Isuprel or Plendil, or Imdur with Inderal or K-Dur.

FIXED-COMBINATION(S)

BiDil: isosorbide/hydralazine, (a vasodilator): 20 mg/37.5 mg.

CLASSIFICATION

PHARMACOTHERAPEUTIC: Nitrate. **CLINICAL:** Antianginal (see p. 114C).

ACTION

A nitrate that stimulates intracellular cyclic guanosine monophosphate. **Therapeutic Effect:** Relaxes vascular smooth muscle of both arterial and venous vasculature. Decreases preload and afterload.

PHARMACOKINETICS

Route	Onset	Peak	Duration
Dinitrate			
Sublingual	2–5 min	N/A	1–2 hr
Oral (Chewable)	2–5 min	N/A	1–2 hr
Oral	15–40 min	N/A	4–6 hr
Oral (Sustained-Release)	30 min	N/A	12 hr
Mononitrate			
Oral (Extended-Release)	60 min	N/A	N/A

Dinitrate poorly absorbed and metabolized in the liver to its activate metabolite isosorbide mononitrate. Mononitrate well absorbed after PO administration. Excreted in urine and feces. **Half-life:** Dinitrate, 1–4 hr; mononitrate, 4 hr.

USES

Prophylaxis, treatment of angina pectoris. **OFF-LABEL:** CHF, dysphagia, pain relief, relief of esophageal spasm with gastroesophageal reflux.

PRECAUTIONS

CONTRAINDICATIONS: Closed-angle glaucoma, GI hypermotility or malabsorption (extended-release tablets), head trauma, hypersensitivity to nitrates, increased intracranial pressure, orthostatic hypotension, severe anemia (extended-release tablets). **CAUTIONS:** Acute MI, hepatic or renal disease, glaucoma (contraindicated in closed-angle glaucoma), blood volume depletion from diuretic therapy, systolic BP less than 90 mm Hg.

⧖ **LIFESPAN CONSIDERATIONS: Pregnancy/Lactation:** Unknown if drug crosses placenta or is distributed in breast milk. **Pregnancy Category C. Children:** Safety and efficacy not established. **Elderly:** May be more sensitive to hypotensive effects. Age-related renal impairment may require dosage adjustment.

INTERACTIONS

DRUG: Alcohol, antihypertensives, vasodilators: May increase risk of orthostatic hypotension. **HERBAL:** None known. **FOOD:** None known. **LAB VALUES:** May increase urine

---

🖊 see color pill atlas   🌿 herb   underlined – top prescribed drug

catecholamine and urine vanillylmandelic acid levels.

AVAILABILITY (Rx)

CAPSULES (SUSTAINED-RELEASE [DILATRATE, ISORDIL TEMBIDS]): 40 mg. **TABLETS:** 5 mg (ISDN, Isordil, Isordil Titradose), 10 mg (ISDN, ISMO, Isordil, Isordil Titradose, Monoket), 20 mg (ISDN, ISMO, Isordil, Isordil Titradose, Monoket), 30 mg (ISDN, Isordil, Isordil Titradose), 40 mg (ISDN, Isordil, Isordil Titradose). **TABLETS (CHEWABLE [SORBITRATE]):** 5 mg, 10 mg. **TABLETS (EXTENDED-RELEASE [IMDUR]):** 30 mg, 60 mg, 120 mg. **TABLETS (SUBLINGUAL [ISORDIL]):** 2.5 mg, 5 mg, 10 mg.

ADMINISTRATION/HANDLING

PO
• Best if taken on an empty stomach. • Oral tablets may be crushed. • Do not crush or break sublingual or extended-release form. • Do not crush chewable form before administering.

SUBLINGUAL
• Do not crush or chew sublingual tablets. • Dissolve tablets under tongue; do not swallow.

INDICATIONS/ROUTES/DOSAGE

ANGINA
PO (ISOSORBIDE DINITRATE): ADULTS, ELDERLY: 5–40 mg 4 times a day. **Sustained-release:** 40 mg q8–12h. **PO (ISOSORBIDE MONONITRATE):** ADULTS, ELDERLY: 5–10 mg twice a day given 7 hr apart. **Sustained-release:** Initially, 30–60 mg/day in morning as a single dose. May increase dose at 3 day intervals. **Maximum:** 240 mg/day.

SIDE EFFECTS

FREQUENT: Burning and tingling at oral point of dissolution (sublingual), headache (possibly severe) occurs mostly in early therapy, diminishes rapidly in intensity, and usually disappears during continued treatment, transient flushing of face and neck, dizziness (especially if patient is standing immobile or is in a warm environment), weakness, orthostatic hypotension, nausea, vomiting, restlessness. **OCCASIONAL:** GI upset, blurred vision, dry mouth.

ADVERSE REACTIONS/ TOXIC EFFECTS

Blurred vision or dry mouth may occur (drug should be discontinued). Isosorbide administration may cause severe orthostatic hypotension manifested by fainting, pulselessness, cold or clammy skin, and diaphoresis. Tolerance may occur with repeated, prolonged therapy, but may not occur with the extended-release form. Minor tolerance may be seen with intermittent use of sublingual tablets. High dosage tends to produce severe headache.

NURSING CONSIDERATIONS

BASELINE ASSESSMENT
Record onset, type (sharp, dull, squeezing), radiation, location, intensity, duration of anginal pain; precipitating factors (exertion, emotional stress). If headache occurs during management therapy, administer medication with meals.

INTERVENTION/EVALUATION
Assist with ambulation if lightheadedness, dizziness occurs. Assess for facial or neck flushing. Monitor number of anginal episodes, orthostatic BP.

PATIENT/FAMILY TEACHING
• Do not chew or crush sublingual or sustained-release forms. • Take sublingual tablets while sitting down. • Notify physician if angina persists for longer than 20 min. • Rise slowly from lying to sitting position, dangle legs momentarily before standing. • Take oral form on empty stomach (however, if headache occurs during management therapy,

take medication with meals). • Dissolve sublingual tablet under tongue; do not swallow. • Take at first signal of angina. • If pain not relieved within 5 min, dissolve second tablet under tongue. • Repeat if no relief in another 5 min. • If pain continues, contact physician. • Expel from mouth any remaining sublingual tablet after pain is completely relieved. • Do not change from one brand of drug to another. • Avoid alcohol (intensifies hypotensive effect). • If alcohol is ingested soon after taking nitrates, possible acute hypotensive episode (marked drop in BP, vertigo, pallor) may occur.

---

isotretinoin

eye-sew-**tret**-ih-noyn

(Accutane, Amnesteem, Claravis, Sotret)

Do not confuse Accutane with Accupril or Accurbron.

CLASSIFICATION

PHARMACOTHERAPEUTIC: Keratinization stabilizer. **CLINICAL:** Anti-acne, antirosacea agent.

ACTION

Reduces sebaceous gland size, inhibiting its activity. **Therapeutic Effect:** Produces antikeratinizing, anti-inflammatory effects.

USES

Treatment of severe, recalcitrant cystic acne that is unresponsive to conventional acne therapies. **OFF-LABEL:** Treatment of gram-negative folliculitis, severe rosacea, correcting severe keratinization disorders.

PRECAUTIONS

CONTRAINDICATIONS: Hypersensitivity to isotretinoin, parabens (component

of capsules). **CAUTIONS:** Renal/hepatic dysfunction. **Pregnancy Category X.**

INTERACTIONS

DRUG: Etretinate, tretinoin, vitamin A: May increase toxic effects. **Tetracycline:** May increase potential of pseudotumor cerebri. **HERBAL: Dong quai, St. John's wort:** May cause photosensitization. **FOOD:** None known. **LAB VALUES:** May increase serum triglycerides, cholesterol, AST, ALT, alkaline phosphatase, LDH, sedimentation rate, fasting blood glucose, uric acid; may decrease HDL.

AVAILABILITY (Rx)

CAPSULES: Accutane, Amnesteem, Claravis: 10 mg, 20 mg, 40 mg; Sotret: 10 mg, 20 mg, 30 mg, 40 mg.

INDICATIONS/ROUTES/DOSAGE

RECALCITRANT CYSTIC ACNE

PO: ADULTS: Initially, 0.5–2 mg/kg/day divided in 2 doses for 15–20 wk. May repeat after at least 2 mo of therapy.

SIDE EFFECTS

FREQUENT: Cheilitis (inflammation of lips) (90%), skin/mucous membrane dryness (80%), skin fragility, pruritus, epistaxis, dry nose/mouth, conjunctivitis (40%), hypertriglyceridemia (25%), nausea, vomiting, abdominal pain (20%). **OCCASIONAL (3%–2%):** Musculoskeletal symptoms (16%) including bone or joint pain, arthralgia, generalized muscle aches; photosensitivity (10%–5%). **RARE:** Diminished night vision, depression.

ADVERSE REACTIONS/ TOXIC EFFECTS

Inflammatory bowel disease, pseudotumor cerebri (benign intracranial hypertension) have been associated with isotretinoin therapy.

NURSING CONSIDERATIONS

BASELINE ASSESSMENT

Assess baselines for blood glucose, lipids.

INTERVENTION/EVALUATION

Assess acne for decreased cysts. Evaluate skin/mucous membranes for excessive dryness. Monitor blood glucose, lipid levels.

PATIENT/FAMILY TEACHING

• Transient exacerbation of acne may occur during initial period. • May have decreased tolerance to contact lenses during and following therapy. • Do not take vitamin supplements with vitamin A due to additive effects. • Immediately notify physician of onset of abdominal pain, severe diarrhea, rectal bleeding (possible inflammatory bowel disease), headache, nausea/vomiting, visual disturbances (possible pseudotumor cerebri). • Diminished night vision may occur suddenly; take caution with night driving. • Avoid prolonged exposure to sunlight; use sunscreens, protective clothing. • Do not donate blood during or for 1 mo following treatment. • **Women:** Explain the serious risk to fetus if pregnancy occurs (both oral and written warnings are given, with patient acknowledging in writing that she understands the warnings and consents to treatment). • Must have a negative serum pregnancy test within 2 wk before starting therapy; therapy will begin on the second or third day of the next normal menstrual period. • Effective contraception (using 2 reliable forms of contraception simultaneously) must be used for at least 1 mo before, during, and for at least 1 mo after therapy.

isradipine

iss-**rah**-dih-peen
(DynaCirc, DynaCirc CR)

Do not confuse DynaCirc with Dynabac or Dynacin.

CLASSIFICATION

PHARMACOTHERAPEUTIC: Calcium channel blocker. **CLINICAL:** Antihypertensive (see p. 69C).

ACTION

An antihypertensive that inhibits calcium movement across cardiac and vascular smooth-muscle cell membranes. Potent peripheral vasodilator that does not depress SA or AV nodes. **Therapeutic Effect:** Produces relaxation of coronary vascular smooth muscle and coronary vasodilation. Increases myocardial oxygen delivery to those with vasospastic angina.

PHARMACOKINETICS

Route	Onset	Peak	Duration
PO	2–3 hr	2–4 wk (with multiple doses) 8–16 hr (with single dose)	N/A
PO (Controlled-release)	2 hr	8–10 hr	N/A

Well absorbed from the GI tract. Protein binding: 95%. Metabolized in the liver (undergoes first-pass effect). Primarily excreted in urine. Not removed by hemodialysis. **Half-life:** 8 hr.

USES

Management of hypertension. May be used alone or with thiazide-type diuretics. **OFF-LABEL:** Treatment of chronic angina pectoris, Raynaud's phenomenon.

PRECAUTIONS

CONTRAINDICATIONS: Cardiogenic shock, CHF, heart block, hypotension, sinus bradycardia, ventricular tachycardia. **CAUTIONS:** Sick sinus syndrome; severe left ventricular dysfunction; hepatic disease; edema; concurrent therapy with beta-blockers.

⧗ **LIFESPAN CONSIDERATIONS: Pregnancy/Lactation:** Unknown if drug crosses placenta or is distributed in breast milk. **Pregnancy Category C. Children:** Safety and efficacy not established. **Elderly:** Age-related renal impairment may require dosage adjustment.

INTERACTIONS

DRUG: Beta blockers: May have additive effect. **HERBAL:** None known. **FOOD: Grapefruit, grapefruit juice:** May increase the absorption of isradipine. **LAB VALUES:** None known.

AVAILABILITY (Rx)

CAPSULES (DYNACIRC): 2.5 mg, 5 mg.
CAPSULES (CONTROLLED-RELEASE [DYNACIRC-CR]): 5 mg, 10 mg.

ADMINISTRATION/HANDLING

PO
• Do not crush or break capsule.

INDICATIONS/ROUTES/DOSAGE

HYPERTENSION
PO: ADULTS, ELDERLY: Initially 2.5 mg twice a day. May increase by 2.5 mg at 2- to 4-wk intervals. Range: 5–20 mg/day.

SIDE EFFECTS

FREQUENT (7%–4%): Peripheral edema, palpitations (higher frequency in females). **OCCASIONAL (3%):** Facial flushing, cough. **RARE (2%–1%):** Angina, tachycardia, rash, pruritus.

ADVERSE REACTIONS/ TOXIC EFFECTS

Overdose produces nausea, drowsiness, confusion, and slurred speech. CHF occurs rarely.

NURSING CONSIDERATIONS

BASELINE ASSESSMENT

Assess baseline renal and liver function tests. Assess BP, apical pulse immediately before drug is administered (if pulse is 60 beats/min or less or systolic BP is less than 90 mm Hg, withhold medication, contact physician).

INTERVENTION/EVALUATION

Assess for peripheral edema behind medial malleolus (sacral area in bedridden patients). Monitor pulse rate for bradycardia. Monitor BP; observe for signs, symptoms of CHF. Assess skin for flushing.

PATIENT/FAMILY TEACHING

• Do not abruptly discontinue medication. Compliance with therapy regimen is essential to control hypertension.
• To avoid hypotensive effect, rise slowly from lying to sitting position, wait momentarily before standing.
• Contact physician or nurse if palpitations, shortness of breath, pronounced dizziness, nausea occurs. • Avoid grapefruit or grapefruit juice.

itraconazole

eye-tra-**con**-ah-zoll
(Sporanox)
Do not confuse Sporanox with Suprax.

Safety and efficacy not established. **Elderly:** Age-related renal impairment may require dosage adjustment.

CLASSIFICATION

CLINICAL: Antifungal.

ACTION

A fungistatic antifungal that inhibits the synthesis of ergosterol, a vital component of fungal cell formation. **Therapeutic Effect:** Damages the fungal cell membrane, altering its function.

PHARMACOKINETICS

Moderately absorbed from the GI tract. Absorption is increased if the drug is taken with food. Protein binding: 99%. Widely distributed, primarily in the fatty tissue, liver, and kidneys. Metabolized in the liver to active metabolite. Primarily excreted in urine. Not removed by hemodialysis. **Half-life:** 21 hr; metabolite, 12 hr.

USES

Treatment of aspergillosis, blastomycosis, esophageal and oropharyngeal candidiasis, empiric treatment in febrile neutropenia, histoplasmosis, onychomycosis. **OFF-LABEL:** Suppression of histoplasmosis; treatment of disseminated sporotrichosis, fungal pneumonia and septicemia, or ringworm of the hand.

PRECAUTIONS

CONTRAINDICATIONS: Hypersensitivity to fluconazole, ketoconazole, or miconazole. **CAUTIONS:** Hepatitis, HIV-infected patients, patients with achlorhydria, hypochlorhydria (decreases absorption), hepatic impairment.

LIFESPAN CONSIDERATIONS : Pregnancy/Lactation: Distributed in breast milk. **Pregnancy Category C. Children:** Safety and efficacy not established. **Elderly:** Age-related renal impairment may require dosage adjustment.

INTERACTIONS

DRUG: Antacids, didanosine, H$_2$ antagonists: May decrease itraconazole absorption. **Buspirone, cyclosporine, digoxin, lovastatin, simvastatin:** May increase blood concentration of these drugs. **Oral anticoagulants:** May increase the effect of oral anticoagulants. **Phenytoin, rifampin:** May decrease itraconazole blood concentration. **HERBAL:** None known. **FOOD: Grapefruit, grapefruit juice:** May alter itraconazole absorption. **LAB VALUES:** May increase serum LDH serum alkaline phosphatase, serum bilirubin, AST, and ALT levels. May decrease serum potassium level.

AVAILABILITY (Rx)

CAPSULES: 100 mg. **ORAL SOLUTION:** 10 mg/ml. **INJECTION:** 10 mg/ml (25-ml ampule).

ADMINISTRATION/HANDLING

IV

Reconstitution • Use only components provided by manufacturer. • Do not dilute with any other diluent. • Add full contents of ampule (250 mg/10 ml) to infusion bag provided (50 ml 0.9% NaCl). • Mix gently.

Rate of administration • Infuse over 60 min using extension line and infusion set provided. • After administration, flush infusion set with 15–20 ml 0.9% NaCl over 30 sec to 15 min. • Discard entire infusion line.

Storage • Store at room temperature. Do not freeze.

PO

• Give capsules with food (increases absorption). • Give solution on an empty stomach.

▨ IV INCOMPATIBILITIES

◄ ALERT ► Dilution compatibility of itraconazole with any solution other than 0.9% NaCl is unknown. Don't mix with D₅W or lactated Ringer's solution. Not for IV bolus administration. Don't administer any medication in same bag or through same IV line as itraconazole.

INDICATIONS/ROUTES/DOSAGE

BLASTOMYCOSIS, HISTOPLASMOSIS

PO: ADULTS, ELDERLY: Initially, 200 mg once a day. **Maximum:** 400 mg/day in 2 divided doses.

IV: ADULTS, ELDERLY: 200 mg twice a day for 4 doses, then 200 mg once a day.

ASPERGILLOSIS

PO: ADULTS, ELDERLY: 600 mg/day in 3 divided doses for 3–4 days, then 200–400 mg/day in 2 divided doses.

IV: ADULTS, ELDERLY: 200 mg twice a day for 4 doses, then 200 mg once a day.

ESOPHAGEAL CANDIDIASIS

PO: ADULTS, ELDERLY: Swish 100–200 mg (10–20 ml) in mouth for several seconds, then swallow. **Maximum:** 200 mg/day.

OROPHARYNGEAL CANDIDIASIS

PO: ADULTS, ELDERLY: 200 mg (10 ml) oral solution, swish and swallow once a day for 7–14 days.

FEBRILE NEUTROPENIA

IV: ADULTS, ELDERLY: 200 mg twice a day for 4 doses, then 200 mg for up to 14 days. Then give PO 200 mg twice a day until neutropenia resolves.

ONYCHOMYCOSIS (FINGERNAIL)

PO: ADULTS, ELDERLY: 200 mg twice a day for 7 days, off for 21 days, repeat 200 mg twice a day for 7 days.

ONYCHOMYCOSIS (TOENAIL)

PO: ADULTS, ELDERLY: 200 mg once daily for 12 wk.

SIDE EFFECTS

FREQUENT (11%–9%): Nausea, rash. **OCCASIONAL (5%–3%):** Vomiting, headache, diarrhea, hypertension, peripheral edema, fatigue, fever. **RARE (2% or less):** Abdominal pain, dizziness, anorexia, pruritus.

ADVERSE REACTIONS/ TOXIC EFFECTS

Hepatitis (as evidenced by anorexia, abdominal pain, unusual fatigue or weakness, jaundice skin or sclera, and dark urine) occurs rarely.

NURSING CONSIDERATIONS

BASELINE ASSESSMENT

Determine baseline temperature, liver function tests. Assess allergies.

INTERVENTION/EVALUATION

Assess for signs, symptoms of hepatic dysfunction. Monitor hepatic enzyme test results in patients with preexisting hepatic dysfunction.

PATIENT/FAMILY TEACHING

• Take capsules with food, liquids if GI distress occurs. • Therapy will continue for at least 3 mo, until lab tests, clinical presentation indicate infection is controlled. • Immediately report the following: unusual fatigue, yellow skin, dark urine, pale stool, anorexia, nausea, vomiting. • Avoid grapefruits and grapefruit juice.

Ivanz, *see ertapenem*

Kadian, *see morphine*

Kaletra, *see lopinavir and ritonavir*

kaolin/pectin

kay-oh-lyn

(Kaodene, Kao-Spen, Kapectolin)

Do not confuse kaolin, Kaodene, or Kapectolin with Kayexalate.

FIXED-COMBINATION(S)

Parepectolin: kaolin/pectin/opium: 5.5 g/162 mg/15 mg.

•CLASSIFICATION

PHARMACOTHERAPEUTIC: Magnesium/aluminum silicate. **CLINICAL:** Antidiarrheal (see p. 43C).

ACTION

Adsorbent, protectant. **Therapeutic Effect:** Adsorbs bacteria, toxins; reduces water loss.

PHARMACOKINETICS

Not absorbed orally. Up to 90% of pectin decomposed in GI tract.

USES

Symptomatic treatment of mild to moderate acute diarrhea.

PRECAUTIONS

CONTRAINDICATIONS: None known. **CAUTIONS:** None known.

⧗ LIFESPAN CONSIDERATIONS: **Pregnancy/Lactation:** Unknown if drug crosses placenta or is distributed in breast milk. **Pregnancy Category C.**

Children: Not recommended in those younger than 3 yr. **Elderly:** More sensitive to fluid and electrolyte loss; use caution.

INTERACTIONS

DRUG: Digoxin: Absorption of this drug may decrease when given concurrently with kaolin. **HERBAL:** None known. **FOOD:** None known. **LAB VALUES:** None known.

AVAILABILITY (OTC)

ORAL SUSPENSION.

ADMINISTRATION/HANDLING

PO

• Shake suspension well before administration.

INDICATIONS/ROUTES/DOSAGE

ANTIDIARRHEAL

PO: ADULTS, ELDERLY: 60–120 ml after each loose bowel movement (LBM). CHILDREN 12 YR AND OLDER: 60 ml after each LBM. CHILDREN 6–12 YR: 30–60 ml after each LBM. CHILDREN 3–5 YR: 15–30 ml after each LBM.

SIDE EFFECTS

RARE: Constipation.

ADVERSE REACTIONS/ TOXIC EFFECTS

None known.

NURSING CONSIDERATIONS

INTERVENTION/EVALUATION

Encourage adequate fluid intake. Assess bowel sounds for peristalsis and stools for frequency, consistency.

PATIENT/FAMILY TEACHING

• Do not use for more than 2 days or in presence of high fever.

K

kava kava

Also known as ava, kew, sakau, tonga, yagona.

◄ **ALERT** ► May be removed from market.

◆CLASSIFICATION

HERBAL: See Appendix G.

ACTION

Exact mechanism of action unknown, but possesses CNS effects. **Effect:** Anxiolytic, sedative, analgesic effects.

USES

Treatment of anxiety disorders, stress, restlessness. Also used for sedation, sleep enhancement.

PRECAUTIONS

CONTRAINDICATIONS: Pregnancy, lactation (may cause loss of uterine tone). **CAUTIONS:** Depression, history of recurrent hepatitis.

⧗ **LIFESPAN CONSIDERATIONS: Pregnancy/Lactation:** Contraindicated. **Children:** Safety and efficacy not established. **Elderly:** No age-related precautions noted.

INTERACTIONS

DRUG: Alcohol, benzodiazepines: May increase risk of drowsiness. **HERBAL: Chamomile, goldenseal, melatonin, St. John's wort, ginseng, valerian:** May increase risk of excessive drowsiness. **FOOD:** None known. **LAB VALUES:** May increase hepatic function tests.

AVAILABILITY (OTC)

CAPSULES: 140 mg, 150 mg, 250 mg, 300 mg, 425 mg, 500 mg. **LIQUID. EXTRACT. TINCTURE.**

INDICATIONS/ROUTES/DOSAGE

USUAL DOSAGE

PO: ADULTS, ELDERLY: 100 mg 3 times a day or 1 cup of the tea 3 times a day.

SIDE EFFECTS

GI upset, headache, dizziness, vision changes (blurred vision, red eyes), allergic skin reactions, dermopathy (dry, flaky skin), yellowing, skin, hair, nails, sclera of the eyes, nausea, vomiting, weight loss, shortness of breath.

ADVERSE REACTIONS/ TOXIC EFFECTS

None known.

NURSING CONSIDERATIONS

BASELINE ASSESSMENT

Assess if patient is pregnant or breastfeeding (contraindicated). Determine baseline liver function tests. Assess for use of other CNS depressants.

INTERVENTION/EVALUATION

Monitor liver function tests. Assess for allergic skin reactions.

PATIENT/FAMILY TEACHING

• Avoid use if pregnant, planning to become pregnant, or breast-feeding; not for use in children 12 yr and younger. • Avoid tasks that require alertness, motor skills until response to herbal is established. • Do not use for more than 3 mo (may be habit forming).

Keflex, *see cephalexin*

Kefzol, *see cefazolin*

Keppra, *see levetiracetam*

ketamine

key-tah-meen
(Ketalar)

◆CLASSIFICATION
CLINICAL: Rapid-acting general anesthetic (see p. 2C).

ACTION
A rapidly acting general anesthetic that selectively blocks afferent impulses and interacts with CNS transmitter systems. **Therapeutic Effect:** Produces an anesthetic state characterized by profound analgesia and normal pharyngeal-laryngeal reflexes.

PHARMACOKINETICS

Route	Onset	Peak	Duration
IM (anesthetic)	3–4 min	N/A	12–25 min
IM (analgesic)	30 min	N/A	15–30 min
IV (anesthetic)	30 sec	N/A	5–10 min
IV (analgesic)	10–15 min	N/A	N/A

Rapidly distributed. Metabolized in the liver. Primarily excreted in urine. **Half-life:** Distribution: 10–15 min, elimination: 2–3 hr.

USES
Induction and maintenance of general anesthesia (especially when cardiovascular depression to be avoided), sedation.

PRECAUTIONS
CONTRAINDICATIONS: Aneurysms, angina, CHF, elevated intracranial pressure (ICP), hypertension, psychotic disorders, thyrotoxicosis. **CAUTIONS:** Gastroesophageal reflux disease (GERD), hepatic impairment, patients with a full stomach, chronic alcoholics, acutely intoxicated patients.

⌛ **LIFESPAN CONSIDERATIONS: Pregnancy/Lactation:** Not recommended; safety not established. **Pregnancy Category B. Children/Elderly:** No age-related precautions noted.

INTERACTIONS
DRUG: Antihypertensives, CNS depressants: May increase the risk of hypotension and respiratory depression. **HERBAL:** None known. **FOOD:** None known. **LAB VALUES:** May increase intraocular pressure (IOP).

AVAILABILITY (Rx)
INJECTION: 10 mg/ml, 50 mg/ml, 100 mg/ml.

ADMINISTRATION/HANDLING
🔲 **IV**

Reconstitution • For induction anesthesia using IV push, dilute 100 mg/ml with equal volume sterile water for injection, D₅W, or 0.9% NaCl. • For maintenance IV infusion, dilute 50 mg/ml vial (10 ml) or 100 mg/ml vial (5 ml) to 250–500 ml D₅W or 0.9% NaCl to provide a concentration of 1–2 mg/ml.

Rate of administration • Administer IV push slowly over 60 sec (too rapid IV may produce severe hypotension, respiratory depression). • Administer IV infusion at rate of 0.5 mg/kg/min.

IM
• Use 10 mg/ml vial.

▦ IV INCOMPATIBILITIES
No information available for Y-site administration.

IV COMPATIBILITIES
Bupivacaine (Marcaine), clonidine (Duraclon), fentanyl (Sublimaze), lidocaine, morphine, propofol (Diprivan).

K

INDICATIONS/ROUTES/DOSAGE

INDUCTION AND MAINTENANCE OF GENERAL ANESTHESIA (ESPECIALLY WHEN CARDIOVASCULAR DEPRESSION IS TO BE AVOIDED), SEDATION, ANALGESIA

IV: ADULTS, ELDERLY: 1–4.5 mg/kg. Usual induction dose: 1–2 mg/kg. CHILDREN: 0.5–2 mg/kg. Usual induction dose: 1–2 mg/kg.
IM: ADULTS, ELDERLY: 3–8 mg/kg. CHILDREN: 3–7 mg/kg.

SIDE EFFECTS

FREQUENT: Increased BP and pulse rate; emergence reaction (marked by dreamlike state, delirium, hallucinations, and vivid imagery and occasionally accompanied by confusion, excitement, and irrational behavior; lasts from few hours to 24 hours after ketamine administration). **OCCASIONAL:** Pain at injection site. **RARE:** Rash.

ADVERSE REACTIONS/ TOXIC EFFECTS

Continuous or repeated intermittent infusion may result in extreme somnolence and circulatory or respiratory depression. Too-rapid IV administration of ketamine may produce severe hypotension, respiratory depression, and irregular muscle movements.

NURSING CONSIDERATIONS

BASELINE ASSESSMENT
Resuscitative equipment, O$_2$ must be available. Obtain vital signs before induction.

INTERVENTION/EVALUATION
Monitor vital signs q3–5min during and after administration until recovery is achieved. Assess for emergence reaction (hypnotic or barbiturate may be needed). Keep verbal, tactile, visual stimulation at minimum during recovery.

PATIENT/FAMILY TEACHING
• Avoid tasks that require alertness, motor skills for 24 hr after anesthesia.

Ketek, see telithromycin

ketoconazole

kee-toe-**koe**-na-zole
(Apo-Ketocomazole ✿, Nizoral, Nizoral AD, Nizoral Topical)
Do not confuse Nizoral with Nasarel.

CLASSIFICATION

PHARMACOTHERAPEUTIC: Imidazole derivative. **CLINICAL:** Antifungal (see p. 44C).

ACTION

A fungistatic antifungal that inhibits the synthesis of ergosterol, a vital component of fungal cell formation. **Therapeutic Effect:** Damages the fungal cell membrane, altering its function.

PHARMACOKINETICS

Well absorbed from GI tract following PO administration. Protein binding: 91%–99%. Metabolized in liver. Primarily excreted in bile with minimal elimination in urine. Negligible systemic absorption following topical absorption. Ketoconazole is not detected in plasma after shampooing or topical administration. **Half-life:** 2–12 hr.

USES

Oral: Treatment of histoplasmosis, blastomycosis, candidiasis, chronic mucocutaneous candidiasis, coccidioidomycosis, paracoccidioidomycosis, chromomycosis, seborrheic dermatitis, tineas (ringworm): corporis, capitis, manus, cruris, pedis, unguium (onychomycosis), oral thrush, candiduria. **Shampoo:** Reduces scaling due to dandruff. Treatment of tinea versicolor. **Topical:** Treatment of tineas, pityriasis versicolor, cutaneous candidiasis, seborrhea dermatitis, dandruff. OFF-LABEL: Systemic: Treatment of fungal pneumonia, prostate cancer, septicemia.

PRECAUTIONS

CONTRAINDICATIONS: None known. **CAUTIONS:** Hepatic impairment.

⧗ LIFESPAN CONSIDERATIONS: Pregnancy/Lactation: Oral form distributed in breast milk. Unknown if topical form crosses placena or is distributed in breast milk. **Pregnancy Category C. Children: Cream, shampoo:** Safety and efficacy not established. **Oral form:** Safety and efficacy not established in those younger than 2 yr. **Elderly:** No age-related precautions noted.

INTERACTIONS

DRUG: **Alcohol, hepatotoxic medications:** May increase hepatotoxicity of ketoconazole. **Antacids, anticholinergics, H₂ antagonists, omeprazole:** May decrease ketoconazole absorption. **Cyclosporine, lovastatin, simvastatin:** May increase blood concentration and risk of toxicity of these drugs. **Isoniazid, rifampin:** May decrease blood concentration of ketoconazole. HERBAL: **Echinacea:** May have additive hepatotoxic effects. FOOD: None known. LAB VALUES: May increase serum alkaline phosphatase, serum bilirubin, AST, and ALT levels. May decrease serum corticosteroid and testosterone concentrations.

AVAILABILITY (Rx)

TABLETS (NIZORAL): 200 mg. **CREAM (NIZORAL TOPICAL):** 2%. **SHAMPOO (Nizoral Ad [OTC]):** 1%.

ADMINISTRATION/HANDLING

PO
• Give with food to minimize GI irritation. • Tablets may be crushed. • Ketoconazole requires acidity; give antacids, anticholinergics, H₂ blockers at least 2 hr following dosing.

SHAMPOO
• Apply to wet hair, massage for 1 min, rinse thoroughly, reapply for 3 min, rinse.

TOPICAL
• Apply, rub gently into affected/surrounding area.

INDICATIONS/ROUTES/DOSAGE

HISTOPLASMOSIS, BLASTOMYCOSIS, SYSTEMIC CANDIDIASIS, CHRONIC MUCOCUTANEOUS CANDIDIASIS, COCCIDIOIDOMYCOSIS, PARACOCCIDIOIDOMYCOSIS, CHROMOMYCOSIS, SEBORRHEIC DERMATITIS, TINEA CORPORIS, TINEA CAPITIS, TINEA MANUS, TINEA CRURIS, TINEA PEDIS, TINEA UNGUIUM (ONYCHOMYCOSIS), ORAL THRUSH, CANDIDURIA

PO: ADULTS, ELDERLY: 200–400 mg/day. CHILDREN: 3.3–6.6 mg/kg/day. **Maximum:** 800 mg/day in 2 divided doses.
TOPICAL: ADULTS, ELDERLY: Apply to affected area 1–2 times a day for 2–4 wk.
SHAMPOO: ADULTS, ELDERLY: Use twice weekly for 4 wk, allowing at least 3 days between shampooing. Use intermittently to maintain control.

K

SIDE EFFECTS

OCCASIONAL (10%–3%): Nausea, vomiting. **RARE (less than 2%):** Abdominal pain, diarrhea, headache, dizziness, photophobia, pruritus. **Topical:** Itching, burning, irritation.

ADVERSE REACTIONS/ TOXIC EFFECTS

Hematologic toxicity (as evidenced by thrombocytopenia, hemolytic anemia, and leukopenia) occurs occasionally. Hepatotoxicity may occur within 1 wk to several months after starting therapy. Anaphylaxis occurs rarely.

NURSING CONSIDERATIONS

BASELINE ASSESSMENT

Confirm that a culture or histologic test was done for accurate diagnosis; therapy may begin before results known.

INTERVENTION/EVALUATION

Monitor liver function tests; be alert for hepatotoxicity: dark urine, pale stools, jaundice, fatigue, anorexia, nausea, or vomiting (unrelieved by giving medication with food). Monitor CBC for evidence of hematologic toxicity. Determine pattern of bowel activity and stool consistency. Assess for dizziness, provide assistance as needed. Evaluate skin for rash, urticaria, itching. **Topical:** Check for localized burning, itching, irritation.

PATIENT/FAMILY TEACHING

• Prolonged therapy (weeks or months) is usually necessary. • Do not miss a dose; continue therapy as long as directed. • Avoid alcohol (potential for hepatotoxicity). • May cause dizziness; avoid tasks that require alertness, motor skills until response to drug is established. • Take antacids and antiulcer medications at least 2 hr after ketoconazole. • Notify physician of dark urine, pale stool, yellow skin or eyes, increased irritation in topical use, onset of other new symptoms. • **Topical:** Rub well into affected areas. • Avoid contact with eyes. • Keep skin clean, dry; wear light clothing for ventilation. • Separate personal items in direct contact with affected area. • **Shampoo:** Initially, use 2 times a wk for 4 wk with at least 3 days between shampooing; frequency then determined by response to medication.

ketoprofen

kee-toe-**proe**-fen
(Apo-Keto ❖, Novo-Keto-EC ❖, Orudis KT, Oruvail, Rhodis ❖)

CLASSIFICATION

PHARMACOTHERAPEUTIC: Nonsteroidal anti-inflammatory. **CLINICAL:** Antirheumatic, analgesic, antidysmenorrheal, vascular headache suppressant (see p. 117C).

ACTION

An NSAID that produces analgesic and anti-inflammatory effects by inhibiting prostaglandin synthesis. **Therapeutic Effect:** Reduces the inflammatory response and intensity of pain.

PHARMACOKINETICS

Immediate-release capsules are rapidly and well-absorbed following PO administration; extended-release capsules are also well-absorbed. Protein binding: 99%. Metabolized in liver. Excreted in urine; less than 10% excreted as unchanged (unconjugated) drug. **Half-life:** 2.4 hr.

USES

Symptomatic treatment of acute and chronic rheumatoid arthritis, osteoarthritis. Relief of mild to moderate pain, primary dysmenorrhea. **OFF-LABEL:** Treatment of acute gouty arthritis, psoriatic arthritis, ankylosing spondylitis, vascular headache.

PRECAUTIONS

CONTRAINDICATIONS: Active peptic ulcer disease, chronic inflammation of the GI tract, GI bleeding or ulceration, history of hypersensitivity to aspirin or NSAIDs. **CAUTIONS:** Renal or hepatic impairment, history of GI tract disease, predisposition to fluid retention.

⏳ **LIFESPAN CONSIDERATIONS: Pregnancy/Lactation:** Crosses placenta; unknown if distributed in breast milk. Avoid during late pregnancy (ductus arteriosis). **Pregnancy Category B (D if used in third trimester or near delivery). Children:** Safety and efficacy not established. **Elderly:** Age-related renal impairment may require dosage adjustment.

INTERACTIONS

DRUG: Antihypertensives, diuretics: May decrease the effects of these drugs. **Aspirin, other salicylates:** May increase the risk of GI side effects such as bleeding. **Bone marrow depressants:** May increase the risk of hematologic reactions. **Heparin, oral anticoagulants, thrombolytics:** May increase the effects of these drugs. **Lithium:** May increase the blood concentration and risk of toxicity of lithium. **Methotrexate:** May increase the risk of methotrexate toxicity. **Probenecid:** May increase the ketoprofen blood concentration. **HERBAL: Feverfew:** May decrease the effects of feverfew. **Ginkgo biloba:** May increase the risk of bleeding. **FOOD:** None known. **LAB VALUES:** May prolong bleeding time. May increase serum alkaline phosphatase and levels and liver function test results. May decrease Hct, blood Hgb, and serum sodium levels.

AVAILABILITY (OTC)

CAPSULES: 25 mg, 50 mg, 75 mg. **CAPSULES (EXTENDED-RELEASE [ORUVAIL]):** 100 mg, 150 mg, 200 mg. **TABLETS (ORUDIS KT):** 12.5 mg (OTC).

ADMINISTRATION/HANDLING
PO
• May give with food, milk, full glass (8 oz) of water (minimizes potential GI distress). • Do not break, chew extended-release capsules.

INDICATIONS/ROUTES/DOSAGE
ACUTE OR CHRONIC RHEUMATOID ARTHRITIS AND OSTEOARTHRITIS
PO: ADULTS: Initially, 75 mg 3 times a day or 50 mg 4 times a day. ELDERLY: Initially, 25–50 mg 3–4 times a day. Maintenance: 150–300 mg/day in 3–4 divided doses.

PO (EXTENDED-RELEASE): ADULTS, ELDERLY: 100–200 mg once a day.

MILD TO MODERATE PAIN, DYSMENORRHEA
PO: ADULTS, ELDERLY: 25–50 mg q6–8h. **Maximum:** 300 mg/day.

OVER-THE-COUNTER (OTC) DOSAGE
PO: ADULTS, ELDERLY: 12.5 mg q4–6h. **Maximum:** 6 tabs/day.

DOSAGE IN RENAL IMPAIRMENT
Mild: 150 mg/day maximum. **Severe:** 100 mg/day maximum.

SIDE EFFECTS
FREQUENT (11%): Dyspepsia. **OCCASIONAL (more than 3%):** Nausea, diarrhea or constipation, flatulence, abdominal cramps, headache. **RARE (less than 2%):** Anorexia, vomiting, visual disturbances, fluid retention.

ADVERSE REACTIONS/ TOXIC EFFECTS

Rare reactions with long-term use include peptic ulcer disease, GI bleeding, gastritis, and severe hepatic reactions (cholestasis, jaundice), nephrotoxicity (dysuria, hematuria, proteinuria, nephrotic syndrome), and severe hypersensitivity reaction (bronchospasm, angioedema).

NURSING CONSIDERATIONS

BASELINE ASSESSMENT
Assess onset, type, location, duration of pain/inflammation. Inspect appearance of affected joints for immobility, deformities, skin condition.

INTERVENTION/EVALUATION
Monitor for evidence of nausea, dyspepsia. Monitor for therapeutic response (relief of pain, improved range of motion, grip strength, mobility). Monitor renal and liver function tests, mental status.

PATIENT/FAMILY TEACHING
• Avoid aspirin, alcohol during therapy (increases risk of GI bleeding). • If GI upset occurs, take with food, milk. • Swallow capsule whole; do not crush or chew.

ketorolac tromethamine

key-**tore**-oh-lack

(Acular, Acular LS, Acular PF, <u>Toradol</u>, Toradol IM, Toradol IV/ IM)

Do not confuse Acular with Acthar or Ocular.

◆ **CLASSIFICATION**

PHARMACOTHERAPEUTIC: Nonsteroidal anti-inflammatory. **CLINICAL:** Analgesic, intraocular anti-inflammatory (see p. 117C).

ACTION

An NSAID that inhibits prostaglandin synthesis and reduces prostaglandin levels in the aqueous humor. **Therapeutic Effect:** Relieves pain stimulus and reduces intraocular inflammation.

PHARMACOKINETICS

Route	Onset	Peak	Duration
PO	30–60 min	1.5–4 hr	4–6 hr
IV/IM	30 min	1–2 hr	4–6 hr

Readily absorbed from the GI tract, after IM administration. Protein binding: 99%. Largely metabolized in the liver. Primarily excreted in urine. Not removed by hemodialysis. **Half-life:** 3.8–6.3 hr (increased with impaired renal function and in the elderly).

USES

Short-term relief of mild to moderate pain. **Ophthalmic:** Relief of ocular itching due to seasonal allergic conjunctivitis. Treatment postop for inflammation following cataract extraction, pain following incisional refractive surgery. **OFF-LABEL:** Prevention or treatment of ocular inflammation (ophthalmic form).

PRECAUTIONS

CONTRAINDICATIONS: Active peptic ulcer disease, chronic inflammation of GI tract, GI bleeding or ulceration, history of hypersensitivity to aspirin or NSAIDs. **CAUTIONS:** Renal or hepatic impairment, history of GI tract disease, predisposition to fluid retention.

⏳ **LIFESPAN CONSIDERATIONS: Pregnancy/Lactation:** Unknown if drug is excreted in breast milk. Avoid use during third trimester (may adversely affect fetal cardiovascular system: premature closure of ductus arteriosus). **Pregnancy Category C (D if used in third trimester). Children:** Safety and efficacy not established, but doses of 0.5 mg/kg have been used. **Elderly:** GI bleeding or ulceration more likely to cause serious adverse effects. Age-related renal impairment may increase risk of hepatic/renal toxicity; decreased dosage recommended.

INTERACTIONS

DRUG: Antihypertensives, diuretics: May decrease the effects of these drugs. **Aspirin, other salicylates:** May increase the risk of GI side effects such as bleeding. **Bone marrow depressants:** May increase the risk of hematologic reactions. **Heparin, oral anticoagulants, thrombolytics:** May increase the effects of these drugs. **Lithium:** May increase the blood concentration and risk of toxicity of lithium. **Methotrexate:** May increase the risk of methotrexate toxicity. **Probenecid:** May increase ketorolac blood concentration. **HERBAL: Feverfew:** May decrease the effects of feverfew. **Ginkgo biloba:** May increase the risk of bleeding. **FOOD:** None known. **LAB VALUES:** May prolong bleeding time. May increase liver function test results.

AVAILABILITY (Rx)

TABLETS (TORADOL): 10 mg. **INJECTION (TORADOL, TORADOL IM, TORADOL IV/ IM):** 15 mg/ml, 30 mg/ml. **OPHTHALMIC**

SOLUTION: 0.4% (Acular LS), 0.5% (Acular, Acular PF).

ADMINISTRATION/HANDLING

🖐 **IV**
• Give undiluted as IV push. • Give over at least 15 sec.

IM
• Give deep IM slowly into large muscle mass.

PO
• Give with food, milk, antacids if GI distress occurs.

OPHTHALMIC
• Place finger on lower eyelid, pull out until pocket is formed between eye and lower lid. Hold dropper above pocket, place prescribed number of drops in pocket. • Close eye gently. Apply digital pressure to lacrimal sac for 1–2 min (minimized drainage into nose and throat, reducing risk of systemic effects). • Remove excess solution with tissue.

▦ **IV INCOMPATIBILITY**
Promethazine (Phenergan).

IV COMPATIBILITIES

Fentanyl (Sublimaze), hydromorphone (Dilaudid), morphine, nalbuphine (Nubain).

INDICATIONS/ROUTES/DOSAGE

SHORT-TERM RELIEF OF MILD TO MODERATE PAIN (MULTIPLE DOSES)
PO: ADULTS, ELDERLY: 10 mg q4–6h. **Maximum:** 40 mg/24 hr.
IV, IM: ADULTS YOUNGER THAN 65 YR: 30 mg q6h. **Maximum:** 120 mg/24 hr. ADULTS 65 YR AND OLDER, THOSE WITH RENAL IMPAIRMENT, THOSE WEIGHING LESS THAN 50 KG: 15 mg q6h. **Maximum:** 60 mg/24 hr. CHILDREN 2–16 YR: 0.5 mg/kg q6h.

K

SHORT-TERM RELIEF OF MILD TO MODERATE PAIN (SINGLE DOSE)

IV: ADULTS YOUNGER THAN 65 YR, CHILDREN 17 YR AND OLDER WEIGHING MORE THAN 50 KG: 30 mg. ADULTS 65 YR AND OLDER, WITH RENAL IMPAIRMENT, WEIGHING LESS THAN 50 KG: 15 mg. CHILDREN 2–16 YR: 0.5 mg/kg. **Maximum:** 15 mg.

IM: ADULTS YOUNGER THAN 65 YR, CHILDREN 17 YR AND OLDER, WEIGHING MORE THAN 50 KG: 60 mg. ADULTS 65 YR AND OLDER, WITH RENAL IMPAIRMENT, WEIGHING LESS THAN 50 KG: 30 mg. CHILDREN 2–16 YR: 1 mg/kg. **Maximum:** 15 kg.

ALLERGIC CONJUNCTIVITIS

OPHTHALMIC: ADULTS, ELDERLY, CHILDREN 3 YR AND OLDER: 1 drop 4 times a day.

CATARACT EXTRACTION

OPHTHALMIC: ADULTS, ELDERLY: 1 drop 4 times a day. Begin 24 hr after surgery and continue for 2 wk.

REFRACTIVE SURGERY

OPHTHALMIC: ADULTS, ELDERLY: 1 drop 4 times a day for 3 days.

SIDE EFFECTS

FREQUENT (17%–12%): Headache, nausea, abdominal cramps or pain, dyspepsia. **OCCASIONAL (9%–3%):** Diarrhea. **Ophthalmic:** Transient stinging and burning. **RARE (3%–1%):** Constipation, vomiting, flatulence, stomatitis, dizziness. **Ophthalmic:** Ocular irritation, allergic reactions, superficial ocular infection, keratitis.

ADVERSE REACTIONS/ TOXIC EFFECTS

Rare reactions with long-term use include peptic ulcer disease, GI bleeding, gastritis, severe hepatic reactions (cholestasis, jaundice), nephrotoxicity (glomerular nephritis, interstitial nephritis, nephrotic syndrome), and an acute hypersensitivity reaction (including fever, chills, and joint pain).

NURSING CONSIDERATIONS

BASELINE ASSESSMENT

Assess onset, type, location, duration of pain.

INTERVENTION/EVALUATION

Monitor renal and liver function tests, occult blood loss, urine output. Evaluate for therapeutic response: relief of pain, stiffness, swelling; increased joint mobility, reduced joint tenderness, improved grip strength. Be alert to signs of bleeding (may also occur with ophthalmic route due to systemic absorption).

PATIENT/FAMILY TEACHING

• Avoid aspirin, alcohol during therapy with oral or ophthalmic ketorolac (increases tendency to bleed). • If GI upset occurs, take with food, milk. • Avoid tasks that require alertness, motor skills until response to drug is established. • **Ophthalmic:** Transient stinging, burning may occur upon instillation. • Do not administer while wearing soft contact lenses.

Klonopin, *see clonazepam*

Klor-Con, *see potassium chloride*

Kytril, *see granisetron*

---

labetalol hydrochloride

lah-**bet**-ah-lol

(Normodyne, Trandate)

Do not confuse Trandate with tramadol or Trental.

FIXED-COMBINATION(S)

Normozide: labetalol/hydrochloro-thiazide (a diuretic): 100 mg/25 mg; 200 mg/25 mg; 300 mg/25 mg.

CLASSIFICATION

PHARMACOTHERAPEUTIC: Alpha-, beta-adrenergic blocker. **CLINICAL:** Antihypertensive.

ACTION

An antihypertensive that blocks alpha$_1$-, beta$_1$-, and beta$_2$-(large doses) adrenergic receptor sites. Large doses increase airway resistance. **Therapeutic Effect:** Slows sinus heart rate; decreases peripheral vascular resistance, cardiac output, and BP.

PHARMACOKINETICS

Route	Onset	Peak	Duration
PO	0.5–2 hr	2–4 hr	8–12 hr
IV	2–5 min	5–15 min	2–4 hr

Completely absorbed from the GI tract. Protein binding: 50%. Undergoes first-pass metabolism. Metabolized in the liver. Primarily excreted in urine. Not removed by hemodialysis. **Half-life:** PO, 6–8 hr; IV, 5.5 hr.

USES

Management of mild, moderate, severe hypertension. May be used alone or in combination with other antihypertensives. **OFF-LABEL:** Control of hypotension during surgery, treatment of chronic angina pectoris.

PRECAUTIONS

CONTRAINDICATIONS: Bronchial asthma, cardiogenic shock, overt cardiac failure, second- or third-degree heart block, severe bradycardia, uncontrolled CHF, other conditions associated with severe and prolonged hypotension. **CAUTIONS:** Medication-controlled CHF, nonallergic bronchospastic disease (chronic bronchitis, emphysema), hepatic or cardiac impairment, pheochromocytoma, diabetes mellitus.

LIFESPAN CONSIDERATIONS: **Pregnancy/Lactation:** Drug crosses placenta. Small amount distributed in breast milk. **Pregnancy Category C (D if used in second or third trimester). Children:** Safety and efficacy not established. **Elderly:** Age-related peripheral vascular disease may increase susceptibility to decreased peripheral circulation.

INTERACTIONS

DRUG: Diuretics, other antihypertensives: May increase hypotensive effect. **Insulin, oral hypoglycemics:** May mask symptoms of hypoglycemia and prolong hypoglycemic effect of these drugs. **MAOIs:** May produce hypertension. **Sympathomimetics, xanthines:** May mutually inhibit effects. **HERBAL:** None known. **FOOD:** None known. **LAB VALUES:** May increase serum antinuclear antibody titer and BUN, serum LDH, lipoprotein, alkaline phosphatase, bilirubin, creatinine, potassium, triglyceride, uric acid, AST, and ALT levels.

AVAILABILITY (Rx)

TABLETS (NORMODYNE, TRANDATE): 100 mg, 200 mg, 300 mg. **INJECTION (TRANDATE):** 5 mg/ml.

ADMINISTRATION/HANDLING

▪ **IV**

◀ **ALERT** ▶ Patient must be in supine position for IV administration and for

3 hr after receiving medication (substantial drop in BP upon standing should be expected).

Reconstitution • For IV infusion, dilute 200 mg in 160 ml D5W, 0.9% NaCl, lactated Ringer's, or any combination thereof to provide concentration of 1 mg/ml.

Rate of administration • For IV push, give over 2 min at 10-min intervals. • For IV infusion, administer at rate of 2 mg/min (2 ml/min) initially. Rate is adjusted according to BP. • Monitor BP immediately before and q5–10min during IV administration (maximum effect occurs within 5 min).

Storage • Store at room temperature. • After dilution, IV solution is stable for 24 hr. • Solution appears clear, colorless to light yellow. • Discard if precipitate forms or discoloration occurs.

PO

• Give without regard to food. • Tablets may be crushed.

☒ IV INCOMPATIBILITIES

Amphotericin B complex (Abelcet, AmBisome, Amphotec), ceftriaxone (Rocephin), furosemide (Lasix), heparin, nafcillin (Nafcil), thiopental.

IV COMPATIBILITIES

Aminophylline, amiodarone (Cordarone), calcium gluconate, diltiazem (Cardizem), dobutamine (Dobutrex), dopamine (Intropin), enalapril (Vasotec), fentanyl (Sublimaze), hydromorphone (Dilaudid), lidocaine, lorazepam (Ativan), magnesium sulfate, midazolam (Versed), milrinone (Primacor), morphine, nitroglycerin, norepinephrine (Levophed), potassium chloride, potassium phosphate, propofol (Diprivan).

INDICATIONS/ROUTES/DOSAGE

HYPERTENSION

PO: ADULTS: Initially, 100 mg twice a day adjusted in increments of 100 mg

twice a day q2–3 days. Maintenance: 200–400 mg twice a day. **Maximum:** 2.4 g/day. ELDERLY: Initially, 100 mg 1–2 times a day. May increase as needed.

SEVERE HYPERTENSION, HYPERTENSIVE EMERGENCY

IV: ADULTS: Initially, 20 mg. Additional doses of 20–80 mg may be given at 10-min intervals, up to total dose of 300 mg.

IV INFUSION: ADULTS: Initially, 2 mg/min up to total dose of 300 mg.

PO (AFTER IV THERAPY): ADULTS: Initially, 200 mg; then, 200–400 mg in 6–12 hr. Increase dose at 1-day intervals to desired level.

SIDE EFFECTS

FREQUENT: Drowsiness, difficulty sleeping, unusual fatigue or weakness, diminished sexual ability, transient scalp tingling. **OCCASIONAL:** Dizziness, dyspnea, peripheral edema, depression, anxiety, constipation, diarrhea, nasal congestion, nausea, vomiting, abdominal discomfort. **RARE:** Altered taste, dry eyes, increased urination, paresthesia.

ADVERSE REACTIONS/ TOXIC EFFECTS

Labetalol administration may precipitate or aggravate CHF because of decreased myocardial stimulation. Abrupt withdrawal may precipitate ischemic heart disease, producing sweating, palpitations, headache, and tremor. May mask signs and symptoms of acute hypoglycemia (tachycardia, BP changes) in patients with diabetes.

NURSING CONSIDERATIONS

BASELINE ASSESSMENT

Assess baseline renal and liver function tests. Assess BP, apical pulse immediately before drug administration (if pulse is 60/min or less or systolic BP is lower than 90 mm Hg, withhold medication, contact physician).

🖊 see color pill atlas   🌿 herb   underlined – top prescribed drug

INTERVENTION/EVALUATION

Monitor BP for hypotension. Assess pulse for quality, irregular rate, bradycardia. Monitor EKG for cardiac arrhythmias. Monitor pattern of bowel activity and stool consistency. Assist with ambulation if dizziness occurs. Assess for evidence of CHF: dyspnea (particularly on exertion or lying down), night cough, peripheral edema, distended neck veins. Monitor I&O (increase in weight, decrease in urine output may indicate CHF).

PATIENT/FAMILY TEACHING

• Do not discontinue drug except upon advice of physician (abrupt discontinuation may precipitate heart failure). • Compliance with therapy regimen is essential to control hypertension, arrhythmias. • Avoid tasks that require alertness, motor skills until response to drug is established. • Report shortness of breath, excessive fatigue, weight gain, prolonged dizziness or headache. • Do not use nasal decongestants, OTC cold preparations (stimulants) without physician approval.

lactulose

lak-tyoo-lose
(Acilac ✹, Cholac, Constilac, Constulose, Duphalac ✹, Enulose, Generlac, Kristalose, Laxilose ✹)

Do not confuse Cholac with diclofenac or lactulose with lactose.

◆ CLASSIFICATION

PHARMACOTHERAPEUTIC: Lactose derivative. **CLINICAL:** Hyperosmotic laxative, ammonia detoxicant (see p. 110C).

ACTION

A lactose derivative that retains ammonia in colon and decreases serum ammonia concentration, producing osmotic effect. **Therapeutic Effect:** Promotes increased peristalsis and bowel evacuation, which expels ammonia from the colon.

PHARMACOKINETICS

Route	Onset	Peak	Duration
PO	24–48 hr	N/A	N/A
Rectal	30–60 min	N/A	N/A

Poorly absorbed from the GI tract. Extensively metabolized in the colon. Primarily excreted in feces.

USES

Prevention and treatment of portal systemic encephalopathy (including hepatic precoma, coma); treatment of constipation.

PRECAUTIONS

CONTRAINDICATIONS: Abdominal pain, appendicitis, nausea, patients on a galactose-free diet, vomiting. **CAUTIONS:** Diabetes mellitus.

⧗ LIFESPAN CONSIDERATIONS: **Pregnancy/Lactation:** Unknown if drug crosses placenta or is distributed in breast milk. **Pregnancy Category B. Children:** Avoid use in children younger than 6 yr (usually unable to describe symptoms). **Elderly:** No age-related precautions noted.

INTERACTIONS

DRUG: Oral medication: May decrease transit time of concurrently administered oral medications, decreasing lactulose absorption. **HERBAL:** None known. **FOOD:** None known. **LAB VALUES:** May decrease serum potassium level.

AVAILABILITY (Rx)

SYRUP (CHOLAC, CONSTILAC, CONSTULOSE, ENULOSE, GENERLAC): 10 g/15 ml. **PACKETS (KRISTALOSE):** 10 g, 20 g.

ADMINISTRATION/HANDLING

PO

• Store solution at room temperature.
• Solution appears pale yellow to yellow, viscous liquid. Cloudiness, darkened solution does not indicate potency loss.
• Drink water, juice, milk with each dose (aids stool softening, increases palatability).

RECTAL

• Lubricate anus with petroleum jelly before enema insertion. • Insert carefully (prevents damage to rectal wall) with nozzle toward navel. • Squeeze container until entire dose expelled.
• Retain until definite lower abdominal cramping felt.

INDICATIONS/ROUTES/DOSAGE

CONSTIPATION

PO: ADULTS, ELDERLY: 15–30 ml (10–20 g)/day, up to 60 ml (40 g)/day. CHILDREN: 7.5 ml (5 g)/day after breakfast.

PORTAL-SYSTEMIC ENCEPHALOPATHY

PO: ADULTS, ELDERLY: Initially, 30–45 ml every hr to induce rapid laxation. Then, 30–45 ml (20–30 g) 3–4 times a day. Adjust dose q1–2 days to produce 2–3 soft stools a day. Usual daily dose: 90–150 ml (60–100 g). CHILDREN: 40–90 ml/day in divided doses 3–4 times a day. INFANTS: 2.5–10 ml/day in 3–4 divided doses.

RECTAL (AS RETENTION ENEMA): ADULTS, ELDERLY: 300 ml (200 g) with 700 ml water or saline solution; patient should retain 30–60 min. Repeat q4–6h. If evacuation occurs too promptly, repeat immediately.

SIDE EFFECTS

OCCASIONAL: Abdominal cramping, flatulence, increased thirst, abdominal discomfort. **RARE:** Nausea, vomiting.

ADVERSE REACTIONS/TOXIC EFFECTS

Diarrhea indicates overdose. Long-term use may result in laxative dependence, chronic constipation, and loss of normal bowel function.

NURSING CONSIDERATIONS

INTERVENTION/EVALUATION

Encourage adequate fluid intake. Assess bowel sounds for peristalsis. Monitor daily bowel activity, stool consistency; record time of evacuation. Assess for abdominal disturbances. Monitor serum electrolytes in patients exposed to prolonged, frequent, or excessive use of medication.

PATIENT/FAMILY TEACHING

• Evacuation occurs in 24–48 hr of initial dose. • Institute measures to promote defecation: increase fluid intake, exercise, high-fiber diet.

Lamictal, *see lamotrigine*

Lamisil Oral, *see terbinafine*

---

lamivudine

lah-**mih**-view-deen

(Epivir, Epivir-HBV, Heptovir ✽)

Do not confuse lamivudine with lamotrigine.

FIXED-COMBINATION(S)

Combivir: lamivudine/zidovudine (an antiviral): 150 mg/300 mg.

Epzicom: lamivudine/abacavir (an antiviral): 300 mg/600 mg. **Trizivir:** lamivudine/zidovudine/abacavir (an antiviral): 150 mg/300 mg/300 mg.

CLASSIFICATION

PHARMACOTHERAPEUTIC: Nucleoside reverse transcriptase inhibitors. **CLINICAL:** Antiviral (see pp. 61C, 103C).

ACTION

An antiviral that inhibits HIV reverse transcriptase by viral DNA chain termination. Also inhibits RNA- and DNA-dependent DNA polymerase, an enzyme necessary for HIV replication. **Therapeutic Effect:** Interrupts HIV replication, slowing the progression of HIV infection.

PHARMACOKINETICS

Rapidly and completely absorbed from the GI tract. Protein binding: less than 36%. Widely distributed (crosses the blood-brain barrier). Primarily excreted unchanged in urine. Not removed by hemodialysis or peritoneal dialysis. **Half-life:** 11–15 hr (intracellular), 2–11 hr (serum, adults), 1.7–2 hr (serum, children). (increased in impaired renal function).

USES

Epivir: Treatment of HIV infection in combination with other antiretroviral agents. **Epivir HBV:** Treatment for chronic hepatitis B. **OFF-LABEL:** Prophylaxis in health care workers at risk of acquiring HIV after occupational exposure.

PRECAUTIONS

CONTRAINDICATIONS: None known. **CAUTIONS:** Peripheral neuropathy or history of peripheral neuropathy, history of pancreatitis in children, renal impairment.

⧗ **LIFESPAN CONSIDERATIONS: Pregnancy/Lactation:** Drug crosses placenta. Unknown if distributed in breast milk. Breast-feeding not recommended (possibility of HIV transmission). **Pregnancy Category C. Children:** Safety and efficacy not established in those younger than 3 mo. **Elderly:** Age-related renal impairment may require dosage adjustment.

INTERACTIONS

DRUG: Co-trimoxazole: Increases lamivudine blood concentration. **HERBAL: St. John's wort:** May decrease lamivudine blood concentration and effect. **FOOD:** None known. **LAB VALUES:** May increase blood Hgb values, neutrophil count, and serum amylase, AST, and ALT levels.

AVAILABILITY (Rx)

ORAL SOLUTION: 5 mg/ml (Epivir-HBV), 10 mg/ml (Epivir). **TABLETS:** 100 mg (Epivir-HBV), 150 mg (Epivir), 300 mg (Epivir).

ADMINISTRATION/HANDLING

PO
- Give without regard to meals.

INDICATIONS/ROUTES/DOSAGE

HIV INFECTION (IN COMBINATION WITH OTHER ANTIRETROVIRALS)

PO: ADULTS, CHILDREN 12–16 YR, WEIGHING 50 KG (100 LB) OR MORE: 150 mg twice a day or 300 mg once a day. ADULTS WEIGHING LESS THAN 50 KG: 2 mg/kg twice a day. CHILDREN 3 MO–11 YR: 4 mg/kg twice a day (up to 150 mg/dose).

CHRONIC HEPATITIS B

PO: ADULTS, CHILDREN 17 YR AND OLDER: 100 mg/day. CHILDREN YOUNGER THAN 17 YR: 3 mg/kg/day. **Maximum:** 100 mg/day.

DOSAGE IN RENAL IMPAIRMENT

Dosage and frequency are modified based on creatinine clearance.

Creatinine Clearance (ml/min)	Dosage
50 ml/min or higher	150 mg twice a day
30–49 ml/min	150 mg once a day
15–29 ml/min	150 mg first dose, then 100 mg once a day
5–14 ml/min	150 mg first dose, then 50 mg once a day
Less than 5 ml/min	50 mg first dose, then 25 mg once a day

SIDE EFFECTS

FREQUENT: Headache (35%), nausea (33%), malaise and fatigue (27%), nasal disturbances (20%), diarrhea, cough (18%), musculoskeletal pain, neuropathy (12%), insomnia (11%), anorexia, dizziness, fever or chills (10%). **OCCASIONAL:** Depression (9%); myalgia (8%); abdominal cramps (6%); dyspepsia, arthralgia (5%).

ADVERSE REACTIONS/ TOXIC EFFECTS

Lactic acidosis and severe hepatomegaly with steatosis, including fatal cases, have been reported. Pancreatitis occurs in 13% of pediatric patients. Anemia, neutropenia, and thrombocytopenia occur rarely.

NURSING CONSIDERATIONS

BASELINE ASSESSMENT

Establish baseline lab values, especially renal function.

INTERVENTION/EVALUATION

Monitor serum creatinine, amylase, lipase, BUN. Assess for headache, nausea, cough. Monitor pattern of bowel activity and stool consistency. Modify diet or administer laxative as needed. Assess for dizziness, sleep pattern. If pancreatitis in children occurs, movement aggravates abdominal pain; sitting up, flexing at the waist relieves the pain.

PATIENT/FAMILY TEACHING

• Continue therapy for full length of treatment. • Doses should be evenly spaced. • Inform patient lamivudine is not a cure for HIV/AIDS nor does it reduce risk of transmission to others; patient may continue to experience illnesses, including opportunistic infections. • Avoid tasks requiring alertness, motor skills until response to drug is established. • Advise parents to closely monitor pediatric patients for symptoms of pancreatitis (severe, steady abdominal pain often radiating to the back, clammy skin, hypotension; nausea or vomiting may accompany abdominal pain).

lamotrigine

lam-**oh**-trih-jeen

(Apo-Lamotrigine 🍃 , <u>Lamictal</u>, Lamictal CD)

Do not confuse lamotrigine with lamivudine.

CLASSIFICATION

CLINICAL: Anticonvulsants (see p. 34C).

ACTION

An anticonvulsant whose exact mechanism is unknown. May block voltage-sensitive sodium channels, thus stabilizing neuronal membranes and regulating presynaptic transmitter release of excitatory amino acids. **Therapeutic Effect:** Reduces seizure activity.

USES

Adjunctive therapy in adults and children with partial seizures, treatment of adults and children with generalized seizures of Lennox-Gastaut syndrome. Conversion to monotherapy in adults treated with another enzyme-inducing antiepileptic drug (EIAED). Long-term maintenance treatment of bipolar disorder.

PRECAUTIONS

CONTRAINDICATIONS: None known. **CAUTIONS:** Renal/hepatic/cardiac impairment. **Pregnancy Category C.**

INTERACTIONS

DRUG: **Carbamazepine, phenobarbital, phenytoin, primidone, valproic acid:** Decrease lamotrigine blood concentration. **Carbamazepine, valproic acid:** May increase serum levels of these drugs. **HERBAL:** None known. **FOOD:** None known. **LAB VALUES:** None known.

AVAILABILITY (Rx)

TABLETS: 25 mg, 100 mg, 150 mg, 200 mg. **TABLETS (CHEWABLE):** 2 mg, 5 mg, 25 mg.

ADMINISTRATION/HANDLING

PO
• Give without regard to food.

INDICATIONS/ROUTES/DOSAGE

SEIZURE CONTROL IN PATIENTS RECEIVING ENZYME-INDUCING ANTIEPILEPTIC DRUG (EIAEDS), BUT NOT VALPROIC ACID
PO: ADULTS, ELDERLY, CHILDREN OLDER THAN 12 YR: Recommended as add-on therapy: 50 mg once a day for 2 wk, followed by 100 mg/day in 2 divided doses for 2 wk. Maintenance: Dosage may be increased by 100 mg/day every week, up to 300–500 mg/day in 2 divided doses. CHILDREN 2–12 YR: 0.6 mg/kg/day in 2 divided doses for 2 wk, then 1.2 mg/kg/day in 2 divided doses for wk 3 and 4. Maintenance: 5–15 mg/kg/day. **Maximum:** 400 mg/day.

SEIZURE CONTROL IN PATIENTS RECEIVING COMBINATION THERAPY OF EIAEDS AND VALPROIC ACID
PO: ADULTS, ELDERLY, CHILDREN OLDER THAN 12 YR: 25 mg every other day for 2 wk,

followed by 25 mg once a day for 2 wk. Maintenance: Dosage may be increased by 25–50 mg/day q1–2wk, up to 150 mg/day in 2 divided doses. CHILDREN 2–12 YR: 0.15 mg/kg/day in 2 divided doses for 2 wk, then 0.3 mg/kg/day in 2 divided doses for wk 3 and 4. Maintenance: 1–5 mg/kg/day in 2 divided doses. **Maximum:** 200 mg/day.

CONVERSION TO MONOTHERAPY FOR PATIENTS RECEIVING EIAED
PO: ADULTS, ELDERLY, CHILDREN 16 YR AND OLDER: 500 mg/day in 2 divided doses. Titrate to desired dose while maintaining EIAED at fixed level, then withdraw EIAED by 20% each wk over a 4-wk period.

CONVERSION TO MONOTHERAPY FOR PATIENTS RECEIVING VALPROIC ACID
PO: ADULTS, ELDERLY, CHILDREN 16 YR AND OLDER: Titrate lamotrigine to 200 mg/day, maintaining valproic acid dose. Maintain lamotrigine dose and decrease valproic acid to 500 mg/day, no greater than 500 mg/day/wk, then maintain 500 mg/day for 1 wk. Increase lamotrigine to 300 mg/day and decrease valproic acid to 250 mg/day. Maintain for 1 wk, then discontinue valproic acid and increase lamotrigine by 100 mg/day each wk until maintenance dose of 500 mg/day reached.

BIPOLAR DISORDER IN PATIENTS RECEIVING EIAED
PO: ADULTS, ELDERLY: 50 mg/day for 2 wk, then 100 mg/day for 2 wk, then 200 mg/day for 1 wk, then 300 mg/day for 1 wk, then up to usual maintenance dose 400 mg/day in divided doses.

BIPOLAR DISORDER IN PATIENTS RECEIVING VALPROIC ACID
PO: ADULTS, ELDERLY: 25 mg/day every other day for 2 wk, then 25 mg/day for 2 wk, then 50 mg/day for 1 wk, then 100 mg/day. Usual maintenance dose with valproic acid: 100 mg/day.

DISCONTINUATION THERAPY
ADULTS, CHILDREN OLDER THAN 12 YR: A dosage reduction of approximately

L

50% per week over at least 2 wk is recommended.

SIDE EFFECTS

FREQUENT: Dizziness (38%), headache (29%), diplopia (28%), ataxia (22%), nausea (19%), blurred vision (16%), somnolence, rhinitis (14%). **OCCASIONAL (10%–5%):** Rash, pharyngitis, vomiting, cough, flu-like symptoms, diarrhea, dysmenorrhea, fever, insomnia, dyspepsia. **RARE:** Constipation, tremor, anxiety, pruritus, vaginitis, hypersensitivity reaction.

ADVERSE REACTIONS/ TOXIC EFFECTS

Abrupt withdrawal may increase seizure frequency. Serious rashes, including Stevens-Johnson syndrome, requiring hospitalization and discontinuation of treatment have been reported.

NURSING CONSIDERATIONS

BASELINE ASSESSMENT

Review history of seizure disorder (type, onset, intensity, frequency, duration, level of consciousness [LOC]), drug history (especially other anticonvulsants), other medical conditions (e.g., renal impairment). Provide safety precautions, quiet, dark environment.

INTERVENTION/EVALUATION

Report to physician promptly if evidence of rash occurs (drug discontinuation may be necessary). Assist with ambulation if dizziness, ataxia occurs. Assess for clinical improvement (decreased intensity/frequency of seizures). Assess for visual abnormalities, headache.

PATIENT/FAMILY TEACHING

• Take medication only as prescribed; do not abruptly withdraw medication after long-term therapy. • Avoid alcohol, tasks that require alertness, motor skills until response to drug is established. • Carry identification card/ bracelet to note anticonvulsant therapy. • Strict maintenance of drug therapy is essential for seizure control. • Report any rash, fever, swelling of glands to physician. • May cause photosensitivity reaction; avoid exposure to sunlight, artificial light.

Lanoxin, *see digoxin*

lansoprazole

lan-so-**prah**-zoll

(Prevacid, Prevacid IV, Prevacid Solu-Tab)

Do not confuse Prevacid with Pepcid, Pravachol, or Prevpac.

FIXED-COMBINATION(S)

Prevacid NapraPac: lansoprazole/ naproxen (an NSAID): 15 mg/375 mg; 15 mg/500 mg.

◆CLASSIFICATION

CLINICAL: Proton pump inhibitor (see p. 134C).

ACTION

A proton pump inhibitor that selectively inhibits the parietal cell membrane enzyme system (hydrogen-potassium adenosine triphosphatase) or proton pump. **Therapeutic Effect:** Suppresses gastric acid secretion.

PHARMACOKINETICS

Route	Onset	Peak	Duration
PO (15 mg)	2–3 hr	N/A	24 hr
PO (30 mg)	1–2 hr	N/A	Longer than 24 hr

Rapid and complete absorption (food may decrease absorption) once drug has left stomach. Protein binding: 97%. Distributed primarily to gastric parietal cells and converted to two active metabolites. Extensively metabolized in the liver. Eliminated in bile and urine. Not removed by hemodialysis. Half-life: 1.5 hr (increased in the elderly and in those with hepatic impairment).

USES

Short-term treatment (4 wk and less) for healing, symptomatic relief of active duodenal ulcer, short-term treatment (8 wk and less) for healing, symptomatic relief of erosive esophagitis. Long-term treatment of pathologic hypersecretory conditions, including Zollinger-Ellison syndrome. Short-term treatment (8 wk and less) of active gastric ulcer, *H. pylori*–associated duodenal ulcer, maintenance treatment for healed duodenal ulcer. Treatment for gastroesophageal reflux disease (GERD), NSAID-associated gastric ulcer. **IV:** Short-term treatment of erosive esophagitis.

PRECAUTIONS

CONTRAINDICATIONS: None known. **CAUTIONS:** Hepatic impairment.

⏳ **LIFESPAN CONSIDERATIONS: Pregnancy/Lactation:** Unknown if distributed in breast milk. **Pregnancy Category B. Children:** Safety and efficacy not established. **Elderly:** No age-related precautions noted but doses greater than 30 mg not recommended.

INTERACTIONS

DRUG: Ampicillin, digoxin, iron salts, ketoconazole: May interfere with the absorption of ampicillin, digoxin, iron salts, and ketoconazole. **Sucralfate:** May delay the absorption of lansoprazole. **HERBAL:** None known. **FOOD:** None known. **LAB VALUES:** May increase LDH, serum alkaline phosphatase, bilirubin, cholesterol, creatinine, AST, ALT, triglyceride, and uric acid levels. May produce abnormal albumin/globulin ratio, electrolyte balance, and platelet, RBC, and WBC counts. May increase Hgb and Hct.

AVAILABILITY (Rx)

CAPSULES (DELAYED-RELEASE [PREVACID]): 15 mg, 30 mg. **GRANULES FOR ORAL SUSPENSION (PREVACID):** 15 mg/pack; 30 mg/pack. **INJECTION POWDER FOR RECONSTITUTION (PREVACID IV):** 30 mg. **ORALLY-DISINTEGRATING TABLETS (PREVACID SOLU-TAB):** 15 mg, 30 mg.

ADMINISTRATION/HANDLING

 IV

• Store at room temperature. • Infuse over 30 min.

PO

• Give while fasting or before meals (food diminishes absorption). • Do not chew or crush delayed-release capsules. • If patient has difficulty swallowing capsules, open capsules, sprinkle granules on 1 tbsp of applesauce, swallow immediately.

PO (SOLU-TAB)

• May give via oral syringe or nasogastric tube. • May dissolve in 4 ml water (15 mg) or 10 ml (30 mg).

INDICATIONS/ROUTES/DOSAGE

DUODENAL ULCER

PO: ADULTS, ELDERLY: 15 mg/day, before eating, preferably in the morning, for up to 4 wk. Maintenance: 15 mg/day.

EROSIVE ESOPHAGITIS

PO: ADULTS, ELDERLY: 30 mg/day, before eating, for up to 8 wk. If healing does not occur within 8 wk (in 5%–10% of cases), may give for additional 8 wk. Maintenance: 15 mg/day.

IV: ADULTS, ELDERLY: 30 mg once a day for up to 7 days. Switch to oral lansoprazole therapy as soon as patient can tolerate oral route.

GASTRIC ULCER

PO: ADULTS: 30 mg/day for up to 8 wk.

NSAID GASTRIC ULCER

PO: ADULTS, ELDERLY: (Healing): 30 mg/day for up to 8 wk. (Prevention): 15 mg/day for up to 12 wk.

HEALED DUODENAL ULCER, GASTROESOPHAGEAL REFLUX DISEASE

PO: ADULTS: 15 mg/day.

USUAL PEDIATRIC DOSAGE

CHILDREN 3 MO–14 YR, WEIGHING MORE THAN 20 KG: 30 mg once daily. CHILDREN 3 MO–14 YR, WEIGHING 10–20 KG: 15 mg once daily. CHILDREN 3 MO–14 YR, WEIGHING LESS THAN 10 KG: 7.5 mg once daily.

H. PYLORI INFECTION

PO: ADULTS, ELDERLY: (triple drug therapy) 30 mg q12h for 10–14 days. (dual drug therapy) 30 mg q8h for 14 days.

PATHOLOGIC HYPERSECRETORY CONDITIONS (INCLUDING ZOLLINGER-ELLISON SYNDROME)

PO: ADULTS, ELDERLY: 60 mg/day. Individualize dosage according to patient needs and for as long as clinically indicated. Administer up to 120 mg/day in divided doses.

SIDE EFFECTS

OCCASIONAL (3%–2%): Diarrhea, abdominal pain, rash, pruritus, altered appetite. **RARE (1%):** Nausea, headache.

ADVERSE REACTIONS/ TOXIC EFFECTS

Bilirubinemia, eosinophilia, and hyperlipemia occur rarely.

NURSING CONSIDERATIONS

BASELINE ASSESSMENT

Obtain baseline lab values. Assess drug history, especially use of sucralfate.

INTERVENTION/EVALUATION

Monitor ongoing laboratory results. Assess for therapeutic response (i.e., relief of GI symptoms). Question if diarrhea, abdominal pain, nausea occurs.

PATIENT/FAMILY TEACHING

• Do not chew or crush delayed-release capsules. • For patients who have difficulty swallowing capsules, open capsules, sprinkle granules on 1 tbsp of applesauce, swallow immediately.

lanthanum carbonate

lan-**thah**-num
(Fosrenol)

CLASSIFICATION

CLINICAL: Phosphate regulator.

ACTION

Dissociates in the acidic environment of the upper GI tract to lanthanum ions that bind to dietary phosphate released from food during digestion, forming highly insoluble lanthanum phosphate complexes. **Therapeutic Effect:** Phosphate complexes are eliminated by urinary excretion, reducing phosphate absorption.

PHARMACOKINETICS

Very low absorption following oral administration. Protein binding: greater than 99%. Not metabolized. Phosphate complexes are eliminated in urine. **Half-Life:** 53 hr (in plasma); 2–3.6 yr (from bone).

USES

To reduce serum phosphate levels in patients with end-stage renal disease.

PRECAUTIONS

CONTRAINDICATIONS: None known. **CAUTIONS:** Acute peptic ulcer disease, ulcerative colitis, Crohn's disease, bowel obstruction.

⌛ LIFESPAN CONSIDERATIONS: Pregnancy/Lactation: Unknown if drug crosses placenta or is distributed in breast milk; do not breastfeed. **Pregnancy Category C. Children:** Safety and efficacy not established; not recommended for children. **Elderly:** No age-related precautions noted.

INTERACTIONS

DRUG: **Antacids:** Interacts with lanthanum carbonate; separate administration by 2 hr. HERBAL: None known. FOOD: **Meals:** Medication should be taken with or immediately after a meal. LAB VALUES: None known.

AVAILABILITY (Rx)

TABLETS, CHEWABLE: 250 mg, 500 mg, 750 mg, 1 g. (Fosrenol).

ADMINISTRATION/HANDLING

PO

• Tablets should be chewed thoroughly before swallowing and given during or immediately after meals.

INDICATIONS/ROUTES/DOSAGE

PHOSPHATE CONTROL

PO: ADULTS, ELDERLY: 750 mg–1,500 mg in divided doses, taken with or immediately after a meal. Dose can be titrated at 2- to 3-wk intervals in 750 mg increment, based on serum phosphate levels.

SIDE EFFECTS

FREQUENT: Nausea (11%), vomiting (9%), dialysis graft occlusion (8%), abdominal pain (5%). Nausea and vomiting decreases over time.

ADVERSE REACTIONS/ TOXIC EFFECTS

Dialysis graft occlusion has been reported.

BASELINE ASSESSMENT

Obtain baseline serum phosphorus level.

INTERVENTION/EVALUATION

Monitor serum phosphate concentration (target concentration is less than 6 mg/dL).

PATIENT/FAMILY TEACHING

• Take with or immediately after a meal.
• Do not take lanthanum within 2 hr of antacids. • Nausea or vomiting usually diminish over time.

Lantus, *see insulin*

Lasix, *see furosemide*

latanoprost

See Antiglaucoma agents (p. 47C)

leflunomide

lee-**flew**-no-mide
(Arava)

◆ **CLASSIFICATION**

PHARMACOTHERAPEUTIC: Immunomodulatory agent. **CLINICAL:** Anti-inflammatory.

ACTION

An immunomodulatory agent that inhibits dihydroorotate dehydrogenase, the enzyme involved in autoimmune process that leads to rheumatoid arthritis. **Therapeutic Effect:** Reduces signs and symptoms of rheumatoid arthritis and slows structural damage.

PHARMACOKINETICS

Well absorbed after PO administration. Protein binding: greater than 99%. Metabolized to active metabolite in the GI wall and liver. Excreted through both renal and biliary systems. Not removed by hemodialysis. Half-life: 16 days.

USES

Treatment of active rheumatoid arthritis. Improve physical function in patients with rheumatoid arthritis.

PRECAUTIONS

CONTRAINDICATIONS: Pregnancy or plans to become pregnant. **CAUTIONS:** Hepatic or renal impairment, positive hepatitis B or C serology, those with immunodeficiency or bone marrow dysplasias, breast-feeding mothers.

⏳ LIFESPAN CONSIDERATIONS: **Pregnancy/Lactation:** Can cause fetal harm. Unknown if excreted in breast milk. Avoid use in breast-feeding mothers. **Pregnancy Category X. Children:** Safety and efficacy not established in those younger than 18 yr. **Elderly:** No age-related precautions noted.

INTERACTIONS

DRUG: **Rifampin:** Increases the blood concentration of leflunomide. **Warfarin:** May increase the effects of warfarin. HERBAL: None known. FOOD: None known. LAB VALUES: May increase hepatic enzyme levels, especially AST, and ALT.

AVAILABILITY (Rx)

TABLETS: 10 mg, 20 mg.

ADMINISTRATION/HANDLING

PO
• Give without regard to food.

INDICATIONS/ROUTES/DOSAGE

RHEUMATOID ARTHRITIS
PO: ADULTS, ELDERLY: Initially, 100 mg/day for 3 days, then 10–20 mg/day.

SIDE EFFECTS

FREQUENT (20%–10%): Diarrhea, respiratory tract infection, alopecia, rash, nausea.

ADVERSE REACTIONS/ TOXIC EFFECTS

Transient thrombocytopenia and leukopenia occur rarely. Rare cases of severe hepatic injury, including cases with fatal outcome, have been reported during treatment.

NURSING CONSIDERATIONS

BASELINE ASSESSMENT

Question for possibility of pregnancy (Pregnancy Category X). Assess limitations in activities of daily living due to rheumatoid arthritis.

INTERVENTION/EVALUATION

Monitor tolerance to medication. Assess symptomatic relief of rheumatoid arthritis (relief of pain; improved range of motion, grip strength, mobility). Monitor liver function tests.

PATIENT/FAMILY TEACHING

• May take without regard to food. • Improvement may take longer than 8 wk. • Avoid pregnancy (Pregnancy Category X).

lenalidomide

len-ah-**lid**-oh-mide
(Revlimid)

◆**CLASSIFICATION**

PHARMACOTHERAPEUTIC: Immunomodulator. CLINICAL: Immunosuppressive.

ACTION

Inhibits the secretion of pro-inflammatory cytokines, increases the secretion of anti-inflammatory cytokines. **Therapeutic Effect:** Prevents growth of B-cell lymphoma cell line, myeloblastic cell line.

PHARMACOKINETICS

Well absorbed following oral administration. Protein binding: 30%. Eliminated in the urine. **Half-life:** 3 hr (increased with renal impairment).

USES

Treatment of transfusion-dependent anemia due to myelodysplastic syndromes.

PRECAUTIONS

CONTRAINDICATIONS: Pregnancy **(Pregnancy Category X)**, women capable of becoming pregnant. **CAUTIONS:** Renal function impairment.

⧗ **LIFESPAN CONSIDERATIONS: Pregnancy/Lactation:** Contraindicated in women who are or may become pregnant and who are not using two required types of birth control or who are not continually abstaining from heterosexual sexual contact. Can cause severe birth defects, fetal death. Unknown if distributed in breast milk; do not breast-feed. **Pregnancy Category X. Children:** Safety and efficacy not established in children younger than 18 yr. **Elderly:** Age-related renal impairment may require care in dosage selection. Risk of toxic reactions is greater in those with renal insufficiency.

INTERACTIONS

DRUG: None known. **HERBAL:** None known. **FOOD:** None known. **LAB VALUES:** May decrease WBC count, Hgb, Hct, thrombocytes, troponin I, serum creatinine, sodium, T_3, T_4. May decrease bilirubin, glucose, potassium, magnesium.

AVAILABILITY (Rx)

CAPSULES: 5 mg, 10 mg.

ADMINISTRATION/HANDLING

• Store at room temperature. • Do not crush or open capsules.

INDICATIONS/ROUTES/DOSAGE

PO: ADULTS, ELDERLY: 10 mg once daily.

SIDE EFFECTS

FREQUENT (49%–31%): Diarrhea, pruritus, rash, fatigue. **OCCASIONAL (24%–12%):** Constipation, nausea, arthralgia, fever, back pain, peripheral edema, cough, dizziness, headache, muscle cramps, epistaxis, asthenia, dry skin, abdominal pain. **RARE (10%–5%):** Limb pain, vomiting, generalized edema, anorexia, insomnia, night sweats, myalgia, dry mouth, ecchymosis, rigors, depression, dysgeusia, palpitations.

ADVERSE REACTIONS/ TOXIC EFFECTS

Significant increased risk of deep vein thrombosis and pulmonary embolism. Thrombocytopenia occurs in 62% of patients, neutropenia in 59% of patients, and anemia in 12% of patients. Upper respiratory infection characterized as nasopharyngitis, pneumonia, sinusitis, bronchitis, rhinitis, and UTI occur occasionally. Cellulitis, peripheral neuropathy, hypertension, hypothyroidism occurs in approximately 6% of patients.

L

NURSING CONSIDERATIONS

BASELINE ASSESSMENT

Due to high potential for human birth defects/fetal death, female patients are to avoid pregnancy 4 wk before therapy, during therapy, during dose interruptions and 4 wk following therapy. Contraception must also be used even if there is a history of infertility unless it is due to hysterectomy or menopause that has occurred for at least 24 consecutive mo. Two reliable forms of contraception must be used. Females of childbearing potential must have two negative pregnancy tests before therapy initiation.

INTERVENTION/EVALUATION

Perform pregnancy tests on women of childbearing potential. Perform the test weekly during the first 4 wk of use, then at 4-wk intervals in women with regular menstrual cycles or q2wk in women with irregular menstrual cycles. Monitor for hematologic toxicity by obtaining a CBC weekly during the first 8 wk of therapy and at least monthly thereafter. Be observant for signs and symptoms of thromboembolism (shortness of breath, chest pain, leg or arm pain, swelling).

PATIENT/FAMILY TEACHING

• Two approved birth control methods must be used before, during, and after therapy for female patients. • A pregnancy test must be performed within 10–14 days and 24 hr before therapy begins. • Males must always use a latex condom during any sexual contact with females of childbearing potential even if they have undergone a successful vasectomy.

---

lepirudin

leh-**peer**-u-din
(Refludan)

◆CLASSIFICATION

PHARMACOTHERAPEUTIC: Thrombin inhibitor. **CLINICAL:** Anticoagulant.

ACTION

An anticoagulant that inhibits thrombogenic action of thrombin (independent of antithrombin II and not inhibited by platelet factor 4). One molecule of lepirudin binds to one molecule of thrombin.

Therapeutic Effect: Produces dose-dependent increases in aPTT.

PHARMACOKINETICS

Distributed primarily in extracellular fluid. Primarily eliminated by the kidneys. Half-life: 1.3 hr (increased in impaired renal function).

USES

Anticoagulant in patients with heparin-induced thrombocytopenia, associated thromboembolic disease to prevent further thromboembolic complications. OFF-LABEL: Acute coronary syndromes with history of heparin-induced thrombocytopenia; acute MI; percutaneous coronary intervention with history of heparin-induced thrombocytopenia; prevention/reduction of ischemic complications associated with unstable angina.

PRECAUTIONS

CONTRAINDICATIONS: Hypersensitivity to hirudins or to any of the components in Refludan [lepirudin (rDNA)] for injection. **CAUTIONS:** Conditions associated with increased risk of bleeding (e.g., bacterial endocarditis, recent major bleeding, cerebrovascular accident (CVA), stroke, intracerebral surgery, hemorrhagic diathesis, severe hypertension, severe renal or hepatic function impairment, recent major surgery).

⧗ LIFESPAN CONSIDERATIONS: **Pregnancy/Lactation:** Unknown if drug is distributed in breast milk or crosses placenta. **Pregnancy Category B. Children:** Safety and efficacy not established. **Elderly:** Age-related renal impairment may require dosage adjustment.

INTERACTIONS

DRUG: **Platelet aggregation inhibitors, thrombolytics, warfarin:** May increase the risk of bleeding complications. HERBAL: **Ginkgo biloba:** May increase the risk of bleeding.

FOOD: None known. **LAB VALUES:** Increases aPTT and thrombin time.

AVAILABILITY (Rx)
POWDER FOR INJECTION: 50 mg.

ADMINISTRATION/HANDLING
IV

Reconstitution • Add 1 ml sterile water for injection or 0.9% NaCl to 50-mg vial. • Shake gently. • Produces a clear, colorless solution (do not use if cloudy). • For IV push, further dilute by transferring to syringe and adding sufficient sterile water for injection, 0.9% NaCl, or D_5W to produce concentration of 5 mg/ml. • For IV infusion, add contents of 2 vials (100 mg) to 250 ml or 500 ml 0.9% NaCl or D_5W, providing a concentration of 0.4 or 0.2 mg/ml, respectively.

Rate of administration • IV push given over 15–20 sec. • Adjust IV infusion based on aPTT or patient's body weight.

Storage • Store unreconstituted vials at room temperature. • Reconstituted solution to be used immediately. • IV infusion stable for up to 24 hr at room temperature.

IV INCOMPATIBILITIES
Do not mix with other medications.

INDICATIONS/ROUTES/DOSAGE
HEPARIN-INDUCED THROMBOCYTOPENIA AND ASSOCIATED THROMBOEMBOLIC DISEASE TO PREVENT FURTHER THROMBOEMBOLIC COMPLICATIONS
IV, IV INFUSION: ADULTS, ELDERLY: 0.2–0.4 mg/kg, IV slowly over 15–20 sec, followed by IV infusion of 0.1–0.15 mg/kg/hr for 2–10 days or longer.

DOSAGE IN RENAL IMPAIRMENT
Initial dose is decreased to 0.2 mg/kg, with infusion rate adjusted based on creatinine clearance.

Creatinine Clearance (ml/min)	% of Standard Infusion Rate	Infusion Rate (mg/kg/hr)
45–60	50	0.075
30–44	30	0.045
15–29	15	0.0225

SIDE EFFECTS
FREQUENT (14%–5%): Bleeding from gums, puncture sites, or wounds, hematuria, fever, GI and rectal bleeding. **OCCASIONAL (3%–1%):** Epistaxis; allergic reaction, such as rash and pruritus; vaginal bleeding.

ADVERSE REACTIONS/ TOXIC EFFECTS
Overdose is characterized by excessively high aPTT. Intracranial bleeding occurs rarely. Abnormal hepatic function occurs in 6% of patients.

NURSING CONSIDERATIONS

BASELINE ASSESSMENT
Assess CBC, including platelet count. Determine initial BP. Assess renal and hepatic function.

INTERVENTION/EVALUATION
Monitor aPTT diligently. Assess Hct, platelet count, urine and stool specimen for occult blood, AST, ALT, renal function studies. Assess for decrease in BP, increase in pulse rate, complaint of abdominal/back pain, severe headache (may be evidence of hemorrhage). Question for increased discharge during menses. Check peripheral pulses; skin for ecchymosis, petechiae. Check for excessive bleeding from minor cuts, scratches. Assess gums for erythema, gingival bleeding. Assess urine output for hematuria.

PATIENT/FAMILY TEACHING
• Report bleeding, bruising, dizziness or lightheadedness, rash, itching, fever, edema, breathing difficulty.

Lescol, *see fluvastatin*

Lescol XL, *see fluvastatin*

letrozole ⚑

leh-troe-zoll
(Femara)
Do not confuse Femara with Femhrt.

◆CLASSIFICATION

PHARMACOTHERAPEUTIC: Aromatase inhibitor, hormone. **CLINICAL:** Antineoplastic (see p. 76C).

ACTION

Decreases the level of circulating estrogen by inhibiting aromatase, an enzyme that catalyzes the final step in estrogen production. **Therapeutic Effect:** Inhibits the growth of breast cancers that are stimulated by estrogens.

PHARMACOKINETICS

Rapidly and completely absorbed. Metabolized in the liver. Primarily eliminated by the kidneys. Unknown if removed by hemodialysis. **Half-life:** Approximately 2 days.

USES

Extended adjuvant treatment of early breast cancer in post-menopausal women who have received 5 yr of adjuvant tamoxifen therapy. First line treatment of post-menopausal women with hormone receptor positive or hormone receptor unknown locally advanced or metastatic breast cancer. Treatment of advanced breast cancer in post-menopausal women with disease progression following anti-estrogen therapy. Post-surgical treatment for post-menopausal women with hormone sensitive early breast cancer.

PRECAUTIONS

CONTRAINDICATIONS: None known.
CAUTIONS: Renal or hepatic impairment.
⧗ **LIFESPAN CONSIDERATIONS: Pregnancy/Lactation:** Unknown if distributed in breast milk. **Pregnancy Category D. Children:** Safety and efficacy not established. **Elderly:** No age-related precautions noted.

INTERACTIONS

DRUG: Tamoxifen: May reduce letrozole serum concentration. **HERBAL:** None known. **FOOD:** None known. **LAB VALUES:** May increase serum calcium, cholesterol, GGT, AST, and ALT levels.

AVAILABILITY (Rx)

TABLETS: 2.5 mg.

ADMINISTRATION/HANDLING

PO
• Give without regard to food.

INDICATIONS/ROUTES/DOSAGE

BREAST CANCER
PO: ADULTS, ELDERLY: 2.5 mg/day. Continue until tumor progression is evident.

SIDE EFFECTS

FREQUENT (21%–9%): Musculoskeletal pain (back, arm, leg), nausea, headache. **OCCASIONAL (8%–5%):** Constipation, arthralgia, fatigue, vomiting, hot flashes, diarrhea, abdominal pain, cough, rash, anorexia, hypertension, peripheral edema. **RARE (4%–1%):** Asthenia, somnolence, dyspepsia, weight gain, pruritus.

ADVERSE REACTIONS/TOXIC EFFECTS

Pleural effusion, pulmonary embolism, bone fracture, thromboembolic disorder, and MI have been reported.

NURSING CONSIDERATIONS

INTERVENTION/EVALUATION

Monitor for, assist with ambulation if asthenia or dizziness occurs. Assess for headache. Offer antiemetic for nausea and vomiting. Monitor CBC, thyroid function, electrolytes, liver and renal function tests. Monitor for evidence of musculoskeletal pain; offer analgesics for pain relief.

PATIENT/FAMILY TEACHING

• Notify physician if nausea, asthenia, hot flashes become unmanageable.

---

leucovorin calcium (folinic acid, citrovorum factor)

loo-**koe**-vor-in

(Lederle Leucovorin ♣, Well-covorin)

Do not confuse Wellcovorin with Wellbutrin or Wellferon.

◆CLASSIFICATION

PHARMACOTHERAPEUTIC: Folic acid antagonist. **CLINICAL:** Antidote.

ACTION

An antidote to folic acid antagonists that may limit methotrexate action on normal cells by competing with methotrexate for the same transport processes into the cells. **Therapeutic Effect:** Reverses toxic effects of folic acid antagonists. Reverses folic acid deficiency.

PHARMACOKINETICS

Readily absorbed from the GI tract. Widely distributed. Primarily concentrated in the liver. Metabolized in the liver and intestinal mucosa to active metabolite. Primarily excreted in urine. **Half-life:** 15 min; metabolite, 30–35 min.

USES

Antidote for folic acid antagonists (methotrexate, trimethoprim, pyrimethamine). Treatment of megaloblastic anemias when folate deficient (e.g., infancy, sprue, pregnancy, when oral therapy not possible). Treatment of colon cancer (with fluorouracil). Methotrexate rescue, after high dose methotrexate for osteosarcoma. **OFF-LABEL:** Treatment of Ewing's sarcoma, gestational trophoblastic neoplasms, or non-Hodgkin's lymphoma; treatment adjunct for head and neck carcinoma.

PRECAUTIONS

CONTRAINDICATIONS: Pernicious anemia, other megaloblastic anemias secondary to vitamin B_{12} deficiency. **CAUTIONS:** History of allergies, bronchial asthma. **With 5-fluorouracil:** Those with GI toxicities (more common/severe).

⧗ LIFESPAN CONSIDERATIONS: **Pregnancy/Lactation:** Unknown if drug crosses placenta or is distributed in breast milk. **Pregnancy Category C. Children:** May increase risk of seizures by counteracting anticonvulsant effects of barbiturate, hydantoins. **Elderly:** Age-related renal impairment may require dosage adjustment when used in rescue from effects of high-dose methotrexate therapy.

INTERACTIONS

DRUG: Anticonvulsants: May decrease the effects of anticonvulsants. **Chemotherapeutic agents:** May increase the effects and toxicity of these drugs when taken in combination. **HERBAL:** None known. **FOOD:** None known. **LAB VALUES:** None known.

AVAILABILITY (Rx)

TABLETS: 5 mg, 10 mg, 15 mg, 25 mg.
POWDER FOR INJECTION: 50 mg, 100 mg, 200 mg, 350 mg, 500 mg.

ADMINISTRATION/HANDLING

📋 IV

Reconstitution • Reconstitute each 50-mg vial with 5 ml sterile water for injection or bacteriostatic water for injection containing benzyl alcohol to provide concentration of 10 mg/ml. • Due to benzyl alcohol in 1-mg ampule and in bacteriostatic water for injection, reconstitute doses greater than 10 mg/m^2 with sterile water for injection. • Further dilute with D$_5$W or 0.9% NaCl.

Rate of administration • Do not exceed 160 mg/min if given by IV infusion (because of calcium content).

Storage • Store vials for parenteral use at room temperature. • Injection appears as clear, yellowish solution. • Use immediately if reconstituted with sterile water for injection; is stable for 7 days if reconstituted with bacteriostatic water for injection.

PO
• Scored tablets may be crushed.

▦ IV INCOMPATIBILITIES

Amphotericin B complex (Abelcet, AmBisome, Amphotec), droperidol (Inapsine), foscarnet (Foscavir).

IV COMPATIBILITIES

Cisplatin (Platinol AQ), cyclophosphamide (Cytoxan), doxorubicin (Adriamycin), etoposide (VePesid), filgrastim (Neupogen), 5-fluorouracil, gemcitabine (Gemzar), granisetron (Kytril), heparin, methotrexate, metoclopramide (Reglan), mitomycin (Mutamycin), piperacillin and tazobactam (Zosyn), vinblastine (Velban), vincristine (Oncovin).

INDICATIONS/ROUTES/DOSAGE

CONVENTIONAL RESCUE DOSAGE IN HIGH-DOSE METHOTREXATE THERAPY
PO, IV, IM: ADULTS, ELDERLY, CHILDREN: 10 mg/m^2 IM or IV one time, then PO q6h until serum methotrexate level is less than 10^{-8} M. If 24-hr serum creatinine level increases by 50% or greater over baseline or methotrexate level exceeds 5 × 10^{-6} M or 48-hr level exceeds 9 × 10^{-7} M, increase to 100 mg/m^2 IV q3h until methotrexate level is less than 10^{-8} M.

FOLIC ACID ANTAGONIST OVERDOSE
PO: ADULTS, ELDERLY, CHILDREN: 2–15 mg/day for 3 days or 5 mg every 3 days.

MEGALOBLASTIC ANEMIA SECONDARY TO FOLATE DEFICIENCY
IM: ADULTS, ELDERLY, CHILDREN: 1 mg/day.

COLON CANCER
IV: ADULTS, ELDERLY: 200 mg/m^2 followed by 370 mg/m^2 fluorouracil daily for 5 days. Repeat course at 4-wk intervals for 2 courses then 4–5 wk intervals or 20 mg/m^2 followed by 425 mg/m^2 fluorouracil daily for 5 days. Repeat course at 4-wk intervals for 2 courses then 4–5 wk intervals.

SIDE EFFECTS

FREQUENT: When combined with chemotherapeutic agents: Diarrhea, stomatitis, nausea, vomiting, lethargy or malaise or fatigue, alopecia, anorexia. **OCCASIONAL:** Urticaria, dermatitis.

ADVERSE REACTIONS/ TOXIC EFFECTS

Excessive dosage may negate chemotherapeutic effects of folic acid antagonists. Anaphylaxis occurs rarely. Diarrhea may cause rapid clinical deterioration.

NURSING CONSIDERATIONS

BASELINE ASSESSMENT

Give as soon as possible, preferably within 1 hr, for treatment of accidental overdosage of folic acid antagonists.

INTERVENTION/EVALUATION

Monitor for vomiting—may need to change from oral to parenteral therapy. Observe elderly, debilitated closely because of risk of severe toxicities. Assess CBC, differential, platelet count (also electrolytes and liver function tests if used in combination with chemotherapeutic agents).

PATIENT/FAMILY TEACHING

• Explain purpose of medication in treatment of cancer. • Report allergic reaction, vomiting.

leuprolide acetate ⚑

loo-proe-lide

(Lupron, <u>Lupron Depot</u>, Lupron Depot-Gyn, Lupron Depot-Ped, Viadur)

Do not confuse leuprolide or Lupron with Lopurin or Nuprin.

◆CLASSIFICATION

PHARMACOTHERAPEUTIC: Gonadotropin-releasing hormone analogue. **CLINICAL:** Antineoplastic (see pp. 76C, 93C).

ACTION

A gonadotropin-releasing hormone analogue and antineoplastic agent that stimulates the release of luteinizing hormone (LH) and follicle-stimulating hormone (FSH) from the anterior pituitary gland. Therapeutic Effect: Produces pharmacologic castration and decreases the growth of abnormal prostate tissue in males; causes endometrial tissue to become inactive and atrophic in females; and decreases the rate of pubertal development in children with central precocious puberty.

PHARMACOKINETICS

Rapidly and well absorbed after subcutaneous administration. Absorbed slowly after IM administration. Protein binding: 43%–49%. Half-life: 3–4 hr.

USES

Palliative treatment of advanced prostate carcinoma. Management of endometriosis as initial or treatment of recurrent symptoms. Pre-operative treatment of anemia caused by uterine leiomyomata (fibroids). Treatment of central precocious puberty.

PRECAUTIONS

CONTRAINDICATIONS: Lactation, pernicious anemia, pregnancy, undiagnosed vaginal bleeding. Eligard 7.5 mg is contraindicated in patients with hypersensitivity to GnRH, GnRH agonist analogs or any of the components, 30 mg Lupron Depot contraindicated in women, the implant form is contraindicated in women and children. **CAUTIONS:** Long-term use in children.

⧗ **LIFESPAN CONSIDERATIONS: Pregnancy/Lactation: Depot:** Contraindicated in pregnancy. May cause spontaneous abortion. **Pregnancy Category X. Children:** Long-term safety not established. **Elderly:** No age-related precautions noted.

INTERACTIONS

DRUG: None known. **HERBAL:** None known. **FOOD:** None known. **LAB VALUES:** May increase serum prostatic acid phosphatase (PAP) levels. Initially increases, then decreases, serum testosterone concentration.

AVAILABILITY (Rx)

IMPLANT (VIADUR): 65 mg. **INJECTION DEPOT FORMULATION:** 3.75 mg (Lupron

Depot), 7.5 mg (Eligard, Lupron Depot, Lupron Depot-Ped), 11.25 mg (Lupron Depot, Lupron Depot-Ped, Lupron Depot-Gyn), 15 mg (Lupron Depot-Ped), 22.5 mg (Eligard, Lupron Depot), 30 mg (Lupron Depot). **INJECTION SOLUTION (LUPRON):** 5 mg/ml.

ADMINISTRATION/HANDLING

◀ **ALERT** ▶ May be carcinogenic, mutagenic, teratogenic. Handle with extreme care during preparation/administration.

IM

Lupron Depot • Store at room temperature. • Protect from light, heat. • Do not freeze vials. • Reconstitute only with diluent provided. Follow instructions for mixing provided by the manufacturer. • Do not use needles less than 22 gauge; use syringes provided by the manufacturer (0.5 ml low-dose insulin syringes may be used as an alternative). • Administer immediately.

Eligard • Refrigerate. • Allow to warm to room temperature before reconstitution. • Follow instructions for mixing provided by the manufacturer. • Following reconstitution, administer within 30 min.

SUBCUTANEOUS

Lupron • Refrigerate vials. • Injection appears clear, colorless. • Discard if precipitate forms or solution appears discolored. • Administer into deltoid muscle, anterior thigh, or abdomen.

INDICATIONS/ROUTES/DOSAGE

ADVANCED PROSTATIC CARCINOMA

IM (LUPRON DEPOT): ADULTS, ELDERLY: 7.5 mg every month or 22.5 mg q3mo or 30 mg q4mo.
SUBCUTANEOUS (ELIGARD): ADULTS, ELDERLY: 7.5 mg every month or 22.5 mg q3mo or 30 mg q4mo.
SUBCUTANEOUS (LUPRON): ADULTS, ELDERLY: 1 mg/day.

SUBCUTANEOUS (VIADUR): ADULTS, ELDERLY: 65 mg implanted q12mo.

ENDOMETRIOSIS

IM (LUPRON DEPOT): ADULTS, ELDERLY: 3.75 mg/mo for up to 6 mo or 11.25 mg q3mo for up to 2 doses.

UTERINE LEIOMYOMATA

IM (WITH IRON [LUPRON DEPOT]): ADULTS, ELDERLY: 3.75 mg/mo for up to 3 mo or 11.25 mg as a single injection.

PRECOCIOUS PUBERTY

IM (LUPRON DEPOT): CHILDREN: 0.3 mg/kg/dose every 28 days. Minimum: 7.5 mg. If down regulation is not achieved, titrate upward in 3.75-mg increments q4wk.
SUBCUTANEOUS (LUPRON): CHILDREN: 20–45 mcg/kg/day. Titrate upward by 10 mcg/kg/day if down regulation is not achieved.

SIDE EFFECTS

FREQUENT: Hot flashes (ranging from mild flushing to diaphoresis). **Females:** Amenorrhea, spotting. **OCCASIONAL:** Arrhythmias; palpitations; blurred vision; dizziness; edema; headache; burning or itching, or swelling at injection site; nausea; insomnia; weight gain. **Females:** Deepening voice, hirsutism, decreased libido, increased breast tenderness, vaginitis, altered mood. **Males:** Constipation, decreased testicle size, gynecomastia, impotence, decreased appetite, angina. **RARE: Males:** Thrombophlebitis.

ADVERSE REACTIONS/TOXIC EFFECTS

Signs and symptoms of metastatic prostatic carcinoma (such as bone pain, dysuria or hematuria, and weakness or paresthesia of the lower extremities) occasionally worsen 1–2 wk after the initial dose but then subside with continued therapy. Pulmonary embolism and MI occur rarely.

✐ see color pill atlas   🌿 herb   underlined – top prescribed drug

NURSING CONSIDERATIONS

BASELINE ASSESSMENT

Question for possibility of pregnancy before initiating therapy (Pregnancy Category X). Obtain serum testosterone, PAP levels periodically during therapy. Serum testosterone and PAP levels should increase during first week of therapy. Testosterone level then should decrease to baseline level or less within 2 wk, PAP level within 4 wk.

INTERVENTION/EVALUATION

Monitor for arrhythmias, palpitations. Assess for peripheral edema. Assess sleep pattern. Monitor for visual difficulties. Assist with ambulation if dizziness occurs. Offer antiemetics if nausea occurs.

PATIENT/FAMILY TEACHING

• Hot flashes tend to decrease during continued therapy. • Temporary exacerbation of signs and symptoms of disease may occur during first few wk of therapy. • Use contraceptive measures during therapy. • Inform physician if regular menstruation persists, pregnancy occurs. • Avoid tasks that require alertness, motor skills until response to drug is established (potential for dizziness).

---

levalbuterol

lee-val-**bwet**-err-all

(Xopenex, Xopenex HFA)

Do not confuse Xopenex with Xanax.

◆ CLASSIFICATION

PHARMACOTHERAPEUTIC: Sympathomimetic. **CLINICAL:** Bronchodilator (see p. 66C).

ACTION

A sympathomimetic that stimulates beta$_2$-adrenergic receptors in the lungs resulting in relaxation of bronchial smooth muscle. **Therapeutic Effect:** Relieves bronchospasm and reduces airway resistance.

PHARMACOKINETICS

Route	Onset	Peak	Duration
Inhalation	10–17 min	1.5 hr	5–6 hr

Metabolized in the liver to inactive metabolite. **Half-life:** 3.3–4 hr.

USES

Treatment, prevention of bronchospasm due to reversible obstructive airway disease.

PRECAUTIONS

CONTRAINDICATIONS: History of hypersensitivity to sympathomimetics. **CAUTIONS:** Cardiovascular disorders (e.g., cardiac arrhythmias), seizures, hypertension, hyperthyroidism, diabetes mellitus. ⧖ **LIFESPAN CONSIDERATIONS: Pregnancy/Lactation:** Crosses placenta. Unknown if distributed in breast milk. **Pregnancy Category C. Children:** Safety and efficacy not established in those younger than 12 yr. **Elderly:** Lower initial dosages recommended.

INTERACTIONS

DRUG: Beta blockers: Antagonize the effects of levalbuterol. **Digoxin:** May increase the risk of arrhythmias. **MAOIs, tricyclic antidepressants:** May potentiate cardiovascular effects. **HERBAL:** None known. **FOOD:** None known. **LAB VALUES:** May increase serum potassium level.

AVAILABILITY (Rx)

SOLUTION FOR NEBULIZATION: 0.31 in 3-ml vials, 0.63 mg in 3-ml vials, 1.25 mg in 3-ml vials. **INHALATION AEROSOL:** 45 mcg/activation.

ADMINISTRATION/HANDLING

NEBULIZATION

• No diluent necessary. • Protect from light and excessive heat. Store at room temperature. • Once foil is opened, use within 2 wk. • Discard if solution is not colorless. • Do not mix with other medications. • Give over 5–15 min.

INDICATIONS/ROUTES/DOSAGE

TREATMENT AND PREVENTION OF BRONCHOSPASM

NEBULIZATION: ADULTS, ELDERLY, CHILDREN 12 YR AND OLDER: Initially, 0.63 mg 3 times a day 6–8 hr apart. May increase to 1.25 mg 3 times a day with dose monitoring. CHILDREN 3–11 YR: Initially 0.31 mg 3 times a day. **Maximum:** 0.63 mg 3 times a day.

INHALATION: ADULTS, ELDERLY, CHILDREN 4 YR AND OLDER: 1–2 inhalations q4–6h.

SIDE EFFECTS

FREQUENT: Tremor, nervousness, headache, throat dryness and irritation. **OCCASIONAL:** Cough, bronchial irritation. **RARE:** Somnolence, diarrhea, dry mouth, flushing, diaphoresis, anorexia.

ADVERSE REACTIONS/ TOXIC EFFECTS

Excessive sympathomimetic stimulation may produce palpitations, extrasystoles, tachycardia, chest pain, a slight increase in BP followed by a substantial decrease, chills, diaphoresis, and blanching of skin. Too-frequent or excessive use may lead to decreased bronchodilating effectiveness and severe, paradoxical bronchoconstriction.

NURSING CONSIDERATIONS

BASELINE ASSESSMENT

Offer emotional support (high incidence of anxiety due to difficulty in breathing, sympathomimetic response to drug).

INTERVENTION/EVALUATION

Monitor rate, depth, rhythm, type of respiration; quality and rate of pulse, EKG, serum potassium, ABG determinations. Assess lung sounds for wheezing (bronchoconstriction), rales.

PATIENT/FAMILY TEACHING

• Increase fluid intake (decreases lung secretion viscosity). • Rinsing mouth with water immediately after inhalation may prevent mouth/throat dryness. • Avoid excessive use of caffeine derivatives (chocolate, coffee, tea, cola, cocoa). • Notify physician if palpitations, tachycardia, chest pain, tremors, dizziness, headache occurs.

Levaquin, *see levofloxacin*

---

levetiracetam

leva-tir-**ass** eh-tam
(Keppra)
Do not confuse Keppra with Kaletra.

CLASSIFICATION

CLINICAL: Anticonvulsant.

ACTION

An anticonvulsant that inhibits burst firing without affecting normal neuronal excitability. **Therapeutic Effect:** Prevents seizure activity.

USES

Adjunctive therapy in treatment of partial-onset seizures in adults and children with epilepsy.

PRECAUTIONS

CONTRAINDICATIONS: None known. **CAUTIONS:** Renal impairment. **Pregnancy Category C.**

INTERACTIONS

DRUG: None known. HERBAL: **Ginkgo biloba:** May decrease anticonvulsant effectiveness. FOOD: None known. LAB VALUES: May increase blood Hgb level, Hct, and RBC and WBC counts.

AVAILABILITY (Rx)

ORAL SOLUTION: 100 mg/ml. TABLETS: 250 mg, 500 mg, 750 mg.

ADMINISTRATION/HANDLING

PO
• Give without regard to food.

INDICATIONS/ROUTES/DOSAGE

PARTIAL-ONSET SEIZURES

PO: ADULTS, ELDERLY: Initially, 500 mg q12h. May increase by 1,000 mg/day q2wk. **Maximum:** 3,000 mg/day. CHILDREN 4–16 YR: 10–20 mg/kg/day in 2 divided doses. May increase at weekly intervals by 10–20 mg/kg. **Maximum:** 60 mg/kg.

DOSAGE IN RENAL IMPAIRMENT

Dosage is modified based on creatinine clearance.

Creatinine Clearance Dosage (ml/min)

Higher than 80 ml/min	500–1,500 mg q12h
50–80 ml/min	500–1,000 mg q12h
30–50 ml/min	250–750 mg q12h
Less than 30 ml/min	250–500 mg q12h
End stage renal disease using dialysis	500–1,000 mg q12h, after dialysis, a 250- to 500-mg supplemental dose is recommended.

SIDE EFFECTS

FREQUENT (15%–10%): Somnolence, asthenia, headache, infection. OCCASIONAL (9%–3%): Dizziness, pharyngitis, pain, depression, nervousness, vertigo, rhinitis, anorexia. RARE (less than 3%): Amnesia, anxiety, emotional lability, cough, sinusitis, anorexia, diplopia.

ADVERSE REACTIONS/TOXIC EFFECTS

Acute psychosis and seizures have been reported. Sudden discontinuance increases the risk of seizure activity.

NURSING CONSIDERATIONS

BASELINE ASSESSMENT

Review history of seizure disorder (intensity, frequency, duration, level of consciousness [LOC]). Initiate seizure precautions. Assess for hypersensitivity to levetiracetam, renal function tests.

INTERVENTION/EVALUATION

Observe for recurrence of seizure activity. Assess for clinical improvement (decrease in intensity/frequency of seizures). Monitor renal function tests. Assist with ambulation if dizziness occurs.

PATIENT/FAMILY TEACHING

• Somnolence, drowsiness usually diminish with continued therapy. • Avoid tasks that require alertness, motor skills until response to drug is established. • Do not abruptly discontinue medication (may precipitate seizures). • Strict maintenance of drug therapy is essential for seizure control.

levobunolol hydrochloride

(Betagan Liquifilm)
See Antiglaucoma agents (p. 48C)

levobupivacaine

(Chirocaine)
See Anesthetics: local

levofloxacin

levo-**flox**-a-sin

(Iquix, Levaquin, Levaquin Leva-Pak, Quixin)

CLASSIFICATION

PHARMACOTHERAPEUTIC: Fluoroquinolone. **CLINICAL:** Antibiotic (see p. 24C).

ACTION

A fluoroquinolone that inhibits the DNA enzyme gyrase in susceptible microorganisms, interfering with bacterial cell replication and repair. Therapeutic Effect: Bactericidal.

PHARMACOKINETICS

Well absorbed after both PO and IV administration. Protein binding: 24%–8%. Penetrates rapidly and extensively into leukocytes, epithelial cells, and macrophages. Lung concentrations are 2–5 times higher than those of plasma. Eliminated unchanged in the urine. Partially removed by hemodialysis. Half-life: 8 hr.

USES

Treatment of acute bacterial exacerbation of chronic bronchitis, acute bacterial sinusitus, community-acquired pneumonia, nosocomial pneumonia, acute maxillary sinusitis, complicated UTIs, acute pyelonephritis, uncomplicated mild to moderate skin and skin-structure infections, prostatitis. **Ophthalmic:** Treatment of superficial infections to conjunctiva (0.5%), cornea (1.5%). Treatment of susceptible infections due to *S. pneumoniae, S. aureus, E. faecalis, H. influenzae, M. catarrhalis, serratia marcescens, K. pneumoniae, E. coli, P. mirabilis, P. aeruginosa, C. pneumoniae, Legionella pneumophila, Mycoplasma pneumoniae* including acute bacterial sinusitis. **OFF-LABEL:** Anthrax, gonorrhea, pelvic inflammatory disease (PID).

PRECAUTIONS

CONTRAINDICATIONS: Hypersensitivity to other fluoroquinolones or nalidixic acid. **CAUTIONS:** Suspected CNS disorders, seizure disorder, renal impairment, bradycardia, cardiomyopathy, hypokalemia, hypomagnesemia.

⏳ **LIFESPAN CONSIDERATIONS: Pregnancy/Lactation:** Excreted in breast milk. Avoid use in pregnancy. **Pregnancy Category C. Children:** Safety and efficacy not established in those younger than 18 yr. **Elderly:** Age-related renal impairment may require dosage adjustment.

INTERACTIONS

DRUG: Antacids, iron preparations, sucralfate, zinc: Decrease levofloxacin absorption. **NSAIDs:** May increase the risk of CNS stimulation or seizures. **HERBAL:** None known. **FOOD:** None known. **LAB VALUES:** May alter blood glucose levels.

AVAILABILITY (Rx)

ORAL SOLUTION: 25 mg/ml. **TABLETS (LEVAQUIN, LEVAQUIN LEVA-PAK):** 250 mg, 500 mg, 750 mg. **INJECTION (LEVAQUIN):** 500-mg/20-ml vials. **PRE-MIXED SOLUTION (LEVAQUIN):** 25 mg/ml, 250 mg/50 ml, 500 mg/100 ml, 750 mg/150 ml. **OPHTHALMIC SOLUTION:** 0.5% (Iquix), 1.5% (Quixin).

ADMINISTRATION/HANDLING

 IV

Reconstitution ● For infusion using single-dose vial, withdraw desired amount (10 ml for 250 mg, 20 ml for 500 mg). Dilute each 10 ml (250 mg) with minimum 40 ml 0.9% NaCl, D_5W.

Rate of administration ● Administer slowly, over not less than 60 min.

Storage • Available in single-dose 20-ml (500-mg) vials and premixed with D$_5$W, ready to infuse.

PO
• Do not administer antacids (aluminum, magnesium), sucralfate, iron or multivitamin preparations with zinc within 2 hr of levofloxacin administration (significantly reduces levofloxacin absorption). • Encourage intake of cranberry juice, citrus fruits (acidifies urine). • Give without regard to food.

OPHTHALMIC
• Place a gloved finger on lower eyelid, pull out until a pocket is formed between eye and lower lid. Hold dropper above pocket, place correct number of drops into pocket. • Close eye gently. Apply digital pressure to lacrimal sac for 1–2 min (minimizes drainage into nose and throat, reducing risk of systemic effects).

▨ IV INCOMPATIBILITIES
Furosemide (Lasix), heparin, insulin, nitroglycerin, propofol (Diprivan).

IV COMPATIBILITIES
Aminophylline, dobutamine (Dobutrex), dopamine (Intron), fentanyl (Sublimaze), lidocaine, lorazepam (Ativan), morphine.

INDICATIONS/ROUTES/DOSAGE
BACTERIAL SINUSITIS
PO: ADULTS, ELDERLY: 500 mg once daily for 10 days or 750 mg once daily for 5 days.

BRONCHITIS
PO, IV: ADULTS, ELDERLY: 500 mg q24h for 7 days.

COMMUNITY-ACQUIRED PNEUMONIA
PO: ADULTS, ELDERLY: 750 mg/day for 5 days or 500 mg for 7–14 days.

PNEUMONIA, NOSOCOMIAL
PO, IV: ADULTS, ELDERLY: 750 mg q24h for 7–14 days.

ACUTE MAXILLARY SINUSITIS
PO, IV: ADULTS, ELDERLY: 500 mg q24h for 10–14 days.

SKIN AND SKIN-STRUCTURE INFECTIONS
PO, IV: ADULTS, ELDERLY: (Uncomplicated) 500 mg q24h for 7–10 days. (Complicated) 750 mg q24h for 7–14 days.

PROSTATITIS
IV, PO: ADULTS, ELDERLY: 500 mg q24h for 28 days.

UNCOMPLICATED UTI
IV, PO: ADULTS, ELDERLY: 250 mg q24h for 3 days.

UTIs, ACUTE PYELONEPHRITIS
PO, IV: ADULTS, ELDERLY: 250 mg q24h for 10 days.

BACTERIAL CONJUNCTIVITIS
OPHTHALMIC: ADULTS, ELDERLY, CHILDREN 1 YR AND OLDER: 1–2 drops q2h for 2 days (up to 8 times a day), then 1–2 drops q4h for 5 days.

CORNEAL ULCER
OPHTHALMIC: ADULTS, ELDERLY, CHILDREN OLDER THAN 5 YR: Days 1–3: Instill 1–2 drops q30min to 2 hours while awake and 4–6 hours after retiring. Days 4 through completion: 1–2 drops q1–4h while awake.

DOSAGE IN RENAL IMPAIRMENT
For bronchitis, pneumonia, sinusitis, and skin and skin-structure infections, dosage and frequency are modified based on creatinine clearance.

Creatinine Clearance	Dosage
50–80 ml/min	No change
20–49 ml/min	500 mg initially, then 250 mg q24h
10–19 ml/min	500 mg initially, then 250 mg q48h

Dialysis 500 mg initially, then 250 mg q48h. For UTIs and pyelonephritis, dosage and frequency are modified based on creatinine clearance.

Creatinine Clearance	Dosage
20 ml/min	No change
10–19 ml/min	250 mg initially, then 250 mg q48h

SIDE EFFECTS

OCCASIONAL   **(3%–1%):** Diarrhea, nausea, abdominal pain, dizziness, drowsiness, headache, light-headedness. **Ophthalmic:** Local burning or discomfort, margin crusting, crystals or scales, foreign body sensation, ocular itching, altered taste. **RARE (less than 1%):** Flatulence; altered taste; pain; inflammation or swelling in calves, hands, or shoulder; chest pain; difficulty breathing; palpitations; edema; tendon pain. **Ophthalmic:** Corneal staining, keratitis, allergic reaction, eyelid swelling, tearing, reduced visual acuity.

ADVERSE REACTIONS/ TOXIC EFFECTS

Antibiotic-associated colitis and other superinfections may occur from altered bacterial balance. Hypersensitivity reactions, including photosensitivity (as evidenced by rash, pruritus, blisters, edema, and burning skin), have occurred in patients receiving fluoroquinolones.

NURSING CONSIDERATIONS

BASELINE ASSESSMENT

Question for hypersensitivity to levofloxacin, other fluoroquinolones.

INTERVENTION/EVALUATION

Monitor blood glucose, renal and liver function tests. Report hypersensitivity reaction: skin rash, urticaria, pruritus, photosensitivity promptly. Be alert for superinfection (e.g., genital or anal pruritus, ulceration or changes in oral mucosa, moderate to severe diarrhea, new or increased fever). Provide symptomatic relief for nausea. Evaluate food tolerance, altered taste.

PATIENT/FAMILY TEACHING

• Drink 6–8 glasses of fluid a day (citrus, cranberry juice acidifies urine). • Avoid tasks that require alertness, motor skills until response to drug is established (may cause dizziness, drowsiness). • Notify physician if tendon pain or swelling, palpitations, chest pain, difficulty breathing, persistent diarrhea occurs.

levorphanol tartrate

leh-**vor**-phan-ole
(Levo-Dromoran)
See Opioid analgesics (p. 128C)

Levothroid, *see* *levothyroxine*

levothyroxine

lee-voe-thye-**rox**-een

(Eltroxin ✦, Levo-T, Levothroid, Levoxyl, Novothyrox ✦, Synthroid, Unithroid)
Do not confuse levothyroxine with liothyronine.

FIXED-COMBINATION(S)

With liothyronine, T_3 **(Thyrolar).**

CLASSIFICATION

PHARMACOTHERAPEUTIC: Synthetic isomer of thyroxine. **CLINICAL:** Thyroid hormone (T4) (see p. 143C).

ACTION

A synthetic isomer of thyroxine involved in normal metabolism, growth, and development, especially of the CNS in infants. Possesses catabolic and anabolic effects. **Therapeutic Effect:** Increases basal metabolic rate, enhances gluconeogenesis and stimulates protein synthesis.

PHARMACOKINETICS

Variable, incomplete absorption from the GI tract. Protein binding: greater than 99%. Widely distributed. Deiodinated in peripheral tissues, minimal metabolism in the liver. Eliminated by biliary excretion. **Half-life:** 6–7 days.

USES

Treatment of hypothyroidism, myxedema coma, pituitary thyroid-stimulating hormone (TSH) suppression.

PRECAUTIONS

CONTRAINDICATIONS: Hypersensitivity to tablet components, such as tartrazine; allergy to aspirin; lactose intolerance; MI and thyrotoxicosis uncomplicated by hypothyroidism; treatment of obesity. **CAUTIONS:** Elderly, angina pectoris, hypertension, other cardiovascular disease.

⌛ **LIFESPAN CONSIDERATIONS: Pregnancy/Lactation:** Drug does not cross placenta. Minimal excretion in breast milk. **Pregnancy Category A. Children:** No age-related precautions noted. Caution in neonates in interpreting thyroid function tests. **Elderly:** May be more sensitive to thyroid effects; individualized dosage recommended.

INTERACTIONS

DRUG: Cholestyramine, colestipol: May decrease the absorption of levothyroxine. **Estrogens:** May cause a decrease in serum-free thyroxine concentration. **Oral anticoagulants:** May alter the effects of oral anticoagulants.

Sympathomimetics: May increase the risk of coronary insufficiency and the effects of levothyroxine. **HERBAL:** None known. **FOOD:** None known. **LAB VALUES:** None known.

AVAILABILITY (Rx)

TABLETS: (LEVO-T, LEVOTHROID, LEVO-XYL, SYNTHROID, UNITHROID): 0.025 mg, 0.05 mg, 0.075 mg, 0.088 mg, 0.1 mg, 0.112 mg, 0.125 mg, 0.137 mg, 0.15 mg, 0.175 mg, 0.2 mg, 0.3 mg. **INJECTION (SYNTHROID):** 200 mcg, 500 mcg.

ADMINISTRATION/HANDLING

◄ **ALERT** ► Do not interchange brands (problems with bioequivalence between manufacturers).

 IV

Reconstitution • Reconstitute 200-mcg or 500-mcg vial with 5 ml 0.9% NaCl to provide a concentration of 40 or 100 mcg/ml, respectively; shake until clear.

Rate of administration • Use immediately and discard unused portions. • Give each 100 mcg or less over 1 min.

Storage • Store vials at room temperature.

PO
• Give at same time each day to maintain hormone levels. • Administer before breakfast to prevent insomnia. • Tablets may be crushed.

▦ IV INCOMPATIBILITIES

Do not use or mix with other IV solutions.

INDICATIONS/ROUTES/DOSAGE

HYPOTHYROIDISM

PO: ADULTS, ELDERLY, CHILDREN OLDER THAN 12 YR, GROWTH AND PUBERTY COMPETE: 1.7 mcg/kg/day as single daily dose. Usual maintenance: 100–200 mcg/day. CHILDREN OLDER THAN 12 YR, GROWTH AND PUBERTY INCOMPLETE: 2–3 mcg/kg/day. CHILDREN 6–12

YR: 4–5 mcg/kg/day. CHILDREN 1–5 YR: 5–6 mcg/kg/day. CHILDREN 6–12 MO: 6–8 mcg/kg/day. CHILDREN 3-6 MO: 8–10 mcg/kg/day. CHILDREN YOUNGER THAN 3 MO: 10–15 mcg/kg/day.

MYXEDEMA COMA

IV: ADULTS, ELDERLY: Initially, 300–500 mcg. Maintenance: 75–100 mcg/day.

PITUITARY TSH SUPPRESSION

PO: ADULTS, ELDERLY: Doses greater than 2 mcg/kg/day usually required to suppress TSH below 0.1 milliunits/liter.

SIDE EFFECTS

OCCASIONAL: Reversible hair loss at the start of therapy (in children). **RARE:** Dry skin, GI intolerance, rash, hives, pseudotumor cerebri or severe headache in children.

ADVERSE REACTIONS/ TOXIC EFFECTS

Excessive dosage produces signs and symptoms of hyperthyroidism, including weight loss, palpitations, increased appetite, tremors, nervousness, tachycardia, hypertension, headache, insomnia, and menstrual irregularities. Cardiac arrhythmias occur rarely.

NURSING CONSIDERATIONS

BASELINE ASSESSMENT

Question for hypersensitivity to tartrazine, aspirin, lactose. Obtain baseline weight, vital signs. Signs and symptoms of diabetes mellitus, diabetes insipidus, adrenal insufficiency, hypopituitarism may become intensified. Treat with adrenocortical steroids before thyroid therapy in coexisting hypothyroidism and hypoadrenalism.

INTERVENTION/EVALUATION

Monitor pulse for rate, rhythm (report pulse of 100 or marked increase). Observe for tremors, anxiety. Assess appetite, sleep pattern.

PATIENT/FAMILY TEACHING

• Do not discontinue drug therapy; replacement for hypothyroidism is lifelong. • Follow-up office visits, thyroid function tests are essential. • Take medication at the same time each day, preferably in the morning. • Monitor pulse for rate, rhythm; report irregular rhythm or pulse rate over 100 beats/min. • Do not change brands. • Notify physician promptly of chest pain, weight loss, anxiety or tremors, insomnia. • Children may have reversible hair loss, increased aggressiveness during the first few months of therapy. • Full therapeutic effect may take 1–3 wk.

Levoxyl, *see levothyroxine*

Lexapro, *see escitalopram*

Lexiva, *see fosamprenavir*

lidocaine hydrochloride 🏳

lye-doe-kane

(Anestacaine, Anestacon, Ela-Max, Ela-Max Plus, Laryng-O-Jet Spray, L-Caine, Lida Mantle, Lidoderm, Lidoject 1, Lidoject 2, LidoSite, LMX 4, LMX 4 with Tegaderm, LMX 5, Truxacaine, UAD Caine, Xylocaine, Xylocaine 10% Oral, Xylocaine Dental Cartridges, Xylocaine HCl For Spinal, Xylocaine Jelly, Xylocaine-MPF, Xylocaine Topical,

---

✐ see color pill atlas   ◢ herb   underlined – top prescribed drug

Xylocaine Viscous, Xylocaine Viscous Topical Solution ✽, Xylocard ✽, Zilactin-L ✽)

FIXED-COMBINATION(S)

EMLA: lidocaine/prilocaine (an anesthetic): 2.5%/2.5%. **Lidocaine with epinephrine:** lidocaine/epinephrine (a sympathomimetic): 2%/1:50,000; 1%/1:100,000; 1%/1:200,000; 0.5%/1:200,000. **Lidosite:** lidocaine/epinephrine, (a sympathomimetic): 10%/0.1%.

◆CLASSIFICATION

PHARMACOTHERAPEUTIC: Amide anesthetic. **CLINICAL:** Antiarrhythmic, anesthetic (see pp. 5C, 14C).

ACTION

An amide anesthetic that inhibits conduction of nerve impulses. Therapeutic Effect: Causes temporary loss of feeling and sensation. Also an antiarrhythmic that decreases depolarization, automaticity, excitability of the ventricle during diastole by direct action. Therapeutic Effect: Inhibits ventricular arrhythmias.

PHARMACOKINETICS

Route	Onset	Peak	Duration
IV	30–90 sec	N/A	10–20 min
Local anesthetic	2.5 min	N/A	30–60 min

Completely absorbed after IM administration. Protein binding: 60% to 80%. Widely distributed. Metabolized in the liver. Primarily excreted in urine. Minimally removed by hemodialysis. Half-life: 1–2 hr.

USES

Antiarrhythmic: Rapid control of acute ventricular arrhythmias following MI, cardiac catheterization, cardiac surgery, digitalis-induced ventricular arrhythmias.

Local Anesthetic: Infiltration/nerve block for dental or surgical procedures, childbirth. **Topical Anesthetic:** Local skin disorders (minor burns, insect bites, prickly heat, skin manifestations of chickenpox, abrasions). Mucous membranes (local anesthesia of oral, nasal, laryngeal mucous membranes; local anesthesia of respiratory, urinary tracts; relief of discomfort of pruritus ani, hemorrhoids, pruritus vulvae). **Dermal Patch:** Treatment of shingles-related skin pain.

PRECAUTIONS

CONTRAINDICATIONS: Adams-Stokes syndrome, hypersensitivity to amide-type local anesthetics, septicemia (spinal anesthesia), supraventricular arrhythmias, Wolff-Parkinson-White syndrome. **CAUTIONS:** Hepatic disease, marked hypoxia, severe respiratory depression, hypovolemia, heart block, bradycardia, atrial fibrillation.

⌛ LIFESPAN CONSIDERATIONS: **Pregnancy/Lactation:** Crosses placenta. Distributed in breast milk. **Pregnancy Category B. Children:** No age-related precautions noted. **Elderly:** More sensitive to adverse effects. Dose, rate of infusion should be reduced. Age-related renal impairment may require dosage adjustment.

INTERACTIONS

DRUG: **Anticonvulsants:** May increase cardiac depressant effects. **Beta-adrenergic blockers:** May increase risk of toxicity. **Local anesthetics:** Amount absorbed from all formulations may be increased. **Other antiarrhythmics:** May increase cardiac effects. HERBAL: None known. FOOD: None known. LAB VALUES: IM lidocaine may increase creatine kinase (CK) level (used to diagnose acute MI). Therapeutic serum level is 1.5 to 6 mcg/ml; toxic serum level is greater than 6 mcg/ml.

AVAILABILITY (Rx)

INJECTION (FOR CONTINUOUS INFUSION [XYLOCAINE]): 4% w/v (40 mg/ml), 10% w/v (100 mg/ml), 20% w/v (200 mg/ml). **INJECTION (WITH DEXTROSE FOR CONTINUOUS INFUSION):** 0.1% w/v (1 mg/ml), 0.2% w/v (2 mg/ml), 0.4% w/v (4 mg/ml), 0.8% w/v (8 mg/ml). **INJECTION (FOR DIRECT INJECTION [XYLOCAINE]):** 1% w/v (10 mg/ml), 2% w/v (20 mg/ml). **INJECTABLE SOLUTION:** 0.5% (Xylocaine HCl), 1% (Anestacaine, L-Caine, Lidoject 1, Truxacaine, UAD Caine, Xylocaine HCl, Xylocaine-MPF), 1.5% (Xylocaine HCl, Xylocaine-MPF), 2% (Anestacaine, Lidoject 2, Truxacaine, Xylocaine Dental Cartridges, Xylocaine HCl, Xylocaine-MPF), 4% (Xylocaine HCl, Xylocaine-MPF), 10% (Xylocaine), 20% (Xylocaine). **OINTMENT (XYLOCAINE TOPICAL):** 5%. **CREAM:** 3% (Lida Mantle), 4% (Ela-Max, Ela-Max Plus, LMX 4, LMX 4 with Tegaderm), 5% (LMX 5). **GEL (ANESTACON, XYLOCAINE JELLY, XYLOCAINE TOPICAL):** 2%. **TOPICAL SPRAY (XYLOCAINE 10% ORAL):** 10%. **TOPICAL SOLUTION:** 2% (Xylocaine Viscous), 4% (Xylocaine Topical). **TOPICAL FILM (LIDODERM):** 5%. **TOPICAL LOTION (LIDA MANTLE):** 3%. **DERMAL PATCH (LIDODERM):** 5%. **KIT (LARYNG-O-JET SPRAY):** 4%.

ADMINISTRATION/HANDLING

◄ **ALERT** ► Resuscitative equipment, drugs (including O_2) must always be readily available when administering lidocaine by any route.

IV

◄ **ALERT** ► Use only lidocaine without preservative, clearly marked **for IV use**.

Reconstitution • For IV infusion, prepare solution by adding 1 g to 1 L D_5W to provide concentration of 1 mg/ml (0.1%). • Commercially available preparations of 0.2%, 0.4%, and 0.8% may be used for IV infusion. **Maximum concentration:** 4 g/250 ml.

Rate of administration • For IV push, use 1% (10 mg/ml) or 2% (20 mg/ml). • Administer IV push at rate of 25–50 mg/min. • Administer for IV infusion at rate of 1–4 mg/min (1–4 ml); use volume control IV set.

Storage • Store at room temperature.

IM
• Use 10% (100 mg/ml); clearly identify lidocaine that is **for IM use**. • Give in deltoid muscle (serum level is significantly higher than if injection is given in gluteus muscle or lateral thigh).

TOPICAL
• Not for ophthalmic use. • For skin disorders, apply directly to affected area or put on gauze or bandage, which is then applied to the skin. • For mucous membrane use, apply to desired area as per manufacturer's insert. • Administer the lowest dosage possible that still provides anesthesia.

❖ IV INCOMPATIBILITIES

Amphotericin B complex (Abelcet, AmBisome, Amphotec), thiopental.

IV COMPATIBILITIES

Aminophylline, amiodarone (Cordarone), calcium gluconate, digoxin (Lanoxin), diltiazem (Cardizem), dobutamine (Dobutrex), dopamine (Intropin), enalapril (Vasotec), furosemide (Lasix), heparin, insulin, nitroglycerin, potassium chloride.

INDICATIONS/ROUTES/DOSAGE

RAPID CONTROL OF ACUTE VENTRICULAR ARRHYTHMIAS AFTER AN MI, CARDIAC CATHETERIZATION, CARDIAC SURGERY, OR DIGITALIS-INDUCED VENTRICULAR ARRHYTHMIAS
IM: ADULTS, ELDERLY: 300 mg (or 4.3 mg/kg). May repeat in 60–90 min.

IV: ADULTS, ELDERLY: Initially, 50–100 mg (1 mg/kg) IV bolus at rate of 25–50 mg/min. May repeat in 5 min. Give no more than 200–300 mg in 1 hr. Maintenance: 20–50 mcg/kg/min (1–4 mg/min) as IV infusion. CHILDREN, INFANTS: Initially, 0.5–1 mg/kg IV bolus; may repeat but total dose not to exceed 3–5 mg/kg. Maintenance: 10–50 mcg/kg/min as IV infusion.

DENTAL OR SURGICAL PROCEDURES, CHILDBIRTH

INFILTRATION, NERVE BLOCK: ADULTS: Local anesthetic dosage varies with procedure, degree of anesthesia, vascularity, duration. **Maximum dose:** 4.5 mg/kg. Do not repeat within 2 hr.

LOCAL SKIN DISORDERS (MINOR BURNS, INSECT BITES, PRICKLY HEAT, SKIN MANIFESTATIONS OF CHICKENPOX, ABRASIONS), AND MUCOUS MEMBRANE DISORDERS (LOCAL ANESTHESIA OF ORAL, NASAL, AND LARYNGEAL MUCOUS MEMBRANES; LOCAL ANESTHESIA OF RESPIRATORY, URINARY TRACT; RELIEF OF DISCOMFORT OF PRURITUS ANI, HEMORRHOIDS, PRURITUS VULVAE)
TOPICAL: ADULTS, ELDERLY: Apply to affected areas as needed.

TREATMENT OF SHINGLES-RELATED SKIN PAIN

TOPICAL (DERMAL PATCH): ADULTS, ELDERLY: Apply to intact skin over most painful area (up to 3 applications once for up to 12 hr in a 24-hr period).

SIDE EFFECTS

CNS effects are generally dose-related and of short duration. **OCCASIONAL: IM:** Pain at injection site. **Topical:** Burning, stinging, tenderness at application site. **RARE:** Generally with high dose: Drowsiness; dizziness; disorientation; light-headedness; tremors; apprehension; euphoria; sensation of heat, cold, or numbness; blurred or double vision; ringing or roaring in ears (tinnitus); nausea.

ADVERSE REACTIONS/ TOXIC EFFECTS

Although serious adverse reactions to lidocaine are uncommon, high dosage by any route may produce cardiovascular depression, bradycardia, hypotension, arrhythmias, heart block, cardiovascular collapse, and cardiac arrest. There is a potential for malignant hyperthermia. CNS toxicity may occur, especially with regional anesthesia use, progressing rapidly from mild side effects to tremors, somnolence, seizures, vomiting, and respiratory depression. Methemoglobinemia (evidenced by cyanosis) has occurred following topical application of lidocaine for teething discomfort and laryngeal anesthetic spray.

NURSING CONSIDERATIONS

BASELINE ASSESSMENT

Question for hypersensitivity to lidocaine, amide anesthetics. Obtain baseline BP, pulse, respirations, EKG, serum electrolytes.

INTERVENTION/EVALUATION

Monitor EKG, vital signs closely during and following drug administration for cardiac performance. If EKG shows arrhythmias, prolongation of PR interval or QRS complex, inform physician immediately. Assess pulse for irregularity, quality, bradycardia. Assess BP for evidence of hypotension. Monitor therapeutic serum level (1.5–6 mcg/ml). For lidocaine given by all routes, monitor vital signs, patient's level of consciousness (LOC). Drowsiness should be considered a warning sign of high serum levels of lidocaine. Therapeutic serum level: 1.5–6 mcg/ml; toxic serum level: greater than 6 mcg/ml.

PATIENT/FAMILY TEACHING

• **Local anesthesia:** Ensure that patient understands loss of feeling or

L

sensation, need for protection until anesthetic wears off (e.g., no ambulation, including special positions for some regional anesthesia). • **Oral mucous membrane anesthesia:** Do not eat, drink, chew gum for 1 hr after application (swallowing reflex may be impaired, increasing risk of aspiration; numbness of tongue or buccal mucosa may lead to bite trauma).

Lidoderm, *see lidocaine*

---

linezolid

lyn-eh-**zoe**-lid
(<u>Zyvox</u>, Zyvoxam ✦)
Do not confuse Zyvox with Zoverax.

◆CLASSIFICATION
PHARMACOTHERAPEUTIC: Oxalodinone. **CLINICAL:** Antibiotic.

ACTION
An oxalodinone anti-infective that binds to a site on bacterial 23S ribosomal RNA, preventing the formation of a complex that is essential for bacterial translation. **Therapeutic Effect:** Bacteriostatic against enterococci and staphylococci; bactericidal against streptococci.

PHARMACOKINETICS
Rapidly and extensively absorbed after PO administration. Protein binding: 31%. Metabolized in the liver by oxidation. Excreted in urine. **Half-life:** 4–5.4 hr.

USES
Treatment of susceptible infections due to aerobic and facultative, gram positive micro-organisms, including *E. faecium* (vancomycin resistant strains only), *S. aureus* (including methicillin-resistant strains), *S. agalactiae, S. pneumoniae* (including multidrug resistant strains) and *S. pyogenes* including pneumonia, skin and soft tissue infections (including diabetic foot infections), bacteremia caused by susceptible vancomycin-resistant organisms.

PRECAUTIONS
CONTRAINDICATIONS: None known. **CAUTIONS:** Uncontrolled hypertension, pheochromocytoma, carcinoid syndrome, severe renal or hepatic impairment, untreated hyperthyroidism.

⌛ LIFESPAN CONSIDERATIONS: **Pregnancy/Lactation:** Unknown if distributed in breast milk. **Pregnancy Category C. Children:** Safety and efficacy not established. **Elderly:** No age-related precautions noted.

INTERACTIONS
DRUG: **Adrenergic agents (sympathomimetics):** Increase the effects of linezolid. **MAOIs:** Decrease the effects of MAOIs. HERBAL: None known. FOOD: **Tyramine-containing foods and beverages:** Excessive amounts may cause significant hypertension. LAB VALUES: May decrease blood Hgb, platelet count, WBC count, and ALT levels.

AVAILABILITY (Rx)
TABLETS: 400 mg, 600 mg. **INJECTION:** 2 mg/ml in 100-ml, 200-ml, 300-ml bags. **POWDER FOR ORAL SUSPENSION:** 100 mg/5 ml.

ADMINISTRATION/HANDLING
📖 IV

Rate of administration • Infuse over 30–120 min.

Storage • Store at room temperature. • Protect from light. • Yellow color does not affect potency.

PO

• Give without regard to meals. • Use suspension within 21 days after reconstitution.

▨ IV INCOMPATIBILITIES

Amphotericin B complex (Abelcet, AmBisome, Amphotec), chlorpromazine (Thorazine), co-trimoxazole (Bactrim), diazepam (Valium), erythromycin (Erythrocin), pentamidine (Pentam IV), phenytoin (Dilantin), total parenteral nutrition (TPN).

INDICATIONS/ROUTES/DOSAGE

VANCOMYCIN-RESISTANT INFECTIONS (VRE)

PO, IV: ADULTS, ELDERLY, CHILDREN OLDER THAN 11 YR: 600 mg q12h for 14–28 days. CHILDREN 11 YR AND YOUNGER: 10 mg/kg q8–12h for 14–28 days.

PNEUMONIA, COMPLICATED SKIN AND SKIN STRUCTURE INFECTIONS

PO, IV: ADULTS, ELDERLY, CHILDREN OLDER THAN 11 YR: 600 mg q12h for 10–14 days. CHILDREN 11 YR AND YOUNGER: 10 mg/kg q8h for 10–14 days.

UNCOMPLICATED SKIN AND SKIN STRUCTURE INFECTIONS

PO: ADULTS, ELDERLY: 400 mg q12h for 10–14 days. CHILDREN OLDER THAN 11 YR: 600 mg q12h for 10–14 days. CHILDREN 5–11 YR: 10 mg/kg/dose q12h for 10–14 days. CHILDREN YOUNGER THAN 5 YR: 10 mg/kg q8h for 10–14 days.

USUAL NEONATE DOSAGE

PO IV: NEONATES: 10 mg/kg/dose q8–12h.

SIDE EFFECTS

OCCASIONAL (5%–2%): Diarrhea, nausea, headache. **RARE (less than 2%):** Altered taste, vaginal candidiasis, fungal infection, dizziness, tongue discoloration.

ADVERSE REACTIONS/ TOXIC EFFECTS

Thrombocytopenia and myelosuppression occur rarely. Antibiotic-associated colitis and other superinfections may result from altered bacterial balance.

NURSING CONSIDERATIONS

INTERVENTION/EVALUATION

Monitor pattern of bowel activity and stool consistency carefully; mild GI effects may be tolerable, but increasing severity may indicate onset of antibiotic-associated colitis. Be alert for super-infection: severe genital or anal pruritus, abdominal pain, severe mouth soreness, moderate to severe diarrhea. Monitor CBC weekly.

PATIENT/FAMILY TEACHING

• Continue therapy for full length of treatment. • Doses should be evenly spaced. • May cause GI upset (may take with food, milk). • Excessive amounts of tyramine-containing foods (e.g., red wine, aged cheese) may cause severe reaction (severe headache, neck stiffness, diaphoresis, palpitations).

---

liothyronine (T₃)

lye-oh-**thye**-roe-neen

(Cytomel, Triostat)

Do not confuse liothyronine with levothyroxine.

FIXED-COMBINATION(S)

With levothyroxine, T₄ **(Thyrolar).**

◆CLASSIFICATION

PHARMACOTHERAPEUTIC: Synthetic form thyroid hormone T₃. **CLINICAL:** Thyroid hormone (see p. 143C).

ACTION

A synthetic form of triiodothyronine (T₃), a thyroid hormone involved in normal metabolism, growth, and development, especially of the CNS in infants. Possesses catabolic and anabolic effects.

Therapeutic Effect: Increases basal metabolic rate, enhances gluconeogenesis, and stimulates protein synthesis.

PHARMACOKINETICS

Almost completely absorbed following PO administration. Absorption is reduced to 43% in congestive heart failure (CHF) patients. Not firmly bound to serum protein. Excreted in urine. Half-life: 25 hr.

USES

PO: Replacement in decreased, absent thyroid function (partial, complete absence of gland; primary atrophy; functional deficiency; effects of surgery, radiation, antithyroid agents; pituitary, hypothalamic hypothyroidism). Management of simple (nontoxic) goiter; diagnostically in T$_3$ suppression test (differentiates hyperthyroidism from euthyroidism). **IV:** Myxedema coma, precoma.

PRECAUTIONS

CONTRAINDICATIONS: MI and thyrotoxicosis uncomplicated by hypothyroidism; obesity, uncorrected adrenal cortical insufficiency. **CAUTIONS:** Cardiovascular disease, adrenal insufficiency, coronary artery disease, diabetes mellitus, diabetes insipidus.

⚖ LIFESPAN CONSIDERATIONS: **Pregnancy/Lactation:** Does not cross placenta; is distributed in breast milk. Avoid during late pregnancy (ductus arteriosis). **Pregnancy Category A. Children:** Safety and efficacy not established. **Elderly:** Age-related increased sensitivity to thyroid effects may require dosage adjustment.

INTERACTIONS

DRUG: Cholestyramine, colestipol: May decrease the absorption of liothyronine. **Oral anticoagulants:** May alter the effects of these drugs. **Sympathomimetics:** May increase the risk of coronary insufficiency and the effects of liothyronine. **HERBAL:** None known. **FOOD:** None known. **LAB VALUES:** None known.

AVAILABILITY (Rx)

TABLETS (CYTOMEL): 5 mcg, 25 mcg, 50 mcg. **INJECTION (TRIOSTAT):** 10 mcg/ml.

ADMINISTRATION/HANDLING

◀ **ALERT** ▶ Initial and subsequent dosages are based on the patient's clinical status and response.

◀ **ALERT** ▶ Do not use different brands of liothyronine interchangeably because of problems with bioequivalence among manufacturers.

 IV

• Administer IV dose over 4 hr but no longer than 12 hr apart.

INDICATIONS/ROUTES/DOSAGE

HYPOTHYROIDISM

PO: ADULTS, ELDERLY: Initially, 25 mcg/day. May increase in increments of 12.5–25 mcg/day q1–2wk. **Maximum:** 100 mcg/day. CHILDREN: Initially, 5 mcg/day. May increase by 5 mcg/day q3–4wk. Maintenance: 100 mcg/day (children older than 3 yr); 50 mcg/day (children 1–3 yr); 20 mcg/day (infants).

MYXEDEMA

PO: ADULTS, ELDERLY: Initially, 5 mcg/day. Increase by 5–10 mcg q1–2wk (after 25 mcg/day has been reached, may increase in 12.5-mcg increments). Maintenance: 50–100 mcg/day.

NONTOXIC GOITER

PO: ADULTS, ELDERLY: Initially, 5 mcg/day. Increase by 5–10 mcg/day q1–2wk. When 25 mcg/day has been reached, may increase by 12.5–25 mcg/day q1–2wk. Maintenance: 75 mcg/day. CHILDREN: 5 mcg/day. May increase by 5 mcg q1–2wk. Maintenance: 15–20 mcg/day.

CONGENITAL HYPOTHYROIDISM

PO: CHILDREN: Initially, 5 mcg/day. Increase by 5 mcg/day q3–4 days. Maintenance: Full adult dosage (children older than 3 yr); 50 mcg/day (children 1–3 yr); 20 mcg/day (infants).

T₃ SUPPRESSION TEST

PO: ADULTS, ELDERLY: 75–100 mcg/day for 7 days; then repeat I¹³¹ thyroid uptake test.

MYXEDEMA COMA, PRECOMA

IV: ADULTS, ELDERLY: Initially, 25–50 mcg (10–20 mcg in patients with cardiovascular disease). Total dose at least 65 mcg/day.

SIDE EFFECTS

OCCASIONAL: Reversible hair loss at start of therapy (in children). **RARE:** Dry skin, GI intolerance, rash, hives, pseudotumor cerebri or severe headache in children.

ADVERSE REACTIONS/ TOXIC EFFECTS

Excessive dosage produces signs and symptoms of hyperthyroidism, including weight loss, palpitations, increased appetite, tremors, nervousness, tachycardia, hypertension, headache, insomnia, and menstrual irregularities. Cardiac arrhythmias occur rarely.

NURSING CONSIDERATIONS

BASELINE ASSESSMENT

Question for hypersensitivity to tartrazine, aspirin. Obtain baseline weight, vital signs. Signs and symptoms of diabetes mellitus, diabetes insipidus, adrenal insufficiency, hypopituitarism may become intensified. Treat with adrenocortical steroids before thyroid therapy in coexisting hypothyroidism and hypoadrenalism.

INTERVENTION/EVALUATION

Monitor pulse for rate, rhythm. Report irregular pulse or rate over 100 beats/min. Assess for tremors, anxiety. Assess appetite, sleep pattern.

PATIENT/FAMILY TEACHING

• Do not discontinue drug therapy; replacement for hypothyroidism is lifelong. • Follow-up office visits, thyroid function tests are essential. • Take medication at the same time each day, preferably in morning. • Teach patient and family to take pulse correctly, report marked increase, pulse of 100 beats/min or over, change of rhythm. • Notify physician promptly of chest pain, weight loss, anxiety or tremors, insomnia. • Children may have reversible hair loss, increased aggressiveness during first few mo of therapy.

Lipitor, *see atorvastatin*

L

---

lisinopril

ly-**sin** oh-pril
(Apo-Lisinopril ♣, Prinivil, Zestril)
Do not confuse lisinopril with fosinopril; Prinivil with Desyrel, Plendil, Proventil, or Restoril; Fibsol with Lioresal; or Zestril with Zostrix. Do not confuse lisinopril's combination form Zestoretic with Prilosec.

FIXED-COMBINATION(S)

Prinzide/Zestoretic: lisinopril/hydrochlorothiazide (a diuretic): 10 mg/12.5 mg; 20 mg/12.5 mg; 20 mg/25 mg.

◆CLASSIFICATION

PHARMACOTHERAPEUTIC: Angiotensin-converting enzyme (ACE) inhibitor. **CLINICAL:** Antihypertensive (see p. 7C).

ACTION

This ACE inhibitor suppresses the renin-angiotensin-aldosterone system and prevents conversion of angiotensin I to angiotensin II, a potent vasoconstrictor; may also inhibit angiotensin II at local vascular and renal sites. Decreases plasma angiotensin II, increases plasma renin activity, and decreases aldosterone secretion. Therapeutic Effect: Reduces peripheral arterial resistance, BP, afterload, pulmonary capillary wedge pressure (preload), and pulmonary vascular resistance. In those with heart failure, also decreases heart size, increases cardiac output, and exercise tolerance time.

PHARMACOKINETICS

Route	Onset	Peak	Duration
PO	1 hr	6 hr	24 hr

Incompletely absorbed from the GI tract. Protein binding: 25%. Primarily excreted unchanged in urine. Removed by hemodialysis. Half-life: 12 hr (half-life is prolonged in those with impaired renal function).

USES

Treatment of hypertension. Used alone or in combination with other antihypertensives. Adjunctive therapy in management of heart failure. Improves survival in patients who had an MI. OFF-LABEL: Treatment of hypertension or renal crises with scleroderma.

PRECAUTIONS

CONTRAINDICATIONS: History of angioedema from previous treatment with ACE inhibitors. CAUTIONS: Renal impairment, those with sodium depletion or on diuretic therapy, dialysis, hypovolemia, coronary/cerebrovascular insufficiency, severe CHF.

⌛ LIFESPAN CONSIDERATIONS: Pregnancy/Lactation: Crosses placenta. Unknown if distributed in breast milk. Pregnancy Category C (D if used in second or third trimester). Children: Safety and efficacy not established. Elderly: May be more sensitive to hypotensive effects.

INTERACTIONS

DRUG: Alcohol, diuretics, hypotensive agents: May increase the effects of lisinopril. Lithium: May increase lithium blood concentration and risk of toxicity. NSAIDs: May decrease the effects of lisinopril. Potassium-sparing diuretics, potassium supplements: May cause hyperkalemia. HERBAL: None known. FOOD: None known. LAB VALUES: May increase BUN, serum alkaline phosphatase, serum bilirubin, serum creatinine, serum potassium, AST, and ALT levels. May decrease serum sodium levels. May cause positive ANA titer.

AVAILABILITY (Rx)

TABLETS (PRINIVIL, ZESTRIL): 2.5 mg, 5 mg, 10 mg, 20 mg, 30 mg, 40 mg.

ADMINISTRATION/HANDLING

PO
• Give without regard to food. • Tablets may be rushed.

INDICATIONS/ROUTES/DOSAGE

HYPERTENSION (USED ALONE)
PO: ADULTS: Initially, 10 mg/day. May increase by 5–10 mcg/day at 1–2 wk intervals. Maximum: 40 mg/day. ELDERLY: Initially, 2.5–5 mg/day. May increase by 2.5–5 mg/day at 1- to 2-wk intervals. Maximum: 40 mg/day.

HYPERTENSION (USED IN COMBINATION WITH OTHER ANTIHYPERTENSIVES)
PO: ADULTS: Initially, 2.5–5 mg/day titrated to patient's needs.

ADJUNCTIVE THERAPY FOR MANAGEMENT OF HEART FAILURE

PO: ADULTS, ELDERLY: Initially, 2.5–5 mg/day. May increase by no more than 10 mg/day at intervals of at least 2 wk. Maintenance: 5–40 mg/day.

IMPROVE SURVIVAL IN PATIENTS AFTER A MYOCARDIAL INFARCTION (MI)

PO: ADULTS, ELDERLY: Initially, 5 mg, then 5 mg after 24 hr, 10 mg after 48 hr, then 10 mg/day for 6 wk. For patients with low systolic BP, give 2.5 mg/day for 3 days, then 2.5–5 mg/day.

DOSAGE IN RENAL IMPAIRMENT

Titrate to patient's needs after giving the following initial dose:

Creatinine Clearance	% Normal Dose
10–50 ml/min	50–75
Less than 10 ml/min	25–50

SIDE EFFECTS

FREQUENT (12%–5%): Headache, dizziness, postural hypotension. **OCCASIONAL (4%–2%):** Chest discomfort, fatigue, rash, abdominal pain, nausea, diarrhea, upper respiratory infection. **RARE (1% or less):** Palpitations, tachycardia, peripheral edema, insomnia, paresthesia, confusion, constipation, dry mouth, muscle cramps.

ADVERSE REACTIONS/ TOXIC EFFECTS

Excessive hypotension may occur in patients with CHF and severe salt and volume depletion. Angioedema (swelling of face and lips) and hyperkalemia occurs rarely. Agranulocytosis and neutropenia may be noted in patients with collagen vascular disease, including scleroderma and systemic lupus erythematosus, and impaired renal function. Nephrotic syndrome may be noted in patients with history of renal disease.

NURSING CONSIDERATIONS

BASELINE ASSESSMENT

Obtain BP, apical pulse immediately before each dose, in addition to regular monitoring (be alert to fluctuations). If excessive reduction in BP occurs, place patientt in supine position, feet slightly elevated. In patients with renal impairment, autoimmune disease, taking drugs that affect leukocytes or immune response, CBC and differential count should be performed before beginning therapy and q2wk for 3 mo, then periodically thereafter.

INTERVENTION/EVALUATION

Assess for edema. Check lungs for rales. Monitor I&O; weigh daily. Monitor bowel activity/stool consistency. Assist with ambulation if dizziness occurs. Monitor BP, renal function tests, WBC, serum potassium.

PATIENT/FAMILY TEACHING

• To reduce hypotensive effect, rise slowly from lying to sitting position, permit legs to dangle from bed momentarily before standing. • Limit alcohol intake. • Inform physician if vomiting, diarrhea, diaphoresis, swelling of face/lips/tongue, difficulty in breathing occur.

lithium carbonate

lith-ee-um
(Duralith ✤, Eskalith, Eskalith CR, Lithobid)

lithium citrate

(Cibalith-S)

Do not confuse Lithobid with Levbid, Lithostat, or Lithotabs.

⬥CLASSIFICATION

PHARMACOTHERAPEUTIC: Psychotherapeutic. **CLINICAL:** Antimanic, antidepressant, vascular headache prophylactic.

ACTION

A psychotherapeutic agent that affects the storage, release, and reuptake of neurotransmitters. Antimanic effect may result from increased norepinephrine reuptake and serotonin receptor sensitivity. **Therapeutic Effect:** Produces antimanic and antidepressant effects.

PHARMACOKINETICS

Rapidly and completely absorbed from the GI tract. Primarily excreted unchanged in urine. Removed by hemodialysis. **Half-life:** 18–24 hr (increased in elderly).

USES

Prophylaxis, treatment of acute mania, manic phase of bipolar disorder (manic depressive illness). **OFF-LABEL:** Prevention of vascular headache; treatment of depression, neutropenia.

PRECAUTIONS

CONTRAINDICATIONS: Debilitated patients, severe cardiovascular disease, severe dehydration, severe renal disease, severe sodium depletion. **CAUTIONS:** Cardiovascular disease, thyroid disease, elderly.

⌛ **LIFESPAN CONSIDERATIONS: Pregnancy/Lactation:** Freely crosses placenta. Distributed in breast milk. **Pregnancy Category D. Children:** May increase bone formation or density (alter parathyroid hormone concentrations). **Elderly:** More susceptible to develop lithium-induced goiter or clinical hypothyroidism, CNS toxicity. Increased

thirst, urination more frequent; lower dosage recommended.

INTERACTIONS

DRUG: Antithyroid medications, iodinated glycerol, potassium iodide: May increase the effects of these drugs. **Diuretics, NSAIDs:** May increase lithium serum concentration and risk of toxicity. **Haloperidol:** May increase extrapyramidal symptoms and the risk of neurologic toxicity. **Molindone:** May increase the risk of neurotoxicity. **Phenothiazines:** May decrease the absorption of phenothiazines, increase the intracellular concentration and renal excretion of lithium, and increase delirium and extrapyramidal symptoms. Antiemetic effect of some phenothiazines may mask early signs of lithium toxicity. **HERBAL:** None known. **FOOD:** None known. **LAB VALUES:** May increase blood glucose, immunoreactive parathyroid hormone, and serum calcium levels. Therapeutic serum level is 0.6–1.2 mEq/L; toxic serum level is greater than 1.5 mEq/L.

AVAILABILITY (Rx)

CAPSULES: 150 mg, 300 mg, 600 mg. **SYRUP:** 300 mg/ml. **TABLETS:** 300 mg. **TABLETS (CONTROLLED-RELEASE):** 450 mg. **TABLETS (SLOW-RELEASE):** 300 mg.

ADMINISTRATION/HANDLING

PO
• Preferable to administer with meals or milk. • Do not crush, chew, or break slow-release or film-coated tablets.

INDICATIONS/ROUTES/DOSAGE

◄ **ALERT** ► During acute phase, a therapeutic serum lithium concentration of 1–1.4 mEq/L is required. For long-term control, the desired level is 0.5–1.3 mEq/L. Monitor serum drug concentration and clinical response to determine proper dosage.

PREVENTION OR TREATMENT OF ACUTE MANIA, MANIC PHASE OF BIPOLAR DISORDER (MANIC-DEPRESSIVE ILLNESS)

PO: ADULTS: 300 mg 3–4 times a day or 450–900 mg slow-release form twice a day. **Maximum:** 2.4 g/day. ELDERLY: 900–1,200 mg/day. Maintenance: 300 mg twice a day. May increase by 300 mg/day q1wk. CHILDREN 12 YR AND OLDER: 600–1,800 mg/day in 3–4 divided doses (2 doses/day for slow-release). CHILDREN YOUNGER THAN 12 YR:. 15–60 mg/kg/day in 3–4 divided doses not to exceed usual adult dose.

SIDE EFFECTS

◀ ALERT ▶ Side effects are dose related and seldom occur at lithium serum levels less than 1.5 mEq/L.
OCCASIONAL: Fine hand tremor, polydipsia, polyuria, mild nausea. **RARE:** Weight gain, bradycardia or tachycardia, acne, rash, muscle twitching, cold and cyanotic extremities, pseudotumor cerebri (eye pain, headache, tinnitus, vision disturbances).

ADVERSE REACTIONS/ TOXIC EFFECTS

A lithium serum concentration of 1.5–2.0 mEq/L may produce vomiting, diarrhea, drowsiness, confusion, incoordination, coarse hand tremor, muscle twitching, and T-wave depression on EKG. A lithium serum concentration of 2.0–2.5 mEq/L may result in ataxia, giddiness, tinnitus, blurred vision, clonic movements, and severe hypotension. Acute toxicity may be characterized by seizures, oliguria, circulatory failure, coma, and death.

NURSING CONSIDERATIONS

BASELINE ASSESSMENT

Serum lithium levels should be tested q3–4 days during initial phase of therapy, q1–2mo thereafter, and weekly if there is no improvement of disorder or adverse effects occur.

INTERVENTION/EVALUATION

Serum lithium testing should be performed as close as possible to 12th hr following last dose. Besides serum lithium concentration levels, clinical assessment of therapeutic effect, tolerance to drug effect is necessary for correct dosing-level management. Assess behavior, appearance, emotional status, response to environment, speech pattern, thought content. Monitor serum lithium concentrations, differential count, urinalysis, creatinine clearance. Assess for increased urine output, persistent thirst. Report polyuria, prolonged vomiting, diarrhea, fever to physician (may need to temporarily reduce or discontinue dosage). Monitor for signs of lithium toxicity. Assess for therapeutic response (interest in surroundings, improvement in self-care, increased ability to concentrate, relaxed facial expression). Monitor lithium levels q3–4 days at initiation of therapy (then q1–2mo). Levels obtained 8–12 hr postdose. Monitor renal, hepatic, thyroid, cardiovascular function; CBC with differential; serum electrolytes. Therapeutic serum level: 0.6–1.2 mEq/L; toxic serum level: greater than 1.5 mEq/L.

PATIENT/FAMILY TEACHING

• Limit alcohol, caffeine intake. • Avoid tasks requiring coordination until CNS effects of drug are known. • May cause dry mouth. • Maintain steady salt and fluid intake (avoid dehydration). • Inform physician if vomiting, diarrhea, muscle weakness, tremors, drowsiness, ataxia occurs. • Serum level monitoring is necessary to determine proper dose.

lomefloxacin hydrochloride

low-meh-**flocks**-ah-sin
(Maxaquin)

◆CLASSIFICATION

PHARMACOTHERAPEUTIC: Quinolone. **CLINICAL:** Antibiotic (see p. 24C).

ACTION

A quinolone that inhibits the enzyme DNA gyrase in susceptible microorganisms, interfering with bacterial cell replication and repair. **Therapeutic Effect:** Bactericidal.

PHARMACOKINETICS

Well absorbed from the GI tract. Protein binding: 10%. Widely distributed. Metabolized in the liver. Primarily excreted in urine. Not removed by hemodialysis. **Half-life:** 4–6 hr (increased with impaired renal function and in the elderly).

USES

Treatment of susceptible infecitons due to *H. influenzae, M. catarrhalis, E. coli, K. pneumoniae, P. mirabilis, S. saprophyticus, P. aeruginosa* including urinary tract, lower respiratory tract infections; postop prophylaxis in patients undergoing transurethral procedures.

PRECAUTIONS

◄ **ALERT** ► Moderate to severe phototoxic reactions have occurred in patients exposed to direct or indirect sunlight or to artificial ultraviolet light during and following therapy.
CONTRAINDICATIONS: Hypersensitivity to quinolones. **CAUTIONS:** Renal impairment, CNS disorders, seizures, those taking theophylline, caffeine.

⌛ **LIFESPAN CONSIDERATIONS: Pregnancy/Lactation:** Unknown if distributed in breast milk. If possible, do not use during pregnancy/lactation (risk of arthropathy to fetus/infant). **Pregnancy Category C. Children:** Safety and efficacy not established. **Elderly:** Age-related renal impairment may require dosage adjustment.

INTERACTIONS

DRUG: Antacids, iron preparations, sucralfate: May decrease lomefloxacin absorption. **Caffeine, oral anticoagulants:** May increase the effects of these drugs. **Theophylline:** Decreases clearance and may increase blood concentration and risk of toxicity of theophylline. **HERBAL:** None known. **FOOD:** None known. **LAB VALUES:** May increase BUN and serum alkaline phosphatase, bilirubin, creatinine, LDH, AST, and ALT levels.

AVAILABILITY (Rx)

TABLETS: 400 mg.

ADMINISTRATION/HANDLING

PO
• May be given without regard to meals (preferred dosing time: 2 hr after meals). • Do not administer antacids (aluminum, magnesium) within 2 hr of lomefloxacin. • Encourage intake of cranberry juice, citrus fruits (acidifies urine).

INDICATIONS/ROUTES/DOSAGE

COMPLICATED UTIs

PO: ADULTS, ELDERLY: 400 mg/day for 10–14 days.

UNCOMPLICATED UTIs

PO: ADULTS (FEMALES): 400 mg/day for 3 days.

LOWER RESPIRATORY TRACT INFECTIONS

PO: ADULTS, ELDERLY: 400 mg/day for 10 days.

✎ see color pill atlas   ⌇ herb   <u>underlined</u> – top prescribed drug

SURGICAL PROPHYLAXIS
PO: ADULTS, ELDERLY: 400 mg 2–6 hr before surgery.

DOSAGE IN RENAL IMPAIRMENT
Dosage and frequency are modified based on creatinine clearance.

Creatinine Clearance	Dosage
41 ml/min and higher	No change
10–40 ml/min	400 mg initially, then 200 mg/day for 10–14 days

SIDE EFFECTS

OCCASIONAL (3%–2%): Nausea, headache, photosensitivity, dizziness. **RARE (1%):** Diarrhea.

ADVERSE REACTIONS/ TOXIC EFFECTS

Antibiotic-associated colitis and other superinfections may result from altered bacterial balance. Hypersensitivity reactions, including photosensitivity (as evidenced by rash, pruritus, blisters, edema, and burning skin), have occurred in patients receiving fluoroquinolones. Arthropathy may occur if the drug is given to children younger than 18 yr.

NURSING CONSIDERATIONS

BASELINE ASSESSMENT
Question for history of hypersensitivity to lomefloxacin, quinolones.

INTERVENTION/EVALUATION
Monitor signs, symptoms of infection, WBC count, mental status. Check for dizziness, headache. Be alert for superinfection (e.g., genital pruritus, vaginitis, fever, oral candidiasis).

PATIENT/FAMILY TEACHING
• Do not skip doses; take full course of therapy. • Do not take antacids (reduces/destroys effectiveness). • Avoid sunlight/ultraviolet exposure; wear sunscreen, protective clothing if photosensitivity develops.

Lomotil, *see diphenoxylate with atropine*

---

lomustine

low-**meuw**-steen
(CeeNU)

• **CLASSIFICATION**
PHARMACOTHERAPEUTIC: Alkylating agent (nitrosourea). **CLINICAL:** Antineoplastic (see p. 76C).

ACTION

An alkylating agent and nitrosourea that inhibits DNA and RNA protein synthesis by cross-linking with DNA and RNA strands, preventing cell division. Cell cycle–phase nonspecific. Therapeutic Effect: Interferes with DNA and RNA function.

PHARMACOKINETICS

Rapidly absorbed following oral administration. Highly lipid soluble. Metabolized in liver. Excreted in urine. Half-life: 16 hr.

USES

Treatment of primary brain tumors, Hodgkin's lymphomas. OFF-LABEL: Breast, colorectal, GI, non–small cell lung, renal carcinomas; malignant melanoma, multiple myeloma.

PRECAUTIONS

CONTRAINDICATIONS: Pregnancy. **CAUTIONS:** Depressed platelet, leukocyte, erythrocyte counts.

⌛ LIFESPAN CONSIDERATIONS: Pregnancy/Lactation: May be harmful to fetus. Distributed in breast milk. Avoid breast-feeding. Pregnancy Category D. Children: Safety and efficacy not established. Elderly: Age-related renal impairment may require dosage adjustment.

INTERACTIONS

DRUG: Bone marrow depressants: May increase myelosuppression. Live virus vaccines: May potentiate virus replication, increase vaccine side effects, and decrease the patient's antibody response to the vaccine. HERBAL: None known. FOOD: None known. LAB VALUES: May increase liver function test results.

AVAILABILITY (Rx)

CAPSULES: 10 mg, 40 mg, 100 mg.

ADMINISTRATION/HANDLING

◀ ALERT ▶ Lomustine dosage is individualized based on the patient's clinical response and tolerance of the drug's adverse effects. When administering this drug in combination therapy, consult specific protocols for optimum dosage and sequence of drug administration.

INDICATIONS/ROUTES/DOSAGE

DISSEMINATED HODGKIN'S DISEASE, PRIMARY AND METASTATIC BRAIN TUMORS

PO: ADULTS, ELDERLY: 100–130 mg/m^2 as single dose. Repeat dose at intervals of at least 6 wk but not until circulating blood elements have returned to acceptable levels. Adjust dose based on hematologic response to previous dose. CHILDREN: 75–150 mg/m^2 as a single dose every 6 wk.

SIDE EFFECTS

FREQUENT: Nausea, vomiting (occurring 45 min–6 hr after dose and lasting 12–24 hr); anorexia (often follows for 2–3 days). OCCASIONAL: Neurotoxicity (confusion, slurred speech), stomatitis, darkening of skin, diarrhea, rash, pruritus, alopecia.

ADVERSE REACTIONS/ TOXIC EFFECTS

Myelosuppression may result in hematologic toxicity, manifested principally as leukopenia, mild anemia, and thrombocytopenia. Leukopenia occurs about 6 wk after a dose, thrombocytopenia about 4 wk after a dose; both persist for 1–2 wk. Refractory anemia and thrombocytopenia occur commonly if lomustine therapy continues for more than 1 yr. Hepatotoxicity occurs infrequently. Large cumulative doses of lomustine may result in renal damage.

NURSING CONSIDERATIONS

BASELINE ASSESSMENT

Manufacturer recommends weekly blood counts; experts recommend first blood count obtained 2–3 wk following initial therapy, subsequent blood counts indicated by prior toxicity. Antiemetics can reduce duration, frequency of nausea, vomiting.

INTERVENTION/EVALUATION

Monitor CBC with differential; platelet count; liver, renal, pulmonary function tests. Monitor for stomatitis. Monitor for hematologic toxicity (fever, sore throat, signs of local infection, unusual ecchymosis or bleeding from any site), symptoms of anemia (excessive fatigue, weakness).

PATIENT/FAMILY TEACHING

• Nausea, vomiting generally abates in less than 1 day. • Fasting before therapy can reduce frequency/duration of GI effects. • Maintain fastidious oral hygiene. • Do not have immunizations without physician's approval (drug lowers body's resistance). • Avoid crowds, those with known illness. • Promptly report fever, sore throat, signs of local infection, unusual bruising or bleeding from any site, swelling of legs or feet, jaundice.

loperamide hydrochloride

loe-**per**-a-mide
(Apo-Loperamide ✢, Diarr-Eze ✢, Imodium, Imodium A-D, Loperacap ✢, Novo-Loperamide ✢)
Do not confuse Imodium with Indocin or Ionamin.

FIXED-COMBINATION(S)

Imodium Advanced: loperamide/simethicone (an antiflatulant): 2 mg/125 mg.

CLASSIFICATION

CLINICAL: Antidiarrheal (see p. 43C).

ACTION

An antidiarrheal that directly affects the intestinal wall muscles. **Therapeutic Effect:** Slows intestinal motility and prolongs transit time of intestinal contents by reducing fecal volume, diminishing loss of fluid and electrolytes, and increasing viscosity and bulk of stool.

PHARMACOKINETICS

Poorly absorbed from the GI tract. Protein binding: 97%. Metabolized in the liver. Eliminated in feces and excreted in urine. Not removed by hemodialysis. **Half-life:** 9.1–14.4 hr.

USES

Controls, provides symptomatic relief of acute nonspecific diarrhea, chronic diarrhea associated with inflammatory bowel disease, traveler's diarrhea.

PRECAUTIONS

CONTRAINDICATIONS: Acute ulcerative colitis (may produce toxic megacolon), diarrhea associated with pseudomembranous enterocolitis due to broad-spectrum antibiotics or to organisms that invade intestinal mucosa (such as *Escherichia coli,* shigella, and salmonella), patients who must avoid constipation. **CAUTIONS:** Those with fluid or electrolyte depletion, hepatic impairment.

▨ **LIFESPAN CONSIDERATIONS: Pregnancy/Lactation:** Unknown if drug crosses placenta or is distributed in breast milk. **Pregnancy Category B. Children:** Not recommended in those younger than 6 yr (infants younger than 3 mo more susceptible to CNS effects). **Elderly:** May mask dehydration, electrolyte depletion.

INTERACTIONS

DRUG: Opioid (narcotic) analgesics: May increase the risk of constipation. **HERBAL:** None known. **FOOD:** None known. **LAB VALUES:** None known.

AVAILABILITY (Rx)

CAPSULES: 2 mg. **LIQUID:** 1 mg/5 ml (OTC). **TABLETS:** 2 mg (OTC).

ADMINISTRATION/HANDLING

ORAL LIQUID
• When administering the drug to children, use the accompanying plastic dropper to measure the liquid.

INDICATIONS/ROUTES/DOSAGE

ACUTE DIARRHEA
PO (CAPSULES): ADULTS, ELDERLY: Initially, 4 mg; then 2 mg after each unformed stool. **Maximum:** 16 mg/day. CHILDREN 9–12 YR, WEIGHING MORE THAN 30 KG: Initially, 2 mg 3 times a day

L

---

for 24 hr. CHILDREN 6–8 YR, WEIGHING 20–30 KG: Initially, 2 mg twice a day for 24 hr. CHILDREN 2–5 YR, WEIGHING 13–20 KG: Initially, 1 mg 3 times a day for 24 hr. Maintenance: 1 mg/10 kg only after loose stool.

CHRONIC DIARRHEA

PO: ADULTS, ELDERLY: Initially, 4 mg; then 2 mg after each unformed stool until diarrhea is controlled. CHILDREN: 0.08–0.24 mg/kg/day in 2–3 divided doses. **Maximum:** 2 mg/dose.

TRAVELER'S DIARRHEA

PO: ADULTS, ELDERLY: Initially, 4 mg; then 2 mg after each loose bowel movement (LBM). **Maximum:** 8 mg/day for 2 days. CHILDREN 9–11 YR: Initially, 2 mg; then 1 mg after each LBM. **Maximum:** 6 mg/day for 2 days. CHILDREN 6–8 YR: Initially, 1 mg; then 1 mg after each LBM. **Maximum:** 4 mg/day for 2 days.

SIDE EFFECTS

RARE: Dry mouth, somnolence, abdominal discomfort, allergic reaction (such as rash and itching).

ADVERSE REACTIONS/ TOXIC EFFECTS

Toxicity results in constipation, GI irritation, including nausea and vomiting, and CNS depression. Activated charcoal is used to treat loperamide toxicity.

NURSING CONSIDERATIONS

BASELINE ASSESSMENT

Do not administer in presence of bloody diarrhea, temperature greater than 101°F.

INTERVENTION/EVALUATION

Encourage adequate fluid intake. Assess bowel sounds for peristalsis. Monitor pattern of bowel activity and stool consistency. Withhold drug, notify physician promptly in event of abdominal pain or distention, fever.

PATIENT/FAMILY TEACHING

• Do not exceed prescribed dose. • May cause dry mouth. • Avoid alcohol. • Avoid tasks that require alertness, motor skills until response to drug is established. • Notify physician if diarrhea does not stop within 3 days, abdominal distention or pain occurs, fever develops.

lopinavir/ritonavir

low-**pin**-ah-veer/rih-**ton**-ah-veer
(Kaletra)
Do not confuse Kaletra with Keppra.

CLASSIFICATION

PHARMACOTHERAPEUTIC: Protease inhibitor combination. CLINICAL: Antiretroviral (see pp. 61C, 105C).

ACTION

A protease inhibitor combination drug in which lopinavir inhibits the activity of the enzyme protease late in the HIV replication process and ritonavir increases plasma levels of lopinavir. Therapeutic Effect: Formation of immature, noninfectious viral particles.

PHARMACOKINETICS

Readily absorbed after PO administration (absorption increased when taken with food). Protein binding: 98%–99%. Metabolized in the liver. Eliminated primarily in feces. Not removed by hemodialysis. Half-life: 5–6 hr.

USES

In combination with other antiretroviral agents for the treatment of HIV infection.

PRECAUTIONS

CONTRAINDICATIONS: Concomitant use

✎ see color pill atlas   🌿 herb   underlined – top prescribed drug of ergot derivatives (causes peripheral ischemia of extremities and vasospasm), flecainide, midazolam, pimozide, propafenone (increases the risk of serious cardiac arrhythmias), or triazolam (increases sedation or respiratory depression); hypersensitivity to lopinavir or ritonavir. **CAUTIONS:** Hepatic impairment, hepatitis B or C. High-dose itraconazole, ketoconazole not recommended. Metronidazole may cause disulfiram-type reaction with oral solution (contains alcohol).

⌛ **LIFESPAN CONSIDERATIONS: Pregnancy/Lactation:** Unknown if excreted in breast milk. Not recommended that HIV-infected mothers breast-feed. **Pregnancy Category C. Children:** Safety and efficacy not established in those younger than 6 mo. **Elderly:** Age-related renal/hepatic/cardiac impairment requires caution.

INTERACTIONS

DRUG: Atorvastatin: May increase lopinavir and ritonavir blood concentration and risk of myopathy. **Atovaquone, methadone, oral contraceptives:** May decrease blood concentration and effects of these drugs. **Carbamazepine, corticosteroids, efavirenz, nevirapine, phenobarbital, phenytoin, rifampin:** May decrease blood concentration and effects of lopinavir and ritonavir. **Clarithromycin, felodipine, immunosuppressants, nicardipine, nifedipine, rifabutin:** May increase blood concentration and effects of these drugs. **Itraconzole, ketoconazole:** May increase blood concentration of these drugs. **Metronidazole:** May produce a disulfiram-like reaction. **Sildenafil, tadalafil, vardenafil:** May increase the adverse effects of these drugs. **HERBAL: St. John's wort:** May decrease blood concentration and effects of lopinavir and ritonavir. **FOOD:** None known. **LAB VALUES:** May increase blood glucose, GGT, total cholesterol, and serum uric acid, AST, ALT, and triglyceride levels.

AVAILABILITY (Rx)

TABLETS: 200 mg lopinavir/50 mg ritonavir. **ORAL SOLUTION:** 80 mg/ml lopinavir/20 mg/ml ritonavir.

ADMINISTRATION/HANDLING

PO
- Swallow whole, do not chew, break, or crush. • Does not require refrigeration. • May take with or without food.
- Solution must be taken with food.

INDICATIONS/ROUTES/DOSAGE

HIV INFECTION
PO: ADULTS: 2 tablets (400 mg lopinavir/100 mg ritonavir) or 5 ml twice a day. Increase to 3 tablets (600 mg lopinavir/100 mg ritonavir) or 6.5 ml when taken with efavirenz or nevirapine. CHILDREN WEIGHING 15–40 KG WHO ARE NOT TAKING EFAVIRENZ OR NEVIRAPINE: 10 mg/kg twice a day. CHILDREN WEIGHING 7–14 KG WHO ARE NOT TAKING ALPRENAVIR, EFAVIRENZ, NELFINAVIR, NEVIRAPINE: 12 mg/kg twice a day. CHILDREN WEIGHING 15–40 KG WHO ARE TAKING EFAVIRENZ OR NEVIRAPINE: 11 mg/kg twice a day. CHILDREN WEIGHING 7–14 KG WHO ARE TAKING EFAVIRENZ OR NEVIRAPINE: 13 mg/kg twice a day.
PO (ONCE DAILY) ◀ ALERT ▶ Once daily dosing is not recommended in therapy-experienced patients and has not been evaluated in children. ADULTS: 4 tablets (800 mg lopinavir/200 mg ritonavir) or 10 ml once daily.

SIDE EFFECTS

FREQUENT (14%): Mild to moderate diarrhea. **OCCASIONAL (6%–2%):** Nausea, asthenia, abdominal pain, headache, vomiting. **RARE (less than 2%):** Insomnia, rash.

ADVERSE REACTIONS/ TOXIC EFFECTS

Anemia, leukopenia, lymphadenopathy, deep vein thrombosis, Cushing's syndrome, pancreatitis, and hemorrhagic colitis occur rarely.

NURSING CONSIDERATIONS

BASELINE ASSESSMENT

Obtain baseline CBC, renal/liver function tests, weight.

INTERVENTION/EVALUATION

Monitor bowel activity and stool consistency. Assess for opportunistic infections: onset of fever, oral mucosa changes, cough, other respiratory symptoms. Check weight at least 2 times a wk. Assess for nausea, vomiting. Monitor for signs/symptoms of pancreatitis (nausea, vomiting, abdominal pain), electrolytes, blood glucose, serum cholesterol, hepatic function, CBC with differential, platelets, CD4 cell count, viral load.

PATIENT/FAMILY TEACHING

• Explain correct administration of medication. • Eat small, frequent meals to offset nausea, vomiting. • Medication is not a cure for HIV infection, nor does it reduce risk of transmission to others.

Lopressor, *see metoprolol*

---

loracarbef

lor-a-**kar**-bef

(Lorabid, Lorabid Pulvules)

Do not confuse loracarbef or Lorabid with Lortab.

◆CLASSIFICATION

PHARMACOTHERAPEUTIC: Cephalosporin. **CLINICAL:** Antibiotic (see p. 22C).

ACTION

A second-generation cephalosporin that binds to bacterial cell membranes and inhibits cell wall synthesis. **Therapeutic Effect:** Bactericidal.

PHARMACOKINETICS

Well absorbed from GI tract. Protein binding: 25%. Widely distributed. Primarily excreted unchanged in urine. Moderately removed by hemodialysis. **Half-life:** 1 hr (increased in impaired renal function).

USES

Treatment of bronchitis, otitis media, pharyngitis, pneumonia, sinusitis, skin and soft tissue infections, UTIs (uncomplicated cystitis, pyelonephritis).

PRECAUTIONS

CONTRAINDICATIONS: History of anaphylactic reaction to penicillins or hypersensitivity to cephalosporins. **CAUTIONS:** Renal impairment, history of colitis.

⏳ **LIFESPAN CONSIDERATIONS: Pregnancy/Lactation:** Drug readily crosses the placenta; is distributed in breast milk. **Pregnancy Category B. Children:** Safety and efficacy not established in children younger than 6 mo. **Elderly:** Age-related renal impairment may require a dosage adjustment in the elderly.

INTERACTIONS

DRUG: Probenecid: Increases serum concentration and half-life of loracarbef. **HERBAL:** None known. **FOOD:** None known. **LAB VALUES:** May increase BUN level and serum alkaline phosphatase, creatinine, AST, and ALT levels. May

---

decrease blood leukocyte and platelet counts.

AVAILABILITY (Rx)

CAPSULES (LORABID PULVULES): 200 mg, 400 mg. **POWDER FOR ORAL SUSPENSION (LORABID):** 100 mg/5 ml, 200 mg/5 ml.

ADMINISTRATION/HANDLING

PO

• Give 1 hr before or 2 hr after meal. • After reconstitution, powder for suspension may be kept at room temperature for 14 days. Discard unused portion after 14 days. • Shake oral suspension well before using.

INDICATIONS/ROUTES/DOSAGE

BRONCHITIS

PO: ADULTS, ELDERLY, CHILDREN 12 YR AND OLDER: 200–400 mg q12h for 7 days.

PHARYNGITIS

PO: ADULTS, ELDERLY, CHILDREN 12 YR AND OLDER: 200 mg q12h for 10 days. CHILDREN 6 MO–11 YR: 7.5 mg/kg q12h for 10 days.

PNEUMONIA

PO: ADULTS, ELDERLY, CHILDREN 12 YR AND OLDER: 400 mg q12h for 14 days.

SINUSITIS

PO: ADULTS, ELDERLY, CHILDREN 12 YR AND OLDER: 400 mg q12h for 10 days. CHILDREN 6 MO–11 YR: 15 mg/kg q12h for 10 days.

SKIN AND SOFT-TISSUE INFECTIONS

PO: ADULTS, ELDERLY, CHILDREN 12 YR AND OLDER: 200 mg q12h for 7 days. CHILDREN 6 MO–11 YR: 7.5 mg/kg q12h for 7 days.

UTIs

PO: ADULTS, ELDERLY, CHILDREN 6 MO–12 YR: 200–400 mg q12h for 7–14 days.

OTITIS MEDIA

PO: CHILDREN 6 MO–12 YR: 15 mg/kg q12h for 10 days.

SIDE EFFECTS

FREQUENT: Abdominal pain, anorexia, nausea, vomiting, diarrhea. **OCCASIONAL:** Rash, pruritus. **RARE:** Dizziness, headache, vaginitis.

ADVERSE REACTIONS/TOXIC EFFECTS

Antibiotic-associated colitis and other superinfections may result from altered bacterial balance. Hypersensitivity reactions (ranging from rash, urticaria, and fever to anaphylaxis) occur in fewer than 5% of patients, most commonly in patients with a history of drug allergies, especially to penicillins.

NURSING CONSIDERATIONS

BASELINE ASSESSMENT

Question for history of allergies, particularly loracarbef, cephalosporins, penicillins.

INTERVENTION/EVALUATION

Assess for nausea, vomiting. Monitor pattern of bowel activity and stool consistency. Assess skin for rash (diaper area in infants, toddlers). Monitor I&O, urinalysis, renal function reports for nephrotoxicity. Be alert for superinfection: genital or anal pruritus, moniliasis, abdominal pain, sore mouth/tongue, moderate to severe diarrhea.

PATIENT/FAMILY TEACHING

• Continue antibiotic therapy for full length of treatment. • Doses should be evenly spaced, given at least 1 hr before or 2 hr after a meal.

---

loratadine

low-**rah**-tah-deen

(Alavert, Claritin, Claritin RediTab, Dimetapp, Tavist ND)

FIXED-COMBINATION(S)

Claritin-D: loratadine/pseudoephedrine (a sympathomimetic): 5 mg/120 mg; 10 mg/240 mg.

◆ CLASSIFICATION

PHARMACOTHERAPEUTIC: H$_1$ antagonist. **CLINICAL:** Antihistamine (see p. 51C).

ACTION

A long-acting antihistamine that competes with histamine for H$_1$ receptor sites on effector cells. **Therapeutic Effect:** Prevents allergic responses mediated by histamine, such as rhinitis, urticaria, and pruritus.

PHARMACOKINETICS

Route	Onset	Peak	Duration
PO	1–3 hr	8–12 hr	Longer than 24 hr

Rapidly and almost completely absorbed from the GI tract. Protein binding: 97%; metabolite, 73%–77%. Distributed mainly to the liver, lungs, GI tract, and bile. Metabolized in the liver to active metabolite; undergoes extensive first-pass metabolism. Eliminated in urine and feces. Not removed by hemodialysis. **Half-life:** 8.4 hr; metabolite, 28 hr (increased in elderly and hepatic impairment).

USES

Relief of nasal and non-nasal symptoms of seasonal allergic rhinitis (hayfever). Treatment of idiopathic chronic urticaria (hives). **OFF-LABEL:** Adjunct treatment of bronchial asthma.

PRECAUTIONS

CONTRAINDICATIONS: Hypersensitivity to loratadine or its ingredients. **CAUTIONS:** Hepatic impairment, breastfeeding women. Safety in children unknown.

⌛ **LIFESPAN CONSIDERATIONS: Pregnancy/Lactation:** Excreted in breast milk. **Pregnancy Category B.**

Children/Elderly: More sensitive to anticholinergic effects (e.g., dry mouth, nose, throat).

INTERACTIONS

DRUG: Clarithromycin, erythromycin, fluconazole, ketoconazole: May increase the loratadine blood concentration. **HERBAL:** None known. **FOOD: All foods:** Delay the absorption of loratadine. **LAB VALUES:** May suppress wheal and flare reactions to antigen skin testing unless the drug is discontinued 4 days before testing.

AVAILABILITY (Rx)

SYRUP (CLARITIN): 10 mg/10 ml. **TABLETS (ALAVERT, CLARITIN, TAVIST ND):** 10 mg. **TABLETS (RAPIDLY-DISINTEGRATING [ALAVERT, CLARITIN REDITAB]):** 10 mg.

ADMINISTRATION/HANDLING

PO
• Preferably give on an empty stomach (food delays absorption).

INDICATIONS/ROUTES/DOSAGE

ALLERGIC RHINITIS, URTICARIA
PO: ADULTS, ELDERLY, CHILDREN 6 YR AND OLDER: 10 mg once a day. CHILDREN 2–5 YR: 5 mg once a day.

DOSAGE IN RENAL AND HEPATIC IMPAIRMENT
PO: ADULTS, ELDERLY, CHILDREN 6 YR AND OLDER: 10 mg every other day. CHILDREN 2–5 YR: 5 mg every other day.

SIDE EFFECTS

FREQUENT (12%–8%): Headache, fatigue, somnolence. **OCCASIONAL (3%):** Dry mouth, nose, or throat. **RARE:** Photosensitivity.

ADVERSE REACTIONS/ TOXIC EFFECTS

Abnormal hepatic function, including jaundice, hepatitis, and hepatic necrosis; alopecia; anaphylaxis; breast enlargement; erythema multiforme; peripheral edema; and seizures have been reported.

NURSING CONSIDERATIONS

BASELINE ASSESSMENT

Assess lung sounds for wheezing, skin for urticaria, other allergy symptoms.

INTERVENTION/EVALUATION

For upper respiratory allergies, increase fluids to decrease viscosity of secretions, offset thirst, replenish loss of fluids from increased diaphoresis. Monitor symptoms for therapeutic response.

PATIENT/FAMILY TEACHING

• Drink plenty of water (may cause dry mouth). • Avoid alcohol. • Avoid tasks that require alertness, motor skills until response to drug is established (may cause drowsiness). • May cause photosensitivity reactions (avoid direct exposure to sunlight.)

---

lorazepam

low-**raz**-ah-pam
(Apo-Lorazepam ✢, <u>Ativan</u>, Lorazepam Intensol, Novo-Lorazem ✢)
Do not confuse lorazepam with Alprazolam.

◆CLASSIFICATION

PHARMACOTHERAPEUTIC: Benzodiazepine **(Schedule IV). CLINICAL:** Antianxiety, sedative-hypnotic, antiemetic, skeletal muscle relaxant, amnesiac, anticonvulsant, antitremor (see p. 12C).

ACTION

A benzodiazepine that enhances the action of the inhibitory neurotransmitter gamma-aminobutyric acid in the CNS,

affecting memory, as well as motor, sensory, and cognitive function. **Therapeutic Effect:** Produces anxiolytic, anticonvulsant, sedative, muscle relaxant, and antiemetic effects.

PHARMACOKINETICS

Route	Onset	Peak	Duration
PO	60 min	N/A	8–12 hr
IV	15–30 min	N/A	8–12 hr
IM	30–60 min	N/A	8–12 hr

Well absorbed after PO and IM administration. Protein binding: 85%. Widely distributed. Metabolized in the liver. Primarily excreted in urine. Not removed by hemodialysis. **Half-life:** 10–20 hr.

USES

Management of anxiety, seizures, status epilepticus, preanesthesia for desired amnesia. **OFF-LABEL:** Treatment of alcohol withdrawal, panic disorders, skeletal muscle spasms, chemotherapy-induced nausea or vomiting, tension headache, tremors; adjunctive treatment before endoscopic procedures (diminishes patient recall).

PRECAUTIONS

CONTRAINDICATIONS: Angle-closure glaucoma, preexisting CNS depression, severe hypotension, severe uncontrolled pain. **CAUTIONS:** Neonates, renal or hepatic impairment, compromised pulmonary function, concomitant CNS depressant use.

⧗ LIFESPAN CONSIDERATIONS: Pregnancy/Lactation: May cross placenta. May be distributed in breast milk. May increase risk of fetal abnormalities if administered during first trimester of pregnancy. Chronic ingestion during pregnancy may produce fetal toxicity, withdrawal symptoms, CNS depression in neonates. **Pregnancy Category D. Children:** Safety and efficacy not established in those younger than 12 yr. **Elderly:** Use small initial doses with gradual increases to avoid ataxia or excessive sedation.

INTERACTIONS

DRUG: Alcohol, other CNS depressants: May increase CNS depression. **HERBAL: Kava kava, valerian:** May increase CNS depression. **FOOD:** None known. **LAB VALUES:** None known. Therapeutic serum drug level is 50–240 ng/ml; toxic serum drug level is unknown.

AVAILABILITY (Rx)

TABLETS: 0.5 mg, 1 mg, 2 mg. **INJECTION:** 2 mg/ml, 4 mg/ml. **ORAL SOLUTION (LORAZEPAM INTENSOL):** 2 mg/ml.

ADMINISTRATION/HANDLING

 IV

Reconstitution • Dilute with equal volume of sterile water for injection, To dilute prefilled 0.9% NaCl, or D₅W. syringe, remove air from half-filled syringe, aspirate equal volume of diluent, pull plunger back slightly to allow for mixing, gently invert syringe several times (do not shake vigorously).

Rate of administration • Give by IV push into tubing of free-flowing IV infusion (0.9% NaCl, D₅W) at a rate not to exceed 2 mg/min.

Storage • Refrigerate parenteral form. • Do not use if precipitate forms or solution appears discolored. • Avoid freezing.

IM
• Give deep IM into large muscle mass.

PO
• Give with food. • Tablets may be crushed.

▨ IV INCOMPATIBILITIES

Aldesleukin (Proleukin), aztreonam (Azactam), idarubicin (Idamycin), ondansetron (Zofran), sufentanil (Sufenta).

IV COMPATIBILITIES

Bumetanide (Bumex), cefepime (Maxipime), diltiazem (Cardizem), dobutamine (Dobutrex), dopamine (Intropin), heparin, labetalol (Normodyne, Trandate), milrinone (Primacor), norepinephrine (Levophed), piperacillin and tazobactam (Zosyn), potassium, propofol (Diprivan).

INDICATIONS/ROUTES/DOSAGE

ANXIETY
PO: ADULTS: 1–10 mg/day in 2–3 divided doses. Average: 2–6 mg/day. ELDERLY: Initially, 0.5–1 mg/day. May increase gradually. Range: 0.5–4 mg.
IV: ADULTS, ELDERLY: 0.02–0.06 mg/kg q2–6h.
IV INFUSION: ADULTS, ELDERLY: 0.01–0.1 mg/kg/h.
PO, IV: CHILDREN: 0.05 mg/kg/dose q4–8h. Range: 0.02–0.1 mg/kg. **Maximum:** 2 mg/dose.

INSOMNIA DUE TO ANXIETY
PO: ADULTS: 2–4 mg at bedtime. ELDERLY: 0.5–1 mg at bedtime.

PREOPERATIVE SEDATION
IV: ADULTS, ELDERLY: 0.044 mg/kg 15–20 min before surgery. **Maximum total dose:** 2 mg.
IM: ADULTS, ELDERLY: 0.05 mg/kg 2 hr before procedure. **Maximum total dose:** 4 mg.

STATUS EPILEPTICUS
IV: ADULTS, ELDERLY: 4 mg over 2–5 min. May repeat in 10–15 min. **Maximum:** 8 mg in 12-hr period. CHILDREN: 0.1 mg/kg over 2–5 min. May give second dose of 0.05 mg/kg in 15–20 min. **Maximum:** 4 mg. NEONATES: 0.05 mg/kg. May repeat in 10–15 min.

SIDE EFFECTS

FREQUENT: Somnolence (initially in the morning), ataxia, confusion. **OCCASIONAL:** Blurred vision, slurred speech, hypotension, headache. **RARE:** Paradoxical CNS restlessness or excitement in elderly or debilitated.

ADVERSE REACTIONS/ TOXIC EFFECTS
Abrupt or too-rapid withdrawal may result in pronounced restlessness, irritability, insomnia, hand tremor, abdominal or muscle cramps, diaphoresis, vomiting, and seizures. Overdose results in somnolence, confusion, diminished reflexes, and coma.

NURSING CONSIDERATIONS

BASELINE ASSESSMENT
Offer emotional support to anxious patient. Patient must remain recumbent for up to 8 hr (individualized) following parenteral administration to reduce hypotensive effect. Assess motor responses (agitation, trembling, tension), autonomic responses (cold or clammy hands, diaphoresis).

INTERVENTION/EVALUATION
Monitor BP, respiratory rate, heart rate, CBC with differential, liver function tests. For those on long-term therapy, liver and renal function tests, blood counts should be performed periodically. Assess for paradoxical reaction, particularly during early therapy. Evaluate for therapeutic response: calm facial expression, decreased restlessness, insomnia. Therapeutic serum level: 50–240 ng/ml; toxic serum level: N/A.

PATIENT/FAMILY TEACHING
• Drowsiness usually disappears during continued therapy. • Avoid tasks that require alertness, motor skills until response to drug is established. • Smoking reduces drug effectiveness. • Do not abruptly withdraw medication after long-term therapy. • Do not use alcohol, CNS depressants. • Contraception recommended for long-term therapy. • Notify physician at once if pregnancy is suspected.

losartan

lo-**sar** tan

(Cozaar)

Do not confuse Cozaar with Zocor.

FIXED-COMBINATION(S)
Hyzaar: losartan/hydrochlorothiazide (a diuretic): 50 mg/12.5 mg; 100 mg/12.5 mg; 100 mg/25 mg.

CLASSIFICATION
PHARMACOTHERAPEUTIC: Angiotensin II receptor antagonist. **CLINICAL:** Antihypertensive (see p. 8C).

ACTION
An angiotensin II receptor, type AT_1, antagonist that blocks vasoconstrictor and aldosterone-secreting effects of angiotensin II, inhibiting the binding of angiotensin II to the AT_1 receptors. **Therapeutic Effect:** Causes vasodilation, decreases peripheral resistance, and decreases BP.

PHARMACOKINETICS

Route	Onset	Peak	Duration
PO	N/A	6 hr	24 hr

Well absorbed after PO administration. Protein binding: 98%. Undergoes first-pass metabolism in the liver to active metabolites. Excreted in urine and via the biliary system. Not removed by hemodialysis. **Half-life:** 2 hr, metabolite: 6–9 hr.

USES
Treatment of hypertension. Used alone or in combination with other

antihypertensives. Treatment of diabetic nephropathy, prevention of stroke. OFF-LABEL: CHF, erythrocytosis.

PRECAUTIONS

CONTRAINDICATIONS: None known. **CAUTIONS:** Renal/hepatic impairment, renal arterial stenosis.

⌛ LIFESPAN CONSIDERATIONS: **Pregnancy/Lactation:** Has caused fetal/neonatal morbidity, mortality. Potential for adverse effects on breast-fed infant. Do not breast-feed. **Pregnancy Category C (D if used in second or third trimesters). Children:** Safety and efficacy not established. **Elderly:** No age-related precautions noted.

INTERACTIONS

DRUG: **Cimetidine:** May increase the effects of losartan. **Ketoconazole, troleandomycin:** May inhibit the effects of these drugs. **Lithium:** May increase lithium blood concentration and risk of lithium toxicity. **Phenobarbital, rifampin:** May decrease the effects of losartan. HERBAL: None known. FOOD: **Grapefruit, grapefruit juice:** May alter the absorption of losartan. LAB VALUES: May increase BUN, serum alkaline phosphatase, serum bilirubin, serum creatinine, AST, and ALT levels. May decrease blood Hgb and Hct levels.

AVAILABILITY (Rx)

TABLETS: 25 mg, 50 mg, 100 mg.

ADMINISTRATION/HANDLING

PO
• May give without regard to food. • Do not crush or break tablets.

INDICATIONS/ROUTES/DOSAGE

HYPERTENSION
PO: ADULTS, ELDERLY: Initially, 50 mg once a day. **Maximum:** May be given once or twice a day, with total daily doses ranging from 25–100 mg.

NEPHROPATHY
PO: ADULTS, ELDERLY: Initially, 50 mg/day. May increase to 100 mg/day based on BP response.

STROKE REDUCTION
PO: ADULTS, ELDERLY: 50 mg/day. **Maximum:** 100 mg/day.

HYPERTENSION IN PATIENTS WITH IMPAIRED HEPATIC FUNCTION
PO: ADULTS, ELDERLY: Initially, 25 mg/day.

SIDE EFFECTS

FREQUENT (8%): Upper respiratory tract infection. **OCCASIONAL (4%–2%):** Dizziness, diarrhea, cough. **RARE (1% or less):** Insomnia, dyspepsia, heartburn, back and leg pain, muscle cramps, myalgia, nasal congestion, sinusitis.

ADVERSE REACTIONS/ TOXIC EFFECTS

Overdosage may manifest as hypotension and tachycardia. Bradycardia occurs less often.

NURSING CONSIDERATIONS

BASELINE ASSESSMENT
Obtain BP, apical pulse immediately before each dose, in addition to regular monitoring (be alert to fluctuations). If excessive reduction in BP occurs, place patient in supine position, feet slightly elevated. Question for possibility of pregnancy (see Pregnancy/Lactation). Assess medication history (especially diuretic).

INTERVENTION/EVALUATION
Maintain hydration (offer fluids frequently). Assess for evidence of upper respiratory infection, cough. Assist with ambulation if dizziness occurs. Monitor bowel activity and stool consistency. Monitor BP, pulse.

✐ see color pill atlas   ⬧ herb   underlined – top prescribed drug

• Inform female patient regarding consequences of second- and third-trimester exposure to losartan. • Report pregnancy to physician as soon as possible. • Avoid tasks that require alertness, motor skills until response to drug is established (possible dizziness effect). • Report any sign of infection (sore throat, fever), chest pain. • Do not take OTC cold preparations, nasal decongestants. • Do not stop taking medication.

Lotensin, *see benazepril*

Lotensin HCT,
see benazepril and hydrochlorothiazide

Lotrel, *see amlodipine and benazepril*

---

lovastatin

lo-va-**sta**-tin

(Altocor, Mevacor)

Do not confuse lovastatin with Leustatin or Livostin, or Mevacor with Mivacron.

FIXED-COMBINATION(S)

Advicor: lovastatin/niacin: 20 mg/500 mg; 20 mg/750 mg; 20 mg/1,000 mg.

♦CLASSIFICATION

PHARMACOTHERAPEUTIC: HMG-CoA reductase inhibitor. **CLINICAL:** Anti-hyperlipidemic (see p. 52C).

ACTION

An antihyperlipidemic that inhibits HMG-CoA reductase, the enzyme that catalyzes the early step in cholesterol synthesis. **Therapeutic Effect:** Decreases LDL cholesterol, VLDL cholesterol, plasma triglycerides; increases HDL cholesterol.

PHARMACOKINETICS

Route	Onset	Peak	Duration
PO	3 days	4–6 wk	N/A

Incompletely absorbed from the GI tract (increased on empty stomach). Protein binding: 95%. Hydrolyzed in the liver to active metabolite. Primarily eliminated in feces. Not removed by hemodialysis. **Half-life:** 1.1–1.7 hr.

USES

Decreases elevated serum total and LDL cholesterol in primary hypercholesterolemia; primary prevention of coronary artery disease. Adjunct to diet in adolescent patients (10–17 yr) with heterozygous familial hypercholesterolemia. Slows progression of coronary atherosclerosis in patients with coronary heart disease.

PRECAUTIONS

CONTRAINDICATIONS: Active liver disease, pregnancy, unexplained elevated liver function tests. **CAUTIONS:** History of heavy or chronic alcohol use; renal impairment; concomitant use of cyclosporine, fibrates, niacin.

⧗ **LIFESPAN CONSIDERATIONS: Pregnancy/Lactation:** Contraindicated in pregnancy (suppression of cholesterol biosynthesis may cause fetal toxicity) and lactation. Unknown if drug is distributed in breast milk. **Pregnancy Category X. Children:** Safety and efficacy not established. **Elderly:** No age-related precautions noted.

INTERACTIONS

DRUG: Cyclosporine, erythromycin, gemfibrozil, immunosuppressants, niacin: Increases the risk of acute renal failure and rhabdomyolysis. **Erythromycin, itraconazole, ketoconazole:** May increase lovastatin blood concentration causing severe muscle inflammation, myalgia, and weakness. **HERBAL:** None known. **FOOD: Grapefruit juice:** Large amounts of grapefruit juice may increase risk of side effects, such as myalgia and weakness. **LAB VALUES:** May increase serum creatine kinase and serum transaminase concentrations.

AVAILABILITY (Rx)

TABLETS (MEVACOR): 10 mg, 20 mg, 40 mg. **TABLETS (EXTENDED-RELEASE [ALTOCOR]):** 20 mg, 40 mg, 60 mg.

ADMINISTRATION/HANDLING
PO
• Give with meals.

INDICATIONS/ROUTES/DOSAGE
ATHEROSCLEROSIS, CORONARY ARTERY DISEASE
PO: ADULTS, ELDERLY: Initially, 20 mg/day. Maintenance: 10–80 mg once daily or in 2 divided doses. **Maximum:** 80 mg/day.

HYPERCHOLESTEROLEMIA
PO: ADULTS, ELDERLY: Initially, 20 mg/day. Maintenance: 10–80 mg once daily or in 2 divided doses. **Maximum:** 80 mg/day.

PO (EXTENDED-RELEASE): ADULTS, ELDERLY: Initially, 20–60 mg once daily at bedtime. Maintenance: 10–60 mg once daily at bedtime.

HETEROZYGOUS FAMILIAL HYPERCHOLESTEROLEMIA
PO: CHILDREN 10–17 YR: Initially, 10 mg/day. May increase to 20 mg/day after 8 wk and 40 mg/day after 16 wk if needed.

SIDE EFFECTS

Generally well tolerated. Side effects usually mild and transient. **FREQUENT (9%–5%):** Headache, flatulence, diarrhea, abdominal pain or cramps, rash and pruritus. **OCCASIONAL (4%–3%):** Nausea, vomiting, constipation, dyspepsia. **RARE (2%–1%):** Dizziness, heartburn, myalgia, blurred vision, eye irritation.

ADVERSE REACTIONS/ TOXIC EFFECTS

There is a potential for cataract development. Lovastatin occasionally produces myopathy manifested as muscle pain, tenderness or weakness with elevated creatine kinase. Myopathy may take the form of rhabdomyolysis fatalities.

NURSING CONSIDERATIONS

BASELINE ASSESSMENT

Question for possibility of pregnancy before initiating therapy (Pregnancy Category X). Assess baseline lab results: serum cholesterol, triglycerides, liver function tests.

INTERVENTION/EVALUATION

Determine pattern of bowel activity. Monitor for headache, dizziness, blurred vision. Assess for rash, pruritus. Monitor serum cholesterol, triglyceride levels for therapeutic response. Be alert for malaise, muscle cramping/weakness.

PATIENT/FAMILY TEACHING
• Take with meals. • Follow special diet (important part of treatment). • Periodic lab tests are essential part of therapy. • Avoid grapefruit juice. • Inform physician of severe gastric upset, vision changes, myalgia or weakness, changes in color of urine/stool, yellowing of eyes or skin, unusual bruising.

Lovenox, *see enoxaparin*

---

loxapine hydrochloride

lox-ah-peen
(Apo-Loxapine ♣, Loxapac ♣, Loxitane)

loxapine succinate

(Loxitane)
See Antipsychotics (p. 58C)

Lupron, *see leuprolide*

---

lymphocyte immune globulin N

lym-phow-site ih-**mewn glah**-byew-lin **N**
(Atgam, Thymoglobulin)

Do not confuse Atgam with Ativan.

◆CLASSIFICATION
PHARMACOTHERAPEUTIC: Biologic response modifier. **CLINICAL:** Immunosuppressant.

ACTION
A biological response modifier that acts as a lymphocyte selective immunosuppressant, reducing the number and altering the function of T lymphocytes, which are responsible for cell-mediated and humoral immunity. Lymphocyte immune globulin N also stimulates the release of hematopoietic growth factors. **Therapeutic Effect:** Prevents allograft rejection; treats aplastic anemia.

PHARMACOKINETICS
Unknown absorption, metabolism, and elimination. **Half-life:** Approximately 5–7 days.

USES
Prevention and/or treatment of renal allograft rejection. Treatment of moderate to severe aplastic anemia in patients not candidates for bone marrow transplant. **OFF-LABEL:** Immunosuppressant in bone marrow, heart, and liver transplants, treatment of pure red cell aplasia, multiple sclerosis, myasthenia gravis, and scleroderma.

PRECAUTIONS
CONTRAINDICATIONS: Systemic hypersensitivity reaction to previous injection of lymphocyte immune globulin N. **CAUTIONS:** Concurrent immunosuppressive therapy.

⧗ **LIFESPAN CONSIDERATIONS: Pregnancy/Lactation:** Unknown if drug crosses placenta; or is distributed in breast milk. **Pregnancy Category C. Children:** Safety and efficacy not

L

established.   **Elderly:** No age-related precautions noted.

INTERACTIONS

DRUG: Corticosteroids, other immunosuppresants: Masks reaction to lymphocyte immune globulin. **HERBAL:** None known. **FOOD:** None known. **LAB VALUES:** May alter renal function test results.

AVAILABILITY

INJECTION: 250 mg/5 ml.

ADMINISTRATION/HANDLING

🖙 IV

Reconstitution • Total daily dose must be further diluted with 0.9% NaCl (do not use D_5W). • Gently rotate diluted solution. Do not shake. • Final concentration must not exceed 4 mg/ml.

Rate of administration • Use 0.2- to 1-micron filter. • Give total daily dose over minimum of 4 hr.

Storage • Keep refrigerated before and after dilution. • Discard diluted solution after 24 hr.

▨ IV INCOMPATIBILITIES

No information is available for Y-site administration.

INDICATIONS/ROUTES/DOSAGE

TO DELAY ONSET OF RENAL ALLOGRAFT REJECTION
IV: ADULTS, ELDERLY, CHILDREN: 15 mg/kg/day for 14 days, then every other day for 14 days. First dose within 24 hr before or after transplantation.

TREATMENT OF RENAL ALLOGRAFT REJECTION
IV: ADULTS, ELDERLY, CHILDREN: 10–15 mg/kg/day for 14 days, then every other day for 14 more days. **Maximum:** 21 doses.

APLASTIC ANEMIA
IV: ADULTS, ELDERLY, CHILDREN: 10–20 mg/kg once a day for 8–14 days, then every other day. **Maximum:** 21 doses.

SIDE EFFECTS

FREQUENT: Fever (51%), thrombocytopenia (30%), rash (2%), chills (16%), leukopenia (14%), systemic infection (13%). **OCCASIONAL (10%–5%):** Serum sickness-like reaction, dyspnea, apnea, arthralgia, chest pain, back pain, flank pain, nausea, vomiting, diarrhea, phlebitis.

ADVERSE REACTIONS/ TOXIC EFFECTS

Thrombocytopenia may occur but is generally transient. A severe hypersensitivity reaction, including anaphylaxis, occurs rarely.

NURSING CONSIDERATIONS

BASELINE ASSESSMENT
Use of high-flow vein (CVL, PICC, Groshong catheter) may prevent chemical phlebitis that may occur if peripheral vein is used.

INTERVENTION/EVALUATION
Monitor frequently for chills, fever, erythema, itching. Obtain order for prophylactic antihistamines or corticosteroids.

Lyrica, *see pregabalin*

Macrobid, *see*
nitrofurantoin

---

magnesium 🏴

mag-**knee**-see-um

magnesium chloride

(Mag-Delay SR, Slow-Mag)

magnesium citrate

(Citrate of Magnesia, Citro-Mag ❀)

magnesium hydroxide

(Phillips Milk of Magnesia)

magnesium oxide

(Mag-Ox 400, Uro-Mag)

magnesium protein complex

(Mg-PLUS)

magnesium sulfate

(Epsom salt, magnesium sulfate injection, Sulfamag)

Do not confuse magnesium sulfate with manganese sulfate.

FIXED-COMBINATION(S)

With aluminum, an antacid (**Aludrox, Delcid, Gaviscon, Maalox**); with aluminum and simethicone, an antiflatulent (**Di-Gel, Gelusil, Maalox Plus, Mylanta**); with aluminum and calcium, an antacid (**Camalox**); with mineral oil, a lubricant laxative (**Haley's MO**); with magnesium oxide and aluminum oxide, an antacid (**Riopan**).

◆CLASSIFICATION

CLINICAL: Antacid, anticonvulsant, electrolyte, laxative (see pp. 10C, 109C).

ACTION

An antacid, laxative, electrolyte, and anticonvulsant. As an antacid, acts in the stomach to neutralize gastric acid. Therapeutic Effect: Increases pH. As a laxative, has an osmotic effect, primarily in the small intestine, and draws water into the intestinal lumen. Therapeutic Effect: Produces distention and promotes peristalsis and bowel evacuation. As a systemic dietary supplement and electrolyte replacement, is found primarily in intracellular fluids and is essential for enzyme activity, nerve conduction, and muscle contraction. As an anticonvulsant, blocks neuromuscular transmission and the amount of acetylcholine released at the motor end plate. Therapeutic Effect: Controls seizure. Maintains and restores magnesium levels.

PHARMACOKINETICS

Antacid, laxative: Minimal absorption through the intestine. Absorbed dose primarily excreted in urine. **Systemic:** Widely distributed. Primarily excreted in urine.

USES

Magnesium Chloride: Dietary supplement. **Magnesium Citrate:** Evacuation of bowel before surgical or diagnostic procedures. **Magnesium Hydroxide:** Short-term treatment of constipation, symptoms of hyperacidity, magnesium replacement. **Magnesium Oxide:** Magnesium replacement. **Magnesium Sulfate:** Treatment and prevention of hypomagnesemia, prevention of seizures, treatment of cardiac arrhythmias, treatment of constipation.

M

❀ Canadian trade name   ℮ see **evolve**   🏴 High Alert drug

OFF-LABEL: **Magnesium sulfate:** Premature labor, torsades de pointes, acute asthma, MI, tocolysis.

PRECAUTIONS

CONTRAINDICATIONS: Antacid: Appendicitis or symptoms of appendicitis, ileostomy, intestinal obstruction, severe renal impairment. **Laxative:** Appendicitis, CHF, colostomy, hypersensitivity, ileostomy, intestinal obstruction, undiagnosed rectal bleeding. **Systemic:** Heart block, myocardial damage, renal failure. **CAUTIONS:** Safety in children younger than 6 yr not known. **Antacids:** Undiagnosed GI or rectal bleeding, ulcerative colitis, colostomy, diverticulitis, chronic diarrhea. **Laxative:** Diabetes mellitus or patients on low-salt diet (some products contain sugar, sodium). **Systemic:** Severe renal impairment.

⏳ **LIFESPAN CONSIDERATIONS: Pregnancy/Lactation: Antacid:** Unknown if distributed in breast milk. **Parenteral:** Readily crosses placenta. Distributed in breast milk for 24 hr after magnesium therapy is discontinued. Continuous IV infusion increases risk of magnesium toxicity in neonate. IV administration should not be used 2 hr preceding delivery. **Pregnancy Category B. Children:** No age-related precautions noted. **Elderly:** Increased risk of developing magnesium deficiency (e.g., poor diet, decreased absorption, medications).

INTERACTIONS

DRUG: **Antacid: Ketoconazole, tetracyclines:** May decrease the absorption of ketoconazole and tetracyclines. **Methenamine:** May decrease the effects of methenamine. **Antacid, laxative: Digoxin, oral anticoagulants, phenothiazines:** May decrease the effects of these drugs. **Tetracyclines:** May form nonabsorbable complex with tetracyclines. **Systemic (dietary supplement, electrolyte replacement): Calcium:** May neutralize the effects of magnesium. **CNS depression-producing medications:** May increase CNS depression. **Digoxin:** May cause changes in cardiac conduction or heart block with digoxin. **HERBAL:** None known. **FOOD:** None known. **LAB VALUES: Antacid:** May increase gastrin production and pH. **Laxative:** May decrease serum potassium level. **Systemic (dietary supplement, electrolyte replacement):** None known.

AVAILABILITY

MAGNESIUM CHLORIDE
TABLETS (MAG DELAY SR, SLO-MAG): 64 mg.
MAGNESIUM CITRATE
ORAL SOLUTION (CITRATE OF MAGNESIA): 290 mg/5 ml.
MAGNESIUM HYDROXIDE
ORAL LIQUID (PHILLIPS MILK OF MAGNESIA): 400 mg/5 ml, 800 mg/5 ml. **TABLETS (CHEWABLE [PHILLIPS MILK OF MAGNESIA]):** 311 mg.
MAGNESIUM OXIDE
TABLETS (MAG-OX 400): 400 mg. **CAPSULES (URO-MAG):** 140 mg.
MAGNESIUM SULFATE
PREMIX INFUSION SOLUTION: 10 mg/ml, 20 mg/ml, 40 mg/ml, 80 mg/ml. **INJECTION:** 125 mg/ml, 500 mg/ml.

ADMINISTRATION/HANDLING

🖥 **IV**

Reconstitution • Must dilute (do not exceed 20 mg/ml concentration).

Rate of administration • For IV infusion, do not exceed magnesium sulfate concentration 200 mg/ml (20%). • Do not exceed IV infusion rate of 150 mg/min.

Storage • Store at room temperature.

IM
• For adults, elderly, use 250 mg/ml (25%) or 500 mg/ml (50%) magnesium

M

sulfate concentration. • For infants, children, do not exceed 200 mg/ml (20%).

PO (ANTACID)
• Shake suspension well before use.
• Chewable tablets should be chewed thoroughly before swallowing, followed with full glass of water.

PO (LAXATIVE)
• Drink full glass of liquid (8 oz) with each dose (prevents dehydration).
• Flavor may be improved by following with fruit juice, citrus carbonated beverage. • Refrigerate citrate of magnesia (retains potency, palatability).

▦ IV INCOMPATIBILITIES
Amphotericin B complex (Abelcet, AmBisome, Amphotec), cefepime (Maxipime).

IV COMPATIBILITIES
Amikacin (Amikin), cefazolin (Ancef), ciprofloxacin (Cipro), dobutamine (Dobutrex), enalapril (Vasotec), gentamicin, heparin, hydromorphone (Dilaudid), insulin, milrinone (Primacor), morphine, piperacillin/tazobactam (Zosyn), potassium chloride, propofol (Diprivan), tobramycin (Nebcin), vancomycin (Vancocin).

INDICATIONS/ROUTES/DOSAGE
HYPOMAGNESEMIA
PO (MAGNESIUM SULFATE): ADULTS, ELDERLY: 3 g q6h for 4 doses as needed.
IV, IM: ADULTS, ELDERLY: 1–12 g/day in divided doses. CHILDREN: 25–50 mg/kg/dose q4–6h for 3–4 doses. Maintenance: 30–60 mg/kg/day.

HYPERTENSION, SEIZURES
IV, IM (MAGNESIUM SULFATE): CHILDREN: 20–100 mg/kg/dose q4–6h as needed.
IV: ADULTS: Initially, 4 g then 1–4 g/hr by continuous infusion.

ARRHYTHMIAS
IV (MAGNESIUM SULFATE): ADULTS, ELDERLY: Initially, 1–2 g then infusion of 1–2 g/hr.

CONSTIPATION
PO (MAGNESIUM SULFATE): ADULTS, ELDERLY, CHILDREN 12 YR AND OLDER: 10–30 g/day in divided doses. CHILDREN 6-11 YR: 5–10 g/day in divided doses. CHILDREN 2-5 YR: 2.5–5 g/kg/day in divided doses.
PO (MAGNESIUM HYDROXIDE): ADULTS, ELDERLY, CHILDREN 12 YR AND OLDER: 6–8 tablets or 30–60 ml/day. CHILDREN 6-11 YR: 3–4 tablets or 7.5–15 ml/day. CHILDREN 2-5 YR: 1–2 tablets or 2.5–7.5 ml/day.

HYPERACIDITY
PO (MAGNESIUM HYDROXIDE): ADULTS, ELDERLY: 2–4 tablets or 5–15 ml as needed up to 4 times a day. CHILDREN 7-14 YR: 1 tablet or 2.5–5 ml as needed up to 4 times a day.

MAGNESIUM DEFICIENCY
PO (MAGNESIUM OXIDE): ADULTS, ELDERLY: 1–2 tablets 2–3 times a day.

DIETARY SUPPLEMENT
PO (MAGNESIUM CHLORIDE): ADULTS, ELDERLY: 54–483 mg/day in 2–4 divided doses.

CATHARTIC
PO (MAGNESIUM CITRATE): ADULTS, ELDERLY, CHILDREN 12 YR AND OLDER: 120–300 ml. CHILDREN 6-11 YR: 100–150 ml. CHILDREN YOUNGER THAN 6 YR: 0.5 ml/kg up to maximum of 200 ml.

SIDE EFFECTS
FREQUENT: Antacid: Chalky taste, diarrhea, laxative effect. **OCCASIONAL: Antacid:** Nausea, vomiting, stomach cramps. **Antacid, laxative:** With prolonged use or large doses in renal impairment, possible hypermagnesemia, marked by dizziness, irregular heartbeat, mental changes, fatigue, and weakness. **Laxative:** Cramping, diarrhea, increased thirst, flatulence. **Systemic (dietary supplement, electrolyte replacement):** Reduced respiratory rate, decreased reflexes, flushing, hypotension, decreased heart rate.

M

ADVERSE REACTIONS/ TOXIC EFFECTS

Magnesium as an antacid or laxative has no known serious reactions. Systemic use of magnesium may produce prolonged PR interval and widening of QRS interval. Magnesium toxicity may cause loss of deep tendon reflexes, heart block, respiratory paralysis, and cardiac arrest. The antidote for toxicity is 10–20 ml 10% calcium gluconate (5–10 mEq of calcium).

NURSING CONSIDERATIONS

BASELINE ASSESSMENT

Assess if patient is sensitive to magnesium. **Antacid:** Assess GI pain (duration, location, quality, time of occurrence, relief with food, causative/ excacerbative factors). **Laxative:** Assess pattern of bowel activity and stool consistency, bowel sounds for peristalsis. Assess patient for weight loss, nausea, vomiting, history of recent abdominal surgery. **Systemic:** Assess renal function, serum magnesium level.

INTERVENTION/EVALUATION

Antacid: Assess for relief of gastric distress. Monitor renal function (especially if dosing is long-term or frequent). **Laxative:** Monitor pattern of bowel activity and stool consistency. Maintain adequate fluid intake. **Systemic:** Monitor renal function, magnesium levels, EKG for cardiac function. Test patellar reflexes (knee jerk reflexes) before giving repeat parenteral doses (used as indication of CNS depression; suppressed reflexes may be sign of impending respiratory arrest). Patellar reflex must be present, respiratory rate should be 16/min or over before each parenteral dose. Provide seizure precautions.

PATIENT/FAMILY TEACHING

• **Antacid:** Give at least 2 hr apart from other medication. • Do not take longer than 2 wk unless directed by physician. • For peptic ulcer, take 1 and 3 hr after meals and at bedtime for 4–6 wk. • Chew tablets thoroughly, followed with glass of water; shake suspensions well. Repeat dosing or large doses may have laxative effect. • **Laxative:** Drink full glass (8 oz) liquid to aid stool softening. • Use only for short term. Do not use if abdominal pain, nausea, vomiting is present. • **Systemic:** Inform physician of any signs of hypermagnesemia (confusion, palpitations, cramping, unusual fatigue, weakness, lightheadedness, dizziness).

mannitol

man-i-tall
(Osmitrol, Resectisol)

CLASSIFICATION

CLINICAL: Osmotic diuretic, antiglaucoma, antihemolytic.

ACTION

An osmotic diuretic, antiglaucoma, and antihemolytic agent that elevates osmotic pressure of the glomerular filtrate, inhibiting tubular reabsorption of water and electrolytes, resulting in increased flow of water into interstitial fluid and plasma. **Therapeutic Effect:** Produces diuresis; reduces IOP; reduces ICP and cerebral edema.

PHARMACOKINETICS

Route	Onset	Peak	Duration
IV (diuresis)	15–30 min	N/A	2–8 hr
IV (reduced ICP)	15–30 min	N/A	3–8 hr
IV (reduced IOP)	N/A	30–60 min	4–8 hr

Remains in extracellular fluid. Primarily excreted in urine. Removed by hemodialysis. **Half-life:** 100 min.

USES

Prevention, treatment of oliguric phase of acute renal failure (before evidence of permanent renal failure). Reduces increased intracranial pressure (ICP) due to cerebral edema, spinal cord edema, intraocular pressure (IOP) due to acute glaucoma. Promotes urinary excretion of toxic substances (aspirin, bromides, imipramine, barbiturates).

PRECAUTIONS

CONTRAINDICATIONS: Dehydration, intracranial bleeding, severe pulmonary edema and congestion; several renal disease (anuria), increasing oliguria and azotemia. **CAUTIONS:** None known.

⧗ **LIFESPAN CONSIDERATIONS: Pregnancy/Lactation:** Unknown if drug crosses placenta or is distributed in breast milk. **Pregnancy Category C. Children:** Safety and efficacy not established in those younger than 12 yr. **Elderly:** Age-related renal impairment may require dosage adjustment.

INTERACTIONS

DRUG: Digoxin: May increase the risk of digoxin toxicity associated with mannitol-induced hypokalemia. **HERBAL:** None known. **FOOD:** None known. **LAB VALUES:** May decrease serum phosphate, potassium, and sodium levels.

AVAILABILITY (Rx)

INJECTION (OSMITROL): 5%, 10%, 15%, 20%, 25%. **IRRIGATION SOLUTION (RESECTISOL):** 5%.

ADMINISTRATION/HANDLING

◀ ALERT ▶ Assess IV site for patency before each dose. Pain, thrombosis noted with extravasation.

 IV

Rate of administration • In-line filter (less than 5 microns) used for concentrations over 20%. • Administer test dose for patients with oliguria. • Give IV push over 3–5 min; over 20–30 min for cerebral edema, elevated ICP. Maximum concentration: 25%. • Do not add KCl or NaCl to mannitol 20% or greater. Do not add to whole blood for transfusion.

Storage • Store at room temperature. • If crystals are noted in solution, warm bottle in hot water, shake vigorously at intervals. Cool to body temperature before administration. Do not use if crystals remain after warming procedure.

IV INCOMPATIBILITIES

Cefepime (Maxipime), doxorubicin liposomal (Doxil), filgrastim (Neupogen).

IV COMPATIBILITIES

Cisplatin (Platinol), ondansetron (Zofran), propofol (Diprivan).

INDICATIONS/ROUTES/DOSAGE

ICP
IV: ADULTS, ELDERLY: 0.25–1 g/kg q6–8h. **Maximum:** 6 g/24 hr. CHILDREN: 0.25–1 g/kg as needed. **Maximum:** 2 g/kg/dose.

IOP
IV: ADULTS, ELDERLY: 1.5–2 g/kg as a 15%–20% solution. **Maximum:** 6 g/24 hr. CHILDREN: 1–2 g/kg. **Maximum:** 2 g/kg/dose.

RENAL IMPAIRMENT, OLIGURIA
IV: ADULTS, ELDERLY: Use test dose. 300–400 mg/kg or up to 100 g given as a single dose. CHILDREN: 0.25–2 g/kg. **Maximum:** 6 g/24 hr.

TOXICITY, POISONING
IV: ADULTS, ELDERLY: Continuous infusion as a 5%–20% solution. CHILDREN: Up to 2 g/kg as 5%–10% solution.

SIDE EFFECTS

FREQUENT: Dry mouth, thirst. **OCCASIONAL:** Blurred vision, increased urinary frequency and urine volume, headache, arm pain, backache, nausea, vomiting, urticaria, dizziness, hypotension or hypertension, tachycardia, fever, angina-like chest pain.

ADVERSE REACTIONS/ TOXIC EFFECTS

Fluid and electrolyte imbalance may occur from rapid administration of large doses or inadequate urine output resulting in overexpansion of extracellular fluid. Circulatory overload may produce pulmonary edema and CHF. Excessive diuresis may produce hypokalemia and hyponatremia. Fluid loss in excess of electrolyte excretion may produce hypernatremia and hyperkalemia.

NURSING CONSIDERATIONS

BASELINE ASSESSMENT

Check BP, pulse before giving medication. Assess skin turgor, mucous membranes, mental status, muscle strength. Obtain baseline weight. Assess I&O.

INTERVENTION/EVALUATION

Monitor urinary output to ascertain therapeutic response. Monitor serum electrolytes, BUN, renal and hepatic reports. Assess vital signs, skin turgor, mucous membranes. Weigh daily. Signs of hyponatremia include confusion, drowsiness, thirst and dry mouth, cold or clammy skin. Signs of hypokalemia include changes in muscle strength, tremors, muscle cramps, altered mental status, cardiac arrhythmias. Signs of hyperkalemia include colic, diarrhea, muscle twitching followed by weakness and paralysis, arrhythmias.

PATIENT/FAMILY TEACHING

* Expect increased frequency, volume of urination. * May cause dry mouth.

maprotiline hydrochloride

(Ludiomil)
See Antidepressants

Mavik, *see trandolapril*

Maxalt, *see rizatriptan*

Maxipine, *see cefepime*

mecasermin

meh-cah-**sir**-min
(Increlex)

◆ CLASSIFICATION

PHARMACOTHERAPEUTIC: Human insulin-like growth factor-1. **CLINICAL:** Growth hormone.

ACTION

A recombinant-DNA-engineered human insulin-like growth factor-1 (rhIGF-1), designed to replace natural IGF-1 in pediatric patients who are deficient, leading to decreased growth (skeletal, cell and organ). **Therapeutic Effect:** Promotes normalized statural growth, cartilage and organ growth.

PHARMACOKINETICS

Extensively bound to albumin. Protein binding: greater than 80%. Metabolized in liver and kidney. **Half-life:** 5.8 hr.

USES

Long-term treatment of growth failure in children with severe primary IGF-1 deficiency or with growth hormone (GH) gene deletions who have developed neutralizing antibodies to GH.

PRECAUTIONS

CONTRAINDICATIONS: Closed epiphyses; active or suspected neoplasia. **CAUTIONS:** Uncorrected thyroid or nutritional deficiencies.

⌛ LIFESPAN CONSIDERATIONS: **Pregnancy/Lactation:** Unknown if distributed in breast milk. **Pregnancy Category C. Children:** Safety and efficacy not established in children younger than 2 yr. **Elderly:** Safety and efficacy not established.

INTERACTIONS

DRUG: None known. HERBAL: None known. FOOD: None known. LAB VALUES: May increase AST, ALT, cholesterol, triglycerides, LDH. May decrease serum glucose.

AVAILABILITY (Rx)

INJECTION: 10 mg/ml (40 mg vial) (Increlex).

ADMINISTRATION/HANDLING

SUBCUTANEOUS

◄ ALERT ► Must be administered within 20 min before or after a meal or snack. Omit dose and do not make up for omitted dose if patient is unable to eat. Rotate injection sites. May be given in thigh, abdomen, or upper arm.

Storage • Refrigerate vials. • After initial needle entry, refrigerated vial is stable for 30 days only. • Discard if cloudy or contains a precipitate.

INDICATIONS/ROUTES/DOSAGE

◄ ALERT ► Give subcutaneous only; do not give IM or IV. Assess preprandial glucose during treatment initiation and dosage adjustment until a well-tolerated dose is established.

INITIAL DOSE

SUBCUTANEOUS: CHILDREN 2 YR AND OLDER: Initial dose is 0.04–0.08 mg/kg (40–80 mcg/kg) twice a day. If tolerated for 7 days, dose can be increased in 0.04 mg/kg/dose (40 mcg/kg/dose)-increments, to a maximum dose of 0.12 mg/kg (120 mcg/kg) twice a day. Reduce dose if hypoglycemia occurs despite adequate food intake.

SIDE EFFECTS

FREQUENT (42%): Hypoglycemia. **OCCASIONAL (15%):** Snoring, tonsillar hypertrophy. **RARE (5% or greater):** Vomiting, injection site bruising, arthralgia, extremity pain, otitis media with associated ear pain, headache, dizziness.

ADVERSE REACTIONS/ TOXIC EFFECTS

Intracranial hypertension has been reported. Thickening of soft facial tissue occurs rarely. Hypoglycemic seizure has occurred.

NURSING CONSIDERATIONS

BASELINE ASSESSMENT

Must be administered within 20 min before or after a meal or snack. If patient is unable to eat, omit dose; drug must be given within 20 min parameter. Obtain preprandial blood glucose level. Patients should avoid high-risk activities within 2–3 hr of dosing until a tolerated dose is established.

INTERVENTION/EVALUATION

Monitor blood glucose for hypoglycemia and take appropriate measures to maintain patient within glucose parameters. Monitor small children closely due to potentially erratic food intake. Monitor facial features, growth.

PATIENT/FAMILY TEACHING

• Contact physician or nurse if limp or complaint of hip or knee pain occurs.

M

mechlorethamine hydrochloride

(Mustargen)

See Cancer chemotherapeutic agents (p. 76C)

meclizine

mek-li-zeen

(Antivert, Bonamine 🍁, Bonine, Meclicot, Meni-D)

Do not confuse Antivert with Axert.

CLASSIFICATION

PHARMACOTHERAPEUTIC: Anticholinergic. **CLINICAL:** Antiemetic, antivertigo.

ACTION

An anticholinergic that reduces labyrinthine excitability and diminishes vestibular stimulation of the labyrinth, affecting the chemoreceptor trigger zone. Therapeutic Effect: Reduces nausea, vomiting, and vertigo.

PHARMACOKINETICS

Route	Onset	Peak	Duration
PO	30–60 min	N/A	12–24 hr

Well absorbed from the GI tract. Widely distributed. Metabolized in the liver. Primarily excreted in urine. Half-life: 6 hr.

USES

Prevention and treatment of nausea, vomiting, vertigo due to motion sickness. Treatment of vertigo associated with diseases affecting vestibular system.

PRECAUTIONS

CONTRAINDICATIONS: None known. **CAUTIONS:** Narrow-angle glaucoma, obstructive diseases of the GI or GU tract.

⧖ LIFESPAN CONSIDERATIONS: **Pregnancy/Lactation:** Unknown if drug crosses placenta or is distributed in breast milk (may produce irritability in nursing infants). **Pregnancy Category B. Children/Elderly:** May be more sensitive to anticholinergic effects (e.g., dry mouth).

INTERACTIONS

DRUG: **Alcohol, CNS depression-producing medications:** May increase CNS depressant effect. HERBAL: None known. FOOD: None known. LAB VALUES: May produce false-negative results in antigen skin testing unless meclizine is discontinued 4 days before testing.

AVAILABILITY (Rx)

TABLETS (ANTIVERT, MECLICOT, MENI-D): 12.5 mg, 25 mg, 50 mg. **TABLETS (CHEWABLE [BONINE]):** 25 mg.

ADMINISTRATION/HANDLING

PO
• Give without regard to meals.
• Scored tablets may be crushed. • Do not crush or break capsules.

INDICATIONS/ROUTES/DOSAGE

MOTION SICKNESS
PO: ADULTS, ELDERLY, CHILDREN 12 YR AND OLDER: 12.5–25 mg 1 hr before travel. May repeat q12–24h. May require a dose of 50 mg.

VERTIGO
PO: ADULTS, ELDERLY, CHILDREN 12 YR AND OLDER: 25–100 mg/day in divided doses, as needed.

SIDE EFFECTS

FREQUENT: Drowsiness. **OCCASIONAL:** Blurred vision; dry mouth, nose, or throat.

ADVERSE REACTIONS/ TOXIC EFFECTS

A hypersensitivity reaction, marked by eczema, pruritus, rash, cardiac disturbances, and photosensitivity, may occur. Overdose may produce CNS depression (manifested as sedation, apnea, cardiovascular collapse, or death) or severe paradoxical reactions (such as hallucinations, tremor, and seizures). Children may experience paradoxical reactions, including restlessness, insomnia, euphoria, nervousness, and tremors. Overdose in children may result in hallucinations, seizures, and death.

NURSING CONSIDERATIONS

INTERVENTION/EVALUATION

Monitor BP, especially in elderly (increased risk of hypotension). Monitor children closely for paradoxical reaction. Monitor serum electrolytes in those with severe vomiting. Assess skin turgor, mucous membranes to evaluate hydration status.

PATIENT/FAMILY TEACHING

• Tolerance to sedative effect may occur. • Avoid tasks that require alertness, motor skills until response to drug is established. • Dry mouth, drowsiness, dizziness may be an expected response of drug. • Avoid alcoholic beverages during therapy. • Sugarless gum, sips of tepid water may relieve dry mouth. • Coffee, tea may help reduce drowsiness.

---

meclofenamate sodium

(Meclodium, Meclomen)
See Nonsteroidal Anti-Inflammatory Drugs (NSAIDs)

---

*medroxy-PROGESTERone acetate

me-**drox**-ee-proe-**jess**-te-rone
(Depo-Provera, Depo-Provera Contraceptive, Depo-SubQ-Provera 104, Novo-Medrone ✤, Provera)
Do not confuse medroxyprogesterone with hydroxyprogesterone, methylprednisolone, or methyltestosterone.

FIXED-COMBINATION(S)

Prempro, Premphase: medroxyprogesterone/conjugated estrogens: 1.5 mg/0.3 mg; 1.5 mg/0.45 mg; 2.5 mg/0.625 mg; 5 mg/0.625 mg.

◆CLASSIFICATION

PHARMACOTHERAPEUTIC: Hormone. **CLINICAL:** Progestin, antineoplastic.

ACTION

A hormone that transforms endometrium from proliferative to secretory in an estrogen-primed endometrium. Inhibits secretion of pituitary gonadotropins. **Therapeutic Effect:** Prevents follicular maturation and ovulation. Stimulates growth of mammary alveolar tissue and relaxes uterine smooth muscle. Corrects hormonal imbalance.

PHARMACOKINETICS

Slowly absorbed after IM administration. Protein binding: 90%. Metabolized in the liver. Primarily excreted in urine. Half-life: 30 days.

USES

PO: Prevention of endometrial hyperplasia (concurrently given with estrogen to women with intact uterus), treatment of secondary amenorrhea, abnormal uterine bleeding. **IM:** Adjunctive therapy,

---

palliative treatment of inoperable, recurrent, metastatic endometrial carcinoma, renal carcinoma; prevention of pregnancy. OFF-LABEL: Hormone replacement therapy in estrogen-treated menopausal women, treatment of endometriosis.

PRECAUTIONS

CONTRAINDICATIONS: Carcinoma of the breast; estrogen-dependent neoplasm; history of or active thrombotic disorders, such as cerebral apoplexy, thrombophlebitis, or thromboembolic disorders; hypersensitivity to progestins; known or suspected pregnancy; missed abortion; severe hepatic dysfunction; undiagnosed abnormal genital bleeding; use as pregnancy test. **CAUTIONS:** Those with conditions aggravated by fluid retention (asthma, seizures, migraine, cardiac or renal dysfunction), diabetes, history of mental depression.

⌛ LIFESPAN CONSIDERATIONS: **Pregnancy/Lactation:** Avoid use during pregnancy, especially first 4 mo (congenital heart, limb reduction defects may occur). Distributed in breast milk. **Pregnancy Category X. Children:** Safety and efficacy not established. **Elderly:** No age-related precautions noted.

INTERACTIONS

DRUG: **Aminoglutethimide:** May reduce medroxyprogesterone serum concentration. **Bromocriptine:** May interfere with the effects of bromocriptine. HERBAL: None known. FOOD: None known. LAB VALUES: May alter results for serum thyroid and liver function tests, prothrombin time, and metapyrone test.

AVAILABILITY (Rx)

TABLETS (PROVERA): 2.5 mg, 5 mg, 10 mg. **INJECTION:** 104 mg/0.65 ml prefilled syringe (Depo-SubQ Provera 104), 150 mg/ml (Depo-Provera 400 mg/ml (Depo-Provera).

Contraceptive), 400 mg/ml (Depo-Provera).

ADMINISTRATION/HANDLING
IM
• Shake vial immediately before administering (ensures complete suspension). • Rarely, a residual lump, change in skin color, sterile abscess occurs at injection site. • Inject IM only in upper arm, upper outer aspect of buttock.

PO
• Give without regard to meals.

INDICATIONS/ROUTES/DOSAGE
HORMONE REPLACEMENT THERAPY
PO: ADULTS: 5–10 mg for 12–14 consecutive days a month, beginning on day 1 or 16 of cycle given as part of regimen with conjugated estrogens.

ENDOMETRIAL HYPERPLASIA
PO: ADULTS: 2.5–10 mg/day for 14 days.

SECONDARY AMENORRHEA
PO: ADULTS: 5–10 mg/day for 5–10 days, beginning at any time during menstrual cycle or 2.5 mg/day.

ABNORMAL UTERINE BLEEDING
PO: ADULTS: 5–10 mg/day for 5–10 days, beginning on calculated day 16 or day 21 of menstrual cycle.

ENDOMETRIAL, RENAL CARCINOMA
IM: ADULTS, ELDERLY: Initially, 400–1,000 mg; repeat at 1-wk intervals. If improvement occurs and disease is stabilized, begin maintenance with as little as 400 mg/mo.

PREGNANCY PREVENTION
IM (DEPO-PROVERA): ADULTS: 150 mg q3mo.
SUBCUTANEOUS (DEPO-SUBQ PROVERA 104): ADULTS: 104 mg q3mo (q12–14wk).

SIDE EFFECTS

FREQUENT: Transient menstrual abnormalities (including spotting, change in menstrual flow or cervical secretions, and amenorrhea) at initiation of

---

* "Tall Man" lettering   ✎ see color pill atlas   ✎ herb   <u>underlined</u> – top prescribed drug therapy. **OCCASIONAL:** Edema, weight change, breast tenderness, nervousness, insomnia, fatigue, dizziness. **RARE:** Alopecia, depression, dermatologic changes, headache, fever, nausea.

ADVERSE REACTIONS/ TOXIC EFFECTS

Thrombophlebitis, pulmonary or cerebral embolism, and retinal thrombosis occur rarely. Women who use medroxyprogesterone injection may lose significant bone mineral density.

NURSING CONSIDERATIONS

BASELINE ASSESSMENT

Question for hypersensitivity to progestins, possibility of pregnancy before initiating therapy (Pregnancy Category X). Obtain baseline weight, serum glucose, BP.

INTERVENTION/EVALUATION

Check weight daily; report weekly gain of 5 lb or more. Check BP periodically. Assess skin for rash, hives. Report immediately the development of chest pain, sudden shortness of breath, sudden decrease in vision, migraine headache, pain (especially with swelling, warmth, redness) in calves, numbness of an arm or leg (thrombotic disorders).

PATIENT/FAMILY TEACHING

• Inform physician of sudden loss of vision, severe headache, chest pain, coughing up of blood (hemoptysis), numbness in arm or leg, severe pain/swelling in calf, unusual heavy vaginal bleeding, severe abdominal pain/tenderness. • Depo-Provera Contraceptive injection should be used as a long-term birth control method (e.g. longer than 2 yr) only if other birth control methods are inadequate.

megestrol acetate

me-**jess**-trole

(Apo-Megestrol ✦, Megace, Megace ES, Megace OS ✦)

CLASSIFICATION

PHARMACOTHERAPEUTIC: Hormone. **CLINICAL:** Antineoplastic (see p. 76C).

ACTION

A hormone and antineoplastic agent that suppresses the release of luteinizing hormone from the anterior pituitary gland by inhibiting pituitary function. Therapeutic Effect: Shrinks tumors. Also increases appetite by an unknown mechanism.

PHARMACOKINETICS

Well absorbed from the GI tract. Metabolized in the liver; excreted in urine. Half-life: 13–105 hr (mean 34 hr).

USES

Palliative management of recurrent, inoperable, metastatic endometrial or breast carcinoma. Treatment of anorexia, cachexia, unexplained significant weight loss in patients with AIDS. OFF-LABEL: Appetite stimulant, treatment of hormone-dependent or advanced prostate carcinoma, treatment of uterine bleeding.

PRECAUTIONS

CONTRAINDICATIONS: Suspension: Known or suspected pregnancy. **CAUTIONS:** History of thrombophlebitis. LIFESPAN CONSIDERATIONS: Pregnancy/Lactation: If possible, avoid use during pregnancy, especially first 4 mo. Breast-feeding not recommended. **Pregnancy Category X (for suspension), D (for tablets). Children:** Safety and efficacy not established. **Elderly:** No age-related precautions noted.

INTERACTIONS

DRUG: Dofetilide: May increase the risk of cardiotoxicity (QT prolongation, torsades de pointes, cardiac arrest). **HERBAL:** None known. **FOOD:** None known. **LAB VALUES:** May increase blood glucose level.

AVAILABILITY (Rx)

TABLETS (MEGACE): 20 mg, 40 mg. **SUSPENSION:** 40 mg/ml (Megace), 625 mg/5 ml (equivalent to 800 mg/20 ml) (Megace ES).

ADMINISTRATION/HANDLING

PO
• Store tablets and oral suspension at room temperature. • Shake suspension container well before use.

INDICATIONS/ROUTES/DOSAGE

PALLIATIVE TREATMENT OF ADVANCED BREAST CANCER
PO: ADULTS, ELDERLY: 160 mg/day in 4 equally divided doses.

PALLIATIVE TREATMENT OF ADVANCED ENDOMETRIAL CARCINOMA
PO: ADULTS, ELDERLY: 40–320 mg/day in divided doses. **Maximum:** 800 mg/day in 1–4 divided doses.

ANOREXIA, CACHEXIA, WEIGHT LOSS
PO: ADULTS, ELDERLY: 800 mg (20 ml)/day. **PO (MEGACE ES):** ADULTS, ELDERLY: 625 mg/day.

SIDE EFFECTS

FREQUENT: Weight gain secondary to increased appetite. **OCCASIONAL:** Nausea, breakthrough bleeding, backache, headache, breast tenderness, carpal tunnel syndrome. **RARE:** Feeling of coldness.

ADVERSE REACTIONS/ TOXIC EFFECTS

Thrombophlebitis and pulmonary embolism occur rarely.

BASELINE ASSESSMENT

Question for possibility of pregnancy before initiating therapy (Pregnancy Category X [suspension], D [tablets]). Provide support to patient and family, recognizing this drug is palliative, not curative.

INTERVENTION/EVALUATION

Monitor for tumor response.

PATIENT/FAMILY TEACHING

• Contraception is imperative. • Report any calf pain, difficulty breathing, vaginal bleeding. • May cause headache, nausea, vomiting, breast tenderness, backache.

melatonin

Also known as pineal hormone.

◆CLASSIFICATION

HERBAL: See Appendix G.

ACTION

Hormone synthesized endogenously by the pineal gland. Interacts with melatonin receptors in the brain. **Effect:** Regulates the body's circadian rhythm, sleep patterns. Acts as an antioxidant, protecting cells from oxidative damage by free radicals.

USES

Treatment for insomnia, jet lag. Also used as an antioxidant.

PRECAUTIONS

CONTRAINDICATIONS: Pregnancy or lactation. **CAUTIONS:** Depression (may worsen dysphoria), seizures (may increase incidence), cardiovascular/hepatic disease.

⏳ **LIFESPAN CONSIDERATIONS: Pregnancy/Lactation:** Contraindicated.

Children: Safety and efficacy not established. **Elderly:** No age-related precautions noted.

INTERACTIONS

DRUG: Alcohol, benzodiazepines: May have additive effects. **Immunosuppressants:** Melatonin may interfere with the effects of these drugs. **Isoniazid:** May have enhanced effects. **HERBAL: Chamomile, ginseng, goldenseal, kava kava, valerian:** May increase sedative effects. **FOOD:** None known. **LAB VALUES:** May increase human growth hormone levels. May decrease luteinizing hormone (LH) levels.

AVAILABILITY (OTC)

LOZENGES: 3 mg. **POWDER. TABLETS:** 0.5 mg, 3 mg.

INDICATIONS/ROUTES/DOSAGE

INSOMNIA
PO: ADULTS, ELDERLY: 0.5–5 mg at bedtime.

JET LAG
PO: ADULTS, ELDERLY: 5 mg a day beginning 3 days before flight and 3 days after flight.

SIDE EFFECTS

Headache, transient depression, fatigue, drowsiness, dizziness, abdominal cramps/irritability, decreased alertness, hypersensitivity reaction, tachycardia, nausea, vomiting, anorexia, altered sleep patterns, confusion.

ADVERSE REACTIONS/ TOXIC EFFECTS

None known.

NURSING CONSIDERATIONS

BASELINE ASSESSMENT
Assess if patient is pregnant or breastfeeding (avoid use). Determine whether patient has history of seizures, depression. Assess sleep patterns if used for insomnia. Determine medication usage (especially CNS depressants).

INTERVENTION/EVALUATION
Monitor effectiveness in improving insomnia. Assess for hypersensitivity reactions, CNS effects.

PATIENT/FAMILY TEACHING
• Do not use if pregnant, planning to become pregnant, breast-feeding.
• Avoid tasks that require mental alertness or motor skills (e.g., driving).

---

meloxicam

meh-**locks**-ih-cam
(Mobic)

◆CLASSIFICATION
PHARMACOTHERAPEUTIC: Nonsteroidal anti-inflammatory. **CLINICAL:** Anti-inflammatory, analgesic (see p. 117C).

M

ACTION

An NSAID that produces analgesic and anti-inflammatory effects by inhibiting prostaglandin synthesis. **Therapeutic Effect:** Reduces the inflammatory response and intensity of pain.

PHARMACOKINETICS

Route	Onset	Peak	Duration
PO (analgesic)	30 min	4–5 hr	N/A

Well absorbed after PO administration. Protein binding: 99%. Metabolized in the liver. Eliminated in urine and feces. Not removed by hemodialysis. **Half-life:** 15–20 hr.

USES

Relief of signs and symptoms of osteoarthritis, rheumatoid arthritis. Treatment of juvenile rheumatoid arthritis. **OFF-LABEL:** Ankylosing spondylitis.

PRECAUTIONS

CONTRAINDICATIONS: Aspirin-induced nasal polyps associated with broncho-spasm. **CAUTIONS:** History of GI disease (e.g., ulcers), renal or hepatic impairment, CHF, dehydration, hypertension, asthma, hemostatic disease. Concurrent use of anticoagulants.

⧗ **LIFESPAN CONSIDERATIONS: Pregnancy/Lactation:** Excreted in breast milk. **Pregnancy Category C (D if used in third trimester or near delivery). Children:** Safety and efficacy not established. **Elderly:** Age-related renal impairment may require dosage adjustment. More susceptible to GI toxicity; lower dosage recommended.

INTERACTIONS

DRUG: Aspirin: May increase the risk of epigastric distress, such as heartburn and indigestion. **Lithium:** May increase the plasma concentration and risk of toxicity of lithium. **HERBAL: Ginkgo biloba:** May increase the risk of bleeding. **FOOD:** None known. **LAB VALUES:** May increase serum creatinine, AST, and ALT levels.

AVAILABILITY (Rx)

TABLETS: 7.5 mg, 15 mg. **ORAL SUSPENSION:** 7.5 mg/5 ml.

ADMINISTRATION/HANDLING

PO
• Give without regard to meals.

INDICATIONS/ROUTES/DOSAGE

OSTEOARTHRITIS, RHEUMATOID ARTHRITIS
PO: ADULTS: Initially, 7.5 mg/day. **Maximum:** 15 mg/day.

JUVENILE RHEUMATOID ARTHRITIS
PO: CHILDREN, 2 YR AND OLDER: 0.125 mg/kg once daily. **Maximum:** 7.5 mg.

SIDE EFFECTS

FREQUENT (9%–7%): Dyspepsia, headache, diarrhea, nausea. **OCCASIONAL (4%–3%):** Dizziness, insomnia, rash, pruritus, flatulence, constipation, vomiting. **RARE (less than 2%):** Somnolence, urticaria, photosensitivity, tinnitus.

ADVERSE REACTIONS/ TOXIC EFFECTS

Rare reactions with long-term use include peptic ulcer disease, GI bleeding, gastritis, severe hepatic reaction (jaundice), nephrotoxicity (hematuria, dysuria, proteinuria), and a severe hypersensitivity reaction (bronchospasm, angioedema).

NURSING CONSIDERATIONS

BASELINE ASSESSMENT

Assess onset, type, location, duration of pain or inflammation. Inspect appearance of affected joints for immobility, deformities, skin condition.

INTERVENTION/EVALUATION

Monitor CBC, liver and renal function tests. Evaluate for therapeutic response: relief of pain, stiffness, swelling, increased joint mobility, reduced joint tenderness, improved grip strength.

PATIENT/FAMILY TEACHING

• Take with food, milk to reduce GI upset. • Inform physician of ringing in ears, persistent abdominal pain or cramping, severe nausea or vomiting, difficulty breathing, unusual bruising or bleeding, rash, peripheral edema, chest pain, palpitations.

melphalan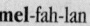

mel-fah-lan
(Alkeran, Alkeran I.V.)

Do not confuse Alkeran with Leukeran, or melphalan with Mephyton or Myleran.

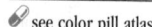

◆ **CLASSIFICATION**

PHARMACOTHERAPEUTIC: Alkylating agent. **CLINICAL:** Antineoplastic (see p. 76C).

ACTION

An alkylating agent that inhibits protein synthesis primarily by cross-linking with strands of DNA and RNA, producing cell death. Cell cycle–phase nonspecific. **Therapeutic Effect:** Disrupts nucleic acid function.

PHARMACOKINETICS

Oral administration is highly variable. Incomplete intestinal absorption, variable first-pass metabolism, or rapid hydrolysis may result. Protein binding: 60%–90%. Extensively metabolized in blood. Eliminated from plasma primarily by chemical hydrolysis. Partially excreted in feces and minimal elimination in urine. **Half-life:** 38–108 min.

USES

Treatment of epithelial ovarian carcinoma, multiple myeloma. **OFF-LABEL:** Treatment of breast, endometrial, testicular carcinoma; chronic myelocytic leukemia, Hodgkin's lymphoma, malignant melanoma, neuroblastoma, rhabdomyosarcoma.

PRECAUTIONS

CONTRAINDICATIONS: Pregnancy, severe myelosuppression. **CAUTIONS:** Leukocyte count less than 3,000/mm^3 or platelet count less than 100,000/mm^3, bone marrow suppression, renal impairment.

⧗ **LIFESPAN CONSIDERATIONS:** **Pregnancy/Lactation:** May cause fetal harm. Unknown if distributed in breast milk. **Pregnancy Category D. Children:** Safety and efficacy not established. **Elderly:** Age-related renal impairment may require dosage adjustment.

INTERACTIONS

DRUG: **Antigout medications:** May decrease the effects of these drugs. **Bone marrow depressants:** May increase myelosuppression. **Live virus vaccines:** May potentiate virus replication, increase vaccine side effects, and decrease the patient's antibody response to the vaccine. **HERBAL:** None known. **FOOD:** None known. **LAB VALUES:** May increase serum uric acid level and cause a positive direct Coombs' test.

AVAILABILITY (Rx)

TABLETS (ALKERAN): 2 mg. **POWDER FOR INJECTION (ALKERAN I.V.):** 50 mg.

ADMINISTRATION/HANDLING

💉 **IV**

Reconstitution • Reconstitute 50-mg vial with diluent supplied by manufacturer to yield a 5 mg/ml solution. • Further dilute with 0.9% NaCl to final concentration, not to exceed 2 mg/ml (central line) or 0.45 mg/ml (peripheral line).

Rate of administration • Infuse over 15–30 min at a rate not to exceed 10 mg/min.

Storage • Store at room temperature; protect from light. • Once reconstituted, stable for 90 min at room temperature (do not refrigerate).

PO
• Store tablets in refrigerator; protect from light.

▦ IV INCOMPATIBILITIES

Don't mix melphalan with any other medications.

INDICATIONS/ROUTES/DOSAGE

OVARIAN CARCINOMA

PO: ADULTS, ELDERLY: 0.2 mg/kg/day for 5 successive days. Repeat at 4- to 6-wk intervals.

MULTIPLE MYELOMA

PO: ADULTS: Initially, 6 mg once a day, adjusted as indicated; or 0.15 mg/kg/day for 7 days or 0.25 mg/kg/day for 4 days. Repeat at 4- to 6-wk intervals.
IV: ADULTS: 16 mg/m²/dose every 2 wk for 4 doses, then repeated monthly according to protocol.

DOSAGE IN RENAL IMPAIRMENT

PO, IV: BUN LEVEL GREATER THAN 30 MG/DL: Decrease melphalan dosage by 50%. SERUM CREATININE LEVEL GREATER THAN 1.5 MG/DL: Decrease the melphalan dosage by 50%.

SIDE EFFECTS

FREQUENT: Nausea, vomiting (may be severe with large dose). **OCCASIONAL:** Diarrhea, stomatitis, rash, pruritus, alopecia.

ADVERSE REACTIONS/ TOXIC EFFECTS

Myelosuppression may cause hematologic toxicity, manifested principally as leukopenia and thrombocytopenia and to lesser extent, anemia, pancytopenia, and agranulocytosis. Leukopenia may occur as early as 5 days after drug initiation. WBC and platelet counts return to normal levels during the 5th week of therapy, but leukopenia and thrombocytopenia may last more than 6 wk after the drug is discontinued. Hyperuricemia, marked by hematuria, crystalluria, and flank pain, may occur.

NURSING CONSIDERATIONS

BASELINE ASSESSMENT

Obtain CBC weekly. Dosage may be decreased or discontinued if WBC falls below 3,000/mm³ or platelet count falls below 100,000/mm³. Antiemetics may be effective in preventing, treating nausea, vomiting.

INTERVENTION/EVALUATION

Monitor CBC with differential, platelet count, serum electrolytes, Hgb. Monitor for stomatitis. Monitor for hematologic toxicity (fever, sore throat, signs of local infection, unusual ecchymosis or bleeding from any site), symptoms of anemia (excessive fatigue, weakness), signs of hyperuricemia (hematuria, flank pain). Avoid IM injections, rectal temperatures, other traumas that may induce bleeding.

PATIENT/FAMILY TEACHING

• Increase fluid intake (may protect against hyperuricemia). • Maintain fastidious oral hygiene. • Alopecia is reversible, but new hair growth may have different color, texture. • Avoid crowds, those with infections. • Inform physician if fever, shortness of breath, cough, sore throat, bleeding, bruising occurs.

memantine hydrochloride

meh-**man**-teen
(Namenda)

◆CLASSIFICATION

PHARMACOTHERAPEUTIC: Neurotransmitter inhibitor. **CLINICAL:** Anti-Alzheimer's agent.

ACTION

A neurotransmitter inhibitor that decreases the effects of glutamate, the principle excitatory neurotransmitter in the brain. Persistent CNS excitation by glutamate is thought to cause the symptoms of Alzheimer's disease. **Therapeutic Effect:** May reduce clinical deterioration in moderate to severe Alzheimer's disease.

PHARMACOKINETICS

Rapidly and completely absorbed after PO administration. Protein binding: 45%. Undergoes little metabolism; most of the dose is excreted unchanged in urine. **Half-life:** 60–80 hr.

USES

Treatment of moderate to severe Alzheimer's disease.

PRECAUTIONS

CONTRAINDICATIONS: Severe renal impairment. **CAUTIONS:** Moderately renal impairment, seizure disorder, GU conditions that raise urine pH level.

LIFESPAN CONSIDERATIONS: Pregnancy/Lactation: Unknown if drug crosses placenta or is distributed in breast milk. **Pregnancy Category B. Children:** Not prescribed for this patient population. **Elderly:** No age-related precautions noted, but use is not recommended in those with severe renal impairment (creatinine clearance less than 9 ml/min).

INTERACTIONS

DRUG: Carbonic anhydrase inhibitors, sodium bicarbonate: May decrease the renal elimination of memantine. **Cimetidine, hydrochlorothiazide, nicotine, quinidine, ranitidine:** May alter plasma levels of both memantine and precipitant drugs. **HERBAL:** None known. **FOOD:** None known. **LAB VALUES:** None known.

AVAILABILITY (Rx)

TABLETS: 5 mg, 10 mg. **ORAL SOLUTION:** 2 mg/ml.

ADMINISTRATION/HANDLING

PO
- Give without regard to food.

INDICATIONS/ROUTES/DOSAGE

ALZHEIMER'S DISEASE
PO: ADULTS, ELDERLY: Initially, 5 mg once a day. May increase dosage at intervals of at least 1 wk in 5-mg increments to 10 mg/day (5 mg twice a day), then 15 mg/day (5 mg and 10 mg as separate doses), and

finally 20 mg/day (10 mg twice a day). Target dose: 20 mg/day.

SIDE EFFECTS

OCCASIONAL (7%–4%): Dizziness, headache, confusion, constipation, hypertension, cough. **RARE (3%–2%):** Back pain, nausea, fatigue, anxiety, peripheral edema, arthralgia, insomnia.

ADVERSE REACTIONS/ TOXIC EFFECTS

None known.

NURSING CONSIDERATIONS

BASELINE ASSESSMENT

Assess cognitive, behavioral, functional deficits of patient. Assess renal function.

INTERVENTION/EVALUATION

Monitor cognitive, behavioral, functional status of patient. Monitor urine pH (alterations of urine pH toward the alkaline condition may lead to accumulation of the drug with possible increase in side effects). Monitor BUN, creatinine clearance lab values.

PATIENT/FAMILY TEACHING

- Do not reduce or stop medication; do not increase dosage without physician direction. - Ensure adequate fluid intake. - If therapy is interrupted for several days, restart at lowest dose, titrate to current dose at minimum of 1-wk intervals. - Inform family of local chapter of Alzheimer's Disease Association (provides a guide to services for these patients).

menotropins

(Humegon, Pergonal, Repronex)
See Fertility agents (p. 94C)

M

meperidine hydrochloride

me-**per**-i-deen
(Demerol)

Do not confuse with Demulen or Dymelor.

◆ CLASSIFICATION
PHARMACOTHERAPEUTIC: Narcotic agonist. **CLINICAL:** Opiate analgesic **(Schedule II)** (see p. 128C).

ACTION
An opioid agonist that binds to opioid receptors in the CNS. Therapeutic Effect: Alters the perception of and emotional response to pain.

PHARMACOKINETICS

Route	Onset	Peak	Duration
PO	15 min	60 min	2–4 hr
IV	Less than 5 min	5–7 min	2–3 hr
IM	10–15 min	30–50 min	2–4 hr
Subcutaneous	10–15 min	30–50 min	2–4 hr

Variably absorbed from the GI tract; well absorbed after IM administration. Protein binding: 60%–80%. Widely distributed. Metabolized in the liver to active metabolite. Primarily excreted in urine. Not removed by hemodialysis. Half-life: 2.4–4 hr; metabolite 8–16 hr (increased in hepatic impairment and disease).

USES
Relief of moderate to severe pain.

PRECAUTIONS
CONTRAINDICATIONS: Delivery of premature infant, diarrhea due to poisoning, use within 14 days of MAOIs. **CAUTIONS:** Renal or hepatic impairment, elderly or debilitated, supraventricular tachycardia, cor pulmonale, history of seizures, acute abdominal conditions, increased intracranial pressure (ICP), respiratory abnormalities.

⌛ **LIFESPAN CONSIDERATIONS: Pregnancy/Lactation:** Crosses placenta. Distributed in breast milk. Respiratory depression may occur in neonate if mother received opiates during labor. Regular use of opiates during pregnancy may produce withdrawal symptoms in neonate (irritability, excessive crying, tremors, hyperactive reflexes, fever, vomiting, diarrhea, yawning, sneezing, seizures). **Pregnancy Category B (D if used for prolonged periods or at high dosages at term). Children:** Paradoxical excitement may occur. Those younger than 2 yr more susceptible to respiratory depressant effects. **Elderly:** More susceptible to respiratory depressant effects. Age-related renal impairment may increase risk of urinary retention.

INTERACTIONS
DRUG: Alcohol, other CNS depressants: May increase CNS or respiratory depression and hypotension. **MAOIs:** May produce a severe, sometimes fatal reaction. Meperidine use is contraindicated. **HERBAL: Kava kava, valerian:** May increase CNS depression. **St. John's wort:** May increase sedation. **FOOD:** None known. **LAB VALUES:** May increase serum amylase and lipase levels. Therapeutic serum level is 100–550 ng/ml; toxic serum level is greater than 1,000 ng/ml.

AVAILABILITY (Rx)
SYRUP: 50 mg/5 ml. **TABLETS:** 50 mg, 100 mg. **INJECTION:** 10 mg/ml, 25 mg/ml, 50 mg/ml, 75 mg/ml, 100 mg/ml.

ADMINISTRATION/HANDLING
💧 IV

◀ **ALERT** ▶ Give by slow IV push or IV infusion.

Reconstitution • May give undiluted or may dilute in D_5W, dextrosesaline combination (2.5%, 5%, or 10% dextrose in water—0.45% or 0.9% NaCl), Ringer's, lactated Ringer's, or molar sodium lactate diluent for IV injection or infusion.

Rate of administration • IV dosage must always be administered very slowly, over 2–3 min. • Rapid IV increases risk of severe adverse reactions (chest wall rigidity, apnea, peripheral circulatory collapse, anaphylactoid effects, cardiac arrest).

Storage • Store at room temperature.

IM, SUBCUTANEOUS
◀ **ALERT** ▶ IM preferred over subcutaneous route (subcutaneous produces pain, local irritation, induration). • Administer slowly. • Those with circulatory impairment at higher risk for overdosage due to delayed absorption of repeated administration.

PO
• Give without regard to meals. • Dilute syrup in glass of water (prevents anesthetic effect on mucous membranes).

▓ IV INCOMPATIBILITIES

Allopurinol (Aloprim), amphotericin B complex (Abelcet, AmBisome, Amphotec), cefepime (Maxipime), cefoperazone (Cefobid), doxorubicin liposomal (Doxil), furosemide (Lasix), idarubicin (Idamycin), nafcillin (Nafcil).

IV COMPATIBILITIES

Atropine, bumetanide (Bumex), diltiazem (Cardizem), diphenhydramine (Benadryl), dobutamine (Dobutrex), dopamine (Intropin), glycopyrrolate (Robinul), heparin, hydroxyzine (Vistaril), insulin, lidocaine, magnesium, midazolam (Versed), oxytocin (Pitocin), potassium, total parenteral nutrition (TPN).

INDICATIONS/ROUTES/DOSAGE
ANALGESIA
PO, IM, SUBCUTANEOUS: ADULTS, ELDERLY: 50–150 mg q3–4h. CHILDREN: 1.1–1.5 mg/kg q3–4h. Don't exceed single dose of 100 mg.

PATIENT-CONTROLLED ANALGESIA (PCA)
IV: ADULTS: **Loading dose:** 50–100 mg. **Intermittent bolus:** 5–30 mg. **Lockout interval:** 10–20 min. **Continuous infusion:** 5–40 mg/hr. **Maximum (4-hr):** 200–300 mg.

DOSAGE IN RENAL IMPAIRMENT
Dosage is based on creatinine clearance.

Creatinine Clearance	Dosage
10–50 ml/min	75% of usual dose
Less than 10 ml/min	50% of usual dose

SIDE EFFECTS

FREQUENT: Sedation, hypotension (including orthostatic hypotension), diaphoresis, facial flushing, dizziness, nausea, vomiting, constipation. **OCCASIONAL:** Confusion, arrhythmias, tremors, urine retention, abdominal pain, dry mouth, headache, irritation at injection site, euphoria, dysphoria. **RARE:** Allergic reaction (rash, pruritus), insomnia.

ADVERSE REACTIONS/ TOXIC EFFECTS

Overdose results in respiratory depression, skeletal muscle flaccidity, cold or clammy skin, cyanosis, and extreme somnolence progressing to seizures, stupor, and coma. The antidote is 0.4 mg naloxone. The patient who uses meperidine repeatedly may develop a tolerance to the drug's analgesic effect and physical dependence.

NURSING CONSIDERATIONS

BASELINE ASSESSMENT
Patient should be in recumbent position before drug is administered by parenteral

M

route. Assess onset, type, location, duration of pain. Obtain vital signs before giving medication. If respirations are 12/min or less (20/min or less in children), withhold medication, contact physician. Effect of medication is reduced if full pain recurs before next dose.

INTERVENTION/EVALUATION

Monitor vital signs 15–30 min after subcutaneous/IM dose, 5–10 min after IV dose (monitor for decreased BP, change in rate and quality of pulse). Monitor pain level, sedation response. Monitor patterns of bowel activity and stool consistency; avoid constipation. Check for adequate voiding. Initiate deep breathing, coughing exercises, particularly in patients with pulmonary impairment. Therapeutic serum level: 100–550 ng/ml; toxic serum level: higher than 1,000 ng/ml.

PATIENT/FAMILY TEACHING

* Medication should be taken before pain fully returns, within ordered intervals. * Discomfort may occur with injection. * Change positions slowly to avoid orthostatic hypotension. * Increase fluids, bulk to prevent constipation. * Tolerance or dependence may occur with prolonged use of high doses. * Avoid alcohol and other CNS depressants. * Avoid tasks requiring mental alertness, motor control until response to drug is established.

mepivacaine hydrochloride

(Carbocaine, Polocaine)

FIXED-COMBINATION(S)

With levonordefrin, a vasoconstrictor
(Isocaine)
See Anesthetics: local (p. 5C)

mercaptopurine

(Purinethol)
See Cancer chemotherapeutic agents (p. 76C)

meropenem

murr-oh-**peh**-nem
(Merrem IV)

◆CLASSIFICATION

PHARMACOTHERAPEUTIC: Carbapenem. **CLINICAL:** Antibiotic.

ACTION

A carbapenem that binds to penicillin-binding proteins and inhibits bacterial cell wall synthesis. **Therapeutic Effect:** Produces bacterial cell death.

PHARMACOKINETICS

After IV administration, widely distributed into tissues and body fluids, including CSF. Protein binding: 2%. Primarily excreted unchanged in urine. Removed by hemodialysis. **Half-life:** 1 hr.

USES

Treatment of intra-abdominal infections caused by *viridans group streptococci, E. coli, K. pneumoniae, P. aeruginosa, B. fragilis*, peptostreptococcus species; bacterial meningitis caused by *S. pneumoniae, H. influenzae, N. meningitidis*. OFF-LABEL: Lower respiratory tract infections, febrile neutropenia, gynecologic and obstetric infections, sepsis.

PRECAUTIONS

CONTRAINDICATIONS: History of seizures or CNS abnormality, hypersensitivity to penicillins. **CAUTIONS:** Hypersensitivity to penicillins, cephalosporins, other allergens; renal function impairment; CNS disorders, particularly with history of seizures, concurrent probenecid use.

⧖ LIFESPAN CONSIDERATIONS: **Pregnancy/Lactation:** Unknown if distributed in breast milk. **Pregnancy Category B. Children:** Safety and efficacy not established in those younger than 3 mo. **Elderly:** Age-related renal impairment may require dosage adjustment.

INTERACTIONS

DRUG: **Probenecid:** May increase the concentration and risk of toxicity of meropenem. Reduces the renal excretion of meropenem. HERBAL: None known. FOOD: None known. LAB-VALUES: May increase BUN level and serum alkaline phosphatase, bilirubin, creatinine, LDH, AST, and ALT levels. May decrease blood Hct and Hgb levels and serum potassium levels.

AVAILABILITY (Rx)

POWDER FOR INJECTION: 500 mg, 1 g.

ADMINISTRATION/HANDLING

 IV

Reconstitution • Reconstitute each 500 mg with 10 ml sterile water for injection to provide a concentration of 50 mg/ml. • Shake to dissolve until clear. • May further dilute with 100 ml 0.9% NaCl or D_5W.

Rate of administration • May give by IV push or IV intermittent infusion (piggyback). • If administering as IV intermittent infusion (piggyback), give over 15–30 min; if administered by IV push (5–20 ml), give over 3–5 min.

Storage • Store vials at room temperature. • After reconstitution with 0.9% NaCl, stable for 2 hr at room temperature, or 18 hr if refrigerated (with D_5W, stable for 1 hr at room temperature, 8 hr if refrigerated).

IV INCOMPATIBILITIES
Acyclovir (Zovirax), amphotericin B (Fungizone), diazepam (Valium), doxycycline (Vibramycin), metronidazole (Flagyl), ondansetron (Zofran).

IV COMPATIBILITIES
Dobutamine (Dobutrex), dopamine (Intropin), heparin, magnesium.

INDICATIONS/ROUTES/DOSAGE
INTRA-ABDOMINAL INFECTIONS
IV: ADULTS, ELDERLY, CHILDREN WEIGHING MORE THAN 50 KG: 1 g q8h. CHILDREN 3 MO AND OLDER, WEIGHING 50 KG AND LESS: 20 mg/kg q8h. **Maximum:** 1 g q8h.

MENINGITIS
IV: ADULTS, ELDERLY, CHILDREN WEIGHING 50 KG OR MORE: 2 g q8h. CHILDREN 3 MO AND OLDER WEIGHING LESS THAN 50 KG: 40 mg/kg q8h. **Maximum:** 2 g/dose.

DOSAGE IN RENAL IMPAIRMENT
Dosage and frequency are modified based on creatinine clearance.

Creatinine Clearance	Dosage	Interval
26–49 ml/min	Recommended dose (1,000 mg)	q12h
10–25 ml/min	½ of recommended dose	q12h
Less than 10 ml/min	½ of recommended dose	q24h

SIDE EFFECTS
FREQUENT (5%–3%): Diarrhea, nausea, vomiting, headache, inflammation at injection site. **OCCASIONAL (2%):** Oral candidiasis, rash, pruritus. **RARE (less than 2%):** Constipation, glossitis.

ADVERSE REACTIONS/ TOXIC EFFECTS
Antibiotic-associated colitis and other superinfections may occur. Anaphylactic reactions have been reported. Seizures may occur in those with CNS disorders (including brain lesions and a history of seizures), bacterial meningitis, or impaired renal function.

M

NURSING CONSIDERATIONS

BASELINE ASSESSMENT
Inquire about history of seizures.

INTERVENTION/EVALUATION
Monitor daily bowel activity and stool consistency. Monitor for nausea, vomiting. Evaluate for inflammation at IV injection site. Assess skin for rash. Evaluate hydration status. Monitor I&O, renal function tests. Check mental status; be alert to tremors, possible seizures. Assess temperature, BP 2 times/day, more often if necessary. Monitor serum electrolytes, especially potassium.

Merrem, *see meropenem*

---

mesalamine (5 aminosalicylic acid, 5-ASA)

mez-**al**-a-meen

(Asacol, Canasa, FIV-ASA, Mesasal ✦, Pentasa, Rowasa, Salofalk ✦)

Do not confuse Asacol with Os-Cal.

◆CLASSIFICATION

PHARMACOTHERAPEUTIC: Salicylic acid derivative. **CLINICAL:** Anti-inflammatory agent.

ACTION

A salicylic acid derivative that locally inhibits arachidonic acid metabolite production, which is increased in patients with chronic inflammatory bowel disease. **Therapeutic Effect:** Blocks prostaglandin production and diminishes inflammation in the colon.

PHARMACOKINETICS

Poorly absorbed from the colon. Moderately absorbed from the GI tract. Metabolized in the liver to active metabolite. Unabsorbed portion eliminated in feces; absorbed portion excreted in urine. Unknown if removed by hemodialysis. **Half-life:** 0.5–1.5 hr; metabolite, 5–10 hr.

USES

Oral: Treatment and maintenance of remission of mild-moderate active ulcerative colitis. **Rectal:** Treatment of active mild-moderate distal ulcerative colitis, proctosigmoiditis or proctitis.

PRECAUTIONS

CONTRAINDICATIONS: None known. **CAUTIONS:** Preexisting renal disease, sulfasalazine sensitivity.

⧗ **LIFESPAN CONSIDERATIONS: Pregnancy/Lactation:** Unknown if drug crosses placenta or is distributed in breast milk. **Pregnancy Category B. Children:** Safety and efficacy not established. **Elderly:** Age-related renal impairment may require dosage adjustment.

INTERACTIONS

DRUG: Anticoagulants: May increase the risk of bleeding. **Varicella virus vaccine:** May increase the risk of developing Reye's syndrome. **HERBAL:** None known. **FOOD:** None known. **LAB VALUES:** May increase BUN, serum alkaline phosphatase, creatinine, AST, and ALT levels.

AVAILABILITY (Rx)

TABLETS (DELAYED-RELEASE [ASACOL]): 400 mg. **CAPSULES (CONTROLLED-RELEASE [PENTASA]):** 250 mg. **RECTAL SUSPENSION (ROWASA):** 4 g/60 ml. **SUPPOSITORIES (CANASA):** 500 mg, 1 g.

ADMINISTRATION/HANDLING

◀ **ALERT** ▶ Store rectal suspension, suppository, oral forms at room temperature.

PO

• Have patient swallow whole; do not break outer coating of tablet. • Give without regard to food.

RECTAL

• Shake bottle well. • Instruct patient to lie on left side with lower leg extended, upper leg flexed forward. • Knee-chest position may also be used. • Insert applicator tip into rectum, pointing toward umbilicus. • Squeeze bottle steadily until contents are emptied.

INDICATIONS/ROUTES/DOSAGE

TREATMENT OF ULCERATIVE COLITIS

PO (CAPSULE): ADULTS, ELDERLY: 1 g 4 times a day. CHILDREN: 50 mg/kg/day divided q6–12h.
PO (TABLET): ADULTS, ELDERLY: 800 mg 3 times a day. CHILDREN: 50 mg/kg/day divided q8–12h.

MAINTENANCE OF REMISSION IN ULCERATIVE COLITIS

PO (CAPSULE): ADULTS, ELDERLY: 1 g 4 times a day.
PO (TABLET): ADULTS, ELDERLY: 1.6 g/day in divided doses.

DISTAL ULCERATIVE COLITIS, PROCTOSIGMOIDITIS, PROCTITIS

RECTAL (RETENTION ENEMA): ADULTS, ELDERLY: 60 ml (4 g) at bedtime; retained overnight for approximately 8 hr for 3–6 wk.
RECTAL: (500 MG SUPPOSITORY) ADULTS, ELDERLY: Twice a day. May increase to 3 times a day.
RECTAL (1,000 MG SUPPOSITORY): ADULTS, ELDERLY: Once daily at bedtime. Continue therapy for 3–6 wk.

SIDE EFFECTS

Mesalamine is generally well tolerated, with only mild and transient effects.
FREQUENT (greater than 6%): PO: Abdominal cramps or pain, diarrhea, dizziness, headache, nausea, vomiting, rhinitis, unusual fatigue. **Rectal:** Abdominal or stomach cramps, flatulence, headache, nausea. **OCCASIONAL (6%–2%): PO:** Hair loss, decreased appetite, back or joint pain, flatulence, acne. **Rectal:** Hair loss. **RARE (less than 2%): Rectal:** Anal irritation.

ADVERSE REACTIONS/ TOXIC EFFECTS

Sulfite sensitivity may occur in susceptible patients, manifested by cramping, headache, diarrhea, fever, rash, hives, itching, and wheezing. Discontinue drug immediately. Hepatitis, pancreatitis, and pericarditis occur rarely with oral forms.

NURSING CONSIDERATIONS

INTERVENTION/EVALUATION

Encourage adequate fluid intake. Assess bowel sounds for peristalsis. Monitor patterns of daily bowel activity and stool consistency; record time of evacuation. Assess for abdominal disturbances. Assess skin for rash, hives. Discontinue medication if rash, fever, cramping, diarrhea occurs.

PATIENT/FAMILY TEACHING

• Avoid tasks that require alertness, motor skills until response to drug is established. • May discolor urine yellow-brown. • Suppositories stain fabrics.

mesna

mess-na
(Mesnex, Uromitexan ✦)

◆CLASSIFICATION

PHARMACOTHERAPEUTIC: Cytoprotective agent. **CLINICAL:** Antineoplastic adjunct, antidote.

M

ACTION

An antineoplastic adjunct and cytoprotective agent that binds with and detoxifies urotoxic metabolites of ifosfamide and cyclophosphamide. **Therapeutic Effect:** Inhibits ifosfamide-and cyclophosphamide-induced hemorrhagic cystitis.

PHARMACOKINETICS

Rapidly metabolized after IV administration to mesna disulfide, which is reduced to mesna in kidney. Excreted in urine. **Half-life:** 24 min.

USES

Detoxifying agent used as a protectant against hemorrhagic cystitis induced by ifosamide, cyclophosphamide.

PRECAUTIONS

CONTRAINDICATIONS: None known.
CAUTIONS: None known.
⧗ **LIFESPAN CONSIDERATIONS: Pregnancy/Lactation:** Unknown if drug crosses placenta or is distributed in breast milk. **Pregnancy Category B. Children:** Safety and efficacy not established. **Elderly:** Information not available.

INTERACTIONS

DRUG: Warfarin: May increase risk of bleeding. **HERBAL:** None known. **FOOD:** None known. **LAB VALUES:** May produce false-positive test result for urinary ketones.

AVAILABILITY (Rx)

TABLETS: 400 mg. **INJECTION:** 100 mg/ml.

ADMINISTRATION/HANDLING

🖧 IV

Reconstitution • May dilute with D$_5$W or 0.9% NaCl to concentration of 1–20 mg/ml. • May add to solutions containing ifosfamide or cyclophosphamide.

Rate of administration • Administer by IV infusion over 15–30 min or by continuous infusion.

Storage • Store parenteral form at room temperature. • After dilution, is stable for 24 hr at room temperature (recommended use within 6 hr). Discard unused medication.

PO
• Dilute mesna solution before oral administration to decrease sulfur odor. Can be diluted in carbonated cola drinks, fruit juices, milk.

⚙ IV INCOMPATIBILITIES

Amphotericin B complex (Abelcet, AmBisome, Amphotec).

IV COMPATIBILITIES

Allopurinol (Aloprim), docetaxel (Taxotere), doxorubicin (Adriamycin), etoposide (VePesid), gemcitabine (Gemzar), granisetron (Kytril), methotrexate, ondansetron (Zofran), paclitaxel (Taxol), vinorelbine (Navelbine).

INDICATIONS/ROUTES/DOSAGE

PREVENTION OF HEMORRHAGIC CYSTITIS IN PATIENTS RECEIVING IFOSFAMIDE
IV: ADULTS, ELDERLY: 20% of ifosfamide dose at time of ifosfamide administration and 4 and 8 hr after each dose of ifosfamide. Total dose: 60% of ifosfamide dosage. Range: 60%–160% of the daily ifosfamide dose.

HEMORRHAGIC CYSTITIS (CHRONIC LOW-DOSE CYCLOPHOSPHAMIDE)
PO: ADULTS, ELDERLY: 20 mg/kg q3–4h.

HEMORRHAGIC CYSTITIS (HIGH-DOSE CYCLOPHOSPHAMIDE)
IV: ADULTS, ELDERLY: 40% of cyclophosphamide dose at 0, 3, 6, 9 hr and IV fluids.

SIDE EFFECTS

FREQUENT (more than 17%): Bad taste, soft stools. **Large doses:** Diarrhea, myalgia, headache, fatigue, nausea, hypotension, allergic reaction.

ADVERSE REACTIONS/ TOXIC EFFECTS

Hematuria occurs rarely.

BASELINE ASSESSMENT
◀ ALERT ▶ Each dose must be administered with ifosfamide.

INTERVENTION/EVALUATION
Assess morning urine specimen for hematuria. If such occurs, dosage reduction or discontinuation may be necessary. Monitor pattern of daily bowel activity and stool consistency; record time of evacuation. Monitor BP for hypotension.

PATIENT/FAMILY TEACHING
• Inform physician or nurse if headache, myalgia, nausea occurs.

mesoridazine besylate

mez-oh-**rid**-a-zeen

(Serentil)

Do not confuse Serentil with Proventil, Serevent, or sertraline.

CLASSIFICATION

PHARMACOTHERAPEUTIC: Phenothiazine. **CLINICAL:** Antipsychotic (see p. 58C).

ACTION

A phenothiazine that blocks dopamine at postsynaptic receptor sites in the brain. Therapeutic Effect: Diminishes schizophrenic behavior. Also has anticholinergic and sedative effects.

PHARMACOKINETICS

Absorption may be erratic. Protein binding: 75%–91%. Undergoes first-pass metabolism. Small portions are metabolized in liver. Excreted in urine and feces. Half-life: Unknown.

USES

Treatment of schizophrenia in patients who fail to respond to other antipsychotic medication. Treatment of behavioral problems.

PRECAUTIONS

CONTRAINDICATIONS: Coma, concurrent administration of drugs that cause QTc-interval prolongation, myelosuppression, severe cardiovascular disease, severe CNS depression, subcortical brain damage. **CAUTIONS:** Respiratory, hepatic, renal, or cardiac impairment, alcohol withdrawal, history of seizures, urinary retention, glaucoma, prostatic hypertrophy.

LIFESPAN CONSIDERATIONS: **Pregnancy/Lactation:** Crosses placenta; distributed in breast milk. **Pregnancy Category C. Children:** Increased risk of developing extrapyramidal symptoms (EPS), dystonias. **Elderly:** Increased risk of anticholinergic effects, EPS, orthostatic hypotension, sedation symptoms.

INTERACTIONS

DRUG: **Alcohol, other CNS depressants:** May increase CNS and respiratory depression and the hypotensive effects of mesoridazine. **Antithyroid agents:** May increase the risk of agranulocytosis. **EPS-producing medications:** May increase EPS. **Hypotension-producing medications:** May increase hypotension. **Levodopa:** May decrease the effects of levodopa. **Lithium:** May decrease mesoridazine absorption and produce adverse neurologic effects. **MAOIs, tricyclic antidepressants:** May increase the anticholinergic and sedative effects of mesoridazine. HERBAL: None known. FOOD: None known. LAB VALUES: May produce false-positive pregnancy and phenylketonuria test results. May produce EKG changes, including prolonged QT and QTc intervals and T-wave depression or inversion.

AVAILABILITY (Rx)

ORAL SOLUTION: 25 mg/ml. **TABLETS:** 10 mg, 25 mg, 50 mg, 100 mg. **INJECTION:** 25 mg/ml.

ADMINISTRATION/HANDLING

• Avoid skin contact with the oral solution because it may cause contact dermatitis.

INDICATIONS/ROUTES/DOSAGE

SCHIZOPHRENIA

PO: ADULTS, ELDERLY: 25–50 mg 3 times a day. **Maximum:** 400 mg/day.

IM: ADULTS, ELDERLY: Initially, 25 mg. May repeat in 30–60 min. Range: 25–200 mg.

SEVERE BEHAVIORAL PROBLEMS (COMBATIVENESS OR EXPLOSIVE, HYPEREXCITABLE BEHAVIOR) ASSOCIATED WITH NEUROLOGIC DISEASES

PO: ELDERLY: Initially, 10 mg once or twice a day. May increase at 4–7 day intervals. **Maximum:** 250 mg.

IM: ADULTS, ELDERLY: Initially, 25 mg. May repeat in 30–60 min. Range: 25–200 mg.

SIDE EFFECTS

FREQUENT: Orthostatic hypotension, dizziness, syncope (occur frequently after first injection, occasionally after subsequent injections, and rarely with oral form). **OCCASIONAL:** Somnolence (during early therapy), dry mouth, blurred vision, lethargy, constipation or diarrhea, nasal congestion, peripheral edema, urine retention. **RARE:** Ocular changes, altered skin pigmentation (in those taking high doses for prolonged periods), darkening of urine.

ADVERSE REACTIONS/ TOXIC EFFECTS

Abrupt withdrawal after long-term therapy may precipitate nausea, vomiting, gastritis, dizziness, and tremors. Blood dyscrasias, particularly agranulocytosis and mild leukopenia may occur. Mesoridazine use may lower the seizure threshold.

NURSING CONSIDERATIONS

BASELINE ASSESSMENT

Avoid skin contact with solution (contact dermatitis). Assess behavior, appearance, emotional status, response to environment, speech pattern, thought content.

INTERVENTION/EVALUATION

Assess for orthostatic hypotension. Monitor pattern of daily bowel activity and stool consistency. Supervise suicidal-risk patient closely during early therapy (as depression lessens, energy level improves, increasing suicide potential). Assess for therapeutic response (interest in surroundings, improvement in self-care, increased ability to concentrate, relaxed facial expression).

PATIENT/FAMILY TEACHING

• Full therapeutic effect may take up to 6 wk. • Urine may become dark. • Do not abruptly withdraw from long-term drug therapy. • Report visual disturbances. • Drowsiness generally subsides during continued therapy. • Do not use alcohol, other CNS depressants.

metaproterenol sulfate

met-a-proe-**ter**-e-nole
(Alupent)

Do not confuse metaproterenol with metipranolol or metoprolol, or Alupent with Atrovent.

🖊 see color pill atlas   🌿 herb   underlined – top prescribed drug

CLASSIFICATION

PHARMACOTHERAPEUTIC: Sympathomimetic (an adrenergic agonist). **CLINICAL:** Bronchodilator (see p. 67C).

ACTION

A sympathomimetic that stimulates beta$_2$-adrenergic receptors, resulting in relaxation of bronchial smooth muscle. **Therapeutic Effect:** Relieves bronchospasm and reduces airway resistance.

PHARMACOKINETICS

Systemic absorption is rapid following aerosol administration; however, serum concentrations at recommended doses are very low. Metabolized in liver. Excreted in urine primarily as glucoside metabolite. **Half-life:** Unknown.

USES

Treatment of reversible airway obstruction caused by asthma or chronic obstructive pulmonary disease (COPD).

PRECAUTIONS

CONTRAINDICATIONS: Angle-closure glaucoma, preexisting arrhythmias associated with tachycardia. **CAUTIONS:** Ischemic heart disease, hypertension, hyperthyroidism, seizure disorder, CHF, diabetes, arrhythmias.

LIFESPAN CONSIDERATIONS: Pregnancy/Lactation: Unknown if drug crosses placenta or is distributed in breast milk. **Pregnancy Category C. Children:** Safety and efficacy not established. **Elderly:** No age-related precautions noted.

INTERACTIONS

DRUG: Beta blockers: May decrease the effects of beta blockers. **Digoxin, other sympathomimetics:** May increase the risk of arrhythmias. **MAOIs:** May increase the risk of

hypertensive crisis. **Tricyclic antidepressants:** May increase cardiovascular effects. **HERBAL:** None known. **FOOD:** None known. **LAB VALUES:** May decrease serum potassium level.

AVAILABILITY (Rx)

SYRUP: 10 mg/5 ml. **TABLETS:** 10 mg, 20 mg. **AEROSOL ORAL INHALATION:** 0.65 mg/inhalation. **SOLUTION FOR ORAL INHALATION:** 0.4%, 0.6%, 5%.

INDICATIONS/ROUTES/DOSAGE
TREATMENT OF BRONCHOSPASM

PO: ADULTS, CHILDREN 10 YR AND OLDER: 20 mg 3–4 times a day. ELDERLY: 10 mg 3–4 times a day. May increase to 20 mg/dose. CHILDREN 6–9 YR: 10 mg 3–4 times a day. CHILDREN 2–5 YR: 1.3–2.6 mg/kg/day in 3–4 divided doses. CHILDREN YOUNGER THAN 2 YR: 0.4 mg/kg 3–4 times a day.

INHALATION: ADULTS, ELDERLY, CHILDREN 12 YR AND OLDER: 2–3 inhalations q3–4h. **Maximum:** 12 inhalations/24 hr.

NEBULIZATION: ADULTS, ELDERLY, CHILDREN 12 YR AND OLDER: 10–15 mg (0.2–0.3 ml) of 5% q4–6h. CHILDREN YOUNGER THAN 12 YR, INFANTS: 0.5–1 mg/kg (0.01–0.02 ml/kg) of 5% q4–6h.

SIDE EFFECTS

FREQUENT (over 10%): Rigors, tremors, anxiety, nausea, dry mouth. **OCCASIONAL (9%–1%):** Dizziness, vertigo, asthenia, headache, GI distress, vomiting, cough, dry throat. **RARE (less than 1%):** Somnolence, diarrhea, altered taste.

ADVERSE REACTIONS/ TOXIC EFFECTS

Excessive sympathomimetic stimulation may cause palpitations, extrasystoles, tachycardia, chest pain, a slight increase in BP followed by a substantial decrease, chills, diaphoresis, and blanching of skin. Too-frequent or excessive use may lead decreased drug effectiveness and severe, paradoxical bronchoconstriction.

M

NURSING CONSIDERATIONS

BASELINE ASSESSMENT
Offer emotional support (high incidence of anxiety because of difficulty in breathing, sympathomimetic response to drug).

INTERVENTION/EVALUATION
Monitor rate, depth, rhythm, type of respiration; quality and rate of pulse. Assess lung sounds for rhonchi, wheezing, rales. Monitor ABGs, pulmonary function tests. Observe lips, fingernails for cyanosis (blue or dusky color in light-skinned patients; gray in dark-skinned patients). Evaluate for clinical improvement (quieter, slower respirations; relaxed facial expression; cessation of clavicular, sternal, intercostal retractions).

PATIENT/FAMILY TEACHING
• Increase fluid intake (decreases lung secretion viscosity). • Do not exceed recommended dosage. • May cause anxiety, restlessness, insomnia. • Inform physician if palpitations, tachycardia, chest pain, tremors, dizziness, headache, flushing, difficulty in breathing persists. • Avoid excessive use of caffeine derivatives (chocolate, coffee, tea, cola, cocoa).

metformin hydrochloride 🖉 ▶

met-**for**-min

(Fortamet, <u>Glucophage</u>, Glucophage XL, Glumetza, Glycon ✣, Novo-Metformin ✣, Riomet)

FIXED-COMBINATION(S)

Actoplus Met: metformin/pioglitazone (an antidiabetic): 500 mg/15 mg, 850 mg/15 mg. **Avandamet:** metformin/rosiglitazone (an antidiabetic): 500 mg/1 mg; 500 mg/2 mg; 500 mg/4 mg; 1,000 mg/2 mg; 1,000 mg/4 mg. **Glucovance:** metformin/glyburide (an antidiabetic): 250 mg/1.25 mg; 500 mg/2.5 mg; 500 mg/5 mg. **Metaglip:** metformin/glipizide (an antidiabetic): 250 mg/2.5 mg; 500 mg/2.5 mg; 500 mg/5 mg.

◆CLASSIFICATION

PHARMACOTHERAPEUTIC: Antihyperglycemic. **CLINICAL:** Antidiabetic (see p. 42C).

ACTION
An antihyperglycemic that decreases hepatic production of glucose. Decreases absorption of glucose and improves insulin sensitivity. **Therapeutic Effect:** Improves glycemic control, stabilizes or decreases body weight, and improves lipid profile.

PHARMACOKINETICS
Slowly, incompletely absorbed after oral administration. Food delays or decreases the extent of absorption. Protein binding: Negligible. Primarily distributed to intestinal mucosa and salivary glands. Primarily excreted unchanged in urine. Removed by hemodialysis. **Half-life:** 3–6 hr.

USES
Management of type 2 diabetes mellitus as monotherapy or concomitantly with an oral sulfonylurea or insulin. **OFF-LABEL:** Treatment of HIV liopodystrophy syndrome, metabolic complications of AIDS, polycystic ovary syndrome, prediabetes, weight reduction.

PRECAUTIONS
◂ **ALERT** ▸ Lactic acidosis is a rare but potentially severe consequence of metformin therapy. Withhold in patients with conditions that may predispose to lactic acidosis (e.g., hypoxemia, dehydration, hypoperfusion, sepsis).

CONTRAINDICATIONS: Acute CHF, MI, cardiovascular collapse, renal disease or dysfunction, respiratory failure, septicemia. **CAUTIONS:** Conditions delaying food absorption (e.g., diarrhea, high fever, malnutrition, gastroparesis, vomiting), causing hyperglycemia or hypoglycemia, uncontrolled hypothyroidism or hyperthyroidism, cardiovascular patients, concurrent drugs that affect renal function, hepatic impairment, elderly, malnourished or debilitated patients with renal impairment, CHF, excessive alcohol intake, chronic respiratory difficulty.

⏳ **LIFESPAN CONSIDERATIONS:** **Pregnancy/Lactation:** Insulin is drug of choice during pregnancy. Distributed in breast milk in animals. **Pregnancy Category B. Children:** Safety and efficacy not established. **Elderly:** Age-related renal impairment or peripheral vascular disease may require dosage adjustment or discontinuation.

INTERACTIONS

DRUG: **Alcohol, amiloride, cimetidine, digoxin, furosemide, morphine, nifedipine, procainamide, quinidine, quinine, ranitidine, triamterene, trimethoprim, vancomycin:** Increase metformin blood concentration. **Furosemide, hypoglycemia-causing medications:** May require a decrease in metformin dosage. **Iodinated contrast studies:** May cause acute renal failure and increased risk of lactic acidosis. **HERBAL:** None known. **FOOD:** None known. **LAB VALUES:** None known.

AVAILABILITY (Rx)

ORAL SOLUTION (RIOMET): 100 mg/ml. **TABLETS (GLUCOPHAGE):** 500 mg, 850 mg, 1,000 mg. **TABLETS (EXTENDED-RELEASE):** 500 mg (Fortamet, Glucophage XL, Glumetza), 750 mg (Glucophage XL), 1,000 mg (Fortamet, Glumetza).

ADMINISTRATION/HANDLING

PO
* Do not crush film-coated tablets.
* Give with meals.

INDICATIONS/ROUTES/DOSAGE

DIABETES MELLITUS
PO (IMMEDIATE-RELEASE TABLETS, SOLUTION): ADULTS, ELDERLY: Initially, 500 mg twice a day or 850 mg once daily. Maintenance: 1–2.55 g/day in 2–3 divided doses. **Maximum:** 2,500 mg/day. CHILDREN 10–16 YR: Initially, 500 mg twice a day. Maintenance: Titrate in 500 mg increments weekly. **Maximum:** 2,000 mg/day.
PO (EXTENDED-RELEASE TABLETS [GLUCOPHAGE XL]): ADULTS, ELDERLY: Initially, 500 mg once daily. Maintenance: 1–2 g daily. **Maximum:** 2,000 mg/day.
PO (EXTENDED-RELEASE TABLETS [FORTAMET, GLUMETZA]): ADULTS, ELDERLY: 500 mg–1 g once daily. Maintenance: 1–2.5 g once daily. **Maximum:** 2,500 mg/day.

SIDE EFFECTS

OCCASIONAL (greater than 3%): GI disturbances (including diarrhea, nausea, vomiting, abdominal bloating, flatulence, and anorexia) that are transient and resolve spontaneously during therapy. **RARE (3%–1%):** Unpleasant or metallic taste that resolves spontaneously during therapy.

ADVERSE REACTIONS/ TOXIC EFFECTS

Lactic acidosis occurs rarely but is a fatal complication in 50% of cases. Lactic acidosis is characterized by an increase in blood lactate levels (greater than 5 mmol/L), a decrease in blood pH, and electrolyte disturbances. Signs and symptoms of lactic acidosis include unexplained hyperventilation, myalgia, malaise, and somnolence, which may advance to cardiovascular collapse

M

(shock), acute CHF, acute MI, and prerenal azotemia.

NURSING CONSIDERATIONS

BASELINE ASSESSMENT
Inform patient of potential risks/advantages of therapy and of alternative modes of therapy. Before initiation of therapy and annually thereafter, assess Hgb, Hct, RBC, serum creatinine.

INTERVENTION/EVALUATION
Monitor fasting blood glucose, Hgb A, renal function. Monitor folic acid, renal function tests for evidence of early lactic acidosis. If patient is on concurrent oral sulfonylureas, assess for hypoglycemia (cool or wet skin, tremors, dizziness, anxiety, headache, tachycardia, numbness in mouth, hunger, diplopia). Be alert to conditions that alter glucose requirements: fever, increased activity or stress, surgical procedure.

PATIENT/FAMILY TEACHING
• Discontinue metformin, contact physician immediately if evidence of lactic acidosis appears (unexplained hyperventilation, muscle aches, extreme fatigue, unusual drowsiness). • Prescribed diet is principal part of treatment; do not skip or delay meals. • Diabetes mellitus requires lifelong control. • Avoid alcohol. • Inform physician if headache, nausea, vomiting, diarrhea persist or skin rash, unusual bruising or bleeding, change in color of urine or stool occurs.

methadone ⚑ hydrochloride

meth-a-done

(Dolophine, Metadol ✦, Methadone Intensol, Methadose)

◆CLASSIFICATION
PHARMACOTHERAPEUTIC: Narcotic agonist. CLINICAL: Opioid analgesic (Schedule II) (see p. 128C).

ACTION
An opioid agonist that binds with opioid receptors in the CNS. Therapeutic Effect: Alters the perception of and emotional response to pain; reduces withdrawal symptoms from other opioid drugs.

PHARMACOKINETICS

Route	Onset	Peak	Duration
Oral	0.5–1 hr	1.5–2 hr	6–8 hr
IM	10–20 min	1–2 hr	4–5 hr
IV	N/A	15–30 min	3–4 hr

Well absorbed after IM injection. Protein binding: 80%–85%. Metabolized in the liver. Primarily excreted in urine. Not removed by hemodialysis. Half-life: 15–25 hr.

USES
Relief of severe pain, detoxification, temporary maintenance treatment of narcotic abstinence syndrome.

PRECAUTIONS
CONTRAINDICATIONS: Delivery of premature infant, diarrhea due to poisoning, hypersensitivity to narcotics, labor. EXTREME CAUTION: Renal/hepatic impairment, elderly/debilitated, supraventricular tachycardia, cor pulmonale, history of seizures, acute abdominal conditions, increased intracranial pressure (ICP), respiratory abnormalities. ⌛ LIFESPAN CONSIDERATIONS: Pregnancy/Lactation: Crosses placenta. Distributed in breast milk. Respiratory depression may occur in neonate if mother received opiates during labor. Regular use of opiates during

pregnancy may produce withdrawal symptoms in neonate (irritability, excessive crying, tremors, hyperactive reflexes, fever, vomiting, diarrhea, yawning, sneezing, seizures). **Pregnancy Category B (D if used for prolonged periods or at high dosages at term). Children:** Paradoxical excitement may occur. Those younger than 2 yr more susceptible to respiratory depressant effects. **Elderly:** More susceptible to respiratory depressant effects. Age-related renal impairment may increase risk of urinary retention.

INTERACTIONS

DRUG: **Alcohol, other CNS depressants:** May increase CNS or respiratory depression and hypotension. **MAOIs:** May produce a severe, sometimes fatal reaction; plan to administer ¼ of usual methadone dose. HERBAL: **Valerian:** May increase CNS depression. FOOD: None known. LAB VALUES: May increase serum amylase and lipase levels.

AVAILABILITY (Rx)

ORAL CONCENTRATE (METHADONE INTENSOL, METHADOSE): 10 mg/ml. **ORAL SOLUTION:** 5 mg/5 ml, 10 mg/5 ml. **TABLETS (DOLPHINE, METHADOSE):** 5 mg, 10 mg. **TABLETS (DISPERSIBLE [METHADOSE]):** 40 mg. **INJECTION (DOLPHINE):** 10 mg/ml.

ADMINISTRATION/HANDLING

IM, SUBCUTANEOUS
◄ ALERT ► IM preferred over subcutaneous route (subcutaneous produces pain, local irritation, induration).
• Do not use if solution appears cloudy or contains a precipitate. • Administer slowly. • Those with circulatory impairment experience higher risk of overdosage due to delayed absorption of repeated administration.

PO
• Give without regard to meals. • Dilute syrup in glass of H_2O (prevents anesthetic effect on mucous membranes).

INDICATIONS/ROUTES/DOSAGE

ANALGESIA
PO: ADULTS, ELDERLY: Initially, 5–10 mg q3–4h. CHILDREN: 0.1–0.2 mg/kg q6h as needed. **Maximum:** 10 mg/dose.
IV, IM, SUBCUTANEOUS: ADULTS, ELDERLY: Initially, 2.5–10 mg q3–4h.

NARCOTIC ADDICTION
IM, PO: ADULTS, ELDERLY: 15–40 mg once daily or as needed. Reduce dose at 1–2 day intervals based on patient response. Maintenance: Individualized.

SIDE EFFECTS

FREQUENT: Sedation, decreased BP (including orthostatic hypotension), diaphoresis, facial flushing, constipation, dizziness, nausea, vomiting. **OCCASIONAL:** Confusion, urine retention, palpitations, abdominal cramps, visual changes, dry mouth, headache, decreased appetite, anxiety, insomnia. **RARE:** Allergic reaction (rash, pruritus).

ADVERSE REACTIONS/ TOXIC EFFECTS

Overdose results in respiratory depression, skeletal muscle flaccidity, cold or clammy skin, cyanosis, and extreme somnolence progressing to seizures, stupor, and coma. The antidote is 0.4 mg naloxone. The patient who uses methadone long term may develop a tolerance to the drug's analgesic effect and physical dependence.

NURSING CONSIDERATIONS

BASELINE ASSESSMENT
Patient should be in recumbent position before drug administration by parenteral route. Obtain vital signs before giving medication. If respirations are 12/min or less (20/min or less in

children), withhold medication, contact physician.

INTERVENTION/EVALUATION

Monitor vital signs 15–30 min after subcutaneous/IM dose, 5–10 min following IV dose. Oral medication is 50% as potent as parenteral. Assess for adequate voiding. Assess for clinical improvement, record onset of relief of pain. Provide support to patient in detoxification program; monitor for withdrawal symptoms.

PATIENT/FAMILY TEACHING

• Methadone may produce drug dependence and has the potential for being abused. • Avoid alcohol. • Do not stop taking abruptly after prolonged use. • May cause dry mouth, drowsiness; avoid tasks that require alertness, motor skills until response to drug is established.

methimazole

meth-**im**-a-zole
(Tapazole)

• CLASSIFICATION

PHARMACOTHERAPEUTIC: Thiomidazole derivative. **CLINICAL:** Antithyroid.

ACTION

A thiomidazole derivative that inhibits synthesis of thyroid hormone by interfering with the incorporation of iodine into tyrosyl residues. **Therapeutic Effect:** Effectively treats hyperthyroidism by decreasing thyroid hormone levels.

USES

Treatment of hyperthyroidism. Used to attain a normal metabolic state before thyroidectomy, to control thyrotoxic crisis that may accompany thyroidectomy.

PRECAUTIONS

CONTRAINDICATIONS: None known. **CAUTIONS:** Patients older than 40 yr or in combination with other agranulocytosis-inducing drugs, hepatic impairment. ⧖ **LIFESPAN CONSIDERATIONS: Pregnancy/Lactation:** Crosses placenta; distributed in breast milk. Avoid breastfeeding. **Pregnancy Category D. Children:** Safety and efficacy not established. **Elderly:** No age-related precautions noted.

INTERACTIONS

DRUG: Amiodarone, iodinated glycerol, iodine, potassium iodide: May decrease response to methimazole. **Digoxin:** May increase the blood concentration of digoxin as patient becomes euthyroid. I^{131}: May decrease thyroid uptake of I^{131}. **Oral anticoagulants:** May decrease the effects of oral anticoagulants. **HERBAL:** None known. **FOOD:** None known. **LAB VALUES:** May increase LDH, serum alkaline phosphatase, bilirubin, AST, and ALT levels and prothrombin time. May decrease prothrombin level and WBC count.

AVAILABILITY (Rx)

TABLETS: 5 mg, 10 mg, 20 mg.

ADMINISTRATION/HANDLING

• Store at room temperature in a light-resistant container. • Administer with food if GI symptoms occur.

INDICATIONS/ROUTES/DOSAGE

HYPERTHYROIDISM

PO: ADULTS, ELDERLY: Initially, 15–60 mg/day in 3 divided doses. Maintenance: 5–15 mg/day. CHILDREN: Initially, 0.4 mg/kg/day in 3 divided doses. Maintenance: One-half the initial dose.

SIDE EFFECTS

FREQUENT (5%–4%): Fever, rash, pruritus. **OCCASIONAL (3%–1%):** Dizziness, loss of taste, nausea, vomiting, stomach pain, peripheral neuropathy or numbness in fingers, toes, face. **RARE (less than 1%):** Swollen lymph nodes or salivary glands.

ADVERSE REACTIONS/ TOXIC EFFECTS

Agranulocytosis as long as 4 mo after therapy, pancytopenia, and hepatitis have occurred.

NURSING CONSIDERATIONS

BASELINE ASSESSMENT
Obtain baseline weight, pulse.

INTERVENTION/EVALUATION
Monitor pulse; weigh daily. Assess skin for rash, pruritus, lymphadenopathy. Monitor CBC with differential, hepatic function, prothrombin time. Assess for signs of infection, bleeding.

PATIENT/FAMILY TEACHING
• Do not exceed ordered dose. • Space doses evenly around the clock. • Take resting pulse daily to monitor therapeutic results. • Seafood, iodine products may be restricted. • Report illness, unusual bleeding or bruising immediately.

methocarbamol
(Robaxin)

FIXED-COMBINATION(S)
With aspirin, a salicylate
(Robaxisal)
See Skeletal muscle relaxants.

methohexital sodium
(Brevital)
See Anesthetics: general (p. 2C)

methotrexate sodium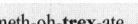

meth-oh-**trex**-ate
(Apo-Methotrexate ✤, Rheumatrex, Trexall)
Do not confuse Trexall with Trexan.

◆ CLASSIFICATION
PHARMACOTHERAPEUTIC: Antimetabolite. **CLINICAL:** Antineoplastic, antiarthritic, antipsoriatic (see p. 76C).

ACTION
An antimetabolite that competes with enzymes necessary to reduce folic acid to tetrahydrofolic acid, a component essential to DNA, RNA, and protein synthesis. This action inhibits DNA, RNA, and protein synthesis. Therapeutic Effect: Causes death of cancer cells.

PHARMACOKINETICS
Variably absorbed from the GI tract. Completely absorbed after IM administration. Protein binding: 50%–60%. Widely distributed. Metabolized intracellularly in the liver. Primarily excreted in urine. Removed by hemodialysis but not by peritoneal dialysis. Half-life: 8–12 hr (large doses, 8–15 hr).

USES
Treatment of breast, head and neck, non–small lung, small cell lung carcinomas, trophoblastic tumors, acute lymphocytic, meningeal leukemias, non-Hodgkin's lymphomas (lymphosarcoma, Burkitt's lymphoma), mycosis fungoides, osteosarcoma, psoriasis, rheumatoid arthritis. OFF-LABEL: Treatment of acute myelocytic leukemia; bladder, cervical, ovarian, prostatic, renal, and testicular carcinomas; psoriatic arthritis; systemic dermatomyositis.

M

PRECAUTIONS

CONTRAINDICATIONS: Hepatic disease or renal impairment, preexisting myelosuppression, psoriasis or rheumatoid arthritis with alcoholism. **CAUTIONS:** Peptic ulcer, ulcerative colitis, bone marrow suppression, ascites, pleural effusion.

⏳ **LIFESPAN CONSIDERATIONS: Pregnancy/Lactation:** Avoid pregnancy during methotrexate therapy and minimum 3 mo after therapy in males or at least one ovulatory cycle after therapy in females. May cause fetal death, congenital anomalies. Drug is distributed in breast milk. Breast-feeding not recommended. **Pregnancy Category D (X for patients with psoriasis or rheumatoid arthritis). Children/Elderly:** Renal or hepatic impairment may require dosage adjustment.

INTERACTIONS

DRUG: Acyclovir (parenteral): May increase the risk of neurotoxicity. **Alcohol, hepatotoxic medications:** May increase the risk of hepatotoxicity. **Asparaginase:** May decrease the effects of methotrexate. **Bone marrow depressants:** May increase myelosuppression. **Live virus vaccines:** May potentiate virus replication, increase vaccine side effects, and decrease the patient's antibody response to the vaccine. **NSAIDs:** May increase the risk of methotrexate toxicity. **Probenecid, salicylates:** May increase blood methotrexate concentration and risk of toxicity. **HERBAL:** None known. **FOOD:** None known. **LAB VALUES:** May increase serum uric acid and AST levels.

AVAILABILITY (Rx)

TABLETS: 2.5 mg (Rheumatrex), 5 mg (Trexall), 7.5 mg (Trexall), 10 mg (Trexall), 15 mg (Trexall). **INJECTION SOLUTION:** 25 mg/ml. **INJECTION POWDER FOR RECONSTITUTION:** 20 mg, 50 mg, 1 g.

ADMINISTRATION/HANDLING

◀ **ALERT** ▶ May be carcinogenic, mutagenic, or teratogenic. Handle with extreme care during preparation and administration. Wear gloves when preparing solution. If powder or solution comes in contact with skin, wash immediately, thoroughly with soap, water. May give IM, IV, intra-arterially, intrathecally.

 IV

Reconstitution • Reconstitute each 5 mg with 2 ml sterile water for injection or 0.9% NaCl to provide a concentration of 2.5 mg/ml. Maximum concentration 25 mg/ml. • May further dilute with D_5W or 0.9% NaCl. • For intrathecal use, dilute with preservative-free 0.9% NaCl to provide a 1 mg/ml concentration.

Rate of administration • Give IV push at rate of 10 mg/min. • Give IV infusion over 30 min–4 hr.

Storage • Store vials at room temperature.

🔲 IV INCOMPATIBILITIES

Chlorpromazine (Thorazine), droperidol (Inapsine), gemcitabine (Gemzar), idarubicin (Idamycin), midazolam (Versed), nalbuphine (Nubain).

IV COMPATIBILITIES

Cisplatin (Platinol AQ), cyclophosphamide (Cytoxan), daunorubicin (DaunoXome), doxorubicin (Adriamycin), etoposide (VePesed), 5-fluorouracil, granisetron (Kytril), leucovorin, mitomycin (Mutamycin), ondansetron (Zofran), paclitaxel (Taxol), vinblastine (Velban), vincristine (Oncovin), vinorelbine (Navelbine).

INDICATIONS/ROUTES/DOSAGE

TROPHOBLASTIC NEOPLASMS

PO, IM: ADULTS, ELDERLY: 15–30 mg/day for 5 days; repeat in 7 days for 3–5 courses.

HEAD AND NECK CANCER

PO, IV, IM: ADULTS, ELDERLY: 25–50 mg/m²
once weekly.

CHORIOCARCINOMA, CHORIOADENOMA DESTRUENS, HYDATIDIFORM MOLE

PO, IV: ADULTS, ELDERLY: 15–30 mg/day for
5 days; repeat 3–5 times with 1–2 wk
between courses.

BREAST CANCER

IV: ADULTS, ELDERLY: 30–60 mg/m² days
1 and 8 q3–4wk.

ACUTE LYMPHOCYTIC LEUKEMIA

PO, IV, IM: ADULTS, ELDERLY: Induction:
3.3 mg/m²/day in combination with other
chemotherapeutic agents. Maintenance:
30 mg/m²/wk PO or IM in divided doses
or 2.5 mg/kg IV every 14 days.

BURKITT'S LYMPHOMA

PO: ADULTS: 10–25 mg/day for 4–8 days;
repeat with 7- to 10-day rest between
courses.

LYMPHOSARCOMA

PO: ADULTS, ELDERLY: 0.625–2.5 mg/kg/
day.

MYCOSIS FUNGOIDES

PO: ADULTS, ELDERLY: 2.5–10 mg/day.
IM: ADULTS, ELDERLY: 50 mg/wk or 25 mg
twice a week.

RHEUMATOID ARTHRITIS

PO: ADULTS, ELDERLY: 7.5 mg once weekly
or 2.5 mg q12h for 3 doses once weekly.
Maximum: 20 mg/wk.

JUVENILE RHEUMATOID ARTHRITIS

PO, IM, SUBCUTANEOUS: CHILDREN:
5–15 mg/m²/wk as a single dose or in
3 divided doses given q12h.

PSORIASIS

PO: ADULTS, ELDERLY: 10–25 mg once
weekly or 2.5–5 mg q12h for 3 doses
once weekly.
IM: ADULTS, ELDERLY: 10–25 mg once
weekly.

ANTINEOPLASTIC DOSAGE FOR CHILDREN

PO, IM: CHILDREN: 7.5–30 mg/m²/wk or
q2wk.

IV: CHILDREN: 10–33,000 mg/m² bolus
or continuous infusion over 6–42 hr.

DOSAGE IN RENAL IMPAIRMENT

Creatinine clearance 61–80 ml/min;
Reduce dose by 25%. **Creatinine clearance 51–60 ml/min;** Reduce dose by
33%. **Creatinine clearance 10–50 ml/min;** Reduce dose by 50%–70%.

SIDE EFFECTS

FREQUENT (10%–3%): Nausea, vomiting,
stomatitis; burning and erythema at
psoriatic site (in patients with psoriasis).
OCCASIONAL (3%–1%): Diarrhea, rash,
dermatitis, pruritus, alopecia, dizziness,
anorexia, malaise, headache, drowsiness, blurred vision.

ADVERSE REACTIONS/ TOXIC EFFECTS

GI toxicity may produce gingivitis, glossitis, pharyngitis, stomatitis, enteritis, and
hematemesis. Hepatotoxicity is more
likely to occur with frequent small
doses than with large intermittent
doses. Pulmonary toxicity may be characterized by interstitial pneumonitis.
Hematologic toxicity, which may develop
rapidly from marked myelosuppression,
may be manifested as leukopenia, thrombocytopenia, anemia, and hemorrhage.
Dermatologic toxicity may produce a
rash, pruritus, urticaria, pigmentation,
photosensitivity, petechiae, ecchymosis,
and pustules. Severe nephrotoxicity may
produce azotemia, hematuria, and renal
failure.

NURSING CONSIDERATIONS

BASELINE ASSESSMENT

Question for possibility of pregnancy
before initiating therapy (Pregnancy
Category X) in patients with psoriasis,
rheumatoid arthritis. Obtain all functional tests before therapy, repeat
throughout therapy. Antiemetics may
prevent nausea, vomiting.

M

INTERVENTION/EVALUATION

Monitor liver and renal function tests, Hgb, Hct, WBC, differential, platelet count, urinalysis, chest x-rays, serum uric acid level. Monitor for hematologic toxicity (fever, sore throat, signs of local infection, unusual ecchymosis or bleeding from any site), symptoms of anemia (excessive fatigue, weakness). Assess skin for evidence of dermatologic toxicity. Keep patient well hydrated, urine alkaline. Avoid IM injections, rectal temperatures, traumas that induce bleeding. Apply 5 full min of pressure to IV sites.

PATIENT/FAMILY TEACHING

• Maintain fastidious oral hygiene. • Do not have immunizations without physician's approval (drug lowers body's resistance). • Avoid crowds, those with infection. • Avoid alcohol, salicylates. • Avoid sunlamp or sunlight exposure. • Use contraceptive measures during therapy and for 3 mo (males) or 1 ovulatory cycle (females) after therapy. • Promptly report fever, sore throat, signs of local infection, unusual bruising or bleeding from any site. • Alopecia is reversible, but new hair growth may have different color, texture. • Contact physician if nausea or vomiting continues at home.

---

methylcellulose

meth-ill-**cell**-you-los
(Citrucel, Cologel)
Do not confuse Citrucel with Citracal.

◆ CLASSIFICATION

CLINICAL: Bulk-forming laxative.

ACTION

A bulk-forming laxative that dissolves and expands in water. **Therapeutic Effect:** Provides increased bulk and moisture content in stool, increasing peristalsis and bowel motility.

PHARMACOKINETICS

Route	Onset	Peak	Duration
PO	12–24 hr	N/A	N/A

Acts in small and large intestines. Full effect may not be evident for 2–3 days.

USES

Prophylaxis in those who should not strain during defecation. Facilitates defecation in those with diminished colonic motor response.

PRECAUTIONS

CONTRAINDICATIONS: Abdominal pain, dysphagia, nausea, partial bowel obstruction, symptoms of appendicitis, vomiting. **CAUTIONS:** None known.

⧗ **LIFESPAN CONSIDERATIONS: Pregnancy/Lactation:** Safe for use in pregnancy. **Pregnancy Category C. Children:** Safety and efficacy not established in those younger than 6 yr. Not recommended in this age group. **Elderly:** No age-related precautions noted.

INTERACTIONS

DRUG: Digoxin, oral anticoagulants, salicylates: May decrease the effects of digoxin, oral anticoagulants, and salicylates by decreasing absorption of these drugs. **Potassium-sparing diuretics, potassium supplements:** May interfere with the effects of potassium-sparing diuretics and potassium supplements. **HERBAL:** None known. **FOOD:** None known. **LAB VALUES:** May increase blood glucose level. May decrease serum potassium level.

AVAILABILITY (OTC)

POWDER (CITRUCEL, COLOGEL).

ADMINISTRATION/HANDLING

PO

• Instruct patient to drink 6–8 glasses of water a day (aids stool softening). • Do not swallow in dry form; mix with at least 1 full glass (8 oz) of liquid.

INDICATIONS/ROUTES/DOSAGE

CONSTIPATION

PO: ADULTS, ELDERLY: 1 tbsp (15 ml) in 8 oz water 1–3 times a day. CHILDREN. 6–12 YR: 1 tsp (5 ml) in 4 oz water 3–4 times a day.

SIDE EFFECTS

RARE: Some degree of abdominal discomfort, nausea, mild cramps, griping, faintness.

ADVERSE REACTIONS/ TOXIC EFFECTS

Esophageal or bowel obstruction may occur if administered with less than 250 ml or 1 full glass of liquid.

NURSING CONSIDERATIONS

INTERVENTION/EVALUATION

Encourage adequate fluid intake. Assess bowel sounds for peristalsis. Monitor pattern of daily bowel activity and stool consistency; record time of evacuation. Monitor serum electrolytes in those exposed to prolonged, frequent, excessive use of medication.

PATIENT/FAMILY TEACHING

• Institute measures to promote defecation: increase fluid intake, exercise, high-fiber diet.

methyldopa

meth-ill-**doe**-pa

(Aldomet, Apo-Methyldopa ✤, Methyldopate, Novomedopa ✤)

Do not confuse Aldomet with Anzemet.

FIXED-COMBINATION(S)

Aldoril: methyldopa/hydrochlorothiazide (a diuretic): 250 mg/15 mg; 250 mg/25 mg; 500 mg/30 mg; 500 mg/50 mg.

CLASSIFICATION

PHARMACOTHERAPEUTIC: Alpha-adrenergic agonist. **CLINICAL:** Antihypertensive (see p. 54C).

ACTION

An antihypertensive agent that stimulates central inhibitory alpha-adrenergic receptors, lowers arterial pressure, and reduces plasma renin activity. **Therapeutic Effect:** Reduces BP.

PHARMACOKINETICS

Absorption from GI tract is variable. Protein binding: Negligible. Metabolized in liver. Excreted in urine. Removed by hemodialysis. **Half-life:** 1.7 hr.

USES

Management of moderate to severe hypertension.

PRECAUTIONS

CONTRAINDICATIONS: Hepatic disease, hepatic disorders previously associated with methyldopa therapy, MAOIs, pheochromocytoma. **CAUTIONS:** Renal impairment.

⧗ LIFESPAN CONSIDERATIONS: **Pregnancy/Lactation:** Unknown if drug crosses placenta; distributed in breast milk. **Pregnancy Category B. Children:** Safety and efficacy not established. **Elderly:** Age-related renal impairment may require dosage adjustment.

INTERACTIONS

DRUG: **Hypotensive-producing medications, such as antihypertensives and diuretics:** May increase the effects of methyldopa. **Lithium:** May increase

M

the risk of lithium toxicity. **MAOIs:** May cause hyperexcitability. **NSAIDs, tricyclic antidepressants:** May decrease the effects of methyldopa. **Other sympathomimetics:** May decrease the effects of sympathomimetics. HERBAL: None known. FOOD: None known. LAB VALUES: May increase BUN and serum prolactin, alkaline phosphatase, bilirubin, creatinine, potassium, sodium, uric acid, AST, and ALT levels. May produce false-positive Coombs' test and prolong PT.

AVAILABILITY (Rx)

TABLETS (ALDOMET): 125 mg, 250 mg, 500 mg. ORAL SUSPENSION (METHYLDOPATE): 250 mg/5 ml. INJECTION: 50 mg/ml.

ADMINISTRATION/HANDLING

IV

• Inspect the drug vial for particulate matter and discoloration and discard if present. • For IV infusion, add the prescribed dose to 100 ml D₅W and infuse over 30–60 min. • Alternatively, add the prescribed dose to D₅W to make a final concentration of 100 mg per 10 ml and infuse over 30–60 min.

INDICATIONS/ROUTES/DOSAGE

HYPERTENSION
IV: ADULTS, ELDERLY: 250–500 mg q6h. **Maximum:** 1 g q6h. CHILDREN: 5–10 mg/kg/dose q6–8h. **Maximum:** 65 mg/kg/day or 3 g/24 hr.
PO: ADULTS, ELDERLY: Initially, 250 mg 2–3 times a day. May increase at 2-day intervals up to 3 g/day. Range: 250–1,000 mg/day in 2 divided doses. CHILDREN: Initially, 10 mg/kg/day in 2–4 divided doses. May increase at 2-day intervals up to 65 mg/kg/day. **Maximum:** 3 g/day.

SIDE EFFECTS

FREQUENT: Peripheral edema, somnolence, headache, dry mouth. **OCCASIONAL:** Mental changes (such as anxiety, depression), decreased sexual function or libido, diarrhea, swelling of breasts, nausea, vomiting, light-headedness, paraesthesia, rhinitis.

ADVERSE REACTIONS/ TOXIC EFFECTS

Hepatotoxicity (abnormal liver function test results, jaundice, hepatitis), hemolytic anemia, unexplained fever and flu-like symptoms may occur. If these conditions appear, discontinue the medication and contact the physician.

NURSING CONSIDERATIONS

BASELINE ASSESSMENT
Obtain baseline BP, pulse, weight.

INTERVENTION/EVALUATION
Monitor BP, pulse closely q30min until stabilized. Monitor weight daily during initial therapy. Monitor liver function tests. Assess for peripheral edema.

PATIENT/FAMILY TEACHING
• Avoid alcohol; may cause drowsiness.
• Avoid tasks requiring mental alertness, motor skills until response to drug is established.

methylergonovine

meth-ill-er-goe-**noe**-veen
(Methergine)

◆ CLASSIFICATION
PHARMACOTHERAPEUTIC: Ergot alkaloid. CLINICAL: Uterine stimulant.

ACTION

An ergot alkaloid that stimulates alpha-adrenergic and serotonin receptors, producing arterial vasoconstriction. Causes vasospasm of coronary arteries and directly stimulates uterine muscle. **Therapeutic Effect:** Increases strength and frequency of uterine contractions. Decreases uterine bleeding.

PHARMACOKINETICS

Route	Onset	Peak	Duration
PO	5–10 min	N/A	N/A
IV	Immediate	N/A	3 hr
IM	2–5 min	N/A	N/A

Rapidly absorbed from the GI tract after IM administration. Distributed rapidly to plasma, extracellular fluid, and tissues. Metabolized in the liver and undergoes first-pass effect. Primarily excreted in urine. **Half-life:** IV (alpha phase), 2–3 min or less; IV (beta phase), 20–30 min or longer.

USES

Prevention and treatment of postpartum, postabortion hemorrhage due to atony or involution (not for induction, augmentation of labor). OFF-LABEL: Treatment of incomplete abortion.

PRECAUTIONS

CONTRAINDICATIONS: Hypertension, pregnancy, toxemia, untreated hypocalcemia. **CAUTIONS:** Renal or hepatic impairment, coronary artery disease, occlusive peripheral vascular disease, sepsis.

LIFESPAN CONSIDERATIONS: **Pregnancy/Lactation:** Contraindicated during pregnancy. Small amounts distributed in breast milk. **Pregnancy Category C. Children/Elderly:** No information available.

INTERACTIONS

DRUG: **Azole antifungals, macrolide antibiotics, protease inhibitors:** May increase risk of vasospasm leading to cerebral ischemia and ischemia of the extremities. **Vasoconstrictors, vasopressors:** May increase the effects of methylergonovine. HERBAL: None known. FOOD: None known. LAB VALUES: May decrease serum prolactin concentration.

AVAILABILITY (Rx)

TABLETS: 0.2 mg. **INJECTION:** 0.2 mg/ml.

ADMINISTRATION/HANDLING

◄ ALERT ► May give IV, IM, or PO.

Reconstitution • Dilute to volume of 5 ml with 0.9% NaCl.

Rate of administration • Give over at least 1 min, carefully monitoring BP.

Storage • Refrigerate ampules. • Initial dose may be given parenterally, followed by oral regimen. • IV use in life-threatening emergencies only.

IV INCOMPATIBILITIES

No information available for Y-site administration.

IV COMPATIBILITIES

Heparin, potassium.

INDICATIONS/ROUTES/DOSAGE

PREVENTION AND TREATMENT OF POSTPARTUM AND POSTABORTION HEMORRHAGE DUE TO ATONY OR INVOLUTION
PO: ADULTS: 0.2 mg 3–4 times a day. Continue for up to 7 days.
IV, IM: ADULTS: Initially, 0.2 mg. May repeat q2–4h for no more than a total of 5 doses.

SIDE EFFECTS

FREQUENT: Nausea, uterine cramping, vomiting. **OCCASIONAL:** Abdominal pain, diarrhea, dizziness, diaphoresis, tinnitus, bradycardia, chest pain. **RARE:** Allergic reaction, such as rash and itching; dyspnea; severe or sudden hypertension.

ADVERSE REACTIONS/ TOXIC EFFECTS

Severe hypertensive episodes may result in cerebrovascular accident (CVA), serious arrhythmias, and seizures.

M

Hypertensive effects are more frequent with patient susceptibility, rapid IV administration, and concurrent use of regional anesthesia or vasoconstrictors. Peripheral ischemia may lead to gangrene.

NURSING CONSIDERATIONS

BASELINE ASSESSMENT

Determine baseline serum calcium level, BP, pulse. Assess bleeding before administration.

INTERVENTION/EVALUATION

Monitor uterine tone, bleeding, BP, pulse q15min until stable (about 1–2 hr). Assess extremities for color, warmth, movement, pain. Report chest pain promptly. Provide support with ambulation if dizziness occurs.

PATIENT/FAMILY TEACHING

• Avoid smoking because of added vasoconstriction. • Report increased cramping, bleeding, foul-smelling lochia. • Pale, cold hands/feet should be reported (possibility of diminished circulation).

methylphenidate hydrochloride

meth-ill-**fen**-i-date

(<u>Concerta</u>, Daytrana, Metadate CD, Metadate ER, Methylin, Methylin ER, PMS-Methylphenidate ❧, Riphenidate ❧, Ritalin, Ritalin LA, Ritalin SR)

Do not confuse Ritalin with Rifadin.

❧CLASSIFICATION

CLINICAL: (Schedule II) CNS stimulant.

ACTION

A CNS stimulant that blocks the reuptake of norepinephrine and dopamine into presynaptic neurons. **Therapeutic Effect:** Decreases motor restlessness and fatigue; increases motor activity, attention span, and mental alertness; produces mild euphoria.

PHARMACOKINETICS

Onset	Peak	Duration
Immediate-release	2 hr	3–5 hr
Sustained-release	4–7 hr	3–8 hr
Extended-release	N/A	8–12 hr

Slowly and incompletely absorbed from the GI tract. Protein binding: 15%. Metabolized in the liver. Eliminated in urine and in feces by biliary system. Unknown if removed by hemodialysis. **Half-life:** 2–4 hr.

USES

Adjunct to treatment of attention deficit hyperactivity disorder (ADHD) with moderate to severe distractibility, short attention spans, hyperactivity, emotional impulsivity in children older than 6 yr. Management of narcolepsy in adults. **OFF-LABEL:** Treatment of disease-related fatigue, secondary mental depression.

PRECAUTIONS

CONTRAINDICATIONS: Use within 14 days of MAOIs. **CAUTIONS:** Hypertension, seizures, acute stress reaction, emotional instability, history of drug dependence, heart failure, recent MI, hyperthyroidism.

⧖ **LIFESPAN CONSIDERATIONS: Pregnancy/Lactation:** Unknown if drug crosses placenta or is distributed in breast milk. **Pregnancy Category C. Children:** May be more susceptible to develop anorexia, insomnia, stomach pain, decreased weight. Chronic use may inhibit growth. **Elderly:** No age-related precautions noted.

INTERACTIONS

DRUG: MAOIs: May increase the effects of methylphenidate. **Other CNS stimulants:** May have an additive effect. **HERBAL:** None known. **FOOD:** None known. **LAB VALUES:** None known.

AVAILABILITY (Rx)

CAPSULES (EXTENDED-RELEASE [METADATE CD]): 10 mg, 20 mg, 30 mg, 40 mg, 50 mg, 60 mg. **CAPSULES (EXTENDED-RELEASE [RITALIN LA]):** 10 mg, 20 mg, 30 mg, 40 mg. **TABLETS (RITALIN):** 5 mg, 10 mg, 20 mg. **TABLETS (EXTENDED-RELEASE [MENTADATE ER, METHYLIN ER]):** 10 mg, 20 mg. **TABLETS (EXTENDED-RELEASE [CONCERTA]): 18 mg, 27 mg, 36 mg, 54 mg, 72 mg. TABLETS (SUSTAINED-RELEASE [RITALIN SR]):** 20 mg. **TABLETS (CHEWABLE [METHYLIN]):** 2.5 mg, 5 mg, 10 mg. **ORAL SOLUTION (METHYLIN):** 5 mg/5 ml, 10 mg/5 ml. **TOPICAL PATCH (DAYTRANA):** 10 mg/9 hr, 16 mg/9 hr, 20 mg/9 hr, 27 mg/9 hr.

ADMINISTRATION/HANDLING

PO
• Do not give drug in afternoon or evening (drug may cause insomnia). • Do not crush, break sustained-release capsules. • Tablets may be crushed. • Give dose 30–45 min before meals.
• **METADATE CD:** May be opened, sprinkled on applesauce.

PATCH
• To be worn daily for 9 hr. • Replace daily in morning.

◄ **ALERT** ► Sustained-release and extended-release tablets may be given in place of regular tablets, once the daily dose is titrated using the regular tablets, and the titrated dosage corresponds to the sustained-release or extended-release tablet strength.

INDICATIONS/ROUTES/DOSAGE

ADHD
PO: CHILDREN 6 YR AND OLDER: **Immediate release:** Initially, 2.5–5 mg before breakfast and lunch. May increase by 5–10 mg/day at weekly intervals. **Maximum:** 60 mg/day.
PO (CONCERTA): CHILDREN 6 YR AND OLDER: Initially, 18 mg once a day; may increase by 18 mg/day at weekly intervals. **Maximum:** 72 mg/day.
PO (METADATE CD): CHILDREN 6 YR AND OLDER: Initially, 20 mg/day. May increase by 20 mg/day at weekly intervals. **Maximum:** 60 mg/day.
PO (RITALIN LA): CHILDREN 6 YR AND OLDER: Initially, 20 mg/day. May increase by 10 mg/day at weekly intervals. **Maximum:** 60 mg/day.
PO (METADATE ER, METHYLIN ER, RITALIN SR): CHILDREN 6 YR AND OLDER: May replace regular tablets after daily dose is titrated and 8-hr dosage corresponds to sustained-release or extended-release tablet size.
PATCH (DAYTRANA): CHILDREN: 10–27 daily (apply and worn for 9 hr).

NARCOLEPSY
PO: ADULTS, ELDERLY: 10 mg 2–3 times a day. Range: 10–60 mg/day.

SIDE EFFECTS

FREQUENT: Anxiety, insomnia, anorexia. **OCCASIONAL:** Dizziness, drowsiness, headache, nausea, abdominal pain, fever, rash, arthralgia, vomiting. **RARE:** Blurred vision, Tourette syndrome (marked by uncontrolled vocal outbursts, repetitive body movements, and tics), palpitations.

ADVERSE REACTIONS/ TOXIC EFFECTS

Prolonged administration to children with ADHD may delay growth. Overdose may produce tachycardia, palpitations, arrhythmias, chest pain, psychotic episode, seizures, and coma. Hypersensitivity reactions and blood dyscrasias occur rarely.

NURSING CONSIDERATIONS

INTERVENTION/EVALUATION
CBC with differential, platelet count

M

should be performed routinely during therapy. If paradoxical return of attention deficit occurs, dosage should be reduced or discontinued. Monitor growth.

PATIENT/FAMILY TEACHING

• Avoid tasks that require alertness, motor skills until response to drug is established. • Sugarless gum, sips of tepid water may relieve dry mouth. • Report any increase in seizures. • Take daily dose early in morning to avoid insomnia. • Report anxiety, palpitations, fever, vomiting, skin rash. • Avoid caffeine. • Do not abruptly stop taking after prolonged use.

---

*methylPREDNISolone

(Medrol)

*methylPREDNISolone acetate

(DepoMedrol, Dep Medalone, Depoject, Depopred, Duralone, Medralon, M-Prednisol)

*methylPREDNISolone sodium succinate

(A-Methapred, Solu-Medrol)

meth-il-pred-**niss**-oh-lone

Do not confuse methylprednisolone with medroxyprogesterone or Medrol with Mebaral.

•CLASSIFICATION

PHARMACOTHERAPEUTIC: Adrenal corticosteroid. **CLINICAL:** Glucocorticoid (see p. 84C).

ACTION

An adrenocortical steroid that suppresses migration of polymorphonuclear leukocytes and reverses increased capillary permeability. **Therapeutic Effect:** Decreases inflammation.

PHARMACOKINETICS

Route	Onset	Peak	Duration
PO	N/A	1–2 hr	30–36 hr
IM	N/A	4–8 days	1–4 wk

Well absorbed from the GI tract after IM administration. Widely distributed. Metabolized in the liver. Excreted in urine. Removed by hemodialysis. **Half-life:** 3.5 hr.

USES

Substitution therapy of deficiency states, e.g., acute or chronic adrenal insufficiency, congenital adrenal hyperplasia, adrenal insufficiency secondary to pituitary insufficiency. **Nonendocrine Disorders:** Arthritis; rheumatic carditis; allergic reaction; collagen, intestinal tract, hepatic, ocular, renal, skin diseases; bronchial asthma; cerebral edema; malignancies, spinal cord injury.

PRECAUTIONS

CONTRAINDICATIONS: Administration of live virus vaccines, systemic fungal infection. **CAUTIONS:** Hypothyroidism, cirrhosis, hypertension, diabetes, CHF, ulcerative colitis, thromboembolic disorders.

⏳ **LIFESPAN CONSIDERATIONS: Pregnancy/Lactation:** Crosses placenta. Distributed in breast milk. May cause cleft palate (chronic use first trimester). Breast-feeding contraindicated. **Pregnancy Category C. Children:** Prolonged treatment or high dosages may decrease short-term growth rate, cortisol secretion. **Elderly:** No age-related precaution noted.

INTERACTIONS

DRUG: Amphotericin: May increase hypokalemia. **Digoxin:** May increase the risk of digoxin toxicity caused by

---

hypokalemia. **Diuretics, insulin, oral hypoglycemics, potassium supplements:** May decrease the effects of these drugs. **Hepatic enzyme inducers:** May decrease the effects of methylprednisolone. **Live virus vaccines:** May decrease the patient's antibody response to vaccine, increase vaccine side effects, and potentiate virus replication. HERBAL: None known. FOOD: None known. LAB VALUES: May increase blood cholesterol, glucose and serum lipid, amylase, and sodium levels. May decrease serum calcium, potassium, and thyroxine levels.

AVAILABILITY (Rx)

TABLETS (MEDROL, MEDROL DOSEPAK, METHYLPRED DP): 2 mg, 4 mg, 8 mg, 16 mg, 32 mg. **INJECTION POWDER FOR RECONSTITUTION (A-METHAPRED, SOLU-MEDROL):** 40 mg, 125 mg, 500 mg, 1 g. **INJECTION SUSPENSION:** 20 mg/ml (Depo-Medrol), 40 mg/ml (Adlone-40, Depo-Medrol, Depopred, Depmedalone, Med-Jec-40, Methylcotol), 80 mg/ml (Adlone-80, Depmedalone, Dep Medalone 80, Depoject-80, Depopred, Depo-Medrol, Medralone 80, Methacort 80, Methylcotolone).

ADMINISTRATION/HANDLING

 IV

Reconstitution • Follow directions with Mix-o-vial. • For infusion, add to D₅W, 0.9% NaCl.

Rate of administration • Give IV push over 2–3 min. • Give IV piggyback over 10–20 min. • Do **not** give methylprednisolone acetate IV.

Storage • Store vials at room temperature.

IM
• Methylprednisolone acetate should not be further diluted. • Methylprednisolone sodium succinate should be reconstituted with bacteriostatic water for injection. • Give deep IM in gluteus maximus.

PO
• Give with food, milk. • Give single doses before 9 AM; give multiple doses at evenly spaced intervals.

IV INCOMPATIBILITIES

Ciprofloxacin (Cipro), diltiazem (Cardizem), docetaxel (Taxotere), etoposide (VePesid), filgrastim (Neupogen), gemcitabine (Gemzar), paclitaxel (Taxol), potassium chloride, propofol (Diprivan), vinorelbine (Navelbine).

IV COMPATIBILITIES

Dopamine (Intropin), heparin, midazolam (Versed), theophylline.

INDICATIONS/ROUTES/DOSAGE

ANTI-INFLAMMATORY, IMMUNOSUPPRESSIVE

IV: ADULTS, ELDERLY: 10–40 mg. May repeat as needed. CHILDREN: 0.5–1.7 mg/kg/day or 5–25 mg/m²/day in 2–4 divided doses. **PO:** ADULTS, ELDERLY: 2–60 mg/day in 1–4 divided doses. CHILDREN: 0.5–1.7 mg/kg/day or 5–25 mg/m²/day in 2–4 divided doses.

STATUS ASTHMATICUS

IV: ADULTS, ELDERLY, CHILDREN: Initially, 2 mg/kg/dose, then 0.5–1 mg/kg/dose q6h for up to 5 days.

SPINAL CORD INJURY

IV BOLUS: ADULTS, ELDERLY: 30 mg/kg over 15 min. Maintenance dose: 5.4 mg/kg/h over 23 hr, to be given within 45 min of bolus dose.

IM (METHYLPREDNISOLONE ACETATE): ADULTS, ELDERLY: 10–80 mg/day. CHILDREN: 0.5–1.7 mg/kg/day or 5–25 mg/m²/day in 2–4 divided doses.

INTRA-ARTICULAR, INTRALESIONAL: ADULTS, ELDERLY: 4–40 mg, up to 80 mg q1–5wk.

SIDE EFFECTS

FREQUENT: Insomnia, heartburn, anxiety, abdominal distention, diaphoresis, acne, mood swings, increased appetite, facial flushing, GI distress, delayed wound healing, increased susceptibility to

M

infection, diarrhea or constipation. **OCCASIONAL:** Headache, edema, tachycardia, change in skin color, frequent urination, depression. **RARE:** Psychosis, increased blood coagulability, hallucinations.

ADVERSE REACTIONS/ TOXIC EFFECTS

Long-term therapy may cause hypocalcemia, hypokalemia, muscle wasting (especially in arms and legs), osteoporosis, spontaneous fractures, amenorrhea, cataracts, glaucoma, peptic ulcer disease, and CHF. Abruptly withdrawing the drug after long-term therapy may cause anorexia, nausea, fever, headache, sudden severe myalgia, rebound inflammation, fatigue, weakness, lethargy, dizziness, and orthostatic hypotension.

NURSING CONSIDERATIONS

BASELINE ASSESSMENT

Question for hypersensitivity to any of the corticosteroids, components. Obtain baselines for height, weight, BP, blood glucose, electrolytes. Check results of initial tests (e.g., tuberculosis [TB] skin test, x-rays, EKG).

INTERVENTION/EVALUATION

Monitor I&O, daily weights; assess for edema. Evaluate bowel activity. Check vital signs at least 2 times a day. Be alert for infection: sore throat, fever, vague symptoms. Monitor serum electrolytes. Monitor for hypocalcemia (muscle twitching, cramps, positive Trousseau's or Chvostek's signs), hypokalemia (weakness or muscle cramps, numbness or tingling [especially lower extremities], nausea or vomiting, irritability, EKG changes). Assess emotional status, ability to sleep. Check lab results for blood coagulability, clinical evidence of thromboembolism.

PATIENT/FAMILY TEACHING

• Take oral dose with food, milk. • Do not change dose or schedule or stop taking drug; must taper off gradually under medical supervision. • Notify physician of fever, sore throat, muscle aches, sudden weight gain or edema. • Maintain fastidious personal hygiene, avoid exposure to disease, trauma. • Severe stress (serious infection, surgery, trauma) may require increased dosage. • Follow-up visits, lab tests are necessary. • Children must be assessed for growth retardation. • Inform dentist, other physicians of methylprednisolone therapy now or within past 12 mo.

methysergide maleate

(Sansert)
See Antimigraine agents

metipranolol

(OptiPranolol)
See Antiglaucoma agents (p. 48C)

metoclopramide

meh-tah-**klo**-prah-myd
(Apo-Metoclop , Reglan)
Do not confuse Reglan with Renagel.

◆CLASSIFICATION

PHARMACOTHERAPEUTIC: Dopamine receptor antagonist. **CLINICAL:** GI emptying adjunct, peristaltic stimulant, antiemetic.

ACTION

A dopamine receptor antagonist that stimulates motility of the upper GI tract

---

* "Tall Man" lettering   🔎 see color pill atlas   🌿 herb   <u>underlined</u> – top prescribed drug and decreases reflux into the esophagus. Also raises the threshold of activity in the chemoreceptor trigger zone. **Therapeutic Effect:** Accelerates intestinal transit and gastric emptying; relieves nausea and vomiting.

PHARMACOKINETICS

Route	Onset	Peak	Duration
PO	30–60 min	N/A	N/A
IV	1–3 min	N/A	N/A
IM	10–15 min	N/A	N/A

Well absorbed from the GI tract. Metabolized in the liver. Protein binding: 30%. Primarily excreted in urine. Not removed by hemodialysis. **Half-life:** 4–6 hr.

USES

Facilitate intestinal intubation, stimulate gastric emptying and intestinal transit in conjunction with radiography, treatment of gastroparesis, gastroesophageal reflux disease (GERD), prevent cancer chemotherapy induced nausea and vomiting, postoperative nausea and vomiting. **OFF-LABEL:** Prevention of aspiration pneumonia; treatment of drug-related postoperative nausea and vomiting, gastric stasis in preterm infants, persistent hiccups, slow gastric emptying, vascular headaches.

PRECAUTIONS

CONTRAINDICATIONS: Concurrent use of medications likely to produce extrapyramidal reactions, GI hemorrhage, GI obstruction or perforation, history of seizure disorders, pheochromocytoma. **CAUTIONS:** Renal impairment, CHF, cirrhosis.

⏳ **LIFESPAN CONSIDERATIONS: Pregnancy/Lactation:** Crosses placenta. Distributed in breast milk. **Pregnancy Category B. Children:** More susceptible to having dystonia reactions. **Elderly:** More likely to have parkinsonism, dyskinesias after long-term therapy.

INTERACTIONS

DRUG: **Alcohol, other CNS suppressants:** May increase CNS depressant effect. HERBAL: None known. FOOD: None known. LAB VALUES: May increase serum aldosterone and prolactin concentrations.

AVAILABILITY (Rx)

SYRUP: 5 mg/5 ml. **TABLETS:** 5 mg, 10 mg. **INJECTION:** 5 mg/ml.

ADMINISTRATION/HANDLING

 IV

Reconstitution • Dilute doses greater than 10 mg in 50 ml D_5W, 0.9% NaCl, or lactated Ringer's.

Rate of administration • Infuse over 15 min. • May give slow IV push at rate of 10 mg over 1–2 min. • A too rapid IV injection may produce intense feeling of anxiety or restlessness, followed by drowsiness.

Storage • Store vials at room temperature. • After dilution, IV infusion (piggyback) is stable for 48 hr.

PO
• Give 30 min before meals and at bedtime. • Tablets may be crushed.

▨ IV INCOMPATIBILITIES

Allopurinol (Aloprim), cefepime (Maxipime), doxorubicin liposomal (Doxil), furosemide (Lasix), propofol (Diprivan).

IV COMPATIBILITIES

Dexamethasone, diltiazem (Cardizem), diphenhydramine (Benadryl), fentanyl (Sublimaze), heparin, hydromorphone (Dilaudid), morphine, potassium chloride, total parenteral nutrition (TPN).

INDICATIONS/ROUTES/DOSAGE

PREVENTION OF CHEMOTHERAPY-INDUCED NAUSEA AND VOMITING
IV: ADULTS, ELDERLY, CHILDREN: 1–2 mg/kg 30 min before chemotherapy; repeat

M

q2h for 2 doses, then q3h as needed for total of 5 doses/day.

POST OPERATIVE NAUSEA, VOMITING
IV: ADULTS, ELDERLY: 10–20 mg q4–6h as needed. CHILDREN: 0.25 mg/kg/dose q6–8h as needed.

DIABETIC GASTROPARESIS
PO, IV: ADULTS: 10 mg 30 min before meals and at bedtime for 2–8 wk.
PO: ELDERLY: Initially, 5 mg 30 min before meals and at bedtime. May increase to 10 mg.
IV: ELDERLY: 5 mg over 1–2 min. May increase to 10 mg.

SYMPTOMATIC GASTROESOPHAGEAL REFLUX
PO: ADULTS: 10–15 mg up to 4 times a day, or single doses up to 20 mg as needed. ELDERLY: Initially, 5 mg 4 times a day. May increase to 10 mg. CHILDREN: 0.4–0.8 mg/kg/day in 4 divided doses.

TO FACILITATE SMALL BOWEL INTUBATION (SINGLE DOSE)
IV: ADULTS, ELDERLY: 10 mg as a single dose. CHILDREN 6–14 YR: 2.5–5 mg as a single dose. CHILDREN YOUNGER THAN 6 YR: 0.1 mg/kg as a single dose.

DOSAGE IN RENAL IMPAIRMENT
Dosage is modified based on creatinine clearance.

Creatinine Clearance	% of normal dose
40–50 ml/min	75%
10–40 ml/min	50%
Less than 10 ml/min	25%–50%

SIDE EFFECTS

FREQUENT (10%): Somnolence, restlessness, fatigue, lethargy. **OCCASIONAL (3%):** Dizziness, anxiety, headache, insomnia, breast tenderness, altered menstruation, constipation, rash, dry mouth, galactorrhea, gynecomastia. **RARE (less than 3%):** Hypotension or hypertension, tachycardia.

ADVERSE REACTIONS/ TOXIC EFFECTS

Extrapyramidal reactions occur most commonly in children and young adults (18–30 yr) receiving large doses (2 mg/kg) during chemotherapy and are usually limited to akathisia (involuntary limb movement and facial grimacing).

NURSING CONSIDERATIONS

BASELINE ASSESSMENT
Antiemetic: Assess for dehydration (poor skin turgor, dry mucous membranes, longitudinal furrows in tongue).

INTERVENTION/EVALUATION
Monitor for anxiety, restlessness, extrapyramidal symptoms (EPS) during IV administration. Monitor pattern of daily bowel activity and stool consistency. Assess skin for rash. Evaluate for therapeutic response from gastroparesis (nausea, vomiting, bloating). Monitor renal function, BP, heart rate.

PATIENT/FAMILY TEACHING
• Avoid tasks that require alertness, motor skills until drug response is established. • Report involuntary eye, facial, limb movement (extrapyramidal reaction). • Avoid alcohol.

metolazone

me-**toh**-lah-zone
(Mykrox, <u>Zaroxolyn</u>)

Do not confuse metolazone with methazolamide or metoprolol, or Zaroxolyn with Zarontin.

◆ CLASSIFICATION
PHARMACOTHERAPEUTIC: Thiazide-like. **CLINICAL:** Diuretic, antihypertensive (see p. 88C).

ACTION

A thiazide-like diuretic and antihypertensive. As a diuretic, blocks reabsorption of sodium, potassium, and chloride at the distal convoluted tubule, increasing renal excretion of sodium and water. As an antihypertensive, reduces plasma and extracellular fluid volume and peripheral vascular resistance. **Therapeutic Effect:** Promotes diuresis and reduces BP.

PHARMACOKINETICS

Route	Onset	Peak	Duration
PO (diuretic)	1 hr	2 hr	12–24 hr

Incompletely absorbed from the GI tract. Protein binding: 95%. Primarily excreted unchanged in urine. Not removed by hemodialysis. **Half-life:** 14 hr.

USES

Zaroxolyn: Treatment of mild to moderate essential hypertension, edema of renal disease, edema due to CHF. **Mykrox:** Treatment of mild to moderate hypertension.

PRECAUTIONS

CONTRAINDICATIONS: Anuria, hepatic coma or precoma, history of hypersensitivity to sulfonamides or thiazide diuretics, renal decompensation. **CAUTIONS:** Severe renal disease, hepatic impairment, gout, lupus erythematosus, diabetes, elevated serum cholesterol or triglyceride levels.

⌛ **LIFESPAN CONSIDERATIONS: Pregnancy/Lactation:** Crosses placenta. Small amount distributed in breast milk; breast-feeding not advised. **Pregnancy Category B (D if used in pregnancy-induced hypertension). Children:** No age-related precautions noted. **Elderly:** May be more sensitive to hypotensive or electrolyte effects. Age-related renal impairment may require dosage adjustment.

INTERACTIONS

DRUG: Cholestyramine, colestipol: May decrease the absorption and effects of metolazone. **Digoxin:** May increase the risk of digoxin toxicity associated with metolazone-induced hypokalemia. **Lithium:** May increase the risk of lithium toxicity. **HERBAL:** None known. **FOOD:** None known. **LAB VALUES:** May increase blood glucose and serum cholesterol, LDL, bilirubin, calcium, creatinine, uric acid, and triglyceride levels. May decrease urinary calcium, and serum magnesium, potassium, and sodium levels.

AVAILABILITY (Rx)

TABLETS (PROMPT-RELEASE [MYKROX]): 0.5 mg. **TABLETS (EXTENDED-RELEASE [ZAROXOLYN]):** 2.5 mg, 5 mg, 10 mg.

ADMINISTRATION/HANDLING

PO
• May give with food, milk if GI upset occurs, preferably with breakfast (may prevent nocturia).

INDICATIONS/ROUTES/DOSAGE

EDEMA
PO (ZAROXOLYN): ADULTS, ELDERLY: 5–10 mg/day. May increase to 20 mg/day in edema associated with renal disease or heart failure. CHILDREN: 0.2–0.4 mg/kg/day in 1–2 divided doses.

HYPERTENSION
PO (ZAROXOLYN): ADULTS, ELDERLY: 2.5–5 mg/day.
PO (MYKROX): ADULTS, ELDERLY: Initially, 0.5 mg/day. May increase up to 1 mg/day.

SIDE EFFECTS

EXPECTED: Increase in urinary frequency and urine volume. **FREQUENT (10%–9%):** Dizziness, light-headedness, headache. **OCCASIONAL (6%–4%):** Muscle cramps and spasm, fatigue, lethargy. **RARE (less than 2%):** Asthenia, palpitations, depression, nausea, vomiting,

M

abdominal bloating, constipation, diarrhea, urticaria.

ADVERSE REACTIONS/ TOXIC EFFECTS

Vigorous diuresis may lead to profound water and electrolyte depletion, resulting in hypokalemia, hyponatremia, and dehydration. Acute hypotensive episodes may occur. Hyperglycemia may occur during prolonged therapy. Pancreatitis, paresthesia, blood dyscrasias, pulmonary edema, allergic pneumonitis, and dermatologic reactions occur rarely. Overdose can lead to lethargy and coma without changes in electrolytes or hydration.

NURSING CONSIDERATIONS

BASELINE ASSESSMENT

Check vital signs, especially BP for hypotension, before administration. Assess baseline serum electrolytes, particularly check for hypokalemia. Assess skin turgor, mucous membranes for hydration status. Assess for peripheral edema. Assess muscle strength, mental status. Note skin temperature, moisture. Obtain baseline weight. Monitor I&O.

INTERVENTION/EVALUATION

Continue to monitor BP, vital signs, serum electrolytes, I&O, weight. Note extent of diuresis. Monitor for electrolyte disturbances (hypokalemia may result in weakness, tremors, muscle cramps, nausea, vomiting, altered mental status, tachycardia; hyponatremia may result in confusion, thirst, cold or clammy skin).

PATIENT/FAMILY TEACHING

• Expect increased frequency and volume of urination. • To reduce hypotensive effect, rise slowly from lying to sitting position, permit legs to dangle momentarily before standing. • Eat foods high in potassium, such as whole grains (cereals), legumes, meat, bananas, apricots, orange juice, potatoes (white, sweet), raisins.

metoprolol tartrate

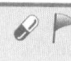

me-**toe** pro-lole

(Apo-Metoprolol ✽, Betaloc ✽, Nu-Metop ✽, PMS-Metoprolol ✽, Toprol XL)

Do not confuse metoprolol with metaproterenol or metolazone, or Toprol XL with Topamax, Tegretol, or Tegretol XR.

FIXED-COMBINATION(S)

Lopressor HCT: metoprolol/hydrochlorothiazide (a diuretic): 50 mg/ 25 mg; 100 mg/25 mg; 100 mg/ 50 mg.

◆CLASSIFICATION

PHARMACOTHERAPEUTIC: Beta$_1$-adrenergic blocker. **CLINICAL:** Antianginal, antihypertensive, MI adjunct (see p. 64C).

ACTION

An antianginal, antihypertensive, and MI adjunct that selectively blocks beta$_1$-adrenergic receptors; high dosages may block beta$_2$-adrenergic receptors. Decreases oxygen requirements. Large doses increase airway resistance. **Therapeutic Effect:** Slows sinus node heart rate, decreases cardiac output, and reduces BP. Also decreases myocardial ischemia severity.

PHARMACOKINETICS

Route	Onset	Peak	Duration
PO	10–15 min	N/A	6 hr
PO (extended release)	N/A	6–12 hr	24 hr
IV	Immediate	20 min	5–8 hr

Well absorbed from the GI tract. Protein binding: 12%. Widely distributed. Metabolized in the liver (undergoes significant first-pass metabolism). Primarily excreted in urine. Removed by hemodialysis. Half-life: 3–7 hr.

USES

Lopressor: Treatment of acute myocardial infarction (AMI), angina pectoris, hypertension. **Toprol XL:** Treatment of angina pectoris, CHF, hypertension. OFF-LABEL: To increase survival rate in diabetic patients with coronary artery disease (CAD); treatment or prevention of anxiety; cardiac arrhythmias; hypertrophic cardiomyopathy; mitral valve prolapse syndrome; pheochromocytoma; tremors; thyrotoxicosis; vascular headache.

PRECAUTIONS

CONTRAINDICATIONS: Cardiogenic shock, MI with a heart rate less than 45 beats/min or systolic BP less than 100 mm Hg, overt heart failure, second- or third-degree heart block, sinus bradycardia. **CAUTIONS:** Bronchospastic disease, renal impairment, peripheral vascular disease, hyperthyroidism, diabetes mellitus, inadequate cardiac function.

LIFESPAN CONSIDERATIONS: **Pregnancy/Lactation:** Crosses placenta. Distributed in breast milk. Avoid use during first trimester. May produce bradycardia, apnea, hypoglycemia, hypothermia during delivery, low birth-weight infants. **Pregnancy Category C (D if used in second or third trimester). Children:** Safety and efficacy not established. **Elderly:** Age-related peripheral vascular disease may increase susceptibility to decreased peripheral circulation.

INTERACTIONS

DRUG: **Cimetidine:** May increase metoprolol blood concentration. **Diuretics,** **other antihypertensives:** May increase hypotensive effect. **Insulin, oral hypoglycemics:** May mask symptoms of hypoglycemia and prolong hypoglycemic effect of these drugs. **NSAIDs:** May decrease antihypertensive effect. **Sympathomimetics, xanthines:** May mutually inhibit effects. HERBAL: None known. FOOD: None known. LAB VALUES: May increase serum antinuclear antibody titer and BUN, serum lipoprotein, serum LDH, serum alkaline phosphatase, serum bilirubin, serum creatinine, serum potassium, serum uric acid, AST levels, ALT levels, and serum triglyceride levels.

AVAILABILITY (Rx)

TABLETS (LOPRESSOR): 25 mg, 50 mg, 100 mg. **TABLETS (EXTENDED-RELEASE [TOPROL XL]):** 25 mg, 50 mg, 100 mg, 200 mg. **INJECTION (LOPRESSOR):** 1 mg/ml.

ADMINISTRATION/HANDLING

 IV

Rate of administration • May give undiluted. • Administer IV injection over 1 min. • Monitor EKG, BP, during administration.

Storage • Store at room temperature.

PO
• Tablets may be crushed; do not crush or break extended-release tablets. • Give at same time each day. • May be given with or immediately after meals (enhances absorption).

IV INCOMPATIBILITIES

Amphotericin B complex (Abelcet, AmBisome, Amphotec).

IV COMPATIBILITY

Alteplase (Activase).

INDICATIONS/ROUTES/DOSAGE

MILD TO MODERATE HYPERTENSION
PO: ADULTS: Initially, 100 mg/day as single or divided dose. Increase at weekly (or longer) intervals.

Maintenance: 100–450 mg/day. ELDERLY: Initially, 25 mg/day. Range: 25–300 mg/day.

PO (EXTENDED-RELEASE): ADULTS: 50–100 mg/day as single dose. May increase at least at weekly intervals until optimum BP attained. **Maximum:** 200 mg/day. ELDERLY: Initially, 25–50 mg/day as a single dose. May increase at 1–2 wk intervals.

CHRONIC, STABLE ANGINA PECTORIS

PO: ADULTS: Initially, 100 mg/day as single or divided dose. Increase at weekly (or longer) intervals. Maintenance: 100–450 mg/day.

PO (EXTENDED-RELEASE): ADULTS: Initially, 100 mg/day as single dose. May increase at least at weekly intervals until optimum clinical response achieved. **Maximum:** 200 mg/day.

CHF

PO (EXTENDED-RELEASE): ADULTS: Initially, 25 mg/day. May double dose q2wk. **Maximum:** 200 mg/day.

EARLY TREATMENT OF MI

IV: ADULTS: 5 mg q2min for 3 doses, followed by 50 mg orally q6h for 48 hr. Begin oral dose 15 min after last IV dose. Or, in patients who do not tolerate full IV dose, give 25–50 mg orally q6h, 15 min after last IV dose.

LATE TREATMENT AND MAINTENANCE AFTER AN MI

PO: ADULTS: 100 mg twice a day for at least 3 mo.

SIDE EFFECTS

Metoprolol is generally well tolerated, with transient and mild side effects. **FREQUENT:** Diminished sexual function, drowsiness, insomnia, unusual fatigue or weakness. **OCCASIONAL:** Anxiety, nervousness, diarrhea, constipation, nausea, vomiting, nasal congestion, abdominal discomfort, dizziness, difficulty breathing, cold hands or feet. **RARE:** Altered taste, dry eyes, nightmares, paraesthesia, allergic reaction (rash, pruritus).

ADVERSE REACTIONS/ TOXIC EFFECTS

Overdose may produce profound bradycardia, hypotension, and bronchospasm. Abrupt withdrawal of metoprolol may result in diaphoresis, palpitations, headache, tremulousness, exacerbation of angina, MI, and ventricular arrhythmias. Metoprolol administration may precipitate CHF and MI in patients with heart disease; thyroid storm in those with thyrotoxicosis; and peripheral ischemia in those with existing peripheral vascular disease. Hypoglycemia may occur in patients with previously controlled diabetes mellitus.

NURSING CONSIDERATIONS

BASELINE ASSESSMENT

Assess baseline renal/liver function tests. Assess BP, apical pulse immediately before drug administration (if pulse is 60/min or less or systolic BP is less than 90 mm Hg, withhold medication, contact physician). **Antianginal:** Record onset, type (sharp, dull, squeezing), radiation, location, intensity, duration of anginal pain, precipitating factors (exertion, emotional stress).

INTERVENTION/EVALUATION

Assess for paradoxical reactions. Measure BP near end of dosing interval (determines whether BP is controlled throughout day). Monitor BP for hypotension, respiration for shortness of breath. Assess pulse for quality, irregular rate, bradycardia. Assess for evidence of CHF: dyspnea (particularly on exertion, lying down), night cough, peripheral edema, distended neck veins. Monitor I&O (increased weight, decreased urine output may indicate CHF). Therapeutic response to hypertension noted in 1–2 wk.

PATIENT/FAMILY TEACHING

• Do not abruptly discontinue medication. • Compliance with therapy regimen is essential to control hypertension, arrhythmias. • If a dose is missed, take next scheduled dose (do not double dose). • To avoid hypotensive effect, rise slowly from lying to sitting position, wait momentarily before standing. • Report excessive fatigue, dizziness. • Avoid tasks that require alertness, motor skills until response to drug is established. • Do not use nasal decongestants, OTC cold preparations (stimulants) without physician approval. • Monitor BP, pulse before taking medication. • Restrict salt, alcohol intake.

MetroGel-Vaginal,

see metronidazole

---

metronidazole hydrochloride

me-troe-**ni**-da-zole

(Apo-Metronidazole ✤, Flagyl, Flagyl 375, Flagyl ER, Flagyl I.V. RTU, MetroCream, MetroGel, MetroGel-Vaginal, Metro I.V., MetroLotion, Metronidazole Benzoate, NidaGel ✤, Noritate, Novonidazol ✤, Protostat, Rozex, Vandazole)

FIXED-COMBINATION(S)

Helidac: metronidazole/bismuth/tetracycline (an anti-infective): 250 mg/262 mg/500 mg.

CLASSIFICATION

PHARMACOTHERAPEUTIC: Nitroimidazole derivative. **CLINICAL:** Antibacterial, antiprotozoal.

ACTION

A nitroimidazole derivative that disrupts bacterial and protozoal DNA, inhibiting nucleic acid synthesis. **Therapeutic Effect:** Produces bactericidal, antiprotozoal, amebicidal, and trichomonacidal effects. Produces anti-inflammatory and immunosuppressive effects when applied topically.

PHARMACOKINETICS

Well absorbed from the GI tract; minimally absorbed after topical application. Protein binding: less than 20%. Widely distributed; crosses blood-brain barrier. Metabolized in the liver to active metabolite. Primarily excreted in urine; partially eliminated in feces. Removed by hemodialysis. **Half-life:** 8 hr (increased in alcoholic hepatic disease and in neonates).

USES

Treatment of anaerobic infections (skin and skin-structure, CNS, lower respiratory tract, bone and joints, intra-abdominal, gynocologic, endocarditis, septicemia). Treatment of trichomoniasis, amebiasis, antibiotic-associated pseudomembranous colitis (AAPC). **OFF-LABEL:** Treatment of bacterial vaginosis, grade III-IV decubitus ulcers with anaerobic infection, *H. pylori*-associated gastritis and duodenal ulcer, inflammatory bowel disease; topical treatment of acne rosacea.

PRECAUTIONS

CONTRAINDICATIONS: Hypersensitivity to other nitroimidazole derivatives (also parabens with topical application). **CAUTIONS:** Blood dyscrasias, severe hepatic dysfunction, CNS disease, predisposition to edema, concurrent corticosteroid therapy. Safety and efficacy of topical administration in those younger than 21 yr not established.

⧗ **LIFESPAN CONSIDERATIONS:** Pregnancy/Lactation: Readily crosses placenta. Distributed in breast milk. Contraindicated during first trimester in those with trichomoniasis. Topical use during pregnancy or lactation discouraged. **Pregnancy Category B. Children:** No age-related precautions noted. **Elderly:** Age-related liver impairment may require dosage adjustment.

INTERACTIONS

DRUG: Alcohol: May cause a disulfiram-type reaction. **Disulfiram:** May increase the risk of toxicity. **Oral anticoagulants:** May increase the effects of these drugs. **HERBAL:** None known. **FOOD:** None known. **LAB VALUES:** May increase serum LDH, AST, and ALT levels.

AVAILABILITY (Rx)

CAPSULES (FIAGYL 375): 375 mg. **TABLETS (FIAGYL, PROTOSTAT):** 250 mg, 500 mg. **TABLETS (EXTENDED-RELEASE [FLAGYL ER]):** 750 mg. **INJECTION (INFUSION [FIAGYL I.V. RTU]):** 500 mg/100 ml. **TOPICAL CREAM:** 0.75% (MetroCream, Rozex), 1% (Noritate). **TOPICAL GEL (METROGEL):** 0.75%, 1%. **TOPICAL LOTION (METROLOTION):** 0.75%. **VAGINAL GEL (METROGEL-VAGINAL, VANDAZOLE):** 0.75%.

ADMINISTRATION/HANDLING

 IV

Rate of administration • Infuse IV over 30–60 min. Do not give by IV bolus. • Avoid prolonged use of indwelling catheters.

Storage • Store at room temperature (ready-to-use infusion bags).

PO

• Give without regard to meals. Give with food to decrease GI irritation.

▦ IV INCOMPATIBILITIES

Amphotericin B complex (Abelcet, AmBisome, Amphotec), filgrastim (Neupogen), total parenteral nutrition (TPN).

IV COMPATIBILITIES

Diltiazem (Cardizem), dopamine (Intropin), heparin, hydromorphone (Dilaudid), lorazepam (Ativan), magnesium sulfate, midazolam (Versed), morphine.

INDICATIONS/ROUTES/DOSAGE

ANAEROBIC INFECTIONS

PO, IV: ADULTS, ELDERLY, CHILDREN: Initially, 15 mg/kg once, then 7.5 mg/kg/dose q6h. **Maximum:** 4 g/day.

AMEBIC DYSENTERY

PO: ADULTS, ELDERLY: 750 mg 3 times a day for 5–10 days. CHILDREN: 35–50 mg/kg/day in 3 divided doses for 10 days. **Maximum:** 750 mg/dose.

AMEBIC LIVER ABSCESS

PO: ADULTS, ELDERLY: 500–750 mg 3 times a day for 5–10 days. CHILDREN: 50 mg/kg/day in 3 divided doses. **Maximum:** 750 mg/dose.

GIARDIASIS

PO: ADULTS, ELDERLY: 250 mg 3 times a day for 5 days. CHILDREN: 15 mg/kg/day in 3 divided doses for 7–10 days. **Maximum:** 250 mg/dose.

PSEUDOMEMBRANOUS COLITIS

PO: ADULTS, ELDERLY: 500–750 mg 3 times a day or 250–500 mg 4 times a day. CHILDREN: 7.5 mg/kg q6h for 7–10 days.

TRICHOMONIASIS

PO: ADULTS, ELDERLY: 250 mg 3 times a day or 375 mg twice a day or 500 mg twice a day or 2 g as a single dose. CHILDREN: 15 mg/kg/day in 3 divided doses for 7 days.

BACTERIAL VAGINOSIS

PO: ADULTS: (NON-PREGNANT): 500 mg twice a day for 7 days or 750 mg (extended-release) once daily for 7 days or 2 g as a single dose. (PREGNANT): 250 mg 3 times a day for 7 days.

INTRAVAGINAL: ADULTS: (PREGNANT, NON-PREGNANT): 0.75% apply twice a day for 5 days. Center for Disease Control (CDC) does not recommend the use of topical agents during pregnancy.

ROSACEA

TOPICAL: ADULTS, ELDERLY: (1%): Apply to affected area once daily. (0.75%): Apply to affected area twice a day.

SIDE EFFECTS

FREQUENT: Systemic: Anorexia, nausea, dry mouth, metallic taste. **Vaginal:** Symptomatic cervicitis and vaginitis, abdominal cramps, uterine pain. **OCCASIONAL: Systemic:** Diarrhea or constipation, vomiting, dizziness, erythematous rash, urticaria, reddish brown urine. **Topical:** Transient erythema, mild dryness, burning, irritation, stinging, tearing when applied too close to eyes. **Vaginal:** Vaginal, perineal, or vulvar itching; vulvar swelling. **RARE:** Mild, transient leukopenia; thrombophlebitis with IV therapy.

ADVERSE REACTIONS/ TOXIC EFFECTS

Oral therapy may result in furry tongue, glossitis, cystitis, dysuria, pancreatitis, and flattening of T waves on EKG readings. Peripheral neuropathy, manifested as numbness and tingling in hands or feet, is usually reversible if treatment is stopped immediately after neurologic symptoms appear. Seizures occur occasionally.

NURSING CONSIDERATIONS

BASELINE ASSESSMENT

Question for history of hypersensitivity to metronidazole or other nitroimidazole derivatives (and parabens with topical). Obtain specimens for diagnostic tests, cultures before giving first dose (therapy may begin before results are known).

INTERVENTION/EVALUATION

Determine pattern of bowel activity. Monitor I&O, assess for urinary problems. Be alert to neurologic symptoms: dizziness; paresthesia of extremities. Assess for rash, urticaria. Watch for onset of superinfection: ulceration/ change of oral mucosa, furry tongue, vaginal discharge, genital or anal pruritus.

PATIENT/FAMILY TEACHING

• Urine may be red-brown or dark. • Avoid alcohol, alcohol-containing preparations (e.g., cough syrups, elixirs). • Avoid tasks that require alertness, motor skills until response to drug established (may cause dizziness). • If taking metronidazole for trichomoniasis, refrain from sexual intercourse until full treatment is completed. • For amebiasis, frequent stool specimen checks will be necessary. • **Topical:** Avoid contact with eyes. • May apply cosmetics after application. • Metronidazole acts on erythema, papules, pustules but has no effect on rhinophyma (hypertrophy of nose), telangiectasia, ocular problems (conjunctivitis, keratitis, blepharitis). • Other recommendations for rosacea include avoidance of hot or spicy foods, alcohol, extremes of hot or cold temperatures, excessive sunlight.

M

Mevacor, see lovastatin

mexiletine hydrochloride

(Mexitil)

See Antiarrhythmics (p. 14C)

Miacalcin, see calcitonin

Miacalcin Nasal,

see calcitonin

micafungin sodium

my-cah-**fun**-gin
(Mycamine)

◆CLASSIFICATION
CLINICAL: Antifungal.

ACTION

Inhibits synthesis of glucan (vital component of fungal cell formation), damaging fungal cell membrane. **Therapeutic Effect:** Decreased glucon content leads to cellular lysis.

PHARMACOKINETICS

Extensively bound to albumin. Protein binding: greater than 99%. Slowly metabolized in liver to active metabolite. Primarily excreted in feces and to a lesser extent, in urine. Not removed by hemodialysis. **Half-life:** 11–21 hr.

USES

Treatment of esophageal candidiasis, prophylaxis of *Candida* infection in patients undergoing hematopoietic stem cell transplant.

PRECAUTIONS

CONTRAINDICATIONS: None known. **CAUTIONS:** Hepatic function impairment, impaired renal function.

⧖ **LIFESPAN CONSIDERATIONS: Pregnancy/Lactation:** May produce decreased sperm count. May be embryotoxic. Unknown if distributed in breast milk. **Pregnancy Category C. Children:** Safety and efficacy not established. **Elderly:** No age-related precautions noted.

INTERACTIONS

DRUG: Nifedipine, sirolimus: Concentrations of these drugs may be increased. **HERBAL:** None known.

FOOD: None known. **LAB VALUES:** May increase AST, ALT, alkaline phosphatase, LDH, bilirubin, creatinine, transaminase, BUN, creatinine. May decrease serum albumin, calcium, magnesium, phosphorus, potassium, Hgb, Hct, WBCs, platelet count.

AVAILABILITY (Rx)

POWDER FOR INJECTION: 50 mg vials (Mycamine).

ADMINISTRATION/HANDLING

 IV

Reconstitution • Add 5 ml 0.9% NaCl (without a bacteriostatic agent) to each 50 mg vial to yield micafungin 10 mg/ml. • Gently swirl to dissolve; do not shake. • Further dilute 50–150 mg micafungin to 100 ml 0.9% NaCl and give as a piggyback. • Alternatively, D₅W may be used for reconstitution and dilution. • Flush existing IV line with 0.9% NaCl or D₅W before infusion.

Rate of administration • Infuse over 60 min.

Storage • Reconstituted solution is stable for 24 hr at room temperature. • Discard if precipitate is present.

▨ IV INCOMPATIBILITIES
Do not mix with any other medication.

INDICATIONS/ROUTES/DOSAGE
ESOPHAGEAL CANDIDIASIS
IV: ADULTS, ELDERLY: Give 150 mg a day as a single dose.

CANDIDA PROPHYLAXIS IN STEM CELL PATIENTS
IV: ADULTS, ELDERLY: Give 50 mg a day as a single dose.

SIDE EFFECTS

OCCASIONAL (3%–2%): Nausea, headache, diarrhea, vomiting, pyrexia. **RARE (1%):** Dizziness, somnolence, pruritus, abdominal pain, dyspepsia.

ADVERSE REACTIONS/ TOXIC EFFECTS

Hypersensitivity reaction characterized by rash, pruritus, facial edema occurs rarely. Anaphylaxis, hemoglobinuria, hemolytic anemia has been reported.

NURSING CONSIDERATIONS

BASELINE ASSESSMENT

Determine baseline liver and renal function tests and periodically thereafter.

INTERVENTION/EVALUATION

Monitor serum chemistry results for evidence of hepatic dysfunction, renal impairment.

Micardis, see telmisartan

---

miconazole nitrate

mih-**kon**-nah-zoll

(Micatin, Micozole ✤, Mitrazol, Monistat ✤, Monistat 3, Monistat 7, Monistat-Derm)

Do not confuse miconazole with Micronase, or Mitrazol with Micronor.

CLASSIFICATION

PHARMACOTHERAPEUTIC: Imidazole derivative. **CLINICAL:** Antifungal (see p. 44C).

ACTION

Inhibits synthesis of ergosterol (vital component of fungal cell formation), damaging fungal cell membrane. **Therapeutic Effect:** Fungistatic; may be fungicidal, depending on concentration.

PHARMACOKINETICS

Small amounts absorbed systemically after vaginal administration. Protein binding: 91%–93%. Primarily excreted in feces. Half-life: 24 hr.

USES

Vaginal: Vulvovaginal candidiasis. **Topical:** Cutaneous candidiasis, tinea cruris, t. corporis, t. pedis, t. versicolor.

PRECAUTIONS

CONTRAINDICATIONS: Avoid vaginal preparations during first trimester of pregnancy. **CAUTIONS:** Sensitivity to other antifungals (e.g., clotrimazole, ketoconazole).

⌛ LIFESPAN CONSIDERATIONS: **Pregnancy/Lactation:** Unknown if drug crosses placenta or is distributed in breast milk. **Pregnancy Category C. Children:** Safety in those younger than 1 yr not established. **Elderly:** No age-related precautions noted.

INTERACTIONS

DRUG: **Isoniazid, rifampin:** May decrease miconazole concentrations. **Oral anticoagulants, oral hypoglycemics:** May increase the effects of these drugs. HERBAL: None known. FOOD: None known. LAB VALUES: None known.

AVAILABILITY (Rx)

CREAM (TOPICAL): Micatin, Monistat-Derm: 2%; **CREAM (VAGINAL):** Monistat-7: 2%; Monistat-3: 4%; **TOPICAL POWDER:** Mitrazol: 2%; **VAGINAL SUPPOSITORY:** Monistat-7: 100 mg; Monistat-3: 200 mg, 1,200 mg.

INDICATIONS/ROUTES/DOSAGE

VULVOVAGINAL CANDIDIASIS
INTRAVAGINAL SUPPOSITORY:
ADULTS, ELDERLY: 100 mg suppository at bedtime for 7 days, or 200 mg suppository at bedtime for 3 days, or 1,200 mg suppository once at bedtime or during the day.

INTRAVAGINAL CREAM: ADULTS, ELDERLY: 2% cream: 1 applicatorful at bedtime for 7 days. 4% cream: 1 applicatorful at bedtime for 3 days.

TOPICAL FUNGAL INFECTIONS, CUTANEOUS CANDIDIASIS

TOPICAL: ADULTS, ELDERLY: Apply liberally twice a day, morning and evening.

SIDE EFFECTS

Topical: Itching, burning, stinging, erythema, urticaria. **Vaginal (2%):** Vulvovaginal burning, itching, irritation; headache; skin rash.

ADVERSE REACTIONS/ TOXIC EFFECTS

None known.

NURSING CONSIDERATIONS

BASELINE ASSESSMENT

Topical: Avoid occlusive dressings. Apply only a small amount to cover area completely. **Spray:** Shake well before using.

INTERVENTION/EVALUATION

Topical/Vaginal: Assess for burning, itching, irritation.

PATIENT/FAMILY TEACHING

• **Vaginal Preparation:** Base interacts with certain latex products such as contraceptive diaphragm. • Ask physician about douching, sexual intercourse. • **Topical:** Rub well into affected areas. • Avoid getting in eyes. • Keep areas clean, dry; wear light clothing for ventilation. • Separate personal items in contact with affected areas.

---

midazolam hydrochloride ⚐

my-**dah**-zoe-lam
(Apo-Midazolam ✤, Versed)
Do not confuse Versed with VePesid.

◆CLASSIFICATION

PHARMACOTHERAPEUTIC: Benzodiazepine (**Schedule IV**). **CLINICAL:** Sedative (see p. 3C).

ACTION

A benzodiazepine that enhances the action of gamma-aminobutyric acid, one of the major inhibitory neurotransmitters in the brain. Therapeutic Effect: Produces anxiolytic, hypnotic, anticonvulsant, muscle relaxant, and amnestic effects.

PHARMACOKINETICS

Route	Onset	Peak	Duration
PO	10–20 min	N/A	N/A
IV	1–5 min	5–7 min	20–30 min
IM	5–15 min	15–60 min	2–6 hr

Well absorbed after IM administration. Protein binding: 97%. Metabolized in the liver to active metabolite. Primarily excreted in urine. Not removed by hemodialysis. Half-life: 1–5 hr.

USES

Sedation, anxiolytic, amnesia before procedure or induction of anesthesia, conscious sedation before diagnostic/radiographic procedure, continuous IV sedation of intubated or mechanically ventilated patients, status epilepticus. OFF-LABEL: Anxiety, status epilepticus.

PRECAUTIONS

CONTRAINDICATIONS: Acute alcohol intoxication, acute angle-closure glaucoma, allergies to cherries, coma, shock. **CAUTIONS:** Acute illness, severe fluid or electrolyte imbalance, renal, hepatic, pulmonary impairment, CHF, treated open-angle glaucoma.

⧖ LIFESPAN CONSIDERATIONS: Pregnancy/Lactation: Crosses placenta. Unknown if drug is distributed in breast milk. **Pregnancy Category D.**

M

Children: Neonates more likely to have respiratory depression. **Elderly:** Age-related renal impairment may require dosage adjustment.

INTERACTIONS

DRUG: **Alcohol, other CNS depressants:** May increase CNS and respiratory depression and hypotensive effects of midazolam. **Hypotension-producing medications:** May increase hypotensive effects of midazolam. HERBAL: **Kava kava, valerian:** May increase CNS depression. FOOD: **Grapefruit, grapefruit juice:** Increases the oral absorption and systemic availability of midazolam. LAB VALUES: None known.

AVAILABILITY (Rx)

SYRUP: 2 mg/ml. INJECTION: 1 mg/ml, 5 mg/ml. INJECTION (PRESERVATIVE-FREE): 1 mg/ml, 5 mg/ml.

ADMINISTRATION/HANDLING

IV

Rate of administration • May give undiluted or as infusion. • Resuscitative equipment, O_2 must be readily available before IV administration. • Administer by slow IV injection, in incremental dosages: Give each incremental dose over 2 min or longer at intervals of at least 2 min. • Reduce IV rate in those older than 60 yr, debilitated patients with chronic disease states, pulmonary impairment. • A too rapid IV rate, excessive doses, or a single large dose increases risk of respiratory depression/arrest.

Storage • Store vials at room temperature.

IM
• Give deep IM into large muscle mass.

IV INCOMPATIBILITIES

Albumin, ampicillin and sulbactam (Unasyn), amphotericin B complex (Abelcet, AmBisome, Amphotec), ampicillin (Polycillin), bumetanide (Bumex), co-trimoxazole (Bactrim), dexamethasone (Decadron), fosphenytoin (Cerebyx), furosemide (Lasix), hydrocortisone (Solu-Cortef), methotrexate, nafcillin (Nafcil), sodium bicarbonate, sodium pentothal (Thiopental).

IV COMPATIBILITIES

Amiodarone (Cordarone), atropine, calcium gluconate, diltiazem (Cardizem), diphenhydramine (Benadryl), dobutamine (Dobutrex), dopamine (Intropin), etomidate (Amidate), fentanyl (Sublimaze), glycopyrrolate (Robinul), heparin, hydromorphone (Dilaudid), hydroxyzine (Vistaril), insulin, lorazepam (Ativan), milrinone (Primacor), morphine, nitroglycerin, norepinephrine (Levophed), potassium chloride, propofol (Diprivan).

INDICATIONS/ROUTES/DOSAGE
PREOPERATIVE SEDATION
PO: CHILDREN: 0.25–0.5 mg/kg. **Maximum:** 20 mg.
IV: ADULTS, ELDERLY: 0.02–0.04 mg/kg. CHILDREN 6–12 YR: 0.025–0.05 mg/kg. CHILDREN 6 MO–5 YR: 0.05–0.1 mg/kg.
IM: ADULTS, ELDERLY: 0.07–0.08 mg/kg 30–60 min before surgery. CHILDREN: 0.1–0.15 mg/kg 30–60 min before surgery. **Maximum:** 10 mg.

CONSCIOUS SEDATION FOR DIAGNOSTIC, THERAPEUTIC, AND ENDOSCOPIC PROCEDURES
IV: ADULTS, ELDERLY: 1–2.5 mg over 2 min. Titrate as needed. **Maximum total dose:** 2.5–5 mg. CHILDREN 6–12 YR: 0.025–0.05 mg/kg. Total dose of 0.4 mg/kg may be necessary. **Maximum total dose:** 10 mg. CHILDREN 6 MO–5 YR: 0.05–0.1 mg/kg. Total dose of 0.6 mg/kg may be necessary. **Maximum total dose:** 6 mg.

CONSCIOUS SEDATION DURING MECHANICAL VENTILATION
IV: ADULTS, ELDERLY: Initially, 0.02–0.08 mg/kg. May repeat at 5- to 15-min

M

intervals or continuous infusion rate of 0.04–0.2 mg/kg/hr and titrated to desired effect. CHILDREN: Initially, 0.05–0.2 mg/kg followed by a continuous infusion of 0.06–0.12 mg/kg/hr (1–2 mcg/kg/min) titrated to desired effect.

STATUS EPILEPTICUS

IV: CHILDREN OLDER THAN 2 MO: Loading dose of 0.15 mg/kg followed by continuous infusion of 1 mcg/kg/min. Titrate as needed. Range: 1–18 mcg/kg/min.

SIDE EFFECTS

FREQUENT (10%–4%): Decreased respiratory rate, tenderness at IM or IV injection site, pain during injection, oxygen desaturation, hiccups. **OCCASIONAL (3%–2%):** Hypotension, paradoxical CNS reaction. **RARE (less than 2%):** Nausea, vomiting, headache, coughing.

ADVERSE REACTIONS/ TOXIC EFFECTS

Inadequate or excessive dosage or improper administration may result in cerebral hypoxia, agitation, involuntary movements, hyperactivity, and combativeness. A too-rapid IV rate, excessive doses, or a single large dose increases the risk of respiratory depression or arrest. Respiratory depression or apnea may produce hypoxia and cardiac arrest.

NURSING CONSIDERATIONS

BASELINE ASSESSMENT

Resuscitative equipment, oxygen must be available. Obtain vital signs before administration.

INTERVENTION/EVALUATION

Monitor respiratory rate and oxygen saturation continuously during parenteral administration for underventilation, apnea. Monitor vital signs, level of sedation q3–5min during recovery period.

midodrine

my-doe-dreen
(Amatine ✦, ProAmatine)

Do not confuse Amatine or ProAmatine with amantadine or protamine.

◆ CLASSIFICATION

PHARMACOTHERAPEUTIC: Vasopressor. **CLINICAL:** Orthostatic hypotension adjunct.

ACTION

A vasopressor that forms the active metabolite desglymidodrine, an alpha$_1$-agonist, activating alpha receptors of the arteriolar and venous vasculature. **Therapeutic Effect:** Increases vascular tone and BP.

PHARMACOKINETICS

Rapid absorption from the GI tract following PO administration. Protein binding: Low. Undergoes enzymatic hydrolysis (deglycination) in the systemic circulation. Excreted in urine. **Half-life:** 0.5 hr.

USES

Treatment of symptomatic orthostatic hypotension. **OFF-LABEL:** Infection-related hypotension, intradialytic hypotension, psychotropic agent-induced hypotension, urinary incontinence.

PRECAUTIONS

CONTRAINDICATIONS: Acute renal function impairment, persistent hypertension, pheochromocytoma, severe cardiac disease, thyrotoxicosis, urine retention. **CAUTIONS:** Renal or hepatic impairment, history of visual problems.
⧗ **LIFESPAN CONSIDERATIONS:** Pregnancy/Lactation: Unknown if drug crosses placenta or is distributed is breast milk. **Pregnancy Category C.**

Children: Safety and efficacy not established. **Elderly:** Age-related renal impairment may require dosage adjustment.

INTERACTIONS

DRUG: Digoxin: May have additive bradycardia effects. **Sodium-retaining steroids (such as fludrocortisone):** May increase sodium retention. **Vasoconstrictors:** May have an additive vasocontricting effect. **HERBAL:** None known. **FOOD:** None known. **LAB VALUES:** None known.

AVAILABILITY (Rx)

TABLETS: 2.5 mg, 5 mg, 10 mg.

ADMINISTRATION/HANDLING

• Give midodrine with or without food.
• The last dose of the day should be given 3–4 hr before bedtime.

INDICATIONS/ROUTES/DOSAGE

ORTHOSTATIC HYPOTENSION

PO: ADULTS, ELDERLY: 10 mg 3 times a day. Give during the day when patient is upright, such as upon arising, midday, and late afternoon. Do not give later than 6 PM.

DOSAGE IN RENAL IMPAIRMENT

For adults and elderly patients, give 2.5 mg 3 times a day; increase gradually, as tolerated.

SIDE EFFECTS

FREQUENT (20%–7%): Paresthesia, piloerection, pruritus, dysuria, supine hypertension. **OCCASIONAL (less than 7%–1%):** Pain, rash, chills, headache, facial flushing, confusion, dry mouth, anxiety.

ADVERSE REACTIONS/ TOXIC EFFECTS

Increased systolic arterial pressure has been reported.

BASELINE ASSESSMENT

Assess sensitivity to midodrine, other medications (especially digoxin, sodium-retaining vasoconstrictors). Assess medical history, especially renal impairment, severe hypertension, cardiac disease.

INTERVENTION/EVALUATION

Monitor BP, renal, hepatic, cardiac function.

PATIENT/FAMILY TEACHING

• Do not take last dose of the day after evening meal or less than 4 hr before bedtime. • Do not give if patient will be supine. • Use caution with OTC medications that may affect BP (e.g., cough and cold, diet medications).

mifepristone

miff-eh-**pris**-tone
(Mifeprex)

Do not confuse Mifeprex with Mirapex or mifepristone with misoprostol.

CLASSIFICATION

CLINICAL: Abortifacient.

ACTION

An abortifacient that has antiprogestational activity resulting from competitive interaction with progesterone. Inhibits the activity of endogenous or exogenous progesterone. Also has antiglucocorticoid and weak antiandrogenic activity. **Therapeutic Effect:** Terminates pregnancy.

PHARMACOKINETICS

Protein binding: 98%. Metabolized in liver. Primarily eliminated in feces; minimal excretion in urine. **Half-life:** 20–54 hr.

USES

Termination of intrauterine pregnancy. OFF-LABEL: Breast or ovarian cancer, Cushing's syndrome, endometriosis, intrauterine fetal death or nonviable early pregnancy, postcoital contraception or contragestation, unresectable meningioma.

PRECAUTIONS

CONTRAINDICATIONS: Chronic adrenal failure, concurrent long-term steroid or anticoagulant therapy, confirmed or suspected ectopic pregnancy, intrauterine device (IUD) in place, hemorrhagic disorders or concurrent anticoagulant therapy, inherited porphyria, hypersensitivity to misoprostol or other prostaglandins. CAUTIONS: Treatment of women older than 35 yr, smoke more than 10 cigarettes/day, cardiovascular disease, hypertension, hepatic/renal impairment, diabetes, severe anemia. Pregnancy Category X.

INTERACTIONS

DRUG: Carbamazepine, phenobarbital, phenytoin, rifampin: May increase the metabolism of mifepristone. Erythromycin, itraconazole, ketoconazole: May inhibit the metabolism of mifepristone. HERBAL: St. John's wort: May increase the metabolism of mifepristone. FOOD: Grapefruit, grapefruit juice: May inhibit the metabolism of mifepristone. LAB VALUES: May decrease Hgb level and Hct and RBC count.

AVAILABILITY (Rx)

TABLETS: 200 mg.

INDICATIONS/ROUTES/DOSAGE

TERMINATION OF PREGNANCY

PO: ADULTS: Day 1: 600 mg as single dose. Day 3: 400 mcg misoprostol. Day 14: Post-treatment examination.

SIDE EFFECTS

FREQUENT (greater than 10%): Headache, dizziness, abdominal pain, nausea, vomiting, diarrhea, fatigue. OCCASIONAL (10%–3%): Uterine hemorrhage, insomnia, vaginitis, dyspepsia, back pain, fever, viral infections, rigors. RARE (2%–1%): Anxiety, syncope, anemia, asthenia, leg pain, sinusitis, leukorrhea.

ADVERSE REACTIONS/ TOXIC EFFECTS

None known.

NURSING CONSIDERATIONS

BASELINE ASSESSMENT

Assess for use of ketoconazole, itraconazole, erythromycin, rifampin, anticonvulsants (inhibits metabolism).

INTERVENTION/EVALUATION

◄ ALERT ► If mifepristone results in an incomplete abortion, surgical intervention may be necessary. Monitor Hgb/Hct. Confirm pregnancy is completely terminated at approximately 14 days after drug administration. Assess degree of vaginal bleeding.

PATIENT/FAMILY TEACHING

• Advise patients of treatment procedure and effects, need for follow-up visit. • Vaginal bleeding or uterine cramping may occur.

milrinone lactate ▷

mill-re-none
(Primacor, Primacor I.V.)

◆ CLASSIFICATION

PHARMACOTHERAPEUTIC: Cardiac inotropic agent. CLINICAL: Vasodilator (see p. 80C).

✎ see color pill atlas   ✦ herb   underlined – top prescribed drug

ACTION

A cardiac inotropic agent that inhibits phosphodiesterase, which increases cyclic adenosine monophosphate and potentiates the delivery of calcium to myocardial contractile systems. Therapeutic Effect: Relaxes vascular muscle, causing vasodilation. Increases cardiac output; decreases pulmonary capillary wedge pressure and vascular resistance.

PHARMACOKINETICS

Route	Onset	Peak	Duration
IV	5–15 min	N/A	N/A

Protein binding: 70%. Primarily excreted unchanged in urine. Half-life: 2.4 hr.

USES

Short-term management of CHF.

PRECAUTIONS

CONTRAINDICATIONS: None known. **CAUTIONS:** Severe obstructive aortic or pulmonic valvular disease, history of ventricular arrhythmias, atrial fibrillation/flutter, renal impairment.

LIFESPAN CONSIDERATIONS: **Pregnancy/Lactation:** Unknown if drug crosses placenta or is distributed in breast milk. **Pregnancy Category C. Children:** Safety and efficacy not established. **Elderly:** Age-related renal impairment may require dosage adjustment.

INTERACTIONS

DRUG: **Other cardiac glycosides:** Produces additive inotropic effects. HERBAL: None known. FOOD: None known. LAB VALUES: None known.

AVAILABILITY (Rx)

INJECTION (PRIMACOR, PRIMACOR I.V.): 1 mg/ml, 10-ml single-dose vial, 20-ml single-dose vial, 50-ml single-dose vial, 5-ml sterile cartridge unit. **INJECTION (PREMIX [PRIMACOR]):** 200 mcg/ml.

ADMINISTRATION/HANDLING

IV

Reconstitution • For IV infusion, dilute 20-mg (20-ml) vial with 80 or 180 ml diluent (0.9% NaCl, D_5W) to provide concentration of 200 or 100 mcg/ml, respectively. Maximum concentration: 100 mg/250 ml.

Rate of administration • For IV injection (loading dose), administer undiluted slowly over 10 min. • Monitor for arrhythmias, hypotension during IV therapy; reduce or temporarily discontinue infusion until condition stabilizes.

Storage • Store at room temperature.

IV INCOMPATIBILITY

Furosemide (Lasix).

IV COMPATIBILITIES

Calcium gluconate, digoxin (Lanoxin), diltiazem (Cardizem), dobutamine (Dobutrex), dopamine (Intropin), heparin, lidocaine, magnesium, midazolam (Versed), nitroglycerin, potassium, propofol (Diprivan).

INDICATIONS/ROUTES/DOSAGE

SHORT-TERM MANAGEMENT OF CHF

IV: ADULTS: Initially, 50 mcg/kg over 10 min. Continue with maintenance infusion rate of 0.375–0.75 mcg/kg/min based on hemodynamic and clinical response. Total daily dosage: 0.59–1.13 mg/kg.

DOSAGE IN RENAL IMPAIRMENT

For patients with severe renal impairment, reduce dosage to 0.2–0.43 mcg/kg/min.

SIDE EFFECTS

OCCASIONAL (3%–1%): Headache, hypotension. **RARE (less than 1%):** Angina, chest pain.

M

ADVERSE REACTIONS/ TOXIC EFFECTS

Supraventricular and ventricular arrhythmias (12%), nonsustained ventricular tachycardia (2%), and sustained ventricular tachycardia (1%) may occur.

NURSING CONSIDERATIONS

BASELINE ASSESSMENT

Offer emotional support (difficulty breathing may produce anxiety). Assess BP, apical pulse rate before treatment begins and during IV therapy. Assess lung sounds; observe for edema.

INTERVENTION/EVALUATION

Monitor BP, heart rate, cardiac output, EKG, serum potassium, renal function, signs and symptoms of CHF.

minocycline hydrochloride

mi-noe-**sye**-kleen

(Arestin, Dynacin, Minocin, Myrac, Novo Minocycline ✤, Vectrin)

Do not confuse Dynacin with Dynabac or Minocin with Mithracin or niacin.

◆CLASSIFICATION

PHARMACOTHERAPEUTIC: Tetracycline. **CLINICAL:** Antibiotic.

ACTION

A tetracycline antibiotic that inhibits bacterial protein synthesis by binding to ribosomes. **Therapeutic Effect:** Bacteriostatic.

PHARMACOKINETICS

Protein binding: 76%. Partial elimination in feces; minimal excretion in urine. Not removed by hemodialysis. **Half-life:** 11–12 hr (oral capsule).

USES

Treatment of susceptible infections due to *Rickettsiae, M. pneumoniae, C. trachomatis, C. psittaci, H. ducreyi, Yersinia pestis, Francisella tularensis, Bivrio cholerae,* Brucella species, gram-negative organisms including prostate, urinary tract, CNS infections (not meningitis), uncomplicated gonorrhea, inflammatory acne, brucellosis, skin granulomas, cholera, trachoma, nocardiasis, yaws, syphilis when penicillins are contraindicated. **OFF-LABEL:** Treatment of atypical mycobacterial infections, rheumatoid arthritis, scleroderma.

PRECAUTIONS

CONTRAINDICATIONS: Children younger than 8 yr, hypersensitivity to tetracyclines, last half of pregnancy. **CAUTIONS:** Renal impairment, sun or ultraviolet exposure (severe photosensitivity reaction).

⧖ **LIFESPAN CONSIDERATIONS: Pregnancy/Lactation:** Readily crosses placenta; distributed in breast milk. May inhibit fetal skeletal growth. **Pregnancy Category D. Children:** May cause permanent discoloration of teeth, enamel hypoplasia. Not recommended in children younger than 8 yr. **Elderly:** No age-related precautions noted.

INTERACTIONS

DRUG: Carbamazepine, phenytoin: May decrease minocycline blood concentration. **Cholestyramine, colestipol:** May decrease minocycline absorption. **Ergot:** May increase risk of ergotism. **Oral contraceptives:** May decrease the effects of oral contraceptives. **HERBAL: St. John's wort:** May increase the risk of photosensitivity. **FOOD:** None known. **LAB VALUES:** May increase serum alkaline phosphatase, amylase, bilirubin, AST, and ALT levels.

AVAILABILITY (Rx)

CAPSULES (DYNACIN, MINOCIN, VECTRIN): 50 mg, 75 mg, 100 mg. **CAPSULES**

(PELLET-FILLED [MINOCIN]): 50 mg, 100 mg. **TABLETS (MINOCIN, MYRAC):** 50 mg, 75 mg, 100 mg. **POWDER FOR INJECTION (MINOCIN, MYRAC):** 100 mg.

ADMINISTRATION/HANDLING

🝆 IV

Reconstitution • For intermittent IV infusion (piggyback), reconstitute each 100-mg vial with 5–10 ml sterile water for injection to provide concentration of 20 or 10 mg/ml, respectively. • Further dilute with 500–1,000 ml D₅W or 0.9 % NaCl.

Rate of administration • Infuse over 6 hr.

Storage • IV solution is stable for 24 hr at room temperature. • Use IV infusion (piggyback) immediately after reconstitution. • Discard if precipitate forms.

PO
• Store at room temperature. • Give capsules, tablets with full glass of water.

▧ IV INCOMPATIBILITIES
Piperacillin and tazobactam (Zosyn).

IV COMPATIBILITIES
Heparin, magnesium, potassium.

INDICATIONS/ROUTES/DOSAGE

MILD, MODERATE, OR SEVERE PROSTATE, URINARY TRACT, AND CNS INFECTIONS (EXCLUDING MENINGITIS); UNCOMPLICATED GONORRHEA; INFLAMMATORY ACNE; BRUCELLOSIS; SKIN GRANULOMAS; CHOLERA; TRACHOMA; NOCARDIASIS; YAWS; AND SYPHILIS WHEN PENICILLINS ARE CONTRAINDICATED

PO: ADULTS, ELDERLY: Initially, 100–200 mg, then 100 mg q12h or 50 mg q6h.
IV: ADULTS, ELDERLY: Initially, 200 mg, then 100 mg q12h up to 400 mg/day.
PO, IV: CHILDREN OLDER THAN 8 YR: Initially, 4 mg/kg, then 2 mg/kg q12h.

SIDE EFFECTS

FREQUENT: Dizziness, light-headedness, diarrhea, nausea, vomiting, abdominal cramps, possibly severe photosensitivity, drowsiness, vertigo. **OCCASIONAL:** Altered pigmentation of skin or mucous membranes, rectal or genital pruritus, stomatitis.

ADVERSE REACTIONS/ TOXIC EFFECTS

Superinfection (especially fungal), anaphylaxis, and benign intracranial hypertension may occur. Bulging fontanelles occur rarely in infants.

NURSING CONSIDERATIONS

BASELINE ASSESSMENT
Question for history of allergies, especially tetracyclines, sulfite.

INTERVENTION/EVALUATION
Assess ability to ambulate (may cause vertigo, dizziness). Monitor pattern of bowel activity and stool consistency. Assess skin for rash. Observe for signs of increased intracranial pressure (ICP), e.g., altered level of consciousness, widened pulse pressure. Be alert for superinfection: diarrhea, stomatitis, anal or genital pruritus.

PATIENT/FAMILY TEACHING
• Continue antibiotic for full length of treatment. • Space doses evenly. • Drink full glass of water with capsules or tablets, avoid bedtime doses. • Avoid tasks that require alertness, motor skills until response to drug is established. • Notify physician if diarrhea, rash, other new symptom occurs. • Protect skin from sun exposure.

M

minoxidil

min-**ox**-i-dill

(Apo-Gain ⚘, Loniten, Milnox ⚘, Rogaine, Rogaine Extra Strength)

Do not confuse Loniten with Lotensin.

CLASSIFICATION

CLINICAL: Antihypertensive, hair growth stimulant (see p. 55C).

ACTION

An antihypertensive and hair growth stimulant that has direct action on vascular smooth muscle, producing vasodilation of arterioles. **Therapeutic Effect:** Decreases peripheral vascular resistance and BP; increases cutaneous blood flow; stimulates hair follicle epithelium and hair follicle growth.

PHARMACOKINETICS

Route	Onset	Peak	Duration
PO	0.5 hr	2–8 hr	2–5 days

Well absorbed from the GI tract; minimal absorption after topical application. Protein binding: None. Widely distributed. Metabolized in the liver to active metabolite. Primarily excreted in urine. Removed by hemodialysis. **Half-life:** 4.2 hr.

USES

Treatment of severe symptomatic hypertension or hypertension associated with organ damage. Used for patients who fail to respond to maximal therapeutic dosages of diuretic and two other antihypertensive agents. Treatment of alopecia androgenetica (**males:** baldness of vertex of scalp; **females:** diffuse hair loss or thinning of frontoparietal areas).

PRECAUTIONS

CONTRAINDICATIONS: Pheochromocytoma. **CAUTIONS:** Severe renal impairment, chronic CHF, coronary artery disease, recent MI (1 mo).

⧗ **LIFESPAN CONSIDERATIONS: Pregnancy/Lactation:** Crosses placenta. Distributed in breast milk. **Pregnancy Category C. Children:** No age-related precautions noted. **Elderly:** More sensitive to hypotensive effects. Age-related renal impairment may require dosage adjustment.

INTERACTIONS

DRUG: NSAIDs: May decrease the hypotensive effects of minoxidil. **Parenteral antihypertensives:** May increase hypotensive effect. **HERBAL:** None known. **FOOD:** None known. **LAB VALUES:** May increase plasma renin activity and BUN, serum alkaline phosphatase, serum creatinine, and serum sodium levels. May decrease blood Hgb and Hct levels and erythrocyte count.

AVAILABILITY

TABLETS (LONITEN): 2.5 mg, 10 mg. **TOPICAL SOLUTION (OTC):** 2% (20 mg/ml) (Rogaine), 5% (50 mg/ml) (Rogaine ExtraStrength).

ADMINISTRATION/HANDLING

PO

• Give without regard to food. Give with food if GI upset occurs. • Tablets may be crushed.

TOPICAL

• Shampoo, dry hair before applying medication. • Wash hands immediately after application. • Do not use hair dryer after application (reduces effectiveness).

INDICATIONS/ROUTES/DOSAGE

SEVERE SYMPTOMATIC HYPERTENSION, HYPERTENSION ASSOCIATED WITH ORGAN DAMAGE, HYPERTENSION THAT HAS FAILED TO RESPOND TO MAXIMAL THERAPEUTIC DOSAGES OF A DIURETIC OR TWO OTHER ANTIHYPERTENSIVES

PO: ADULTS, CHILDREN 12 YR AND OLDER: Initially, 5 mg/day. Increase with at least 3-day intervals to 10 mg, then 20 mg, then up to 40 mg/day in 1–2 doses. ELDERLY: Initially, 2.5 mg/day. May increase gradually. Maintenance: 10–40 mg/day. Maximum: 100 mg/day. CHILDREN YOUNGER THAN 12 YR: Initially, 0.1–0.2 mg/kg (5 mg maximum) daily. Gradually increase at a minimum of 3-day intervals. Maintenance: 0.25–1 mg/kg/day in 1–2 doses. **Maximum:** 50 mg/day.

HAIR REGROWTH

TOPICAL: ADULTS: 1 ml to affected areas of scalp 2 times a day. Total daily dose not to exceed 2 ml.

SIDE EFFECTS

FREQUENT: PO: Edema with concurrent weight gain, hypertrichosis (elongation, thickening, increased pigmentation of fine body hair; develops in 80% of patients within 3–6 wk after beginning therapy). **OCCASIONAL: PO:** T-wave changes (usually revert to pretreatment state with continued therapy or drug withdrawal). **Topical:** Pruritus, rash, dry or flaking skin, erythema. **RARE: PO:** Breast tenderness, headache, photosensitivity reaction. **Topical:** Allergic reaction, alopecia, burning sensation at scalp, soreness at hair root, headache, visual disturbances.

ADVERSE REACTIONS/ TOXIC EFFECTS

Tachycardia and angina pectoris may occur because of increased oxygen demands associated with increased heart rate and cardiac output. Fluid and electrolyte imbalance and CHF may occur, especially if a diuretic is not given concurrently with minoxidil. Too rapid reduction in BP may result in syncope, cerebrovascular accident (CVA), MI, and ocular or vestibular ischemia. Pericardial effusion and tamponade may be seen in patients with impaired renal function who are not on dialysis.

BASELINE ASSESSMENT

Assess BP on both arms and take pulse for 1 full min immediately before giving medication. If pulse increases 20 beats or more/min over baseline or systolic or diastolic BP decreases more than 20 mm Hg, withhold drug, contact physician.

INTERVENTION/EVALUATION

Monitor fluids and electrolytes, body weight, BP. Assess for peripheral edema. Assess for signs of CHF (cough, rales at base of lungs, cool extremities, dyspnea on exertion). Monitor fluid, serum electrolyte levels. Assess for distant or muffled heart sounds by auscultation (pericardial effusion, tamponade).

PATIENT/FAMILY TEACHING

• Maximum BP response occurs in 3–7 days. • Reversible growth of fine body hair may begin 3–6 wk following initiation of treatment. • When used topically for stimulation of hair growth, treatment must continue on a permanent basis—cessation of treatment will begin reversal of new hair growth. • Avoid exposure to sunlight, artificial light sources.

mirtazapine

mir-**taz**-a-peen

(Remeron, Remeron Soltab)

Do not confuse Remeron with Premarin.

◆CLASSIFICATION

PHARMACOTHERAPEUTIC: Tetracyclic compound. **CLINICAL:** Antidepressant (see p. 38C).

ACTION

A tetracyclic compound that acts as an antagonist at presynaptic

M

alpha$_2$-adrenergic receptors, increasing both norepinephrine and serotonin neurotransmission. Has low anticholinergic activity. Therapeutic Effect: Relieves depression and produces sedative effects.

PHARMACOKINETICS

Rapidly and completely absorbed after PO administration; absorption not affected by food. Protein binding: 85%. Metabolized in the liver. Primarily excreted in urine. Unknown if removed by hemodialysis. Half-life: 20–40 hr (longer in males [37 hr] than females [26 hr]).

USES

Treatment of depression.

PRECAUTIONS

CONTRAINDICATIONS: Use within 14 days of MAOIs. CAUTIONS: Cardiovascular or GI disorders, prostatic hyperplasia, urinary retention, narrow-angle glaucoma, renal or hepatic impairment.

⧗ LIFESPAN CONSIDERATIONS: Pregnancy/Lactation: Unknown if distributed in breast milk. Pregnancy Category C. Children: Safety and efficacy not established. Elderly: Age-related renal impairment may require dosage adjustment.

INTERACTIONS

DRUG: Alcohol, diazepam: May increase impairment of cognition and motor skills. MAOIs: May increase the risk of neuroleptic malignant syndrome, hypertensive crisis, and severe seizures. HERBAL: None known. FOOD: None known. LAB VALUES: May increase serum cholesterol, triglyceride, AST, and ALT levels.

AVAILABILITY (Rx)

TABLETS (REMERON): 15 mg, 30 mg, 45 mg. TABLETS (ORALLY-DISINTE-GRATING [REMERON SOLTAB]): 15 mg, 30 mg, 45 mg.

ADMINISTRATION/HANDLING

PO
• Give without regard to food. • May crush or break scored tablets.

INDICATIONS/ROUTES/DOSAGE

DEPRESSION
PO: ADULTS: Initially, 15 mg at bedtime. May increase by 15 mg/day q1–2wk. Maximum: 45 mg/day. ELDERLY: Initially, 7.5 mg at bedtime. May increase by 7.5–15 mg/day q1–2wk. Maximum: 45 mg/day.

SIDE EFFECTS

FREQUENT: Somnolence (54%), dry mouth (25%), increased appetite (17%), constipation (13%), weight gain (12%). OCCASIONAL: Asthenia (8%), dizziness (7%), flu-like symptoms (5%), abnormal dreams (4%). RARE: Abdominal discomfort, vasodilation, paresthesia, acne, dry skin, thirst, arthralgia.

ADVERSE REACTIONS/ TOXIC EFFECTS

Mirtazapine poses a higher risk of seizures than tricyclic antidepressants, especially in those with no previous history of seizures. Overdose may produce cardiovascular effects, such as severe orthostatic hypotension, dizziness, tachycardia, palpitations, and arrhythmias. Abrupt discontinuation after prolonged therapy may produce headache, malaise, nausea, vomiting, and vivid dreams. Agranulocytosis occurs rarely.

NURSING CONSIDERATIONS

BASELINE ASSESSMENT

For patients on long-term therapy, liver and renal function tests, blood counts should be performed periodically.

INTERVENTION/EVALUATION

Supervise suicidal-risk patient closely during early therapy (as depression lessens, energy level improves, increasing suicide potential). Children and adolescents are at an increased risk for suicidal thoughts and behavior and worsening of depression, especially during the first few months of therapy. Assess appearance, behavior, speech pattern, level of interest, mood. Monitor for hypotension, arrhythmias.

PATIENT/FAMILY TEACHING

• Take as a single bedtime dose. • Avoid alcohol, depressant or sedating medications. • Avoid tasks requiring mental alertness, motor skills until response to drug established.

misoprostol

mis-oh-**pros**-toll

(Cytotec)

Do not confuse misoprostol with mifepristone, or Cytotec with Cytoxan.

FIXED-COMBINATION(S)

Arthrotec: misoprostol/diclofenac (an NSAID): 200 mcg/50 mg; 200 mcg/75 mg.

CLASSIFICATION

PHARMACOTHERAPEUTIC: Prostaglandin. **CLINICAL:** Antisecretory, gastric protectant.

ACTION

Gastric antisecretory agent that replaces the protective prostaglandins consumed with prostaglandin-inhibiting therapies (e.g., NSAIDs). **Therapeutic Effect:** Reduces acid secretion from the gastric parietal cell, stimulates bicarbonate production from gastric/duodenal mucosa.

PHARMACOKINETICS

Route	Onset	Peak	Duration
PO	30 min	1–1.5 hr	3–6 hr min

Rapidly absorbed from GI tract. Protein binding: 80%–90%. Rapidly converted to active metabolite. Primarily excreted in urine. Unknown if removed by hemodialysis. **Half-life:** 20–40 min.

USES

Prevention of NSAID-induced gastric ulcers and in patients at high risk of developing gastric ulcer/gastric ulcer complications. **OFF-LABEL:** Treatment of therapeutic, second trimester abortion, cervical ripening, duodenal ulcer, treatment and prevention of NSAID-associated gastric ulcer, induction of labor.

PRECAUTIONS

CONTRAINDICATIONS: Pregnancy (produces uterine contractions). **CAUTIONS:** Renal impairment.

⏳ **LIFESPAN CONSIDERATIONS: Pregnancy/Lactation:** Unknown if distributed in breast milk. Produces uterine contractions, uterine bleeding, expulsion of products of conception (abortifacient property). **Pregnancy Category X. Children:** Safety and efficacy not established. **Elderly:** No age-related precautions noted.

INTERACTIONS

DRUG: Magnesium antacids: Enhance diarrhea associated with misoprostol. **HERBAL:** None known. **FOOD:** None known. **LAB VALUES:** None known.

AVAILABILITY (Rx)

TABLETS: 100 mcg, 200 mcg.

ADMINISTRATION/HANDLING
PO
• Give with or after meals (minimizes diarrhea).

INDICATIONS/ROUTES/DOSAGE
PREVENTION OF NSAID-INDUCED GASTRIC ULCER
PO: ADULTS: 200 mcg 4 times a day with food (last dose at bedtime). Continue for duration of NSAID therapy. May reduce

dosage to 100 mcg if 200-mcg dose is not tolerated. ELDERLY: 100–200 mcg 4 times a day with food.

SIDE EFFECTS

FREQUENT (40%–20%): Abdominal pain, diarrhea. **OCCASIONAL (3%–2%):** Nausea, flatulence, dyspepsia, headache. **RARE (1%):** Vomiting, constipation.

ADVERSE REACTIONS/ TOXIC EFFECTS

Overdosage may produce sedation, tremor, seizures, dyspnea, palpitations, hypotension, bradycardia.

NURSING CONSIDERATIONS

BASELINE ASSESSMENT

Question for possibility of pregnancy before initiating therapy (Pregnancy Risk Category X).

PATIENT/FAMILY TEACHING

• Avoid magnesium-containing antacids (minimizes potential for diarrhea). • Women of childbearing potential must not be pregnant before or during medication therapy (may result in hospitalization, surgery, infertility, fetal death). • Incidence of diarrhea may be lessened by taking immediately following meals.

---

mitomycin   ⚑

my-toe-**my**-sin
(Mutamycin)

◆CLASSIFICATION

PHARMACOTHERAPEUTIC: Antibiotic. **CLINICAL:** Antineoplastic (see p. 76C).

ACTION

An antibiotic that acts similar to an alkylating agent, cross-linking with strands of DNA. Therapeutic Effect: Inhibits DNA and RNA synthesis.

PHARMACOKINETICS

Widely distributed. Does not cross the blood-brain barrier. Primarily metabolized in the liver and excreted in urine. Half-life: 50 min.

USES

Treatment of disseminated adenocarcinoma of stomach, pancreas. OFF-LABEL: Treatment of biliary, bladder, breast, cervical, colorectal, head and neck, and lung carcinomas; chronic myelocytic leukemia, esophageal cancer.

PRECAUTIONS

CONTRAINDICATIONS: Coagulation disorders and bleeding tendencies, platelet count less than 75,000/mm^3, serious infection, serum creatinine level greater than 1.7 mg/dl, WBC count less than 3,000/mm^3. **CAUTIONS:** Myelosuppression, renal or hepatic impairment.

⏳ LIFESPAN CONSIDERATIONS: **Pregnancy/Lactation:** If possible, avoid use during pregnancy, especially first trimester. Breast-feeding not recommended. Safety in pregnancy not established. **Pregnancy Category: Safety in pregnancy has not been established. Children:** No age-related precautions noted. **Elderly:** Age-related renal impairment may require dosage adjustment.

INTERACTIONS

DRUG: **Bone marrow depressants:** May increase myelosuppression. **Live-virus vaccines:** May potentiate virus replication, increase vaccine side effects, and decrease the patient's antibody response to the vaccine. HERBAL: None known. FOOD: None known. LAB VALUES: May increase BUN and serum creatinine levels.

AVAILABILITY (Rx)

POWDER FOR INJECTION: 5 mg, 20 mg, 40 mg.

ADMINISTRATION/HANDLING

◄ **ALERT** ► May be carcinogenic, mutagenic, or teratogenic. Handle with extreme care during preparation and administration. Give via IV push, IV infusion. Extremely irritating to vein. May produce pain with induration on injection, thrombophlebitis, paresthesia.

 IV

Reconstitution • Reconstitute 5-mg vial with 10 ml sterile water for injection (40 ml for 20-mg vial) to provide solution containing 0.5 mg/ml. • Do not shake vial to dissolve. • Allow vial to stand at room temperature until complete dissolution occurs. • For IV infusion, further dilute with 50–100 ml D_5W or 0.9% NaCl.

Rate of administration • Give IV push over 5–10 min. • Give IV through tubing of functional IV catheter or running IV infusion. • Extravasation may produce cellulitis, ulceration, tissue sloughing. Terminate administration immediately, inject ordered antidote. Apply ice intermittently for up to 72 hr; keep area elevated.

Storage • Use only clear, blue-gray solutions. • Concentration of 0.5 mg/ml is stable for 7 days at room temperature or 2 wk if refrigerated. Further diluted solution with D_5W is stable for 3 hr, 24 hr if diluted with 0.9% NaCl.

IV INCOMPATIBILITIES

Aztreonam (Azactam), bleomycin (Blenoxane), cefepime (Maxipime), filgrastim (Neupogen), heparin, piperacillin/tazobactam (Zosyn), sargramostin (Leukine), vinorelbine (Navelbine).

IV COMPATIBILITIES

Cisplatin (Platinol AQ), cyclophosphamide (Cytoxan), doxorubicin (Adriamycin), 5-fluorouracil, granisetron (Kytril), leucovorin, methotrexate, ondansetron (Zofran), vinblastine (Velban), vincristine (Oncovin).

INDICATIONS/ROUTES/DOSAGE

DISSEMINATED ADENOCARCINOMA OF PANCREAS AND STOMACH

IV: ADULTS, ELDERLY, CHILDREN: Initially, 10–20 mg/m² as single dose. Repeat q6–8wk. Give additional courses only after platelet and WBC counts are within acceptable levels, as shown below.

Leukocytes/ mm³	Platelets/ mm³	% of Prior Dose to Give
4,000	More than 100,000	100%
3,000–3,999	75,000–99,000	100%
2,000–2,999	25,000–74,999	70%
1,999 or less	Less than 25,000	50%

DOSAGE IN RENAL IMPAIRMENT

Patients with creatinine clearance less than 10 ml/min should receive 75% of normal dose.

SIDE EFFECTS

FREQUENT (greater than 10%): Fever, anorexia, nausea, vomiting. **OCCASIONAL (10%–2%):** Stomatitis, paraesthesia, purple color bands on nails, rash, alopecia, unusual fatigue. **RARE (less than 1%):** Thrombophlebitis, cellulitis, extravasation.

ADVERSE REACTIONS/ TOXIC EFFECTS

Marked myelosuppression may result in hematologic toxicity (manifested as leukopenia, thrombocytopenia and to a lesser extent, anemia), usually within 2–4 wk after the start of therapy. Renal toxicity (manifested as increased BUN and serum creatinine levels) and pulmonary toxicity (manifested as dyspnea, cough, hemoptysis, and pneumonia) may occur. Long-term therapy may produce hemolytic uremic syndrome, characterized by hemolytic anemia, thrombocytopenia, renal failure, and hypertension.

M

NURSING CONSIDERATIONS

BASELINE ASSESSMENT

Obtain CBC with differential, PT, bleeding time, before and periodically during therapy. Antiemetics before and during therapy may alleviate nausea and vomiting.

INTERVENTION/EVALUATION

Monitor hematologic status, renal function studies. Assess IV site for phlebitis, extravasation. Monitor for hematologic toxicity (fever, sore throat, signs of local infection, unusual ecchymosis or bleeding from any site), symptoms of anemia (excessive fatigue, weakness). Assess for renal toxicity (foul odor from urine, elevated BUN, serum creatinine).

PATIENT/FAMILY TEACHING

• Maintain fastidious oral hygiene. • Immediately report any stinging, burning, pain at injection site. • Do not have immunizations without physician's approval (drug lowers body's resistance to infection). • Avoid contact with those who have recently received live virus vaccine. • Alopecia is reversible, but new hair growth may have different color, texture. • Contact physician if nausea or vomiting, fever, sore throat, bruising, bleeding, shortness of breath, painful urination occur.

mitotane

(Lysodren)
See Cancer chemotherapeutic agents (p. 76C)

mitoxantrone

my-toe-**zan**-trone
(Novantrone)

◆ CLASSIFICATION

PHARMACOTHERAPEUTIC: Anthracenedione. **CLINICAL:** Nonvesicant, antineoplastic (see p. 77C).

ACTION

An anthracenedione that inhibits B-cell, T-cell, and macrophage proliferation and DNA and RNA synthesis. Active throughout the entire cell cycle. **Therapeutic Effect:** Causes cell death.

PHARMACOKINETICS

Protein binding: 78%. Widely distributed. Metabolized in the liver. Primarily eliminated in feces by the biliary system. Not removed by hemodialysis. **Half-life:** 2.3–13 days.

USES

Treatment of acute, nonlymphocytic leukemia (monocytic, myelogenous, promyelocytic), late-stage hormone-resistant prostate cancer, multiple sclerosis. **OFF-LABEL:** Treatment of acute lymphocytic leukemia, breast or hepatic carcinoma, non-Hodgkin's lymphoma.

PRECAUTIONS

CONTRAINDICATIONS: Baseline left ventricular ejection fraction less than 50%, cumulative lifetime mitoxantrone dose of 140 mg/m^2 or more, multiple sclerosis with hepatic impairment. **CAUTIONS:** Preexisting bone marrow suppression, previous treatment with cardiotoxic medications, hepatobiliary impairment.

⧗ **LIFESPAN CONSIDERATIONS: Pregnancy/Lactation:** If possible, avoid use during pregnancy, especially first trimester. May cause fetal harm. Breastfeeding not recommended. **Pregnancy Category D. Children:** Safety and efficacy not established. **Elderly:** No age-related precautions noted.

 see color pill atlas ⬧ herb underlined – top prescribed drug

INTERACTIONS

DRUG: **Antigout medications:** May decrease the effects of these drugs. **Bone marrow depressants:** May increase myelosuppression. **Live virus vaccines:** May potentiate virus replication, increase vaccine side effects, and decrease the patient's antibody response to the vaccine. HERBAL: None known. FOOD: None known. LAB VALUES: May increase serum bilirubin and uric acid, AST, and ALT levels.

AVAILABILITY (Rx)

INJECTION: 2 mg/ml.

ADMINISTRATION/HANDLING

◄ ALERT ► May be carcinogenic, mutagenic, teratogenic. Handle with extreme care during preparation/administration. Give by IV injection, IV infusion. Must dilute before administration.

 IV

Reconstitution • Dilute with at least 50 ml D_5W or 0.9% NaCl.

Rate of administration • Do not administer by subcutaneous, IM, intrathecal, or intra-arterial injection. • Do not give IV push over less than 3 min. • Give IV bolus over at least 3 min, IV intermittent infusion over 15–60 min, or IV continuous infusion (0.02–0.5 mg/ml) in D_5W or 0.9% NaCl.

Storage • Store vials at room temperature.

▓ IV INCOMPATIBILITIES

Aztreonam (Azactam), cefepime (Maxipime), heparin, paclitaxel (Taxol), piperacillin and tazobactam (Zosyn).

IV COMPATIBILITIES

Allopurinol (Aloprim), etoposide (VePesid), gemcitabine (Gemzar), granisetron (Kytril), ondansetron (Zofran), potassium chloride.

INDICATIONS/ROUTES/DOSAGE

LEUKEMIAS

IV: ADULTS, ELDERLY, CHILDREN 2 YR AND OLDER: 12 mg/m^2 once a day for 2–3 days. CHILDREN YOUNGER THAN 2 YR: 0.4 mg/kg once a day for 3–5 days.

ACUTE LEUKEMIA IN RELAPSE

IV: ADULTS, ELDERLY, CHILDREN OLDER THAN 2 YR: 8–12 mg/m^2 once a day for 4–5 days.

ACUTE NONLYMPHOCYTIC LEUKEMIA

IV: ADULTS, ELDERLY, CHILDREN OLDER THAN 2 YR: 10 mg/m^2 once a day for 3–5 days.

SOLID TUMORS

IV: ADULTS, ELDERLY: 12–14 mg/m^2 once q3–4wk. CHILDREN: 18–20 mg/m^2 once q3–4 wk.

PROSTATE CANCER

IV: ADULTS, ELDERLY: 12–14 mg/m^2 every 21 days.

MULTIPLE SCLEROSIS

IV: ADULTS, ELDERLY: 12 mg/m^2/dose q3mo.

SIDE EFFECTS

FREQUENT (greater than 10%): Nausea, vomiting, diarrhea, cough, headache, stomatitis, abdominal discomfort, fever, alopecia. **OCCASIONAL (9%–4%):** Ecchymosis, fungal infection, conjunctivitis, UTI. **RARE (3%):** Arrhythmias.

ADVERSE REACTIONS/ TOXIC EFFECTS

Myelosuppression may be severe, resulting in GI bleeding, hematologic toxicity, sepsis, and pneumonia. Renal failure, seizures, jaundice, and CHF may occur. Cardiotoxicity has been reported during therapy.

NURSING CONSIDERATIONS

BASELINE ASSESSMENT

Offer emotional support. Establish baseline for CBC with differential, temperature, pulse rate/quality, respiratory status.

M

INTERVENTION/EVALUATION

Monitor hematologic status, pulmonary function studies, liver/renal function tests. Monitor for stomatitis, fever, signs of local infection, unusual ecchymosis/bleeding from any site. Extravasation produces swelling, pain, burning, blue discoloration of skin.

PATIENT/FAMILY TEACHING

• Urine will appear blue/green for 24 hr after administration. Blue tint to sclera may also appear. • Maintain adequate daily fluid intake (may protect against renal impairment). • Do not have immunizations without physician's approval (drug lowers body's resistance to infection). • Avoid crowds, those with infection. • Contraceptive measures recommended during therapy.

mivacurium chloride

(Mivacron)

See Neuromuscular blockers (p. 112C)

Mobic, *see meloxicam*

modafinil

mode-ah-**feen**-awl

(Alertec ✤, Provigil, Sparlon)

◆ CLASSIFICATION

PHARMACOTHERAPEUTIC: Alpha₁-agonist. **CLINICAL:** Wakefulness-promoting agent, antinarcoleptic.

ACTION

An alpha₁-agonist that may bind to dopamine reuptake carrier sites, increasing alpha activity and decreasing delta, theta, and beta brain wave activity. **Therapeutic Effect:** Reduces the number of sleep episodes and total daytime sleep.

PHARMACOKINETICS

Well absorbed. Protein binding: 60%. Widely distributed. Metabolized in the liver. Excreted by the kidneys. Unknown if removed by hemodialysis. **Half-life:** 8–10 hr.

USES

Treatment of excessive daytime sleepiness associated with narcolepsy, other sleep disorders. **OFF-LABEL:** Treatment of attention deficit hyperactivity disorder, brain injury–related underarousal, depression, endozepine stupor, multiple sclerosis–related fatigue, parkinson-related fatigue, seasonal affective disorder.

PRECAUTIONS

CONTRAINDICATIONS: None known. **CAUTIONS:** History of clinically significant manifestation of mitral valve prolapse, left ventricular hypertrophy, hepatic impairment, history of seizures.

⧗ **LIFESPAN CONSIDERATIONS: Pregnancy/Lactation:** Unknown if drug is excreted in breast milk. Use caution if given to pregnant women. **Pregnancy Category C. Children:** Safety and efficacy not established in those younger than 16 yr. **Elderly:** Age-related renal or hepatic impairment may require decreased dosage.

INTERACTIONS

DRUG: **Cyclosporine, oral contraceptives, theophylline:** May decrease plasma concentrations of these drugs. **Diazepam, phenytoin, propranolol, tricyclic antidepressants,**

🖉 see color pill atlas   ▱ herb   underlined – top prescribed drug

warfarin: May increase plasma concentrations of these drugs. **Other CNS stimulants:** May increase CNS stimulation. HERBAL: None known. FOOD: None known. LAB VALUES: None known.

AVAILABILITY (Rx)

TABLETS: 100 mg, 200 mg. **SPARLON:** 85 mg, 170 mg, 255 mg, 340 mg, 425 mg.

ADMINISTRATION/HANDLING

PO
- Give without regard to meals.

INDICATIONS/ROUTES/DOSAGE

NARCOLEPSY, OTHER SLEEP DISORDERS
PO: ADULTS, ELDERLY: 200 mg/day. **(SPARLON):** 85–425 mg once daily.

SIDE EFFECTS

FREQUENT: Anxiety, insomnia, nausea. **OCCASIONAL:** Anorexia, diarrhea, dizziness, dry mouth or skin, muscle stiffness, polydipsia, rhinitis, paraesthesia, tremor, headache, vomiting.

ADVERSE REACTIONS/ TOXIC EFFECTS

Agitation, excitation, hypertension, and insomnia may occur.

NURSING CONSIDERATIONS

BASELINE ASSESSMENT
Obtain baseline evidence of narcolepsy or other sleep disorders, including pattern, environmental situations, length of sleep episodes. Question for sudden loss of muscle tone (cataplexy) precipitated by strong emotional responses before sleep episode. Assess frequency/severity of sleep episodes before drug therapy.

INTERVENTION/EVALUATION
Monitor sleep pattern, evidence of restlessness during sleep, length of insomnia episodes at night. Assess for dizziness, anxiety; initiate fall precautions. Sugarless gum, sips of tepid water may relieve dry mouth.

PATIENT/FAMILY TEACHING
- Avoid tasks that require alertness, motor skills until response to drug is established. • Do not increase dose without physician approval. • Use alternative contraceptives during therapy and 1 mo after discontinuing modafinil (reduces effectiveness of oral contraceptives).

moexipril hydrochloride

moe-**ex**-a-prile
(Univasc)

FIXED-COMBINATION(S)

Uniretic: moexipril/hydrochlorothiazide (a diuretic): 7.5 mg/12.5 mg, 15 mg/12.5 mg, 15 mg/25 mg.

◆CLASSIFICATION

PHARMACOTHERAPEUTIC: Angiotensin-converting enzyme (ACE) inhibitor. **CLINICAL:** Antihypertensive (see p. 7C).

ACTION

An ACE inhibitor that suppresses the renin-angiotensin-aldosterone system and prevents conversion of angiotensin I to angiotensin II, a potent vasoconstrictor; may also inhibit angiotensin II at local vascular and renal sites. Therapeutic Effect: Reduces peripheral arterial resistance and lowers BP.

PHARMACOKINETICS

Route	Onset	Peak	Duration
PO	1 hr	3–6 hr	24 hr

Incompletely absorbed from the GI tract. Food decreases drug absorption. Rapidly converted to active metabolite. Protein binding: 50%. Primarily recovered in feces, partially excreted in urine.

M

Unknown if removed by dialysis. **Half-life:** 1 hr, metabolite 2–9 hr.

USES

Treatment of hypertension. Used alone or in combination with thiazide diuretics.

PRECAUTIONS

CONTRAINDICATIONS: History of angioedema from previous treatment with ACE inhibitors. **CAUTIONS:** Renal impairment, dialysis, hypovolemia, coronary or cerebrovascular insufficiency, hyperkalemia, aortic stenosis, ischemic heart disease, angina, severe CHF, cerebrovascular disease, those with sodium depletion or on diuretic therapy.

⧗ **LIFESPAN CONSIDERATIONS: Pregnancy/Lactation:** Crosses placenta. Unknown if distributed in breast milk. **Pregnancy Category C (D if used in second or third trimesters). Children:** Safety and efficacy not established. **Elderly:** Age-related renal impairment may require dosage adjustment.

INTERACTIONS

DRUG: Alcohol, antihypertensives, diuretics: May increase the effects of moexipril. **Lithium:** May increase lithium blood concentration and risk of lithium toxicity. **NSAIDs:** May decrease the effects of moexipril. **Potassium-sparing diuretics, potassium supplements:** May cause hyperkalemia. **HERBAL:** None known. **FOOD:** None known. **LAB VALUES:** May increase BUN, serum alkaline phosphatase, serum bilirubin, serum creatinine, serum potassium, AST, and ALT levels. May decrease serum sodium levels. May cause positive serum ANA titer.

AVAILABILITY (Rx)

TABLETS: 7.5 mg, 15 mg.

ADMINISTRATION/HANDLING

PO

• Give 1 hr before meals. • Tablets may be crushed.

INDICATIONS/ROUTES/DOSAGE

HYPERTENSION

PO: ADULTS, ELDERLY: For patients not receiving diuretics, initial dose is 7.5 mg once a day 1 hr before meals. Adjust according to BP effect. Maintenance: 7.5–30 mg a day in 1–2 divided doses 1 hr before meals.

HYPERTENSION IN PATIENTS WITH IMPAIRED RENAL FUNCTION

PO: ADULTS, ELDERLY: 3.75 mg once a day in patients with creatinine clearance of 40 ml/min. **Maximum:** May titrate up to 15 mg/day.

SIDE EFFECTS

OCCASIONAL: Cough, headache (6%); dizziness (4%); fatigue (3%). **RARE:** Flushing, rash, myalgia, nausea, vomiting.

ADVERSE REACTIONS/ TOXIC EFFECTS

Excessive hypotension ("first-dose syncope") may occur in patients with CHF and in those who are severely salt or volume depleted. Angioedema (swelling of face and lips) and hyperkalemia occur rarely. Agranulocytosis and neutropenia may be noted in those with collagen vascular disease, including scleroderma and systemic lupus erythematosus, and impaired renal function. Nephrotic syndrome may be noted in those with history of renal disease.

NURSING CONSIDERATIONS

BASELINE ASSESSMENT

Obtain BP, apical pulse immediately before each dose, in addition to regular monitoring (be alert to fluctuations). If excessive reduction in BP occurs, place patient in supine position, feet slightly elevated. Renal function tests should be performed before therapy begins. In patients with renal impairment, autoimmune disease, taking drugs that affect leukocytes or immune response, CBC

M

with differential count should be performed before therapy, q2wk for 3 mo, then periodically thereafter.

INTERVENTION/EVALUATION

Monitor BP, serum potassium, renal function, WBC count. Observe for hypotensive effect within 1–3 hr of first dose or increase in dose. Assist with ambulation if dizziness occurs.

PATIENT/FAMILY TEACHING

• Do not abruptly stop medication. • Inform physician of sore throat, fever, difficulty breathing, chest pain, cough. • Notify physician of signs of angioedema. • Arrhythmias may occur. • To reduce hypotensive effect, rise slowly from lying to sitting position, permit legs to dangle momentarily before standing.

---

molindone hydrochloride

(Moban)

See Antipsychotics

---

mometasone

mo-**met**-a-sone

(Elocon)

mometasone furoate monohydrate

(Asmanex Twisthaler, Nasonex)

◆ CLASSIFICATION

PHARMACOTHERAPEUTIC: Adrenocorticosteroid. **CLINICAL:** Anti-inflammatory.

ACTION

An adrenocorticosteroid that inhibits the release of inflammatory cells into nasal tissue, preventing early activation of the allergic reaction. **Therapeutic Effect:** Decreases response to seasonal and perennial rhinitis.

PHARMACOKINETICS

Undetectable in plasma. Protein binding: 98%–99%. The swallowed portion undergoes extensive metabolism. Excreted primarily through bile and, to a lesser extent, urine. **Half-life:** 5.8 hr (nasal).

USES

Treatment of nasal symptoms of seasonal/perennial allergic rhinitis in adults, children over 2 yr. Prophylaxis of nasal symptoms of seasonal allergic rhinitis in adults, adolescents over 12 yr. Treatment of nasal polyps.

PRECAUTIONS

CONTRAINDICATIONS: Hypersensitivity to any corticosteroid, persistently positive sputum cultures for *Candida albicans*, status asthmaticus (inhalation), systemic fungal infections, untreated localized infection involving nasal mucosa. **CAUTIONS:** Adrenal insufficiency, cirrhosis, glaucoma, hypothyroidism, untreated infection, osteoporosis, tuberculosis.

⧗ **LIFESPAN CONSIDERATIONS: Pregnancy/Lactation:** Unknown if drug crosses placenta or is distributed in breast milk. **Pregnancy Category C. Children:** Prolonged treatment/high doses may decrease short-term growth rate, cortisol secretion. **Elderly:** No age-related precautions noted.

INTERACTIONS

DRUG: Ketoconazole: May increase mometasone plasma concentrations (inhalation). **HERBAL:** None known. **FOOD:** None known. **LAB VALUES:** None known.

AVAILABILITY (Rx)

NASAL SPRAY (NASONEX): 50 mcg/spray. **CREAM (ELOCON):** 0.1%. **LOTION (ELOCON):** 0.1%. **OINTMENT (ELOCON):** 0.1%. **ORAL INHALER (ASMANEX TWISTHALER):** 220 mcg.

ADMINISTRATION/HANDLING

INHALATION

• Each actuation contains 220 mcg of mometasone. • Tell the patient to hold the twistinhaler straight up with the pink portion (base) on the bottom, then remove the cap. • Instruct the patient to exhale fully. • Instruct the patient to bring the mouthpiece up to the mouth and firmly close his or her lips around the mouthpiece and take in a fast, deep breath. • Tell the patient to remove the twisthaler and hold his or her breath for 10 seconds. • Remind the patient to wipe twisthaler mouthpiece dry and to replace the cap. • Instruct the patient to rinse his or her mouth with water without swallowing after every dose.

INTRANASAL

• Shake well before each use. • Clear nasal passages as much as possible before administration of nasal spray. • Insert spray tip into nostril, pointing toward nasal passages, away from nasal septum. • Spray into nostril while holding other nostril closed, concurrently inspire through nose to permit medication as high into nasal passages as possible.

TOPICAL

• Apply a thin layer of cream, lotion, or ointment to cover the affected area. Rub it in gently. • Do not cover area with occlusive dressing.

INDICATIONS/ROUTES/DOSAGE

ALLERGIC RHINITIS

NASAL SPRAY: ADULTS, ELDERLY, CHILDREN 12 YR AND OLDER: 2 sprays in each nostril once a day. CHILDREN 2–11 YR: 1 spray in each nostril once a day.

ASTHMA

INHALATION: ADULTS, ELDERLY, CHILDREN 12 YR AND OLDER: Initially, inhale 220 mcg (1 puff) once a day. **Maximum:** 880 mcg once a day.

SKIN DISEASE

TOPICAL: ADULTS, ELDERLY, CHILDREN 12 YR AND OLDER: Apply cream, lotion, or ointment to affected area once a day.

NASAL POLYP

NASAL SPRAY: ADULTS, ELDERLY: 2 sprays in each nostril twice a day.

SIDE EFFECTS

OCCASIONAL: Inhalation: Headache, allergic rhinitis, upper respiratory infection, muscle pain, fatigue. **Nasal:** Nasal irritation, stinging. **Topical:** Burning. **RARE: Inhalation:** Abdominal pain, dyspepsia, nausea. **Nasal:** Nasal or pharyngeal candidiasis. **Topical:** Pruritus.

ADVERSE REACTIONS/ TOXIC EFFECTS

An acute hypersensitivity reaction, including urticaria, angioedema, and severe bronchospasm, occurs rarely. Transfer from systemic to local steroid therapy may unmask previously suppressed bronchial asthma condition.

NURSING CONSIDERATIONS

BASELINE ASSESSMENT

Question for hypersensitivity to any corticosteroids.

INTERVENTION/EVALUATION

Teach proper use of nasal spray. Clear nasal passages before use. Contact physician if no improvement in symptoms, sneezing, nasal irritation occur.

PATIENT/FAMILY TEACHING

• Do not change dose schedule or stop taking drug; must taper off gradually under medical supervision. • Contact physician if symptoms do not improve; sneezing, nasal irritation occur. • Clear nasal passages prior to use. • Inhale rapidly and deeply and rinse mouth after inhalation. • With topical form, don't cover affected area with bandage or dressing.

Monopril, *see fosinopril*

---

montelukast

mon-**tee**-leu-cast
(Singulair)

CLASSIFICATION
PHARMACOTHERAPEUTIC: Leukotriene receptor inhibitor. **CLINICAL:** Antiasthmatic (see p. 68C).

ACTION
An antiasthmatic that binds to cysteinyl leukotriene receptors, inhibiting the effects of leukotrienes on bronchial smooth muscle. **Therapeutic Effect:** Decreases bronchoconstriction, vascular permeability, mucosal edema, and mucus production.

PHARMACOKINETICS

Route	Onset	Peak	Duration
PO	N/A	N/A	24 hr
PO (chewable)	N/A	N/A	24 hr

Rapidly absorbed from the GI tract. Protein binding: 99%. Extensively metabolized in the liver. Excreted almost exclusively in feces. **Half-life:** 2.7–5.5 hr (slightly longer in the elderly).

USES
Prophylaxis, chronic treatment of asthma. Not for use in reversal of bronchospasm in acute asthma attacks, status asthmaticus, exercise-induced bronchospasm. Treatment of seasonal allergic rhinitis (hay fever). Relief of perennial allergic rhinitis.

PRECAUTIONS
CONTRAINDICATIONS: None known. **CAUTIONS:** Systemic corticosteroid treatment reduction during montelukast therapy, hepatic impairment.

⏳ **LIFESPAN CONSIDERATIONS: Pregnancy/Lactation:** Unknown if excreted in breast milk. Use during pregnancy only if necessary. **Pregnancy Category B. Children/Elderly:** No age-related precautions noted in those older than 6 yr or the elderly.

INTERACTIONS
DRUG: Phenobarbital, rifampin: May decrease the duration of action of montelukast. **Prednisone:** May decrease the bioavailability of montelukast. **HERBAL:** None known. **FOOD:** None known. **LAB VALUES:** May increase AST and ALT levels.

AVAILABILITY (Rx)
ORAL GRANULES: 4 mg. **TABLETS:** 10 mg. **TABLETS (CHEWABLE):** 4 mg, 5 mg.

ADMINISTRATION/HANDLING
PO
• Administer in the evening without regard to meals.

INDICATIONS/ROUTES/DOSAGE
BRONCHIAL ASTHMA, PERENNIAL ALLERGIC RHINITIS, SEASONAL ALLERGIC RHINITIS
PO: ADULTS, ELDERLY, ADOLESCENTS OLDER THAN 14 YR: One 10-mg tablet a day, taken in the evening. CHILDREN 6–14 YR: One 5-mg chewable tablet a day, taken in the evening. CHILDREN 1–5 YR: One 4-mg chewable tablet a day, taken in the evening.

SIDE EFFECTS
ADULTS, ADOLESCENTS 15 YR AND OLDER: FREQUENT (18%): Headache. **OCCASIONAL (4%):** Influenza. **RARE (3%–2%):** Abdominal pain, cough,

---

M

dyspepsia, dizziness, fatigue, dental pain. **CHILDREN 6–14 YR: RARE (less than 2%):** Diarrhea, laryngitis, pharyngitis, nausea, otitis media, sinusitis, viral infection.

ADVERSE REACTIONS/ TOXIC EFFECTS

None known.

NURSING CONSIDERATIONS

BASELINE ASSESSMENT

Chewable tablet contains phenylalanine (a component of aspartame); parents of phenylketonuric patients should be informed. Montelukast should not be abruptly substituted for inhaled or oral corticosteroids.

INTERVENTION/EVALUATION

Monitor rate, depth, rhythm, type of respirations; quality and rate of pulse. Assess lung sounds for rhonchi, wheezing, rales. Observe lips, fingernails for cyanosis (blue/dusky color in light-skinned patients, gray in dark-skinned patients).

PATIENT/FAMILY TEACHING

• Increase fluid intake (decreases lung secretion viscosity). • Take as prescribed, even during symptom-free periods as well as during exacerbations of asthma. • Do not alter/stop other asthma medications. • Drug is not for treatment of acute asthma attacks. • Patients with aspirin sensitivity should avoid aspirin, NSAIDs while taking montelukast.

moricizine hydrochloride

(Ethmozine)
See Antiarrhythmics (p. 15C)

---

morphine sulfate ⚐

mor-feen

(Astramorph PF, Avinza, DepoDur, Duramorph PF, Infumorph, Kadian, M-Eslon, <u>MS Contin</u>, MSIR, MS/S, Oramorph SR, Rapi-Ject, RMS, Roxanol, Roxanol-T, Statex ✦)

Do not confuse morphine with hydromorphone, or Roxanol with Roxicet.

◆CLASSIFICATION

PHARMACOTHERAPEUTIC: Narcotic agonist. **CLINICAL:** Opiate analgesic (**Schedule II**) (see p. 128C).

ACTION

An opioid agonist that binds with opioid receptors in the CNS. **Therapeutic Effect:** Alters the perception of and emotional response to pain; produces generalized CNS depression.

PHARMACOKINETICS

Route	Onset	Peak	Duration
Oral Solution	N/A	1 hr	3–5 hr
Tablets	N/A	1 hr	3–5 hr
Tablets (ER)	N/A	3–4 hr	8–12 hr
IV	Rapid	0.3 hr	3–5 hr
IM	5–30 min	0.5–1 hr	3–5 hr
Epidural	N/A	1 hr	12–20 hr
Subcutaneous	N/A	1.1–5 hr	3–5 hr
Rectal	N/A	0.5–1 hr	3–7 hr

Variably absorbed from the GI tract. Readily absorbed after IM or subcutaneous administration. Protein binding: 20%–35%. Widely distributed. Metabolized in the liver. Primarily excreted in urine. Removed by hemodialysis. **Half-life:** 2–3 hr. (Increased in patients with hepatic disease.)

USES

Relief of severe, acute, or chronic pain, analgesia during labor. Drug of choice for pain due to MI, dyspnea from pulmonary edema not resulting from chemical respiratory irritant.

PRECAUTIONS

CONTRAINDICATIONS: Acute or severe asthma, GI obstruction, paralytic ileus, severe hepatic or renal impairment, severe respiratory depression. **EXTREME CAUTION:** Chronic obstructive pulmonary disease (COPD), cor pulmonale, hypoxia, hypercapnia preexisting respiratory depression, head injury, increased intracrania pressure (ICP), severe hypotension. **CAUTIONS:** Biliary tract disease, pancreatitis, Addison's disease, hypothyroidism, urethral stricture, prostatic hypertrophy, debilitated patients, those with CNS depression, toxic psychosis, seizure disorders, alcoholism.

⧖ **LIFESPAN CONSIDERATIONS: Pregnancy/Lactation:** Crosses placenta. Distributed in breast milk. May prolong labor if administered in latent phase of first stage of labor or before cervical dilation of 4–5 cm has occurred. Respiratory depression may occur in neonate if mother received opiates during labor. Regular use of opiates during pregnancy may produce withdrawal symptoms in neonate (irritability, excessive crying, tremors, hyperactive reflexes, fever, vomiting, diarrhea, yawning, sneezing, seizures). **Pregnancy Category C (D if used for prolonged periods or at high dosages at term). Children:** Paradoxical excitement may occur; those younger than 2 yr are more susceptible to respiratory depressant effects. **Elderly:** Paradoxical excitement may occur. Age-related renal impairment may increase risk of urinary retention.

INTERACTIONS

DRUG: Alcohol, other CNS depressants: May increase CNS or respiratory depression and hypotension. **MAOIs:** May produce a severe, sometimes fatal reaction; expect to administer ¼ of usual morphine dose. **HERBAL:** None known. **FOOD:** None known. **LAB VALUES:** May increase serum amylase and lipase levels.

AVAILABILITY (Rx)

CAPSULES (EXTENDED-RELEASE): 20 mg (Kadian), 30 mg (Avinza, Kadian), 50 mg (Kadian), 60 mg (Avinza, Kadian), 90 mg (Avinza), 100 mg (Kadian), 120 mg (Avinza). **CAPSULES (MSIR):** 15 mg, 30 mg. **SOLUTION FOR INJECTION:** 0.5 mg/ml, 1 mg/ml, 2 mg/ml, 4 mg/ml, 5 mg/ml, 8 mg/ml, 10 mg/ml, 15 mg/ml, 25 mg/ml, 50 mg/ml. **SOLUTION FOR INJECTION:** 5% dextrose-20 mg morphine/100 ml, 5% dextrose-100 mg morphine/100 ml. **SOLUTION FOR INJECTION (PRESERVATIVE-FREE):** 0.5 mg/ml (Astramorph PF, Duramorph PF), 1 mg/ml (Astramorph PF, Duramorph PF), 10 mg/ml (Infumorph), 15 mg/ml, 25 mg/ml (Infumorph), 50 mg/ml. **EPIDURAL AND INTRATHECAL VIA INFUSION DEVICE (INFUMORPH):** 10 mg/ml, 25 mg/ml. **ORAL SOLUTION:** 10 mg/ml (MSIR), 20 mg/ml (MSIR, Roxanol), 100 mg/ml (Roxanol). **SUPPOSITORIES (RMS):** 5 mg, 10 mg, 20 mg, 30 mg. **TABLETS (MSIR):** 15 mg, 30 mg. **TABLETS (EXTENDED-RELEASE):** 15 mg (MS Contin, Oramorph SR), 30 mg (MS Contin, Oramorph SR), 60 mg (MS Contin, Oramorph SR), 100 mg (MS Contin, Oramorph SR), 200 mg (MS Contin). **LIPOSOMAL INJECTION (DEPODUR):** 10 mg/ml, 15 mg/1.5 ml, 20 mg/2 ml.

ADMINISTRATION/HANDLING

 IV

Reconstitution • May give undiluted. • For IV injection, may dilute 2.5–15 mg morphine in 4–5 ml sterile water for injection. • For continuous IV infusion, dilute to concentration of 0.1–1 mg/ml in D_5W and give through controlled infusion device.

M

Rate of administration • Always administer very slowly. Rapid IV increases risk of severe adverse reactions (apnea, chest wall rigidity, peripheral circulatory collapse, cardiac arrest, anaphylactoid effects).

Storage • Store at room temperature.

IM, SUBCUTANEOUS

• Administer slowly, rotating injection sites. • Patients with circulatory impairment experience higher risk of overdosage due to delayed absorption of repeated administration.

PO

• Mix liquid form with fruit juice to improve taste. • Do not crush, break extended-release capsule. • **Kadian:** May mix with applesauce immediately prior to administration.

RECTAL

• If suppository is too soft, chill for 30 min in refrigerator or run cold water over foil wrapper. • Moisten suppository with cold water before inserting well into rectum.

✷ IV INCOMPATIBILITIES

Amphotericin B complex (Abelcet, AmBisome, Amphotec), cefepime (Maxipime), doxorubicin liposomal (Doxil), thiopental.

IV COMPATIBILITIES

Amiodarone (Cordarone), atropine, bumetanide (Bumex), bupivacaine (Marcaine, Sensorcaine), diltiazem (Cardizem), diphenhydramine (Benadryl), dobutamine (Dobutrex), dopamine (Intropin), glycopyrrolate (Robinul), heparin, hydroxyzine (Vistaril), lidocaine, lorazepam (Ativan), magnesium, midazolam (Versed), milrinone (Primacor), nitroglycerin, potassium, propofol (Diprivan), total parenteral nutrition (TPN).

INDICATIONS/ROUTES/DOSAGE

◀ ALERT ▶ Dosage should be titrated to desired effect.

ANALGESIA

PO (PROMPT-RELEASE): ADULTS, ELDERLY: 10–30 mg q3–4h as needed. CHILDREN: 0.2–0.5 mg/kg q3–4h as needed.

◀ ALERT ▶ For the Avinza dosage below, be aware that this drug is to be administered once a day only.

◀ ALERT ▶ For the Kadian dosage information below, be aware that this drug is to be administered q12h or once a day only.

◀ ALERT ▶ Be aware that pediatric dosages of extended-release preparations Kadian and Avinza have not been established.

◀ ALERT ▶ For the MSContin and Oramorph SR dosage information below, be aware that the daily dosage is divided and given q8h or q12h.

PO (EXTENDED-RELEASE [AVINZA]): ADULTS, ELDERLY: Dosage requirement should be established using prompt-release formulations and is based on total daily dose. Avinza is given once a day only.

PO (EXTENDED-RELEASE [KADIAN]): ADULTS, ELDERLY: Dosage requirement should be established using prompt-release formulations and is based on total daily dose. Dose is given once a day or divided and given q12h.

PO (EXTENDED-RELEASE [MSCONTIN, ORAMORPH SR]): ADULTS, ELDERLY: Dosage requirement should be established using prompt-release formulations and is based on total daily dose. Daily dose is divided and given q8h or q12h. CHILDREN: 0.3–0.6 mg/kg/dose q12h.

IV: ADULTS, ELDERLY: 2.5–5 mg q3–4h as needed. Note: Repeated doses (e.g., 1–2 mg) may be given more frequently (e.g., every hour) if needed. CHILDREN: 0.05–0.1 mg/kg q3–4h as needed.

IV CONTINUOUS INFUSION: ADULTS, ELDERLY: 0.8–10 mg/hr. Range: Up to 80 mg/hr. CHILDREN: 10–30 mcg/kg/hr.

IM: ADULTS, ELDERLY: 5–10 mg q3–4h as needed. CHILDREN: 0.1 mg/kg q3–4h as needed.

EPIDURAL: ADULTS, ELDERLY: Initially, 1–6 mg bolus, infusion rate: 0.1–1 mg/h. **Maximum:** 10 mg/24 h.

INTRATHECAL: ADULTS, ELDERLY: One-tenth of the epidural dose: 0.2–1 mg/dose.

PCA

IV: ADULTS, ELDERLY: **Loading dose:** 5–10 mg. **Intermittent bolus:** 0.5–3 mg. **Lockout interval:** 5–12 min. **Continuous infusion:** 1–10 mg/hr. **4-hr limit:** 20–30 mg.

SIDE EFFECTS

FREQUENT: Sedation, decreased BP (including orthostatic hypotension), diaphoresis, facial flushing, constipation, dizziness, somnolence, nausea, vomiting. **OCCASIONAL:** Allergic reaction (rash, pruritus), dyspnea, confusion, palpitations, tremors, urine retention, abdominal cramps, vision changes, dry mouth, headache, decreased appetite, pain or burning at injection site. **RARE:** Paralytic ileus.

ADVERSE REACTIONS/ TOXIC EFFECTS

Overdose results in respiratory depression, skeletal muscle flaccidity, cold or clammy skin, cyanosis, and extreme somnolence progressing to seizures, stupor, and coma. The patient who uses morphine repeatedly may develop a tolerance to the drug's analgesic effect and physical dependence. The drug may have a prolonged duration of action and cumulative effect in those with hepatic and renal impairment.

NURSING CONSIDERATIONS

BASELINE ASSESSMENT

Patient should be in a recumbent position before drug is given by parenteral route. Assess onset, type, location, duration of pain. Obtain vital signs before giving medication. If respirations are 12/min or less (20/min or less in children), withhold medication, contact physician. Effect of medication is reduced if full pain recurs before next dose.

INTERVENTION/EVALUATION

Monitor vital signs 5–10 min after IV administration, 15–30 min after subcutaneous, IM. Be alert for decreased respirations, BP. Check for adequate voiding. Monitor bowel activity; avoid constipation. Initiate deep breathing, coughing exercises, particularly in those with pulmonary impairment. Assess for clinical improvement, record onset of pain relief. Consult physician if pain relief is not adequate.

PATIENT/FAMILY TEACHING

• Discomfort may occur with injection. • Change positions slowly to avoid orthostatic hypotension. • Avoid tasks that require alertness, motor skills until response to drug is established. • Avoid alcohol, CNS depressants. • Tolerance or dependence may occur with prolonged use of high doses.

Motrin, *see ibuprofen*

---

moxifloxacin hydrochloride

moks-i-**floks**-a-sin

(Avelox, Avelox IV, Vigamox)

Do not confuse Avelox with Avonex.

CLASSIFICATION

PHARMACOTHERAPEUTIC: Fluoroquinolone. **CLINICAL:** Antibacterial (see p. 24C).

ACTION

A fluoroquinolone that inhibits two enzymes, topoisomerase II and IV, in susceptible microorganisms. **Therapeutic Effect:** Interferes with bacterial DNA replication. Prevents or delays emergence of resistant organisms. Bactericidal.

PHARMACOKINETICS

Well absorbed from the GI tract after PO administration. Protein binding: 50%. Widely distributed throughout body with tissue concentration often exceeding plasma concentration. Metabolized in liver. Primarily excreted in urine with a lesser amount in feces. **Half-life:** 10.7–13.3 hr.

USES

Treatment of susceptible infections due to *S. pneumoniae, S. pyogenes, S. aureus, H. influenzae, M. catarrhalis, K. pneumoniae, M. pneumoniae, C. pneumoniae* including acute bacterial exacerbation of chronic bronchitis, acute bacterial sinusitis, intra-abdominal infection, community-acquired pneumonia, uncomplicated skin and skin-structure infections. **Ophthalmic:** Topical treatment of bacterial conjunctivitis due to susceptible strains of bacteria.

PRECAUTIONS

CONTRAINDICATIONS: Hypersensitivity to quinolones. **CAUTIONS:** Renal or hepatic impairment, CNS disorders, cerebral arthrosclerosis, seizures, those with prolonged QT interval, uncorrected hypokalemia, those receiving quinidine, procainamide, amiodarone, sotalol.

⧗ LIFESPAN CONSIDERATIONS: **Pregnancy/Lactation:** May be distributed in breast milk. May produce teratogenic effects. **Pregnancy Category C. Children:** Safety and efficacy not established. **Elderly:** No age-related precautions noted.

INTERACTIONS

DRUG: **Antacids, didanosine chewable, buffered tablets or pediatric powder for oral solution, iron preparations, sucralfate:** May decrease moxifloxacin absorption. HERBAL: None known. FOOD: None known. LAB VALUES: None known.

AVAILABILITY (Rx)

TABLETS (AVELOX): 400 mg. **INJECTION (AVELOX IV):** 400 mg. **OPHTHALMIC SOLUTION (VIGAMOX):** 0.5%.

ADMINISTRATION/HANDLING

 IV

Reconstitution • N/A. Available in ready-to-use containers.

Rate of administration • Give by IV infusion only. • Avoid rapid or bolus IV infusion. • Infuse over 60 min.

Storage • Store at room temperature. • Do not refrigerate.

PO

• Give without regard to meals. • Oral moxifloxacin should be administered 4 hr before or 8 hr after antacids, multivitamins, iron preparations, sucralfate, didanosine chewable/buffered tablets, pediatric powder for oral solution.

OPHTHALMIC

• Tilt patient's head backward, have patient look up. • Gently pull lower eyelid down until pocket formed. • Hold dropper above pocket. • Without touching eyelid or conjunctival sac place drops into center of pocket. • Close eyes gently, apply gentle finger pressure to lacrimal sac at inner canthus. • Remove excess solution around eye with a tissue.

▨ IV INCOMPATIBILITIES

Do not add or infuse other drugs simultaneously through the same IV line. Flush line before and after use if same IV line is used with other medications.

✎ see color pill atlas   ✐ herb   underlined – top prescribed drug

INDICATIONS/ROUTES/DOSAGE

ACUTE BACTERIAL SINUSITIS
PO, IV: ADULTS, ELDERLY: 400 mg q24h
for 10 days.

**ACUTE BACTERIAL EXACERBATION
OF CHRONIC BRONCHITIS**
PO, IV: ADULTS, ELDERLY: 400 mg q24h
for 5 days.

COMMUNITY ACQUIRED PNEUMONIA
PO, IV: ADULTS, ELDERLY: 400 mg q24h for
7–14 days.

SKIN AND SKIN-STRUCTURE INFECTION
PO, IV: ADULTS, ELDERLY: 400 mg once
a day for 7 days.

**TOPICAL TREATMENT OF BACTERIAL
CONJUNCTIVITIS DUE TO SUSCEPTIBLE
STRAINS OF BACTERIA**
OPHTHALMIC: ADULTS, ELDERLY CHILDREN
OLDER THAN 1 YR: 1 drop 3 times a day for
7 days.

SIDE EFFECTS

FREQUENT (8%–6%): Nausea, diarrhea.
OCCASIONAL: PO, IV (3%–2%): Dizziness, headache, abdominal pain,
vomiting. **Ophthalmic (6%–1%):**
conjunctival irritation, reduced visual
acuity, dry eye, keratitis, eye pain, ocular
itching, swelling of tissue around cornea,
eye discharge, fever, cough, pharyngitis,
rash, rhinitis. **RARE (1%):** Change in
sense of taste, dyspepsia (heartburn,
indigestion), photosensitivity.

ADVERSE REACTIONS/
TOXIC EFFECTS

Pseudomembranous colitis as evidenced
by fever, severe abdominal cramps or
pain, and severe watery diarrhea may
occur. Superinfection manifested as anal
or genital pruritus, moderate to severe
diarrhea, and stomatitis may occur.

NURSING CONSIDERATIONS

BASELINE ASSESSMENT
Question for history of hypersensitivity to moxifloxacin, quinolones.

INTERVENTION/EVALUATION
Determine pattern of bowel activity
and stool consistency. Assist with ambulation if dizziness occurs. Assess for
headache, abdominal pain, vomiting,
altered taste, dyspepsia (heartburn,
indigestion). Monitor WBC, signs of
infection.

PATIENT/FAMILY TEACHING
• May be taken without regard to food.
• Drink plenty of fluids. • Avoid exposure to direct sunlight; may cause
photosensitivity reaction. • Do not take
antacids 4 hr before or 8 hr after
dosing. • Take full course of therapy.

MS Contin, *see morphine*

---

mupirocin

mew-pie-ro-sin

(Bactroban, Bactroban Nasal, Centany)

**Do not confuse Bactroban or
Bactroban Nasal with bacitracin,
baclofen, or Bactrim.**

CLASSIFICATION

PHARMACOTHERAPEUTIC: Anti-infective. **CLINICAL:** Topical antibacterial.

ACTION

Inhibits bacterial protein, RNA synthesis.
Less effective on DNA synthesis. **Nasal:**
Eradicates nasal colonization of methicillin-resistant *Staphylococcus aureus*
(MRSA). **Therapeutic Effect:** Prevents
bacterial growth, replication. Bacteriostatic.

PHARMACOKINETICS

Following topical administration, penetrates outer layer of skin (minimal

through intact skin). Protein binding: 95%. Metabolized in liver; excreted in urine. **Half-life:** 17–36 min.

USES

Ointment: Topical treatment of impetigo caused by *S. aureus, S. pyogenes;* treatment of folliculitis, furunculosis, minor wounds, burns, ulcers caused by susceptible organisms. **Cream:** Treatment of traumatic skin lesions due to *S. aureus, S. pyogenes,* prophylactic agent applied to IV catheter exit sites. **Intranasal ointment:** Eradication of *S. aureus* from nasal, perineal carriage sites. **OFF-LABEL:** Treatment of infected eczema, folliculitis, minor bacterial skin infections.

PRECAUTIONS

CONTRAINDICATIONS: None known. **CAUTIONS:** Renal impairment, burn patients.

LIFESPAN CONSIDERATIONS: Pregnancy/Lactation: Unknown if distributed in breast milk. Temporarily discontinue breast-feeding while using mupirocin. **Pregnancy Category B. Children:** Safety and efficacy not established. **Elderly:** No age-related precautions noted.

INTERACTIONS

DRUG: None known. **HERBAL:** None known. **FOOD:** None known. **LAB VALUES:** None known.

AVAILABILITY (Rx)

CREAM (BACTROBAN): 2%. **OINTMENT (BACTROBAN, CENTANY):** 2%. **NASAL OINTMENT (BACTROBAN NASAL):** 2%.

ADMINISTRATION/HANDLING
TOPICAL

CREAM, OINTMENT • For topical use only. • Do not apply into the eyes. • May cover with gauze dressing.

INTRANASAL
• Avoid contact with eyes. • Apply ½ ointment from single-use tube into each nostril.

INDICATIONS/ROUTES/DOSAGE
USUAL TOPICAL DOSAGE
TOPICAL: ADULTS, ELDERLY, CHILDREN: **Cream:** Apply small amount 3 times a day for 10 days. **Ointment:** Apply small amount 3–5 times a day for 5–14 days.

USUAL NASAL DOSAGE
INTRANASAL: ADULTS, ELDERLY, CHILDREN: Apply small amount 2–4 times a day for 5–14 days.

SIDE EFFECTS

FREQUENT: Nasal (9%–3%): Headache, rhinitis, upper respiratory congestion, pharyngitis, altered taste. **OCCASIONAL: Nasal (2%):** Burning, stinging, cough. **Topical (2%–1%):** Pain, burning, stinging, itching. **RARE: Nasal (less than 1%):** Pruritus, diarrhea, dry mouth, epistaxis, nausea, rash. **Topical (less than 1%):** Rash, nausea, dry skin, contact dermatitis.

ADVERSE REACTIONS/ TOXIC EFFECTS

Superinfection may result in bacterial, fungal infections, especially with prolonged, repeated therapy.

NURSING CONSIDERATIONS
BASELINE ASSESSMENT
Assess skin for type, extent of lesions.

INTERVENTION/EVALUATION
Keep neonates or patients with poor hygiene isolated. Wear gloves, gown if necessary when contact with discharges is likely; continue until 24 hr after therapy is effective. Cleanse/dispose of articles soiled with discharge according to institutional guidelines. In event of skin reaction, stop applications, cleanse area gently, notify physician.

• For external use only. • Avoid contact with eyes. • Explain precautions to avoid spread of infection; teach how to apply medication. • If skin reaction, irritation develops, notify physician. • If no improvement is noted in 3–5 days, patient should be reevaluated.

muromonab-CD3

mur-oo-**mon**-ab
(Orthoclone OKT3)

◆CLASSIFICATION
PHARMACOTHERAPEUTIC: Murine monoclonal antibody. **CLINICAL:** Immunosuppressant.

ACTION
A monoclonal antibody derived from purified IgG_2 that reacts with a T-3 (CD3) antigen of human T-cell membranes, blocking the production and function of T cells, which play a major role in acute organ rejection. **Therapeutic Effect:** Reverses organ rejection.

PHARMACOKINETICS
Binds to lymphocytes. **Half-life:** approximately 18 hr.

USES
Treatment of acute allograft rejection in renal transplant patients; steroid-resistant acute allograft rejection in cardiac, hepatic transplant patients.

PRECAUTIONS
CONTRAINDICATIONS: History of hypersensitivity to any murine-derived product, fluid overload (as evidenced by chest x-ray or weight gain of more than 3%) in the week before initial treatment. **CAUTIONS:** Hepatic, renal, cardiac impairment.

 LIFESPAN CONSIDERATIONS: Pregnancy/Lactation: Crosses placenta; unknown if distributed in breast milk. **Pregnancy Category C. Children:** Safety and efficacy not established. **Elderly:** No age-related precautions noted.

INTERACTIONS
DRUG: Live virus vaccines: May potentiate virus replication, increase the vaccine's side effects, and decrease the patient's response to the vaccine. **Other immunosuppressants:** May increase the risk of infection or lymphoproliferative disorders. **HERBAL: Echinacea:** May decrease the effects of muromonab-CD3. **FOOD:** None known. **LAB VALUES:** None known.

AVAILABILITY (Rx)
INJECTION: 1 mg/ml.

ADMINISTRATION/HANDLING
IV
Reconstitution • Draw solution into syringe through 0.22-micron filter. Discard filter; use needle for IV administration.

Rate of administration • Administer IV push over less than 1 min. • Give methylprednisolone 1 mg/kg before and 100 mg hydrocortisone 30 min after dose (decreases adverse reaction to first dose).

Storage • Refrigerate ampule. Do not use if left out of refrigerator for over 4 hr. • Do not shake ampule before using. • Fine translucent particles may develop; does not affect potency.

▓ IV INCOMPATIBILITIES
Do not mix muromonab with any other medications.

M

INDICATIONS/ROUTES/DOSAGE

TREATMENT OF ACUTE RENAL ALLOGRAFT REJECTION

IV: ADULTS, ELDERLY, CHILDREN 12 YR AND OLDER: 5 mg/day for 10–14 days, beginning as soon as acute renal rejection is diagnosed. CHILDREN YOUNGER THAN 12 YR: 0.1 mg/kg/day for 10–14 days, beginning as soon as acute renal rejection is diagnosed.

SIDE EFFECTS

FREQUENT: Fever, chills, dyspnea, malaise frequently occur 30 min–6 hr after first dose. This reaction markedly diminishes after the second day of treatment. **OCCASIONAL:** Chest pain, nausea, vomiting, diarrhea, tremor.

ADVERSE REACTIONS/ TOXIC EFFECTS

Symptoms of cytokine release syndrome, a common reaction, may range from mild flu-like symptoms to a life-threatening, shock-like reaction. Infection due to immunosuppression generally occurs within 45 days after initial treatment. Cytomegalovirus occurs in 19% of patients, and herpes simplex occurs in 27% of patients. A severe, life-threatening infection occurs in fewer than 5% of patients. Severe pulmonary edema occurs in fewer than 2% of patients. Fatal hypersensitivity reactions occur occasionally.

NURSING CONSIDERATIONS

BASELINE ASSESSMENT

Chest x-ray must be taken within 24 hr of initiation of therapy and be clear of fluid. Weight should be at least 3% above minimum weight the week before beginning treatment (pulmonary edema occurs when fluid overload is present before treatment). Have resuscitative drugs, equipment immediately available.

INTERVENTION/EVALUATION

Monitor WBC, differential, platelet count, renal and liver function tests, immunologic tests (plasma levels, quantitative T lymphocyte surface phenotyping) before and during therapy. If fever exceeds 100°F, antipyretics should be instituted. Monitor for fluid overload by chest x-ray and weight gain of more than 3% over weight before treatment. Assess lung sounds for evidence of fluid overload. Monitor I&O. Assess pattern of bowel activity and stool consistency.

PATIENT/FAMILY TEACHING

• Inform patient of first-dose reaction (fever, chills, chest tightness, wheezing, nausea, vomiting, diarrhea). • Avoid crowds, those with infections. • Do not receive immunizations.

Mycamine, see
micafungin

mycophenolate mofetil

my-co-**feno**-late
(CellCept)

◆CLASSIFICATION

PHARMACOTHERAPEUTIC: Immunologic agent. **CLINICAL:** Immunosuppressant (see p. 107C).

ACTION

An immunologic agent that suppresses the immunologically mediated inflammatory response by inhibiting inosine monophosphate dehydrogenase, an enzyme that deprives lymphocytes of nucleotides necessary for DNA and RNA synthesis, thus inhibiting the proliferation of T and B lymphocytes. Therapeutic Effect: Prevents transplant rejection.

PHARMACOKINETICS

Rapidly and extensively absorbed after PO administration (food decreases drug plasma concentration but doesn't affect absorption). Protein binding: 97%. Completely hydrolyzed to active metabolite mycophenolic acid. Primarily excreted in urine. Not removed by hemodialysis. Half-life: 17.9 hr.

USES

Prophylaxis of organ rejection in patients receiving allogeneic hepatic/renal/cardiac transplants. Should be used concurrently with cyclosporine and corticosteroids. OFF-LABEL: Treatment of liver transplantation rejection, mild heart transplant rejection, moderate to severe psoriasis.

PRECAUTIONS

CONTRAINDICATIONS: Hypersensitivity to mycophenolic acid or polysorbate 80 (IV formulation). CAUTIONS: Active serious digestive disease, renal impairment, neutropenia, women of childbearing potential.

LIFESPAN CONSIDERATIONS: Pregnancy/Lactation: Unknown if drug crosses placenta or is distributed in breast milk. Avoid breast-feeding. Pregnancy Category C. Children: Safety and efficacy not established. Elderly: Age-related renal impairment may require dosage adjustment.

INTERACTIONS

DRUG: Acyclovir, ganciclovir: May increase plasma concentrations of both drugs in patients with renal impairment. Antacids (aluminum and magnesium-containing), cholestyramine: May decrease the absorption of mycophenolate. Live virus vaccines: May potentiate virus replication, increase vaccine side effects, and decrease the patient's antibody response to the vaccine. Other immunosuppressants: May increase the risk of infection or lymphomas. Probenecid: May increase mycophenolate plasma concentration. HERBAL: Echinacea: May decrease the effects of mycophenolate. FOOD: All foods: May decrease mycophenolate plasma concentration. LAB VALUES: May increase serum cholesterol, alkaline phosphatase, creatinine, AST, and ALT levels. May increase or decrease blood glucose as well as serum lipid, calcium, potassium, phosphate, and uric acid levels.

AVAILABILITY (Rx)

CAPSULES (CELLCEPT): 250 mg. ORAL SUSPENSION (CELLCEPT): 200 mg/ml. TABLETS (CELLCEPT): 500 mg. TABLETS (DELAYED-RELEASE [MYFORTIC]): 180 mg, 360 mg. INJECTION (CELLCEPT): 500 mg.

ADMINISTRATION/HANDLING

 IV

Reconstitution • Reconstitute each 500-mg vial with 14 ml D_5W. Gently agitate. • For 1-g dose, further dilute with 140 ml D_5W; for 1.5-g dose further dilute with 210 ml D_5W, providing a concentration of 6 mg/ml.

Rate of administration • Infuse over at least 2 hr.

Storage • Store at room temperature.

PO
• Give on an empty stomach. • Do not open or crush capsules. Avoid inhalation of powder in capsules, direct contact of powder on skin/mucous membranes. If contact occurs, wash thoroughly with soap and water. Rinse eyes profusely with plain water. • Store reconstituted suspension in refrigerator or at room temperature. • Suspension is stable for 60 days after reconstitution.

• Suspension can be administered orally or via a nasogastric tube (minimum size 8 French).

▧ IV INCOMPATIBILITIES

Mycophenolate is compatible only with D_5W. Do not infuse it concurrently with other drugs or IV solutions.

INDICATIONS/ROUTES/DOSAGE

PREVENTION OF RENAL TRANSPLANT REJECTION

PO, IV (CELLCEPT): ADULTS, ELDERLY: 1 g twice a day.
PO (MYFORTIC): ADULTS, ELDERLY: 720 mg twice a day. CHILDREN 5–16 YR: 400 mg/m^2 twice a day. **Maximum:** 720 mg twice a day.

PREVENTION OF HEART TRANSPLANT REJECTION

PO, IV (CELLCEPT): ADULTS, ELDERLY: 1.5 g twice a day.

PREVENTION OF LIVER TRANSPLANT REJECTION

PO (CELLCEPT): ADULTS, ELDERLY: 1.5 g twice a day.
IV (CELLCEPT): ADULTS, ELDERLY: 1 g twice a day.

USUAL PEDIATRIC DOSAGE

PO (CELLCEPT): CHILDREN: 600 mg/m^2/dose twice a day. **Maximum:** 2 g/day.

SIDE EFFECTS

FREQUENT (37%–20%): UTI, hypertension, peripheral edema, diarrhea, constipation, fever, headache, nausea.
OCCASIONAL (18%–10%): Dyspepsia; dyspnea; cough; hematuria; asthenia; vomiting; edema; tremors; abdominal, chest, or back pain; oral candidiasis; acne. **RARE (9%–6%):** Insomnia, respiratory tract infection, rash, dizziness.

ADVERSE REACTIONS/ TOXIC EFFECTS

Significant anemia, leukopenia, thrombocytopenia, neutropenia, and leukocytosis may occur, particularly in those undergoing reanl transplant rejection. Sepsis and infection occur occasionally. GI tract hemorrhage occurs rarely. Patients receiving mycophenolate have an increased risk of developing neoplasms. Immunosuppression may result in an increased susceptibility to infection and the development of lymphoma.

BASELINE ASSESSMENT

Women of childbearing potential should have a negative serum or urine pregnancy test within 1 wk before initiation of drug therapy. Assess medical history, especially renal function, existence of active digestive system disease, drug history, especially other immunosuppressants.

INTERVENTION/EVALUATION

CBC should be performed weekly during first month of therapy, twice monthly during second and third months of treatment, then monthly throughout the first year. If rapid fall in WBC occurs, dosage should be reduced or discontinued. Assess particularly for delayed bone marrow suppression. Report any major change in assessment of patient.

PATIENT/FAMILY TEACHING

• Effective contraception should be used before, during, and for 6 wk after discontinuing therapy, even if patient has a history of infertility, other than hysterectomy. • Two forms of contraception must be used concurrently unless abstinence is absolute. • Contact physician if unusual bleeding/bruising, sore throat, mouth sores, abdominal pain, fever occurs. • Inform patients of need for laboratory follow-up while taking medication. • Inform patients of risk of malignancies that may occur.

🖉 see color pill atlas   ◢ herb   underlined – top prescribed drug

nabumetone

na-**byu**-me-tone
(Apo-Nabumetone, Relafen)

◆CLASSIFICATION

PHARMACOTHERAPEUTIC: Nonsteroidal anti-inflammatory. **CLINICAL:** Analgesic, anti-inflammatory (see p. 117C).

ACTION

An NSAID that produces analgesic and anti-inflammatory effects by inhibiting prostaglandin synthesis. Therapeutic Effect: Reduces the inflammatory response and intensity of pain.

PHARMACOKINETICS

Readily absorbed from the GI tract. Protein binding: 99%. Widely distributed. Metabolized in the liver to active metabolite. Primarily excreted in urine. Not removed by hemodialysis. Half-life: 22–30 hr.

USES

Acute, chronic treatment of osteoarthritis, rheumatoid arthritis.

PRECAUTIONS

CONTRAINDICATIONS: Active peptic ulcer disease, chronic inflammation of GI tract, GI bleeding or ulceration, history of hypersensitivity to aspirin or NSAIDs, history of significant renal impairment. **CAUTIONS:** CHF, hypertension, decreased hepatic or renal function, concurrent use of anticoagulants.

⧗ LIFESPAN CONSIDERATIONS: **Pregnancy/Lactation:** Distributed in low concentration in breast milk. Avoid use during last trimester (may adversely affect fetal cardiovascular system: premature closing of ductus arteriosus). **Pregnancy Category C (D if used in third trimester or near delivery).**

Children: Safety and efficacy not established. **Elderly:** Age-related renal impairment may increase risk of hepatic or renal toxicity; reduced dosage recommended. More likely to have serious adverse effects with GI bleeding or ulceration.

INTERACTIONS

DRUG: **Antihypertensives, diuretics:** May decrease the effects of these drugs. **Aspirin, other salicylates:** May increase the risk of GI side effects such as bleeding. **Bone marrow depressants:** May increase the risk of hematologic reactions. **Heparin, oral anticoagulants, thrombolytics:** May increase the effects of these drugs. **Lithium:** May increase the blood concentration and risk of toxicity of lithium. **Methotrexate:** May increase the risk of methotrexate toxicity. **Probenecid:** May increase the nabumetone blood concentration. HERBAL: **Feverfew:** May decrease the effects of feverfew. **Ginkgo biloba:** May increase the risk of bleeding. FOOD: None known. LAB VALUES: May increase BUN level; urine protein levels; and serum LDH, alkaline phosphatase, creatinine, potassium, AST, and ALT levels. May decrease serum uric acid level.

AVAILABILITY (Rx)

TABLETS (RELAFEN): 500 mg, 750 mg.

ADMINISTRATION/HANDLING

PO
• Give with food, milk, antacids if GI distress occurs. • Do not crush; swallow whole.

INDICATIONS/ROUTES/DOSAGE

ACUTE OR CHRONIC RHEUMATOID ARTHRITIS AND OSTEOARTHRITIS
PO: ADULTS, ELDERLY: Initially, 1,000 mg as a single dose or in 2 divided doses. May increase up to 2,000 mg/day as a single or in 2 divided doses.

N

SIDE EFFECTS

FREQUENT (14%–12%): Diarrhea, abdominal cramps or pain, dyspepsia. **OCCASIONAL (9%–4%):** Nausea, constipation, flatulence, dizziness, headache. **RARE (3%–1%):** Vomiting, stomatitis, confusion.

ADVERSE REACTIONS/ TOXIC EFFECTS

Overdose may result in acute hypotension and tachycardia. Rare reactions with long-term use include peptic ulcer disease, GI bleeding, gastritis, nephrotoxicity (dysuria, cystitis, hematuria, proteinuria, nephrotic syndrome), severe hepatic reactions (cholestasis, jaundice), and severe hypersensitivity reactions (bronchospasm, angioedema).

NURSING CONSIDERATIONS

BASELINE ASSESSMENT

Assess onset, type, location, duration of pain or inflammation. Inspect appearance of affected joints for immobility, deformities, skin condition.

INTERVENTION/EVALUATION

Assist with ambulation if somnolence, drowsiness, or dizziness occurs. Monitor for evidence of dyspepsia, pattern of daily bowel activity and stool consistency. Evaluate for therapeutic response: relief of pain, stiffness, swelling. Assess for increase in joint mobility, reduced joint tenderness; improved grip strength.

PATIENT/FAMILY TEACHING

• May cause serious GI bleeding with or without pain. • Avoid aspirin. • May take with food if GI upset occurs. • Avoid tasks requiring mental alertness, motor skills until response to drug is established (may cause dizziness, confusion).

nadolol ⚑

nay-**doe**-lole

(Apo-Nadol 🍁, Corgard, Novo-Nadolol 🍁)

FIXED-COMBINATION(S)

Corzide: nadolol/bendroflumethiazide (a diuretic): 40 mg/5 mg, 80 mg/5 mg.

•CLASSIFICATION

PHARMACOTHERAPEUTIC: Betaadrenergic blocker. **CLINICAL:** Antianginal, antihypertensive (see p. 64C).

ACTION

A nonselective beta-blocker that blocks beta$_1$- and beta$_2$-adrenergic receptors. Large doses increase airway resistance. Therapeutic Effect: Slows sinus heart rate, decreases cardiac output and BP. Decreases myocardial ischemia severity by decreasing oxygen requirements.

PHARMACOKINETICS

Variable absorption after PO administration. Protein binding: 28%–30%. Not metabolized. Excreted unchanged in feces. Half-life: 20–24 hr.

USES

Management of mild to moderate hypertension. Used alone or in combination with diuretics, especially thiazide type. Management of chronic stable angina pectoris. OFF-LABEL: Treatment of arrhythmias, hypertrophic cardiomyopathy, MI, mitral valve prolapse syndrome, neuroleptic-induced akathisia, pheochromocytoma, tremors, thyrotoxicosis, vascular headaches.

PRECAUTIONS

CONTRAINDICATIONS: Bronchial asthma, cardiogenic shock, CHF secondary to tachyarrhythmias, chronic obstructive pulmonary disease (COPD), patients

SIDE EFFECTS

COMMON (90%): Hot flashes. **OCCASIONAL (22%–10%):** Decreased libido, vaginal dryness, headache, emotional lability, acne, myalgia, decreased breast size, nasal irritation. **RARE (8%–2%):** Insomnia, edema, weight gain, seborrhea, depression.

ADVERSE REACTIONS/ TOXIC EFFECTS

None known.

NURSING CONSIDERATIONS

BASELINE ASSESSMENT

Inquire about menstrual cycle; therapy should begin between days 2 and 4 of cycle.

INTERVENTION/EVALUATION

Check for pain relief as result of therapy. Inquire about menstrual cessation, other decreased estrogen effects.

PATIENT/FAMILY TEACHING

• Patient should use nonhormonal contraceptive during therapy. • Do not take drug if pregnancy is suspected **(Pregnancy Category X)**. • Discuss importance of full length of therapy, regular visits to physician's office. • Notify physician if regular menstruation continues (menstruation should stop with therapy).

---

nafcillin sodium

naf-**sill**-in

(Nallpen ✤, Unipen ✤)

Do not confuse Unipen with Unicap.

◆CLASSIFICATION

PHARMACOTHERAPEUTIC: Penicillinase-resistant penicillin. **CLINICAL:** Antibiotic (see p. 27C).

ACTION

Binds to bacterial membranes. **Therapeutic Effect:** Inhibits cell wall synthesis. Bactericidal.

USES

Treatment of respiratory tract, skin/skin structure infections, osteomyelitis, endocarditis; meningitis, perioperatively, especially in cardiovascular, orthopedic procedures. Predominant treatment of infections caused by penicillinase-producing staphylococci.

PRECAUTIONS

CONTRAINDICATIONS: Hypersensitivity to any penicillin. **CAUTIONS:** History of allergies, particularly cephalosporins, severe renal/hepatic impairment. **Pregnancy Category B.**

INTERACTIONS

DRUG: Probenecid: May increase concentration, toxicity risk. **HERBAL:** None known. **FOOD:** None known. **LAB VALUES:** May cause positive Coombs' test.

AVAILABILITY (Rx)

POWDER FOR INJECTION: 1 g, 2 g.

ADMINISTRATION/HANDLING

◀ ALERT ▶ Space doses evenly around the clock.

 IV

Reconstitution • For IV push, reconstitute each vial with 15–30 ml sterile water for injection or 0.9% NaCl. Administer over 5–10 min. • For intermittent IV infusion (piggyback), further dilute with 50–100 ml D_5W, $D_{10}W$, 0.9% NaCl, 0.45% NaCl, 0.2% NaCl, Ringer's solution, lactated Ringer's solution, or any combination thereof.

Rate of administration • Infuse over 30–60 min. • Because of potential for hypersensitivity/anaphylaxis, start initial dose at few drops per min, increase

N

slowly to ordered rate; stay with patient first 10–15 min, then check q10min.
• Limit IV therapy to less than 48 hr, if possible. Stop infusion if patient complains of pain at IV site.

Storage [IV Infusion (piggyback)]
• Stable for 24 hr at room temperature, 96 hr if refrigerated. • Discard if precipitate forms.

IM
• Reconstitute each 500 mg with 1.7 ml sterile water for injection or 0.9% NaCl to provide concentration of 250 mg/ml.
• Inject IM into large muscle mass.

⊞ IV INCOMPATIBILITIES

Diltiazem (Cardizem), droperidol (Inapsine), fentanyl, insulin, labetalol (Normodyne, Trandate), midazolam (Versed), nalbuphine (Nubain), vancomycin (Vancocin), verapamil (Isoptin).

IV COMPATIBILITIES

Heparin, lidocaine, magnesium, potassium chloride, propofol (Diprivan).

INDICATIONS/ROUTES/DOSAGE

USUAL DOSAGE

IV: ADULTS, ELDERLY: 0.5–2 g q4–6h. CHILDREN: 50–200 mg/kg/day in divided doses q4–6h. **Maximum:** 12 g a day. NEONATES: 40–60 mg/kg/day in divided doses q8–12h.

IM: ADULTS, ELDERLY: 500 mg q4–6h. CHILDREN: 50–200 mg/kg/day in divided doses q4–6h. **Maximum:** 12 g a day.

SIDE EFFECTS

FREQUENT: Mild hypersensitivity reaction (fever, rash, pruritus), GI effects (nausea, vomiting, diarrhea). **OCCASIONAL:** Hypokalemia with high IV dosages, phlebitis, thrombophlebitis (common in elderly). **RARE:** Extravasation with IV administration.

ADVERSE REACTIONS/ TOXIC EFFECTS

Superinfections, potentially fatal antibiotic-associated colitis may result from altered bacterial balance. Hematologic effects (especially involving platelets, WBCs), severe hypersensitivity reactions, anaphylaxis occur rarely.

NURSING CONSIDERATIONS

BASELINE ASSESSMENT

Question for history of allergies, especially penicillins, cephalosporins.

INTERVENTION/EVALUATION

Hold medication, promptly report rash (possible hypersensitivity), diarrhea (fever, abdominal pain, mucus/blood in stool may indicate antibiotic-associated colitis). Evaluate IV site frequently for phlebitis (heat, pain, red streaking over vein), infiltration (potential extravasation). Monitor periodic CBC, urinalysis, serum potassium, renal/hepatic function. Be alert for superinfection: increased fever, onset of sore throat, vomiting, diarrhea, stomatitis, anal/genital pruritus. Check hematology reports (especially WBCs), periodic serum renal/hepatic reports in prolonged therapy.

PATIENT/FAMILY TEACHING

• Continue antibiotic for full length of treatment. • Doses should be evenly spaced. • Discomfort may occur with IM injection. • Report IV discomfort immediately. • Notify physician in event of diarrhea, rash, other new symptoms.

naftifine hydrochloride
(Naftin)
See Antifungals: topical

---

nalbuphine hydrochloride

nal-**byoo**-feen

(Nubain)

Do not confuse Nubain with Navane.

•CLASSIFICATION

PHARMACOTHERAPEUTIC: Narcotic agonist, antagonist. **CLINICAL:** Opioid analgesic (see p. 128C).

ACTION

A narcotic agonist-antagonist that binds with opioid receptors in the CNS. May displace opioid agonists and competitively inhibit their action; may precipitate withdrawal symptoms. Therapeutic Effect: Alters the perception of and emotional response to pain.

PHARMACOKINETICS

Route	Onset	Peak	Duration
IV	2–3 min	30 min	3–6 hr
IM	Less than 15 min	60 min	3–6 hr
Subcu-taneous	Less than 15 min	N/A	3–6 hr

Well absorbed after IM or subcutaneous administration. Protein binding: 50%. Metabolized in the liver. Primarily eliminated in feces by biliary secretion. Half-life: 3.5–5 hr.

USES

Relief of moderate to severe pain, preop sedation, obstetric analgesia, adjunct to anesthesia.

PRECAUTIONS

CONTRAINDICATIONS: Respiratory rate less than 12 breaths/min. **CAUTIONS:** Hepatic or renal impairment, respiratory depression, recent MI, recent biliary tract surgery, head trauma, increased intracranial pressure (ICP), pregnancy, those suspected to be opioid dependent.

⧗ LIFESPAN CONSIDERATIONS: **Pregnancy/Lactation:** Readily crosses placenta. Distributed in breast milk (breast-feeding not recommended). May cause fetal and neonatal adverse effects during labor and delivery (e.g., fetal bradycardia). **Pregnancy Category B (D if used for prolonged periods or at high dosages at term). Children:** Paradoxical excitement may occur. Those younger than 2 yr more susceptible to respiratory depression. **Elderly:** More susceptible to respiratory depression. Age-related renal impairment may increase risk of urinary retention.

INTERACTIONS

DRUG: **Alcohol, other CNS depressants:** May increase CNS or respiratory depression and hypotension. **Buprenorphine:** May decrease the effects of nalbuphine. **MAOIs:** May produce a severe, possibly fatal reaction; plan to administer 25% of the usual nalbuphine dose. HERBAL: None known. FOOD: None known. LAB VALUES: May increase serum amylase and lipase levels.

AVAILABILITY (Rx)

INJECTION: 10 mg/ml, 20 mg/ml.

ADMINISTRATION/HANDLING

◄ ALERT ► Store parenteral form at room temperature.

 IV

Reconstitution • May give undiluted.

Rate of administration • For IV push, administer each 10 mg over 3–5 min.

Storage • Store at room temperature.

IM
• Rotate IM injection sites.

⬛ IV INCOMPATIBILITIES

Amphotericin B complex (Abelcet, AmBisome, Amphotec), cefepime (Maxipime), docetaxel (Doxil), methotrexate, nafcillin (Nafcil), piperacillin and tazobactam (Zosyn), sargramostim (Leukine, Prokine), sodium bicarbonate.

IV COMPATIBILITIES

Diphenhydramine (Benadryl), droperidol (Inapsine), glycopyrrolate (Robinul), hydroxyzine (Vistaril), ketorolac (Toradol), lidocaine, midazolam (Versed), propofol (Diprivan).

INDICATIONS/ROUTES/DOSAGE

ANALGESIA

IV, IM, SUBCUTANEOUS: ADULTS, ELDERLY: 10 mg q3–6h as needed. Don't exceed maximum single dose of 20 mg or daily dose of 160 mg. For patients receiving long-term narcotic analgesics of similar duration of action, give 25% of usual dose. CHILDREN: 0.1–0.15 mg/kg q3–6h as needed.

SUPPLEMENT TO ANESTHESIA

IV: ADULTS, ELDERLY: Induction: 0.3–3 mg/kg over 10–15 min. Maintenance: 0.25–0.5 mg/kg as needed.

SIDE EFFECTS

FREQUENT (35%): Sedation. **OCCASIONAL (9%–3%):** Diaphoresis, cold and clammy skin, nausea, vomiting, dizziness, vertigo, dry mouth, headache. **RARE (less than 1%):** Restlessness, emotional lability, paresthesia, flushing, paradoxical reaction.

ADVERSE REACTIONS/ TOXIC EFFECTS

Abrupt withdrawal after prolonged use may produce symptoms of narcotic withdrawal, such as abdominal cramping, rhinorrhea, lacrimation, anxiety, fever, and piloerection (goose bumps). Overdose results in severe respiratory depression, skeletal muscle flaccidity, cyanosis, and extreme somnolence progressing to seizures, stupor, and coma. Repeated use may result in drug tolerance and physical dependence.

NURSING CONSIDERATIONS

BASELINE ASSESSMENT

Raise bed rails. Obtain vital signs before giving medication. If respirations are 12/min or less (20/min or less in children), withhold medication, contact physician. Assess onset, type, location, duration of pain. Effect of medication is reduced if full pain recurs before next dose. Low abuse potential.

INTERVENTION/EVALUATION

Monitor for change in respirations, BP, rate and quality of pulse. Monitor pattern of daily bowel activity and stool consistency. Initiate deep breathing, coughing exercises, particularly in patients with pulmonary impairment. Assess for clinical improvement, record onset of relief of pain. Consult physician if pain relief is not adequate.

PATIENT/FAMILY TEACHING

• Avoid alcohol. • Avoid tasks that require alertness, motor skills until response to drug is established. • May cause dry mouth. • May be habit forming.

---

naloxone hydrochloride

nay-**lox**-own

(Narcan)

Do not confuse naltrexone or Narcan with Norcuron.

CLASSIFICATION

PHARMACOTHERAPEUTIC: Narcotic antagonist. **CLINICAL:** Antidote.

ACTION

A narcotic antagonist that displaces opioids at opioid-occupied receptor sites in the CNS. **Therapeutic Effect:** Reverses opioid-induced sleep or sedation, increases respiratory rate, raises BP to normal range.

PHARMACOKINETICS

Route	Onset	Peak	Duration
IV	1–2 min	N/A	20–60 min
IM	2–5 min	N/A	20–60 min
Subcutaneous	2–5 min	N/A	20–60 min

Well absorbed after IM or subcutaneous administration. Metabolized in the liver. Primarily excreted in urine. **Half-life:** 60–100 min.

USES

Diagnosis, treatment of opioid toxicity, treatment of opioid-induced respiratory depression, other effects (e.g., sedation, coma, seizures). Used in neonates to reverse respiratory depression caused by opioids given to mother during labor or delivery. **OFF-LABEL:** Treatment of ethanol ingestion, *Pneumocystitis carinii* pneumonia (PCP).

PRECAUTIONS

CONTRAINDICATIONS: Respiratory depression due to nonopioid drugs. **CAUTIONS:** Chronic cardiac or pulmonary disease, coronary artery disease. Those suspected of being opioid dependent, postop patients (to avoid cardiovascular changes).

⧗ LIFESPAN CONSIDERATIONS: **Pregnancy/Lactation:** Unknown if drug crosses placenta or is distributed in breast milk. **Pregnancy Category B. Children/Elderly:** No age-related precautions noted.

INTERACTIONS

DRUG: Butorphanol, nalbuphine, opioid agonist analgesics, **pentazocine:** Reverses the analgesic and adverse effects of these drugs and may precipitate withdrawal symptoms. **HERBAL:** None known. **FOOD:** None known. **LAB VALUES:** None known.

AVAILABILITY (Rx)

INJECTION: 0.02 mg/ml, 0.4 mg/ml, 1 mg/ml.

ADMINISTRATION/HANDLING

 IV

Reconstitution • May dilute 1 mg/ml with 50 ml sterile water for injection to provide a concentration of 0.02 mg/ml. • For continuous IV infusion, dilute each 2 mg of naloxone with 500 ml of D_5W in water or 0.9% NaCl, producing solution containing 0.004 mg/ml.

Rate of administration • May administer undiluted. • Give each 0.4 mg as IV push over 15 sec. • Use the 0.4 mg/ml and 1 mg/ml for injection for adults, the 0.02 mg/ml concentration for neonates.

Storage • Store parenteral form at room temperature. • Use mixture within 24 hr; discard unused solution. • Protect from light. Stable in D_5W or 0.9% NaCl at 4 mcg/ml for 24 hr.

IM
• Give deep IM in large muscle mass.

▓ IV INCOMPATIBILITIES

Amphotericin B complex (Abelcet, AmBisome, Amphotec).

IV COMPATIBILITIES

Heparin, ondansetron (Zofran), propofol (Diprivan).

INDICATIONS/ROUTES/DOSAGE

OPIOID TOXICITY

IV, IM, SUBCUTANEOUS: ADULTS, ELDERLY: 0.4–2 mg q2–3min as needed. May repeat q20–60min. CHILDREN 5 YR AND OLDER AND WEIGHING 20 KG AND MORE: 2 mg/dose; if no response, may repeat q2–3min. May need to repeat dose q20–60min. CHILDREN YOUNGER THAN 5 YR AND WEIGHING LESS THAN 20 KG: 0.1 mg/kg; if no response, repeat q2–3min. May need to repeat dose q20–60min.

POSTANESTHESIA NARCOTIC REVERSAL

IV: CHILDREN: 0.01 mg/kg; may repeat q2–3min.

NEONATAL OPIOID-INDUCED DEPRESSION

IV: NEONATES: May repeat q2–3min as needed. May need to repeat dose q1–2h.

SIDE EFFECTS

None known; little or no pharmacologic effect in absence of narcotics.

ADVERSE REACTIONS/ TOXIC EFFECTS

Too-rapid reversal of narcotic-induced respiratory depression may result in nausea, vomiting, tremors, increased BP, and tachycardia. Excessive dosage in postop patients may produce significant excitement, tremors, and reversal of analgesia. Patients with cardiovascular disease may experience hypotension or hypertension, ventricular tachycardia and fibrillation, and pulmonary edema.

NURSING CONSIDERATIONS

BASELINE ASSESSMENT

Maintain clear airway. Obtain weight of children to calculate drug dosage.

INTERVENTION/EVALUATION

Monitor vital signs, especially rate, depth, rhythm of respiration, during and frequently following administration. Carefully observe patient after satisfactory response (duration of opiate may exceed duration of naloxone, resulting in recurrence of respiratory depression). Assess for increased pain with reversal of opiate.

Naprosyn, *see naproxen*

---

naproxen

na-**prox**-en

(EC-Naprosyn, Naprelan, Naprelan 375, Naprelan 500)

naproxen sodium

(Aflaxen, Aleve, Anaprox, Anaprox DS, Apo-Naprosyn ✦, Novo-Naprox ✦, Nu-Naprox ✦, Pamprin)

Do not confuse Aleve with Allese or Anaprox with Anaspaz.

FIXED-COMBINATION(S)

Prevacid NapraPac: naproxen/ lansoprazole (proton pump inhibitor): 375 mg/15 mg, 500 mg/15 mg.

CLASSIFICATION

PHARMACOTHERAPEUTIC: Nonsteroidal anti-inflammatory. **CLINICAL:** Analgesic, anti-inflammatory (see p. 117C).

ACTION

An NSAID that produces analgesic and anti-inflammatory effects by inhibiting prostaglandin synthesis. Therapeutic Effect: Reduces the inflammatory response and intensity of pain.

PHARMACOKINETICS

Route	Onset	Peak	Duration
PO (analgesic)	Less than 1 hr	N/A	7 hr or less
PO (anti-rheumatic)	Less than 14 days	2–4 wk	N/A

Completely absorbed from the GI tract. Protein binding: 99%. Metabolized in the liver. Primarily excreted in urine. Not removed by hemodialysis. Half-life: 13 hr.

USES

Treatment of acute or long-term mild to moderate pain, primary

---

dysmenorrhea, rheumatoid arthritis, juvenile rheumatoid arthritis, osteoarthritis, ankylosing spondylitis, acute gouty arthritis, bursitis, tendinitis. **OFF-LABEL:** Treatment of vascular headaches.

PRECAUTIONS

CONTRAINDICATIONS: Hypersensitivity to aspirin, naproxen, or other NSAIDs. **CAUTIONS:** GI or cardiac disease, renal or hepatic impairment. Concurrent use of anticoagulants.

⧗ **LIFESPAN CONSIDERATIONS: Pregnancy/Lactation:** Crosses placenta. Distributed in breast milk. Avoid use during third trimester (may adversely affect fetal cardiovascular system: premature closing of ductus arteriosus). **Pregnancy Category B (D if used in third trimester or near delivery). Children:** Safety and efficacy not established in those younger than 2 yr. Children older than 2 yr at increased risk of skin rash. **Elderly:** Age-related renal impairment may increase risk of hepatic and renal toxicity; reduced dosage recommended. More likely to have serious adverse effects with GI bleeding/ulceration.

INTERACTIONS

DRUG: Antihypertensives, diuretics: May decrease the effects of these drugs. **Aspirin, other salicylates:** May increase the risk of GI side effects such as bleeding. **Bone marrow depressants:** May increase the risk of hematologic reactions. **Heparin, oral anticoagulants, thrombolytics:** May increase the effects of these drugs. **Lithium:** May increase the blood concentration and risk of toxicity of lithium. **Methotrexate:** May increase the risk of methotrexate toxicity. **Probenecid:** May increase the naproxen blood concentration. **HERBAL: Feverfew:** May decrease the effects of feverfew. **Ginkgo biloba:** May increase the risk of bleeding.

FOOD: None known. **LAB VALUES:** May prolong bleeding time and alter blood glucose level. May increase serum hepatic function test results. May decrease serum sodium and uric acid levels.

AVAILABILITY (Rx)

GELCAPS (ALEVE [OTC]): 220 mg naproxen sodium (equivalent to 200 mg naproxen). **ORAL SUSPENSION (NAPROSYN):** 125 mg/5 ml naproxen. **TABLETS:** 220 mg naproxen (Aleve [OTC]), 250 mg (Naprosyn), 275 mg naproxen sodium (equivalent to 250 mg naproxen) (Anaprox), 550 mg naproxen sodium (equivalent to 500 mg naproxen) (Aflaxen, Anaprox DS). **TABLETS (CONTROLLED-RELEASE):** 375 mg naproxen (EC-Naprosyn), 421 mg naproxen (Naprelan), 500 mg naproxen (EC-Naprosyn), 550 mg naproxen sodium (equivalent to 500 mg naproxen) (Naprelan).

ADMINISTRATION/HANDLING

PO

• Swallow enteric-coated form whole; scored tablets may be broken or crushed. • May give with food, milk, antacids if GI distress occurs.

INDICATIONS/ROUTES/DOSAGE

RHEUMATOID ARTHRITIS, OSTEOARTHRITIS, ANKYLOSING SPONDYLITIS
PO: ADULTS, ELDERLY: 250–500 mg naproxen (275–550 mg naproxen sodium) twice a day or 250 mg naproxen (275 mg naproxen sodium) in morning and 500 mg naproxen (550 mg naproxen sodium) in evening. **Naprelan:** 750–1,000 mg once a day.

ACUTE GOUTY ARTHRITIS
PO: ADULTS, ELDERLY: Initially, 750 mg naproxen (825 mg naproxen sodium), then 250 mg naproxen (275 mg naproxen sodium) q8h until attack subsides. **Naprelan:** Initially, 1,000–1,500 mg, then 1,000 mg once a day until attack subsides.

MILD TO MODERATE PAIN, DYSMENORRHEA, BURSITIS, TENDINITIS
PO: ADULTS, ELDERLY: Initially, 500 mg naproxen (550 mg naproxen sodium), then 250 mg naparoxen (275 mg naproxen sodium) q6–8h as needed. **Maximum:** 1.25 g/day naproxen (1.375 g/day naproxen sodium). **Naprelan:** 1,000 mg once a day.

JUVENILE RHEUMATOID ARTHRITIS
PO (NAPROXEN ONLY): CHILDREN: 10–15 mg/kg/day in 2 divided doses. **Maximum:** 1,000 mg/day.

OTC USES
PO: ADULTS 65 YR AND YOUNGER, CHILDREN 12 YR AND OLDER: 220 mg (200 mg naproxen sodium) q8–12h. May take 440 mg (200 mg naproxen sodium) as initial dose. ADULTS OLDER THAN 65 YR: 220 mg (200 mg naproxen sodium) q12h.

SIDE EFFECTS

FREQUENT (9%–4%): Nausea, constipation, abdominal cramps or pain, heartburn, dizziness, headache, somnolence. **OCCASIONAL (3%–1%):** Stomatitis, diarrhea, indigestion. **RARE (less than 1%):** Vomiting, confusion.

ADVERSE REACTIONS/ TOXIC EFFECTS

Rare reactions with long-term use include peptic ulcer disease, GI bleeding, gastritis, severe hepatic reactions (cholestasis, jaundice), nephrotoxicity (dysuria, hematuria, proteinuria, nephrotic syndrome), and a severe hypersensitivity reaction (fever, chills, bronchospasm).

NURSING CONSIDERATIONS

BASELINE ASSESSMENT

Assess onset, type, location, duration of pain or inflammation. Inspect appearance of affected joints for immobility, deformities, skin condition.

INTERVENTION/EVALUATION

Assist with ambulation if dizziness occurs. Monitor CBC, platelet count, serum renal and liver function tests, Hgb, pattern of daily bowel activity and stool consistency. Evaluate for therapeutic response: relief of pain, stiffness, swelling; increased joint mobility; reduced joint tenderness; improved grip strength.

PATIENT/FAMILY TEACHING

• Avoid tasks that require alertness, motor skills until response to drug is established. • If GI upset occurs, take with food, milk. • Avoid aspirin, alcohol during therapy (increases risk of GI bleeding). • Report headache, rash, visual disturbances, weight gain, black or tarry stools, persistent headache.

naratriptan

nare-a-**trip**-tan
(Amerge)
Do not confuse Amerge with Amaryl.

CLASSIFICATION

PHARMACOTHERAPEUTIC: Serotonin receptor agonist. **CLINICAL:** Antimigraine (see p. 56C).

ACTION

A serotonin receptor agonist that binds selectively to vascular receptors producing a vasoconstrictive effect on cranial blood vessels. **Therapeutic Effect:** Relieves migraine headache.

PHARMACOKINETICS

Well absorbed after PO administration. Protein binding: 28%–31%. Metabolized by the liver to inactive metabolite. Eliminated primarily in urine and, to

---

a lesser extent, in feces. **Half-life:** 6 hr (increased in hepatic or renal impairment).

USES

Treatment of acute migraine headache with or without aura in adults.

PRECAUTIONS

CONTRAINDICATIONS: Basilar or hemiplegic migraine, cerebrovascular or peripheral vascular disease, coronary artery disease, ischemic heart disease (including angina pectoris, history of MI, silent ischemia, and Prinzmetal's angina), severe hepatic impairment (Child-Pugh grade C), severe renal impairment (serum creatinine less than 15 ml/min), uncontrolled hypertension, use within 24 hr of ergotamine-containing preparations or another serotonin receptor agonist, use within 14 days of MAOIs. **CAUTIONS:** Mild to moderate renal or hepatic impairment, patient profile suggesting cardiovascular risks.

⧗ LIFESPAN CONSIDERATIONS: **Pregnancy/Lactation:** Unknown if drug is excreted in breast milk. **Pregnancy Category C. Children:** Safety and efficacy not established. **Elderly:** Not recommended in the elderly.

INTERACTIONS

DRUG: **Ergotamine-containing medications:** May produce a vasospastic reaction. **Fluoxetine, fluvoxamine, paroxetine, sertraline:** May produce hyperreflexia, incoordination, and weakness. **Oral contraceptives:** Decrease naratriptan clearance and volume of distribution. HERBAL: None known. FOOD: None known. LAB VALUES: None known.

AVAILABILITY (Rx)

TABLETS: 1 mg, 2.5 mg.

ADMINISTRATION/HANDLING

PO
- Give without regard to food.

INDICATIONS/ROUTES/DOSAGE

ACUTE MIGRAINE ATTACK
PO: ADULTS: 1 mg or 2.5 mg. If headache improves but then returns, dose may be repeated after 4 hr. **Maximum:** 5 mg/24 hr.

DOSAGE IN MILD TO MODERATE HEPATIC OR RENAL IMPAIRMENT
A lower starting dose is recommended. Don't exceed 2.5 mg/24 hr.

SIDE EFFECTS

OCCASIONAL (5%): Nausea. RARE (2%): Paresthesia; dizziness; fatigue; somnolence; jaw, neck, or throat pressure.

ADVERSE REACTIONS/ TOXIC EFFECTS

Corneal opacities and other ocular defects may occur. Cardiac reactions (including ischemia, coronary artery vasospasm, and MI) and noncardiac vasospasm-related reactions (such as hemorrhage and cerebrovascular accident [CVA]), occur rarely, particularly in patients with hypertension, diabetes, or a strong family history of coronary artery disease; obese patients; smokers; males older than 40 yr; and postmenopausal women.

NURSING CONSIDERATIONS

BASELINE ASSESSMENT
Question for history of peripheral vascular disease, renal or hepatic impairment, possibility of pregnancy. Question patient regarding onset, location, duration of migraine; possible precipitating symptoms.

INTERVENTION/EVALUATION
Assess for relief of migraine headache; potential for photophobia, phonophobia (sound sensitivity), nausea, vomiting.

N

PATIENT/FAMILY TEACHING

• Do not crush, chew tablet; swallow whole with water. • May repeat dose after 4 hr (maximum of 5 mg/24 hr). • May cause dizziness, fatigue, drowsiness. • Avoid tasks that require alertness, motor skills until response to drug is established. • Inform physician of any chest pain, palpitations, tightness in throat, rash, hallucinations, anxiety, panic.

Nasacort AQ, see
triamcinolone

Nasonex, see *mometasone*

---

natamycin

(Natacyn)
See Antifungals: topical

---

nateglinide

nah-**teh**-glih-nide
(Starlix)

◆**CLASSIFICATION**

PHARMACOTHERAPEUTIC: Antihyperglycemic. **CLINICAL:** Antidiabetic (see p. 42C).

ACTION

An antihyperglycemic that stimulates release of insulin from beta cells of the pancreas by depolarizing beta cells, leading to an opening of calcium channels. Resulting calcium influx induces insulin secretion. Therapeutic Effect: Lowers blood glucose concentration.

PHARMACOKINETICS

Absolute bioavailability is approximately 73%. Protein binding: 98%. Extensive metabolism in liver. Primarily excreted in urine; minimal elimination in feces. Half-life: 1.5 hr.

USES

Treatment of type 2 diabetes mellitus in patients whose disease cannot be adequately controlled with diet and exercise and in patients who have not been chronically treated with other antidiabetic agents. Used as monotherapy or in combination with other drugs.

PRECAUTIONS

CONTRAINDICATIONS: Diabetic ketoacidosis, type 1 diabetes mellitus. **CAUTIONS:** Hepatic or renal impairment.

⧗ LIFESPAN CONSIDERATIONS: **Pregnancy/Lactation:** Unknown if drug crosses placenta or is distributed is breast milk. **Pregnancy Category C. Children:** Safety and efficacy not established. **Elderly:** Increased susceptibility to hypoglycemia.

INTERACTIONS

DRUG: **Beta blockers, MAOIs, NSAIDs, salicylates:** May increase hypoglycemic effect of nateglinide. **Corticosteroids, thiazide diuretics, thyroid medication, sympathomimetics:** May decrease hypoglycemic effect of nateglinide. HERBAL: None known. FOOD: **Liquid meal:** Peak plasma levels may be significantly reduced if administered 10 min before a liquid meal. LAB VALUES: None known.

AVAILABILITY (Rx)

TABLETS: 60 mg, 120 mg.

ADMINISTRATION/HANDLING

PO

• Ideally, give within 15 min of a meal, but may be given immediately before a meal to as long as 30 min before a meal.

INDICATIONS/ROUTES/DOSAGE
DIABETES MELLITUS
PO: ADULTS, ELDERLY: 120 mg 3 times a day before meals. Initially, 60 mg may be given.

SIDE EFFECTS
FREQUENT (10%): Upper respiratory tract infection. **OCCASIONAL (4%–3%):** Back pain, flu symptoms, dizziness, arthropathy, diarrhea. **RARE (3% or less):** Bronchitis, cough.

ADVERSE REACTIONS/ TOXIC EFFECTS
Hypoglycemia occurs in less than 2% of patients.

NURSING CONSIDERATIONS
BASELINE ASSESSMENT
Check fasting blood glucose, glycosylated Hgb (HbA$_{1C}$) periodically to determine minimum effective dose. Discuss lifestyle to determine extent of learning, emotional needs. Ensure follow-up instruction if patient and amily do not thoroughly understand diabetes management or glucose-testing technique. At least 1 wk should elapse to assess response to drug before new dose adjustment is made.

INTERVENTION/EVALUATION
Monitor blood glucose, food intake. Assess for hypoglycemia (cool, wet skin, tremors, dizziness, anxiety, headache, tachycardia, numbness in mouth, hunger, diplopia), hyperglycemia (polyuria, polyphagia, polydipsia, nausea, vomiting, dim vision, fatigue, deep rapid breathing). Be alert to conditions that alter glucose requirements: fever, increased activity or stress, surgical procedures.

PATIENT/FAMILY TEACHING
• Diabetes mellitus requires lifelong control. • Prescribed diet, exercise are principal parts of treatment; do not skip or delay meals. • Continue to adhere to dietary instructions, a regular exercise program, regular testing of blood glucose.

Natrecor, *see nesiritide*

Nebcin, *see tobramycin*

---

nedocromil sodium

ned-oh-**crow**-mil
(Alocril, Mireze ✹, Tilade)

◆CLASSIFICATION
PHARMACOTHERAPEUTIC: Mast cell stabilizer. **CLINICAL:** Respiratory inhalant anti-inflammatory (see p. 68C).

ACTION
A mast cell stabilizer that prevents the activation and release of inflammatory mediators, such as histamine, leukotrienes, mast cells, eosinophils, and monocytes. Therapeutic Effect: Prevents both early and late asthmatic responses.

USES
Inhalation: Maintenance therapy for preventing airway inflammation, bronchoconstriction in patients with mild to moderate bronchial asthma. **Ophthalmic:** Treatment of itching associated with allergic conjunctivitis. OFF-LABEL: Prevention of bronchospasm in patients with reversible obstructive airway disease.

PRECAUTIONS
CONTRAINDICATIONS: None known. **CAUTIONS:** Not used for reversing acute bronchospasm.

N

⌛ **LIFESPAN CONSIDERATIONS: Pregnancy/Lactation:** Unknown if distributed in breast milk. **Pregnancy Category B. Children:** Safety and efficacy of ophthalmic form not established in children younger than 3 yr; safety and efficacy of inhaled form not established in children younger than 6 yr. **Elderly:** No age-related precautions noted.

INTERACTIONS

DRUG: None known. **HERBAL:** None known. **FOOD:** None known. **LAB VALUES:** None known.

AVAILABILITY (Rx)

AEROSOL FOR INHALATION (TILADE): 1.75 mg/activation. **OPHTHALMIC SOLUTION (ALOCRIL):** 2%.

INDICATIONS/ROUTES/DOSAGE

MILD TO MODERATE ASTHMA
ORAL INHALATION: ADULTS, ELDERLY, CHILDREN 6 YR AND OLDER: 2 inhalations 4 times a day. May decrease to 3 times a day then twice a day as asthma becomes controlled.

ALLERGIC CONJUNCTIVITIS
OPHTHALMIC: ADULTS, ELDERLY, CHILDREN 3 YR AND OLDER: 1–2 drops in each eye twice a day.

SIDE EFFECTS

FREQUENT (10%–6%): Inhalation: Cough, pharyngitis, bronchospasm, headache, altered taste. **Ophthalmic:** Burning sensation in eye. **OCCASIONAL (5%–1%): Inhalation:** Rhinitis, upper respiratory tract infection, abdominal pain, fatigue. **RARE (less than 1%): Inhalation:** Diarrhea, dizziness. **Ophthalmic:** Conjunctivitis, light intolerance.

ADVERSE REACTIONS/TOXIC EFFECTS

None known.

NURSING CONSIDERATIONS

INTERVENTION/EVALUATION

Evaluate therapeutic response: reduced dependence on antihistamine, less frequent or less severe asthmatic attacks.

PATIENT/FAMILY TEACHING

• Increase fluid intake (decreases lung secretion viscosity). • Must be administered at regular intervals (even when symptom free) to achieve optimal results of therapy. • Unpleasant taste after inhalation may be relieved by rinsing mouth with water immediately.

nelarabine ⚑

nel-**ay**-reh-bean
(Arranon)

CLASSIFICATION

PHARMACOTHERAPEUTIC: DNA demethylation agent. **CLINICAL:** Antineoplastic; antimetabolite.

ACTION

Incorporates into DNA, leading to inhibition of DNA synthesis. Exerts cytotoxic effect on rapidly dividing cells by causing demethylation of DNA. Therapeutic Effect: Produces cell death.

PHARMACOKINETICS

Rapidly eliminated from plasma. Extensive distribution. Protein binding: Less than 25%. Partially eliminated in urine. Half-Life: 30 min.

USES

Treatment of T-cell acute lymphoblastic leukemia and T-cell lymphoblastic lymphoma in patients whose disease has not responded to or has relapsed following treatment with at least two chemotherapy regimens.

PRECAUTIONS

CONTRAINDICATIONS: None known. **CAUTIONS:** Previous or current intrathecal chemotherapy, craniospinal radiation therapy, hepatic disease, renal impairment.

⌛ **LIFESPAN CONSIDERATIONS: Pregnancy/Lactation:** May cause developmental abnormalities of the fetus. Mothers should avoid breast-feeding. **Pregnancy Category D. Children:** No age-related precautions noted. **Elderly:** Increased risk of neurologic toxicities.

INTERACTIONS

DRUG: None known. **HERBAL:** None known. **FOOD:** None known. **LAB VALUES:** May decrease Hgb, Hct, WBCs, RBCs, platelets, albumin, calcium, glucose, magnesium, potassium. May increase bilirubin, transaminase, creatinine, AST.

AVAILABILITY (Rx)

INJECTION: 250 mg (5 mg/ml) in 50 ml vials (Arranon).

ADMINISTRATION/HANDLING

 IV

Reconstitution • Do not dilute before administration. • Transfer appropriate dose into polyvinylchloride infusion bag or glass container before administration.

Rate of administration • Administer as a 2-hr infusion for adults, a 1-hr infusion for pediatric patients.

Storage • Store vials at room temperature. • Solution should appear colorless, free of precipitate.

INDICATIONS/ROUTES/DOSAGE

T-CELL LEUKEMIA, LYMPHOMA
IV: ADULTS, ELDERLY: $1,500$ mg/m^2 infused over 2 hr on day 1, 3, and 5 repeated q21days. CHILDREN 21 YR AND YOUNGER: 650 mg/m^2 infused over 1 hr daily for 5 consecutive days repeated q21days.

SIDE EFFECTS

ADULTS
FREQUENT (50%–41%): Fatigue, nausea. **OCCASIONAL (25%–11%):** Cough, fever, somnolence, vomiting, dyspnea, diarrhea, constipation, dizziness, asthenia (loss of strength, energy), peripheral edema, paresthesia, headache, peripheral neuropathy, myalgia, petechiae, generalized edema. **RARE (9%–4%):** Anorexia, abdominal pain, arthralgia, hypertension, tachycardia, confusion, rigors, stomatitis, back pain, epistaxis, insomnia, dehydration, extremity pain, depression, abdominal distension, blurred vision.

CHILDREN
FREQUENT (17%): Headache. **OCCASIONAL (10%–6%):** Vomiting, somnolence, asthenia (loss of strength, energy), peripheral neuropathy. **RARE (4%–2%):** Paresthesia, tremor, ataxia.

ADVERSE REACTIONS/ TOXIC EFFECTS

Overdosage may result in severe neurotoxicity, myelosuppression. Hematologic toxicity manifested as thrombocytopenia, neutropenia, anemia occur in most cases. Pleural effusion, pneumonia occur in 10% and 8% respectively. Seizures occur in 6% of patients.

NURSING CONSIDERATIONS

BASELINE ASSESSMENT

Give emotional support to patient and family. Use strict asepsis and protect patient from infection. Hydration, urine alkalization, prophylaxis with allopurinol must be given to prevent hyperuricemia of tumor lysis syndrome. Perform blood counts as needed to monitor response and toxicity but particularly before each dosing cycle.

INTERVENTION/EVALUATION

Monitor for hematologic toxicity (fever, sore throat, signs of local infections, easy bruising, unusual bleeding), symptoms of anemia (excessive fatigue, weakness). Assess response to medication; monitor and report nausea, vomiting, diarrhea. Avoid rectal temperatures, other traumas that may induce bleeding.

PATIENT/FAMILY TEACHING

• Do not have immunizations without physician's approval (drug lowers body's resistance). • Avoid crowds, persons with known infections. • Report signs of infection at once (fever, flu-like symptoms). • Contact physician if nausea or vomiting continues at home. • Advise men to use barrier contraception while receiving treatment. • Women should use effective contraceptive measures to avoid pregnancy. • Contact physician or nurse if new or worsening symptoms of peripheral neuropathy occur.

nelfinavir

nel-**fin**-eh-veer
(Viracept)

CLASSIFICATION

PHARMACOTHERAPEUTIC: Protease inhibitor. **CLINICAL:** Antiviral (see pp. 61C, 105C).

ACTION

Inhibits the activity of HIV-1 protease, the enzyme necessary for the formation of infectious HIV. Therapeutic Effect: Formation of immature noninfectious viral particles rather than HIV replication.

PHARMACOKINETICS

Well absorbed after PO administration (absorption increased with food). Protein binding: 98%. Metabolized in the liver. Highly bound to plasma proteins. Eliminated primarily in feces. Unknown if removed by hemodialysis. Half-life: 3.5–5 hr.

USES

Treatment of HIV infection in combination with other antiretrovirals. OFF-LABEL: HIV, postexposure prophylaxis.

PRECAUTIONS

CONTRAINDICATIONS: Concurrent administration with midazolam, rifampin, or triazolam. **CAUTIONS:** Hepatic impairment.

⧗ LIFESPAN CONSIDERATIONS: **Pregnancy/Lactation:** Unknown if distributed in breast milk. **Pregnancy Category B. Children:** No age-related precautions noted in those older than 2 yr. **Elderly:** No information available.

INTERACTIONS

DRUG: **Alcohol, psychoactive drugs:** May produce additive CNS effects. **Anticonvulsants, rifabutin, rifampin:** Decrease nelfinavir plasma concentration. **Indinavir, saquinavir:** Increases plasma concentration of these drugs. **Oral contraceptives:** Decreases the effects of these drugs. **Ritonavir:** Increases nelfinavir plasma concentration. HERBAL: **St. John's wort:** May decrease plasma concentration and effects of nelfinavir. FOOD: **All foods:** Increase nelfinavir plasma concentration. LAB VALUES: May decrease Hgb values and neutrophil and WBC counts. May increase serum creatine kinase (CK), AST, and ALT levels.

AVAILABILITY (Rx)

POWDER FOR ORAL SUSPENSION: 50 mg/g. **TABLETS:** 250 mg, 625 mg.

ADMINISTRATION/HANDLING

PO

• Give with food (light meal, snack). • Mix oral powder with small amount of water, milk, formula, soy formula, soy milk, dietary supplement. • Entire contents must be consumed in order to ingest full dose. • Do not mix with acidic food, orange juice, apple juice, applesauce (bitter taste), or with water in original oral powder container.

INDICATIONS/ROUTES/DOSAGE

HIV INFECTION

PO: ADULTS: 750 mg (three 250-mg tablets) 3 times a day or 1,250 mg twice a day in combination with nucleoside analogues (enhances antiviral activity). CHILDREN 2–13 YR: 45–55 mg/kg twice a day or 25–30 mg/kg 3 times a day. **Maximum:** 2,500 mg/day.

SIDE EFFECTS

FREQUENT (20%): Diarrhea. **OCCASIONAL (7%–3%):** Nausea, rash. **RARE (2%–1%):** Flatulence, asthenia.

ADVERSE REACTIONS/ TOXIC EFFECTS

Diabetes mellitus and hyperglycemia occur rarely.

NURSING CONSIDERATIONS

BASELINE ASSESSMENT

Check hematology, liver function tests for accurate baseline.

INTERVENTION/EVALUATION

Monitor pattern of bowel activity and stool consistency. Monitor hepatic enzyme studies for abnormalities. Be alert to development of opportunistic infections, (e.g., fever, chills, cough, myalgia).

PATIENT/FAMILY TEACHING

• Take with food (optimizes absorption). • Take medication every day as prescribed. • Doses should be evenly spaced around the clock. • Do not alter dose or discontinue medication without informing physician. • Medication is not a cure for HIV infection nor does it reduce risk of transmission to others; patient may continue to experience illnesses, including opportunistic infections.

neomycin sulfate

nee-oh-**mye**-sin

(Myciguent, Neo-Fradin, Neo-Rx, Neo-Tab)

FIXED-COMBINATION(S)

Neosporin GU Irrigant: neomycin/polymyxin B: 40 mg/200,000 units/ml. **Neosporin Ointment, Triple Antibiotic:** neomycin/polymyxin B/bacitracin: 3.5 mg/5,000 units/400 units/g; 3.5 mg/10,000 units/400 units/g.

CLASSIFICATION

PHARMACOTHERAPEUTIC: Aminoglycoside. **CLINICAL:** Antibiotic (see p. 19C).

ACTION

An aminoglycoside antibiotic that binds to bacterial microorganisms. **Therapeutic Effect:** Interferes with bacterial protein synthesis.

PHARMACOKINETICS

Poorly absorbed from the GI tract following PO administration. Protein binding: Low. Primarily eliminated unchanged in the feces; minimal excretion in urine. Removed by hemodialysis. **Half-life:** 3 hr.

USES

Preparation of GI tract for surgery. Treatment of minor skin infections, diarrhea caused by *E. coli*. Adjunct in treatment of hepatic encephalopathy.

PRECAUTIONS

CONTRAINDICATIONS: Hypersensitivity to neomycin, other aminoglycosides (cross-sensitivity), or their components. **CAUTIONS:** Elderly, infants with renal insufficiency or immaturity; neuromuscular disorders, prior hearing loss, vertigo, renal impairment.

N

⌛ LIFESPAN CONSIDERATIONS: Pregnancy/Lactation: Unknown if distributed in breast milk. Avoid breast-feeding. Pregnancy Category C. Children: Safety and efficacy not established in children younger than 18 yr. Elderly: Age-related renal impairment may require dosage adjustment.

INTERACTIONS

DRUG: Nephrotoxic medications, other aminoglycosides, ototoxic medications: May increase nephrotoxicity and ototoxicity if significant systemic absorption occurs. HERBAL: None known. FOOD: None known. LAB VALUES: None known.

AVAILABILITY

TABLETS (NEO-TAB): 500 mg. OINTMENT (MYCIGUENT): 0.5%. CREAM (MYCIGUENT): 0.5% (OTC). ORAL SOLUTION (NEO-FRADIN): 125 mg/5 ml. POWDER FOR COMPOUNDING (NEO-RX): 100%.

INDICATIONS/ROUTES/DOSAGE

PREOPERATIVE BOWEL ANTISEPSIS

PO: ADULTS, ELDERLY: 1 g/hr for 4 doses; then 1 g q4h for 5 doses or 1 g at 1 PM, 2 PM, and 10 PM. (with erythromycin) on day before surgery. CHILDREN: 90 mg/kg/day in divided doses q4h for 2 days or 25 mg/kg at 1 PM, 2 PM, and 10 PM. on day before surgery.

HEPATIC ENCEPHALOPATHY

PO: ADULTS, ELDERLY: 4–12 g/day in divided doses q4–6h. CHILDREN: 2.5–7 g/m^2/day in divided doses q4–6h.

DIARRHEA CAUSED BY ESCHERICHIA COLI

PO: ADULTS, ELDERLY: 3 g/day in divided doses q6h. CHILDREN: 50 mg/kg/day in divided doses q6h.

MINOR SKIN INFECTIONS

TOPICAL: ADULTS, ELDERLY, CHILDREN: Usual dosage, apply to affected area 1–3 times a day.

SIDE EFFECTS

FREQUENT: Systemic: Nausea, vomiting, diarrhea, irritation of mouth or rectal area. Topical: Itching, redness, swelling, rash. RARE: Systemic: Malabsorption syndrome, neuromuscular blockade (difficulty breathing, drowsiness, weakness).

ADVERSE REACTIONS/ TOXIC EFFECTS

Nephrotoxicity (as evidenced by increased BUN and serum creatinine levels and decreased creatinine clearance) may be reversible if the drug is stopped at the first sign of nephrotoxic symptoms. Irreversible ototoxicity (manifested as tinnitus, dizziness, and impaired hearing) and neurotoxicity (as evidenced by headache, dizziness, lethargy, tremor, and visual disturbances) occur occasionally. Severe respiratory depression and anaphylaxis occur rarely. Superinfections, particularly fungal infections, may occur.

NURSING CONSIDERATIONS

BASELINE ASSESSMENT

Dehydration must be treated before aminoglycoside therapy. Establish patient's baseline hearing acuity before beginning therapy.

INTERVENTION/EVALUATION

Be alert to ototoxic, neurotoxic symptoms. Assess for hypersensitivity reaction (topical: assess for rash, redness, itching). Be alert for superinfection, particularly genital or anal pruritus, stomatitis, diarrhea.

PATIENT/FAMILY TEACHING

• Continue antibiotic for full length of treatment. • Space doses evenly. • Topical: Cleanse area gently before application; report redness, itching. • Inform physician if ringing in the ears, impaired hearing, dizziness occurs.

neostigmine

nee-oh-**stig**-meen
(Prostigmin, Prostigmin Bromide)

Do not confuse neostigmine with physostigmine.

CLASSIFICATION

PHARMACOTHERAPEUTIC: Cholinergic. **CLINICAL:** Antimyasthenic, antidote (see p. 82C).

ACTION

A cholinergic that prevents destruction of acetylcholine by inhibiting the enzyme acetylcholinesterase, thus enhancing impulse transmission across the myoneural junction. **Therapeutic Effect:** Improves intestinal and skeletal muscle tone; stimulates salivary and sweat gland secretions.

USES

Improvement of muscle strength in control of myasthenia gravis, diagnosis of myasthenia gravis, prevention or treatment of postop distention and urinary retention, antidote for reversal of effects of nondepolarizing neuromuscular blocking agents after surgery.

PRECAUTIONS

CONTRAINDICATIONS: GI or GU obstruction, history of hypersensitivity reaction to bromides, peritonitis. **CAUTIONS:** Epilepsy, asthma, bradycardia, hyperthyroidism, arrhythmias, peptic ulcer, recent coronary occlusion. **Pregnancy Category C.**

INTERACTIONS

DRUG: Anticholinergics: Reverse or prevent the effects of neostigmine. **Cholinesterase inhibitors:** May increase the risk of toxicity. **Neuromuscular blockers:** Antagonizes the effects of these drugs. **Procainamide, quinidine:** May antagonize the action of neostigmine. **HERBAL:** None known. **FOOD:** None known. **LAB VALUES:** None known.

AVAILABILITY (Rx)

TABLETS (PROSTIGMIN BROMIDE): 15 mg. **INJECTION (PROSTIGMIN):** 0.25 mg/ml, 0.5 mg/ml, 1 mg/ml.

ADMINISTRATION/HANDLING

◀ **ALERT** ▶ Discontinue all anticholinesterase therapy at least 8 hr before testing, as prescribed.
• Plan to give 0.011 mg/kg atropine sulfate IV simultaneously with neostigmine or IM 30 min before administering neostigmine to prevent adverse effects.
• Expect to give larger doses when the patient is most tired.

IV INCOMPATIBILITY

None known.

IV COMPATIBILITIES

Glycopyrrolate (Robinul), heparin, ondansetron (Zofran), potassium chloride, thiopental (Pentothal).

INDICATIONS/ROUTES/DOSAGE

MYASTHENIA GRAVIS
PO: ADULTS, ELDERLY: Initially, 15–30 mg 3–4 times a day. Increase as necessary. Maintenance: 150 mg/day (range of 15–375 mg). CHILDREN: 2 mg/kg/day or 60 mg/m^2/day divided q3–4h.
IV, IM, SUBCUTANEOUS: ADULTS: 0.5–2.5 mg as needed. CHILDREN: 0.01–0.04 mg/kg q2–4h.

DIAGNOSIS OF MYASTHENIA GRAVIS
IM: ADULTS, ELDERLY: 0.022 mg/kg. If cholinergic reaction occurs, discontinue tests and administer 0.4–0.6 mg or more atropine sulfate IV. CHILDREN: 0.025–0.04 mg/kg preceded by atropine sulfate 0.011 mg/kg subcutaneously.

PREVENTION OF POSTOPERATIVE URINARY RETENTION
IM, SUBCUTANEOUS: ADULTS, ELDERLY: 0.25 mg q4–6h for 2–3 days.

N

POSTOPERATIVE ABDOMINAL DISTENTION AND URINE RETENTION
IM, SUBCUTANEOUS: ADULTS, ELDERLY: 0.5–1 mg. Catheterize patient if voiding does not occur within 1 hr. After voiding, administer 0.5 mg q3h for 5 injections.

REVERSAL OF NEUROMUSCULAR BLOCKADE
IV: ADULTS, ELDERLY: 0.5–2.5 mg given slowly. CHILDREN: 0.025–0.08 mg/kg/dose. INFANTS: 0.025–0.1 mg/kg/dose.

SIDE EFFECTS

FREQUENT: Muscarinic effects (diarrhea, diaphoresis, increased salivation, nausea, vomiting, abdominal cramps or pain). **OCCASIONAL:** Muscarinic effects (urinary urgency or frequency, increased bronchial secretions, miosis, lacrimation).

ADVERSE REACTIONS/ TOXIC EFFECTS

Overdose produces a cholinergic crisis manifested as abdominal discomfort or cramps, nausea, vomiting, diarrhea, flushing, facial warmth, excessive salivation, diaphoresis, lacrimation, pallor, bradycardia or tachycardia, hypotension, bronchospasm, urinary urgency, blurred vision, miosis, and fasciculation (involuntary muscular contractions visible under the skin).

NURSING CONSIDERATIONS

BASELINE ASSESSMENT
Larger doses should be given at time of greatest fatigue. Avoid large doses in those with megacolon, reduced GI motility.

INTERVENTION/EVALUATION
Monitor muscle strength, vital signs. Monitor for therapeutic response to medication (increased muscle strength, decreased fatigue, improved chewing, swallowing functions).

PATIENT/FAMILY TEACHING
• Report nausea, vomiting, diarrhea, diaphoresis, increased salivary secretions, palpitations, muscle weakness, severe abdominal pain, difficulty breathing.

Neo-Synephrine, *see* *phenylephrine*

nesiritide

ness-**ear**-ih-tide
(Natrecor)

◆ CLASSIFICATION

PHARMACOTHERAPEUTIC: Brain natriuretic peptide. **CLINICAL:** Endogenous hormone.

ACTION

A brain natriuretic peptide that facilitates cardiovascular homeostasis and fluid status through counterregulation of the renin-angiotensin-aldosterone system, stimulating cyclic guanosine monophosphate, thereby leading to smooth-muscle cell relaxation. **Therapeutic Effect:** Promotes vasodilation, natriuresis, and diuresis, correcting CHF.

PHARMACOKINETICS

Route	Onset	Peak	Duration
IV	15–30 min	1–2 hr	4 hr

Excreted primarily in the heart by the left ventricle. Metabolized by the natriuretic neutral endopeptidase enzymes on the vascular luminal surface. **Half-life:** 18–23 min.

USES

Treatment of acutely decompensated CHF in patients who have dyspnea at rest or with minimal activity.

PRECAUTIONS

CONTRAINDICATIONS: Cardiogenic shock, systolic BP less than 90 mm Hg. **CAUTIONS:** Significant valvular stenosis, restrictive/obstructive cardiomyopathy, constrictive pericarditis, pericardial tamponade, suspected low cardiac filling pressures, atrial/ventricular arrhythmias/conduction defects, hypotension, hepatic/renal insufficiency.

LIFESPAN CONSIDERATIONS: Pregnancy/Lactation: Unknown if drug crosses placenta or is distributed in breast milk. **Pregnancy Category C. Children:** Safety and efficacy not established. **Elderly:** No age-related precautions noted.

INTERACTIONS

DRUG: ACE inhibitors, IV nitroglycerin, milrinone, nitroprusside: May increase risk of hypotension. **Arsenic trioxide:** May increase the risk of QT prolongation. **HERBAL:** None known. **FOOD:** None known. **LAB VALUES:** None known.

AVAILABILITY (Rx)

INJECTION POWDER FOR RECONSTITUTION: 1.5 mg/5-ml vial.

ADMINISTRATION/HANDLING

◀ **ALERT** ▶ Do not mix with other injections or infusions. Do not give IM.

IV

Reconstitution • Reconstitute one 1.5-mg vial with 5 ml D_5W or 0.9% NaCl, 0.2% NaCl or any combination thereof. Swirl or rock gently, add to 250-ml bag D_5W or 0.9% NaCl, 0.2% NaCl, or any combination thereof yielding a solution of 6 mcg/ml.

Rate of administration • Give as an IV bolus over approx. 60 sec initially, followed by continuous IV infusion.

Storage • Store vial at room temperature. Once reconstituted, use within 24 hr at room temperature or refrigerated.

IV INCOMPATIBILITIES

Sodium metabisulfite, bumetanide (Bumex), enalapril (Vasotec), ethacrynic acid (Edecrin), furosemide (Lasix), heparin, hydralazine (Apresoline), insulin.

INDICATIONS/ROUTES/DOSAGE

TREATMENT OF ACUTELY DECOMPENSATED CHF IN PATIENTS WITH DYSPNEA AT REST OR WITH MINIMAL ACTIVITY

IV BOLUS: ADULTS, ELDERLY: 2 mcg/kg followed by a continuous IV infusion of 0.01 mcg/kg/min. At intervals of 3 hr or longer, may be increased by 0.005 mcg/kg/min (preceded by a bolus of 1 mcg/kg), up to a maximum of 0.03 mcg/kg/min.

SIDE EFFECTS

FREQUENT (11%): Hypotension. **OCCASIONAL (8%–2%):** Headache, nausea, bradycardia. **RARE (1% or less):** Confusion, paresthesia, somnolence, tremor.

ADVERSE REACTIONS/TOXIC EFFECTS

Ventricular arrhythmias, including ventricular tachycardia, atrial fibrillation, AV node conduction abnormalities, and angina pectoris occur rarely.

NURSING CONSIDERATIONS

BASELINE ASSESSMENT

Obtain BP immediately before each dose, in addition to regular monitoring (be alert to fluctuations). If excessive reduction in BP occurs, place patient in supine position with legs elevated.

INTERVENTION/EVALUATION

Monitor BP, pulse rate for hypotension frequently during therapy. Hypotension is dose-limiting and dose-dependent. With physician, establish parameters for adjusting rate or stopping infusion. Maintain accurate I&O; measure urine output frequently. Immediately notify physician of decreased urine output, cardiac arrhythmias, significant decrease in BP or heart rate.

PATIENT/FAMILY TEACHING

• Report chest pain, palpitations.

netilmicin sulfate

(Netromycin)

See Antibiotic: aminoglycosides (p. 19C)

Neulasta, see

pegfilgrastim

Neupogen, see *filgrastim*

Neurontin, see *gabapentin*

nevirapine

neh-**veer**-a-peen

(Viramune)

◆CLASSIFICATION

PHARMACOTHERAPEUTIC: Non-nucleoside reverse transcriptase inhibitor. **CLINICAL:** Antiviral (see p. 104C).

ACTION

A non-nucleoside reverse transcriptase inhibitor that binds directly to HIV-1 reverse transcriptase, thus changing the shape of this enzyme and blocking RNA- and DNA-dependent polymerase activity. **Therapeutic Effect:** Interferes with HIV replication, slowing the progression of HIV infection.

PHARMACOKINETICS

Readily absorbed after PO administration. Protein binding: 60%. Widely distributed. Extensively metabolized in the liver. Excreted primarily in urine. **Half-life:** 45 hr (single dose), 25–30 hr (multiple doses).

USES

Used in combination with other antiretroviral agents for treatment of HIV-1 infected adults who have experienced clinical and immunologic deterioration. **OFF-LABEL:** To reduce the risk of transmitting HIV from infected mother to newborn.

PRECAUTIONS

CONTRAINDICATIONS: None known. **CAUTIONS:** Renal/hepatic dysfunction, elevated AST or ALT levels, history of chronic hepatitis (B or C), higher CD4+ cell counts.

⧗ **LIFESPAN CONSIDERATIONS: Pregnancy/Lactation:** Crosses placenta. Distributed in breast milk. Breast-feeding not recommended (possibility of HIV transmission). **Pregnancy Category C. Children:** Granulocytopenia occurs more frequently. **Elderly:** No information available.

INTERACTIONS

DRUG: Ketoconazole, oral contraceptives, protease inhibitors: May decrease the plasma concentrations of these drugs. **Rifabutin, rifampin:** May decrease nevirapine blood concentration. **HERBAL: St. John's wort:** May decrease blood concentration and effects of nevirapine. FOOD: None known. LAB VALUES: May significantly increase serum bilirubin, GGT, AST, and ALT levels. May significantly decrease Hgb level and neutrophil and platelet counts.

AVAILABILITY (Rx)

TABLETS: 200 mg. **ORAL SUSPENSION:** 50 mg/5 ml.

ADMINISTRATION/HANDLING

PO
• Give without regard to meals.

INDICATIONS/ROUTES/DOSAGE

HIV INFECTION
PO: ADULTS: 200 mg once a day for 14 days (to reduce the risk of rash). Maintenance: 200 mg twice a day in combination with nucleoside analogues. CHILDREN OLDER THAN 8 YR: 4 mg/kg once a day for 14 days; then 4 mg/kg twice a day. **Maximum:** 400 mg/day. CHILDREN 2 MO–8 YR: 4 mg/kg once a day for 14 days; then 7 mg/kg twice a day.

SIDE EFFECTS

FREQUENT (8%–3%): Rash, fever, headache, nausea, granulocytopenia (more common in children). **OCCASIONAL (3%–1%):** Stomatitis (burning, erythema, or ulceration of the oral mucosa; dysphagia). **RARE (less than 1%):** Paresthesia, myalgia, abdominal pain.

ADVERSE REACTIONS/ TOXIC EFFECTS

Hepatitis and rash may become severe and life-threatening.

NURSING CONSIDERATIONS

BASELINE ASSESSMENT
Establish baseline lab values, especially liver function tests, before initiating therapy and at intervals during therapy. Obtain medication history (especially use of oral contraceptives).

INTERVENTION/EVALUATION
Closely monitor for evidence of rash (usually appears on trunk, face, extremities; occurs within first 6 wk of drug initiation). Observe for rash accompanied by fever, blistering, oral lesions, conjunctivitis, swelling, muscle/joint aches, general malaise.

PATIENT/FAMILY TEACHING
• If nevirapine therapy is missed for longer than 7 days, restart by using one 200 mg tablet daily for first 14 days, followed by one 200 mg tablet 2 times/ day. • Continue therapy for full length of treatment. • Doses should be evenly spaced. • Nevirapine is not a cure for HIV infection, nor does it reduce risk of transmission to others. • If rash appears, contact physician before continuing therapy.

Nexium, *see esomeprazole*

---

niacin, nicotinic acid

nye-a-sin
(Niacor, <u>Niaspan</u>, Nicotinex, Slo-Niacin)

Do not confuse niacin, Niacor, or Niaspan with minocin or Nitro-Bid.

FIXED-COMBINATION(S)

Advicor: niacin/lovastatin: 500 mg/ 20 mg; 750 mg/20 mg; 1,000 mg/ 20 mg.

◆ CLASSIFICATION

CLINICAL: Antihyperlipidemic, water-soluble vitamin (see pp. 53C, 145C).

ACTION

An antihyperlipidemic, water-soluble vitamin that is a component of two coenzymes needed for tissue respiration, lipid metabolism, and glycogenolysis. Inhibits synthesis of VLDLs. **Therapeutic Effect:** Reduces total, LDL, and VLDL cholesterol levels and triglyceride levels; increases HDL cholesterol concentration.

PHARMACOKINETICS

Readily absorbed from the GI tract. Widely distributed. Metabolized in the liver. Primarily excreted in urine. **Half-life:** 45 min.

USES

Adjunct in treatment of hyperlipidemias, peripheral vascular disease; treatment of pellagra; dietary supplement.

PRECAUTIONS

CONTRAINDICATIONS: Active peptic ulcer disease, arterial hemorrhaging, hepatic dysfunction, hypersensitivity to niacin or tartrazine (frequently seen in patients sensitive to aspirin), severe hypotension. **CAUTIONS:** Diabetes mellitus, gallbladder disease, gout, history of jaundice/hepatic disease.

⚱ **LIFESPAN CONSIDERATIONS: Pregnancy/Lactation:** Not recommended for use during pregnancy/lactation. Distributed in breast milk. **Pregnancy Category A (C if used at dosages above the recommended daily allowance). Children:** No age-related precautions noted. Not recommended in those younger than 2 yr. **Elderly:** No age-related precautions noted.

INTERACTIONS

DRUG: Alcohol: May increase risk of niacin side effects, such as flushing. **Lovastatin, pravastatin, simvastatin:** May increase the risk of acute renal failure and rhabdomyolysis. **HERBAL:** None known. **FOOD:** None known. **LAB VALUES:** May increase serum uric acid level.

AVAILABILITY (OTC)

CAPSULES (TIMED-RELEASE): 125 mg, 250 mg, 400 mg, 500 mg. **TABLETS (NIACOR):** 50 mg, 100 mg, 250 mg, 500 mg. **TABLETS (TIMED-RELEASE [SLO-NIACIN]):** 250 mg, 500 mg, 750 mg. **TABLETS (TIMED-RELEASE [NIASPAN]):** 500 mg, 750 mg, 1,000 mg. **ELIXIR (NICOTINEX):** 50 mg/5 ml.

ADMINISTRATION/HANDLING

PO

• For patients switching from immediate-release niacin to extended-release niacin, therapy with extended-release niacin should be initiated with low doses and titrated to therapeutic response.
• Take at bedtime after a low-fat snack.
• Give aspirin 30 min before taking extended-release niacin to minimize flushing.

INDICATIONS/ROUTES/DOSAGE

HYPERLIPIDEMIA

PO (IMMEDIATE-RELEASE): ADULTS, ELDERLY: Initially, 50–100 mg twice a day for 7 days. Increase gradually by doubling dose qwk up to 1–1.5 g/day in 2–3 doses. **Maximum:** 3 g/day. CHILDREN: Initially, 100–250 mg/day (**maximum:** 10 mg/kg/day) in 3 divided doses. May increase by 100 mg/wk or 250 mg q2–3wk. **Maximum:** 2,250 mg/day.

PO (TIMED-RELEASE): ADULTS, ELDERLY: Initially, 500 mg/day in 2 divided doses for 1 wk; then increase to 500 mg twice a day. Maintenance: 2 g/day.

NUTRITIONAL SUPPLEMENT

PO: ADULTS, ELDERLY: 10–20 mg/day. **Maximum:** 100 mg/day.

PELLEGRA

PO (IMMEDIATE-RELEASE): ADULTS, ELDERLY: 50–100 mg 3–4 times a day. **Maximum:** 500 mg/day. CHILDREN: 50–100 mg 3 times a day.

SIDE EFFECTS

FREQUENT: Flushing (especially of the face and neck) occurring within 20 min of drug administration and lasting for 30–60 min GI upset, pruritus. **OCCASIONAL:** Dizziness, hypotension, headache, blurred vision, burning or tingling of skin, flatulence, nausea, vomiting, diarrhea. **RARE:** Hyperglycemia, glycosuria, rash, hyperpigmentation, dry skin.

ADVERSE REACTIONS/ TOXIC EFFECTS

Arrhythmias occur rarely.

NURSING CONSIDERATIONS

BASELINE ASSESSMENT

Question for history of hypersensitivity to niacin, tartrazine, aspirin. Assess serum baselines: cholesterol, triglyceride, glucose, hepatic function tests.

INTERVENTION/EVALUATION

Evaluate flushing, degree of GI discomfort. Check for headache, dizziness, blurred vision. Determine pattern of bowel activity. Monitor hepatic function, serum cholesterol, triglycerides. Check blood glucose levels carefully in those on insulin, oral antihyperglycemics. Assess skin for rash, dryness. Monitor serum uric acid levels.

PATIENT/FAMILY TEACHING

• Transient flushing of the skin, sensation of warmth, itching, tingling may occur. • Notify physician if dizziness occurs (avoid sudden changes in posture). • Inform physician if nausea, vomiting, loss of appetite, yellowing of skin, dark urine, feeling of weakness occurs. • Advise the patient to take aspirin 30 min before taking extended-release niacin to minimize flushing.

Niaspan, *see nicotinic acid*

*niCARdipine hydrochloride

nigh-**car**-dih-peen
(Cardene, Cardene IV, Cardene SR)

Do not confuse nicardipine with nifedipine, Cardene with codeine, or Cardene SR with Cardizem SR or codeine.

CLASSIFICATION

PHARMACOTHERAPEUTIC: Calcium channel blocker. **CLINICAL:** Antianginal, antihypertensive (see p. 69C).

ACTION

An antianginal and antihypertensive agent that inhibits calcium ion movement across cell membranes, depressing contraction of cardiac and vascular smooth muscle. **Therapeutic Effect:** Increases heart rate and cardiac output. Decreases systemic vascular resistance and BP.

PHARMACOKINETICS

Route	Onset	Peak	Duration
PO	N/A	1–2 hr	8 hr

Rapidly, completely absorbed from the GI tract. Protein binding: 95%. Undergoes first-pass metabolism in the liver. Primarily excreted in urine. Not removed by hemodialysis. **Half-life:** 2–4 hr.

USES

PO: Treatment of chronic stable (effort-associated) angina, essential hypertension. **Sustained-Release:** Treatment

N

of essential hypertension. **Parenteral:** Short-term treatment of hypertension when oral therapy not feasible or desirable. OFF-LABEL: Treatment of associated neurologic deficits, Raynaud's phenomenon, subarachnoid hemorrhage, vasospastic angina.

PRECAUTIONS

CONTRAINDICATIONS: Atrial fibrillation or flutter associated with accessory conduction pathways, cardiogenic shock, CHF, second- or third-degree heart block, severe hypotension, sinus bradycardia, ventricular tachycardia, within several hours of IV beta-blocker therapy. **CAUTIONS:** Sick sinus syndrome, severe left ventricular dysfunction, renal or hepatic impairment, cardiomyopathy, edema, concomitant beta-blocker or digoxin therapy.

⧗ LIFESPAN CONSIDERATIONS: **Pregnancy/Lactation:** Unknown if distributed in breast milk. **Pregnancy Category C. Children:** Safety and efficacy not established. **Elderly:** Age-related renal impairment may require dosage adjustment.

INTERACTIONS

DRUG: **Beta blockers:** May have additive effect. **Digoxin:** May increase nicardipine blood concentration. **Hypokalemia-producing agents (such as furosemide and certain other diuretics):** May increase risk of arrhythmias. **Procainamide, quinidine:** May increase risk of QT-interval prolongation. HERBAL: None known. FOOD: **Grapefruit, grapefruit juice:** May alter absorption of nicardipine. LAB VALUES: None known.

AVAILABILITY (Rx)

CAPSULES (CARDENE): 20 mg, 30 mg.
CAPSULES (SUSTAINED-RELEASE [CARDENE SR]): 30 mg, 45 mg, 60 mg.
INJECTION (CARDENE IV): 2.5 mg/ml.

ADMINISTRATION/HANDLING

 IV

Reconstitution • Dilute each 25-mg ampule with 250 ml D₅W, 0.9% NaCl, 0.45% NaCl, or any combination thereof to provide a concentration of 1 mg/ 10 ml. Maximum Concentration: 4 mg/ 10 ml.

Rate of administration • Give by slow IV infusion. • Change IV site q12h if administered peripherally.

Storage • Store at room temperature. • Diluted IV solution is stable for 24 hr at room temperature.

PO
• Do not crush or break oral, sustained-release capsules. • Give without regard to food.

▦ IV INCOMPATIBILITIES

Furosemide (Lasix), heparin, thiopental (Pentothal).

IV COMPATIBILITIES

Diltiazem (Cardizem), dobutamine (Dobutrex), dopamine (Intropin), epinephrine, hydromorphone (Dilaudid), labetalol (Trandate), lorazepam (Ativan), midazolam (Versed), milrinone (Primacor), morphine, nitroglycerin, norepinephrine (Levophed).

INDICATIONS/ROUTES/DOSAGE

CHRONIC STABLE (EFFORT-ASSOCIATED) ANGINA

PO: ADULTS, ELDERLY: Initially, 20 mg 3 times a day. Range: 20–40 mg 3 times a day.

ESSENTIAL HYPERTENSION

PO: ADULTS, ELDERLY: Initially, 20 mg 3 times a day. Range: 20–40 mg 3 times a day.

PO (SUSTAINED-RELEASE): ADULTS, ELDERLY: Initially, 30 mg twice a day. Range: 30–60 mg twice a day.

SHORT-TERM TREATMENT OF HYPERTENSION WHEN ORAL THERAPY ISN'T FEASIBLE OR DESIRABLE (SUBSTITUTE FOR ORAL NICARDIPINE)

IV: ADULTS, ELDERLY: 0.5 mg/hr (for patient receiving 20 mg PO q8h); 1.2 mg/hr (for patient receiving 30 mg PO q8h); 2.2 mg/hr (for patient receiving 40 mg PO q8h).

PATIENTS NOT ALREADY RECEIVING NICARDIPINE

IV: ADULTS, ELDERLY (GRADUAL BP DECREASE): Initially, 5 mg/hr. May increase by 2.5 mg/hr q15min. After BP goal is achieved, decrease rate to 3 mg/hr. ADULTS, ELDERLY (RAPID BP DECREASE): Initially, 5 mg/hr. May increase by 2.5 mg/hr q5min. **Maximum:** 15 mg/hr until desired BP attained. After BP goal achieved, decrease rate to 3 mg/hr.

CHANGING FROM IV TO ORAL ANTIHYPERTENSIVE THERAPY

ADULTS, ELDERLY: Begin antihypertensives other than nicardipine when IV has been discontinued; for nicardipine, give first dose 1 hr before discontinuing IV.

DOSAGE IN HEPATIC IMPAIRMENT

For adults and elderly patients, initially give 20 mg twice a day; then titrate.

DOSAGE IN RENAL IMPAIRMENT

For adults and elderly patients, initially give 20 mg q8h (30 mg twice a day [sustained-release capsules]); then titrate.

SIDE EFFECTS

FREQUENT (10%–7%): Headache, facial flushing, peripheral edema, light-headedness, dizziness. **OCCASIONAL (6%–3%):** Asthenia (loss of strength, energy), palpitations, angina, tachycardia. **RARE (less than 2%):** Nausea, abdominal cramps, dyspepsia, dry mouth, rash.

ADVERSE REACTIONS/ TOXIC EFFECTS

Overdose produces confusion, slurred speech, somnolence, marked hypotension, and bradycardia.

NURSING CONSIDERATIONS

BASELINE ASSESSMENT

Concurrent therapy of sublingual nitroglycerin may be used for relief of anginal pain. Record onset, type (sharp, dull, squeezing), radiation, location, intensity, duration of anginal pain, precipitating factors (exertion, emotional stress).

INTERVENTION/EVALUATION

Monitor BP during and following IV infusion. Assess for peripheral edema behind medial malleolus. Assess skin for facial flushing, dermatitis, rash. Question for asthenia, headache. Monitor serum hepatic enzyme results. Assess EKG, pulse for tachycardia.

PATIENT/FAMILY TEACHING

• Take sustained-release with food; do not crush. • Avoid alcohol, limit caffeine. • Inform physician if angina pains not relieved or palpitations, shortness of breath, swelling, dizziness, constipation, nausea, hypotension occurs.

nicotine

nik-o-teen

(Commit, Habitrol ◆, NicoDerm ◆, NicoDerm CQ, NicoDerm CQ Clear, Nicorette, Nicorette Plus ◆, Nicotrol, Nictrol Inhaler, Nicotrol NS, Nicotrol Patch ◆)

Do not confuse Nicoderm with Nitroderm.

• CLASSIFICATION

PHARMACOTHERAPEUTIC: Cholinergic-receptor agonist. **CLINICAL:** Smoking deterrent.

ACTION

A cholinergic-receptor agonist that binds to acetylcholine receptors, producing both stimulating and depressant effects on the peripheral and central nervous systems. **Therapeutic Effect:** Provides a source of nicotine during nicotine withdrawal and reduces withdrawal symptoms.

PHARMACOKINETICS

Absorbed slowly after transdermal administration. Protein binding: 5%. Metabolized in the liver. Excreted primarily in urine. **Half-life:** 4 hr.

USES

An alternative, less potent form of nicotine (without tar, carbon monoxide, carcinogenic substances of tobacco) used as part of a smoking cessation program.

PRECAUTIONS

CONTRAINDICATIONS: Immediate post-MI period, life-threatening arrhythmias, severe or worsening angina. **CAUTIONS:** Hyperthyroidism, pheochromocytoma, insulin-dependent diabetes mellitus, severe renal impairment, eczematous dermatitis, oral or pharyngeal inflammation, esophagitis, peptic ulcer (delays healing in peptic ulcer disease).

⧗ **LIFESPAN CONSIDERATIONS:** **Pregnancy/Lactation:** Passes freely into breast milk. Use of cigarettes, nicotine gum associated with decrease in fetal breathing movements. **Pregnancy Category D (transdermal). Children:** Not recommended. **Elderly:** Age-related decrease in cardiac function may require dosage adjustment.

INTERACTIONS

DRUG: **Beta-adrenergic blockers, bronchodilators (such as theophylline), insulin, propoxyphene:** May increase the effects of these drugs. **HERBAL:** None known. **FOOD:** None known. **LAB VALUES:** None known.

AVAILABILITY (OTC)

CHEWING GUM (NICORETTE): 2 mg, 4 mg. **LOZENGE (COMMIT):** 2 mg, 4 mg.

TRANSDERMAL PATCH (NICODERM CQ, NICOTROL): 5 mg/16 hr, 7 mg/24 hr, 10 mg/16 hr, 14 mg/24 hr, 21 mg/24 hr mg. **NASAL SPRAY (NICOTROL NS):** 0.5 mg/spray. **INHALATION (NICOTROL INHALER):** 10 mg cartridge.

ADMINISTRATION/HANDLING

GUM
• Do not swallow. • Chew 1 piece when urge to smoke present. • Chew slowly and intermittently for 30 min. • Chew until distinctive nicotine taste (peppery) or slight tingling in mouth perceived, then stop; when tingling almost gone (about 1 min) repeat chewing procedure (this allows constant slow buccal absorption). • Too rapid chewing may cause excessive release of nicotine, resulting in adverse effects similar to oversmoking (e.g., nausea, throat irritation).

INHALER
• Insert cartridge into mouthpiece. • Puff on nicotine cartridge mouthpiece for 20 min.

TRANSDERMAL
• Apply promptly upon removal from protective pouch (prevents evaporation, loss of nicotine). Use only intact pouch. Do not cut patch. • Apply only once/day to hairless, clean, dry skin on upper body or outer arm. • Replace daily; rotate sites; do not use same site within 7 days; do not use same patch longer than 24 hr. • Wash hands with water alone after applying patch (soap may increase nicotine absorption). • Discard used patch by folding patch in half (sticky side together), placing in pouch of new patch, and throwing away in such a way as to prevent child or pet accessibility.

INDICATIONS/ROUTES/DOSAGE

SMOKING CESSATION AID TO RELIEVE NICOTINE WITHDRAWAL SYMPTOMS
PO (CHEWING GUM): ADULTS, ELDERLY: Usually, 10–12 pieces/day. **Maximum:** 30 pieces/day.
PO (LOZENGE): ◂ **ALERT** ▸ For those who smoke the first cigarette within

30 min of waking, administer the 4-mg lozenge; otherwise administer the 2-mg lozenge. ADULTS, ELDERLY: One 4-mg or 2-mg lozenge q1–2h for the first 6 wk; 1 lozenge q2–4h for wk 7–9; and 1 lozenge q4–8h for wk 10–12. **Maximum:** 1 lozenge at a time, 5 lozenges/6 hr, 20 lozenges/day.

TRANSDERMAL: ADULTS, ELDERLY WHO SMOKE 10 CIGARETTES OR MORE PER DAY: Follow the guidelines below. **Step 1:** 21 mg/day for 4–6 wk. **Step 2:** 14 mg/day for 2 wk. **Step 3:** 7 mg/day for 2 wk. ADULTS, ELDERLY WHO SMOKE LESS THAN 10 CIGARETTES PER DAY: Follow the guidelines below. **Step 1:** 14 mg/day for 6 wk. **Step 2:** 7 mg/day for 2 wk. PATIENTS WEIGHING LESS THAN 100 LB, PATIENTS WITH A HISTORY OF CARDIOVASCULAR DISEASE: Initially, 14 mg/day for 4–6 wk, then 7 mg/day for 2–4 wk.

TRANSDERMAL (NICOTROL): ADULTS, ELDERLY: One patch a day for 6 wk.

NASAL: ADULTS, ELDERLY: 1–2 doses/hr (1 dose = 2 sprays [1 in each nostril] = 1 mg). **Maximum:** 5 doses (5 mg)/hr; 40 doses (40 mg)/day.

INHALER (NICOTROL): ADULTS, ELDERLY: Puff on nicotine cartridge mouthpiece for about 20 min as needed.

SIDE EFFECTS

FREQUENT: All forms: Hiccups, nausea. **Gum:** Mouth or throat soreness, nausea, hiccups. **Transdermal:** Erythema, pruritus, or burning at application site. **OCCASIONAL: All forms:** Eructation, GI upset, dry mouth, insomnia, diaphoresis, irritability. **Gum:** Hiccups, hoarseness. **Inhaler:** Mouth or throat irritation, cough. **RARE: All forms:** Dizziness, myalgia, arthralgia.

ADVERSE REACTIONS/ TOXIC EFFECTS

Overdose produces palpitations, tachyarrhythmias, seizures, depression, confusion, diaphoresis, hypotension, rapid or weak pulse, and dyspnea. Lethal dose

for adults is 40–60 mg. Death results from respiratory paralysis.

NURSING CONSIDERATIONS

BASELINE ASSESSMENT
Screen, evaluate those with coronary heart disease (history of MI, angina pectoris), serious cardiac arrhythmias, Buerger's disease, Prinzmetal's variant angina.

INTERVENTION/EVALUATION
Monitor smoking habit, BP, pulse, sleep pattern, skin for erythema, pruritus, burning at application site if transdermal system used.

PATIENT/FAMILY TEACHING
• Instruct patient on proper application of transdermal system. • Inform patient to chew gum slowly to avoid jaw ache and maximize benefit. • Inform physician if persistent rash, itching occurs with patch. • Do not smoke while wearing patches.

N

*NIFEdipine

nye-**fed**-i-peen
(Adalat CC, Adalat FT ✤, Adalat P.A. ✤, Apo-Nifed ✤, Nifedical XL, Novo-Nifedin ✤, Procardia, Procardia XL)

Do not confuse nifedipine with nicardipine or nimodipine.

CLASSIFICATION

PHARMACOTHERAPEUTIC: Calcium channel blocker. **CLINICAL:** Antianginal, antihypertensive (see p. 69C).

ACTION

An antianginal and antihypertensive agent that inhibits calcium ion movement across cell membranes, depressing contraction of cardiac and vascular smooth muscle. **Therapeutic Effect:** Increases heart rate and cardiac output. Decreases systemic vascular resistance and BP.

PHARMACOKINETICS

Route	Onset	Peak	Duration
Sublingual	1–5 min	N/A	N/A
PO	20–30 min	N/A	4–8 hr
PO (extended release)	2 hr	N/A	24 hr

Rapidly, completely absorbed from the GI tract. Protein binding: 92%–98%. Undergoes first-pass metabolism in the liver. Primarily excreted in urine. Not removed by hemodialysis. **Half-life:** 2–5 hr.

USES

Treatment of angina due to coronary artery spasm (Prinzmetal's variant angina), chronic stable angina (effort-associated angina). **Extended-Release:** Treatment of essential hypertension. OFF-LABEL: Treatment of Raynaud's phenomenon.

PRECAUTIONS

CONTRAINDICATIONS: Advanced aortic stenosis, severe hypotension. **CAUTIONS:** Renal or hepatic impairment.

⌛ LIFESPAN CONSIDERATIONS: **Pregnancy/Lactation:** Insignificant amount distributed in breast milk. **Pregnancy Category C. Children:** Safety and efficacy not established. **Elderly:** Age-related renal impairment may require dosage adjustment.

INTERACTIONS

DRUG: **Beta blockers:** May have additive effect. **Digoxin:** May increase digoxin blood concentration. **Hypokalemia-producing agents (such as furosemide and certain other diuretics):** May increase risk of arrhythmias. HERBAL: None known. FOOD: **Grapefruit, grapefruit**

juice: May increase nifedipine plasma concentration. LAB VALUES: May cause positive ANA and direct Coombs' test.

AVAILABILITY (Rx)

CAPSULES (PROCARDIA): 10 mg. **TABLETS (EXTENDED-RELEASE):** 30 mg (Adalat CC, Nifedical XL, Procardia XL), 60 mg (Adalat CC, Nifedical XL, Procardia XL), 90 mg (Adalat CC, Procardia XL).

ADMINISTRATION/HANDLING

PO
• Do not crush or break extended-release tablet. • Give without regard to meals. • Grapefruit juice may alter absorption.

SUBLINGUAL
• Capsule must be punctured, chewed, and/or squeezed to express liquid into mouth.

INDICATIONS/ROUTES/DOSAGE

PRINZMETAL'S VARIANT ANGINA, CHRONIC STABLE (EFFORT-ASSOCIATED) ANGINA
PO: ADULTS, ELDERLY: Initially, 10 mg 3 times a day. Increase at 7- to 14-day intervals. Maintenance: 10 mg 3 times a day up to 30 mg 4 times a day.
PO (EXTENDED-RELEASE): ADULTS, ELDERLY: Initially, 30–60 mg/day. Maintenance: Up to 120 mg/day.

ESSENTIAL HYPERTENSION
PO (EXTENDED-RELEASE): ADULTS, ELDERLY: Initially, 30–60 mg/day. Maintenance: Up to 120 mg/day.

SIDE EFFECTS

FREQUENT (30%–11%): Peripheral edema, headache, flushed skin, dizziness. **OCCASIONAL (12%–6%):** Nausea, shakiness, muscle cramps and pain, somnolence, palpitations, nasal congestion, cough, dyspnea, wheezing. **RARE (5%–3%):** Hypotension, rash, pruritus, urticaria, constipation, abdominal discomfort, flatulence, sexual difficulties.

ADVERSE REACTIONS/ TOXIC EFFECTS

Nifedipine may precipitate CHF and MI in patients with cardiac disease and peripheral ischemia. Overdose produces nausea, somnolence, confusion, and slurred speech.

NURSING CONSIDERATIONS

BASELINE ASSESSMENT

Concurrent therapy of sublingual nitroglycerin may be used for relief of anginal pain. Record onset, type (sharp, dull, squeezing), radiation, location, intensity, duration of anginal pain; precipitating factors (exertion, emotional stress). Check BP for hypotension immediately before giving medication.

INTERVENTION/EVALUATION

Assist with ambulation if lightheadedness, dizziness occurs. Assess for peripheral edema. Assess skin for flushing. Monitor serum hepatic enzyme tests.

PATIENT/FAMILY TEACHING

• Rise slowly from lying to sitting position, permit legs to dangle from bed momentarily before standing to reduce hypotensive effect. • Contact physician or nurse if palpitations, shortness of breath, pronounced dizziness, nausea occurs. • Avoid alcohol, concomitant grapefruit or grapefruit juice use.

---

nilutamide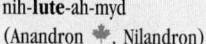

nih-**lute**-ah-myd
(Anandron ♣, Nilandron)

◆CLASSIFICATION

PHARMACOTHERAPEUTIC: Hormone. **CLINICAL:** Antineoplastic (see p. 77C).

ACTION

An antiandrogen hormone and antineoplastic agent that competitively inhibits androgen action by binding to androgen receptors in target tissue. Therapeutic Effect: Decreases growth of abnormal prostate tissue.

PHARMACOKINETICS

Well absorbed following PO administration. Protein binding: 80%–84%. Metabolized in liver. Primarily excreted in urine. Half-life: 38–59 hr.

USES

Treatment of metastatic prostatic carcinoma (stage D_2) in combination with surgical castration. For maximum benefit, begin on same day or day after surgical castration.

PRECAUTIONS

CONTRAINDICATIONS: Severe hepatic impairment, severe respiratory insufficiency. **CAUTIONS:** Hepatitis, marked increase in serum hepatic enzymes.

⌛ LIFESPAN CONSIDERATIONS: **Pregnancy/Lactation:** Unknown if drug crosses placenta or is distributed in breast milk. **Pregnancy Category C. Children:** Safety and efficacy not established. **Elderly:** No age-related precautions noted.

INTERACTIONS

DRUG: **Fosphenytoin, phenytoin, theophylline:** May increase the risk of toxicity of these drugs. **Warfarin:** May increase the risk of bleeding. HERBAL: None known. FOOD: None known. LAB VALUES: May increase serum bilirubin, creatinine, AST, and ALT levels.

AVAILABILITY (Rx)

TABLETS: 150 mg.

INDICATIONS/ROUTES/DOSAGE

PROSTATIC CARCINOMA

PO: ADULTS, ELDERLY: 300 mg once a day for 30 days, then 150 mg once a day.

N

---

* "Tall Man" lettering   ♣ Canadian trade name   ⓔ see **evolve**   ▷ High Alert drug

Begin on day of, or day after, surgical castration.

SIDE EFFECTS

FREQUENT (greater than 10%): Hot flashes, delay in recovering vision after bright illumination (such as sun, television, bright lights), decreased libido, diminished sexual function, mild nausea, gynecomastia, alcohol intolerance. **OCCASIONAL (less than 10%):** Constipation, hypertension, dizziness, dyspnea, UTIs.

ADVERSE REACTIONS/ TOXIC EFFECTS

Interstitial pneumonitis occurs rarely.

NURSING CONSIDERATIONS

BASELINE ASSESSMENT

Baseline chest x-ray, hepatic enzyme levels should be obtained before beginning therapy

INTERVENTION/EVALUATION

Monitor BP periodically and liver function tests in long-term therapy.

PATIENT/FAMILY TEACHING

• Contact physician if any side effects occur at home, especially signs of hepatic toxicity (jaundice, dark urine, fatigue, abdominal pain). • Caution about driving at night (tinted glasses may help).

nimodipine

nye-**mode**-i-peen
(Nimotop)

Do not confuse nimodipine with nifedipine.

◆CLASSIFICATION

PHARMACOTHERAPEUTIC: Calcium channel blocker. **CLINICAL:** Cerebral vasospasm agent (see p. 69C).

ACTION

A cerebral vasospasm agent that inhibits movement of calcium ions across vascular smooth-muscle cell membranes. **Therapeutic Effect:** Produces favorable effect on severity of neurologic deficits due to cerebral vasospasm. Exerts greatest effect on cerebral arteries; may prevent cerebral spasm.

PHARMACOKINETICS

Rapidly absorbed from the GI tract. Protein binding: 95%. Metabolized in the liver. Excreted in urine; eliminated in feces. Not removed by hemodialysis. **Half-life:** terminal, 3 hr.

USES

Improvement of neurologic deficits due to cerebral vasospasm following subarachnoid hemorrhage from ruptured congenital intracranial aneurysms in patients in satisfactory neurologic condition. **OFF-LABEL:** Treatment of chronic and classic migraine, chronic cluster headaches.

PRECAUTIONS

CONTRAINDICATIONS: Atrial fibrillation or flutter, cardiogenic shock, CHF, heart block, sinus bradycardia, ventricular tachycardia, within several hours of IV beta-blocker therapy. **CAUTIONS:** Renal or hepatic impairment.

⧖ **LIFESPAN CONSIDERATIONS: Pregnancy/Lactation:** Unknown if drug crosses placenta or is distributed in breast milk. **Pregnancy Category C. Children:** Safety and efficacy not established. **Elderly:** Age-related renal impairment may require dosage adjustment. May experience greater hypotensive response, constipation.

INTERACTIONS

DRUG: Beta blockers: May prolong SA and AV conduction, which may lead to severe hypotension, bradycardia, and cardiac failure. **Erythromycin,**

N

itraconazole, ketoconazole, protease inhibitors: May inhibit the metabolism of nimodipine. **Rifabutin, rifampin:** May increase the metabolism of nimodipine. HERBAL: **Garlic:** May increase antihypertensive effect. **Ginseng, yohimbe:** May worsen hypertension. FOOD: **Grapefruit juice:** May increase nimodipine blood concentration and risk of toxicity. LAB VALUES: None known.

AVAILABILITY (Rx)

CAPSULES: 30 mg.

ADMINISTRATION/HANDLING

PO
• If patient unable to swallow, place hole in both ends of capsule with 18-gauge needle to extract contents into syringe.
• Empty into NG tube; flush tube with 30 ml normal saline.

INDICATIONS/ROUTES/DOSAGE

IMPROVEMENT OF NEUROLOGIC DEFICITS AFTER SUBARACHNOID HEMORRHAGE FROM RUPTURED CONGENITAL ANEURYSMS
PO: ADULTS, ELDERLY: 60 mg q4h for 21 days. Begin within 96 hr of subarachnoid hemorrhage.

SIDE EFFECTS

OCCASIONAL   (6%–2%): Hypotension, peripheral edema, diarrhea, headache. RARE (less than 2%): Allergic reaction (rash, hives), tachycardia, flushing of skin.

ADVERSE REACTIONS/ TOXIC EFFECTS

Overdose produces nausea, weakness, dizziness, somnolence, confusion, and slurred speech.

NURSING CONSIDERATIONS

BASELINE ASSESSMENT
Assess level of consciousness (LOC), neurologic response, initially and throughout therapy. Monitor baseline liver function tests. Assess BP, apical pulse immediately before drug administration (if pulse is 60/min or less or systolic BP is less than 90 mm Hg, withhold medication, contact physician).

INTERVENTION/EVALUATION
Monitor CNS response, heart rate, BP for evidence of hypotension, signs and symptoms of CHF.

PATIENT/FAMILY TEACHING
• Do not crush or chew capsules.
• Inform physician if palpitations, shortness of breath, swelling, constipation, nausea, dizziness occurs.

nisoldipine
(Sular)
See Calcium channel blockers

nitazoxanide

nye-tay-**zocks**-ah-nide
(Alinia)

CLASSIFICATION
PHARMACOTHERAPEUTIC: Antiparasitic. CLINICAL: Antiprotozoal.

ACTION
An antiparasitic that interferes with the body's reaction to pyruvate ferredoxin oxidoreductase, an enzyme essential for anaerobic energy metabolism. Therapeutic Effect: Produces antiprotozoal activity, reducing or terminating diarrheal episodes.

PHARMACOKINETICS
Rapidly hydrolyzed to an active metabolite. Protein binding: 99%. Excreted in the urine, bile, and feces. Half-life: 2–4 hr.

N

USES

Treatment of diarrhea caused by *Cryptosporidium parvum* and *Giardia lamblia* in children 12 mo and older and adults.

PRECAUTIONS

CONTRAINDICATIONS: History of sensitivity to aspirin and salicylates. **CAUTIONS:** GI disorders, hepatic/biliary disease, renal impairment.

⧖ LIFESPAN CONSIDERATIONS: **Pregnancy/Lactation:** Unknown if distributed in breast milk. **Pregnancy Category B. Children:** Safety and efficacy in children older than 11 yr has not been established. **Elderly:** Not for use in this age group.

INTERACTIONS

DRUG: None known. HERBAL: None known. FOOD: None known. LAB VALUES: May increase serum creatinine and ALT levels.

AVAILABILITY (Rx)

POWDER FOR ORAL SUSPENSION: 100 mg/5 ml. **TABLETS:** 500 mg.

ADMINISTRATION/HANDLING

PO, ORAL SUSPENSION
• Store unreconstituted powder at room temperature. • Reconstitute oral suspension with 48 ml water to provide a concentration of 100 mg/5 ml. • Shake vigorously to suspend powder. • Reconstituted solution is stable for 7 days at room temperature. • Give with food.

PO (TABLETS)
• Do not crush or cut film-coated tablets. • Give with food.

INDICATIONS/ROUTES/DOSAGE

DIARRHEA CAUSED BY *C. PARVUM*
PO: CHILDREN 4–11 YR: 200 mg q12h for 3 days. CHILDREN 12–47 MO: 100 mg q12h for 3 days.

DIARRHEA CAUSED BY *G. LAMBIA*
PO: ADULTS, ELDERLY, CHILDREN 12 YR AND OLDER: 500 mg q12h for 3 days. CHILDREN 4–11 YR: 200 mg q12h for 3 days. CHILDREN 12–47 MO: 100 mg q12h for 3 days.

SIDE EFFECTS

OCCASIONAL (8%): Abdominal pain. **RARE (2%–1%):** Diarrhea, vomiting, headache.

ADVERSE REACTIONS/ TOXIC EFFECTS

None known.

BASELINE ASSESSMENT
Establish baseline BP, weight, blood glucose, electrolytes. Assess for dehydration.

INTERVENTION/EVALUATION
Evaluate blood glucose levels in diabetics, electrolytes (therapy generally reduces abnormalities). Weigh patient daily. Encourage adequate fluid intake. Assess bowel sounds for peristalsis. Monitor bowel activity/stool consistency.

PATIENT/FAMILY TEACHING
• Parents of children with diabetes should be aware that the oral suspension contains 1.48 g of sucrose per 5 ml. • Therapy should provide significant improvement of diarrhea.

nitrofurantoin sodium

ny-tro-feur-**an**-toyn
(Apo-Nitrofurantoin ✦, Furadantin, Macrobid, Macrodantin, Nitro Macro, Novo-Furan ✦)

◆CLASSIFICATION

PHARMACOTHERAPEUTIC: Antibacterial. **CLINICAL:** UTI prophylaxis.

ACTION

An antibacterial UTI agent that inhibits the synthesis of bacterial DNA, RNA, proteins, and cell walls by altering or inactivating ribosomal proteins. **Therapeutic Effect:** Bacteriostatic (bactericidal at high concentrations).

PHARMACOKINETICS

Microcrystalline form rapidly and completely absorbed; macrocrystalline form more slowly absorbed. Food increases absorption. Protein binding: 40%. Primarily concentrated in urine and kidneys. Metabolized in most body tissues. Primarily excreted in urine. Removed by hemodialysis. Half-life: 20–60 min.

USES

Treatment of UTIs, initial and chronic. OFF-LABEL: Prevention of bacterial UTIs.

PRECAUTIONS

CONTRAINDICATIONS: Anuria, oliguria, substantial renal impairment (creatinine clearance less than 40 ml/min); infants younger than 1 mo old because of the risk of hemolytic anemia. **CAUTIONS:** Renal impairment, diabetes mellitus, electrolyte imbalance, anemia, vitamin B deficiency, debilitated (greater risk of peripheral neuropathy), G6PD deficiency (greater risk of hemolytic anemia).

⧗ LIFESPAN CONSIDERATIONS: Pregnancy/Lactation: Readily crosses placenta. Distributed in breast milk. Contraindicated at term and during lactation when infant suspected of having G6PD deficiency. **Pregnancy Category B. Children:** No age-related precautions noted in those older than 1 mo. **Elderly:** More likely to develop acute pneumonitis and peripheral neuropathy. Age-related renal impairment may require dosage adjustment.

INTERACTIONS

DRUG: **Hemolytics:** May increase the risk of nitrofurantoin toxicity. **Neurotoxic medications:** May increase the risk of neurotoxicity. **Probenecid:** May increase blood concentration and toxicity of nitrofurantoin. HERBAL: None known. FOOD: None known. LAB VALUES: None known.

AVAILABILITY (Rx)

CAPSULES (MACROCRYSTALLINE, MONOHYDRATE [MACROBID]): 100 mg. **CAPSULES (MACROCRYSTALLINE [MACRODANTIN, NITRO MACRO]):** 25 mg, 50 mg, 100 mg. **ORAL SUSPENSION (MICROCRYSTALLINE [FURADANTIN]):** 25 mg/5 ml.

ADMINISTRATION/HANDLING

PO
• Give with food, milk to enhance absorption, reduce GI upset.

INDICATIONS/ROUTES/DOSAGE

UTIs
PO (FURADANTIN, MACRODANTIN): ADULTS, ELDERLY: 50–100 mg q6h. **Maximum:** 400 mg/day. CHILDREN: 5–7 mg/kg/day in divided doses q6h. **Maximum:** 400 mg/day.
PO (MACROBID): ADULTS, ELDERLY: 100 mg twice a day. **Maximum:** 400 mg/day.

LONG-TERM PREVENTION OF UTIs
PO: ADULTS, ELDERLY: 50–100 mg at bedtime. CHILDREN: 1–2 mg/kg/day as a single dose. **Maximum:** 100 mg/day.

SIDE EFFECTS

FREQUENT: Anorexia, nausea, vomiting, dark urine. **OCCASIONAL:** Abdominal pain, diarrhea, rash, pruritus, urticaria, hypertension, headache, dizziness, drowsiness. **RARE:** Photosensitivity, transient alopecia, asthmatic exacerbation in those with history of asthma.

N

ADVERSE REACTIONS/ TOXIC EFFECTS

Superinfection, hepatotoxicity, peripheral neuropathy (may be irreversible), Stevens-Johnson syndrome, permanent pulmonary function impairment, and anaphylaxis occur rarely.

NURSING CONSIDERATIONS

BASELINE ASSESSMENT

Question for history of asthma. Evaluate lab test results for renal and hepatic baseline values.

INTERVENTION/EVALUATION

Monitor I&O, renal function results. Determine pattern of bowel activity. Assess skin for rash, urticaria. Be alert for numbness or tingling, especially of lower extremities (may signal onset of peripheral neuropathy). Observe for signs of hepatotoxicity (fever, rash, arthralgia, hepatomegaly). Perform respiratory assessment: auscultate lungs, check for cough, chest pain, difficulty breathing.

PATIENT/FAMILY TEACHING

• Urine may become dark yellow/ brown. • Take with food, milk for best results and to reduce GI upset. • Complete full course of therapy. • Avoid sun and ultraviolet light; use sunscreens, wear protective clothing. • Notify physician if cough, fever, chest pain, difficult breathing, numbness or tingling of fingers or toes occurs. • Rare occurrence of alopecia is transient.

nitroglycerin

nye-troe-**gli**-ser-in

(Minitran, Nitrek, Nitro-Bid, Nitro-Bid IV, Nitrocot, Nitro-Dur, Nitrogard, Nitroglyn E-R, Nitroject ✤, Nitrol Appli-Kit, Nitrolingual, Nitrong, Nitrong-SR ✤,

NitroQuick, Nitrostat, Nitro-Tab, Nitro TD Patch-A, Nitro-Time, Tridil, Trinipatch ✤)

Do not confuse nitroglycerin with nitroprusside; Nitro-Bid with Nicobid; Nitro-Dur with Nicoderm; Nitrostat with Hyperstat, Nilstat, or Nystatin; or Nitrong-SR with Nizoral.

◆CLASSIFICATION

PHARMACOTHERAPEUTIC: Nitrate. **CLINICAL:** Antianginal, antihypertensive, coronary vasodilator (see p. 114C).

ACTION

A nitrate that decreases myocardial oxygen demand. Reduces left ventricular preload and afterload. **Therapeutic Effect:** Dilates coronary arteries and improves collateral blood flow to ischemic areas within myocardium. IV form produces peripheral vasodilation.

PHARMACOKINETICS

Route	Onset	Peak	Duration
Sublingual	1–3 min	4–8 min	30–60 min
Translingual spray	2 min	4–10 min	30–60 min
Buccal tablet	2–5 min	4–10 min	2 hr
PO (extended-release)	20–45 min	45–120 min	4–8 hr
Topical	15–60 min	30–120 min	2–12 hr
Transdermal patch	40–60 min	60–180 min	18–24 hr
IV	1–2 min	Immediate	3–5 min

Well absorbed after PO, sublingual, and topical administration. Undergoes extensive first-pass metabolism. Metabolized in the liver and by enzymes in the bloodstream. Primarily excreted in urine. Not removed by hemodialysis. **Half-life:** 1–4 min.

USES

Lingual, sublingual, buccal dose used for acute relief of angina pectoris. Extended-release, topical forms used for prophylaxis, long-term angina management. IV form used in treatment of CHF associated with acute MI.

PRECAUTIONS

CONTRAINDICATIONS: Allergy to adhesives (transdermal), closed-angle glaucoma, constrictive pericarditis (IV), early MI (sublingual), GI hypermotility or malabsorption (extended-release), head trauma, hypotension (IV), inadequate cerebral circulation (IV), increased intracranial pressure (ICP), nitrates, orthostatic hypotension, pericardial tamponade (IV), severe anemia, uncorrected hypovolemia (IV). **CAUTIONS:** Acute MI, hepatic or renal disease, glaucoma (contraindicated in closed-angle glaucoma), blood volume depletion from diuretic therapy, systolic BP less than 90 mm Hg.

⧗ LIFESPAN CONSIDERATIONS: **Pregnancy/Lactation:** Unknown if drug crosses placenta or is distributed in breast milk. **Pregnancy Category B. Children:** Safety and efficacy not established. **Elderly:** More susceptible to hypotensive effects. Age-related renal impairment may require dosage adjustment.

INTERACTIONS

DRUG: **Alcohol, other antihypertensives, vasodilators:** May increase risk of orthostatic hypotension. **Sildenafil, tadalafil, vardenafil:** Concurrent use of these drugs produces significant hypotension. HERBAL: None known. FOOD: None known. LAB VALUES: May increase blood methemoglobin, urine catecholamine, and urine vanillylmandelic acid concentrations.

AVAILABILITY (Rx)

CAPSULES (EXTENDED-RELEASE [NITRO-BID, NITROCOT, NITROGLYN E-R, **NITRO-TIME]):** 2.5 mg, 6.5 mg, 9 mg. **TABLETS (EXTENDED-RELEASE, ORAL TRANSMUCOSAL):** 1 mg (Nitrogard), 2.6 mg (Nitrong), 3 mg (Nitrogard), 6.5 mg (Nitrong). **TABLETS (SUBLINGUAL [NITROQUICK, NITROSTAT, NITRO-TAB]):** 0.3 mg, 0.4 mg, 0.6 mg. **SPRAY (TRANSLINGUAL [NITROLINGUAL]):** 0.4 mg/spray. **INFUSION SOLUTION:** 0.1 mg/ml, 0.2 mg/ml, 0.4 mg/ml. **INTRAVENOUS SOLUTION (NITRO-BID IV, TRIDIL):** 5 mg/ml. **INTRAVENOUS SOLUTION:** 5% dextrose-10 mg nitroglycerin/100 ml, 5% dextrose-20 mg nitroglycerin/100 ml, 5% dextrose-40 mg nitroglycerin/100 ml. **TOPICAL OINTMENT (NITRO-BID, NITROL, NITROL APPL-KIT):** 2%. **TRANSDERMAL PATCH (MINITRAN):** 0.1 mg/h (Minitran, Nitro-Dur), 0.2 mg/h (Minitran, Nitrek, Nitro-Dur), 0.3 mg/h (Minitran, Nitro-Dur), 0.4 mg/h (Minitran, Nitrek, Nitro-Dur), 0.6 mg/h (Nitrek, Nitro-Dur), 0.8 mg/h (Nitro-Dur).

ADMINISTRATION/HANDLING

◀ ALERT ▶ Cardioverter or defibrillator must not be discharged through paddle electrode overlying nitroglycerin system (may cause burns to patient or damage to paddle via arcing).

 IV

Reconstitution • Available in ready-to-use injectable containers. • Dilute vials in 250 or 500 ml D_5W or 0.9% NaCl. Maximum concentration: 250 mg/250 ml.

Rate of administration • Use microdrop or infusion pump.

Storage • Store at room temperature.

PO
• Do not chew extended-release form.
• Do not shake oral aerosol canister before lingual spraying.

SUBLINGUAL
• Do not swallow; dissolve under the tongue. • Administer while seated.

• Slight burning sensation under tongue may be lessened by placing tablet in buccal pouch. • Keep sublingual tablets in original container.

TOPICAL
• Spread thin layer on clean, dry, hairless skin of upper arm or body (not below knee or elbow), using applicator or dose-measuring papers. Do not use fingers; do not rub or massage into skin.

TRANSDERMAL
• Apply patch on clean, dry, hairless skin of upper arm or body (not below knee or elbow).

▦ IV INCOMPATIBILITY
Alteplase (Activase).

IV COMPATIBILITIES
Amiodarone (Cordarone), diltiazem (Cardizem), dobutamine (Dobutrex), dopamine (Intropin), epinephrine, famotidine (Pepcid), fentanyl (Sublimaze), furosemide (Lasix), heparin, hydromorphone (Dilaudid), insulin, labetalol (Trandate), lidocaine, lorazepam (Ativan), midazolam (Versed), milrinone (Primacor), morphine, nicardipine (Cardene), nitroprusside (Nipride), norepinephrine (Levophed), propofol (Diprivan).

INDICATIONS/ROUTES/DOSAGE
ACUTE RELIEF OF ANGINA PECTORIS, ACUTE PROPHYLAXIS
LINGUAL SPRAY: ADULTS, ELDERLY: 1 spray onto or under tongue q3–5min until relief is noted (no more than 3 sprays in 15-min period).
SUBLINGUAL: ADULTS, ELDERLY: 0.4 mg q5min until relief is noted (no more than 3 doses in 15-min period). Use prophylactically 5–10 min before activities that may cause an acute attack.

LONG-TERM PROPHYLAXIS OF ANGINA
PO (EXTENDED-RELEASE): ADULTS, ELDERLY: 2.5–9 mg 2–4 times a day. **Maximum:** 26 mg 4 times a day.

TOPICAL: ADULTS, ELDERLY: Initially, ½ inch q8h. Increase by ½ inch with each application. Range: 1–2 inches q8h up to 4–5 inches q4h.
TRANSDERMAL PATCH: ADULTS, ELDERLY: Initially, 0.2–0.4 mg/hr. Maintenance: 0.4–0.8 mg/hr. Consider patch on for 12–14 hr, patch off for 10–12 hr (prevents tolerance).

CHF ASSOCIATED WITH ACUTE MI
IV: ADULTS, ELDERLY: Initially, 5 mcg/min via infusion pump. Increase in 5-mcg/min increments at 3- to 5-min intervals until BP response is noted or until infusion reaches 20 mcg/min; then increase as needed by 10 mcg/min. Dosage may be further titrated according to clinical, therapeutic response up to 200 mcg/min. CHILDREN: Initially, 0.25–0.5 mcg/kg/min; titrate by 0.5–1 mcg/kg/min up to 20 mcg/kg/min.

SIDE EFFECTS
FREQUENT: Headache (possibly severe; occurs mostly in early therapy, diminishes rapidly in intensity, and usually disappears during continued treatment), transient flushing of face and neck, dizziness (especially if patient is standing immobile or is in a warm environment), weakness, orthostatic hypotension. **Sublingual:** Burning, tingling sensation at oral point of dissolution. **Ointment:** Erythema, pruritus. **OCCASIONAL:** GI upset. **Transdermal:** Contact dermatitis.

ADVERSE REACTIONS/ TOXIC EFFECTS
Nitroglycerin should be discontinued if blurred vision or dry mouth occurs. Severe orthostatic hypotension may occur, manifested by fainting, pulselessness, cold or clammy skin, and diaphoresis. Tolerance may occur with repeated, prolonged therapy; minor tolerance may occur with intermittent use of sublingual tablets. High doses of nitroglycerin tend to produce severe headache.

N

NURSING CONSIDERATIONS

BASELINE ASSESSMENT

Record onset, type (sharp, dull, squeezing), radiation, location, intensity, duration of anginal pain; and precipitating factors (exertion, emotional stress). Assess BP, apical pulse before administration and periodically following dose. Patient must have continuous EKG monitoring for IV administration.

INTERVENTION/EVALUATION

Monitor BP, heart rate. Assess for facial or neck flushing. Cardioverter or defibrillator must not be discharged through paddle electrode overlying nitroglycerin system (may cause burns to patient or damage to paddle via arcing).

PATIENT/FAMILY TEACHING

• Rise slowly from lying to sitting position, dangle legs momentarily before standing. • Take oral form on empty stomach (however, if headache occurs during therapy, take medication with meals). • Use spray only when lying down. • Dissolve sublingual tablet under tongue; do not swallow. • Take at first sign of angina. • If not relieved within 5 min, contact physician or immediately go to emergency room. • May take another dose q5min if needed up to a total of 3 doses. • Do not change brands. • Keep container away from heat, moisture. • Do not inhale lingual aerosol but spray onto or under tongue (avoid swallowing after spray is administered). • Expel from mouth any remaining lingual, sublingual, or intrabuccal tablet after pain is completely relieved. • Place transmucosal tablets under upper lip or buccal pouch (between cheek and gum); do not chew or swallow tablet. • Avoid alcohol (intensifies hypotensive effect). If alcohol is ingested soon after taking nitroglycerin, possible acute hypotensive episode (marked drop in BP, vertigo, diaphoresis, pallor) may occur.

nitroprusside sodium ⚑

nye-troe-**pruss**-ide
(Nipride ✤, Nitropress)
Do not confuse nitroprusside with nitroglycerin or Nitrostat.

◆CLASSIFICATION

PHARMACOTHERAPEUTIC: Hypertensive emergency agent. **CLINICAL:** Antihypertensive, vasodilator, CHF/MI adjunct, antidote.

ACTION

A potent vasodilator used to treat emergent hypertensive conditions; acts directly on arterial and venous smooth muscle. Decreases peripheral vascular resistance, preload and afterload; improves cardiac output. **Therapeutic Effect:** Dilates coronary arteries, decreases oxygen consumption, and relieves persistent chest pain.

PHARMACOKINETICS

Route	Onset	Peak	Duration
IV	1–10 min	Dependent on infusion rate	Dissipates rapidly after stopping IV

Reacts with Hgb in erythrocytes, producing cyanmethemoglobin, and cyanide ions. Primarily excreted in urine. **Half-life:** less than 10 min.

USES

Immediate reduction of BP in hypertensive crisis. Produces controlled hypotension in surgical procedures to reduce bleeding. Treatment of acute CHF. **OFF-LABEL:** Control of paroxysmal hypertension before and during surgery for pheochromocytoma, peripheral vasospasm caused by ergot alkaloid overdose, treatment adjunct for MI, valvular regurgitation.

N

PRECAUTIONS

CONTRAINDICATIONS: Compensatory hypertension (AV shunt or coarctation of aorta), congenital (Leber's) optic atrophy, inadequate cerebral circulation, moribund patients, tobacco amblyopia. **CAUTIONS:** Severe hepatic or renal impairment, hypothyroidism, hyponatremia, elderly.

 LIFESPAN CONSIDERATIONS: **Pregnancy/Lactation:** Unknown if drug crosses placenta or is distributed in breast milk. **Pregnancy Category C. Children:** Safety and efficacy not established. **Elderly:** More sensitive to hypotensive effect. Age-related renal impairment may require dosage adjustment.

INTERACTIONS

DRUG: Dobutamine: May increase cardiac output and decrease pulmonary wedge pressure. **Hypotension-producing medications:** May increase hypotensive effect. **HERBAL:** None known. **FOOD:** None known. **LAB VALUES:** None known.

AVAILABILITY (Rx)

INJECTION: 25 mg/ml. **POWDER FOR INJECTION:** 50 mg.

ADMINISTRATION/HANDLING

 IV

Reconstitution • Reconstitute 50-mg vial with 2–3 ml D$_5$W or sterile water for injection without preservative. • Further dilute with 250–1,000 ml D$_5$W to provide concentration of 200 mcg, 50 mcg/ml, respectively. Maximum concentration: 200 mg/250 ml. • Wrap infusion bottle in aluminum foil immediately after mixing.

Rate of administration • Give by IV infusion only using infusion rate chart provided by manufacturer or protocol. • Administer using IV infusion pump and lock in rate. • Be alert for extravasation (produces severe pain, sloughing).

Storage • Protect solution from light. • Solution should appear very faint brown. • Use only freshly prepared solution. Once prepared, do not keep or use longer than 24 hr. • Deterioration evidenced by color change from brown to blue, green, dark red. • Discard unused portion.

IV INCOMPATIBILITY

Cisatracurium (Nimbex).

IV COMPATIBILITIES

Diltiazem (Cardizem), dobutamine (Dobutrex), dopamine (Intropin), enalapril (Vasotec), heparin, insulin, labetalol (Normodyne, Trandate), lidocaine, midazolam (Versed), milrinone (Primacor), nitroglycerin, propofol (Diprivan).

INDICATIONS/ROUTES/DOSAGE

IMMEDIATE REDUCTION OF BP IN HYPERTENSIVE CRISIS; TO PRODUCE CONTROLLED HYPOTENSION IN SURGICAL PROCEDURES TO REDUCE BLEEDING; TREATMENT OF ACUTE CHF
IV INFUSION: ADULTS, ELDERLY: Initially, 0.3–0.5 mcg/kg/min. May increase by 0.5 mcg/kg/min to desired hemodynamic effect or appearance of headache or nausea. Usual dose: 3 mcg/kg/min. **Maximum:** 10 mcg/kg/min.

SIDE EFFECTS

OCCASIONAL: Flushing of skin, increased intracranial pressure, rash, pain or redness at injection site.

ADVERSE REACTIONS/ TOXIC EFFECTS

A too-rapid IV infusion rate reduces BP too quickly. Nausea, vomiting, diaphoresis, apprehension, headache, restlessness, muscle twitching, dizziness, palpitations, retrosternal pain, and abdominal pain may occur. Symptoms disappear rapidly if rate of administration is slowed or drug is temporarily discontinued. Overdose produces metabolic acidosis and tolerance to therapeutic effect.

NURSING CONSIDERATIONS

BASELINE ASSESSMENT
Monitor EKG, BP continuously. Check with physician for desired BP parameters (BP is normally maintained about 30%–40% below pretreatment levels). Medication should be discontinued if therapeutic response is not achieved within 10 min after IV infusion at 10 mcg/kg/min.

INTERVENTION/EVALUATION
Monitor rate of infusion frequently. Monitor blood acid-base balance, electrolytes, laboratory results, I&O. Assess for metabolic acidosis (weakness, disorientation, headache, nausea, hyperventilation, vomiting). Assess for therapeutic response to medication. Monitor BP for potential rebound hypertension after infusion is discontinued.

nizatidine

ni-**za**-ti-deen

(Apo-Nizatidine ♣, Axid, Axid AR)

Do not confuse Axid with Ansaid.

◆CLASSIFICATION

PHARMACOTHERAPEUTIC: H_2 receptor antagonist. **CLINICAL:** Antiulcer, gastric acid secretion inhibitor (see p. 96C).

ACTION
An antiulcer agent and gastric acid secretion inhibitor that inhibits histamine action at histamine 2 receptors of parietal cells. **Therapeutic Effect:** Inhibits basal and nocturnal gastric acid secretion.

PHARMACOKINETICS
Rapidly, well absorbed from the GI tract. Protein binding: 35%. Metabolized in the liver. Primarily excreted in urine. Not removed by hemodialysis. **Half-life:** 1–2 hr (increased with impaired renal function).

USES
Short-term treatment of active duodenal ulcer, active benign gastric ulcer. Prevention of duodenal ulcer recurrence. Treatment of gastroesophageal reflux disease (GERD), including erosive esophagitis. OTC for prevention of meal induced heartburn, acid indigestion, and sour stomach. **OFF-LABEL:** Gastric hypersecretory conditions, multiple endocrine adenoma, Zollinger-Ellison syndrome, weight gain reduction in patients taking Zyprexa.

PRECAUTIONS
CONTRAINDICATIONS: Hypersensitivity to other H_2-antagonists. **CAUTIONS:** Renal/hepatic impairment.

⌛ **LIFESPAN CONSIDERATIONS: Pregnancy/Lactation:** Unknown if drug crosses placenta or is distributed in breast milk. **Pregnancy Category B. Children:** Safety and efficacy not established in those younger than 12 yr. **Elderly:** No age-related precautions noted.

INTERACTIONS
DRUG: Antacids: May decrease the absorption of nizatidine. **Ketoconazole:** May decrease the absorption of ketoconazole. **HERBAL:** None known.

N

FOOD: None known. **LAB VALUES:** Interferes with skin tests using allergen extracts. May increase serum alkaline phosphatase, AST, and ALT levels.

AVAILABILITY (Rx)

CAPSULES: 75 mg (Axid AR [OTC]), 150 mg (Axid), 300 mg (Axid). **ORAL SOLUTION (AXID):** 15 mg/ml.

ADMINISTRATION/HANDLING

PO
• Give without regard to meals. Best given after meals or at bedtime. • Do not administer within 1 hr of magnesium- or aluminum-containing antacids (decreases absorption). • May give right before eating for heartburn prevention.

INDICATIONS/ROUTES/DOSAGE

ACTIVE DUODENAL ULCER
PO: ADULTS, ELDERLY: 300 mg at bedtime or 150 mg twice a day.

PREVENTION OF DUODENAL ULCER RECURRENCE
PO: ADULTS, ELDERLY: 150 mg at bedtime.

GASTROESOPHAGEAL REFLUX DISEASE
PO: ADULTS, ELDERLY: 150 mg twice a day.

ACTIVE BENIGN GASTRIC ULCER
PO: ADULTS, ELDERLY: 150 mg twice a day or 300 mg at bedtime.
PO, ORAL SOLUTION: CHILDREN 12 YR AND OLDER: 2 tsp twice a day.

DYSPEPSIA
PO: ADULTS, ELDERLY: 75 mg 30–60 min before meals; no more than 2 tablets a day.

DOSAGE IN RENAL IMPAIRMENT
Dosage adjustment is based on creatinine clearance.

Creatinine Clearance	Active Ulcer	Maintenance Therapy
20–50 ml/min	150 mg at bedtime	150 mg every other day
Less than 20 ml/min	150 mg every other day	150 mg q3days

SIDE EFFECTS

OCCASIONAL (2%): Somnolence, fatigue.
RARE (1%): Diaphoresis, rash.

ADVERSE REACTIONS/ TOXIC EFFECTS

Asymptomatic ventricular tachycardia, hyperuricemia not associated with gout, and nephrolithiasis occur rarely.

NURSING CONSIDERATIONS

INTERVENTION/EVALUATION
Assess for abdominal pain, GI bleeding (overt blood in emesis/stool, tarry stools). Monitor blood tests for elevated AST, ALT, serum alkaline phosphatase (hepatocellular injury).

PATIENT/FAMILY TEACHING
• Avoid tasks that require alertness, motor skills until drug response is established. • Avoid alcohol, aspirin, smoking. • Inform physician if symptoms of heartburn, acid indigestion, sour stomach persist after 2 wk of continuous use of nizatidine.

Nolvadex, *see tamoxifen*

norepinephrine bitartrate ▷

nor-eh-pih-**nef**-rin
(Levophed)
Do not confuse Levophed with Levid, or norepinephrine with epinephrine.

◆CLASSIFICATION

PHARMACOTHERAPEUTIC: Sympathomimetic. **CLINICAL:** Vasopressor (see p. 142C).

ACTION

A sympathomimetic that stimulates beta$_1$-adrenergic receptors and alpha-adrenergic receptors, increasing peripheral resistance. Enhances contractile myocardial force, increases cardiac output. Constricts resistance and capacitance vessels. Therapeutic Effect: Increases systemic BP and coronary blood flow.

PHARMACOKINETICS

Route	Onset	Peak	Duration
IV	Rapid	1–2 min	N/A

Localized in sympathetic tissue. Metabolized in the liver. Primarily excreted in urine.

USES

Corrects hypotension unresponsive to adequate fluid volume replacement, as part of shock syndrome, caused by MI, bacteremia, open heart surgery, renal failure.

PRECAUTIONS

CONTRAINDICATIONS: Hypovolemic states (unless as an emergency measure), mesenteric or peripheral vascular thrombosis, profound hypoxia. **CAUTIONS:** Severe cardiac disease, hypertensive or hypothyroid patients, those on MAOIs.

⧗ **LIFESPAN CONSIDERATIONS: Pregnancy/Lactation:** Readily crosses placenta. May produce fetal anoxia due to uterine contraction, constriction of uterine blood vessels. **Pregnancy**

Category C. Children/Elderly: No age-related precautions noted.

INTERACTIONS

DRUG: Beta blockers: May have mutually inhibitory effects. **Digoxin:** May increase risk of arrhythmias. **Ergonovine, oxytocin:** May increase vasoconstriction. **MAOIs:** May cause prolonged hypertension. **Maprotiline, tricyclic antidepressants:** May increase cardiovascular effects. **Methyldopa:** May decrease the effects of methyldopa. **HERBAL:** None known. **FOOD:** None known. **LAB VALUES:** None known.

AVAILABILITY (Rx)

INJECTION: 1-mg/ml ampules.

ADMINISTRATION/HANDLING

◄ **ALERT** ► Blood, fluid volume depletion should be corrected before drug is administered.

 IV

Reconstitution • Add 4 ml (4 mg) to 250 ml (16 mcg/ml). Maximum concentration: 32 ml (32 mg) to 250 ml (128 mcg/ml).

Rate of administration • Avoid catheter tie in technique (encourages stasis, increases local drug concentration). • Closely monitor IV infusion flow rate (use microdrip or infusion pump). • Monitor BP q2min during IV infusion until desired therapeutic response is achieved, then q5min during remaining IV infusion. • Never leave patient unattended. • Maintain BP at 80–100 mm Hg in previously normotensive patients, and 30–40 mm Hg below preexisting BP in previously hypertensive patients. • Reduce IV infusion gradually. Avoid abrupt withdrawal. • If using peripherally inserted catheter, it is imperative to check the IV site

N

frequently for free flow and infused vein for blanching, hardness to vein, coldness, pallor to extremity. • If extravasation occurs, area should be infiltrated with 10–15 ml sterile saline containing 5–10 mg phentolamine (does not alter pressor effects of norepinephrine).

Storage • Do not use if brown or contains precipitate. • Store ampules at room temperature.

⁜ IV INCOMPATIBILITY
Regular insulin.

IV COMPATIBILITIES

Amiodarone (Cordarone), calcium gluconate, diltiazem (Cardizem), dobutamine (Dobutrex), dopamine (Intropin), epinephrine, esmolol (Brevibloc), fentanyl (Sublimaze), furosemide (Lasix), haloperidol (Haldol), heparin, hydromorphone (Dilaudid), labetalol (Trandate), lorazepam (Ativan), magnesium, midazolam (Versed), milrinone (Primacor), morphine, nicardipine (Cardene), nitroglycerin, potassium chloride, propofol (Diprivan).

INDICATIONS/ROUTES/DOSAGE

ACUTE HYPOTENSION UNRESPONSIVE TO FLUID VOLUME REPLACEMENT

IV: ADULTS, ELDERLY: Initially, administer at 0.5–1 mcg/min. Adjust rate of flow to establish and maintain desired BP (40 mm Hg below preexisting systolic pressure). Average maintenance dose: 8–30 mcg/min. CHILDREN: Initially, 0.05–0.1 mcg/kg/min; titrate to desired effect. **Maximum:** 1–2 mcg/kg/min. Range: 0.5–3 mcg/min.

SIDE EFFECTS

Norepinephrine produces less pronounced and less frequent side effects than epinephrine. **OCCASIONAL (5%–3%):** Anxiety, bradycardia, palpitations. **RARE (2%–1%):** Nausea, anginal pain, shortness of breath, fever.

ADVERSE REACTIONS/ TOXIC EFFECTS

Extravasation may produce tissue necrosis and sloughing. Overdose is manifested as severe hypertension with violent headache (which may be the first clinical sign of overdose), arrhythmias, photophobia, retrosternal or pharyngeal pain, pallor, excessive sweating, and vomiting. Prolonged therapy may result in plasma volume depletion. Hypotension may recur if plasma volume is not restored.

NURSING CONSIDERATIONS

BASELINE ASSESSMENT

Assess EKG, BP continuously (be alert to precipitous BP drop). Never leave patient alone during IV infusion. Be alert to patient complaint of headache.

INTERVENTION/EVALUATION

Monitor IV flow rate diligently. Assess for extravasation characterized by blanching of skin over vein, coolness (results from local vasoconstriction); color and temperature of IV site extremity (pallor, cyanosis, mottling). Assess nailbed capillary refill. Monitor I&O; measure output hourly, and report urine output less than 30 ml/hr. IV should not be reinstated unless systolic BP falls below 70–80 mm Hg.

norfloxacin ⓔ

nor-**flox**-a-sin

(Apo-Norflox ✢, INorfloxacine ✢, Noroxin, Novo-Norfloxacin ✢, PMS-Norfloxacin ✢)

CLASSIFICATION

PHARMACOTHERAPEUTIC: Quinolone. **CLINICAL:** Anti-infective (see p. 24C).

ACTION

A quinolone that inhibits DNA gyrase in susceptible microorganisms, interfering with bacterial cell replication and repair. **Therapeutic Effect:** Bactericidal.

USES

Treatment of susceptible infections due to *E. faecalis, E. coli, K. pneumoniae, P. mirabilis, P. aeruginosa, S. epidermidis. S. saprophyticus* including UTIs, uncomplicated gonococcal infections, acute or chronic prostatitis.

PRECAUTIONS

CONTRAINDICATIONS: Children younger than 18 yr because of risk of arthropathy; hypersensitivity to other quinolones or their components. **CAUTIONS:** Renal impairment; predisposition to seizures.

⧗ LIFESPAN CONSIDERATIONS: **Pregnancy/Lactation:** Unknown if drug crosses placenta or is distributed in breast milk. **Pregnancy Category C. Children:** Safety and efficacy not established. **Elderly:** Age-related renal impairment may require dosage adjustment.

INTERACTIONS

DRUG: **Antacids, sucralfate:** May decrease norfloxacin absorption. **Oral anticoagulants:** May increase effects of oral anticoagulants. **Theophylline:** Decreases clearance and may increase blood concentration and risk of toxicity of theophylline. HERBAL: None known. FOOD: None known. LAB VALUES: May increase BUN level and serum alkaline phosphatase, bilirubin, creatinine, LDH, AST, and ALT levels.

AVAILABILITY (Rx)

TABLETS: 400 mg.

ADMINISTRATION/HANDLING

PO

• Give 1 hr before or 2 hr after meals, with 8 oz of water. • Encourage additional glasses of water between meals. • Do not administer antacids with or within 2 hr of norfloxacin dose. • Encourage cranberry juice, citrus fruits (to acidify urine).

INDICATIONS/ROUTES/DOSAGE

UTIs
PO: ADULTS, ELDERLY: 400 mg twice a day for 3–21 days.

PROSTATITIS
PO: ADULTS: 400 mg twice a day for 28 days.

DOSAGE IN RENAL IMPAIRMENT
Dosage and frequency are modified based on creatinine clearance.

Creatinine Clearance	Dosage
30 ml/min or higher	400 mg twice a day
Less than 30 ml/min	400 mg once a day

SIDE EFFECTS

FREQUENT: Nausea, headache, dizziness. **RARE:** Vomiting, diarrhea, dry mouth, bitter taste, nervousness, drowsiness, insomnia, photosensitivity, tinnitus, crystalluria, rash, fever, seizures.

ADVERSE REACTIONS/ TOXIC EFFECTS

Superinfection, anaphylaxis, Stevens-Johnson syndrome, and arthropathy occur rarely. Hypersensitivity reactions, including photosensitivity (as evidenced by rash, pruritus, blisters, edema, and burning skin), have occurred in patients receiving fluoroquinolones.

NURSING CONSIDERATIONS

BASELINE ASSESSMENT

Question for history of hypersensitivity to norfloxacin, quinolones.

INTERVENTION/EVALUATION

Assess for nausea, headache, dizziness. Evaluate food tolerance. Assess for chest, joint pain.

PATIENT/FAMILY TEACHING

- Take 1 hr before or 2 hr after meals.
- Complete full course of therapy.
- Take with 8 oz of water; drink several glasses of water between meals. • May cause dizziness, drowsiness. • Do not take antacids with or within 2 hr of norfloxacin dose (reduces or destroys effectiveness).

Normodyne, *see labetalol*

---

nortriptyline hydrochloride ©

nor-**trip**-ti-leen

(Apo-Nortriptyline ✺, Aventyl, Norventyl, Novo-Nortriptyline ✺, Pamelor)

Do not confuse nortriptyline with amitriptyline, or Aventyl with Ambenyl or Bentyl.

◆ CLASSIFICATION

PHARMACOTHERAPEUTIC: Tricyclic compound. **CLINICAL:** Antidepressant (see p. 37C).

ACTION

A tricyclic antidepressant that blocks reuptake of the neurotransmitters norepinephrine and serotonin at neuronal presynaptic membranes, increasing their availability at postsynaptic receptor sites. Therapeutic Effect: Relieves depression.

USES

Treatment of various forms of depression, often in conjunction with psychotherapy. Treatment of nocturnal enuresis. OFF-LABEL: Treatment of neurogenic pain, panic disorder; prevention of migraine headache.

PRECAUTIONS

CONTRAINDICATIONS: Acute recovery period after MI, use within 14 days of MAOIs. **CAUTIONS:** Prostatic hypertrophy, history of urinary retention/ obstruction, glaucoma, diabetes mellitus, history of seizures, hyperthyroidism, cardiac/hepatic/renal disease, schizophrenia, increased intraocular pressure (IOP), hiatal hernia. **Pregnancy Category D.**

INTERACTIONS

DRUG: **Alcohol, other CNS depressants:** May increase CNS and respiratory depression and the hypotensive effects of nortriptyline. **Antithyroid agents:** May increase the risk of agranulocytosis. **Cimetidine:** May increase the blood

---

concentration and risk of toxicity of nortriptyline. **Clonidine, guanadrel:** May decrease the effects of these drugs. **MAOIs:** May increase the risk of neuroleptic malignant syndrome, seizures, hyperpyrexia, and hypertensive crisis. **Phenothiazines:** May increase the anticholinergic and sedative effects of nortriptyline. **Sympathomimetics:** May increase the risk of cardiac effects. HERBAL: None known. FOOD: None known. LAB VALUES: May alter blood glucose level and EKG readings. The therapeutic peak serum level is 6–10 mcg/ml; the therapeutic trough serum level is 0.5–2 mcg/ml. The toxic peak serum level is greater than 12 mcg/ml; the toxic trough serum level is greater than 2 mcg/ml.

AVAILABILITY (Rx)

CAPSULES (AVENTYL): 10 mg, 25 mg. **CAPSULES (PAMELOR):** 10 mg, 25 mg, 50 mg, 75 mg. **ORAL SOLUTION (AVENTYL, PAMELOR):** 10 mg/5 ml.

ADMINISTRATION/HANDLING

‹ ALERT › Make sure at least 14 days elapse between the use of MAOIs and nortriptyline.

PO
• Give with food or milk if GI distress occurs.

INDICATIONS/ROUTES/DOSAGE

DEPRESSION
PO: ADULTS: 75–100 mg/day in 1–4 divided doses until therapeutic response is achieved. Reduce dosage gradually to effective maintenance level. ELDERLY: Initially, 10–25 mg at bedtime. May increase by 25 mg every 3–7 days. **Maximum:** 150 mg/day. CHILDREN 12 YR AND OLDER: **Maximum:** 30–50 mg/day in 3–4 divided doses. **Maximum:** 150 mg/day. CHILDREN 6–11 YR: 10–20 mg/day in 3–4 divided doses.

ENURESIS
PO: CHILDREN 12 YR AND OLDER: 25–35 mg/day. CHILDREN 8–11 YR: 10–20 mg/day. CHILDREN 6–7 YR: 10 mg/day.

SIDE EFFECTS

FREQUENT: Somnolence, fatigue, dry mouth, blurred vision, constipation, delayed micturition, orthostatic hypotension, diaphoresis, impaired concentration, increased appetite, urine retention. **OCCASIONAL:** GI disturbances (nausea, GI distress, metallic taste), photosensitivity. **RARE:** Paradoxical reactions (agitation, restlessness, nightmares, insomnia), extrapyramidal symptoms (particularly fine hand tremor).

ADVERSE REACTIONS/ TOXIC EFFECTS

Overdose may produce seizures; cardiovascular effects, such as severe orthostatic hypotension, dizziness, tachycardia, palpitations, and arrhythmias; and altered temperature regulation, such as hyperpyrexia or hypothermia. Abrupt discontinuation after prolonged therapy may produce headache, malaise, nausea, vomiting, and vivid dreams.

N

NURSING CONSIDERATIONS

BASELINE ASSESSMENT
For patients on long-term therapy, liver/renal function tests, blood counts should be performed periodically.

INTERVENTION/EVALUATION
Supervise suicidal-risk patient closely during early therapy (as depression lessens, energy level improves, increasing suicide potential). Assess appearance, behavior, speech pattern, level of interest, mood. Monitor stool consistency; avoid constipation with increased fluids, bulky foods. Monitor BP, pulse

for hypotension, arrhythmias. Assess for urinary retention, including output estimate and bladder palpation if indicated. Therapeutic serum level: Peak: 6–10 mcg/ml; trough: 0.5–2 mcg/ml. Toxic serum level: Peak: over 12 mcg/ml; trough: over 2 mcg/ml.

PATIENT/FAMILY TEACHING

• Change positions slowly to avoid hypotensive effect. • Tolerance to postural hypotension, sedative, anticholinergic effects usually develops during early therapy. • Avoid tasks that require alertness, motor skills until response to drug is established. • Therapeutic effect may be noted in 2 wk or longer. • Photosensitivity to sun may occur. • Use sunscreens, protective clothing. • Dry mouth may be relieved by sugarless gum, sips of tepid water. • Report visual disturbances. • Do not abruptly discontinue medication.

Norvasc, *see amlodipine*

Novantrone, *see mitoxantrone*

---

nystatin

nye-**stat**-in

(Bio-Statin, Mycostatin, Mycostatin Pastilles, Mycostatin Topical, Nilstat ♣, Nyaderm, Nystat-Rx, Nystex, Nystop, Pedi-Dri)

Do not confuse nystatin or Mycostatin with Nitrostat.

FIXED-COMBINATION(S)

Mycolog, Myco-Triacet: nystatin/ triamcinolone (a steroid): 100,000 units/0.1%.

CLASSIFICATION

CLINICAL: Antifungal (see p. 45C).

ACTION

A fungistatic antifungal that binds to sterols in the fungal cell membrane. Therapeutic Effect: Increases fungal cell-membrane permeability, allowing loss of potassium and other cellular components.

PHARMACOKINETICS

PO: Poorly absorbed from the GI tract. Eliminated unchanged in feces. **Topical:** Not absorbed systemically from intact skin.

USES

Treatment of cutaneous, oral cavity, and vaginal fungal infections. OFF-LABEL: Prophylaxis and treatment of oropharyngeal candidiasis, tinea barbae, tinea capitis.

PRECAUTIONS

CONTRAINDICATIONS: None known. **CAUTIONS:** None known.

⧗ LIFESPAN CONSIDERATIONS: **Pregnancy/Lactation:** Unknown if distributed in breast milk. Vaginal applicators may be contraindicated, requiring manual insertion of tablets during pregnancy. **Pregnancy Category C. Children:** No age-related precautions noted for suspension or topical use. Lozenges not recommended in those younger than 5 yr. **Elderly:** No age-related precautions noted.

INTERACTIONS

DRUG: None known. **HERBAL**: None known. **FOOD**: None known. **LAB VALUES**: None known.

AVAILABILITY (Rx)

ORAL SUSPENSION (MYCOSTATIN): 100,000 units/ml. **TABLETS (MYCOSTATIN)**: 500,000 units. **CAPSULES (BIO-STATIN)**: 500,000 units, 1,000,000 units. **ORAL LOZENGE (MYCOSTATIN PASTILLES)**: 200,000 units. **VAGINAL TABLETS**: 100,000 units. **CREAM (MYCOSTATIN TOPICAL)**: 100,000 units/g. **OINTMENT**: 100,000 units/g. **TOPICAL POWDER (MYCOSTATIN TOPICAL, NYSTOP, PEDI-DRI)**: 100,000 units/g. **POWDER (COMPOUNDING)**: 50,000,000 units (Nystat-Rx), 150,000,000 units (Bio-Statin, Nystat-Rx), 500,000,000 units (Nystat-Rx), 1,000,000,000 units, 2,000,000,000 units (Bio-Statin, Nystat-Rx).

ADMINISTRATION/HANDLING

PO

• Dissolve lozenges (troches) slowly and completely in mouth (optimal therapeutic effect). Do not chew or swallow lozenges whole. • Shake suspension well before administration. • Place and hold suspension in mouth or swish throughout mouth as long as possible before swallowing.

INDICATIONS/ROUTES/DOSAGE

INTESTINAL INFECTIONS

PO: ADULTS, ELDERLY: 500,000–1,000,000 units q8h.

ORAL CANDIDIASIS

PO: ADULTS, ELDERLY, CHILDREN: 400,000–600,000 units 4 times/day. INFANTS: 200,000 units 4 times/day.

VAGINAL INFECTIONS

VAGINAL: ADULTS, ELDERLY, ADOLESCENTS: 1 tablet/day at bedtime for 14 days.

CUTANEOUS CANDIDAL INFECTIONS

TOPICAL: ADULTS, ELDERLY, CHILDREN: Apply 2–4 times/day.

SIDE EFFECTS

OCCASIONAL: **PO**: None known. **Topical**: Skin irritation. **Vaginal**: Vaginal irritation.

ADVERSE REACTIONS/ TOXIC EFFECTS

High dosages of oral form may produce nausea, vomiting, diarrhea, and GI distress.

NURSING CONSIDERATIONS

BASELINE ASSESSMENT

Confirm that cultures or histologic tests were done for accurate diagnosis.

INTERVENTION/EVALUATION

Assess for increased irritation with topical, increased vaginal discharge with vaginal application.

PATIENT/FAMILY TEACHING

• Do not miss doses; complete full length of treatment (continue vaginal use during menses). • Notify physician if nausea, vomiting, diarrhea, stomach pain develops. • **Vaginal**: Insert high in vagina. • Check with physician regarding douching, sexual intercourse. • **Topical**: Rub well into affected areas. • Must not contact eyes. • Use cream (sparingly) or powder on erythematous areas. • Keep areas clean, dry; wear light clothing for ventilation. • Separate personal items in contact with affected areas.

N

octreotide acetate

ok-**tree**-oh-tide

(Sandostatin, Sandostatin LAR Depot)

Do not confuse octreotide with OctreoScan, or Sandostatin with Sandimmune or Sandoglobulin.

CLASSIFICATION

CLINICAL: Secretory inhibitory, growth hormone suppressant.

ACTION

An antidiarrheal and growth hormone suppressant that suppresses the secretion of serotonin and gastroenteropancreatic peptides and enhances fluid and electrolyte absorption from the GI tract. **Therapeutic Effect:** Prolongs intestinal transit time.

PHARMACOKINETICS

Route	Onset	Peak	Duration
Subcutaneous	N/A	N/A	Up to 12 hr

Rapidly and completely absorbed from injection site. Excreted in urine. Removed by hemodialysis. **Half-life:** 1.5 hr.

USES

Controls diarrhea in patients with metastatic carcinoid tumors, vasoactive intestinal peptic-secreting tumors (VIPomas), secretory diarrhea, acromegaly. **OFF-LABEL:** Control of bleeding esophageal varices, treatment of AIDS-associated secretory diarrhea, chemotherapy-induced diarrhea, insulinomas, small-bowel fistulas, control of bleeding esophageal varices.

PRECAUTIONS

CONTRAINDICATIONS: None known. **CAUTIONS:** Insulin-dependent diabetes, renal failure.

⌛ **LIFESPAN CONSIDERATIONS: Pregnancy/Lactation:** Unknown if excreted in breast milk. **Pregnancy Category B. Children:** Dosage not established in children. **Elderly:** No age-related precautions noted.

INTERACTIONS

DRUG: Cyclosporine: May decrease the effectiveness of cyclosporine. **Glucagon, growth hormone, insulin, oral antidiabetics:** May alter glucose concentrations. **HERBAL:** None known. **FOOD:** None known. **LAB VALUES:** May decrease serum thyroxine (T_4) concentration.

AVAILABILITY (Rx)

INJECTION (SANDOSTATIN): 0.05 mg/ml, 0.1 mg/ml, 0.2 mg/ml, 0.5 mg/ml, 1 mg/ml. **SUSPENSION FOR INJECTION (SANDOSTATIN LAR DEPOT):** 10-mg, 20-mg, 30-mg vials.

ADMINISTRATION/HANDLING

◀ **ALERT** ▶ Sandostatin may be given IV, IM, subcutaneous. Sandostatin LAR Depot may be given only IM.

IM
• Give immediately after mixing. • Administer deep IM in large muscle mass at 4-wk intervals. • Avoid deltoid injections.

SUBCUTANEOUS
• Do not use if particulates or discoloration is noted. • Avoid multiple injections at the same site within short periods.

INDICATIONS/ROUTES/DOSAGE

DIARRHEA

IV (SANDOSTATIN): ADULTS, ELDERLY: Initially, 50–100 mcg q8h. May increase by 100 mcg/dose q48h. **Maximum:** 500 mcg q8h.

SUBCUTANEOUS (SANDOSTATIN): ADULTS, ELDERLY: 50 mcg 1–2 times a day. **IV, SUBCUTANEOUS (SANDOSTATIN):** CHILDREN: 1–10 mcg/kg q12h.

O

CARCINOID TUMORS
IV, SUBCUTANEOUS (SANDOSTA-TIN): ADULTS, ELDERLY: 100–600 mcg/day in 2–4 divided doses.
IM (SANDOSTATIN LAR DEPOT): ADULTS, ELDERLY: 20 mg q4wk.

VIPOMAS
IV, SUBCUTANEOUS (SANDOSTA-TIN): ADULTS, ELDERLY: 200–300 mcg/day in 2–4 divided doses.
IM (SANDOSTATIN LAR DEPOT): ADULTS, ELDERLY: 20 mg q4wk.

ESOPHAGEAL VARICES
IV (SANDOSTATIN): ADULTS, ELDERLY: Bolus of 25–50 mcg followed by IV infusion of 25–50 mcg/hr for 48 hr.

ACROMEGALY
IV, SUBCUTANEOUS (SANDOSTA-TIN): ADULTS, ELDERLY: 50 mcg 3 times a day. Increase as needed. **Maximum:** 500 mcg 3 times a day.
IM (SANDOSTATIN LAR DEPOT): ADULTS, ELDERLY: 20 mg q4wk for 3 mo. **Maximum:** 40 mg q4wk.

SIDE EFFECTS

FREQUENT (10%–6%, 58%–30% in acromegaly patients): Diarrhea, nausea, abdominal discomfort, headache, injection site pain. **OCCASIONAL (5%–1%):** Vomiting, flatulence, constipation, alopecia, facial flushing, pruritus, dizziness, fatigue, arrhythmias, ecchymosis, blurred vision. **RARE (less than 1%):** Depression, diminished libido, vertigo, palpitations, dyspnea.

ADVERSE REACTIONS/ TOXIC EFFECTS

Patients using octreotide may develop cholelithiasis or, with prolonged high dosages, hypothyroidism. GI bleeding, hepatitis, and seizures occur rarely.

NURSING CONSIDERATIONS

BASELINE ASSESSMENT
Establish baseline BP, weight, blood glucose, electrolytes.

INTERVENTION/EVALUATION
Monitor blood glucose, serum thyroid function tests, fluid and electrolyte balance, fecal fat. In acromegaly, monitor growth hormone levels. Weigh every 2–3 days, report ⏺ lb gain per wk. Monitor BP, pulse, respirations periodically during treatment. Be alert for decreased urinary output, peripheral edema (especially ankles). Monitor pattern of bowel activity and stool consistency.

PATIENT/FAMILY TEACHING
• Therapy should provide significant improvement of severe, watery diarrhea.

Ocuflox, *see ofloxacin*

---

ocular lubricant

ock-you-lar **lube**-rih-cant
(Hypotears, Lacrilube, Tears Naturale)

◆ CLASSIFICATION
PHARMACOTHERAPEUTIC: Topical ophthalmic. **CLINICAL:** Lubricant, toner, buffer, viscosity agent.

ACTION
Forms an occlusive film on eye surface. **Therapeutic** **Effect:** Lubricates/protects eye from drying.

USES
Protection/lubrication of the eye in exposure keratitis, decreased corneal sensitivity, recurrent corneal erosions, keratitis sicca (particularly for nighttime use), after removal of a foreign body, during and following surgery.

PRECAUTIONS

CONTRAINDICATIONS: None known.
CAUTIONS: None known. **Pregnancy Category Unknown.**

INTERACTIONS

DRUG: None known. **HERBAL:** None known. **FOOD:** None known. **LAB VALUES:** None known.

AVAILABILITY (OTC)

OPHTHALMIC OINTMENT. SOLUTION.

ADMINISTRATION/HANDLING

OPHTHALMIC (OINTMENT)
• Do not use with contact lenses. • Hold tube in hand for a few minutes to warm ointment. • Avoid touching tip of tube or dropper to any surface. • Gently pull lower lid down to form pouch between eye and lower lid (conjunctival sac). • Place ordered amount of ointment into pouch with a sweeping motion. • Instruct patient to close the eye for 1–2 min and roll the eyeball around in all directions. • Inform patient of temporary blurred vision. If possible, apply just before bedtime.

OPHTHALMIC (DROPS)
• Do not use with contact lenses. • Instruct patient to lie down or tilt head backward and look up. • Gently pull lower lid down to form pouch between eye and lower lid (conjunctival sac). • Hold dropper above pouch. Instill drop(s); have patient close eye gently for 1–2 min (placing drops directly onto eye may cause a sudden squeezing of eyelid, with subsequent loss of solution). • Apply gentle pressure with fingers to bridge of nose (inside corner of eye) for 1–2 min (promotes absorption, minimizes drainage into nose/throat).

INDICATIONS/ROUTES/DOSAGE

USUAL OPHTHALMIC DOSAGE
OPHTHALMIC: ADULTS, ELDERLY: Small amount in conjunctival sac as needed.

SIDE EFFECTS

FREQUENT: Temporary blurring after administration, especially with ointment.

ADVERSE REACTIONS/ TOXIC EFFECTS

None known.

NURSING CONSIDERATIONS

PATIENT/FAMILY TEACHING
• Teach proper application. • Do not use with contact lenses. • Do not touch tip of tube or dropper to any surface (may contaminate). • Temporary blurring will occur, especially with administration of ointment. • Avoid activities requiring visual acuity until blurring clears. • If eye pain, change of vision, worsening of condition occurs, or if condition is unchanged after 72 hr, notify physician.

ofloxacin

o-**flox**-a-sin
(Apo-Oflox ✦, Floxin, Floxin Otic, Ocuflox)

Do not confuse Floxin with Flexeril or Flexon, or Ocuflox with Ocufen.

◆CLASSIFICATION

PHARMACOTHERAPEUTIC: Fluoroquinolone. **CLINICAL:** Antibiotic (see p. 24C).

ACTION

A fluoroquinolone antibiotic that inhibits DNA gyrase in susceptible microorganisms, interfering with bacterial cell replication and repair. **Therapeutic Effect:** Bactericidal.

PHARMACOKINETICS

Rapidly and well absorbed from the GI tract. Protein binding: 20%–25%.

---

*see color pill atlas   ✦ herb   underlined – top prescribed drug

Widely distributed (including to cerebrospinal fluid [CSF]). Metabolized in the liver. Primarily excreted in urine. Removed by hemodialysis. Half-life: 4.7–7 hr (increased in impaired renal function, cirrhosis, and the elderly).

USES

Treatment of susceptible infections due to *S. pneumoniae, S. aureus, S. pyogenes, H. influenzae, P. mirabilis, N. gonorrhoeae, C. trachomatis, E. coli, K. pneumoniae, P. aeruginosa* including infections of urinary tract, lower respiratory tract, skin and skinstructure; sexually transmitted diseases; prostatitis due to *Escherichia coli;* pelvic inflammatory disease (PID). **Ophthalmic:** Bacterial conjunctivitis, corneal ulcers. **Otic:** Otitis externa, acute or chronic otitis media.

PRECAUTIONS

CONTRAINDICATIONS: Children 18 yr and younger, hypersensitivity to any quinolones. **CAUTIONS:** Renal impairment, CNS disorders, seizures, those taking theophylline or caffeine. May mask or delay symptoms of syphilis; serologic test for syphilis should be done at diagnosis and 3 mo after treatment.

⌛ LIFESPAN CONSIDERATIONS: **Pregnancy/Lactation:** Distributed in breast milk; potentially serious adverse reactions in breast-feeding infants. Risk of arthropathy to fetus. **Pregnancy Category C. Children:** Safety and efficacy not established (otic not established in those younger than 1 yr). **Elderly:** No age-related precautions for otic. Age-related renal impairment may require dosage adjustment for oral administration.

INTERACTIONS

DRUG: **Antacids, sucralfate:** May decrease absorption and effects of ofloxacin. **Caffeine:** May increase the effects of caffeine. **Theophylline:** May increase theophylline blood concentration and risk of toxicity. HERBAL: None known. FOOD: None known. LAB VALUES: None known.

AVAILABILITY (Rx)

TABLETS (FLOXIN): 200 mg, 300 mg, 400 mg. **OPHTHALMIC SOLUTION (OCUFLOX):** 0.3%. **OTIC SOLUTION (FLOXIN):** 0.3%.

ADMINISTRATION/HANDLING

PO
• Do not give with food; preferred dosing time: 1 hr before or 2 hr following meals. • Do not administer antacids (aluminum, magnesium) or iron or zinc-containing products within 2 hr of ofloxacin. • Encourage cranberry juice, citrus fruits (to acidify urine). • Give with 8 oz of water, encourage fluid intake.

OPHTHALMIC
• Tilt patient's head back; place solution in conjunctival sac. • Have patient close eyes; press gently on lacrimal sac for 1 min. • Do not use ophthalmic solutions for injection. • Unless infection very superficial, systemic administration generally accompanies ophthalmic.

OTIC
• Instruct patient to lie down with head turned so affected ear is upright. • Instill toward canal wall, not directly on eardrum. • Pull the auricle down and posterior in children; up and posterior in adults.

INDICATIONS/ROUTES/DOSAGE

UTIs
PO: ADULTS: 200 mg q12h.

PID
PO: ADULTS: 400 mg q12h for 10–14 days.

LOWER RESPIRATORY TRACT, SKIN AND SKIN-STRUCTURE INFECTIONS
PO: ADULTS: 400 mg q12h for 10 days.

PROSTATITIS, SEXUALLY TRANSMITTED DISEASES (CERVICITIS, URETHRITIS)
PO: ADULTS: 300 mg q12h.

ACUTE, UNCOMPLICATED GONORRHEA
PO: ADULTS: 400 mg 1 time.

USUAL ELDERLY DOSAGE
PO: ELDERLY: 200–400 mg q12–24h for 7 days up to 6 wk.

BACTERIAL CONJUNCTIVITIS
OPHTHALMIC: ADULTS, ELDERLY: 1–2 drops q2–4h for 2 days, then 4 times a day for 5 days.

CORNEAL ULCERS
OPHTHALMIC: ADULTS: 1–2 drops q30min while awake for 2 days, then q60min while awake for 5–7 days, then 4 times a day.

ACUTE OTITIS MEDIA
OTIC: CHILDREN 1–12 YR: 5 drops into the affected ear 2 times/day for 10 days.

OTITIS EXTERNA
OTIC: ADULTS, ELDERLY, CHILDREN 12 YR AND OLDER: 10 drops into the affected ear once a day for 7 days. CHILDREN 6 MO–11 YR: 5 drops into the affected ear once a day for 7 days.

DOSAGE IN RENAL IMPAIRMENT
After a normal initial dose, dosage and frequency are based on creatinine clearance.

Creatinine Clearance	Adjusted Dose	Dosage Interval
Greater than 50 ml/min	None	q12h
10–50 ml/min	None	q24h
Less than 10 ml/min		q24h

SIDE EFFECTS

FREQUENT (10%–7%): Nausea, headache, insomnia. **OCCASIONAL (5%–3%):** Abdominal pain, diarrhea, vomiting, dry mouth, flatulence, dizziness, fatigue, drowsiness, rash, pruritus, fever. **RARE (less than 1%):** Constipation, paraesthesia.

ADVERSE REACTIONS/ TOXIC EFFECTS

Antibiotic-associated colitis and other superinfections may occur from altered bacterial balance. Hypersensitivity reactions, including photosensitivity (as evidenced by rash, pruritus, blisters, edema, and burning skin), have occurred in patients receiving fluoroquinolones. Arthropathy (swelling, pain, and clubbing of fingers and toes, degeneration of stress-bearing portion of a joint) may occur if the drug is given to children. There is a risk of peripheral neuropathy, tendon rupture, and torsades de pointes.

NURSING CONSIDERATIONS

BASELINE ASSESSMENT
Question for history of hypersensitivity to ofloxacin, other quinolones.

INTERVENTION/EVALUATION
Monitor signs and symptoms of infection, WBC, mental status. Assess skin, discontinue medication at first sign of rash or other allergic reaction. Monitor pattern of bowel activity and stool consistency. Assess for insomnia. Check for dizziness, headache, visual difficulties, tremors; provide assistance with ambulation as needed. Be alert for superinfection (genital pruritus, vaginitis, fever, stomatitis).

PATIENT/FAMILY TEACHING
• Do not take antacids within 6 hr before or 2 hr after taking oflaxocan. • Best taken 1 hr before or 2 hr after meals. • May cause insomnia, headache, drowsiness, dizziness. • Avoid tasks requiring alertness, motor skills until response to drug is established.

olanzapine

oh-**lan**-za-peen

(Zyprexa, Zyprexa Intramuscular, Zyprexa Zydis)

Do not confuse olanzapine with olsalazine, or Zyprexa with Zyrtec.

FIXED-COMBINATION(S)

Symbyax: olanzapine/fluoxetine (an antidepressant): 6 mg/25 mg, 6 mg/50 mg, 12 mg/25 mg, 12 mg/50 mg.

◆CLASSIFICATION

PHARMACOTHERAPEUTIC: Dibenzapin derivative. **CLINICAL:** Antipsychotic (see p. 58C).

ACTION

A thienobenzodiazepine derivative that antagonizes alpha$_1$-adrenergic, dopamine, histamine, muscarinic, and serotonin receptors. Produces anticholinergic, histaminic, and CNS depressant effects. **Therapeutic Effect:** Diminishes manifestations of psychotic symptoms.

PHARMACOKINETICS

Well absorbed after PO administration. Protein binding: 93%. Extensively distributed throughout the body. Undergoes extensive first-pass metabolism in the liver. Excreted primarily in urine and, to a lesser extent, in feces. Not removed by dialysis. Half-life: 21–54 hr.

USES

Oral: Management of manifestations of psychotic disorders. Treatment of acute mania associated with bipolar disorder. **IM:** Controls agitation in schizophrenia or bipolar disorder. OFF-LABEL: Treatment of anorexia, apathy, borderline personality disorder, Huntington's disease; maintenance of long-term treatment response in schizophrenic patients; nausea; vomiting.

PRECAUTIONS

CONTRAINDICATIONS: None known.

CAUTIONS: Hypersensitivity to clozapine, patients who should avoid anticholinergics (e.g., patients with benign prostatic hypertrophy), hepatic impairment, elderly, concurrent use of potentially hepatotoxic drugs, dose escalation, known cardiovascular disease (history of MI, ischemia, heart failure, conduction abnormalities), cerebrovascular disease, conditions predisposing patients to hypotension (dehydration, hypovolemia, hypertensive medications), history of seizures, conditions lowering seizure threshold (e.g., Alzheimer's dementia), those at risk of aspiration pneumonia.

LIFESPAN CONSIDERATIONS: Pregnancy/Lactation: Unknown if drug crosses placenta or is distributed in breast milk. **Pregnancy Category C. Children:** Safety and efficacy not established. **Elderly:** No age-related precautions noted.

INTERACTIONS

DRUG: **Alcohol, other CNS depressants:** May increase CNS depressant effects. **Antihypertensives:** May increase the hypotensive effects of these drugs. **Carbamazepine:** Increases olanzapine clearance. **Ciprofloxacin, fluvoxamine:** May increase the olanzapine blood concentration. **Dopamine agonists, levodopa:** May antagonize the effects of these drugs. **Imipramine, theophylline:** May inhibit the metabolism of these drugs. HERBAL: None known. FOOD: None known. LAB VALUES: May significantly increase serum GGT, prolactin, AST, and ALT levels.

AVAILABILITY (Rx)

TABLETS (ZYPREXA): 2.5 mg, 5 mg, 7.5 mg, 10 mg, 15 mg, 20 mg. **TABLETS (ORALLY-DISINTEGRATING [ZYPREXA ZYDIS]):** 5 mg, 10 mg, 15 mg, 20 mg. **INJECTION (ZYPREXA INTRAMUSCULAR):** 10 mg.

ADMINISTRATION/HANDLING

PO

• Give without regard to meals.

INDICATIONS/ROUTES/DOSAGE

SCHIZOPHRENIA

PO: ADULTS: Initially, 5–10 mg once daily. May increase by 10 mg/day at 5–7 day intervals. If further adjustments are indicated, may increase by 5–10 mg/day at 7 day intervals. Range: 10–30 mg/day. ELDERLY: Initially, 2.5 mg/day. May increase as indicated. Range: 2.5–10 mg/day. CHILDREN: Initially, 2.5 mg/day. Titrate as necessary up to 20 mg/day.

BIPOLAR MANIA

PO: ADULTS: Initially, 10–15 mg/day. May increase by 5 mg/day at intervals of at least 24 hr. **Maximum:** 20 mg/day. CHILDREN: Initially, 2.5 mg/day. Titrate as necessary up to 20 mg/day.

DOSAGE FOR ELDERLY OR DEBILITATED PATIENTS AND THOSE PREDISPOSED TO HYPOTENSIVE REACTIONS

The initial dosage for these patients is 5 mg/day.

CONTROL AGITATION IN SCHIZOPHRENIC OR BIPOLAR PATIENTS

IM: ADULTS, ELDERLY: 2.5–10 mg. May repeat 2 hr after first dose and 4 hr after 2nd dose. **Maximum:** 30 mg/day.

SIDE EFFECTS

FREQUENT: Somnolence (26%), agitation (23%), insomnia (20%), headache (17%), nervousness (16%), hostility (15%), dizziness (11%), rhinitis (10%). **OCCASIONAL:** Anxiety, constipation (9%); nonaggressive atypical behavior (8%); dry mouth (7%); weight gain (6%); orthostatic hypotension, fever, arthralgia, restlessness, cough, pharyngitis, visual changes (dim vision) (5%). **RARE:** Tachycardia; back, chest, abdominal, or extremity pain; tremor.

ADVERSE REACTIONS/ TOXIC EFFECTS

Rare reactions include seizures and neuroleptic malignant syndrome, a potentially fatal syndrome characterized by hyperpyrexia, muscle rigidity, irregular pulse or BP, tachycardia, diaphoresis, and cardiac arrhythmias. Extrapyramidal symptoms and dysphagia may also occur. Overdose (300 mg) produces drowsiness and slurred speech.

NURSING CONSIDERATIONS

BASELINE ASSESSMENT

Obtain baseline liver function lab values before initiating treatment. Assess behavior, appearance, emotional status, response to environment, speech pattern, thought content.

INTERVENTION/EVALUATION

Monitor BP. Assess for tremors, changes in gait, abnormal muscular movements, behavior. Supervise suicidal-risk patient closely during early therapy (as depression lessens, energy level improves, increasing suicide potential). Assess for therapeutic response (interest in surroundings, improvement in self-care, increased ability to concentrate, relaxed facial expression). Assist with ambulation if dizziness occurs. Assess sleep pattern. Notify physician if extrapyramidal symptoms (EPS) occur.

PATIENT/FAMILY TEACHING

• Avoid dehydration, particularly during exercise, exposure to extreme heat, concurrent use of medication causing dry mouth, other drying effects. • Sugarless gum, sips of tepid water may relieve dry mouth. • Notify physician if pregnancy occurs or if there is intention to become pregnant during olanzapine therapy. • Take medication as ordered; do not stop taking or increase dosage. • Drowsiness generally subsides during continued therapy. • Avoid tasks that require alertness, motor skills until response to drug is established. • Monitor diet and exercise program to prevent weight gain.

olmesartan medoxomil

ol-**mess**-er-tan

(Benicar)

CLASSIFICATION

PHARMACOTHERAPEUTIC: Angiotensin II receptor antagonist. **CLINICAL:** Antihypertensive (see p. 8C).

ACTION

An angiotensin II receptor, type AT_1, antagonist that blocks the vasoconstrictor and aldosterone-secreting effects of angiotensin II, inhibiting the binding of angiotensin II to the AT_1 receptors. **Therapeutic Effect:** Causes vasodilation, decreases peripheral resistance, and decreases BP.

PHARMACOKINETICS

Rapidly and completely absorbed after PO administration. Metabolized in the liver. Recovered primarily in feces and, to a lesser extent, in urine. Not removed by hemodialysis. **Half-life:** 13 hr.

USES

Treatment of hypertension alone or in combination with other antihypertensives (diuretics, calcium channel blockers).

PRECAUTIONS

CONTRAINDICATIONS: Bilateral renal artery stenosis. **CAUTIONS:** Renal/hepatic impairment, renal arterial stenosis.

LIFESPAN CONSIDERATIONS: Pregnancy/Lactation: Unknown if distributed in breast milk. **Pregnancy Category C (D if used in second or third trimester). Children:** Safety and efficacy not established. **Elderly:** No age-related precautions noted.

INTERACTIONS

DRUG: Diuretics: Further reduce BP. **HERBAL:** None known. **FOOD:** None known. **LAB VALUES:** May increase blood Hgb and Hct levels.

AVAILABILITY (Rx)

TABLETS: 5 mg, 20 mg, 40 mg.

ADMINISTRATION/HANDLING

PO
- Give without regard to meals.

INDICATIONS/ROUTES/DOSAGE

HYPERTENSION

PO: ADULTS, ELDERLY: Patients with mildly impaired hepatic or renal function. 20 mg once a day in patients who are not volume depleted. After 2 wk of therapy, if further reduction in BP is needed, may increase dosage to 40 mg/day.

SIDE EFFECTS

OCCASIONAL (3%): Dizziness. **RARE (less than 2%):** Headache, diarrhea, upper respiratory tract infection.

ADVERSE REACTIONS/TOXIC EFFECTS

Overdosage may manifest as hypotension and tachycardia. Bradycardia occurs less often. Rare cases of rhabdomyolysis have been reported.

NURSING CONSIDERATIONS

BASELINE ASSESSMENT

Obtain BP, apical pulse immediately before each dose in addition to regular monitoring (be alert to fluctuations). If excessive reduction in BP occurs, place patient in supine position, feet slightly elevated. Question for possibility of pregnancy (see Pregnancy Category). Assess medication history (especially diuretics).

INTERVENTION/EVALUATION

Maintain hydration (offer fluids frequently). Assess for evidence of upper respiratory infection. Assist with ambulation if dizziness occurs. Monitor serum chemistry levels. Assess BP for hypertension and hypotension.

PATIENT/FAMILY TEACHING

• Inform female patients regarding consequences of second- and third-trimester exposure to olmesartan. • Avoid tasks that require alertness, motor skills until response to drug is established (possible dizziness effect). • Report any signs of infection (sore throat, fever). • Discuss need for life-long control, importance of diet and exercise. • Caution against exercise during hot weather (risk of dehydration, hypotension).

---

olsalazine sodium

ohl-**sal**-ah-zeen

(Dipentum)

Do not confuse olsalazine with olanzapine.

◆CLASSIFICATION

PHARMACOTHERAPEUTIC: Salicylic acid derivative. **CLINICAL:** Anti-inflammatory.

ACTION

A salicylic acid derivative that is converted to mesalamine in the colon by bacterial action. Blocks prostaglandin production in bowel mucosa. **Therapeutic Effect:** Reduces colonic inflammation in inflammatory bowel disease.

PHARMACOKINETICS

Small amount absorbed. Protein binding: 99%. Metabolized by bacteria in the colon. Minimal elimination in urine and feces. **Half-life:** 0.9 hr.

USES

Maintenance of remission of ulcerative colitis in patients intolerant of sulfasalazine medication. **OFF-LABEL:** Treatment of inflammatory bowel disease.

PRECAUTIONS

CONTRAINDICATIONS: History of hypersensitivity to salicylates. **CAUTIONS:** Pre-existing renal disease.

⧗ **LIFESPAN CONSIDERATIONS: Pregnancy/Lactation:** Crosses placenta; distributed in breast milk. **Pregnancy Category C. Children:** Safety and efficacy not established. **Elderly:** Age-related renal impairment may require dosage adjustment.

INTERACTIONS

DRUG: Warfarin: May increase prothrombin time. **HERBAL:** None known. **FOOD:** None known. **LAB VALUES:** May increase AST and ALT levels.

AVAILABILITY (Rx)

CAPSULES: 250 mg.

ADMINISTRATION/HANDLING

PO

• Give with food in evenly divided doses.

INDICATIONS/ROUTES/DOSAGE

MAINTENANCE OF CONTROLLED ULCERATIVE COLITIS

PO: ADULTS, ELDERLY: 1 g/day in 2 divided doses, preferably q12h.

SIDE EFFECTS

FREQUENT (10%–5%): Headache, diarrhea, abdominal pain or cramps, nausea. **OCCASIONAL (5%–1%):** Depression, fatigue, dyspepsia, upper respiratory tract infection, decreased appetite, rash, itching, arthralgia. **RARE (1%):** Dizziness, vomiting, stomatitis.

ADVERSE REACTIONS/ TOXIC EFFECTS

Sulfite sensitivity may occur in susceptible patients manifested by cramping, headache, diarrhea, fever, rash, hives, itching, and wheezing may occur. Discontinue drug immediately. Excessive diarrhea associated with extreme fatigue is noted rarely.

INTERVENTION/EVALUATION

Encourage adequate fluid intake. Assess bowel sounds for peristalsis. Monitor pattern of daily bowel activity and stool consistency; record time of evacuation. Assess for abdominal disturbances. Assess skin for rash, hives. Medication should be discontinued if rash, fever, cramping, diarrhea occurs.

PATIENT/FAMILY TEACHING

• Notify physician if diarrhea, cramping continues or worsens or if rash, fever, or pruritus occurs.

omalizumab

oh-mah-**liz**-uw-mab
(Xolair)

◆ CLASSIFICATION

PHARMACOTHERAPEUTIC: Monoclonal antibody. **CLINICAL:** Antiasthmatic.

ACTION

A monoclonal antibody that selectively binds to human immunoglobulin E (IgE) preventing it from binding to the surface of mast cells and basophiles. **Therapeutic Effect:** Prevents or reduces the number of asthmatic attacks.

PHARMACOKINETICS

Absorbed slowly after subcutaneous administration, with peak concentration in 7–8 days. Excreted in the liver, reticuloendothelial system, and endothelial cells. **Half-life:** 26 days.

USES

Treatment of moderate to severe persistent asthma in patients reactive to a perennial allergen and inadequately controlled asthma symptoms with inhaled corticosteroids. **OFF-LABEL:** Treatment of seasonal allergic rhinitis.

PRECAUTIONS

CONTRAINDICATIONS: None known. **CAUTIONS:** Not for use in reversing acute bronchospasm, status asthmaticus.
☒ **LIFESPAN CONSIDERATIONS: Pregnancy/Lactation:** Because IgE is present in breast milk, is it expected omalizumab is present in breast milk. Use only if clearly needed. **Pregnancy Category B. Children:** Safety and efficacy not established in children younger than 12 yr. **Elderly:** No age-related precautions noted.

INTERACTIONS

DRUG: None known. **HERBAL:** None known. **FOOD:** None known. **LAB VALUES:** May increase serum IgE levels.

AVAILABILITY (Rx)

POWDER FOR INJECTION: 202.5 mg/1.2 ml or 150 mg/1.2 ml after reconstitution.

ADMINISTRATION/HANDLING

SUBCUTANEOUS

Reconstitution • Use only sterile water for injection to prepare for subcutaneous administration. • Medication takes 15–20 min to dissolve. • Draw 1.4 ml sterile water for injection into a 3-ml syringe with a 1-inch, 18-gauge needle; inject contents into powdered vial. • Swirl vial for approx. 1 min (do not shake) and again swirl vial for 5–10 sec every 5 min until no gel-like particles appear in the solution. • Do not

O

use if contents do not dissolve completely within 40 min. • Invert the vial for 15 sec (allows solution to drain toward the stopper). • Using a new 3-ml syringe with a 1-inch 18-gauge needle, obtain the required 1.2-ml dose, replace 18-gauge needle with a 25-gauge needle for subcutaneous administration.

Rate of administration • Subcutaneous administration may take 5–10 sec to administer due to its viscosity.

Storage • Use only clear or slightly opalescent solution; solution is slightly viscous. • Refrigerate. Reconstituted solution is stable for 8 hr if refrigerated or within 4 hr of reconstitution when stored at room temperature.

INDICATIONS/ROUTES/DOSAGE

MODERATE TO SEVERE PERSISTENT ASTHMA IN PATIENTS WHO ARE REACTIVE TO A PERENNIAL ALLERGEN AND WHOSE ASTHMA SYMPTOMS HAVE BEEN INADEQUATELY CONTROLLED WITH INHALED CORTICOSTEROIDS

SUBCUTANEOUS: ADULTS, ELDERLY, CHILDREN 12 YR AND OLDER: 150–375 mg every 2 or 4 wk; dose and dosing frequency are individualized based on weight and pretreatment IgE level (as shown below).

4-WK DOSING TABLE

Pretreatment Serum IgE Levels (units/ml)	Weight 30–60 kg	Weight 61–70 kg	Weight 71–90 kg	Weight 91–150 kg
30–100	150 mg	150 mg	150 mg	300 mg
101–200	300 mg	300 mg	300 mg	See next table
201–300	300 mg	See next table	See next table	See next table

2-WEEK DOSING TABLE

Pretreatment Serum IgE Levels (units/ml)	Weight 30–60 kg	Weight 61–70 kg	Weight 71–90 kg	Weight 91–150 kg
101–200	See preceding table	See preceding table	See preceding table	225 mg
201–300	See previous table	225 mg	225 mg	300 mg
301–400	225 mg	225 mg	300 mg	Do not dose
401–500	300 mg	300 mg	375 mg	Do not dose
501–600	300 mg	375 mg	Do not dose	Do not dose
601–700	375 mg	Do not dose	Do not dose	Do not dose

SIDE EFFECTS

FREQUENT (45%–11%): Injection site ecchymosis, redness, warmth, stinging, and urticaria; viral infections; sinusitis; headache; pharyngitis. **OCCASIONAL (8%–3%):** Arthralgia, leg pain, fatigue, dizziness. **RARE (2%):** Arm pain, earache, dermatitis, pruritus.

ADVERSE REACTIONS/ TOXIC EFFECTS

Anaphylaxis occurs within 2 hr of the first dose or subsequent doses in 0.1% of patients. Malignant neoplasms occur in 0.5% of patients.

NURSING CONSIDERATIONS

BASELINE ASSESSMENT

Obtain baseline serum total IgE levels before initiation of treatment (dosage is based on pretreatment levels). Drug is not for treatment of acute exacerbations of asthma, acute bronchospasm, status asthmaticus.

INTERVENTION/EVALUATION

Monitor rate, depth, rhythm, type of respirations, quality and rate of pulse. Assess lung sounds for rhonchi, wheezing, rales. Observe lips, fingernails for cyanosis (blue/dusky color in light-skinned patients, gray in dark-skinned patients).

PATIENT/FAMILY TEACHING

• Increase fluid intake (decreases viscosity of pulmonary secretions). • Do not alter or stop other asthma medications.

omega-3 acid ethyl esters

oh-**meg**-ah 3 **ah**-sid **eth**-ill **eh**-stirs (Omacor)
Do not confuse with Amicar.

◆CLASSIFICATION

PHARMACOTHERAPEUTIC: Omega-3 fatty acid. **CLINICAL:** Antihypertriglyceridemia.

ACTION

Inhibits the esterification of fatty acids, prevents hepatic enzymes from catalyzing the final step of triglyceride synthesis. **Therapeutic Effect:** Reduces triglyceride serum level.

PHARMACOKINETICS

Well absorbed following PO administration. Incorporated into phospholipids. **Half-life:** N/A.

USES

Adjunct to diet to reduce very high (500 mg/dL or higher) triglyceride levels in adult patients.

PRECAUTIONS

CONTRAINDICATIONS: None known.

CAUTIONS: Known sensitivity or allergy to fish.

⌛ **LIFESPAN CONSIDERATIONS: Pregnancy/Lactation:** Unknown if distributed in breast milk. **Pregnancy Category C. Children:** Safety and efficacy in children younger than 18 yr not established. **Elderly:** No age-related precautions noted.

INTERACTIONS

DRUG: Anticoagulants: May increase bleeding time. **Atenolol, chlorothiazide, chlorthalidone, estradiol, hydrochlorothiazide, indapamide, metolazone, metoprolol, propranolol:** May increase triglyceride levels; discontinue or change before therapy. **HERBAL:** None known. **FOOD:** None known. **LAB VALUES:** May increase ALT, LDL.

AVAILABILITY (Rx)

CAPSULES, SOFT GELATIN (OIL-FILLED): 1 gram.

ADMINISTRATION/HANDLING

PO
• Give without regard to meals.

INDICATIONS/ROUTES/DOSAGE

◀ **ALERT** ▶ Before initiating therapy, patient should be on standard cholesterol-lowering diet for minimum of 3–6 mo. Continue diet throughout therapy.
USUAL DOSAGE
PO: ADULTS, ELDERLY: 4 g/day, given as a single dose (4 capsules) or 2 capsules twice daily.

SIDE EFFECTS

OCCASIONAL (5%–3%): Eructation, altered taste, dyspepsia. **RARE (2%–1%):** Rash, back pain.

ADVERSE REACTIONS/TOXIC EFFECTS

None known.

NURSING CONSIDERATIONS

BASELINE ASSESSMENT
Assess baseline serum triglyceride level, liver function tests. Obtain a diet history.

INTERVENTION/EVALUATION
Monitor serum triglyceride level for therapeutic response. Monitor ALT, LDL periodically during therapy. Discontinue therapy if no response after 2 mo of treatment.

PATIENT/FAMILY TEACHING
• Continue to adhere to lipid-lowering diet (important part of treatment).
• Periodic lab tests are essential part of therapy to determine drug effectiveness.

---

omeprazole

oh-**mep**-rah-zole
(Losec ✢, <u>Prilosec</u>, Prilosec OTC, Zegerid)

Do not confuse Prilosec with prilocaine, Prinivil, or Prozac.

CLASSIFICATION
PHARMACOTHERAPEUTIC: Benzimidazole. **CLINICAL:** Gastric acid pump inhibitor (see p. 134C).

ACTION
A benzimidazole that is converted to active metabolites that irreversibly bind to and inhibit hydrogen-potassium adenosine triphosphatase, an enzyme on the surface of gastric parietal cells. Inhibits hydrogen ion transport into gastric lumen. Therapeutic Effect: Increases gastric pH, reduces gastric acid production.

PHARMACOKINETICS

Route	Onset	Peak	Duration
PO	1 hr	2 hr	72 hr

Rapidly absorbed from the GI tract. Protein binding: 99%. Primarily distributed into gastric parietal cells. Metabolized extensively in the liver. Primarily excreted in urine. Unknown if removed by hemodialysis. Half-life: 0.5–1 hr (increased in patients with hepatic impairment).

USES
Short-term treatment (4–8 wk) of erosive esophagitis (diagnosed by endoscopy), symptomatic gastroesophageal reflux disease (GERD) poorly responsive to other treatment. Long-term treatment of pathologic hypersecretory conditions; treatment of active duodenal ulcer. Maintenance healing of erosive esophagitis. OFF-LABEL: *H. pylori*–associated duodenal ulcer (with amoxicillin and clarithromycin), prevention and treatment of NSAID-induced ulcers, treatment of active benign gastric ulcers.

PRECAUTIONS
CONTRAINDICATIONS: None known. **CAUTIONS:** None known.

⧗ LIFESPAN CONSIDERATIONS: **Pregnancy/Lactation:** Unknown if drug crosses placenta or is distributed in breast milk. **Pregnancy Category C. Children:** Safety and efficacy not established. **Elderly:** No age-related precautions noted.

INTERACTIONS
DRUG: **Diazepam, oral anticoagulants, phenytoin:** May increase the blood concentration of diazepam, oral anticoagulants, and phenytoin. HERBAL: **Ginkgo biloba:** May decrease omeprazole effectiveness. **St. John's wort:** May decrease omeprazole serum concentration. FOOD: None known. LAB VALUES: May increase serum alkaline phosphatase, AST, and ALT levels.

✐ see color pill atlas   🍃 herb   <u>underlined</u> – top prescribed drug

AVAILABILITY (Rx)

CAPSULES (DELAYED-RELEASE [PRILOSEC]): 10 mg, 20 mg, 40 mg. **(ZEGERID):** 20 mg, 40 mg. **ORAL SUSPENSION (ZEGERID):** 20 mg, 40 mg.

ADMINISTRATION/HANDLING

PO

• Give before meals. • Do not crush or chew capsule; swallow whole.

INDICATIONS/ROUTES/DOSAGE

EROSIVE ESOPHAGITIS, POORLY RESPONSIVE GERD, ACTIVE DUODENAL ULCER, PREVENTION AND TREATMENT OF NSAID-INDUCED ULCERS
PO: ADULTS, ELDERLY: 20 mg/day.

TO MAINTAIN HEALING OF EROSIVE ESOPHAGITIS
PO: ADULTS, ELDERLY: 20 mg/day.

PATHOLOGIC HYPERSECRETORY CONDITIONS
PO: ADULTS, ELDERLY: Initially, 60 mg/day up to 120 mg 3 times a day.

H. PYLORI DUODENAL ULCER
PO: ADULTS, ELDERLY: 20 mg once daily or 40 mg/day as a single or in 2 divided doses in combination therapy with antibiotics. Dose varies with regimen used.

ACTIVE BENIGN GASTRIC ULCER
PO: ADULTS, ELDERLY: 40 mg/day for 4–8 wk.

OTC USE (FREQUENT HEARTBURN)
PO: ADULTS, ELDERLY: 20 mg/day for 14 days. May repeat after 4 mo if needed.

USUAL PEDIATRIC DOSAGE
CHILDREN OLDER THAN 2 YR, WEIGHING 20 KG AND MORE: 20 mg/day. CHILDREN OLDER THAN 2 YR, WEIGHING LESS THAN 20 KG: 10 mg/day.

SIDE EFFECTS

FREQUENT (7%): Headache. **OCCASIONAL (3%–2%):** Diarrhea, abdominal pain, nausea. **RARE (2%):** Dizziness, asthenia or loss of strength, vomiting, constipation, upper respiratory tract infection, back pain, rash, cough.

ADVERSE REACTIONS/TOXIC EFFECTS

Pancreatitis, hepatotoxicity, and interstitial nephritis have been reported.

NURSING CONSIDERATIONS

INTERVENTION/EVALUATION

Evaluate for therapeutic response: relief of GI symptoms. Question if GI discomfort, nausea, diarrhea occurs.

PATIENT/FAMILY TEACHING

• Report headache. • Swallow capsules whole; do not chew or crush. • Take before eating.

Omnicef, *see cefdinir*

---

ondansetron hydrochloride

on-**dan**-sah-tron
(Zofran, Zofran ODT)
Do not confuse Zofran with Zantac or Zosyn.

◆ **CLASSIFICATION**

PHARMACOTHERAPEUTIC: Selective receptor antagonist. **CLINICAL:** Antinausea, antiemetic.

ACTION

An antiemetic that blocks serotonin, both peripherally on vagal nerve terminals and centrally in the chemoreceptor trigger zone. **Therapeutic Effect:** Prevents nausea and vomiting.

PHARMACOKINETICS

Readily absorbed from the GI tract. Protein binding: 70%–76%. Metabolized in the liver. Primarily excreted in urine. Unknown if removed by hemodialysis. Half-life: 4 hr.

USES

Prevention, treatment of nausea/vomiting due to cancer chemotherapy, including high-dose cisplatin. Prevention of postop nausea/vomiting. Prevention of radiation-induced nausea/vomiting. OFF-LABEL: Treatment of postoperative nausea and vomiting.

PRECAUTIONS

CONTRAINDICATIONS: None known. **CAUTIONS:** None known.

⏳ LIFESPAN CONSIDERATIONS: **Pregnancy/Lactation:** Unknown if drug crosses placenta or is distributed in breast milk. **Pregnancy Category B. Children:** Safety and efficacy not established. **Elderly:** No age-related precautions noted.

INTERACTIONS

DRUG: **Apomorphine:** May cause profound hypotension and alter consciousness. HERBAL: None known. FOOD: None known. LAB VALUES: May transiently increase serum bilirubin, AST, and ALT levels.

AVAILABILITY (Rx)

ORAL SOLUTION (ZOFRAN): 4 mg/5 ml. **TABLETS (ZOFRAN):** 4 mg, 8 mg, 24 mg. **TABLETS (ORALLY DISINTEGRATING [ZOFRAN ODT]):** 4 mg, 8 mg. **INJECTION (ZOFRAN):** 2 mg/ml. **INJECTION (PREMIX):** 32 mg/50 ml.

ADMINISTRATION/HANDLING

💧 IV

Reconstitution • May give undiluted. • For IV infusion, dilute with 50 ml D₅W or 0.9% NaCl before administration.

Rate of administration • Give IV push over 2–5 min. • Give IV infusion over 15 min.

Storage • Store at room temperature. • Stable for 48 hr following dilution.

IM
• Inject into large muscle mass.

PO
• Give without regard to food.

▦ IV INCOMPATIBILITIES

Acyclovir (Zovirax), allopurinol (Aloprim), aminophylline, amphotericin B (Fungizone), amphotericin B complex (Abelcet, AmBisome, Amphotec), ampicillin (Polycillin), ampicillin and sulbactam (Unasyn), cefepime (Maxipime), cefoperazone (Cefobid), 5-fluorouracil, lorazepam (Ativan), meropenem (Merrem IV), methylprednisolone (Solu-Medrol).

IV COMPATIBILITIES

Carboplatin (Paraplatin), cisplatin (Platinol), cyclophosphamide (Cytoxan), cytarabine (Cytosar), dacarbazine (DTIC-Dome), daunorubicin (Cerubidine), dexamethasone (Decadron), diphenhydramine (Benadryl), docetaxel (Taxotere), dopamine (Intropin), etoposide (VePesid), gemcitabine (Gemzar), heparin, hydromorphone (Dilaudid), ifosfamide (Ifex), magnesium, mannitol, mesna (Mesnex), methotrexate, metoclopramide (Reglan), mitomycin (Mutamycin), mitoxantrone (Novantrone), morphine, paclitaxel (Taxol), potassium chloride, teniposide (Vumon), topotecan (Hycamtin), vinblastine (Velban), vincristine (Oncovin), vinorelbine (Navelbine).

INDICATIONS/ROUTES/DOSAGE

CHEMOTHERAPY-INDUCED EMESIS

IV: ADULTS, ELDERLY: 0.15 mg/kg 3 times a day beginning 30 min before chemotherapy or 0.45 mg/kg once daily or 8–10 mg 1–2 times/day or 24–32 mg once daily. CHILDREN 4–18 YR: 0.15 mg/kg 3 times a day beginning 30 min before chemotherapy and again 4 and 8 hr after first dose or 0.45 mg/kg as a single dose.

O

PO: ADULTS, ELDERLY: (highly emetogenic) 24 mg 30 min before start of chemotherapy, (moderately emetogenic) 8 mg q12h beginning 30 min before chemotherapy and continuing for 1–2 days after completion of chemotherapy.

PREVENTION OF POST-OPERATIVE NAUSEA AND VOMITING

IV, IM: ADULTS, ELDERLY: 4 mg as a single dose. CHILDREN 2–12 YR, WEIGHING MORE THAN 40 KG: 4 mg. CHILDREN 2–12 YR, WEIGHING 40 KG AND LESS: 0.1 mg/kg.

PO: ADULTS, ELDERLY: 16 mg 1 hr before induction of anesthesia.

PREVENTION OF RADIATION-INDUCED NAUSEA AND VOMITING

PO: ADULTS, ELDERLY: (total body irradiation) 8 mg 1–2 hr daily before each fraction of radiotherapy, (single high-dose radiotherapy to abdomen) 8 mg 1–2 hr before irradiation, then 8 mg q8h after first dose for 1–2 days after completion of radiotherapy, (daily fractionated radiotherapy to abdomen) 8 mg 1–2 hr before irradiation, then 8 mg 8 hr after first dose for each day of radiotherapy.

SIDE EFFECTS

FREQUENT (13%–5%): Anxiety, dizziness, somnolence, headache, fatigue, constipation, diarrhea, hypoxia, urine retention. **OCCASIONAL (4%–2%):** Abdominal pain, xerostomia, fever, feeling of cold, redness and pain at injection site, paresthesia, asthenia. **RARE (1%):** Hypersensitivity reaction (including rash and pruritus), blurred vision.

ADVERSE REACTIONS/ TOXIC EFFECTS

Overdose may produce a combination of CNS stimulant and depressant effects.

NURSING CONSIDERATIONS

BASELINE ASSESSMENT

Assess for dehydration if excessive vomiting occurs (poor skin turgor, dry mucous membranes, longitudinal furrows in tongue). Provide emotional support.

INTERVENTION/EVALUATION

Monitor patient in environment. Assess bowel sounds for peristalsis. Provide supportive measures. Assess mental status. Monitor daily bowel activity/stool consistency; record time of evacuation.

PATIENT/FAMILY TEACHING

• Relief from nausea/vomiting generally occurs shortly after drug administration. • Avoid alcohol, barbiturates. • Report persistent vomiting (may cause drowsiness, dizziness). • Avoid tasks that require alertness, motor skills until response to drug is established.

Onxol, *see paclitaxel*

oprelvekin (interleukin-2, IL-2)

oh-**prel**-vee-kinn

(Neumega)

Do not confuse Neumega with Neupogen.

CLASSIFICATION

PHARMACOTHERAPEUTIC: Hematopoietic. **CLINICAL:** Platelet growth factor.

ACTION

A hematopoietic that stimulates production of blood platelets, essential to the blood-clotting process. **Therapeutic Effect:** Increases platelet production.

PHARMACOKINETICS

Renal elimination. **Half-life:** 6.9 + 1.7 hr.

O

USES
Prevents severe thrombocytopenia, reduces need for platelet transfusions following myelosuppressive chemotherapy in patients with nonmyeloid malignancies.

PRECAUTIONS
CONTRAINDICATIONS: None known. **CAUTIONS:** CHF, those susceptible to developing CHF, history of heart failure, history of atrial arrhythmia.

⏳ **LIFESPAN CONSIDERATIONS: Pregnancy/Lactation:** Unknown if drug crosses placenta or is distributed is breast milk. **Pregnancy Category C. Children:** Safety and efficacy not established. **Elderly:** No age-related precautions noted.

INTERACTIONS
DRUG: None known. HERBAL: None known. FOOD: None known. LAB VALUES: May decrease Hgb and Hct, usually within 3–5 days of initiation of therapy; reverses about 1 wk after discontinuance of therapy.

AVAILABILITY (Rx)
INJECTION: 5 mg.

ADMINISTRATION/HANDLING
SUBCUTANEOUS

Reconstitution • Add 1 ml sterile water for injection on side of vial; swirl contents gently (avoid excessive agitation) to provide concentration of 5 mg/ml oprelvekin). • Discard unused portion.

Storage • Store in refrigerator. Once reconstituted, use within 3 hr. • Give single injection in abdomen, thigh, hip, upper arm.

INDICATIONS/ROUTES/DOSAGE
PREVENTION OF THROMBOCYTOPENIA
SUBCUTANEOUS: ADULTS: 50 mcg/kg once a day. CHILDREN: 75–100 mcg/kg once a day. Continue for 10–21 days or until platelet count reaches 50,000 cells/mcL after its nadir.

SIDE EFFECTS
FREQUENT: Nausea or vomiting (77%); fluid retention (59%); neutropenic fever (48%); diarrhea (43%); rhinitis (42%); headache (41%); dizziness (38%); fever (36%); insomnia (33%); cough (29%); rash, pharyngitis (25%); tachycardia (20%); vasodilation (19%).

ADVERSE REACTIONS/TOXIC EFFECTS
Transient atrial fibrillation or flutter occurs in 10% of patients and may be caused by increased plasma volume; oprelvekin is not directly arrhythmogenic. Arrhythmias usually are brief in duration and spontaneously convert to normal sinus rhythm. Papilledema may occur in children.

NURSING CONSIDERATIONS

BASELINE ASSESSMENT
Obtain CBC before to chemotherapy and at regular intervals thereafter.

INTERVENTION/EVALUATION
Monitor platelet counts. Closely monitor fluid and electrolyte status, particularly in patients receiving diuretic therapy. Assess for fluid retention evidenced by peripheral edema, dyspnea on exertion (DOE) (generally occurs during first week of therapy and continues for duration of treatment). Monitor platelet count periodically to assess therapeutic duration of therapy. Dosing should continue until postnadir platelet count is more than 50,000 cells/mcL. Treatment should be stopped longer than 2 days before starting next round of chemotherapy.

Orapred, *see prednisolone*

---

orlistat

ohr-lih-stat
(Xenical)
Do not confuse Xenical with Xeloda.

◆CLASSIFICATION

PHARMACOTHERAPEUTIC: Gastric/pancreatic lipase inhibitor. **CLINICAL:** Obesity management agent (see p. 125C).

ACTION

A gastric and pancreatic lipase inhibitor that inhibits absorption of dietary fats by inactivating gastric and pancreatic enzymes. **Therapeutic Effect:** Resulting caloric deficit may positively affect weight control.

PHARMACOKINETICS

Minimal absorption after administration. Protein binding: 99%. Primarily eliminated unchanged in feces. Unknown if removed by hemodialysis. **Half-life:** 1–2 hr.

USES

Management of obesity, including weight loss and maintenance, when used in conjunction with a reduced-calorie diet. **OFF-LABEL:** Type 2 diabetes.

PRECAUTIONS

CONTRAINDICATIONS: Cholestasis, chronic malabsorption syndrome. **CAUTIONS:** None known.

⌛ **LIFESPAN CONSIDERATIONS:** Pregnancy/Lactation: Unknown if excreted in breast milk. Not recommended during pregnancy or in breast-feeding women. **Pregnancy Category B. Children:** Safety and efficacy not established. **Elderly:** No age-related precautions noted.

INTERACTIONS

DRUG: Pravastatin: May increase the blood concentration of pravastatin and risk of rhabdomyolysis. **HERBAL:** None known. **FOOD:** None known. **LAB VALUES:** Decreases blood glucose, total serum cholesterol, and serum LDL levels. Decreases absorption and levels of vitamins A and E.

AVAILABILITY (Rx)

CAPSULES: 120 mg.

ADMINISTRATION/HANDLING

PO
• Give without regard to food.

INDICATIONS/ROUTES/DOSAGE

WEIGHT REDUCTION
PO: ADULTS, ELDERLY, CHILDREN 12–16 YR: 120 mg 3 times a day with each main meal containing fat (omit if meal is occasionally missed or contains no fat).

SIDE EFFECTS

FREQUENT (30%–20%): Headache, abdominal discomfort, flatulence, fecal urgency, fatty or oily stool. **OCCASIONAL (14%–5%):** Back pain, menstrual irregularity, nausea, fatigue, diarrhea, dizziness. **RARE (less than 4%):** Anxiety, rash, myalgia, dry skin, vomiting.

ADVERSE REACTIONS/ TOXIC EFFECTS

Hypersensitivity reaction occurs rarely.

NURSING CONSIDERATIONS

INTERVENTION/EVALUATION

Monitor serum cholesterol, LDL, glucose, changes in coagulation parameters.

PATIENT/FAMILY TEACHING

• Maintain nutritionally balanced, reduced-calorie diet. • Daily intake of fat, carbohydrates, protein to be distributed over the 3 main meals.

orphenadrine citrate

(Norflex)
See Skeletal muscle relaxants

---

oseltamivir

ah-suhl-**tahm**-ah-veer
(Tamiflu)

CLASSIFICATION

PHARMACOTHERAPEUTIC: Neuraminidase inhibitor. **CLINICAL:** Antiviral (see p. 61C).

ACTION

A selective inhibitor of influenza virus neuraminidase, an enzyme essential for viral replication. Acts against both influenza A and B viruses. **Therapeutic Effect:** Suppresses the spread of infection within the respiratory system and reduces the duration of clinical symptoms.

PHARMACOKINETICS

Readily absorbed. Protein binding: 3%. Extensively converted to active drug in the liver. Primarily excreted in urine. **Half-life:** 6–10 hr.

USES

Symptomatic treatment of uncomplicated acute illness caused by influenza A or B virus in adults and children 1 yr and older who are symptomatic no longer than 2 days. Prevention of influenza in adults, children 1 yr and older.

PRECAUTIONS

CONTRAINDICATIONS: None known. **CAUTIONS:** Renal impairment.

⧗ **LIFESPAN CONSIDERATIONS: Pregnancy/Lactation:** Unknown if excreted in breast milk. **Pregnancy Category C. Children:** Safety and efficacy not established in those younger than 1 yr.

Elderly: No age-related precautions noted.

INTERACTIONS

DRUG: Probenecid: Increases oseltamivir concentration. **HERBAL:** None known. **FOOD:** None known. **LAB VALUES:** None known.

AVAILABILITY (Rx)

CAPSULES: 75 mg. **ORAL SUSPENSION:** 12 mg/ml.

ADMINISTRATION/HANDLING
PO
• Give without regard to food.

INDICATIONS/ROUTES/DOSAGE
INFLUENZA

PO: ADULTS, ELDERLY: 75 mg 2 times a day for 5 days. CHILDREN WEIGHING MORE THAN 40 KG: 75 mg twice a day. CHILDREN WEIGHING 24–40 KG: 60 mg twice a day. CHILDREN WEIGHING 15–23 KG: 45 mg twice a day. CHILDREN WEIGHING LESS THAN 15 KG: 30 mg twice a day.

PREVENTION OF INFLUENZA

PO: ADULTS, ELDERLY, CHILDREN 13 YR AND OLDER: 75 mg once daily for at least 7 days. CHILDREN 1–12 YR: 30–60 mg once daily for 10 days.

DOSAGE IN RENAL IMPAIRMENT

PO: For adult and elderly patients, dosage is decreased to 75 mg once a day for at least 7 days and possibly up to 6 wk.

SIDE EFFECTS

FREQUENT (10%–7%): Nausea, vomiting, diarrhea. **RARE (2%–1%):** Abdominal pain, bronchitis, dizziness, headache, cough, insomnia, fatigue, vertigo.

ADVERSE REACTIONS/ TOXIC EFFECTS

Colitis, pneumonia, tympanic membrane disorder, and pyrexia occur rarely.

NURSING CONSIDERATIONS

INTERVENTION/EVALUATION

Monitor serum glucose, renal function, in patients with diabetes.

PATIENT/FAMILY TEACHING

• Begin as soon as possible from first appearance of flu symptoms. • Avoid contact with those who are at high risk for influenza. • Not a substitute for flu shot.

oxacillin

(Prostaphlin)
See Antibiotic: penicillins (p. 27C)

oxaliplatin

ox-**ale**-ee-plah-tin
(Eloxatin)

◆CLASSIFICATION

PHARMACOTHERAPEUTIC: Platinum-containing complex. **CLINICAL:** Antineoplastic (see p. 77C).

ACTION

A platinum-containing complex that cross-links with DNA strands, preventing cell division. Cell cycle–phase nonspecific. Therapeutic Effect: Inhibits DNA replication.

PHARMACOKINETICS

Rapidly distributed. Protein binding: 90%. Undergoes rapid, extensive non-enzymatic biotransformation. Excreted in urine. Half-life: 70 hr.

USES

Combination treatment of metastatic carcinoma of the colon or rectum with 5-fluorouracil (5-FU)/leucovorin in patients whose disease has recurred or progressed during or within 6 mo of completion of first-line therapy with bolus 5-FU/leucovorin and irinotecan. OFF-LABEL: Treatment of germ cell cancer, ovarian cancer, pancreatic cancer, renal cell cancer, solid tumors.

PRECAUTIONS

CONTRAINDICATIONS: History of allergy to other platinum compounds. **CAUTIONS:** Previous therapy with other antineoplastic agents, radiation, renal impairment, infection, pregnancy, immunosuppression, presence or history of peripheral neuropathy.

⧗ LIFESPAN CONSIDERATIONS: **Pregnancy/Lactation:** If possible, avoid use during pregnancy, especially first trimester. May cause fetal harm. Breast-feeding not recommended. **Pregnancy Category D. Children:** Safety and efficacy not established. **Elderly:** Increased incidence of diarrhea, dehydration, hypokalemia, fatigue.

INTERACTIONS

DRUG: Live virus vaccines: May potentiate virus replication, increase vaccine side effects, and decrease the patient's antibody response to the vaccine. **Nephrotic medications:** May decrease the clearance of oxaliplatin. **HERBAL:** None known. **FOOD:** None known. **LAB VALUES:** May alter serum bilirubin, AST, and ALT levels. May decrease blood Hgb and Hct levels and platelet count.

AVAILABILITY (Rx)

INJECTION SOLUTION: 50-mg, 100-mg vials 5 mg/ml.

ADMINISTRATION/HANDLING

◀ ALERT ▶ Pretreat the patient with antiemetics (5-HT₃ antagonists), if ordered. Know that repeat courses should not be given more frequently than every 2 wk.
◀ ALERT ▶ Wear protective gloves during handling of oxaliplatin. If solution

comes in contact with skin, wash skin immediately with soap, water. Do not use aluminum needles or administration sets that may come in contact with drug; may cause degradation of platinum compounds.

◀ **ALERT** ▶ Patient to avoid ice or drinking, touching cold objects during infusion (can exacerbate acute neuropathy).

 IV

Rate of administration • Administer differing infusion rates as a 2-hr or 22-hr rate, according to protocol orders.

▓ IV INCOMPATIBILITIES

Don't infuse oxaliplatin with alkaline medications.

INDICATIONS/ROUTES/DOSAGE

METASTATIC COLON OR RECTAL CANCER IN PATIENTS WHOSE DISEASE HAS RECURRED OR PROGRESSED DURING OR WITHIN 6 MO OF COMPLETING FIRST-LINE THERAPY WITH BOLUS 5-FU, LEUCOVORIN, AND IRINOTECAN

IV: ADULTS: Day 1: Oxaliplatin 85 mg/m^2 in 250–500 ml D$_5$W and leucovorin 200 mg/m^2, both given simultaneously over more than 2 hr in separate bags using a Y-line, followed by 5-FU 400 mg/m^2 IV bolus given over 2–4 min, followed by 5-FU 600 mg/m^2 in 500 ml D$_5$W as a 22-hr continuous IV infusion. Day 2: Leucovorin 200 mg/m^2 IV infusion given over more than 2 hr, followed by 5-FU 400 mg/m^2 IV bolus given over 2–4 min, followed by 5-FU 600 mg/m^2 in 500 ml D$_5$W as a 22-hr continuous IV infusion.

OVARIAN CANCER

IV: ADULTS: Cisplatin 100 mg/m^2 and oxaliplatin 130 mg/m^2 q3wk.

SIDE EFFECTS

FREQUENT (76%–20%): Peripheral or sensory neuropathy (usually occurs in hands, feet, perioral area, and throat but may present as jaw spasm, abnormal tongue sensation, eye pain, chest pressure, or difficulty walking, swallowing, or writing), nausea (64%), fatigue, diarrhea, vomiting, constipation, abdominal pain, fever, anorexia. **OCCASIONAL (14%–10%):** Stomatitis, earache, insomnia, cough, difficulty breathing, backache, edema. **RARE (7%–3%):** Dyspepsia, dizziness, rhinitis, flushing, alopecia.

ADVERSE REACTIONS/ TOXIC EFFECTS

Peripheral or sensory neuropathy can occur, sometimes precipitated or exacerbated by drinking or holding a glass of cold liquid during the IV infusion. Pulmonary fibrosis, characterized by a nonproductive cough, dyspnea, crackles, and radiologic pulmonary infiltrates, may require drug discontinuation. Hypersensitivity reaction (rash, urticaria, pruritus) occurs rarely.

NURSING CONSIDERATIONS

BASELINE ASSESSMENT

Patient to avoid ice or drinking, holding a glass of cold liquid during IV infusion; can precipitate/exacerbate neurotoxicity (occurs within hours or 1–2 days of dosing, lasts up to 14 days). Assess baseline BUN, serum creatinine, WBC, platelet count.

INTERVENTION/EVALUATION

Monitor for decrease in WBC or platelets (myelosuppression is minimal). Monitor for diarrhea, GI bleeding (bright red or tarry stool). Maintain strict I&O. Assess oral mucosa for stomatitis.

PATIENT/FAMILY TEACHING

• Promptly report fever, sore throat, signs of local infection, unusual bruising or bleeding from any site. • Do not have immunizations without physician's approval (lowers body's resistance). • Avoid contact with those who have recently taken oral polio vaccine.

• Avoid cold drinks, ice, cold objects (may produce neuropathy).

oxaprozin

ox-a-**pro**-zin

(Daypro)

Do not confuse oxaprozin with oxazepam.

◆ CLASSIFICATION

PHARMACOTHERAPEUTIC: Nonsteroidal anti-inflammatory. **CLINICAL:** Analgesic, anti-inflammatory (see p. 117C).

ACTION

An NSAID that produces analgesic and anti-inflammatory effects by inhibiting prostaglandin synthesis. **Therapeutic Effect:** Reduces the inflammatory response and intensity of pain.

PHARMACOKINETICS

Well absorbed from the GI tract. Protein binding: 99%. Widely distributed. Metabolized in the liver. Primarily excreted in urine; partially eliminated in feces. Not removed by hemodialysis. **Half-life:** 42–50 hr.

USES

Acute, chronic treatment of osteoarthritis, juvenile rheumatoid arthritis, rheumatoid arthritis.

PRECAUTIONS

CONTRAINDICATIONS: Active peptic ulcer disease, chronic inflammation of GI tract, GI bleeding or ulceration, history of hypersensitivity to aspirin or NSAIDs. **CAUTIONS:** Renal or hepatic impairment, history of GI tract disease, predisposition to fluid retention.

⌛ **LIFESPAN CONSIDERATIONS: Pregnancy/Lactation:** Unknown if drug is excreted in breast milk. Avoid use during third trimester (may adversely affect fetal cardiovascular system: premature closure of ductus arteriosus). **Pregnancy Category C (D if used in third trimester or near delivery). Children:** Safety and efficacy not established. **Elderly:** Age-related renal impairment may increase risk of hepatic or renal toxicity; decreased dosage recommended. GI bleeding or ulceration more likely to cause serious adverse effects.

INTERACTIONS

DRUG: Antihypertensives, diuretics: May decrease the effects of these drugs. **Aspirin, other salicylates:** May increase the risk of GI side effects such as bleeding. **Bone marrow depressants:** May increase the risk of hematologic reactions. **Heparin, oral anticoagulants, thrombolytics:** May increase the effects of these drugs. **Lithium:** May increase the blood concentration and risk of toxicity of lithium. **Methotrexate:** May increase the risk of methotrexate toxicity. **Probenecid:** May increase the oxaprozin blood concentration. **HERBAL: Feverfew:** May decrease the effects of feverfew. **Ginkgo biloba:** May increase the risk of bleeding. **FOOD:** None known. **LAB VALUES:** May increase BUN, serum creatinine, AST, and ALT levels.

AVAILABILITY (Rx)

TABLETS: 600 mg.

ADMINISTRATION/HANDLING

PO

• May give with food, milk, antacids if GI distress occurs.

INDICATIONS/ROUTES/DOSAGE

OSTEOARTHRITIS

PO: ADULTS, ELDERLY: 1,200 mg once a day (600 mg in patients with low body weight or mild disease). **Maximum:** 1,800 mg/day.

RHEUMATOID ARTHRITIS
PO: ADULTS, ELDERLY: 1,200 mg once a day. Range: 600–1,800 mg/day.

JUVENILE RHEUMATOID ARTHRITIS
PO: CHILDREN WEIGHING MORE THAN 54 KG: 1,200 mg/day. CHILDREN WEIGHING 32–54 KG: 900 mg/day. CHILDREN WEIGHING 22–31 KG: 600 mg/day.

DOSAGE IN RENAL IMPAIRMENT
For adults and elderly patients with renal impairment, the recommended initial dose is 600 mg/day; may be increased up to 1,200 mg/day.

SIDE EFFECTS
OCCASIONAL (9%–3%): Nausea, diarrhea, constipation, dyspepsia, edema. **RARE (less than 3%):** Vomiting, abdominal cramps or pain, flatulence, anorexia, confusion, tinnitus, insomnia, somnolence.

ADVERSE REACTIONS/ TOXIC EFFECTS
Hypertension, acute renal failure, respiratory depression, GI bleeding, and coma occur rarely.

NURSING CONSIDERATIONS

BASELINE ASSESSMENT
Assess onset, type, location, duration of pain or inflammation.

INTERVENTION/EVALUATION
Observe for weight gain, edema, bleeding, ecchymoses, mental confusion. Monitor renal and liver function tests. Evaluate for therapeutic response: relief of pain, stiffness, swelling; increased joint mobility; reduced joint tenderness; improved grip strength.

PATIENT/FAMILY TEACHING
• Avoid aspirin, alcohol during therapy (increases risk of GI bleeding). • If gastric upset occurs, take with food, milk, antacids. • If GI effects persist, inform physician. • Avoid tasks that require alertness, motor skills until

response to drug is established (may cause drowsiness, confusion).

oxazepam

ox-**az**-eh-pam

(Apo-Oxazepam ✦, Serax)

Do not confuse oxazepam with oxaprozin, or Serax with Eurax or Xerac.

CLASSIFICATION
PHARMACOTHERAPEUTIC: Benzodiazepine (**Schedule IV**). **CLINICAL:** Antianxiety (see p. 12C).

ACTION
A benzodiazepine that potentiates the effects of gamma-aminobutyric acid and other inhibitory neurotransmitters by binding to specific receptors in the CNS. **Therapeutic Effect:** Produces anxiolytic effect and skeletal muscle relaxation.

PHARMACOKINETICS
Well absorbed from the GI tract. Protein binding: 97%. Metabolized in the liver. Primarily excreted in urine. Not removed by hemodialysis. **Half-life:** 5–20 hr.

USES
Management of acute alcohol withdrawal symptoms (tremors, anxiety on withdrawal). Treatment of anxiety associated with depressive symptoms.

PRECAUTIONS
CONTRAINDICATIONS: Angle-closure glaucoma; preexisting CNS depression; severe, uncontrolled pain. **CAUTIONS:** History of drug dependence.

⚖ **LIFESPAN CONSIDERATIONS: Pregnancy/Lactation:** Drug crosses placenta; is distributed in breast milk.

May produce CNS depression in the neonate. **Pregnancy Category D. Children:** Safety and efficacy not established. **Elderly:** May produce excessive sedation, ataxia.

INTERACTIONS

DRUG: **Alcohol, other CNS depressants:** May potentiate CNS depression. **HERBAL:** **Kava kava, valerian:** May increase CNS depression. **FOOD:** None known. **LAB VALUES:** May elevate serum alkaline phosphatase, bilirubin, LDH, AST, and ALT levels. May produce abnormal renal function test results. Therapeutic serum drug level is 0.2–1.4 mcg/ml; toxic serum drug level has not been established.

AVAILABILITY (Rx)

CAPSULES: 10 mg, 15 mg, 30 mg. **TABLETS:** 15 mg.

INDICATIONS/ROUTES/DOSAGE

ANXIETY

PO: ADULTS: 10–30 mg 3–4 times a day. ELDERLY: 10 mg 2–3 times a day. CHILDREN: 1 mg/kg/day.

ALCOHOL WITHDRAWAL

PO: ADULTS, ELDERLY: 15–30 mg 3–4 times a day.

SIDE EFFECTS

FREQUENT: Mild, transient somnolence at beginning of therapy. **OCCASIONAL:** Dizziness, headache. **RARE:** Paradoxical CNS reactions, such as hyperactivity or nervousness in children and excitement or restlessness in the elderly or debilitated (generally noted during the first 2 wk of therapy).

ADVERSE REACTIONS/ TOXIC EFFECTS

Abrupt or too-rapid withdrawal may result in pronounced restlessness, irritability, insomnia, hand tremor, abdominal or muscle cramps, diaphoresis, vomiting, and seizures. Overdose results in somnolence, confusion, diminished reflexes, and coma.

NURSING CONSIDERATIONS

BASELINE ASSESSMENT

Offer emotional support to anxious patient. Assess motor responses (agitation, trembling, tension), autonomic responses (cold and clammy hands, diaphoresis).

INTERVENTION/EVALUATION

For those on long-term therapy, liver and renal function tests, blood counts should be performed periodically. Assess for paradoxical reaction, particularly during early therapy. Assist with ambulation if drowsiness, lightheadedness occurs. Evaluate for therapeutic response: a calm facial expression, decreased restlessness, diminished insomnia. Therapeutic serum level: 0.2–1.4 mcg/ml; toxic serum level: Not established.

PATIENT/FAMILY TEACHING

• Avoid alcohol, other CNS depressants. • Avoid tasks requiring alertness, motor skills until response to drug is established (may cause drowsiness). • Avoid abrupt discontinuation.

oxcarbazepine

ox-car-**bah**-zeh-peen

(Trileptal)

◆CLASSIFICATION

CLINICAL: Anticonvulsant (see p. 34C).

ACTION

An anticonvulsant that blocks sodium channels, resulting in stabilization of hyperexcited neural membranes, inhibition of repetitive neuronal firing, and diminishing synaptic impulses. **Therapeutic Effect:** Prevents seizures.

PHARMACOKINETICS

Completely absorbed from GI tract and extensively metabolized in the liver to active metabolite. Protein binding: 40%. Primarily excreted in urine. **Half-life:** 2 hr; metabolite, 6–10 hr.

USES

Monotherapy and adjunctive therapy in adults, children 2 yr of age and older for treatment of partial seizures. **OFF-LABEL:** Atypical panic disorder, bipolar disorders, neuralgia/neuropathy.

PRECAUTIONS

CONTRAINDICATIONS: None known. **CAUTIONS:** Renal impairment, sensitivity to carbamazepine.

LIFESPAN CONSIDERATIONS: Pregnancy/Lactation: Crosses placenta. Distributed in breast milk. **Pregnancy Category C. Children:** No age-related precautions in those older than 4 yr. **Elderly:** Age-related renal impairment may require dosage adjustment.

INTERACTIONS

DRUG: Carbamazepine, phenobarbital, phenytoin, valproic acid, verapamil: May decrease the blood concentration and effects of oxcarbazepine. **Felodipine, oral contraceptives:** May decrease the effectiveness of these drugs. **Phenobarbital, phenytoin:** May increase the blood concentration and risk of toxicity of these drugs. **HERBAL:** None known. **FOOD:** None known. **LAB VALUES:** May increase GGT level and other hepatic function test results. May increase or decrease blood glucose level. May decrease serum calcium, potassium, and sodium levels.

AVAILABILITY (Rx)

ORAL SUSPENSION: 300 mg/5 ml. **TABLETS:** 150 mg, 300 mg, 600 mg.

ADMINISTRATION/HANDLING
PO
• Give without regard to food.

INDICATIONS/ROUTES/DOSAGE
ADJUNCTIVE TREATMENT OF SEIZURES
PO: ADULTS, ELDERLY: Initially, 600 mg/day in 2 divided doses. May increase by up to 600 mg/day at weekly intervals. **Maximum:** 2,400 mg/day. CHILDREN 4–16 YR: 8–10 mg/kg. **Maximum:** 600 mg/day. Maintenance (based on weight): 1,800 mg/day for children weighing more than 39 kg; 1,200 mg/day for children weighing 29.1–39 kg; and 900 mg/day for children weighing 20–29 kg.

CONVERSION TO MONOTHERAPY
PO: ADULTS, ELDERLY: 600 mg/day in 2 divided doses (while decreasing concomitant anticonvulsant over 3–6 wk). May increase by 600 mg/day at weekly intervals up to 2,400 mg/day. CHILDREN: Initially, 8–10 mg/kg/day in 2 divided doses with simultaneous initial reduction of dose of concomitant antiepileptic.

INITIATION OF MONOTHERAPY
PO: ADULTS, ELDERLY: 600 mg/day in 2 divided doses. May increase by 300 mg/day every 3 days up to 1,200 mg/day. CHILDREN: Initially, 8–10 mg/kg/day in 2 divided doses. Increase at 3 day intervals by 5 mg/kg/day to achieve maintenance dose by weight; (70 kg): 1,500–2,100 mg/day; (60–69 kg): 1,200–2,100 mg/day; (50–59 kg): 1,200–1,800 mg/day; (41–49 kg): 1,200–1,500 mg/day; (35–40 kg): 900–1,500 mg/day;

(25–34 kg): 900–1,200 mg/day; (20–24 kg): 600–900 mg/day.

oxiconazole

(Oxistat)

See Antifungals: topical (p. 45C)

DOSAGE IN RENAL IMPAIRMENT

For patients with creatinine clearance less than 30 ml/min, give 50% of normal starting dose, then titrate slowly to desired dose.

SIDE EFFECTS

FREQUENT   (22%–13%): Dizziness, nausea, headache. **OCCASIONAL (7%–5%):** Vomiting, diarrhea, ataxia, nervousness, heartburn, indigestion, epigastric pain, constipation. **RARE (4%):** Tremor, rash, back pain, epistaxis, sinusitis, diplopia.

ADVERSE REACTIONS/ TOXIC EFFECTS

Clinically significant hyponatremia may occur.

NURSING CONSIDERATIONS

BASELINE ASSESSMENT

Review history of seizure disorder (type, onset, intensity, frequency, duration, level of consciousness [LOC]), drug history (especially other anticonvulsants). Provide safety precautions; quiet, dark environment.

INTERVENTION/EVALUATION

Assist with ambulation if dizziness, ataxia occurs. Assess for visual abnormalities, headache. Monitor serum sodium levels. Assess for signs of hyponatremia (nausea, malaise, headache, lethargy, confusion). Assess for clinical improvement (decrease in intensity and frequency of seizures).

PATIENT/FAMILY TEACHING

• Do not abruptly stop taking medication (may increase seizure activity). • Inform physician if rash, nausea, headache, dizziness occurs. • May need periodic blood tests.

oxybutynin

ox-i-**byoo**-ti-nin

(Ditropan, Ditropan XL, Oxytrol, Urotrol)

Do not confuse oxybutynin with OxyContin, or Ditropan with diazepam.

CLASSIFICATION

PHARMACOTHERAPEUTIC: Anticholinergic. **CLINICAL:** Antispasmodic.

ACTION

An anticholinergic that exerts antispasmodic (papaverine-like) and antimuscarinic (atropine-like) action on the detrusor smooth muscle of the bladder. **Therapeutic Effect:** Increases bladder capacity and delays desire to void.

PHARMACOKINETICS

Route	Onset	Peak	Duration
PO	0.5–1 hr	3–6 hr	6–10 hr

Rapidly absorbed from the GI tract. Metabolized in the liver. Primarily excreted in urine. Unknown if removed by hemodialysis. **Half-life:** 1–2.3 hr.

USES

Relief of symptoms (urgency, incontinence, frequency, nocturia, urge incontinence) associated with uninhibited neurogenic bladder, reflex neurogenic bladder.

PRECAUTIONS

CONTRAINDICATIONS: GI or GU obstruction, glaucoma, myasthenia gravis, toxic megacolon, ulcerative colitis. **CAUTIONS:** Renal or hepatic impairment, cardiovascular disease, hyperthyroidism, reflux esophagitis, hypertension, prostatic hypertrophy, neuropathy.

⧗ **LIFESPAN CONSIDERATIONS: Pregnancy/Lactation:** Unknown if drug crosses placenta or is distributed in breast milk. **Pregnancy Category B. Children:** No age-related precautions noted in those older than 5 yr. **Elderly:** May be more sensitive to anticholinergic effects (e.g., dry mouth, urinary retention).

INTERACTIONS

DRUG: Medications with anticholinergic effects (such as antihistamines): May increase the anticholinergic effects of oxybutynin. **HERBAL:** None known. **FOOD:** None known. **LAB VALUES:** None known.

AVAILABILITY (Rx)

SYRUP (DITROPAN): 5 mg/5 ml. **TABLETS (DITROPAN, UROTROL):** 5 mg. **TABLETS (EXTENDED-RELEASE [DITRO-PAN XL]):** 5 mg, 10 mg, 15 mg. **TRANSDERMAL (OXYTROL):** 3.9 mg.

ADMINISTRATION/HANDLING

PO
* Give without regard to meals.

TRANSDERMAL
* Apply patch to dry, intact skin on the abdomen, hip, or buttock. * Use a new application site for each new patch; avoid reapplication to the same site within 7 days.

INDICATIONS/ROUTES/DOSAGE

NEUROGENIC BLADDER
PO: ADULTS: 5 mg 2–3 times a day up to 5 mg 4 times a day. ELDERLY: 2.5–5 mg twice a day. May increase by 2.5 mg/day every 1–2 days. CHILDREN 5 YR AND OLDER: 5 mg twice a day up to 5 mg 4 times a day. CHILDREN 1–4 YR: 0.2 mg/kg/dose 2–4 times a day.
PO (EXTENDED-RELEASE): ADULTS. ELDERLY: 5–10 mg/day up to 30 mg/day. CHILDREN 6 YR AND OLDER: Initially, 5–10 mg once daily. May increase in 5–10 mg increments. **Maximum:** 30 mg/day.
TRANSDERMAL: ADULTS: 3.9 mg applied twice a week. Apply every 3–4 days.

SIDE EFFECTS

FREQUENT: Constipation, dry mouth, somnolence, decreased perspiration. **OCCASIONAL:** Decreased lacrimation or salivation, impotence, urinary hesitancy and retention, suppressed lactation, blurred vision, mydriasis, nausea or vomiting, insomnia.

ADVERSE REACTIONS/ TOXIC EFFECTS

Overdose produces CNS excitation (including nervousness, restlessness, hallucinations, and irritability), hypotension or hypertension, confusion, tachycardia, facial flushing, and respiratory depression.

NURSING CONSIDERATIONS

BASELINE ASSESSMENT
Assess dysuria, urgency, frequency, incontinence.

INTERVENTION/EVALUATION
Monitor for symptomatic relief. Monitor I&O; palpate bladder for retention. Monitor pattern of bowel activity and stool consistency.

PATIENT/FAMILY TEACHING
* Avoid alcohol. * May cause dry mouth. * Avoid tasks that require alertness, motor skills until response to drug is established (may cause drowsiness).

oxycodone

ox-ee-**koe**-done

(M-Oxy, <u>OxyContin</u>, Oxydose, Oxy-Fast, OxyIR, Percolone, Roxicodone, Roxicodone Intensol, Supeudol ✦)

Do not confuse oxycodone with oxybutynin.

FIXED-COMBINATION(S)

Combunox: oxycodone/ibuprofen (an NSAID): 5 mg/400 mg. **Percocet, Roxicet, Tylox:** oxycodone/acetaminophen (a non-narcotic analgesic): 5 mg/500 mg. **Percocet:** oxycodone/acetaminophen: 2.5 mg/325 mg; 5 mg/325 mg; 5 mg/500 mg; 7.5 mg/325 mg; 7.5 mg/500 mg; 10 mg/325 mg; 10 mg/650 mg. **Percodan:** oxycodone/aspirin (a non-narcotic analgesic): 2.25 mg/325 mg; 4.5 mg/325 mg.

◆CLASSIFICATION

PHARMACOTHERAPEUTIC: Opioid analgesic (**Schedule II**). **CLINICAL:** Narcotic analgesic (see p. 128C).

ACTION

An opioid analgesic that binds with opioid receptors in the CNS. **Therapeutic Effect:** Alters the perception of and emotional response to pain.

PHARMACOKINETICS

Route	Onset	Peak	Duration
PO, Immediate-release	N/A	N/A	4–5 hr
PO, Controlled-release	N/A	N/A	12 hr

Moderately absorbed from the GI tract. Protein binding: 38%–45%. Widely distributed. Metabolized in the liver.

Excreted in urine. Unknown if removed by hemodialysis. **Half-life:** 2–3 hr (3.2 hr controlled-release).

USES

Relief of mild to moderately severe pain.

PRECAUTIONS

CONTRAINDICATIONS: Acute bronchial asthma or hypercarbia, paralytic ileus, respiratory depression. **EXTREME CAUTION:** CNS depression, anoxia, hypercapnia, respiratory depression, seizures, acute alcoholism, shock, untreated myxedema, respiratory dysfunction. **CAUTIONS:** Increased intracranial pressure (ICP), hepatic impairment, acute abdominal conditions, hypothyroidism, prostatic hypertrophy, Addison's disease, urethral stricture, chronic obstructive pulmonary disease (COPD).

⧗ **LIFESPAN CONSIDERATIONS: Pregnancy/Lactation:** Readily crosses placenta. Distributed in breast milk. Respiratory depression may occur in neonate if mother received opiates during labor. Regular use of opiates during pregnancy may produce withdrawal symptoms in neonate (irritability, excessive crying, tremors, hyperactive reflexes, fever, vomiting, diarrhea, yawning, sneezing, seizures. **Pregnancy Category B (D if used for prolonged periods or at high dosages at term). Children:** Paradoxical excitement may occur. Those younger than 2 yr are more susceptible to respiratory depressant effects. **Elderly:** Age-related renal impairment may increase risk of urinary retention. May be more susceptible to respiratory depressant effects.

INTERACTIONS

DRUG: Alcohol, other CNS depressants: May increase CNS or respiratory depression and hypotension.

MAOIs: May produce a severe, sometimes fatal reaction; expect to administer ¼ of usual oxycodone dose. **HERBAL:** None known. **FOOD:** None known. **LAB VALUES:** May increase serum amylase and lipase levels.

AVAILABILITY (Rx)

CAPSULES (IMMEDIATE-RELEASE [OXYIR]): 5 mg. **ORAL CONCENTRATE (OXYDOSE, OXYFAST, ROXICODONE INTENSOL):** 20 mg/ml. **ORAL SOLUTION (ROXICODONE):** 5 mg/5 ml. **TABLETS (M-OXY, PERCOLONE, ROXICODONE):** 5 mg, 15 mg, 30 mg. **TABLETS (EXTENDED-RELEASE [OXY-CONTIN]):** 10 mg, 20 mg, 40 mg, 80 mg, 160 mg.

ADMINISTRATION/HANDLING

PO
• Give without regard to meals. • Tablets may be crushed. • **Controlled-release:** Swallow whole; do not crush, break, chew.

INDICATIONS/ROUTES/DOSAGE

ANALGESIA
PO (CONTROLLED-RELEASE): ADULTS, ELDERLY: Initially, 10 mg q12h. May increase every 1–2 days by 25%–50%. Usual: 40 mg/day (100 mg/day for cancer pain).
PO (IMMEDIATE-RELEASE): ADULTS, ELDERLY: Initially, 5 mg q6h as needed. May increase up to 30 mg q4h. Usual: 10–30 mg q4h as needed. CHILDREN: 0.05–0.15 mg/kg/dose q4–6h.

SIDE EFFECTS

FREQUENT: Somnolence, dizziness, hypotension (including orthostatic hypotension), anorexia. **OCCASIONAL:** Confusion, diaphoresis, facial flushing, urine retention, constipation, dry mouth, nausea, vomiting, headache. **RARE:** Allergic reaction, depression, paradoxical CNS hyperactivity or nervousness in children, paradoxical excitement and restlessness in elderly or debilitated patients.

ADVERSE REACTIONS/TOXIC EFFECTS

Overdose results in respiratory depression, skeletal muscle flaccidity, cold or clammy skin, cyanosis, and extreme somnolence progressing to seizures, stupor, and coma. Hepatotoxicity may occur with overdose of the acetaminophen component of fixed-combination products. The patient who uses oxycodone repeatedly may develop a tolerance to the drug's analgesic effect and physical dependence.

NURSING CONSIDERATIONS

BASELINE ASSESSMENT
Assess onset, type, location, duration of pain. Effect of medication is reduced if full pain recurs before next dose. Obtain vital signs before giving medication. If respirations are 12/min or less (20/min or less in children), withhold medication, contact physician.

INTERVENTION/EVALUATION
Palpate bladder for urinary retention. Monitor pattern of daily bowel activity and stool consistency. Initiate deep breathing, coughing exercises, particularly in patients with pulmonary impairment. Monitor pain relief, respiratory rate, mental status, BP.

PATIENT/FAMILY TEACHING
• May cause dry mouth, drowsiness. • Avoid tasks that require alertness, motor skills until response to drug is established. • Avoid alcohol. • May be habit forming. • Do not crush, chew, break controlled-release tablets.

OxyContin, *see oxycodone*

OxyFast, *see oxycodone*

OxyIR, *see oxycodone*

oxytocin

ox-ee-**toe**-sin
(Pitocin, Syntocinon)
Do not confuse Pitocin with Pitressin.

◆ CLASSIFICATION
PHARMACOTHERAPEUTIC: Uterine smooth muscle stimulant. **CLINICAL:** Oxytocic.

ACTION
An oxytocic that affects uterine myofibril activity and stimulates mammary smooth muscle. **Therapeutic Effect:** Contracts uterine smooth muscle. Enhances lactation.

PHARMACOKINETICS

Route	Onset	Peak	Duration
IV	Immediate	N/A	1 hr
IM	3–5 min	N/A	2–3 hr

Rapidly absorbed through nasal mucous membranes. Protein binding: 30%. Distributed in extracellular fluid. Metabolized in the liver and kidney. Primarily excreted in urine. **Half-life:** 1–6 min.

USES
Induction of labor at term, control postpartum bleeding. Adjunct in management of abortion.

PRECAUTIONS
CONTRAINDICATIONS: Adequate uterine activity that fails to progress, cephalopelvic disproportion, fetal distress without imminent delivery, grand multiparity, hyperactive or hypertonic uterus, obstetric emergencies that favor surgical intervention, prematurity, unengaged fetal head, unfavorable fetal position or presentation, when vaginal delivery is contraindicated, such as active genital herpes infection, placenta previa, or cord presentation. **CAUTIONS:** Induction of labor should be for medical, not elective, reasons.

⧖ **LIFESPAN CONSIDERATIONS: Pregnancy/Lactation:** Used as indicated, not expected to present risk of fetal abnormalities. Small amounts in breast milk; breast-feeding not recommended. **Pregnancy Category X. Children/Elderly:** Not used in these patient populations.

INTERACTIONS
DRUG: Caudal block anesthetics, vasopressors: May increase pressor effects. **Other oxytocics:** May cause cervical lacerations, uterine hypertonus, or uterine rupture. **HERBAL:** None known. **FOOD:** None known. **LAB VALUES:** None known.

AVAILABILITY (Rx)
INJECTION (PITOCIN): 10 units/ml. **NASAL SPRAY (SYNTOCINON):** 40 units/ml.

ADMINISTRATION/HANDLING
📳 **IV**

Reconstitution • Dilute 10–40 units (1–4 ml) in 1,000 ml of 0.9% NaCl, lactated Ringer's, or D_5W to provide a concentration of 10–40 milliunits/ml solution.

Rate of administration • Give by IV infusion (use infusion device to carefully control rate of flow as ordered by physician).

Storage • Store at room temperature.

INTRANASAL

• Store at room temperature. • Use before breast-feeding or pumping of breasts. • Insert the spray tip into the patient's nostril, pointing toward the nasal passages, away from the nasal septum. • Spray oxytocin into the nostril while holding the patient's other nostril closed and at the same time, have the patient inhale through nose to deliver the medication as high into the nasal passages as possible.

▨ IV INCOMPATIBILITIES

No known incompatibilities via Y-site administration.

IV COMPATIBILITIES

Heparin, insulin, multivitamins, potassium chloride.

INDICATIONS/ROUTES/DOSAGE

INDUCTION OR STIMULATION OF LABOR
IV: ADULTS: 0.5–1 milliunit/min. May gradually increase in increments of 1–2 milliunit/min. Rates of 9–10 milliunit/min are rarely required.

ABORTION
IV: ADULTS: 10–20 milliunit/min. **Maximum:** 30 unit/12h dose.

CONTROL OF POSTPARTUM BLEEDING
IV INFUSION: ADULTS: 10–40 units in 1,000 ml IV fluid at a rate sufficient to control uterine atony.
IM: ADULTS: 10 units (total dose) after delivery.

LACTATION STIMULANT
INTRANASAL: ADULTS: One spray into one or both nostrils 2–3 min before breast-feeding or pumping of the breasts.

SIDE EFFECTS

OCCASIONAL: Tachycardia, premature ventricular contractions, hypotension, nausea, vomiting. **RARE: Nasal:** Lacrimation or tearing, nasal irritation, rhinorrhea, unexpected uterine bleeding or contractions.

ADVERSE REACTIONS/ TOXIC EFFECTS

Hypertonicity may occur with tearing of the uterus, increased bleeding, abruptio placentae (i.e., placental abruption), and cervical and vaginal lacerations. In the fetus, bradycardia, CNS or brain damage, trauma due to rapid propulsion, low Apgar score at 5 min, and retinal hemorrhage occur rarely. Prolonged IV infusion of oxytocin with excessive fluid volume has caused severe water intoxication with seizures, coma, and death.

NURSING CONSIDERATIONS

BASELINE ASSESSMENT

Assess baselines for vital signs, BP, fetal heart rate. Determine frequency, duration, strength of contractions.

INTERVENTION/EVALUATION

Monitor BP, pulse, respirations, fetal heart rate, intrauterine pressure, contractions (duration, strength, frequency) q15min. Notify physician of contractions that last longer than 1 min, occur more frequently than every 2 min, or stop. Maintain careful I&O; be alert to potential water intoxication. Check for blood loss.

PATIENT/FAMILY TEACHING

• Keep patient, family informed of labor progress.

Pacerone, *see*
amiodarone

paclitaxel

pass-leh-**tax**-ell
(Abraxane, Onxol, <u>Taxol</u>)
**Do not confuse paclitaxel with
Paxil, or Taxol with Taxotere.**

◆ CLASSIFICATION

PHARMACOTHERAPEUTIC: Taxoid,
antimitotic agent. **CLINICAL:** Antineoplastic (see p. 77C).

ACTION

An antimitotic agent in the taxoid family
that disrupts the microtubular cell
network, which is essential for cellular
function. Blocks cells in the late G_2
phase and M phase of the cell cycle.
Therapeutic Effect: Inhibits cellular
mitosis and replication.

PHARMACOKINETICS

Does not readily cross the blood-brain
barrier. Protein binding: 89%–98%.
Metabolized in the liver to active metabolites; eliminated by bile. Not removed
by hemodialysis. **Half-life:** 1.3–8.6 hr.

USES

First-line treatment of advanced ovarian
cancer, treatment of metastatic ovarian
cancer following failure of first-line or
subsequent chemotherapy. Treatment of
breast cancer, AIDS-related Kaposi's
sarcoma, non–small-cell lung cancer.
OFF-LABEL: Treatment of upper GI
tract adenocarcinoma, head and neck
cancer, hormone-refractory prostate
cancer, metastic breast cancer, non–
Hodgkin's lymphoma, small-cell lung
cancer, transitional cell cancer of
urothelium.

PRECAUTIONS

CONTRAINDICATIONS: Baseline neutropenia (neutrophil count 1,500 cells/
mm³), hypersensitivity to drugs developed with Cremophor EL (polyoxyethylated castor oil). **CAUTIONS:**
Hepatic impairment, severe neutropenia,
peripheral neuropathy.

⧗ **LIFESPAN CONSIDERATIONS: Preg-
nancy/Lactation:** May produce fetal
harm. Unknown if distributed in breast
milk. Avoid use in pregnancy.
Pregnancy Category D. Children: Safety
and efficacy not established.
Elderly: No age-related precautions
noted.

INTERACTIONS

DRUG: Bone marrow depressants:
May increase myelosuppression. **Live
virus vaccines:** May potentiate virus
replication, increase vaccine side effects,
and decrease the patient's antibody
response to the vaccine. **HERBAL:** None
known. **FOOD:** None known. **LAB
VALUES:** May elevate serum alkaline
phosphatase, bilirubin, AST, and ALT
levels. Decreases blood Hgb and Hct
levels and platelet, RBC, and WBC counts.

AVAILABILITY (Rx)

INJECTION (ABRAXANE): 100-mg vial.
INJECTION (ONXOL, TAXOL): 6 mg/ml.

ADMINISTRATION/HANDLING

◻ **IV**

◀ **ALERT** ▶ Wear gloves during handling; if contact with skin occurs, wash
hands thoroughly with soap, water. If
contact with mucous membranes occurs,
flush with water.

Reconstitution • Dilute with 0.9%
NaCl, D_5W to final concentration of
0.3–1.2 mg/ml.

Rate of administration • Administer
at rate as ordered by physician through
in-line filter not greater than 0.22
microns. • Monitor vital signs during

P

infusion, especially during first hour.
• Discontinue administration if severe hypersensitivity reaction occurs.

Storage • Refrigerate unopened vials.
• Prepared solution is stable at room temperature for 24 hr. • Store diluted solutions in bottles or plastic bags and administer through polyethylene-lined administration sets (avoid plasticized PVC equipment or devices).

▩ IV INCOMPATIBILITIES

Amphotericin B complex (Abelcet, AmBisome, Amphotec), chlorpromazine (Thorazine), doxorubicin liposomal (Doxil), hydroxyzine (Vistaril), methylprednisolone (Solu-Medrol), mitoxantrone (Novantrone).

IV COMPATIBILITIES

Carboplatin (Paraplatin), cisplatin (Platinol AQ), cyclophosphamide (Cytoxan), cytarabine (Cytosar), dacarbazine (DTIC-Dome), dexamethasone (Decadron), diphenhydramine (Benadryl), doxorubicin (Adriamycin), etoposide (VePesid), gemcitabine (Gemzar), granisetron (Kytril), hydromorphone (Dilaudid), magnesium sulfate, mannitol, methotrexate, morphine, ondansetron (Zofran), potassium chloride, vinblastine (Velban), vincristine (Oncovin).

INDICATIONS/ROUTES/DOSAGE

OVARIAN CANCER

IV: ADULTS: 135–175 mg/m²/dose over 1–24 hr q3wk.

BREAST CARCINOMA

IV (ONXOL, TAXOL): ADULTS, ELDERLY: 175 mg/m² over 3 hr q3wk.
PO (ABRAXANE): ADULTS, ELDERLY: 260 mg/m² over 30 min q3wk.

NON–SMALL-CELL LUNG CARCINOMA

IV: ADULTS, ELDERLY: 135 mg/m² over 24 hr, followed by cisplatin 75 mg/m² q3wk.

KAPOSI'S SARCOMA

IV: ADULTS, ELDERLY: 135 mg/m²/dose over 3 hr q3wk or 100 mg/m²/dose over 3 hr q2wk.

DOSAGE IN HEPATIC IMPAIRMENT

Total Bilirubin	Total Dose
More than 3 mg/dl	Less than 50 mg/m²
1.6–3 mg/dl	Less than 75 mg/m²
1.5 mg/dl or less	Less than 135 mg/m²

SIDE EFFECTS

EXPECTED (90%–70%): Diarrhea, alopecia, nausea, vomiting. **FREQUENT (48%–46%):** Myalgia or arthralgia, peripheral neuropathy. **OCCASIONAL (20%–13%):** Mucositis, hypotension during infusion, pain or redness at injection site. **RARE (3%):** Bradycardia.

ADVERSE REACTIONS/ TOXIC EFFECTS

Neutropenic nadir occurs at approximately day 11 of paclitaxel therapy. Anemia and leukopenia are common reactions. Thrombocytopenia occurs occasionally. A severe hypersensitivity reaction, including dyspnea, severe hypotension, angioedema, and generalized urticaria, occurs rarely.

NURSING CONSIDERATIONS

BASELINE ASSESSMENT

Give emotional support to patient, family. Use strict asepsis, protect patient from infection. Check blood counts, particularly neutrophil, platelet count before each course of therapy or as clinically indicated.

INTERVENTION/EVALUATION

Monitor CBC, platelets, vital signs, hepatic enzymes. Monitor for hematologic toxicity (fever, sore throat, signs of local infections, unusual bleeding/ ecchymosis), symptoms of anemia (excessive fatigue, weakness). Assess response to medication; monitor, report diarrhea. Avoid IM injections, rectal temperatures, other traumas that may induce bleeding. Put pressure to injection sites for full 5 min.

P

PATIENT/FAMILY TEACHING

• Explain that alopecia is reversible, but new hair may have different color, texture. • Do not have immunizations without physician's approval (drug lowers body's resistance). • Avoid crowds, persons with known infections. • Report signs of infection at once (fever, flu-like symptoms). • Contact physician if nausea/vomiting continues at home. • Teach signs of peripheral neuropathy. • Avoid pregnancy during therapy.

palifermin

pal-ih-**fur**-min
(Kepivance)

◆CLASSIFICATION

PHARMACOTHERAPEUTIC: Keratinocyte growth factor. **CLINICAL:** Antineoplastic adjunct.

ACTION

An antineoplastic adjunct that binds to the keratinocyte growth factor receptor, present on epithelial cells of the buccal mucosa and tongue, resulting in the proliferation, differentiation, and migration of epithelial cells. **Therapeutic Effect:** Reduces incidence and duration of severe oral mucositis.

PHARMACOKINETICS

Clearance is higher in cancer patients compared to healthy subjects. **Half-life:** 4.5 hr.

USES

Reduces incidence, duration, severity of severe stomatitis in patients with hematologic malignancies receiving myelotoxic therapy requiring hematopoietic stem cell support.

PRECAUTIONS

CONTRAINDICATIONS: Patients allergic to *Escherichia coli*–derived proteins. **CAUTIONS:** Pregnant and breast-feeding patients.

⧗ **LIFESPAN CONSIDERATIONS: Pregnancy/Lactation:** It is unknown if palifermin crosses the placenta or is excreted in breast milk. Use palifermin only if the potential benefit justifies fetal risk. **Pregnancy Category C. Children:** Safety and effectiveness have not been established.   **Elderly:** No   age-related precaution.

INTERACTIONS

DRUG: Heparin: Palifermin binds to heparin. **Myelotoxic chemotherapy:** Administration of palifermin during or within 24 hr before or after myelotoxic chemotherapy results in increased severity and duration of oral mucositis. **HERBAL:** None known. **FOOD:** None known. **LAB VALUES:** May elevate serum lipase and amylase levels.

AVAILABILITY (Rx)

INJECTION: 6.25-mg vials.

ADMINISTRATION/HANDLING

 IV

Reconstitution • Reconstitute only with 1.2 ml sterile water for injection, using aseptic technique. • Swirl gently to dissolve. Dissolution takes less than 3 min. Do not shake or agitate solution. • Yields a final concentration of 5 mg/ml.

Rate of administration • If heparin is being used to maintain an IV line, use 0.9% NaCl to rinse the IV line before and after palifermin administration. • Administer by IV bolus injection.

Storage • If reconstituted solution is not used immediately, may be stored refrigerated for up to 24 hr. • Before administration, may be warmed to room temperature for up to 1 hr. • Discard if left at room temperature for more than 1 hr or if discoloration or particulate matter is observed. • Protect from light.

INDICATIONS/ROUTES/DOSAGE

MUCOSITIS (PREMYELOTOXIC THERAPY)
IV: ADULTS, ELDERLY: 60 mcg/kg/day for 3 consecutive days, with the 3rd dose 24–48 hr before chemotherapy.

MUCOSITIS (POSTMYELOTOXIC THERAPY)
IV: ADULTS, ELDERLY: The last 3 doses should be administered after myelotoxic therapy; the first of these doses should be administered after, but on the same day of, hematopoietic stem cell infusion and at least 4 days after the most recent administration of palifermin.

SIDE EFFECTS

FREQUENT: Rash (62%), fever (39%), pruritus (35%), erythema (32%), edema (28%). **OCCASIONAL:** Mouth and tongue thickness or discoloration (17%), altered taste (16%), dysesthesia manifested as hyperesthesia, hypoesthesia, paresthesia (12%), arthralgia (10%).

ADVERSE REACTIONS/ TOXIC EFFECTS

Transient hypertension occurs occasionally.

BASELINE ASSESSMENT
Assess oral mucous membranes for stomatitis (i.e., erythema, white patches, ulceration, bleeding).

INTERVENTION/EVALUATION
Assess for oral inflammation, difficulty swallowing, mucosal bleeding. Offer sponge sticks to wash mouth with water. Monitor patient's pain level and medicate as necessary for improved pain control. Offer the patient and family emotional support.

PATIENT/FAMILY TEACHING
• Offer bland meals and advise against eating any spicy food. • Rinse mouth often with tepid water and avoid either hot or cold liquids. • Advise the female patient to notify the physician if she is pregnant or breast-feeding.

palivizumab

pal-**iv**-ih-zoo-mab
(Synagis)

Do not confuse Synagis with Synalgos-DC.

CLASSIFICATION

PHARMACOTHERAPEUTIC: Monoclonal antibody. **CLINICAL:** Pediatric lower respiratory tract infection agent.

ACTION

Exhibits neutralizing activity against respiratory syncytial virus (RSV) in infants. **Therapeutic Effect:** Inhibits RSV replication in the lower respiratory tract.

USES

Prevention of serious lower respiratory tract disease caused by RSV in pediatric patients at high risk for RSV disease (e.g., hemodynamically significant congenital heart disease).

PRECAUTIONS

CONTRAINDICATIONS: Children with cyanotic congenital heart disease. **CAUTIONS:** Thrombocytopenia, any coagulation disorder. Not to be used for treatment of established RSV disease. **Pregnancy Category C.**

INTERACTIONS

DRUG: None known. **HERBAL:** None known. **FOOD:** None known. **LAB VALUES:** None known.

AVAILABILITY (Rx)

INJECTION, SOLUTION: 50 mg/0.5 ml, 100 mg/ml.

INDICATIONS/ROUTES/DOSAGE

RSV PREVENTION
IM: CHILDREN: 15 mg/kg once/mo during RSV season.

SIDE EFFECTS

FREQUENT (49%–22%): Upper respiratory tract infection, otitis media, rhinitis, rash. **OCCASIONAL (10%–2%):** Pain, pharyngitis. **RARE (less than 2%):** Cough, diarrhea, vomiting, injection site reaction.

ADVERSE REACTIONS/ TOXIC EFFECTS

Anaphylaxis, severe acute hypersensitivity reaction occur very rarely.

NURSING CONSIDERATIONS

BASELINE ASSESSMENT
Assess for sensitivity to palivizumab.

INTERVENTION/EVALUATION
Monitor potential side effects, especially otitis media, rhinitis, skin rash, upper respiratory tract infection.

PATIENT/FAMILY TEACHING
• Discuss with family the purpose and potential side effects of medication.

---

palonosetron hydrochloride

pal-oh-**noe**-seh-tron
(Aloxi)

• CLASSIFICATION

PHARMACOTHERAPEUTIC: 5-HT$_3$ receptor antagonist. **CLINICAL:** Antinauseant, antiemetic.

ACTION

A 5-HT$_3$ receptor antagonist that acts centrally in the chemoreceptor trigger zone and peripherally at the vagal nerve terminals. **Therapeutic Effect:** Prevents nausea and vomiting associated with chemotherapy.

PHARMACOKINETICS

Protein binding: 52%. Metabolized in liver. Eliminated in urine. **Half-life:** 40 hr.

USES

Prevention of acute, delayed nausea and vomiting associated with initial, repeated courses of moderately or highly emetogenic cancer chemotherapy. **OFF-LABEL:** Prevention of postop bleeding.

PRECAUTIONS

CONTRAINDICATIONS: None known. **CAUTIONS:** History of cardiovascular disease.

⧖ **LIFESPAN CONSIDERATIONS: Pregnancy/Lactation:** Unknown if excreted in breast milk. **Pregnancy Category B. Children:** Safety and efficacy not established. **Elderly:** No age-related precautions noted.

INTERACTIONS

DRUG: Apomorphine: May cause profound hypotension, altered consciousness. **HERBAL:** None known. **FOOD:** None known. **LAB VALUES:** May transiently increase serum bilirubin, AST, and ALT levels.

AVAILABILITY (Rx)

INJECTION: 0.25 mg/5 ml.

ADMINISTRATION/HANDLING

IV

Reconstitution • Give undiluted as an IV push.

Rate of administration • Give IV push over 30 sec. • Flush infusion line

---

with 0.9% NaCl before and following administration.

Storage • Store at room temperature. Solution should appear colorless, clear. Discard if precipitate is present or solution appears cloudy.

▦ IV INCOMPATIBILITIES
Dont mix palonosetron with any other drugs.

INDICATIONS/ROUTES/DOSAGE
CHEMOTHERAPY-INDUCED NAUSEA AND VOMITING
IV: ADULTS, ELDERLY: 0.25 mg as a single dose 30 min before starting chemotherapy.

SIDE EFFECTS
OCCASIONAL (9%–5%): Headache, constipation. **RARE (less than 1%):** Diarrhea, dizziness, fatigue, abdominal pain, insomnia.

ADVERSE REACTIONS/ TOXIC EFFECTS
Overdose may produce a combination of CNS stimulant and depressant effects. Cardiac dysrhythmia has been reported.

NURSING CONSIDERATIONS

BASELINE ASSESSMENT
Assess for dehydration if excessive vomiting occurs (poor skin turgor, dry mucous membranes, longitudinal furrows in tongue). Provide emotional support.

INTERVENTION/EVALUATION
Monitor patient in environment. Provide supportive measures. Assess mental status. Monitor pattern of daily bowel activity and stool consistency; record time of evacuation.

PATIENT/FAMILY TEACHING
• Relief from nausea or vomiting generally occurs shortly after drug administration. • Avoid alcohol, barbiturates. • Report persistent vomiting.

pamidronate disodium

pam-id-**drow**-nate
(Aredia, Pamidronate Disodium Novaplus)
Do not confuse Aredia with Adriamcyin.

◆ CLASSIFICATION
PHARMACOTHERAPEUTIC: Bisphosphonate. **CLINICAL:** Hypocalcemic.

ACTION
A bisphosphate that binds to bone and inhibits osteoclast-mediated calcium resorption. **Therapeutic Effect:** Lowers serum calcium concentrations.

PHARMACOKINETICS

Route	Onset	Peak	Duration
IV	24–48 hr	5–7 days	N/A

After IV administration, rapidly absorbed by bone. Slowly excreted unchanged in urine. Unknown if removed by hemodialysis. **Half-life:** bone, 300 days; unmetabolized, 2.5 hr.

USES
Treatment of moderate to severe hypercalcemia associated with malignancy (with or without bone metastases). Treatment of moderate to severe Paget's disease, osteolytic bone lesions of multiple myeloma, breast cancer.

PRECAUTIONS
CONTRAINDICATIONS: Hypersensitivity to other bisphosphonates, such as etidronate, tiludronate, risedronate, and alendronate. **CAUTIONS:** Cardiac failure, renal impairment.

⌛ **LIFESPAN CONSIDERATIONS: Pregnancy/Lactation:** There are no adequate and well-controlled studies in

P

pregnant women; unknown if fetal harm can occur. Unknown if excreted in breast milk. **Pregnancy Category D. Children:** Safety and efficacy not established. **Elderly:** May become overhydrated. Careful monitoring of fluid and electrolytes; recommend diluted in smaller volume.

INTERACTIONS

DRUG: Calcium-containing medications, vitamin D: May antagonize effects of pamidronate in treatment of hypercalcemia. **HERBAL:** None known. **FOOD:** None known. **LAB VALUES:** May decrease serum phosphate, magnesium, calcium, and potassium levels.

AVAILABILITY (Rx)

POWDER FOR INJECTION (AREDIA, PAMIDRONATE DISODIUM NOVAPLUS): 30 mg, 90 mg. **INJECTION SOLUTION:** 3 mg/ml, 6 mg/ml, 9 mg/ml.

ADMINISTRATION/HANDLING

 IV

Reconstitution • Reconstitute each 30-mg vial with 10 ml sterile water for injection to provide concentration of 3 mg/ml. • Allow drug to dissolve before withdrawing. • Further dilute with 1,000 ml sterile 0.45% or 0.9% NaCl or D₅W.

Rate of administration • Adequate hydration is essential in conjunction with pamidronate therapy (avoid overhydration in patients with potential for cardiac failure). • Administer as IV infusion over 2–24 hr for treatment of hypercalcemia; over 2–4 hr for other indications.

Storage • Store parenteral form at room temperature. • Reconstituted vial is stable for 24 hr refrigerated; IV solution is stable for 24 hr after dilution.

IV INCOMPATIBILITIES

Calcium-containing IV fluids.

INDICATIONS/ROUTES/DOSAGE

HYPERCALCEMIA

IV INFUSION: ADULTS, ELDERLY: Moderate hypercalcemia (corrected serum calcium level 12–13.5 mg/dl): 60–90 mg. Severe hypercalcemia (corrected serum calcium level greater than 13.5 mg/dl): 90 mg.

PAGET'S DISEASE

IV INFUSION: ADULTS, ELDERLY: 30 mg/day for 3 days.

OSTEOLYTIC BONE LESION

IV INFUSION: ADULTS, ELDERLY: 90 mg over 2–4 hr once a month.

SIDE EFFECTS

FREQUENT (greater than 10%): Temperature elevation (at least 1°C) 24–48 hr after administration (27%); redness, swelling, induration, pain at catheter site with in patients receiving 90 mg (18%); anorexia, nausea, fatigue. **OCCASIONAL (10%–1%):** Constipation, rhinitis.

ADVERSE REACTIONS/ TOXIC EFFECTS

Hypophosphatemia, hypokalemia, hypomagnesemia, and hypocalcemia occur more frequently with higher dosages. Anemia, hypertension, tachycardia, atrial fibrillation, and somnolence occur more frequently with 90-mg doses. GI hemorrhage occurs rarely.

NURSING CONSIDERATIONS

INTERVENTION/EVALUATION

Monitor serum calcium, potassium, magnesium, creatinine, Hgb, Hct, CBC. Provide adequate hydration; avoid overhydration. Monitor I&O carefully; check lungs for rales, dependent body parts for edema. Monitor BP, temperature, pulse. Assess catheter site for redness, swelling, pain. Monitor food intake, pattern of bowel activity and stool consistency. Be alert for potential GI hemorrhage with 90-mg dosage.

P

pancreatin ℮

pan-kree-**ah**-tin

(Ku-Zyme, Pancreatin)

pancrelipase

pan-kree-**lie**-pace

(Cotazym 🍃, Cotazym-65 B 🍃, Cotazym-S, Creon 5, Creon 10, Creon 20, Ilozyme, Kutrase, Ku-Zyme, Ku-Zyme HP, Lipram, Lipram-CR, Lipram-CR 5, Lipram-CR 20, Lipram-PN, Lipram-UL 12, Lipram-UL 18, Lipram-UL 20, Panase, Pancrease, Pancrease MT 4, Pancrease MT 10 🍃, Pancrease MT 16 🍃, Pancrease MT 20, Pancreatic EC, Pancreatil-UL 12, Pancrecarb MS-4, Pancrecarb MS-8, Pangestyme CN 10, Pangestyme CN 20, Pangestyme EC, Pangestyme MT 16, Pangestyme NL 18, Panokase, Plaretase, Protilase, Ultrase, Ultrase MT 12, Ultrase MT 18, Ultrase MT 20, Viokase, Viokase 8, Viokase 16, Zymase)

◆CLASSIFICATION

PHARMACOTHERAPEUTIC: Digestive enzyme. **CLINICAL:** Pancreatic enzyme replenisher.

ACTION

Digestive enzymes that replace endogenous pancreatic enzymes. **Therapeutic Effect:** Assist in digestion of protein, starch, and fats.

USES

Pancreatic enzyme replacement or supplement when enzymes are absent or deficient (chronic pancreatitis, cystic fibrosis, ductal obstruction from pancreatic cancer, common bile duct). Treatment of steatorrhea associated with postgastrectomy syndrome, bowel resection; reduces malabsorption. **OFF-LABEL:** Treatment of occluded feeding tubes.

PRECAUTIONS

CONTRAINDICATIONS: Acute pancreatitis, exacerbation of chronic pancreatitis, hypersensitivity to pork protein. **CAUTIONS:** Inhalation of powder may cause asthmatic attack. **Pregnancy Category C.**

INTERACTIONS

DRUG: Antacids: May decrease the effects of pancreatin and pancrelipase. **Iron supplements:** May decrease the absorption of iron supplements. **HERBAL:** None known. **FOOD:** None known. **LAB VALUES:** May increase serum uric acid level.

AVAILABILITY (Rx)

CAPSULES: 15,000 units-12,000 units-15,000 units (Ku-Zyme), 30,000 units-24,000 units-30,000 units (Kutrase), 30,000 units-8,000 units-30,000 units (Panokase, Cotazym, Ku-Zyme HP). **CAPSULES (EXTENDED-RELEASE):** 33,200 units-10,000 units-37,500 units (Creon 10, Lipram-CR), 30,000 units-10,000 units-30,000 units (Pangestyme CN 10, Lipram, Pancrease MT 10), 39,000 units-12,000 units-39,000 units (Lipram-UL 12, Pancreatil-UL 12, Ultrase MT 12), 12,000 units-4,000 units-12,000 units (Pancrease MT 4), 48,000 units-16,000 units-48,000 units (Lipram-PN, Pancrease MT 16, Pangestyme MT 16), 16,600 units-5,000 units-18,750 units (Creon 5, Lipram-CR5), 59,000 units-18,000 units-59,000 units (Pangestyme NL 18, Lipram-UL 18, Ultrase MT 18), 20,000 units-5,000 units-20,000 units (Cotazym-S), 66,400 units-20,000 units-75,000 units (Creon 20, Lipram-CR 20), 20,000 units-4,500 units-25,000 units (Lipram, Pancrease, Pangestyme EC, Ultrase), 56,000 units-20,000 units-44,000 units (Lipram-PN,

Pancrease MT 20), 65,000 units-20,000 units-65,000 units (Lipram-UL 20, Pangestyme NL 18, Pangestyme CN 20, Ultrase MT 20), 20,000 units-4,000 units-25,000 units (Panase, Pancreatic EC, Protilase), 25,000 units-4,000 units-25,000 units (Pancrecarb MS-4), 40,000 units-8,000 units-45,000 units (Pancrecarb MS-8). **POWDER FOR RECONSTITUTION, ORAL (VIOKASE):** 70,000 units-16,800 units-70,000 units/0.7 gm. **TABLETS:** 30,000 units-11,000 units-30,000 units (Ilozyme), 60,000 units-16,000 units-60,000 units (Viokase 16), 30,000 units-8,000 units-30,000 units (Panokase, Plaretase, Viokase 8).

ADMINISTRATION/HANDLING

◆ **ALERT** ▶ Spilling powder on hands (Viokase) may irritate skin.
◆ **ALERT** ▶ Inhaling powder may irritate mucous membranes, produce bronchospasm.

PO
• Give before or with meals, snacks.
• Tablets may be crushed. Do not crush enteric-coated form. • Instruct patient not to chew (minimizes irritation to mouth, lips, tongue). • May open capsule and spread over applesauce, mashed fruit, rice cereal.

INDICATIONS/ROUTES/DOSAGE

PANCREATIC ENZYME REPLACEMENT OR SUPPLEMENT WHEN ENZYMES ARE ABSENT OR DEFICIENT, SUCH AS WITH CHRONIC PANCREATITIS, CYSTIC FIBROSIS, OR DUCTAL OBSTRUCTION FROM CANCER OF THE PANCREAS OR COMMON BILE DUCT; TO REDUCE MALABSORPTION; TREATMENT OF STEATORRHEA ASSOCIATED WITH BOWEL RESECTION AND POSTGASTRECTOMY SYNDROME
PO: ADULTS, ELDERLY: 1–3 capsules or tablets before or with meals or snacks. May increase to 8 tablets/dose. CHILDREN: 1–2 tablets with meals or snacks.

SIDE EFFECTS
RARE: Allergic reaction, mouth irritation, shortness of breath, wheezing.

ADVERSE REACTIONS/ TOXIC EFFECTS

Excessive dosage may produce nausea, cramping, and diarrhea. Hyperuricosuria and hyperuricemia have occurred with extremely high dosages.

NURSING CONSIDERATIONS

INTERVENTION/EVALUATION
Question for therapeutic relief from GI symptoms. Do not change brands without consulting physician.

PATIENT/FAMILY TEACHING
• Do not chew capsules or tablets.
• Instruct patients with trouble swallowing to open capsules and spread contents over applesauce, mashed fruit, or rice cereal.

pancuronium bromide

(Pavulon)
See Neuromuscular blockers (p. 112C)

pantoprazole

pan-toe-**pra**-zole
(Protonix, Protonix IV, Pantoloc ✦)

Do not confuse Protonix with Lotronex.

◆ **CLASSIFICATION**
PHARMACOTHERAPEUTIC: Benzimidazole. **CLINICAL:** Proton pump inhibitor (see p. 134C).

P

ACTION

A benzimidazole that is converted to active metabolites that irreversibly bind to and inhibit hydrogen-potassium adenosine triphosphate, an enzyme on the surface of gastric parietal cells. Inhibits hydrogen ion transport into gastric lumen. **Therapeutic Effect:** Increases gastric pH and reduces gastric acid production.

PHARMACOKINETICS

Route	Onset	Peak	Duration
PO	N/A	N/A	24 hr

Rapidly absorbed from the GI tract. Protein binding: 98%. Primarily distributed into gastric parietal cells. Metabolized extensively in the liver. Primarily excreted in urine. Not removed by hemodialysis. **Half-life:** 1 hr.

USES

Oral: Treatment and maintenance of healing or erosive esophagitis associated with gastroesophageal reflux disease (GERD). Treatment of hypersecretory conditions including Zollinger-Ellison syndrome. **IV:** Short-term treatment of erosive esophagitis associated with GERD, treatment of hypersecretory conditions. **OFF-LABEL:** Peptic ulcer disease, active ulcer bleeding (injection), adjunct in treatment of *H. pylori.*

PRECAUTIONS

CONTRAINDICATIONS: None known. **CAUTIONS:** History of chronic or current hepatic disease.

⌛ **LIFESPAN CONSIDERATIONS: Pregnancy/Lactation:** Unknown if drug crosses placenta or is distributed in breast milk. **Pregnancy Category B. Children:** Safety and efficacy not established. **Elderly:** No age-related precautions noted.

INTERACTIONS

DRUG: None known. **HERBAL:** None known. **FOOD:** None known. **LAB VALUES:** May increase serum creatinine, cholesterol, and uric acid levels.

AVAILABILITY (Rx)

TABLETS (DELAYED-RELEASE [PROTONIX]): 20 mg, 40 mg. **POWDER FOR INJECTION (PROTONIX IV):** 40 mg.

ADMINISTRATION/HANDLING

💧 IV

Reconstitution • Mix 40-mg vial with 10 ml 0.9% NaCl injection. • May be further diluted with 100 ml D₅W, 0.9% NaCl, or lactated Ringer's.

Rate of administration • Infuse 10 ml solution over at least 2 min. • Infuse 100 ml solution over at least 15 min.

Storage • Store at room temperature. • Once diluted with 10 ml 0.9% NaCl, stable for 2 hr at room temperature; when further diluted with 100 ml, stable for 22 hr at room temperature.

PO
• Give without regard to meals. • Do not crush, chew, split tablets; swallow whole.

▦ IV INCOMPATIBILITIES

Do not mix with other medications. Flush IV with D₅W, 0.9% NaCl, or lactated Ringer's solution before and after administration.

INDICATIONS/ROUTES/DOSAGE
EROSIVE ESOPHAGITIS

PO: ADULTS, ELDERLY: 40 mg/day for up to 8 wk. If not healed after 8 wk, may continue an additional 8 wk.
IV: ADULTS, ELDERLY: 40 mg/day for 7–10 days.

HYPERSECRETORY CONDITIONS

PO: ADULTS, ELDERLY: Initially, 40 mg twice a day. May increase to 240 mg/day.
IV: ADULTS, ELDERLY: 80 mg twice a day. May increase to 80 mg q8h.

SIDE EFFECTS

RARE (less than 2%): Diarrhea, headache, dizziness, pruritus, rash.

ADVERSE REACTIONS/ TOXIC EFFECTS

Hyperglycemia occurs rarely.

NURSING CONSIDERATIONS

BASELINE ASSESSMENT

Obtain baseline lab values, including serum creatinine, cholesterol.

INTERVENTION/EVALUATION

Evaluate for therapeutic response (i.e., relief of GI symptoms). Question if GI discomfort, nausea occur.

PATIENT/FAMILY TEACHING

• Report headache. • Swallow tablets whole; do not chew, crush. • Take before eating.

Paraplatin, see

carboplatin

paroxetine hydrochloride

par-**ox**-e-teen

(Paxeva, <u>Paxil</u>, <u>Paxil CR</u>)

Do not confuse paroxetine with pyridoxine, or Paxil with Doxil or Taxol.

◆CLASSIFICATION

PHARMACOTHERAPEUTIC: Serotonin uptake inhibitor. **CLINICAL:** Antidepressant, antiobsessive-compulsive, antianxiety (see pp. 12C, 38C).

ACTION

An antidepressant, anxiolytic, and antiobsessional agent that selectively blocks uptake of the neurotransmitter serotonin at neuronal presynaptic membranes, thereby increasing its availability at postsynaptic receptor sites. **Therapeutic Effect:** Relieves depression, reduces obsessive-compulsive behavior, decreases anxiety.

PHARMACOKINETICS

Well absorbed from the GI tract. Protein binding: 95%. Widely distributed. Metabolized in the liver. Excreted in urine. Not removed by hemodialysis. **Half-life:** 24 hr.

USES

Treatment of major depression exhibited as persistent, prominent dysphoria (occurring nearly every day for at least 2 wk) manifested by 4 of 8 symptoms: change in appetite, change in sleep pattern, increased fatigue, impaired concentration, feelings of guilt/worthlessness, loss of interest in usual activities, psychomotor agitation/retardation, suicidal tendencies. Treatment of panic disorder, obsessive-compulsive disorder (OCD) manifested as repetitive tasks producing marked distress, time-consuming, or significant interference with social/occupational behavior. Treatment of social anxiety disorder (SAD), generalized anxiety disorder (GAD), premenstrual dysphoric disorder, post-traumatic stress disorder (PTSD). **OFF-LABEL:** Eating disorders, impulse disorders, menopause symptoms, premenstrual disorders, treatment of depression and OCD in children.

PRECAUTIONS

CONTRAINDICATIONS: Use within 14 days of MAOIs. **CAUTIONS:** History of seizures, mania, renal/hepatic impairment, cardiac disease, patients with suicidal tendencies, impaired platelet aggregation. Those who are volume depleted or using diuretics.

⧗ **LIFESPAN CONSIDERATIONS: Pregnancy/Lactation:** May impair reproductive function. Not distributed in breast milk. May increase risk of congenital malformations. **Pregnancy Category D. Children:** Safety and efficacy not established. **Elderly:** Age-related renal impairment may require dosage adjustment.

INTERACTIONS

DRUG: Cimetidine: May increase paroxetine blood concentration. **MAOIs:** May cause serotonin syndrome, marked by excitement, diaphoresis, rigidity, hyperthermia, autonomic hyperactivity, and coma, and neuroleptic malignant syndrome. **Phenytoin:** May decrease paroxetine blood concentration. **Risperidone:** May increase risperidone blood concentration and cause extrapyramidal symptoms. **HERBAL: St. John's wort:** May increase paroxetine's pharmacologic effects and risk of toxicity. **FOOD:** None known. **LAB VALUES:** May increase serum hepatic enzyme levels. May decrease blood Hgb level, Hct, and WBC count.

AVAILABILITY (Rx)

ORAL SUSPENSION (PAXIL): 10 mg/5 ml. **TABLETS (PAXIL, PEXEVA):** 10 mg, 20 mg, 30 mg, 40 mg. **TABLETS (CONTROLLED-RELEASE [PAXIL CR]):** 12.5 mg, 25 mg, 37.5 mg.

ADMINISTRATION/HANDLING

PO
• Give with food, milk if GI distress occurs. • Scored tablet may be crushed. • Best if given as single morning dose.

INDICATIONS/ROUTES/DOSAGE

DEPRESSION
PO: ADULTS: Initially, 20 mg/day. May increase by 10 mg/day at intervals of more than 1 wk. **Maximum:** 50 mg/day.

PO (CONTROLLED-RELEASE): ADULTS: Initially, 25 mg/day. May increase by 12.5 mg/day at intervals of more than 1 wk. **Maximum:** 62.5 mg/day.

GAD
PO: ADULTS: Initially, 20 mg/day. May increase by 10 mg/day at intervals of more than 1 wk. Range: 20–50 mg/day.

OCD
PO: ADULTS: Initially, 20 mg/day. May increase by 10 mg/day at intervals of more than 1 wk. Range: 20–60 mg/day.

PANIC DISORDER
PO: ADULTS: Initially, 10–20 mg/day. May increase by 10 mg/day at intervals of more than 1 wk. Range: 10–60 mg/day.

SAD
PO: ADULTS: Initially 20 mg/day. Range: 20–60 mg/day.

PTSD
PO: ADULTS: Initially, 20 mg/day. May increase by 10 mg/day at intervals of more than 1 wk. Range: 20–50 mg/day.

PREMENSTRUAL DYSPHORIC DISORDER
PO (PAXIL CR): ADULTS: Initially, 12.5 mg/day. May increase by 12.5 mg at weekly intervals to a maximum of 25 mg/day.

USUAL ELDERLY DOSAGE
PO: Initially, 10 mg/day. May increase by 10 mg/day at intervals of more than 1 wk. **Maximum:** 40 mg/day.

PO (CONTROLLED-RELEASE): Initially, 12.5 mg/day. May increase by 12.5 mg/day at intervals of more than 1 wk. **Maximum:** 50 mg/day.

SIDE EFFECTS

FREQUENT: Nausea (26%); somnolence (23%); headache, dry mouth (18%); asthenia (15%); constipation (15%); dizziness, insomnia (13%); diarrhea (12%); diaphoresis (11%); tremor (8%). **OCCASIONAL:** Decreased appetite, respiratory disturbance (such as increased cough) (6%); anxiety, nervousness (5%); flatulence, paresthesia, yawning (4%); decreased libido, sexual dysfunction, abdominal discomfort (3%). **RARE**: Palpitations, vomiting, blurred vision, altered taste, confusion.

ADVERSE REACTIONS/ TOXIC EFFECTS

Abnormal bleeding, hyponatremia, seizures, hypomania, and suicidal thoughts have been reported.

NURSING CONSIDERATIONS

BASELINE ASSESSMENT

Assess appearance, behavior, speech pattern, level of interest, mood.

INTERVENTION/EVALUATION

For those on long-term therapy, liver/ renal function tests, blood counts should be performed periodically. Supervise suicidal-risk patient closely during early therapy (as depression lessens, energy level improves, increasing suicide potential). Assess appearance, behavior, speech pattern, level of interest, mood.

PATIENT/FAMILY TEACHING

• May cause dry mouth. • Avoid alcohol, St. John's wort. • Therapeutic effect may be noted within 1–4 wk. • Do not abruptly discontinue medication. • Avoid tasks that require alertness, motor skills until response to drug is established. • Inform physician of intention for pregnancy or if pregnancy occurs.

Paxil, *see paroxetine*

Paxil CR, *see paroxetine*

---

pegaspargase

(Oncaspar)
See Cancer chemotherapeutic agents (p. 77C)

Pegasys, *see peginterferon alfa-2a*

---

pegfilgrastim

pehg-phil-**gras**-tim
(Neulasta)
Do not confuse Neulasta with Neumega.

• CLASSIFICATION

PHARMACOTHERAPEUTIC: Colony-stimulating factor. **CLINICAL:** Hematopoietic, antineutropenic.

ACTION

A colony-stimulating factor that regulates production of neutrophils within bone marrow. Also a glycoprotein that primarily affects neutrophil progenitor proliferation, differentiation, and selected end-cell functional activation. **Therapeutic Effect:** Increases phagocytic ability and antibody-dependent destruction; decreases incidence of infection.

PHARMACOKINETICS

Readily absorbed after subcutaneous administration. **Half-life:** 15–80 hr.

USES

Fights infection manifested by febrile neutropenia in cancer patients receiving moderately myelosuppressive chemotherapy. Stimulates WBC production in patients receiving myelosuppressive chemotherapy.

✤ Canadian trade name   ℮ see **evolve**   ☞ High Alert drug

PRECAUTIONS

CONTRAINDICATIONS: Hypersensitivity to *Escherichia coli*–derived proteins, do not administer within 14 days before and 24 hr after cytotoxic chemotherapy. **CAUTIONS:** Concurrent use with medications having mycoloid properties, sickle cell disease.

⌛ **LIFESPAN CONSIDERATIONS: Pregnancy/Lactation:** Unknown if drug crosses placenta or is distributed in breast milk. **Pregnancy Category C. Children:** Safety and efficacy not established. **Elderly:** No age-related precautions noted.

INTERACTIONS

DRUG: Lithium: May potentiate the release of neutrophils. **HERBAL:** None known. **FOOD:** None known. **LAB VALUES:** May increase LDH concentrations, leukocyte alkaline phosphatase scores, and serum alkaline phosphatase and uric acid levels.

AVAILABILITY (Rx)

SOLUTION FOR INJECTION: 6 mg/0.6 ml syringe.

ADMINISTRATION/HANDLING

SUBCUTANEOUS

Storage • Store in refrigerator, but may warm to room temperature up to a maximum of 48 hr before use. Discard if left at room temperature for more than 48 hr. • Protect from light. • Avoid freezing; but if accidentally frozen, may allow to thaw in refrigerator before administration. Discard if freezing takes place a second time. • Discard if discoloration, precipitate is present.

INDICATIONS/ROUTES/DOSAGE

MYELOSUPPRESSION

SUBCUTANEOUS: ADULTS, ELDERLY: Give as a single 6-mg injection once per chemotherapy cycle.

SIDE EFFECTS

FREQUENT (72%–15%): Bone pain, nausea, fatigue, alopecia, diarrhea, vomiting, constipation, anorexia, abdominal pain, arthralgia, generalized weakness, peripheral edema, dizziness, stomatitis, mucositis, neutropenic fever.

ADVERSE REACTIONS/ TOXIC EFFECTS

Allergic reactions, such as anaphylaxis, rash, and urticaria, occur rarely. Cytopenia resulting from an antibody response to growth factors occurs rarely. Splenomegaly occurs rarely; assess for left upper abdominal or shoulder pain. Adult respiratory distress syndrome (ARDS) may occur in patients with sepsis. Severe sickle cell crisis has been reported.

NURSING CONSIDERATIONS

BASELINE ASSESSMENT

CBC, platelet count should be obtained before initiating therapy and routinely thereafter.

INTERVENTION/EVALUATION

Monitor for allergic-type reactions. Assess for peripheral edema, particularly behind medial malleolus (usually first area showing peripheral edema). Assess mucous membranes for evidence of stomatitis, mucositis (red mucous membranes, white patches, extreme mouth soreness). Assess muscle strength. Monitor pattern of daily bowel activity and stool consistency. ARDS may occur in septic patients.

PATIENT/FAMILY TEACHING

• Inform patient of possible side effects, signs and symptoms of allergic reactions. • Counsel patient on importance of compliance with pegfilgrastim treatment, including regular monitoring of blood counts.

---

peginterferon alfa-2a

peg-inn-ter-**fear**-on
(Pegasys)

◆CLASSIFICATION

PHARMACOTHERAPEUTIC: Immunomodulator. **CLINICAL:** Immunologic agent.

ACTION

An immunomodulator that binds to specific membrane receptors on the cell surface, inhibiting viral replication in virus-infected cells, suppressing cell proliferation, and producing reversible decreases in leukocyte and platelet counts. **Therapeutic Effect:** Inhibits hepatitis C virus.

PHARMACOKINETICS

Readily absorbed after subcutaneous administration. Excreted by the kidneys. **Half-life:** 80 hr.

USES

Treatment of chronic hepatitis C alone or in combination with ribavirin in patients who have compensated hepatic disease.

PRECAUTIONS

CONTRAINDICATIONS: Autoimmune hepatitis, decompensated hepatic disease, infants, neonates. **EXTREME CAUTION:** History of neuropsychiatric disorders. **CAUTIONS:** Renal impairment (creatinine clearance less than 50 ml/min), elderly, pulmonary disorders, compromised CNS function, cardiac diseases, autoimmune disorders, endocrine abnormalities, colitis, ophthalmologic disorders, myelosuppression.

⌛ LIFESPAN CONSIDERATIONS: **Pregnancy/Lactation:** May have abortifacient potential. Unknown if distributed in breast milk. **Pregnancy Category C.**

Children: Safety and efficacy not established in those younger than 18 yr. **Elderly:** CNS, cardiac, systemic effects may be more severe in the elderly, particularly in those with renal impairment.

INTERACTIONS

DRUG: Bone marrow depressants: May increase myelosuppression. **Theophylline:** May increase the serum level of theophylline. **HERBAL:** None known. **FOOD:** None known. **LAB VALUES:** May increase ALT level. May decrease the absolute neutrophil, platelet, and WBC counts. May cause a slight decrease in blood Hgb level and Hct.

AVAILABILITY (Rx)

INJECTION SOLUTION: 180 mcg/ml. **INJECTION, PREFILLED SYRINGE:** 180 mcg/0.5 ml.

ADMINISTRATION/HANDLING

SUBCUTANEOUS
• Refrigerate. • Vials are for single use only; discard unused portion. • Give subcutaneous in the abdomen, thigh.

INDICATIONS/ROUTES/DOSAGE

HEPATITIS C
SUBCUTANEOUS: ADULTS 18 YR AND OLDER, ELDERLY: 180 mcg (1 ml) injected in abdomen or thigh once weekly for 48 wk.

DOSAGE IN RENAL IMPAIRMENT
For patients who require hemodialysis, dosage is 135 mg injected in abdomen or thigh once weekly for 48 wk.

DOSAGE IN HEPATIC IMPAIRMENT
For patients with progressive ALT increases above baseline values, dosage is 90 mcg injected in abdomen or thigh once weekly for 48 wk.

SIDE EFFECTS

FREQUENT (54%): Headache. **OCCASIONAL (23%–13%):** Alopecia, nausea, insomnia, anorexia, dizziness, diarrhea,

P

---

abdominal pain, flu-like symptoms, psychiatric reactions (depression, irritability, anxiety), injection site reaction. **RARE (8%–5%):** Impaired concentration, diaphoresis, dry mouth, nausea, vomiting.

ADVERSE REACTIONS/ TOXIC EFFECTS

Serious, acute hypersensitivity reactions, such as urticaria, angioedema, bronchoconstriction, and anaphylaxis, may occur. Other rare reactions include pancreatitis, colitis, endocrine disorders (e.g., diabetes mellitus), hyperthyroidism or hypothyroidism, ophthalmologic neuropsychiatric, autoimmune, ischemic, infectious, and pulmonary disorders.

NURSING CONSIDERATIONS

BASELINE ASSESSMENT

CBC, platelet count, blood chemistry, urinalysis, renal and liver function tests, EKG should be performed before initial therapy and routinely thereafter. Patients with diabetes or hypertension should have an ophthalmologic exam before treatment begins.

INTERVENTION/EVALUATION

Monitor for evidence of depression. Offer emotional support. Monitor for abdominal pain, bloody diarrhea as evidence of colitis. Monitor chest x-ray for pulmonary infiltrates. Assess for pulmonary impairment. Encourage ample fluid intake, particularly during early therapy. Assess serum hepatitis C virus RNA levels after 24 wk of treatment.

PATIENT/FAMILY TEACHING

• Clinical response occurs in 1–3 mo. • Flu-like symptoms tend to diminish with continued therapy. • Immediately report symptoms of depression, suicidal ideation. • Avoid tasks requiring mental alertness, motor skills until response to drug is established.

peginterferon alfa-2b

peg-inn-ter-**fear**-on
(PEG-Intron)

CLASSIFICATION

PHARMACOTHERAPEUTIC: Immunomodulator. **CLINICAL:** Immunologic agent.

ACTION

An immunomodulator that inhibits viral replication in virus-infected cells, suppresses cell proliferation, increases phagocytic action of macrophages, and augments specific cytotoxicity of lymphocytes for target cells. **Therapeutic Effect:** Inhibits hepatitis C virus.

PHARMACOKINETICS

The bioavailability of peginterferon alfa-2b is increased after multiple weekly dosing. Metabolized in liver. Excreted in urine. **Half-life:** 22–60 hr.

USES

As monotherapy or in combination with ribavirin for treatment of chronic hepatitis C in patients not previously treated with interferon alfa who have compensated hepatic disease and are older than 18 yr.

PRECAUTIONS

CONTRAINDICATIONS: Autoimmune hepatitis, decompensated hepatic disease, history of psychiatric disorders. **CAUTIONS:** Renal impairment (creatinine clearance less than 50 ml/min), elderly, pulmonary disorders, compromised CNS function, cardiac diseases, autoimmune disorders, endocrine disorders (e.g., diabetes, hyper- or hypothyroidism), ophthalmologic disorders, myelosuppression.

P

⌛ **LIFESPAN CONSIDERATIONS: Pregnancy/Lactation:** May have abortifacient potential. Unknown if distributed in breast milk. **Pregnancy Category C. Children:** Safety and efficacy not established in those younger than 18 yr. **Elderly:** CNS, cardiac, systemic effects may be more severe in the elderly, particularly in those with renal impairment.

INTERACTIONS

DRUG: Bone marrow depressants: May increase myelosuppression. **HERBAL:** None known. **FOOD:** None known. **LAB VALUES:** May increase blood glucose and ALT levels. May decrease neutrophil and platelet counts.

AVAILABILITY (Rx)

INJECTION POWDER FOR RECONSTITUTION: 50 mcg, 80 mcg, 120 mcg, 150 mcg.

ADMINISTRATION/HANDLING

SUBCUTANEOUS

Reconstitution • To reconstitute, add 0.7 ml sterile water for injection (supplied) to the vial. Use immediately or after reconstituted; may be refrigerated for up to 24 hr before use.

Storage • Store at room temperature.

INDICATIONS/ROUTES/DOSAGE

CHRONIC HEPATITIS C, MONOTHERAPY

SUBCUTANEOUS: ADULTS 18 YR AND OLDER, ELDERLY: Administer appropriate dosage (see chart below) once weekly for 1 yr on the same day each wk.

Vial Strength	Weight (kg)	mcg*	ml*
100 mcg/ml	37–45	40	0.4
	46–56	50	0.5
160 mcg/ml	57–72	64	0.4
	73–88	80	0.5
240 mcg/ml	89–106	96	0.4
	107–136	120	0.5
300 mcg/ml	137–160	150	0.5

*Of peginterferon alfa-2b to administer.

CHRONIC HEPATITIS C

SUBCUTANEOUS: COMBINATION THERAPY WITH RIBAVIRIN (400 MG TWICE A DAY): Initially, 1.5 mcg/kg/wk.

SIDE EFFECTS

FREQUENT (50%–47%): Flu-like symptoms; inflammation, bruising, pruritus, and irritation at injection site. **OCCASIONAL (29%–18%):** Psychiatric reactions (depression, anxiety, emotional lability, irritability), insomnia, alopecia, diarrhea. **RARE:** Rash, diaphoresis, dry skin, dizziness, flushing, vomiting, dyspepsia.

ADVERSE REACTIONS/ TOXIC EFFECTS

Serious, acute hypersensitivity reactions (such as urticaria, angioedema, bronchoconstriction, and anaphylaxis), pulmonary disorders, endocrine disorders (e.g., diabetes mellitus), hypothyroidism, hyperthyroidism, and pancreatitis occur rarely. Ulcerative colitis may occur within 12 wk of starting treatment.

NURSING CONSIDERATIONS

BASELINE ASSESSMENT

CBC, platelet count, blood chemistry, urinalysis, renal and liver hepatic function tests, EKG should be performed before initial therapy and routinely thereafter. Patients with diabetes or hypertension should have an ophthalmologic exam before treatment begins.

INTERVENTION/EVALUATION

Monitor for evidence of depression; offer emotional support. Monitor for abdominal pain, bloody diarrhea as evidence of colitis. Monitor chest x-ray for pulmonary infiltrates. Assess for pulmonary impairment. Encourage adequate fluid intake, particularly during early therapy. Assess serum hepatitis C virus RNA levels after 24 wk of treatment.

P

PATIENT/FAMILY TEACHING

• Maintain adequate hydration, avoid alcohol. • May experience flu-like syndrome: nausea, body aches, headache. • Inform physician of persistent abdominal pain, bloody diarrhea, fever, signs of depression or infection, unusual bruising or bleeding.

Peg-Intron, see
peginterferon alfa-2b

pegvisomant

peg-**vis**-oh-mant
(Somavert)

Do not confuse Somavert with somatrem or somatropin.

♦ CLASSIFICATION

PHARMACOTHERAPEUTIC: Protein.
CLINICAL: Acromegaly agent.

ACTION

A protein that selectively binds to growth hormone (GH) receptors on cell surfaces, blocking the binding of endogenous growth hormones and interfering with growth hormone signal transduction. **Therapeutic Effect:** Decreases serum concentrations of insulin-like growth factor 1 (IGF-1) and other GH-responsive serum proteins.

PHARMACOKINETICS

Not distributed extensively into tissues after subcutaneous administration. Less than 1% excreted in urine. **Half-life:** 6 days.

USES

Treatment of acromegaly in patients with inadequate response to surgery, radiation, other medical therapies or for whom these therapies are inappropriate.

PRECAUTIONS

CONTRAINDICATIONS: Latex allergy (stopper on vial contains latex). **CAUTIONS:** Elderly, diabetes mellitus.
⏳ **LIFESPAN CONSIDERATIONS: Pregnancy/Lactation:** Unknown if excreted in breast milk. **Pregnancy Category B. Children:** Safety and efficacy not established. **Elderly:** Initiation of treatment should begin at the low end of the dosage range.

INTERACTIONS

DRUG: Insulin, oral antidiabetics: May enhance effects of these drugs, possibly resulting in hypoglycemia. Dosage should be decreased when initiating pegvisomant therapy. **Opioids:** Decrease serum pegvisomant level. **HERBAL:** None known. **FOOD:** None known. **LAB VALUES:** Interferes with measurement of serum growth hormone concentration. May increase AST, ALT, and transaminase levels. Decreases effect of insulin on carbohydrate metabolism.

AVAILABILITY (Rx)

POWDER FOR INJECTION: 10-mg, 15-mg, 20-mg vials.

ADMINISTRATION/HANDLING
SUBCUTANEOUS

Reconstitution • Withdraw 1 ml sterile water for injection, inject into the vial of pegvisomant, aiming the stream against the glass wall. • Hold the vial between the palms of both hands, roll to dissolve the powder (do not shake).

Rate of administration • Administer subcutaneously only 1 dose from each vial.

Storage • Refrigerate unreconstituted vials. • Administer within 6 hr following reconstitution. • Solution should appear clear after reconstitution. Discard if particulate is present or solution appears cloudy.

INDICATIONS/ROUTES/DOSAGE

ACROMEGALY

SUBCUTANEOUS: ADULTS, ELDERLY: Initially, 40 mg, as a loading dose, then 10 mg daily. After 4–6 wk, adjust dosage in 5-mg increments if serum IGF-1 level is still elevated, or in 5-mg decrements if IGF-1 level has decreased below the normal range. **Maximum:** 30 mg daily.

SIDE EFFECTS

FREQUENT (23%): Infection (cold symptoms, upper respiratory tract infection, blister, ear infection). **OCCASIONAL (8%–5%):** Back pain, dizziness, injection site reaction, peripheral edema, sinusitis, nausea. **RARE (less than 4%):** Diarrhea, paresthesia.

ADVERSE REACTIONS/ TOXIC EFFECTS

Pegvisomant use may markedly elevate liver function test results, including serum transaminase levels. Substantial weight gain occurs rarely.

NURSING CONSIDERATIONS

BASELINE ASSESSMENT

Obtain baseline AST, ALT, serum alkaline phosphatase, total bilirubin levels.

INTERVENTION/EVALUATION

Monitor all patients with tumors that secrete growth hormone with periodic imaging scans of sella turcica for progressive tumor growth. Monitor diabetic patients for hypoglycemia. Obtain IGF-1 serum concentrations 4–6 wk after therapy begins and periodically thereafter; dosage adjustment based on results; dosage adjustment should not be based on growth hormone assays.

PATIENT/FAMILY TEACHING

• Inform patient that routine monitoring of liver function tests is essential during treatment. • Contact physician if jaundice (yellowing of eyes, skin) occurs.

pemetrexed

pem-eh-**trex**-ed
(Alimta)

◆CLASSIFICATION

PHARMACOTHERAPEUTIC: Antimetabolite. **CLINICAL:** Antineoplastic.

ACTION

An antimetabolite that disrupts folate-dependent enzymes essential for cell replication. Therapeutic Effect: Inhibits the growth of mesothelioma cell lines.

PHARMACOKINETICS

Protein binding: 81%. Not metabolized. Excreted in urine. Half-life: 3.5 hr.

USES

Combination chemotherapy with cisplatin for treatment of malignant pleural mesothelioma. Single agent in treatment of locally advanced or metastatic non–small-cell lung cancer after prior chemotherapy. OFF-LABEL: Treatment of bladder, breast, cervical, colorectal, esophageal, gastric, head and neck, ovarian, pancreatic, and renal cell carcinoma.

PRECAUTIONS

CONTRAINDICATIONS: None known. **CAUTIONS:** Hepatic or renal impairment.

LIFESPAN CONSIDERATIONS: **Pregnancy/Lactation:** Unknown if drug crosses placenta or is distributed in breast milk. May cause fetal harm. Not recommended during pregnancy. **Pregnancy Category D. Children:** Safety and efficacy not established in children younger than 18 yr. **Elderly:** Higher incidence of fatigue, leukopenia, neutropenia, thrombocytopenia in those 65 yr and older.

P

INTERACTIONS

DRUG: **Nephrotoxic agents, probenecid:** May delay pemetrexed clearance. **NSAIDs (particularly ibuprofen):** Increase the risk of myelosuppression and GI and renal toxicity. HERBAL: None known. FOOD: None known. LAB VALUES: May decrease platelet, RBC, and WBC counts.

AVAILABILITY (Rx)

POWDER FOR INJECTION: 500 mg.

ADMINISTRATION/HANDLING

IV INFUSION

Reconstitution • Dilute 500-mg vial with 20 ml 0.9% NaCl to provide a concentration of 25 mg/ml. • Gently swirl each vial until powder is completely dissolved. • Solution appears clear and ranges in color from colorless to yellow or green-yellow. • Further dilute reconstituted solution with 100 ml 0.9% NaCl.

Rate of administration • Infuse over 10 min.

Storage • Store at room temperature. • Diluted solution is stable for up to 24 hr at room temperature or if refrigerated.

IV INCOMPATIBILITIES

Use only 0.9% NaCl to reconstitute; flush the line before and after the infusion. Don't add any other medications to the IV line.

INDICATIONS/ROUTES/DOSAGE

◀ ALERT ▶ Pretreatment with dexamethasone (or equivalent) will reduce the risk and severity of a cutaneous reaction; treatment with folic acid and vitamin B_{12} beginning 1 wk before treatment and continuing for 21 days after the last pemetrexed dose will reduce the risk of side effects.

MALIGNANT PLEURAL MESOTHELIOMA
IV: ADULTS, ELDERLY: 600 mg/m^2 q3wk when used as a single agent; 500 mg/m^2 q3wk when used in combination with cisplatin 75 mg/m^2.

NON–SMALL-CELL LUNG CANCER
IV: ADULTS, ELDERLY: 500 mg/m^2 q3wk.

SIDE EFFECTS

FREQUENT (12%–10%): Fatigue, nausea, vomiting, rash or desquamation. **OCCASIONAL (8%–4%):** Stomatitis, pharyngitis, diarrhea, anorexia, hypertension, chest pain. **RARE (less than 3%):** Constipation, depression, dysphagia.

ADVERSE REACTIONS/ TOXIC EFFECTS

Myelosuppression, manifested as neutropenia, thrombocytopenia, or anemia, may occur.

NURSING CONSIDERATIONS

BASELINE ASSESSMENT

Question for possibility of pregnancy before initiating therapy (Pregnancy Category D). Do not breast-feed once treatment has been initiated. Obtain CBC, serum chemistry tests before therapy and repeat throughout therapy.

INTERVENTION/EVALUATION

Monitor Hgb, Hct, WBC, differential, platelet count. Monitor for hematologic toxicity (fever, sore throat, signs of local infection, ecchymosis, unusual bleeding from any site), symptoms of anemia (excessive fatigue, weakness). Assess skin for evidence of dermatologic toxicity. Keep patient well hydrated, urine alkaline. Monitor WBC count for nadir and recovery.

PATIENT/FAMILY TEACHING

• Maintain fastidious oral hygiene. • Do not have immunizations without physician's approval (drug lowers body's resistance). • Avoid crowds, those with infection. • Use contraceptive measures during therapy. • Promptly report fever, sore throat, signs of local infection, unusual bruising or bleeding from any site.

---

penbutolol

(Levatol)

See Beta-adrenergic blockers (p. 64C)

penciclovir

pen-**sigh**-klo-vear
(Denavir)

CLASSIFICATION

PHARMACOTHERAPEUTIC: Anti-infective. CLINICAL: Topical antiviral.

ACTION

Inhibits antiviral activity against herpes simplex virus (HSV). Therapeutic Effect: Prevents DNA synthesis, HSV replication.

USES

Treatment of recurrent herpes labialis (cold sores).

PRECAUTIONS

CONTRAINDICATIONS: None known. CAUTIONS: None known. Pregnancy Category B.

INTERACTIONS

DRUG: None known. HERBAL: None known. FOOD: None known. LAB VALUES: None known.

AVAILABILITY (Rx)

CREAM: 1%.

ADMINISTRATION/HANDLING

TOPICAL
• Store at room temperature. Do not freeze.

INDICATIONS/ROUTES/DOSAGE

◄ ALERT ► Begin treatment as soon as possible (as soon as symptom indicating immediate onset of virus is evident or when lesions appear).

HERPES LABIALIS (COLD SORES)
TOPICAL: ADULTS, ELDERLY: Apply q2h during waking hours for 4 days.

SIDE EFFECTS

FREQUENT (greater than 5%): Headache, mild erythema. OCCASIONAL (5%–1%): Application site reaction. RARE (less than 1%): Altered taste, rash.

ADVERSE REACTIONS/ TOXIC EFFECTS

None known.

NURSING CONSIDERATIONS

BASELINE ASSESSMENT
Use only on lips/face. Do not apply to oral mucous membranes. Avoid application in, near eyes (produces irritation).

PATIENT/FAMILY TEACHING
• Observe precautions to avoid exposure of cold sores to direct sunlight.

penicillamine

pen-ih-**sill**-ah-mine
(Cuprimine, Depen)

Do not confuse penicillamine with penicillin.

CLASSIFICATION

PHARMACOTHERAPEUTIC: Heavy metal antagonist. CLINICAL: Chelating agent, anti-inflammatory.

ACTION

Chelates with lead, copper, mercury, iron to form soluble complexes; depresses circulating IgM rheumatoid factor levels; depresses T-cell activity; combines with cystine to form more soluble compound. Therapeutic Effect: Promotes excretion of heavy metals, acts as anti-inflammatory drug, prevents renal calculi, may dissolve existing stones.

USES

Promotes excretion of copper in treatment of Wilson's disease, decreases excretion of cystine, prevents renal calculi in cystinuria associated with nephrolithiasis. Treatment of active rheumatoid arthritis not controlled with conventional therapy. OFF-LABEL: Treatment of rheumatoid vasculitis, heavy metal toxicity.

PRECAUTIONS

CONTRAINDICATIONS: History of penicillamine-related aplastic anemia or agranulocytosis, rheumatoid arthritis patients with history or evidence of renal insufficiency, pregnancy, breastfeeding. **CAUTIONS:** Elderly, debilitated, renal/hepatic impairment, penicillin allergy. **Pregnancy Category D.**

INTERACTIONS

DRUG: **Antacids, iron supplements:** May decrease absorption. **Bone marrow depressants, gold compounds, immunosuppressants:** May increase risk of hematologic, renal adverse effects. HERBAL: None known. FOOD: **All foods:** May decrease absorption. LAB VALUES: None known.

AVAILABILITY (Rx)

CAPSULES   (CUPRIMINE): 125   mg, 250 mg. **TABLETS (DEPEN):** 250 mg.

INDICATIONS/ROUTES/DOSAGE

RHEUMATOID ARTHRITIS

PO: ADULTS, ELDERLY: 125–250 mg/day. **Maximum (adults):** May increase at 1- to 3-mo intervals up to 1–1.5 g/day. **Maximum (elderly):** 750 mg/day. ◀ ALERT ▶ Dose more than 500 mg/day should be in divided doses. CHILDREN: Initially, 3 mg/kg/day (**Maximum:** 250 mg) for 3 mo, then 6 mg/kg/day

(**Maximum:** 500 mg) in 2 divided doses for 3 mo. **Maximum:** 10 mg/kg/day (750 mg/day) in 3–4 divided doses.

WILSON'S DISEASE

PO: ADULTS, CHILDREN, 12 YR AND OLDER: 1 g/day in 4 divided doses. **Maximum:** 2 g/day. ELDERLY: 750 mg/day in 3–4 divided doses. CHILDREN: 20 mg/kg/day in 2–4 doses. **Maximum:** 1 g/day.
◀ ALERT ▶ Titrate to maintain urinary copper excretion more than 1 mg/day.

CYSTINURIA

◀ ALERT ▶ Doses titrated to maintain urinary cystine excretion at 100–200 mg/day.
PO: ADULTS, ELDERLY: Initially, 2 g/day in divided doses q6h. Range: 1–4 g/day. CHILDREN: 30 mg/kg/day in 4 divided doses. **Maximum:** 4 g/day.

SIDE EFFECTS

FREQUENT: Rash (pruritic, erythematous, maculopapular, morbilliform), reduced/altered sense of taste (hypogeusia), GI disturbances (anorexia, epigastric pain, nausea, vomiting, diarrhea) oral ulcers, glossitis. **OCCASIONAL:** Proteinuria, hematuria, hot flashes, drug fever. **RARE:** Alopecia, tinnitus, pemphigoid rash (water blisters).

ADVERSE REACTIONS/ TOXIC EFFECTS

Aplastic anemia, agranulocytosis, thrombocytopenia, leukopenia, myasthenia gravis, bronchiolitis, erythematous-like syndrome, evening hypoglycemia, skin friability at sites of pressure/trauma producing extravasation or white papules at venipuncture, surgical sites reported. Iron deficiency (particularly children, menstruating women) may develop.

NURSING CONSIDERATIONS

BASELINE ASSESSMENT

Baseline WBC, differential, Hgb, platelet count should be performed before

---

beginning therapy, q2wk thereafter for first 6 mo, then monthly during therapy. Liver function tests (GGT, AST, ALT, LDH) and CT scan for renal stones should also be ordered. A 2-hr interval is necessary between iron and penicillamine therapy. In event of upcoming surgery, dosage should be reduced to 250 mg a day until wound healing is complete.

INTERVENTION/EVALUATION

Encourage copious amounts of water in patients with cystinuria. Monitor WBC, differential, platelet count. If WBC less than 3,500, neutrophils less than 2,000/mm^3, monocytes more than 500/mm^3, or platelet counts less than 100,000, or if a progressive fall in either platelet count or WBC in 3 successive determinations noted, inform physician (drug withdrawal necessary). Assess for evidence of hematuria. Monitor urinalysis for hematuria, proteinuria (if proteinuria exceeds 1 g/24 hr, inform physician).

PATIENT/FAMILY TEACHING

• Promptly report any missed menstrual periods/other indications of pregnancy. • Report fever, sore throat, chills, bruising, bleeding, difficulty breathing on exertion, unexplained cough or wheezing. • Take medication 1 hr before or 2 hr after meals or at least 1 hr from any other drug, food, or milk.

penicillin G benzathine

pen-ih-**sil**-lin G **benz**-ah-thene (Bicillin C-R, Bicillin LA, Isoject Permapen, Wycillin)

Do not confuse penicillin G benzathine with penicillin G potassium or penicillin G procaine.

FIXED-COMBINATION(S)

Bicillin CR: penicillin G benzathine/penicillin procaine: 600,000 units benzathine/600,000 units procaine.

◆CLASSIFICATION

PHARMACOTHERAPEUTIC: Penicillin. **CLINICAL:** Antibiotic (see p. 27C)

ACTION

A penicillin that inhibits bacterial cell wall synthesis by binding to one or more of the penicillin-binding proteins of bacteria. **Therapeutic Effect:** Bactericidal.

USES

Treatment of mild to moderate severe infections caused by organisms susceptible to low concentrations of penicillin including streptococcal (Group A) upper respiratory infections, syphilis, yaws. Prophylaxis of infections caused by susceptible organisms (e.g., rheumatic fever prophylaxis).

PRECAUTIONS

CONTRAINDICATIONS: Hypersensitivity to any penicillin. **CAUTIONS:** Renal or cardiac impairment, seizure disorder, hypersensitivity to cephalosporins.

⧖ LIFESPAN CONSIDERATIONS: **Pregnancy/Lactation:** Readily crosses placenta; distributed in breast milk. **Pregnancy Category B. Children:** May delay renal excretion in neonates, young infants. **Elderly:** Age-related renal impairment may require dosage adjustment.

INTERACTIONS

DRUG: **Erythromycin:** May antagonize effects of penicillin. **Probenecid:** Increases serum concentration of penicillin. HERBAL: None known. FOOD: None known. LAB VALUES: May cause a positive Coombs' test.

P

AVAILABILITY (Rx)

INJECTION (PREFILLED SYRINGE [BICILLIN LA, ISOJECT PERMAPEN]): 300,000 units/ml, 600,000 units/ml. **INJECTION (BICILLIN C-R):** 150,000 units G benzathine-150,000 units procaine/ml, 900,000 units G benzathine-300,000 units procaine/2 ml. **INJECTION, G PROCAINE (WYCILLIN):** 600,000 units/ml.

ADMINISTRATION/HANDLING

◄ **ALERT** ► Do not give IV, intra-arterially, or subcutaneously (may cause thrombosis, severe neurovascular damage, cardiac arrest, death).

IM
• Store in refrigerator. Do not freeze.
• Administer undiluted by deep IM injection.

INDICATIONS/ROUTES/DOSAGE

GROUP A STREPTOCOCCAL INFECTIONS
IM: ADULTS, ELDERLY: 1.2 million units as a single dose. CHILDREN: 25,000–50,000 units/kg as a single dose.

PREVENTION OF RHEUMATIC FEVER
IM: ADULTS, ELDERLY: 1.2 million units q3–4wk or 600,000 units twice monthly. CHILDREN: 25,000–50,000 units/kg q3–4wk.

EARLY SYPHILIS
IM: ADULTS, ELDERLY: 2.4 million units divided and administered in two separate injection sites.

CONGENITAL SYPHILIS
IM: CHILDREN: 50,000 units/kg weekly for 3 wk.

SYPHILIS OF MORE THAN 1 YR DURATION
IM: ADULTS, ELDERLY: 2.4 million units divided and administered in two separate injection sites weekly for 3 wk. CHILDREN: 50,000 units/kg weekly for 3 wk.

SIDE EFFECTS

OCCASIONAL: Lethargy, fever, dizziness, rash, pain at injection site. **RARE:** Seizures, interstitial nephritis.

ADVERSE REACTIONS/ TOXIC EFFECTS

Hypersensitivity reactions, ranging from chills, fever, and rash to anaphylaxis, may occur.

NURSING CONSIDERATIONS

BASELINE ASSESSMENT
Question for history of allergies, particularly penicillins, cephalosporins.

INTERVENTION/EVALUATION
Monitor CBC, urinalysis, renal function tests.

penicillin G potassium

pen-ih-**sil**-lin G
(Megacillin ♣, Novepen-G ♣, Pfizerpen)

Do not confuse penicillin G potassium with penicillin G benzathine or penicillin G procaine.

CLASSIFICATION

PHARMACOTHERAPEUTIC: Penicillin. **CLINICAL:** Antibiotic (see p. 27C).

ACTION

A penicillin that inhibits bacterial cell wall synthesis by binding to one or more of the penicillin-binding proteins of bacteria. **Therapeutic Effect:** Bactericidal.

PHARMACOKINETICS

Protein binding: 60%. Widely distributed. Metabolized in the liver. Primarily excreted in urine. **Half-life:** 0.5 hr (increased in impaired renal function).

USES

Treatment of susceptible infections due to gram positive organisms, gram negative organisms, actinomycosis, clostridium, diphtheria, Listeria, *N. meningitidis,* pasteurella including anthrax, endocarditis, respiratory tract infections, meningitis, neurosyphilis, skin and skin-structure infections.

PRECAUTIONS

CONTRAINDICATIONS: Hypersensitivity to any penicillin. **CAUTIONS:** Renal or hepatic impairment, seizure disorder, hypersensitivity to cephalosporins.

LIFESPAN CONSIDERATIONS: Pregnancy/Lactation: Readily crosses placenta; distributed in breast milk. **Pregnancy Category B. Children:** May delay renal excretion in neonates, young infants. **Elderly:** Age-related renal impairment may require dosage adjustment.

INTERACTIONS

DRUG: Erythromycin: May antagonize effects of penicillin. **Probenecid:** Increases serum concentration of penicillin. **HERBAL:** None known. **FOOD: Food, milk:** Decrease penicillin absorption. **LAB VALUES:** May cause a positive Coombs' test.

AVAILABILITY (Rx)

INJECTION: 5 million units. **INTRAVENOUS SOLUTION:** 1 million units/50 ml, 2 million units/50 ml, 3 million units/ 50 ml. **POWDER FOR INJECTION:** 1 million units, 5 million units (Pfizerpen), 20 million units (Pfizerpen). **PREMIXED DEXTROSE SOLUTION:** 1 million units, 2 million units, 3 million units.

ADMINISTRATION/HANDLING

 IV

Reconstitution • Follow dilution guide per manufacturer. • After reconstitution, further dilute with 50–100 ml D$_5$W or 0.9% NaCl for a final concentration of 100–500,000 units/ml (50,000 units/ml for infants and neonates).

Rate of administration • Infuse over 15–60 min.

Storage • Reconstituted solution is stable for 7 days if refrigerated.

IV INCOMPATIBILITIES

Amikacin (Amikin), aminophylline, amphotericin B, dopamine (Intropin).

IV COMPATIBILITIES

Amiodarone (Cordarone), calcium gluconate, diltiazem (Cardizem), diphenhydramine (Benadryl), furosemide (Lasix), heparin, hydromorphone (Dilaudid), lidocaine, magnesium sulfate, methylprednisolone (Solu-Medrol), morphine, potassium chloride, total parenteral nutrition (TPN).

INDICATIONS/ROUTES/DOSAGE

SEPSIS, MENINGITIS, PERICARDITIS, ENDOCARDITIS, PNEUMONIA DUE TO SUSCEPTIBLE GRAM-POSITIVE ORGANISMS (NOT STAPHYLOCOCCUS AUREUS) AND SOME GRAM-NEGATIVE ORGANISMS
IV, IM: ADULTS, ELDERLY: 2–24 million units/day in divided doses q4–6h. CHILDREN: 100,000–400,000 units/kg/day in divided doses q4–6h.

DOSAGE IN RENAL IMPAIRMENT
Dosage interval is modified based on creatinine clearance.

Creatinine Clearance	Dosage Interval
10–30 ml/min	Usual dose q8–12h
Less than 10 ml/min	Usual dose q12–18h

SIDE EFFECTS

OCCASIONAL: Lethargy, fever, dizziness, rash, electrolyte imbalance, diarrhea, thrombophlebitis. **RARE:** Seizures, interstitial nephritis.

ADVERSE REACTIONS/ TOXIC EFFECTS

Hypersensitivity reactions ranging from rash, fever, and chills to anaphylaxis occur.

P

NURSING CONSIDERATIONS

BASELINE ASSESSMENT
Question for history of allergies, particularly penicillins, cephalosporins.

INTERVENTION/EVALUATION
Monitor CBC, urinalysis electrolytes, renal function tests.

penicillin V potassium

pen-ih-**sil**-in V

(Apo-Pen-VK ✦, Beepen-VK, Novo-Pen-VK ✦, PC Pen VK, Pen-V, Truxcillin VK, Veetids)

◆ CLASSIFICATION
PHARMACOTHERAPEUTIC: Penicillin. **CLINICAL:** Antibiotic (see p. 27C).

ACTION
A penicillin that inhibits cell wall synthesis by binding to bacterial cell membranes. **Therapeutic Effect:** Bactericidal.

PHARMACOKINETICS
Moderately absorbed from the GI tract. Protein binding: 80%. Widely distributed. Metabolized in the liver. Primarily excreted in urine. **Half-life:** 1 hr (increased in impaired renal function).

USES
Treatment of mild to moderate infections of respiratory tract and skin and skin-structure, otitis media, necrotizing ulcerative gingivitis; prophylaxis for rheumatic fever, dental procedures.

PRECAUTIONS
CONTRAINDICATIONS: Hypersensitivity to any penicillin. **CAUTIONS:** Renal impairment, history of allergies (particularly cephalosporins), history of seizures.

⌛ **LIFESPAN CONSIDERATIONS: Pregnancy/Lactation:** Readily crosses placenta; appears in cord blood, amniotic fluid. Distributed in breast milk in low concentrations. May lead to allergic sensitization, diarrhea, candidiasis, skin rash in infant. **Pregnancy Category B. Children:** Use caution in neonates and young infants (may delay renal elimination). **Elderly:** Age-related renal impairment may require dosage adjustment.

INTERACTIONS
DRUG: Probenecid: May increase penicillin blood concentration and risk of toxicity. **HERBAL:** None known. **FOOD:** None known. **LAB VALUES:** May cause positive a Coombs' test.

AVAILABILITY (Rx)
TABLETS: 250 mg (PC Pen VK, Pen-V, Veetids), 500 mg (Pen-V, Veetids, Truxcillin VK). **POWDER FOR ORAL SOLUTION:** 125 mg/5 ml (Veetids), 250 mg/5 ml (Beepen-VK, Veetids).

ADMINISTRATION/HANDLING
PO
• Store tablets at room temperature. Oral solution, after reconstitution, is stable for 14 days if refrigerated.
• Space doses evenly around the clock.
• Give without regard to meals.

INDICATIONS/ROUTES/DOSAGE
MILD TO MODERATE RESPIRATORY TRACT OR SKIN OR SKIN-STRUCTURE INFECTIONS, OTITIS MEDIA, NECROTIZING ULCERATIVE GINGIVITIS
PO: ADULTS, ELDERLY, CHILDREN 12 YR AND OLDER: 125–500 mg q6–8h. CHILDREN YOUNGER THAN 12 YR: 25–50 mg/kg/day in divided doses q6–8h. **Maximum:** 3 g/day.

PRIMARY PREVENTION OF RHEUMATIC FEVER
PO: ADULTS, ELDERLY: 500 mg 2–3 times

a day for 10 days. CHILDREN: 250 mg 2–3 times a day for 10 days.

PRIMARY PREVENTION OF RHEUMATIC FEVER
PO: ADULTS, ELDERLY, CHILDREN: 250 mg twice a day.

SIDE EFFECTS

FREQUENT: Mild hypersensitivity reaction (chills, fever, rash), nausea, vomiting, diarrhea. **RARE:** Bleeding, allergic reaction.

ADVERSE REACTIONS/ TOXIC EFFECTS

Severe hypersensitivity reactions, including anaphylaxis, may occur. Nephrotoxicity, antibiotic-associated colitis, and other superinfections may result from high dosages or prolonged therapy.

NURSING CONSIDERATIONS

BASELINE ASSESSMENT
Question for history of allergies, particularly penicillins, cephalosporins.

INTERVENTION/EVALUATION
Hold medication, promptly report rash (hypersensitivity) or diarrhea (with fever, abdominal pain, mucus or blood in stool may indicate antibiotic-associated colitis). Monitor I&O, urinalysis, renal function tests for nephrotoxicity. Be alert for superinfection: increased fever, sore throat, nausea, vomiting, diarrhea, stomatitis, vaginal discharge, anal or genital pruritus. Review Hgb levels; check for bleeding: overt bleeding, ecchymosis, swelling of tissue.

PATIENT/FAMILY TEACHING
• Continue antibiotic for full length of treatment. • Space doses evenly. • Notify physician immediately in event of rash, diarrhea, bleeding, bruising, other new symptoms.

pentaerythritol tetranitrate (P.E.T.N.)

(Duotrate, Peritrate)
See Nitrates

pentamidine isethionate

pen-**tam**-i-deen
(NebuPent, Pentacarinat ✤, Pentam-300)

◆CLASSIFICATION

PHARMACOTHERAPEUTIC: Anti-infective. **CLINICAL:** Antiprotozoal.

ACTION

An anti-infective that interferes with nuclear metabolism and incorporation of nucleotides, inhibiting DNA, RNA, phospholipid, and protein synthesis. **Therapeutic Effect:** Produces antibacterial and antiprotozoal effects.

PHARMACOKINETICS

Well absorbed after IM administration; minimally absorbed after inhalation. Widely distributed. Primarily excreted in urine. Minimally removed by hemodialysis. **Half-life:** 6.5 hr (increased in impaired renal function).

USES

Treatment of pneumonia caused by *Pneumocystis carinii* (PCP). Prevention of PCP in high-risk HIV-infected patients. **OFF-LABEL:** Treatment of African trypanosomiasis, cutaneous or visceral leishmaniasis.

PRECAUTIONS

CONTRAINDICATIONS: Concurrent use with didanosine. **CAUTIONS:** Diabetes

P

mellitus, renal or hepatic impairment, hypertension/hypotension.

⌛ **LIFESPAN CONSIDERATIONS: Pregnancy/Lactation:** Unknown if drug crosses placenta or is distributed in breast milk. **Pregnancy Category C. Children:** No age-related precautions noted. **Elderly:** No age-related information available.

INTERACTIONS

DRUG: Blood dyscrasia-producing medications, bone marrow depressants: May increase the abnormal hematologic effects of pentamidine. **Didanosine:** May increase the risk of pancreatitis. **Foscarnet:** May increase the risk of hypocalcemia, hypomagnesemia, and nephrotoxicity of pentamidine. **Nephrotoxic medications:** May increase the risk of nephrotoxicity. **HERBAL:** None known. **FOOD:** None known. **LAB VALUES:** May increase BUN and serum alkaline phosphatase, bilirubin, creatinine, AST, and ALT levels. May decrease serum calcium and magnesium levels. May alter blood glucose levels.

AVAILABILITY (Rx)

INJECTION (PENTAM-300): 300 mg. **POWDER FOR NEBULIZATION (NEBUPENT):** 300 mg.

ADMINISTRATION/HANDLING

◀ **ALERT** ▶ Patient must be in supine position during administration, with frequent BP checks until stable (potential for life-threatening hypotensive reaction). Have resuscitative equipment immediately available.

💧 **IV**

Reconstitution • For intermittent IV infusion (piggyback), reconstitute each vial with 3–5 ml D_5W or sterile water for injection. • Withdraw desired dose and further dilute with 50–250 ml D_5W.

Rate of administration • Infuse over 60 min. • Do not give by IV injection or

rapid IV infusion (increases potential for severe hypotension).

Storage • Store vials at room temperature. • After reconstitution, IV solution is stable for 48 hr at room temperature. • Discard unused portion.

IM
• Reconstitute 300-mg vial with 3 ml sterile water for injection to provide concentration of 100 mg/ml.

AEROSOL (NEBULIZER)
• Aerosol stable for 48 hr at room temperature. • Reconstitute 300-mg vial with 6 ml sterile water for injection. Avoid NaCl (may cause precipitate). • Do not mix with other medication in nebulizer reservoir.

▨ IV INCOMPATIBILITIES

Cefazolin (Ancef), cefotaxime (Claforan), ceftazidime (Fortaz), ceftriaxone (Rocephin), fluconazole (Diflucan), foscarnet (Foscavir), interleukin (Proleukin).

IV COMPATIBILITIES

Diltiazem (Cardizem), zidovudine (Retrovir), total parenteral nutrition (TPN).

INDICATIONS/ROUTES/DOSAGE
PCP

IV, IM: ADULTS, ELDERLY: 4 mg/kg/day once a day for 14–21 days. CHILDREN: 4 mg/kg/day once a day for 10–14 days.

PREVENTION OF PCP

INHALATION: ADULTS, ELDERLY: 300 mg once q4wk. CHILDREN 5 YR AND OLDER: 300 mg q3–4wk. CHILDREN YOUNGER THAN 5 YR: 8 mg/kg/dose once q3–4wk.

SIDE EFFECTS

FREQUENT: Injection (greater than 10%): Abscess, pain at injection site. **Inhalation (greater than 5%):** Fatigue, metallic taste, shortness of breath, decreased appetite, dizziness, rash, cough, nausea, vomiting, chills.

OCCASIONAL: Injection (10%–1%): Nausea, decreased appetite, hypotension, fever, rash, altered taste, confusion. **Inhalation (5%–1%):** Diarrhea, headache, anemia, muscle pain. **RARE: Injection (less than 1%):** Neuralgia, thrombocytopenia, phlebitis, dizziness.

ADVERSE REACTIONS/ TOXIC EFFECTS

Rare reactions include life-threatening or fatal hypotension, arrhythmias, hypoglycemia, leukopenia, nephrotoxicity or renal failure, anaphylactic shock, Stevens-Johnson syndrome, and toxic epidural necrolysis. Hyperglycemia and insulin-dependent diabetes mellitus (often permanent) may occur even months after therapy has stopped.

NURSING CONSIDERATIONS

BASELINE ASSESSMENT

Avoid concurrent use of nephrotoxic drugs. Establish baseline for BP, blood glucose. Obtain specimens for diagnostic tests before giving first dose.

INTERVENTION/EVALUATION

Monitor BP during administration until stable for both IM and IV administration (patient should remain supine). Check serum glucose levels and clinical signs for hypoglycemia (diaphoresis, nervousness, tremor, tachycardia, palpitations, lightheadedness, headache, numbness of lips, double vision, incoordination), hyperglycemia (polyuria, polyphagia, polydipsia, malaise, visual changes, abdominal pain, headache, nausea/vomiting). Evaluate IM sites for pain, redness, induration; IV sites for phlebitis (heat, pain, red streaking over vein). Monitor renal, liver, hematology test results. Assess skin for rash. Evaluate equilibrium during ambulation. Be alert for respiratory difficulty when administering by inhalation route.

PATIENT/FAMILY TEACHING

• Remain flat in bed during administration of medication; get up slowly with assistance only when BP stable. • Notify nurse immediately of diaphoresis, shakiness, lightheadedness, palpitations. • Drowsiness, increased urination, thirst, anorexia may develop in the months following therapy. • Maintain adequate fluid intake. • Inform physician if fever, cough, shortness of breath occurs. • Avoid alcohol.

Pentasa, *see mesalamine*

pentazocine

(Talwin)
See Opioid analgesics

pentobarbital

(Nembutal)
See Sedative-hypnotics

pentostatin

(Nipent)
See Cancer chemotherapeutic agents (p. 77C)

pentoxifylline

pen-tox-ih-**fill**-in

(Albert ✤, Apo-Pentoxifylline SR ✤, Pentopak, Pentoxifylline ✤, Pentoxil, Trental)
Do not confuse Trental with Tegretol or Trandate.

◆CLASSIFICATION

PHARMACOTHERAPEUTIC: Blood viscosity-reducing agent. **CLINICAL:** Hemorheologic.

ACTION

A blood viscosity-reducing agent that alters the flexibility of RBCs; inhibits production of tumor necrosis factor, neutrophil activation, and platelet aggregation. **Therapeutic Effect:** Reduces blood viscosity and improves blood flow.

PHARMACOKINETICS

Well absorbed after oral administration. Undergoes first-pass metabolism in the liver. Primarily excreted in urine. Unknown if removed by hemodialysis. **Half-life:** 24–48 min; metabolite, 60–90 min.

USES

Symptomatic treatment of intermittent claudication associated with occlusive peripheral vascular disease, diabetic angiopathies. **OFF-LABEL:** Diabetic neuropathy, gangrene, hemodialysis shunt thrombosis, septic shock, sickle cell syndrome, vascular impotence.

PRECAUTIONS

CONTRAINDICATIONS: History of intolerance to xanthine derivatives, such as caffeine, theophylline, or theobromine; recent cerebral or retinal hemorrhage. **CAUTIONS:** Renal or hepatic impairment, insulin-treated diabetes, chronic occlusive arterial disease, recent surgery, peptic ulcer disease.

⧗ LIFESPAN CONSIDERATIONS: **Pregnancy/Lactation:** Unknown if drug crosses placenta. Distributed in breast milk. **Pregnancy Category C. Children:** Safety and efficacy not established. **Elderly:** Age-related renal impairment may require dosage adjustment.

INTERACTIONS

DRUG: **Antihypertensives:** May increase the effects of antihypertensives. HERBAL: None known. FOOD: None known. LAB VALUES: None known.

AVAILABILITY (Rx)

TABLETS (CONTROLLED-RELEASE [PENTOPAK, PENTOXIL, TRENTAL]): 400 mg.

ADMINISTRATION/HANDLING

PO
• Do not crush or break film-coated tablets. • Give with meals to avoid GI upset.

INDICATIONS/ROUTES/DOSAGE

INTERMITTENT CLAUDICATION
PO: ADULTS, ELDERLY: 400 mg 3 times a day. Decrease to 400 mg twice a day if GI or CNS adverse effects occur. Continue for at least 8 wk.

SIDE EFFECTS

OCCASIONAL (5%–2%): Dizziness, nausea, altered taste, dyspepsia, marked by heartburn, epigastric pain, and indigestion. **RARE (less than 2%):** Rash, pruritus, anorexia, constipation, dry mouth, blurred vision, edema, nasal congestion, anxiety.

ADVERSE REACTIONS/ TOXIC EFFECTS

Angina and chest pain occur rarely and may be accompanied by palpitations, tachycardia, and arrhythmias. Signs and symptoms of overdose, such as flushing, hypotension, nervousness, agitation, hand tremor, fever, and somnolence, appear 4–5 hr after ingestion and last for 12 hr.

NURSING CONSIDERATIONS

INTERVENTION/EVALUATION
Assist with ambulation if dizziness occurs. Assess for hand tremor. Monitor for relief of symptoms of intermittent

---

claudication (pain, aching, cramping in calf muscles, buttocks, thigh, feet). Symptoms generally occur while walking or exercising and not at rest or with weight bearing in absence of walking or exercising.

PATIENT/FAMILY TEACHING

• Therapeutic effect generally noted in 2–4 wk. • Avoid tasks requiring alertness, motor skills until response to drug is established. • Do not smoke (causes constriction, occlusion of peripheral blood vessels). • Limit caffeine.

Pepcid, *see famotidine*

Percocet, *see acetaminophen and oxycodone*

---

pergolide mesylate

per-go-lide
(Permax)

Do not confuse Permax with Pentrax or Pernox.

◆**CLASSIFICATION**

PHARMACOTHERAPEUTIC: Dopamine agonist. **CLINICAL:** Antidyskinetic.

ACTION

A centrally active dopamine agonist that directly stimulates dopamine receptors. **Therapeutic Effect:** Decreases signs and symptoms of Parkinson's disease.

PHARMACOKINETICS

Well absorbed from the GI tract. Protein binding: 90%. Undergoes extensive first-pass metabolism in the liver. Primarily excreted in urine. Unknown if removed by hemodialysis.

USES

Adjunctive treatment with levodopa/carbidopa in patients with Parkinson's disease. OFF-LABEL: Chronic motor or vocal tic disorder, Tourette's disorder.

PRECAUTIONS

CONTRAINDICATIONS: Hypersensitivity to other ergot derivatives. **CAUTIONS:** Cardiac arrhythmias, history of confusion, hallucinations.

⌛ LIFESPAN CONSIDERATIONS: **Pregnancy/Lactation:** Unknown if drug crosses placenta or is distributed in breast milk. May interfere with lactation. **Pregnancy Category B. Children:** Safety and efficacy not established. **Elderly:** No age-related precautions noted.

INTERACTIONS

DRUG: **Haloperidol, loxapine, methyldopa, metoclopramide, phenothiazines:** May decrease the effectiveness of pergolide. **Hypotension-producing medications:** May increase the hypotensive effect. HERBAL: None known. FOOD: None known. LAB VALUES: May increase the serum growth hormone level.

AVAILABILITY (Rx)

TABLETS: 0.05 mg, 0.25 mg, 1 mg.

ADMINISTRATION/HANDLING

PO

• Scored tablets may be crushed. • Give without regard to meals.

INDICATIONS/ROUTES/DOSAGE

PARKINSONISM

PO: ADULTS, ELDERLY: Initially, 0.05 mg/day for 2 days. May increase by 0.1–0.15 mg/day every 3 days over the next 12 days; afterward may increase by 0.25 mg/day every 3 days. Range: 2–3 mg/day in 3 divided doses. **Maximum:** 5 mg/day.

P

SIDE EFFECTS

FREQUENT (24%–10%): Nausea, dizziness, hallucinations, constipation, rhinitis, dystonia, confusion, somnolence. **OCCASIONAL (9%–3%):** Orthostatic hypotension, insomnia, dry mouth, peripheral edema, anxiety, diarrhea, dyspepsia, abdominal pain, headache, abnormal vision, anorexia, tremor, depression, rash. **RARE (less than 2%):** Urinary frequency, vivid dreams, neck pain, hypotension, vomiting.

ADVERSE REACTIONS/ TOXIC EFFECTS

Symptoms of overdose may vary from CNS depression, characterized by sedation, apnea, cardiovascular collapse, and death, to severe paradoxical reactions, such as hallucinations, tremor, and seizures.

NURSING CONSIDERATIONS

INTERVENTION/EVALUATION

Be alert to neurologic effects: headache, lethargy, mental confusion, agitation. Monitor BP. Monitor for evidence of dyskinesia (difficulty with movement). Assess for clinical reversal of Parkinson symptoms (improvement of tremor of head and hands at rest, mask-like facial expression, shuffling gait, muscular rigidity).

PATIENT/FAMILY TEACHING

• Tolerance to feeling of lightheadedness develops during therapy. • To reduce hypotensive effect, rise slowly from lying to sitting position, permit legs to dangle momentarily before standing. • Dry mouth, drowsiness, dizziness may be expected responses of drug. • Avoid tasks that require alertness, motor skills until response to drug is established. • Avoid alcoholic beverages during therapy.

perindopril erbumine

(Aceon)

See Angiotensin-converting enzyme (ACE) inhibitors (p. 7C)

perphenazine

(Trilafon)

See Antipsychotics

phenazopyridine hydrochloride

fen-az-o-**peer**-i-deen

(Azo-Gesic, Azo-Standard, Eridium, Phenazo ♣, Prodium, Pyridiate, Pyridium, Uristat, Urodol, Urogesic)

Do not confuse phenazopyridine with pyridoxine, or Prodium with Perdiem.

◆CLASSIFICATION

PHARMACOTHERAPEUTIC: Interstitial cystitis agent. **CLINICAL:** Urinary tract analgesic.

ACTION

An interstitial cystitis agent that exerts topical analgesic effect on urinary tract mucosa. **Therapeutic Effect:** Relieves urinary pain, burning, urgency, and frequency.

PHARMACOKINETICS

Well absorbed from the GI tract. Partially metabolized in the liver. Primarily excreted in urine. **Half-life:** Unknown.

USES

Symptomatic relief of pain, burning, urgency, frequency resulting from lower urinary tract mucosa irritation (may be caused by infection, trauma, surgery).

PRECAUTIONS

CONTRAINDICATIONS: Hepatic or renal insufficiency. **CAUTIONS:** None known.

⌛ **LIFESPAN CONSIDERATIONS: Pregnancy/Lactation:** Unknown if drug crosses placenta or is distributed in breast milk. **Pregnancy Category B. Children:** No age-related precautions noted in those older than 6 yr. **Elderly:** Age-related renal impairment may increase toxicity.

INTERACTIONS

DRUG: None known. **HERBAL:** None known. **FOOD:** None known. **LAB VALUES:** May interfere with urinalysis tests based on color reactions, such as urinary glucose, ketones, protein, and 17-ketosteroids.

AVAILABILITY (Rx)

TABLETS: 95 mg (Pyridium), 100 mg (Azo-Gesic, Azo-Standard, Prodium, Uristat), 200 mg (Azo-Gesic, Azo-Standard, Prodium, Uristat).

ADMINISTRATION/HANDLING

PO
• Give with meals.

INDICATIONS/ROUTES/DOSAGE

URINARY ANALGESIC
PO: ADULTS: 100–200 mg 3–4 times a day. CHILDREN 6 YR AND OLDER: 12 mg/kg/day in 3 divided doses for 2 days.

DOSAGE IN RENAL IMPAIRMENT
Dosage interval is modified based on creatinine clearance.

Creatinine Clearance	Interval
50–80 ml/min	Usual dose q8–16h
Less than 50 ml/min	Avoid use

SIDE EFFECTS

OCCASIONAL: Headache, GI disturbance, rash, pruritus.

ADVERSE REACTIONS/ TOXIC EFFECTS

Overdose may lead to hemolytic anemia, nephrotoxicity, or hepatotoxicity. Patients with renal impairment or severe hypersensitivity to the drug may also develop these reactions. A massive and acute overdose may result in methemoglobinemia.

NURSING CONSIDERATIONS

INTERVENTION/EVALUATION
Assess for therapeutic response: relief of dysuria (pain, burning), urgency, frequency of urination.

PATIENT/FAMILY TEACHING
• A reddish orange discoloration of urine should be expected. • May stain fabric. • Take with meals (reduces possibility of GI upset).

---

phenelzine sulfate ⓔ

fen-ell-zeen
(Nardil)

◆ CLASSIFICATION

PHARMACOTHERAPEUTIC: MAOI. **CLINICAL:** Antidepressant (see p. 37C).

ACTION

An MAOI that inhibits the activity of the enzyme monoamine oxidase at CNS storage sites, leading to increased levels of the neurotransmitters epinephrine, norepinephrine, serotonin, and dopamine at neuronal receptor sites. **Therapeutic Effect:** Relieves depression.

USES

Treatment of depression refractory to other antidepressants, electroconvulsive therapy. **OFF-LABEL:** Treatment of panic disorder, selective mutism, vascular or tension headaches.

PRECAUTIONS

CONTRAINDICATIONS: Cardiovascular or cerebrovascular disease, hepatic or renal impairment, pheochromocytoma. **CAUTIONS:** Ingestion of tyramine-containing foods, cardiac arrhythmias, severe/frequent headaches, hypertension, suicidal tendencies.

⧗ **LIFESPAN CONSIDERATIONS:** **Pregnancy/Lactation:** Crosses placenta. Minimally distributed in breast milk. **Pregnancy Category C. Children:** Not recommended for children (increased risk of suicidal ideation). **Elderly:** Increased risk of drug toxicity may require dosage adjustment.

INTERACTIONS

DRUG: Alcohol, other CNS depressants: May increase CNS depression. **Buspirone:** May increase BP. **Caffeine-containing medications:** May increase the risk of cardiac arrhythmias and hypertension. **Carbamazepine, cyclobenzaprine, maprotiline, other MAOIs:** May precipitate hypertensive crisis. **Dopamine, tryptophan:** May cause sudden, severe hypertension. **Fluoxetine, trazodone, tricyclic antidepressants:** May cause serotonin syndrome. **Insulin, oral antidiabetics:** May increase the effects of these drugs. **Meperidine, other opioid analgesics:** May produce diaphoresis, immediate excitation, rigidity, and severe hypertension or hypotension, sometimes leading to severe respiratory distress, vascular collapse, seizures, coma, and death. **Methylphenidate:** May increase the CNS stimulant effects of methylphenidate. **Sympathomimetics:** May increase the cardiac stimulant and vasopressor effects of phenelzine. **HERBAL:** None known. **FOOD: Caffeine, chocolate, tyramine-containing foods (such as aged cheese):** May cause sudden, severe hypertension. **LAB VALUES:** None known.

AVAILABILITY (Rx)

TABLETS: 15 mg.

ADMINISTRATION/HANDLING

PO
• Store tablets at room temperature. Don't freeze. • Give with food or milk if GI distress occurs. • May crush tablets and give with food or fluids if patient has difficulty swallowing.

INDICATIONS/ROUTES/DOSAGE

DEPRESSION REFRACTORY TO OTHER ANTIDEPRESSANTS OR ELECTROCONVULSIVE THERAPY
PO: ADULTS: 15 mg 3 times a day. May increase to 60–90 mg/day. ELDERLY: Initially, 7.5 mg/day. May increase by 7.5–15 mg/day q3–4wk up to 60 mg/day in divided doses.

SIDE EFFECTS

FREQUENT: Orthostatic hypotension, restlessness, GI upset, insomnia, dizziness, headache, lethargy, asthenia, dry mouth, peripheral edema. **OCCASIONAL:** Flushing, diaphoresis, rash, urinary frequency, increased appetite, transient impotence. **RARE:** Visual disturbances.

ADVERSE REACTIONS/ TOXIC EFFECTS

Hypertensive crisis occurs rarely and is marked by severe hypertension, occipital headache radiating frontally, neck stiffness or soreness, nausea, vomiting, diaphoresis, fever or chilliness, clammy skin, dilated pupils, palpitations, tachycardia or bradycardia, and constricting chest pain. Intracranial bleeding has been reported in association with severe hypertension.

NURSING CONSIDERATIONS

BASELINE ASSESSMENT

Periodic liver function tests should be performed for patients requiring high dosage who are undergoing prolonged therapy.

INTERVENTION/EVALUATION

Assess appearance, behavior, speech pattern, level of interest, mood. Monitor for occipital headache radiating frontally and/or neck stiffness/soreness (may be first signal of impending hypertensive crisis). Monitor BP, heart rate, diet, weight, change in mood.

PATIENT/FAMILY TEACHING

• Antidepressant relief may be noted during first week of therapy; maximum benefit noted in 2–6 wk. • Report headache, neck stiffness/soreness immediately. • Avoid foods that require bacteria/molds for their preparation/preservation or those that contain tyramine (e.g., cheese, sour cream, beer, wine, figs, raisins, bananas, avocados, soy sauce, yeast extracts, yogurt, papaya, broad beans, meat tenderizers, excessive amounts of caffeine [coffee, tea, chocolate]) or OTC preparations for hay fever, colds, weight reduction.

phenobarbital

fee-noe-**bar**-bi-tal

(Luminal)

Do not confuse phenobarbital with pentobarbital, or Luminal with Tuinal.

FIXED-COMBINATION(S)

Bellergal-S: phenobarbital/ergotamine/belladonna (an anticholinergic): 40 mg/0.6 mg/0.2 mg. **Dilantin with PB:** phenobarbital/phenytoin (an anticonvulsant): 15 mg/100 mg; 30 mg/100 mg. **Donnatal:** phenobarbital/atropine (an anticholinergic)/hyoscyamine (an anticholinergic)/scopolamine (an anticholinergic): 16.2 mg/0.0194 mg/0.1037 mg/0.0065 mg.

CLASSIFICATION

PHARMACOTHERAPEUTIC: Barbiturate **(Schedule IV). CLINICAL:** Anticonvulsant, hypnotic (see p. 34C).

ACTION

A barbiturate that enhances the activity of gamma-aminobutyric acid (GABA) by binding to the GABA receptor complex. **Therapeutic Effect:** Depresses CNS activity.

PHARMACOKINETICS

Route	Onset	Peak	Duration
PO	20–60 min	N/A	6–10 hr
IV	5 min	30 min	4–10 hr

Well absorbed after PO or parenteral administration. Protein binding: 35%–50%. Rapidly and widely distributed. Metabolized in the liver. Primarily excreted in urine. Removed by hemodialysis. **Half-life:** 53–118 hr.

USES

Management of generalized tonic-clonic (grand mal) seizures, partial seizures, control of acute seizure episodes (status epilepticus, eclampsia, febrile seizures). Used as a sedative, hypnotic. **OFF-LABEL:** Prevention and treatment of febrile seizures in children and hyperbilirubinemia, management of sedative or hypnotic withdrawal.

PRECAUTIONS

CONTRAINDICATIONS: Hypersensitivity to other barbiturates, porphyria, pre-existing CNS depression, severe pain, severe respiratory disease. **CAUTIONS:** Renal or hepatic impairment.

P

⏳ **LIFESPAN CONSIDERATIONS: Pregnancy/Lactation:** Readily crosses placenta. Distributed in breast milk. Produces respiratory depression in neonates during labor. May cause postpartum hemorrhage, hemorrhagic disease in newborn. Withdrawal symptoms may appear in neonates born to women receiving barbiturates during last trimester of pregnancy. Lowers serum bilirubin concentration in neonates. **Pregnancy Category D. Children:** May cause paradoxical excitement. **Elderly:** May exhibit excitement, confusion, mental depression.

INTERACTIONS

DRUG: Alcohol, other CNS depressants: May increase the effects of phenobarbital. **Carbamazepine:** May increase the metabolism of carbamazepine. **Digoxin, glucocorticoids, metronidazole, oral anticoagulants, quinidine, tricyclic antidepressants:** May decrease the effects of these drugs. **Valproic acid:** Increases the blood concentration and risk of toxicity of phenobarbital. **HERBAL:** None known. **FOOD:** None known. **LAB VALUES:** May decrease serum bilirubin level. Therapeutic serum level is 10–40 mcg/ml; toxic serum level is greater than 40 mcg/ml.

AVAILABILITY (Rx)

ELIXIR: 15 mg/5 ml, 20 mg/5 ml. **TABLETS:** 15 mg, 30 mg, 32.4 mg, 60 mg, 64.8 mg, 97.2 mg, 100 mg. **INJECTION:** 30 mg/ml, 60 mg/ml, 65 mg/ml, 130 mg/ml.

ADMINISTRATION/HANDLING
💉 **IV**

Reconstitution • May give undiluted or may dilute with NaCl, D₅W, lactated Ringer's.

Rate of administration • Adequately hydrate patient before and immediately after (decreases risk of adverse renal effects). • Do not inject IV faster than 1 mg/kg/min and a maximum of 30 mg/min for children and 60 mg/min for adults. Too rapid IV may produce severe hypotension, marked respiratory depression. • Inadvertent intra-arterial injection may result in arterial spasm with severe pain, tissue necrosis. Extravasation in subcutaneous tissue may produce redness, tenderness, tissue necrosis. If either occurs, treat with 0.5% procaine solution into affected area, apply moist heat.

Storage • Store vials at room temperature.

IM
• Do not inject more than 5 ml in any one IM injection site (produces tissue irritation). • Inject deep IM into large muscle mass.

PO
• Give without regard to meals. • Tablets may be crushed. • Elixir may be mixed with water, milk, fruit juice.

▨ IV INCOMPATIBILITIES
Amphotericin B complex (Abelcet, AmBisome, Amphotec), hydrocortisone (Solu-Cortef), hydromorphone (Dilaudid), insulin.

IV COMPATIBILITIES
Calcium gluconate, enalapril (Vasotec), fentanyl (Sublimaze), fosphenytoin (Cerebyx), morphine, propofol (Diprivan).

INDICATIONS/ROUTES/DOSAGE
STATUS EPILEPTICUS
IV: ADULTS, ELDERLY: Initially, 300–800 mg, then 120–240 mg/dose at 20 min intervals until seizures are controlled or total dose of 1–2 g administered. CHILDREN, INFANTS: 10–20 mg/kg. May administer additional 5 mg/kg/dose q15–30min until seizures controlled or total dose of 40 mg/kg administered.

SEIZURE CONTROL

PO, IV: ADULTS, ELDERLY, CHILDREN OLDER THAN 12 YR: 1–3 mg/kg/day. Or 50–100 mg 2–3 times a day. CHILDREN 6–12 YR: 4–6 mg/kg/day. CHILDREN 1–5 YR: 6–8 mg/kg/day. CHILDREN YOUNGER THAN 1 YR: 5–6 mg/kg/day. NEONATES: 3–4 mg/kg/day.

SEDATION

PO, IM: ADULTS, ELDERLY: 30–120 mg/day in 2–3 divided doses. CHILDREN: 2 mg/kg 3 times a day.

HYPNOTIC

PO, IV, IM, SUBCUTANEOUS: ADULTS, ELDERLY: 100–320 mg at bedtime. CHILDREN: 3–5 mg/kg at bedtime.

SIDE EFFECTS

OCCASIONAL **(3%–1%):** Somnolence. **RARE (less than 1%):** Confusion; paradoxical CNS reactions, such as hyperactivity or nervousness in children and excitement or restlessness in the elderly (generally noted during first 2 wk of therapy, particularly in presence of uncontrolled pain).

ADVERSE REACTIONS/ TOXIC EFFECTS

Abrupt withdrawal after prolonged therapy may produce increased dreaming, nightmares, insomnia, tremor, diaphoresis, and vomiting, hallucinations, delirium, seizures, and status epilepticus. Skin eruptions may be a sign of a hypersensitivity reaction. Blood dyscrasias, hepatic disease, and hypocalcemia occur rarely. Overdose produces cold or clammy skin, hypothermia, severe CNS depression, cyanosis, tachycardia, and Cheyne-Stokes respirations. Toxicity may result in severe renal impairment.

NURSING CONSIDERATIONS

BASELINE ASSESSMENT

Assess BP, pulse, respirations immediately before administration. **Hypnotic:** Raise bed rails, provide environment conducive to sleep (back rub, quiet environment, low lighting). **Seizures:** Review history of seizure disorder (length, presence of auras, level of consciousness [LOC]). Observe frequently for recurrence of seizure activity. Initiate seizure precautions.

INTERVENTION/EVALUATION

Monitor CNS status, seizure activity, liver and renal function, respiratory rate, heart rate, BP. Monitor for therapeutic serum level (10–30 mcg/ml). Therapeutic serum level: 10–40 mcg/ml; toxic serum level: greater than 40 mcg/ml.

PATIENT/FAMILY TEACHING

• Avoid alcohol, limit caffeine. • May be habit forming. • Do not discontinue abruptly. • May cause dizziness/drowsiness; impair ability to perform tasks requiring mental alertness, coordination.

phentolamine

fen-**toll**-ah-mean

(Regitine ✤)

Do not confuse phentolamine with phentermine.

◆CLASSIFICATION

PHARMACOTHERAPEUTIC: Alpha-adrenergic blocking agent. **CLINICAL:** Pheochromocytoma agent.

ACTION

Blocks presynaptic (alpha$_2$) and postsynaptic (alpha$_1$) adrenergic receptors, acting on both arterial tree and venous bed. **Therapeutic Effect:** Decreases total peripheral resistance, diminishes venous return to heart.

PHARMACOKINETICS

Onset	Peak	Duration
IM		
15–20 min	20 min	30–45 min
IV		
Immediate	2 min	15–30 min

Metabolized in the liver. Excreted in urine. Half-life: 19 min.

USES

Diagnosis of pheochromocytoma. Control/prevention of hypertensive episodes immediately before, during surgical excision. Prevention/treatment of dermal necrosis, sloughing after IV administration of alpha adrenergic drugs (e.g., norepinephrine/dopamine). OFF-LABEL: Treatment of CHF.

PRECAUTIONS

CONTRAINDICATIONS: Epinephrine, MI, coronary insufficiency, angina, coronary artery disease. **CAUTIONS:** Gastritis, peptic ulcer, history of arrhythmias.

LIFESPAN CONSIDERATIONS: Pregnancy/Lactation: Unknown if drug crosses placenta or is distributed in breast milk. **Pregnancy Category C. Children:** Safety and efficacy not established. **Elderly:** No age-related precautions noted.

INTERACTIONS

DRUG: **Sympathomimetics (e.g., dopamine, phenylephrine):** Effects of these drugs may be decreased when given with phentolamine. HERBAL: None known. FOOD: None known. LAB VALUES: None known.

AVAILABILITY (Rx)

INJECTION, POWDER FOR RECONSTITUTION: 5-mg vials.

ADMINISTRATION/HANDLING

◂ ALERT ▸ Maintain patient in supine position (preferably in quiet, darkened room) during pheochromocytoma testing. Decrease in BP generally noted in less than 2 min.

 IV

Reconstitution • Reconstitute 5-mg vial with 1 ml sterile water for injection to provide concentration of 5 mg/ml.

Rate of administration • Inject rapidly. Monitor BP immediately after injection, q30sec for 3 min, then q60sec for 7 min.

Storage • Store vials at room temperature. • After reconstitution, is stable for 48 hr at room temperature or 1 wk if refrigerated.

IV INCOMPATIBILITIES

Do not mix with any other medications.

IV COMPATIBILITIES

Amiodarone (Cordarone), dobutamine (Dobutrex).

INDICATIONS/ROUTES/DOSAGE

DIAGNOSIS OF PHEOCHROMOCYTOMA

IM, IV: ADULTS, ELDERLY: 2.5–5 mg. CHILDREN: 0.05–0.1 mg/kg/dose. **Maximum:** 5 mg.

CONTROL/PREVENTION OF HYPERTENSION IN PHEOCHROMOCYTOMA

IV: ADULTS, ELDERLY: 5 mg 1–2 hr before surgery. May repeat q2–4h. CHILDREN: 0.05–0.1 mg/kg/dose 1–2 hr before surgery. May repeat.

PREVENTION/TREATMENT OF NECROSIS/ SLOUGHING

Infiltrate area with 1 ml of solution (reconstituted by diluting 5–10 mg in 0.9% NaCl) within 12 hr of extravasation. **Maximum:** 0.1–0.2 mg/kg or 5 mg total.

SIDE EFFECTS

OCCASIONAL (3%–2%): Weakness, dizziness, flushing, nausea, vomiting, diarrhea, orthostatic hypotension.

ADVERSE REACTIONS/ TOXIC EFFECTS

Tachycardia, arrhythmias, acute/prolonged hypotension may occur. Do not use epinephrine (will produce further drop in BP).

NURSING CONSIDERATIONS

BASELINE ASSESSMENT

Positive pheochromocytoma test indicated by decrease in BP greater than 35 mm Hg systolic, greater than 25 mm Hg diastolic pressure. Negative test indicated by no change in BP or elevation of BP. BP generally returns to baseline within 15–30 min following administration.

INTERVENTION/EVALUATION

Monitor BP, heart rate. Assess for orthostatic hypotension. Monitor for extravasation (skin color streaking).

---

phenylephrine ⚑ *hydrochloride*

fen-ill-**eh**-frin

(AK-Dilate, AD-Nephrin, Despec-SF, Mydfrin, Neo-Synephrine, Neo-Synephrine Ophthalmic, Ocu-Phrin, Phenoptic, Prefrin, Rectasol, Sudafed PE Nasal Decongestant)

◆ CLASSIFICATION

PHARMACOTHERAPEUTIC: Sympathomimetic, alpha receptor stimulant. **CLINICAL:** Nasal decongestant, mydriatic, vasopressor (see p. 142C).

ACTION

A sympathomimetic, alpha receptor stimulant that acts on the alpha-adrenergic receptors of vascular smooth muscle. Causes vasoconstriction of arterioles of nasal mucosa or conjunctiva, activates dilator muscle of the pupil to cause contraction, produces systemic arterial vasoconstriction. Therapeutic Effect: Decreases mucosal blood flow and relieves congestion and increases systolic BP.

PHARMACOKINETICS

Route	Onset	Peak	Duration
IV	Immediate	N/A	15–20 min
IM	10–15 min	N/A	0.5–2 hr
Sub-cutaneous	10–15 min	N/A	1 hr

Minimal absorption after intranasal and ophthalmic administration. Metabolized in the liver and GI tract. Primarily excreted in urine. Half-life: 2.5 hr.

USES

Nasal: Topical application to nasal mucosa reduces nasal secretion, promoting drainage of sinus secretions. **Ophthalmic:** Topical application to conjunctiva relieves congestion, itching, minor irritation; whitens sclera of eye. **Parenteral:** Vascular failure in shock, drug-induced hypotension.

PRECAUTIONS

CONTRAINDICATIONS: Acute pancreatitis, heart disease, hepatitis, narrow-angle glaucoma, pheochromocytoma, severe hypertension, thrombosis, ventricular tachycardia. **CAUTIONS:** Hyperthyroidism, bradycardia, heart block, severe arteriosclerosis.

🔖 LIFESPAN CONSIDERATIONS: **Pregnancy/Lactation:** Crosses placenta. Distributed in breast milk. **Pregnancy Category C. Children:** May exhibit increased absorption, toxicity with nasal preparation. No age-related precautions noted with systemic use. **Elderly:** More likely to experience adverse effects.

INTERACTIONS

DRUG: **Beta blockers:** May have mutually inhibitory effects. **Digoxin:** May

P

---

increase risk of arrhythmias. **Ergonovine, oxytocin:** May increase vasoconstriction. **MAOIs:** May increase vasopressor effects. **Maprotiline, tricyclic antidepressants:** May increase cardiovascular effects. **Methyldopa:** May decrease effects of methyldopa. HERBAL: None known. FOOD: None known. LAB VALUES: None known.

AVAILABILITY (OTC)

INJECTION: 1% (10 mg/ml). **NASAL SOLUTION DROPS (NEO-SYNEPHRINE):** 0.5%, 1%. **NASAL SPRAY (NEO-SYNEPHRINE):** 0.25%, 0.5%, 1%. **OPHTHALMIC SOLUTION:** 0.12% (AK-Nephrin), 2.5% (AK-Dilate, Mydfrin, Neofrin, Neo-Synephrine Ophthalmic, Ocu-Phrin, Phenoptic), 10% (AK-Dilate, Ocu-Phrin, Neo-Synephrine). **ORAL LIQUID (DESPEC-SF):** 5 mg/5 ml. **TABLETS (SUDAFED PE NASAL DECONGESTANT):** 10 mg.

ADMINISTRATION/HANDLING
IV

Reconstitution • For IV push, dilute 1 ml of 10 mg/ml solution with 9 ml sterile water for injection to provide a concentration of 1 mg/ml. • For IV infusion, dilute 10-mg vial with 500 ml D_5W or 0.9% NaCl to provide a concentration of 2 mcg/ml. Maximum concentration: 500 mg/250 ml.

Rate of administration • For IV push, give over 20–30 sec. • For IV infusion, give as per physician order.

Storage • Store vials at room temperature.

NASAL
• Instruct the patient to blow his or her nose before administering medication. • Tilt the patient's head, apply drops in 1 nostril. Keep the patient in the same position and wait 5 min before applying drops in other nostril. • Sprays should be administered into each nostril with head erect. • The patient should sniff briskly while squeezing container and wait 3–5 min before blowing nose gently. • Rinse tip of spray bottle.

OPHTHALMIC
• Instruct patient to tilt head backward, look up. • Gently pull lower lid down to form pouch and instill medication. • Do not touch tip of applicator to lids or any surface. • When lower lid is released, have patient keep eye open without blinking for at least 30 sec. • Apply gentle finger pressure to lacrimal sac (bridge of the nose, inside corner of the eye) for 1–2 min. • Remove excess solution around eye with tissue. • Wash hands immediately to remove medication on hands.

⊞ IV INCOMPATIBILITY
Thiopentothal (Pentothal).

IV COMPATIBILITIES
Amiodarone (Cordarone), dobutamine (Dobutrex), lidocaine, potassium chloride, propofol (Diprivan).

INDICATIONS/ROUTES/DOSAGE
NASAL DECONGESTANT
NASAL SPRAY, NASAL SOLUTION, NASAL TABLET: ADULTS, ELDERLY, CHILDREN 12 YR AND OLDER: 2–3 drops or 1–2 sprays of 0.25%–0.5% solution into each nostril q4h as needed, or 1 tablet q4h as needed (not more than 6 doses/24 hr. CHILDREN 6–11 YR: 2–3 drops or 1–2 sprays of 0.25% solution into each nostril q4h as needed. CHILDREN YOUNGER THAN 6 YR: 1 drop of 0.125% solution (dilute 0.5% solution with 0.9% NaCl to achieve 0.125%) in each nostril. Repeat q2–4h as needed. Do not use for more than 3 days.

CONJUNCTIVAL CONGESTION, ITCHING, AND MINOR IRRITATION; WHITENING OF SCLERA
OPHTHALMIC: ADULTS, ELDERLY, CHILDREN 12 YR AND OLDER: 1–2 drops of 0.12% solution q3–4h.

HYPOTENSION, SHOCK
IM, SUBCUTANEOUS: ADULTS, ELDERLY:
2–5 mg/dose q1–2h. CHILDREN: 0.1 mg/
kg/dose q1–2h. **Maximum: 5 mg.**
IV BOLUS: ADULTS, ELDERLY: 0.1–0.5 mg/
dose q10–15min as needed. CHILDREN:
5–20 mcg/kg/dose q10–15min.
IV INFUSION: ADULTS, ELDERLY: 100–180
mcg/min. When BP is stabilized, maintenance rate: 40–60 mcg/min. CHILDREN:
0.1–0.5 mcg/kg/min. Titrate to desired
effect.

SIDE EFFECTS

FREQUENT: Nasal: Rebound nasal congestion due to overuse, especially when
used longer than 3 days. **OCCASIONAL:**
Mild CNS stimulation (restlessness,
nervousness, tremors, headache, insomnia, particularly in those hypersensitive
to sympathomimetics, such as elderly
patients). **Nasal:** Stinging, burning,
drying of nasal mucosa. **Ophthalmic:**
Transient burning or stinging, brow
ache, blurred vision.

**ADVERSE REACTIONS/
TOXIC EFFECTS**

Large doses may produce tachycardia
and palpitations (particularly in those
with cardiac disease), light-headedness,
nausea, and vomiting. Overdose in those
older than 60 yr may result in hallucinations, CNS depression, and seizures.
Prolonged nasal use may produce
chronic swelling of nasal mucosa and
rhinitis.

NURSING CONSIDERATIONS

BASELINE ASSESSMENT
If phenylephine 10% ophthalmic is instilled into denuded or damaged corneal
epithelium, corneal clouding may result.

INTERVENTION/VALUATION
Monitor BP, heart rate.

PATIENT/FAMILY TEACHING
• Discontinue drug if adverse reactions
occur. • Do not use for nasal

decongestion for longer than 5 days,
(rebound congestion). • Discontinue
drug if insomnia, dizziness, weakness,
tremor, palpitations occur. • **Nasal:**
Stinging or burning of nasal mucosa may
occur. • **Opthalmic:** Blurring of vision
with eye instillation generally subsides
with continued therapy. • Discontinue
medication if redness or swelling of
eyelids, itching appears.

phenytoin

phen-ih-toyn
(Dilantin, Dilantin-125, Dilantin In-
fatabs, Dilantin Kapseals, Di-Phen,
Epamin, Phenytek, Phenytoin, Extended Release)

phenytoin sodium

(Dilantin)
**Do not confuse phenytoin with
mephenytoin, or Dilantin with
Dilaudid.**

FIXED-COMBINATION(S)
Dilantin with PB: phenytoin/phe-
nobarbital (a barbiturate): 100 mg/
15 mg; 100 mg/30 mg.

CLASSIFICATION
PHARMACOTHERAPEUTIC: Hydantoin. **CLINICAL:** Anticonvulsant, antiarrhythmic (see p. 34C).

ACTION
A hydantoin anticonvulsant that stabilizes
neuronal membranes in the motor cortex
by decreasing sodium and calcium ion
influx into the neurons. Also acts as an
antiarrhythmic agent by decreasing
abnormal ventricular automaticity and
shortening the refractory period, QT
interval, and action potential duration.
Therapeutic Effect: Limits the spread

of seizure activity. Restores normal cardiac rhythm.

PHARMACOKINETICS

Slowly and variably absorbed after PO administration; slowly but completely absorbed after IM administration. Protein binding: 90%–95%. Widely distributed. Metabolized in the liver. Primarily excreted in urine. Not removed by hemodialysis. Half-life: 22 hr.

USES

Management of generalized tonic-clonic seizures (grand mal), complex partial seizures (psychomotor), cortical focal seizures, status epilepticus. Ineffective in absence seizures, myoclonic seizures, atonic epilepsy when used alone. Treatment of cardiac arrhythmias including those due to digoxin intoxication. OFF-LABEL: Adjunctive treatment of tricyclic antidepressant toxicity; treatment of muscle hyperirritability, digoxin-induced arrhythmias, and trigeminal neuralgia.

PRECAUTIONS

CONTRAINDICATIONS: Hypersensitivity to hydantoins, seizures due to hypoglycemia. **IV:** Adam-Stokes syndrome, second- and third-degree AV block, sinoatrial block, sinus bradycardia. **EXTREME CAUTION: IV Route Only:** Respiratory depression, MI, CHF, damaged myocardium. **CAUTIONS:** Hepatic or renal impairment, severe myocardial insufficiency, hypotension, hyperglycemia.

LIFESPAN CONSIDERATIONS: Pregnancy/Lactation: Crosses placenta. Is distributed in small amount in breast milk. Fetal hydantoin syndrome (craniofacial abnormalities, nail or digital hypoplasia, prenatal growth deficiency) has been reported. Increased frequency of seizures in pregnant women due to altered absorption or metabolism of phenytoin. May increase risk of hemorrhage in neonate, maternal bleeding during delivery. **Pregnancy Category D. Children:** More susceptible to gingival hyperplasia, coarsening of facial hair; excess body hair. **Elderly:** No age-related precautions noted but lower dosages recommended.

INTERACTIONS

DRUG: **Alcohol, other CNS depressants:** May increase CNS depression. **Amiodarone, anticoagulants, cimetidine, disulfiram, fluoxetine, isoniazid, sulfonamides:** May increase phenytoin blood concentration, effects, and risk of toxicity. **Antacids:** May decrease phenytoin absorption. **Fluconazole, ketoconazole, miconazole:** May increase phenytoin blood concentration. **Glucocorticoids:** May decrease the effects of glucocorticoids. **Lidocaine, propranolol:** May increase cardiac depressant effects. **Valproic acid:** May decrease the metabolism and increase the blood concentration of phenytoin. **Xanthine:** May increase the metabolism of these drugs. HERBAL: None known. FOOD: None known. LAB VALUES: May increase blood glucose level and serum GGT and alkaline phosphatase levels. Therapeutic serum level is 10–20 mcg/ml; toxic serum level is greater than 20 mcg/ml.

AVAILABILITY (Rx)

CAPSULES (PROMPT-RELEASE [DILANTIN]): 100 mg. **CAPSULES (EXTENDED-RELEASE [DILANTIN]):** 30 mg (Dilantin Kapseals), 100 mg (Dilantin Kapseals, Phenytoin, Extended Release), 200 mg (Phenytek), 300 mg (Phenytek). **ORAL SUSPENSION (DILANTIN-125):** 125 mg/5 ml. **TABLETS (CHEWABLE [DILANTIN INFATABS]):** 50 mg. **INJECTION:** 50 mg/ml.

ADMINISTRATION/HANDLING

 IV

‹ ALERT › Give by IV push.

Reconstitution • May give undiluted or may dilute with 0.9% NaCl.

Rate of administration • Administer 50 mg over 2–3 min for elderly. In neonates, administer at rate not exceeding 1–3 mg/kg/min. • Severe hypotension, cardiovascular collapse occurs if rate of IV injection exceeds 50 mg/min for adults. IV push very painful (chemical irritation of vein due to alkalinity of solution). To minimize effect, flush vein with sterile saline solution through same IV needle and catheter after each IV push. • IV toxicity characterized by CNS depression, cardiovascular collapse.

Storage • Precipitate may form if parenteral form is refrigerated (will dissolve at room temperature). • Slight yellow discoloration of parenteral form does not affect potency, but do not use if solution is not clear or if precipitate is present.

PO
• Give with food if GI distress occurs. • Do not chew or break capsules. Tablets may be chewed. • Shake oral suspension well before using.

▧ IV INCOMPATIBILITIES
Diltiazem (Cardizem), dobutamine (Dobutrex), enalapril (Vasotec), heparin, hydromorphone (Dilaudid), insulin, lidocaine, morphine, nitroglycerin, norepinephrine (Levophed), potassium chloride, propofol (Diprivan).

INDICATIONS/ROUTES/DOSAGE
STATUS EPILEPTICUS
IV: ADULTS, ELDERLY, CHILDREN: 15–18 mg/kg. Maintenance dose: 300 mg/day or 4–6 mg/kg/day in 2–3 divided doses for adults and elderly; 6–7 mg/kg/day for children 10–16 yr; 7–8 mg/kg/day for children 7–9 yr; 7.5–9 mg/kg/day for children 4–6 yr; 8–10 mg/kg/day for children 6 mo–3 yr. NEONATES: Loading dose: 15–20 mg/kg. Maintenance dose: 5–8 mg/kg/day.

SEIZURE CONTROL
PO: ADULTS, ELDERLY, CHILDREN: Loading dose: 15–20 mg/kg in 3 divided doses 2–4 hr apart. Maintenance dose: Same as for status epilepticus.

ARRHYTHMIAS
PO: ADULTS, ELDERLY: Loading dose: 250 mg 4 times a day for 1 day, then 250 mg twice a day for 2 days. Maintenance Dose: 300–400 mg/day 1–4 times a day. CHILDREN: Maintenance dose: 5–10 mg/kg/day in 2–3 divided doses.
IV: ADULTS, ELDERLY, CHILDREN: Loading dose: 1.25 mg/kg q5min. May repeat up to total dose of 15 mg/kg. CHILDREN: Maintenance dose: 5–10 mg/kg/day in 2–3 divided doses.

SIDE EFFECTS
FREQUENT: Drowsiness, lethargy, confusion, slurred speech, irritability, gingival hyperplasia, hypersensitivity reaction (including fever, rash, and lymphadenopathy), constipation, dizziness, nausea.
OCCASIONAL: Headache, hirsutism, coarsening of facial features, insomnia, muscle twitching.

ADVERSE REACTIONS/ TOXIC EFFECTS
Abrupt withdrawal may precipitate status epilepticus. Blood dyscrasias, lymphadenopathy, and osteomalacia (caused by impaired vitamin D metabolism) may occur. Toxic phenytoin blood concentration (25 mcg/ml or more) may produce ataxia, nystagmus, or diplopia. As the level increases, extreme lethargy may lead to coma.

NURSING CONSIDERATIONS

BASELINE ASSESSMENT
Anticonvulsant: Review history of seizure disorder (intensity, frequency, duration, level of consciousness [LOC]). Initiate seizure precautions. Liver function tests, CBC, platelet count should be performed before beginning therapy and

P

periodically during therapy. Repeat CBC, platelet count 2 wk following initiation of therapy and 2 wk following administration of maintenance dose.

INTERVENTION/EVALUATION

Observe frequently for recurrence of seizure activity. Assess for clinical improvement (decrease in intensity and frequency of seizures). Monitor CBC with differential, liver and renal function tests, BP (with IV use). Assist with ambulation if drowsiness, lethargy occurs. Monitor for therapeutic serum level (10–20 mcg/ml). Therapeutic serum level: 10–20 mcg/ml; toxic serum level: greater than 20 mcg/ml.

PATIENT/FAMILY TEACHING

• Pain may occur with IV injection. • To prevent gingival hyperplasia (bleeding, tenderness, swelling of gums), encourage good oral hygiene care, gum massage, regular dental visits. • CBC should be performed every month for 1 yr after maintenance dose is established and q3mo thereafter. • Report sore throat, fever, glandular swelling, skin reaction (hematologic toxicity). • Drowsiness usually diminishes with continued therapy. • Avoid tasks that require alertness, motor skills until response to drug is established. • Do not abruptly withdraw medication after long-term use (may precipitate seizures). • Strict maintenance of drug therapy is essential for seizure control, arrhythmias. • Avoid alcohol.

PhosLo, *see calcium acetate*

---

phosphates

fos-fates

(Fleet Enema, Fleet Phospho-Soda, K-Phos MF, K-Phos Neutral, Neutra-Phos, Neutra-Phos-K, Uro-KP-Neutral)

◆ CLASSIFICATION

PHARMACOTHERAPEUTIC: Electrolyte. **CLINICAL:** Mineral.

ACTION

Electrolytes that participate in bone deposition, calcium metabolism, and utilization of B complex vitamins and act as a buffer in maintaining acid-base balance. Also exert an osmotic effect in small intestine, producing distention and promoting peristalsis. **Therapeutic Effect:** Correct hypophosphatemia, acidify urine in UTIs, help prevent calcium deposits in urinary tract, and promote evacuation of the bowel.

PHARMACOKINETICS

Poorly absorbed after PO administration. PO form excreted in feces; IV form excreted in urine.

USES

Prophylactic treatment of hypophosphatemia. Short-term treatment of constipation, for evacuation of colon for exams; urinary acidifier for reduction of formation of calcium stones. **OFF-LABEL:** Prevention of calcium renal calculi.

PRECAUTIONS

CONTRAINDICATIONS: Abdominal pain or fecal impaction (from rectal dosage form), ascitic conditions, CHF, hyperkalemia, hypernatremia, hyperphosphatemia, hypocalcemia, hypomagnesemia, paralytic ileus, phosphate renal calculi, severe renal impairment. **CAUTIONS:** Renal impairment, concomitant use of potassium-sparing drugs, adrenal insufficiency, cirrhosis.

⧗ **LIFESPAN CONSIDERATIONS:** **Pregnancy/Lactation:** Unknown if drug crosses placenta or is distributed in breast milk. **Pregnancy Category C.** **Children:** Increased risk of dehydration in children younger than 12 yr. **Elderly:** No age-related precautions noted.

INTERACTIONS

DRUG: **Angiotensin-converting enzyme (ACE) inhibitors, NSAIDs, potassium-containing medications, potassium-sparing diuretics, salt substitutes containing potassium phosphate:** May increase potassium blood concentration. **Antacids:** May decrease the absorption of phosphates. **Calcium-containing medications:** May increase the risk of calcium deposition in soft tissues and decrease phosphate absorption. **Digoxin:** May increase the risk of heart block caused by hyperkalemia when given with potassium phosphates. **Glucocorticoids:** May cause edema when given with sodium phosphate. **Phosphate-containing medications:** May increase the risk of hyperphosphatemia. **Sodium-containing medications:** May increase the risk of edema when given with sodium phosphate. **HERBAL:** None known. **FOOD:** None known. **LAB VALUES:** None known.

AVAILABILITY (Rx)

ORAL SOLUTION (FLEET PHOSPHA-SODA): 4 mmol phosphate per ml. **POWDER (NEUTRA-PHOS, NEUTRA-PHOS-K):** 250 mg (8 mmol) phosphate. **TABLETS:** 125 mg (4 mmol) phosphate, 250 mg (8 mmol) phosphate (K-Phos MF, K-Phos Neutral, Uro-KP-Neutral). **ENEMA (FLEET ENEMA):** 2.25 oz, 4.5 oz. **INJECTION (POTASSIUM PHOSPHATE):** 3 mmol phosphate and 4.4 mEq potassium per ml. **INJECTION (SODIUM PHOSPHATE):** 3 mmol phosphate and 4 mEq sodium per ml.

ADMINISTRATION/HANDLING

 IV

Reconstitution • Must be diluted. Soluble in all commonly used IV solutions.

Rate of administration • Maximum rate of infusion: 0.06 mmol phosphate/kg/hr.

Storage • Store at room temperature.
PO
• Dissolve tablets in water. • Take after meals or with food (decreases GI upset).
• Maintain high fluid intake (prevents kidney stones).

RECTAL
• Use enema at room temperature.
• Remove orange protective shield from tip before using. • Have patient lie on his or her left side with the knee slightly bent and right leg drawn up or in knee-chest position. • Insert tube pointing toward navel. • Slowly squeeze and empty contents into rectum. Rubber diaphragm at the base of the tube prevents accidental leakage and assures controlled flow of the enema solution.
• Remove tube from patient's rectum.
• Have the patient remain in one position until defecation impulse felt (usually 2–5 min).

▓ IV INCOMPATIBILITY
Dobutamine (Dobutrex).

IV COMPATIBILITIES
Diltiazem (Cardizem), enalapril (Vasotec), famotidine (Pepcid), magnesium sulfate, metoclopramide (Reglan).

INDICATIONS/ROUTES/DOSAGE
HYPOPHOSPHATEMIA
PO (NEUTRA-PHOS, NEUTRA-PHOS-K, K-PHOS MF, K-PHOS-NEUTRAL, URO-KP-NEUTRAL): ADULTS, ELDERLY: 50–150 mmol/day. CHILDREN: 2–3 mmol/kg/day.

P

IV: ADULTS, ELDERLY: 50–70 mmol/day.
CHILDREN: 0.5–1.5 mmol/kg/day.

LAXATIVE

PO (NEUTRA-PHOS, NEUTRA-PHOS-K, URO-KP-NEUTRAL): ADULTS, ELDERLY CHILDREN 4 YR AND OLDER: 1–2 capsules/packets 4 times a day. CHILDREN YOUNGER THAN 4 YR: 1 capsule/packet 4 times a day. **RECTAL:** ADULTS, ELDERLY, CHILDREN 12 YR AND OLDER: 4.5-oz enema as single dose. May repeat. CHILDREN YOUNGER THAN 12 YR: 2.25-oz enema as single dose. May repeat.

URINE ACIDIFICATION

PO: ADULTS, ELDERLY: 8 mmol 4 times a day.

SIDE EFFECTS

FREQUENT: Mild laxative effect (in first few days of therapy). **OCCASIONAL:** Diarrhea, nausea, abdominal pain, vomiting. **RARE:** Headache; dizziness; confusion; heaviness of lower extremities; fatigue; muscle cramps; paraesthesia; peripheral edema; arrhythmias; weight gain; thirst.

ADVERSE REACTIONS/ TOXIC EFFECTS

Hyperphosphatemia may produce extraskeletal calcification.

NURSING CONSIDERATIONS

INTERVENTION/EVALUATION

Monitor serum calcium, phosphorus, potassium, sodium, AST, ALT, alkaline phosphatase, bilirubin levels routinely.

PATIENT/FAMILY TEACHING

• Report diarrhea, nausea, vomiting.

physostigmine

fi-zoe-**stig**-meen
(Antilirium)

Do not confuse physostigmine with Prostigmin or pyridostigmine.

♦CLASSIFICATION

PHARMACOTHERAPEUTIC: Parasympathomimetic (cholinergic). **CLINICAL:** Anticholinesterase agent (see p. 46C).

ACTION

A cholinergic that inhibits destruction of acetylcholine by enzyme acetylcholinesterase, thus enhancing impulse transmission across the myoneural junction. **Therapeutic Effect:** Improves skeletal muscle tone, stimulates salivary and sweat gland secretions.

PHARMACOKINETICS

Penetrates blood-brain barrier. Rapidly hydrolyzed by cholinesterases. Small amount eliminated in urine; largely destroyed in body by hydrolysis. **Half-life:** Unknown.

USES

Antidote for reversal of toxic CNS effects due to anticholinergic drugs, tricyclic antidepressants. **OFF-LABEL:** Treatment of hereditary ataxia.

PRECAUTIONS

CONTRAINDICATIONS: Active uveal inflammation, angle-closure glaucoma before iridectomy, asthma, cardiovascular disease, concurrent use of ganglionic-blocking agents, diabetes, gangrene, glaucoma associated with iridocyclitis, hypersensitivity to cholinesterase inhibitors or their components, mechanical obstruction of intestinal or urogenital tract, vagotonic state. **CAUTIONS:** Bronchial asthma, GI disturbances, peptic ulcer, bradycardia, hypotension, recent MI, epilepsy, parkinsonism, other disorders that may respond adversely to vagotonic effects. Use ophthalmic physostigmine only when shorter-acting miotics are not adequate, except in aphakics.

 LIFESPAN CONSIDERATIONS: Pregnancy/Lactation: Unknown if drug crosses placenta or is distributed in breast milk. **Pregnancy Category C. Children:** No age-related precautions noted. **Elderly:** No age-related precautions noted.

INTERACTIONS

DRUG: Cholinesterase agents, including bethanechol and carbachol: May increase the effects of these drugs. **Succinylcholine:** May prolong the action of succinylcholine. **HERBAL:** None known. **FOOD:** None known. **LAB VALUES:** None known.

AVAILABILITY (Rx)

INJECTION: 1 mg/ml.

ADMINISTRATION/HANDLING

🖥 **IV**

• For adults, administer at a rate not exceeding 1 mg/min. • For children, administer no more than 0.02 mg/kg over at least 1 min.

INDICATIONS/ROUTES/DOSAGE

TO REVERSE CNS EFFECTS OF ANTICHOLINERGIC DRUGS AND TRICYCLIC ANTIDEPRESSANTS
IV, IM: ADULTS, ELDERLY: Initially, 0.5–2 mg. If no response, repeat q20min until response or adverse cholinergic effects occur. If initial response occurs, may give additional doses of 1–4 mg q30–60min as life-threatening signs, such as arrhythmias, seizures, and deep coma, recur. CHILDREN: 0.01–0.03 mg/kg. May give additional doses q5–10min until response or adverse cholinergic effects occur or total dose of 2 mg given.

SIDE EFFECTS

EXPECTED: Miosis, increased GI and skeletal muscle tone, bradycardia. **OCCASIONAL:** Marked drop in BP (hypertensive patients). **RARE:** Allergic reaction.

ADVERSE REACTIONS/ TOXIC EFFECTS

Parenteral overdose produces a cholinergic crisis manifested as abdominal discomfort or cramps, nausea, vomiting, diarrhea, flushing, facial warmth, excessive salivation, diaphoresis, urinary urgency, and blurred vision. If overdose occurs, stop all anticholinergic drugs and immediately and administer 0.6–1.2 mg atropine sulfate IM or IV for adults, or 0.01 mg/kg for infants and children younger than 12 yr.

NURSING CONSIDERATIONS

BASELINE ASSESSMENT
Have tissues readily available at patient's bedside.

INTERVENTION/EVALUATION
Parenteral: Assess vital signs immediately before and q15–30min following administration. Monitor diligently for cholinergic reaction (diaphoresis, palpitations, muscle weakness, abdominal pain, dyspnea, hypotension).

PATIENT/FAMILY TEACHING
• Adverse effects often subside after the first few days of therapy. • Avoid night driving, activities requiring visual acuity in dim light.

pimecrolimus

pim-eh-**crow**-leh-mus
(Elidel)
Do not confuse Elidel with Elavil.

CLASSIFICATION

PHARMACOTHERAPEUTIC: Immuno-modulator. **CLINICAL:** Anti-inflammatory.

ACTION

Inhibits release of cytokine, an enzyme that produces an inflammatory reaction. **Therapeutic Effect:** Produces anti-inflammatory activity.

USES

Treatment of mild to moderate atopic dermatitis (eczema).

PRECAUTIONS

CONTRAINDICATIONS: None known. **CAUTIONS:** Potential cancer risk. **Pregnancy Category C.**

INTERACTIONS

DRUG: None known. **HERBAL:** None known. **FOOD:** None known. **LAB VALUES:** None known.

AVAILABILITY (Rx)

TOPICAL: 1% cream.

INDICATIONS/ROUTES/DOSAGE

ATOPIC DERMATITIS (ECZEMA)
TOPICAL: ADULTS, ELDERLY, CHILDREN 2–17 YR: Apply to affected area twice a day for up to 3 wk (up to 6 wk in children 2–17 yr). Rub in gently, completely. Reevaluate if symptoms persist for more than 6 wk.

SIDE EFFECTS

RARE: Transient sensation of burning/feeling of heat at application site.

ADVERSE REACTIONS/ TOXIC EFFECTS

Lymphadenopathy, phototoxicity occur rarely.

NURSING CONSIDERATIONS

PATIENT/FAMILY TEACHING
• Wash hands after application. • May cause a mild to moderate feeling of warmth, sensation of burning at the application site. • Inform physician if application site reaction is severe or lasts for longer than 1 wk. • Avoid artificial sunlight, tanning beds. • Contact physician if no improvement in the atopic dermatitis is seen following 6 wk of treatment or if condition worsens.

pindolol

(Novo-Pindol ♣, Visken)
Do not confuse with Panadol, Parlodel, Plendil.
See Beta-adrenergic blockers (p. 64C).

pioglitazone

pie-oh-**glit**-ah-zone
(Actos)

FIXED-COMBINATION(S)

Actoplus Met: pioglitazone/metformin, (an antidiabetic): 15 mg/500 mg, 15 mg/850 mg.

CLASSIFICATION

CLINICAL: Antidiabetic (see p. 42C).

ACTION

An antidiabetic that improves target-cell response to insulin without increasing pancreatic insulin secretion. Decreases hepatic glucose output and increases insulin-dependent glucose utilization in skeletal muscle. **Therapeutic Effect:** Lowers blood glucose concentration.

PHARMACOKINETICS

Rapidly absorbed. Highly protein bound (99%), primarily to albumin. Metabolized in the liver. Excreted in urine. Unknown if removed by hemodialysis. Half-life: 16–24 hr.

USES

Adjunct to diet, exercise to lower blood glucose in those with type 2 non–insulin-dependent diabetes mellitus (NIDDM). Used as monotherapy or in combination with a sulfonylurea, metformin, or insulin to improve glycemic control.

PRECAUTIONS

CONTRAINDICATIONS: Active hepatic disease; diabetic ketoacidosis; increased serum transaminase levels, including ALT greater than 2.5 times normal serum level; type 1 diabetes mellitus. **CAUTIONS:** Hepatic impairment, CHF, edematous patients.

⏳ **LIFESPAN CONSIDERATIONS: Pregnancy/Lactation:** Unknown if drug crosses placenta or is distributed in breast milk. Not recommended in pregnant or breast-feeding women. **Pregnancy Category C. Children:** Safety and efficacy not established. **Elderly:** No age-related precautions noted.

INTERACTIONS

DRUG: Gemfibrizol: May increase the effect and toxicity of pioglitazone. **Ketoconazole:** May significantly inhibit metabolism of pioglitazone. **Oral contraceptives:** May alter the effects of oral contraceptives. **FOOD:** None known. **HERBAL:** None known. **LAB VALUES:** May increase creatine kinase (CK) level. May decrease Hgb levels by 2% to 4% and serum alkaline phosphatase, bilirubin, and ALT levels. Less than 1% of patients experience ALT values 3 times the normal level.

AVAILABILITY (Rx)

TABLETS: 15 mg, 30 mg, 45 mg.

ADMINISTRATION/HANDLING

PO
• Give without regard to meals.

INDICATIONS/ROUTES/DOSAGE

DIABETES MELLITUS, COMBINATION THERAPY

PO: ADULTS, ELDERLY: **With insulin:** Initially, 15–30 mg once a day. Initially, continue current insulin dosage; then decrease insulin dosage by 10%–25% if hypoglycemia occurs or plasma glucose level decreases to less than 100 mg/dl. **Maximum:** 45 mg/day. **With sulfonylureas:** Initially, 15–30 mg/day. Decrease sulfonylurea dosage if hypoglycemia occurs. **With metformin:** Initially, 15–30 mg/day. **As monotherapy:** Monotherapy is not to be used if patient is well controlled with diet and exercise alone. Initially, 15–30 mg/day. May increase dosage in increments until 45 mg/day is reached.

SIDE EFFECTS

FREQUENT (13%–9%): Headache, upper respiratory tract infection. **OCCASIONAL (6%–5%):** Sinusitis, myalgia, pharyngitis, aggravated diabetes mellitus.

ADVERSE REACTIONS/ TOXIC EFFECTS

Hepatotoxicity occurs rarely.

NURSING CONSIDERATIONS

BASELINE ASSESSMENT

Obtain hepatic enzyme levels before initiating therapy and periodically thereafter. Ensure follow-up instruction if patient and family do not thoroughly understand diabetes management or glucose-testing technique.

INTERVENTION/EVALUATION

Monitor blood glucose, Hgb, liver function tests, especially AST, ALT. Assess for hypoglycemia (cool, wet skin, tremors, dizziness, anxiety, headache, tachycardia, numbness in mouth,

P

hunger, diplopia), hyperglycemia (polyuria, polyphagia, polydipsia, nausea, vomiting, dim vision, fatigue, deep rapid breathing). Be alert to conditions that alter serum glucose requirements: fever, increased activity or stress, surgical procedures.

PATIENT/FAMILY TEACHING

• Understand signs and symptoms of hypoglycemia and its management. • Avoid alcohol. • Inform physician of chest pain, palpitations, abdominal pain, fever, rash, hypoglycemic reactions, yellowing of skin/eyes, dark urine, light stool, nausea, vomiting.

pipecuronium

(Arduan)
See Neuromuscular blockers

piperacillin sodium

(Pipracil)
See Antibiotic: penicillins

piperacillin sodium/ tazobactam sodium

pip-ur-ah-**sill**-in/tay-zoe-**back**-tam
(Tazocin ✦, Zosyn)
Do not confuse Zosyn with Zofran or Zyvox.

◆ CLASSIFICATION

PHARMACOTHERAPEUTIC: Penicillin. **CLINICAL:** Antibiotic (see p. 28C).

ACTION

Piperacillin inhibits cell wall synthesis by binding to bacterial cell membranes.

Tazobactam inactivates bacterial beta-lactamase. **Therapeutic Effect:** Piperacillin is bactericidal in susceptible organisms. Tazobactam protects piperacillin from enzymatic degradation, extends its spectrum of activity, and prevents bacterial overgrowth.

PHARMACOKINETICS

Protein binding: 16%–30%. Widely distributed. Primarily excreted unchanged in urine. Removed by hemodialysis. **Half-life:** 0.7–1.2 hr (increased in hepatic cirrhosis and impaired renal function).

USES

Treatment of appendicitis (complicated by rupture, abscess); peritonitis; uncomplicated and complicated skin and skin-structure infections, including cellulitis, cutaneous abscesses, ischemic or diabetic foot infections; postpartum endometritis; pelvic inflammatory disease (PID); community-acquired pneumonia (moderate severity only); moderate to severe nosocomial pneumonia.

PRECAUTIONS

CONTRAINDICATIONS: Hypersensitivity to any penicillin, cephalosporins, or beta-lactamase inhibitors. **CAUTIONS:** History of allergies, especially cephalosporins, other drugs, renal impairment, preexisting seizure disorder.

⧖ **LIFESPAN CONSIDERATIONS: Pregnancy/Lactation:** Readily crosses placenta; appears in cord blood, amniotic fluid. Distributed in breast milk in low concentrations. May lead to allergic sensitization, diarrhea, candidiasis, skin rash in infant. **Pregnancy Category B. Children:** Dosage not established for those younger than 12 yr. **Elderly:** Age-related renal impairment may require dosage adjustment.

INTERACTIONS

DRUG: Hepatotoxic medications: May increase the risk of hepatotoxicity.

Probenecid: May increase piperacillin blood concentration and risk of toxicity. **HERBAL:** None known. **FOOD:** None known. **LAB VALUES:** May increase serum sodium, alkaline phosphatase, bilirubin, LDH, AST, and ALT levels. May decrease serum potassium level. May cause a positive Coombs' test.

AVAILABILITY (Rx)

◀ **ALERT** ▶ Piperacillin/tazobactam is a combination product in an 8:1 ratio of piperacillin to tazobactam.
POWDER FOR INJECTION: 2.25 g, 3.375 g, 4.5 g. **PREMIX READY TO USE:** 2.25 g, 3.375 g, 4.5 g.

ADMINISTRATION/HANDLING
 IV

Reconstitution • Reconstitute each 1 g with 5 ml D_5W or 0.9% NaCl. Shake vigorously to dissolve. • Further dilute with at least 50 ml D_5W, 0.9% NaCl, D_5W 0.9% NaCl, or lactated Ringer's.

Rate of administration • Infuse over 30 min.

Storage • Reconstituted vial is stable for 24 hr at room temperature or 48 hr if refrigerated. • After further dilution, is stable for 24 hr at room temperature or 7 days if refrigerated.

▦ IV INCOMPATIBILITIES

Amphotericin B (Fungizone), amphotericin B complex (Abelcet, AmBisome, Amphotec), chlorpromazine (Thorazine), dacarbazine (DTIC), daunorubicin (Cerubidine), dobutamine (Dobutrex), doxorubicin (Adriamycin), doxorubicin liposomal (Doxil), droperidol (Inapsine), famotidine (Pepcid), haloperidol (Haldol), hydroxyzine (Vistaril), idarubicin (Idamycin), minocycline (Minocin), nalbuphine (Nubain), prochlorperazine (Compazine), promethazine (Phenergan), vancomycin (Vancocin).

IV COMPATIBILITIES

Aminophylline, bumetanide (Bumex), calcium gluconate, diphenhydramine (Benadryl), dopamine (Intropin), enalapril (Vasotec), furosemide (Lasix), granisetron (Kytril), heparin, hydrocortisone (Solu-Cortef), hydromorphone (Dilaudid), lorazepam (Ativan), magnesium sulfate, methylprednisolone (Solu-Medrol), metoclopramide (Reglan), morphine, ondansetron (Zofran), potassium chloride, total parenteral nutrition (TPN).

INDICATIONS/ROUTES/DOSAGE

SEVERE INFECTIONS
IV: ADULTS, ELDERLY, CHILDREN 12 YR AND OLDER: 4 g/0.5 g q8h or 3 g/0.375 g q6h. **Maximum:** 18 g/2.25 g daily.

MODERATE INFECTIONS
IV: ADULTS, ELDERLY, CHILDREN 12 YR AND OLDER: 2 g/0.225g q6–8h.

DOSAGE IN RENAL IMPAIRMENT
Dosage and frequency are modified based on creatinine clearance.

Creatinine Clearance	Dosage
20–40 ml/min	8 g/1 g/day (2.25 g q6h)
Less than 20 ml/min	6 g/0.75 g/day (2.25 g q8h)

DOSAGE IN HEMODIALYSIS PATIENTS
IV: ADULTS, ELDERLY: 2.25 g q8h with additional dose of 0.75 g after each dialysis session.

SIDE EFFECTS

FREQUENT: Diarrhea, headache, constipation, nausea, insomnia, rash. **OCCASIONAL:** Vomiting, dyspepsia, pruritus, fever, agitation, candidiasis, dizziness, abdominal pain, edema, anxiety, dyspnea, rhinitis.

ADVERSE REACTIONS/ TOXIC EFFECTS

Antibiotic-associated colitis and other superinfections may result from altered

P

---

bacterial balance. Seizures and other neurologic reactions are more likely to occur in patients with renal impairment and those who have received an overdose. Severe hypersensitivity reactions, including anaphylaxis, occur rarely.

NURSING CONSIDERATIONS

BASELINE ASSESSMENT
Question for history of allergies, especially to penicillins, cephalosporins.

INTERVENTION/EVALUATION
Monitor pattern of bowel activity and stool consistency; mild GI effects may be tolerable, but increasing severity may indicate onset of antibiotic-associated colitis. Be alert for superinfection: severe genital or anal pruritus, abdominal pain, stomatitis, moderate to severe diarrhea. Monitor I&O, urinalysis. Monitor serum electrolytes, especially potassium, renal function tests.

piroxicam

peer-**ox**-i-kam
(Apo-Piroxicam ✦, Feldene, Fexicam ✦, Novopirocam ✦)
Do not confuse Feldene with Seldane.

CLASSIFICATION

PHARMACOTHERAPEUTIC: Nonsteroidal anti-inflammatory. **CLINICAL:** Anti-inflammatory, analgesic (see p. 117C).

ACTION

An NSAID that produces analgesic and anti-inflammatory effects by inhibiting prostaglandin synthesis. Therapeutic Effect: Reduces inflammatory response and intensity of pain.

PHARMACOKINETICS

Well absorbed following oral administration. Protein binding: 99%. Extensively metabolized in liver. Primarily excreted in urine; small amount eliminated in feces. Half-life: 50 hr.

USES

Symptomatic treatment of acute or chronic rheumatoid arthritis, osteoarthritis. OFF-LABEL: Treatment of acute gouty arthritis, ankylosing spondylitis, dysmenorrhea.

PRECAUTIONS

CONTRAINDICATIONS: Active peptic ulcer disease, chronic inflammation of the GI tract, GI bleeding or ulceration, history of hypersensitivity to aspirin or NSAIDs. **CAUTIONS:** Renal or cardiac impairment, hypertension, GI disease, concomitant use of anticoagulants.

⧖ LIFESPAN CONSIDERATIONS: **Pregnancy/Lactation:** Crosses placenta; distributed in breast milk. Avoid use during third trimester (may adversely affect fetal cardiovascular system: premature closing of ductus arteriosus). **Pregnancy Category C (D if used in third trimester or near delivery). Children:** Safety and efficacy not established. **Elderly:** Age-related renal impairment may increase the risk of hepatotoxicity, renal toxicity; reduced dosage recommended. More likely to have serious adverse effects with GI bleeding/ulceration.

INTERACTIONS

DRUG: **Antihypertensives, diuretics:** May decrease the effects of these drugs. **Aspirin, other salicylates:** May increase the risk of GI side effects such as bleeding. **Bone marrow depressants:** May increase the risk of hematologic reactions. **Heparin, oral anticoagulants, thrombolytics:** May increase the effects of these drugs. **Lithium:** May increase the blood concentration and risk of toxicity of lithium. **Methotrexate:** May increase the risk of methotrexate toxicity. **Probenecid:** May increase the piroxicam blood concentration. HERBAL: **Feverfew:** May decrease the effects of feverfew. **Ginkgo biloba:** May increase the risk of bleeding. **St. John's wort:** May increase the risk of phototoxicity. FOOD: None known. LAB VALUES: May increase AST and ALT levels. May decrease serum uric acid levels.

AVAILABILITY (Rx)

CAPSULES: 10 mg, 20 mg.

ADMINISTRATION/HANDLING

PO
• Do not crush or break capsules.
• May give with food, milk, antacids if GI distress occurs.

INDICATIONS/ROUTES/DOSAGE

ACUTE OR CHRONIC RHEUMATOID ARTHRITIS AND OSTEOARTHRITIS
PO: ADULTS, ELDERLY: Initially, 10–20 mg/day as a single dose or in divided doses. Some patients may require up to 30–40 mg/day. CHILDREN: 0.2–0.3 mg/kg/day. **Maximum:** 15 mg/day.

SIDE EFFECTS

FREQUENT (9%–4%): Dyspepsia, nausea, dizziness. OCCASIONAL (3%–1%): Diarrhea, constipation, abdominal cramps or pain, flatulence, stomatitis. RARE (less than 1%): Hypertension, urticaria, dysuria, ecchymosis, blurred vision, insomnia, phototoxicity.

ADVERSE REACTIONS/TOXIC EFFECTS

Rare reactions with long-term use include peptic ulcer disease, GI bleeding, gastritis, severe hepatic reaction (cholestasis, jaundice), nephrotoxicity (dysuria, hematuria, proteinuria, nephrotic syndrome), hematologic sensitivity (anemia, leukopenia, eosinophilia,

thrombocytopenia), and a severe hypersensitivity reaction (fever, chills, bronchospasm).

NURSING CONSIDERATIONS

BASELINE ASSESSMENT

Assess onset, type, location, duration of pain/inflammation. Inspect appearance of affected joints for immobility, deformities, skin condition.

INTERVENTION/EVALUATION

Monitor pattern of daily bowel activity and stool consistency. Monitor for evidence of nausea, GI distress. Evaluate for therapeutic response (relief of pain, stiffness, swelling; increased joint mobility; reduced joint tenderness; improved grip strength). Monitor CBC, renal and liver function tests.

PATIENT/FAMILY TEACHING

• Avoid aspirin, alcohol during therapy (increases risk of GI bleeding). • If GI upset occurs, take with food, milk, antacids. • Avoid tasks that require alertness until response to drug is established.

Pitocin, *see oxytocin*

Plavix, *see clopidogrel*

Plenaxis, *see abarelix*

Plendil, *see felodipine*

plicamycin

ply-kah-**my**-sin
(Mithracin)

Do not confuse Mithracin with Minocin.

CLASSIFICATION

PHARMACOTHERAPEUTIC: Antibiotic. **CLINICAL:** Antihypercalcemic, antineoplastic (see p. 77C).

ACTION

Forms complexes with DNA, inhibiting DNA-directed RNA synthesis. **Therapeutic Effect:** Lowers serum calcium, phosphate levels.

USES

Treatment of malignant testicular tumors, hypercalcemia, hypercalcuria associated with advanced neoplasms. **OFF-LABEL:** Treatment of Paget's disease refractory to other therapy.

PRECAUTIONS

CONTRAINDICATIONS: Existing thrombocytopenia, thrombocytopathy, coagulation disorders, myelosuppression. **EXTREME CAUTION:** Renal/hepatic impairment. **CAUTIONS:** Electrolyte imbalance. **Pregnancy Category X.**

INTERACTIONS

DRUG: Aspirin, dipyridamole, NSAIDs, sulfinpyrazone, valproic acid: May increase the risk of hemorrhage. **Bone marrow depressants, hepatotoxic and nephrotoxic medications:** May increase toxicity. **Calcium-containing medications, vitamin D:** May decrease effect. **Heparin, oral anticoagulants, thrombolytics:** Effects may be increased. **Live virus vaccines:** May potentiate virus replication **HERBAL:** None known. **FOOD:** None known. **LAB VALUES:** None known.

AVAILABILITY(Rx)

POWDER FOR INJECTION: 2,500 mcg.

ADMINISTRATION/HANDLING

 IV

Rate of administration • Infuse over 4–6 hr. • Extravasation produces painful inflammation, induration.

Storage • Refrigerate vials. • Solution must be freshly prepared before use; discard unused portions.

IV INCOMPATIBILITY

Cefepime (Maxipime).

IV COMPATIBILITY

Granisetron (Kytril).

INDICATIONS/ROUTES/DOSAGE

◄ **ALERT** ▶ Dose based on actual body weight. Use ideal body weight for obese or edematous patients. Do not exceed 30 mcg/kg/day or more than 10 daily doses (increases potential for hemorrhage).

TESTICULAR TUMORS

IV: ADULTS, ELDERLY: 25–30 mcg/kg/day for 8–10 days. Repeat monthly.

HYPERCALCEMIA/HYPERURICEMIA

IV: ADULTS, ELDERLY: 15–25 mcg/kg/day for 3–4 days. Repeat at weekly or longer intervals. Reduce dose to 12.5 mcg/kg in patients with renal or hepatic impairment.

PAGET'S DISEASE

IV: ADULTS, ELDERLY: 15 mcg/kg/day for 10 days.

SIDE EFFECTS

FREQUENT: Nausea, vomiting, anorexia, diarrhea, stomatitis. **OCCASIONAL:** Fever, drowsiness, weakness, lethargy, malaise, headache, mental depression, nervousness, dizziness, rash, acne.

ADVERSE REACTIONS/ TOXIC EFFECTS

Hematologic toxicity noted by marked facial flushing, nosebleeds, ecchymoses, and neutropenia.

NURSING CONSIDERATIONS

BASELINE ASSESSMENT

Question for possibility of pregnancy (Pregnancy Category X). Discontinue therapy if platelet count falls below 150,000/mm^3, WBC falls below 4,000/mm^3, or if prothrombin time is 4 sec higher than control test.

INTERVENTION/EVALUATION

Monitor for stomatitis, thrombocytopenia. Avoid IM injections, rectal temperatures, any trauma that may induce bleeding.

PATIENT/FAMILY TEACHING

• Maintain fastidious oral hygiene. • Do not have immunizations without physician's approval (drug lowers body's resistance). • Avoid crowds, those with infection.

polycarbophil

polly-**car**-bow-fill
(Fibercon, Replens ✤)

◆CLASSIFICATION

CLINICAL: Bulk-forming laxative, antidiarrheal (see p. 109C).

ACTION

A bulk-forming laxative and antidiarrheal. As a laxative, retains water in the intestine and opposes dehydrating forces of the bowel. **Therapeutic Effect:** Promotes well-formed stools. As an antidiarrheal, absorbs fecal-free water, restores normal moisture level, and provides bulk. **Therapeutic Effect:** Forms gel and produces formed stool.

PHARMACOKINETICS

Route	Onset	Peak	Duration
PO	12–72 hr	N/A	N/A

Polycarbophil is not absorbed following oral administration. Acts in small and large intestines.

USES

Treatment of diarrhea associated with irritable bowel syndrome (IBS), diverticulosis, acute nonspecific diarrhea. Relieves constipation associated with irritable or spastic bowel.

PRECAUTIONS

CONTRAINDICATIONS: Abdominal pain, dysphagia, fecal impaction, nausea, partial bowel obstruction, symptoms of appendicitis, vomiting. **CAUTIONS:** None known.

⧗ **LIFESPAN CONSIDERATIONS: Pregnancy/Lactation:** Safe for use in pregnancy. **Pregnancy Category C. Children:** Not recommended in those younger than 6 yr. **Elderly:** No age-related precautions noted.

INTERACTIONS

DRUG: Digoxin, oral anticoagulants, salicylates, tetracyclines: May decrease the effects of digoxin, salicylates, and tetracyclines. **Potassium-sparing diuretics, potassium supplements:** May interfere with the effects of potassium-sparing diuretics and potassium supplements. **HERBAL:** None known. **FOOD:** None known. **LAB VALUES:** May increase blood glucose level. May decrease serum potassium levels.

AVAILABILITY (OTC)

TABLETS: 500 mg, 625 mg. **TABLETS (CHEWABLE):** 500 mg.

INDICATIONS/ROUTES/DOSAGE

CONSTIPATION, DIARRHEA
PO: ADULTS, ELDERLY, CHILDREN 12 YR AND

P

OLDER: 1 g 1–4 times a day, or as needed. **Maximum:** 4 g/24 hr. CHILDREN 6–11 YR: 500 mg 1–4 times a day, or as needed. **Maximum:** 2 g/24 hr. CHILDREN YOUNGER THAN 6 YR: Consult product labeling.

SIDE EFFECTS

OCCASIONAL: Epigastric fullness, flatulence. **RARE:** Some degree of abdominal discomfort, nausea, mild cramps, griping, syncope/near syncope.

ADVERSE REACTIONS/ TOXIC EFFECTS

Esophageal or bowel obstruction may occur if administered with less than 250 ml or 1 full glass of liquid.

NURSING CONSIDERATIONS

INTERVENTION/EVALUATION

Encourage adequate fluid intake. Assess bowel sounds for peristalsis. Monitor pattern of daily bowel activity and stool consistency, record time of evacuation. Monitor serum electrolytes in those exposed to prolonged, frequent, excessive use of medication.

PATIENT/FAMILY TEACHING

• Institute measures to promote defecation (increase fluid intake, exercise, high-fiber diet). • Drink 6–8 glasses of water a day when used as laxative (aids stool softening).

polyethylene glycol-electrolyte solution (PEG-ES)

poly-**eth**-ah-leen

(CoLyte, CoLyte 4 Flavor, CoLyte Flavored, GlycoLax, GoLYTELY, Klean-Prep ✦, <u>MiraLax</u>, NuLytely, NuLytely Cherry, NuLytely Lemon Lime, NuLytely Orange, Peglyte ✦, Pro-Lax ✦, TriLyte)

◆CLASSIFICATION

PHARMACOTHERAPEUTIC: Laxative. **CLINICAL:** Bowel evacuant (see p. 110C).

ACTION

A laxative that has an osmotic effect. **Therapeutic Effect:** Induces diarrhea and cleanses bowel without depleting electrolytes.

PHARMACOKINETICS

Route	Onset	Peak	Duration
PO (Bowel cleansing)	1–2 hr	N/A	N/A
PO (Constipation)	2–4 days	N/A	N/A

USES

Bowel cleansing before GI examination, colon surgery. **MiraLax:** Treatment of occasional constipation.

PRECAUTIONS

CONTRAINDICATIONS: Bowel perforation, gastric retention, GI obstruction, megacolon, toxic colitis, toxic ileus. **CAUTIONS:** Ulcerative colitis.
⏳ **LIFESPAN CONSIDERATIONS: Pregnancy/Lactation:** Unknown if drug crosses placenta or is distributed in breast milk. **Pregnancy Category C. Children/Elderly:** No age-related precautions noted.

INTERACTIONS

DRUG: **Oral medications:** May decrease the absorption of oral medications if given within 1 hr because they may be flushed from GI tract. HERBAL: None known. FOOD: None known. LAB VALUES: None known.

AVAILABILITY (Rx)

POWDER FOR RECONSTITUTION: (CoLyte, CoLyte Flavored, Colyte 4 Flavor, GlycoLax, GoLytely, MiraLax, NuLytely, NuLytely

---

✐ see color pill atlas   ✦ herb   <u>underlined</u> – top prescribed drug

Cherry, NuLytely Lemon Lime, NuLytely Orange, TriLyte).

ADMINISTRATION/HANDLING
PO
• Refrigerate reconstituted solutions; use within 48 hr. • May use tap water to prepare solution. Shake vigorously for several min to ensure complete dissolution of powder. • Fasting should occur for more than 3 hr before ingestion of solution (solid food should always be avoided for less than 2 hr before administration). • Only clear liquids permitted after administration. • May give via NG tube. • Rapid drinking preferred. Chilled solution is more palatable.

INDICATIONS/ROUTES/DOSAGE
BOWEL CLEANSING
PO: ADULTS, ELDERLY: Before GI examination: 240 ml (8 oz) q10min until 4 liters consumed or rectal effluent clear. NG tube: 20–30 ml/min until 4 liters given. CHILDREN: 25–40 ml/kg/hr until rectal effluent clear.

CONSTIPATION
PO (MIRALAX): ADULTS: 17 g or 1 heaping tbsp a day.

SIDE EFFECTS
FREQUENT (50%): Some degree of abdominal fullness, nausea, bloating. **OCCASIONAL (10%–1%):** Abdominal cramping, vomiting, anal irritation. **RARE (less than 1%):** Urticaria, rhinorrhea, dermatitis.

ADVERSE REACTIONS/ TOXIC EFFECTS
Cases of urticaria, rhinorrhea, dermatitis, and rarely anaphylaxis, angioedema, tongue edema, and face edema have been reported which may represent allergic reactions.

NURSING CONSIDERATIONS

BASELINE ASSESSMENT
Do not give oral medication within 1 hr of start of therapy (may not adequately be absorbed before GI cleansing).

INTERVENTION/EVALUATION
Assess bowel sounds for peristalsis. Monitor pattern of bowel activity and stool consistency; record time of evacuation. Assess for abdominal disturbances. Monitor serum electrolytes, BUN, glucose, urine osmolality.

poly-L-lactic acid

polly-el-**lack**-tic
(Sculptra)

CLASSIFICATION
PHARMACOTHERAPEUTIC: Physical adjunct. **CLINICAL:** Lipoatrophy agent.

ACTION
A lipoatrophy agent containing microparticles of a synthetic polymer that is used as an injectable implant. **Therapeutic Effect:** Restores facial fat.

PHARMACOKINETICS
Biodegradable, biocompatible synthetic polymer.

USES
Treatment for restoration and/or correction of facial lipatropy in people with HIV.

PRECAUTIONS
CONTRAINDICATIONS: None known. **CAUTIONS:** Tendency to keloid formation.

 LIFESPAN CONSIDERATIONS: Pregnancy/Lactation: Safety and efficacy not established. **Pregnancy Category not established. Children:** Safety and efficacy not established in children younger than 18 yr. **Elderly:** No age-related precautions noted.

P

INTERACTIONS

DRUG: None known. **HERBAL:** None known. **FOOD:** None known. **LAB VALUES:** None known.

AVAILABILITY (Rx)

POWDER FOR INJECTION (FREEZE-DRIED): Each carton contains 2 vials.

ADMINISTRATION/HANDLING

🛢 IV INFUSION

Reconstitution • Draw 3–5 ml sterile water for injection. • Using an 18-gauge sterile needle, slowly add all sterile water for injection into the vial. • Let vial stand for at least 2 hr; do not shake during this period. • After 2 hr, agitate vial until a uniform translucent suspension is obtained. • Withdraw amount of the suspension (usually 1 ml) into a syringe using a new, 18-gauge needle and replace with a 26-gauge needle before injecting the product into the deep dermis or subcutaneous layer.

Storage • Store at room temperature. • Reconstituted product is stable for up to 72 hr at room temperature.

INDICATIONS/ROUTES/DOSAGE

FACIAL LIPOATROPHY

SUBCUTANEOUS: ADULTS, ELDERLY: For severe facial fat loss, one vial usually injected into multiple points of each cheek during each injection session. Volume of drug for each injection and number of injection sessions depend on severity of condition. Typically, 3–6 injection sessions, separated by intervals of at least 2 wk, are required.

SIDE EFFECTS

FREQUENT: Ecchymosis. **OCCASIONAL:** Discomfort, edema. **RARE:** Erythema.

ADVERSE REACTIONS/ TOXIC EFFECTS

Subcutaneous papules at injection sites and hematoma occur occasionally.

BASELINE ASSESSMENT

Defer use if skin inflammation or infection occurs in or near the treatment area until the inflammatory or infectious process has been controlled.

INTERVENTION/EVALUATION

Apply ice packs to the treatment area to reduce inflammation. Treatment area should be massaged daily for several days following injection session.

PATIENT/FAMILY TEACHING

• Potential for redness, swelling, or bruising typically resolves in hours to 1 wk. • Full therapeutic effect noted in weeks to months. • Avoid excessive sunlight or UV lamp exposure until initial swelling and redness has resolved.

poractant alfa

poor-**ak**-tant
(Curosurf)

◆ **CLASSIFICATION**

CLINICAL: Pulmonary surfactant.

ACTION

A pulmonary surfactant that reduces alveolar surface tension during ventilation and stabilizes the alveoli against collapse that may occur at resting transpulmonary pressures. **Therapeutic Effect:** Improves lung compliance and respiratory gas exchange.

PHARMACOKINETICS

The pharmacokinetics of poractant alfa are not fully understood.

USES

Treatment (rescue) of respiratory distress syndrome (RDS—hyaline membrane disease) in premature infants. OFF-LABEL: Adult RDS due to viral pneumonia or near-drowning, *Pneumocystis carinii* pneumonia in HIV-infected patients, prevention of RDS.

PRECAUTIONS

CONTRAINDICATIONS: None known. **CAUTIONS:** Patients at risk for circulatory overload. Acidosis, hypotension, anemia, hypoglycemia, hypothermia should be corrected before administration.

⧖ **LIFESPAN CONSIDERATIONS: Neonate:** No age-related precautions noted for neonate. **Pregnancy Category:** This drug is not indicated for use in pregnant women.

INTERACTIONS

DRUG: None known. **HERBAL:** None known. **FOOD:** None known. **LAB VALUES:** None known.

AVAILABILITY (Rx)

INTRATRACHEAL SUSPENSION: 1.5 ml (120 mg), 3 ml (240 mg).

ADMINISTRATION/HANDLING

INTRATRACHEAL

Administration • Attach syringe to catheter and instill through catheter inserted into infant's endotracheal tube. • Monitor for bradycardia, decreased O_2 saturation during administration. Stop dosing procedure if these effects occur; begin appropriate measures before reinstituting therapy.

Storage • Refrigerate vials. • Warm by standing vial at room temperature for 20 min or warm in hand 8 min. • To obtain uniform suspension, turn upside down gently, swirl vial (do not shake). • After warming, may return to refrigerator one time only. • Withdraw entire contents of vial into a 3- or 5-ml plastic syringe through large-gauge needle (20 gauge or larger).

INDICATIONS/ROUTE/DOSAGE

RDS

INTRATRACHEAL: INFANTS: Initially, 2.5 ml/kg of birth weight. May give up to 2 subsequent doses of 1.25 ml/kg of birth weight at 12-hr intervals. **Maximum:** 5 ml/kg (total dose).

SIDE EFFECTS

FREQUENT: Transient bradycardia, oxygen (O_2) desaturation, increased carbon dioxide (CO_2) retention. **OCCASIONAL:** Endotracheal tube reflux. **RARE:** Hypotension or hypertension, pallor, vasoconstriction.

ADVERSE REACTIONS/ TOXIC EFFECTS

Desaturation of blood, blocked endotracheal tube, apnea occur rarely.

NURSING CONSIDERATIONS

BASELINE ASSESSMENT

Immediately before administration, change ventilator setting to 40–60 breaths/min, inspiratory time 0.5 sec, supplemental O_2 sufficient to maintain SaO_2 over 92%. Drug must be administered in highly supervised setting. Clinicians caring for neonate must be experienced with intubation, ventilator management. Offer emotional support to parents.

INTERVENTION/EVALUATION

Monitor infant with arterial or transcutaneous measurement of systemic O_2 and CO_2. Assess lung sounds for rales, moist breath sounds. Monitor heart rate.

P

porfimer

(Photofrin)
See Cancer chemotherapeutic agents

---

potassium ⚑
acetate

potassium
bicarbonate/citrate

(Effer K, Klor-Con EF, K-Lyte, K-Lyte DS)

potassium 🖉
chloride

(Apo-K ✦, Cena K, Ed K+10, K+Care, K-8, K-10, Kaochlor, Kaon-Cl, Kaon-CL 10, Kaon-CL 20%, Kato, Kay Ciel, KCl-20, KCl-40, K-Dur, K-Dur 10, K-Dur 20, K-Lor, K-Lor-Con M 15, <u>Klor-Con</u>, Klor-Con 8, Klor-Con 10, Klor-Con/25, Klor-Con M10, Klor-Con M15, Klor-Con M20, Klotrix, K-Norm, K-Sol, K-Tab, Kaon-Cl, Micro-K, Micro-K 10, Rum-K)

potassium
gluconate

(Kaon)

poe-**tah**-see-um

Do not confuse K-dur with Cardura.

◆ CLASSIFICATION

PHARMACOTHERAPEUTIC: Electrolyte. **CLINICAL:** Potassium replenisher.

ACTION

An electrolyte that is necessary for multiple cellular metabolic processes. Primary action is intracellular. Therapeutic Effect: Needed for nerve impulse conduction and contraction of cardiac, skeletal, and smooth muscle; maintains normal renal function and acid-base balance.

PHARMACOKINETICS

Well absorbed from the GI tract. Enters cells by active transport from extracellular fluid. Primarily excreted in urine.

USES

Treatment of potassium deficiency found in severe vomiting, diarrhea, loss of GI fluid, malnutrition, prolonged diuresis, debilitated, poor GI absorption, metabolic alkalosis, prolonged parenteral alimentation. Prevention of hypokalemia in at-risk patients.

PRECAUTIONS

CONTRAINDICATIONS: Concurrent use of potassium-sparing diuretics, digitalis toxicity, heat cramps, hyperkalemia, postop oliguria, severe burns, severe renal impairment, shock with dehydration or hemolytic reaction, untreated Addison's disease. **CAUTIONS:** Cardiac disease, tartrazine sensitivity (mostly noted in those with aspirin hypersensitivity).

⧗ LIFESPAN CONSIDERATIONS: **Pregnancy/Lactation:** Unknown if drug crosses placenta or is distributed in breast milk. **Pregnancy Category C (A for potassium chloride). Children:** No age-related precautions noted. **Elderly:** May be at increased risk for hyperkalemia. Age-related ability to excrete potassium is reduced.

INTERACTIONS

DRUG: **Angiotensin-converting enzyme (ACE) inhibitors, beta-adrenergic blockers, heparin, NSAIDs, potassium-containing medications, potassium-sparing diuretics, salt substitutes:** May increase potassium blood concentration. **Anticholinergics:** May increase the risk of GI lesions. HERBAL: None known. FOOD: None known. LAB VALUES: None known.

P

AVAILABILITY (Rx)

POTASSIUM ACETATE
INJECTION: 2 mEq/ml.
POTASSIUM BICARBONATE AND
POTASSIUM CITRATE
TABLETS FOR SOLUTION: 25 mEq (Klor-Con EF, Effer-K, K-Lyte), 50 mEq (K-Lyte DS).
POTASSIUM CHLORIDE
CAPSULES (CONTROLLED-RELEASE [MICRO-K]): 8 mEq, 10 mEq. **LIQUID:** 20 mEq/15 ml (Kaochlor), 40 mEq/15 ml (Kaon-Cl). **POWDER FOR ORAL SOLUTION (K-LOR):** 20 mEq. **POWDER FOR RECONSTITUTION (K+CARE):** 20 mEq. **INJECTION:** 2 mEq/ml. **TABLETS (EXTENDED-RELEASE):** 8 mEq (K-8, Klor-Con, Klor-Con 8, Klor-Con M10, Micro-K, Micro-K10), 10 mEq (K-8, Kaon-CL, Kaon-CL 10, K-Dur, Klor-Con, Klor-Con 8, Klor-Con M10, Klotrix, K-Tab, Micro-K, Micro-K 10), 20 mEq (K-Dur).
POTASSIUM GLUCONATE
ELIXIR (KAON): 20 mEq/15 ml.

ADMINISTRATION/HANDLING

IV

Reconstitution • For IV infusion only, must dilute before administration, mix well, infuse slowly. • Avoid adding potassium to hanging IV.

Rate of administration • Give at rate no more than 40 mEq/L; no faster than 20 mEq/hr. (Higher concentrations or faster rates may sometimes be necessary.) • Check IV site closely during infusion for evidence of phlebitis (heat, pain, red streaking of skin over vein, hardness to vein), extravasation (swelling, pain, cool skin, little or no blood return).

Storage • Store at room temperature.

PO
• Take with or after meals and with full glass of water (decreases GI upset).
• Liquids, powder, effervescent tablets: Mix, dissolve with juice, water before administering. • Do not chew, crush tablets; swallow whole.

IV INCOMPATIBILITIES

Amphotericin B complex (Abelcet, AmBisome, Amphotec), methylprednisolone (Solu-Medrol), phenytoin (Dilantin).

IV COMPATIBILITIES

Aminophylline, amiodarone (Cordarone), atropine, aztreonam (Azactam), calcium gluconate, cefepime (Maxipime), ciprofloxacin (Cipro), clindamycin (Cleocin), dexamethasone (Decadron), digoxin (Lanoxin), diltiazem (Cardizem), diphenhydramine (Benadryl), dobutamine (Dobutrex), dopamine (Intropin), enalapril (Vasotec), famotidine (Pepcid), fluconazole (Diflucan), furosemide (Lasix), granisetron (Kytril), heparin, hydrocortisone (Solu-Cortef), insulin, lidocaine, lorazepam (Ativan), magnesium sulfate, methylprednisolone (Solu-Medrol), metoclopramide (Reglan), midazolam (Versed), milrinone (Primacor), morphine, norepinephrine (Levophed), ondansetron (Zofran), oxytocin (Pitocin), piperacillin and tazobactam (Zosyn), procainamide (Pronestyl), propofol (Diprivan), propranolol (Inderal).

INDICATIONS/ROUTES/DOSAGE

PREVENTION OF HYPOKALEMIA (IN PATIENTS ON DIURETIC THERAPY)
PO: ADULTS, ELDERLY: 20–40 mEq/day in 1–2 divided doses. CHILDREN: 1–2 mEq/kg/day in 1–2 divided doses.

TREATMENT OF HYPOKALEMIA
PO: ADULTS, ELDERLY: 40–80 mEq/day; further doses based on laboratory values. CHILDREN: 2–5 mEq/day; further doses based on laboratory values.
IV: ADULTS, ELDERLY: 5–10 mEq/hr. **Maximum:** 400 mEq/day. CHILDREN: 1 mEq/kg over 1–2 hr.

P

SIDE EFFECTS

OCCASIONAL: Nausea, vomiting, diarrhea, flatulence, abdominal discomfort with distention, phlebitis with IV administration (particularly when potassium concentration of greater than 40 mEq/L is infused). **RARE:** Rash.

ADVERSE REACTIONS/ TOXIC EFFECTS

Hyperkalemia (more common in elderly patients and those with impaired renal function) may be manifested as paresthesia, feeling of heaviness in the lower extremities, cold skin, grayish pallor, hypotension, confusion, irritability, flaccid paralysis, and cardiac arrhythmias.

NURSING CONSIDERATIONS

BASELINE ASSESSMENT

PO should be given with food or after meals with full glass of water, fruit juice (minimizes GI irritation).

INTERVENTION/EVALUATION

Monitor serum potassium level (particularly in renal impairment). If GI disturbance is noted, dilute preparation further or give with meals. Be alert to decrease in urinary output (may be indication of renal insufficiency). Monitor pattern of daily bowel activity and stool consistency. Assess I&O diligently during diuresis, IV site for extravasation, phlebitis. Be alert to evidence of hyperkalemia (skin pallor/coldness, complaints of paraesthesia, feeling of heaviness of lower extremities).

PATIENT/FAMILY TEACHING

• Foods rich in potassium include beef, veal, ham, chicken, turkey, fish, milk, bananas, dates, prunes, raisins, avocados, watermelon, cantaloupe, apricots, molasses, beans, yams, broccoli, Brussels sprouts, lentils, potatoes, spinach. • Report paraesthesia, feeling of heaviness of lower extremities.

pramipexole

pram-eh-**pex**-ol
(Mirapex)
Do not confuse Mirapex with Mifeprex or MiraLax.

◆CLASSIFICATION

PHARMACOTHERAPEUTIC: Dopamine receptor agonist. **CLINICAL:** Antiparkinson agent.

ACTION

An antiparkinson agent that stimulates dopamine receptors in the striatum. **Therapeutic Effect:** Relieves signs and symptoms of Parkinson's disease.

PHARMACOKINETICS

Rapidly and extensively absorbed after PO administration. Protein binding: 15%. Widely distributed. Steady-state concentrations achieved within 2 days. Primarily eliminated in urine. Not removed by hemodialysis. **Half-life:** 8 hr (12 hr in patients older than 65 yr).

USES

Treatment of signs and symptoms of idiopathic Parkinson's disease. **OFF-LABEL:** Depression (due to bipolar disorder), fibromyalgia, restless legs syndrome.

PRECAUTIONS

CONTRAINDICATIONS: History of hypersensitivity to pramipexole. **CAUTIONS:** History of orthostatic hypotension, syncope, hallucinations, renal impairment, concomitant use of CNS depressants.

⧗ **LIFESPAN CONSIDERATIONS: Pregnancy/Lactation:** Unknown if drug is distributed in breast milk. **Pregnancy Category C. Children:** Safety and efficacy not established. **Elderly:** Increased risk of hallucinations.

✎ see color pill atlas   ⚕ herb   <u>underlined</u> – top prescribed drug

INTERACTIONS

DRUG: **Carbidopa and levodopa, levodopa:** May increase plasma level of levodopa. **Cimetidine:** Increases pramipexole plasma concentration and half-life. May decrease pramipexole clearance. **Diltiazem, quinidine, quinine, ranitidine, triamterene, verapamil:** May decrease pramipexole clearance. HERBAL: None known. FOOD: **All foods:** Delay peak drug plasma levels by 1 hr but don't affect drug absorption. LAB VALUES: None known.

AVAILABILITY (Rx)

TABLETS: 0.125 mg, 0.25 mg, 0.5 mg, 1 mg, 1.5 mg.

ADMINISTRATION/HANDLING

PO
• Give without regard to food.

INDICATIONS/ROUTES/DOSAGE

PARKINSON'S DISEASE
PO: ADULTS, ELDERLY: Initially, 0.375 mg/day in 3 divided doses. Don't increase dosage more frequently than every 5–7 days. Maintenance: 1.5–4.5 mg/day in 3 equally divided doses.

DOSAGE IN RENAL IMPAIRMENT
Dosage and frequency are modified based on creatinine clearance.

Creatinine Clearance	Initial Dose	Maximum Dose
Greater than 60 ml/min	0.125 mg 3 times a day	1.5 mg 3 times a day
35–60 ml/min	0.125 mg twice a day	1.5 mg twice a day
15–34 ml/min	0.125 mg once a day	1.5 mg once a day

SIDE EFFECTS

FREQUENT: **Early Parkinson's disease (28%–10%):** Nausea, asthenia, dizziness, somnolence, insomnia, constipation. **Advanced Parkinson's disease (53%–17%):** Orthostatic hypoten-sion, extrapyramidal reactions, insomnia, dizziness, hallucinations. OCCASIONAL: **Early Parkinson's disease (5%–2%):** Edema, malaise, confusion, amnesia, akathisia, anorexia, dysphagia, peripheral edema, vision changes, impotence. **Advanced Parkinson's disease (10%–7%):** Asthenia, somnolence, confusion, con-stipation, abnormal gait, dry mouth. RARE: **Advanced Parkinson's disease (6%–2%):** General edema, malaise, chest pain, amnesia, tremor, urinary frequency or incontinence, dyspnea, rhinitis, vision changes.

ADVERSE REACTIONS/ TOXIC EFFECTS

Vascular disease, MI, angina pectoris, atrial fibrillation, heart failure, arrhythmia, atrial arrhythmia, and pulmonary embolism have been reported.

NURSING CONSIDERATIONS

INTERVENTION/EVALUATION

Instruct patient to rise from lying to sitting or sitting to standing position slowly to prevent risk of postural hypotension. Assess for clinical improvement. Assist with ambulation if dizziness occurs. Assess for con-stipation; encourage fiber, fluids, exercise.

PATIENT/FAMILY TEACHING

• Inform patient that hallucinations may occur, especially in the elderly. • Postural hypotension may occur more frequently during initial therapy. • Avoid tasks that require alertness, motor skills until response to drug is established. • If nausea occurs, take medication with food. • Avoid abrupt withdrawal.

P

pramlintide acetate

pram-lin-tide
(Symlin)

CLASSIFICATION

PHARMACOTHERAPEUTIC: Antihyperglycemic. **CLINICAL:** Antidiabetic.

ACTION

Co-secreted with insulin by pancreatic beta cells, reduces postprandial glucose increases by the following mechanisms: slows gastric emptying time, reduces postprandial glucagon secretion, reduces caloric intake through centrally-mediated appetite suppression. **Therapeutic Effect:** Improves glycemic control by reducing postprandial glucose concentrations in patients with type 1 and type 2 diabetes mellitus.

PHARMACOKINETICS

	Onset	Peak	Duration
Sub-cutaneous	NA	20 min	3 hr

Metabolized primarily by the kidneys. Protein binding: 60%. Excreted in the urine. Half-life: 48 min.

USES

Adjunctive treatment with mealtime insulin in type 1 and type 2 diabetes mellitus patients who have failed to achieve desired glucose control despite optimal insulin therapy and with or without concurrent sulfonylurea and/or metformin in type 2 diabetes mellitus.

PRECAUTIONS

CONTRAINDICATIONS: Diagnosed gastroparesis, presence of hypoglycemia or recurrent severe hypoglycemic episodes in the past 6 mo, poor compliance with insulin monitoring or current insulin therapy, those with a hemoglobin A_{1c} greater than 9%, patients with conditions or taking concurrent medications likely to impair gastric motility (e.g., anticholinergics), in patients requiring medication to stimulate gastric emptying. **CAUTIONS:** Coadministration with insulin may induce severe hypoglycemia (usually with 3 hr following administration); concurrent use of other glucose-lowering agents may increase risk of hypoglycemia.

LIFESPAN CONSIDERATIONS: Pregnancy/Lactation: Unknown if distributed in breast milk. **Pregnancy Category C. Children:** Safety and efficacy not established. **Elderly:** No age related precautions noted.

INTERACTIONS

DRUG: Acarbose, anticholinergics, miglitol: Alter GI motility or slow intestinal absorption and may delay absorption of concomitantly administered medication due to increased gastric emptying time. **Agents in which a rapid onset of action is desired (e.g., analgesics):** Coadministration may delay drug response; separate by at least 1 hr before or 2 hr after pramlinitide administration. **Alpha-blockers, anabolic steroids, angiotensin-converting enzyme (ACE) inhibitors, clofibrate, clonidine, disopyramide, fenfluramine, fibrates, fluoxetine, guanethidine, MAOIs, pentamidine, pentoxifylline, phenylbutazone, propoxyphene, reserpine, salicylates, sulfinpyrazone, sulfonamides, tetracyclines:** May induce or exacerbate hypoglycemia. **Beta-blockers:** May delay recovery from hypoglycemic episodes and mask signs and symptoms of hypoglycemia. **HERBAL: Garlic, chromium, gymnema:** Increase the risk of hypoglycemia. **FOOD: Ethanol:** Increases the risk of hypoglycemia. **LAB VALUES:** Decreases glucose serum levels.

AVAILABILITY (Rx)

SOLUTION FOR INJECTION: 0.6 mg/ml in 5 ml vials (Symlin).

ADMINISTRATION/HANDLING

SUBCUTANEOUS

• Administer immediately before each major meal (350 or more kcal or containing 30 g or more carbohydrate). • Give in abdomen or thigh; do not give in arm (variable absorption). • Injection site should be distinct from insulin injection site. • Rotation of injection sites is essential. • Use U-100 insulin syringe for accuracy. • Always give pramlintide and insulin as separate injections.

Storage • Store unopened vials in refrigerator. • Discard if freezing occurs. • Vials that have been opened (punctured) may be stored in refrigerator or kept at room temperature for up to 28 days.

INDICATIONS/ROUTES/DOSAGE

◀ **ALERT** ▶ Initially, current insulin dosage in all patients with both type 1 and type 2 diabetes mellitus should be reduced by 50%. This includes preprandial, rapid-acting, short-acting, fixed-mixed (70/30) insulins.

TYPE 1 DIABETES MELLITUS

SUBCUTANEOUS: ADULTS, ELDERLY: Initially, 15 mcg immediately before a major meal. Titrate in 15 mcg increments every 3 days (if no significant nausea occurs) to target dose of 30–60 mcg.

TYPE 2 DIABETES MELLITUS

SUBCUTANEOUS: ADULTS, ELDERLY: Initially, 60 mcg immediately before a major meal. After 3–7 days, increase to 120 mcg if no significant nausea occurs (if nausea occurs at 120 mcg dose, reduce to 60 mcg).

SIDE EFFECTS

TYPE 1 DIABETES MELLITUS

FREQUENT (48%): Nausea. **OCCASIONAL (17%–11%):** Anorexia, vomiting. **RARE (7%–5%):** Fatigue, arthralgia, allergic reaction, dizziness.

TYPE 2 DIABETES MELLITUS

FREQUENT (28%): Nausea. **OCCASIONAL (13%–8%):** Headache, anorexia, vomiting, abdominal pain. **RARE (7%–5%):** Fatigue, dizziness, cough, pharyngitis.

ADVERSE REACTIONS/ TOXIC EFFECTS

Overdose produces severe nausea, vomiting, diarrhea, vasodilation, dizziness. No hypoglycemia was reported. When given concurrently with nontitrated insulin, there is an increased risk of severe hypoglycemia.

NURSING CONSIDERATIONS

BASELINE ASSESSMENT

Check blood glucose concentration before administration, both pre- and post-meals and at bedtime. Discuss lifestyle to determine extent of learning, emotional needs. Ensure follow-up instruction if patient or family does not thoroughly understand diabetes management or glucose-testing technique.

INTERVENTION/EVALUATION

Risk for hypoglycemia occurs within the first 3 hr following drug administration if given concurrently with insulin. Assess for hypoglycemia (diaphoresis, tremors, dizziness, anxiety, headache, tachycardia, numbness in mouth, hunger, diplopia, difficulty concentrating). Be alert to conditions that alter glucose requirements: fever, increased activity or stress, surgical procedures.

PATIENT/FAMILY TEACHING

• Diabetes mellitus requires lifelong control. • Prescribed diet and exercise is principal part of treatment; do not skip or delay meals. • Continue to adhere to dietary instructions, a regular exercise program, and regular testing of blood glucose. • When taking

P

combination drug therapy, have a source of glucose available to treat symptoms of low blood sugar.

Prandin, *see repaglinide*

Pravachol, *see pravastatin*

pravastatin

pra-vah-sta-tin
(Pravachol)
Do not confuse pravastatin with Prevacid, or Pravachol with propranolol.

FIXED-COMBINATION(S)

Pravigard: pravastatin/aspirin (anticoagulant): 20 mg/81 mg; 40 mg/81 mg; 80 mg/81 mg; 20 mg/325 mg; 40 mg/325 mg; 80 mg/325 mg.

◆CLASSIFICATION

PHARMACOTHERAPEUTIC: Hydroxymethylglutaryl CoA (HMG-CoA) reductase inhibitor. **CLINICAL:** Antihyperlipidemic (see p. 52C).

ACTION

An HMG-CoA reductase inhibitor that interferes with cholesterol biosynthesis by preventing the conversion of HMG-CoA reductase to mevalonate, a precursor to cholesterol. **Therapeutic Effect:** Lowers serum LDL and VLDL cholesterol and plasma triglyceride levels; increases serum HDL concentration.

PHARMACOKINETICS

Poorly absorbed from the GI tract. Protein binding: 50%. Metabolized in the liver (minimal active metabolites). Primarily excreted in feces via the biliary system. Not removed by hemodialysis. **Half-life:** 2.7 hr.

USES

Primary prevention of coronary events in patients with hypercholesterol without established coronary heart disease to reduce risk of MI, coronary revascularization procedures. Secondary prevention of coronary events in patients with established coronary heart disease to slow progression of coronary atherosclerosis, reduce risk of MI, coronary vascular procedures, stroke, transient ischemic attacks (TIAs). Treatment of hyperlipidemias to reduce total cholesterol, LDL-C, apolipoprotein B and triglycerides. Treatment of heterozygous familial hypercholesterolemia in pediatric patients 8–18 yr of age.

PRECAUTIONS

CONTRAINDICATIONS: Active hepatic disease or unexplained, persistent elevations of liver function test results. **CAUTIONS:** History of hepatic disease, substantial alcohol consumption. Withholding or discontinuing pravastatin may be necessary when patient is at risk for renal failure secondary to rhabdomyolysis. Severe metabolic, endocrine, electrolyte disorders.

⧖ **LIFESPAN CONSIDERATIONS: Pregnancy/Lactation:** Contraindicated in pregnancy (suppression of cholesterol biosynthesis may cause fetal toxicity) and lactation. Unknown if drug is distributed in breast milk, but there is risk of serious adverse reactions in breastfeeding infants. **Pregnancy Category X. Children:** Safety and efficacy not established. **Elderly:** No age-related precautions noted.

INTERACTIONS

DRUG: Cyclosporine, erythromycin, gemfibrozil, immunosuppressants, niacin: Increases the risk of acute renal failure and rhabdomyolysis. **HERBAL:** None known. **FOOD:** None known. **LAB VALUES:** May increase serum creatine kinase (CK) and transaminase concentrations.

AVAILABILITY (Rx)

TABLETS: 10 mg, 20 mg, 40 mg, 80 mg.

ADMINISTRATION/HANDLING

PO
• Give without regard to meals.
• Administer in evening.

INDICATIONS/ROUTES/DOSAGE

HYPERLIPIDEMIA, PRIMARY AND SECONDARY PREVENTION OF CARDIOVASCULAR EVENTS IN PATIENT WITH ELEVATED CHOLESTEROL LEVELS
PO: ADULTS, ELDERLY: Initially, 40 mg/day. Titrate to desired response. Range: 10–80 mg/day. CHILDREN 14–18 YR: 40 mg/day. CHILDREN 8–13 YR: 20 mg/day.

DOSAGE IN HEPATIC AND RENAL IMPAIRMENT
For adults, give 10 mg/day initially. Titrate to desired response.

SIDE EFFECTS

Pravastatin is generally well tolerated. Side effects are usually mild and transient. **OCCASIONAL (7%–4%):** Nausea, vomiting, diarrhea, constipation, abdominal pain, headache, rhinitis, rash, pruritus. **RARE (3%–2%):** Heartburn, myalgia, dizziness, cough, fatigue, flu-like symptoms.

ADVERSE REACTIONS/ TOXIC EFFECTS

Malignancy and cataracts may occur. Hypersensitivity occurs rarely. Myopathy and rhabdomyolysis have been reported.

BASELINE ASSESSMENT
Question for possibility of pregnancy before initiating therapy (Pregnancy Category X). Assess baseline serum lab results: cholesterol, triglycerides, liver function tests.

INTERVENTION/EVALUATION
Monitor serum cholesterol, triglyceride lab results for therapeutic response. Monitor liver function tests. Determine pattern of bowel activity. Check for headache, dizziness (provide assistance as needed). Assess for rash, pruritus. Be alert for malaise, muscle cramping or weakness; if accompanied by fever, may require discontinuation of medication.

PATIENT/FAMILY TEACHING
• Follow special diet (important part of treatment). • Periodic lab tests are essential part of therapy. • Report promptly any muscle pain/weakness, especially if accompanied by fever, malaise. • Avoid tasks that require alertness, motor skills until response to drug is established (potential for dizziness). • Use nonhormonal contraception.

prazosin hydrochloride

pra-zoe-sin
(Minipress)

FIXED-COMBINATION(S)

Minizide: prazosin/polythiazide (a diuretic): 1 mg/0.5 mg; 2 mg/0.5 mg; 5 mg/0.5 mg.

•CLASSIFICATION

PHARMACOTHERAPEUTIC: Alpha-adrenergic blocker. **CLINICAL:** Antihypertensive, antidote, vasodilator (see p. 55C).

ACTION

An antidote, antihypertensive, and vasodilator that selectively blocks alpha$_1$-adrenergic receptors, decreasing peripheral vascular resistance. **Therapeutic Effect:** Produces vasodilation of veins and arterioles, decreases total peripheral resistance, and relaxes smooth muscle in bladder neck and prostate.

PHARMACOKINETICS

Well absorbed following oral administration. Protein binding: 92%–97%. Metabolized in liver. Primarily excreted in feces. **Half-life:** 2–4 hr.

USES

Treatment of mild to moderate hypertension. Used alone or in combination with other antihypertensives. **OFF-LABEL:** Treatment of benign prostate hyperplasia, CHF, ergot alkaloid toxicity, pheochromocytoma, Raynaud's phenomenon.

PRECAUTIONS

CONTRAINDICATIONS: Hypersensitivity to quinazolines. **CAUTIONS:** Chronic renal failure, hepatic impairment.

⧗ LIFESPAN CONSIDERATIONS: **Pregnancy/Lactation:** Unknown if drug crosses placenta; is distributed in breast milk. **Pregnancy Category C. Children:** Safety and efficacy not established. **Elderly:** May be more sensitive to hypotensive effects.

INTERACTIONS

DRUG: Estrogen, NSAIDs, other sympathomimetics: May decrease the effects of prazosin. **Hypotension-producing medications, such as antihypertensives and diuretics:** May increase the effects of prazosin. **HERBAL: Licorice:** Causes sodium and water retention, potassium loss. **FOOD:** None known. **LAB VALUES:** None known.

AVAILABILITY (Rx)

CAPSULES: 1 mg, 2 mg, 5 mg.

ADMINISTRATION/HANDLING

PO
• Give without regard to food.
• Administer first dose at bedtime (minimizes risk of fainting due to "first-dose syncope").

INDICATIONS/ROUTES/DOSAGE

MILD TO MODERATE HYPERTENSION

PO: ADULTS, ELDERLY: Initially, 1 mg 2–3 times a day. Maintenance: 3–15 mg/day in divided doses. **Maximum:** 20 mg/day. CHILDREN: 5 mcg/kg/dose q6h. Gradually increase up to 25 mcg/kg/dose.

SIDE EFFECTS

FREQUENT (10%–7%): Dizziness, somnolence, headache, asthenia (loss of strength, energy). **OCCASIONAL (5%–4%):** Palpitations, nausea, dry mouth, nervousness. **RARE (less than 1%):** Angina, urinary urgency.

ADVERSE REACTIONS/TOXIC EFFECTS

First-dose syncope (hypotension with sudden loss of consciousness) may occur 30–90 min following initial dose of more than 2 mg, a too-rapid increase in dosage, or addition of another antihypertensive agent to therapy. First-dose syncope may be preceded by tachycardia (pulse rate of 120–160 beats/min).

NURSING CONSIDERATIONS

BASELINE ASSESSMENT

Give first dose at bedtime. If initial dose is given during daytime, patient must remain recumbent for 3–4 hr. Assess BP, pulse immediately before each dose and q15–30min until stabilized (be alert to BP fluctuations).

INTERVENTION/EVALUATION

Monitor BP, pulse diligently (first-dose syncope may be preceded by tachycardia). Monitor pattern of daily bowel activity and stool consistency. Assist with ambulation if dizziness occurs.

PATIENT/FAMILY TEACHING

• Avoid tasks that require alertness, motor skills until response to drug is established. • Use caution when rising from sitting or lying position. • Report continued dizziness or palpitations.

---

prednicarbate

(Dermatop)
See Corticosteroids: topical (p. 87C)

---

*prednisoLONE   @

pred-**niss**-oh-lone

(AK-Pred, AK-Tate 🍁, Cotolone, Depo-Predate, Hydeltrasol, Inflamase Forte, Inflamase Mild, Key-Pred, Key-Pred SP, Minims-Prednisolone 🍁, Novo-Prednisolone 🍁, <u>Orapred</u>, Pediapred, Predacort 50, Predaject-50, Predate-50, Pred Forte, Pred-Ject-50, Pred Mild, Prednisolone Acetate, Prelone)

Do not confuse prednisolone with prednisone or primidone.

FIXED-COMBINATION(S)

Blephamide: prednisolone/sulfacetamide (an anti-infective): 0.2%/10%. **Vasocidin:** prednisolone/sulfacetamide: 0.25%/10%.

◆CLASSIFICATION

PHARMACOTHERAPEUTIC: Adrenal corticosteroid. **CLINICAL:** Glucocorticoid (see p. 84C).

ACTION

An adrenocortical steroid that inhibits accumulation of inflammatory cells at inflammation sites, phagocytosis, lysosomal enzyme release and synthesis, and release of mediators of inflammation. **Therapeutic Effect:** Prevents or suppresses cell-mediated immune reactions. Decreases or prevents tissue response to inflammatory process.

USES

Substitution Therapy in Deficiency States: Acute or chronic adrenal insufficiency, congenital adrenal hyperplasia, adrenal insufficiency secondary to pituitary insufficiency. **Nonendocrine Disorders:** Allergic, collagen, intestinal tract, hepatic, ocular, renal, skin diseases; bronchial asthma; arthritis; rheumatic carditis; cerebral edema; malignancies. **Ophthalmic:** Treatment conjunctivitis, corneal injury (from chemical or thermal burns, foreign body).

PRECAUTIONS

CONTRAINDICATIONS: Acute superficial herpes simplex keratitis, systemic fungal infections, varicella. **CAUTIONS:** Hyperthyroidism, cirrhosis, ocular herpes simplex, peptic ulcer disease, osteoporosis, myasthenia gravis, hypertension, CHF, ulcerative colitis, thromboembolic disorders. **Pregnancy Category C. (D if used in first trimester).**

INTERACTIONS

DRUG: Amphotericin: May increase hypokalemia. **Digoxin:** May increase the risk of digoxin toxicity caused by hypokalemia. **Diuretics, insulin, oral hypoglycemics, potassium supplements:** May decrease the effects of these drugs. **Hepatic enzyme inducers:** May decrease the effects of prednisolone. **Live virus vaccines:** May decrease the patient's antibody response to vaccine, increase vaccine side effects, and potentiate virus replication. **HERBAL:** None known. **FOOD:** None known. **LAB VALUES:** May increase blood glucose and serum lipid, amylase, and sodium levels. May decrease serum calcium, potassium, and thyroxine levels.

AVAILABILITY (Rx)

TABLETS: 5 mg. **SYRUP:** 5 mg/5 ml (Prelone), 15 mg/5 ml (Prednisolone Acetate, Prelone). **ORAL LIQUID, SODIUM PHOSPHATE:** 5 mg/5 ml (Orapred, Pediapred), 15 mg/5 ml (Orapred). **INJECTABLE SOLUTION, SODIUM PHOS-PHATE (HYDELTRASOL, KEY-PRED SP):** 20 mg/ml. **INJECTABLE SUSPENSION, ACETATE:** 25 mg/ml (Cotolone, Key-Pred), 40 mg/ml (Depo-Predate), 50 mg/ml (Cotolone, Predacort 50, Predaject-50, Predate-50, Pred-Ject-50), 80 mg/ml (Depo-Predate). **OPHTHALMIC SOLUTION, SODIUM PHOSPHATE:** 0.125% (Inflamase Mild), 1% (AK-Pred, Inflamase Forte). **OPHTHALMIC SUSPENSION, ACETATE:** 0.12% (Pred Mild), 1% (Pred Forte).

ADMINISTRATION/HANDLING

IM, INTRA-ARTICULAR, INTRALESIONAL

• Do not administer prednisolone intravenously. • Shake well before using. • Inject into joint, lesion, or muscle as needed.

PO

• Give without regard to meals; give with food if GI upset occurs.

OPHTHALMIC

• For ophthalmic solution, shake well before using. • Instill drops into conjunctival sac, as prescribed. • Avoid touching the applicator tip to the conjunctiva to avoid contamination.

▩ IV INCOMPATIBILITIES

Do not mix with other medications.

INDICATIONS/ROUTES/DOSAGE

SUBSTITUTION THERAPY FOR DEFICIENCY STATES; ACUTE OR CHRONIC ADRENAL INSUFFICIENCY, CONGENITAL ADRENAL HYPERPLASIA, AND ADRENAL INSUFFICIENCY SECONDARY TO PITUITARY INSUFFICIENCY; NONENDOCRINE DISORDERS: ARTHRITIS; RHEUMATIC CARDITIS; ALLERGIC, COLLAGEN, INTESTINAL TRACT, LIVER, OCULAR, RENAL, SKIN DISEASES; BRONCHIAL ASTHMA; CEREBRAL EDEMA; MALIGNANCIES

PO: ADULTS, ELDERLY: 5–60 mg/day in divided doses. CHILDREN: 0.1–2 mg/kg/day in 1–4 divided doses.

INTRA-ARTICULAR, INTRALESIONAL (ACETATE): ADULTS, ELDERLY: 4–100 mg, repeated as needed.

INTRA-ARTICULAR, INTRALESIONAL (SODIUM PHOSPHATE): ADULTS, ELDERLY: 2–30 mg, repeated at 3-day to 3-wk intervals, as needed.

IM (ACETATE, SODIUM PHOSPHATE): ADULTS, ELDERLY: 4–60 mg a day.

TREATMENT OF CONJUCTIVITIS AND CORNEAL INJURY

OPHTHALMIC: ADULTS, ELDERLY: 1–2 drops every hr during day and q2h during night. After response, decrease dosage to 1 drop q4h, then 1 drop 3–4 times a day.

SIDE EFFECTS

FREQUENT: Insomnia, heartburn, nervousness, abdominal distention, increased sweating, acne, mood swings, increased appetite, facial flushing, delayed wound healing, increased susceptibility to infection, diarrhea or constipation. **OCCASIONAL:** Headache, edema, change in skin color, frequent urination. **RARE:** Tachycardia, allergic reaction (such as rash and hives), psychological changes, hallucinations, depression. **Ophthalmic:** stinging or burning, posterior subcapsular cataracts.

ADVERSE REACTIONS/ TOXIC EFFECTS

Long-term therapy may cause hypocalcemia, hypokalemia, muscle wasting (especially in the arms and legs), osteoporosis, spontaneous fractures, amenorrhea, cataracts, glaucoma, peptic ulcer disease, and CHF. Abruptly withdrawing the drug after long-term therapy may cause anorexia, nausea, fever, headache, severe or sudden joint pain, rebound inflammation, fatigue, weakness, lethargy, dizziness, and orthostatic hypotension. Suddenly discontinuing prednisolone may be fatal.

NURSING CONSIDERATIONS

BASELINE ASSESSMENT

Obtain baselines for height, weight, BP, serum glucose, electrolytes. Check results of initial tests (e.g., tuberculosis (TB) skin test, x-rays, EKG). Never give live virus vaccine (e.g., smallpox).

INTERVENTION/EVALUATION

Monitor BP, weight, serum electrolytes, glucose, height, weight in children. Be alert to infection (sore throat, fever, vague symptoms); assess oral cavity daily for signs of candida infection (white patches, painful tongue or mucous membranes).

PATIENT/FAMILY TEACHING

• Notify physician of fever, sore throat, muscle aches, sudden weight gain/ swelling. • Avoid alcohol, minimize use of caffeine. • Do not abruptly discontinue without physician's approval. • Avoid exposure to chickenpox, measles.

---

*predniSONE

pred-ni-sone
(Apo-Prednisone ♣, Deltasone, Liquid Pred, Meticorten, Prednicen-M, Prednicot, Prednisone Intensol, Sterapred, Sterapred DS, Winpred ♣)

Do not confuse prednisone with prednisolone or primidone.

CLASSIFICATION

PHARMACOTHERAPEUTIC: Adrenal corticosteroid. **CLINICAL:** Glucocorticoid (see p. 84C).

ACTION

An adrenocortical steroid that inhibits accumulation of inflammatory cells at inflammation sites, phagocytosis, lysosomal enzyme release and synthesis, and release of mediators of inflammation. Therapeutic Effect: Prevents or suppresses cell-mediated immune reactions. Decreases or prevents tissue response to inflammatory process.

PHARMACOKINETICS

Well absorbed from the GI tract. Protein binding: 70%-90%. Widely distributed. Metabolized in the liver and converted to prednisolone. Primarily excreted in urine. Not removed by hemodialysis. Half-life: 3.4-3.8 hr.

USES

Substitution Therapy in Deficiency States: Acute or chronic adrenal insufficiency, congenital adrenal hyperplasia, adrenal insufficiency secondary to pituitary insufficiency. **Nonendocrine Disorders:** Arthritis; rheumatic carditis; allergic, collagen, intestinal tract, liver, ocular, renal, skin diseases; bronchial asthma; cerebral edema; malignancies.

P

PRECAUTIONS

CONTRAINDICATIONS: Acute superficial herpes simplex keratitis, systemic fungal infections, varicella. **CAUTIONS:** Hyperthyroidism, cirrhosis, ocular herpes simplex, peptic ulcer disease, osteoporosis, myasthenia gravis, hypertension, CHF, ulcerative colitis, thromboembolic disorders.

⧗ **LIFESPAN CONSIDERATIONS: Pregnancy/Lactation:** Crosses placenta. Distributed in breast milk. Cleft palate generally occurs with chronic use, first trimester. **Pregnancy Category C (D if used in first trimester). Children:** Prolonged treatment or high dosages may decrease short-term growth rate, cortisol secretion. **Elderly:** May be more susceptible to developing hypertension or osteoporosis.

INTERACTIONS

DRUG: Amphotericin: May increase hypokalemia. **Digoxin:** May increase the risk of digoxin toxicity caused by hypokalemia. **Diuretics, insulin, oral hypoglycemics, potassium supplements:** May decrease the effects of these drugs. **Hepatic enzyme inducers:** May decrease the effects of prednisone. **Live virus vaccines:** May decrease the patient's antibody response to vaccine, increase vaccine side effects, and potentiate virus replication. **HERBAL:** None known. **FOOD:** None known. **LAB VALUES:** May increase blood glucose and serum lipid, amylase, and sodium levels. May decrease serum calcium, potassium, and thyroxine levels.

AVAILABILITY (Rx)

ORAL CONCENTRATE (PREDNISONE INTENSOL): 5 mg/ml. **ORAL SOLUTION (LIQUID PRED):** 5 mg/5 ml. **TABLETS:** 1 mg (Sterapred), 2.5 mg (Deltasone), 5 mg (Deltasone, Prednicen-M, Sterapred), 10 mg (Deltasone, Sterapred), 20 mg (Deltasone), 50 mg (Deltasone).

ADMINISTRATION/HANDLING

PO
• Give without regard to meals (give with food if GI upset occurs). • Give single doses before 9 AM, multiple doses at evenly spaced intervals.

INDICATIONS/ROUTES/DOSAGE

SUBSTITUTION THERAPY IN DEFICIENCY STATES: ACUTE OR CHRONIC ADRENAL INSUFFICIENCY, CONGENITAL ADRENAL HYPERPLASIA, AND ADRENAL INSUFFICIENCY SECONDARY TO PITUITARY INSUFFICIENCY; NONENDOCRINE DISORDERS: ARTHRITIS; RHEUMATIC CARDITIS; ALLERGIC, COLLAGEN, INTESTINAL TRACT, LIVER, OCULAR, RENAL, SKIN DISEASES; BRONCHIAL ASTHMA; CEREBRAL EDEMA; MALIGNANCIES
PO: ADULTS, ELDERLY: 5–60 mg/day in divided doses. CHILDREN: 0.05–2 mg/kg/day in 1–4 divided doses.

SIDE EFFECTS

FREQUENT: Insomnia, heartburn, nervousness, abdominal distention, increased sweating, acne, mood swings, increased appetite, facial flushing, delayed wound healing, increased susceptibility to infection, diarrhea or constipation. **OCCASIONAL:** Headache, edema, change in skin color, frequent urination. **RARE:** Tachycardia, allergic reaction (including rash and hives), psychological changes, hallucinations, depression.

ADVERSE REACTIONS/ TOXIC EFFECTS

Long-term therapy may cause muscle wasting in the arms and legs, osteoporosis, spontaneous fractures, amenorrhea, cataracts, glaucoma, peptic ulcer disease, and CHF. Abruptly withdrawing the drug following long-term therapy may cause anorexia, nausea, fever, headache, sudden or severe joint pain, rebound inflammation, fatigue, weakness, lethargy, dizziness, and orthostatic

---

* "Tall Man" lettering   ✐ see color pill atlas   ◢ herb   underlined – top prescribed drug

hypotension. Suddenly discontinuing prednisone may be fatal.

NURSING CONSIDERATIONS

BASELINE ASSESSMENT
Obtain baselines for height, weight, BP, serum glucose, electrolytes. Check results of initial tests (e.g., tuberculosis (TB) skin test, x-rays, EKG). Never give live virus vaccine (e.g., smallpox).

INTERVENTION/EVALUATION
Monitor BP, weight, serum electrolytes, glucose, height, weight. Be alert to infection (sore throat, fever, vague symptoms); assess oral cavity daily for signs of candida infection (white patches, painful tongue or mucous membranes).

PATIENT/FAMILY TEACHING
• Notify physician of fever, sore throat, muscle aches, sudden weight gain or swelling. • Avoid alcohol, minimize use of caffeine. • Do not abruptly discontinue without physician's approval. • Avoid exposure to chickenpox, measles.

pregabalin

pre-**gab**-ah-lin
(Lyrica)

◆CLASSIFICATION

CLINICAL: Anticonvulsant, antineuralgic, analgesic (**Schedule V**).

ACTION

Binds to alpha2-delta site (a subunit of calcium channels) in CNS tissue, inhibiting excitatory neurotransmitter release. Exerts anti-nociceptive and anticonvulsant activity. **Therapeutic Effect:** Decreases symptoms of painful peripheral neuropathy; decreases the frequency of partial seizures.

PHARMACOKINETICS

Well absorbed following oral administration. Eliminated in the urine. **Half-life:** 6 hr.

USES

Adjunctive therapy in treatment of partial onset seizures. Management of neuropathic pain associated with diabetic peripheral neuropathy. Management of postherpetic neuralgia.

PRECAUTIONS

CONTRAINDICATIONS: None known.
CAUTIONS: CHF, renal impairment.
⚱ **LIFESPAN CONSIDERATIONS: Pregnancy/Lactation:** Increased risk of fetal skeletal abnormalities. Unknown if distributed in breast milk. **Pregnancy Category C. Children:** Safety and efficacy not established. **Elderly:** Age-related renal function impairment may require dosage adjustment.

INTERACTIONS

DRUG: Alcohol, barbiturates, narcotic analgesics, other sedative agents: May increase sedative effect. **Pioglitazone, rosiglitazone:** Effect on weight gain or edema may be additive with these drugs. **HERBAL: Gotu kola, kava kava, St. John's wort, valerian:** May increase CNS depression. **FOOD:** None known. **LAB VALUES:** May increase CPK, mild PR interval prolongation. May decrease glucose, platelet count.

AVAILABILITY (Rx)

CAPSULES: 25 mg, 50 mg, 75 mg, 100 mg, 150 mg, 200 mg, 225 mg, 300 mg (Lyrica).

ADMINISTRATION/HANDLING
• Give without regard to food. • Do not open or crush capsule.

INDICATIONS/ROUTES/DOSAGE
PARTIAL ONSET SEIZURES
PO: ADULTS, ELDERLY: Initially, 75 mg twice a day or 50 mg 3 times a day.

P

Dosage may be increased to maximum 600 mg a day.

NEUROPATHIC PAIN

PO: ADULTS, ELDERLY: Initially, 50 mg 3 times a day. Dosage may be increased to maximum 300 mg a day, based on efficacy and tolerability.

POSTHERPETIC NEURALGIA

PO: ADULTS, ELDERLY: Initially, 75 mg twice a day or 50 mg 3 times a day. Dosage may be increased to maximum 300 mg a day.

DOSAGE IN RENAL IMPAIRMENT

Creatinine Clearance	Dosage (mg/day)
Greater than 60 ml/min	150–300 mg in 2 to 3 divided daily doses
30–60 ml/min	75–150 mg in 2 to 3 divided daily doses
15–29 ml/min	25–50 mg in single or 2 divided daily doses
Less than 15 ml/min	25–50 mg in single divided dose

DOSAGE FOR HEMODIALYSIS

◀ **ALERT** ▶ Take supplemental dose immediately following dialysis.

Daily Dosage	Supplemental Dosage
25 mg	Single dose of 25 mg or 50 mg
25–50 mg	Single dose of 50 mg or 75 mg
75 mg	Single dose of 100 mg or 150 mg

SIDE EFFECTS

FREQUENT (32%–12%): Dizziness, somnolence, ataxia, peripheral edema. **OCCASIONAL (12%–5%):** Weight gain, blurred vision, diplopia, difficulty with concentration, attention, cognition; tremor, dry mouth, headache, constipation, asthenia (loss of strength, energy). **RARE (4%–2%):** Abnormal gait, confusion, incoordination, twitching, flatulence, vomiting, edema.

ADVERSE REACTIONS/ TOXIC EFFECTS

Abrupt withdrawal increases risk of seizure frequency in patients with seizure disorders; withdraw gradually over a minimum of 1 wk.

NURSING CONSIDERATIONS

BASELINE ASSESSMENT

Seizure: Review history of seizure disorder (type, onset, intensity, frequency, duration, level of consciousness [LOC]). **Pain:** Assess onset, type, location, and duration of pain.

INTERVENTION/EVALUATION

Provide safety measures as needed. Assess for seizure activity. Assess for clinical improvement and record onset of relief of pain. Assess for evidence of peripheral edema behind medial malleolus (usually first area of edema). Question for changes in visual acuity.

PATIENT/FAMILY TEACHING

• Do not abruptly stop taking drug because seizure frequency may be increased. • Do not drive, operate machinery, or perform activities requiring mental acuity due to potential dizziness, somnolence, ataxia. • Avoid alcohol. • Carry identification card or bracelet to note anticonvulsant therapy. • If noncompliance is an issue in causing acute seizures, discuss reasons for noncompliance and address them.

Premarin, *see conjugated estrogens*

Prempro, *see estrogen and medroxyprogesterone*

Prevacid, *see lansoprazole*

Prilosec, *see omeprazole*

Primacor, *see milrinone*

Primaxin, *see imipenem and cilastatin*

primidone

pri-mi-done

(Apo-Primidone ✤, Mysoline)

Do not confuse primidone with prednisone.

◆ CLASSIFICATION

PHARMACOTHERAPEUTIC: Barbiturate. **CLINICAL:** Anticonvulsant (see p. 35C).

ACTION

A barbiturate that decreases motor activity from electrical and chemical stimulation and stabilizes the seizure threshold against hyperexcitability. **Therapeutic Effect:** Reduces seizure activity.

PHARMACOKINETICS

Rapidly and usually completely absorbed following oral administration. Protein binding: 20%–30%. Extensively metabolized in liver to phenobarbital and phenylethylmalonamide (PEMA). Minimal excretion in urine. **Half-life:** 3.3–7 hr.

USES

Management of partial seizures with complex symptomatology (psychomotor seizures), generalized tonic-clonic (grand mal) seizures. **OFF-LABEL:** Treatment of essential tremor.

PRECAUTIONS

CONTRAINDICATIONS: History of bronchopneumonia, hypersensitivity to phenobarbital, porphyria. **CAUTIONS:** Renal/hepatic impairment.

⌛ **LIFESPAN CONSIDERATIONS: Pregnancy/Lactation:** Crosses placenta; is distributed in breast milk. **Pregnancy Category D. Children, Elderly:** May produce paradoxical excitement, restlessness.

INTERACTIONS

DRUG: Alcohol, other CNS depressants: May increase the effects of primidone. **Carbamazepine:** May increase the metabolism of carbamazepine. **Digoxin, glucocorticoids, metronidazole, oral anticoagulants, quinidine, tricyclic antidepressants:** May decrease the effects of these drugs. **Valproic acid:** Increases the blood concentration and risk of toxicity of primidone. **HERBAL:** None known. **FOOD:** None known. **LAB VALUES:** May decrease serum bilirubin level. Therapeutic serum level is 4–12 mcg/ml; toxic serum level is greater than 12 mcg/ml.

AVAILABILITY (Rx)

TABLETS: 50 mg, 250 mg. **ORAL SUSPENSION:** 250 mg/5 ml.

INDICATIONS/ROUTES/DOSAGE

SEIZURE CONTROL

PO: ADULTS, ELDERLY, CHILDREN 8 YR AND OLDER: 125–150 mg/day at bedtime. May increase by 125–250 mg/day every 3–7 days. **Maximum:** 2 g/day. CHILDREN YOUNGER THAN 8 YR: Initially, 50–125 mg/day at bedtime. May increase by 50–125

P

✤ Canadian trade name   ⓔ see **evolve**   ▶ High Alert drug mg/day every 3–7 days. Usual dose: 10–25 mg/kg/day in divided doses. NEONATES: 12–20 mg/kg/day in divided doses.

SIDE EFFECTS

FREQUENT: Ataxia, dizziness. **OCCASIONAL:** Anorexia, drowsiness, mental changes, nausea, vomiting, paradoxical excitement. **RARE:** Rash.

ADVERSE REACTIONS/ TOXIC EFFECTS

Abrupt withdrawal after prolonged therapy may produce effects ranging from increased dreaming, nightmares, insomnia, tremor, diaphoresis, and vomiting to hallucinations, delirium, seizures, and status epilepticus. Skin eruptions may be a sign of a hypersensitivity reaction. Blood dyscrasias, hepatic disease, and hypocalcemia occur rarely. Overdose produces cold or clammy skin, hypothermia, and severe CNS depression, followed by high fever and coma.

NURSING CONSIDERATIONS

BASELINE ASSESSMENT

Review history of seizure disorder (intensity, frequency, duration, level of consciousness [LOC]). Observe frequently for recurrence of seizure activity. Initiate seizure precautions.

INTERVENTION/EVALUATION

Monitor serum concentrations; CBC; neurologic status: frequency, duration, severity of seizures. Monitor for therapeutic serum level: 4–12 mcg/ml; toxic serum level: more than 12 mcg/ml.

PATIENT/FAMILY TEACHING

• Do not abruptly withdraw medication after long-term use (may precipitate seizures). • Strict maintenance of drug therapy is essential for seizure control. • Drowsiness usually disappears during continued therapy. • If dizziness occurs, change positions slowly from recumbent to sitting position before standing. • Avoid tasks that require alertness, motor skills until response to drug is established. • Avoid alcohol.

Prinivil, *see lisinopril*

probenecid

proe-**ben**-e-sid
(Benuryl ✦)
Do not confuse probenecid with procainamide.

CLASSIFICATION

PHARMACOTHERAPEUTIC: Uricosuric. **CLINICAL:** Antigout.

ACTION

A uricosuric that competitively inhibits reabsorption of uric acid at the proximal convoluted tubule. Also, inhibits renal tubular secretion of weak organic acids, such as penicillins. **Therapeutic Effect:** Promotes uric acid excretion, reduces serum uric acid level, and increases plasma levels of penicillins and cephalosporins.

PHARMACOKINETICS

Rapidly and completely absorbed following oral administration. Protein binding: High. Extensively metabolized in liver. Excreted in urine. Excretion is dependent upon urinary pH and is increased in alkaline urine. **Half-life:** 3–8 hr (dose-dependent).

USES

Treatment of hyperuricemia associated with gout, gouty arthritis. Adjunctive therapy with penicillins or cephalosporins to elevate or prolong antibiotic plasma levels.

PRECAUTIONS

CONTRAINDICATIONS: Blood dyscrasias, children younger than 2 yr, concurrent high-dose aspirin therapy, severe renal impairment, uric acid calculi. **CAUTIONS:** Peptic ulcer, hematuria, renal colic.

⧗ **LIFESPAN CONSIDERATIONS: Pregnancy/Lactation:** Unknown if drug crosses placenta or is distributed in breast milk. **Pregnancy Category C. Children:** Safety and efficacy not established in children younger than 2 yr. **Elderly:** No age-related precautions noted.

INTERACTIONS

DRUG: Alcohol: May increase serum urate level. **Antineoplastics:** May increase the risk of uric acid nephropathy. **Cephalosporins, methotrexate, nitrofurantoin, NSAIDs, penicillins, zidovudine:** May increase blood concentrations of these drugs. **Heparin:** May increase and prolong the effects of heparin. **Salicylates:** May decrease uricosuric effect. **HERBAL:** None known. **FOOD:** None known. **LAB VALUES:** May inhibit renal excretion of serum PSP (phenolsulfonphthalein), 17-ketosteroids, and BSP (sulfobromophthalein).

AVAILABILITY (Rx)

TABLETS: 500 mg.

ADMINISTRATION/HANDLING

PO
• Give with or immediately after meals or milk. • Instruct patient to drink at least 6–8 glasses (8 oz) of water a day (prevents kidney stone development).

INDICATIONS/ROUTES/DOSAGE

GOUT
PO: ADULTS, ELDERLY: Initially, 250 mg twice a day for 1 wk; then 500 mg twice a day. May increase by 500 mg q4wk. **Maximum:** 2–3 g/day.

Maintenance: Dosage that maintains normal uric acid level.

AS ADJUNCT TO PENICILLIN OR CEPHALOSPORIN THERAPY TO PROLONG ANTIBIOTIC PLASMA LEVELS
PO: ADULTS, ELDERLY: 2 g/day in divided doses. **CHILDREN WEIGHING MORE THAN 50 KG:** Receive adult dosage. **CHILDREN 2–14 YR:** Initially, 25 mg/kg. Maintenance: 40 mg/kg/day in 4 divided doses.

GONORRHEA
PO: ADULTS, ELDERLY: 1 g 30 min before penicillin, ampicillin, or amoxicillin. **CHILDREN WEIGHING LESS THAN 45 KG:** 25 mg/kg 30 min before penicillin, ampicillin, amoxicillin. **Maximum:** 1 g.

SIDE EFFECTS

FREQUENT (10%–6%): Headache, anorexia, nausea, vomiting. **OCCASIONAL (5%–1%):** Lower back or side pain, rash, hives, itching, dizziness, flushed face, frequent urge to urinate, gingivitis.

ADVERSE REACTIONS/ TOXIC EFFECTS

Severe hypersensitivity reactions, including anaphylaxis, occur rarely and usually within a few hours after administration following previous use. If severe hypersensitivity reactions develop, discontinue the drug immediately and contact the physician. Pruritic maculopapular rash, possibly accompanied by malaise, fever, chills, arthralgia, nausea, vomiting, leukopenia, and aplastic anemias should be considered a toxic reaction.

NURSING CONSIDERATIONS

BASELINE ASSESSMENT
Do not initiate therapy until acute gouty attack has subsided. Question for hypersensitivity to probenecid or if taking penicillin or cephalosporin antibiotics.

INTERVENTION/EVALUATION
If exacerbation of gout recurs after therapy, use other agents for gout.

Discontinue medication immediately if rash or other evidence of allergic reaction appears. Encourage high fluid intake (3,000 ml/day). Monitor I&O (output should be at least 2,000 ml/day). Assess CBC, serum uric acid levels. Assess urine for cloudiness, unusual color, odor. Assess for therapeutic response (reduced joint tenderness, swelling, redness, limitation of motion).

PATIENT/FAMILY TEACHING

• Drink plenty of fluids to decrease risk of uric acid kidney stones. • Avoid alcohol, large doses of aspirin or other salicylates. • Encourage low-purine food intake (reduce or omit meat, fowl, fish; use eggs, cheese, vegetables). • Foods high in purine: kidney, liver, sweetbreads, sardines, anchovies, meat extracts. • May take over 1 wk for full therapeutic effect. • Drink 6–8 glasses (8 oz) of fluid daily while on medication.

---

procainamide hydrochloride

pro-**cane**-ah-myd
(Apo-Procainamide ✤, Procanbid, Procan-SR, Pronestyl, Pronestyl-SR)
Do not confuse with Procanbid with probenecid, or Pronestyl with Ponstel.

CLASSIFICATION

CLINICAL: Antiarrhythmic (see p. 14C).

ACTION

An antiarrhythmic that increases the electrical stimulation threshold of the ventricles and His-Purkinje system. Decreases myocardial excitability and conduction velocity and depresses myocardial contractility. Exerts direct cardiac effects. **Therapeutic Effect:** Suppresses arrhythmias.

PHARMACOKINETICS

Rapidly, completely absorbed from the GI tract. Protein binding: 15%–20%. Widely distributed. Metabolized in the liver to active metabolite. Primarily excreted in urine. Removed by hemodialysis. **Half-life:** 2.5–4.5 hr; metabolite, 6 hr.

USES

Prophylactic therapy to maintain normal sinus rhythm after conversion of atrial fibrillation or flutter. Treatment of premature ventricular contractions, paroxysmal atrial tachycardia, atrial fibrillation, ventricular tachycardia. **OFF-LABEL:** Conversion and management of atrial fibrillation.

PRECAUTIONS

CONTRAINDICATIONS: Complete heart block, myasthenia gravis, preexisting QT prolongation, second-degree heart block, systemic lupus erythematosus, torsades de pointes. **CAUTIONS:** Marked AV conduction disturbances, bundle-branch block, severe digoxin toxicity, CHF, supraventricular tachyarrhythmias, renal or hepatic impairment.

⧗ **LIFESPAN CONSIDERATIONS: Pregnancy/Lactation:** Crosses placenta. Unknown if distributed in breast milk. **Pregnancy Category C. Children:** No age-related precautions noted. **Elderly:** More susceptible to hypotensive effect. Age-related renal impairment may require dosage adjustment.

INTERACTIONS

DRUG: Antihypertensives (IV procainamide), neuromuscular blockers: May increase the effects of these drugs. May decrease antimyasthenic effect on skeletal muscle. **Other antiarrhythmics, pimozide:** May increase cardiac effects. **HERBAL:** None known.

FOOD: None known. **LAB VALUES:** May cause EKG changes and positive ANA titers and Coombs' test. May increase AST, ALT, serum alkaline phosphatase, serum bilirubin, and serum LDH levels. Therapeutic serum level is 4–8 mcg/ml; toxic serum level is greater than 10 mcg/ml.

AVAILABILITY (Rx)

CAPSULES (PRONESTYL): 250 mg, 500 mg. **TABLETS (PRONESTYL):** 250 mg, 375 mg, 500 mg. **TABLETS (EXTENDED-RELEASE):** 500 mg (Procanbid, Pronestyl-SR), 750 mg (Procanbid), 1,000 mg (Procanbid). **INJECTION (PRONESTYL):** 100 mg/ml, 500 mg/ml.

ADMINISTRATION/HANDLING

🖉 IV, IM

◀ **ALERT** ▶ May give by IM injection, IV push, IV infusion.

Reconstitution • For IV push, dilute with 5–10 ml D5W. • For initial loading infusion, add 1 g to 50 ml D5W to provide a concentration of 20 mg/ml. • For IV infusion, add 1 g to 250–500 ml D5W to provide concentration of 2–4 mg/ml. Maximum concentration: 4 g/250 ml.

Rate of administration • For IV push, with patient in supine position, administer at rate not exceeding 25–50 mg/min. • For initial loading infusion, infuse 1 ml/min for up to 25–30 min. • For IV infusion, infuse at 1–3 ml/min. • Check BP q5–10min during infusion. If fall in BP exceeds 15 mm Hg, discontinue drug, contact physician. • Monitor EKG for cardiac changes, particularly widening of QRS, prolongation of PR and QT intervals. Notify physician of any significant interval changes. • BP, EKG should be monitored continuously during IV administration and rate of infusion adjusted to eliminate arrhythmias.

Storage • Solution appears clear, colorless to light yellow. • Discard if solution darkens or appears discolored or if precipitate forms. • When diluted with D5W, solution is stable for 24 hr at room temperature or for 7 days if refrigerated.

PO

• Do not crush or break extended-release tablets.

▦ IV INCOMPATIBILITY

Milrinone (Primacor).

IV COMPATIBILITIES

Amiodarone (Cordarone), dobutamine (Dobutrex), heparin, lidocaine, potassium chloride.

INDICATIONS/ROUTES/DOSAGE

MAINTENANCE OF NORMAL SINUS RHYTHM AFTER CONVERSION OF ATRIAL FIBRILLATION OR FLUTTER; TREATMENT OF PREMATURE VENTRICULAR CONTRACTIONS, PAROXYSMAL ATRIAL TACHYCARDIA, ATRIAL FIBRILLATION, AND VENTRICULAR TACHYCARDIA

PO: ADULTS, ELDERLY: 250–500 mg of immediate-release tablets q3–6h. 0.5–1 g of extended-release tablets q6h. 1–2 g of Procanbid q12h. CHILDREN: 15–50 mg/kg/day of immediate-release tablets in divided doses q3–6h. **Maximum:** 4 g/day.

IV: ADULTS, ELDERLY: Loading dose: 50–100 mg. May repeat q5–10min or 15–18 mg/kg (**maximum:** 1–1.5 g). Then maintenance infusion of 3–4 mg/min. Range: 1–6 mg/min. CHILDREN: Loading dose: 3–6 mg/kg over 5 min (**maximum:** 100 mg). May repeat q5–10min to maximum total dose of 15 mg/kg. Then maintenance dose of 20–80 mcg/kg/min. **Maximum:** 2 g/day.

DOSAGE IN RENAL IMPAIRMENT

Dosage interval is modified based on creatinine clearance.

Creatinine Clearance	Dosage Interval
10–50 ml/min	q6–12h
Less than 10 ml/min	q8–24h

SIDE EFFECTS

FREQUENT: PO: Abdominal pain or cramping, nausea, diarrhea, vomiting. **OCCASIONAL:** Dizziness, giddiness, weakness, hypersensitivity reaction (rash, urticaria, pruritus, flushing). **IV:** Transient, but at times, marked hypotension. **RARE:** Confusion, mental depression, psychosis.

ADVERSE REACTIONS/ TOXIC EFFECTS

Paradoxical, extremely rapid ventricular rate may occur during treatment of atrial fibrillation or flutter. Systemic lupus erythematosus-like syndrome (fever, myalgia, pleuritic chest pain) may occur with prolonged therapy. Cardiotoxic effects occur most commonly with IV administration and appear as conduction changes (50% widening of QRS complex, frequent ventricular premature contractions, ventricular tachycardia, and complete AV block). Prolonged PR and QT intervals and flattened T waves occur less frequently.

NURSING CONSIDERATIONS

BASELINE ASSESSMENT

Check BP, pulse for 1 full min (unless patient is on continuous monitor) before giving medication.

INTERVENTION/EVALUATION

Monitor EKG for cardiac changes, particularly widening of QRS, prolongation of PR and QT intervals. Assess pulse for strength or weakness, irregular rate. Monitor I&O, serum electrolyte level (potassium, chloride, sodium). Assess for complaints of GI upset, headache, arthralgia. Monitor pattern of daily bowel activity and stool consistency. Assess for dizziness. Monitor BP for hypotension. Assess skin for evidence of hypersensitivity reaction (especially in patients on high-dose therapy). Monitor for therapeutic serum level (3–10 mcg/ml). Therapeutic serum level: 4–8 mcg/

ml; toxic serum level: greater than 10 mcg/ml.

PATIENT/FAMILY TEACHING

• Take medication at evenly spaced doses around the clock. • Contact physician if fever, joint pain or stiffness, signs of upper respiratory infection occur. • Avoid tasks that require alertness, motor skills until response to drug is established (potential for dizziness). • Do not abruptly discontinue medication. • Compliance with therapy regimen is essential to control arrhythmias. • Do not use nasal decongestants, OTC cold preparations (stimulants) without physician approval. • Restrict salt, alcohol intake.

procaine hydrochloride

(Novocaine)
See Anesthetics: local (p. 4C)

procarbazine hydrochloride   ⚑

pro-**car**-bah-zeen
(Matulane, Natulan ✦)
Do not confuse procarbazine with dacarbazine.

◆ CLASSIFICATION

PHARMACOTHERAPEUTIC: Methylhydrazine derivative. **CLINICAL:** Antineoplastic (see p. 77C).

ACTION

A methylhydrazine derivative that inhibits DNA, RNA, and protein synthesis. May also directly damage DNA. Cell cycle–phase specific for S phase of cell division. Therapeutic Effect: Causes cell death.

PHARMACOKINETICS

Rapidly and completely absorbed from the GI tract. Crosses blood-brain barrier. Metabolized primarily in liver and kidneys. Excreted in urine and feces. Half-life: 10 min.

USES

Treatment of advanced Hodgkin's disease. OFF-LABEL: Treatment of lung carcinoma, malignant melanoma, multiple myeloma, non-Hodgkin's lymphoma, polycythemia vera, primary brain tumors.

PRECAUTIONS

CONTRAINDICATIONS: Myelosuppression. **CAUTIONS:** Renal or hepatic impairment.

⧗ LIFESPAN CONSIDERATIONS: Pregnancy/Lactation: Unknown if distributed in breast milk. May cause fetal harm. Pregnancy Category D. Children: Safety and efficacy not established. Elderly: Age-related renal impairment may require dosage adjustment.

INTERACTIONS

DRUG: **Alcohol:** May cause a disulfiram-like reaction. **Anticholinergics, antihistamines:** May increase the anticholinergic effects of these drugs. **Bone marrow depressants:** May increase myelosuppression. **Buspirone, caffeine-containing medications:** May increase BP. **Carbamazepine, cyclobenzaprine, MAOIs, maprotiline:** May cause hyperpyretic crisis, seizures, or death. **CNS depressants:** May increase CNS depression. **Insulin, oral antidiabetics:** May increase the effects of these drugs. **Meperidine:** May produce coma, seizures, immediate excitation, rigidity, severe hypertension or hypotension, severe respiratory distress, diaphoresis, and vascular collapse.

Sympathomimetics: May increase cardiac stimulant and vasopressor effects. **Tricyclic antidepressants:** May increase anticholinergic effects; may cause seizures and hyperpyretic crisis. HERBAL: None known. FOOD: **Caffeine-containing beverages:** May increase BP. LAB VALUES: None known.

AVAILABILITY (Rx)

CAPSULES: 50 mg.

INDICATIONS/ROUTES/DOSAGE
ADVANCED HODGKIN'S DISEASE

PO: ADULTS, ELDERLY: Initially, 2–4 mg/kg/day as a single dose or in divided doses for 1 wk, then 4–6 mg/kg/day. Maintenance: 1–2 mg/kg/day. CHILDREN: 50–100 mg/m^2/day for 10–14 days of a 28-day cycle. Continue until maximum response occurs, leukocyte count falls below 4,000/mm^3, or platelet count falls below 100,000/mm^3. Maintenance: 100 mg/m^2/day for 14 days and repeat q4wk.

SIDE EFFECTS

FREQUENT: Severe nausea, vomiting, respiratory disorders (cough, effusion), myalgia, arthralgia, drowsiness, nervousness, insomnia, nightmares, diaphoresis, hallucinations, seizures. **OCCASIONAL:** Hoarseness, tachycardia, nystagmus, retinal hemorrhage, photophobia, photosensitivity, urinary frequency, nocturia, hypotension, diarrhea, stomatitis, paraesthesia, unsteadiness, confusion, decreased reflexes, foot drop. **RARE:** Hypersensitivity reaction (dermatitis, pruritus, rash, urticaria), hyperpigmentation, alopecia.

ADVERSE REACTIONS/ TOXIC EFFECTS

Procarbazine's major toxic effects are myelosuppression manifested as hematologic toxicity (mainly leukopenia, thrombocytopenia, and anemia) and hepatotoxicity manifested as jaundice and ascites. UTIs may occur secondary to leukopenia.

P

🍁 Canadian trade name   ℮ see *evolve*   ➤ High Alert drug

NURSING CONSIDERATIONS

BASELINE ASSESSMENT

Obtain bone marrow tests, Hgb, Hct, leukocyte, differential, reticulocyte, platelet, urinalysis, serum transaminase, serum alkaline phosphatase, BUN results before therapy and periodically thereafter. Therapy should be interrupted if WBC falls below 4,000/mm³ or platelet count falls below 100,000/mm³.

INTERVENTION/EVALUATION

Monitor hematologic status, renal, liver function studies. Assess for stomatitis. Monitor for hematologic toxicity (fever, sore throat, signs of local infection, unusual ecchymosis or bleeding from any site), symptoms of anemia (excessive fatigue, weakness).

PATIENT/FAMILY TEACHING

• Inform physician of fever, sore throat, bleeding, bruising. • Avoid alcohol (may cause disulfiram reaction: nausea, vomiting, headache, sedation, visual disturbances).

---

prochlorperazine

proe-klor-**per**-a-zeen

(Compazine, Compazine Spansule, Compro, Procot, Stemetil ✤)

Do not confuse prochlorperazine with chlorpromazine, or Compazine with Copaxone.

◆CLASSIFICATION

PHARMACOTHERAPEUTIC: Phenothiazine. **CLINICAL:** Antiemetic.

ACTION

A phenothiazine that acts centrally to inhibit or block dopamine receptors in the chemoreceptor trigger zone and peripherally to block the vagus nerve in the GI tract. **Therapeutic** **Effect:** Relieves nausea and vomiting and improves psychotic conditions.

PHARMACOKINETICS

Route	Onset*	Peak	Duration
Tablets, oral solution	30–40 min	N/A	3–4 hr
Capsules (Extended-release)	30–40 min	N/A	10–12 hr
Rectal	60 min	N/A	3–4 hr

*As an antiemetic.

Variably absorbed after PO administration. Widely distributed. Metabolized in the liver and GI mucosa. Primarily excreted in urine. Unknown if removed by hemodialysis. **Half-life:** 23 hr.

USES

Management of nausea and vomiting. Treatment of acute or chronic psychosis. **OFF-LABEL:** Behavior syndromes in dementia.

PRECAUTIONS

CONTRAINDICATIONS: Angle-closure glaucoma, CNS depression, coma, myelosuppression, severe cardiac or hepatic impairment, severe hypotension or hypertension. **CAUTIONS:** Seizures, Parkinson's disease, children younger than 2 yr.

⌛ **LIFESPAN CONSIDERATIONS: Pregnancy/Lactation:** Crosses placenta. Distributed in breast milk. **Pregnancy Category C. Children:** Safety and efficacy not established in those weighing less than 9 kg or younger than 2 yr. **Elderly:** More susceptible to orthostatic hypotension, anticholinergic effects (e.g., dry mouth), sedation, extrapyramidal symptoms (EPS); lower dosage recommended.

INTERACTIONS

DRUG: Alcohol, other CNS depressants: May increase CNS and respiratory depression and the hypotensive effects of prochlorperazine. **Antihypertensives:** May increase hypotension. **Antithyroid agents:** May increase the risk of agranulocytosis. **EPS–producing medications:** May increase EPS. **Levodopa:** May decrease the effects of levodopa. **Lithium:** May decrease the absorption of prochlorperazine and produce adverse neurologic effects. **MAOIs, tricyclic antidepressants:** May increase the anticholinergic and sedative effects of prochlorperazine. HERBAL: None known. FOOD: None known. LAB VALUES: None known.

AVAILABILITY (Rx)

CAPSULES (EXTENDED-RELEASE [COMPAZINE SPANSULE]): 10 mg, 15 mg. **ORAL SOLUTION (COMPAZINE):** 5 mg/5ml. **TABLETS (COMPAZINE):** 5 mg, 10 mg. **SUPPOSITORIES (COMPAZINE):** 2.5 mg, 5 mg, 25 mg. **INJECTION (COMPAZINE, PROCOT):** 5 mg/ml.

ADMINISTRATION/HANDLING

 IV

Rate of administration • May give by IV push slowly over 5–10 min. • May give by IV infusion over 30 min.

Storage • Store at room temperature. • Protect from light. • Clear or slightly yellow solutions may be used.

PO

• Give without regard to meals.

RECTAL

• Moisten suppository with cold water before inserting well into rectum.

IV INCOMPATIBILITIES

Atropine, furosemide (Lasix), midazolam (Versed).

IV COMPATIBILITIES

Calcium gluconate, diphenhydramine (Benadryl), fentanyl, glycopyrrolate (Robinul), heparin, hydromorphone (Dilaudid), morphine, metoclopramide (Reglan), nalbuphine (Nubain), potassium chloride, promethazine (Phenergan), propofol (Diprivan).

INDICATIONS/ROUTES/DOSAGE

NAUSEA AND VOMITING

PO: ADULTS, ELDERLY: 5–10 mg 3–4 times a day. CHILDREN: 0.4 mg/kg/day in 3–4 divided doses.

PO (EXTENDED-RELEASE): ADULTS, ELDERLY: 10 mg twice a day or 15 mg once a day.

IV: ADULTS, ELDERLY: 2.5–10 mg. May repeat q3–4h.

IM: ADULTS, ELDERLY: 5–10 mg q3–4h. CHILDREN: 0.1–0.15 mg/kg/dose q8–12h. **Maximum:** 40 mg/day.

RECTAL: ADULTS, ELDERLY: 25 mg twice a day. CHILDREN: 0.4 mg/kg/day in 3–4 divided doses.

PSYCHOSIS

PO: ADULTS, ELDERLY: 5–10 mg 3–4 times a day. **Maximum:** 150 mg/day. CHILDREN: 2.5 mg 2–3 times a day. **Maximum:** 25 mg for children 6–12 yr; 20 mg for children 2–5 yr.

IM: ADULTS, ELDERLY: 10–20 mg q4h. CHILDREN: 0.13 mg/kg/dose.

SIDE EFFECTS

FREQUENT: Somnolence, hypotension, dizziness, fainting (commonly occurring after first dose, occasionally after subsequent doses, and rarely with oral form). **OCCASIONAL:** Dry mouth, blurred vision, lethargy, constipation, diarrhea, myalgia, nasal congestion, peripheral edema, urine retention.

ADVERSE REACTIONS/TOXIC EFFECTS

EPS appear to be dose related and are divided into three categories: akathisia (marked by inability to sit still, tapping of feet), parkinsonian symptoms (including mask-like face, tremors, shuffling gait, hypersalivation), and acute dystonias (such as torticollis, opisthotonos, and oculogyric crisis. A dystonic reaction may

P

also produce diaphoresis or pallor. Tardive dyskinesia, manifested as tongue protrusion, puffing of the cheeks, and puckering of the mouth, is a rare reaction that may be irreversible. Abrupt withdrawal after long-term therapy may precipitate nausea, vomiting, gastritis, dizziness, and tremors. Blood dyscrasias, particularly agranulocytosis and mild leukopenia, may occur. Prochlorperazine use may lower the seizure threshold.

NURSING CONSIDERATIONS

BASELINE ASSESSMENT

Avoid skin contact with solution (contact dermatitis). **Antiemetic:** Assess for dehydration (poor skin turgor, dry mucous membranes, longitudinal furrows in tongue). **Antipsychotic:** Assess behavior, appearance, emotional status, response to environment, speech pattern, thought content.

INTERVENTION/EVALUATION

Monitor BP for hypotension. Assess for EPS. Monitor WBC, differential count for blood dyscrasias. Monitor for fine tongue movement (may be early sign of tardive dyskinesia). Supervise suicidal-risk patient closely during early therapy (as depression lessens, energy level improves, increasing suicide potential). Assess for therapeutic response (interest in surroundings, improvement in self-care, increased ability to concentrate, relaxed facial expression).

PATIENT/FAMILY TEACHING

• Limit caffeine. • Avoid alcohol. • May cause drowsiness, impair ability to perform tasks requiring mental alertness, coordination.

Procrit, *see epoetin alfa*

---

progesterone

proe-**jess**-ter-one
(Crinone, First Progesterone MC10, First Progesterone MC5, Prochieve, Prometrium)

CLASSIFICATION

PHARMACOTHERAPEUTIC: Progestin.
CLINICAL: Hormone.

ACTION

A natural steroid hormone that promotes mammary gland development and relaxes uterine smooth muscle. **Therapeutic Effect:** Decreases abnormal uterine bleeding; transforms endometrium from proliferative to secretory in an estrogen-primed endometrium.

PHARMACOKINETICS

Oral: Maximum serum concentrations attained within 3 hr. Protein binding: 96%–99%. Metabolized in liver. Excreted in bile and urine. **Half-life:** 18.3 hr. **IM:** Rapidly absorbed. Undergoes rapid metabolism. **Half-life:** Few min. **Long-acting form:** Approximately 10 wk. **Vaginal Gel:** Rate limited by absorption rather than by elimination. Protein binding: 96%–99%. Undergoes both biliary and renal elimination. **Half-life:** 5–20 hr.

USES

Oral: Prevent endometrial hyperplasia, secondary amenorrhea. **IM:** Amenorrhea, abnormal uterine bleeding. **Vaginal Gel (8%):** Treatment of infertility. **OFF-LABEL:** Treatment of corpus luteum dysfunction.

PRECAUTIONS

CONTRAINDICATIONS: Allergy to peanut oil (oral), breast cancer, history of active cerebral apoplexy, thromboembolic disorders or thrombophlebitis, missed abortion, severe hepatic dysfunction,

P

undiagnosed vaginal bleeding, use as a pregnancy test. **CAUTIONS:** Diabetes, conditions aggravated by fluid retention (e.g., asthma, epilepsy, migraine, cardiac or renal dysfunction), history of mental depression.

⌛ **LIFESPAN CONSIDERATIONS: Pregnancy/Lactation:** Distributed in breast milk. Avoid use during pregnancy. **Pregnancy Category D. Children:** Safety and efficacy not established. **Elderly:** No age-related precautions noted.

INTERACTIONS

DRUG: Bromocriptine: May interfere with the effects of bromocriptine. **HERBAL: Red clover:** May decrease progesterone effectiveness. **FOOD:** None known. **LAB VALUES:** May increase serum LDL and serum alkaline phosphatase levels. May decrease glucose tolerance and HDL concentrations. May cause abnormal serum thyroid, metapyrone, hepatic, and endocrine function test results.

AVAILABILITY (Rx)

CAPSULES (PROMETRIUM): 100 mg, 200 mg. **INJECTION:** 50 mg/ml. **VAGINAL GEL (CRINONE, PROCHIEVE):** 4% (45 mg), 8% (90 mg). **TOPICAL CREAM:** 5% (First Progesterone MC5), 10% (First Progesterone MC10).

ADMINISTRATION/HANDLING
IM
• Store at room temperature. • Administer only deep IM in large muscle mass.

PO
• If given in morning, administer 2 hr after eating breakfast.

VAGINAL GEL
• Administer at bedtime (may cause drowsiness).

VAGINAL (CRINONE)
• Remove applicator from sealed wrapper. Do not remove twist-off tab at this time. • Hold applicator by the thick end.

Shake down several times like a thermometer to ensure that contents are at the thin end. • Hold the applicator by the flat section of the thick end. Twist off and throw away the tab at other end. Do not squeeze thick end while twisting the tab (could force some gel to be released before insertion). • Insert applicator into vagina while the patient is in a sitting position or lying on the back with knees bent. • Gently insert thin end well into vagina. • Squeeze thick end of the applicator to deposit the gel. • Remove applicator and discard.

INDICATIONS/ROUTES/DOSAGE
AMENORRHEA
PO: ADULTS: 400 mg daily in evening for 10 days.
IM: ADULTS: 5–10 mg for 6–8 days. Withdrawal bleeding expected in 48–72 hr if ovarian activity produced proliferative endometrium.
VAGINAL: ADULTS: Apply 45 mg (4% gel) every other day for 6 or fewer doses.

ABNORMAL UTERINE BLEEDING
IM: ADULTS: 5–10 mg for 6 days. When estrogen given concomitantly, begin progesterone after 2 wk of estrogen therapy; discontinue when menstrual flow begins.

PREVENTION OF ENDOMETRIAL HYPERPLASIA
PO: ADULTS: 200 mg in evening for 12 days per 28-day cycle in combination with daily conjugated estrogen.

INFERTILITY
VAGINAL: ADULTS: 90 mg (8% gel) once a day (twice a day in women with partial or complete ovarian failure).

SIDE EFFECTS
FREQUENT: Breakthrough bleeding or spotting at beginning of therapy, amenorrhea, change in menstrual flow, breast tenderness. **Gel:** Drowsiness. **OCCASIONAL:** Edema, weight gain or loss, rash, pruritus, photosensitivity, skin pigmentation. **RARE:** Pain or

P

swelling at injection site, acne, depression, alopecia, hirsutism.

ADVERSE REACTIONS/ TOXIC EFFECTS

Thrombophlebitis, cerebrovascular disorders, retinal thrombosis, and pulmonary embolism occur rarely.

NURSING CONSIDERATIONS

BASELINE ASSESSMENT

Question for possibility of pregnancy or hypersensitivity to progestins before initiating therapy. Obtain baseline weight, blood glucose level, BP.

INTERVENTION/EVALUATION

Check weight daily; report weekly gain over 5 lbs. Assess skin for rash, hives. Immediately report the development of chest pain, sudden shortness of breath, sudden decrease in vision, migraine headache, pain (especially with swelling, warmth, redness) in calves, numbness of an arm or leg (thrombotic disorders). Check BP periodically. Note progesterone therapy on pathology specimens.

PATIENT/FAMILY TEACHING

• Use sunscreens, protective clothing to protect from sunlight or ultraviolet light until tolerance determined. • Notify physician of abnormal vaginal bleeding, other symptoms. • Stop taking medication and contact physician at once if pregnancy suspected. • If using vaginal gel, avoid tasks that require alertness, motor skills until response to drug is established.

Prograf, *see tacrolimus*

Proleukin, *see aldesleukin*

---

promethazine hydrochloride

proe-**meth**-a-zeen
(Adgan, Anergan 50, Antinaus 50, Pentazine, Phenadoz, Phenergan, Phenoject-50, Promacot, Promethegan)

Do not confuse promethazine with promazine.

FIXED-COMBINATION(S)

Phenergan with codeine: promethazine/codeine (a cough suppressant): 6.25 mg/10 mg/5 ml. **Phenergan VC:** promethazine/phenylephrine (a vasoconstrictor): 6.25 mg/5 mg/5 ml. **Phenergan VC with codeine:** promethazine/phenylephrine/codeine: 6.25 mg/5 mg/ 10 mg/5 ml.

•CLASSIFICATION

PHARMACOTHERAPEUTIC: Phenothiazine. **CLINICAL:** Antihistamine, antiemetic, sedative-hypnotic (see p. 51C).

ACTION

A phenothiazine that acts as an antihistamine, antiemetic, and sedative-hypnotic. As an antihistamine, inhibits histamine at histamine receptor sites. As an antiemetic, diminishes vestibular stimulation, depresses labyrinthine function, and act on the chemoreceptor trigger zone. As a sedative-hypnotic, produces CNS depression by decreasing stimulation to the brain stem reticular formation. **Therapeutic Effect:** Prevents allergic responses mediated by histamine, such as rhinitis, urticaria, and pruritus. Prevents and relieves nausea and vomiting.

P

PHARMACOKINETICS

Route	Onset	Peak	Duration
PO	20 min	N/A	2–8 hr
IV	3–5 min	N/A	2–8 hr
IM	20 min	N/A	2–8 hr
Rectal	20 min	N/A	2–8 hr

Well absorbed from the GI tract after IM administration. Widely distributed. Metabolized in the liver. Primarily excreted in urine. Not removed by hemodialysis. Half-life: 16–19 hr.

USES

Treatment of allergic conditions, motion sickness, nausea, vomiting. May be used as mild sedative.

PRECAUTIONS

CONTRAINDICATIONS: Angle-closure glaucoma, children 2 yr and younger, GI or GU obstruction, hypersensitivity to phenothiazines, severe CNS depression or coma. **CAUTIONS:** Impaired cardiovascular disease, hepatic impairment, asthma, peptic ulcer, history of seizures, sleep apnea, patients suspected of Reye's syndrome.

LIFESPAN CONSIDERATIONS: Pregnancy/Lactation: Readily crosses placenta. Unknown if drug is excreted in breast milk. May inhibit platelet aggregation in neonates if taken within 2 wk of birth. May produce jaundice, extrapyramidal symptoms (EPS) in neonates if taken during pregnancy. **Pregnancy Category C. Children:** May experience increased excitement. Not recommended for those younger than 2 yr. **Elderly:** More sensitive to dizziness, sedation, confusion, hypotension, hyperexcitability, anticholinergic effects (e.g., dry mouth).

INTERACTIONS

DRUG: Alcohol, other CNS depressants: May increase CNS depressant effects. **Anticholinergics:** May increase anticholinergic effects. **MAOIs:** May intensify and prolong the anticholinergic and CNS depressant effects of promethazine. **HERBAL:** None known. **FOOD:** None known. **LAB VALUES:** May suppress wheal and flare reactions to antigen skin testing unless the drug is discontinued 4 days before testing.

AVAILABILITY (Rx)

SYRUP (PENTAZINE, PHENERGAN): 6.25 mg/ml. **TABLETS (PHENERGAN, PROMACOT):** 12.5 mg, 25 mg, 50 mg. **INJECTION:** 25 mg/ml (Phenergan), 50 mg/ml (Adgan, Anergan 50, Antinaus 50, Phenergan, Phenoject-50, Promacot). **SUPPOSITORIES:** 12.5 mg (Phenergan, Promethegan), 25 mg (Phenadoz, Phenergan, Promethegan), 50 mg (Phenergan, Promethegan).

ADMINISTRATION/HANDLING

◀ **ALERT** ▶ Significant tissue necrosis may occur if given subcutaneously. Inadvertent intra-arterial injection may produce severe arteriospasm, resulting in severe circulation impairment.

 IV

Reconstitution • May be given undiluted or dilute with 0.9% NaCl. Final dilution should not exceed 25 mg/ml.

Rate of administration • Administer at 25 mg/min rate through IV infusion tube. • A too rapid rate of infusion may result in transient fall in BP, producing orthostatic hypotension, reflex tachycardia.

Storage • Store at room temperature.

IM
• Inject deep IM.

PO
• Give without regard to meals. • Scored tablets may be crushed.

RECTAL
• Refrigerate suppository. • Moisten suppository with cold water before inserting well into rectum.

▨ IV INCOMPATIBILITIES

Allopurinol (Aloprim), amphotericin B complex (Abelcet, AmBisome, Amphotec), heparin, ketorolac (Toradol), nalbuphine (Nubain), piperacillin and tazobactam (Zosyn).

IV COMPATIBILITIES

Atropine, diphenhydramine (Benadryl), glycopyrrolate (Robinul), hydromorphone (Dilaudid), hydroxyzine (Vistaril), meperidine (Demerol), midazolam (Versed), morphine, prochlorperazine (Compazine).

INDICATIONS/ROUTES/DOSAGE

◀ ALERT ▶ Contraindicated in children 2 yr and younger.

ALLERGIC SYMPTOMS
PO: ADULTS, ELDERLY: 6.25–12.5 mg 3 times a day plus 25 mg at bedtime. CHILDREN: 0.1 mg/kg/dose (**maximum:** 12.5 mg) 3 times a day plus 0.5 mg/kg/dose (**maximum:** 25 mg) at bedtime.
IV, IM: ADULTS, ELDERLY: 25 mg. May repeat in 2 hr.

MOTION SICKNESS
PO: ADULTS, ELDERLY: 25 mg 30–60 min before departure; may repeat in 8–12 hr, then every morning on rising and before evening meal. CHILDREN: 0.5 mg/kg 30–60 min before departure; may repeat in 8–12 hr, then every morning on rising and before evening meal.

PREVENTION OF NAUSEA, AND VOMITING
PO, IV, IM, RECTAL: ADULTS, ELDERLY: 12.5–25 mg q4–6h as needed. CHILDREN: 0.25–1 mg/kg q4–6h as needed.

PREOP AND POSTOP SEDATION; ADJUNCT TO ANALGESICS
IV, IM: ADULTS, ELDERLY: 25–50 mg. CHILDREN: 12.5–25 mg.

SEDATIVE
PO, IV, IM, RECTAL: ADULTS, ELDERLY: 25–50 mg/dose. May repeat q4–6h as needed. CHILDREN: 0.5–1 mg/kg/dose q6h as needed. **Maximum:** 50 mg/dose.

SIDE EFFECTS

EXPECTED: Somnolence, disorientation; in elderly, hypotension, confusion, syncope. **FREQUENT:** Dry mouth, nose, or throat; urine retention; thickening of bronchial secretions. **OCCASIONAL:** Epigastric distress, flushing, visual disturbances, hearing disturbances, wheezing, paraesthesia, diaphoresis, chills. **RARE:** Dizziness, urticaria, photosensitivity, nightmares.

ADVERSE REACTIONS/TOXIC EFFECTS

Children may experience paradoxical reactions, such as excitation, nervousness, tremor, hyperactive reflexes, and seizures. Infants and young children have experienced CNS depression manifested as respiratory depression, sleep apnea, and sudden infant death syndrome. Long-term therapy may produce extrapyramidal symptoms, such as dystonia (abnormal movements), pronounced motor restlessness (most frequently in children), and parkinsonian (most frequently in elderly patients). Blood dyscrasias, particularly agranulocytosis, occur rarely.

NURSING CONSIDERATIONS

BASELINE ASSESSMENT
Assess BP, pulse for bradycardia or tachycardia if patient is given parenteral form. If used as an antiemetic, assess for dehydration (poor skin turgor, dry mucous membranes, longitudinal furrows in tongue).

INTERVENTION/EVALUATION
Monitor serum electrolytes in patients with severe vomiting. Assist with ambulation if drowsiness, lightheadedness occurs.

PATIENT/FAMILY TEACHING
• Drowsiness, dry mouth may be an expected response to drug. • Avoid tasks that require alertness, motor

skills until response to drug is established. • Sugarless gum, sips of tepid water may relieve dry mouth. • Coffee or tea may help reduce drowsiness. • Report visual disturbances. • Avoid alcohol, other CNS depressants.

Prometrium, *see* *progesterone*

propafenone hydrochloride

proe-**pa**-fen-one
(Rythmol, Rythmol SR)

◆CLASSIFICATION
CLINICAL: Antiarrhythmic (see p. 15C).

ACTION
An antiarrhythmic that decreases the fast sodium current in Purkinje or myocardial cells. Decreases excitability and automaticity; prolongs conduction velocity and the refractory period. **Therapeutic Effect:** Suppresses arrhythmias.

PHARMACOKINETICS
Nearly completely absorbed following oral administration. Protein binding: 85%–97%. Metabolized in liver; undergoes first pass metabolism. Primarily excreted in feces. **Half-life:** 2–10 hr.

USES
Treatment of documented, life-threatening ventricular arrhythmias (e.g., sustained ventricular tachycardias). **Rythmol SR:** Maintenance of normal sinus rhythm in patients with symptomatic atrial fibrillation. **OFF-LABEL:** Treatment of supraventricular arrhythmias.

PRECAUTIONS
CONTRAINDICATIONS: Bradycardia; bronchospastic disorders; cardiogenic shock; electrolyte imbalance; sinoatrial, AV, and intraventricular impulse generation or conduction disorders, such as sick sinus syndrome or AV block, without the presence of a pacemaker; uncontrolled CHF. **CAUTIONS:** Renal or hepatic impairment, recent MI, CHF, conduction disturbances.

⏳ **LIFESPAN CONSIDERATIONS: Pregnancy/Lactation:** Unknown if drug crosses placenta or is distributed in breast milk. **Pregnancy Category C. Children:** Safety and efficacy not established. **Elderly:** No age-related precautions noted.

INTERACTIONS
DRUG: Cyclosporine: May increase risk of cyclosporine toxicity. **Desipramine:** May increase risk of cardiotoxicity. **Digoxin, propranolol:** May increase concentrations of these drugs. **Local anesthetics:** May increase risk of CNS side effects. **Rifampin:** May decrease propafenone effectiveness. **Warfarin:** May increase warfarin effects. **HERBAL:** None known. **FOOD:** None known. **LAB VALUES:** May cause EKG changes, such as QRS widening and PR interval prolongation, and positive ANA titers.

AVAILABILITY (Rx)
TABLETS (RYTHMOL): 150 mg, 225 mg, 300 mg. **CAPSULES (EXTENDED-RELEASE [RYTHMOL SR]):** 225 mg, 325 mg, 425 mg.

INDICATIONS/ROUTES/DOSAGE
DOCUMENTED, LIFE-THREATENING VENTRICULAR ARRHYTHMIAS, SUCH AS SUSTAINED VENTRICULAR TACHYCARDIA
PO: ADULTS, ELDERLY: Initially, 150 mg q8h;

may increase at 3- to 4-day intervals to 225 mg q8h, then to 300 mg q8h. **Maximum:** 900 mg/day.
PO (EXTENDED-RELEASE): ADULTS, ELDERLY: Initially, 225 mg q12h. May increase at 5 day intervals. **Maximum:** 425 mg q12h.

SIDE EFFECTS

FREQUENT (13%–7%): Dizziness, nausea, vomiting, altered taste, constipation. **OCCASIONAL (6%–3%):** Headache, dyspnea, blurred vision, dyspepsia (heartburn, indigestion, epigastric pain). **RARE (less than 2%):** Rash, weakness, dry mouth, diarrhea, edema, hot flashes.

ADVERSE REACTIONS/ TOXIC EFFECTS

Propafenone may produce or worsen existing arrhythmias. Overdose may produce hypotension, somnolence, bradycardia, and atrioventricular conduction disturbances.

NURSING CONSIDERATIONS

BASELINE ASSESSMENT

Correct electrolyte imbalance before administering medication.

INTERVENTION/EVALUATION

Assess pulse for quality, irregular rate. Monitor EKG for cardiac performance and changes, particularly widening of QRS, prolongation of PR interval. Question for visual disturbances, headache, GI upset. Monitor fluid, serum electrolyte levels. Monitor pattern of daily bowel activity and stool consistency. Assess for dizziness, unsteadiness. Monitor hepatic enzymes results Monitor for therapeutic serum level (0.06–1 mcg/ml).

PATIENT/FAMILY TEACHING

* Compliance with therapy regimen is essential to control arrhythmias.
* Altered taste sensation may occur.
* Report headache, blurred vision.
* Avoid tasks that require alertness, motor skills until response to drug is established.

propofol ⚑

pro-poe-**fall**
(Diprivan)

◆CLASSIFICATION

PHARMACOTHERAPEUTIC: Rapid-acting general anesthetic. **CLINICAL:** Sedative-hypnotic (see p. 3C).

ACTION

A rapidly acting general anesthetic that inhibits sympathetic vasoconstrictor nerve activity and decreases vascular resistance. Therapeutic Effect: Produces hypnosis rapidly.

PHARMACOKINETICS

Route	Onset	Peak	Duration
IV	40 sec	N/A	3–10 min

Rapidly and extensively distributed. Protein binding: 97%–99%. Metabolized in the liver. Primarily excreted in urine. Unknown if removed by hemodialysis. Half-life: 3–12 hr.

USES

Induction and maintenance of anesthesia. Continuous sedation in intubated and respiratory controlled adult patients in ICU.

PRECAUTIONS

CONTRAINDICATIONS: Impaired cerebral circulation, increased intracranial pressure (ICP). **CAUTIONS:** Debilitated; impaired respiratory, circulatory, renal, hepatic, lipid metabolism disorders; history of epilepsy or seizure disorder.

⌛ LIFESPAN CONSIDERATIONS: **Pregnancy/Lactation:** Unknown if drug crosses placenta. Distributed in breast milk. Not recommended for obstetrics, breast-feeding mothers. **Pregnancy Category B. Children:** Safety and efficacy not established. FDA approved for use in those 2 mo and older. **Elderly:** No age-related precautions noted; lower dosages recommended.

INTERACTIONS

DRUG: **Alcohol, other CNS depressants:** May increase hypotensive and CNS and respiratory depressant effects of propofol. HERBAL: None known. FOOD: None known. LAB VALUES: None known.

AVAILABILITY (Rx)

INJECTION: 10 mg/ml.

ADMINISTRATION/HANDLING

◊ IV

◀ ALERT ▶ Do not give through same IV line with blood or plasma.

Reconstitution • May give undiluted, Do not dilute or dilute only with D₅W. • Do not dilute to concentration less than 2 mg/ml (4 ml D₅W to 1 ml propofol yields 2 mg/ml).

Rate of administration • A too rapid IV may produce marked severe hypotension, respiratory depression, irregular muscular movements. • Observe for signs of intra-arterial injection (pain, discolored skin patches, white or blue color to peripheral IV site area, delayed onset of drug action).

Storage • Store at room temperature. • Discard unused portions. • Do not use if emulsion separates. • Shake well before using.

🔆 IV INCOMPATIBILITIES

Amikacin (Amikin), amphotericin B complex (Abelcet, AmBisome, Amphotec), bretylium (Bretylol), calcium chloride, ciprofloxacin (Cipro), diazepam (Valium), digoxin (Lanoxin), doxorubicin (Adriamycin), gentamicin (Garamycin), methylprednisolone (Solu-Medrol), minocycline (Minocin), phenytoin (Dilantin), tobramycin (Nebcin), verapamil (Isoptin).

IV COMPATIBILITIES

Acyclovir (Zovirax), bumetanide (Bumex), calcium gluconate, ceftazidime (Fortaz), dobutamine (Dobutrex), dopamine (Intropin), enalapril (Vasotec), fentanyl, heparin, insulin, labetalol (Normodyne, Trandate), lidocaine, lorazepam (Ativan), magnesium, milrinone (Primacor), nitroglycerin, norepinephrine (Levophed), potassium chloride, vancomycin (Vancocin).

INDICATIONS/ROUTES/DOSAGE

ANESTHESIA

IV: ADULTS, ELDERLY: Induction, 20–40 mg every 10 sec until induction onset, then infusion of 50–200 mcg/kg/min with 20–50 mg bolus as needed. CHILDREN 3–16 YR: Induction, 2.5–3.5 mg/kg over 20–30 sec, then infusion of 125–300 mcg/kg/min.

INTENSIVE CARE UNIT (ICU) SEDATION

IV: ADULTS, ELDERLY: Initially, 5 mcg/kg/min for 5 min, then titrate to 5–50 mcg/kg/min in 5–10 mcg/kg/min increments allowing a minimum of 5 min between dose adjustments.

SIDE EFFECTS

FREQUENT: Involuntary muscle movements, apnea (common during induction; lasts longer than 60 sec), hypotension, nausea, vomiting, IV site burning or stinging. OCCASIONAL: Twitching, bucking, jerking, thrashing, headache, dizziness, bradycardia, hypertension, fever, abdominal cramps, paresthesia, coldness, cough, hiccups, facial flushing, greenish-colored urine. RARE: Rash, dry mouth, agitation, confusion, myalgia, thrombophlebitis.

P

ADVERSE REACTIONS/ TOXIC EFFECTS

A continuous infusion or repeated intermittent infusions of propofol may result in extreme somnolence, respiratory depression, and circulatory depression. Too-rapid IV administration may produce severe hypotension, respiratory depression, and involuntary muscle movements. The patient may experience an acute allergic reaction, characterized by abdominal pain, anxiety, restlessness, dyspnea, erythema, hypotension, pruritus, rhinitis, and urticaria.

NURSING CONSIDERATIONS

BASELINE ASSESSMENT

Resuscitative equipment, suction, O₂ must be available. Obtain vital signs before administration.

INTERVENTION/EVALUATION

Monitor respiratory rate, BP, heart rate, O₂ saturation, ABGs, depth of sedation, lipid and triglycerides if used longer than 24 hr. May change urine color to green.

---

propoxyphene hydrochloride

(Darvon, PP-Cap)

propoxyphene napsylate

(Darvon-N)

pro-**pox**-ih-feen

Do not confuse Darvon with Diovan.

FIXED-COMBINATION(S)

Balacet 325: propoxyphene/ acetaminophen: 100 mg/325 mg. **Darvocet-N:** propoxyphene/ acetamino-phen: 50 mg/325 mg; 100 mg/650 mg. **Darvocet A500:** propoxyphene/acetaminophen: 100 mg/500 mg.

♦CLASSIFICATION

PHARMACOTHERAPEUTIC: Opioid agonist. **(Schedule IV). CLINICAL:** Analgesic (see p. 128C).

ACTION

An opioid agonist that binds with opioid receptors in the CNS. Therapeutic Effect: Alters the perception of and emotional response to pain.

PHARMACOKINETICS

Route	Onset	Peak	Duration
PO	15–60 min	N/A	4–6 hr

Well absorbed from the GI tract. Protein binding: High. Widely distributed. Metabolized in the liver. Primarily excreted in urine. Not removed by hemodialysis. Half-life: 6–12 hr; metabolite: 30–36 hr.

USES

Relief of mild to moderate pain.

PRECAUTIONS

CONTRAINDICATIONS: None known. **CAUTIONS:** Renal or hepatic impairment, substitution for opiates in narcotic-dependent patients.

⧗ **LIFESPAN CONSIDERATIONS: Pregnancy/Lactation:** Crosses placenta. Minimal amount distributed in breast milk. Respiratory depression may occur in neonate if mother received opiates during labor. Regular use of opiates during pregnancy may produce withdrawal symptoms in neonate (irritability, excessive crying, tremors, hyperactive reflexes, fever, vomiting, diarrhea, yawning, sneezing, seizures). **Pregnancy Category C (D if used for prolonged**

---

periods). **Children:** Dosage not established. **Elderly:** May be more susceptible to CNS effects, constipation. Avoid use if possible.

INTERACTIONS

DRUG: **Alcohol, other CNS depressants:** May increase CNS or respiratory depression and risk of hypotension. **Buprenorphine:** May decrease the effects of propoxyphene. **Carbamazepine:** May increase the blood concentration and risk of toxicity of carbamazepine. **MAOIs:** May produce a severe, sometimes fatal reaction; plan to administer 25% of usual propoxyphene dose. HERBAL: None known. FOOD: None known. LAB VALUES: May increase serum alkaline phosphatase, lipase, amylase, bilirubin, LDH, AST, and ALT levels. Therapeutic serum drug level is 100–400 ng/ml; toxic serum drug level is greater than 500 ng/ml.

AVAILABILITY (Rx)

CAPSULES (HYDROCHLORIDE [DARVON, PP-CAP]): 65 mg. **TABLETS (NAPSYLATE [DARVON-N]):** 100 mg.

ADMINISTRATION/HANDLING

PO
• Give without regard to meals. • Capsules may be emptied and mixed with food. • Do not crush or break film-coated tablets.

INDICATIONS/ROUTES/DOSAGE

MILD TO MODERATE PAIN
PO (PROPOXYPHENE HYDROCHLORIDE): ADULTS, ELDERLY: 65 mg q4h as needed. **Maximum:** 390 mg/day.
PO (PROPOXYPHENE NAPSYLATE): ADULTS, ELDERLY: 100 mg q4h as needed. **Maximum:** 600 mg/day.

SIDE EFFECTS

FREQUENT: Dizziness, somnolence, dry mouth, euphoria, hypotension (including orthostatic hypotension), nausea, vomiting, fatigue. **OCCASIONAL:** Allergic reaction (including decreased BP), diaphoresis, flushing, and wheezing), trembling, urine retention, vision changes, constipation, headache. **RARE:** Confusion, increased BP, depression, abdominal cramps, anorexia.

ADVERSE REACTIONS/ TOXIC EFFECTS

Overdose results in respiratory depression, skeletal muscle flaccidity, cold or clammy skin, cyanosis, and extreme somnolence progressing to seizures, stupor, and coma. Hepatotoxicity may occur with overdose of the acetaminophen component of fixed-combination products. The patient who uses propoxyphene repeatedly may develop a tolerance to the drug's analgesic effect and physical dependence.

NURSING CONSIDERATIONS

BASELINE ASSESSMENT

Obtain vital signs vefore giving medication. If respirations are 12/min or less (20/min or less in children), withhold medication, contact physician. Assess onset, type, location, duration of pain. Effect of medication is reduced if full pain recurs before next dose.

INTERVENTION/EVALUATION

Palpate bladder for urinary retention. Monitor pattern of daily bowel activity and stool consistency. Initiate deep breathing and coughing exercises, particularly in patients with pulmonary impairment. Assess for clinical improvement, record onset of relief of pain. Contact physician if pain is not adequately relieved. Therapeutic serum level: 100–400 ng/ml; toxic serum level: greater than 500 ng/ml.

PATIENT/FAMILY TEACHING

• Avoid alcohol. • May be habit forming. • May cause drowsiness, impair ability to perform tasks requiring mental alertness, coordination. • Do not discontinue abruptly.

P

propranolol hydrochloride

proe-**pran**-oh-lole
(Apo-Propranolol ✤, Inderal, Inderal LA, InnoPran XL, Nu-Propranolol ✤, Propranolol Intensol)

Do not confuse Inderal with Adderall or Isordil, or propranolol with Pravachol.

FIXED-COMBINATION(S)

Inderide: propranolol/hydrochlorothiazide (a diuretic): 40 mg/25 mg; 80 mg/25 mg. **Inderide LA:** propranolol/hydrochlorothiazide (a diuretic): 80 mg/50 mg; 120 mg/50 mg; 160 mg/50 mg.

CLASSIFICATION

PHARMACOTHERAPEUTIC: Beta-adrenergic blocker. **CLINICAL:** Antihypertensive, antianginal, antiarrhythmic, antimigraine (see pp. 15C, 64C).

ACTION

An antihypertensive, antianginal, antiarrhythmic, and antimigraine agent that blocks $beta_1$- and $beta_2$-adrenergic receptors. Decreases oxygen requirements. Slows AV conduction and increases refractory period in AV node. Large doses increase airway resistance. Therapeutic Effect: Slows sinus heart rate; decreases cardiac output, BP, and myocardial ischemia severity. Exhibits antiarrhythmic activity.

PHARMACOKINETICS

Route	Onset	Peak	Duration
PO	1–2 hr	N/A	6 hr

Well absorbed from the GI tract. Protein binding: 93%. Widely distributed.

Metabolized in the liver. Primarily excreted in urine. Not removed by hemodialysis. Half-life: 3–5 hr.

USES

Treatment of angina pectoris, arrhythmias, essential tremors, hypertension, hypertrophic subaortic stenosis, migraine headache, pheochromocytoma, post-MI. OFF-LABEL: Treatment adjunct for anxiety, mitral valve prolapse syndrome, thyrotoxicosis.

PRECAUTIONS

CONTRAINDICATIONS: Asthma, bradycardia, cardiogenic shock, chronic obstructive pulmonary disease (COPD), heart block, Raynaud's syndrome, uncompensated CHF. **CAUTIONS:** Diabetes, renal or hepatic impairment, concurrent use of calcium blockers when using IV form.

⏳ LIFESPAN CONSIDERATIONS: **Pregnancy/Lactation:** Crosses placenta. Distributed in breast milk. Avoid use during first trimester. May produce low birth-weight infants, bradycardia, apnea, hypoglycemia, hypothermia during delivery. **Pregnancy Category C (D if used in second or third trimester). Children:** No age-related precautions noted. **Elderly:** Age-related peripheral vascular disease may increase susceptibility to decreased peripheral circulation.

INTERACTIONS

DRUG: **Diuretics, other antihypertensives:** May increase hypotensive effect. **Insulin, oral hypoglycemics:** May mask symptoms of hypoglycemia and prolong the hypoglycemic effect of insulin and oral hypoglycemics. **IV phenytoin:** May increase cardiac depressant effect. **NSAIDs:** May decrease antihypertensive effect. **Sympathomimetics, xanthines:** May mutually inhibit effects. HERBAL: None known. FOOD: None known. LAB VALUES: May increase serum antinuclear antibody titer and BUN, serum LDH, serum lipoprotein, serum alkaline phosphatase, serum bilirubin, serum creatinine, serum potassium, serum uric acid, AST, ALT, and serum triglyceride levels.

AVAILABILITY (Rx)

TABLETS (INDERAL): 10 mg, 20 mg, 40 mg, 60 mg, 80 mg. **CAPSULES (EXTENDED-RELEASE):** 60 mg (Inderal LA), 80 mg (Inderal LA, InnoPran XL), 120 mg (Inderal LA, InnoPran XL), 160 mg (Inderal LA). **ORAL SOLUTION (INDERAL):** 20 mg/5 ml, 40 mg/5 ml. **ORAL CONCENTRATE (PROPRANOLOL INTENSOL):** 80 mg/ml. **INJECTION (INDERAL):** 1 mg/ml.

ADMINISTRATION/HANDLING

 IV

Reconstitution • Give undiluted for IV push. • For IV infusion, may dilute each 1 mg in 10 ml D₅W.

Rate of administration • Do not exceed 1 mg/min injection rate. • For IV infusion, give 1 mg over 10–15 min.

Storage • Store at room temperature.

PO
• May crush scored tablets. • Give at same time each day.

🔲 IV INCOMPATIBILITIES

Amphotericin B complex (Abelcet, AmBisome, Amphotec).

IV COMPATIBILITIES

Alteplase (Activase), heparin, milrinone (Primacor), potassium chloride, propofol (Diprivan).

INDICATIONS/ROUTES/DOSAGE

HYPERTENSION

PO: ADULTS, ELDERLY: Initially, 40 mg twice a day. May increase dose q3–7 days. Range: Up to 320 mg/day in divided doses. **Maximum:** 640 mg/day. CHILDREN: Initially, 0.5–1 mg/kg/day in divided doses q6–12h. May increase at 3- to 5-day intervals. Usual dose: 1–5 mg/kg/day. **Maximum:** 16 mg/kg/day.

ANGINA

PO: ADULTS, ELDERLY: 80–320 mg/day in divided doses.
PO (LONG ACTING): Initially, 80 mg/day. **Maximum:** 320 mg/day.

ARRHYTHMIAS

IV: ADULTS, ELDERLY: 1 mg/dose. May repeat q5min. **Maximum:** 5 mg total dose. CHILDREN: 0.01–0.1 mg/kg. **Maximum:** infants, 1 mg; children, 3 mg.
PO: ADULTS, ELDERLY: Initially, 10–20 mg q6-8h. May gradually increase dose. Range: 40–320 mg/day. CHILDREN: Initially, 0.5–1 mg/kg/day in divided doses q6–8h. May increase q3–5days. Usual dosage: 2–4 mg/kg/day. **Maximum:** 16 mg/kg/day or 60 mg/day.

LIFE-THREATENING ARRHYTHMIAS

IV: ADULTS, ELDERLY: 0.5–3 mg. Repeat once in 2 min. Give additional doses at intervals of at least 4 hr. CHILDREN: 0.01–0.1 mg/kg.

HYPERTROPHIC SUBAORTIC STENOSIS

PO: ADULTS, ELDERLY: 20–40 mg in 3–4 divided doses. Or 80–160 mg/day as extended-release capsule.

ADJUNCT TO ALPHA-BLOCKING AGENTS TO TREAT PHEOCHROMOCYTOMA

PO: ADULTS, ELDERLY: 60 mg/day in divided doses with alpha-blocker for 3 days before surgery. Maintenance (inoperable tumor): 30 mg/day with alpha-blocker.

MIGRAINE HEADACHE

PO: ADULTS, ELDERLY: 80 mg/day in divided doses. Or 80 mg once daily as extended-release capsule. Increase up to 160–240 mg/day in divided doses. CHILDREN: 0.6–1.5 mg/kg/day in divided doses q8h. **Maximum:** 4 mg/kg/day.

REDUCTION OF CARDIOVASCULAR MORTALITY AND REINFARCTION IN PATIENTS WITH PREVIOUS MI

PO: ADULTS, ELDERLY: 180–240 mg/day in divided doses.

P

ESSENTIAL TREMOR

PO: ADULTS, ELDERLY: Initially, 40 mg twice a day increased up to 120–320 mg/day in 3 divided doses.

SIDE EFFECTS

FREQUENT: Diminished sexual ability, drowsiness, difficulty sleeping, unusual fatigue or weakness. **OCCASIONAL:** Bradycardia, depression, sensation of coldness in extremities, diarrhea, constipation, anxiety, nasal congestion, nausea, vomiting. **RARE:** Altered taste, dry eyes, pruritus, paraesthesia.

ADVERSE REACTIONS/ TOXIC EFFECTS

Overdose may produce profound bradycardia and hypotension. Abrupt withdrawal may result in sweating, palpitations, headache, and tremors. Propranolol administration may precipitate CHF and MI in patients with cardiac disease; thyroid storm in those with thyrotoxicosis; and peripheral ischemia in those with existing peripheral vascular disease. Hypoglycemia may occur in patients with previously controlled diabetes.

NURSING CONSIDERATIONS

BASELINE ASSESSMENT

Assess baseline renal and liver function tests. Assess BP, apical pulse immediately before administering the drug (if pulse is 60/min or less or systolic BP is less than 90 mm Hg, withhold medication, contact physician). **Anginal:** Record onset, quality, radiation, location, intensity, duration of anginal pain, precipitating factors (exertion, emotional stress).

INTERVENTION/EVALUATION

Assess pulse for quality, irregular rate, bradycardia. Monitor EKG for cardiac arrhythmias. Assess fingers for color, numbness (Raynaud's). Assess for evidence of CHF (dyspnea [particularly on exertion or lying down], night cough, peripheral edema, distended neck veins). Monitor I&O (increase in weight, decrease in urine output may indicate CHF). Assess for rash, fatigue, behavioral changes. Therapeutic response ranges from a few days to several weeks. Measure BP near end of dosing interval (determines if BP is controlled throughout day).

PATIENT/FAMILY TEACHING

• Do not abruptly discontinue medication. Compliance with therapy regimen is essential to control hypertension, arrhythmia, anginal pain. • To avoid hypotensive effect, rise slowly from lying to sitting position, wait momentarily before standing. • Avoid tasks that require alertness, motor skills until response to drug is established. • Report excessively slow pulse rate (less than 60 beats/min), peripheral numbness, dizziness. • Do not use nasal decongestants, OTC cold preparations (stimulants) without physician approval. • Restrict salt, alcohol intake.

propylthiouracil

proe-pill-thye-oh-**yoor**-a-sill
(Propylthiouracil, Propyl-Thyracil ✦)

CLASSIFICATION

PHARMACOTHERAPEUTIC: Thiourea derivative. **CLINICAL:** Antithyroid.

ACTION

A thiourea derivative that blocks oxidation of iodine in the thyroid gland and blocks synthesis of thyroxine and triiodothyronine. **Therapeutic**

Effect: Inhibits synthesis of thyroid hormone.

PHARMACOKINETICS

Readily absorbed from GI tract. Protein binding: 80%. Metabolized in liver. Excreted in urine. Half-life: 1–4 hr.

USES

Palliative treatment of hyperthyroidism; adjunct to ameliorate hyperthyroidism in preparation for surgical treatment, radioactive iodine therapy.

PRECAUTIONS

CONTRAINDICATIONS: Breast-feeding mothers. **CAUTIONS:** Patients older than 40 yr or in combination with other agranulocytosis-inducing drugs. **Pregnancy Category D.**

INTERACTIONS

DRUG: **Amiodarone, iodinated glycerol, iodine, potassium iodide:** May decrease response of propylthiouracil. **Digoxin:** May increase digoxin blood concentration as patient becomes euthyroid. **I^{131}:** May decrease thyroid uptake of I^{131}. **Oral anticoagulants:** May decrease the effects of oral anticoagulants. HERBAL: None known. FOOD: None known. LAB VALUES: May increase LDH, serum alkaline phosphatase, bilirubin, AST, and ALT levels and prothrombin time.

AVAILABILITY (Rx)

TABLETS: 50 mg.

INDICATIONS/ROUTES/DOSAGE
HYPERTHYROIDISM

PO: ADULTS, ELDERLY: Initially: 300–450 mg/day in divided doses q8h. Maintenance: 100–150 mg/day in divided doses q8–12h. CHILDREN: Initially: 5–7 mg/kg/day in divided doses q8h. Maintenance: 33%–66% of initial dose in divided doses q8–12h. NEONATES: 5–10 mg/kg/day in divided doses q8h.

SIDE EFFECTS

FREQUENT: Urticaria, rash, pruritus, nausea, skin pigmentation, hair loss, headache, paraesthesia. **OCCASIONAL:** Somnolence, lymphadenopathy, vertigo. **RARE:** Drug fever, lupus-like syndrome.

ADVERSE REACTIONS/ TOXIC EFFECTS

Agranulocytosis as long as 4 mo after therapy, pancytopenia, and fatal hepatitis have occurred.

NURSING CONSIDERATIONS

BASELINE ASSESSMENT
Obtain baseline weight, pulse.

INTERVENTION/EVALUATION
Monitor pulse, weight daily. Check for skin eruptions, pruritus, swollen lymph glands. Be alert to hepatitis (nausea, vomiting, drowsiness, jaundice). Monitor hematology results for bone marrow suppression; check for signs of infection and bleeding.

PATIENT/FAMILY TEACHING
• Space evenly around the clock. • Teach patient and family to take resting pulse daily. • Report pulse rate less than 60 beats/min. • Seafood, iodine products may be restricted. • Report illness, unusual bleeding or bruising immediately. • Inform physician of sudden or continuous weight gain, cold intolerance, depression.

Proscar, *see finasteride*

protamine sulfate

proe-ta-meen
(Protamine ✦, Protamine sulfate)

Do not confuse protamine with ProAmatine, Protopam, or Protropin.

◆CLASSIFICATION

PHARMACOTHERAPEUTIC: Protein.
CLINICAL: Heparin antagonist.

ACTION

A protein that complexes with heparin to form a stable salt. **Therapeutic Effect:** Reduces anticoagulant activity of heparin.

PHARMACOKINETICS

Metabolized by fibrinolysin. **Half-life:** 7.4 min.

USES

Treatment of severe heparin overdose (causing hemorrhage). Neutralizes effects of heparin administered during extracorporeal circulation. **OFF-LABEL:** Treatment of low molecular weight heparin toxicity.

PRECAUTIONS

CONTRAINDICATIONS: None known. **CAUTIONS:** History of allergy to fish or seafood; vasectomized or infertile men; those on isophane (NPH), insulin, or previous protamine therapy (propensity to hypersensitivity reaction).

⏳ **LIFESPAN CONSIDERATIONS: Pregnancy/Lactation:** Unknown if drug crosses placenta or is distributed in breast milk. **Pregnancy Category C. Children:** Safety and efficacy not established. **Elderly:** No age-related precautions noted.

INTERACTIONS

DRUG: None known. **HERBAL:** None known. **FOOD:** None known. **LAB VALUES:** None known.

AVAILABILITY (Rx)

INJECTION: 10 mg/ml.

ADMINISTRATION/HANDLING

 IV

Rate of administration • May give undiluted over 10 min. Do not exceed 5 mg/min (50 mg in any 10-min period).

Storage • Store vials at room temperature.

INDICATIONS/ROUTES/DOSAGE

HEPARIN OVERDOSE (ANTIDOTE AND TREATMENT)
IV: ADULTS, ELDERLY: 1–1.5 mg protamine neutralizes 100 units heparin. Heparin disappears rapidly from circulation, reducing the dosage demand for protamine as time elapses.

SIDE EFFECTS

FREQUENT: Decreased BP, dyspnea. **OCCASIONAL:** Hypersensitivity reaction (urticaria, angioedema); nausea and vomiting, which generally occur in those sensitive to fish and seafood, vasectomized men, infertile men, those on isophane (NPH) insulin, or those previously on protamine therapy. **RARE:** Back pain.

ADVERSE REACTIONS/ TOXIC EFFECTS

Too rapid IV administration may produce acute hypotension, bradycardia, pulmonary hypertension, dyspnea, transient flushing, and feeling of warmth. Heparin rebound may occur several hours after heparin has been neutralized (usually 8–9 hr after protamine administration). Heparin rebound occurs most often after arterial or cardiac surgery.

NURSING CONSIDERATIONS

BASELINE ASSESSMENT
Check PT, aPTT, Hct; assess for bleeding.

INTERVENTION/EVALUATION

Monitor coagulation tests, aPTT or ACT, BP, cardiac function.

Protonix, *see pantoprazole*

---

protriptyline hydrochloride

(Vivactil)

See Antidepressants (p. 37C)

Proventil HFA, *see albuterol*

Provigil, *see modafinil*

Prozac, *see fluoxetine*

---

pseudoephedrine

soo-doe-e-**fed**-rin

(Balminil Decongestant ♣, BioContac Cold 12 Hour Relief Non Drowsy ♣, Biofed, Decofed, Dimetapp 12 Hour Non Drowsy Extentabs, Dimetapp Decongestant, Dimetapp Decongestant Infant Drops, Genaphed, PMS-Pseudoephedrine ♣, Robidrine ♣, Sudafed, Sudafed 12h ♣, Sudafed 12 Hour, Sudafed 24 Hour)

FIXED-COMBINATION(S)

Advil Cold, Motrin Cold: pseudoephedrine/ibuprofen (NSAID): 30 mg/200 mg; 15 mg/100 mg per 5 ml. **Allegra-D:** pseudoephedrine/fexofenadine (an antihistamine): 120 mg/60 mg. **Allegra D 24 Hour:** pseudoephedrine/fexofenadine: 240 mg/180 mg. **Claritin-D:** pseudoephedrine/loratadine (an antihistamine): 120 mg/5 mg; 240 mg/10 mg. **Clarinex-D 24-Hour:** pseudoephedrine/desloratadine (an antihistamine): 240 mg/5 mg. **Clarinex-D 12-Hour:** pseudoephedrine/desloratadine: 120 mg/2.5 mg. **Zyrtec-D:** pseudoephedrine/cetirizine (an antihistamine): 120 mg/5 mg.

◆CLASSIFICATION

PHARMACOTHERAPEUTIC: Sympathomimetic. **CLINICAL:** Nasal decongestant.

ACTION

A sympathomimetic that directly stimulates alpha-adrenergic and beta-adrenergic receptors. **Therapeutic Effect:** Produces vasoconstriction of respiratory tract mucosa; shrinks nasal mucous membranes; reduces edema, and nasal congestion.

PHARMACOKINETICS

Route	Onset	Peak	Duration
PO (tablets, syrup)	15–30 min	N/A	4–6 hr
PO (extended-release)	N/A	N/A	8–12 hr

Well absorbed from the GI tract. Partially metabolized in the liver. Primarily excreted in urine. Not removed by hemodialysis. **Half-life:** 9–16 hr (children, 3.1 hr).

P

USES

Temporary relief of nasal congestion due to the common cold, upper respiratory allergies, sinusitis. Enhances nasal, sinus drainage.

PRECAUTIONS

CONTRAINDICATIONS: Breast-feeding women, coronary artery disease, severe hypertension, use within 14 days of MAOIs. Sustained release: children younger than 12 yr. **CAUTIONS:** Elderly, hyperthyroidism, diabetes, ischemic heart disease, prostatic hypertrophy.

⏳ **LIFESPAN CONSIDERATIONS: Pregnancy/Lactation:** Crosses placenta. Distributed in breast milk. **Pregnancy Category C. Children:** Safety and efficacy not established in those younger than 2 yr. **Elderly:** Age-related prostatic hypertrophy may require dosage adjustment.

INTERACTIONS

DRUG: Antihypertensive, beta blockers, diuretics: May decrease the effects of these drugs. **MAOIs:** May increase cardiac stimulant and vasopressor effects. **HERBAL:** None known. **FOOD:** None known. **LAB VALUES:** None known.

AVAILABILITY (OTC)

GELCAPS (DIMETAPP DECONGESTANT): 30 mg. **LIQUID:** 15 mg/5 ml. **ORAL DROPS (DIMETAPP DECONGESTANT INFANT DROPS):** 7.5 mg/0.8 ml. **SYRUP (BIOFED, DECOFED):** 30 mg/5 ml. **TABLETS (GENAPHED, SUDAFED):** 30 mg. **TABLETS (CHEWABLE [SUDAFED]):** 15 mg. **TABLETS (EXTENDED-RELEASE):** 120 mg (Dimetapp 12 Hour Non Drowsy Extentabs, Sudafed 12 Hour), 240 mg (Sudafed 24 Hour).

◀ **ALERT** ▶ Pseudoephedrine is a key ingredient in synthesizing methamphetamine. Many pharmacies have moved pseudoephedrine behind the counter due to concerns about its purchase and theft for the purposes of methamphetamine manufacture.

ADMINISTRATION/HANDLING
PO
• Do not crush, chew extended-release tablets; swallow whole.

INDICATIONS/ROUTES/DOSAGE
DECONGESTANT
PO: ADULTS, CHILDREN 12 YR AND OLDER: 60 mg q4–6h. **Maximum:** 240 mg/day. CHILDREN 6–11 YR: 30 mg q6h. **Maximum:** 120 mg/day. CHILDREN 2–5 YR: 15 mg q6h. **Maximum:** 60 mg/day. CHILDREN YOUNGER THAN 2 YR: 4 mg/kg/day in divided doses q6h. ELDERLY: 30–60 mg q6h as needed.
PO (EXTENDED-RELEASE): ADULTS, CHILDREN 12 YR AND OLDER: 120 mg q12h or 240 mg once daily.

SIDE EFFECTS

OCCASIONAL (10%–5%): Nervousness, restlessness, insomnia, tremor, headache. **RARE (4%–1%):** Diaphoresis, weakness.

ADVERSE REACTIONS/ TOXIC EFFECTS

Large doses may produce tachycardia, palpitations (particularly in patients with cardiac disease), light-headedness, nausea, and vomiting. Overdose in patients older than 60 yr may result in hallucinations, CNS depression, and seizures.

NURSING CONSIDERATIONS

PATIENT/FAMILY TEACHING
• Discontinue drug if adverse reactions occur. • Report insomnia, dizziness, tremors, tachycardia, palpitations.

psyllium

sill-ee-yum

(Fiberall, Hydrocil, Konsyl, Metamucil, Novo-Mucilax ✤, Perdiem)

CLASSIFICATION

PHARMACOTHERAPEUTIC: Bulk-forming laxative (see p. 109C).

ACTION

A bulk-forming laxative that dissolves and swells in water providing increased bulk and moisture content in stool. Therapeutic Effect: Promotes peristalsis and bowel motility.

PHARMACOKINETICS

Route	Onset	Peak	Duration
PO	12–24 hr	2–3 days	N/A

Acts in small and large intestines.

USES

Treatment of chronic constipation, constipation associated with rectal disorders, management of irritable bowel syndrome (IBS).

PRECAUTIONS

CONTRAINDICATIONS: Fecal impaction, GI obstruction, undiagnosed abdominal pain. **CAUTIONS:** Esophageal strictures, ulcers, stenosis, intestinal adhesions.

⌛ LIFESPAN CONSIDERATIONS: **Pregnancy/Lactation:** Safe for use in pregnancy. **Pregnancy Category B. Children:** Safety and efficacy not established for those younger than 6 yr. **Elderly:** No age-related precautions noted.

INTERACTIONS

DRUG: **Digoxin, oral anticoagulants, salicylates:** May decrease the effects of digoxin, oral anticoagulants, and salicylates by decreasing absorption. **Potassium-sparing diuretics, potassium supplements:** May interfere with the effects of potassium-sparing diuretics and potassium supplements. HERBAL: None known. FOOD: None known. LAB VALUES: May increase blood glucose level. May decrease serum potassium level.

AVAILABILITY (OTC)

POWDER (FIBERALL, HYDROCIL, KONSYL, METAMUCIL). WAFER (METAMUCIL): 3.4 g/dose. **CAPSULES (METAMUCIL):** 0.52 g. **GRANULES (PERDIEM):** 4 g/5 ml.

ADMINISTRATION/HANDLING

PO

• Administer at least 2 hr before or after other medication. • All doses should be followed with 8 oz liquid • Drink 6–8 glasses of water/day (aids stool softening) • Do not swallow in dry form; mix with at least 1 full glass (8 oz) of liquid.

INDICATIONS/ROUTES/DOSAGE

CONSTIPATION, IRRITABLE BOWEL SYNDROME

PO: ◀ ALERT ▶ 3.4 g powder equals 1 rounded tsp, 1 packet, or 1 wafer. ADULTS, ELDERLY: 2–5 capsules/dose 1–3 times a day. 1–2 tsp granules 1–2 times a day. 1 rounded tsp or 1 tbsp of powder 1–3 times a day. 2 wafers 1–3 times a day. CHILDREN 6–11 YR: ½–1 tsp powder in water 1–3 times a day.

SIDE EFFECTS

RARE: Some degree of abdominal discomfort, nausea, mild abdominal cramps, griping, faintness.

ADVERSE REACTIONS/ TOXIC EFFECTS

Esophageal or bowel obstruction may occur if administered less than 250 ml of liquid.

P

NURSING CONSIDERATIONS

INTERVENTION/EVALUATION

Encourage adequate fluid intake. Assess bowel sounds for peristalsis. Monitor pattern of daily bowel activity and stool consistency. Monitor serum electrolytes in patients exposed to prolonged, frequent, excessive use of medication.

PATIENT/FAMILY TEACHING

• Take each dose with a full glass (250 ml) of water. • Inadequate fluid intake may cause GI obstruction. • Institute measures to promote defecation (increase fluid intake, exercise, high-fiber diet).

Pulmicort Respules,
see budesonide

Pulmicort Turbuhaler, *see budesonide*

pyrazinamide

pye-ra-**zin**-a-mide
(Pyrazinamide, Tebrazid ✦)

FIXED-COMBINATION(S)

Rifater: pyrazinamide/isoniazid/rifampin (an antitubercular): 300 mg/50 mg/120 mg.

⬩CLASSIFICATION

CLINICAL: Antitubercular.

ACTION

An antitubercular whose exact mechanism of action is unknown. Therapeutic Effect: Either bacteriostatic or bactericidal, depending on the drugs concentration at the infection site and the susceptibility of infecting bacteria.

PHARMACOKINETICS

Nearly completely absorbed from GI tract. Protein binding: 5%–10%. Excreted in urine. Half-life: 9–23 hr.

USES

In conjunction with at least one other antitubercular agent in treatment of clinical tuberculosis after failure of primary agents (isoniazid, rifampin).

PRECAUTIONS

CONTRAINDICATIONS: Severe hepatic dysfunction. CAUTIONS: Diabetes mellitus, renal impairment, history of gout, children (safety not established). Possible cross-sensitivity with isoniazid, ethionamide, niacin.

⧗ LIFESPAN CONSIDERATIONS: Pregnancy/Lactation: Unknown if drug crosses placenta or is distributed in breast milk. Pregnancy Category C. Children: Safety and efficacy not established. Elderly: No age-related precautions noted.

INTERACTIONS

DRUG: **Allopurinol, colchicine, probenecid, sulfinpyrazone:** May decrease the effects of these drugs. HERBAL: None known. FOOD: None known. LAB VALUES: May increase AST, ALT, and serum uric acid concentrations.

AVAILABILITY (Rx)

TABLETS: 500 mg.

INDICATIONS/ROUTES/DOSAGE

TUBERCULOSIS (IN COMBINATION WITH OTHER ANTITUBERCULARS)

PO: ADULTS: 15–30 mg/kg/day in 1–4 doses. **Maximum:** 3 g/day. CHILDREN: 20–40 mg/kg/day in 1 or 2 doses. **Maximum:** 2 g/day.

SIDE EFFECTS

FREQUENT: Arthralgia, myalgia (usually mild and self-limiting). **RARE:** Hypersensitivity reaction (rash, pruritus, urticaria), photosensitivity, gouty arthritis.

ADVERSE REACTIONS/ TOXIC EFFECTS

Hepatotoxicity, gouty arthritis, thrombocytopenia, and anemia occur rarely.

NURSING CONSIDERATIONS

BASELINE ASSESSMENT

Question for hypersensitivity to pyrazinamide, isoniazid, ethionamide, niacin. Ensure collection of specimens for culture, sensitivity. Evaluate results of initial CBC, liver function tests, serum uric acid levels.

INTERVENTION/EVALUATION

Monitor liver function test results; be alert for hepatic reactions: jaundice, malaise, fever, liver tenderness, anorexia, nausea, vomiting (stop drug, notify physician promptly). Check serum uric acid levels; assess for hot, painful, swollen joints, especially big toe, ankle, knee (gout). Evaluate serum blood sugar levels, diabetic status carefully (pyrazinamide makes management difficult). Assess for rash, skin eruptions. Monitor CBC for thrombocytopenia, anemia.

PATIENT/FAMILY TEACHING

• Do not skip doses; complete full length of therapy (may be months or years). • Office visits, lab tests are essential part of treatment. • Take with food to reduce GI upset. • Avoid excessive exposure to sun, ultraviolet light until photosensitivity is determined. • Notify physician of any new symptom, immediately for jaundice (yellow sclera of eyes/skin); unusual fatigue; fever; loss of appetite; hot, painful, swollen joints.

pyridostigmine bromide

peer-id-oh-**stig**-meen
(Mestinon, Mestinon SR ✦, Mestinon Timespan)
Do not confuse pyridostigmine with physostigmine or Mesitonin with Mesantoin or Metatensin.

◆ CLASSIFICATION

PHARMACOTHERAPEUTIC: Anticholinesterase. **CLINICAL:** Cholinergic muscle stimulant (see p. 82C).

ACTION

A cholinergic that prevents destruction of acetylcholine by inhibiting the enzyme acetylcholinesterase, thus enhancing impulse transmission across the myoneural junction. **Therapeutic Effect:** Produces miosis; increases tone of intestinal, skeletal muscle tone; stimulates salivary and sweat gland secretions.

PHARMACOKINETICS

Not protein bound. Excreted unchanged in urine. **Half-life:** Unknown.

USES

Improvement of muscle strength in control of myasthenia gravis, reversal of effects of nondepolarizing neuromuscular blocking agents after surgery.

PRECAUTIONS

CONTRAINDICATIONS: Mechanical GI or urinary tract obstruction, hypersensitivity to anticholinesterase agents. **CAUTIONS:** Bronchial asthma, bradycardia, epilepsy, recent coronary occlusion, vagotonia, hyperthyroidism, cardiac arrhythmias, peptic ulcer.

⧗ **LIFESPAN CONSIDERATIONS:** Pregnancy/Lactation: Unknown if drug crosses placenta or is distributed in breast milk. **Pregnancy Category C. Children:** Safety and efficacy not established. **Elderly:** No age-related precautions noted.

INTERACTIONS

DRUG: Anticholinergics: Prevent or reverse the effects of pyridostigmine. **Cholinesterase inhibitors:** May increase the risk of toxicity. **Neuromuscular blockers:** Antagonizes the effects of these drugs. **Procainamide, quinidine:** May antagonize the action of pyridostigmine. **HERBAL:** None known. **FOOD:** None known. **LAB VALUES:** None known.

AVAILABILITY (Rx)

SYRUP (MESTINON): 60 mg/5 ml. **TABLETS (MESTINON):** 60 mg. **TABLETS (EXTENDED-RELEASE [MESTINON TIMESPAN]):** 180 mg. **INJECTION (MESTINON):** 5 mg/ml.

ADMINISTRATION/HANDLING

▽ **IV, IM**

• Give large parenteral doses concurrently with 0.6–1.2 mg atropine sulfate IV to minimize side effects.

PO

• Give with food, milk. • Tablets may be crushed; do not chew, crush extended-release tablets (may be broken). • Give

larger dose at times of increased fatigue (e.g., for those with difficulty in chewing, 30–45 min before meals).

▨ IV INCOMPATIBILITIES

Don't mix pyridostigmine with any other medications.

INDICATIONS/ROUTES/DOSAGE

MYASTHENIA GRAVIS

PO: ADULTS, ELDERLY: Initially, 60 mg 3 times a day. Dosage increased at 48 hr intervals. Maintenance: 60 mg–1.5 g a day.

PO (EXTENDED-RELEASE): ADULTS, ELDERLY: 180–540 mg once or twice a day with at least a 6 hr interval between doses.

IV, IM: ADULTS, ELDERLY: 2 mg q2–3h. CHILDREN, NEONATES: 0.05–0.15 mg/kg/dose. **Maximum single dose:** 10 mg.

REVERSAL OF NONDEPOLARIZING NEUROMUSCULAR BLOCKADE

IV: ADULTS, ELDERLY: 10–20 mg with, or shortly after, 0.6–1.2 mg atropine sulfate or 0.3–0.6 mg glycopyrrolate. CHILDREN: 0.1–0.25 mg/kg/dose preceded by atropine or glycopyrrolate.

SIDE EFFECTS

FREQUENT: Miosis, increased GI and skeletal muscle tone, bradycardia, constriction of bronchi and ureters, diaphoresis, increased salivation. **OCCASIONAL:** Headache, rash, temporary decrease in diastolic BP with mild reflex tachycardia, short periods of atrial fibrillation (in hyperthyroid patients), marked drop in BP (in hypertensive patients).

ADVERSE REACTIONS/TOXIC EFFECTS

Overdose may produce a cholinergic crisis, manifested as increasingly severe muscle weakness that appears first in muscles involving chewing and swallowing and is followed by muscle weakness of the shoulder girdle and upper extremities, respiratory muscle paralysis, and pelvis girdle and leg muscle paralysis. If overdose occurs, stop all cholinergic drugs and immediately administer 1–4 mg atropine sulfate IV for adults or 0.01 mg/kg for infants and children younger than 12 yr.

NURSING CONSIDERATIONS

BASELINE ASSESSMENT

Larger doses should be given at time of greatest fatigue. Assess muscle strength before testing for diagnosis of myasthenia gravis and following drug administration. Avoid large doses in patients with megacolon or reduced GI motility.

INTERVENTION/EVALUATION

Have tissues readily available at patient's bedside. Monitor respirations closely during myasthenia gravis testing or if dosage is increased. Assess diligently for cholinergic reaction, as well as bradycardia in the myasthenic patient in crisis. Coordinate dosage time with periods of fatigue and increased or decreased muscle strength. Monitor for therapeutic response to medication (increased muscle strength, decreased fatigue, improved chewing and swallowing functions).

PATIENT/FAMILY TEACHING

• Report nausea, vomiting, diarrhea, diaphoresis, profuse salivary secretions, palpitations, muscle weakness, severe abdominal pain, difficulty breathing.

pyridoxine hydrochloride (vitamin B₆)

peer-i-**dox**-een

(Aminoxin, Beesix, Doxine, Nestrex, Pryi, Rodex, Vitabee 6, Vitamin B₆)

Do not confuse pyridoxine with paroxetine, pralidoxime, or Pyridium.

◆CLASSIFICATION

PHARMACOTHERAPEUTIC: Coenzyme. **CLINICAL:** Vitamin (B₆) (see p. 145C).

ACTION

Acts as a coenzyme for various metabolic functions, including metabolism of proteins, carbohydrates, and fats. Aids in the breakdown of glycogen and in the synthesis of gamma-aminobutyric acid in the CNS. **Therapeutic Effect:** Prevents pyridoxine deficiency. Increases the excretion of certain drugs, such as isoniazid, that are pyridoxine antagonists.

PHARMACOKINETICS

Readily absorbed primarily in jejunum. Stored in the liver, muscle, and brain. Metabolized in the liver. Primarily excreted in urine. Removed by hemodialysis. **Half-life:** 15–20 days.

USES

Prevention and treatment of vitamin B₆ deficiency, pyridoxine-dependent seizures in infants, drug-induced neuritis (e.g., isoniazid).

PRECAUTIONS

CONTRAINDICATIONS: None known. **CAUTIONS:** None known.

⧖ **LIFESPAN CONSIDERATIONS: Pregnancy/Lactation:** Crosses placenta.

P

Distributed in breast milk. High dosages in utero may produce seizures in neonates. **Pregnancy Category A. Children/Elderly:** No age-related precautions noted.

INTERACTIONS

DRUG: **Immunosuppressants, isoniazid, penicillamine:** May antagonize pyridoxine, causing anemia or peripheral neuritis. **Levodopa:** Reverses the effects of levodopa. HERBAL: None known. FOOD: None known. LAB VALUES: None known.

AVAILABILITY (OTC)

CAPSULES: 250 mg. **TABLETS:** 25 mg, 50 mg, 100 mg, 250 mg, 500 mg. **TABLETS (ENTERIC-COATED [AMINOXIN]):** 20 mg. **INJECTION (VITAMIN B$_6$):** 100 mg/ml.

ADMINISTRATION/HANDLING

◀ ALERT ▶   Give PO unless nausea, vomiting, malabsorption occurs. Avoid IV use in cardiac patients.

IV
• Give undiluted or add to IV solutions and give as infusion.

▓ IV INCOMPATIBILITIES

Don't mix pyridoxine with any other medications.

INDICATIONS/ROUTES/DOSAGE

PYRIDOXINE DEFICIENCY
PO: ADULTS, ELDERLY: Initially, 2.5–10 mg/day; then 2.5 mg/day when clinical signs are corrected. CHILDREN: Initially, 5–25 mg/day for 3 wk, then 1.5–2.5 mg/day.

PYRIDOXINE DEPENDENT SEIZURES
PO, IV, IM: INFANTS: Initially, 10–100 mg/day. Maintenance: **PO:** 50–100 mg/day.

DRUG-INDUCED NEURITIS
PO (TREATMENT): ADULTS, ELDERLY: 100–300 mg/day in divided doses. CHILDREN: 10–50 mg/day.
PO (PROPHYLAXIS): ADULTS, ELDERLY: 25–100 mg/day. CHILDREN: 1–2mg/kg/day.

SIDE EFFECTS

OCCASIONAL: Stinging at IM injection site. **RARE:** Headache, nausea, somnolence; sensory neuropathy (paraesthesia, unstable gait, clumsiness of hands) with high doses.

ADVERSE REACTIONS/ TOXIC EFFECTS

Long-term megadoses (2–6 g over more than 2 mo) may produce sensory neuropathy (reduced deep tendon reflexes, profound impairment of sense of position in distal limbs, gradual sensory ataxia). Toxic symptoms subside when drug is discontinued. Seizures have occurred after IV megadoses.

INTERVENTION/EVALUATION
Observe for improvement of deficiency symptoms and glossitis. Evaluate for nutritional adequacy.

PATIENT/FAMILY TEACHING
• Discomfort may occur with IM injection. • Encourage intake of foods rich in pyridoxine (legumes, soybeans, eggs, sunflower seeds, hazelnuts, organ meats, tuna, shrimp, carrots, avocado, banana, wheat germ, bran).

quazepam

(Doral)
See Sedative-hypnotics (p. 136C)

quetiapine

kwe-**tye**-a-peen
(Seroquel)

◆ CLASSIFICATION

PHARMACOTHERAPEUTIC: Dibenzapine derivative. **CLINICAL:** Antipsychotic (see p. 59C).

ACTION

A dibenzothiazepine derivative that antagonizes dopamine, serotonin, histamine, and alpha1-adrenergic receptors. Therapeutic Effect: Diminishes manifestations of psychotic disorders. Produces moderate sedation, few extrapyramidal effects, and no anticholinergic effects.

PHARMACOKINETICS

Well absorbed after PO administration. Protein binding: 83%. Widely distributed in tissues; CNS concentration exceeds plasma concentration. Undergoes extensive first-pass metabolism in the liver. Primarily excreted in urine. Half-life: 6 hr.

USES

Management of manifestations of psychotic disorders. Short-term treatment of acute manic episodes associated with bipolar disorder. OFF-LABEL: Autism, psychosis (children).

PRECAUTIONS

CONTRAINDICATIONS: None known. **CAUTIONS:** Alzheimer's dementia, history of breast cancer, cardiovascular disease (e.g., CHF, history of MI), cerebrovascular disease, hepatic impairment, dehydration, hypovolemia, history of drug abuse or dependence, seizures, hypothyroidism.

🖅 LIFESPAN CONSIDERATIONS: **Pregnancy/Lactation:** Unknown if drug is distributed in breast milk. Not recommended for breast-feeding mothers. **Pregnancy Category C. Children:** Safety and efficacy not established. **Elderly:** No age-related precautions noted, but lower initial and target dosages may be necessary.

INTERACTIONS

DRUG: Alcohol, other CNS depressants: May increase CNS depression. **Antihypertensives:** May increase the hypotensive effects of these drugs. **Hepatic enzyme inducers (such as phenytoin):** May increase quetiapine clearance. HERBAL: None known. FOOD: None known. LAB VALUES: May decrease serum total and free thyroxine (T_4) serum levels. May increase serum cholesterol, triglyceride, AST, and ALT levels. May produce a false-positive pregnancy test result.

AVAILABILITY (Rx)

TABLETS: 25 mg, 50 mg, 100 mg, 200 mg, 300 mg, 400 mg.

ADMINISTRATION/HANDLING

PO

• Adjust dosage at 2-day intervals. • Initial dose and dosage titration should occur at a lower dosage in elderly, patients with hepatic impairment, debilitated, or those predisposed to hypotensive reactions. • When restarting patients who have been off quetiapine for less than 1 wk, titration is not required and maintenance dose can be reinstituted. • When restarting patients who have been off quetiapine for longer than 1 wk, follow initial titration schedule. • Give without regard to food.

INDICATIONS/ROUTES/DOSAGE

TO MANAGE MANIFESTATIONS OF PSYCHOTIC DISORDERS

PO: ADULTS, ELDERLY: Initially, 25 mg twice a day, then 25–50 mg 2–3 times a day on the second and third days, up to 300–400 mg/day in divided doses 2–3 times a day by the fourth day. Further adjustments of 25–50 mg twice a day may be made at intervals of 2 days or longer. Maintenance: 300–800 mg/day (adults); 50–200 mg/day (elderly).

MANIA IN BIPOLAR DISORDER

PO: ADULTS, ELDERLY: Initially, 50 mg twice a day for 1 day. May increase in increments of 100 mg/day to 200 mg twice a day on day 4. May increase in increments of 200 mg/day to 800 mg/day on day 6. Range: 400–800 mg/day.

DOSAGE IN HEPATIC IMPAIRMENT, ELDERLY OR DEBILITATED PATIENTS, AND THOSE PREDISPOSED TO HYPOTENSIVE REACTIONS

These patients should receive a lower initial dose and lower dosage increases.

SIDE EFFECTS

FREQUENT (19%–10%): Headache, somnolence, dizziness. **OCCASIONAL (9%–3%):** Constipation, orthostatic hypotension, tachycardia, dry mouth, dyspepsia, rash, asthenia, abdominal pain, rhinitis. **RARE (2%):** Back pain, fever, weight gain.

ADVERSE REACTIONS/ TOXIC EFFECTS

Overdose may produce heart block hypotension, hypokalemia, and tachycardia.

NURSING CONSIDERATIONS

BASELINE ASSESSMENT

Assess behavior, appearance, emotional status, response to environment, speech pattern, thought content. Obtain baseline CBC, hepatic enzyme levels before initiating treatment and periodically thereafter.

INTERVENTION/EVALUATION

Assist with ambulation if dizziness occurs. Supervise suicidal-risk patient closely during early therapy (as psychosis, depression lessens, energy level improves, increasing suicide potential). Monitor BP for hypotension. Assess pulse for tachycardia (especially with rapid increase in dosage). Assess bowel activity for evidence of constipation. Assess for therapeutic response (improved thought content, increased ability to concentrate, improvement in self-care). Eye exam to detect cataract formation should be obtained q6mo during treatment.

PATIENT/FAMILY TEACHING

• Avoid exposure to extreme heat. • Drink fluids often, especially during physical activity. • Take medication as ordered; do not stop taking or increase dosage. • Drowsiness generally subsides during continued therapy. • Avoid tasks that require alertness, motor skills until response to drug is established. • Avoid alcohol. • Change positions slowly to reduce hypotensive effect.

quinapril hydrochloride

kwin-na-pril

(Accupril)

Do not confuse Accupril with Accolate or Accutane.

FIXED-COMBINATION(S)

Accuretic: quinapril/hydrochlorothiazide (a diuretic): 10 mg/12.5 mg; 20 mg/12.5 mg; 20 mg/25 mg.

CLASSIFICATION

PHARMACOTHERAPEUTIC: Angiotensin-converting enzyme (ACE) inhibitor. **CLINICAL:** Antihypertensive (see p. 7C).

ACTION

An ACE inhibitor that suppresses the renin-angiotensin-aldosterone system and prevents the conversion of angiotensin I to angiotensin II, a potent vasoconstrictor; may also inhibit angiotensin II at local vascular and renal sites. Therapeutic Effect: Reduces peripheral arterial resistance, BP, and pulmonary capillary wedge pressure; improves cardiac output.

PHARMACOKINETICS

Route	Onset	Peak	Duration
PO	1 hr	N/A	24 hr

Readily absorbed from the GI tract. Protein binding: 97%. Metabolized in the liver, GI tract, and extravascular tissue to active metabolite. Primarily excreted in urine. Minimal removal by hemodialysis. Half-life: 1–2 hr; metabolite, 3 hr (increased in those with impaired renal function).

USES

Treatment of hypertension. Used alone or in combination with other antihypertensives. Adjunctive therapy in management of heart failure. OFF-LABEL: Treatment of hypertension and renal crisis in scleroderma, treatment of left ventricular dysfunction following MI.

PRECAUTIONS

CONTRAINDICATIONS: Bilateral renal artery stenosis, history of angioedema from previous treatment with ACE inhibitors. **CAUTIONS:** Renal impairment, CHF, collagen vascular disease, hypovolemia, renal stenosis, hyperkalemia.

LIFESPAN CONSIDERATIONS: **Pregnancy/Lactation:** Crosses placenta. Unknown if distributed in breast milk. May cause fetal or neonatal mortality or morbidity. **Pregnancy Category C (D if used in second or third trimester).** **Children:** Safety and efficacy not established. **Elderly:** May be more sensitive to hypotensive effects.

INTERACTIONS

DRUG: **Alcohol, antihypertensives, diuretics:** May increase the effects of quinapril. **Lithium:** May increase lithium blood concentration and risk of lithium toxicity. **NSAIDs:** May decrease the effects of quinapril. **Potassium-sparing diuretics, potassium supplements:** May cause hyperkalemia. HERBAL: **Garlic:** May increase antihypertensive effect. **Ginseng, yohimbe:** May worsen hypertension. FOOD: None known. LAB VALUES: May increase BUN, serum alkaline phosphatase, serum bilirubin, serum creatinine, serum potassium, AST, and ALT levels. May decrease serum sodium levels. May cause positive antinuclear antibody titer.

AVAILABILITY (Rx)

TABLETS: 5 mg, 10 mg, 20 mg, 40 mg.

ADMINISTRATION/HANDLING

PO
• Give without regard to food. • Tablets may be crushed.

INDICATIONS/ROUTES/DOSAGE

HYPERTENSION (MONOTHERAPY)
PO: ADULTS: Initially, 10–20 mg/day. May adjust dosage at intervals of at least 2 wk or longer. Maintenance: 20–80 mg/day as single dose or 2 divided doses. **Maximum:** 80 mg/day. ELDERLY: Initially, 2.5–5 mg/day. May increase by 2.5–5 mg q1–2wk.

Q

HYPERTENSION (COMBINATION THERAPY)

PO: ADULTS: Initially, 5 mg/day titrated to patient's needs. **ELDERLY:** Initially, 2.5–5 mg/day. May increase by 2.5–5 mg q1–2wk.

ADJUNCT TO MANAGE HEART FAILURE

PO: ADULTS, ELDERLY: Initially, 5 mg twice a day. Range: 20–40 mg/day.

DOSAGE IN RENAL IMPAIRMENT

Dosage is titrated to the patient's needs after the following initial doses:

Creatinine Clearance	Initial Dose
More than 60 ml/min	10 mg
30–60 ml/min	5 mg
10–29 ml/min	2.5 mg

SIDE EFFECTS

FREQUENT (7%–5%): Headache, dizziness. **OCCASIONAL (4%–2%):** Fatigue, vomiting, nausea, hypotension, chest pain, cough, syncope. **RARE (less than 2%):** Diarrhea, cough, dyspnea, rash, palpitations, impotence, insomnia, drowsiness, malaise.

ADVERSE REACTIONS/ TOXIC EFFECTS

Excessive hypotension ("first-dose syncope") may occur in patients with CHF and in those who are severely salt or volume depleted. Angioedema and hyperkalemia occur rarely. Agranulocytosis and neutropenia may be noted in those with collagen vascular disease, including scleroderma and systemic lupus erythematosus, and impaired renal function. Nephrotic syndrome may be noted in those with history of renal disease.

NURSING CONSIDERATIONS

BASELINE ASSESSMENT

Obtain BP immediately before each dose in addition to regular monitoring (be alert to fluctuations). If excessive reduction in BP occurs, place patient in supine position with legs slightly elevated. Renal function tests should be performed before beginning therapy. In patients with prior renal disease, urine test for protein by dipstick method should be made with first urine of day before beginning therapy and periodically thereafter. In those with renal impairment, autoimmune disease or in those taking drugs that affect leukocytes or immune response, CBC, differential count should be performed before beginning therapy and q2wk for 3 mo, then periodically thereafter.

INTERVENTION/EVALUATION

Monitor renal function, serum potassium, WBC. Assist with ambulation if dizziness occurs. Question for evidence of headache. Non-cola carbonated beverage, unsalted crackers, dry toast may relieve nausea.

PATIENT/FAMILY TEACHING

• To reduce hypotensive effect, rise slowly from lying to sitting position, permit legs to dangle from bed momentarily before standing. • Full therapeutic effect may take 1–2 wk. • Report any sign of infection (sore throat, fever). • Skipping doses or voluntarily discontinuing drug may produce severe rebound hypertension. • Avoid tasks that require alertness, motor skills until response to drug is established.

quinidine

kwin-ih-deen

(Apo-Quin-G ✤, Apo-Quinidine ✤, BioQuin Durules ✤, Quinaglute Dura-Tabs, Quinate ✤, Quinidex Extentabs)

Do not confuse quinidine with clonidine or quinine.

CLASSIFICATION

CLINICAL: Antiarrhythmic (see p. 14C).

ACTION

An antiarrhythmic that decreases sodium influx during depolarization, potassium efflux during repolarization, and reduces calcium transport across the myocardial cell membrane. Decreases myocardial excitability, conduction velocity, and contractility. **Therapeutic Effect:** Suppresses arrhythmias.

PHARMACOKINETICS

Almost completely absorbed after PO administration. Protein binding: 80%–90%. Metabolized in liver. Excreted in urine. Removed by hemodialysis. Half-life: 6–8 hr.

USES

Prophylactic therapy to maintain normal sinus rhythm following conversion of atrial fibrillation or flutter. Prevention of premature atrial, AV, ventricular contractions, paroxysmal atrial tachycardia, paroxysmal AV junctional rhythm, atrial fibrillation, atrial flutter, paroxysmal ventricular tachycardia not associated with complete heart block. OFF-LABEL: Treatment of malaria (IV only).

PRECAUTIONS

CONTRAINDICATIONS: Complete AV block, development of thrombocytopenic purpura during prior therapy with quinidine or quinine, intraventricular conduction defects (widening of QRS complex). **CAUTIONS:** Myocardial depression, sick sinus syndrome, incomplete AV block, digoxin toxicity, renal or hepatic impairment, myasthenia gravis.

LIFESPAN CONSIDERATIONS: Pregnancy/Lactation: Crosses placenta; distributed in breast milk. **Pregnancy Category C. Children:** Safety and efficacy not established. **Elderly:** No age-related precautions noted.

INTERACTIONS

DRUG: **Antimyasthenics:** May decrease effects of these drugs on skeletal muscle. **Digoxin:** May increase digoxin serum concentration. **Other antiarrhythmics, pimozide:** May increase cardiac effects. **Neuromuscular blockers, oral anticoagulants:** May increase effects of these drugs. **Urinary alkalizers such as antacids:** May decrease quinidine renal excretion. HERBAL: None known. FOOD: None known. LAB VALUES: None known. Therapeutic serum level is 2–5 mcg/ml; toxic serum level is greater than 5 mcg/ml.

AVAILABILITY (Rx)

INJECTION: 80 mg/ml. **TABLETS:** 200 mg, 300 mg. **TABLETS (EXTENDED-RELEASE):** 300 mg (Quinidex Extentabs), 324 mg (Quinaglute Dura-Tabs).

ADMINISTRATION/HANDLING

IV

‹ ALERT › BP, EKG should be monitored continuously during IV administration and rate of infusion adjusted to minimize arrhythmias and hypotension.

Reconstitution • For IV infusion, dilute 800 mg with 40 ml D_5W to provide concentration of 16 mg/ml.

Rate of administration • Administer with patient in supine position. • For IV infusion, give at rate of 1 ml (16 mg)/min (a too rapid rate may markedly decrease arterial pressure). • Monitor EKG for cardiac changes, particularly prolongation of PR, QT intervals, widening of QRS complex. Notify

Q

physician of any significant interval changes.

Storage • Use only clear, colorless solution. • Solution is stable for 24 hr at room temperature when diluted with D₅W.

PO
• Do not crush or chew extended-release tablets. • GI upset can be reduced if given with food.

◼ IV INCOMPATIBILITIES
Furosemide (Lasix), heparin.

IV COMPATIBILITY
Milrinone (Primacor).

INDICATIONS/ROUTES/DOSAGE
MAINTENANCE OF NORMAL SINUS RHYTHM AFTER CONVERSION OF ATRIAL FIBRILLATION OR FLUTTER; PREVENTION OF PREMATURE ATRIAL, AV, AND VENTRICULAR CONTRACTIONS; PAROXYSMAL ATRIAL TACHYCARDIA; PAROXYSMAL AV JUNCTIONAL RHYTHM; ATRIAL FIBRILLATION; ATRIAL FLUTTER; PAROXYSMAL VENTRICULAR TACHYCARDIA NOT ASSOCIATED WITH COMPLETE HEART BLOCK
PO: ADULTS, ELDERLY: 100–600 mg q4–6h. (Long-acting): 324–972 mg q8–12h. CHILDREN: 30 mg/kg/day in divided doses q4–6h.
IV: ADULTS, ELDERLY: 200–400 mg. CHILDREN: 2–10 mg/kg.

SIDE EFFECTS
FREQUENT: Abdominal pain and cramps, nausea, diarrhea, vomiting (can be immediate, intense). **OCCASIONAL:** Mild cinchonism (ringing in ears, blurred vision, hearing loss) or severe cinchonism (headache, vertigo, diaphoresis, light-headedness, photophobia, confusion, delirium). **RARE:** Hypotension (particularly with IV administration),

hypersensitivity reaction (fever, anaphylaxis, photosensitivity reaction).

ADVERSE REACTIONS/ TOXIC EFFECTS
Cardiotoxic effects occur most commonly with IV administration, particularly at high concentrations, and are observed as conduction changes (50% widening of QRS complex, prolonged QT interval, flattened T waves, and disappearance of P wave), ventricular tachycardia or flutter, frequent premature ventricular contractions (PVCs), or complete AV block. Quinidine-induced syncope may occur with the usual dosage. Severe hypotension may result from high dosages. Patients with atrial flutter and fibrillation may experience a paradoxical, extremely rapid ventricular rate that may be prevented by prior digitalization. Hepatotoxicity with jaundice due to drug hypersensitivity may occur.

NURSING CONSIDERATIONS

BASELINE ASSESSMENT
Check BP, pulse (for 1 full min unless patient is on continuous monitor) before giving medication. For those on long-term therapy, CBC, liver and renal function tests should be performed periodically.

INTERVENTION/EVALUATION
Monitor EKG for cardiac changes, particularly prolongation of PR, QT intervals, widening of QRS complex. Monitor I&O, CBC, serum potassium, liver and renal function tests. Monitor pattern of daily bowel activity and stool consistency. Monitor BP for hypotension (especially in patients on high-dose therapy). If cardiotoxic effect occurs (see Adverse Reactions/Toxic Effects), notify physician immediately. Therapeutic serum level: 2–5 mcg/ml; toxic serum level: greater than 5 mcg/ml.

Q

quinine sulfate ℮

kwye-nine

(Quinine, Quinine-Odan ✦)

Do not confuse quinine with quinidine.

FIXED-COMBINATION(S)

With vitamin E for nocturnal leg cramps (**M-KYA, Q-vel**).

CLASSIFICATION

PHARMACOTHERAPEUTIC: Cinchona alkaloid. **CLINICAL:** Antimalarial, antimyotonic.

ACTION

Myotonia: Increases the refractory period, decreases excitability of motor end plates, affects distribution of calcium within the muscle fiber. **Therapeutic Effect:** Relaxes skeletal muscle. **Anti-malaria:** Depresses O_2 uptake, carbohydrate metabolism, elevates pH in intracellular organelles of parasites. **Therapeutic Effect:** Produces parasitic death.

USES

Treatment or suppression of chloroquine resistant *P. falciparum* malaria, treatment of babesiosis, prevention and treatment of nocturnal recumbency leg cramps.

PRECAUTIONS

CONTRAINDICATIONS: Tinnitus, optic neuritis, G6PD deficiency, pregnancy. **CAUTIONS:** Arrhythmias, myasthenia gravis, hepatic impairment. **Pregnancy Category X.**

INTERACTIONS

DRUG: Digoxin: The concentration of this drug may be increased when taken with quinine. **Mefloquine:** May increase seizures, EKG abnormalities. **HERBAL:** None known. **FOOD:** None known. **LAB VALUES:** May interfere with 17-OH steroid determinations.

AVAILABILITY (Rx)

CAPSULES: 200 mg, 325 mg. **TABLETS:** 260 mg.

INDICATIONS/ROUTES/DOSAGE

MALARIA TREATMENT
PO: ADULTS, ELDERLY: 650 mg q8h for 3–7 days (in combination). CHILDREN: 30 mg/kg/day in divided doses for 3–7 days (in combination). **Maximum:** 2 g a day.

MALARIA SUPPRESSION
PO: ADULTS, ELDERLY: 325 mg twice a day for up to 6 wk.

BABESIOSIS
PO: ADULTS, ELDERLY: 600 mg q6–8h for 7 days. CHILDREN: 25 mg/kg/day in divided doses for 7 days. **Maximum:** 650 mg/dose.

LEG CRAMPS
PO: ADULTS, ELDERLY: 200–300 mg at bedtime.

SIDE EFFECTS

FREQUENT: Nausea, headache, tinnitus, slight visual disturbances (mild cinchonism). **OCCASIONAL:** Extreme flushing of skin with intense generalized pruritus is most typical hypersensitivity reaction; also rash, wheezing, dyspnea, angioedema. Prolonged therapy: cardiac conduction disturbances, diminished hearing.

Q

ADVERSE REACTIONS/ TOXIC EFFECTS

Overdosage may produce severe cinchonism: cardiovascular effects, severe headache, intestinal cramps with vomiting/diarrhea, apprehension, confusion, seizures, blindness, respiratory depression. Hypoprothrombinemia, thrombocytopenic purpura, hemoglobinuria, asthma, agranulocytosis, hypoglycemia, deafness, optic atrophy occur rarely.

NURSING CONSIDERATIONS

BASELINE ASSESSMENT

Question for possibility of pregnancy before initiating therapy (Pregnancy Category X). Question for hypersensitivity to quinine, quinidine. Evaluate initial EKG, CBC results.

INTERVENTION/EVALUATION

Check for hypersensitivity: flushing, rash/urticaria, pruritus, dyspnea, wheezing. Assess level of hearing, visual acuity, presence of headache/tinnitus, nausea. Report adverse effects promptly (possible cinchonism). Monitor CBC results for blood dyscrasias. Be alert to infection (fever, sore throat), bleeding/ecchymosis, unusual fatigue/weakness. Assess pulse, EKG for arrhythmias. Check fasting blood sugar levels; watch for hypoglycemia (diaphoresis, tremors, tachycardia, hunger, anxiety).

PATIENT/FAMILY TEACHING

* Report tinnitus, hearing loss, rash, any visual disturbances. * Discuss the need for periodic lab tests as a part of therapy.

---

quinupristin-dalfopristin

kwin-yoo-pris-tin **dal**-foh-pris-tin
(Synercid)

◆ CLASSIFICATION

PHARMACOTHERAPEUTIC: Streptogramin. **CLINICAL:** Antimicrobial.

ACTION

Two chemically distinct compounds that, when given together, bind to different sites on bacterial ribosomes, inhibiting protein synthesis. **Therapeutic Effect:** Bactericidal.

PHARMACOKINETICS

After IV administration, both are extensively metabolized in the liver, with dalfopristin to active metabolite. Protein binding: quinupristin, 23%–32%; dalfopristin, 50%–56%. Primarily eliminated in feces. **Half-life:** quinupristin, 0.85 hr; dalfopristin, 0.7 hr.

USES

Treatment of serious or life-threatening infections caused by vancomycin-resistant *Enterococcus faecium* (VRE), complicated skin and skin-structure infections caused by *S. aureus* and *S. pyogenes.*

PRECAUTIONS

CONTRAINDICATIONS: Hypersensitivity to pristinamycin, virginiamycin. **CAUTIONS:** Hepatic or renal dysfunction.
⏳ **LIFESPAN CONSIDERATIONS: Pregnancy/Lactation:** Unknown if drug crosses placenta or is distributed in breast milk. **Pregnancy Category B. Children:** Safety and efficacy not established. **Elderly:** No age-related precautions noted.

INTERACTIONS

DRUG: Pimozide: May increase risk of cardiotoxicity. **HERBAL:** None known. **FOOD:** None known. **LAB VALUES:** May increase serum bilirubin, creatinine, LDH, AST, and ALT levels.

Q

AVAILABILITY (Rx)
INJECTION: 500-mg vial (150 mg quinupristin/350 mg dalfopristin).

ADMINISTRATION/ HANDLING
 IV

Reconstitution • Reconstitute vial by slowly adding 5 ml D₅W or sterile water for injection to make a 100 mg/ml solution. • Gently swirl vial contents to minimize foaming. • Further dilute with D₅W to final concentration of 2 mg/ml (5 mg/ml using central line).

Rate of administration • Infuse over 60 min. • After infusion, flush line with D₅W to minimize vein irritation. Do not flush with 0.9% NaCl (incompatible).

Storage • Refrigerate unopened vials. • Reconstituted vials are stable for 1 hr at room temperature. Diluted infusion bag is stable for 6 hr at room temperature or 54 hr if refrigerated.

IV INCOMPATIBILITIES
Heparin, sodium chloride.

IV COMPATIBILITIES
Aztreonam (Azactam), ciprofloxacin (Cipro), fluconazole (Diflucan), haloperidol (Haldol), metoclopramide (Reglan), morphine, potassium chloride.

INDICATIONS/ROUTES/ DOSAGE
INFECTIONS DUE TO VANCOMYCIN-RESISTANT *ENTEROCOCCUS FAECIUM*
IV: ADULTS, ELDERLY: 7.5 mg/kg/dose q8h.

SKIN AND SKIN-STRUCTURE INFECTIONS
IV: ADULTS, ELDERLY: 7.5 mg/kg/dose q12h.

SIDE EFFECTS
FREQUENT: Mild erythema, pruritus, pain, or burning at infusion site (with doses greater than 7 mg/kg). **OCCASIONAL:** Headache, diarrhea. **RARE:** Vomiting, arthralgia, myalgia.

ADVERSE REACTIONS/ TOXIC EFFECTS
Antibiotic-associated colitis and other superinfections may result from bacterial imbalance. Hepatic function abnormalities and severe venous pain and inflammation may occur.

NURSING CONSIDERATIONS

BASELINE ASSESSMENT
Assess temperature, BP, respiratory rate, pulse. Obtain baseline liver function tests, BUN, CBC, urinalysis.

INTERVENTION/EVALUATION
Monitor CBC, liver function tests. Observe infusion site for redness, vein irritation. Hold medication and promptly inform physician of diarrhea (with fever, abdominal pain, mucus or blood in stool may indicate antibiotic-associated colitis). Evaluate IV site for erythema, pruritus, pain, burning. Be alert for superinfection: increased fever, onset of sore throat, nausea, vomiting, diarrhea, stomatitis, anal or genital pruritus.

Q

rabeprazole sodium

rah-**bep**-rah-zole

(Aciphex, Pariet ✦)

Do not confuse Aciphex with Accupril or Aricept.

◆ CLASSIFICATION

PHARMACOTHERAPEUTIC: Proton pump inhibitor. **CLINICAL:** Gastric acid inhibitor (see p. 135C).

ACTION

A proton pump inhibitor that converts to active metabolites that irreversibly bind to and inhibit hydrogen-potassium adenosine triphosphate, an enzyme on the surface of gastric parietal cells. Actively secretes hydrogen ions for potassium ions, resulting in an accumulation of hydrogen ions in gastric lumen. Therapeutic Effect: Increases gastric pH, reducing gastric acid production.

PHARMACOKINETICS

Rapidly absorbed from the GI tract after passing through the stomach relatively intact. Protein binding: 96%. Metabolized extensively in the liver. Primarily excreted in urine. Unknown if removed by hemodialysis. Half-life: 1–2 hr (increased with hepatic impairment).

USES

Short-term treatment (4–8 wk) in healing and maintenance of erosive or ulcerative gastroesophageal reflux disease (GERD). Treatment of daytime and nighttime heartburn, other symptoms of GERD. Short-term treatment (4 wk or less) in healing, symptomatic relief of duodenal ulcers. Long-term treatment of pathologic hypersecretory conditions, including Zollinger-Ellison syndrome. Treatment of NSAID-induced ulcers. Treatment of *H. pylori* (in combination with other medication).

PRECAUTIONS

CONTRAINDICATIONS: None known. **CAUTIONS:** Hepatic impairment.

⧗ **LIFESPAN CONSIDERATIONS: Pregnancy/Lactation:** Unknown if drug crosses placenta or is distributed in breast milk. **Pregnancy Category B. Children:** Safety and efficacy not established. **Elderly:** No age-related precautions noted.

INTERACTIONS

DRUG: Digoxin: May increase the plasma concentration of digoxin. **Ketoconazole:** May decrease the blood concentration of ketoconazole. **HERBAL:** None known. **FOOD:** None known. **LAB VALUES:** May increase serum alkaline phosphatase, AST, and ALT levels.

AVAILABILITY (Rx)

TABLETS (DELAYED-RELEASE): 20 mg.

ADMINISTRATION/HANDLING

PO

• Give before meals. • Do not crush, chew, split tablet; swallow whole.

INDICATIONS/ROUTES/DOSAGE

GASTROESOPHAGEAL REFLUX DISEASE
PO: ADULTS, ELDERLY: 20 mg/day for 4–8 wk. Maintenance: 20 mg/day.

DUODENAL ULCER
PO: ADULTS, ELDERLY: 20 mg/day after morning meal for 4 wk.

NSAID-INDUCED ULCER
PO: ADULTS, ELDERLY: 20 mg/day.

PATHOLOGIC HYPERSECRETORY CONDITIONS
PO: ADULTS, ELDERLY: Initially, 60 mg once a day. May increase to 60 mg twice a day.

H. PYLORI INFECTION
PO: ADULTS, ELDERLY: 20 mg twice a day for 7 days (given with amoxicillin 1,000 mg and clarithromycin 500 mg).

SIDE EFFECTS

RARE (less than 2%): Headache, nausea, dizziness, rash, diarrhea, malaise.

✎ see color pill atlas   ◢ herb   underlined – top prescribed drug

ADVERSE REACTIONS/ TOXIC EFFECTS

Hyperglycemia, hypokalemia, hyponatremia, and hyperlipemia occur rarely.

NURSING CONSIDERATIONS

BASELINE ASSESSMENT

Obtain baseline lab values, especially serum chemistries.

INTERVENTION/EVALUATION

Monitor ongoing laboratory results. Evaluate for therapeutic response (i.e., relief of GI symptoms). Question if GI discomfort, nausea, diarrhea, headache occurs. Assess skin for evidence of rash. Observe for evidence of dizziness; utilize appropriate safety precautions.

PATIENT/FAMILY TEACHING

• Swallow tablets whole; do not chew, split, crush tablets. • Report headache.

---

raloxifene

ra-**lox**-i-feen
(Evista)

Do not confuse raloxifene with propoxyphene.

◆CLASSIFICATION

PHARMACOTHERAPEUTIC: Selective estrogen receptor modulator. **CLINICAL:** Osteoporosis preventive.

ACTION

A selective estrogen receptor modulator that affects some receptors like estrogen. **Therapeutic Effect:** Like estrogen, prevents bone loss and improves lipid profiles.

PHARMACOKINETICS

Rapidly absorbed after PO administration. Highly bound to plasma proteins (greater than 95%) and albumin. Undergoes extensive first-pass metabolism in liver. Excreted mainly in feces and, to a lesser extent, in urine. Unknown if removed by hemodialysis. **Half-life:** 27.7 hr.

USES

Prevention and treatment of osteoporosis in postmenopausal women. **OFF-LABEL:** Prevention of fractures, treatment of breast cancer in postmenopausal women.

PRECAUTIONS

CONTRAINDICATIONS: Active or history of venous thromboembolic events, such as deep vein thrombosis (DVT), pulmonary embolism, and retinal vein thrombosis; women who are or may become pregnant. **CAUTIONS:** Cardiovascular disease, history of cervical or uterine cancer, renal or hepatic impairment.

⧗ **LIFESPAN CONSIDERATIONS: Pregnancy/Lactation:** Unknown if distributed in breast milk. Not recommended for breast-feeding mothers. **Pregnancy Category X. Children:** Not used in this population. **Elderly:** No age-related precautions noted.

INTERACTIONS

DRUG: Ampicillin, cholestyramine: Reduce raloxifene absorption. **Hormone replacement therapy, systemic estrogen:** Don't use raloxifene concurrently with these drugs. **Warfarin:** May decrease PT and the effects of warfarin. **HERBAL:** None known. **FOOD:** None known. **LAB VALUES:** Lowers serum total cholesterol and LDL levels, but does not affect HDL or triglyceride levels. Slightly decreases platelet count and serum inorganic phosphate, albumin, calcium, and protein levels.

AVAILABILITY (Rx)

TABLETS: 60 mg.

R

ADMINISTRATION/HANDLING

PO

• Give at any time of day without regard to meals.

INDICATIONS/ROUTES/DOSAGE

PREVENTION OR TREATMENT OF OSTEOPOROSIS

PO: ADULTS, ELDERLY: 60 mg a day.

SIDE EFFECTS

FREQUENT (25%–10%): Hot flashes, flu-like symptoms, arthralgia, sinusitis. **OCCASIONAL (9%–5%):** Weight gain, nausea, myalgia, pharyngitis, cough, dyspepsia, leg cramps, rash, depression. **RARE (4%–3%):** Vaginitis, UTI, peripheral edema, flatulence, vomiting, fever, migraine, diaphoresis.

ADVERSE REACTIONS/ TOXIC EFFECTS

Pneumonia, gastroenteritis, chest pain, vaginal bleeding, and breast pain occur rarely.

NURSING CONSIDERATIONS

BASELINE ASSESSMENT

Question for possibility of pregnancy (Pregnancy Category X). Drug should be discontinued 72 hr before and during prolonged immobilization (postop recovery, prolonged bed rest). Therapy may be resumed only after patient is fully ambulatory. Determine serum total and LDL cholesterol levels before therapy and routinely thereafter.

INTERVENTION/EVALUATION

Monitor serum total and LDL cholesterol, total calcium, inorganic phosphate, total protein, albumin, bone mineral density, platelet count.

PATIENT/FAMILY TEACHING

• Avoid prolonged restriction of movement during travel (increased risk of venous thromboembolic events). • Take supplemental calcium, vitamin D if daily dietary intake is inadequate. • Encourage regular exercise. • Recommend modification and discontinuation of cigarette smoking, alcohol consumption.

ramelteon

rah-**mel**-tea-on

(Rozerem)

Do not confuse Rozerem with Razadyne.

CLASSIFICATION

PHARMACOTHERAPEUTIC: Melatonin receptor agonist. **CLINICAL:** Hypnotic.

ACTION

A nonscheduled sleep medication; no evidence of abuse or dependence. Selectively targets melatonin receptors, thought to be involved in the maintenance of the circadian rhythm underlying the normal sleep-wake cycle. **Therapeutic Effect:** Prevents insomnia characterized by difficulty with sleep onset.

PHARMACOKINETICS

Rapidly absorbed following PO administration. Protein binding: 82%. Substantial tissue distribution. Metabolized in the liver. Excreted mainly in urine with a small amount eliminated in the feces. **Half-life:** 2–5 hr.

USES

Long-term treatment of insomnia in patients who experience difficulty with sleep onset.

PRECAUTIONS

CONTRAINDICATIONS: Severe hepatic impairment, concurrent fluvoxamine therapy. **CAUTIONS:** Clinical depression, alcohol consumption, moderate hepatic impairment.

⧗ **LIFESPAN CONSIDERATIONS: Pregnancy/Lactation:** Unknown if distributed in breast milk; breast-feeding not recommended. **Pregnancy Category C. Children:** Safety and efficacy not established. **Elderly:** Age-related hepatic impairment may require dosage adjustment.

INTERACTIONS

DRUG: Alcohol: Concurrent use with ramelteon produces additive effect. **Fluconazole, ketoconazole:** May increase the serum levels, effects of ramelteon. **Fluvoxamine:** May cause severe increase in ramelteon serum level, toxicity. **Rifampin:** May decrease the levels and effects of ramelteon. **HERBAL:** None known. **FOOD: Heavy meals:** The onset of action may be reduced if taken with or immediately after a heavy meal. **LAB VALUES:** May decrease testosterone levels. May increase prolactin levels.

AVAILABILITY (Rx)

TABLETS, FILM-COATED: 8 mg (Rozerem).

ADMINISTRATION/HANDLING

PO
• Should be administered within 30 min before bedtime. • Do not give with, or immediately following, a high-fat meal. • Do not crush or break tablet.

INDICATIONS/ROUTES/DOSAGE

INSOMNIA
PO: ADULTS, ELDERLY: 8 mg before bedtime.

SIDE EFFECTS

FREQUENT (7%–5%): Headache, dizziness, somnolence. **OCCASIONAL (4%–3%):** Fatigue, nausea, exacerbated insomnia. **RARE (2%):** Diarrhea, myalgia, depression, altered taste sensation, arthralgia.

ADVERSE REACTIONS/ TOXIC EFFECTS

There is an association with an effect on reproductive hormones in adults, e.g. decreased testosterone levels and increased prolactin levels resulting in unexplained amenorrhea, galactorrhea, decreased libido, or problems with fertility.

NURSING CONSIDERATIONS

BASELINE ASSESSMENT

Assess BP, pulse, respirations. Raise bed rails, provide call light. Provide environment conducive to sleep (quiet environment, low or no lighting, TV off).

INTERVENTION/EVALUATION

Assess sleep pattern of patient. Evaluate for therapeutic response: rapid induction of sleep onset, decrease in number of nocturnal awakenings.

PATIENT/FAMILY TEACHING

• Take within 30 min before going to bed and confine activities to those necessary to prepare for bed. • Avoid engaging in any hazardous activities after taking medication. • Do not take medication with or immediately after a high fat meal.

ramipril

ram-i-pril
(Altace)

Do not confuse Altace with Alteplase or Artane.

◆CLASSIFICATION

PHARMACOTHERAPEUTIC: Renin-angiotensin system antagonist. **CLINICAL:** Antihypertensive (see p. 7C).

ACTION

An angiotensin-converting enzyme (ACE) inhibitor that suppresses the renin-angiotensin-aldosterone system. Decreases plasma angiotensin II, increases plasma renin activity, and decreases aldosterone secretion.

❦ Canadian trade name   © see **evolve**   ▷ High Alert drug

Therapeutic Effect: Reduces peripheral arterial resistance and BP.

PHARMACOKINETICS

Route	Onset	Peak	Duration
PO	1–2 hr	3–6 hr	24 hr

Well absorbed from the GI tract. Protein binding: 73%. Metabolized in the liver to active metabolite. Primarily excreted in urine. Not removed by hemodialysis. **Half-life:** 5.1 hr.

USES

Treatment of hypertension. Used alone or in combination with other antihypertensives. Treatment of CHF. Prevention of heart attack, stroke. OFF-LABEL: Treatment of hypertension and renal crisis in scleroderma.

PRECAUTIONS

CONTRAINDICATIONS: Bilateral renal artery stenosis. **CAUTIONS:** Renal impairment, CHF, collagen vascular disease, hypovolemia, renal stenosis, hyperkalemia.

⧖ **LIFESPAN CONSIDERATIONS: Pregnancy/Lactation:** Crosses placenta. Distributed in breast milk. May cause fetal or neonatal mortality or morbidity. **Pregnancy Category C (D if used in second or third trimester). Children:** Safety and efficacy not established. **Elderly:** May be more sensitive to hypotensive effects.

INTERACTIONS

DRUG: **Alcohol, antihypertensives, diuretics:** May increase the effects of ramipril. **Lithium:** May increase lithium blood concentration and risk of lithium toxicity. **NSAIDs:** May decrease the effects of ramipril. **Potassium-sparing diuretics, potassium supplements:** May cause hyperkalemia. HERBAL: **Garlic:** May increase antihypertensive effect. **Ginseng,**

yohimbe: May worsen hypertension. FOOD: None known. LAB VALUES: May increase BUN, serum alkaline phosphatase, serum bilirubin, serum creatinine, serum potassium, AST, and ALT levels. May decrease serum sodium levels. May cause positive antinuclear antibody titer.

AVAILABILITY (Rx)

CAPSULES: 1.25 mg, 2.5 mg, 5 mg, 10 mg.

ADMINISTRATION/HANDLING

PO
• Give without regard to food. • Do not chew or break capsules. • May mix with water, apple juice or sauce.

INDICATIONS/ROUTES/DOSAGE

HYPERTENSION (MONOTHERAPY)
PO: ADULTS, ELDERLY: Initially, 2.5 mg/day. Maintenance: 2.5–20 mg/day as single dose or in 2 divided doses.

HYPERTENSION (IN COMBINATION WITH OTHER ANTIHYPERTENSIVES)
PO: ADULTS, ELDERLY: Initially, 1.25 mg/day titrated to patient's needs.

CHF
PO: ADULTS, ELDERLY: Initially, 1.25–2.5 mg twice a day. **Maximum:** 5 mg twice a day.

RISK REDUCTION FOR MI STROKE
PO: ADULTS, ELDERLY: Initially, 2.5 mg/day for 7 days, then 5 mg/day for 21 days, then 10 mg/day as a single dose or in divided doses.

DOSAGE IN RENAL IMPAIRMENT
Creatinine clearance equal to or less than 40 ml/min: 25% of normal dose.
HYPERTENSION: Initially, 1.25 mg/day titrated upward.
CHF: Initially, 1.25 mg/day, titrated up to 2.5 mg twice a day.

SIDE EFFECTS

FREQUENT (12%–5%): Cough, headache. **OCCASIONAL (4%–2%):** Dizziness, fatigue, nausea, asthenia (loss of strength). **RARE (less than 2%):** Palpitations, insomnia, nervousness, malaise, abdominal pain, myalgia.

ADVERSE REACTIONS/ TOXIC EFFECTS

Excessive hypotension ("first-dose syncope") may occur in patients with CHF and in those who are severely salt or volume depleted. Angioedema and hyperkalemia occur rarely. Agranulocytosis and neutropenia may be noted in those with collagen vascular disease, including scleroderma and systemic lupus erythematosus, and impaired renal function. Nephrotic syndrome may be noted in those with history of renal disease.

BASELINE ASSESSMENT

Obtain BP immediately before each dose, in addition to regular monitoring (be alert to fluctuations). If excessive reduction in BP occurs, place patient in supine position with legs elevated. Renal function tests should be performed before beginning therapy. In patients with prior renal disease, urine test for protein (by dipstick method) should be made with first urine of day before beginning therapy and periodically thereafter. In those with renal impairment, autoimmune disease, or taking drugs that affect leukocytes or immune response, CBC, differential count should be performed before beginning therapy and q2wk for 3 mo, then periodically thereafter.

INTERVENTION/EVALUATION

Monitor renal function, serum potassium, WBC. Assess for cough (frequent effect). Assist with ambulation if dizziness occurs. Assess lung sounds for rales, wheezing in patients with CHF. Monitor urinalysis for proteinuria. Monitor serum potassium levels in those on concurrent diuretic therapy.

PATIENT/FAMILY TEACHING

• Do not discontinue medication without physician approval. • Report palpitations, cough, chest pain. • Dizziness, lightheadedness may occur in the first few days. • Avoid tasks that require alertness, motor skills until response to drug is established.

ranitidine hydrochloride

(Apo-Ranitidine ✚, Novo-Ranitidine ✚, Zantac, Zantac-75, Zantac-150, Zantac-300, Zantac EFFERdose, Zantac-25 EFFERdose, Zantac-150 EFFERdose, Zantac-150 Maximum Strength)

ranitidine bismuth citrate

ra-**ni**-ti-deen

(Tritec)

Do not confuse Zantac with Xanax, Ziac, or Zyrtec.

CLASSIFICATION

PHARMACOTHERAPEUTIC: Histamine H_2 receptor antagonist. **CLINICAL:** Antiulcer (see p. 96C).

ACTION

An antiulcer agent that inhibits histamine action at histamine 2 receptors of gastric parietal cells. **Therapeutic Effect:** Inhibits gastric acid secretion when fasting, at night, or when stimulated by food, caffeine, or insulin. Reduces volume and hydrogen ion concentration of gastric juice.

PHARMACOKINETICS

Rapidly absorbed from the GI tract. Protein binding: 15%. Widely distributed.

Metabolized in the liver. Primarily excreted in urine. Not removed by hemodialysis. **Half-life:** PO, 2.5 hr; IV, 2–2.5 hr (increased with impaired renal function).

USES

Short-term treatment of active duodenal ulcer. Prevention of duodenal ulcer recurrence. Treatment of active benign gastric ulcer, pathologic GI hypersecretory conditions, acute gastroesophageal reflux disease (GERD), including erosive esophagitis. Maintenance of healed erosive esophagitis. Part of regimen for *H. pylori* eradication to reduce risk of duodenal ulcer recurrence. OTC: Relieve heartburn, acid indigestion, sour stomach. OFF-LABEL: Prevention of aspiration pneumonia, treatment of recurrent postop ulcer, upper GI bleeding, prevention of acid aspiration pneumonitis during surgery, prevention of stress-induced ulcers.

PRECAUTIONS

CONTRAINDICATIONS: History of acute porphyria. **CAUTIONS:** Renal/hepatic impairment, elderly.

⧗ LIFESPAN CONSIDERATIONS: **Pregnancy/Lactation:** Unknown if drug crosses placenta or is distributed in breast milk. **Pregnancy Category B. Children:** No age-related precautions noted. **Elderly:** Confusion more likely in patients with hepatic/renal impairment.

INTERACTIONS

DRUG: **Antacids:** May decrease the absorption of ranitidine. **Ketoconazole:** May decrease the absorption of ketoconazole. HERBAL: None known. FOOD: None known. LAB VALUES: Interferes with skin tests using allergen extracts. May increase hepatic function enzyme, gamma-glutamyl transpeptidase, and serum creatinine levels.

AVAILABILITY (Rx)

TABLETS (EFFERVESCENT): 25 mg (Zantac-25 EFFERdose), 150 mg (Zantac-150 EFFERdose). **CAPSULES (ZANTAC):** 150 mg, 300 mg. **GRANULES (ZANTAC EFFERDOSE):** 150 mg. **SYRUP (ZANTAC):** 15 mg/ml. **TABLETS (HYDROCHLORIDE):** 75 mg (Zantac-75 [OTC]), 150 mg (Zantac-150, Zantac 150 Maximum Strength), 300 mg (Zantac-300). **TABLETS (BISUMUTH CITRATE [TRITEC]):** 400 mg. **INJECTION (ZANTAC):** 25 mg/ml.

ADMINISTRATION/HANDLING

💉 IV

Reconstitution • For IV push, dilute each 50 mg with 20 ml 0.9% NaCl, D₅W. • For intermittent IV infusion (piggyback), dilute each 50 mg with 50 ml 0.9% NaCl, D₅W. • For IV infusion, dilute with 250–1,000 ml 0.9% NaCl, D₅W.

Rate of administration • Administer IV push over minimum of 5 min (prevents arrhythmias, hypotension). • Infuse IV piggyback over 15–20 min. • Infuse IV infusion over 24 hr.

Storage • IV solutions appear clear, colorless to yellow (slight darkening does not affect potency). • IV infusion (piggyback) is stable for 48 hr at room temperature (discard if discolored or precipitate forms).

IM
• May be given undiluted. • Give deep IM into large muscle mass.

PO
• Give without regard to meals. Best given after meals or at bedtime. • Do not administer within 1 hr of magnesium- or aluminum-containing antacids (decreases absorption by 33%).

▦ IV INCOMPATIBILITIES

Amphotericin B complex (Abelcet, AmBisome, Amphotec).

IV COMPATIBILITIES

Diltiazem (Cardizem), dobutamine (Dobutrex), dopamine (Intropin), heparin, hydromorphone (Dilaudid), insulin, lidocaine, lorazepam (Ativan), morphine, norepinephrine (Levophed), potassium chloride, propofol (Diprivan).

INDICATIONS/ROUTES/DOSAGE

DUODENAL ULCERS, GASTRIC ULCERS, GERD

PO: ADULTS, ELDERLY: 150 mg twice a day or 300 mg at bedtime. Maintenance: 150 mg at bedtime. CHILDREN: 2–4 mg/kg/day in divided doses twice a day. **Maximum:** 300 mg/day.

DUODENAL ULCERS ASSOCIATED WITH *H. PYLORI* INFECTION

PO: ADULTS, ELDERLY: 400 mg twice a day for 4 wk in combination with clarithromycin 500 mg 2–3 times a day for the first 2 wk.

EROSIVE ESOPHAGITIS

PO: ADULTS, ELDERLY: 150 mg 4 times a day. Maintenance: 150 mg twice a day or 300 mg at bedtime. CHILDREN: 4–10 mg/kg/day in 2 divided doses. **Maximum:** 600 mg/day.

HYPERSECRETORY CONDITIONS

PO: ADULTS, ELDERLY: 150 mg twice a day. May increase up to 6 g/day.

OTC USE

PO: ADULTS, ELDERLY: 75 mg 30–60 min before eating food or drinking beverages that cause heartburn. **Maximum:** 150 mg per 24 hr period and/or longer than 14 days.

USUAL PARENTERAL DOSAGE

IV, IM: ADULTS, ELDERLY: 50 mg/dose q6–8h. **Maximum:** 400 mg/day. CHILDREN: 2–4 mg/kg/day in divided doses q6–8h. **Maximum:** 200 mg/day.

USUAL NEONATAL DOSAGE

PO: NEONATES: 2 mg/kg/day in divided doses q12h.
IV: NEONATES: Initially, 1.5 mg/kg/dose; then 1.5–2 mg/kg/day in divided doses q12h.

DOSAGE IN RENAL IMPAIRMENT

For patients with creatinine clearance less than 50 ml/min, give 150 mg PO q24h or 50 mg IV or IM q18–24h.

SIDE EFFECTS

OCCASIONAL (2%): Diarrhea. **RARE (1%):** Constipation, headache (may be severe).

ADVERSE REACTIONS/ TOXIC EFFECTS

Reversible hepatitis and blood dyscrasias occur rarely.

NURSING CONSIDERATIONS

BASELINE ASSESSMENT

Obtain baseline liver/renal function tests.

INTERVENTION/EVALUATION

Monitor serum AST, ALT levels. Assess mental status in elderly.

PATIENT/FAMILY TEACHING

• Smoking decreases effectiveness of medication. • Do not take medicine within 1 hr of magnesium- or aluminum-containing antacids. • Transient burning/itching may occur with IV administration. • Report headache. • Avoid alcohol, aspirin.

Raptiva, *see efalizumab*

Rebetol, *see ribavirin*

Reglan, *see metoclopramide*

Remeron, *see mirtazipine*

R

Remicade, *see infliximab*

remifentanil hydrochloride

(Ultiva)
See Opioid analgesics

RenaGel, *see sevelamer*

ReoPro, *see abciximab*

repaglinide   ⚐

reh-**pah**-glih-nide
(GlucoNorm ✦, Prandin)

◆ CLASSIFICATION

PHARMACOTHERAPEUTIC: Antihyperglycemic. **CLINICAL:** Antidiabetic (see p. 42C).

ACTION

An antihyperglycemic that stimulates release of insulin from beta cells of the pancreas by depolarizing beta cells, leading to an opening of calcium channels. Resulting calcium influx induces insulin secretion. **Therapeutic Effect:** Lowers blood glucose concentration.

PHARMACOKINETICS

Rapidly, completely absorbed from the GI tract. Protein binding: 98%. Metabolized in the liver to inactive metabolites. Excreted primarily in feces with a lesser amount in urine. Unknown if removed by hemodialysis. **Half-life:** 1 hr.

USES

Adjunct to diet and exercise to lower blood glucose in patients with type 2 diabetes mellitus. Used as monotherapy or in combination with metformin, pioglitazone, or rosiglitazone.

PRECAUTIONS

CONTRAINDICATIONS: Diabetic ketoacidosis, type 1 diabetes mellitus. **CAUTIONS:** Hepatic and renal impairment.

⧗ **LIFESPAN CONSIDERATIONS: Pregnancy/Lactation:** Unknown if drug is distributed in breast milk. **Pregnancy Category C. Children:** Safety and efficacy not established. **Elderly:** No age-related precautions noted, but hypoglycemia more difficult to recognize.

INTERACTIONS

DRUG: Beta blockers, chloramphenicol, gemfibrozil, MAOIs, NSAIDs, probenecid, salicylates, sulfonamides, warfarin: May increase the effects of repaglinide. **HERBAL:** None known. **FOOD: All food:** Decreases repaglinide plasma concentration. **LAB VALUES:** None known.

AVAILABILITY (Rx)

TABLETS: 0.5 mg, 1 mg, 2 mg.

ADMINISTRATION/HANDLING

PO
• Ideally, give within 15 min of a meal but may be given immediately before a meal to as long as 30 min before a meal.

INDICATIONS/ROUTES/DOSAGE

DIABETES MELLITUS
PO: ADULTS, ELDERLY: 0.5–4 mg 2–4 times a day. **Maximum:** 16 mg/day.

SIDE EFFECTS

FREQUENT (10%–6%): Upper respiratory tract infection, headache, rhinitis, bronchitis, back pain. **OCCASIONAL (5%– 3%):** Diarrhea, dyspepsia, sinusitis, nausea, arthralgia, UTI. **RARE (2%):** Constipation, vomiting, paresthesia, allergy.

ADVERSE REACTIONS/ TOXIC EFFECTS

Hypoglycemia occurs in 16% of patients. Chest pain occurs rarely.

NURSING CONSIDERATIONS

BASELINE ASSESSMENT

Check fasting blood glucose and glycosylated Hgb (HbA$_1$C) levels periodically to determine minimum effective dose. Ensure follow-up instruction if patient and family do not thoroughly understand diabetes management or glucose-testing technique. At least 1 wk should elapse to assess response to drug before new dosage adjustment is made.

INTERVENTION/EVALUATION

Monitor fasting blood glucose, glycosylated Hgb (HbA$_1$C) levels, food intake. Assess for hypoglycemia (cool, wet skin, tremors, dizziness, anxiety, headache, tachycardia, numbness in mouth, hunger, diplopia), hyperglycemia (polyuria, polyphagia, polydipsia, nausea, vomiting, dim vision, fatigue, deep or rapid breathing). Be alert to conditions that alter glucose requirements: fever, increased activity/stress, surgical procedures.

PATIENT/FAMILY TEACHING

• Diabetes mellitus requires lifelong control. • Prescribed diet and exercise is principal part of treatment; do not skip, delay meals. • Continue to adhere to dietary instructions, a regular exercise program, regular testing of urine or blood glucose. • When taking combination drug therapy with a sulfonylurea or insulin, have a source of glucose available to treat symptoms of low blood sugar.

Requip, *see ropinirole*

---

respiratory syncytial immune globulin

res-purr-ah-tore-ee sin-**sish**-ee-al ih-**mewn glah**-byew-lin

(RespiGam)

◆CLASSIFICATION

PHARMACOTHERAPEUTIC: Immuneserum. **CLINICAL:** Respiratory agent.

ACTION

An immune serum with a high concentration of neutralizing and protective antibodies specific for respiratory syncytial virus (RSV). **Therapeutic Effect:** Provides protection against RSV infection and decreases the severity of existing infection.

USES

Prevents serious lower respiratory tract infections caused by RSV in children younger than 24 mo with bronchopulmonary dysplasia, history of premature birth.

PRECAUTIONS

CONTRAINDICATIONS: IgA deficiency, hypersensitivity to other human immunoglobulins. **CAUTIONS:** Pulmonary disease.

   LIFESPAN CONSIDERATIONS: **Pregnancy/Lactation:** Unknown if distributed in breast milk. **Pregnancy Category C. Children:** Safety and efficacy not established. **Elderly:** No age-related precautions noted.

INTERACTIONS

DRUG: Live virus vaccines: May decrease the patient's antibody response

R

---

to the vaccine. **HERBAL:** None known. **FOOD:** None known. **LAB VALUES:** None known.

AVAILABILITY (Rx)

INJECTION: 2,500 mcg RSV immune globulin.

ADMINISTRATION/HANDLING
IV

Rate of administration • Initial infusion rate of 1.5 ml/kg/hr for first 15 min, then increase to 3 ml/kg/hr next 15 min. Infusion rate of 6 ml/kg/hr 30 min to end of infusion. • Maximum infusion rate: 6 ml/kg/hr.

Storage • Refrigerate vials. Do not freeze. • Do not shake. • Start infusion within 6 hr and complete within 12 hr of vial entry.

INDICATIONS/ROUTES/DOSAGE

PREVENTION OF RSV IN CHILDREN WITH BRONCHOPULMONARY DYSPLASIA AND HISTORY OF PREMATURE BIRTH

IV: CHILDREN YOUNGER THAN 24 MO: 750 mg/kg (15 ml/kg) administered at a rate of 1.5 ml/kg/hr for the first 15 min, then 3.6 ml/kg/hr for remainder of infusion. Given once monthly for 5 doses beginning in September or October.

SIDE EFFECTS

OCCASIONAL (6%–2%): Fever, vomiting, wheezing. **RARE (less than 1%):** Diarrhea, rash, tachycardia, hypertension, hypoxia, injection site inflammation.

ADVERSE REACTIONS/ TOXIC EFFECTS

Hypersensitivity reactions, characterized by dizziness, flushing, anxiety, palpitations, pruritus, myalgia, and arthralgia, occur rarely.

NURSING CONSIDERATIONS

INTERVENTION/EVALUATION
Monitor heart rate, BP, temperature, respiratory rate. Observe for rales, wheezing, retractions.

Restoril, *see temazepam*

---

reteplase, recombinant

reh-te-place
(Retavase)

Do not confuse reteplase or Retavase with Restasis.

CLASSIFICATION

PHARMACOTHERAPEUTIC: Tissue plasminogen activator. **CLINICAL:** Thrombolytic (see p. 32C).

ACTION

A tissue plasminogen activator that activates the fibrinolytic system by directly cleaving plasminogen to generate plasmin, an enzyme that degrades the fibrin of the thrombus. **Therapeutic Effect:** Exerts thrombolytic action.

PHARMACOKINETICS

Rapidly cleared from plasma. Eliminated primarily by the liver and kidney. **Half-life:** 13–16 min.

USES

Management of acute myocardial infarction (AMI), improvement of ventricular function following AMI, reduction of incidence of CHF, reduction of mortality associated with AMI. **OFF-LABEL:** Occluded catheters.

PRECAUTIONS

CONTRAINDICATIONS: Active internal bleeding, AV malformation or aneurysm, bleeding diathesis, history of cerebrovascular accident (CVA), intracranial neoplasm, recent intracranial or intraspinal surgery or trauma, severe uncontrolled hypertension. **CAUTIONS:** Recent major surgery (coronary artery bypass graft, OB delivery, organ biopsy), cerebrovascular disease, recent GI/GU bleeding, hypertension, mitral stenosis with atrial fibrillation, acute pericarditis, bacterial endocarditis, hepatic or renal impairment, diabetic retinopathy, ophthalmic hemorrhage, septic thrombophlebitis, occluded AV cannula at an infected site, advanced age, patients receiving oral anticoagulants.

🗶 LIFESPAN CONSIDERATIONS: **Pregnancy/Lactation:** Unknown if drug is distributed in breast milk. **Pregnancy Category C. Children:** Safety and efficacy not established. **Elderly:** More susceptible to bleeding; caution advised.

INTERACTIONS

DRUG: **Heparin, platelet aggregation antagonists (such as abciximab, aspirin, dipyridamole), warfarin:** Increase the risk of bleeding. HERBAL: **Ginkgo biloba:** May increase the risk of bleeding. FOOD: None known. LAB VALUES: May decrease fibrinogen and serum plasminogen levels.

AVAILABILITY (Rx)

POWDER FOR INJECTION: 10.4 units (18.1 mg).

ADMINISTRATION/HANDLING

🖫 IV

Reconstitution • Reconstitute only with sterile water for injection immediately before use. • Reconstituted solution contains 1 unit/ml. • Do not shake. • Slight foaming may occur; let stand

for a few minutes to allow bubbles to dissipate.

Rate of administration • Give through a dedicated IV line. • Give as a 10 unit plus 10 unit double bolus, with each IV bolus administered over 2-min period. • Give the second bolus 30 min after the first bolus injection. • Do not add other medications to the bolus injection solution. • Do not give second bolus if serious bleeding occurs after first IV bolus is given.

Storage • Use within 4 hr of reconstitution. • Discard any unused portion.

▨ IV INCOMPATIBILITIES

Do not mix with other medications.

INDICATIONS/ROUTES/DOSAGE

ACUTE MI, CHF
IV BOLUS: ADULTS, ELDERLY: 10 units over 2 min; repeat in 30 min.

SIDE EFFECTS

FREQUENT: Bleeding at superficial sites, such as venous injection sites, catheter insertion sites, venous cutdowns, arterial punctures, and sites of recent surgical procedures, gingival bleeding.

ADVERSE REACTIONS/TOXIC EFFECTS

Bleeding at internal sites may occur, including intracranial, retroperitoneal, GI, GU, and respiratory sites. Lysis or coronary thrombi may produce atrial or ventricular arrhythmias and stroke.

NURSING CONSIDERATIONS

BASELINE ASSESSMENT
Obtain baseline BP, apical pulse. Evaluate 12-lead EKG, CPK, CPK-MB, serum electrolytes. Assess Hct, platelet count, thrombin (TT), aPTT, PT, serum plasminogen, fibrinogen level before therapy is instituted. Type, hold blood.

R

 Canadian trade name   ℮ see **evolve**   ☞ High Alert drug

INTERVENTION/EVALUATION

Carefully monitor all needle puncture sites, catheter insertion sites for bleeding. Continuous cardiac monitoring for arrhythmias, BP, pulse, respiration is essential until patient is stable. Check peripheral pulses, lung sounds. Monitor for chest pain relief; notify physician of continuation/recurrence of chest pain (note location, type, intensity). Avoid any trauma that may increase risk of bleeding (injections, shaving).

Rh₀ (D) immune globulin

row D ih-**mewn glah**-byew-lin

(BayRHo, BayRho-D Full Dose, BayRho Mini-dose, MICRhogam, RhoGAM, Rhophylac, WinRho SDF)

CLASSIFICATION

CLINICAL: Immune globulin.

ACTION

Rh₀(D) immune globulin contains anti-Rh₀(D) antibody to the RBC antigen Rh₀(D). Rh₀(D) immune globulin suppresses the active antibody response and formation of anti-Rh₀(D) in Rh₀(D)-negative women exposed to Rh₀-positive blood from a pregnancy with an Rh₀(D)-positive fetus or transfusion with Rh₀(D)-positive blood. The anti-Rh₀(D) antibody in Rh₀(D) immune globulin may bind to Rh₀(D) antigen in maternal circulation, preventing stimulation of the primary immune response to Rh₀(D) and subsequent active production of anti-Rh₀(D). Injection of Rh₀(D) immune globulin into an Rh-positive patient with idiopathic thrombocytopenic purpura (ITP) may result in the formation of anti-Rh₀(D)-coated RBC complexes; as the RBCs are cleared by the spleen, they saturate the capacity of the spleen to clear antibody-coated cells, sparing antibody-coated platelets. **Therapeutic Effect:** Prevents antibody response and hemolytic disease of the newborn in women who have previously conceived an Rh₀(D)-positive fetus. Prevents Rh₀(D) sensitization in patients who have received Rh₀(D)-positive blood. Decreases bleeding in patients with ITP.

PHARMACOKINETICS

Half-life: 24 days (IV); 30 days (IM).

USES

Treatment of Rh₀(D)-positive children and adults (without splenectomy) with chronic ITP, children with acute ITP, children and adults with ITP secondary to HIV infection; prevention of isoimmunization in Rh-negative individuals exposed to Rh-positive blood during delivery of an Rh-positive infant, within 72 hr of an abortion, following amniocentesis or abdominal trauma, following a transfusion accident; prevention of hemolytic disease of the newborn if there is a subsequent pregnancy with an Rh-positive infant.

PRECAUTIONS

CONTRAINDICATIONS: Hypersensitivity to any component, IgA deficiency, mothers whose Rh group or immune status is uncertain, prior sensitization to Rh₀(D), Rh₀(D)-positive mother or pregnant woman, transfusion of Rh₀(D)-positive blood in previous 3 mo. **CAUTIONS:** Thrombocytopenia, bleeding disorders. Hgb less than 8 g/dl.

⧗ **LIFESPAN CONSIDERATIONS: Pregnancy/Lactation:** Does not appear to harm fetus. **Pregnancy Category C. Children/Elderly:** No age-related precautions noted.

INTERACTIONS

DRUG: Live virus vaccines: May interfere with the patient's immune response to the vaccine. **HERBAL:** None known. **FOOD:** None known. **LAB VALUES:** None known.

AVAILABILITY (Rx)

INJECTION, POWDER FOR RECONSTITUTION (WINRHO SDF): 120 mcg, 300 mcg. **INJECTION SOLUTION:** 50 mcg (BayRho D Mini-dose, MICRORhoGAM), 300 mcg (BayRho D Full Dose, RhoGAM), 300 mcg/2 ml (Rhophylac).

ADMINISTRATION/HANDLING

 IV

Reconstitution • Reconstitute 120 mcg and 300 mcg with 2.5 ml NaCl (8.5 ml for 1,000-mcg vial). • Gently swirl; do not shake.

Rate of administration • Infuse over 3–5 min.

Storage • Refrigerate vials (do not freeze). • Once reconstituted, stable for 12 hr at room temperature.

IM

• Reconstitute 120 mcg and 300 mcg with 2.5 ml NaCl (8.5 ml for 1,000-mcg vial). • Administer into deltoid muscle of upper arm or anterolateral aspect of upper thigh.

INDICATIONS/ROUTES/DOSAGE

ITP

IV (WINRHO SDF): ADULTS, ELDERLY, CHILDREN: Initially, 50 mcg/kg as single dose (reduce to 25–40 mcg/kg if Hgb is less than 10 g/dl). Maintenance: 25–60 mcg/kg based on platelet count and Hgb level.

SUPPRESSION OF THE ACTIVE ANTIBODY RESPONSE AND FORMATION OF ANTI-RH₀(D) IN RH₀(D)-NEGATIVE WOMEN EXPOSED TO RH₀-POSITIVE BLOOD FROM A PREGNANCY WITH AN RH₀(D)-POSITIVE FETUS

IM (BAYRHO-D FULL DOSE, RHOGAM): ADULTS: 300 mcg preferably within 72 hr of delivery.

IV, IM (WINRHO SDF): ADULTS: 300 mcg at 28 wk gestation. After delivery: 120 mcg preferably within 72 hr.

SUPPRESSION OF ACTIVE ANTIBODY RESPONSE AND FORMATION OF ANTI-RH₀(D) IN RH₀(D)-NEGATIVE WOMEN EXPOSED TO RH₀-POSITIVE BLOOD FROM A MISCARRIAGE WITH AN RH₀(D)-POSITIVE FETUS

IM (BAYRHO-D FULL DOSE, RHOGAM): ADULTS: 300 mcg as soon as possible.

SUPPRESSON OF THE ACTIVE ANTIBODY RESPONSE AND FORMATION OF ANTI-RH₀(D) IN RH₀(D)-NEGATIVE WOMEN EXPOSED TO RH₀-POSITIVE BLOOD FROM AN ABORTION, MISCARRIAGE, OR TERMINATION OF AN ECTOPIC PREGNANCY WITH AN RH₀(D)-POSITIVE FETUS

IM (BAYRHO-D, RHOGAM): ADULTS: 300 mcg if more than 13 wk gestation, 50 mcg if less than 13 wk gestation. **IV, IM (WINRHO SDF):** ADULTS: 120 mcg after 34 wk gestation.

TRANSFUSION INCOMPATIBILITY

IV: ADULTS: 3,000 units (600 mcg) q8h until total dose given. **IM:** ADULTS: 6,000 units (1,200 mcg) q12h until total dose given.

SIDE EFFECTS

Hypotension, pallor, vasodilation (IV formulation), fever, headache, chills, dizziness, somnolence, lethargy, rash, pruritus, abdominal pain, diarrhea, discomfort and swelling at injection site, back pain, myalgia, arthralgia, asthenia.

ADVERSE REACTIONS/ TOXIC EFFECTS

Acute renal failure has been reported.

NURSING CONSIDERATIONS

BASELINE ASSESSMENT

Determine existence of bleeding disorders. Assess the patient's Hgb level, give

R

this drug cautiously to patients with an Hgb level less than 8 g/dl.

INTERVENTION/EVALUATION

Monitor CBC (especially Hgb and platelet count), BUN and serum creatinine levels, reticulocyte count, and urinalysis results. Assess for signs and symptoms of hemolysis.

PATIENT/FAMILY TEACHING

• Inform the patient this drug is given only by injection, which may be painful. • Notify the physician if chills, dizziness, fever, headache, or rash occur.

Rhinocort Aqua, see
budesonide

---

ribavirin

rye-ba-**vye** rin
(Copegus, Rebetol, Rebetron, Virazole)

Do not confuse ribavirin with riboflavin.

FIXED-COMBINATION(S)

With interferon, alfa 2b (**Rebetron**). Individually packaged.

◆CLASSIFICATION

PHARMACOTHERAPEUTIC: Synthetic nucleoside. **CLINICAL:** Antiviral (see p. 61C).

ACTION

A synthetic nucleoside that inhibits influenza virus RNA polymerase activity and interferes with expression of messenger RNA. **Therapeutic Effect:** Inhibits viral protein synthesis and replication of viral RNA and DNA.

USES

Inhalation: Treatment of respiratory syncytial virus (RSV) infections (especially in patients with underlying compromising conditions such as chronic lung disorders, congenital heart disease, recent transplant recipients). **Capsule/Tablet/Oral Solution:** Treatment of chronic hepatitis C in patients with compensated hepatic disease. **OFF-LABEL:** Treatment of influenza A or B and west Nile virus.

PRECAUTIONS

CONTRAINDICATIONS: Autoimmune hepatitis, creatinine clearance less than 50 ml/min, hemoglobinopathies, hepatic decompensation, hypersensitivity to ribavirin products, pregnancy, significant or unstable cardiac disease, women of childbearing age who won't use contraception reliably **CAUTIONS: Inhalation:** Patients requiring assisted ventilation, chronic obstructive pulmonary disease (COPD), asthma. **Oral:** Cardiac, pulmonary disease, elderly, history of psychiatric disorders. **Pregnancy Category X.**

INTERACTIONS

DRUG: Didanosine: May increase the risk of pancreatitis and peripheral neuropathy and decrease the effects of didanosine. **Nucleoside analogues (including adefovir, didanosine, lamivudine, stavudine, zalcitabine, zidovudine):** May increase the risk of lactic acidosis. **HERBAL:** None known. **FOOD:** None known. **LAB VALUES:** None known.

AVAILABILITY (Rx)

CAPSULES (REBETOL, REBETRON COMBINATION THERAPY WITH ALFA-2B INJECTION): 200 mg. **TABLETS (CEPEGUS):** 200 mg. **POWDER FOR RECONSTITUTION (AEROSOL [VIRAZOLE]):** 6 g. **ORAL SOLUTION (REBETOL):** 40 mg/ml.

✐ see color pill atlas   ✐ herb   <u>underlined</u> – top prescribed drug

ADMINISTRATION/HANDLING

PO

• Store Rebetron combination package in the refrigerator. Store oral solution in the refrigerator or at room temperature. • Capsules may be taken without regard to food. • Tablets should be given with food.

INHALATION

◀ ALERT ▶ May be given via nasal or oral inhalation.

• Solution appears clear and colorless, is stable for 24 hr at room temperature. • Discard solution for nebulization after 24 hr. • Discard solution if discolored or cloudy. • Add 50–100 ml sterile water for injection or inhalation to 6-g vial. • Transfer to a flask, serving as reservoir for aerosol generator. • Further dilute to final volume of 300 ml, giving a solution concentration of 20 mg/ml. • Use only aerosol generator available from manufacturer of drug. • Do not give concomitantly with other drug solutions for nebulization. • Discard reservoir solution when fluid levels are low and at least q24h. • Controversy over safety in ventilator-dependent patients; only experienced personnel should administer drug.

INDICATIONS/ROUTES/DOSAGE

CHRONIC HEPATITIS C

PO (CAPSULE OR ORAL SOLUTION IN COMBINATION WITH INTERFERON ALFA-2B): ADULTS, ELDERLY: 1,000–1,200 mg/day in 2 divided doses. CHILDREN WEIGHING 60 KG OR MORE: Use adult dosage (51–60 kg): 400 mg 2 times/day. (37–50 kg): 200 mg in morning, 400 mg in evening. (24–36 kg): 200 mg 2 times/day.

PO (CAPSULES IN COMBINATION WITH PEGINTERFERON ALFA-2B): ADULTS, ELDERLY: 800 mg/day in 2 divided doses.

PO (TABLETS IN COMBINATION WITH PEGINTERFERON ALFA-2B): ADULTS, ELDERLY: 800–1,200 mg/day in 2 divided doses.

SEVERE LOWER RESPIRATORY TRACT INFECTION CAUSED BY RSV

INHALATION: CHILDREN, INFANTS: Use with Viratek small-particle aerosol generator at a concentration of 20 mg/ml (6 g reconstituted with 300 ml sterile water) over 12–18 hr/day for 3–7 days.

SIDE EFFECTS

FREQUENT (greater than 10%): Dizziness, headache, fatigue, fever, insomnia, irritability, depression, emotional lability, impaired concentration, alopecia, rash, pruritus, nausea, anorexia, dyspepsia, vomiting, decreased hemoglobin, hemolysis, arthralgia, musculoskeletal pain, dyspnea, sinusitis, flu-like symptoms. **OCCASIONAL (1%–10%):** Nervousness, altered taste, weakness.

ADVERSE REACTIONS/ TOXIC EFFECTS.

Cardiac arrest, apnea and ventilator dependence, bacterial pneumonia, pneumonia, and pneumothorax occur rarely. Anemia may occur if ribavirin therapy exceeds 7 days.

NURSING CONSIDERATIONS

BASELINE ASSESSMENT

Obtain sputum specimens before giving first dose or at least during first 24 hr of therapy. Assess respiratory status for baseline. **Oral:** CBC with differential, pretreatment and monthly pregnancy test for women of childbearing age.

INTERVENTION/EVALUATION

Monitor I&O, fluid balance carefully. Check hematology reports for anemia due to reticulocytosis when therapy exceeds 7 days. For ventilator-assisted patients, watch for "rainout" in tubing and empty frequently; be alert to impaired ventilation/gas exchange due to drug precipitate. Assess skin for rash. Monitor BP, respirations; assess lung sounds.

R

PATIENT/FAMILY TEACHING
• Report immediately any difficulty breathing, itching/swelling/redness of eyes. • Educate females about prevention of pregnancy and need for pregnancy testing. • Educate males about protection of female partners from pregnancy.

rifabutin

rye-fah-**byew**-tin
(Mycobutin)
Do not confuse rifabutin with rifampin.

CLASSIFICATION

PHARMACOTHERAPEUTIC: Antitubercular. **CLINICAL:** Antibacterial (antimycobacterial).

ACTION

An antitubercular that inhibits DNA-dependent RNA polymerase, an enzyme in susceptible strains of *Escherichia coli* and *Bacillus subtilis*. Rifabutin has a broad spectrum of antimicrobial activity, including against mycobacteria such as *Mycobacterium avium* complex (MAC). **Therapeutic Effect:** Prevents MAC disease.

PHARMACOKINETICS

Readily absorbed from the GI tract (high-fat meals delay absorption). Protein binding: 85%. Widely distributed. Crosses the blood-brain barrier. Extensive intracellular tissue uptake. Metabolized in the liver to active metabolite. Excreted in urine; eliminated in feces. Unknown if removed by hemodialysis. **Half-life:** 16–69 hr.

USES

Prevention of disseminated MAC disease in those with advanced HIV infection.

OFF-LABEL: Part of multidrug regimen for treatment of MAC.

PRECAUTIONS

CONTRAINDICATIONS: Active tuberculosis; hypersensitivity to other rifamycins, including rifampin. **CAUTIONS:** Safety in children not established. Renal or hepatic impairment.

⏳ **LIFESPAN CONSIDERATIONS: Pregnancy/Lactation:** Unknown if drug crosses placenta or is excreted in breast milk. **Pregnancy Category B.** **Children/Elderly:** No age-related precautions noted.

INTERACTIONS

DRUG: Oral contraceptives: May decrease contraceptive effectiveness. **Zidovudine:** May decrease blood concentration of zidovudine, but does not affect the drug's inhibition of HIV. **HERBAL:** None known. **FOOD:** None known. **LAB VALUES:** May increase serum alkaline phosphatase, AST, and ALT levels.

AVAILABILITY (Rx)

CAPSULES: 150 mg.

ADMINISTRATION/HANDLING

PO
• Give without regard to food. Give with food if GI irritation occurs. • May mix with applesauce if patient is unable to swallow capsules whole.

INDICATIONS/ROUTES/DOSAGE

PREVENTION OF MAC DISEASE (FIRST EPISODE)
PO: ADULTS, ELDERLY: 300 mg as a single dose or in 2 divided doses if GI upset occurs.

PREVENTION OF RECURRENT MAC DISEASE
PO: ADULTS, ELDERLY: 300 mg/day (in combination).

DOSAGE IN RENAL IMPAIRMENT

Dosage is modified based on creatinine clearance. If creatinine clearance is less than 30 ml/min, reduce dosage by 50%.

SIDE EFFECTS

FREQUENT (30%): Red-orange or red-brown discoloration of urine, feces, saliva, skin, sputum, sweat, or tears. **OCCASIONAL (11%–3%):** Rash, nausea, abdominal pain, diarrhea, dyspepsia, belching, headache, altered taste, uveitis, corneal deposits. **RARE (less than 2%):** Anorexia, flatulence, fever, myalgia, vomiting, insomnia.

ADVERSE REACTIONS/ TOXIC EFFECTS

Hepatitis and thrombocytopenia occur rarely. Anemia and neutropenia may also occur.

NURSING CONSIDERATIONS

BASELINE ASSESSMENT

Obtain chest x-ray, sputum and blood cultures. Biopsy of suspicious node(s) must be done to rule out active tuberculosis. Obtain baseline CBC, serum liver function tests.

INTERVENTION/EVALUATION

Monitor serum liver function tests, CBC, platelet count, Hgb, Hct. Avoid IM injections, rectal temperatures, other trauma that may induce bleeding. Check temperature; notify physician of flu-like syndrome, rash, GI intolerance.

PATIENT/FAMILY TEACHING

• Urine, feces, saliva, sputum, perspiration, tears, skin may be discolored brown-orange. • Soft contact lenses may be permanently discolored. • Rifabutin may decrease efficacy of oral contraceptives; nonhormonal methods should be considered. • Avoid crowds, those with infection. • Report flu-like symptoms, nausea, vomiting, dark urine, unusual bruising or bleeding from any site, any visual disturbances.

rifampin

rif-**am**-pin

(Rifadin, Rifadin IV, Rimactane, Rofact ✤)

Do not confuse rifampin with rifabutin, Rifamate, rifapentine, or Ritalin.

FIXED-COMBINATION(S)

Rifamate: rifampin/isoniazid (an antitubercular): 300 mg/150 mg. **Rifater:** rifampin/isoniazid/pyrazinamide (an antitubercular): 120 mg/50 mg/300 mg.

CLASSIFICATION

PHARMACOTHERAPEUTIC: Antitubercular.

ACTION

An antitubercular that interferes with bacterial RNA synthesis by binding to DNA-dependent RNA polymerase, thus preventing its attachment to DNA and blocking RNA transcription. **Therapeutic Effect:** Bactericidal in susceptible microorganisms.

PHARMACOKINETICS

Well absorbed from the GI tract (food delays absorption). Protein binding: 80%. Widely distributed. Metabolized in the liver to active metabolite. Primarily eliminated by the biliary system. Not removed by hemodialysis. **Half-life:** 3–5 hr (increased in hepatic impairment).

USES

In conjunction with at least one other antitubercular agent for initial treatment and retreatment of clinical tuberculosis. Eliminates *Neisseria* meningococci from the nasopharynx of asymptomatic carriers in situations with high risk of meningococcal meningitis (prophylaxis, not cure). **OFF-LABEL:** Prophylaxis of

R

H. influenzae type b infection; treatment of atypical mycobacterial infection and serious infections caused by *Staphylococcus* species.

PRECAUTIONS

CONTRAINDICATIONS: Concomitant therapy with amprenavir, hypersensitivity to other rifamycins. **CAUTIONS:** Hepatic dysfunction, active or treated alcoholism.

⧗ LIFESPAN CONSIDERATIONS: Pregnancy/Lactation: Crosses placenta. Distributed in breast milk. **Pregnancy Category C. Children/Elderly:** No age-related precautions noted.

INTERACTIONS

DRUG: Alcohol, hepatotoxic medications, ritonavir, saquinavir: May increase the risk of hepatotoxicity. **Aminophylline, theophylline:** May increase clearance of these drugs. **Chloramphenicol, digoxin, disopyramide, fluconazole, methadone, mexiletine, oral anticoagulants, oral antidiabetics, phenytoin, quinidine, tocainide, verapamil:** May decrease the effects of these drugs. **Oral contraceptives:** May decrease oral contraceptive effectiveness. **HERBAL:** None known. **FOOD:** None known. **LAB VALUES:** May increase serum alkaline phosphatase, bilirubin, uric acid, AST, and ALT levels.

AVAILABILITY (Rx)

CAPSULES: 150 mg (Rifadin), 300 mg (Rifadin, Rimactane). **INJECTION, POWDER FOR RECONSTITUTION (RIFADIN IV):** 600 mg.

ADMINISTRATION/HANDLING

▯ IV

Reconstitution • Reconstitute 600-mg vial with 10 ml sterile water for injection to provide concentration of 60 mg/ml. • Withdraw desired dose and further dilute with 500 ml D$_5$W.

Rate of administration • For IV infusion only. Avoid IM, subcutaneous administration. • Avoid extravasation (local irritation, inflammation). • Infuse over 3 hr (may dilute with 100 ml D$_5$W and infuse over 30 min).

Storage • Reconstituted vial is stable for 24 hr. • Once reconstituted vial is further diluted, it is stable for 4 hr in D$_5$W or 24 hrs in 0.9% NaCl.

PO
• Preferably give 1 hr before or 2 hr following meals with 8 oz of water (may give with food to decrease GI upset; will delay absorption). • For those unable to swallow capsules, contents may be mixed with applesauce, jelly. • Administer at least 1 hr before antacids, especially those containing aluminum.

INDICATIONS/ROUTES/DOSAGE
TUBERCULOSIS
PO, IV: ADULTS, ELDERLY: 10 mg/kg/day. **Maximum:** 600 mg/day. CHILDREN: 10–20 mg/kg/day in divided doses q12–24h.

PREVENTION OF MENINGOCOCCAL INFECTIONS
PO, IV: ADULTS, ELDERLY: 600 mg q12h for 2 days. CHILDREN 1 MO AND OLDER: 20 mg/kg/day in divided doses q12–24h. **Maximum:** 600 mg/dose. INFANTS YOUNGER THAN 1 MO: 10 mg/kg/day in divided doses q12h for 2 days.

STAPHYLOCOCCAL INFECTIONS
PO, IV: ADULTS, ELDERLY: 600 mg once a day. CHILDREN: 15 mg/kg/day in divided doses q12h.

STAPHYLOCOCCUS AUREUS INFECTIONS (IN COMBINATION WITH OTHER ANTI-INFECTIVES)
PO: ADULTS, ELDERLY: 300–600 mg twice a day. NEONATES: 5–20 mg/kg/day in divided doses q12h.

PREVENTION OF *HAEMOPHILUS INFLUENZAE* INFECTION
PO: ADULTS, ELDERLY: 600 mg/day for 4 days. CHILDREN 1 MO AND OLDER: 20 mg/kg/day in divided doses q12h for

5–10 days. CHILDREN YOUNGER THAN 1 MO: 10 mg/kg/day in divided doses q12h for 2 days.

⬛ IV INCOMPATIBILITY

Diltiazem (Cardizem).

SIDE EFFECTS

EXPECTED: Red-orange or red-brown discoloration of urine, feces, saliva, skin, sputum, sweat, or tears. **OCCASIONAL (5%–2%):** Hypersensitivity reaction (such as flushing, pruritus, or rash). **RARE (2%–1%):** Diarrhea, dyspepsia, nausea, candida as evidenced by sore mouth or tongue.

ADVERSE REACTIONS/ TOXIC EFFECTS

Rare reactions include hepatotoxicity (risk is increased when rifampin is taken with isoniazid), hepatitis, blood dyscrasias, Stevens-Johnson syndrome, and antibiotic-associated colitis.

NURSING CONSIDERATIONS

BASELINE ASSESSMENT

Question for hypersensitivity to rifampin, rifamycins. Ensure collection of diagnostic specimens. Evaluate initial serum liver or renal function, CBC results.

INTERVENTION/EVALUATION

Assess IV site at least hourly during infusion; restart at another site at the first sign of irritation or inflammation. Monitor liver function tests and assess for hepatitis: jaundice, anorexia, nausea, vomiting, fatigue, weakness (hold rifampin and inform physician at once). Report hypersensitivity reactions promptly: any type of skin eruption, pruritus, flu-like syndrome with high dosage. Monitor pattern of daily bowel activity and stool consistency (potential for antibiotic-associated colitis). Monitor CBC results for blood dyscrasias, be alert for infection (fever, sore throat), bleeding or ecchymosis, unusual fatigue/weakness.

PATIENT/FAMILY TEACHING

• Preferably take on empty stomach with 8 oz of water 1 hr before or 2 hr after meal (with food if GI upset). • Avoid alcohol during treatment. • Do not take **any** other medications without consulting physician, including antacids; must take rifampin at least 1 hr before antacid. • Urine, feces, sputum, sweat, tears may become red-orange; soft contact lenses may be permanently stained. • Notify physician of **any** new symptom, immediately for yellow eyes or skin, fatigue, weakness, nausea or vomiting, sore throat, fever, flu, unusual bruising or bleeding. • If taking oral contraceptives, check with physician (reliability may be affected).

rifapentine

rif-a-**pen**-teen
(Priftin)
Do not confuse rifapentine with rifampin.

◆CLASSIFICATION

PHARMACOTHERAPEUTIC: Antitubercular.

ACTION

An antitubercular that inhibits bacterial RNA synthesis by binding to DNA-dependent RNA polymerase in *Mycobacterium tuberculosis*. This action prevents the enzyme from attaching to DNA, thereby blocking RNA transcription. **Therapeutic Effect:** Bactericidal.

PHARMACOKINETICS

Rapidly and well absorbed from the GI tract. Protein binding: 97.7%. Metabolized in liver. Primarily eliminated in feces; partial excretion in urine. Not removed by hemodialysis. **Half-life:** 14–17 hr.

R

🍁 Canadian trade name   ℮ see **evolve**   ☞ High Alert drug

USES

Treatment of pulmonary tuberculosis in combination with at least one other antituberculosis medication.

PRECAUTIONS

CONTRAINDICATIONS: History of hypersensitivity to any rifamycins (e.g., rifampin and rifabutin). **CAUTIONS:** Alcoholism, hepatic function impairment.

⌛ **LIFESPAN CONSIDERATIONS: Pregnancy/Lactation:** Unknown if drug crosses placenta or is distributed is breast milk. Since rifapentine may produce a red-orange discoloration of body fluids, there is a potential for discoloration of breast milk. **Pregnancy Category C. Children:** Safety and efficacy not established in children under 12 yr. **Elderly:** Age-related renal or hepatic impairment may require dosage adjustment.

INTERACTIONS

DRUG: Alcohol: May increase the risk of hepatotoxicity. **Oral contraceptives, warfarin:** May decrease the effects of these drugs. **HERBAL:** None known. **FOOD:** None known. **LAB VALUES:** May increase serum AST, ALT, and bilirubin levels.

AVAILABILITY (Rx)

TABLETS: 150 mg.

INDICATIONS/ROUTES/DOSAGE

TUBERCULOSIS

PO: ADULTS, ELDERLY: Intensive phase: 600 mg twice weekly for 2 mo (interval between doses no less than 3 days). Continuation phase: 600 mg weekly for 4 mo.

SIDE EFFECTS

RARE (less than 4%): Red-orange or red-brown discoloration of urine, feces, saliva, skin, sputum, sweat, or tears; arthralgia, pain, nausea, vomiting, headache, dyspepsia, hypertension, dizziness, diarrhea.

ADVERSE REACTIONS/ TOXIC EFFECTS

Hyperuricemia, neutropenia, proteinuria, hematuria, and hepatitis occur rarely.

NURSING CONSIDERATIONS

BASELINE ASSESSMENT

Evaluate initial serum liver function, CBC results.

INTERVENTION/EVALUATION

Monitor serum liver function tests, pattern of bowel activity and stool consistency. Assess for nausea, vomiting, GI upset, diarrhea.

PATIENT/FAMILY TEACHING

• Urine, feces, sputum, sweat, tears may become red-orange; soft contact lenses may be permanently stained. • If taking oral contraceptives, check with physician (reliability may be affected). • Report fever, decreased appetite, nausea, vomiting, dark urine, pain or swelling of joints.

rifaximin

rye-**fax**-ih-min
(Xifaxan)

CLASSIFICATION

PHARMACOTHERAPEUTIC: Anti-infective. **CLINICAL:** Site-specific antibiotic.

ACTION

An anti-infective that inhibits bacterial RNA synthesis by binding to a subunit of bacterial DNA-dependent RNA polymerase. **Therapeutic Effect:** Bactericidal.

PHARMACOKINETICS

Less than 0.4% absorbed after PO administration. Primarily eliminated in feces; minimal excretion in urine. Half-life: 5.85 hr.

USES

Treatment of traveler's diarrhea caused by noninvasive strains of *E. Coli*. OFF-LABEL: Treatment of hepatic encephalopathy.

PRECAUTIONS

CONTRAINDICATIONS: Hypersensitivity to other rifamycin antibiotics. CAUTIONS: Pseudomembranous colitis.

⌛ LIFESPAN CONSIDERATIONS: Pregnancy/Lactation: Unknown if drug is excreted in breast milk. Pregnancy Category C. Children: Safety and efficacy not established in children younger than 12 yr. Elderly: No age-related precautions noted.

INTERACTIONS

DRUG: None known. HERBAL: None known. FOOD: None known. LAB VALUES: None known.

AVAILABILITY (Rx)

TABLETS: 200 mg.

ADMINISTRATION/HANDLING

PO

• Give without regard to food. • Store at room temperature. • Do not break or crush film-coated tablets.

INDICATIONS/ROUTES/DOSAGE

TRAVELER'S DIARRHEA

PO: ADULTS, ELDERLY, CHILDREN 12 YR AND OLDER: 200 mg 3 times a day for 3 days.

HEPATIC ENCEPHALOPATHY

PO: ADULTS, ELDERLY: 1,200 mg/day for 15–21 days.

SIDE EFFECTS

OCCASIONAL (11%–5%): Flatulence, headache, abdominal discomfort, rectal tenesmus, defecation urgency, nausea. RARE (4%–2%): Constipation, fever, vomiting.

ADVERSE REACTIONS/ TOXIC EFFECTS

Hypersensitivity reactions, including dermatitis, angioneurotic edema, pruritus, rash, and urticaria may occur. Superinfection occurs rarely.

NURSING CONSIDERATIONS

BASELINE ASSESSMENT

Check baseline hydration status: skin turgor, mucous membranes for dryness, urinary status.

INTERVENTION/EVALUATION

Encourage adequate fluid intake. Assess bowel sounds for peristalsis. Monitor pattern of bowel activity and stool consistency. Assess for GI disturbances.

PATIENT/FAMILY TEACHING

• Notify physician if diarrhea worsens or within 48 hr, blood occurs in the stool, or fever develops.

rimantadine hydrochloride

ri-**man**-ti-deen

(Flumadine)

Do not confuse rimantadine with ranitidine, or Flumadine with flunisolide or flutamide.

R

◆CLASSIFICATION

CLINICAL: Antiviral.

ACTION

An antiviral that appears to exert an inhibitory effect early in the viral replication cycle. May inhibit uncoating of the virus. Therapeutic Effect: Prevents replication of influenza A virus.

PHARMACOKINETICS

Well absorbed following PO administration. Protein binding: 40%. Metabolized in liver. Excreted in urine. Half-life: 19–36 hr.

USES

Adults: Prophylaxis or treatment of illness due to influenza A virus. **Children:** Prophylaxis against influenza A virus.

PRECAUTIONS

CONTRAINDICATIONS: Hypersensitivity to amantadine. **CAUTIONS:** Hepatic disease, seizures, history of recurrent eczematoid dermatitis, uncontrolled psychosis, renal impairment, concomitant use of CNS stimulant medications.

⏳ LIFESPAN CONSIDERATIONS: **Pregnancy/Lactation:** Unknown if drug crosses placenta or is distributed in breast milk. **Pregnancy Category C. Children:** Safety and efficacy not established in infants. **Elderly:** May be more susceptible to CNS side effects.

INTERACTIONS

DRUG: Acetaminophen, aspirin: May decrease rimantadine blood concentration. **Anticholinergics, CNS stimulants:** May increase side effects of rimantadine. **Cimetidine:** May increase rimantadine blood concentration. HERBAL: None known. FOOD: None known. LAB VALUES: None known.

AVAILABILITY (Rx)

SYRUP: 50 mg/5 ml. **TABLETS:** 100 mg.

ADMINISTRATION/HANDLING

PO
- Give without regard to food.

INDICATIONS/ROUTES/DOSAGE

INFLUENZA A VIRUS
PO: ADULTS, ELDERLY: 100 mg twice a day for 7 days. ELDERLY NURSING HOME PATIENTS, PATIENTS WITH SEVERE HEPATIC OR RENAL IMPAIRMENT: 100 mg once a day for 7 days.

PREVENTION OF INFLUENZA A VIRUS
PO: ADULTS, ELDERLY, CHILDREN 10 YR AND OLDER: 100 mg twice a day for at least 10 days after known exposure (usually for 6–8 wk). CHILDREN YOUNGER THAN 10 YR: 5 mg/kg once a day. **Maximum:** 150 mg. ELDERLY NURSING HOME PATIENTS, PATIENTS WITH SEVERE HEPATIC OR RENAL IMPAIRMENT: 100 mg once a day.

SIDE EFFECTS

OCCASIONAL (3%–2%): Insomnia, nausea, nervousness, impaired concentration, dizziness. **RARE (less than 2%):** Vomiting, anorexia, dry mouth, abdominal pain, asthenia, fatigue.

ADVERSE REACTIONS/ TOXIC EFFECTS

None known.

NURSING CONSIDERATIONS

INTERVENTION/EVALUATION

Assess for anxiety and nervousness, evaluate sleep pattern for insomnia. Provide assistance if dizziness occurs.

PATIENT/FAMILY TEACHING

- Avoid contact with those who are at high risk for influenza A (rimantadine-resistant virus may be shed during therapy). • Avoid tasks that require alertness, motor skills until response to drug is established. • Do not take aspirin, acetaminophen, compounds containing these drugs. • May cause dry mouth.

risedronate sodium

rize-droe-nate
(Actonel)

FIXED-COMBINATION(S)

Actonel with Calcium: Risedronate/Calcium: 35 mg/6 × 500 mg.

CLASSIFICATION

PHARMACOTHERAPEUTIC: Bisphosphonate. **CLINICAL:** Calcium regulator.

ACTION

A bisphosphonate that binds to bone hydroxyapatite and inhibits osteoclasts. **Therapeutic Effect:** Reduces bone turnover (the number of sites at which bone is remodeled) and bone resorption.

PHARMACOKINETICS

Rapidly absorbed following PO administration. Bioavailability is decreased when administered with food. Protein binding: 24%. Not metabolized. Excreted unchanged in urine and feces. Not removed by hemodialysis. **Half-life:** 1.5 hr (initial); 480 hr (terminal).

USES

Treatment of Paget's disease of bone (osteitis deformans). Treatment/prophylaxis for postmenopausal, glucocorticoid-induced osteoporosis.

PRECAUTIONS

CONTRAINDICATIONS: Hypersensitivity to other bisphosphonates, including etidronate, tiludronate, risedronate, and alendronate; hypocalcemia; inability to stand or sit upright for at least 20 minutes; renal impairment when serum creatinine clearance is greater than 5 mg/dl. **CAUTIONS:** GI diseases (duodenitis, dysphagia, esophagitis, gastritis, ulcers [drug may exacerbate these conditions]), severe renal impairment. **Pregnancy Category C.**

INTERACTIONS

DRUG: Antacids containing aluminum, calcium, magnesium; vitamin D: May decrease the absorption of risedronate. **HERBAL:** None known. **FOOD:** None known. **LAB VALUES:** None known.

AVAILABILITY (Rx)

TABLETS: 5 mg, 30 mg, 35 mg.

ADMINISTRATION/HANDLING

PO
• Administer 30–60 min before taking any food, drink, other medications orally to avoid interference with absorption. • Take on empty stomach with full glass of water (not mineral water). • Avoid lying down for 30 min after swallowing tablet (assists with delivery to stomach, reduces risk of esophageal irritation).

INDICATIONS/ROUTES/DOSAGE

PAGET'S DISEASE
PO: ADULTS, ELDERLY: 30 mg/day for 2 mo. Retreatment may occur after 2-mo post-treatment observation period.

PREVENTION AND TREATMENT OF POSTMENOPAUSAL OSTEOPOROSIS
PO: ADULTS, ELDERLY: 5 mg/day or 35 mg once weekly.

GLUCOCORTICOID-INDUCED OSTEOPOROSIS
PO: ADULTS, ELDERLY: 5 mg/day.

SIDE EFFECTS

FREQUENT (30%): Arthralgia. **OCCASIONAL (12%–8%):** Rash, flu-like symptoms, peripheral edema. **RARE (5%–3%):** Bone pain, sinusitis, asthenia, dry eye, tinnitus.

ADVERSE REACTIONS/ TOXIC EFFECTS

Overdose causes hypocalcemia, hypophosphatemia, and significant GI disturbances.

NURSING CONSIDERATIONS

BASELINE ASSESSMENT
Hypocalcemia, vitamin D deficiency must be corrected before therapy. Obtain lab baselines, especially serum electrolytes, renal function.

INTERVENTION/EVALUATION
Check serum electrolytes (especially calcium, alkaline phosphatase levels). Monitor I&O, BUN, creatinine in patients with renal impairment.

R

PATIENT/FAMILY TEACHING
• Instruct patient that expected benefits occur only when medication is taken with full glass (6–8 oz) of plain water, first thing in the morning and at least 30 min before first food, beverage, medication of the day. Any other beverage (mineral water, orange juice, coffee) significantly reduces absorption of medication. • Do not lie down for at least 30 min after taking medication (potentiates delivery to stomach, reduces risk of esophageal irritation). • Consider weight-bearing exercises, modify behavioral factors (e.g., cigarette smoking, alcohol consumption).

Risperdal, *see risperidone*

---

risperidone

ris-**per**-i-done

(Risperdal, Risperdal Consta, Risperdol M-Tabs)

Do not confuse risperidone with reserpine.

◆ CLASSIFICATION

PHARMACOTHERAPEUTIC: Benzisoxazole derivative. **CLINICAL:** Antipsychotic (see p. 59C).

ACTION

A benzisoxazole derivative that may antagonize dopamine and serotonin receptors. **Therapeutic Effect:** Suppresses psychotic behavior.

PHARMACOKINETICS

Well absorbed from the GI tract; unaffected by food. Protein binding: 90%. Extensively metabolized in the liver to active metabolite. Primarily excreted in urine. **Half-life:** 3–20 hr; metabolite: 21–30 hr (increased in elderly).

USES

Management of manifestations of psychotic disorders (e.g., schizophrenia). Treatment of acute mania associated with bipolar disorder. **OFF-LABEL:** Autism in children, behavioral symptoms associated with dementia, Tourette's disorder.

PRECAUTIONS

CONTRAINDICATIONS: None known. **CAUTIONS:** Renal or hepatic impairment, seizure disorders, cardiac disease, recent MI, breast cancer, suicidal patients, those at risk for aspiration pneumonia. May increase risk of stroke in patients with dementia. May increase risk of hyperglycemia.

⌛ **LIFESPAN CONSIDERATIONS: Pregnancy/Lactation:** Unknown if drug crosses placenta or is excreted in breast milk. Recommend against breastfeeding. **Pregnancy Category C. Children:** Safety and efficacy not established. **Elderly:** More susceptible to postural hypotension. Age-related renal or hepatic impairment may require dosage adjustment.

INTERACTIONS

DRUG: Alcohol, other CNS depressants: May increase CNS depression. **Carbamazepine:** May decrease the risperidone blood concentration. **Clozapine:** May increase the risperidone blood concentration. **Dopamine agonists, levodopa:** May decrease the effects of these drugs. **Paroxetine:** May increase the risperidone blood concentration and the risk of extrapyramidal symptoms. **HERBAL:** None known. **FOOD:** None known. **LAB VALUES:** May increase serum prolactin, creatinine, alkaline phosphatase, uric acid, AST, ALT, and triglyceride levels.

May increase blood glucose, decrease serum potassium, protein, and sodium levels. May cause EKG changes.

AVAILABILITY (Rx)

ORAL SOLUTION (RISPERDAL) 1 mg/ml. **TABLETS (RISPERDAL):** 0.25 mg, 0.5 mg, 1 mg, 2 mg, 3 mg, 4 mg. **TABLETS (ORALLY-DISINTEGRATING [RISPERDAL M-TABS]):** 0.5 mg, 1 mg, 2 mg. **INJECTION (RISPERDAL CONSTA):** 25 mg, 37.5 mg, 50 mg.

ADMINISTRATION/HANDLING

◄ ALERT ► Do not administer risperidone via IV route.

IM

Reconstitution • Use only the diluent and needle supplied in the dose pack. • All the components in the dose pack are required for administration. Don't substitute any components. • Prepare the suspension according to the manufacturer's directions. • The drug may be given up to 6 hr after reconstitution, but immediate administration is recommended. • If 2 min pass before the injection, reconstitute the solution by shaking the upright vial vigorously back and forth for as long as it takes to resuspend the microspheres.

Rate of administration • Inject the drug IM into the upper outer quadrant of the gluteus maximus.

Storage • Store the drug below 77°F (25°C) once it is in suspension.

PO

• Give without regard to food. • May mix oral solution with water, coffee, orange juice, low-fat milk. Do not mix with cola, tea.

INDICATIONS/ROUTES/DOSAGE

PSYCHOTIC DISORDER

PO: ADULTS: 0.5–1 mg twice a day. May increase dosage slowly. Range: 2–6 mg/day. ELDERLY: Initially, 0.25–2 mg/day in 2 divided doses. May increase dosage slowly. Range: 2–6 mg/day.

IM: ADULTS, ELDERLY: 25 mg q2wk. **Maximum:** 50 mg q2wk.

MANIA

PO: ADULTS, ELDERLY: Initially, 2–3 mg as a single daily dose. May increase at 24 hr intervals of 1 mg/day. Range: 2–6 mg/day.

DOSAGE IN RENAL IMPAIRMENT

Initial dosage for adults and elderly patients is 0.25–0.5 mg twice a day. Dosage is titrated slowly to desired effect.

SIDE EFFECTS

FREQUENT (26%–13%): Agitation, anxiety, insomnia, headache, constipation. **OCCASIONAL (10%–4%):** Dyspepsia, rhinitis, somnolence, dizziness, nausea, vomiting, rash, abdominal pain, dry skin, tachycardia. **RARE (3%–2%):** Visual disturbances, fever, back pain, pharyngitis, cough, arthralgia, angina, aggressive behavior, orthostatic hypotension, breast swelling.

ADVERSE REACTIONS/TOXIC EFFECTS

Rare reactions include tardive dyskinesia (characterized by tongue protrusion, puffing of the cheeks, and chewing or puckering of the mouth) and neuroleptic malignant syndrome (marked by hyperpyrexia, muscle rigidity, change in mental status, irregular pulse or BP, tachycardia, diaphoresis, cardiac arrhythmias, rhabdomyolysis, and acute renal failure). Hyperglycemia, in some cases extreme and associated with ketoacidosis or hyperosmolar coma or death, has been reported.

NURSING CONSIDERATIONS

BASELINE ASSESSMENT

Serum renal and liver function tests should be performed before therapy. Assess behavior, appearance, emotional status, response to environment, speech pattern, thought content. Obtain fasting blood glucose value.

R

INTERVENTION/EVALUATION

Monitor BP, heart rate, weight, liver function tests, EKG. Monitor for fine tongue movement (may be first sign of tardive dyskinesia, which may be irreversible). Supervise suicidal-risk patient closely during early therapy (as depression lessens, energy level improves, increasing suicide potential). Assess for therapeutic response (greater interest in surroundings, improved self-care, increased ability to concentrate, relaxed facial expression). Monitor for potential neuroleptic malignant syndrome: fever, muscle rigidity, irregular BP or pulse, altered mental status. Monitor fasting blood glucose periodically during therapy.

PATIENT/FAMILY TEACHING

• Avoid tasks that may require alertness, motor skills until response to drug is established (may cause dizziness/drowsiness). • Avoid alcohol. • Use caution when changing position from lying or sitting to standing. • Inform physician of trembling in fingers, altered gait, unusual muscle or skeletal movements, palpitations, severe dizziness/fainting, swelling or pain in breasts, visual changes, rash, difficulty in breathing.

Ritalin, *see methylphenidate*

---

ritonavir

ri-**tone**-a-veer
(Norvir, Norvisec ✦)
Do not confuse ritonavir with Retrovir.

◆CLASSIFICATION

PHARMACOTHERAPEUTIC: Protease inhibitor. **CLINICAL:** Antiviral (see pp. 61C, 105C).

ACTION

Inhibits HIV-1 and HIV-2 proteases, rendering these enzymes incapable of processing the polypeptide precursors; this results in the production of noninfectious, immature HIV particles. **Therapeutic Effect:** Impedes HIV replication, slowing the progression of HIV infection.

PHARMACOKINETICS

Well absorbed after PO administration (absorption increased with food). Protein binding: 98%–99%. Extensively metabolized in the liver to active metabolite. Primarily eliminated in feces. Unknown if removed by hemodialysis. **Half-life:** 2.7–5 hr.

USES

Treatment of HIV infection in combination with other antiretroviral agents.

PRECAUTIONS

CONTRAINDICATIONS: Concurrent use of amiodarone, astemizole, bepridil, bupropion, cisapride, clozapine, encainide, flecainide, meperidine, piroxicam, propafenone, propoxyphene, quinidine, rifabutin, or terfenadine (increased risk of serious or life-threatening drug interactions, such as arrhythmias, hematologic abnormalities, and seizures); concurrent use of alprazolam, clorazepate, diazepam, estazolam, flurazepam, midazolam, triazolam, or zolpidem (may produce extreme sedation and respiratory depression). **CAUTIONS:** Hepatic impairment.

⧗ **LIFESPAN CONSIDERATIONS: Pregnancy/Lactation:** Breast-feeding not recommended (possibility of HIV transmission). **Pregnancy Category B. Children:** No age-related precautions noted in those older than 2 yr. **Elderly:** None known.

INTERACTIONS

DRUG: Desipramine, fluoxetine, other antidepressants: May increase the blood concentration of these drugs. **Disulfiram, drugs causing disulfiram-like reaction (such as metronidazole):** May produce a disulfiram-like reaction. **Enzyme inducers (including carbamazepine, dexamethasone, nevirapine, phenobarbital, phenytoin, rifabutin, rifampin):** May increase the metabolism and decrease the efficacy of ritonavir. **Oral contraceptives, theophylline:** May decrease the effectiveness of these drugs. **HERBAL: St. John's wort:** May decrease the blood concentration and effect of ritonavir. **FOOD:** None known. **LAB VALUES:** May alter serum CK, GGT, triglyceride, uric acid, AST, and ALT levels as well as creatinine clearance.

AVAILABILITY (Rx)

ORAL SOLUTION: 80 mg/ml. **SOFT GELATIN CAPSULES:** 100 mg.

ADMINISTRATION/HANDLING
PO
• Store capsules, solution in refrigerator. • Protect from light. • Refrigeration of oral solution is recommended but not necessary if used within 30 days and stored below 77°F. • Give without regard to meals (preferably give with food). • May improve taste of oral solution by mixing with chocolate milk, Ensure, Advera, Boost within 1 hr of dosing.

INDICATIONS/ROUTES/DOSAGE
HIV INFECTION
PO: ADULTS, CHILDREN 12 YR AND OLDER: 600 mg twice a day. If nausea occurs at this dosage, give 300 mg twice a day for 1 day, 400 mg twice a day for 2 days, 500 mg twice a day for 1 day, then 600 mg twice a day thereafter. CHILDREN 1 MO–11 YR: Initially, 250 mg/m^2/dose twice a day. Increase by 50 mg/m^2/dose up to 400 mg/m^2/dose. **Maximum:** 600 mg/dose twice a day.

DOSAGE ADJUSTMENTS IN COMBINATION THERAPY
Amprenavir: Amprenavir 1,200 mg and ritonavir 200 mg once a day or amprenavir 600 mg and ritonavir 100 mg twice a day.
Ampenavir and efavirenz: Amprenavir 1200 mg twice a day and ritonavir 200 mg twice a day with standard dose of efavirenz.
Indinavir: Indinavir 800 mg twice a day and ritonavir 100–200 mg twice a day or indinavir 400 mg twice a day and ritonavir 400 mg twice a day.
Nelfinavir or saquinavir: Ritonavir 400 mg twice a day.
Rifabutin: Decrease rifabutin dosage to 150 mg every other day.

SIDE EFFECTS
FREQUENT: GI disturbances (abdominal pain, anorexia, diarrhea, nausea, vomiting), circumoral and peripheral paresthesias, altered taste, headache, dizziness, fatigue, asthenia. **OCCASIONAL:** Allergic reaction, flu-like symptoms, hypotension. **RARE:** Diabetes mellitus, hyperglycemia.

ADVERSE REACTIONS/ TOXIC EFFECTS
Hepatitis and fatal cases of pancreatitis have been reported.

NURSING CONSIDERATIONS
BASELINE ASSESSMENT
Patients beginning combination therapy with ritonavir and nucleosides may promote GI tolerance by beginning ritonavir alone and subsequently adding nucleosides before completing 2 wk of ritonavir monotherapy. Obtain baseline laboratory testing, especially serum liver function tests, triglycerides before beginning ritonavir therapy and at periodic intervals during therapy. Offer emotional support to patient and family.

INTERVENTION/EVALUATION

Closely monitor for evidence of GI disturbances, neurologic abnormalities (particularly paraesthesias). Monitor serum liver function tests, blood glucose, CD4 cell count, plasma levels of HIV RNA.

PATIENT/FAMILY TEACHING

• Continue therapy for full length of treatment. • Doses should be evenly spaced. • Ritonavir is not a cure for HIV infection, nor does it reduce risk of transmission to others. • Patients may continue to acquire illnesses associated with advanced HIV infection. • If possible, take ritonavir with food. • Taste of solution may be improved when mixed with chocolate milk, Ensure, Advera, Boost. • Inform physician of increased thirst, frequent urination, nausea, vomiting, abdominal pain.

Rituxan, *see rituximab*

---

rituximab ⚑

rye-**tucks**-ih-mab
(Rituxan)

◆CLASSIFICATION

PHARMACOTHERAPEUTIC: Monoclonal antibody. **CLINICAL:** Antineoplastic (see p. 78C).

ACTION

Binds to CD20, the antigen found on the surface of B lymphocytes and B-cell non-Hodgkin's lymphomas. **Therapeutic Effect:** Produces cytotoxicity, reducing tumor size.

PHARMACOKINETICS

Rapidly depletes B cells. **Half-life:** 59.8 hr after first infusion and 174 hr after fourth infusion.

USES

Treatment of relapsed or refractory low-grade or follicular B-cell non-Hodgkin's lymphoma. First line treatment for diffuse large B cell, CD20 positive, non-Hodgkin's lymphoma. Treatment of moderate to severe rheumatoid arthritis.

PRECAUTIONS

CONTRAINDICATIONS: Hypersensitivity to murine proteins. **CAUTIONS:** Those with history of cardiac disease.

⧗ **LIFESPAN CONSIDERATIONS: Pregnancy/Lactation:** Has potential to cause fetal B-cell depletion. Unknown if distributed in breast milk. Those with childbearing potential should use contraceptive methods during treatment and up to 12 mo following therapy. **Pregnancy Category C. Children:** Safety and efficacy not established. **Elderly:** No age-related precautions noted.

INTERACTIONS

DRUG: None known. **HERBAL:** None known. **FOOD:** None known. **LAB VALUES:** None known.

AVAILABILITY (Rx)

INJECTION: 10 mg/ml.

ADMINISTRATION/HANDLING

🖳 IV

Reconstitution • Dilute with 0.9% NaCl or D₅W to provide a final concentration of 1–4 mg/ml into infusion bag.

Rate of administration • Infuse at rate of 50 mg/hr. May increase infusion rate in 50 mg/hr increments q30min to maximum 400 mg/hr. • Subsequent infusion can be given at 100 mg/hr and increased by 100 mg/hr increments q30min to maximum 400 mg/hr.

Storage
◄ ALERT ► Do not give by IV push or bolus.
• Refrigerate vials. • Diluted solution is stable for 24 hr if refrigerated and at room temperature for an additional 12 hr.

R

▨ IV INCOMPATIBILITIES

Don't mix rituximab with any other medications.

INDICATIONS/ROUTES/DOSAGE

NON-HODGKIN'S LYMPHOMA

IV: ADULTS: 375 mg/m^2 once weekly for 4–8 wk. May administer a second 4-wk course.

RHEUMATOID ARTHRITIS

IV: ADULTS: 100 mg every 2 wk times 2 doses.

SIDE EFFECTS

FREQUENT: Fever (49%), chills (32%), asthenia (16%), headache (14%), angioedema (13%), hypotension (10%), nausea (18%), rash or pruritus (10%). **OCCASIONAL (less than 10%):** Myalgia, dizziness, abdominal pain, throat irritation, vomiting, neutropenia, rhinitis, bronchospasm, urticaria.

ADVERSE REACTIONS/ TOXIC EFFECTS

A hypersensitivity reaction marked by hypotension, bronchospasm, and angioedema may occur. Arrhythmias may occur, particularly in those with a history of preexisting cardiac conditions.

NURSING CONSIDERATIONS

BASELINE ASSESSMENT

Pretreatment with acetaminophen and diphenhydramine before each infusion may prevent infusion-related effects. CBC, platelet count should be obtained at regular interval during therapy.

INTERVENTION/EVALUATION

Monitor for an infusion-related symptoms complex consisting mainly of fever, chills, rigors that generally occurs within 30 min–2 hr of beginning first infusion. Slowing infusion resolves symptoms.

rivastigmine tartrate

rye-vah-**stig**-meen
(Exelon)

◆CLASSIFICATION

PHARMACOTHERAPEUTIC: Cholinesterase inhibitor. **CLINICAL:** Anti-Alzheimer's dementia agent.

ACTION

A cholinesterase inhibitor that inhibits the enzyme acetylcholinesterase, thus increasing the concentration of acetylcholine at cholinergic synapses and enhancing cholinergic function in the CNS. **Therapeutic Effect:** Slows the progression of symptoms of Alzheimer's disease.

PHARMACOKINETICS

Rapidly and completely absorbed. Protein binding: 60%. Widely distributed throughout the body. Rapidly and extensively metabolized. Primarily excreted in urine. **Half-life:** 1.5 hr.

USES

Treatment of mild to moderate dementia of the Alzheimer's type.

PRECAUTIONS

CONTRAINDICATIONS: Hypersensitivity to other carbamate derivatives. **CAUTIONS:** Peptic ulcer disease, concurrent use of NSAIDs, sick sinus syndrome, bradycardia, urinary obstruction, seizure disorders, asthma, chronic obstructive pulmonary disease (COPD).

⧗ **LIFESPAN CONSIDERATIONS: Pregnancy/Lactation:** Unknown if distributed in breast milk. **Pregnancy Category B. Children:** Not indicated for use in children. **Elderly:** No age-related precautions.

INTERACTIONS

DRUG: Anticholinergics: May decrease the effects of rivastigmine or anticholinergics. **Bethanechol:** May increase the effects of rivastigmine or bethanechol. **HERBAL:** None known. **FOOD:** None known. **LAB VALUES:** None known.

R

AVAILABILITY (Rx)

CAPSULES: 1.5 mg, 3 mg, 4.5 mg, 6 mg.
ORAL SOLUTION: 2 mg/ml.

ADMINISTRATION/HANDLING

PO
• Give with food in divided doses morning and evening.

ORAL SOLUTION
• Using oral syringe (provided by manufacturer), withdraw prescribed amount rivastigmine from container. • May be swallowed directly from syringe or mixed in small glass of water, cold fruit juice, soda (use within 4 hr of mixing).

INDICATIONS/ROUTES/DOSAGE

ALZHEIMER'S DISEASE
PO: ADULTS, ELDERLY: Initially, 1.5 mg twice a day. May increase at intervals of least 2 wk to 3 mg twice a day, then 4.5 mg twice a day, and finally 6 mg twice a day. **Maximum:** 6 mg twice a day.

SIDE EFFECTS

FREQUENT (47%–17%): Nausea, vomiting, dizziness, diarrhea, headache, anorexia. **OCCASIONAL (13%–6%):** Abdominal pain, insomnia, dyspepsia (heartburn, indigestion, epigastric pain), confusion, UTI, depression. **RARE (5%–3%):** Anxiety, somnolence, constipation, malaise, hallucinations, tremor, flatulence, rhinitis, hypertension, flu-like symptoms, weight loss, syncope.

ADVERSE REACTIONS/ TOXIC EFFECTS

Overdose may result in cholinergic crisis, characterized by severe nausea and vomiting, increased salivation, diaphoresis, bradycardia, hypotension, respiratory depression, and seizures.

NURSING CONSIDERATIONS

BASELINE ASSESSMENT

Obtain baseline vital signs. Assess history for peptic ulcer, urinary obstruction, asthma, COPD. Assess cognitive, behavioral, functional deficits.

INTERVENTION/EVALUATION

Monitor for cholinergic reaction: GI discomfort or cramping, feeling of facial warmth, excessive salivation and diaphoresis, lacrimation, pallor, urinary urgency, dizziness. Monitor for nausea, diarrhea, headache, insomnia.

PATIENT/FAMILY TEACHING

• Take with meals (at breakfast, dinner). • Swallow capsule whole. Do not chew, break, crush capsules. • Report nausea, vomiting, diarrhea, diaphoresis, increased salivary secretions, severe abdominal pain, dizziness.

rizatriptan benzoate

rize-a-**trip**-tan
(Maxalt, Maxalt-MLT)

◆CLASSIFICATION

PHARMACOTHERAPEUTIC: Serotonin receptor agonist. **CLINICAL:** Antimigraine (see p. 56C).

ACTION

A serotonin receptor agonist that binds selectively to vascular receptors, producing a vasoconstrictive effect on cranial blood vessels. **Therapeutic Effect:** Relieves migraine headache.

PHARMACOKINETICS

Well absorbed after PO administration. Protein binding: 14%. Crosses the blood-brain barrier. Metabolized by the liver to inactive metabolite. Eliminated primarily in urine and, to a lesser extent, in feces. **Half-life:** 2–3 hr.

USES

Treatment of acute migraine attack with or without aura.

✏ see color pill atlas   ✒ herb   underlined – top prescribed drug

PRECAUTIONS

CONTRAINDICATIONS: Basilar or hemiplegic migraine, coronary artery disease, ischemic heart disease (including angina pectoris, history of MI, silent ischemia, and Prinzmetal's angina), uncontrolled hypertension, use within 24 hr of ergotamine-containing preparations or another serotonin receptor agonist, use within 14 days of MAOIs. **CAUTIONS:** Mild to moderate renal or hepatic impairment, patient profile suggesting cardiovascular risks.

⏳ **LIFESPAN CONSIDERATIONS:** **Pregnancy/Lactation:** Unknown if drug is distributed in breast milk. **Pregnancy Category C.** **Children:** Safety and efficacy not established. **Elderly:** No age-related precautions noted.

INTERACTIONS

DRUG: **Ergotamine-containing medications:** May produce a vasospastic reaction. **Fluoxetine, fluvoxamine, paroxetine, sertraline:** May produce hyperreflexia, incoordination, and weakness. **MAOIs, propranolol:** May dramatically increase plasma concentration of rizatriptan. **HERBAL:** None known. **FOOD:** **All foods:** Delay peak drug concentration by 1 hr. **LAB VALUES:** None known.

AVAILABILITY (Rx)

TABLETS (MAXALT): 5 mg, 10 mg. **TABLETS (ORALLY-DISINTEGRATING [MAXALT-MLT]):** 5 mg, 10 mg.

ADMINISTRATION/HANDLING

PO

• Oral disintegrating tablet is packaged in an individual aluminum pouch. • Open packet with dry hands. • Place tablet onto tongue; allow to dissolve and swallow dissolved and with saliva. Administration with water is not necessary.

INDICATIONS/ROUTES/DOSAGE

ACUTE MIGRAINE ATTACK
PO: ADULTS OLDER THAN 18 YR, ELDERLY: 5–10 mg. If headache improves, but then returns, dose may be repeated after 2 hr. **Maximum:** 30 mg/24 hr.

SIDE EFFECTS

FREQUENT (9%–7%): Dizziness, somnolence, paraesthesia, fatigue. **OCCASIONAL (6%–3%):** Nausea, chest pressure, dry mouth. **RARE (2%):** Headache; neck, throat, or jaw pressure; photosensitivity.

ADVERSE REACTIONS/ TOXIC EFFECTS

Cardiac reactions (such as ischemia, coronary artery vasospasm, and MI) and noncardiac vasospasm-related reactions (including hemorrhage and cerebrovascular accident [CVA]), occur rarely, particularly in patients with hypertension, diabetes, or a strong family history of coronary artery disease; obese patients; smokers; males older than 40 yr; and postmenopausal women.

NURSING CONSIDERATIONS

BASELINE ASSESSMENT

Question for history of peripheral vascular disease, renal or hepatic impairment. Question patient regarding onset, location, duration of migraine and possible precipitating symptoms.

INTERVENTION/EVALUATION

Monitor for evidence of dizziness. Assess for relief of migraine headache and potential for photophobia, phonophobia (sound sensitivity, nausea, vomiting).

PATIENT/FAMILY TEACHING

• Take a single dose as soon as symptoms of an actual migraine attack appear. • Medication is intended to relieve migraine, not to prevent or reduce number of attacks. • Avoid tasks that require alertness, motor skills until response to drug is established. • If palpitations,

R

pain or tightness in chest/throat, pain or weakness of extremities occurs, contact physician immediately. • Do not remove the blister from the orally disintegrating tablet until just before dosing. • Use protective measures (sunscreen, protective clothing) against exposure to UV light and sunlight.

Rocephin, *see ceftriaxone*

---

rocuronium bromide

(Zemuron)
See Neuromuscular blockers (p. 112C)

---

ropinirole hydrochloride

ro-**pin**-i-role
(Requip)

CLASSIFICATION

PHARMACOTHERAPEUTIC: Dopamine agonist. **CLINICAL:** Antiparkinson agent.

ACTION

An antiparkinson agent that stimulates dopamine receptors in the striatum. **Therapeutic Effect:** Relieves signs and symptoms of Parkinson's disease.

PHARMACOKINETICS

Rapidly absorbed after PO administration. Protein binding: 40%. Extensively distributed throughout the body. Extensively metabolized. Steady-state concentrations achieved within 2 days. Eliminated in urine. Unknown if removed by hemodialysis. **Half-life:** 6 hr.

USES

Treatment of signs/symptoms of idiopathic Parkinson's disease.

PRECAUTIONS

CONTRAINDICATIONS: None known. **CAUTIONS:** History of orthostatic hypotension, syncope, hallucinations, especially in elderly. Concurrent use of CNS depressants.

⏳ **LIFESPAN CONSIDERATIONS: Pregnancy/Lactation:** Distributed in breast milk. Drug activity possible in breast-feeding infant. **Pregnancy Category C. Children:** Safety and efficacy not established. **Elderly:** No age-related precautions noted, but hallucinations appear to occur more frequently.

INTERACTIONS

DRUG: Butyrophenones, metoclopramide, phenothiazines, thioxanthenes: Decrease the effectiveness of ropinirole. **Cimetidine, diltiazem, enoxacin, erythromycin, fluvoxamine, mexiletine, norfloxacin, tacrine:** Alter ropinirole blood concentration. **Ciprofloxacin:** Increases ropinirole blood concentration. **CNS depressants:** May increase CNS depressant effects. **Estrogens:** Reduce the clearance of ropinirole. **Levodopa:** Increases the blood concentration of levodopa. **HERBAL: Kava kava:** May decrease the effectiveness of ropinirole. **FOOD: All foods:** Delay peak plasma levels by 1 hr but don't affect drug absorption. **LAB VALUES:** May increase serum alkaline phosphatase level.

AVAILABILITY (Rx)

TABLETS: 0.25 mg, 0.5 mg, 1 mg, 2 mg, 3 mg, 4 mg, 5 mg.

ADMINISTRATION/HANDLING
PO

• Ascending-dose schedule should increase very gradually at weekly intervals: **Week 1:** 0.25 mg 3 times a day to total

---

daily dose 0.75 mg. **Week 2:** 0.5 mg 3 times a day to total daily dose 1.5 mg. **Week 3:** 0.75 mg 3 times a day to total daily dose 2.25 mg. **Week 4:** 1 mg 3 times a day to total daily dose 3 mg. • Discontinue medication gradually. Decrease frequency from 3 times a day to 2 times a day for 4 days. For the remaining 3 days, decrease frequency to once a day before complete withdrawal.

INDICATIONS/ROUTES/DOSAGE

PARKINSON'S DISEASE

PO: ADULTS, ELDERLY: Initially, 0.25 mg 3 times a day. May increase dosage every 7 days.

RESTLESS LEG SYNDROME

PO: ADULTS, ELDERLY: 0.25 mg for days 1 and 2; 0.5 mg for days 3–7; 1 mg for week 2; 1.5 mg for week 3; 2 mg for week 4; 2.5 mg for week 5; 3 mg for week 6; 4 mg for week 7. All doses to be given 1–3 hours before bedtime.

SIDE EFFECTS

FREQUENT (60%–40%): Nausea, dizziness, somnolence. **OCCASIONAL (12%–5%):** Syncope, vomiting, fatigue, viral infection, dyspepsia, diaphoresis, asthenia, orthostatic hypotension, abdominal discomfort, pharyngitis, abnormal vision, dry mouth, hypertension, hallucinations, confusion. **RARE (less than 4%):** Anorexia, peripheral edema, memory loss, rhinitis, sinusitis, palpitations, impotence.

ADVERSE REACTIONS/ TOXIC EFFECTS

Falling asleep without warning while engaged in activities of daily living, including driving motor vehicles, has been reported.

NURSING CONSIDERATIONS

INTERVENTION/EVALUATION

Assess for clinical improvement, clinical reversal of symptoms (improvement of tremors of head/hands at rest, mask-like facial expression, shuffling gait, muscular rigidity). Assist with ambulation if dizziness occurs.

PATIENT/FAMILY TEACHING

• Drowsiness, dizziness may be an initial response to drug. • Postural hypotension may occur more frequently during initial therapy. Instruct patient to rise from lying to sitting or sitting to standing position slowly to prevent risk of postural hypotension. • Avoid tasks that require alertness, motor skills until response to drug is established. • If nausea occurs, take medication with food. • Inform patient that hallucinations may occur, more so in the elderly than in younger patients with Parkinson's disease.

rosiglitazone maleate

roz-ih-**glit**-a-zone

(<u>Avandia</u>)

Do not confuse Avandia with Avalide, Avinza, or Prandin, or Avandaryl with Benadryl.

FIXED-COMBINATION(S)

Avandamet: rosiglitazone/metformin: 1 mg/500 mg; 2 mg/500 mg; 4 mg/500 mg; 2 mg/1 g; 4 mg/1 g. **Avandaryl:** rosiglitazone/glimepiride (an antidiabetic): 4 mg/1 mg, 4 mg/2 mg, 4 mg/4 mg.

CLASSIFICATION

CLINICAL: Antidiabetic (see p. 42C).

ACTION

An antidiabetic that improves target-cell response to insulin without increasing pancreatic insulin secretion. Decreases hepatic glucose output and increases insulin-dependent glucose utilization in skeletal muscle. **Therapeutic Effect:** Lowers blood glucose concentration.

PHARMACOKINETICS

Rapidly absorbed. Protein binding: 99%. Metabolized in the liver. Excreted primarily in urine, with a lesser amount in feces. Not removed by hemodialysis. **Half-life:** 3–4 hr.

USES

Adjunct to diet/exercise to lower blood glucose in those with type 2 non–insulin-dependent diabetes mellitus (NIDDM). Used as monotherapy or in combination with metformin, sulfonylurea, or insulin to improve glycemic control.

PRECAUTIONS

CONTRAINDICATIONS: Active hepatic disease, diabetic ketoacidosis, increased serum transaminase levels, including ALT greater than 2.5 times the normal serum level, type 1 diabetes mellitus. **CAUTIONS:** Hepatic impairment, CHF, edematous patients. May cause or worsen macular edema.

⧗ **LIFESPAN CONSIDERATIONS: Pregnancy/Lactation:** Unknown if drug crosses placenta or is distributed in breast milk. Not recommended in pregnant or breast-feeding women. **Pregnancy Category C. Children:** Safety and efficacy not established. **Elderly:** No age-related precautions noted in the elderly.

INTERACTIONS

DRUG: Gemfibrozil: May increase plasma concentrations of rosiglitazone. **HERBAL: Bitter melon, eucalyptus, fenugreek, ginseng, guar gum, St. John's wort:** May increase the risk of hypoglycemia. **Glucosamine, licorice:** May reduce the effectiveness of rosiglitazone. **FOOD:** None known. **LAB VALUES:** May decrease Hct and Hgb and serum alkaline phosphatase,

bilirubin, and AST levels. Less than 1% of patients experience ALT values that are 3 times the normal level.

AVAILABILITY (Rx)

TABLETS: 2 mg, 4 mg, 8 mg.

ADMINISTRATION/HANDLING

PO
• Give without regard to meals.

INDICATIONS/ROUTES/DOSAGE

DIABETES MELLITUS, COMBINATION THERAPY
PO (WITH SULFONYLUREAS, METFORMIN): ADULTS, ELDERLY: Initially, 4 mg as a single daily dose or in divided doses twice a day. May increase to 8 mg/day after 12 wk of therapy if fasting glucose level is not adequately controlled.
PO (WITH INSULIN): ADULTS, ELDERLY: Initially, 4 mg/day in 1 or 2 doses and reduce insulin dose by 10%–25%. If hypoglycemia occurs or plasma glucose falls to less than 100 mg/dl, doses of rosiglitazone greater than 4 mg are not recommended.

DIABETES MELLITUS, MONOTHERAPY
ADULTS, ELDERLY: Initially, 4 mg as single daily dose or in divided doses twice a day. May increase to 8 mg/day after 12 wk of therapy.

SIDE EFFECTS

FREQUENT (9%): Upper respiratory tract infection. **OCCASIONAL (4%–2%):** Headache, edema, back pain, fatigue, sinusitis, diarrhea.

ADVERSE REACTIONS/ TOXIC EFFECTS

Hepatotoxicity occurs rarely.

NURSING CONSIDERATIONS

BASELINE ASSESSMENT

Obtain hepatic enzyme levels before initiation of therapy and periodically thereafter. Ensure follow-up instruction if patient or family does not thoroughly understand diabetes management or glucose-testing technique.

INTERVENTION/EVALUATION

Monitor blood glucose, Hgb, serum hepatic function tests, esp. AST, ALT. Assess for hypoglycemia (cool/wet skin, tremors, dizziness, anxiety, headache, tachycardia, numbness in mouth, hunger, diplopia), hyperglycemia (polyuria, polyphagia, polydipsia, nausea, vomiting, dim vision, fatigue, deep/rapid breathing). Be alert to conditions that alter glucose requirements: fever, increased activity/stress, surgical procedures.

PATIENT/FAMILY TEACHING

• Diabetes mellitus requires lifelong control. • Prescribed diet, exercise are principal parts of treatment; do not skip/delay meals. • Wear medical alert identification. • Continue to adhere to dietary instructions, a regular exercise program, regular testing of urine or blood glucose. • When taking combination drug therapy with a sulfonylurea or insulin, have a source of glucose available to treat symptoms of low blood sugar.

---

rosuvastatin calcium

ross-uh-vah-**stah**-tin
(Crestor)

♦CLASSIFICATION

PHARMACOTHERAPEUTIC: Hydroxamethylglutaryl CoA (HMG-CoA) reductase inhibitor. **CLINICAL:** Antihyperlipidemic.

ACTION

An antihyperlipidemic that interferes with cholesterol biosynthesis by inhibiting the conversion of the enzyme HMG-CoA to mevalonate, a precursor to cholesterol. **Therapeutic Effect:** Decreases LDL cholesterol, VLDL, and plasma triglyceride levels, increases HDL concentration.

PHARMACOKINETICS

Protein binding: 88%. Minimal hepatic metabolism. Primarily eliminated in the feces. **Half-life:** 19 hr (increased in patients with severe renal dysfunction).

USES

Adjunct to diet therapy to decrease elevated total and LDL cholesterol concentrations in patients with primary hypercholesterolemia (types IIa and IIb), lowers serum triglyceride levels, increases HDL.

PRECAUTIONS

CONTRAINDICATIONS: Active hepatic disease, breast-feeding, pregnancy, unexplained, persistent elevations of serum transaminase levels. **CAUTIONS:** Anticoagulant therapy, history of hepatic disease, substantial alcohol consumption, major surgery, severe acute infection, trauma, hypotension, severe metabolic or endocrine disorders, severe electrolyte imbalances, uncontrolled seizures.

⌛ **LIFESPAN CONSIDERATIONS: Pregnancy/Lactation:** Contraindicated in pregnancy (suppression of cholesterol biosynthesis may cause fetal toxicity), lactation. Risk of serious adverse reactions in breast-feeding infants. **Pregnancy Category X. Children:** Safety and efficacy not established. **Elderly:** No age-related precautions noted.

INTERACTIONS

DRUG: Cyclosporine, gemfibrozil, niacin: Increases the risk of myopathy with cyclosporine, gemfibrozil, and niacin. **Erythromycin:** Reduces the plasma concentration of erythromycin. **Ethinylestradiol, norgestrel:** Increases the plasma concentrations of ethinylestradiol and norgestrel. **Warfarin:** Enhances anticoagulant effect. **HERBAL:**

R

St. John's wort: May reduce the effectiveness of rosuvastatin. **FOOD:** None known. **LAB VALUES:** May increase serum creatine kinase (CK) and transaminase concentrations. May produce hematuria and proteinuria.

AVAILABILITY (Rx)

TABLETS: 5 mg, 10 mg, 20 mg, 40 mg.

ADMINISTRATION/HANDLING

PO

• Give without regard to meals. Usually administered in the evening.

INDICATIONS/ROUTES/DOSAGE

HYPERLIPIDEMIA, DYSLIPIDEMIA

PO: ADULTS, ELDERLY: 5 to 40 mg/day. Usual starting dosage is 10 mg/day, with adjustments based on lipid levels; monitor q2–4wk until desired level is achieved. Lower starting dose of 5 mg is recommended in Asians. **Maximum:** 40 mg/day.

RENAL IMPAIRMENT (CREATININE CLEARANCE LESS THAN 30 ml/min)

PO: ADULTS, ELDERLY: 5 mg/day; do not exceed 10 mg/day.

CONCURRENT CYCLOSPORINE USE

PO: ADULTS, ELDERLY: 5 mg/day.

CONCURRENT LIPID-LOWERING THERAPY

PO: ADULTS, ELDERLY: 10 mg/day.

SIDE EFFECTS

Rosuvastatin is generally well tolerated. Side effects are usually mild and transient. **OCCASIONAL (9%–3%):** Pharyngitis, headache, diarrhea, dyspepsia, including heartburn and epigastric distress, nausea. **RARE (less than 3%):** Myalgia, asthenia or unusual fatigue and weakness, back pain, jaundice.

ADVERSE REACTIONS/ TOXIC EFFECTS

Cases of rhabdomyolysis have been reported. Lens opacities may occur. Hypersensitivity reaction and hepatitis occur rarely.

NURSING CONSIDERATIONS

BASELINE ASSESSMENT

Question for possibility of pregnancy before initiating therapy (Pregnancy Category X). Assess baseline lab results: serum cholesterol, triglycerides, liver function tests.

INTERVENTION/EVALUATION

Monitor serum cholesterol, triglyceride results for therapeutic response. Lipid levels should be monitored within 2–4 wk of initiation of therapy or change in dosage. Monitor liver function tests. Liver function tests should be performed at 12 wk following the initiation of therapy and any elevation of dose, and periodically (e.g. semiannually) thereafter. Monitor creatine phosphokinase (CPK) if myopathy is suspected. Determine pattern of bowel activity and stool consistency. Assess for headache, sore throat. Be alert for myalgia/weakness.

PATIENT/FAMILY TEACHING

• Use appropriate contraceptive measures (Pregnancy Category X). • Periodic lab tests are essential part of therapy. • Maintain appropriate diet (important part of treatment). • Report side effects (cramps, muscle pain, weakness, especially with fever).

Roxanol, *see morphine*

Roxicet, *see acetaminophen and oxycodone*

Rozerem, *see ramelteon*

---

salmeterol

sal-**met**-er-all

(Serevent Diskus)

Do not confuse Serevent with Serentil.

FIXED-COMBINATION(S)

Advair: salmeterol/fluticasone (a corticosteroid): 50 mcg/100 mcg; 50 mcg/250 mcg; 50 mcg/500 mcg.

◆CLASSIFICATION

PHARMACOTHERAPEUTIC: Sympathomimetic (adrenergic agonist). **CLINICAL:** Bronchodilator (see p. 67C).

ACTION

An adrenergic agonist that stimulates beta$_2$-adrenergic receptors in the lungs, resulting in relaxation of bronchial smooth muscle. **Therapeutic Effect:** Relieves bronchospasm and reduces airway resistance.

PHARMACOKINETICS

Route	Onset	Peak	Duration
Inhalation	10–20 min	3 hr	12 hr

Low systemic absorption; acts primarily in the lungs. Protein binding: 95%. Metabolized by hydroxylation. Primarily eliminated in feces. **Half-life:** 3–4 hr.

USES

Maintenance of asthma; prevention of exercise-induced bronchospasm, bronchospasm in patients with reversible obstructive airway disease. Long-term maintenance treatment of bronchospasm associated with chronic obstructive pulmonary disease (COPD), including emphysema, chronic bronchitis.

PRECAUTIONS

CONTRAINDICATIONS: History of hypersensitivity to sympathomimetics.

CAUTIONS: Not for acute symptoms. May cause paradoxical bronchospasm, severe asthma. Patients with cardiovascular disorders (e.g., coronary insufficiency, arrhythmias, hypertension), seizure disorders, thyrotoxicosis.

⌛ **LIFESPAN CONSIDERATIONS:** Pregnancy/Lactation: Unknown if excreted in breast milk. **Pregnancy Category C. Children:** No age-related precautions in those older than 4 yr. **Elderly:** Lower dosages may be needed due to increased sympathetic sensitivity (may be more susceptible to tachycardia or tremors).

INTERACTIONS

DRUG: Beta blockers: May decrease the effects of beta blockers. **MAOIs, tricyclic antidepressants:** May increase the effects of salmeterol. **HERBAL:** None known. **FOOD:** None known. **LAB VALUES:** May decrease serum potassium level.

AVAILABILITY (Rx)

POWDER FOR ORAL INHALATION: 50 mcg.

ADMINISTRATION/HANDLING

INHALATION

• Shake container well. Instruct the patient to exhale completely through mouth; place mouthpiece into mouth and close lips, holding inhaler upright. • Have the patient inhale deeply through mouth while fully depressing the top of canister. Hold breath as long as possible before exhaling slowly. • Wait 2 min before second dose (allows for deeper bronchial penetration). • Rinse mouth with water immediately after inhalation (prevents mouth/throat dryness).

INDICATIONS/ROUTES/DOSAGE

PREVENTION AND MAINTENANCE TREATMENT OF ASTHMA

INHALATION (DISKUS): ADULTS, ELDERLY, CHILDREN 4 YR AND OLDER: 1 inhalation (50 mcg) q12h.

PREVENTION OF EXERCISE-INDUCED BRONCHOSPASM

INHALATION (DISKUS): ADULTS, ELDERLY, CHILDREN 4 YR AND OLDER: 1 inhalation at least 30 min before exercise.

COPD

INHALATION (DISKUS): ADULTS, ELDERLY: 1 inhalation q12h.

SIDE EFFECTS

FREQUENT (28%): Headache. **OCCASIONAL (7%–3%):** Cough, tremor, dizziness, vertigo, throat dryness or irritation, pharyngitis. **RARE (3%):** Palpitations, tachycardia, nausea, heartburn, GI distress, diarrhea.

ADVERSE REACTIONS/ TOXIC EFFECTS

Salmeterol may prolong the QT interval, which may precipitate ventricular arrhythmias. Hypokalemia and hyperglycemia may occur.

NURSING CONSIDERATIONS

INTERVENTION/EVALUATION

Monitor rate, depth, rhythm, type of respiration; quality and rate of pulse, BP. Assess lungs for wheezing, rales, rhonchi. Periodically evaluate serum potassium levels.

PATIENT/FAMILY TEACHING

• Not for relief of acute episodes. • Keep canister at room temperature (cold decreases effects). • Do not stop medication or exceed recommended dosage. • Notify physician promptly of chest pain, dizziness. • Wait at least 1 full min before second inhalation. • Administer dose 30–60 min before exercise when used to prevent exercise-induced bronchospasm. • Avoid excessive use of caffeine derivatives: coffee, tea, colas, chocolate.

salsalate

sal-sa-late
(Amigesic, Disalcid, Mono-Gesic, Salflex)

◆CLASSIFICATION

PHARMACOTHERAPEUTIC: Nonsteroidal anti-inflammatory. **CLINICAL:** Analgesic, anti-inflammatory.

ACTION

An NSAID that inhibits prostaglandin synthesis, reducing the inflammatory response and the intensity of pain stimuli reaching the sensory nerve endings. **Therapeutic Effect:** Produces analgesic and anti-inflammatory effects.

USES

Treatment of minor pain or fever, arthritis.

PRECAUTIONS

CONTRAINDICATIONS: Bleeding disorders, hypersensitivity to salicylates or NSAIDs. **CAUTIONS:** Platelet or bleeding disorders, hepatic/renal impairment, history of gastric irritation, peptic ulcer, gastritis, asthma. **Pregnancy Category C.**

INTERACTIONS

DRUG: Alcohol, NSAIDs: May increase the risk of GI effects, such as ulceration. **Antacids, urinary alkalinizers:** Increase the excretion of salsalate. **Anticoagulants, heparin, thrombolytics:** Increase the risk of bleeding. **Insulin, oral antidiabetics:** May increase the effects of these drugs (with large doses of salsalate). **Methotrexate, zidovudine:** May increase the toxicity of these drugs. **Ototoxic medications, vancomycin:** May increase the risk of ototoxicity. **Platelet aggregation inhibitors, valproic acid:** May increase the risk of bleeding. **Probenecid,**

sulfinpyrazone: May decrease the effects of these drugs. **HERBAL: Ginkgo biloba:** May increase the risk of bleeding. **FOOD:** None known. **LAB VALUES:** May alter serum alkaline phosphatase, uric acid, AST, and ALT levels. May prolong PT and bleeding time. May decrease serum cholesterol, potassium, T_3, and T_4 levels.

AVAILABILITY (Rx)

TABLETS (AMIGESIC, DISALCID): 500 mg, 750 mg. **TABLETS (MONO-GESIC, SLAFLEX):** 750 mg.

ADMINISTRATION/HANDLING
PO
• Give with food to minimize GI discomfort.

INDICATIONS/ROUTES/DOSAGE
RHEUMATOID ARTHRITIS, OSTEOARTHRITIS PAIN
PO: ADULTS, ELDERLY: Initially, 3 g/day in 2–3 divided doses. Maintenance: 2–4 g/day.

SIDE EFFECTS
OCCASIONAL: Nausea, dyspepsia (including heartburn, indigestion, and epigastric pain).

ADVERSE REACTIONS/ TOXIC EFFECTS
There is an increased risk of cardiovascular events, including MI and cerebrovascular accident, and serious—potentially life-threatening—GI bleeding. Tinnitus may be the first indication that the serum salicylic acid concentration is reaching or exceeding the upper therapeutic range. Salsalate use may also produce vertigo, headache, confusion, drowsiness, diaphoresis, hyperventilation, vomiting, and diarrhea. Reye's syndrome may occur in children with chickenpox or the flu. Severe overdose may result in electrolyte imbalance, hyperthermia, dehydration, and blood pH imbalance. GI bleeding, peptic ulcer, and Reye's syndrome rarely occur.

NURSING CONSIDERATIONS

BASELINE ASSESSMENT
Do not give to children or teenagers who have flu or chickenpox (increases risk of Reye's syndrome). Assess type, location, duration of pain, inflammation. Inspect appearance of affected joints for immobility, deformities, skin condition.

INTERVENTION/EVALUATION
Assess for evidence of nausea, dyspepsia. Evaluate for therapeutic response: relief of pain, stiffness, and swelling, increased joint mobility, reduced joint tenderness, improved grip strength.

PATIENT/FAMILY TEACHING
• Avoid alcohol. • Avoid use of aspirin-containing products. • Use antacids or take with food to relieve stomach upset. • Report tinnitus, persistent GI pain. • Report behavioral changes, vomiting to physician (may be early signs of Reye's syndrome).

Sanctura, see trospium

Sandostatin, see octreotide

saquinavir

sa-**kwin**-a-veer
(Invirase)
Do not confuse saquinavir with Sinequan.

◆CLASSIFICATION

PHARMACOTHERAPEUTIC: Protease inhibitor. **CLINICAL:** Antiretroviral (see pp. 62C, 105C).

ACTION

Inhibits HIV protease, rendering the enzyme incapable of processing the polyprotein precursors needed to generate functional proteins in HIV-infected cells. **Therapeutic Effect:** Interferes with HIV replication, slowing the progression of HIV infection.

PHARMACOKINETICS

Poorly absorbed after PO administration (absorption increased with high-calorie and high-fat meals). Protein binding: 99%. Metabolized in the liver to inactive metabolite. Primarily eliminated in feces. Unknown if removed by hemodialysis. **Half-life:** 13 hr.

USES

Treatment of HIV infection in combination with other antiretroviral agents.

PRECAUTIONS

CONTRAINDICATIONS: Concurrent use with ergot medications, lovastatin, midazolam, simvastatin, or triazolam. **CAUTIONS:** Diabetes mellitus, hepatic impairment.

⏳ **LIFESPAN CONSIDERATIONS: Pregnancy/Lactation:** Breast-feeding not recommended (possibility of HIV transmission). **Pregnancy Category B. Children:** Safety and efficacy not established. **Elderly:** Information not available.

INTERACTIONS

DRUG: Calcium channel blockers, clindamycin, dapsone, quinidine, triazolam: May increase the plasma concentrations of these drugs. **Carbamazepine, dexamethasone, phenobarbital, phenytoin, rifampin:** May reduce saquinavir plasma concentration. **Ketoconazole:** Increases saquinavir plasma concentration. **HERBAL: Garlic, St. John's wort:** May decrease the plasma concentration and effect of saquinavir. **FOOD: Grapefruit, grapefruit juice:** May increase saquinavir plasma concentration. **LAB VALUES:** May alter serum creatine kinase (CK) levels, elevate liver function test results, and lower blood glucose levels.

AVAILABILITY (Rx)

CAPSULES (INVIRASE): 200 mg. **TABLETS (INVIRASE):** 500 mg.

ADMINISTRATION/HANDLING

PO
• Give within 2 hr after a full meal (if taken without food in stomach, may result in no antiviral activity).

INDICATIONS/ROUTES/DOSAGE

HIV INFECTION IN COMBINATION WITH OTHER ANTIRETROVIRALS
PO: ADULTS, ELDERLY: 1,000 mg (5 × 200 mg or 2 × 500 mg) twice a day in combination with ritonavir 100 mg twice a day.

DOSAGE ADJUSTMENTS WHEN GIVEN IN COMBINATION THERAPY
Delavirdine: Fortovase 800 mg 3 times a day.
Lopinavir/ritonavir: Fortovase 800 mg twice a day.
Nelfinavir: Fortovase 800 mg 3 times a day or 1,200 mg twice a day.
Ritonavir: Fortovase or Invirase 1,000 mg twice a day.

SIDE EFFECTS

OCCASIONAL: Diarrhea, abdominal discomfort and pain, nausea, photosensitivity, stomatitis. **RARE:** Confusion, ataxia, asthenia, headache, rash.

✐ see color pill atlas   ✒ herb   <u>underlined</u> – top prescribed drug

ADVERSE REACTIONS/ TOXIC EFFECTS

Ketoacidosis occurs rarely.

BASELINE ASSESSMENT

Obtain baseline laboratory testing, especially liver function tests, before beginning saquinavir therapy and at periodic intervals during therapy. Offer emotional support. Obtain medication history.

INTERVENTION/EVALUATION

Monitor serum liver function tests, triglycerides, glucose, CD4 cell count, HIV RNA levels. Closely monitor for evidence of GI discomfort. Monitor pattern of bowel activity and stool consistency. Inspect mouth for signs of mucosal ulceration. Monitor serum chemistry tests for marked laboratory abnormalities. If serious or severe toxicities occur, interrupt therapy, contact physician.

PATIENT/FAMILY TEACHING

• Report persistent abdominal pain, nausea, vomiting. • Avoid exposure to sunlight, artificial light sources. • Continue therapy for full length of treatment. • Doses should be evenly spaced. • Saquinavir is not a cure for HIV infection, nor does it reduce risk of transmission to others. • Patients may continue to acquire illnesses associated with advanced HIV infection. • Take within 2 hr after a full meal. • Avoid coadministration with grapefruit products.

sargramostim (granulocyte macrophage colony-stimulating factor, GM-CSF)

sar-gra-**moh**-stim
(Leukine)
Do not confuse Leukine with Leukeran.

CLASSIFICATION

PHARMACOTHERAPEUTIC: Colony-stimulating factor. **CLINICAL:** Hematopoietic, antineutropenic.

ACTION

A colony-stimulating factor that stimulates proliferation and differentiation of hematopoietic cells to activate mature granulocytes and macrophages. **Therapeutic Effect:** Assists bone marrow in making new WBCs and increases their chemotactic, antifungal, and antiparasitic activity. Increases cytoneoplastic cells and activates neutrophils to inhibit tumor cell growth.

PHARMACOKINETICS

Effect	Onset	Peak	Duration
Increase WBCs	7–14 days	N/A	1 wk

Detected in serum within 5 min after subcutaneous administration. **Half-life:** IV, 1 hr; subcutaneous, 3 hr.

USES

Accelerates myeloid recovery in patients undergoing autologous or allogeneic bone marrow transplant or in patients who have undergone hematopoietic stem cell transplant following myeloablative chemotherapy. Prolongs survival in patients following bone marrow transplant in whom engraftment has been delayed or has failed. Enhances peripheral progenitor cell yield in autologous hematopoietic stem cell transplant. OFF-LABEL: Treatment of AIDS-related neutropenia; chronic, severe neutropenia; drug-induced neutropenia; myelodysplastic syndrome.

PRECAUTIONS

CONTRAINDICATIONS: 12 hr before or after radiation therapy; 24 hr before or after chemotherapy; excessive leukemic myeloid blasts in bone marrow or peripheral blood (greater than 10%); known hypersensitivity to yeast-derived products. **CAUTIONS:** Preexisting cardiac disease, hypoxia, preexisting fluid retention, pulmonary infiltrates, CHF, renal or hepatic impairment.

LIFESPAN CONSIDERATIONS: Pregnancy/Lactation: Unknown if drug crosses placenta or is distributed in breast milk. **Pregnancy Category C. Children:** Safety and efficacy not established. **Elderly:** No age-related precautions noted.

INTERACTIONS

DRUG: Lithium, steroids: May increase the effects of sargramostim. **HERBAL:** None known. **FOOD:** None known. **LAB VALUES:** May increase serum bilirubin, creatinine, and hepatic enzyme levels. May decrease serum albumin level.

AVAILABILITY (Rx)

INJECTION SOLUTION: 500 mcg/ml. **INJECTION POWDER FOR RECONSTITUTION:** 250 mcg.

ADMINISTRATION/HANDLING

IV

Reconstitution • To 250 mcg/500 mcg vial, add 1 ml sterile water for injection (preservative free). • Direct sterile water for injection to side of vial, gently swirl contents to avoid foaming; do not shake or vigorously agitate. • After reconstitution, further dilute with 0.9% NaCl. If final concentration less than 10 mcg/ml, add 1 mg albumin/ml 0.9% NaCl to provide a final albumin concentration of 0.1%.

◄ **ALERT** ▶ Albumin is added before addition of sargramostim (prevents drug adsorption to components of drug delivery system).

Rate of administration • Give each single dose over 2, 4, or 24 hr as directed by physician.

Storage • Refrigerate powder, reconstituted solution, diluted solution for injection. • Do not shake. • Do not use past expiration date. • Reconstituted solutions are clear, colorless. • Use within 6 hr; discard unused portions. • Use 1 dose per vial; do not reenter vial.

INDICATIONS/ROUTES/DOSAGE

MYELOID RECOVERY FOLLOWING BONE MARROW TRANSPLANT (BMT)

IV INFUSION: ADULTS, ELDERLY: Usual parenteral dosage: 250 mcg/m²/day for 21 days (as 2-hr infusion). Begin 2–4 hr after autologous bone marrow infusion and not less than 24 hr after last dose of chemotherapy or not less than 12 hr after last radiation treatment. Discontinue if blast cells appear or underlying disease progresses.

BONE MARROW TRANSPLANT FAILURE, ENGRAFTMENT DELAY

IV INFUSION: ADULTS, ELDERLY: 250 mcg/m²/day for 14 days. Infuse over 2 hr. May repeat after 7 days off therapy if engraftment has not occurred with 500 mcg/m²/day for 14 days.

STEM CELL TRANSPLANT

IV, SUBCUTANEOUS: ADULTS: 250 mcg/m²/day.

▦ IV INCOMPATIBILITIES

Amphotericin B complex (Abelcet, AmBisome, Amphotec), hydromorphone

(Dilaudid), lorazepam (Ativan), morphine.

IV COMPATIBILITIES

Calcium gluconate, dopamine (Intropin), heparin, magnesium, potassium chloride.

SIDE EFFECTS

FREQUENT: GI disturbances, including nausea, diarrhea, vomiting, stomatitis, anorexia, and abdominal pain; arthralgia or myalgia; headache; malaise; rash; pruritus. **OCCASIONAL:** Peripheral edema, weight gain, dyspnea, asthenia, fever, leukocytosis, capillary leak syndrome (such as fluid retention, irritation at local injection site, and peripheral edema). **RARE:** Rapid or irregular heartbeat, thrombophlebitis.

ADVERSE REACTIONS/ TOXIC EFFECTS

Pleural or pericardial effusion occurs rarely after infusion.

NURSING CONSIDERATIONS

BASELINE ASSESSMENT

Monitor for supraventricular arrhythmias during administration (particularly in patients with history of cardiac arrhythmias). Assess closely for dyspnea during and immediately following infusion (particularly in patients with history of lung disease). If dyspnea occurs during infusion, cut infusion rate by half. If dyspnea continues, stop infusion immediately. If neutrophil count exceeds 20,000 cells/mm^3 or platelet count exceeds 500,000/mm^3, stop infusion or reduce dose by half, based on clinical condition of patient. Blood counts return to normal or baseline 3–7 days after discontinuation of therapy.

INTERVENTION/EVALUATION

Monitor CBC with differential, platelets, serum renal and liver function, pulmonary function, vital signs, weight.

saw palmetto

Also known as American dwarf palm tree, cabbage palm, sabal, zuzhong.

◆CLASSIFICATION

HERBAL: See Appendix G.

ACTION

Appears to inhibit 5-alpha-reductase and prevent conversion of testosterone to dihydrotestosterone (DHT). **Effect:** Reduces prostate growth. Contains antiandrogenic, antiproliferative, antiinflammatory properties.

USES

Symptoms of benign prostate hyperplasia (BPH). Also used as a mild diuretic, sedative, anti-inflammatory agent, antiseptic.

PRECAUTIONS

CONTRAINDICATIONS: Pregnancy, lactation due to antiandrogenic and estrogenic activity. **CAUTIONS:** None known.
⧖ **LIFESPAN CONSIDERATIONS: Pregnancy/Lactation:** Contraindicated. **Children:** Safety and efficacy not established. **Elderly:** No age-related precautions noted.

INTERACTIONS

DRUG: Oral contraceptives, hormone therapy: Saw palmetto may interfere with the effects of these drugs. **HERBAL:** None known. **FOOD:** None known. **LAB VALUES:** None known.

AVAILABILITY (OTC)

CAPSULES: 80 mg, 160 mg, 500 mg. **BERRIES. FLUID EXTRACT. TEA.**

INDICATIONS/ROUTES/DOSAGE

BPH
PO: ADULTS, ELDERLY: 160 mg twice a day

or 320 mg once a day using a liquid extract or 1–2 g of whole berries.

DIURETIC, SEDATIVE, ANTI-INFLAMMATORY, ANTISEPTIC

PO: ADULTS, ELDERLY: 0.6–1.5 ml liquid extract or 0.5–1 g dried berries 3 times a day.

SIDE EFFECTS

Mild anorexia, dizziness, nausea, vomiting, constipation, diarrhea, headache, impotence, hypersensitivity reactions, back pain.

ADVERSE REACTIONS/ TOXIC EFFECTS

None known.

NURSING CONSIDERATIONS

BASELINE ASSESSMENT

Determine use of oral contraceptives, hormone replacement therapy (may interfere). Assess patient's urinary patterns. Obtain a prostate-specific antigen (PSA) level before using.

INTERVENTION/EVALUATION

Assess for hypersensitivity reactions. Monitor symptoms of BHP (e.g., frequent/painful urination, hesitancy, urgency). Observe for decreased nocturia, improved urinary flow, decreased residual urine volume.

PATIENT/FAMILY TEACHING

• Should be taken with food.

scopolamine

skoe-**pol**-a-meen

(Trans-Derm Scop, Transderm-V 🍁)

FIXED-COMBINATION(S)

Donnatal: scopolamine/atropine (anticholinergic)/hyoscyamine (anticholinergic)/phenobarbital (sedative): 0.0065 mg/0.0194 mg/0.1037 mg/16.2 mg.

◆ CLASSIFICATION

PHARMACOTHERAPEUTIC: Anticholinergic. **CLINICAL:** Antinausea, antiemetic.

ACTION

An anticholinergic that reduces excitability of labyrinthine receptors, depressing conduction in the vestibular cerebellar pathway. **Therapeutic Effect:** Prevents motion-induced nausea and vomiting.

USES

Prevention of motion sickness, postop nausea, vomiting.

PRECAUTIONS

CONTRAINDICATIONS: Angle-closure glaucoma, GI or GU obstruction, myasthenia gravis, paralytic ileus, tachycardia, thyrotoxicosis. **CAUTIONS:** Hepatic or renal impairment, cardiac disease, seizures, psychoses.

⧖ **LIFESPAN CONSIDERATIONS: Pregnancy/Lactation:** Crosses placenta; unknown if distributed in breast milk. **Pregnancy Category C. Children:** Safety and efficacy not established. **Elderly:** Dizziness, hallucinations, confusion may require dosage adjustment.

INTERACTIONS

DRUG: Antihistamines, tricyclic antidepressants: May increase the anticholinergic effects of scopolamine. **CNS depressants:** May increase CNS depression. **HERBAL:** None known. **FOOD:** None known. **LAB VALUES:** May interfere with gastric secretion test.

AVAILABILITY (Rx)

TRANSDERMAL SYSTEM (TRANS-DERM SCOP): 1.5 mg.

ADMINISTRATION/HANDLING

TRANSDERMAL
• Apply patch to hairless area behind one ear. • If dislodged or on for more than 72 hr, replace with fresh patch.

INDICATIONS/ROUTES/DOSAGE

PREVENTION OF MOTION SICKNESS
TRANSDERMAL: ADULTS: 1 system q72h.

POSTOP NAUSEA OR VOMITING
TRANSDERMAL: ADULTS, ELDERLY: 1 system no sooner than 1 hr before surgery and removed 24 hr after surgery.

SIDE EFFECTS

FREQUENT (greater than 15%): Dry mouth, somnolence, blurred vision. **RARE (5%–1%):** Dizziness, restlessness, hallucinations, confusion, difficulty urinating, rash.

ADVERSE REACTIONS/ TOXIC EFFECTS

None known.

NURSING CONSIDERATIONS

BASELINE ASSESSMENT
Assess for use of other CNS depressants, drugs with anticholinergic action, history of narrow-angle glaucoma.

INTERVENTION/EVALUATION
Monitor serum hepatic and renal function.

PATIENT/FAMILY TEACHING
• Avoid tasks requiring alertness, motor skills until response to drug is established (may cause drowsiness, disorientation, confusion). • Teach proper application of patch. • Use only 1 patch at a time; do not cut. • Wash hands after administration.

secobarbital sodium

(Seconal)
See Sedative-hypnotics

selegiline hydrochloride

sell-**eh**-geh-leen
(Apo-Selegiline ✦, Eldepryl, Emsam, Novo-Selegiline ✦)
Do not confuse selegiline with Stelazine, or Eldepryl with enalapril.

◆ CLASSIFICATION
CLINICAL: Antiparkinson agent.

ACTION

An antiparkinson agent that irreversibly inhibits the activity of monoamine oxidase type B, the enzyme that breaks down dopamine, thereby increasing dopaminergic action. **Therapeutic Effect:** Relieves signs and symptoms of Parkinson's disease.

PHARMACOKINETICS

Rapidly absorbed from the GI tract. Crosses the blood-brain barrier. Metabolized in the liver to the active metabolites. Primarily excreted in urine. **Half-life:** 17 hr (amphetamine), 20 hr (methamphetamine).

USES

Adjunct to levodopa/carbidopa in treatment of Parkinson's disease. **Transdermal:** Treatment of major depressive disorder (MDD). **OFF-LABEL:** Treatment of Alzheimer's disease, attention deficit hyperactivity disorder, depression, early Parkinson's disease, extrapyramidal symptoms, negative symptoms of schizophrenia.

PRECAUTIONS

CONTRAINDICATIONS: Concurrent use with meperidine. **CAUTIONS:** History of peptic ulcer disease, dementia, psychosis, tardive dyskinesia, profound tremor, cardiac dysrhythmias.

S

⧖ **LIFESPAN CONSIDERATIONS:** Pregnancy/Lactation: Unknown if drug crosses placenta or is distributed in breast milk. **Pregnancy Category C. Children:** Safety and efficacy not established. **Elderly:** No age-related precautions noted.

INTERACTIONS

DRUG: Fluoxetine: May cause serotonin syndrome. **Meperidine:** May cause a diaphoresis, excitation, hypertension or hypotension, coma, and even death. **HERBAL:** None known. **FOOD: Caffeine, tyramine-rich foods:** Large amounts of these substances may produce a severe hypertensive reaction. **LAB VALUES:** None known.

AVAILABILITY (Rx)

CAPSULES: 5 mg. **TABLETS:** 5 mg. **TRANSDERMAL:** 6 mg/24 hr, 9 mg/24 hr, 12 mg/24 hr.

ADMINISTRATION/HANDLING

PO
• Give without regard to meals. • Avoid tyramine-containing foods, large quantities of caffeine-containing beverages.

TRANSDERMAL
• Apply to dry, intact skin on upper torso or thigh, or outer surface of upper arm.

INDICATIONS/ROUTES/DOSAGE

ADJUNCTIVE TREATMENT FOR PARKINSONISM
PO: ADULTS: 10 mg/day in divided doses, such as 5 mg at breakfast and lunch, given concomitantly with each dose of carbidopa and levodopa. ELDERLY: Initially, 5 mg in the morning. May increase up to 10 mg/day.

TRANSDERMAL: ADULTS, ELDERLY: Initially, 6 mg/24 hr. May increase in 3 mg/24 hr increments at minimum of 2 wk. **Maximum:** 12 mg/24 hr.

SIDE EFFECTS

FREQUENT (10%–4%): Nausea, dizziness, light-headedness, syncope, abdominal discomfort. **OCCASIONAL (3%–2%):** Confusion, hallucinations, dry mouth, vivid dreams, dyskinesia. **RARE (1%):** Headache, myalgia, anxiety, diarrhea, insomnia.

ADVERSE REACTIONS/ TOXIC EFFECTS

Symptoms of overdose may vary from CNS depression, characterized by sedation, apnea, cardiovascular collapse, and death, to severe paradoxical reactions, such as hallucinations, tremor, and seizures. Other serious effects may include involuntary movements, impaired motor coordination, loss of balance, blepharospasm, facial grimaces, feeling of heaviness in the lower extremities, depression, nightmares, delusions, overstimulation, sleep disturbance, and anger.

NURSING CONSIDERATIONS

INTERVENTION/EVALUATION
Be alert to neurologic effects (headache, lethargy, mental confusion, agitation). Monitor for evidence of dyskinesia (difficulty with movement). Assess for clinical reversal of symptoms (improvement of tremors of head and hands at rest, mask-like facial expression, shuffling gait, muscular rigidity).

PATIENT/FAMILY TEACHING
• Tolerance to feeling of lightheadedness develops during therapy. • To reduce hypotensive effect, rise slowly from lying to sitting position, permit legs to dangle momentarily before standing. • Avoid tasks that require alertness, motor skills until response to drug is established. • Dry mouth, drowsiness, dizziness may be an expected response of drug. • Avoid alcohol during therapy. • Coffee or tea may help reduce drowsiness.

✎ see color pill atlas   ⬎ herb   underlined – top prescribed drug

senna

sen-na

(Ex-Lax, Senexon, Senna-Gen, Sennatural, Senokot, X-Prep)

FIXED-COMBINATION(S)

Gentlax-S, Senokot-S: senna/docusate (a laxative): 8.6 mg/50 mg.

◆CLASSIFICATION

PHARMACOTHERAPEUTIC: GI stimulant. **CLINICAL:** Laxative (see p. 110C).

ACTION

A GI stimulant that has a direct effect on intestinal smooth musculature by stimulating the intramural nerve plexi. **Therapeutic Effect:** Increases peristalsis and promotes laxative effect.

PHARMACOKINETICS

Route	Onset	Peak	Duration
PO	6–12 hr	N/A	N/A
Rectal	0.5–2 hr	N/A	N/A

Minimal absorption after oral administration. Hydrolyzed to active form by enzymes of colonic flora. Absorbed drug metabolized in the liver. Eliminated in feces via biliary system.

USES

Short-term use in constipation, to evacuate the colon before bowel or rectal examinations.

PRECAUTIONS

CONTRAINDICATIONS: Abdominal pain, appendicitis, intestinal obstruction, nausea, vomiting. **CAUTIONS:** Prolonged use (longer than 1 wk).

⧗ **LIFESPAN CONSIDERATIONS: Pregnancy/Lactation:** Unknown if distributed in breast milk. **Pregnancy Category C. Children:** Safety and efficacy not established in those younger than 6 yr. **Elderly:** No age-related precautions noted; monitor for signs of dehydration and electrolyte loss.

INTERACTIONS

DRUG: Oral medications: May decrease transit time of concurrently administered oral medications, decreasing absorption of senna. **HERBAL:** None known. **FOOD:** None known. **LAB VALUES:** May increase blood glucose level. May decrease serum potassium level.

AVAILABILITY (OTC)

GRANULES (SENOKOT): 15 mg/tsp. **LIQUID (X-PREP):** 8.8 mg/5 ml. **SYRUP (SENOKOT):** 8.8 mg/5 ml. **TABLETS (SENNATURAL, SENOKOT, SENEXON, SENNA-GEN):** 8.6 mg, 15 mg. **TABLETS (EX-LAX):** 15 mg, 90 mg.

ADMINISTRATION/HANDLING

PO

• Give on an empty stomach (decreases time to effect). • Offer at least 6–8 glasses of water a day (aids stool softening). • Avoid giving within 1 hr of other oral medication (decreases drug absorption).

INDICATIONS/ROUTES/DOSAGE

CONSTIPATION

PO (TABLETS): ADULTS, ELDERLY, CHILDREN 12 YR AND OLDER: 2 tablets at bedtime. **Maximum:** 4 tablets twice a day. CHILDREN 6–11 YR: 1 tablet at bedtime. **Maximum:** 2 tablets twice a day. CHILDREN 2–5 YR: $\frac{1}{2}$ tablet at bedtime. **Maximum:** 1 tablet twice a day.

PO (SYRUP): ADULTS, ELDERLY, CHILDREN 12 YR AND OLDER: 10–15 ml at bedtime. **Maximum:** 15 ml twice a day. CHILDREN 6–11 YR: 5–7.5 ml at bedtime. **Maximum:** 7.5 ml twice a day. CHILDREN 2–5 YR: 2.5–3.75 ml at bedtime. **Maximum:** 3.75 ml twice a day.

PO (GRANULES): ADULTS, ELDERLY, CHILDREN 12 YR AND OLDER: 1 tsp at bedtime. **Maximum:** 2 tsp twice a day. CHILDREN

S

6–11 YR: ½ teaspoon at bedtime up to 1 teaspoon 2 times/day. CHILDREN 2–5 YR: ¼ teaspoon at bedtime up to ½ teaspoon 2 times/day.

BOWEL EVACUATION

PO: ADULTS, ELDERLY, CHILDREN OLDER THAN 1 YR: 75 ml between 2 PM and 4 PM on day prior to procedure.

SIDE EFFECTS

FREQUENT: Pink-red, red-violet, red-brown, or yellow-brown discoloration of urine. **OCCASIONAL:** Some degree of abdominal discomfort, nausea, mild cramps, griping, faintness.

ADVERSE REACTIONS/ TOXIC EFFECTS

Long-term use may result in laxative dependence, chronic constipation, and loss of normal bowel function. Prolonged use or overdose may result in electrolyte and metabolic disturbances (such as hypokalemia, hypocalcemia, and metabolic acidosis or alkalosis), vomiting, muscle weakness, persistent diarrhea, malabsorption, and weight loss.

NURSING CONSIDERATIONS

INTERVENTION/EVALUATION

Encourage adequate fluid intake. Assess bowel sounds for peristalsis. Monitor pattern of bowel activity and stool consistency. Assess for GI disturbances. Monitor serum electrolytes in patients exposed to prolonged, frequent, excessive use of medication.

PATIENT/FAMILY TEACHING

• Urine may turn pink-red, red-violet, red-brown, yellow-brown (only temporary and not harmful). • Institute measures to promote defecation (increase fluid intake, exercise, high-fiber diet). • Laxative effect generally occurs in 6–12 hr but may take 24 hr. • Do not take other oral medication within 1 hr of taking this medicine (decreased effectiveness).

Sensipar, *see cinacalcet*

Septra, *see co-trimoxazole*

Serevent Diskus, *see salmeterol*

Seroquel, *see quetiapine*

---

sertraline hydrochloride

sir-trah-leen

(Apo-Sertraline ✦, Novo-Sertraline ✦, PMS-Sertraline ✦, <u>Zoloft</u>)

Do not confuse sertraline with Serentil.

◆ CLASSIFICATION

PHARMACOTHERAPEUTIC: Serotonin reuptake inhibitor. **CLINICAL:** Antidepressant, anxiolytic, obsessive-compulsive disorder adjunct (see p. 38C).

ACTION

An antidepressant, anxiolytic, and obsessive-compulsive disorder adjunct that blocks the reuptake of the neurotransmitter serotonin at CNS neuronal presynaptic membranes, increasing its availability at postsynaptic receptor sites. Therapeutic Effect: Relieves depression, reduces obsessive-compulsive behavior, decreases anxiety.

PHARMACOKINETICS

Incompletely and slowly absorbed from the GI tract; food increases absorption. Protein binding: 98%. Widely distributed. Undergoes extensive first-pass metabolism in the liver to active compound. Excreted in urine and feces. Not removed by hemodialysis. **Half-life:** 26 hr.

USES

Treatment of major depressive disorders, panic disorder, obsessive-compulsive disorder (OCD), post-traumatic stress disorder (PTSD), premenstrual dysphoric disorder (PMDD), social anxiety disorder. **OFF-LABEL:** Eating disorders, generalized anxiety disorder (GAD), impulse control disorders.

PRECAUTIONS

CONTRAINDICATIONS: User within 14 days of MAOIs. **CAUTIONS:** Seizure disorders, cardiac disease, recent MI, hepatic impairment, suicidal patients.

⧖ LIFESPAN CONSIDERATIONS: **Pregnancy/Lactation:** Unknown if drug crosses placenta or is distributed in breast milk. **Pregnancy Category B. Children:** Children and adolescents are at an increased risk of suicidal ideation and behavior or worsening of depression, especially during the first few months of therapy. **Elderly:** No age-related precautions noted, but lower initial dosages recommended.

INTERACTIONS

DRUG: **Highly protein-bound medications (such as, digoxin and warfarin):** May increase the blood concentration and risk of toxicity of these drugs. **MAOIs:** May cause neuroleptic malignant syndrome, hypertensive crisis, hyperpyrexia, seizures, and serotonin syndrome (marked by diaphoresis, diarrhea, fever, mental changes, restlessness, and shivering). **HERBAL:** **St. John's wort:** May increase the risk of adverse effects. **FOOD:** None known.

LAB VALUES: May increase serum total cholesterol, triglyceride, AST, and ALT levels. May decrease serum uric acid level.

AVAILABILITY (Rx)

ORAL CONCENTRATE: 20 mg/ml. **TABLETS:** 25 mg, 50 mg, 100 mg.

ADMINISTRATION/HANDLING

PO
• Give with food, milk if GI distress occurs.

INDICATIONS/ROUTES/DOSAGE

DEPRESSION
PO: ADULTS: Initially, 50 mg/day. May increase by 50 mg/day at 7-day intervals up to 200 mg/day. ELDERLY: Initially, 25 mg/day. May increase by 25–50 mg/day at 7-day intervals up to 200 mg/day.

OCD
PO: ADULTS, CHILDREN 13–17 YR: Initially, 50 mg/day with morning or evening meal. May increase by 50 mg/day at 7-day intervals. ELDERLY, CHILDREN 6–12 YR: Initially, 25 mg/day. May increase by 25–50 mg/day at 7-day intervals. **Maximum:** 200 mg/day.

PANIC DISORDER, PTSD, SOCIAL ANXIETY DISORDER
PO: ADULTS, ELDERLY: Initially, 25 mg/day. May increase by 50 mg/day at 7-day intervals. Range: 50–200 mg/day. **Maximum:** 200 mg/day.

PREMENSTRUAL DYSPHORIC DISORDER
PO: ADULTS: Initially, 50 mg/day. May increase up to 150 mg/day in 50-mg increments.

SIDE EFFECTS

FREQUENT (26%–12%): Headache, nausea, diarrhea, insomnia, somnolence, dizziness, fatigue, rash, dry mouth. **OCCASIONAL (6%–4%):** Anxiety, nervousness, agitation, tremor, dyspepsia, diaphoresis, vomiting, constipation, abnormal ejaculation, visual disturbances, altered taste. **RARE (less than 3%):** Flatulence, urinary frequency, paraesthesia, hot flashes, chills.

ADVERSE REACTIONS/ TOXIC EFFECTS

None known.

NURSING CONSIDERATIONS

BASELINE ASSESSMENT

For those on long-term therapy, serum liver/renal function tests, blood counts should be performed periodically.

INTERVENTION/EVALUATION

Supervise suicidal-risk patients, especially children and adolescents, closely during early therapy (as depression lessens, energy level improves, increasing suicide potential). Assess appearance, behavior, speech pattern, level of interest, mood. Monitor pattern of daily bowel activity/stool consistency. Assist with ambulation if dizziness occurs.

PATIENT/FAMILY TEACHING

• Dry mouth may be relieved by sugarless gum, sips of tepid water. • Report headache, fatigue, tremor, sexual dysfunction. • Avoid tasks that require alertness, motor skills until response to drug is established (may cause dizziness, drowsiness). • Take with food if nausea occurs. • Inform physician if pregnancy occurs. • Avoid alcohol. • Do not take OTC medications without consulting physician.

sevelamer hydrochloride

seh-**vel**-a-mer

(Renagel)

Do not confuse Renagel with Reglan or Regonol.

⁂CLASSIFICATION

PHARMACOTHERAPEUTIC: Polymeric phosphate binder. **CLINICAL:** Antihyperphosphatemia.

ACTION

An antihyperphosphatemia agent that binds with dietary phosphorus in the GI tract, thus allowing phosphorus to be eliminated through the normal digestive process and decreasing the serum phosphorus level. **Therapeutic Effect:** Decreases incidence of hypercalcemic episodes in patients receiving calcium acetate treatment.

PHARMACOKINETICS

Not absorbed systemically. Unknown if removed by hemodialysis.

USES

Reduction of serum phosphorus in patients with end-stage renal disease (ESRD).

PRECAUTIONS

CONTRAINDICATIONS: Bowel obstruction, hypophosphatemia. **CAUTIONS:** Dysphagia, severe GI tract motility disorders, major GI tract surgery, swallowing disorders.

⌛ **LIFESPAN CONSIDERATIONS: Pregnancy/Lactation:** Not distributed in breast milk. **Pregnancy Category C. Children:** Safety and efficacy not established. **Elderly:** No age-related precautions noted.

INTERACTIONS

DRUG: None known. **HERBAL:** None known. **FOOD:** None known. **LAB VALUES:** None known.

AVAILABILITY (Rx)

CAPSULES: 403 mg. **TABLETS:** 400 mg, 800 mg.

ADMINISTRATION/HANDLING

PO

• Give with meals. • Do not break capsule apart before administration (contents expand in water). • Space other medication by at least 1 hr before or 3 hr after sevelamer.

INDICATIONS/ROUTES/DOSAGE

HYPERPHOSPHATEMIA

PO: ADULTS, ELDERLY: 800–1,600 mg with each meal, depending on severity of hyperphosphatemia.

SIDE EFFECTS

FREQUENT (20%–11%): Infection, pain, hypotension, diarrhea, dyspepsia, nausea, vomiting. **OCCASIONAL (10%–1%):** Headache, constipation, hypertension, thrombosis, increased cough.

ADVERSE REACTIONS/ TOXIC EFFECTS

Thrombosis occurs rarely.

BASELINE ASSESSMENT

Obtain baseline serum phosphorus level; assess for bowel obstruction.

INTERVENTION/EVALUATION

Monitor serum phosphorus, bicarbonate, chloride, calcium levels.

PATIENT/FAMILY TEACHING

• Take with meals, swallow whole. • Report persistent headache, nausea, vomiting, diarrhea, hypotension.

---

sibutramine

sigh-**bew**-trah-meen
(Meridia)

See Obesity management (p. 126C)

---

sildenafil citrate

sill-**den**-a-fill
(Revatio, Viagra)
Do not confuse Viagra with Vaniqa.

◆ CLASSIFICATION

CLINICAL: Erectile dysfunction adjunct.

ACTION

An erectile dysfunction agent that inhibits phosphodiesterase type 5, the enzyme responsible for degrading cyclic guanosine monophosphate in the corpus cavernosum of the penis, pulmonary vascular smooth muscle, resulting in smooth muscle relaxation and increased blood flow. **Therapeutic Effect:** Facilitates an erection, produces pulmonary vasodilation.

USES

Viagra: Treatment of male erectile dysfunction. **Revatio:** Treatment of pulmonary arterial hypertension. **OFF-LABEL:** Treatment of diabetic gastroparesis, sexual dysfunction associated with the use of selective serotonin reuptake inhibitors.

PRECAUTIONS

CONTRAINDICATIONS: Concurrent use of sodium nitroprusside or nitrates in any form. **CAUTIONS:** Renal, cardiac, hepatic impairment; anatomic deformation of the penis; patients who may be predisposed to priapism (sickle cell anemia, multiple myeloma, leukemia). **Pregnancy Category B.**

INTERACTIONS

DRUG: Cimetidine, erythromycin, itraconazole, ketoconazole: May increase sildenafil plasma concentration. **Nitrates:** Potentiates the hypotensive

---

S

effects of nitrates. HERBAL: None known. FOOD: **High-fat meals:** Delay drug's maximum effectiveness by 1 hr. LAB VALUES: None known.

AVAILABILITY (Rx)

TABLETS: 20 mg (Revatio), 25 mg (Viagra), 50 mg (Viagra), 100 mg (Viagra).

ADMINISTRATION/HANDLING

PO
• May take approximately 1 hr before sexual activity but may be taken anywhere from 4 hr–30 min before sexual activity.
• Revatio may be given with or without food.

INDICATIONS/ROUTES/DOSAGE

ERECTILE DYSFUNCTION
PO: ADULTS: 50 mg (30 min–4 hr before sexual activity). Range: 25–100 mg. Maximum dosing frequency is once daily. ELDERLY OLDER THAN 65 YR: Consider starting dose of 25 mg.

PULMONARY ARTERIAL HYPERTENSION
PO: ADULTS, ELDERLY: 20 mg 3 times a day.

SIDE EFFECTS

FREQUENT: Headache (16%), flushing (10%). **OCCASIONAL (7%–3%):** Dyspepsia, nasal congestion, UTI, abnormal vision, diarrhea. **RARE (2%):** Dizziness, rash.

ADVERSE REACTIONS/ TOXIC EFFECTS

Prolonged erections (lasting over 4 hr) and priapism (painful erections lasting over 6 hr) occur rarely.

NURSING CONSIDERATIONS

BASELINE ASSESSMENT
Viagra: Determine if patient has other medical conditions, including angina, cardiac disease, and benign prostatic hypertrophy (BPH). Assess the patient's baseline serum renal/hepatic function. **Revatio:** Obtain baseline ABG's,

pulmonary function, cardiovascular status.

PATIENT/FAMILY TEACHING
• Sildenafil has no effect in the absence of sexual stimulation. • Seek treatment immediately if an erection lasts longer than 4 hr. • Avoid nitrate drugs while taking sildenafil.

silver sulfadiazine

sul-fah-**dye**-ah-zeen
(Demazin ❦, Flamazine ❦, Silvadene, SSD, SSD AF, Thermazene)

◆CLASSIFICATION

PHARMACOTHERAPEUTIC: Anti-infective. **CLINICAL:** Burn preparation.

ACTION

Acts on cell wall/cell membrane in concentrations selectively toxic to bacteria. **Therapeutic Effect:** Produces bactericidal effect.

USES

Prevention, treatment of infection in second- and third-degree burns; protection against conversion from partial- to full-thickness wounds (infection causing extended tissue destruction). OFF-LABEL: Treatment of minor bacterial skin infection, dermal ulcer.

PRECAUTIONS

CONTRAINDICATIONS: None known. **CAUTIONS:** Renal/hepatic impairment, G6PD deficiency, premature neonates, infants younger than 2 mo. **Pregnancy Category B.**

INTERACTIONS

DRUG: **Collagenase, papain, sutilains:** May be inactivated when given concurrently with silver sulfadiazine.

HERBAL: None known. **FOOD:** None known. **LAB VALUES:** None known.

AVAILABILITY (Rx)

TOPICAL CREAM (SILVADENE, SSD, SSD AF, THERMAZENE) 1% (10 mg/g).

ADMINISTRATION/HANDLING

TOPICAL

• Apply to cleansed, debrided burns using sterile glove. • Keep burn areas covered with silver sulfadiazine cream at all times; reapply to areas where removed by patient activity. • Dressings may be ordered on individual basis.

INDICATIONS/ROUTES/DOSAGE

USUAL TOPICAL DOSAGE

TOPICAL: ADULTS, ELDERLY, CHILDREN: Apply 1–2 times a day.

SIDE EFFECTS

Side effects characteristic of all sulfonamides may occur when systemically absorbed, (e.g., extensive burn areas [over 20% of body surface]): anorexia, nausea, vomiting, headache, diarrhea, dizziness, photosensitivity, arthralgia. **FREQUENT:** Burning feeling at treatment site. **OCCASIONAL:** Brown-gray skin discoloration, rash, itching. **RARE:** Increased sensitivity of skin to sunlight.

ADVERSE REACTIONS/ TOXIC EFFECTS

Hemolytic anemia, hypoglycemia, diuresis, peripheral neuropathy, Stevens-Johnson syndrome, agranulocytosis, disseminated lupus erythematosus, anaphylaxis, hepatitis, toxic nephrosis possible with significant systemic absorption. Fungal superinfections may occur. Interstitial nephritis occurs rarely.

NURSING CONSIDERATIONS

BASELINE ASSESSMENT

Determine initial CBC, serum renal/liver function test results.

INTERVENTION/EVALUATION

Monitor serum electrolytes, urinalysis, renal function, CBC if burns are extensive, therapy prolonged.

PATIENT/FAMILY TEACHING

• For external use only; may discolor skin.

simethicone

si-**meth**-i-kone

(Alka-Seltzer Gas Relief, Gas-X, Genasyme, Infant Mylicon, Mylanta Gas, Ovol ✤, Phazyme)

FIXED-COMBINATION(S)

Mylanta, Extra Strength Maalox, Aludrox: simethicone/magnesium and aluminum hydroxide (antacids): 20 mg/200 mg/200 mg; 40 mg/400 mg/400 mg.

◆CLASSIFICATION

CLINICAL: Antiflatulent.

ACTION

An antiflatulent that changes surface tension of gas bubbles, allowing easier elimination of gas. **Therapeutic Effect:** Drug dispersal, prevents formation of gas pockets in the GI tract.

PHARMACOKINETICS

Does not appear to be absorbed from GI tract. Excreted unchanged in feces.

USES

Treatment of flatulence, gastric bloating, postop gas pain, when gas retention may be problem (i.e., peptic ulcer, spastic colon, air swallowing). **OFF-LABEL:** Adjunct to bowel radiography and gastroscopy.

S

PRECAUTIONS

CONTRAINDICATIONS: None   known.
CAUTIONS: None known.

⧗ **LIFESPAN CONSIDERATIONS: Pregnancy/Lactation:** Unknown if drug crosses placenta or is distributed in breast milk. **Pregnancy Category C. Children/Elderly:** None known.

INTERACTIONS

DRUG: None   known.   **HERBAL:** None known.   **FOOD:** None   known.   **LAB VALUES:** None known.

AVAILABILITY (OTC)

ORAL DROPS (INFANT MYLICON): 40 mg/0.6 ml. **SOFTGEL:** 125 mg (Alka-Seltzer Gas Relief, Gas-Z, Mylanta Gas), 180 mg (Phazyme). **TABLETS (CHEWABLE):** 80 mg (Gas-X, Genasyme, Mylanta Gas), 125 mg (Gas-X, Mylanta Gas).

ADMINISTRATION/HANDLING

PO

• Give after meals and at bedtime as needed. • Chewable tablets are to be chewed thoroughly before swallowing. • Shake suspension well before using.

INDICATIONS/ROUTES/DOSAGE

ANTIFLATULENT

PO: ADULTS, ELDERLY, CHILDREN 12 YR AND OLDER: 40–360 mg after meals and at bedtime. **Maximum:** 500 mg/day. CHILDREN 2–11 YR: 40 mg 4 times a day. CHILDREN YOUNGER THAN 2 YR: 20 mg 4 times a day.

SIDE EFFECTS

None known.

ADVERSE REACTIONS/ TOXIC EFFECTS

None known.

NURSING CONSIDERATIONS

INTERVENTION/EVALUATION

Evaluate for therapeutic response: relief of flatulence, abdominal bloating.

PATIENT/FAMILY TEACHING

• Avoid carbonated beverages.

simvastatin

sim-vah-**stay**-tin

(Apo-Simvastatin ✦, <u>Zocor</u>)

Do not confuse Zocor with Cozaar.

FIXED-COMBINATION(S)

Vytorin: simvastatin/ezetimibe (a cholesterol absorption inhibitor): 10 mg/10 mg; 20 mg/10 mg; 40 mg/10 mg; 80 mg/10 mg.

CLASSIFICATION

PHARMACOTHERAPEUTIC: Hydroxymethylglutaryl-CoA (HMG-CoA) reductase inhibitor. **CLINICAL:** Antihyperlipidemic (see p. 53C).

ACTION

A HMG-CoA reductase inhibitor that interferes with cholesterol biosynthesis by inhibiting the conversion of the enzyme HMG-CoA to mevalonate. **Therapeutic Effect:** Decreases serum LDL, cholesterol, VLDL, and plasma triglyceride levels; slightly increases serum HDL concentration.

PHARMACOKINETICS

Well absorbed from the GI tract. Protein binding: 95%. Undergoes extensive first-pass metabolism. Hydrolyzed to active metabolite. Primarily eliminated in feces. Unknown if removed by hemodialysis.

Route	Onset	Peak	Duration
PO to reduce cholesterol	3 days	14 days	N/A

USES

Secondary prevention of cardiovascular events in patients with hypercholesterol and coronary heart disease (CHD) or at high risk for CHD. Hyperlipidemias to reduce elevations in total cholesterol. Treatment of homozygous familial hypercholesterol. Treatment of heterozygous familial hypercholesterol in adolescents (10–17 yr, females more than 1 yr postmenarche).

PRECAUTIONS

CONTRAINDICATIONS: Active hepatic disease or unexplained, persistent elevations of liver function test results, age younger than 18 yr, pregnancy. **CAUTIONS:** History of hepatic disease, substantial alcohol consumption. Withholding or discontinuing simvastatin may be necessary when patient is at risk for renal failure secondary to rhabdomyolysis. Severe metabolic, endocrine, electrolyte disorders.

⌛ **LIFESPAN CONSIDERATIONS: Pregnancy/Lactation:** Contraindicated in pregnancy (suppression of cholesterol biosynthesis may cause fetal toxicity), lactation. Risk of serious adverse reactions in breast-feeding infants. **Pregnancy Category X. Children:** Safety and efficacy not established. **Elderly:** No age-related precautions noted.

INTERACTIONS

DRUG: Cyclosporine, erythromycin, gemfibrozil, immunosuppressants, niacin: Increases the risk of acute renal failure and rhabdomyolysis. **Erythromycin, itraconazole, ketoconazole:** May increase simvastatin blood concentration and cause muscle inflammation, myalgia, or weakness. **HERBAL:** None known. **FOOD: Grapefruit, grapefruit juice:** Large amounts of grapefruit juice may increase the risk of side effects, such as particularly myalgia, and weakness. **LAB VALUES:** May increase serum creatine kinase (CK) and serum transaminase concentrations.

AVAILABILITY (Rx)

TABLETS: 5 mg, 10 mg, 20 mg, 40 mg, 80 mg.

ADMINISTRATION/HANDLING

PO
- Give without regard to meals.
- Administer in evening.

INDICATIONS/ROUTES/DOSAGE

PREVENTION OF CARDIOVASCULAR EVENTS, HYPERLIPIDEMIAS
PO: ADULTS, ELDERLY: 20–40 mg once daily. Range: 5–80 mg/day.

HOMOZYGOUS FAMILIAL HYPERCHOLESTEROL
PO: ADULTS, ELDERLY: 40 mg once daily in evening or 80 mg/day in divided doses.

HETEROZYGOUS FAMILIAL HYPERCHOLESTEROL
PO: CHILDREN 10–17 YR: 10 mg once daily in evening. Range: 10–40 mg/day.

SIDE EFFECTS

Simvastatin is generally well tolerated. Side effects are usually mild and transient. **OCCASIONAL (3%–2%):** Headache, abdominal pain or cramps, constipation, upper respiratory tract infection. **RARE (less than 2%):** Diarrhea, flatulence, asthenia (loss of strength and energy), nausea or vomiting.

ADVERSE REACTIONS/TOXIC EFFECTS

Lens opacities may occur. Hypersensitivity reaction and hepatitis occur rarely. Myopathy manifested as muscle pain, tenderness or weakness with elevated CK sometimes taking the form of rhabdomyolysis fatalities, have occurred.

NURSING CONSIDERATIONS

BASELINE ASSESSMENT

Question for possibility of pregnancy before initiating therapy (Pregnancy

Category X). Question for history of hypersensitivity to simvastatin. Assess baseline lab results: serum cholesterol, triglycerides, liver function tests.

INTERVENTION/EVALUATION

Monitor serum cholesterol, triglyceride lab results for therapeutic response. Monitor liver function tests. Determine pattern of bowel activity and stool consistency. Assess for headache.

PATIENT/FAMILY TEACHING

• Use appropriate contraceptive measures (Pregnancy Category X). • Periodic lab tests are essential part of therapy.

Sinemet, see carbidopa and levodopa

Singulair, see montelukast

---

sirolimus

sigh-row-**lie**-mus
(Rapamune)

CLASSIFICATION

CLINICAL: Immunosuppressant (see p. 107C).

ACTION

An immunosuppressant that inhibits T-lymphocyte proliferation induced by stimulation of cell surface receptors, mitogens, alloantigens, and lymphokines. Prevents activation of the enzyme target of rapamycin, a key regulatory kinase in cell cycle progression. **Therapeutic** **Effect:** Inhibits proliferation of T and B cells, essential components of the immune response; prevents organ transplant rejection.

PHARMACOKINETICS

Rapidly absorbed from the GI tract. Protein binding: 92%. Extensively metabolized in liver. Primarily eliminated in feces; minimal excretion in urine. **Half-life:** 57–63 hr.

USES

Prophylaxis of organ rejection in patients after renal transplant in combination with cyclosporine and corticosteroids. **OFF-LABEL:** Immunosuppression of other organ transplants.

PRECAUTIONS

CONTRAINDICATIONS: Malignancy. **CAUTIONS:** Chickenpox, herpes zoster, hepatic impairment, infection.

⏳ **LIFESPAN CONSIDERATIONS: Pregnancy/Lactation:** Unknown if drug crosses placenta or is distributed in breast milk. **Pregnancy Category C. Children:** Safety and efficacy not established in children younger than 13 yr. **Elderly:** No age-related precautions noted.

INTERACTIONS

DRUG: Cyclosporine, diltiazem, ketoconazole: May increase the blood concentration and risk of toxicity of sirolimus. **Rifampin:** May decrease the blood concentration and effects of sirolimus. **HERBAL:** None known. **FOOD: Grapefruit, grapefruit juice:** May decrease the metabolism of sirolimus. **LAB VALUES:** May decrease blood Hgb level, Hct, and platelet count. May increase serum cholesterol, creatinine, and triglyceride levels.

AVAILABILITY (Rx)

ORAL SOLUTION: 1 mg/ml. **TABLETS:** 1 mg, 2 mg, 5 mg.

✎ see color pill atlas   🌿 herb   <u>underlined</u> – top prescribed drug

INDICATIONS/ROUTES/DOSAGE

PREVENTION OF ORGAN TRANSPLANT REJECTION

PO: ADULTS: Loading dose: 6 mg. Maintenance: 2 mg/day. CHILDREN 13 YR AND OLDER WEIGHING LESS THAN 40 KG: Loading dose: 3 mg/m². Maintenance: 1 mg/m²/day.

SIDE EFFECTS

OCCASIONAL: Hypercholesterolemia, hyperlipidemia, hypertension, rash; with high doses (5 mg/day): anemia, arthralgia, diarrhea, hypokalemia, and thrombocytopenia. **RARE:** Peripheral edema, hypertension.

ADVERSE REACTIONS/ TOXIC EFFECTS

Pancytopenia and hepatotoxicity occur rarely.

NURSING CONSIDERATIONS

BASELINE ASSESSMENT

Obtain baseline serum hepatic profile. Assess for pregnancy, lactation. Question for medication usage (especially cyclosporine, diltiazem, ketoconazole, rifampin). Determine if patient has chickenpox, herpes zoster, malignancy, infection.

INTERVENTION/EVALUATION

Monitor serum hepatic function periodically.

PATIENT/FAMILY TEACHING

• Avoid those with colds, other infections. • Avoid grapefruit juice and grapefruit. • Strict monitoring is essential in identifying and preventing symptoms of organ rejection.

---

sodium bicarbonate

sew-dee-um bye-**car**-bon-ate
(Neut)

CLASSIFICATION

PHARMACOTHERAPEUTIC: Alkalinizing agent. **CLINICAL:** Antacid.

ACTION

An alkalinizing agent that dissociates to provide bicarbonate ion. **Therapeutic Effect:** Neutralizes hydrogen ion concentration, raises blood and urinary pH.

PHARMACOKINETICS

Route	Onset	Peak	Duration
PO	15 min	N/A	1–3 hr
IV	Immediate	N/A	8–10 min

After administration, sodium bicarbonate dissociates to sodium and bicarbonate ions. With increased hydrogen ion concentrations bicarbonate ions combine with hydrogen ions to form carbonic acid, which then dissociates to CO_2, which is excreted by the lungs.

USES

Management of metabolic acidosis, antacid, alkalinization of urine, stabilizes acid-base balance, cardiac arrest, life-threatening hyperkalemia.

PRECAUTIONS

CONTRAINDICATIONS: Excessive chloride loss due to diarrhea, diuretics, GI suctioning, or vomiting; hypocalcemia; metabolic or respiratory alkalosis. **CAUTIONS:** CHF, edematous states, renal insufficiency, patients on corticosteroid therapy.

LIFESPAN CONSIDERATIONS: Pregnancy/Lactation: May produce hypernatremia, increase tendon reflexes in neonate or fetus whose mother is administered chronically high doses. May be distributed in breast milk. **Pregnancy Category C. Children:** No age-related precautions noted. Do not use as antacid in those younger than 6 yr.

S

Elderly: Age-related renal impairment may require dosage adjustment.

INTERACTIONS

DRUG: **Calcium-containing products:** May result in milk-alkali syndrome. **Corticosteroids:** May cause edema and hypertension. **Lithium, salicylates:** May increase the excretion of these drugs. **Methenamine:** May decrease the effects of methenamine. HERBAL: None known. FOOD: **Milk, other dairy products:** May result in milk-alkali syndrome. LAB VALUES: May increase serum and urinary pH.

AVAILABILITY (OTC)

TABLETS: 325 mg, 650 mg. **INJECTION:** 4%, 0.5 mEq/ml (4.2%), 0.6 mEq/ml (5%), 0.9 mEq/ml (7.5%), 1 mEq/ml (8.4%).

ADMINISTRATION/HANDLING

🖃 IV

◀ ALERT ▶ For direct IV administration in neonates or infants, use 0.5 mEq/ml concentration.

Reconstitution • May give undiluted.

Rate of administration • For IV push, give up to 1 mEq/kg over 1–3 min for cardiac arrest. • For IV infusion, do not exceed rate of infusion of 50 mEq/hr. • For children younger than 2 yr, premature infants, neonates, administer by slow infusion, up to 8 mEq/min.

Storage • Store at room temperature. **PO**
• Give 1–3 hr after meals.

▨ IV INCOMPATIBILITIES

Ascorbic acid, diltiazem (Cardizem), dobutamine (Dobutrex), dopamine (Intropin), hydromorphone (Dilaudid), magnesium sulfate, midazolam (Versed), morphine, norepinephrine (Levophed), total parenteral nutrition (TPN).

IV COMPATIBILITIES

Aminophylline, calcium chloride, furosemide (Lasix), heparin, insulin, lidocaine, mannitol, milrinone (Primacor), morphine, phenylephrine (Neo-Synephrine), phenytoin (Dilantin), potassium chloride, propofol (Diprivan), vancomycin (Vancocin).

INDICATIONS/ROUTES/DOSAGE

CARDIAC ARREST
IV: ADULTS, ELDERLY: Initially, 1 mEq/kg (as 7.5%–8.4% solution). May repeat with 0.5 mEq/kg q10min during continued cardiopulmonary arrest. Use in the postresuscitation phase is based on arterial blood pH, partial pressure of carbon dioxide in arterial blood ($PaCO_2$) and base deficit calculation. CHILDREN, INFANTS: Initially, 1 mEq/kg.

METABOLIC ACIDOSIS (NOT SEVERE)
IV: ADULTS, ELDERLY, CHILDREN: 2–5 mEq/kg over 4–8 hr. May repeat based on laboratory values.

METABOLIC ACIDOSIS (ASSOCIATED WITH CHRONIC RENAL FAILURE)
PO: ADULTS, ELDERLY: Initially, 20–36 mEq/ day in divided doses.

RENAL TUBULAR ACIDOSIS (DISTAL)
PO: ADULTS, ELDERLY: 0.5–2 mEq/kg/day in 4–6 divided doses. CHILDREN: 2–3 mEq/ kg/day in divided doses.

RENAL TUBULAR ACIDOSIS (PROXIMAL)
PO: ADULTS, ELDERLY, CHILDREN: 5–10 mEq/ kg/day in divided doses.

URINE ALKALINIZATION
PO: ADULTS, ELDERLY: Initially, 4 g, then 1–2 g q4h. **Maximum:** 16 g/day. CHILDREN: 84–840 mg/kg/day in divided doses.

ANTACID
PO: ADULTS, ELDERLY: 300 mg–2 g 1–4 times a day.

HYPERKALEMIA
IV: ADULTS, ELDERLY: 1 mEq/kg over 5 min.

SIDE EFFECTS

FREQUENT: Abdominal distention, flatulence, belching.

ADVERSE REACTIONS/ TOXIC EFFECTS

Excessive or chronic use may produce metabolic alkalosis (characterized by irritability, twitching, paraesthesias, cyanosis, slow or shallow respirations, headache, thirst, and nausea). Fluid overload results in headache, weakness, blurred vision, behavioral changes, incoordination, muscle twitching, elevated BP, bradycardia, tachypnea, wheezing, coughing, and distended neck veins. Extravasation may occur at the IV site, resulting in tissue necrosis and ulceration.

NURSING CONSIDERATIONS

BASELINE ASSESSMENT

Do not give other PO medication within 1–2 hr of antacid administration.

INTERVENTION/EVALUATION

Monitor blood and urine pH, CO_2 level, serum electrolytes, plasma bicarbonate levels. Watch for signs of metabolic alkalosis, fluid overload. Assess for clinical improvement of metabolic acidosis (relief from hyperventilation, weakness, disorientation). Assess pattern of daily bowel activity and stool consistency. Monitor serum phosphate, calcium, uric acid levels. Assess for relief of gastric distress.

---

sodium chloride ▷

sew-dee-um **klor**-eyed

(Muro 128, Nasal Mist, Nasal Moist, Ocean, SalineX, SeaMist, Slo-Salt)

◆ CLASSIFICATION

CLINICAL: Electrolyte, ophthalmic adjunct, bronchodilator.

ACTION

Sodium is a major cation of extracellular fluid that controls water distribution, fluid and electrolyte balance, and osmotic pressure of body fluids; it also maintains acid-base balance.

PHARMACOKINETICS

Well absorbed from the GI tract. Widely distributed. Primarily excreted in urine.

USES

Parenteral: Source of hydration; prevention and treatment of sodium and chloride deficiencies (hypertonic for severe deficiencies). Prevention of muscle cramps and heat prostration occurring with excessive perspiration. **Nasal:** Restores moisture, relieves dry or inflamed nasal membranes. **Ophthalmic:** Therapy in reduction corneal edema, diagnostic aid in ophthalmoscopic exam.

PRECAUTIONS

CONTRAINDICATIONS: Fluid retention, hypernatremia. **CAUTIONS:** CHF, renal impairment, cirrhosis, hypertension. Do not use sodium chloride preserved with benzyl alcohol in neonates.

⧗ **LIFESPAN CONSIDERATIONS: Pregnancy Category C. Children/Elderly:** No age-related precautions noted.

INTERACTIONS

DRUG: Hypertonic saline solution, oxytocics: May cause uterine hypertonus, ruptures, or lacerations. **HERBAL:** None known. **FOOD:** None known. **LAB VALUES:** None known.

AVAILABILITY

TABLETS (OTC): 1 g. **INJECTION (CONCENTRATE):** 23.4% (4 mEq/ml). **INJECTION:** 0.45%, 0.9%, 3%. **IRRIGATION:** 0.45%, 0.9%. **NASAL GEL (NASAL MOIST):** 0.65%. **NASAL**

SOLUTION (OTC): 0.4% (SalineX), 0.65% (Nasal Moist, SeaMist). **OPHTHALMIC SOLUTION (OTC [MURO 128]):** 5%. **OPHTHALMIC OINTMENT (OTC [MURO 128]):** 5%.

ADMINISTRATION/HANDLING

IV

• Hypertonic solutions (3% or 5%) are administered via large vein; avoid infiltration; do not exceed 100 ml/hr. • Vials containing 2.5–4 mEq/ml (concentrated NaCl) must be diluted with D_5W or $D_{10}W$ before administration.

PO

• Do not crush or break enteric-coated or extended-release tablets. • Administer with full glass of water.

NASAL

• Instruct patient to begin inhaling slowly just before releasing medication into nose. • Inhale slowly, then release air gently through mouth. • Continue technique for 20–30 sec.

OPHTHALMIC

• Place finger on lower eyelid, pull out until pocket is formed between eye and lower lid. • Hold dropper above pocket, place prescribed number of drops (or apply thin strip of ointment) in pocket. • Instruct patient to close eyes gently so that medication will not be squeezed out of sac. • When lower lid is released, have patient keep eye open without blinking for at least 30 sec for solution; for ointment have patient close eye, roll eyeball around to distribute medication. • When using drops, apply gentle finger pressure to lacrimal sac (bridge of the nose, inside corner of the eye) for 1–2 min after administration of solution (reduces systemic absorption).

INDICATIONS/ROUTES/DOSAGE

PREVENTION AND TREATMENT OF SODIUM AND CHLORIDE DEFICIENCIES; SOURCE OF HYDRATION

IV: ADULTS, ELDERLY: 1–2 L/day 0.9% or 0.45% or 100 ml 3% or 5% over 1 hr; assess serum electrolyte levels before giving additional fluid.

PREVENTION OF HEAT PROSTRATION AND MUSCLE CRAMPS FROM EXCESSIVE PERSPIRATION

PO: ADULTS, ELDERLY: 1–2 g 3 times a day.

RELIEF OF DRY AND INFLAMED NASAL MEMBRANES

INTRANASAL: ADULTS, ELDERLY: Use as needed.

DIAGNOSTIC AID IN OPHTHALMOSCOPIC EXAM, TREATMENT OF CORNEAL EDEMA

OPHTHALMIC SOLUTION: ADULTS, ELDERLY: Apply 1–2 drops q3–4h.
OPHTHALMIC OINTMENT: ADULTS, ELDERLY: Apply once a day or as directed.

SIDE EFFECTS

FREQUENT: Facial flushing. **OCCASIONAL:** Fever; irritation, phlebitis, or extravasation at injection site. **Ophthalmic:** Temporary burning or irritation.

ADVERSE REACTIONS/ TOXIC EFFECTS

Too rapid administration may produce peripheral edema, CHF, and pulmonary edema. Excessive dosage may cause hypokalemia, hypervolemia, and hypernatremia.

NURSING CONSIDERATIONS

BASELINE ASSESSMENT

Assess fluid balance (I&O, daily weight, lung sounds, edema).

INTERVENTION/EVALUATION

Monitor fluid balance (I&O, daily weight, edema, lung sounds), IV site for extravasation. Monitor serum electrolytes, acid-base balance, BP. Hypernatremia associated with edema, weight gain, elevated BP; hyponatremia associated with muscle cramps, nausea, vomiting, dry mucous membranes.

PATIENT/FAMILY TEACHING

• Temporary burning, irritation may

occur upon instillation of eye medication. ● Discontinue eye medication and contact physician if severe pain, headache, rapid change in vision (side and straight ahead), sudden appearance of floating spots, acute redness of eyes, pain on exposure to light, double vision occurs.

sodium ferric gluconate complex

sew-**dee**-um **fair**-ick **glue**-koe-nate **calm**-plex

(Ferrlecit)

CLASSIFICATION
PHARMACOTHERAPEUTIC: Trace element. **CLINICAL:** Hematinic.

ACTION
A trace element that repletes total iron content in body. Replaces iron found in Hgb, myoglobin, and specific enzymes; allows oxygen transport via Hgb. Therapeutic Effect: Prevents and corrects iron deficiency.

PHARMACOKINETICS
Half-life: 1 hr.

USES
Treatment of iron deficiency anemia in patients undergoing chronic hemodialysis who are receiving supplemental erythropoietin therapy.

PRECAUTIONS
CONTRAINDICATIONS: All anemias not associated with iron deficiency, hypersensitivity to iron products. **CAUTIONS:** Patients with iron overload, significant allergies, asthma, hepatic impairment, rheumatoid arthritis.

⌛ **LIFESPAN CONSIDERATIONS: Pregnancy/Lactation:** Unknown if

distributed in breast milk. **Pregnancy Category B. Children:** Safety and efficacy not established. **Elderly:** No age-related precautions noted; lower initial dosages recommended.

INTERACTIONS
DRUG: **Aluminum, calcium, magnesium containing drugs:** May decrease iron effectiveness. **Ibandronate, levodopa, quinolone antibiotics:** May decrease the effectiveness of these drugs. HERBAL: None known. FOOD: None known. LAB VALUES: None known.

AVAILABILITY (Rx)
AMPULES: 12.5 mg/ml elemental iron.

ADMINISTRATION/HANDLING
▣ IV

Reconstitution ● Must be diluted. ● Test dose: dilute 25 mg (2 ml) with 50 ml 0.9% NaCl. ● Recommended dose: dilute 125 mg (10 ml) with 100 ml 0.9% NaCl.

Rate of administration ● Infuse test dose and recommended dose over 1 hr.

Storage ● Store at room temperature. ● Use immediately after dilution.

▨ **IV INCOMPATIBILITIES**
Do not mix with other medications.

INDICATIONS/ROUTES/DOSAGE
IRON DEFICIENCY ANEMIA
IV INFUSION: ADULTS, ELDERLY: 125 mg in 100 ml 0.9% NaCl infused over 1 hr. Minimum cumulative dose 1 g elemental iron given over 8 sessions at sequential dialysis treatments. May be given during dialysis session. CHILDREN 6 YR AND OLDER: 1.5 mg/kg diluted in 25 ml 0.9% NaCl administered over 60 min at sequential dialysis sessions. **Maximum:** 125 mg/dose.

SIDE EFFECTS
FREQUENT (greater than 3%): Flushing, hypotension, hypersensitivity

S

reaction. **OCCASIONAL** **(3%–1%):** Injection site reaction, headache, abdominal pain, chills, flu-like syndrome, dizziness, leg cramps, dyspnea, nausea, vomiting, diarrhea, myalgia, pruritus, edema.

ADVERSE REACTIONS/ TOXIC EFFECTS

A potentially fatal hypersensitivity reaction occurs rarely, characterized by cardiovascular collapse, cardiac arrest, dyspnea, bronchospasm, angioedema, and urticaria. Rapid administration may cause hypotension associated with flushing, lightheadedness, fatigue, weakness, or severe pain in the chest, back, or groin.

NURSING CONSIDERATIONS

BASELINE ASSESSMENT

Do not give concurrently with oral iron form (excessive iron may produce excessive iron storage [hemosiderosis]). Be alert to patients with rheumatoid arthritis or iron deficiency anemia (acute exacerbation of joint pain, swelling may occur).

INTERVENTION/EVALUATION

Monitor vital signs, lab tests, especially CBC, serum iron concentrations (may not be meaningful for 3 wk after administration).

PATIENT/FAMILY TEACHING

• Stools frequently become black with iron therapy; this is harmless unless accompanied by red streaking, sticky consistency of stool, abdominal pain or cramping, which should be reported to physician.

sodium oxybate (gamma hydroxybutyrate)

(GHB, Xyrem)

♦ CLASSIFICATION

PHARMACOTHERAPEUTIC: Neurotransmitter. **CLINICAL:** Antinarcolepsy.

ACTION

Mechanism of action unknown.

USES

Treatment of adult with cataplexy associated with narcolepsy. Treatment of excessive daytime sleepiness in patients with narcolepsy.

PRECAUTIONS

CONTRAINDICATIONS: Metabolic/respiratory alkalosis, current treatment with sedative-hypnotics, succinic semialdehyde dehydrogenase deficient. **CAUTIONS:** Hepatic insufficiency; history of depression; hypertension; pregnancy; concurrent ingestion of alcohol, other CNS depressants.

INTERACTIONS

DRUG: **Alcohol:** May have additive CNS and respiratory depressant effects. **Barbiturates, benzodiazepines, centrally-acting muscle relaxants, opioid analgesics:** May have additive CNS and respiratory depressant effects. **HERBAL:** None known. **FOOD:** None known. **LAB VALUES:** May increase serum sodium, glucose.

AVAILABILITY (Rx)

ORAL SOLUTION: 500 mg/ml.

ADMINISTRATION/HANDLING

PO

• Store at room temperature. • Give first of two daily dosages at bedtime while patient is in bed and the second dosage 2.5–4 hr later.

INDICATIONS/ROUTES/DOSAGE

NARCOLEPSY

PO: ADULTS, ELDERLY: 4.5 g a day in 2 equal doses of 2.25 g, the first taken at bedtime while in bed and the second 2.5–4 hr later. **Maximum:** 9 g a day in 2 weekly increments of 1.5 g a day.

SIDE EFFECTS

FREQUENT (58%): Mild bradycardia. **OCCASIONAL:** Headache, vertigo, dizziness, restless legs, abdominal pain, muscle weakness. **RARE:** Dreamlike state of confusion.

ADVERSE REACTIONS/ TOXIC EFFECTS

Metabolic alkalosis (irritability, muscle twitching, paraesthesias, cyanosis, slow/ shallow respiration, headache, thirst, nausea) has been noted, particularly in patients with head trauma before treatment. Concurrent use of alcohol may result in respiratory depression, apnea, comatose state. Severe dependence, craving produces a high potential for abuse.

NURSING CONSIDERATIONS

INTERVENTION/EVALUATION

Watch for signs of metabolic alkalosis (irritability, muscle twitching, paraesthesias, cyanosis, slow/shallow respiration, headache, thirst, nausea). Monitor serum glucose, sodium levels.

PATIENT/FAMILY TEACHING

• Avoid alcohol due to high potential for comatose state. • Severe dependence may occur.

sodium polystyrene sulfonate

sew-dee-um pol-ee-**stye**-reen (Kayexelate, Kionex, PMS-Sodium Polystyrene Sulfonate ✦, SPS)

CLASSIFICATION

PHARMACOTHERAPEUTIC: Cation exchange resin. **CLINICAL:** Antihyperkalemic.

ACTION

An ion exchange resin that releases sodium ions in exchange primarily for potassium ions. **Therapeutic Effect:** Moves potassium from the blood into the intestine so it can be expelled from the body.

USES

Treatment of hyperkalemia.

PRECAUTIONS

CONTRAINDICATIONS: Hypokalemia, hypernatremia, intestinal obstruction or perforation. **CAUTIONS:** Severe CHF, hypertension, edema. **Pregnancy Category C.**

INTERACTIONS

DRUG: Cation-donating antacids, laxatives (such as magnesium hydroxide): May decrease effect of sodium polystyrene sulfonate, and cause systemic alkalosis in patients with renal impairment. **HERBAL:** None known. **FOOD:** None known. **LAB VALUES:** May decrease serum calcium and magnesium levels.

AVAILABILITY (Rx)

SUSPENSION (SPS): 15 g/60 ml. **POWDER FOR SUSPENSION (KAYEXALATE, KIONEX):** 454 g. **RECTAL ENEMA:** 15 g/60 ml.

S

ADMINISTRATION/HANDLING

PO

• Give with 20–100 ml sorbitol (facilitates passage of resin through intestinal tract, prevents constipation, aids in potassium removal, increases palatability). • Do not mix with foods, liquids containing potassium.

RECTAL

• After initial cleansing enema, insert large rubber tube into rectum well into sigmoid colon, tape in place. • Introduce suspension (with 100 ml sorbitol) via gravity. • Flush with 50–100 ml fluid and clamp. • Retain for several hr if possible. • Irrigate colon with non–sodium-containing solution to remove resin.

INDICATIONS/ROUTES/DOSAGE

HYPERKALEMIA

PO: ADULTS, ELDERLY: 60 ml (15 g) 1–4 times a day. CHILDREN: 1 g/kg/dose q6h. RECTAL: ADULTS, ELDERLY: 30–50 g as needed q6h. CHILDREN: 1 g/kg/dose q2–6h.

SIDE EFFECTS

FREQUENT: High dosage: Anorexia, nausea, vomiting, constipation. High dosage in elderly: Fecal impaction characterized by severe stomach pain with nausea or vomiting. OCCASIONAL: Diarrhea, sodium retention marked by decreased urination, peripheral edema, and increased weight.

ADVERSE REACTIONS/TOXIC EFFECTS

Potassium deficiency may occur. Early signs of hypokalemia include confusion, delayed thought processes, extreme weakness, irritability, and EKG changes (including prolonged QT interval; widening, flattening, or inversion of T wave; and prominent U waves). Hypocalcemia, manifested by abdominal or muscle cramps, occurs occasionally. Arrhythmias and severe muscle weakness may be noted.

NURSING CONSIDERATIONS

BASELINE ASSESSMENT

Does not rapidly correct severe hyperkalemia (may take hours to days). Consider other measures in medical emergency (IV calcium, IV sodium bicarbonate/glucose/insulin, dialysis).

INTERVENTION/EVALUATION

Monitor serum potassium levels frequently. Assess patient's clinical condition, EKG (valuable in determining when treatment should be discontinued). In addition to checking serum potassium, monitor serum magnesium, calcium levels. Monitor pattern of daily bowel activity and stool consistency (fecal impaction may occur in patients on high dosages, particularly in elderly).

solifenacin

sol-ih-**fen**-ah-sin
(VESIcare)

CLASSIFICATION

PHARMACOTHERAPEUTIC: Muscarinic receptor antagonist. CLINICAL: Urinary antispasmodic.

ACTION

A urinary antispasmodic that acts as a direct antagonist at muscarinic acetylcholine receptors in cholinergically innervated organs. Reduces tonus (elastic tension) of smooth muscle in the bladder and slows parasympathetic contractions. Therapeutic Effect: Decreases urinary bladder contractions, increases residual urine volume, and decreases detrusor muscle pressure.

PHARMACOKINETICS

Well absorbed following PO administration. Protein binding: 98%. Metabolized by liver. Excreted in feces and urine. Half-life: 40–68 hr.

USES

Treatment of overactive bladder with symptoms of urge urinary incontinence, urgency, urinary frequency.

PRECAUTIONS

CONTRAINDICATIONS: Breast-feeding, GI obstruction, uncontrolled angle-closure glaucoma, urine retention. **CAUTIONS:** Bladder outflow obstruction, GI obstructive disorders, decreased GI motility, controlled narrow-angle glaucoma, renal or hepatic impairment, congenital or acquired QT prolongation, pregnancy.

⏳ LIFESPAN CONSIDERATIONS: **Pregnancy/Lactation:** Unknown if drug crosses placenta or is distributed is breast milk. **Pregnancy Category C. Children:** Safety and efficacy not established. **Elderly:** No age-related precautions noted.

INTERACTIONS

DRUG: **Aminoglutethimide, carbamazepine, nafcillin, nevirapine, phenobarbital, phenytoin:** May decrease the effects and serum level of solifenacin. **Azole antifungals, ciprofloxacin, clarithromycin, diclofenac, doxycycline, erythromycin, imatinib, isoniazid, nefazodone, nicardipine, propofol, protease inhibitors, quinidine, verapamil:** May increase the effects and serum level of solifenacin. **Ketoconazole:** May increase the serum level of solifenacin. HERBAL: **St John's wort:** May decrease the effects and serum level of solifenacin. FOOD: **Grapefruit, grapefruit juice:** May increase the effects and serum level of solifenacin. LAB VALUES: None known.

AVAILABILITY (Rx)

TABLETS: 5 mg, 10 mg.

ADMINISTRATION/HANDLING

PO
• Give solifenacin without regard to food. Swallow solifenacin tablets whole.

INDICATIONS/ROUTES/DOSAGE

OVERACTIVE BLADDER
PO: ADULTS, ELDERLY: 5 mg/day; if tolerated, may increase to 10 mg/day.

DOSAGE IN RENAL OR HEPATIC IMPAIRMENT
For patients with severe renal impairment or moderate hepatic impairment, maximum dosage is 5 mg/day.

SIDE EFFECTS

FREQUENT (11%–5%): Dry mouth, constipation, blurred vision. **OCCASIONAL (5%–3%):** UTI, dyspepsia, nausea. **RARE (2%–1%):** Dizziness, dry eyes, fatigue, depression, edema, hypertension, upper abdominal pain, vomiting, urine retention.

ADVERSE REACTIONS/ TOXIC EFFECTS

Angioneurotic edema and GI obstruction occur rarely. Overdose can result in severe central anticholinergic effects.

NURSING CONSIDERATIONS

BASELINE ASSESSMENT
Assess symptoms of overactive bladder before beginning the drug.

INTERVENTION/EVALUATION
Monitor I&O. Assess for a decrease in symptoms.

PATIENT/FAMILY TEACHING
• Avoid tasks requiring mental alertness, motor control until response to the drug is known. • Inform the patient of potential anticholinergic side effects (constipation, urinary retention, blurred vision, heat prostration in a hot environment).

S

Solu-Medrol, *see* *methylprednisolone*

somatrem

soe-ma-trem
(Protopin)

somatropin

soe-mah-**troe**-pin
(Genotropin, Genotropin Miniquick, Humatrope, Norditropin, Norditropin Cartridge, Nutropin, Nutropin AQ, Nutropin Depot, Saizen, Serostim, Zorbitive)

Do not confuse Protopin with Proloprim, Protamine, or Protopam or somatropin with sumatriptan.

◆CLASSIFICATION

PHARMACOTHERAPEUTIC: Polypeptide hormone. **CLINICAL:** Growth hormone.

ACTION

A polypeptide hormone that stimulates cartilaginous growth areas of long bones, increases the number and size of skeletal muscle cells, influences the size of organs, and increases RBC mass by stimulating erythropoietin. Influences the metabolism of carbohydrates (decreases insulin sensitivity), fats (mobilizes fatty acids), minerals (retains phosphorus, sodium, potassium by promotion of cell growth), and proteins (increases protein synthesis). **Therapeutic Effect:** Stimulates growth.

PHARMACOKINETICS

Well absorbed after subcutaneous or IM administration. Localized primarily in the kidneys and liver. **Half-life:** IV, 20–30 min; subcutaneous, IM, 3–5 hr.

USES

Somatrem, somatropin: Long-term treatment of growth failure in children caused by pituitary growth hormone (GH) deficiency. **Somatropin:** Treatment of growth failure in adults caused by GH deficiency, treatment of growth failure in children caused by chronic renal insufficiency, long-term treatment of short stature associated with Turner's syndrome, treatment of AIDS-related cachexia, weight loss, treatment of short bowel syndrome.ʻ

PRECAUTIONS

CONTRAINDICATIONS: Active neoplasia (either newly diagnosed or recurrent), critical illness, hypersensitivity to growth hormone. **CAUTIONS:** Diabetes mellitus, untreated hypothyroidism, malignancy.

⧗ **LIFESPAN CONSIDERATIONS: Pregnancy/Lactation:** Unknown if drug is distributed in breast milk. **Pregnancy Category B (Genotropin, Genotropin Miniquick, Saizen, Serostim, Zorbitive); C (Humatrope, Norditropin, Norditropin Cartridge, Nutropin, Nutropin AQ, Nutropin Depot, Protopin). Children/Elderly:** No age-related precautions noted.

INTERACTIONS

DRUG: Corticosteroids: May inhibit growth response. **HERBAL:** None known. **FOOD:** None known. **LAB VALUES:** May increase serum alkaline phosphatase, inorganic phosphorus, and parathyroid hormone levels. May decrease glucose tolerance. May slightly decrease thyroid function.

AVAILABILITY (Rx)

INJECTION POWDER FOR RECONSTITUTION (SOMATREM [PROTOPIN]): 5 mg.
INJECTION POWDER FOR RECONSTITUTION (SOMATROPIN): 0.4 mg

(Genotropin Miniquick), 0.6 mg (Genotropin Miniquick), 0.8 mg (Genotropin Miniquick), 1 mg (Genotropin Miniquick), 1.2 mg (Genotropin Miniquick), 1.4 mg (Genotropin Miniquick), 1.5 mg (Genotropin, Genotropin Miniquick), 1.6 mg (Genotropin Miniquick), 1.8 mg (Genotropin Miniquick), 2 mg (Genotropin Miniquick), 4 mg (Norditropin, Serostim, Zorbitive) 5 mg (Humatrope, Nutropin, Saizen, Serostim, Zorbitive), 5.8 mg (Genotropin), 6 mg (Humatrope, Serostim, Zorbitive), 8 mg (Norditropin), 8.8 mg (Saizen, Zorbitive), 10 mg (Nutropin), 12 mg (Humatrope), 13.5 mg (Nutropin Depot), 18 mg (Nutropin Depot), 22.5 mg (Nutropin Depot), 24 mg (Humatrope). **SOLUTION FOR INJECTION (SOMATROPIN [NORDITROPIN CARTRIDGE]):** 15 mg/1.5 ml. **INJECTION SOLUTION (SOMATROPIN [NUTROPIN AQ]):** 5 mg/ml.

ADMINISTRATION/HANDLING

SOMATREM

‹ ALERT › **Neonate:** Benzyl alcohol as a preservative has been associated with fatal toxicity, e.g., gasping syndrome, in premature infants. Reconstitute with sterile water for injection only. Use only 1 dose per vial. Discard unused portion.

IM, SUBCUTANEOUS

Reconstitution • Reconstitute each 5 mg vial with 1–5 ml bacteriostatic water for injection (benzyl alcohol preserved) or each 10 mg vial with 1–10 ml bacteriostatic water for injection (benzyl alcohol preserved only). • Aim the stream of diluent against glass wall of the vial. • Swirl contents with a gentle rotary motion until completely dissolved. Do not shake (results in a cloudy solution). The solution should be clear immediately after reconstitution. If the solution is cloudy immediately after reconstitution or refrigeration, contents must not be injected.

Storage • Store in refrigeraton. • Use reconstituted vials within 14 days. • Do not freeze. • Do not use if solution is cloudy.

SOMATROPIN

‹ ALERT › **Neonate:** Benzyl alcohol as a preservative has been associated with fatal toxicity, e.g., gasping syndrome, in premature infants. Reconstitute with sterile water for injection only. Use only 1 dose per vial. Discard unused portion.

Reconstitution **Humatrope:** *Vial:* • Reconstitute with 1.5–5 ml diluent for Humatrope. • Diluent should be injected into vial by aiming stream of liquid against glass wall. • Swirl vial with a gently rotary motion until contents are completely dissolved. Do not shake. *Cartridge* • Reconstitute cartridge using only the diluent syringe and diluent connector. • Do not reconstitute with diluent for Humatrope provided with Humatrope vials.

Nutropin • Reconstitute each 5 mg vial with 1–5 ml bacteriostatic water for injection (benzyl alcohol preserved), or each 10 mg vial with 1–10 ml bacteriostatic water for injection (benzyl alcohol preserved only). • Aim the stream of diluent against glass wall of the vial. • Swirl contents with a gentle rotary motion until completely dissolved. Do not shake (results in a cloudy solution). The solution should be clear immediately after reconstitution. If the solution is cloudy immediately after reconstitution or refrigeration, contents must not be injected.

Storage: Humatrope: Refrigerate vials. • Do not freeze. • Reconstituted solution is stable for 14 days if reconstituted with bacteriostatic water for injection and stored in refrigerator. Reconstituted solution is stable for 24 hr if reconstituted with sterile water for injection and stored in refrigerator. If reconstituted solution is cloudy or contains precipitate, discard.

S

Nutropin • Refrigerate vials. • Do not freeze. • Reconstituted solution is stable for 14 days if reconstituted with bacteriostatic water for injection and stored in refrigerator. If reconstituted solution is cloudy or contains precipitate, discard.

INDICATIONS/ROUTES/DOSAGE

GROWTH HORMONE DEFICIENCY
SUBCUTANEOUS (HUMATROPE): ADULTS: 0.006 mg/kg once daily. CHILDREN: 0.18–0.3 mg/kg weekly divided into alternate-day doses or 6 doses/wk.
SUBCUTANEOUS (NUTROPIN): ADULTS: 0.006 mg/kg once daily. CHILDREN: 0.3–0.7 mg/kg weekly divided into daily doses.
SUBCUTANEOUS (NUTROPIN AQ): ADULTS: 0.006 mg/kg once daily.
SUBCUTANEOUS (GENOTROPIN): ADULTS: 0.04–0.08 mg/kg weekly divided into 6–7 equal doses/wk. CHILDREN: 0.16–0.24 mg/kg weekly divided into daily doses.
SUBCUTANEOUS (PROTOPIN): CHILDREN: 0.3 mg/kg weekly divided into daily doses.
SUBCUTANEOUS (NORDITROPIN): CHILDREN: 0.024–0.036 mg/kg/dose 6–7 times a week.
SUBCUTANEOUS (SAIZEN): CHILDREN: 0.06 mg/kg 3 times a week.
SUBCUTANEOUS ONLY (NUTROPIN DEPOT): CHILDREN: 0.75 mg/kg twice monthly or 1.5 mg/kg once monthly.

CHRONIC RENAL INSUFFICIENCY
SUBCUTANEOUS (NUTROPIN, NUTROPIN AQ): CHILDREN: 0.35 mg/kg weekly divided into daily doses.

TURNER SYNDROME
SUBCUTANEOUS (HUMATROPE, NUTROPIN, NUTROPIN AQ): CHILDREN: 0.375 mg/kg weekly divided into equal doses 3–7 times a week.

AIDS-RELATED WASTING
SUBCUTANEOUS: ADULTS WEIGHING MORE THAN 55 KG: 6 mg once a day at bedtime. ADULTS WEIGHING 45–55 KG: 5 mg once a day at bedtime. ADULTS WEIGHING

35–44 KG: 4 mg once a day at bedtime. ADULTS WEIGHING LESS THAN 35 KG: 0.1 mg/kg once a day at bedtime.

SHORT BOWEL SYNDROME
SUBCUTANEOUS (ZORBTIVE): ADULTS: 0.1 mg/kg/day. **Maximum:** 8 mg/day.

SIDE EFFECTS

FREQUENT: Otitis media, other ear disorders (with Turner's syndrome). **OCCASIONAL:** Carpal tunnel syndrome; gynecomastia; myalgia; swelling of hands, feet, or legs; fatigue; asthenia. **RARE:** Rash, pruritus, altered vision, headache, nausea, vomiting, injection site pain and swelling, abdominal pain, hip or knee pain.

ADVERSE REACTIONS/ TOXIC EFFECTS

Glucose intolerance can occur with overdosage. Long-term overdosage with growth hormone could result in signs and symptoms of acromegaly.

NURSING CONSIDERATIONS

BASELINE ASSESSMENT
Obtain baseline thyroid function, blood glucose level.

INTERVENTION/EVALUATION
Monitor bone growth, growth rate in relation to the patient's age. Monitor serum calcium, glucose, phosphorus levels, renal and parathyroid and thyroid function. Observe for decreased muscle wasting in AIDS patients.

PATIENT/FAMILY TEACHING
• Teach correct procedure to reconstitute drug for administration, safe handling and disposal of needles. • Inform patient of need for regular follow-up with physician. • Report development of severe headache, visual changes, pain in hip or knee, limping.

Sonata, *see zaleplon*

sorafenib

sor-ah-**fen**-ib

(Nexavar)

◆CLASSIFICATION

PHARMACOTHERAPEUTIC: Multikinase inhibitor. **CLINICAL:** Antineoplastic.

ACTION

Decreases tumor cell proliferation by interacting with multiple intracellular and cell surface kinases. **Therapeutic Effect:** Inhibits tumor growth.

PHARMACOKINETICS

Metabolized in liver. Protein binding: 99.5%. Eliminated mainly in feces with a lesser amount excreted in urine. **Half-life:** 25–48 hr.

USES

Treatment of advanced renal cell carcinoma.

PRECAUTIONS

CONTRAINDICATIONS: None known. **CAUTIONS:** Hepatic impairment, dialysis patients, renal impairment.

⌛ **LIFESPAN CONSIDERATIONS: Pregnancy/Lactation:** May cause fetal harm. Adequate contraception should be used during therapy and for at least 2 wk after therapy completion. Unknown if distributed in breast milk; do not breast-feed. **Pregnancy Category D. Children:** Safety and efficacy not established. **Elderly:** No age-related precautions noted.

INTERACTIONS

DRUG: **Carbamazine, dexamethasone, phenobarbital, phenytoin, rifampin:** May decrease sorafenib concentrations. **Doxorubicin:** The concentration of this drug may be increased when taken with sorafenib. **Warfarin:** May increase INR, risk of bleeding. HERBAL: **St John's wort:** May decrease sorafenib concentration. FOOD: **High-fat meals:** Decrease sorafenib effectiveness. LAB VALUES: May increase serum lipase, amylase, bilirubin, alkaline phosphatase. May decrease serum phosphorus, lymphocytes, WBCs, Hgb, Hct.

AVAILABILITY (Rx)

TABLETS, FILM-COATED: 200 mg (Nexavar).

ADMINISTRATION/HANDLING

PO

● Do not crush or break film-coated tablets. ● Give 1 hr before or 2 hr after eating (high-fat meal reduces effectiveness).

INDICATIONS/ROUTES/DOSAGE

RENAL CELL CARCINOMA

PO: ADULTS, ELDERLY: 400 mg (2 tablets) twice a day without food.

SIDE EFFECTS

FREQUENT (43%–16%): Diarrhea, rash, fatigue, exfoliative dermatitis, alopecia, nausea, pruritus hypertension anorexia, vomiting. **OCCASIONAL (15%–10%):** Constipation, minor bleeding, dyspnea, sensory neuropathy, cough, abdominal pain, dry skin, weight, loss, joint pain, headache. **RARE (9%–1%):** Acne, flushing, stomatitis, mucositis, dyspepsia, arthralgia, myalgia, hoarseness.

ADVERSE REACTIONS/ TOXIC EFFECTS

Anemia, neutropenia thrombocytopenia, leukopenia occur in less than 10%

S

of patients. Pancreatitis, gastritis, erectile dysfunction occur occasionally. Hemorrhage, cardiac ischemia/infarction, hypertensive crisis occur rarely.

NURSING CONSIDERATIONS

BASELINE ASSESSMENT
Monitor BP weekly during first 6 wk of therapy and routinely thereafter. CBC, blood chemistries including electrolytes, renal and liver function tests, chest x-ray should be performed before therapy begins and routinely thereafter.

INTERVENTION/EVALUATION
Determine serum amylase, lipase, phosphorus concentration frequently during therapy. Monitor CBC for evidence of bone marrow depression. Monitor for blood dyscrasias (fever, sore throat, signs of local infection, easy bruising, or unusual bleeding from any site), symptoms of anemia (excessive tiredness, weakness). Monitor for signs of neuropathy (gait disturbances, handwriting difficulties, numbness).

PATIENT/FAMILY TEACHING
• Report any episode of chest pain. • Do not have immunizations without physician's approval (drug lowers body resistance); avoid contact with those who have recently taken live virus vaccine. • Promptly report fever, sore throat, signs of local infection, easy bruising or unusual bleeding from any site.

---

sotalol hydrochloride ▷

soe-ta-lole

(Apo-Sotalol ✦, Betapace, Betapace AF, Novo-Sotalol ✦, PMS-Sotalol ✦, Sorine)

Do not confuse sotalol with Stadol.

◆ CLASSIFICATION

PHARMACOTHERAPEUTIC: Beta-adrenergic blocking agent. **CLINICAL:** Antiarrhythmic (see pp. 16C, 65C).

ACTION
A beta-adrenergic blocking agent that prolongs action potential, effective refractory period, and QT interval. Decreases heart rate and AV node conduction; increases AV node refractoriness. Therapeutic Effect: Produces antiarrhythmic activity.

PHARMACOKINETICS
Well absorbed from the GI tract. Protein binding: None. Widely distributed. Primarily excreted unchanged in urine. Removed by hemodialysis. Half-life: 12 hr (increased in the elderly and patients with impaired renal function).

USES
Betapace, Sorine: Treatment of documented, life-threatening ventricular arrhythmias. **Betapace AF:** Maintain normal sinus rhythm in patients with symptomatic atrial fibrillation or flutter. OFF-LABEL: Maintenance of normal heart rhythm in chronic or recurring atrial fibrillation or flutter; treatment of anxiety, chronic angina pectoris, hypertension, hypertrophic cardiomyopathy, MI, mitral valve prolapse syndrome, pheochromocytoma, thyrotoxicosis, tremors.

PRECAUTIONS
CONTRAINDICATIONS: Bronchial asthma, cardiogenic shock, prolonged QT syndrome (unless functioning pacemaker is present), second- and third-degree heart block, sinus bradycardia, uncontrolled cardiac failure. **CAUTIONS:** Patients with history of ventricular tachycardia,

ventricular fibrillation, cardiomegaly, CHF, diabetes mellitus, excessive prolongation of QT interval, hypokalemia, hypomagnesemia. Severe, prolonged diarrhea. Patients with sick sinus syndrome, patients at risk of developing thyrotoxicosis. Avoid abrupt withdrawal.

⌧ LIFESPAN CONSIDERATIONS: **Pregnancy/Lactation:** Crosses placenta. Excreted in breast milk. **Pregnancy Category B (D if used in second or third trimester). Children:** Safety and efficacy not established. **Elderly:** Age-related peripheral vascular disease may increase susceptibility to decreased peripheral circulation. Age-related renal impairment may require dosage adjustment in the elderly.

INTERACTIONS

DRUG: Antiarrhythmics, phenothiazine, tricyclic antidepressants: May prolong QT interval. **Calcium channel blockers:** May increase effect on AV conduction and BP. **Clonidine:** May potentiate rebound hypertension after clonidine is discontinued. **Digoxin:** May increase risk of proarrhythmias. **Insulin, oral hypoglycemics:** May mask signs of hypoglycemia and prolong the effects of insulin and oral hypoglycemics. **Sympathomimetics:** May inhibit the effects of sympathomimetics. **HERBAL:** None known. **FOOD:** None known. **LAB VALUES:** May increase blood glucose, serum alkaline phosphatase, serum LDH, serum lipoprotein, AST, ALT, and serum triglyceride levels.

AVAILABILITY (Rx)

TABLETS: 80 mg (Betapace, Betapace AF Sorine), 120 mg (Betapace, Betapace AF, Sorine), 160 mg (Betapace, Betapace AF, Sorine), 240 mg (Betapace, Sorine).

ADMINISTRATION/HANDLING

◂ ALERT ▸ Some patients may require 480–640 mg a day. Sotalol has a long half-life and administering the drug more than twice a day is usually not necessary. Avoid abrupt withdrawal. To minimize risk of induced arrhythmia, patients initiated or reinitiated on Betapace or Betapace AF should be placed in a facility that can provide continuous EKG monitoring for a minimum of 3 days (on their maintenance dose).

PO
• Give without regard to food.

INDICATIONS/ROUTES/DOSAGE

DOCUMENTED, LIFE-THREATENING ARRHYTHMIAS

PO (BETAPACE, SORINE): ADULTS, ELDERLY: Initially, 80 mg twice a day. May increase gradually at 2- to 3-day intervals. Range: 240–320 mg/day.

ATRIAL FIBRILLATION, ATRIAL FLUTTER

PO (BETAPACE AF): ADULTS, ELDERLY: 80 mg twice a day.

DOSAGE IN RENAL IMPAIRMENT

Dosage interval is modified based on creatinine clearance.

Betapace, Sorine

Creatinine Clearance	Dosage Interval
31–60 ml/min	24 hr
10–30 ml/min	36–48 hr
Less than 10 ml/min	Individualized

Betapace AF

Creatinine Clearance	Dosage Interval
Greater than 60 ml/min	12 hr
40–60 ml/min	24 hr
Less than 40 ml/min	Contraindicated

SIDE EFFECTS

FREQUENT: Diminished sexual function, drowsiness, insomnia, unusual fatigue or weakness. **OCCASIONAL:** Depression, cold hands or feet, diarrhea, constipation, anxiety, nasal congestion, nausea, vomiting. **RARE:** Altered taste, dry eyes, itching, numbness of fingers, toes, or scalp.

ADVERSE REACTIONS/ TOXIC EFFECTS

Bradycardia, CHF, hypotension, bronchospasm, hypoglycemia, prolonged QT interval, torsades de pointes, ventricular tachycardia, and premature ventricular complexes may occur.

NURSING CONSIDERATIONS

BASELINE ASSESSMENT

Patient must be on continuous cardiac monitoring upon initiation of therapy. Do not administer without consulting physician if pulse is 60 beats/min or less. Assess creatinine clearance before dosing.

INTERVENTION/EVALUATION

Diligently monitor for arrhythmias. Assess BP for hypotension, pulse for bradycardia. Assess for CHF: dyspnea, peripheral edema, jugular vein distention, increased weight, rales in lungs, decreased urine output.

PATIENT/FAMILY TEACHING

• Do not discontinue or change dose without physician approval. • Avoid tasks requiring alertness, motor skills until response to drug is established (may cause drowsiness). • Periodic lab tests, EKGs are a necessary part of therapy.

Spectrocef, *see cefditoren*

Spiriva, *see tiotropium*

spironolactone

speer-on-oh-**lak**-tone

(Aldactone, Novospiroton ✦)

Do not confuse Aldactone with Aldactazide.

FIXED-COMBINATION(S)

Aldactazide: spironolactone/hydrochlorothiazide (a thiazide diuretic): 25 mg/25 mg; 50 mg/50 mg.

•CLASSIFICATION

PHARMACOTHERAPEUTIC: Aldosterone antagonist. **CLINICAL:** Potassium-sparing diuretic, antihypertensive, antihypokalemic (see p. 89C).

ACTION

A potassium-sparing diuretic that interferes with sodium reabsorption by competitively inhibiting the action of aldosterone in the distal tubule, thus promoting sodium and water excretion and increasing potassium retention. **Therapeutic Effect:** Produces diuresis; lowers BP; diagnostic aid for primary aldosteronism.

PHARMACOKINETICS

Route	Onset	Peak	Duration
PO	24–48 hr	48–72 hr	48–72 hr

Well absorbed from the GI tract (absorption increased with food). Protein binding: 91%–98%. Metabolized in the liver to active metabolite. Primarily excreted in urine. Unknown if removed by hemodialysis. **Half-life:** 0–24 hr (metabolite, 13–24 hr).

USES

Management of edema associated with CHF, cirrhosis, nephrotic syndrome. Treatment of hypertension, male hirsutism, hypokalemia, CHF. Diagnosis and treatment of primary hyperaldosteronism. OFF-LABEL: Treatment of edema and hypertension in children; female acne, hirsutism, polycystic ovary disease.

PRECAUTIONS

CONTRAINDICATIONS: Acute renal insufficiency, anuria, BUN and serum creatinine levels more than twice normal values, hyperkalemia. **CAUTIONS:** Dehydration, hyponatremia, renal or hepatic impairment, concurrent use of supplemental potassium.

⧗ **LIFESPAN CONSIDERATIONS: Pregnancy/Lactation:** Active metabolite excreted in breast milk; breast-feeding not advised. **Pregnancy Category C (D if used in pregnancy-induced hypertension). Children:** No age-related precautions noted. **Elderly:** May be more susceptible to develop hyperkalemia. Age-related renal impairment may require dosage adjustment.

INTERACTIONS

DRUG: **ACE inhibitors (such as captopril), potassium-containing medications, potassium supplements:** May increase the risk of hyperkalemia. **Anticoagulants, heparin:** May decrease the effects of these drugs. **Digoxin:** May increase the half-life of digoxin. **Lithium:** May decrease the clearance and increase the risk of toxicity of lithium. **NSAIDs:** May decrease the antihypertensive effect of spironolactone. HERBAL: None known. FOOD: None known. LAB VALUES: May increase urinary calcium excretion; BUN and blood glucose levels; serum creatinine, magnesium, potassium, and uric acid levels. May decrease serum sodium level.

AVAILABILITY (Rx)

TABLETS: 25 mg, 50 mg, 100 mg.

ADMINISTRATION/HANDLING

PO

• Oral suspension containing crushed

tablets in cherry syrup is stable for up to 30 days if refrigerated. • Drug absorption enhanced if taken with food. • Scored tablets may be crushed.

INDICATIONS/ROUTES/DOSAGE

EDEMA

PO: ADULTS, ELDERLY: 25–200 mg/day as a single dose or in 2 divided doses. CHILDREN: 1.5–3.3 mg/kg/day in divided doses. NEONATES: 1–3 mg/kg/day in 1–2 divided doses.

HYPERTENSION

PO: ADULTS, ELDERLY: 25–50 mg/day in 1–2 doses/day. CHILDREN: 1.5–3.3 mg/kg/day in divided doses.

HYPOKALEMIA

PO: ADULTS, ELDERLY: 25–200 mg/day as a single dose or in 2 divided doses.

MALE HIRSUTISM

PO: ADULTS, ELDERLY: 50–200 mg/day as a single dose or in 2 divided doses.

PRIMARY ALDOSTERONISM

PO: ADULTS, ELDERLY: 100–400 mg/day as a single dose or in 2 divided doses. CHILDREN: 100–400 mg/m^2/day as a single dose or in 2 divided doses.

CHF

PO: ADULTS, ELDERLY: 25 mg/day adjusted based on patient response and evidence of hyperkalemia.

DOSAGE IN RENAL IMPAIRMENT

Dosage interval is modified based on creatinine clearance.

Creatinine Clearance	Interval
10–50 ml/min	Usual dose q12–24h
Less than 10 ml/min	Avoid use

SIDE EFFECTS

FREQUENT: Hyperkalemia (in patients with renal insufficiency and those taking potassium supplements), dehydration, hyponatremia, lethargy. **OCCASIONAL:** Nausea, vomiting, anorexia, abdominal cramps, diarrhea, headache, ataxia,

---

somnolence, confusion, fever. **Male:** Gynecomastia, impotence, decreased libido. **Female:** Menstrual irregularities (including amenorrhea and postmenopausal bleeding), breast tenderness. **RARE:** Rash, urticaria, hirsutism.

ADVERSE REACTIONS/ TOXIC EFFECTS

Severe hyperkalemia may produce arrhythmias, bradycardia, and EKG changes (tented T waves, widening QRS complex and ST segment depression). These may proceed to cardiac standstill or ventricular fibrillation. Cirrhosis patients are at risk for hepatic decompensation if dehydration or hyponatremia occurs. Patients with primary aldosteronism may experience rapid weight loss and severe fatigue during high-dose therapy.

NURSING CONSIDERATIONS

BASELINE ASSESSMENT

Weigh patient; initiate strict I&O. Evaluate hydration status by assessing mucous membranes, skin turgor. Obtain baseline serum electrolytes, renal and hepatic functions, urinalysis. Assess for edema; note location, extent. Check baseline vital signs, note pulse rate/regularity.

INTERVENTION/EVALUATION

Monitor serum electrolyte values, especially for increased potassium. Monitor BP. Monitor for hyponatremia: mental confusion, thirst, cold or clammy skin, drowsiness, dry mouth. Monitor for hyperkalemia: colic, diarrhea, muscle twitching followed by weakness/paralysis, arrhythmias. Obtain daily weight. Note changes in edema, skin turgor.

PATIENT/FAMILY TEACHING

• Expect increase in volume, frequency of urination. • Therapeutic effect takes several days to begin and can last for several days when drug is discontinued.

This may not apply if patient is on a potassium-losing drug concomitantly (diet and use of supplements should be established by physician). • Notify physician for irregular or slow pulse, electrolyte imbalance (signs noted previously). • Avoid foods high in potassium such as whole grains (cereals), legumes, meat, bananas, apricots, orange juice, potatoes (white, sweet), raisins. • Avoid tasks that require alertness, motor skills until response to drug is established (may cause drowsiness).

Sporanox, *see*
itraconazole

St. John's wort

Also known as amber, demon chaser, goatweed, hardhay, rosin rose, tipton weed.

◆CLASSIFICATION

HERBAL: See Appendix G.

ACTION

Inhibits COMT (catechol-*O*-methyl transferase), MAO (monoamine oxidase); modulates effects of serotonin by inhibiting serotonin reuptake and 5-HT$_3$ andantagonism. **Effect:** Produces 5-HT$_4$ antidepressant effect.

USES

Treatment of depression, including secondary effects of depression (fatigue, loss of appetite, anxiety, nervousness, insomnia).

PRECAUTIONS

CONTRAINDICATIONS: Pregnancy, breast-feeding (may cause increased muscle tone of uterus; infants may experience colic, drowsiness, lethargy). **CAUTIONS:** Bipolar disorder, schizophrenia.

⧖ **LIFESPAN CONSIDERATIONS: Pregnancy/Lactation:** Contraindicated. **Pregnancy Category C. Children:** Safety and efficacy not established. Avoid use. **Elderly:** No age-related precautions noted.

INTERACTIONS

DRUG: **Angiotensin-converting enzyme (ACE) Inhibitors:** May cause hypertension. May decrease concentration/effect of indinavir. **Antidepressants:** May increase therapeutic effect. May decrease effectiveness of cyclosporine, resulting in organ rejection. **Digoxin:** May cause CHF exacerbation. **HERBAL:** **Ginseng, chamomile, goldenseal, kava kava, valerian:** May increase therapeutic and adverse effects. **FOOD:** **Tyramine-containing food:** May cause hypertensive crisis with high doses of St. John's wort. **LAB VALUES:** May increase INR or PT in patients treated with warfarin.

AVAILABILITY (Rx)

CAPSULES: 150 mg, 300 mg. **LIQUID EXTRACT. TINCTURE.**

INDICATIONS/ROUTES/DOSAGE

DEPRESSION
PO: ADULTS, ELDERLY: 300 mg 3 times a day is the most common.

SIDE EFFECTS

Abdominal cramps, insomnia, vivid dreams, restlessness, anxiety, agitation, irritability, fatigue, dry mouth, headache, dizziness, photosensitivity, confusion.

ADVERSE REACTIONS/ TOXIC EFFECTS

None known.

NURSING CONSIDERATIONS

BASELINE ASSESSMENT
Assess if patient is pregnant or breast-feeding, has history of psychiatric disease. Determine medication usage (many potential interactions). Assess mental status: mood, memory, anxiety level.

INTERVENTION/EVALUATION
Monitor changes in depressive state, behavior, signs of side effects.

PATIENT/FAMILY TEACHING
• Do not abruptly discontinue (may increase adverse effects). • Check with physician before taking other medications (many interactions). • Avoid foods high in tyramine (e.g., aged cheese, pickled products, beer, wine). • Therapeutic effect may take 4–6 wk. • Avoid the sun, use sunscreen/protective clothing (increased photosensitivity).

stavudine (d4T)

stay-view-deen
(Zerit)

◆CLASSIFICATION

PHARMACOTHERAPEUTIC: Nucleoside reverse transcriptase inhibitor. **CLINICAL:** Antiviral (see pp. 62C, 103C).

ACTION

Inhibits HIV reverse transcriptase by terminating the viral DNA chain. Also inhibits RNA- and DNA-dependent DNA polymerase, an enzyme necessary for

S

HIV replication. **Therapeutic Effect:** Impedes HIV replication, slowing the progression of HIV infection.

PHARMACOKINETICS

Rapidly and completely absorbed after PO administration. Undergoes minimal metabolism. Excreted in urine. **Half-life:** 1.5 hr (increased in renal impairment).

USES

Treatment of HIV infection, in combination with other agents.

PRECAUTIONS

CONTRAINDICATIONS: None known. **CAUTIONS:** History of peripheral neuropathy, renal or hepatic impairment.

⌛ **LIFESPAN CONSIDERATIONS: Pregnancy/Lactation:** Breast-feeding not recommended (possibility of HIV transmission). **Pregnancy Category C. Children:** No age-related precautions noted. **Elderly:** Information not available.

INTERACTIONS

DRUG: Didanosine, ethambutol, isoniazid, lithium, phenytoin, zalcitabine: May increase the risk of peripheral neuropathy development. **Didanosine, hydroxyurea:** May increase the risk of hepatotoxicity. **Zidovudine:** May have antagonistic antiviral effect. **HERBAL:** None known. **FOOD:** None known. **LAB VALUES:** Commonly increases AST and ALT levels. May decrease neutrophil count.

AVAILABILITY (Rx)

CAPSULES: 15 mg, 20 mg, 30 mg, 40 mg. **ORAL SOLUTION:** 1 mg/ml.

ADMINISTRATION/HANDLING

PO
• Give without regard to meals.

INDICATIONS/ROUTES/DOSAGE

HIV INFECTION

PO: ADULTS, ELDERLY, CHILDREN WEIGHING 60 KG AND MORE: 40 mg q12h. CHILDREN WEIGHING 30–59 KG: 30 mg q12h. NEONATES 14 DAYS AND OLDER, INFANTS, CHILDREN WEIGHING LESS THAN 30 KG: 1 mg/kg/dose q12h. **Maximum:** 30 mg q12h. NEONATES 0–13 DAYS: 0.5 mg/kg/dose q12h.

DOSAGE IN RENAL IMPAIRMENT

Dosage and frequency are modified based on creatinine clearance and patient weight.

Creatinine Clearance	Weight 60 kg or More	Weight Less Than 60 kg
Greater than 50 ml/min	40 mg q12h	30 mg q12h
26–50 ml/min	20 mg q12h	15 mg q12h
10–25 ml/min	20 mg q24h	15 mg q24h

SIDE EFFECTS

FREQUENT: Headache (55%), diarrhea (50%), chills and fever (38%), nausea and vomiting, myalgia (35%), rash (33%), asthenia (28%), insomnia, abdominal pain (26%), anxiety (22%), arthralgia (18%), back pain (20%), diaphoresis (19%), malaise (17%), depression (14%). **OCCASIONAL:** Anorexia, weight loss, nervousness, dizziness, conjunctivitis, dyspepsia, dyspnea. **RARE:** Constipation, vasodilation, confusion, migraine, urticaria, abnormal vision.

ADVERSE REACTIONS/ TOXIC EFFECTS

Peripheral neuropathy, (numbness, tingling, or pain in the hands and feet) occurs in 15%–21% of patients. Ulcerative stomatitis (erythema or ulcers of oral mucosa, glossitis, gingivitis), pneumonia, and benign skin neoplasms occur occasionally. Pancreatitis, hepatomegaly, and lactic acidosis have been reported.

✏ see color pill atlas   🌿 herb   underlined – top prescribed drug

NURSING CONSIDERATIONS

BASELINE ASSESSMENT

Obtain baseline laboratory testing, especially serum liver function testing, before beginning stavudine therapy and at periodic intervals during therapy. Offer emotional support to patient and family. Question for previous history of peripheral neuropathy.

INTERVENTION/EVALUATION

Monitor for peripheral neuropathy (characterized by paraesthesia in extremities). Symptoms resolve promptly if therapy is discontinued (symptoms may worsen temporarily after drug is withdrawn). If symptoms resolve completely, reduced dosage may be resumed. Assess for headache, nausea, vomiting, myalgia. Monitor skin for evidence of rash, signs of fever. Determine pattern of bowel activity and stool consistency. Assess for myalgia, arthralgia, dizziness. Monitor sleep patterns. Assess eating pattern; monitor for weight loss. Check eyes for signs of conjunctivitis. Monitor CBC, Hgb, serum liver and renal function, CD4 cell count, HIV RNA levels.

PATIENT/FAMILY TEACHING

• Continue therapy for full length of treatment. • Doses should be evenly spaced. • Do not take any medications, including OTC drugs, without consulting physician. • Stavudine is not a cure for HIV infection, nor does it reduce risk of transmission to others. • Patient may continue to experience illnesses, including opportunistic infections. • Report tingling, burning, pain, numbness, abdominal discomfort, nausea, vomiting, fatigue, dyspnea, weakness.

Strattera, *see atomoxetine*

streptokinase ⚐

strep-toe-**kye**-nase
(Kabikinase, Streptase)

◆CLASSIFICATION

PHARMACOTHERAPEUTIC: Enzyme.
CLINICAL: Thrombolytic (see p. 32C).

ACTION

An enzyme that activates the fibrinolytic system by converting plasminogen to plasmin, an enzyme that degrades fibrin clots. Acts indirectly by forming a complex with plasminogen, which converts plasminogen to plasmin. Action occurs within the thrombus, on its surface, and in circulating blood. **Therapeutic Effect:** Destroys thrombi.

PHARMACOKINETICS

Rapidly cleared from plasma by antibodies and the reticuloendothelial system. Route of elimination unknown. Duration of action continues for several hours after drug has been discontinued. **Half-life:** 23 min.

USES

Management of acute MI (lyses thrombi obstructing coronary arteries, decreases infarct size, improves ventricular function after MI, decreases CHF, mortality associated with MI). Lysis of diagnosed pulmonary emboli, acute or extensive thrombi of deep veins, acute arterial thrombi or emboli.

PRECAUTIONS

CONTRAINDICATIONS: Carcinoma of the brain, cerebrovascular accident, internal bleeding, intracranial surgery, recent streptococcal infection, severe hypertension. **CAUTIONS:** Major surgery within 10 days, GI bleeding, recent trauma.

S

✽ Canadian trade name   © see   ⚐ High Alert drug

⧗ **LIFESPAN CONSIDERATIONS: Pregnancy/Lactation:** Use only when benefit outweighs potential risk to fetus. Unknown if drug crosses placenta or is distributed in breast milk. **Pregnancy Category C. Children:** Safety and efficacy not established. **Elderly:** May have increased risk of intracranial hemorrhage; caution recommended.

INTERACTIONS

DRUG: Anticoagulants, heparin: May increase the risk of hemorrhage. **Platelet aggregation inhibitors such as aspirin:** May increase the risk of bleeding. **HERBAL:** None known. **FOOD:** None known. **LAB VALUES:** Decreases serum plasminogen and fibrinogen level during infusion, decreasing clotting time and confirming presence of lysis.

AVAILABILITY (Rx)

POWDER FOR INJECTION (KABIKINASE, STREPTASE): 250,000 units, 750,000 units, 1.5 million units.

ADMINISTRATION/HANDLING

◀ **ALERT** ▶ Must be administered within 12–14 hr of clot formation (little effect on older, organized clots).

 IV

Reconstitution • Reconstitute vial with 5 ml D₅W or 0.9% NaCl (preferred). Add diluent slowly to side of vial, roll and tilt to avoid foaming. Do not shake vial. • May further dilute with 50–500 ml in 45-ml in-crements of D₅W or 0.9% NaCl.

Rate of administration

PERIPHERAL IV ADMINISTRATION FOR CORONARY ARTERY THROMBI
• Give 1.5 million international units over 60 min.

DIRECT INTRACORONARY ADMINISTRATION FOR CORONARY ARTERY THROMBI
• Give bolus dose over 25–30 sec using coronary catheter. Follow with 2,000 international units/min for 60 min.

DEEP VEIN THROMBOSIS, PULMONARY ARTERIAL EMBOLISM, ARTERIAL THROMBI
• Give single dose over 25–30 min. Follow with maintenance dose of 100,000 or more every hr for 24–72 hr.
• Monitor BP during infusion (hypotension may be severe, occurs in 1%–10% of patients). Decrease of infusion rate may be necessary • If uncontrolled hemorrhage occurs, discontinue infusion immediately (slowing rate of infusion may produce worsening hemorrhage). Do not use dextran to control hemorrhage.

Storage • Store unopened vials at room temperature. Refrigerate reconstituted solution. Use within 24 hr.

▧ IV INCOMPATIBILITIES

Do not mix with medications other than dobutamine (Dobutrex), dopamine (Intropin), heparin, lidocaine, and nitroglycerin.

IV COMPATIBILITIES

Dobutamine (Dobutrex), dopamine (Intropin), heparin, lidocaine, nitroglycerin.

INDICATIONS/ROUTES/DOSAGE

ACUTE EVOLVING TRANSMURAL MI (GIVEN AS SOON AS POSSIBLE AFTER SYMPTOMS OCCUR)
IV INFUSION: ADULTS, ELDERLY (1.5 MILLION UNITS DILUTED TO 45 ML): 1.5 million units infused over 60 min.
INTRACORONARY INFUSION: ADULTS, ELDERLY (250,000 UNITS DILUTED TO 125 ML): Initially, 20,000-units (10-ml) bolus; then, 2,000 units/min for 60 min. Total dose: 140,000 units.

PULMONARY EMBOLISM, DEEP VEIN THROMBOSIS (DVT), ARTERIAL THROMBOSIS AND EMBOLISM (GIVEN WITHIN 7 DAYS OF ONSET)

S

IV INFUSION: ADULTS, ELDERLY (1.5 MILLION UNITS DILUTED TO 90 ML): Initially, 250,000 units infused over 30 min; then, 100,000 units/hr for 24–72 hr for arterial thrombosis or embolism, and pulmonary embolism, 72 hr for DVT.

INTRA-ATERIAL INFUSION: ADULTS, ELDERLY (1.5 MILLION UNITS DILUTED TO 45 ML): Initially, 250,000 units infused over 30 min; then 100,000 units/hr for maintenance.

SIDE EFFECTS

FREQUENT: Fever, superficial bleeding at puncture sites, decreased BP. **OCCASIONAL:** Allergic reaction, including rash and wheezing; ecchymosis.

ADVERSE REACTIONS/ TOXIC EFFECTS

Severe internal hemorrhage may occur. Lysis of coronary thrombi may produce life-threatening arrhythmias.

NURSING CONSIDERATIONS

BASELINE ASSESSMENT

Assess Hct, platelet count, thrombin, aPTT, PT, fibrinogen level before therapy is instituted. If heparin is component of treatment, discontinue before streptokinase is instituted (PT/aPTT should be less than twice normal value before institution of therapy).

INTERVENTION/EVALUATION

Assess clinical response, vital signs per protocol. Handle patient carefully and as infrequently as possible to prevent ecchymoses and bleeding. Do not obtain BP in lower extremities (possible deep vein thrombi). Monitor thrombin, PT, aPTT, fibrinogen level q4h after initiation of therapy. Check stool for occult blood. Assess for decrease in BP, increase in pulse rate, complaint of abdominal or back pain, severe headache (may be evidence of hemorrhage). Question for increase in amount of discharge during menses. Assess area of peripheral thromboembolus for color, temperature. Assess peripheral pulses, skin for ecchymosis, petechiae. Check for excessive bleeding from minor cuts, scratches. Assess urine for hematuria. Monitor BP, platelets, Hgb, Hct, signs of bleeding.

---

streptomycin sulfate

(Streptomycin)
See Antibiotic: aminoglycosides (p. 20C)

---

succinylcholine chloride

(Anectine, Quelicin)
See Neuromuscular blockers (p. 112C)

---

sucralfate

soo-**kral**-fate
(Apo-Sucralate ✦, Carafate, Novo-Sucralate ✦)
Do not confuse Carafate with Cafergot.

✦CLASSIFICATION
CLINICAL: Antiulcer.

ACTION

An antiulcer agent that forms an ulcer-adherent complex with proteinaceous

---

exudate, such as albumin, at ulcer site. Also forms a viscous, adhesive barrier on the surface of intact mucosa of the stomach or duodenum. **Therapeutic Effect:** Protects damaged mucosa from further destruction by absorbing gastric acid, pepsin, and bile salts.

PHARMACOKINETICS

Minimally absorbed from the GI tract. Eliminated in feces, with small amount excreted in urine. Not removed by hemodialysis.

USES

Short-term treatment (up to 8 wk) of duodenal ulcer. Maintenance therapy of duodenal ulcer after healing of acute ulcers. OFF-LABEL: Prevention and treatment of stress-related mucosal damage, especially in acutely or critically ill patients; treatment of gastric ulcer and rheumatoid arthritis; relief of GI symptoms associated with NSAIDs; treatment of gastroesophageal reflux disease.

PRECAUTIONS

CONTRAINDICATIONS: None known. **CAUTIONS:** None known.

⌛ LIFESPAN CONSIDERATIONS: **Pregnancy/Lactation:** Unknown if drug crosses placenta or is distributed in breast milk. **Pregnancy Category B. Children:** Safety and efficacy not established. **Elderly:** No age-related precautions noted.

INTERACTIONS

DRUG: **Antacids:** May interfere with binding of sucralfate. **Digoxin, phenytoin, quinolones, such as ciprofloxacin, theophylline:** May decrease the absorption of these drugs. HERBAL: None known. FOOD: None known. LAB VALUES: None known.

AVAILABILITY (Rx)

ORAL SUSPENSION: 1 g/10 ml. **TABLETS:** 1 g.

ADMINISTRATION/HANDLING

PO
• Administer 1 hr before meals and at bedtime. • Tablets may be crushed and dissolved in water. • Avoid antacids for 30 min before or after giving sucralfate. Shake suspension well before using.

INDICATIONS/ROUTES/DOSAGE

ACTIVE DUODENAL ULCERS
PO: ADULTS, ELDERLY: 1 g 4 times a day (before meals and at bedtime) for up to 8 wk.

MAINTENANCE THERAPY AFTER HEALING OF ACUTE DUODENAL ULCERS
PO: ADULTS, ELDERLY: 1 g twice a day.

SIDE EFFECTS

FREQUENT (2%): Constipation. **OCCASIONAL (less than 2%):** Dry mouth, backache, diarrhea, dizziness, somnolence, nausea, indigestion, rash, hives, itching, abdominal discomfort.

ADVERSE REACTIONS/ TOXIC EFFECTS

Bezoars (ingested compaction that does not pass into intestine) have been reported in patients treated with sucralfate.

NURSING CONSIDERATIONS

INTERVENTION/EVALUATION
Monitor pattern of bowel activity and stool consistency.

PATIENT/FAMILY TEACHING
• Take medication on an empty stomach. • Antacids may be given as

an adjunct but should not be taken for 30 min before or after sucralfate (formation of sucralfate gel is activated by stomach acid). • Dry mouth may be relieved by sour hard candy, sips of tepid water.

Sudafed, *see*
pseudoephedrine

---

sufentanil citrate

(Sufenta)
See Opioid analgesics

---

sulconazole nitrate

(Exelderm)
See Antifungals: topical

---

sulfacetamide ⓔ
sodium

sul-fah-**see**-tah-mide

(AK-Sulf, Belph-10, Cetamide ✤, Dio-sulf ✤, Ocusulf-10, Sodium Sula-myd ✤, Sulf-10)

◆**CLASSIFICATION**

PHARMACOTHERAPEUTIC: Sulfonamide. **CLINICAL:** Ophthalmic, topical agent.

ACTION

Interferes with synthesis of folic acid that bacteria require for growth. **Therapeutic Effect:** Prevents further bacterial growth. Bacteriostatic.

USES

Treatment and prophylaxis of conjunctivitis, corneal ulcers, superficial ocular infections. **OFF-LABEL:** Treatment of bacterial blepharitis, blepharoconjunctivitis, bacterial keratitis, keratoconjunctivitis.

PRECAUTIONS

CONTRAINDICATIONS: Infants younger than 2 mo, herpes simplex keratitis, varicella, other viral diseases of cornea/conjunctiva, fungal disease. **CAUTIONS:** Severe dry eye, G6PD deficiency. **Pregnancy Category C.**

INTERACTIONS

DRUG: Silver-containing preparations: May cause additive effects. **HERBAL:** None known. **FOOD:** None known. **LAB VALUES:** None known.

AVAILABILITY (Rx)

OPHTHALMIC OINTMENT (AK-SULF, BLEPH-10): 10%. **OPHTHALMIC SOLUTION: (BLEPH-10, OCUSULF-10, SULF-10):** 10%.

INDICATIONS/ROUTES/DOSAGE

USUAL OPHTHALMIC DOSAGE
OPHTHALMIC: ADULTS, ELDERLY, CHILDREN OLDER THAN 2 MO: **Ointment:** Apply small amount in lower conjunctival sac 1–4 times a day and at bedtime. **Solution:** 1–2 drops to lower conjunctival sac q2–3h.

SIDE EFFECTS

FREQUENT: Transient ophthalmic burning, stinging. **OCCASIONAL:** Headache. **RARE:** Hypersensitivity: erythema, rash, itching, swelling, photosensitivity.

ADVERSE REACTIONS/ TOXIC EFFECTS

Superinfection, drug-induced lupus erythematosus, Stevens-Johnson syndrome occur rarely.

NURSING CONSIDERATIONS

BASELINE ASSESSMENT

Question for hypersensitivity to sulfonamides, any ingredients of preparation (e.g., sulfite).

INTERVENTION/EVALUATION

Withhold medication, notify physician at once of hypersensitivity reaction (redness, itching, urticaria, rash). Assess for fever, arthralgia, stomatitis—hold drug, inform physician.

PATIENT/FAMILY TEACHING

• May have transient burning, stinging upon ophthalmic application; may cause sensitivity to light; wear sunglasses, avoid bright light. • Notify physician of **any** new symptom, especially swelling, itching, rash, joint pain, fever.

---

sulfasalazine

sul-fa-**sal**-a-zeen

(Alti-Sulfasalazine ✸, Azulfidine, Azulfidine EN-tabs, Salazopyrin ✸, Salazopyrin EN-Tabs ✸)

Do not confuse Azulfidine with azathioprine, or sulfasalazine with sulfadiazine or sulfisoxazole.

•CLASSIFICATION

PHARMACOTHERAPEUTIC: Sulfonamide. **CLINICAL:** Anti-inflammatory.

ACTION

A sulfonamide that inhibits prostaglandin synthesis, acting locally in the colon. **Therapeutic Effect:** Decreases inflammatory response, interferes with GI secretion.

PHARMACOKINETICS

Poorly absorbed from the GI tract. Cleaved in colon by intestinal bacteria, forming sulfapyridine and mesalamine (5-ASA). Absorbed in colon. Widely distributed. Metabolized in the liver. Primarily excreted in urine. **Half-life:** sulfapyridine, 6–14 hr; 5-ASA, 0.6–1.4 hr.

USES

Treatment of ulcerative colitis, rheumatoid arthritis. **OFF-LABEL:** Treatment of ankylosing spondylitis, collagenous colitis, Chrohn's disease, juvenile chronic arthritis, psoriasis, psoriatic arthritis.

PRECAUTIONS

CONTRAINDICATIONS: Children younger than 2 yr; hypersensitivity to carbonic anhydrase inhibitors, local anesthetics, salicylates, sulfonamides, sulfonylureas, sunscreens containing PABA, or thiazide or loop diuretics; intestinal or urinary tract obstruction; porphyria; pregnancy at term; severe hepatic or renal dysfunction. **CAUTIONS:** Severe allergies, bronchial asthma, impaired hepatic or renal function, G6PD deficiency.

⧗ **LIFESPAN CONSIDERATIONS: Pregnancy/Lactation:** May produce infertility, oligospermia in men while taking medication. Readily crosses placenta; if given near term, may produce jaundice, hemolytic anemia, kernicterus. Excreted in breast milk. Do not breastfeed premature infant or those with hyperbilirubinemia or G6PD deficiency. **Pregnancy Category B (D if given near term). Children/Elderly:** No

---

age-related precautions noted in those older than 2 yr.

INTERACTIONS

DRUG: **Anticonvulsants, methotrexate, oral anticoagulants, oral antidiabetics:** May increase the effects of these drugs. **Hemolytics:** May increase the toxicity of sulfasalazine. **Hepatotoxic medications:** May increase the risk of hepatotoxicity. HERBAL: None known. FOOD: None known. LAB VALUES: None known.

AVAILABILITY (Rx)

TABLETS (AZULFIDINE): 500 mg. **TABLETS (DELAYED-RELEASE [AZULFIDINE EN-TABS]):** 500 mg.

ADMINISTRATION/HANDLING

PO
• Space doses evenly (intervals not to exceed 8 hr). • Administer after meals if possible (prolongs intestinal passage). • Swallow enteric-coated tablets whole; do not chew. • Give with 8 oz of water; encourage several glasses of water between meals.

INDICATIONS/ROUTES/DOSAGE

ULCERATIVE COLITIS
PO: ADULTS, ELDERLY: 1 g 3–4 times a day in divided doses q4–6h. Maintenance: 2 g/day in divided doses q6–12h. **Maximum:** 6 g/day. CHILDREN: 40–75 mg/kg/day in divided doses q4–6h. Maintenance: 30–50 mg/kg/day in divided doses q4–8h. **Maximum:** 2 g/day. **Maximum:** 6 g/day.

RHEUMATOID ARTHRITIS
PO: ADULTS, ELDERLY: Initially, 0.5–1 g/day for 1 wk. Increase by 0.5 g/wk, up to 3 g/day.

JUVENILE RHEUMATOID ARTHRITIS
PO: CHILDREN: Initially, 10 mg/kg/day. May increase by 10 mg/kg/day at weekly intervals. Range: 30–50 mg/kg/day. **Maximum:** 2 g/day.

SIDE EFFECTS

FREQUENT (33%): Anorexia, nausea, vomiting, headache, oligospermia (generally reversed by withdrawal of drug). **OCCASIONAL (3%):** Hypersensitivity reaction (rash, urticaria, pruritus, fever, anemia). **RARE (less than 1%):** Tinnitus, hypoglycemia, diuresis, photosensitivity.

ADVERSE REACTIONS/ TOXIC EFFECTS

Anaphylaxis, Stevens-Johnson syndrome, hematologic toxicity (leukopenia, agranulocytosis), hepatotoxicity, and nephrotoxicity occur rarely.

NURSING CONSIDERATIONS

BASELINE ASSESSMENT
Question for hypersensitivity to medications. Check initial urinalysis, CBC, serum liver and renal function tests.

INTERVENTION/EVALUATION
Monitor I&O, urinalysis, renal function tests; ensure adequate hydration (minimum output 1,500 ml/24 hr) to prevent nephrotoxicity. Assess skin for rash (discontinue drug and notify physician at first sign). Monitor pattern of bowel activity and stool consistency (dosage may need to be increased if diarrhea continues or recurs). Monitor CBC closely; assess for and report immediately any hematologic effects: bleeding, ecchymoses, fever, pharyngitis, pallor, weakness, purpura, jaundice.

PATIENT/FAMILY TEACHING
• May cause orange-yellow discoloration of urine, skin. • Space doses evenly around the clock. • Take after food with 8 oz of water; drink several glasses

of water between meals. • Continue for full length of treatment; may be necessary to take drug even after symptoms relieved. • Follow-up, lab tests are essential. • In event of dental or other surgery, inform dentist or surgeon of sulfasalazine therapy. • Avoid exposure to sun, ultraviolet light until photosensitivity determined (may last for months after last dose).

sulindac

sul-**in**-dak

(Apo-Sulin ✦, Clinoril, Novo-Sundac ✦)

Do not confuse Clinoril with Clozaril.

CLASSIFICATION

PHARMACOTHERAPEUTIC: Nonsteroidal anti-inflammatory. **CLINICAL:** Anti-inflammatory, antigout (see p. 117C).

ACTION

An NSAID that produces analgesic and anti-inflammatory effects by inhibiting prostaglandin synthesis. **Therapeutic Effect:** Reduces inflammatory response and intensity of pain.

PHARMACOKINETICS

Route	Onset	Peak	Duration
PO (Antirheu-matic)	7 days	2–3 wk	N/A

Well absorbed from the GI tract. Metabolized in liver to active metabolite. Primarily excreted in urine. Not removed by hemodialysis. **Half-life:** 7.8 hr; metabolite: 16.4 hr.

USES

Treatment of pain of rheumatoid arthritis, osteoarthritis, ankylosing spondylitis, acute painful shoulder, bursitis or tendinitis, acute gouty arthritis.

PRECAUTIONS

CONTRAINDICATIONS: Active peptic ulcer disease, chronic inflammation of GI tract, GI bleeding or ulceration, history of hypersensitivity to aspirin or NSAIDs. **CAUTIONS:** Renal or hepatic impairment, history of GI tract disease, predisposition to fluid retention, concurrent anticoagulant use.

⧖ **LIFESPAN CONSIDERATIONS: Pregnancy/Lactation:** Unknown if drug is excreted in breast milk. Avoid use during third trimester (may adversely affect fetal cardiovascular system: premature closure of ductus arteriosus). **Pregnancy Category B (D if used in third trimester or near delivery). Children:** Safety and efficacy not established. **Elderly:** GI bleeding or ulceration more likely to cause serious adverse effects. Age-related renal impairment may increase risk of hepatic or renal toxicity; lower dosage recommended.

INTERACTIONS

DRUG: Antacids: May decrease the sulindac blood concentration. **Antihypertensives, diuretics:** May decrease the effects of these drugs. **Aspirin, other salicylates:** May increase the risk of GI side effects such as bleeding. **Bone marrow depressants:** May increase the risk of hematologic reactions. **Heparin, oral anticoagulants, thrombolytics:** May increase the effects of these drugs. **Lithium:** May increase the blood concentration and risk of toxicity of lithium. **Methotrexate:** May increase the risk of methotrexate toxicity. **Probenecid:** May increase the sulindac blood concentration. **HERBAL: Feverfew:** May decrease the effects of feverfew. **Ginkgo biloba:** May increase the risk

---

🔖 see color pill atlas   🌱 herb   <u>underlined</u> – top prescribed drug

of bleeding. **FOOD:** None known. **LAB VALUES:** May increase liver function test results and serum alkaline phosphatase level.

AVAILABILITY (Rx)
TABLETS: 150 mg, 200 mg.

ADMINISTRATION/HANDLING
PO
• Give with food, milk, antacids if GI distress occurs.

INDICATIONS/ROUTES/DOSAGE
RHEUMATOID ARTHRITIS, OSTEOARTHRITIS, ANKYLOSING SPONDYLITIS
PO: ADULTS, ELDERLY: Initially, 150 mg twice a day; may increase up to 400 mg/day.
ACUTE SHOULDER PAIN, GOUTY ARTHRITIS, BURSITIS, TENDINITIS
PO: ADULTS, ELDERLY: 200 mg twice a day.

SIDE EFFECTS
FREQUENT (9%–4%): Diarrhea or constipation, indigestion, nausea, maculopapular rash, dermatitis, dizziness, headache. **OCCASIONAL (3%–1%):** Anorexia, abdominal cramps, flatulence.

ADVERSE REACTIONS/ TOXIC EFFECTS
Rare reactions with long-term use include peptic ulcer disease GI bleeding, gastritis, nephrotoxicity (glomerular nephritis, interstitial nephritis, nephrotic syndrome), severe hepatic reactions (cholestasis, jaundice), and severe hypersensitivity reactions (fever, chills, and joint pain).

NURSING CONSIDERATIONS

BASELINE ASSESSMENT
Assess onset, type, location, duration of pain, fever, inflammation. Inspect appearance of affected joints for immobility, deformities, skin condition.

INTERVENTION/EVALUATION
Assist with ambulation if dizziness occurs. Monitor pattern of daily bowel activity and stool consistency. Assess for evidence of rash. Evaluate for therapeutic response: relief of pain, stiffness, swelling; increased joint mobility; reduced joint tenderness; improved grip strength. Monitor serum hepatic and renal function, CBC, platelets.

PATIENT/FAMILY TEACHING
• Therapeutic antiarthritic effect noted 1–3 wk after therapy begins. • Avoid aspirin, alcohol during therapy (increases risk of GI bleeding). • If GI upset occurs, take with food, milk. • Avoid tasks that require alertness, motor skills until response to drug is established (may cause dizziness).

sumatriptan

soo-ma-**trip**-tan

(Imitrex, Imitrex Nasal, Imitrex Statdose, Imitrex Statdose Refill)
Do not confuse sumatriptan with somatropin.

CLASSIFICATION
PHARMACOTHERAPEUTIC: Serotonin receptor agonist. **CLINICAL:** Antimigraine (see p. 56C).

ACTION
A serotonin receptor agonist that binds selectively to vascular receptors, producing a vasoconstrictive effect on cranial blood vessels. **Therapeutic Effect:** Relieves migraine headache.

PHARMACOKINETICS

Route	Onset	Peak	Duration
Nasal	15 min	N/A	24–48 hr
PO	30 min	2 hr	24–48 hr
Subcutaneous	10 min	1 hr	24–48 hr

Rapidly absorbed after subcutaneous administration. Absorption after PO administration is incomplete, with significant amounts undergoing hepatic metabolism, resulting in low bio-availability (about 14%). Protein binding: 10%–21%. Widely distributed. Undergoes first-pass metabolism in the liver. Excreted in urine. Half-life: 2 hr.

USES

Acute treatment of migraine headache with or without aura; treatment of cluster headaches.

PRECAUTIONS

CONTRAINDICATIONS: Cerebrovascular accident (CVA), ischemic heart disease (including angina pectoris, history of MI, silent ischemia, and Prinzmetal's angina), severe hepatic impairment, transient ischemic attack, uncontrolled hypertension, use within 14 days of MAOIs, use within 24 hr of ergotamine preparations. **CAUTIONS:** Hepatic or renal impairment, epilepsy, hypersensitivity to sulfonamides.

⧗ LIFESPAN CONSIDERATIONS: **Pregnancy/Lactation:** Unknown if distributed in breast milk. **Pregnancy Category C. Children:** Safety and efficacy not established. **Elderly:** No age-related precautions noted.

INTERACTIONS

DRUG: **Ergotamine-containing medications:** May produce vasospastic reaction. **MAOIs:** May increase sumatriptan blood concentration and half-life.

HERBAL: None known. FOOD: None known. LAB VALUES: None known.

AVAILABILITY (Rx)

TABLETS (IMITREX): 25 mg, 50 mg, 100 mg. **INJECTION (IMITREX STATDOSE):** 6 mg/0.5 ml, 4 mg prefilled cartridge. **NASAL SPRAY (IMITREX NASAL):** 5 mg, 20 mg.

ADMINISTRATION/HANDLING

SUBCUTANEOUS
• Follow patient instructions provided by manufacturer using autoinjection device.

PO
• Swallow tablets whole. • Take with full glass of water.

NASAL
• Unit contains only one spray—do not test before use. • Instruct the patient to gently blow nose to clear nasal passages. • With head upright, have the patient close one nostril with index finger and breathe out gently through mouth. • Insert nozzle into open nostril about ½ inch. • Instruct the patient to close mouth, and while taking a breath through nose, release spray dosage by firmly pressing the blue plunger. • Remove nozzle from nose and instruct the patient to gently breathe in through nose and out through mouth for 10–20 sec. Advise the patient not to breathe in deeply.

INDICATIONS/ROUTES/DOSAGE

ACUTE MIGRAINE ATTACK
PO: ADULTS, ELDERLY: 25–50 mg. Dose may be repeated after at least 2 hr. **Maximum:** 100 mg/single dose; 200 mg/24 hr.
SUBCUTANEOUS: ADULTS, ELDERLY: 6 mg. **Maximum:** Two 6-mg injections/24 hr (separated by at least 1 hr).
INTRANASAL: ADULTS, ELDERLY: 5–20 mg; may repeat in 2 hr. **Maximum:** 40 mg/24 hr.

SIDE EFFECTS

FREQUENT: Oral (10%–5%): Tingling, nasal discomfort. **Subcutaneous (greater than 10%):** Injection site reactions, tingling, warm or hot sensation, dizziness, vertigo. **Nasal (greater than 10%):** Bad or unusual taste, nausea, vomiting. **OCCASIONAL: Oral (5%–1%):** Flushing, asthenia, visual disturbances. **Subcutaneous (10%–2%):** Burning sensation, numbness, chest discomfort, drowsiness, asthenia. **Nasal (5%–1%):** Nasopharyngeal discomfort, dizziness. **RARE: Oral (less than 1%):** Agitation, eye irritation, dysuria. **Subcutaneous (less than 2%):** Anxiety, fatigue, diaphoresis, muscle cramps, myalgia. **Nasal (less than 1%):** Burning sensation.

ADVERSE REACTIONS/ TOXIC EFFECTS

Excessive dosage may produce tremor, red extremities, reduced respirations, cyanosis, seizures, and paralysis. Serious arrhythmias occur rarely, especially in patients with hypertension, diabetes, or a strong family history of coronary artery disease; obese patients; and smokers.

NURSING CONSIDERATIONS

BASELINE ASSESSMENT

Question for history of peripheral vascular disease, renal or hepatic impairment, possibility of pregnancy. Question regarding onset, location, duration of migraine and possible precipitating symptoms.

INTERVENTION/EVALUATION

Evaluate for relief of migraine headache and resulting photophobia, phonophobia (sound sensitivity), nausea, vomiting.

PATIENT/FAMILY TEACHING

• Teach patient proper loading of autoinjector, injection technique, and discarding of syringe. • Do not use more than 2 injections during any 24-hr period and allow at least 1 hr between injections. • If wheezing, palpitations, skin rash, facial swelling, pain or tightness in chest or throat occurs, contact physician immediately.

Survanta, *see beractant*

Sustiva, *see efavirenz*

Symlin, *see pramlinitide*

Synagis, *see palivizumab*

Synthroid, *see levothyroxine*

tacrine hydrochloride

tay-crin
(Cognex)

♦CLASSIFICATION
PHARMACOTHERAPEUTIC: Cholinesterase inhibitor. **CLINICAL:** Antidementia.

ACTION
A cholinesterase inhibitor that inhibits the enzyme acetylcholinesterase, thus increasing the concentration of acetylcholine at cholinergic synapses and enhancing cholinergic function in the CNS. **Therapeutic Effect:** Slows the progression of Alzheimer's disease.

PHARMACOKINETICS
Rapidly absorbed following PO administration. Protein binding: 55%. Extensively metabolized in liver. Negligible amounts excreted in urine. **Half-life:** 2–4 hr.

USES
Symptomatic treatment of patients with Alzheimer's disease.

PRECAUTIONS
CONTRAINDICATIONS: Known hypersensitivity to tacrine, patients previously treated with tacrine who developed jaundice. **CAUTIONS:** Known hepatic dysfunction, asthma, chronic obstructive pulmonary disease (COPD), seizure disorders, bradycardia, hyperthyroidism, cardiac arrhythmias, history of gastric or intestinal ulcers, alcohol abuse.

⌛ **LIFESPAN CONSIDERATIONS: Pregnancy/Lactation:** Unknown if distributed in breast milk. **Pregnancy Category C. Children:** Safety and efficacy not established. **Elderly:** No age-related precautions noted.

INTERACTIONS
DRUG: Anticholinergics: May decrease the effects of tacrine or anticholinergics. **Cimetidine:** May increase the tacrine blood concentration. **NSAIDs:** May increase the adverse effects of NSAIDs. **Theophylline:** May increase the theophylline blood concentration. **HERBAL:** None known. **FOOD:** None known. **LAB VALUES:** Increases AST and ALT levels. Alters blood Hgb, Hct, and serum electrolyte levels.

AVAILABILITY (Rx)
CAPSULES: 10 mg, 20 mg, 30 mg, 40 mg.

ADMINISTRATION/HANDLING
PO
• Give without regard to food.

INDICATIONS/ROUTES/DOSAGE
ALZHEIMER'S DISEASE
PO: ADULTS, ELDERLY: Initially, 10 mg 4 times a day for 6 wk, followed by 20 mg 4 times a day for 6 wk, 30 mg 4 times a day for 12 wk, then 40 mg 4 times a day if needed.

DOSAGE IN HEPATIC IMPAIRMENT
For patients with ALT greater than 3–5 times normal, decrease the dose by 40 mg/day and resume the normal dose when ALT returns to normal. For patients with ALT greater than 5 times normal, stop treatment and resume it when ALT returns to normal.

SIDE EFFECTS
FREQUENT (28%–11%): Headache, nausea, vomiting, diarrhea, dizziness. **OCCASIONAL (9%–4%):** Fatigue, chest pain, dyspepsia, anorexia, abdominal pain, flatulence, constipation, confusion, agitation, rash, depression, ataxia, insomnia, rhinitis, myalgia. **RARE (less than 3%):** Weight loss, anxiety, cough, facial flushing, urinary frequency, back pain, tremor.

ADVERSE REACTIONS/ TOXIC EFFECTS

Overdose can cause cholinergic crisis, marked by increased salivation, lacrimation, bradycardia, respiratory depression, hypotension, and increased muscle weakness. Treatment usually consists of supportive measures and an anticholinergic such as atropine.

NURSING CONSIDERATIONS

BASELINE ASSESSMENT
Assess cognitive, behavioral, functional deficits of patient. Assess liver function.

INTERVENTION/EVALUATION
Monitor cognitive, behavioral, functional status of patient. Monitor AST, ALT. EKG evaluation, periodic rhythm strips in patients with underlying arrhythmias. Monitor for symptoms of ulcer, GI bleeding.

PATIENT/FAMILY TEACHING
• Take at regular intervals, between meals (may take with meals if GI upset occurs). • Do not reduce or stop medication; do not increase dosage without physician direction. • Do not smoke (reduces plasma concentration of tacrine). • Inform family of local chapter of Alzheimer's Disease Association (provides a guide to services for these patients).

---

tacrolimus

tack-row-**lee**-mus

(Prograf, Protopic)

Do not confuse Protopic with Protonix, Protopam, Protopin.

◆ CLASSIFICATION

PHARMACOTHERAPEUTIC: Immunologic agent. **CLINICAL:** Immunosuppressant (see p. 107C).

ACTION

An immunologic agent that inhibits T-lymphocyte activation by binding to intracellular proteins, forming a complex, and inhibiting phosphatase activity. **Therapeutic Effect:** Suppresses the immunologically mediated inflammatory response; prevents organ transplant rejection.

PHARMACOKINETICS

Variably absorbed after PO administration (food reduces absorption). Protein binding: 75%–97%. Extensively metabolized in the liver. Excreted in urine. Not removed by hemodialysis. **Half-life:** 11.7 hr.

USES

Oral/injection: Prophylaxis of organ rejection in patients receiving allogeneic liver transplants, kidney transplants, heart transplant. Should be used concurrently with adrenal corticosteroids. **Topical:** Atopic dermatitis. **OFF-LABEL:** Prevention of organ rejection in patients receiving allogeneic bone marrow, heart, pancreas, pancreatic island cell, or small-bowel transplant, treatment of autoimmune disease, severe recalcitrant psoriasis.

PRECAUTIONS

◀ **ALERT** ▶ There is a potential cancer risk in using topical Protoptic ointment. **CONTRAINDICATIONS:** Concurrent use with cyclosporine (increases the risk of nephrotoxicity), hypersensitivity to HCO-60 polyoxyl 60 hydrogenated castor oil (used in solution for injection). **CAUTIONS:** Immunosuppressed patients, renal or hepatic impairment.

⚕ **LIFESPAN CONSIDERATIONS: Pregnancy/Lactation:** Crosses placenta. Neonatal hyperkalemia, renal dysfunction noted in neonates. Excreted in breast milk. Avoid breast-feeding. **Pregnancy Category C. Children:** May require higher dosages (decreased bioavailability, increased clearance). May make post-transplant lymphoproliferative disorder more common (especially in those younger than 3 yr). **Elderly:** Age-related renal impairment may require dosage adjustment.

INTERACTIONS

DRUG: Aminoglycosides, amphotericin B, cisplatin: May increase the risk of renal dysfunction. **Antacids:** May decrease the absorption of tacrolimus. **Antifungals, bromocriptine, calcium channel blockers, cimetidine, clarithromycin, cyclosporine, danazol, diltiazem, erythromycin, methylprednisolone, metoclopramide:** Increase tacrolimus blood concentration. **Carbamazepine, phenobarbital, phenytoin, rifamycin:** Decrease tacrolimus blood concentration. **Cyclosporine:** Increases the risk of nephrotoxicity. **Live virus vaccines:** May potentiate virus replication, increase vaccine side effects, and decrease the patient's antibody response to the vaccine. **Other immunosuppressants:** May increase the risk of infection or lymphomas. **HERBAL: Echinacea:** May decrease the effects of tacrolimus. **FOOD: Grapefruit, grapefruit juice:** May alter the effects of the drug. **LAB VALUES:** May increase blood glucose, BUN, and serum creatinine levels, as well as WBC count. May decrease serum magnesium level and RBC and thrombocyte counts. May alter serum potassium level.

AVAILABILITY (Rx)

CAPSULES (PROGRAF): 0.5 mg, 1 mg, 5 mg. **INJECTION (PROGRAF):** 5 mg/ml. **OINTMENT (PROTOPIC):** 0.03%, 0.1%.

ADMINISTRATION/HANDLING

IV

Reconstitution • Dilute with an appropriate amount (250–1,000 ml, depending on desired dose) 0.9% NaCl or D$_5$W to provide a concentration between 0.004 and 0.02 mg/ml.

Rate of administration • Give as continuous IV infusion. • Continuously monitor patient for anaphylaxis for at least 30 min after start of infusion. • Stop infusion immediately at first sign of hypersensitivity reaction.

Storage • Store diluted infusion solution in glass or polyethylene containers and discard after 24 hr. • Do not store in a PVC container (decreased stability, potential for extraction).

PO
• Administer on empty stomach. • Do not give with grapefruit or grapefruit juice or within 2 hr of antacids.

TOPICAL
• For external use only. • Do not cover with occlusive dressing. • Rub in gently and completely onto clean, dry skin.

IV INCOMPATIBILITIES

No known drug incompatibilities. Do not mix tacrolimus with other medications if possible.

IV COMPATIBILITIES

Calcium gluconate, dexamethasone (Decadron), diphenhydramine (Benadryl), dobutamine (Dobutrex), dopamine (Intropin), furosemide (Lasix), heparin, hydromorphone (Dilaudid), insulin, leucovorin, lorazepam (Ativan), morphine, nitroglycerin, potassium chloride.

INDICATIONS/ROUTES/DOSAGE

PREVENTION OF LIVER TRANSPLANT REJECTION
PO: ADULTS, ELDERLY: 0.1–0.15 mg/kg/day in 2 divided doses 12 hr apart. CHILDREN: 0.15–0.2 mg/kg/day in 2 divided doses 12 hr apart.
IV: ADULTS, ELDERLY, CHILDREN: 0.03–0.05 mg/kg/day as continuous infusion.

PREVENTION OF KIDNEY TRANSPLANT REJECTION

PO: ADULTS, ELDERLY: 0.2 mg/kg/day in 2 divided doses 12 hr apart.
IV: ADULTS, ELDERLY: 0.03–0.05 mg/kg/day as continuous infusion.

ATOPIC DERMATITIS

TOPICAL: ADULTS, ELDERLY, CHILDREN 2 YR AND OLDER: Apply 0.03% ointment to affected area twice a day. 0.1% ointment may be used in adults and the elderly. Continue until 1 wk after symptoms have cleared.

SIDE EFFECTS

FREQUENT (greater than 30%): Headache, tremor, insomnia, paresthesia, diarrhea, nausea, constipation, vomiting, abdominal pain, hypertension. **OCCASIONAL (29%–10%):** Rash, pruritus, anorexia, asthenia, peripheral edema, photosensitivity.

ADVERSE REACTIONS/ TOXIC EFFECTS

Nephrotoxicity (characterized by increased serum creatinine level and decreased urine output), neurotoxicity (including tremor, headache, and mental status changes), and pleural effusion are common adverse reactions. Thrombocytopenia, leukocytosis, anemia, atelectasis, sepsis, and infection occur occasionally.

NURSING CONSIDERATIONS

BASELINE ASSESSMENT

Assess medical history, especially renal function, and drug history, especially other immunosuppressants. Have aqueous solution of epinephrine 1:1,000 available at bedside as well as O_2 before beginning IV infusion. Assess patient continuously for first 30 min following start of infusion and at frequent intervals thereafter.

INTERVENTION/EVALUATION

Closely monitor patients with impaired renal function. Monitor lab values, especially serum creatinine, potassium levels, CBC with differential, serum liver function tests. Monitor I&O closely. CBC should be performed weekly during first month of therapy, twice monthly during second and third months of treatment, then monthly throughout the first year. Report any major change in patient assessment.

PATIENT/FAMILY TEACHING

• Take dose at same time each day.
• Avoid crowds, those with infection.
• Inform physician if decreased urination, chest pain, headache, dizziness, respiratory infection, rash, unusual bleeding or bruising occurs. • Avoid exposure to sun, artificial light (may cause photosensitivity reaction).

tadalafil

tah-**dal**-ah-fill

(Cialis)

CLASSIFICATION

PHARMACOTHERAPEUTIC: Phosphodiesterase inhibitor. **CLINICAL:** Erectile dysfunction adjunct.

ACTION

An erectile dysfunction agent that inhibits phosphodiesterase type 5, the enzyme responsible for degrading cyclic guanosine monophosphate in the corpus cavernosum of the penis, resulting in smooth muscle relaxation and increased blood flow. **Therapeutic Effect:** Facilitates an erection.

PHARMACOKINETICS

Route	Onset	Peak	Duration
PO	16 min	2 hr	36 hr

Rapidly absorbed after PO administration. Drug has no effect on penile blood

T

flow without sexual stimulation. Half-life: 17.5 hr.

USES

Treatment of erectile dysfunction.

PRECAUTIONS

CONTRAINDICATIONS: Concurrent use of alpha-adrenergic blockers (other than the minimum dose tamsulosin), concurrent use of sodium nitroprusside or nitrates in any form, severe hepatic impairment. **CAUTIONS:** Renal/hepatic impairment, anatomical deformation of the penis, patients who may be predisposed to priapism (sickle cell anemia, multiple myeloma, leukemia).

⧗ LIFESPAN CONSIDERATIONS: Pregnancy/Lactation: **Pregnancy Category B. Children:** This drug is not indicated for use in these groups. **Elderly:** No age-related precautions noted.

INTERACTIONS

DRUG: **Alcohol:** Increases the risk of orthostatic hypotension. **Alpha-adrenergic blockers, nitrates:** Potentiate the hypotensive effects of these drugs. **Erythromycin, indinavir, itraconazole, ketoconazole, ritonavir:** May increase tadalafil blood concentration. HERBAL: None known. FOOD: None known. LAB VALUES: None known.

AVAILABILITY (Rx)

TABLETS: 5 mg, 10 mg, 20 mg.

ADMINISTRATION/HANDLING

PO

• May give without regard to food. • Do not crush/break film-coated tablets. • Take before anticipated sexual activity.

INDICATIONS/ROUTES/DOSAGE

ERECTILE DYSFUNCTION

PO: ADULTS, ELDERLY: 10 mg 30 min before sexual activity. Dose may be increased to 20 mg or decreased to 5 mg, based on patient tolerance. Maximum dosing frequency is once daily.

DOSAGE IN RENAL IMPAIRMENT

For patients with a creatinine clearance of 31–50 ml/min: Starting dose is 5 mg before sexual activity once a day and the maximum dose is 10 mg no more frequently than once q48h. **For patients with a creatinine clearance of less than 31 ml/min:** Starting dose is 5 mg before sexual activity once a day.

DOSAGE IN MILD OR MODERATE HEPATIC IMPAIRMENT

Patients with Child-Pugh class A or B hepatic impairment should take no more than 10 mg once a day.

SIDE EFFECTS

OCCASIONAL: Headache, dyspepsia, back pain, myalgia, nasal congestion, flushing.

ADVERSE REACTIONS/ TOXIC EFFECTS

Prolonged erections (lasting over 4 hr) and priapism (painful erections lasting over 6 hr) occur rarely. Angina, chest pain, and MI have been reported.

NURSING CONSIDERATIONS

BASELINE ASSESSMENT

Assess cardiovascular status before initiating treatment for erectile dysfunction.

PATIENT/FAMILY TEACHING

• Has no effect in the absence of sexual stimulation. • Seek treatment immediately if an erection persists for over 4 hr.

Tagamet, *see cimetidine*

Tamiflu, *see oseltamivir*

tamoxifen citrate ▷

tam-**ox**-ih-feen

(Apo-Tamox ♣, Istubol, Nolvadex, Nolvadex-D ♣, Novo-Tamoxifen ♣, Soltamox, Tamofen ♣)

CLASSIFICATION

PHARMACOTHERAPEUTIC: Nonsteroidal antiestrogen. **CLINICAL:** Antineoplastic (see p. 78C).

ACTION

A nonsteroidal antiestrogen that competes with estradiol for estrogen-receptor binding sites in the breasts, uterus, and vagina. Therapeutic Effect: Inhibits DNA synthesis and estrogen response.

PHARMACOKINETICS

Well absorbed from the GI tract. Metabolized in the liver. Primarily eliminated in feces by biliary system. Half-life: 7 days.

USES

Adjunct treatment in advanced breast cancer, reduce risk of breast cancer in patients at high risk, reduce risk of invasive breast cancer in women with ductal carcinoma *in situ* (DCIS), metastatic breast cancer in women and men, treatment of melanoma, desmoid tumors. OFF-LABEL: Induction of ovulation.

PRECAUTIONS

CONTRAINDICATIONS: Concomitant coumarin-type therapy when used in the treatment of breast cancer in high-risk women, history of deep vein thrombosis or pulmonary embolism in high-risk women, pregnancy. **CAUTIONS:** Leukopenia, thrombocytopenia.

⧗ LIFESPAN CONSIDERATIONS: Pregnancy/Lactation: If possible, avoid use during pregnancy, especially first trimester. May cause fetal harm. Unknown if distributed in breast milk.

Breast-feeding not recommended. **Pregnancy Category D. Children:** Safe and effective in girls 2–10 yr with McCune Albright syndrome and precocious puberty. **Elderly:** No age-related precautions noted.

INTERACTIONS

DRUG: **Anticoagulants:** May increase the risk of bleeding. **Estrogens:** May decrease the effects of tamoxifen. HERBAL: **Red clover, St. John's wort:** May decrease tamoxifen's effectiveness. FOOD: None known. LAB VALUES: May increase serum cholesterol, calcium, and triglyceride levels.

AVAILABILITY (Rx)

TABLETS (NOLVADEX): 10 mg, 20 mg.
SOLTAMOX: Oral liquid.

ADMINISTRATION/HANDLING

PO
• Give without regard to food.

INDICATIONS/ROUTES/DOSAGE

ADJUNCTIVE TREATMENT OF BREAST CANCER
PO: ADULTS, ELDERLY: 20–40 mg/day. Give doses greater than 20 mg/day in divided doses.

PREVENTION OF BREAST CANCER IN HIGH-RISK WOMEN
PO: ADULTS, ELDERLY: 20 mg/day.

SIDE EFFECTS

FREQUENT: Women (greater than 10%): Hot flashes, nausea, vomiting. **OCCASIONAL: Women (9%–1%):** Changes in menstruation, genital itching, vaginal discharge, endometrial hyperplasia or polyps. **Men:** Impotence, decreased libido. **Men and women:** Headache, nausea, vomiting, rash, bone pain, confusion, weakness, somnolence.

ADVERSE REACTIONS/TOXIC EFFECTS

Retinopathy, corneal opacity, and decreased visual acuity have been noted

T

---

in patients receiving extremely high dosages (240–320 mg/day) for longer than 17 mo. There have been an increased number of incidences of endometrial changes, thromboembolic events, and uterine malignancies while using tamoxifen.

NURSING CONSIDERATIONS

BASELINE ASSESSMENT

An estrogen receptor assay should be done before therapy is begun. CBC, platelet count, serum calcium levels should be checked before and periodically during therapy.

INTERVENTION/EVALUATION

Be alert to increased bone pain and ensure adequate pain relief. Monitor I&O, weight. Observe for edema, especially of dependent areas. Assess for hypercalcemia (increased urine volume, excessive thirst, nausea, vomiting, constipation, hypotonicity of muscles, deep bone/flank pain, renal stones).

PATIENT/FAMILY TEACHING

• Report vaginal bleeding/discharge/ itching, leg cramps, weight gain, shortness of breath, weakness. • May initially experience increase in bone, tumor pain (appears to indicate good tumor response). • Contact physician if nausea/vomiting continues at home. • Nonhormonal contraceptives are recommended during treatment.

---

tamsulosin hydrochloride

tam-**sool**-o-sin

(Flomax)

Do not confuse Flomax with Fosamax or Volmax.

◆CLASSIFICATION

PHARMACOTHERAPEUTIC: Alpha$_1$-adrenergic blocker. **CLINICAL:** Benign prostatic hyperplasia agent.

ACTION

An alpha$_1$ antagonist that targets receptors around bladder neck and prostate capsule. **Therapeutic Effect:** Relaxes smooth muscle and improves urinary flow and symptoms of prostatic hyperplasia.

PHARMACOKINETICS

Well absorbed and widely distributed. Protein binding: 94%–99%. Metabolized in the liver. Primarily excreted in urine. Unknown if removed by hemodialysis. **Half-life:** 9–13 hr.

USES

Treatment of symptoms of benign prostatic hyperplasia.

PRECAUTIONS

CONTRAINDICATIONS: Concurrent use of sildenafil, tadalafil, or vardenafil. **CAUTIONS:** Renal impairment.

⧖ **LIFESPAN CONSIDERATIONS: Pregnancy/Lactation:** Not indicated for use in women. **Pregnancy Category B (Not indicated for use in women.). Children:** Not indicated in this patient population. **Elderly:** No age-related precautions noted.

INTERACTIONS

DRUG: Other alpha-adrenergic blocking agents (such as cimetidine, doxazosin, prazosin, terazosin): May increase the alpha-blockade effects of both drugs. **Warfarin:** May alter the effects of warfarin. **HERBAL:** None known. **FOOD:** None known. **LAB VALUES:** None known.

T

AVAILABILITY (Rx)
CAPSULES: 0.4 mg.

ADMINISTRATION/HANDLING
PO
• Give at the same time each day, 30 min after the same meal. • Do not crush or open capsule unless directed by physician.

INDICATIONS/ROUTES/DOSAGE
BENIGN PROSTATIC HYPERPLASIA
PO: ADULTS: 0.4 mg once a day, approximately 30 min after same meal each day. May increase dosage to 0.8 mg if inadequate response in 2–4 wk.

SIDE EFFECTS
FREQUENT (9%–7%): Dizziness, somnolence. **OCCASIONAL (5%–3%):** Headache, anxiety, insomnia, orthostatic hypotension. **RARE (less than 2%):** Nasal congestion, pharyngitis, rhinitis, nausea, vertigo, impotence.

ADVERSE REACTIONS/ TOXIC EFFECTS
First-dose syncope (hypotension with sudden loss of consciousness) may occur within 30–90 min after administration of initial dose and may be preceded by tachycardia (pulse rate of 120–160 beats/min).

NURSING CONSIDERATIONS

BASELINE ASSESSMENT
Question for sensitivity to tamsulosin, use of other alpha-adrenergic blocking agents, warfarin.

INTERVENTION/EVALUATION
Assist with ambulation if dizziness occurs. Monitor renal function, BP.

PATIENT/FAMILY TEACHING
• Take at the same time each day, 30 min after the same meal. • Use caution when getting up from sitting or lying position. • Avoid tasks that require alertness, motor skills until response to drug is established. • Do not chew, crush, open capsule.

Taxol, see *paclitaxel*

Taxotere, see *docetaxel*

---

tazarotene

tay-zah-**row**-teen
(Avage, Tazorac)

◆**CLASSIFICATION**
PHARMACOTHERAPEUTIC: Retinoid.
CLINICAL: Antipsoriasis, antiacne.

ACTION
Modulates differentiation/proliferation of epithelial tissue; binds selectively to retinoic acid receptors. **Therapeutic Effect:** Restores normal differentiation of the epidermis, reduces epidermal inflammation.

USES
Treatment of stable plaque psoriasis in patients with at least 20% body surface area involvement. Treatment of mild to moderate facial acne.

⬜ LIFESPAN CONSIDERATIONS: **Pregnancy/Lactation:** Unknown if distributed in breast milk. May cause fetal harm. **Pregnancy Category X. Children:** Safety and efficacy not established. **Elderly:** No age-related precautions noted.

AVAILABILITY (Rx)
CREAM: 0.05% (Tazorac), 0.1% (Avage). **GEL (TAZORAC):** 0.05%, 0.1%.

INDICATIONS/ROUTES/DOSAGE

ACNE

TOPICAL: ADULTS, ELDERLY, CHILDREN 12 YR AND OLDER: *(Cream, gel 0.1%)*: Cleanse face. After skin is dry, apply thin film once a day in the evening.

PSORIASIS

TOPICAL: ADULTS, ELDERLY, CHILDREN 12 YR AND OLDER: *(Gel 0.05%, 0.1%)*: Apply once a day in evening (no more than 20% of body surface area). ADULTS, ELDERLY: *(Cream 0.05%, 0.1%)*: Apply once a day in evening (no more than 20% of body surface area).

SIDE EFFECTS

FREQUENT (30%–10%): Acne: Desquamation, burning/stinging, dry skin, itching, erythema. **Psoriasis:** Itching, burning/stinging, erythema, worsening of psoriasis, irritation, skin pain. **OCCASIONAL (9%–1%): Acne:** Irritation, skin pain, fissuring, localized edema, skin discoloration. **Psoriasis:** Rash, desquamation, contact dermatitis, skin inflammation, fissuring, bleeding, dry skin.

BASELINE ASSESSMENT

Assess for sensitivity to tazarotene. Determine whether patient is taking medications that may increase risk of photosensitivity (e.g., sulfa, fluoroquinolones).

INTERVENTION/EVALUATION

Monitor for improvement of psoriasis, acne. Assess skin for irritation, burning, stinging.

PATIENT/FAMILY TEACHING

• Discontinue if skin irritation, pruritus, skin redness is excessive; contact physician. • For external use only. • Avoid contact with eyes, eyelids, mouth. • Photosensitization may occur; use sunscreen, protective clothing.

tegaserod

teh-**gas**-er-od
(Zelnorm)

CLASSIFICATION

PHARMACOTHERAPEUTIC: 5-HT_4 receptor partial agonist. **CLINICAL:** Anti-irritable bowel syndrome (IBS) agent.

ACTION

An anti-irritable bowel syndrome (IBS) agent that binds to 5-HT_4 receptors in the GI tract. **Therapeutic Effect:** Triggers a peristaltic reflex in the gut, increasing bowel motility.

PHARMACOKINETICS

Rapidly absorbed. Widely distributed. Protein binding: 98%. Metabolized by hydrolysis in the stomach and by oxidation and conjugation of the primary metabolite. Primarily excreted in feces. **Half-life:** 11 hr.

USES

Short-term treatment of women with IBS whose primary bowel symptom is constipation. Treatment of chronic constipation in those younger than 65 yr.

PRECAUTIONS

CONTRAINDICATIONS: Abdominal adhesions, diarrhea, history of bowel obstruction, moderate to severe hepatic impairment, severe renal impairment, suspected sphincter of Oddi dysfunction, symptomatic gallbladder disease. **CAUTIONS:** None known.

⧗ **LIFESPAN CONSIDERATIONS: Pregnancy/Lactation:** Unknown if distributed in breast milk. **Pregnancy Category B. Children:** Safety and efficacy not established. **Elderly:** No age related precautions noted.

INTERACTIONS

DRUG: None known. HERBAL: None known. FOOD: None known. LAB VALUES: None known.

AVAILABILITY (Rx)

TABLETS: 2 mg, 6 mg.

ADMINISTRATION/HANDLING

PO
• Give before meals. • Tablets may crushed.

INDICATIONS/ROUTES/DOSAGE

IBS
PO: ADULTS, ELDERLY WOMEN: 6 mg twice a day for 4–6 wk.

CHRONIC CONSTIPATION
PO: ADULTS: 6 mg twice a day.

SIDE EFFECTS

FREQUENT (greater than 5%): Headache, abdominal pain, diarrhea, nausea, flatulence. OCCASIONAL (5%–2%): Dizziness, migraine, back pain, extremity pain.

ADVERSE REACTIONS/ TOXIC EFFECTS

Ischemic colitis, mesenteric ischemia, gangrenous bowel, rectal bleeding, syncope, hypotension, hypovolemia, electrolyte disorders, suspected sphincter of Oddi spasm, bile duct stone, cholecystitis with elevated transaminases, and hypersensitivity reaction including rash, urticaria, pruritus and serious allergic Type I reactions have been reported.

BASELINE ASSESSMENT

Assess for diarrhea (avoid use in these patients).

INTERVENTION/EVALUATION

Assess for improvement in symptoms (relief from bloating, cramping, urgency, abdominal discomfort).

PATIENT/FAMILY TEACHING

• Take before meals. • Inform physician of new or worsening episodes of abdominal pain, severe diarrhea.

Tegretol, see
carbamazepine

telithromycin

teh-**lith**-row-my-sin
(Ketek, Ketek Pak)

◆CLASSIFICATION

PHARMACOTHERAPEUTIC: Ketolide. CLINICAL: Antibiotic.

ACTION

A ketolide that blocks protein synthesis by binding to ribosomal receptor sites on the bacterial cell wall. Therapeutic Effect: Bactericidal.

PHARMACOKINETICS

Protein binding: 60%–70%. More of drug is concentrated in WBCs than in plasma, and drug is eliminated more slowly from WBCs than from plasma. Partially metabolized by the liver. Minimally excreted in feces and urine. Half-life: 10 hr.

USES

Treatment of susceptible infections due to *S. aureus, S. pneumoniae, H. influenzae, M. catarrhalis, C. pneumoniae, M. pneumoniae* including acute bacterial exacerbation of chronic bronchitis, acute bacterial sinusitis, community-acquired pneumonia. OFF-LABEL: Treatment of tonsillitis and pharyngitis due to *S. pyogenes.*

PRECAUTIONS

CONTRAINDICATIONS: Hypersensitivity to macrolide antibiotics, concurrent use of cisapride or pimozide. **CAUTIONS:** Renal/hepatic impairment, hypokelemia, hypomagnesemia, clinically significant bradycardia, QT prolongation, myasthenia gravis, those receiving class IA or III antiarrhythmics.

⏳ **LIFESPAN CONSIDERATIONS: Pregnancy/Lactation:** Unknown if drug crosses placenta. May be distributed in breast milk. **Pregnancy Category C. Children:** Safety and effectiveness not established. **Elderly:** No age-related precautions noted.

INTERACTIONS

DRUG: Atorvastatin, digoxin, lovastatin, metoprolol, pimozide, simvastatin, theophylline: May increase the blood concentration and toxicity of these drugs. **Carbamazepine, phenobarbital, phenytoin, rifampin:** May decrease the blood concentration of telithromycin. **Cisapride:** Increases blood concentration of cisapride, resulting in significantly increased QT interval. **Itraconazole, ketoconazole:** May increase the blood concentration of telithromycin. **Sotalol:** Decreases the blood concentration of sotalol. **HERBAL:** None known. **FOOD:** None known. **LAB VALUES:** May increase platelet count and AST and ALT levels.

AVAILABILITY (Rx)

TABLETS (KETEK, KETEK PAK): 400 mg.

ADMINISTRATION/HANDLING

PO
• Store at room temperature. • Do not break or crush film-coated tablets. • Give without regard to food.

INDICATIONS/ROUTES/DOSAGE

CHRONIC BRONCHITIS, SINUSITIS
PO: ADULTS, ELDERLY: 800 mg once a day for 5 days.

COMMUNITY-ACQUIRED PNEUMONIA
PO: ADULTS, ELDERLY: 800 mg once a day for 7–10 days.

SIDE EFFECTS

OCCASIONAL (11%–4%): Diarrhea, nausea, headache, dizziness. **RARE (3%–2%):** Vomiting, loose stools, altered taste, dry mouth, flatulence, visual disturbances.

ADVERSE REACTIONS/TOXIC EFFECTS

Hepatic dysfunction, severe hypersensitivity reaction, and atrial arrhythmias occur rarely. Antibiotic-associated colitis and other superinfections may result from altered bacterial balance.

NURSING CONSIDERATIONS

BASELINE ASSESSMENT
Question patient for concurrent use of cisapride or pimozide (contraindicated).

INTERVENTION/EVALUATION
Determine pattern of bowel activity/stool consistency. Give with food if nausea occurs. Assess hepatic function panel for evidence of hepatotoxicity.

PATIENT/FAMILY TEACHING
• Avoid quick changes in viewing between objects in the distance and objects nearby (drug may produce temporary difficulty in focusing that may last several hours after the first or second dose). • Avoid tasks that require alertness, motor skills until response to drug is established.

telmisartan

tel-meh-**sar**-tan
(Micardis)

FIXED-COMBINATION(S)
Micardis HCT: telmisartan/hydrochlorothiazide (a diuretic): 40 mg/12.5 mg; 80 mg/12.5 mg.

⌀ see color pill atlas   🍂 herb   underlined – top prescribed drug

CLASSIFICATION

PHARMACOTHERAPEUTIC: Angiotensin II receptor antagonist. **CLINICAL:** Antihypertensive (see p. 8C).

ACTION

An angiotensin II receptor, type AT_1, antagonist that blocks vasoconstrictor and aldosterone-secreting effects of angiotensin II, inhibiting the binding of angiotensin II to the AT_1 receptors. **Therapeutic Effect:** Causes vasodilation, decreases peripheral resistance, and decreases BP.

PHARMACOKINETICS

Rapidly and completely absorbed after PO administration. Protein binding: greater than 99%. Undergoes metabolism in the liver to inactive metabolite. Excreted in feces. Unknown if removed by hemodialysis. **Half-life:** 24 hr.

USES

Treatment of hypertension alone or in combination with other antihypertensives. **OFF-LABEL:** Treatment of CHF.

PRECAUTIONS

CONTRAINDICATIONS: None known. **CAUTIONS:** Volume-depleted patients, hepatic or renal impairment, renal artery stenosis (unilateral or bilateral).

⧗ **LIFESPAN CONSIDERATIONS: Pregnancy/Lactation:** May cause fetal harm. Unknown if drug is excreted in breast milk. **Pregnancy Category C (D if used in second or third trimester). Children:** Safety and efficacy not established. **Elderly:** No age-related precautions noted.

INTERACTIONS

DRUG: Digoxin: Increases digoxin plasma concentration. **Warfarin:** Slightly decreases warfarin plasma concentration **HERBAL:** None known.

FOOD: None known. **LAB VALUES:** May increase serum creatinine level. May decrease blood Hgb and Hct levels.

AVAILABILITY (Rx)

TABLETS: 20 mg, 40 mg, 80 mg.

ADMINISTRATION/HANDLING

PO
• Give without regard to meals.

INDICATIONS/ROUTES/DOSAGE

HYPERTENSION
PO: ADULTS, ELDERLY: 40 mg once a day. Range: 20–80 mg/day.

SIDE EFFECTS

OCCASIONAL (7%–3%): Upper respiratory tract infection, sinusitis, back or leg pain, diarrhea. **RARE (1%):** Dizziness, headache, fatigue, nausea, heartburn, myalgia, cough, peripheral edema.

ADVERSE REACTIONS/ TOXIC EFFECTS

Overdosage may manifest as hypotension and tachycardia. Bradycardia occurs less often.

NURSING CONSIDERATIONS

BASELINE ASSESSMENT

Obtain BP, apical pulse immediately before each dose, in addition to regular monitoring (be alert to fluctuations). If excessive reduction in BP occurs, place patient in supine position, feet slightly elevated. Assess medication history (especially diuretic). Question for history of hepatic or renal impairment, renal artery stenosis. Obtain BUN, serum creatinine, Hgb, vital signs, particularly BP, pulse rate.

INTERVENTION/EVALUATION

Monitor BP, pulse, serum electrolytes, renal function.

PATIENT/FAMILY TEACHING

• Monitor during initial doses for hypotension. • Avoid tasks that require

T

alertness, motor skills until response to drug is established (possible dizziness effect). • Maintain proper fluid intake. • Inform female patient regarding consequences of second- and third-trimester exposure to telmisartan. • Report pregnancy to physician as soon as possible. • Report any sign of infection (sore throat, fever). • Discuss need for lifelong BP control. • Caution against excessive exertion during hot weather (risk of dehydration, hypotension).

---

temazepam

tem-**az**-eh-pam

(Apo-Temazepam 🍁, Novo-Temazepam 🍁, PMS-Temazepam 🍁, Restoril)

Do not confuse Restoril with Vistaril or Zestril.

CLASSIFICATION

PHARMACOTHERAPEUTIC: Benzodiazepine (**Schedule IV**). **CLINICAL:** Sedative-hypnotic (see p. 136C).

ACTION

A benzodiazepine that enhances the action of the inhibitory neurotransmitter gamma-aminobutyric acid, resulting in CNS depression. Therapeutic Effect: Induces sleep.

PHARMACOKINETICS

Well absorbed from the GI tract. Protein binding: 96%. Widely distributed. Crosses the blood-brain barrier. Metabolized in the liver. Primarily excreted in urine. Not removed by hemodialysis. Half-life: 4–18 hr.

USES

Short-term treatment of insomnia (5 wk or less). Reduces sleep-induction time, number of nocturnal awakenings; increases length of sleep. OFF-LABEL: Treatment of anxiety, depression, panic attacks.

PRECAUTIONS

CONTRAINDICATIONS: Angle-closure glaucoma; CNS depression; pregnancy or breast-feeding; severe, uncontrolled pain; sleep apnea. **CAUTIONS:** Mental impairment, patients with drug dependence potential.

⧗ LIFESPAN CONSIDERATIONS: **Pregnancy/Lactation:** Crosses placenta. May be distributed in breast milk. Chronic ingestion during pregnancy may produce withdrawal symptoms, CNS depression in neonates. **Pregnancy Category X. Children:** Not recommended in those younger than 18 yr. **Elderly:** Use small initial doses with gradual dosage increases to avoid ataxia, excessive sedation.

INTERACTIONS

DRUG: Alcohol, other CNS depressants: May increase CNS depression. **HERBAL: Kava kava, valerian:** May increase CNS depression **FOOD:** None known. **LAB VALUES:** None known.

AVAILABILITY (Rx)

CAPSULES: 7.5 mg, 15 mg, 22.5 mg, 30 mg.

ADMINISTRATION/HANDLING
PO
• Give without regard to meals.
• Capsules may be emptied and mixed with food.

INDICATIONS/ROUTES/DOSAGE
INSOMNIA
PO: ADULTS, CHILDREN 18 YR AND OLDER: 15–30 mg at bedtime. ELDERLY, DEBILITATED: 7.5–15 mg at bedtime.

SIDE EFFECTS

FREQUENT: Somnolence, sedation, rebound insomnia (may occur for

---

✏ see color pill atlas   🍃 herb   underlined – top prescribed drug

1–2 nights after drug is discontinued), dizziness, confusion, euphoria. **OCCASIONAL:** Asthenia, anorexia, diarrhea. **RARE:** Paradoxical CNS excitement or restlessness (particularly in elderly or debilitated patients).

ADVERSE REACTIONS/ TOXIC EFFECTS

Abrupt or too-rapid withdrawal may result in pronounced restlessness, irritability, insomnia, hand tremor, abdominal or muscle cramps, vomiting, diaphoresis, and seizures. Overdose results in somnolence, confusion, diminished reflexes, respiratory depression, and coma.

NURSING CONSIDERATIONS

BASELINE ASSESSMENT

Question for possibility of pregnancy before initiating therapy (Pregnancy Category X). Assess BP, pulse, respirations immediately before administration. Raise bed rails. Provide environment conducive to sleep (back rub, quiet environment, low lighting).

INTERVENTION/EVALUATION

Assess sleep pattern of patient. Assess elderly or debilitated for paradoxical reaction, particularly during early therapy. Monitor respiratory, cardiovascular, mental status. Evaluate for therapeutic response: decrease in number of nocturnal awakenings, increase in length of sleep.

PATIENT/FAMILY TEACHING

• Avoid alcohol, other CNS depressants. • May cause daytime drowsiness. • Avoid tasks that require alertness, motor skills until response to drug is established. • Take about 30 min before bedtime. • Inform physician if pregnant or planning to become pregnant.

Temodar, *see* *temozolomide*

temozolomide

teh-moe-**zoll**-oh-mide
(Temodal ✤, Temodar)

◆CLASSIFICATION

PHARMACOTHERAPEUTIC: Imidazotetrazine derivative. **CLINICAL:** Antineoplastic (see p. 78C).

ACTION

An imidazotetrazine derivative that acts as a prodrug and is converted to a highly active cytotoxic metabolite. Its cytotoxic effect is associated with methylation of DNA. **Therapeutic Effect:** Inhibits DNA replication, causing cell death.

PHARMACOKINETICS

Rapidly and completely absorbed after PO administration. Protein binding: 15%. Peak plasma concentration occurs in 1 hr. Penetrates the blood-brain barrier. Eliminated primarily in urine and, to a much lesser extent, in feces. **Half-life:** 1.6–1.8 hr.

USES

Treatment of adults with refractory anaplastic astrocytoma, newly diagnosed glioblastoma multiforme concomitantly with radiotherapy and then as maintenance therapy. **OFF-LABEL:** Malignant glioma, malignant melanoma.

PRECAUTIONS

CONTRAINDICATIONS: Hypersensitivity to dacarbazine, pregnancy. **CAUTIONS:** Severe renal/hepatic impairment, bacterial/viral infection, elderly.

⌛ **LIFESPAN CONSIDERATIONS: Pregnancy/Lactation:** May cause fetal harm. May produce malformation of external organs, soft tissue, skeleton. If possible, avoid use during pregnancy. Unknown if drug is excreted in breast milk. **Pregnancy Category D. Children:** Safety and efficacy not established. **Elderly:** Those older than 70 yr may experience a higher risk of developing grade 4 neutropenia and grade 4 thrombocytopenia.

INTERACTIONS

DRUG: **Live virus vaccines:** May potentiate virus replication, increase vaccine side effects, and decrease the patient's antibody response to the vaccine. **Valproic acid:** Decreases the clearance of temozolomide. HERBAL: None known. FOOD: **All foods:** Decrease the rate of drug absorption. LAB VALUES: May decrease blood Hgb levels and neutrophil, platelet, and WBC counts.

AVAILABILITY (Rx)

CAPSULES: 5 mg, 20 mg, 100 mg, 250 mg.

ADMINISTRATION/HANDLING

PO
• Food reduces rate, extent of absorption; increases risk of nausea, vomiting. • For best results, administer at bedtime. • Swallow capsule whole with glass of water. If unable to swallow, open capsule and mix with applesauce, apple juice. • Avoid exposure to medication during handling (cytotoxic).

INDICATIONS/ROUTES/DOSAGE

ANAPLASTIC ASTROCYTOMA

PO: ADULTS, ELDERLY: Initially, 150 mg/m^2/day for 5 consecutive days of a 28-day treatment cycle. Subsequent doses based on platelet count and ANC during previous cycle. ANC greater than 1,500 per microliter and platelet: more than 100,000 per microliter. Maintenance: 200 mg/m^2/day for 5 days q4wk.

Continue until disease progression. Minimum: 100 mg/m^2/day for 5 days q4wk.

GLIOBLASTOMA MULTIFORME

PO: ADULTS, ELDERLY: 75 mg/m^2 daily for 42 days. Maintenance: (Cycle 1): 150 mg/m^2 once daily for 5 days followed by 23 days without treatment. (Cycles 2–6): 200 mg/m^2 once daily for 5 days followed by 23 days without treatment.

SIDE EFFECTS

FREQUENT (53%–33%): Nausea, vomiting, headache, fatigue, constipation, seizure. **OCCASIONAL (16%–10%):** Diarrhea, asthenia, fever, dizziness, peripheral edema, incoordination, insomnia. **RARE (9%–5%):** Paraesthesia, drowsiness, anorexia, urinary incontinence, anxiety, pharyngitis, cough.

ADVERSE REACTIONS/ TOXIC EFFECTS

Elderly patients and women are at increased risk for developing severe myelosuppression, characterized by neutropenia and thrombocytopenia and usually occurring within the first few cycles. Neutrophil and platelet counts reach their nadirs approximately 26–28 days after administration and recover within 14 days of the nadir. Opportunistic infection characterized as pneumocystis carinii pneumonia occurs rarely.

NURSING CONSIDERATIONS

BASELINE ASSESSMENT

Before dosing, absolute neutrophil count (ANC) must be greater than 1,500 and platelet count greater than 100,000. Potential for nausea, vomiting readily controlled with antiemetic therapy.

INTERVENTION/EVALUATION

Obtain CBC on day 22 (21 days after the first dose) or within 48 hr of that day and weekly until ANC is greater than 1,500 and platelet count is greater than 100,000. Monitor for hematologic toxicity (fever, sore throat, signs of local infection, unusual ecchymoses/bleeding from any site), symptoms of anemia (excessive fatigue, weakness).

PATIENT/FAMILY TEACHING

• To reduce nausea/vomiting, take temozolomide on an empty stomach. • Do not open capsules. • Promptly report fever, sore throat, signs of local infection, unusual bruising/bleeding from any site. • Avoid crowds, those with infection. • Do not have immunizations without physician's approval. • Avoid pregnancy.

tenecteplase

ten-**eck**-teh-place
(TNKase)

CLASSIFICATION

PHARMACOTHERAPEUTIC: Tissue plasminogen activator. **CLINICAL:** Thrombolytic (see p. 32C).

ACTION

A tissue plasminogen activator produced by recombinant DNA that binds to fibrin and converts plasminogen to plasmin. Initiates fibrinolysis by degrading fibrin clots, fibrinogen, other plasma proteins. **Therapeutic Effect:** Exerts thrombolytic action.

PHARMACOKINETICS

Extensively distributed to tissues. Completely eliminated by hepatic metabolism. **Half-life:** 11–20 min.

USES

Treatment and reduction of mortality associated with acute myocardial infarction (AMI).

PRECAUTIONS

CONTRAINDICATIONS: Active internal bleeding, aneurysm, AV malformation, bleeding diathesis, history of cerebrovascular accident (CVA), intracranial or intraspinal surgery or trauma within past 2 mo, intracranial neoplasm, severe uncontrolled hypertension. **CAUTIONS:** Patients who previously received tenecteplase, severe hepatic impairment.

LIFESPAN CONSIDERATIONS: **Pregnancy/Lactation:** Unknown if distributed in breast milk. **Pregnancy Category C. Children:** Safety and efficacy not established. **Elderly:** May have increased risk of intracranial hemorrhage, stroke, major bleeding; caution advised.

INTERACTIONS

DRUG: **Anticoagulants (such as heparin, warfarin), aspirin, dipyridamole, glycoprotein IIb/IIIa inhibitors:** Increase the risk of bleeding. HERBAL: **Ginkgo biloba:** May increase the risk of bleeding. FOOD: None known. LAB VALUES: Decreases plasminogen and fibrinogen levels during infusion, decreasing clotting time and confirming presence of lysis. Decreases Hct and Hgb.

AVAILABILITY (Rx)

POWDER FOR INJECTION: 50 mg.

ADMINISTRATION/HANDLING

IV

Reconstitution • Add 10 ml sterile water for injection without preservative to vial to provide concentration of 5 mg/ml. • Gently swirl until dissolved. Do not shake. • If foaming occurs, vial should be left undisturbed for several minutes.

Rate of administration • Administer as IV push over 5 sec.

Storage • Store at room temperature. • If possible, use immediately but may refrigerate up to 8 hr after reconstitution. • Appears as colorless to pale yellow solution. Do not use if discolored or contains particulates. • Discard after 8 hr.

⬚ IV INCOMPATIBILITIES
Do not mix with other medications.

INDICATIONS/ROUTES/DOSAGE
ACUTE MI
IV: ADULTS: Dosage is based on patient's weight. Treatment should be initiated as soon as possible after onset of symptoms.

Weight (kg)	(mg)	(ml)
90 or more	50	10
80–less than 90	45	9
70–less than 80	40	8
60–less than 70	35	7
Less than 60	30	6

SIDE EFFECTS
FREQUENT: Bleeding (major, 4.7%; minor, 21.8%).

ADVERSE REACTIONS/ TOXIC EFFECTS
Bleeding at internal sites may occur, including intracranial, retroperitoneal, GI, GU, and respiratory sites. Lysis or coronary thrombi may produce atrial or ventricular arrhythmias and stroke.

NURSING CONSIDERATIONS
BASELINE ASSESSMENT
Obtain baseline BP, apical pulse. Record weight. Evaluate 12-lead EKG, cardiac enzymes, serum electrolytes. Assess Hgb, Hct, platelet count, thrombin (TT), aPTT, PT, fibrinogen level before therapy is instituted. Type and hold blood.

INTERVENTION/EVALUATION
Continuous cardiac monitoring for arrhythmias, BP, pulse, respirations q15min until stable, then hourly. Check peripheral pulses, heart and lung sounds. Monitor chest pain relief; notify physician of continuation/recurrence (note location, type, intensity). Assess for overt or occult blood in any

body substance. Monitor aPTT per protocol. Maintain BP. Avoid any trauma that might increase risk of bleeding (e.g., injections, shaving). Assess neurologic status with vital signs.

teniposide
ten-**ih**-poe-side
(Vumon)
See Cancer chemotherapeutic agents (p. 78C)

tenofovir
ten-**oh**-foh-veer
(Viread)

FIXED-COMBINATION(S)
Truvada: tenofovir/emtricitabine (an antiretroviral agent): 300 mg/ 200 mg.

• CLASSIFICATION
PHARMACOTHERAPEUTIC: Nucleotide analogue. **CLINICAL:** Antiviral (see pp. 62C, 103C).

ACTION
A nucleotide analogue that inhibits HIV reverse transcriptase by being incorporated into viral DNA, resulting in DNA chain termination. **Therapeutic Effect:** Slows HIV replication and reduces HIV RNA levels (viral load).

PHARMACOKINETICS
Bioavailability in fasted patients is approximately 25%. High-fat meals increase the bioavailability. Protein binding: 0.7%–7.2%. Excreted in urine. Removed by hemodialysis. **Half-life:** Unknown.

USES

Treatment of HIV-1 infection in combination with other antiretroviral agents.

PRECAUTIONS

CONTRAINDICATIONS: None known. **CAUTIONS:** Hepatic or renal impairment.

⌛ LIFESPAN CONSIDERATIONS: **Pregnancy/Lactation:** Unknown if drug crosses placenta or is distributed in breast milk. **Pregnancy Category B. Children:** Safety and efficacy not established. **Elderly:** No age-related precautions noted.

INTERACTIONS

DRUG: **Didanosine:** May increase didaosine blood concentration. **Indinavir, lamivudine, lopinavir, ritonavir:** May decrease the blood concentrations of these drugs. HERBAL: None known. FOOD: **High-fat food:** Increases tenofovir bioavailability. LAB VALUES: May elevate liver function test results. May alter serum creatine kinase (CK), GGT, uric acid, AST, ALT, and triglyceride levels as well as creatinine clearance.

AVAILABILITY (Rx)

TABLETS: 300 mg.

ADMINISTRATION/HANDLING

PO
• Give with food.

INDICATIONS/ROUTES/DOSAGE

HIV INFECTION (IN COMBINATION WITH OTHER ANTIRETROVIRALS)
PO: ADULTS, ELDERLY, CHILDREN 18 YR AND OLDER: 300 mg once a day.

DOSAGE IN RENAL IMPAIRMENT

Creatinine Clearance	Dosage
30–49 ml/min	300 mg q48h
10–29 ml/min	300 mg twice a wk
Less than 10 ml/min	Not recommended

SIDE EFFECTS

OCCASIONAL: GI disturbances (diarrhea, flatulence, nausea, vomiting).

ADVERSE REACTIONS/ TOXIC EFFECTS

Lactic acidosis and hepatomegaly with steatosis occur rarely, but may be severe.

NURSING CONSIDERATIONS

BASELINE ASSESSMENT

Obtain baseline laboratory testing, especially serum liver function tests, triglycerides before beginning tenofovir therapy and at periodic intervals during therapy. Offer emotional support to patient and family.

INTERVENTION/EVALUATION

Closely monitor for evidence of GI discomfort. Monitor pattern of bowel activity and stool consistency. Monitor CBC, Hgb, reticulocyte count, serum liver function, CD4 cell count, HIV, RNA plasma levels.

PATIENT/FAMILY TEACHING

• Continue therapy for full length of treatment. • Tenofovir is not a cure for HIV infection, nor does it reduce risk of transmission to others. • Take with a meal (increases absorption). • Inform physician if persistent abdominal pain, nausea, vomiting occurs.

Tenormin, *see atenolol*

T

Tequin, *see gatifloxacin*

---

terazosin hydrochloride

ter-a-zoe-sin

(Apo-Terazosin ✦, Hytrin, Novo-Terazosin ✦)

✦CLASSIFICATION

PHARMACOTHERAPEUTIC: Alpha-adrenergic blocker. **CLINICAL:** Antihypertensive, benign prostatic hyperplasia agent (see p. 55C).

ACTION

An antihypertensive and benign prostatic hyperplasia agent that blocks alpha-adrenergic receptors. Produces vasodilation, decreases peripheral resistance, and targets receptors around bladder neck and prostate. **Therapeutic Effect:** In hypertension, decreases BP. In benign prostatic hyperplasia, relaxes smooth muscle and improves urine flow.

PHARMACOKINETICS

Route	Onset	Peak	Duration
PO	15 min	1–2 hr	12–24 hr

Rapidly, completely absorbed from the GI tract. Protein binding: 90%–94%. Metabolized in the liver to active metabolite. Primarily eliminated in feces via biliary system; excreted in urine. Not removed by hemodialysis. **Half-life:** 12 hr.

USES

Treatment of mild to moderate hypertension. Used alone or in combination with other antihypertensives. Treatment of benign prostatic hypertrophy.

PRECAUTIONS

CONTRAINDICATIONS: None known. **CAUTIONS:** Confirmed or suspected coronary artery disease.

⌛ LIFESPAN CONSIDERATIONS: Pregnancy/Lactation:
Unknown if drug crosses placenta or is distributed in breast milk. **Pregnancy Category C. Children:** Safety and efficacy not established. **Elderly:** No age-related precautions noted but may be more sensitive to hypotensive effects.

INTERACTIONS

DRUG: Estrogen, NSAIDs, other sympathomimetics: May decrease the effects of terazosin. **Hypotension-producing medications, such as antihypertensives and diuretics:** May increase the effects of terazosin. **HERBAL: Dong quai, ginseng, garlic, yohimbe:** May decrease the effects of terazosin. **FOOD:** None known. **LAB VALUES:** May decrease blood Hgb and Hct levels, serum albumin level, total serum protein level, and WBC count.

AVAILABILITY (Rx)

CAPSULES: 1 mg, 2 mg, 5 mg, 10 mg. **TABLETS:** 1 mg, 2 mg, 5 mg, 10 mg.

ADMINISTRATION/HANDLING

PO
• Give without regard to food. • Tablets may be crushed. • Administer first dose at bedtime (minimizes risk of fainting due to "first-dose syncope").

INDICATIONS/ROUTES/DOSAGE

MILD TO MODERATE HYPERTENSION
PO: ADULTS, ELDERLY: Initially, 1 mg at bedtime. Slowly increase dosage to desired levels. Range: 1–5 mg/day as single or 2 divided doses. **Maximum:** 20 mg.

BENIGN PROSTATIC HYPERPLASIA
PO: ADULTS, ELDERLY: Initially, 1 mg at bedtime. May increase up to 10 mg/day. **Maximum:** 20 mg/day.

SIDE EFFECTS

FREQUENT (9%–5%): Dizziness, headache, unusual tiredness. **RARE (less than 2%):** Peripheral edema, orthostatic

---

✐ see color pill atlas   ⬤ herb   <u>underlined</u> – top prescribed drug hypotension, myalgia, arthralgia, blurred vision, nausea, vomiting, nasal congestion, somnolence.

ADVERSE REACTIONS/ TOXIC EFFECTS

First-dose syncope (hypotension with sudden loss of consciousness) may occur 30–90 min after initial dose of 2 mg or more, a too rapid increase in dosage, or addition of another antihypertensive agent to therapy. First-dose syncope may be preceded by tachycardia (pulse rate of 120–160 beats/min).

NURSING CONSIDERATIONS

BASELINE ASSESSMENT

Give first dose at bedtime. If initial dose is given during daytime, patient must remain recumbent for 3–4 hr. Assess BP, pulse immediately before each dose, and q15–30min until stabilized (be alert to BP fluctuations).

INTERVENTION/EVALUATION

Monitor pulse diligently (first-dose syncope may be preceded by tachycardia). Assist with ambulation if dizziness occurs. Assess for peripheral edema. Monitor BP, GU function.

PATIENT/FAMILY TEACHING

• Noncola carbonated beverage, unsalted crackers, dry toast may relieve nausea. • Nasal congestion may occur. • Full therapeutic effect may not occur for 3–4 wk. • Avoid tasks requiring alertness, motor skills until response to drug is established. • Use caution rising from sitting position. • Report dizziness, palpitations.

terbinafine hydrochloride

ter-**been**-a-feen

(Apo-Terbinafine ♣, Lamisil, Lamisil AT, Novo-Terbinafine ♣)

Do not confuse terbinafine with terbutaline or Lamisil with Lamictal.

◆CLASSIFICATION

CLINICAL: Antifungal (see p. 45C).

ACTION

A fungicidal antifungal that inhibits the enzyme squalene epoxidase, thereby interfering with fungal biosynthesis. Therapeutic Effect: Results in death of fungal cells.

PHARMACOKINETICS

Well absorbed following PO administration. Protein binding: 99%. Metabolized by liver. Primarily excreted in urine; minimal elimination in feces. Half-life: (oral): 36 hr, (topical): 22–26 hr.

USES

Systemic: Treatment of onychomycosis (fungal disease of nails due to dermatophytes). **Topical:** Treatment of *tinea cruris* (jock itch), *t. pedis* (athlete's foot), *t. corporis* (ringworm).

PRECAUTIONS

CONTRAINDICATIONS: Oral: Children younger than 12 yr, preexisting hepatic or renal impairment (creatinine clearance of 50 ml/min or less). **CAUTIONS:** None known.

⧗ LIFESPAN CONSIDERATIONS: **Pregnancy/Lactation:** Distributed in breast milk. **Pregnancy Category B. Children:** Safety and efficacy not established. **Elderly:** Age-related renal impairment may require dosage adjustment.

♣ Canadian trade name   @ see **evolve**   ☞ High Alert drug

INTERACTIONS

DRUG: **Alcohol, other hepatotoxic medications:** May increase the risk of hepatotoxicity. **Hepatic enzyme inducers, including rifampin:** May increase terbinafine clearance. **Hepatic enzyme inhibitors, including cimetidine:** May decrease terbinafine clearance. HERBAL: None known. FOOD: None known. LAB VALUES: May increase AST and ALT levels.

AVAILABILITY (Rx)

TABLETS (LAMISIL): 250 mg. **CREAM (LAMISIL AT):** 1%. **TOPICAL SOLUTION (LAMISIL, LAMISIL AT):** 1%. **TOPICAL SPRAY (LAMISIL AT):** 1%.

INDICATIONS/ROUTES/DOSAGE

TINEA PEDIS

TOPICAL: ADULTS, ELDERLY, CHILDREN 12 YR AND OLDER: Apply twice a day until signs and symptoms significantly improve.

TINEA CRURIS, TINEA CORPORIS

TOPICAL: ADULTS, ELDERLY, CHILDREN 12 YR AND OLDER: Apply 1–2 times a day until signs and symptoms significantly improve.

ONYCHOMYCOSIS

PO: ADULTS, ELDERLY, CHILDREN 12 YR AND OLDER: 250 mg/day for 6 wk (fingernails) or 12 wk (toenails).

TINEA VERSICOLOR

TOPICAL SOLUTION: ADULTS, ELDERLY: Apply to the affected area twice a day for 7 days.

SYSTEMIC MYCOSIS

PO: ADULTS, ELDERLY: 250–500 mg/day for up to 16 mo.

SIDE EFFECTS

FREQUENT (13%): Oral: Headache. **OCCASIONAL (6%–3%):** Abdominal pain, flatulence, urticaria, visual disturbance. **Oral:** Diarrhea, rash, dyspepsia, pruritus, taste disturbance, nausea. **Topical:** Irritation, burning, pruritus, dryness.

ADVERSE REACTIONS/ TOXIC EFFECTS

Hepatobiliary dysfunction (including cholestatic hepatitis), serious skin reactions, and severe neutropenia occur rarely. Ocular lens and retinal changes have been noted.

NURSING CONSIDERATIONS

BASELINE ASSESSMENT

Serum liver function tests should be obtained in patients receiving treatment for longer than 6 wk.

INTERVENTION/EVALUATION

Check for therapeutic response. Discontinue medication, notify physician if local reaction occurs (irritation, redness, swelling, itching, oozing, blistering, burning). Monitor serum liver function in patients receiving treatment for longer than 6 wk.

PATIENT/FAMILY TEACHING

• Keep areas clean, dry; wear light clothing to promote ventilation. • Separate personal items. • Avoid topical cream contact with eyes, nose, mouth, other mucous membranes. • Rub well into affected, surrounding area. • Do not cover with occlusive dressing. • Notify physician if skin irritation, diarrhea occurs.

terbutaline sulfate

ter-**byoo**-te-leen
(Brethine, Bricanyl ✦)
Do not confuse terbutaline with tolbutamide or terbinafine, or Brethine with Brethaire.

◆ CLASSIFICATION

PHARMACOTHERAPEUTIC: Sympathomimetic (adrenergic agonist). **CLINICAL:** Bronchodilator, premature labor inhibitor (see p. 67C).

ACTION

An adrenergic agonist that stimulates beta$_2$-adrenergic receptors, resulting in relaxation of uterine and bronchial smooth muscle. **Therapeutic Effect:** Relieves bronchospasm and reduces airway resistance. Also inhibits uterine contractions.

PHARMACOKINETICS

Partially absorbed in GI tract following oral administration. Protein binding: 14%–25%. Metabolized in liver. Excreted in feces and urine. **Half-life:** 3–4 hr.

USES

Symptomatic relief of reversible bronchospasm due to bronchial asthma, bronchitis, emphysema. Delays premature labor in pregnancies between 20 and 34 wk.

PRECAUTIONS

CONTRAINDICATIONS: History of hypersensitivity to sympathomimetics. **CAUTIONS:** Cardiac impairment, diabetes mellitus, hypertension, hyperthyroidism, history of seizures.

⚖ **LIFESPAN CONSIDERATIONS: Pregnancy/Lactation:** Crosses placenta; distributed in breast milk. **Pregnancy Category B. Children:** Safety and efficacy not established in children younger than 6 yr. **Elderly:** Increased risk of tremors, tachycardia due to sympathomimetic sensitivity.

INTERACTIONS

DRUG: Beta blockers: May decrease the effects of beta blockers. **Digoxin, sympathomimetics:** May increase the risk of arrhythmias. **MAOIs:** May increase the risk of hypertensive crisis. **Tricyclic antidepressants:** May increase cardiovascular effects. **HERBAL:** None known. **FOOD:** None known. **LAB VALUES:** May decrease serum potassium level.

AVAILABILITY (Rx)

TABLETS: 2.5 mg, 5 mg. **INJECTION:** 1 mg/ml.

ADMINISTRATION/HANDLING

SUBCUTANEOUS
• Do not use if solution appears discolored. • Inject subcutaneously into lateral deltoid region.

PO
• Give without regard to food (give with food if GI upset occurs). • Tablets may be crushed.

INDICATIONS/ROUTES/DOSAGE

BRONCHOSPASM
PO: ADULTS, ELDERLY, CHILDREN 15 YR AND OLDER: Initially, 2.5 mg 3–4 times a day. Maintenance: 2.5–5 mg 3 times a day q6h while awake. **Maximum:** 15 mg/day. CHILDREN 12–14 YR: 2.5 mg 3 times a day. **Maximum:** 7.5 mg/day. CHILDREN YOUNGER THAN 12 YR: Initially, 0.05 mg/kg/dose q8h. May increase up to 0.15 mg/kg/dose. **Maximum:** 5 mg.

SUBCUTANEOUS: ADULTS, CHILDREN 12 YR AND OLDER: Initially, 0.25 mg. Repeat in 15–30 min if substantial improvement does not occur. **Maximum:** 0.5 mg/4 hr. CHILDREN YOUNGER THAN 12 YR: 0.005–0.01 mg/kg/dose to a maximum of 0.4 mg/dose q15–20min for 2 doses.

PRETERM LABOR
PO: ADULTS: 2.5–10 mg q4–6h.
IV: ADULTS: 2.5–10 mcg/min. May increase gradually q15–20min up to 17.5–30 mcg/min.

SIDE EFFECTS

FREQUENT (23%–18%): Tremor, anxiety. **OCCASIONAL (11%–10%):** Somnolence, headache, nausea, heartburn, dizziness. **RARE (3%–1%):** Flushing, asthenia, mouth and throat dryness or irritation (with inhalation therapy).

ADVERSE REACTIONS/TOXIC EFFECTS

Too-frequent or excessive use may lead to decreased drug effectiveness and

T

---

severe, paradoxical bronchoconstriction. Excessive sympathomimetic stimulation may cause palpitations, extrasystoles, tachycardia, chest pain, a slight increase in BP followed by a substantial decrease, chills, diaphoresis, and blanching of skin.

NURSING CONSIDERATIONS

BASELINE ASSESSMENT

Bronchospasm: Offer emotional support (high incidence of anxiety due to difficulty in breathing, sympathomimetic response to drug). **Preterm labor:** Assess baseline maternal pulse, BP, frequency and duration of contractions, fetal heart rate.

INTERVENTION/EVALUATION

Bronchospasm: Monitor rate, depth, rhythm, type of respiration; quality and rate of pulse. Assess lung sounds for rhonchi, wheezing, rales. Monitor ABGs. Observe lips, fingernails for cyanosis (blue or dusky color in light-skinned patients; gray in dark-skinned patients). Observe for clavicular retractions, hand tremor. Evaluate for clinical improvement (quieter, slower respirations, relaxed facial expression, cessation of clavicular retractions). **Preterm labor:** Monitor for frequency, duration, strength of contractions. Diligently monitor fetal heart rate.

PATIENT/FAMILY TEACHING

• Inform physician if palpitations, chest pain, muscle tremors, dizziness, headache, flushing, breathing difficulties continue. • May cause nervousness, anxiety, shakiness. • Avoid excessive use of caffeine derivatives (chocolate, coffee, tea, cola, cocoa).

terconazole

ter-con-ah-zole
(Terazol ♦, Terazol 7)
Do not confuse terconazole with tioconazole.

CLASSIFICATION

CLINICAL: Antifungal.

ACTION

Disrupts fungal cell membrane permeability. **Therapeutic Effect:** Produces antifungal activity.

PHARMACOKINETICS

Minimal systemic absorption.

USES

Treatment of vulvovaginal candidiasis (moniliasis).

⧗ **LIFESPAN CONSIDERATIONS: Pregnancy/Lactation:** Unknown if distributed in breast milk. **Pregnancy Category C. Children:** Safety and efficacy not established. **Elderly:** No age-related precautions noted.

AVAILABILITY (Rx)

VAGINAL CREAM: 0.4% (Terazol 7), 0.8% (Terazol). **VAGINAL SUPPOSITORY (TERAZOL 3):** 80 mg.

INDICATIONS/ROUTES/DOSAGE

VULVOVAGINAL CANDIDIASIS

TABLET (INTRAVAGINAL): ADULTS, ELDERLY: 1 suppository vaginally at bedtime for 3 days.
CREAM: ADULTS, ELDERLY: (0.4%): 1 applicatorful at bedtime for 7 days; (0.8%): 1 applicatorful at bedtime for 3 days.

SIDE EFFECTS

FREQUENT (over 10%): Headache, vulvovaginal burning. **OCCASIONAL (10%–1%):** Dysmenorrhea, pain in female genitalia, abdominal pain, fever, itching. **RARE (less than 1%):** Chills.

teriparatide acetate

tear-ee-**pear**-ah-tide
(Forteo)

CLASSIFICATION

PHARMACOTHERAPEUTIC: Synthetic hormone. **CLINICAL:** Osteoporosis agent.

ACTION

A synthetic hormone that acts on bone to mobilize calcium; also acts on kidney to reduce calcium clearance and increase phosphate excretion. **Therapeutic Effect:** Increases the rate at which calcium is released from bone into blood; stimulates new bone formation.

PHARMACOKINETICS

Extensively absorbed following subcutaneous injection. Metabolized in the liver. Excreted in urine. **Half-life:** 1 hr.

USES

Treatment of postmenopausal women with osteoporosis who are at increased risk for fractures, increase bone mass in men with primary or hypogonadal osteoporosis who are at high risk for fractures. High-risk patients include those with a history of osteoporotic fractures, those who have failed previous osteoporosis therapy or are intolerant to previous osteoporosis therapy.

PRECAUTIONS

CONTRAINDICATIONS: Conditions that increase the risk of osteosarcoma (including Paget's disease, unexplained elevations of alkaline phosphatase level, open epiphyses, and prior skeletal radiation therapy, implant therapy), hypercalcemia, hypercalcemic disorders (such as hyperparathyroidism). **CAUTIONS:** Bone metastases, history of skeletal malignancies, metabolic bone diseases other than osteoporosis, concurrent therapy with digoxin.

⌛ **LIFESPAN CONSIDERATIONS:** **Pregnancy/Lactation:** Unknown if drug crosses placenta or is distributed in breast milk. **Pregnancy Category C.** **Children:** Safety and efficacy not established. **Elderly:** No age-related precautions noted.

INTERACTIONS

DRUG: **Digoxin:** May increase serum digoxin concentration. **HERBAL:** None known. **FOOD:** None known. **LAB VALUES:** May increase the serum calcium level.

AVAILABILITY (Rx)

INJECTION: 750 mg in 3-ml prefilled pen delivers 20 mcg/dose.

ADMINISTRATION/HANDLING

SUBCUTANEOUS
• Refrigerate, minimizing the time out of the refrigerator. Do not freeze; discard if frozen. • Administer into the thigh or abdominal wall.

INDICATIONS/ROUTES/DOSAGE

OSTEOPOROSIS
SUBCUTANEOUS: ADULTS, ELDERLY: 20 mcg once a day into thigh or abdominal wall.

SIDE EFFECTS

OCCASIONAL: Leg cramps, nausea, dizziness, headache, orthostatic hypotension, tachycardia.

ADVERSE REACTIONS/ TOXIC EFFECTS

Angina pectoris has been reported.

NURSING CONSIDERATIONS

BASELINE ASSESSMENT

Check urinary and serum calcium levels, serum parathyroid hormone levels.

INTERVENTION/EVALUATION

Monitor bone mineral density, urinary and serum calcium levels, serum

T

parathyroid hormone levels. Observe for symptoms of hypercalcemia. Monitor BP for hypotension, pulse for tachycardia.

PATIENT/FAMILY TEACHING

• Immediately sit or lie down if symptoms of orthostatic hypotension occur.
• Inform physician if persistent symptoms of hypercalcemia occur (e.g., nausea, vomiting, constipation, lethargy, asthenia [loss of strength, energy]).

testosterone

tess-**toss**-ter-one

(Andriol ✹, Androderm, AndroGel, Andro LA 200, Andropository ✹, Delatestryl, Depandro 100, Depotest ✹, Depo-Testosterone, Everone ✹, FIRST-Testosterone, FIRST-Testosterone MC, Striant, Testim, Testoderm, Testro AQ, Testro-L.A., Testoprel, Virilon IM ✹)

Do not confuse testosterone with testolactone.

◆ CLASSIFICATION

PHARMACOTHERAPEUTIC: Androgen. **CLINICAL:** Sex hormone.

ACTION

A primary endogenous androgen that promotes growth and development of male sex organs and maintains secondary sex characteristics in androgen-deficient males. **Therapeutic Effect:** Helps relieve androgen deficiency.

PHARMACOKINETICS

Well absorbed after IM administration. Protein binding: 98%. Undergoes first-pass metabolism in the liver. Primarily excreted in urine. Unknown if removed by hemodialysis. **Half-life:** 10–20 min.

USES

Injection: Treatment of delayed male puberty, male hypogonadism, inoperable female breast cancer. **Pellet:** Treatment of delayed male puberty, male hypogonadism. **Buccal, transdermal:** Male hypogonadism.

PRECAUTIONS

CONTRAINDICATIONS: Breast-feeding, cardiac impairment, hypercalcemia, pregnancy, prostate or breast cancer in males, severe hepatic or renal disease. **CAUTIONS:** Renal or hepatic dysfunction, diabetes.

⌛ LIFESPAN CONSIDERATIONS: **Pregnancy/Lactation:** Contraindicated during lactation. **Pregnancy Category X. Children:** Safety and efficacy not established; use with caution. **Elderly:** May increase risk of hyperplasia or stimulate growth of occult prostate carcinoma.

INTERACTIONS

DRUG: **Hepatotoxic medications:** May increase the risk of hepatotoxicity. **Oral anticoagulants:** May increase the effects of oral anticoagulants. HERBAL: None known. FOOD: None known. LAB VALUES: May increase blood Hgb level and Hct, as well as serum LDL, alkaline phosphatase, bilirubin, calcium, potassium, sodium, and AST levels. May decrease serum HDL level.

AVAILABILITY (Rx)

CYPIONATE INJECTION (DEPO-TESTOSTERONE): 100 mg/ml, 200 mg/ml. **ETHANATE INJECTION (ANDRO LA 200, DELATESTRYL, TESTRO-L.A.):** 200 mg/ml. **PROPIONATE INJECTION SOLUTION (DEPANDRO 100):** 100 mg/ml. **INTRAMUSCULAR SOLUTION:** 50 mg/ml (Testro), 100 mg/ml (Testro AQ). **SUBCUTANEOUS PELLETS (TESTOPEL):** 75 mg. **TOPICAL GEL:** 25 mg/2.5 g (AndroGel) 50 mg/5 g (AndroGel, Testim). **TOPICAL CREAM (FIRST-TESTOSTERONE MC):** 2%. **TOPICAL OINTMENT (FIRST-TESTOSTERONE):** 2%. **TRANSDERMAL PATCH:** 2.5 mg/day (Androderm), 4 mg/day (Testoderm), 5 mg/

day (Androderm), 6 mg/day (Testoderm). **BUCCAL (STRIANT):** 30 mg.

ADMINISTRATION/HANDLING
IM
• Give deep in gluteal muscle. • Do not give IV. • Warming or shaking redissolves crystals that may form in long-acting preparations. • Wet needle of syringe may cause solution to become cloudy; this does not affect potency.

BUCCAL (STRIANT)
• Apply to gum area (above incisor tooth). • Not affected by food, tooth brushing, gum, chewing, alcoholic beverages. • Remove before placing new system.

TRANSDERMAL
Testoderm • Apply to clean, dry scrotal skin that has been dry-shaved (optimal skin contact). Testoderm TTS may be applied to arm, back, upper buttock.

Androderm • Apply to clean, dry area on skin on back, abdomen, upper arms, thighs. • Do not apply to bony prominences (e.g., shoulder) or oily, damaged, irritated skin. Do not apply to scrotum. • Rotate application site with 7-day interval to same site.

TRANSDERMAL GEL
(Androgel, Testim) • Apply (morning preferred) to clean, dry, intact skin of shoulder, upper arms (Androgel may also be applied to abdomen). • Upon opening packet(s), squeeze entire contents into palm of hand and immediately to application site. • Allow to dry. • Do not apply to genitals.

INDICATIONS/ROUTES/DOSAGE
MALE HYPOGONADISM
IM: ADULTS: 50–400 mg q2–4wk. ADOLESCENTS: Initially 40–50 mg/m²/dose monthly until growth rate falls to prepubertal levels. 100 mg/m²/dose until growth ceases. Maintenance virilizing

dose: 100 mg/m²/dose twice a mo.

SUBCUTANEOUS (PELLETS): ADULTS, ADOLESCENTS: 150–450 mg q3–6mo.

TRANSDERMAL (PATCH [TESTODERM]): ADULTS, ELDERLY: Start therapy with 6 mg/day patch. Apply patch to scrotal skin.

TRANSDERMAL (PATCH [TESTODERM TTS]): ADULTS, ELDERLY: Apply TTS patch to arm, back, or upper buttocks.

TRANSDERMAL (PATCH [ANDRODERM]): ADULTS, ELDERLY: Start therapy with 5 mg/day patch applied at night. Apply patch to abdomen, back, thighs, or upper arms.

TRANSDERMAL (GEL [ANDROGEL]): ADULTS, ELDERLY: Initial dose of 5 mg delivers 50 mg testosterone and is applied once daily to the abdomen, shoulders, or upper arms. May increase to 7.5 g, then to 10 g, if necessary.

TRANSDERMAL (GEL [TESTIM]): ADULTS, ELDERLY: Initial dose of 5 g delivers 50 mg testosterone and is applied once a day to the shoulders or upper arms. May increase to 10 g.

BUCCAL SYSTEM (STRIANT): ADULTS, ELDERLY: 30 mg q12h.

DELAYED PUBERTY
IM: ADULTS: 50–200 mg q2–4wk. ADOLESCENTS: 40–50 mg/m²/dose every mo for 6 mo.

SUBCUTANEOUS (PELLETS): ADULTS, ADOLESCENTS: 150–450 mg q3–6mo.

BREAST CARCINOMA
IM (TESTOSTERONE AQUEOUS): ADULTS: 50–100 mg 3 times a wk.

IM (TESTOSTERONE CYPIONATE OR TESTOSTERONE ETHANATE): ADULTS: 200–400 mg q2–4wk.

IM (TESTOSTERONE PROPIONATE): ADULTS: 50–100 mg 3 times a wk.

SIDE EFFECTS
FREQUENT: Gynecomastia, acne. **Females:** Hirsutism, amenorrhea or other menstrual irregularities, deepening of voice, clitoral enlargement that

may not be reversible when drug is discontinued. **OCCASIONAL:** Edema, nausea, insomnia, oligospermia, priapism, male-pattern baldness, bladder irritability, hypercalcemia (in immobilized patients or those with breast cancer), hypercholesterolemia, inflammation and pain at IM injection site. **Transdermal:** Pruritus, erythema, skin irritation. **RARE:** Polycythemia (with high dosage), hypersensitivity.

ADVERSE REACTIONS/ TOXIC EFFECTS

Peliosis hepatitis (presence of blood-filled cysts in parenchyma of liver), hepatic neoplasms, and hepatocellular carcinoma have been associated with prolonged high-dose therapy. Anaphylactic reactions occur rarely.

NURSING CONSIDERATIONS

BASELINE ASSESSMENT
Establish baseline weight, BP, Hgb, Hct. Check serum liver function, electrolytes, cholesterol. Wrist x-rays may be ordered to determine bone maturation in children.

INTERVENTION/EVALUATION
Weigh daily and report weekly gain of more than 5 lb; evaluate for edema. Monitor I&O. Check BP at least twice a day. Assess serum electrolytes, cholesterol, Hgb, Hct (periodically for high dosage), liver function test results, radiologic exam of wrist and hand (when using in prepubertal children). With breast cancer or immobility, check for hypercalcemia (lethargy, muscle weakness, confusion, irritability). Ensure adequate intake of protein, calories. Assess for virilization. Monitor sleep patterns. Check injection site for redness, swelling, pain.

PATIENT/FAMILY TEACHING
• Regular visits to physician and monitoring tests are necessary. • Do not take any other medications without consulting physician. • Teach diet high in protein, calories. • Food may be better tolerated in small, frequent feedings. • Weigh daily, report 5 lb/wk gain. • Notify physician if nausea, vomiting, acne, pedal edema occurs. • **Females:** Promptly report menstrual irregularities, hoarseness, deepening of voice. • **Males:** Report frequent erections, difficulty urinating, gynecomastia.

tetracaine

(Pontocaine)
See Anesthetics: local (pp. 4C, 6C)

tetracycline hydrochloride

tet-ra-**sye**-kleen
(Achromycin ♣, Ala-Tet, Apo-Tetra ♣, Novotetra ♣, Nu-Tetra ♣, Panmycin, Sumycin, Tetracon)

◆CLASSIFICATION
PHARMACOTHERAPEUTIC: Tetracycline. **CLINICAL:** Antibiotic.

ACTION

A tetracycline antibiotic that inhibits bacterial protein synthesis by binding to ribosomes. **Therapeutic Effect:** Bacteriostatic.

PHARMACOKINETICS

Readily absorbed from the GI tract. Protein binding: 30%–60%. Widely distributed. Excreted in urine; eliminated in feces through biliary system. Not removed by hemodialysis. **Half-life:** 6–11 hr (increased in impaired renal function).

USES

Treatment of susceptible infections due to *Rickettsiae, M. pneumoniae, C. trachomatis, C. psittaci, H. ducreyi, Yersinia pestis, Francisella tularensis, Bivrio cholerae,* Brucella species, gram-negative organisms including inflammatory acne vulgaris, Lyme disease, mycoplasma disease, *Legionella,* Rocky Mountain spotted fever, chlamydial infection in patients with gonorrhea. Part of multidrug regimen of *H. pylori* eradication to reduce risk of duodenal ulcer recurrence.

PRECAUTIONS

CONTRAINDICATIONS: Children 8 yr and younger, hypersensitivity to sulfites. **CAUTIONS:** Sun, ultraviolet light exposure (severe photosensitivity reaction).

⧖ **LIFESPAN CONSIDERATIONS:** Pregnancy/Lactation: Readily crosses placenta. Distributed in breast milk. Avoid use in women during last half of pregnancy. May produce permanent tooth discoloration and enamel hypoplasia, inhibit fetal skeletal growth in children 8 yr and younger. **Pregnancy Category D (B with topical form). Children:** Not recommended in those 8 yr and younger; may cause permanent staining of teeth, enamel hypoplasia, decreased linear skeletal growth rate. **Elderly:** No age-related precautions noted.

INTERACTIONS

DRUG: **Carbamazepine, phenytoin:** May decrease tetracycline blood concentration. **Cholestyramine, colestipol:** May decrease tetracycline absorption. **Oral contraceptives:** May decrease the effects of oral contraceptives. **HERBAL:** **St. John's wort:** May increase the risk of photosensitivity. **FOOD:** **Dairy products:** Inhibit tetracycline absorption. **LAB VALUES:** May increase BUN and serum alkaline phosphatase, amylase, bilirubin, AST, and ALT levels.

AVAILABILITY (Rx)

CAPSULES: 250 mg (Ala-Tet, Panmycin, Sumycin, Tetracon), 500 mg (Sumycin, Tetracon). **ORAL SUSPENSION (SUMYCIN):** 125 mg/5 ml. **TABLETS (SUMYCIN):** 250 mg, 500 mg. **TOPICAL SOLUTION:** 2.2 mg/ml. **TOPICAL OINTMENT:** 3%.

ADMINISTRATION/HANDLING

PO
• Give capsules, tablets with full glass of water 1 hr before or 2 hr after meals.

TOPICAL
• Cleanse area gently before application.
• Apply only to affected area.

INDICATIONS/ROUTES/DOSAGE

INFLAMMATORY ACNE VULGARIS, LYME DISEASE, MYCOPLASMAL DISEASE, *LEGIONELLA* INFECTIONS, ROCKY MOUNTAIN SPOTTED FEVER, CHLAMYDIAL INFECTIONS IN PATIENTS WITH GONORRHEA
PO: ADULTS, ELDERLY: 250–500 mg q6–12h. CHILDREN 8 YR AND OLDER: 25–50 mg/kg/day in 4 divided doses. **Maximum:** 3 g/day.

H. PYLORI INFECTIONS
PO: ADULTS, ELDERLY: 500 mg 2–4 times a day (in combination).
TOPICAL: ADULTS, ELDERLY: Apply twice a day (once in the morning, once in the evening).

DOSAGE IN RENAL IMPAIRMENT
Dosage interval is modified based on creatinine clearance.

Creatinine Clearance	Dosage Interval
50–80 ml/min	Usual dose q8–12h
10–50 ml/min	Usual dose q12–24h
Less than 10 ml/min	Usual dose q24h

SIDE EFFECTS

FREQUENT: Dizziness, light-headedness, diarrhea, nausea, vomiting, abdominal cramps, possibly severe photosensitivity. **Topical:** Dry, scaly skin; stinging or burning sensation. **OCCASIONAL:** Pigmentation of skin or mucous

T

---

membranes, rectal or genital pruritus, stomatitis. **Topical:** Pain, redness, swelling, or other skin irritation.

ADVERSE REACTIONS/ TOXIC EFFECTS

Superinfection (especially fungal), anaphylaxis, and benign intracranial hypertension may occur. Bulging fontanelles occur rarely in infants.

NURSING CONSIDERATIONS

BASELINE ASSESSMENT

Question for history of allergies, especially tetracyclines, sulfite.

INTERVENTION/EVALUATION

Assess skin for rash. Determine pattern of bowel activity and stool consistency. Monitor food intake, tolerance. Be alert for superinfection: diarrhea, stomatitis, anal or genital pruritus. Monitor BP, level of consciousness (LOC) (potential for increased intracranial pressure [ICP]).

PATIENT/FAMILY TEACHING

• Continue antibiotic for full length of treatment. • Space doses evenly. • Take oral doses on empty stomach (1 hr before or 2 hr after food, beverages). • Drink full glass of water with capsules; avoid bedtime doses. • Notify physician if diarrhea, rash, other new symptom occurs. • Protect skin from sun, ultraviolet light exposure. • Consult physician before taking any other medication. • Avoid tasks that require alertness, motor skills until response to drug is established (may cause dizziness, lightheadedness). • **Topical:** Skin may turn yellow with topical application (washing removes solution); fabrics may be stained by heavy application. • Do not apply to deep or open wounds.

Teveten, *see eprosartan*

thalidomide

thah-**lid**-owe-mide
(Thalomid)

CLASSIFICATION

PHARMACOTHERAPEUTIC: Immunomodulator. **CLINICAL:** Immunosuppressive agent.

ACTION

An immunomodulator whose exact mechanism is unknown. Has sedative, anti-inflammatory, and immunosuppressive activity, which may be due to selective inhibition of the production of tumor necrosis factor-alpha. **Therapeutic Effect:** Improves muscle wasting in HIV patients; reduces local and systemic effects of leprosy.

PHARMACOKINETICS

Protein binding: 55%. Metabolism and elimination are not known. **Half-life:** 5–7 hr.

USES

Treatment of leprosy. **OFF-LABEL:** Prevention and treatment of discoid lupus erythematosus, erythema fultiforme, graft vs host reactions following bone marrow transplantation, rheumatoid arthritis; treatment of Behcet's syndrome, Crohn's disease, GI bleeding, multiple myeloma, pruritus, recurrent aphthous ulcers in HIV patients, wasting syndrome associated with HIV or cancer.

PRECAUTIONS

CONTRAINDICATIONS: Neutropenia, peripheral neuropathy; pregnancy. **CAUTIONS:** History of seizures.

⧗ **LIFESPAN CONSIDERATIONS: Pregnancy/Lactation:** Contraindicated in women who are or may become pregnant and who are not using two required types of birth control or who are not continually abstaining from heterosexual

---

sexual contact. Can cause severe birth defects, fetal death. Unknown if distributed in breast milk. **Pregnancy Category X. Children:** Safety and efficacy not established in children under 12 yr. **Elderly:** No age-related precautions noted.

INTERACTIONS

DRUG: **Alcohol, other CNS depressants:** May increase sedative effects. **Medications associated with peripheral neuropathy (such as isoniazid, lithium, metronidazole, phenytoin):** May increase peripheral neuropathy. **Medications that decrease effectiveness of hormonal contraceptives (such as carbamazepine, protease inhibitors, rifampin):** May decrease the effectiveness of the contraceptive; patient must use two other methods of contraception. HERBAL: None known. FOOD: None known. LAB VALUES: None known.

AVAILABILITY (Rx)

CAPSULES: 50 mg, 100 mg, 200 mg.

ADMINISTRATION/HANDLING

◀ ALERT ▶ Thalidomide may be prescribed only by licensed prescribers who are registered in the S.T.E.P.S. program and understand the risk of teratogenicity if thalidomide is used during pregnancy.
• Administer thalidomide with water at least 1 hr after the evening meal and, if possible, at bedtime because of the risk of developing somnolence.

INDICATIONS/ROUTES/DOSAGE

AIDS-RELATED MUSCLE WASTING
PO: ADULTS: 100–300 mg a day.

LEPROSY
PO: ADULTS, ELDERLY: Initially, 100–300 mg/day as single bedtime dose, at least 1 hr after the evening meal. Continue until active reaction subsides, then reduce dose q2–4wk in 50 mg increments.

SIDE EFFECTS

FREQUENT: Somnolence, dizziness, mood changes, constipation, dry mouth, peripheral neuropathy. OCCASIONAL: Increased appetite, weight gain, headache, loss of libido, edema of face and limbs, nausea, alopecia, dry skin, rash, hypothyroidism.

ADVERSE REACTIONS/ TOXIC EFFECTS

Neutropenia, peripheral neuropathy, and thromboembolism occur rarely.

NURSING CONSIDERATIONS

BASELINE ASSESSMENT
Assess for hypersensitivity to thalidomide. Assess for pregnancy in females 24 hr before beginning thalidomide therapy (contraindicated). Determine use of other medications (many interactions).

INTERVENTION/EVALUATION
Monitor WBC, nerve conduction studies, HIV viral load. Observe for signs and symptoms of peripheral neuropathy. Perform pregnancy tests on women of childbearing potential. Perform the test weekly during the first 4 wk of use, then at 4-wk intervals in women with regular menstrual cycles or q2wk in women with irregular menstrual cycles.

PATIENT/FAMILY TEACHING
• Avoid tasks requiring alertness, motor skills until response to drug is established. • Avoid use of alcoholic beverages, other drugs causing drowsiness. • Pregnancy test within 24 hr before starting thalidomide, then q2–4wk in women of childbearing age. • Discontinue and call physician if symptoms of peripheral neuropathy occur. • Advise male patients receiving thalidomide to always use a latex condom during any sexual contact with women of childbearing potential.

T

Thalomid, *see thalidomide*

---

thiamine hydrochloride (vitamin B₁)

thy-a-min
(Betaxin ✦, Thiamilate, Vitamin B₁)

◆CLASSIFICATION

PHARMACOTHERAPEUTIC: Water-soluble vitamin. **CLINICAL:** Vitamin B complex (see p. 144C).

ACTION

A water-soluble vitamin that combines with adenosine triphosphate in the liver, kidneys, and leukocytes to form thiamine diphosphate, a coenzyme that is necessary for carbohydrate metabolism. **Therapeutic Effect:** Prevents and reverses thiamine deficiency.

PHARMACOKINETICS

Readily absorbed from the GI tract, primarily in duodenum, after IM administration. Widely distributed. Metabolized in the liver. Primarily excreted in urine.

USES

Prevention and treatment of thiamine deficiency (e.g., beriberi, Wernicke's encephalopathy syndrome, peripheral neuritis associated with pellegra, alcoholic patients with altered sensorium), metabolic disorders.

PRECAUTIONS

CONTRAINDICATIONS: None known. **CAUTIONS:** Wernicke's encephalopathy.

⧗ **LIFESPAN CONSIDERATIONS: Pregnancy/Lactation:** Crosses placenta.

Unknown if drug is excreted in breast milk. **Pregnancy Category A (C if used in doses above recommended daily allowance). Children/Elderly:** No age-related precautions noted.

INTERACTIONS

DRUG: None known. **HERBAL:** None known. **FOOD:** None known. **LAB VALUES:** None known.

AVAILABILITY

TABLETS (OTC): 50 mg, 100 mg, 250 mg, 500 mg. **INJECTION (VITAMIN B₁):** 100 mg/ml.

ADMINISTRATION/HANDLING

◄ **ALERT** ► IV, IM administration used only in acutely ill or those unresponsive to PO route (GI malabsorption syndrome). IM route preferred to IV use. Give by IV push, or add to most IV solutions and give as infusion.

▦ IV INCOMPATIBILITY

Sodium bicarbonate.

IV COMPATIBILITIES

Famotidine (Pepcid), multivitamins.

INDICATIONS/ROUTES/DOSAGE

DIETARY SUPPLEMENT
PO: ADULTS, ELDERLY: 1–2 mg/day. CHILDREN: 0.5–1 mg/day. INFANTS: 0.3–0.5 mg/day.

THIAMINE DEFICIENCY
PO: ADULTS, ELDERLY: 5–30 mg/day, as a single dose or in 3 divided doses, for 1 mo. CHILDREN: 10–50 mg/day in 3 divided doses.

THIAMINE DEFICIENCY IN PATIENTS WHO ARE CRITICALLY ILL OR HAVE MALABSORPTION SYNDROME
IV, IM: ADULTS, ELDERLY: 5–100 mg, 3 times a day. CHILDREN: 10–25 mg/day.

METABOLIC DISORDERS
PO: ADULTS, ELDERLY, CHILDREN: 10–20 mg/day; increased up to 4 g/day in divided doses.

SIDE EFFECTS

FREQUENT: Pain, induration, and tenderness at IM injection site.

ADVERSE REACTIONS/ TOXIC EFFECTS

IV administration may result in a rare, severe hypersensitivity reaction marked by a feeling of warmth, pruritus, urticaria, weakness, diaphoresis, nausea, restlessness, tightness in throat, angioedema, cyanosis, pulmonary edema, GI tract bleeding, and cardiovascular collapse.

NURSING CONSIDERATIONS

INTERVENTION/EVALUATION

Monitor lab values for erythrocyte activity, EKG readings. Assess for clinical improvement (improved sense of well-being, weight gain). Observe for reversal of deficiency symptoms (**neurologic:** peripheral neuropathy, hyporeflexia, nystagmus, ophthalmoplegia, ataxia, muscle weakness; **cardiac:** venous hypertension, bounding arterial pulse, tachycardia, edema; **mental:** confused state).

PATIENT/FAMILY TEACHING

• Discomfort may occur with IM injection. • Foods rich in thiamine include pork, organ meats, whole grain and enriched cereals, legumes, nuts, seeds, yeast, wheat germ, rice bran. • Urine may appear bright yellow.

---

thioguanine

thigh-oh-**guan**-een

(Thioguanine)

See Cancer chemotherapeutic agents (p. 78C)

---

thiopental sodium

(Pentothal)

See Anesthetics: general (p. 3C)

---

thioridazine

thye-or-**rid**-a-zeen

(Apo-Thioridazine ✤, Mellaril, Thioridazine Intensol)

Do not confuse thioridazine with thiothixene or Thorazine, or Mellaril with Mebaral.

◆CLASSIFICATION

PHARMACOTHERAPEUTIC: Phenothiazine. **CLINICAL:** Antipsychotic, sedative, antidyskinetic (see p. 59C).

ACTION

A phenothiazine that blocks dopamine at postsynaptic receptor sites. Possesses strong anticholinergic and sedative effects. Therapeutic Effect: Suppresses behavioral response in psychosis; reduces locomotor activity and aggressiveness.

PHARMACOKINETICS

Absorption may be erratic. Protein binding: Very high. Metabolized in liver. Excreted in urine. Half-life: 21–24 hr.

USES

Treatment of refractory schizophrenic patients. OFF-LABEL: Treatment of behavioral problems in children, dementia, depressive neurosis.

PRECAUTIONS

CONTRAINDICATIONS: Angle-closure glaucoma, blood dyscrasias, cardiac arrhythmias, cardiac or hepatic impairment, concurrent use of drugs that prolong QT interval, severe CNS depression. **CAUTIONS:** Seizures, decreased

GI motility, urinary retention, benign prostatic hypertrophy, visual problems.

⏳ **LIFESPAN CONSIDERATIONS: Pregnancy/Lactation:** Drug crosses placenta; is distributed is breast milk. **Pregnancy Category C. Children:** Increased risk for development of extrapyramidal symptoms (EPS), or neuromuscular symptoms, especially dystonias. **Elderly:** Prone to anticholinergic effects (dry mouth, EPS, orthostatic hypotension, sedation).

INTERACTIONS

DRUG: Alcohol, other CNS depressants: May increase respiratory depression and the hypotensive effects of thioridazine. **Antithyroid agents:** May increase the risk of agranulocytosis. **EPS-producing medications:** May increase the risk of EPS. **Hypotension-producing agents:** May increase hypotension. **Levodopa:** May decrease the effects of levodopa. **Lithium:** May decrease the absorption of thioridazine and produce adverse neurologic effects. **MAOIs, tricyclic antidepressants:** May increase the anticholinergic and sedative effects of thioridazine. **HERBAL:** None known. **FOOD:** None known. **LAB VALUES:** May cause EKG changes. Therapeutic serum level is 0.2–2.6 mcg/ml; toxic serum level is not established.

AVAILABILITY (Rx)

ORAL SOLUTION (CONCENTRATE): 30 mg/ml (Mellaril), 100 mg/ml (Thioridazine Intensol). **TABLETS (MELLARIL):** 10 mg, 15 mg, 25 mg, 50 mg, 100 mg, 150 mg, 200 mg.

INDICATIONS/ROUTES/DOSAGE
PSYCHOSIS

PO: ADULTS, ELDERLY, CHILDREN 12 YR AND OLDER: Initially, 25–100 mg 3 times a day; dosage increased gradually. **Maximum:** 800 mg/day. CHILDREN 2–11 YR: Initially,

0.5 mg/kg/day in 2–3 divided doses. **Maximum:** 3 mg/kg/day.

SIDE EFFECTS

OCCASIONAL: Drowsiness during early therapy, dry mouth, blurred vision, lethargy, constipation or diarrhea, nasal congestion, peripheral edema, urine retention. **RARE:** Ocular changes, altered skin pigmentation (in those taking high doses for prolonged periods), photosensitivity, darkening of urine.

ADVERSE REACTIONS/ TOXIC EFFECTS

Prolonged QT interval may produce torsades de pointes, a form of ventricular tachycardia, and sudden death.

NURSING CONSIDERATIONS

BASELINE ASSESSMENT

Avoid skin contact with solution (contact dermatitis). Assess behavior, appearance, emotional status, response to environment, speech pattern, thought content.

INTERVENTION/EVALUATION

Assess for EPS. Monitor EKG, CBC, BP, serum potassium, liver function, eye exams. Monitor for fine tongue movement (may be early sign of tardive dyskinesia). Supervise suicidal-risk patient closely during early therapy (as depression lessens, energy level improves, and suicide potential increases). Assess for therapeutic response (interest in surroundings, improvement in self-care, increased ability to concentrate, relaxed facial expression). Therapeutic serum level: 0.2–2.6 mcg/ml; toxic serum level: not established.

PATIENT/FAMILY TEACHING

• Full therapeutic effect may take up to 6 wk. • Urine may darken. • Do not abruptly withdraw from long-term drug therapy. • Report visual disturbances. • Sugarless gum, sips of tepid water may relieve dry mouth. • Drowsiness generally subsides during continued therapy. • Avoid tasks that require alertness, motor skills until response to drug is established. • Avoid alcohol. • Avoid exposure to sunlight, artificial light.

thiotepa

thigh-oh-**teh**-pah
(Thioplex)

CLASSIFICATION

PHARMACOTHERAPEUTIC: Alkylating agent. **CLINICAL:** Antineoplastic (see p. 78C).

ACTION

An alkylating agent that inhibits DNA and RNA protein synthesis by cross-linking with DNA and RNA strands, preventing cell growth. Cell cycle–phase nonspecific. Therapeutic Effect: Interferes with DNA and RNA function.

PHARMACOKINETICS

Incompletely absorbed from the GI tract. Metabolized in liver. Excreted in urine. Half-life: 2.3–2.4 hr.

USES

Treatment of superficial papillary carcinoma of urinary bladder, adenocarcinoma of breast and ovary, Hodgkin's disease, lymphosarcoma. Intracavitary injection to control pleural, pericardial, peritoneal effusions due to metastatic tumors. OFF-LABEL: Treatment of lung carcinoma.

PRECAUTIONS

CONTRAINDICATIONS: Pregnancy, severe myelosuppression (leukocyte count less than 3,000/mm^3 or platelet count less than 150,000/mm^3). **CAUTIONS:** Hepatic or renal impairment, bone marrow dysfunction.

LIFESPAN CONSIDERATIONS: Pregnancy/Lactation: May cause fetal harm. Unknown if drug is distributed is breast milk. **Pregnancy Category D. Children:** Safety and efficacy not established. **Elderly:** No age-related precautions noted.

INTERACTIONS

DRUG: **Antigout medications:** May decrease the effects of these drugs. **Bone marrow depressants:** May increase myelosuppression. **Live virus vaccines:** May potentiate virus replication, increase vaccine side effects, and decrease the patient's antibody response to the vaccine. HERBAL: None known. FOOD: None known. LAB VALUES: May increase serum uric acid levels.

AVAILABILITY (Rx)

POWDER FOR INJECTION: 15 mg, 30 mg.

ADMINISTRATION/HANDLING

◀ ALERT ▶ May be carcinogenic, mutagenic, teratogenic. Handle with extreme care during preparation/administration.

◀ ALERT ▶ Give by IV, intrapleural, intraperitoneal, intrapericardial, or intratumor injection; intravesical instillation.

 IV

Reconstitution • Reconstitute 15-mg vial with 1.5 ml sterile water for injection to provide concentration of 10 mg/ml. Shake solution gently; let stand to clear.

Rate of administration • Withdraw reconstituted drug through a 0.22-micron filter before administration. • For IV push, give over 5 min at concentration of 10 mg/ml. • Give IV infusion at concentration of 1 mg/ml.

Storage • Refrigerate unopened vials. • Reconstituted solution appears clear to slightly opaque; is stable for 5 days if refrigerated. Discard if solution appears grossly opaque or precipitate forms.

⊞ IV INCOMPATIBILITIES
Cisplatin (Platinol-AQ), filgrastim (Neupogen).

IV COMPATIBILITIES
Allopurinol (Aloprim), bumetanide (Bumex), calcium gluconate, carboplatin (Paraplatin), cyclophosphamide (Cytoxan), dexamethasone (Decadron), diphenhydramine (Benadryl), doxorubicin (Adriamycin), etoposide (VePesid), fluorouracil, gemcitabine (Gemzar), granisetron (Kytril), heparin, hydromorphone (Dilaudid), leucovorin, lorazepam (Ativan), magnesium sulfate, morphine, ondansetron (Zofran), paclitaxel (Taxol), potassium chloride, vincristine (Oncovin), vinorelbine (Navelbine).

INDICATIONS/ROUTES/DOSAGE
ADENOCARCINOMA OF BREAST AND OVARY, HODGKIN'S DISEASE, LYMPHOSARCOMA, SUPERFICIAL PAPILLARY CARCINOMA OF URINARY BLADDER
IV: ADULTS, ELDERLY: Initially, 0.3–0.4 mg/kg every 1–4 wk. Maintenance dose adjusted weekly based on blood counts. CHILDREN: 25–65 mg/m² as a single dose every 3–4 wk.

CONTROL OF PERICARDIAL, PERITONEAL, OR PLEURAL EFFUSIONS DUE TO METASTATIC TUMORS
INTRACAVITARY INJECTION: ADULTS, ELDERLY: 0.6–0.8 mg/kg every 1–4 wk.

SIDE EFFECTS
OCCASIONAL: Pain at injection site, headache, dizziness, urticaria, rash, nausea, vomiting, anorexia, stomatitis. RARE: Alopecia, cystitis, hematuria (after intravesical dose).

ADVERSE REACTIONS/TOXIC EFFECTS
Hematologic toxicity, manifested as leukopenia, anemia, thrombocytopenia, and pancytopenia, may occur from bone marrow depression. Although the WBC count falls to its lowest point 10–14 days after initial therapy, the initial effects on bone marrow may not be evident for 30 days. Stomatitis and ulceration of intestinal mucosa may occur.

NURSING CONSIDERATIONS
BASELINE ASSESSMENT
Obtain hematologic status at least weekly during therapy and for 3 wk after therapy discontinued.

INTERVENTION/EVALUATION
Interrupt therapy if WBC falls below 3,000/mm³, platelet count below 150,000/mm³, WBC or platelet count declines rapidly. Monitor uric acid serum levels, hematology tests. Assess for stomatitis. Monitor for hematologic toxicity: infection (fever, sore throat, signs of local infection), unusual ecchymoses or bleeding from any site, symptoms of anemia (excessive fatigue, weakness). Assess skin for rash, hives.

PATIENT/FAMILY TEACHING
• Maintain fastidious oral hygiene. • Do not have immunizations without physician's approval (drug lowers body's resistance). • Avoid crowds, those with infection. • Promptly report fever, sore throat, signs of local infection, unusual bruising or bleeding from any site.

thiothixene
thye-oh-**thix**-een
(Navane)
Do not confuse thiothixene with thioridazine.

CLASSIFICATION
CLINICAL: Antipsychotic (see p. 59C).

ACTION

An antipsychotic that blocks postsynaptic dopamine receptor sites in brain. Has alpha-adrenergic blocking effects, and depresses the release of hypothalamic and hypophyseal hormones. Therapeutic Effect: Suppresses psychotic behavior.

PHARMACOKINETICS

Well absorbed from the GI tract after IM administration. Widely distributed. Metabolized in the liver. Primarily excreted in urine. Unknown if removed by hemodialysis. Half-life: 34 hr.

USES

Symptomatic management of psychotic disorders.

PRECAUTIONS

CONTRAINDICATIONS: Blood dyscrasias, circulatory collapse, CNS depression, coma, history of seizures. **CAUTIONS:** Severe cardiovascular disorders, alcoholic withdrawal, patient exposure to extreme heat, glaucoma, prostatic hypertrophy.

⏳ **LIFESPAN CONSIDERATIONS: Pregnancy/Lactation:** Drug crosses placent; is distributed in breast milk. **Pregnancy Category C. Children:** May develop neuromuscular or extrapyramidal symptoms (EPS), especially dystonias. **Elderly:** More prone to orthostatic hypotension, anticholinergic effects (e.g., dry mouth), sedation, EPS.

INTERACTIONS

DRUG: Alcohol, other CNS depressants: May increase CNS and respiratory depression and the hypotensive effects of thiothixene. **EPS–producing medications:** May increase the risk of EPS. **Levodopa:** May inhibit the effects of levodopa. **Quinidine:** May increase cardiac effects. **HERBAL: Kava**

kava, St. John's wort, valerian: May increase CNS depression. FOOD: None known. LAB VALUES: May decrease serum uric acid level.

AVAILABILITY (Rx)

CAPSULES: 1 mg, 2 mg, 5 mg, 10 mg, 20 mg. **ORAL CONCENTRATE:** 5 mg/ml. **INJECTION:** 5 mg of thiothixene and 59.6 mg of mannitol per ml when reconstituted with 2.2 ml of sterile water for injection.

ADMINISTRATION/HANDLING

PO
• Give without regard to meals. • Avoid skin contact with oral solution (contact dermatitis).

INDICATIONS/ROUTES/DOSAGE

MILD TO MODERATE PSYCHOSIS
PO: ADULTS, ELDERLY, CHILDREN 12 YR AND OLDER: 2 mg 3 times a day up to 20–30 mg/day.

SEVERE PSYCHOSIS
PO: ADULTS, ELDERLY, CHILDREN 12 YR AND OLDER: Initially, 5 mg twice a day. May increase gradually up to 60 mg/day.

RAPID TRANQUILIZATION OF AGITATED PATIENT
PO: ADULTS, ELDERLY: 5–10 mg q15–30min. **Total dose:** 15–30 mg.

SIDE EFFECTS

EXPECTED: Hypotension, dizziness, syncope (occur frequently after first injection, occasionally after subsequent injections, and rarely with oral form). **FREQUENT:** Transient drowsiness, dry mouth, constipation, blurred vision, nasal congestion. **OCCASIONAL:** Diarrhea, peripheral edema, urine retention, nausea. **RARE:** Ocular changes, altered skin pigmentation (in those taking high doses for prolonged periods), photosensitivity.

T

ADVERSE REACTIONS/ TOXIC EFFECTS

The most common extrapyramidal reaction is akathisia, characterized by motor restlessness and anxiety. Akinesia, marked by rigidity, tremor, increased salivation, mask-like facial expression, and reduced voluntary movements, occurs less frequently. Dystonias, including torticollis, opisthotonos, and oculogyric crisis, occur rarely. Tardive dyskinesia, characterized by tongue protrusion, puffing of the cheeks, and chewing or puckering of the mouth, occurs rarely but may be irreversible. Elderly female patients have a greater risk of developing this reaction. Grand mal seizures may occur in epileptic patients, especially those receiving the drug by IM administration. Neuroleptic malignant syndrome occurs rarely.

NURSING CONSIDERATIONS

BASELINE ASSESSMENT

Assess behavior, appearance, emotional status, response to environment, speech pattern, thought content.

INTERVENTION/EVALUATION

Supervise suicidal-risk patient closely during early therapy (as depression lessens, energy level improves, increasing suicide potential). Monitor BP for hypotension. Assess for peripheral edema. Monitor pattern of bowel activity and stool consistency. Prevent constipation. Monitor for EPS, tardive dyskinesia and potentially fatal, rare neuroleptic malignant syndrome. Assess for therapeutic response (interest in surroundings, improvement in self-care, increased ability to concentrate, relaxed facial expression).

PATIENT/FAMILY TEACHING

• Full therapeutic effect may take up to 6 wk. • Report visual disturbances. • Sugarless gum, sips of tepid water may relieve dry mouth. • Drowsiness generally subsides during continued therapy. • Avoid tasks that require alertness, motor skills until response to drug is established. • Avoid alcohol, other CNS depressants. • Avoid exposure to direct sunlight, artificial light.

thyroid

(Armour Thyroid, S-P-T, Thyrar)
See Thyroid (p. 143C)

tiagabine

tie-**ag**-ah-bean
(Gabitril)

CLASSIFICATION

CLINICAL: Anticonvulsant (see p. 35C).

ACTION

An anticonvulsant that enhances the activity of gamma-aminobutyric acid, the major inhibitory neurotransmitter in the CNS. **Therapeutic Effect:** Inhibits seizures.

USES

Adjunctive therapy for treatment of partial seizures. OFF-LABEL: Bipolar disorder.

PRECAUTIONS

CONTRAINDICATIONS: None known.
CAUTIONS: Hepatic impairment. Concurrent use of alcohol, other CNS depressants may cause seizures. **Pregnancy Category C.**

INTERACTIONS

DRUG: Carbamazepine, phenobarbital, phenytoin: May increase tiagabine clearance. **Valproic acid:** May alter

---

the effects of valproic acid. **HERBAL: Ginkgo biloba:** May increase anticonvulsant effectiveness. **FOOD:** None known. **LAB VALUES:** None known.

AVAILABILITY (Rx)

TABLETS: 2 mg, 4 mg, 12 mg, 16 mg.

ADMINISTRATION/HANDLING

• Give with food.

INDICATIONS/ROUTES/DOSAGE

ADJUNCTIVE TREATMENT OF PARTIAL SEIZURES
PO: ADULTS, ELDERLY: Initially, 4 mg once a day. May increase by 4–8 mg/day at weekly intervals. **Maximum:** 56 mg/day. CHILDREN 12–18 YR: Initially, 4 mg once a day. May increase by 4 mg at week 2 and by 4–8 mg at weekly intervals thereafter. **Maximum:** 32 mg/day.

SIDE EFFECTS

FREQUENT (34%–20%): Dizziness, asthenia, somnolence, nervousness, confusion, headache, infection, tremor. **OCCASIONAL:** Nausea, diarrhea, abdominal pain, impaired concentration.

ADVERSE REACTIONS/ TOXIC EFFECTS

Overdose is characterized by agitation, confusion, hostility, and weakness. Full recovery occurs within 24 hr.

NURSING CONSIDERATIONS

BASELINE ASSESSMENT
Review history of seizure disorder (intensity, frequency, duration, level of consciousness [LOC]). Observe frequently for recurrence of seizure activity. Initiate seizure precautions.

INTERVENTION/EVALUATION
For those on long-term therapy, serum liver and renal function tests, CBC should be performed periodically. Assist with ambulation if dizziness occurs. Assess for clinical improvement (decrease in intensity/frequency of seizures).

PATIENT/FAMILY TEACHING
• If dizziness occurs, change positions slowly from recumbent to sitting position before standing. • Avoid tasks that require alertness, motor skills until response to drug is established. • Avoid alcohol.

Tiazac, *see diltiazem*

ticarcillin disodium

(Ticar)
See Antibiotic: penicillins

ticarcillin disodium/ clavulanate potassium

tie-car-**sill**-in/klah-view-**lan**-ate
(Timentin)

•CLASSIFICATION

PHARMACOTHERAPEUTIC: Penicillin. **CLINICAL:** Antibiotic (see p. 28C).

ACTION

Ticarcillin binds to bacterial cell walls, inhibiting cell wall synthesis. Clavulanate inhibits the action of bacterial beta-lactamase. **Therapeutic Effect:** Ticarcillin is bactericidal in susceptible organisms. Clavulanate protects ticarcillin from enzymatic degradation.

USES

Treatment of susceptible infections due to *P. aeruginosa, E. coli,* Enterobacter,

Proteus, beta-lactamase producing *S. aureus, M. catarrhalis, H. influenzae,* Klebsiella, *B. fragilis* including septicemia, skin and skin-structure, bone, joint, lower respiratory tract, gynecologic, intra-abdominal, urinary tract infections.

PRECAUTIONS

CONTRAINDICATIONS: Hypersensitivity to any penicillin or clavulanic acid. **CAUTIONS:** History of allergies (especially cephalosporins), renal impairment. **Pregnancy Category B.**

INTERACTIONS

DRUG: Anticoagulants, heparin, NSAIDs, thrombolytics: May increase the risk of hemorrhage with high dosages of ticarcillin. **Probenecid:** May increase ticarcillin blood concentration and risk of toxicity. **HERBAL:** None known. **FOOD:** None known. **LAB VALUES:** May increase bleeding time and serum alkaline phosphatase, bilirubin, creatinine, LDH, AST, and ALT levels. May decrease serum potassium, sodium, and uric acid levels. May cause a positive Coombs' test.

AVAILABILITY (Rx)

ADD-VANTAGE VIAL: 3.1 g. **POWDER FOR INJECTION:** 3.1 g. **PREMIXED SOLUTION FOR INFUSION:** 3.1 g/100 ml.

ADMINISTRATION/HANDLING

 IV

Reconstitution • Available in ready-to-use containers. • For IV infusion (piggyback), reconstitute each 3.1-g vial with 13 ml sterile water for injection or 0.9% NaCl to provide concentration of 200 mg ticarcillin and 6.7 mg clavulanic acid per ml. • Shake vial to assist reconstitution. • Further dilute with 50–100 ml D₅W or 0.9% NaCl.

Rate of administration • Infuse over 30 min. • Because of potential for hypersensitivity and anaphylaxis, start

initial dose at few drops/min, increase slowly to ordered rate. • Monitor patient first 10–15 min during initial dose, then check q10min.

Storage • Solution appears colorless to pale yellow (if solution darkens, indicates loss of potency). • Reconstituted IV infusion (piggyback) is stable for 24 hr at room temperature, 3 days if refrigerated. • Discard if precipitate forms.

IV INCOMPATIBILITIES

Amphotericin B complex (Abelcet, AmBisome, Amphotec), vancomycin (Vancocin), total parenteral nutrition (TPN).

IV COMPATIBILITIES

Diltiazem (Cardizem), heparin, insulin, morphine, propofol (Diprivan).

INDICATIONS/ROUTES/DOSAGE

SKIN AND SKIN-STRUCTURE, BONE, JOINT, AND LOWER RESPIRATORY TRACT INFECTIONS; SEPTICEMIA; ENDOMETRIOSIS

IV: ADULTS, ELDERLY: 3.1 g (3 g ticarcillin) q4–6h. **Maximum:** 18–24 g/day. CHILDREN 3 MO AND OLDER: 200–300 mg (as ticarcillin) q4–6h.

UTIs

IV: ADULTS, ELDERLY: 3.1 g q6–8h.

DOSAGE IN RENAL IMPAIRMENT
Dosage interval is modified based on creatinine clearance.

Creatinine Clearance	Dosage Interval
10–30 ml/min	Usual dose q8h
Less than 10 ml/min	Usual dose q12h

SIDE EFFECTS

FREQUENT: Phlebitis or thrombophlebitis (with IV dose), rash, urticaria, pruritus, altered smell or taste. **OCCASIONAL:** Nausea, diarrhea, vomiting. **RARE:** Headache, fatigue, hallucinations, bleeding or ecchymosis.

✎ see color pill atlas   ▰ herb   underlined – top prescribed drug

ADVERSE REACTIONS/ TOXIC EFFECTS

Overdosage may produce seizures and other neurologic reactions. Antibiotic-associated colitis and other superinfections may result from bacterial imbalance. Severe hypersensitivity reactions, including anaphylaxis, occur rarely.

NURSING CONSIDERATIONS

BASELINE ASSESSMENT

Question for history of allergies, especially penicillins, cephalosporins.

INTERVENTION/EVALUATION

Hold medication and promptly report rash (hypersensitivity), diarrhea (fever, abdominal pain, mucus and blood in stool may indicate antibiotic-associated colitis). Assess food tolerance. Provide mouth care, sugarless gum, hard candy to offset altered taste, smell. Evaluate IV site for phlebitis (heat, pain, red streaking over vein). Monitor I&O, urinalysis, renal function tests. Assess for overt bleeding, ecchymoses, swelling. Monitor hematology reports, serum electrolytes, particularly potassium. Be alert for superinfection: increased fever, sore throat, diarrhea, vomiting, stomatitis, anal/genital pruritus.

---

ticlopidine hydrochloride ⚑

tye-**klo**-pa-deen
(Apo-Ticlopidine ✿ , Ticlid)

♦ CLASSIFICATION

PHARMACOTHERAPEUTIC: Aggregation inhibitor. **CLINICAL:** Antiplatelet (see p. 31C).

ACTION

An aggregation inhibitor that inhibits the release of adenosine diphosphate from activated platelets, which prevents fibrinogen from binding to glycoprotein IIb/IIIa receptors on the surface of activated platelets. **Therapeutic Effect:** Inhibits platelet aggregation and thrombus formation.

PHARMACOKINETICS

Rapidly absorbed following PO administration. Protein binding: 98%. Extensively metabolized in liver. Primarily excreted in urine; partially eliminated in feces. **Half-life:** 12.6 hr.

USES

To reduce risk of stroke in those who have experienced stroke-like symptoms (transient ischemic attacks) or those with history of thrombotic stroke. **OFF-LABEL:** Prevention of postop deep vein thrombosis (DVT), protection of aorto-coronary bypass grafts, reduction of graft loss after renal transplant, treatment of intermittent claudication, sickle cell disease, subarachnoid hemorrhage, diabetic microangiopathy, ischemic heart disease.

PRECAUTIONS

CONTRAINDICATIONS: Active pathologic bleeding, such as bleeding peptic ulcer and intracranial bleeding, hematopoietic disorders, including neutropenia and thrombocytopenia; presence of hemostatic disorder; severe hepatic impairment. **CAUTIONS:** Those at increased risk of bleeding, severe hepatic or renal disease.

⌧ LIFESPAN CONSIDERATIONS: **Pregnancy/Lactation:** Unknown if drug crosses placenta or is distributed in breast milk. **Pregnancy Category B. Children:** Safety and efficacy not established. **Elderly:** No age-related precautions noted.

INTERACTIONS

DRUG: Aspirin, heparin, oral anticoagulants, thrombolytics: May increase the risk of bleeding with these drugs. **HERBAL:** None known. **FOOD:** None known. **LAB VALUES:** May increase serum cholesterol, serum alkaline phosphatase, bilirubin, triglyceride, AST, and ALT levels. May prolong bleeding time. May decrease neutrophil and platelet counts.

AVAILABILITY (Rx)

TABLETS: 250 mg.

ADMINISTRATION/HANDLING

PO

• Give with food or just after meals (bioavailability increased, GI discomfort decreased).

INDICATIONS/ROUTES/DOSAGE

PREVENTION OF STROKE
PO: ADULTS, ELDERLY: 250 mg twice a day.

SIDE EFFECTS

FREQUENT (13%–5%): Diarrhea, nausea, dyspepsia, including heartburn, indigestion, GI discomfort, and bloating. **RARE (2%–1%):** Vomiting, flatulence, pruritus, dizziness.

ADVERSE REACTIONS/ TOXIC EFFECTS

Neutropenia occurs in approximately 2% of patients. Thrombotic thrombocytopenia purpura, agranulocytosis, hepatitis, cholestatic jaundice, and tinnitus occur rarely.

NURSING CONSIDERATIONS

BASELINE ASSESSMENT

Drug should be discontinued 10–14 days before surgery if antiplatelet effect is not desired.

INTERVENTION/EVALUATION

Monitor pattern of bowel activity and stool consistency. Assist with ambulation if dizziness occurs. Monitor heart sounds by auscultation. Assess BP for hypotension. Assess skin for flushing, rash. Observe for signs of bleeding. Monitor CBC, serum liver function tests.

PATIENT/FAMILY TEACHING

• Take with food to decrease GI symptoms. • Periodic blood tests are essential. • Inform physician if fever, sore throat, chills, unusual bleeding occurs.

tigecycline

tie-geh-**sigh**-clean
(Tygacil)

CLASSIFICATION

PHARMACOTHERAPEUTIC: Glycylcycline. **CLINICAL:** Antibiotic.

ACTION

Blocks protein synthesis by binding to ribosomal receptor sites of bacterial cell wall. **Therapeutic Effect:** Bacteriostatic effect.

PHARMACOKINETICS

Extensive tissue distribution, minimally metabolized. Eliminated mainly by biliary/fecal route with a lesser amount excreted in the urine. Protein binding: 71%–89%. **Half-life:** Single dose: 27 hr, following multiple doses: 42 hr.

USES

Treatment of susceptible infections due to *E. coli, E. faecalis, S. aureus, S. agalactiae, S. anginosus* group (includes *S. anginosus, S. intermedius, S. constellatus*), *S. pyogenes, B. fragilis, Citrobacter freundii, E. cloacae, K. oxytoca, K. pneumoniae, B. thetaiotaomicron, B. umniformis, B. vulgatus, C. perfringens, Peptostreptococcus micros* including complicated skin and skin structure infections, complicated intra-abdominal infections.

PRECAUTIONS

CONTRAINDICATIONS: Children younger than 18 yr. **CAUTIONS:** Hypersensitivity to tetracyclines, last half of pregnancy, impaired hepatic function.

⏳ **LIFESPAN CONSIDERATIONS: Pregnancy/Lactation:** May cause fetal harm. May be distributed in breast milk. Permanent discoloration of the teeth (brown-gray) may occur if used during tooth development. **Pregnancy Category D. Children:** Safety and effectiveness not established in children younger than 18 yr. **Elderly:** No age-related precautions noted.

INTERACTIONS

DRUG: Oral contraceptives: The effects of these drugs may be decreased. **Warfarin:** May increase the risk of hypoprothrombinemia. **HERBAL:** None known. **FOOD:** None known. **LAB VALUES:** May increase BUN, alkaline phosphatase, amylase, bilirubin, glucose, LDH, ALT, AST. May decrease Hgb, WBCs, thrombocytes, potassium protein.

AVAILABILITY (Rx)

POWDER FOR INJECTION (TYGACIL): 50 mg/5 ml vial.

ADMINISTRATION/HANDLING

 IV

Reconstitution • Add 5.3 ml 0.9% NaCl or D_5W to each 50 mg vial. Swirl gently to dissolve. Resulting solution is 10 mg/ml. • Immediately withdraw 5 ml reconstituted solution and add to 100 ml 0.9% NaCl or D_5W bag for infusion (final concentration should not exceed 1 mg/ml). • Reconstituted solution appears yellow to red-orange.

Rate of administration • Administer over 30–60 min every 12 hr. • May be given through a dedicated line or by Y-site piggyback. If same line is used for sequential infusion of several different drugs, the line should be flushed before

and after infusion of tigecycline with either 0.9% NaCl or D_5W.

Storage • Reconstitution solution is stable for up to 6 hr at room temperature or up to 24 hr if refrigerated. • Discard if solution has particulate matter or discoloration (green, black).

🔲 IV INCOMPATIBILITIES

Amphotericin B, chlorpromazine, methylprednisolone, voriconazole.

IV COMPATIBILITIES

Dobutamine, dopamine, Ringer's lactate, lidocaine, potassium chloride, ranitidine, theophylline.

INDICATIONS/ROUTES/DOSAGE

SKIN AND SKIN STRUCTURE, INTRAABDOMINAL INFECTIONS
IV: ADULTS OVER 18 YR, ELDERLY: Initially, 100 mg, followed by 50 mg every 12 hr for 5–14 days.

SEVERE HEPATIC IMPAIRMENT
IV: ADULTS OVER 18 YR, ELDERLY: Initially, 100 mg, followed by 25 mg every 12 hr.

SIDE EFFECTS

FREQUENT (29%–13%): Nausea, vomiting, diarrhea. **OCCASIONAL (7%–4%):** Headache, hypertension, dizziness, increased cough, abnormal healing. **RARE (3%–2%):** Peripheral edema, pruritus, constipation, dyspepsia, weakness, hypotension, phlebitis, insomnia, rash, diaphoresis.

ADVERSE REACTIONS/TOXIC EFFECTS

Dyspnea, abscess, pseudomembranous colitis (abdominal cramps, watery severe diarrhea, fever) ranging from mild to life-threatening, may result from altered bacterial balance.

NURSING CONSIDERATIONS

BASELINE ASSESSMENT
Question for history of allergies, especially tetracyclines, before therapy.

T

INTERVENTION/EVALUATION

Determine pattern of daily bowel activity and stool consistency. Be alert for signs and symptoms of superinfection: severe diarrhea, changes of oral mucosa (white patches, erythema of gums, tongue, mouth soreness), anal/genital pruritus. Nausea, vomiting may be controlled by antiemetics.

PATIENT/FAMILY TEACHING

• Notify nurse/physician if diarrhea, rash, mouth soreness or other new symptom occurs.

---

tiludronate

ti-**loo**-dro-nate
(Skelid)

◆CLASSIFICATION

PHARMACOTHERAPEUTIC: Bone resorption inhibitor. **CLINICAL:** Calcium regulator.

ACTION

A calcium regulator that inhibits functioning osteoclasts through disruption of cytoskeletal ring structure and inhibition of osteoclastic proton pump. **Therapeutic Effect:** Inhibits bone resorption.

PHARMACOKINETICS

Well absorbed following PO administration. Protein binding: 90%. Not metabolized in liver. **Half-life:** 150 hr.

USES

Treatment of Paget's disease of bone (osteitis deformans).

PRECAUTIONS

CONTRAINDICATIONS: GI disease, such as dysphagia and gastric ulcer, impaired renal function. **CAUTIONS:** Hyperparathyroidism, hypocalcemia, vitamin D deficiency.

⏳ **LIFESPAN CONSIDERATIONS: Pregnancy/Lactation:** Unknown if drug crosses placenta or is distributed is breast milk. **Pregnancy Category C. Children:** Safety and efficacy not established. **Elderly:** No age-related precautions noted.

INTERACTIONS

DRUG: Antacids containing aluminum or magnesium, calcium, salicylates: May interfere with the absorption of tiludronate. **HERBAL:** None known. **FOOD:** None known. **LAB VALUES:** None known.

AVAILABILITY (Rx)

TABLETS: 200 mg.

INDICATIONS/ROUTES/DOSAGE

PAGET'S DISEASE

PO: ADULTS, ELDERLY: 400 mg once a day for 3 mo. Must take with 6–8 ounces plain water. Do not give within 2 hr of food intake. Avoid giving aspirin, calcium supplements, mineral supplements, or antacids within 2 hr of tiludronate administration.

SIDE EFFECTS

FREQUENT (9%–6%): Nausea, diarrhea, generalized body pain, back pain, headache. **OCCASIONAL:** Rash, dyspepsia, vomiting, rhinitis, sinusitis, dizziness.

ADVERSE REACTIONS/ TOXIC EFFECTS

Dysphagia, esophagitis, esophageal ulcer, and gastric ulcer occur rarely.

NURSING CONSIDERATIONS

BASELINE ASSESSMENT

Assess if patient is pregnant, using other medications (especially aluminum, magnesium, calcium, salicylates). Determine baseline renal function. Assess for GI disease.

T

INTERVENTION/EVALUATION

Monitor serum osteocalcin, alkaline phosphatase, adjusted calcium, urinary hydroxyproline to assess effectiveness of medication.

PATIENT/FAMILY TEACHING

• Take with 6–8 oz water. • Avoid other medication for 2 hr before or after taking tiludronate. • Check with physician if calcium and vitamin D supplements are necessary.

Timentin, *see ticarcillin and clavulanate*

---

timolol maleate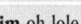

tim-oh-lole

(Apo-Timol ✤, Apo-Timop ✤, Betimol, Blocadren, Gen-Timolol ✤, Istalol, Novo-Timol ✤, PMS-Timolol ✤, Timolol Ophthalmic, Timoptic, Timoptic OccuDose, Timoptic Ocumeter, Timoptic Ocumeter Plus, Timoptic XE).

Do not confuse timolol with atenolol, or Timoptic with Viroptic.

FIXED-COMBINATION(S)

Cosopt: timolol/dorzolamide (a carbonic anhydrase inhibitor): 0.5%/2%. **Timolide:** timolol/hydrochlorothiazide (a diuretic): 10 mg/ 25 mg.

◆CLASSIFICATION

PHARMACOTHERAPEUTIC: Beta-adrenergic blocker. **CLINICAL:** Antihypertensive, antimigraine, antiglaucoma (see pp. 48C, 65C).

ACTION

An antihypertensive, antimigraine, and antiglaucoma agent that blocks beta$_1$- and beta$_2$-adrenergic receptors. **Therapeutic Effect:** Reduces intraocular pressure (IOP) by reducing aqueous humor production, lowers BP, slows the heart rate, and decreases myocardial contractility.

PHARMACOKINETICS

Route	Onset	Peak	Duration
PO	15–45 min	0.5–2.5 hr	4 hr
Ophthalmic	30 min	1–2 hr	12–24 hr

Well absorbed from the GI tract. Protein binding: 60%. Minimal absorption after ophthalmic administration. Metabolized in the liver. Primarily excreted in urine. Not removed by hemodialysis. **Half-life:** 4 hr. Systemic absorption may occur with ophthalmic administration.

USES

Management of mild to moderate hypertension. Used alone or in combination with diuretics, especially thiazide type. Reduces cardiovascular mortality in those with definite or suspected acute MI. Prophylaxis of migraine headache. **Ophthalmic:** Reduces IOP in management of open-angle glaucoma, aphakic glaucoma, ocular hypertension, secondary glaucoma. **OFF-LABEL: Systemic:** Treatment of anxiety, cardiac arrhythmias, chronic angina pectoris, hypertrophic cardiomyopathy, migraine, pheochromocytoma, thyrotoxicosis, tremors. **Ophthalmic:** To decrease IOP in acute or chronic angle-closure glaucoma, treatment of angle-closure glaucoma during and after iridectomy, malignant glaucoma, secondary glaucoma.

PRECAUTIONS

CONTRAINDICATIONS: Bronchial asthma, cardiogenic shock, CHF unless

---

T

secondary to tachyarrhythmias, chronic obstructive pulmonary disorder (COPD), patients receiving MAOI therapy, second- or third-degree heart block, sinus bradycardia, uncontrolled cardiac failure. **CAUTIONS:** Inadequate cardiac function, renal or hepatic impairment, hyperthyroidism. Precautions also apply to ophthalmic administration (due to systemic absorption of ophthalmic solution).

⌛ **LIFESPAN CONSIDERATIONS: Pregnancy/Lactation:** Distributed in breast milk; not for use in breast-feeding women because of potential for serious adverse effect on breast-feeding infant. Avoid use during first trimester. May produce bradycardia, apnea, hypoglycemia, hypothermia during delivery, low birth-weight infants. **Pregnancy Category C (D if used in second or third trimester). Children:** Safety and efficacy not established. **Elderly:** Age-related peripheral vascular disease increases susceptibility to decreased peripheral circulation.

INTERACTIONS

DRUG: Diuretics, other antihypertensives: May increase hypotensive effect. **Insulin, oral hypoglycemics:** May mask symptoms of hypoglycemia and prolong hypoglycemic effects of these drugs. **NSAIDs:** May decrease antihypertensive effect. **Sympathomimetics, xanthines:** May mutually inhibit effects. **HERBAL:** None known. **FOOD:** None known. **LAB VALUES:** May increase antinuclear antibody titer and BUN, serum LDH, serum lipoprotein, serum alkaline phosphatase, serum bilirubin, serum creatinine, serum potassium, serum uric acid, AST, ALT, and serum triglyceride levels.

AVAILABILITY (Rx)

TABLETS (BLOCADREN): 5 mg, 10 mg, 20 mg. **OPHTHALMIC GEL (TIMOPTIC-XE):** 0.25%, 0.5%. **OPHTHALMIC SOLUTION (BETIMOL, TIMOPTIC, TIMOPTIC OCCU-DOSE, TIMOPTIC OCUMETER, TIMOPTIC OCUMETER PLUS):** 0.25%, 0.5%.

ADMINISTRATION/HANDLING

PO
• Give without regard to meals.
• Tablets may be crushed.

OPHTHALMIC
◄ **ALERT** ► When using gel, invert container, shake once before each use.
• Place finger on lower eyelid, pull out until pocket is formed between eye and lower lid. • Hold dropper above pocket, place prescribed number of drops or amount of prescribed gel into pocket.
• Instruct patient to close eyes gently so that medication will not be squeezed out of sac. • Apply gentle finger pressure to the lacrimal sac at inner canthus for 1 min following installation (lessens risk of systemic absorption).

INDICATIONS/ROUTES/DOSAGE

MILD TO MODERATE HYPERTENSION
PO: ADULTS, ELDERLY: Initially, 10 mg twice a day, alone or in combination with other therapy. Gradually increase at intervals of not less than 1 wk. Maintenance: 20–60 mg/day in 2 divided doses.

REDUCTION OF CARDIOVASCULAR MORTALITY IN DEFINITE OR SUSPECTED ACUTE MI
PO: ADULTS, ELDERLY: 10 mg twice a day, beginning 1–4 wk after infarction.

MIGRAINE PREVENTION
PO: ADULTS, ELDERLY: Initially, 10 mg twice a day. Range: 10–30 mg/day.

REDUCTION OF IOP IN OPEN-ANGLE GLAUCOMA, APHAKIC GLAUCOMA, OCULAR HYPERTENSION, AND SECONDARY GLAUCOMA
OPHTHALMIC: ADULTS, ELDERLY, CHILDREN: 1 drop of 0.25% solution in affected eye(s) twice a day. May be increased to 1 drop of 0.5% solution in affected eye(s) twice a day. When IOP is controlled, dosage may be reduced to 1 drop once

a day. If patient is switched to timolol from another antiglaucoma agent, administer concurrently for 1 day. Discontinue other agent on following day.

OPHTHALMIC (TIMOPTIC XE): ADULTS, ELDERLY: 1 drop/day.

OPHTHALMIC (ISTALOL): ADULTS, ELDERLY: Apply once daily.

SIDE EFFECTS

FREQUENT: Diminished sexual function, drowsiness, difficulty sleeping, unusual tiredness or weakness. **Ophthalmic:** Eye irritation, visual disturbances. **OCCASIONAL:** Depression, cold hands or feet, diarrhea, constipation, anxiety, nasal congestion, nausea, vomiting. **RARE:** Altered taste, dry eyes, itching, numbness of fingers, toes, or scalp.

ADVERSE REACTIONS/ TOXIC EFFECTS

Overdose may produce profound bradycardia, hypotension, and bronchospasm. Abrupt withdrawal may result in diaphoresis, palpitations, headache, and tremors. Timolol administration may precipitate CHF and MI in patients with cardiac disease; thyroid storm in those with thyrotoxicosis; and peripheral ischemia in those with existing peripheral vascular disease. Hypoglycemia may occur in patients with previously controlled diabetes. Ophthalmic overdose may produce bradycardia, hypotension, bronchospasm, and acute cardiac failure.

NURSING CONSIDERATIONS

BASELINE ASSESSMENT

Assess BP, apical pulse immediately before drug is administered (if pulse is 60 min or less or systolic BP is less than 90 mm Hg, withhold medication, contact physician).

INTERVENTION/EVALUATION

Assess pulse for quality, irregular rate, bradycardia. Monitor EKG for cardiac arrhythmias, particularly PVCs. Monitor pattern of bowel activity and stool consistency. Monitor heart rate, BP, serum liver and renal function, IOP (ophthalmic preparation).

PATIENT/FAMILY TEACHING

• Do not abruptly discontinue medication. • Compliance with therapy regimen is essential to control glaucoma, hypertension, angina, arrhythmias. • Avoid tasks that require alertness, motor skills until response to drug is established. • Report shortness of breath, excessive fatigue, prolonged dizziness or headache. • Do not use nasal decongestants, OTC cold preparations (stimulants) without physician approval. • Restrict salt, alcohol intake. • **Ophthalmic:** Teach patient how to instill drops correctly, how to take pulse. • Transient stinging, discomfort may occur upon instillation.

Tindamax, *see tinidazole*

tinidazole

tin-**nid**-ah-zole
(Tindamax)

◆CLASSIFICATION

PHARMACOTHERAPEUTIC: Nitroimidazole derivative. **CLINICAL:** Antiprotozoal.

ACTION

A nitroimidazole derivative that is converted to the active metabolite by reduction of cell extracts of *Trichomonas*. The active metabolite causes DNA damage in pathogens. **Therapeutic Effect:** Produces antiprotozoal effect.

T

PHARMACOKINETICS

Rapidly and completely absorbed. Protein binding: 12%. Distributed in all body tissues and fluids; crosses blood-brain barrier. Significantly metabolized. Primarily excreted in urine; partially eliminated in feces. Half-life: 12–14 hr.

USES

Treatment of intestinal amebiasis and amebic hepatic abscess, giardiasis, trichomoniasis.

PRECAUTIONS

CONTRAINDICATIONS: First trimester of pregnancy, hypersensitivity to nitro-imidazole derivatives. **CAUTIONS:** CNS diseases, hepatic impairment, history of blood abnormalities.

⌛ **LIFESPAN CONSIDERATIONS: Pregnancy/Lactation:** Mutagenic, spermatogenic. Readily crosses placenta; distributed in breast milk. Contraindicated during first trimester. **Pregnancy Category C. Children:** Safety and efficacy in children younger than 3 yr not established. **Elderly:** Age-related hepatic impairment may require dosage adjustment.

INTERACTIONS

DRUG: Alcohol: May cause a disulfiram-type reaction. **Cholestyramine, oxytetracycline:** May decrease the effectiveness of tinidazole; separate dosage times. **Cimetidine, fosphenytoin, ketoconazole, phenobarbital, rifampin:** Decreases the metabolism of tinidazole. **Cyclosporine, fluorouracil, lithium, phenytoin (IV), tacrolimus:** May increase blood levels of these drugs. **Disulfiram:** May increase the risk of psychotic reactions (separate dose by 2 wk). **Oral anticoagulants:** Increase the risk of bleeding. **HERBAL:** None known. **FOOD:** None known. **LAB VALUES:** May increase serum LDH, triglyceride, AST, and ALT levels.

AVAILABILITY (Rx)

TABLETS: 250 mg, 500 mg.

ADMINISTRATION/HANDLING
PO

• Store at room temperature. • Scored tablets may be crushed. • Give with food (minimizes incidence of epigastric distress).

INDICATIONS/ROUTES/DOSAGE
INTESTINAL AMEBIASIS

PO: ADULTS, ELDERLY: 2 g/day for 3 days. CHILDREN 3 YR AND OLDER: 50 mg/kg/day (up to 2 g) for 3 days.

AMEBIC HEPATIC ABSCESS

PO: ADULTS, ELDERLY: 2 g/day for 3–5 days. CHILDREN 3 YR AND OLDER: 50 mg/kg/day (up to 2 g) for 3–5 days.

GIARDIASIS

PO: ADULTS, ELDERLY: 2 g as a single dose. CHILDREN 3 YR AND OLDER: 50 mg/kg (up to 2 g) as a single dose.

TRICHOMONIASIS

PO: ADULTS, ELDERLY: 2 g as a single dose.

SIDE EFFECTS

OCCASIONAL (4%–2%): Metallic or bitter taste, nausea, weakness, fatigue or malaise. **RARE (less than 2%):** Epigastric distress, anorexia, vomiting, headache, dizziness, red-brown or darkened urine.

ADVERSE REACTIONS/ TOXIC EFFECTS

Peripheral neuropathy, characterized by paresthesia, is usually reversible if tinidazole treatment is stopped as soon as neurologic symptoms appear. Superinfection, hypersensitivity reaction, and seizures occur rarely.

NURSING CONSIDERATIONS

BASELINE ASSESSMENT

Question for history of hypersensitivity to metronidazole or other nitroimidazole derivatives. Obtain specimens for diagnostic tests before giving first dose

---

T

✐ see color pill atlas   ⚘ herb   underlined – top prescribed drug (therapy may begin before results are known).

INTERVENTION/EVALUATION

Be alert to neurologic symptoms: dizziness, numbness, tingling, paraesthesia of extremities. Assess for nausea, vomiting and initiate appropriate measures. Watch for onset of superinfection: ulceration or change of oral mucosa, furry tongue, vaginal discharge, genital or anal pruritus.

PATIENT/FAMILY TEACHING

• Take medication with food. • Avoid alcoholic beverages during therapy and for 3 days after completion of treatment. • Urine may be red-brown or dark. • Avoid alcohol-containing preparations, e.g., cough syrups, elixirs. • Avoid tasks that require alertness, motor skills until response to drug is established (may cause dizziness).

---

tinzaparin sodium ▷

tin-za-**pair**-in
(Innohep)

◆CLASSIFICATION

PHARMACOTHERAPEUTIC: Low-molecular-weight heparin. **CLINICAL:** Anticoagulant (see p. 30C).

ACTION

A low-molecular-weight heparin that inhibits factor Xa. Causes less inactivation of thrombin, inhibition of platelets, and bleeding than standard heparin. Does not significantly influence bleeding time, PT, aPTT. Therapeutic Effect: Produces anticoagulation.

PHARMACOKINETICS

Well absorbed after subcutaneous administration. Primarily eliminated in urine. Half-life: 3–4 hr.

USES

Treatment of acute symptomatic deep vein thrombosis (DVT) with or without pulmonary embolism, when given in conjunction with warfarin.

PRECAUTIONS

CONTRAINDICATIONS: Active major bleeding, concurrent heparin therapy, hypersensitivity to heparin, sulfites, benzyl alcohol, or pork products, thrombocytopenia associated with positive in vitro test for antiplatelet antibody. **CAUTIONS:** Conditions with increased risk of hemorrhage, history of heparin-induced thrombocytopenia, renal impairment, elderly, uncontrolled arterial hypertension, history of recent GI ulceration or hemorrhage.

⚗ LIFESPAN CONSIDERATIONS: **Pregnancy/Lactation:** Use with caution, particularly during last trimester, immediate postpartum period (increased risk of maternal hemorrhage). Unknown if distributed in breast milk. **Pregnancy Category B. Children:** Safety and efficacy not established. **Elderly:** May be more susceptible to bleeding.

INTERACTIONS

DRUG: Anticoagulants, platelet inhibitors: May increase the risk of bleeding. HERBAL: **Ginkgo biloba:** May increase the risk of bleeding. FOOD: None known. LAB VALUES: Increases (reversible) LDH, serum alkaline phosphatase, AST, and ALT levels.

AVAILABILITY (Rx)

INJECTION: 20,000 anti-Xa international units/ml.

ADMINISTRATION/HANDLING

◀ ALERT ▶ Do not mix with other injections or infusions. Do not give IM.

SUBCUTANEOUS

• Parenteral form appears clear and colorless to pale yellow. • Store at

---

room temperature. • Instruct patient to lie down before administering by deep subcutaneous injection.

INDICATIONS/ROUTES/DOSAGE

DEEP VEIN THROMBOSIS (DVT)
SUBCUTANEOUS: ADULTS, ELDERLY: 175 anti-Xa international units/kg once a day. Continue for at least 6 days and until patient is sufficiently anticoagulated with warfarin (INR of 2 or more for 2 consecutive days).

SIDE EFFECTS

FREQUENT (16%): Injection site reaction, such as inflammation, oozing, nodules, and skin necrosis. **RARE (less than 2%):** Nausea, asthenia, constipation, epistaxis.

ADVERSE REACTIONS/ TOXIC EFFECTS

Overdose may lead to bleeding complications ranging from local ecchymoses to major hemorrhage. Antidote: Dose of protamine sulfate (1% solution) should be equal to dose of tinzaparin injected. One mg protamine sulfate neutralizes 100 units of tinzaparin. A second dose of 0.5 mg tinzaparin per 1 mg protamine sulfate may be given if aPTT tested 2–4 hr after the initial infusion remains prolonged.

NURSING CONSIDERATIONS

BASELINE ASSESSMENT

Assess CBC, including platelet count. Determine initial BP.

INTERVENTION/EVALUATION

Periodically monitor CBC, platelet count. Assess for any sign of bleeding: bleeding at surgical site, hematuria, blood in stool, bleeding from gums, petechiae, bruising, bleeding from injection sites.

PATIENT/FAMILY TEACHING

• Administer only subcutaneously. • May have tendency to bleed easily, use precautions (e.g., use electric razor,

soft toothbrush). • Inform physician if chest pain, unusual bleeding or bruising, pain, numbness, tingling, swelling in joints, injection site reaction (oozing, nodules, inflammation) occurs.

tiotropium bromide

tee-oh-**trow**-pea-um

(Spiriva)

◆CLASSIFICATION

PHARMACOTHERAPEUTIC: Anticholinergic. **CLINICAL:** Bronchodilator.

ACTION

An anticholinergic that binds to recombinant human muscarinic receptors at the smooth muscle, resulting in long-acting bronchial smooth-muscle relaxation. **Therapeutic Effect:** Relieves bronchospasm.

PHARMACOKINETICS

Route	Onset	Peak	Duration
Inhalation	N/A	N/A	24–36 hr

Binds extensively to tissue. Protein binding: 72%. Metabolized by oxidation. Excreted in urine. **Half-life:** 5–6 days.

USES

Long-term maintenance treatment of bronchospasm associated with chronic obstructive pulmonary disease (COPD), including chronic bronchitis, emphysema.

PRECAUTIONS

CONTRAINDICATIONS: History of hypersensitivity to atropine or its derivatives, including ipratropium. **CAUTIONS:** Narrow-angle glaucoma, prostatic hypertrophy, bladder neck obstruction.

⌛ LIFESPAN CONSIDERATIONS: Pregnancy/Lactation: Unknown if distributed in breast milk. **Pregnancy Category C. Children:** Safety and efficacy not established. **Elderly:** Higher frequency of dry mouth, constipation, UTI noted with increasing age.

INTERACTIONS

DRUG: **Ipratropium:** Concurrent administration with this drug is not recommended. HERBAL: None known. FOOD: None known. LAB VALUES: None known.

AVAILABILITY (Rx)

POWDER FOR INHALATION: 18 mcg/capsule (in blister packs containing 6 capsules with inhaler).

ADMINISTRATION/HANDLING
INHALATION
• Open dustcap of *HandiHaler* by pulling it upward, then open the mouthpiece. • Place capsule in the center chamber and firmly close the mouthpiece until a click is heard, leaving the dustcap open. • Hold *HandiHaler* device with the mouthpiece upward, pressing the piercing button completely in once, and release. • Instruct patient to breathe out completely before breathing in slowly and deeply but at a rate sufficient to hear the capsule vibrate. • Have the patient hold breath as long as it is comfortable until exhaling slowly. • To ensure receiving the full dose, instruct patient to repeat once.

Storage • Store at room temperature. Do not expose capsules to extreme temperature or moisture. • Do not store capsules in *HandiHaler* device.

INDICATIONS/ROUTES/DOSAGE
COPD
INHALATION: ADULTS, ELDERLY: 18 mcg (1 capsule)/day via *HandiHaler* inhalation device.

SIDE EFFECTS

FREQUENT (16%–6%): Dry mouth, sinusitis, pharyngitis, dyspepsia, UTI, rhinitis. OCCASIONAL (5%–4%): Abdominal pain, peripheral edema, constipation, epistaxis, vomiting, myalgia, rash, oral candidiasis.

ADVERSE REACTIONS/
TOXIC EFFECTS
Angina pectoris, depression, and flu-like symptoms occur rarely.

NURSING CONSIDERATIONS

BASELINE ASSESSMENT
Offer emotional support (high incidence of anxiety due to difficulty in breathing and sympathomimetic response to drug).

INTERVENTION/EVALUATION
Monitor rate, depth, rhythm, type of respiration; quality and rate of pulse. Assess lung sounds for rhonchi, wheezing, rales. Monitor ABGs. Observe lips, fingernails for cyanosis (blue or dusky color in light-skinned patients; gray in dark-skinned patients). Observe for clavicular retractions, hand tremor. Evaluate for clinical improvement (quieter, slower respirations, relaxed facial expression, cessation of clavicular retractions).

PATIENT/FAMILY TEACHING
• Increase fluid intake (decreases lung secretion viscosity). • Do not use more than 1 capsule for inhalation at any one time. • Rinsing mouth with water immediately after inhalation may prevent mouth and throat dryness, moniliasis. • Avoid excessive use of caffeine derivatives (chocolate, coffee, tea, cola, cocoa).

T

tipranavir

ti-**pran**-ah-veer
(Aptivus)

CLASSIFICATION

PHARMACOTHERAPEUTIC: Antiretroviral. **CLINICAL:** Protease inhibitor.

ACTION

A nonpeptide HIV-1 protease inhibitor that prevents the virus-specific processing of polyproteins and HIV-1 infected cells. **Therapeutic Effect:** Prevents formation of mature viral cells.

PHARMACOKINETICS

Readily absorbed following PO administration. Protein binding: 98%–99%. Metabolized in liver. Eliminated mainly in feces with a lesser amount eliminated in urine. **Half-life:** 6 hr.

USES

Treatment of HIV infection in combination with ritonavir.

PRECAUTIONS

CONTRAINDICATIONS: Moderate or severe hepatic insufficiency, concurrent therapy of tipranavir/ritonavir with alfuzosin, amiodarone, bepridil, cisapride, dihydroergotamine, ergonovine, ergotamine, flecainide, lovastatin, methylergonovine, midazolam, pimozide, propafenone, quinidine, simvastatin, St John's wort, triazolam, voriconazole. **CAUTIONS:** Diabetes mellitus, hemophilia, known sulfonamide allergy, mild hepatic impairment.

⧖ **LIFESPAN CONSIDERATIONS: Pregnancy/Lactation:** Unknown if drug crosses placenta or is distributed in breast milk. **Pregnancy Category C. Children:** Safety and efficacy not established. **Elderly:** Age-related hepatic impairment may require dosage adjustment.

INTERACTIONS

DRUG: Amiodarone, bepridil, ergotamine, lidocaine, midazolam, oral contraceptives, quinidine, triazolam, tricyclic antidepressants: Tipranavir use may interfere with the metabolism of these drugs. **Antiarrhythmics, antihistamines, GI motility agents:** May increase plasma concentration of antiarrhythmics. **Benzodiazepines:** May increase sedation, increase risk of respiratory depression. **Carbamazepine, phenobarbital, phenytoin, rifampin:** May decrease concentration. **Clozapine, HMG-CoA reductase inhibitors, warfarin:** Tipranavir use may increase the concentrations of these drugs. **Ergot derivatives:** May cause ergot toxicity. **HMG-CoA reductase inhibitors:** May increase the risk of myopathy including rhabdomyolysis. **HERBAL: St. John's wort:** May lead to loss of virologic response, potential resistance to tipranavir. **FOOD: High-fat meals:** May increase tipranavir bioavailability. **LAB VALUES:** May increase cholesterol, triglycerides, amylase, ALT, AST. May decrease WBC count.

AVAILABILITY (Rx)

CAPSULES: 250 mg.

ADMINISTRATION/HANDLING

PO
• Give without regard to meals. • Do not crush or open capsules.

INDICATIONS/ROUTES/DOSAGE

HIV INFECTION, CONCURRENT THERAPY WITH RITONAVIR

PO: ADULTS, ELDERLY: 500 mg (2 capsules) administered with 200 mg of ritonavir twice a day.

SIDE EFFECTS

FREQUENT (11%): Diarrhea. **OCCASIONAL (7%–2%):** Nausea, fever, fatigue, headache, depression, vomiting, abdominal pain, weakness, rash. **RARE (less than 2%):** Abdominal distention, anorexia, flatulence, dizziness, insomnia, myalgia.

ADVERSE REACTIONS/ TOXIC EFFECTS

Bronchitis occurs in 3% of patients. Anemia, neutropenia, thrombocytopenia, diabetes mellitus, hepatic failure, hepatitis, peripheral neuropathy, pancreatitis occur rarely.

NURSING CONSIDERATIONS

BASELINE ASSESSMENT

Obtain baseline laboratory testing, especially hepatic function tests, before beginning therapy and at periodic intervals during therapy. Offer emotional support. Obtain medication history.

INTERVENTION/EVALUATION

Closely monitor for evidence of GI discomfort. Monitor stool frequency/consistency. Assess skin for evidence of rash. Monitor serum chemistry tests for marked laboratory abnormalities, particularly hepatic profile. Assess for opportunistic infections: onset of fever, oral mucosa changes, cough, or other respiratory symptoms.

PATIENT/FAMILY TEACHING

• Eat small, frequent meals to offset nausea, vomiting and avoid high-fat meals. • Continue therapy for full length of treatment. • Doses should be evenly spaced. • Medication is not a cure for HIV infection, nor does it reduce risk of transmission to others. • Patient may continue to experience illnesses, including opportunistic infections. • Diarrhea can be controlled with OTC medication.

tirofiban 🏳

tye-**roe**-fye-ban
(Aggrastat)
Do not confuse Aggrastat with Aggrenox.

CLASSIFICATION

PHARMACOTHERAPEUTIC: Glycoprotein (GP) IIb/IIIa inhibitor. **CLINICAL:** Antiplatelet, antithrombotic (see p. 31C).

ACTION

An antiplatelet and antithrombotic agent that binds to platelet receptor glycoprotein IIb/IIIa, preventing binding of fibrinogen. Therapeutic Effect: Inhibits platelet aggregation and thrombus formation.

USES

Antiplatelet in combination with heparin, treatment of acute coronary syndrome, including those to be managed medically and those undergoing percutaneous transluminal coronary angioplasty (PTCA) or atherectomy.

PRECAUTIONS

CONTRAINDICATIONS: Active internal bleeding or a history of bleeding diathesis within previous 30 days, arteriovenous malformation or aneurysm, history of intracranial hemorrhage, history of thrombocytopenia after prior exposure to tirofiban, intracranial neoplasm, major surgical procedure within previous 30 days, severe hypertension, stroke. **CAUTIONS:** Patients with platelets less than $150,000/mm^3$, hemorrhagic retinopathy. Concomitant use of drugs affecting hemostasis (e.g., warfarin), renal impairment. **Pregnancy Category B.**

T

INTERACTIONS

DRUG: **Drugs that affect hemostasis (such as aspirin, heparin, NSAIDs, and warfarin):** May increase the risk of bleeding. **HERBAL:** None known. **FOOD:** None known. **LAB VALUES:** Decreases Hct, Hgb and platelet count.

AVAILABILITY (Rx)

INJECTION PREMIX: 12.5 mg/250 ml, 25 mg/500 ml (50 mcg/ml). **VIAL:** 250 mcg/ml.

ADMINISTRATION/HANDLING

 IV

Reconstitution

◀ **ALERT** ▶ Heparin and tirofiban can be administered through the same IV line.

INJECTION FOR SOLUTION (250 MCG/ML)
• Withdraw and discard 100 ml from a 500-ml bag 0.9% NaCl or D₅W and replace this volume with 100 ml of tirofiban (from two 50-ml vials) or withdraw and discard 50 ml from a 250-ml bag and replace with 50 ml of tirofiban (from one 50-ml vial) to achieve a final concentration of 50 mcg/ml. • Mix well before administration.

INJECTION (50 MCG/ML) PREMIX IN 500-ML INTRAVIA CONTAINER
• To open the IntraVia container, tear off the dust cover. • Check for leaks by squeezing the inner bag firmly; if any leak is found or if the solution is not clear, discard the solution. • Do not add other drugs or remove solution directly from the bag with a syringe. Do not use plastic containers in series connections (may result in air embolism by drawing air from the first container if it is empty of solution).

Rate of administration • For loading dose, give 0.4 mcg/kg/min for 30 min.

• For maintenance infusion, give 0.1 mcg/kg/min.

Storage • Store at room temperature. • Protect from light. • Use only clear solution. • Discard unused solution 24 hr after start of infusion.

IV INCOMPATIBILITIES

Do not mix with other medications.

INDICATIONS/ROUTES/DOSAGE

INHIBITION OF PLATELET AGGREGATION
IV: ADULTS, ELDERLY: Initially, 0.4 mcg/kg/min for 30 min; then continue at 0.1 mcg/kg/min through procedure and for 12–24 hr after procedure.

SEVERE RENAL INSUFFICIENCY (CREATININE CLEARANCE LESS THAN 30 ML/MIN)
IV: ADULTS, ELDERLY: Half the usual rate of infusion.

SIDE EFFECTS

OCCASIONAL **(6%–3%):** Pelvis pain, bradycardia, dizziness, leg pain. **RARE (2%–1%):** Edema and swelling, vasovagal reaction, diaphoresis, nausea, fever, headache.

ADVERSE REACTIONS/ TOXIC EFFECTS

Signs and symptoms of overdose include generally minor mucocutaneous bleeding and bleeding at the femoral artery access site. Thrombocytopenia occurs rarely.

NURSING CONSIDERATIONS

BASELINE ASSESSMENT

Assess platelet count, Hgb, Hct, aPTT, renal function before treatment, within 6 hr following the loading dose, and at least daily thereafter during therapy. If platelet count is less than 90,000/mm³, additional platelet counts should be obtained routinely to avoid thrombocytopenia. If thrombocytopenia occurs, drug therapy and heparin should be discontinued.

INTERVENTION/EVALUATION

Monitor aPTT 6 hr following the beginning of the heparin infusion. Adjust heparin dosage to maintain aPTT at approximately 2 times control. Diligently monitor for potential bleeding, particularly at other arterial and venous puncture sites, IM injection site. If possible, urinary catheters, NG tubes should be avoided. Maintain complete bed rest with head of the bed elevated at 30°.

tizanidine

tye-**zan**-i-deen
(Zanaflex)

◆ CLASSIFICATION

PHARMACOTHERAPEUTIC: Skeletal muscle relaxant. **CLINICAL:** Antispastic.

ACTION

A skeletal muscle relaxant that increases presynaptic inhibition of spinal motor neurons mediated by alpha$_2$-adrenergic agonists, reducing facilitation to postsynaptic motor neurons. Therapeutic Effect: Reduces muscle spasticity.

USES

Acute and intermittent management of muscle spasticity (spasms, stiffness, rigidity). OFF-LABEL: Low back pain, spasticity associated with multiple sclerosis or spinal cord injury, tension headaches, trigeminal neuralgia.

PRECAUTIONS

CONTRAINDICATIONS: None known. **CAUTIONS:** Renal or hepatic disease, hypotension, cardiac disease. **Pregnancy Category C.**

INTERACTIONS

DRUG: Alcohol, other CNS depressants: May increase CNS depressant effects. **Antihypertensives:** May increase tizanidine's hypotensive potential. **Oral contraceptives:** May reduce tizanidine clearance. **Phenytoin:** May increase serum levels and risk of toxicity of phenytoin. HERBAL: None known. FOOD: None known. LAB VALUES: May increase serum alkaline phosphatase, AST, and ALT levels.

AVAILABILITY (Rx)

TABLETS: 2 mg, 4 mg.

INDICATIONS/ROUTES/DOSAGE

MUSCLE SPASTICITY

PO: ADULTS, ELDERLY: Initially 2–4 mg, gradually increased in 2- to 4-mg increments and repeated q6–8h. **Maximum:** 3 doses/day or 36 mg/24 hr.

SIDE EFFECTS

FREQUENT (49%–41%): Dry mouth, somnolence, asthenia. **OCCASIONAL (16%–4%):** Dizziness, UTI, constipation. **RARE (3%):** Nervousness, amblyopia, pharyngitis, rhinitis, vomiting, urinary frequency.

ADVERSE REACTIONS/ TOXIC EFFECTS

Hypotension (a reduction in either diastolic or systolic BP) may be associated with bradycardia, orthostatic hypotension and, rarely, syncope. The risk of hypotension increases as dosage increases; BP may decrease within 1 hr after administration.

NURSING CONSIDERATIONS

BASELINE ASSESSMENT

Record onset, type, location, duration of muscular spasm. Check for immobility, stiffness, swelling. Obtain baseline serum liver function tests, alkaline phosphatase, total bilirubin.

INTERVENTION/EVALUATION

Assist with ambulation at all times. For those on long-term therapy, serum liver

T

and renal function tests should be performed periodically. Evaluate for therapeutic response (decreased intensity of skeletal muscle pain or tenderness, improved mobility, decrease in spasticity). To reduce risk of orthostatic hypotension, instruct patient to rise slowly from lying to sitting and from sitting to supine position.

PATIENT/FAMILY TEACHING

• Avoid tasks that require alertness, motor skills until response to drug is established. • Avoid sudden changes in posture. • May cause hypotension, sedation, impaired coordination.

TNKase, *see tenecteplase*

---

tobramycin sulfate

tow-bra-**my**-sin

(AK-Tob, Apo-Tobramycin ✽, Nebcin, Nebcin Pediatric, PMS-Tobramycin, TOBI, Tobrex)

FIXED-COMBINATION(S)

TobraDex: tobramycin/dexamethasone (a steroid): 0.3%/0.1% per ml or per g. **Zylet:** tobramycin/loteprednol: 0.3%/0.5%.

♦CLASSIFICATION

PHARMACOTHERAPEUTIC: Aminoglycoside. **CLINICAL:** Antibiotic (see p. 20C).

ACTION

An aminoglycoside antibiotic that irreversibly binds to protein on bacterial ribosomes. **Therapeutic Effect:** Interferes with protein synthesis of susceptible microorganisms.

PHARMACOKINETICS

Rapid, complete absorption after IM administration. Protein binding: less than 30%. Widely distributed (doesn't cross the blood-brain barrier; low concentrations in cerebrospinal fluid (CSF). Excreted unchanged in urine. Removed by hemodialysis. Half-life: 2–4 hr (increased in impaired renal function and neonates; decreased in cystic fibrosis and febrile or burn patients).

USES

Treatment of susceptible infections due to *P. aeruginosa*, other gram negative organisms including skin and skin-structure, bone, joint, respiratory tract infections; postop, burn, intra-abdominal infections; complicated UTIs; septicemia; meningitis. **Ophthalmic:** Superficial eye infections: blepharitis, conjunctivitis, keratitis, corneal ulcers. **Inhalation:** Bronchopulmonary infections in patients with cystic fibrosis.

PRECAUTIONS

CONTRAINDICATIONS: Hypersensitivity to other aminoglycosides (cross-sensitivity) and their components. **CAUTIONS:** Renal impairment, preexisting auditory or vestibular impairment, concomitant use of neuromuscular blocking agents.

⏳ LIFESPAN CONSIDERATIONS: **Pregnancy/Lactation:** Drug readily crosses placenta; is distributed in breast milk. May cause fetal nephrotoxicity. Ophthalmic form should not be used in breast-feeding mothers and only when specifically indicated in pregnancy. **Pregnancy Category C (B, ophthalmic form). Children:** Immature renal function in neonates and premature infants may increase risk of toxicity. **Elderly:** Age-related renal impairment may increase risk of toxicity; dosage adjustment recommended.

✎ see color pill atlas   🌿 herb   underlined – top prescribed drug

INTERACTIONS

DRUG: **Nephrotoxic medications, other aminoglycosides, ototoxic medications:** May increase the risk of nephrotoxicity and ototoxicity. **Neuromuscular blockers:** May increase neuromuscular blockade. **HERBAL:** None known. **FOOD:** None known. **LAB VALUES:** May increase serum bilirubin, BUN, serum creatinine, serum LDH, AST, and ALT levels. May decrease serum calcium, magnesium, potassium, and sodium concentrations. Therapeutic peak serum level is 5–20 mcg/ml; therapeutic trough serum level is 0.5–2 mcg/ml. Toxic peak serum level is greater than 20 mcg/ml; toxic trough serum level is greater than 2 mcg/ml.

AVAILABILITY (Rx)

INJECTION SOLUTION: 10 mg/ml (Nebcin Pediatric), 40 mg/ml (Nebcin). **INJECTION POWDER FOR RECONSTITUTION (NEBCIN):** 1.2 g. **OPHTHALMIC OINTMENT (TOBREX):** 0.3%. **OPHTHALMIC SOLUTION (AKTob, TOBREX):** 0.3%. **NEBULIZATION SOLUTION (TOBI):** 60 mg/ml.

ADMINISTRATION/HANDLING

◀ **ALERT** ▶ Coordinate peak and trough lab draws with administration times.

 IV

Reconstitution • Dilute with 50–200 ml D₅W, 0.9% NaCl. Amount of diluent for infants, children depends on individual need.

Rate of administration • Infuse over 20–60 min.

Storage • Store vials at room temperature. • Solutions may be discolored by light or air (does not affect potency).

IM
• To minimize discomfort, give deep IM slowly. • Less painful if injected into gluteus maximus rather than lateral aspect of thigh.

OPHTHALMIC
• Place finger on lower eyelid, pull out until a pocket is formed between eye and lower lid. • Hold dropper above pocket, place correct number of drops (¼–½ inch ointment) into pocket. Have patientt close eye gently. • **Solution:** Apply digital pressure to lacrimal sac for 1–2 min (minimizes drainage into nose and throat, reducing risk of systemic effects). • **Ointment:** Close eye for 1–2 min, rolling eyeball (increases contact area of drug to eye). • Remove excess solution or ointment around eye with tissue.

IV INCOMPATIBILITIES

Amphotericin B complex (Abelcet, AmBisome, Amphotec), heparin, hetastarch (Hespan), indomethacin (Indocin), propofol (Diprivan), sargramostim (Leukine, Prokine).

IV COMPATIBILITIES

Amiodarone (Cordarone), calcium gluconate, diltiazem (Cardizem), furosemide (Lasix), hydromorphone (Dilaudid), insulin, magnesium sulfate, midazolam (Versed), morphine, theophylline, total parenteral nutrition (TPN).

INDICATIONS/ROUTES/DOSAGE

USUAL PARENTERAL DOSAGE
IV: ADULTS, ELDERLY: 3–6 mg/kg/day in 3 divided doses. Once daily dosing: 4–7 mg/kg every 24 hr. CHILDREN 7 DAYS AND OLDER: 6–7.5 mg/kg/day in 3–4 divided doses. CHILDREN YOUNGER THAN 7 DAYS: 2.5–4 mg/kg/day in 2 divided doses.

SUPERFICIAL EYE INFECTIONS, INCLUDING BLEPHARITIS, CONJUNCTIVITIS, KERATITIS, AND CORNEAL ULCERS
OPHTHALMIC OINTMENT: ADULTS, ELDERLY: Usual dosage, apply a thin strip to conjunctiva q8–12h (q3–4h for severe infections).
OPHTHALMIC SOLUTION: ADULTS, ELDERLY: Usual dosage, 1–2 drops in affected eye q4h (2 drops/hr for severe infections).

T

BRONCHOPULMONARY INFECTIONS IN PATIENTS WITH CYSTIC FIBROSIS

INHALATION SOLUTION: ADULTS: Usual dosage, 60–80 mg twice a day for 28 days, then off for 28 days. CHILDREN: 40–80 mg 2–3 times a day.

DOSAGE IN RENAL IMPAIRMENT

Dosage and frequency are modified based on the degree of renal impairment and the serum drug concentration. After a loading dose of 1–2 mg/kg, the maintenance dose and frequency are based on serum creatinine levels and creatinine clearance.

SIDE EFFECTS

OCCASIONAL: IM: Pain, induration. **IV:** Phlebitis, thrombophlebitis. **Topical:** Hypersensitivity reaction (fever, pruritus, rash, urticaria). **Ophthalmic:** Tearing, itching, redness, eyelid swelling. **RARE:** Hypotension, nausea, vomiting.

ADVERSE REACTIONS/ TOXIC EFFECTS

Nephrotoxicity (as evidenced by increased BUN and serum creatinine levels and decreased creatinine clearance) may be reversible if the drug is stopped at the first sign of nephrotoxic symptoms. Irreversible ototoxicity (manifested as tinnitus, dizziness, ringing or roaring in ears, and hearing loss) and neurotoxicity (manifested as headache, dizziness, lethargy, tremor, and visual disturbances) occur occasionally. The risk of these reactions increases with higher dosages or prolonged therapy and when the solution is applied directly to the mucosa. Superinfections, particularly fungal infections, may result from bacterial imbalance with any administration route. Anaphylaxis may occur.

NURSING CONSIDERATIONS

BASELINE ASSESSMENT

Dehydration must be treated before beginning parenteral therapy. Question for history of allergies, especially aminoglycosides and sulfite (and parabens for topical or ophthalmic routes). Establish baseline for hearing acuity.

INTERVENTION/EVALUATION

Monitor I&O (maintain hydration), urinalysis (casts, RBCs, WBCs, decrease in specific gravity). Monitor results of peak/trough blood tests. Therapeutic serum level: Peak: 5–20 mcg/ml; trough: 0.5–2 mcg/ml. Toxic serum level: Peak: over 20 mcg/ml; trough: over 2 mcg/ml. Be alert to ototoxic and neurotoxic symptoms. Evaluate IV site for phlebitis (heat, pain, red streaking over vein). Assess for rash. Be alert for superinfection, particularly genital or anal pruritus, changes of oral mucosa, diarrhea. When treating patients with neuromuscular disorders, assess respiratory response carefully. **Ophthalmic:** Assess for redness, swelling, itching, tearing.

PATIENT/FAMILY TEACHING

• Notify physician in event of any hearing, visual, balance, urinary problems, even after therapy is completed. • **Ophthalmic:** Blurred vision or tearing may occur briefly after application. • Contact physician if tearing, redness, irritation continues.

tocainide hydrochloride

toe-**kay**-nide
(Tonocard)

◆CLASSIFICATION

PHARMACOTHERAPEUTIC: Amide-type local anesthetic. **CLINICAL:** Anti-arrhythmic (see p. 14C).

ACTION

An amide-type local anesthetic that short-ens the action potential duration and decreases the effective refractory period and automaticity in the His-Purkinje system of the myocardium by blocking sodium transport across myocardial cell membranes. **Therapeutic Effect:** Suppresses ventricular arrhythmias.

PHARMACOKINETICS

Very rapidly and completely absorbed following PO administration. Protein binding: 10%. Metabolized in liver. Excreted in urine. **Half-life:** 15 hr.

USES

Suppression, prevention of ventricular arrhythmias, including frequent unifocal/multifocal coupled premature ventricular contractions, paroxysmal ventricular tachycardia. **OFF-LABEL:** Trigeminal neuralgia.

PRECAUTIONS

CONTRAINDICATIONS: Hypersensitivity to local anesthetics, second- or third-degree AV block. **CAUTIONS:** Renal or hepatic impairment, preexisting arrhythmias, bone marrow failure, CHF.

⌛ **LIFESPAN CONSIDERATIONS: Pregnancy/Lactation:** Drug is distributed is breast milk. **Pregnancy Category C. Children:** Safety and efficacy not established. **Elderly:** Age-related renal impairment may require dosage adjustment. Due to increased sensitivity of effects, dosage and rate of infusion should be reduced.

INTERACTIONS

DRUG: Beta-adrenergic blockers: May increase pulmonary wedge pressure and decrease cardiac index. **Other antiarrhythmics:** May increase risk of adverse cardiac effects. **HERBAL:** None known. **FOOD:** None known. **LAB VALUES:** None known.

AVAILABILITY (Rx)

TABLETS: 400 mg, 600 mg.

INDICATIONS/ROUTES/DOSAGE

SUPPRESSION AND PREVENTION OF VENTRICULAR ARRHYTHMIAS
PO: ADULTS, ELDERLY: Initially, 400 mg q8h. Maintenance: 1.2–1.8 g/day in divided doses q8h. **Maximum:** 2,400 mg/day.

SIDE EFFECTS

Tocainide is generally well tolerated. **FREQUENT (10%–3%):** Minor, transient light-headedness, dizziness, nausea, paresthesia, rash, tremor. **OCCASIONAL (3%–1%):** Clammy skin, night sweats, myalgia. **RARE (less than 1%):** Restlessness, nervousness, disorientation, mood changes, ataxia (muscular incoordination), visual disturbances.

ADVERSE REACTIONS/TOXIC EFFECTS

High dosage may produce bradycardia or tachycardia, hypotension, palpitations, increased ventricular arrhythmias, premature ventricular contractions (PVCs), chest pain, and exacerbation of CHF.

NURSING CONSIDERATIONS

BASELINE ASSESSMENT
Assess baseline EKG, pulse for quality, irregular rate.

INTERVENTION/EVALUATION
Monitor EKG for cardiac changes, particularly shortening of QT interval. Notify physician of any significant interval changes. Monitor fluid status and serum electrolyte levels. Assess hand movement for sign of tremor (usually first clinical sign that maximum dose is being reached). Assess sleeping patient for night sweats. Question for paresthesia in hands or feet. Assess skin for rash, clamminess. Observe for CNS disturbances (restlessness, disorientation, mood changes, incoordination).

Assess for evidence of CHF: dyspnea (particularly on exertion or lying down), night cough, peripheral edema, distended neck veins. Monitor I&O (increase in weight, decrease in urine output may indicate CHF). Monitor for therapeutic serum level (3–10 mcg/ml). Therapeutic serum level: 4–10 mcg/ml; toxic serum level: not established.

PATIENT/FAMILY TEACHING

• Avoid tasks that require alertness, motor skills until response to drug is established. • Inform physician if any unusual bleeding, cough, tremors, palpitations, chills, fever, sore throat, breathing difficulties occur. • May take with food. • Side effects generally disappear with continued therapy.

---

*TOLAZamide

(Tolamide, Tolinase)
See Antidiabetics (p. 41C)

---

*TOLBUTamide

(Oramide, Orinase)
See Antidiabetics (p. 41C)

---

tolnaftate

(Aftate, Tinactin)
See Antifungals: topical (p. 45C)

---

tolterodine tartrate

tol-**tare**-oh-deen
(Detrol, Detrol LA)

◆CLASSIFICATION

PHARMACOTHERAPEUTIC: Muscarinic receptor antagonist. **CLINICAL:** Antispasmodic.

ACTION

An antispasmodic that exhibits potent antimuscarinic activity by interceding via cholinergic muscarinic receptors, thereby inhibiting urinary bladder contraction. **Therapeutic Effect:** Decreases urinary frequency, urgency.

PHARMACOKINETICS

Rapidly and well absorbed after PO administration. Protein binding: 96%. Extensively metabolized in the liver to active metabolite. Primarily excreted in urine. Unknown if removed by hemodialysis. **Half-life:** 1.9–3.7 hr.

USES

Treatment of overactive bladder in patients with symptoms of urinary frequency, urgency, incontinence.

PRECAUTIONS

CONTRAINDICATIONS: Gastric retention, uncontrolled angle-closure glaucoma, urine retention. **CAUTIONS:** Renal impairment, clinically significant bladder outflow obstruction (risk of urinary retention), GI obstructive disorders (e.g., pyloric stenosis [risk of gastric retention]), treated narrow-angle glaucoma.

⧗ **LIFESPAN CONSIDERATIONS: Pregnancy/Lactation:** Unknown if drug is distributed in breast milk. Breast-feeding not recommended. **Pregnancy Category C. Children:** Safety and efficacy not established. **Elderly:** No age-related precautions noted.

INTERACTIONS

DRUG: Clarithromycin, erythromycin, itraconazole, ketoconazole,

---

miconazole: May increase tolterodine blood concentration. **Fluoxetine:** May inhibit tolterodine metabolism. HERBAL: None known. FOOD: None known. LAB VALUES: None known.

AVAILABILITY (Rx)

TABLETS (DETROL): 1 mg, 2 mg. CAPSULES (EXTENDED-RELEASE [DETROL LA]): 2 mg, 4 mg.

ADMINISTRATION/HANDLING

PO
• May give without regard to food.

INDICATIONS/ROUTES/DOSAGE

OVERACTIVE BLADDER
PO: ADULTS, ELDERLY: 1–2 mg twice a day.

DOSAGE IN SEVERE RENAL OR HEPATIC IMPAIRMENT
PO: ADULTS, ELDERLY: 1 mg twice a day.
PO (EXTENDED-RELEASE): ADULTS, ELDERLY: 2–4 mg once a day.

SIDE EFFECTS

FREQUENT (40%): Dry mouth. OCCASIONAL (11%–4%): Headache, dizziness, fatigue, constipation, dyspepsia (heartburn, indigestion, epigastric discomfort), upper respiratory tract infection, UTI, dry eyes, abnormal vision (accommodation problems), nausea, diarrhea. RARE (3%): Somnolence, chest or back pain, arthralgia, rash, weight gain, dry skin.

ADVERSE REACTIONS/ TOXIC EFFECTS

Overdose can result in severe anticholinergic effects, including abdominal cramps, facial warmth, excessive salivation or lacrimation, diaphoresis, pallor, urinary urgency, blurred vision, and prolonged QT interval.

NURSING CONSIDERATIONS

INTERVENTION/EVALUATION
Assist with ambulation if dizziness occurs. Question for visual changes.

Monitor incontinence, postvoid residuals.

PATIENT/FAMILY TEACHING
• May cause blurred vision, dry eyes/mouth, constipation. • Inform physician of any confusion, altered mental status.

Topamax, *see topiramate*

---

topiramate

toe-**peer**-a-mate
(Topamax)

Do not confuse topiramate or Topamax with Toprol XL, Tegretol, or Tegretol XL.

◆CLASSIFICATION

CLINICAL: Anticonvulsant (see p. 35C).

ACTION

An anticonvulsant that blocks repetitive, sustained firing of neurons by enhancing the ability of gamma-aminobutyric acid to induce an influx of chloride ions into the neurons; may also block sodium channels. Therapeutic Effect: Decreases seizure activity.

PHARMACOKINETICS

Rapidly absorbed after PO administration. Protein binding: 13%–17%. Not extensively metabolized. Primarily excreted unchanged in urine. Removed by hemodialysis. Half-life: 21 hr.

USES

Adjunctive therapy for the treatment of partial-onset seizures, tonic-clonic seizures, seizures associated with Lennox-Gastaut syndrome. Prevention of migraine. Initial monotherapy in patients 10 yr of age and older with partial or primary generalized tonic-clonic

T

---

seizures. OFF-LABEL: Treatment of alcohol dependence.

PRECAUTIONS

CONTRAINDICATIONS: Bipolar disorder. **CAUTIONS:** Sensitivity to topiramate, hepatic/renal impairment, predisposition to renal calculi.

⧗ LIFESPAN CONSIDERATIONS: **Pregnancy/Lactation:** Unknown if distributed in breast milk. **Pregnancy Category C. Children:** No age-related precautions noted in those older than 2 yr. **Elderly:** Age-related renal impairment may require dosage adjustment.

INTERACTIONS

DRUG: **Alcohol, other CNS depressants:** May increase CNS depression. **Carbamazepine, phenytoin, valproic acid:** May decrease topiramate blood concentration. **Carbonic anhydrase inhibitors:** May increase the risk of renal calculi. **Oral contraceptives:** May decrease the effectiveness of oral. HERBAL: None known. FOOD: None known. LAB VALUES: None known.

AVAILABILITY (Rx)

CAPSULES (SPRINKLE): 15 mg, 25 mg. **TABLETS:** 25 mg, 50 mg, 100 mg, 200 mg.

ADMINISTRATION/HANDLING

PO
• Do not break tablets (bitter taste).
• Give without regard to meals.
• Capsules may be swallowed whole or contents sprinkled on a teaspoonful of soft food and swallowed immediately; do not chew.

INDICATIONS/ROUTES/DOSAGE

ADJUNCTIVE TREATMENT OF PARTIAL SEIZURES, LENNOX-GASTANT SYNDROME, TONIC-CLONIC SEIZURES
PO: ADULTS, ELDERLY, CHILDREN OLDER THAN 17 YR: Initially, 25–50 mg for 1 wk. May

increase by 25–50 mg/day at weekly intervals. **Maximum:** 1,600 mg/day. CHILDREN 2–16 YR: Initially, 1–3 mg/kg/day to maximum of 25 mg. May increase by 1–3 mg/kg/day at weekly intervals. Maintenance: 5–9 mg/kg/day in 2 divided doses.

MONOTHERAPY WITH PARTIAL, TONIC-CLONIC SEIZURES

PO: ADULTS, ELDERLY, CHILDREN 10 YR AND OLDER: Initially, 25 mg twice a day. Increase at weekly intervals up to 400 mg/day according to the following schedule: Week 1, 25 mg twice a day. Week 2, 50 mg twice a day. Week 3, 75 mg twice a day. Week 4, 100 mg twice a day. Week 5, 150 mg twice a day. Week 6, 200 mg twice a day.

MIGRAINE PREVENTION

PO: ADULTS, ELDERLY: Initially, 25 mg/day. May increase by 25 mg/day at 7-day intervals up to a total daily dose of 100 mg/day in 2 divided doses.

DOSAGE IN RENAL IMPAIRMENT

Expect to reduce drug dosage by 50% in patients with tonic-clonic seizures who have a creatinine clearance of less than 70 ml/min.

SIDE EFFECTS

FREQUENT (30%–10%): Somnolence, dizziness, ataxia, nervousness, nystagmus, diplopia, paresthesia, nausea, tremor. OCCASIONAL (9%–3%): Confusion, breast pain, dysmenorrhea, dyspepsia, depression, asthenia, pharyngitis, weight loss, anorexia, rash, musculoskeletal pain, abdominal pain, difficulty with coordination, sinusitis, agitation, flu-like symptoms. RARE (3%–2%): Mood disturbances, such as irritability and depression; dry mouth; aggressive behavior.

ADVERSE REACTIONS/ TOXIC EFFECTS

Psychomotor slowing, impaired concentration, language problems (such as word-finding difficulties), and memory disturbances occur occasionally. These reactions are generally mild to moderate but may be severe enough to require discontinuation of drug therapy.

NURSING CONSIDERATIONS

BASELINE ASSESSMENT
Review history of seizure disorder (intensity, frequency, duration, level of consciousness [LOC]). Initiate seizure precautions. Provide quiet, dark environment. Question for sensitivity to topiramate, pregnancy, use of other anticonvulsant medication (especially carbamazepine, valproic acid, phenytoin, carbonic anhydrase inhibitors). Assess serum renal function. Instruct patient to use alternative/additional means of contraception (topiramate decreases effectiveness of oral contraceptives).

INTERVENTION/EVALUATION
Observe frequently for recurrence of seizure activity. Assess for clinical improvement (decrease in intensity/frequency of seizures). Monitor serum renal function tests (BUN, creatinine). Assist with ambulation if dizziness occurs.

PATIENT/FAMILY TEACHING
• Avoid tasks that require alertness, motor skills until response to drug is established (may cause dizziness, drowsiness, impaired concentration). • Drowsiness usually diminishes with continued therapy. • Avoid use of alcohol, other CNS depressants. • Do not abruptly discontinue drug (may precipitate seizures). • Strict maintenance of drug therapy is essential for seizure control. • Do not break tablets (bitter taste). • Maintain adequate fluid intake (decreases risk of renal stone formation). • Inform physician if blurred vision, eye pain occurs.

topotecan

toe-**poh**-teh-can
(Hycamtin)

CLASSIFICATION
PHARMACOTHERAPEUTIC: DNA topoisomerase inhibitor. **CLINICAL:** Antineoplastic (see p. 78C).

ACTION
A DNA topoisomerase inhibitor that interacts with topoisomerase I, an enzyme that allows DNA replication by producing reversible single-strand breaks in DNA that relieve torsional strain. Topotecan prevents religation of the DNA strand, resulting in damage to double-strand DNA and cell death. **Therapeutic Effect:** Kills cancer cells.

PHARMACOKINETICS
Hydrolyzed to active form after IV administration. Protein binding: 35%. Excreted in urine. **Half-life:** 2–3 hr (increased in impaired renal function).

USES
Treatment of metastatic carcinoma of ovary after failure of initial or recurrent chemotherapy. Treatment of sensitive, relapsed small cell lung cancer. **OFF-LABEL:** Treatment of solid tumors including osteosarcoma, neuroblastoma, pediatric leukemia, rhabdomyosarcoma.

PRECAUTIONS
CONTRAINDICATIONS: Baseline neutrophil count less than 1,500 cells/mm^3, breast-feeding, pregnancy, severe myelosuppression. **CAUTIONS:** Mild bone marrow depression, hepatic or renal impairment.

⧖ **LIFESPAN CONSIDERATIONS: Pregnancy/Lactation:** May cause fetal harm. Avoid pregnancy; breast-feeding not recommended. **Pregnancy Category D. Children:** Safety and efficacy not

T

---

established. **Elderly:** Age-related renal impairment may require dosage adjustment.

INTERACTIONS

DRUG: **Cisplatin:** May increase the severity of myelosuppression. **Live virus vaccines:** May potentiate virus replication, increase vaccine side effects, and decrease the patient's antibody response to the vaccine. **Other bone marrow depressants:** May increase the risk of myelosuppression. HERBAL: None known. FOOD: None known. LAB VALUES: May increase serum bilirubin, AST, and ALT levels. May decrease RBC, leukocyte, neutrophil, and platelet counts.

AVAILABILITY (Rx)

POWDER FOR INJECTION: 4 mg (single-dose vial).

ADMINISTRATION/HANDLING

◀ ALERT ▶ Because topotecan may be carcinogenic, mutagenic, or teratogenic, handle the drug with extreme care during preparation and administration.

 IV

Reconstitution • Reconstitute each 4-mg vial with 4 ml sterile water for injection. • Further dilute with 50–100 ml 0.9% NaCl or D_5W.

Rate of administration • Administer all doses as IV infusion over 30 min. • Extravasation associated with only mild local reactions (erythema, ecchymosis).

Storage • Store vials at room temperature in original cartons. • Reconstituted vials diluted for infusion stable at room temperature, ambient lighting for 24 hr.

▓ IV INCOMPATIBILITIES

Dexamethasone (Decadron), 5-fluorouracil, mitomycin (Mutamycin).

IV COMPATIBILITIES

Carboplatin (Paraplatin), cisplatin (Platinol AQ), cyclophosphamide (Cytoxan), doxorubicin (Adriamycin), etoposide (VePesid), gemcitabine (Gemzar), granisetron (Kytril), ondansetron (Zofran), paclitaxel (Taxol), vincristine (Oncovin).

INDICATIONS/ROUTES/DOSAGE

OVARIAN CARCINOMA, SMALL-CELL LUNG CANCER

IV: ADULTS, ELDERLY: 1.5 mg/m²/day over 30 min for 5 consecutive days, beginning on day 1 of a 21-day course. Minimum of four courses recommended. If severe neutropenia (neutrophil count less than 1,500/mm²) occurs during treatment, reduce dose for subsequent courses by 0.25 mg/m², or administer filgrastim (G-CSF) no sooner than 24 hr after the last dose of topotecan.

DOSAGE IN RENAL IMPAIRMENT

No dosage adjustment is necessary in patients with mild renal impairment (creatinine clearance of 40–60 ml/min). For moderate renal impairment (creatinine clearance of 20–39 ml/min), give 0.75 mg/m².

SIDE EFFECTS

FREQUENT: Nausea (77%); vomiting (58%); diarrhea, total alopecia (42%); headache (21%); dyspnea (21%). OCCASIONAL: Paraesthesia (9%); constipation, abdominal pain (3%). RARE: Anorexia, malaise, arthralgia, asthenia, myalgia.

ADVERSE REACTIONS/ TOXIC EFFECTS

Severe neutropenia (neutrophil count less than 500 cells/mm³) occurs in 60% of patients, usually during the first course of therapy. The neutrophil nadir usually occurs at a median of 11 days after starting therapy. Thrombocytopenia (platelet count less than 25,000/mm³) occurs in 26% of patients, and severe anemia (RBC count less than 8 g/dl) occurs in 40% of patients. The platelet and RBC nadirs usually occur at a median of 15 days after starting the first course of therapy.

NURSING CONSIDERATIONS

BASELINE ASSESSMENT

Offer emotional support to patient and family. Assess CBC with differential, Hgb, platelet count before each dose. Myelosuppression may precipitate life-threatening hemorrhage, infection, anemia. If platelet count drops, minimize trauma to patient (e.g., IM injections, patient positioning). Premedicate with antiemetics on day of treatment, starting at least 30 min before administration.

INTERVENTION/EVALUATION

Assess for bleeding, signs of infection, anemia. Monitor hydration status, I&O, serum electrolytes (diarrhea, vomiting are common side effects). Monitor CBC with differential, Hgb, platelets for evidence of myelosuppression. Assess response to medication and provide interventions (e.g., small, frequent meals and antiemetics for nausea and vomiting). Question for complaints of headache. Assess breathing pattern for evidence of dyspnea.

PATIENT/FAMILY TEACHING

• Explain that alopecia is reversible but that new hair may have different color, texture. • Inform patient of possible late diarrhea causing dehydration, electrolyte depletion. • Provide antiemetic an dantidiarrheal regimen for subsequent use. • Notify physician if diarrhea, vomiting continues at home. • Do not have immunizations without physician's approval (drug lowers body's resistance). • Avoid contact with those who have recently received live virus vaccine.

Toprol XL, *see metoprolol*

Toradol, *see ketorolac*

---

toremifene citrate ▷

tore-mih-feen
(Fareston)

◆ CLASSIFICATION

PHARMACOTHERAPEUTIC: Nonsteroidal antiestrogen. **CLINICAL:** Antineoplastic (see p. 78C).

ACTION

A nonsteroidal antiestrogen and antineoplastic agent that binds to estrogen receptors on tumors, producing a complex that decreases DNA synthesis and inhibits estrogen effects. Therapeutic Effect: Blocks growth-stimulating effects of estrogen in breast cancer.

PHARMACOKINETICS

Well absorbed after PO administration. Metabolized in the liver. Eliminated in feces. Half-life: Approximately 5 days.

USES

Treatment of advanced breast cancer in postmenopausal women with estrogen receptor–positive disease. OFF-LABEL: Treatment of desmoid tumors, endometrial carcinoma.

PRECAUTIONS

CONTRAINDICATIONS: History of thromboembolic disease. **CAUTIONS:** Preexisting endometrial hyperplasia, leukopenia, thrombocytopenia.

LIFESPAN CONSIDERATIONS: **Pregnancy/Lactation:** Unknown if distributed in breast milk. **Pregnancy Category D. Children:** Safety and efficacy not established. Not prescribed in this patient population. **Elderly:** No age-related precautions noted.

T

INTERACTIONS

DRUG: Carbamazepine, phenobarbital, phenytoin: May decrease toremifene blood concentration. **Warfarin:** May increase PT, risk of bleeding. **HERBAL:** None known. **FOOD:** None known. **LAB VALUES:** May increase serum alkaline phosphatase, bilirubin, calcium, and AST levels.

AVAILABILITY (Rx)

TABLETS: 60 mg.

ADMINISTRATION/HANDLING

PO
• Give without regard to food.

INDICATIONS/ROUTES/DOSAGE

BREAST CANCER
PO: ADULTS: 60 mg/day until disease progression is observed.

SIDE EFFECTS

FREQUENT: Hot flashes (35%); diaphoresis (20%); nausea (14%); vaginal discharge (13%); dizziness, dry eyes (9%). **OCCASIONAL (5%–2%):** Edema, vomiting, vaginal bleeding. **RARE:** Fatigue, depression, lethargy, anorexia.

ADVERSE REACTIONS/ TOXIC EFFECTS

Ocular toxicity (cataracts, glaucoma, decreased visual acuity) and hypercalcemia may occur. Overdose may be manifested as an increase of antiestrogenic effects, such as hot flashes; estrogenic effects, such as vaginal bleeding; or nervous system disorders, such as vertigo, dizziness, ataxia, and nausea.

NURSING CONSIDERATIONS

BASELINE ASSESSMENT

An estrogen receptor assay should be done before beginning therapy. CBC, platelet count, serum calcium levels should be checked before and periodically during therapy.

INTERVENTION/EVALUATION

Assess for hypercalcemia (increased urine volume, excessive thirst, nausea, vomiting, constipation, hypotonicity of muscles, deep bone or flank pain, renal stones). Monitor CBC, leukocyte, platelet counts, serum calcium, liver function tests.

PATIENT/FAMILY TEACHING

• May have an initial flare of symptoms (bone pain, hot flashes) that will subside. • Report vaginal bleeding or discharge/itching, leg cramps, weight gain, shortness of breath, weakness. • Contact physician if nausea or vomiting continues. • Nonhormone contraceptives are recommended during treatment.

torsemide

tor-se-mide
(Demadex, Demadex I.V.)
Do not confuse torsemide with furosemide.

CLASSIFICATION

PHARMACOTHERAPEUTIC: Loop diuretic. **CLINICAL:** Antihypertensive, antiedema (see p. 89C).

ACTION

A loop diuretic that enhances excretion of sodium, chloride, potassium, and water at the ascending limb of the loop of Henle; also reduces plasma and extracellular fluid volume. **Therapeutic Effect:** Produces diuresis; lowers BP.

PHARMACOKINETICS

Route	Onset	Peak	Duration
PO	1 hr	1–2 hr	6–8 hr
IV	10 min	1 hr	6–8 hr

Rapidly and well absorbed from the GI tract. Protein binding: 97%–99%. Metabolized in the liver. Primarily excreted in urine. Not removed by hemodialysis. **Half-life:** 3.3 hr.

USES

Treatment of hypertension either alone or in combination with other antihypertensives. Edema associated with CHF, renal disease, hepatic cirrhosis, chronic renal failure.

PRECAUTIONS

CONTRAINDICATIONS: Anuria, hepatic coma, severe electrolyte depletion. **EXTREME CAUTION:** Hypersensitivity to sulfonamides. **CAUTIONS:** Elderly, cardiac patients, patients with history of ventricular arrhythmias, patients with hepatic cirrhosis, ascites. Renal impairment, systemic lupus erythematosus. Safety in children not known.

⧗ **LIFESPAN CONSIDERATIONS: Pregnancy/Lactation:** Unknown if drug is excreted in breast milk. **Pregnancy Category B. Children:** Safety and efficacy not established. **Elderly:** No age-related precautions noted.

INTERACTIONS

DRUG: Amphotericin B, nephrotoxic medications, ototoxic medications: May increase the risk of nephrotoxicity and ototoxicity. **Anticoagulants, heparin, thrombolytics:** May decrease the effects of these drugs. **Digoxin:** May increase the risk of digoxin toxicity associated with torsemide-induced hypokalemia. **Lithium:** May increase the risk of lithium toxicity. **NSAIDs, probenecid:** May decrease the diuretic effect of torsemide. **Other antihypertensives:** May increase the risk of hypotension. **Other hypokalemia-causing medications:** May increase the risk of hypokalemia. **HERBAL:** None known. **FOOD:** None known. **LAB VALUES:** May increase BUN, serum creatinine, and serum uric acid levels. May decrease serum calcium, chloride, magnesium, potassium, and sodium levels.

AVAILABILITY (Rx)

TABLETS (DEMADEX): 5 mg, 10 mg, 20 mg, 100 mg. **INJECTION (DEMADEX I.V.):** 10 mg/ml.

ADMINISTRATION/HANDLING

 IV

Rate of administration

◀ **ALERT** ▶ Flush IV line with 0.9% NaCl before and following administration.
• May give undiluted as IV push over 2 min. • For continuous IV infusion, dilute with 0.9% or 0.45% NaCl or D₅W and infuse over 24 hr. • A too rapid IV rate, high dosages may cause ototoxicity; administer IV rate **slowly.**

Storage • Store at room temperature.

PO

• Give without regard to food. Give with food to avoid GI upset, preferably with breakfast (prevents nocturia).

▦ IV INCOMPATIBILITIES

Don't mix torsemide with any other medications except for milrinone (Primacor).

IV COMPATIBILITY

Milrinone (Primacor).

INDICATIONS/ROUTES/DOSAGE

T

HYPERTENSION

PO: ADULTS, ELDERLY: Initially, 2.5–5 mg/day. May increase to 10 mg/day if no response in 4–6 wk. If no response, additional antihypertensive added.

CHF

PO, IV: ADULTS, ELDERLY: Initially, 10–20 mg/day. May increase by approximately doubling dose until desired therapeutic effect is attained. Doses greater than 200 mg have not been adequately studied.

CHRONIC RENAL FAILURE

PO, IV: ADULTS, ELDERLY: Initially, 20 mg/day. May increase by approximately doubling dose until desired therapeutic effect is attained. Doses greater than 200 mg have not been adequately studied.

HEPATIC CIRRHOSIS

PO, IV: ADULTS, ELDERLY: Initially, 5 mg/day given with aldosterone antagonist or potassium-sparing diuretic. May increase by approximately doubling dose until desired therapeutic effect is attained. Doses greater than 40 mg have not been adequately studied.

SIDE EFFECTS

FREQUENT (10%–4%): Headache, dizziness, rhinitis. **OCCASIONAL (3%–1%):** Asthenia, insomnia, nervousness, diarrhea, constipation, nausea, dyspepsia, edema, EKG changes, pharyngitis, cough, arthralgia, myalgia. **RARE (less than 1%):** Syncope, hypotension, arrhythmias.

ADVERSE REACTIONS/ TOXIC EFFECTS

Ototoxicity may occur with high doses or a too-rapid IV administration. Overdose produces acute, profound water loss; volume and electrolyte depletion; dehydration; decreased blood volume; and circulatory collapse.

NURSING CONSIDERATIONS

BASELINE ASSESSMENT

Check serum electrolyte levels, especially potassium. Obtain baseline weight; check for edema. Assess for rales in lungs.

INTERVENTION/EVALUATION

Monitor BP, serum electrolytes (especially potassium), I&O, weight. Notify physician of any hearing abnormality. Note extent of diuresis. Assess lungs for rales. Check for signs of edema, particularly of dependent areas. Although less potassium is lost with torsemide than with furosemide, assess for signs of hypokalemia (change of muscle strength, tremors, muscle cramps, altered mental status, cardiac arrhythmias).

PATIENT/FAMILY TEACHING

• Take medication in morning to prevent nocturia. • Expect increased frequency and volume of urination. • Report palpitations, muscle weakness, cramps, nausea, dizziness. • Do not take other medications (including OTC drugs) without consulting physician. • Eat foods high in potassium such as whole grains (cereals), legumes, meat, bananas, apricots, orange juice, potatoes (white, sweet), raisins.

tositumomab and iodine ^{131}I-tositumomab

toe-sit-**two**-mo-mab
(Bexxar)

CLASSIFICATION

PHARMACOTHERAPEUTIC: Monoclonal antibody. **CLINICAL:** Antineoplastic.

ACTION

A monoclonal antibody composed of an antibody conjoined with a radiolabeled antitumor antibody. The antibody portion binds specifically to the CD20 antigen, which is found on pre-B and B lymphocytes and on more than 90% of B-cell non-Hodgkin's lymphomas resulting in formation of a complex. Therapeutic Effect: Induces cytotoxicity associated with ionizing radiation from the radioisotope. Depletes circulating CD20-positive cells.

PHARMACOKINETICS

Elimination of iodine 131 (^{131}I) occurs by decay and excretion in urine. Half-life: 8 days. Patients with high tumor burden, splenomegaly, or bone marrow involvement have a faster clearance, shorter half-life, and larger volume of distribution.

USES

Treatment of patients with CD 20 antigen-expressing relapsed or refractory low grade, follicular, or transformed non-Hodgkin's lymphoma, whose disease has relapsed following chemotherapy.

PRECAUTIONS

CONTRAINDICATIONS: Hypersensitivity to murine proteins, pregnancy. **CAUTIONS:** Renal impairment, active systemic infection, immunosuppression.

⚖ LIFESPAN CONSIDERATIONS: Pregnancy/Lactation: The ^{131}I-tositumomab component is contraindicated during pregnancy (severe, possibly irreversible hypothyroidism in neonates). Radioiodine is excreted in breast milk; do not breast-feed. **Pregnancy Category X.** **Children:** Safety and efficacy not established. **Elderly:** The response rate and duration of severe hematologic toxicity is lower in patients older than 65 yr.

INTERACTIONS

DRUG: Anticoagulants, medications that interfere with platelet function: Increase the risk of bleeding and hemorrhage. **HERBAL:** None known. **FOOD:** None known. **LAB VALUES:** May decrease blood Hct and Hgb levels, platelet and WBC counts, and thyroid-stimulating hormone level.

AVAILABILITY (Rx)

KIT (DOSIMETRIC): tositumomab 225 mg/16.1 ml (2 vials), tositumomab 35 mg/2.5 ml (1 vial), and iodine^{131} tositumomab 0.1 mg/ml (1 vial).

KIT (THERAPEUTIC): tositumomab 225 mg/16.1 ml (2 vials), tositumomab 35 mg/2.5 ml (1 vial), and iodine^{131} tositumomab 1.1 mg/ml (1 or 2 vials).

ADMINISTRATION/HANDLING

◄ ALERT ► The regimen consists of 4 components given in 2 separate steps: The dosimetric step, followed 7–14 days later by a therapeutic step. When infusing, use IV tubing with an in-line 0.22-micron filter (use the same tubing throughout the entire dosimetric or therapeutic step; changing the filter results in drug loss). Reduce infusion rate by 50% for mild to moderate infusion toxicity; interrupt infusion for severe infusion toxicity (may resume when resolution of toxicity occurs). Resume at 50% reduction rate of infusion.

 IV

Reconstitution
◄ ALERT ► Reconstitution amounts and rates of administration are the same for both dosimetric and therapeutic steps. TOSITUMOMAB • Reconstitute 450 mg tositumomab in 50 ml 0.9% NaCl. IODINE ^{131}I-TOSITUMOMAB • Reconstitute iodine ^{131}I-tositumomab in 30 ml 0.9% NaCl.

Rate of administration
TOSITUMOMAB • Infuse over 60 min. IODINE ^{131}I-TOSITUMOMAB • Infuse over 20 min.

Storage
TOSITUMOMAB • Refrigerate vials before dilution. Protect from strong light. • Following dilution, solution is stable for 24 hr if refrigerated, up to 8 hr at room temperature. • Discard any unused portion left in the vial. • Do not shake.
IODINE ^{131}I-TOSITUMOMAB • Store frozen until it is removed for thawing before administration. Thawed doses are stable for 8 hr if refrigerated. • Discard any unused portion.

T

INDICATIONS/ROUTES/DOSAGE

NON-HODGKIN'S LYMPHOMA

IV: ADULTS, ELDERLY: Dosage contains 4 components. **Day 0:** tositumomab 450 mg/50 NaCl over 60 min. Then iodine^{131} tositumomab 35 mg in 30 ml NaCl over 20 min. **Day 7:** tositumomab 450 mg/50 NaCl over 60 min. Then, iodine^{131} tositumomab to deliver 65–75 cGy total body irradiation and tositumomab 35 mg over 20 min.

SIDE EFFECTS

FREQUENT (46%–18%): Asthenia, fever, nausea, cough, chills. **OCCASIONAL (17%–10%):** Rash, headache, abdominal pain, vomiting, anorexia, myalgia, diarrhea, pharyngitis, arthralgia, rhinitis, pruritus. **RARE (9%–5%):** Peripheral edema, diaphoresis, constipation, dyspepsia, back pain, hypotension, vasodilation, dizziness, somnolence.

ADVERSE REACTIONS/ TOXIC EFFECTS

◀ **ALERT** ▶ Infusion toxicity, characterized by fever, rigors, diaphoresis, hypotension, dyspnea, and nausea, may occur during or within 48 hr of the infusion. Severe, prolonged myelosuppression, characterized by neutropenia, anemia, and thrombocytopenia, occurs in 71% of patients. Sepsis occurs in 45% of patients. Hemorrhage occurs in 12% of patients. Myelodysplastic syndrome occurs in 8% of patients.

NURSING CONSIDERATIONS

BASELINE ASSESSMENT

Pretreatment with acetaminophen and diphenhydramine before administering infusion may prevent infusion-related effects. Obtain baseline CBC before therapy and at least weekly following administration for a minimum of 10 wk. Use strict aseptic technique to protect patient from infection. Follow radiation safety protocols. Time to nadir is 4–7 wk, duration of cytopenias is approximately 30 days.

INTERVENTION/EVALUATION

Diligently monitor lab values for possibly severe, prolonged thrombocytopenia, neutropenia, anemia. Monitor for hematologic toxicity (fever, chills, unusual ecchymoses/bleeding from any site), symptoms of anemia (excessive fatigue, weakness). Assess for signs of hypothyroidism.

PATIENT/FAMILY TEACHING

• Avoid pregnancy (Pregnancy Category X). • Do not have immunizations without physician's approval (drug lowers body's resistance). • Avoid contact with those who have recently received live virus vaccine. • Promptly report fever, sore throat, signs of local infection, unusual bruising or bleeding from any site.

tramadol hydrochloride

tray-mah-doal

(Ultram)

Do not confuse tramadol with Toradol, or Ultram with Ultane.

FIXED-COMBINATION(S)

Ultracet: tramadol/acetaminophen (a non-narcotic analgesic): 37.5 mg/ 325 mg.

◆CLASSIFICATION

CLINICAL: Analgesic.

ACTION

An analgesic that binds to mu-opioid receptors and inhibits reuptake of norepinephrine and serotonin. Reduces the intensity of pain stimuli reaching sensory nerve endings.

Therapeutic Effect: Alters the perception of and emotional response to pain.

PHARMACOKINETICS

Route	Onset	Peak	Duration
PO	Less than 1 hr	2–3 hr	4–6 hr

Rapidly and almost completely absorbed after PO administration. Protein binding: 20%. Extensively metabolized in the liver to active metabolite (reduced in patients with advanced cirrhosis). Primarily excreted in urine. Minimally removed by hemodialysis. **Half-life:** 6–7 hr.

USES

Management of moderate to moderately severe pain.

PRECAUTIONS

CONTRAINDICATIONS: Acute alcohol intoxication; concurrent use of centrally acting analgesics, hypnotics, opioids, or psychotropic drugs, hypersensitivity to opioids. **EXTREME CAUTION:** CNS depression, anoxia, advanced hepatic cirrhosis, epilepsy, respiratory depression, acute alcoholism, shock. **CAUTIONS:** Sensitivity to opioids, increased intracranial pressure (ICP), hepatic or renal impairment, acute abdominal conditions, opioid-dependent patients.

⌧ **LIFESPAN CONSIDERATIONS:** Pregnancy/Lactation: Crosses placenta. Distributed in breast milk. **Pregnancy Category C. Children:** Safety and efficacy not established. **Elderly:** Age-related renal impairment may require dosage adjustment.

INTERACTIONS

DRUG: Alcohol, other CNS depressants: May increase CNS or respiratory depression and hypotension. **Carbamazepine:** Decreases tramadol blood concentration. **MAOIs:** May increase tramadol blood concentration and increase the risk of seizures. **Selective serotonin reuptake inhibitors (SSRIs), tricyclic antidepressants, opioids, neuroleptics:** May increase the risk of seizures. **HERBAL:** None known. **FOOD:** None known. **LAB VALUES:** May increase serum creatinine, AST, and ALT hepatic levels. May decrease blood Hgb level. May cause proteinuria.

AVAILABILITY (Rx)

TABLETS: 50 mg. **ORALLY-DISINTE-GRATING TABLETS:** 50 mg. **EXTENDED-RELEASE TABLETS:** 100 mg, 200 mg, 300 mg.

ADMINISTRATION/HANDLING

PO
• Give without regard to meals.

INDICATIONS/ROUTES/DOSAGE

MODERATE TO MODERATELY SEVERE PAIN
PO (IMMEDIATE-RELEASE, ORALLY-DISINTEGRATING): ADULTS, ELDERLY: 50–100 mg q4–6h. **Maximum:** 400 mg/day for patients 75 yr and younger; 300 mg/day for patients older than 75 yr. **PO (EXTENDED-RELEASE):** ADULTS, ELDERLY: 100–300 mg once daily.

DOSAGE IN RENAL IMPAIRMENT
For patients with creatinine clearance of less than 30 ml/min, increase dosing interval to q12h. **Maximum:** 200 mg/day.

DOSAGE IN HEPATIC IMPAIRMENT
Dosage is decreased to 50 mg q12h.

SIDE EFFECTS

FREQUENT (25%–15%): Dizziness or vertigo, nausea, constipation, headache, somnolence. **OCCASIONAL (10%–5%):** Vomiting, pruritus, CNS stimulation (such as nervousness, anxiety, agitation, tremor, euphoria, mood swings, and hallucinations), asthenia, diaphoresis, dyspepsia, dry mouth, diarrhea. **RARE (less than 5%):** Malaise, vasodilation, anorexia, flatulence, rash, blurred vision, urine retention or urinary frequency, menopausal symptoms.

ADVERSE REACTIONS/ TOXIC EFFECTS

Seizures have been reported in patients receiving tramadol within the recommended dosage range. Overdose results in respiratory depression and seizures. Tramadol may have a prolonged duration of action and cumulative effect in patients with hepatic or renal impairment.

NURSING CONSIDERATIONS

BASELINE ASSESSMENT

Assess onset, type, location, duration of pain. Effect of medication is reduced if full pain recurs before next dose. Assess drug history, especially carbamazepine, CNS depressant medication, MAOIs. Review past medical history, especially epilepsy or seizures. Assess renal and Liver function lab values.

INTERVENTION/EVALUATION

Monitor pulse, BP. Assist with ambulation if dizziness, vertigo occurs. Dry crackers, cola may relieve nausea. Palpate bladder for urinary retention. Monitor pattern of daily bowel activity and stool consistency. Sips of tepid water may relieve dry mouth. Assess for clinical improvement, record onset of relief of pain.

PATIENT/FAMILY TEACHING

• May cause dependence. • Avoid alcohol, OTC medications (analgesics, sedatives). • May cause drowsiness, dizziness, blurred vision. • Avoid tasks requiring alertness, motor skills until response to drug is established. • Inform physician if severe constipation, difficulty breathing, excessive sedation, seizures, muscle weakness, tremors, chest pain, palpitations occur.

trandolapril

tran-**doe**-la-pril

(<u>Mavik</u>)

Do not confuse trandolapril with tramadol.

FIXED-COMBINATION(S)

Tarka: trandolapril/verapamil (a calcium channel blocker): 1 mg/240 mg; 2 mg/180 mg; 2 mg/240 mg; 4 mg/240 mg.

◆ CLASSIFICATION

PHARMACOTHERAPEUTIC: Angiotensin-converting enzyme (ACE) inhibitor. **CLINICAL:** Antihypertensive, CHF agent (see p. 7C).

ACTION

An ACE inhibitor that suppresses the renin-angiotensin-aldosterone system and prevents the conversion of angiotensin I to angiotensin II, a potent vasoconstrictor; may also inhibit angiotensin II at local vascular and renal sites. Decreases plasma angiotensin II, increases plasma renin activity, and decreases aldosterone secretion. Therapeutic Effect: Reduces peripheral arterial resistance and pulmonary capillary wedge pressure; improves cardiac output and exercise tolerance.

PHARMACOKINETICS

Slowly absorbed from the GI tract. Protein binding: 80%. Metabolized in the liver and GI mucosa to active metabolite. Primarily excreted in urine. Removed by hemodialysis. Half-life: 24 hr.

USES

Treatment of left ventricular dysfunction following MI. Treatment of hypertension. Used alone or in combination with other antihypertensives. **OFF-LABEL:** Treatment of systolic CHF.

PRECAUTIONS

CONTRAINDICATIONS: History of angioedema from previous treatment with ACE inhibitors, pregnancy. **CAUTIONS:** Renal impairment, CHF, hypovolemia, valvular stenosis, hyperkalemia.

⧖ **LIFESPAN CONSIDERATIONS: Pregnancy/Lactation:** Drug crosses placenta; is distributed in breast milk. May cause fetal or neonatal mortality or morbidity. **Pregnancy Category C (D if used in second or third trimester). Children:** Safety and efficacy not established. **Elderly:** No age-related precautions noted.

INTERACTIONS

DRUG: Alcohol, antihypertensives, diuretics: May increase the effects of trandolapril. **Lithium:** May increase lithium blood concentration and risk of lithium toxicity. **NSAIDs:** May decrease the effects of trandolapril. **Potassium-sparing diuretics, potassium supplements:** May cause hyperkalemia. **HERBAL:** None known. **FOOD:** None known. **LAB VALUES:** May increase BUN, serum alkaline phosphatase, serum bilirubin, serum creatinine, serum potassium, AST, and ALT levels. May decrease serum sodium levels. May cause positive antinuclear antibody (ANA) titer.

AVAILABILITY (Rx)

TABLETS: 1 mg, 2 mg, 4 mg.

ADMINISTRATION/HANDLING

PO
• Give without regard to meals.
• Tablets may be crushed.

INDICATIONS/ROUTES/DOSAGE

HYPERTENSION (WITHOUT DIURETIC)
PO: ADULTS, ELDERLY: Initially, 1 mg once a day in nonblack patients, 2 mg once a day in black patients. Adjust dosage at least

at 7-day intervals. Maintenance: 2–4 mg/day. **Maximum:** 8 mg/day.

HEART FAILURE OR LEFT VENTRICULAR DYSFUNCTION POST-MI
PO: ADULTS, ELDERLY: Initially, 0.5–1 mg, titrated to target dose of 4 mg/day.

SIDE EFFECTS

FREQUENT (35%–23%): Dizziness, cough. **OCCASIONAL (11%–3%):** Hypotension, dys-pepsia (heartburn, epigastric pain, indigestion), syncope, asthenia (loss of strength), tinnitus. **RARE (less than 1%):** Palpitations, insomnia, drowsiness, nausea, vomiting, constipation, flushed skin.

ADVERSE REACTIONS/ TOXIC EFFECTS

Excessive hypotension ("first-dose syncope") may occur in patients with CHF and in those who are severely salt or volume depleted. Angioedema and hyperkalemia occur rarely. Agranulocytosis and neutropenia may be noted in those with collagen vascular disease, including scleroderma and systemic lupus erythematosus, and impaired renal function. Nephrotic syndrome may be noted in those with history of renal disease.

NURSING CONSIDERATIONS

BASELINE ASSESSMENT

Obtain BP immediately before each dose, in addition to regular monitoring (be alert to fluctuations). Serum renal function tests should be performed before therapy begins. In patients with renal impairment, autoimmune disease, or taking drugs that affect leukocytes or immune response, CBC and differential count should be performed before therapy begins and q2wk for 3 mo, then periodically thereafter.

INTERVENTION/EVALUATION

If excessive reduction in BP occurs, place patient in supine position with legs

T

elevated. Assist with ambulation if dizziness occurs. Assess for urinary frequency. Auscultate lung sounds for rales, wheezing in those with CHF. Monitor urinalysis for proteinuria. Monitor serum potassium levels in those on concurrent diuretic therapy. Monitor pattern of daily bowel activity and stool consistency.

PATIENT/FAMILY TEACHING

• Do not discontinue medication.
• Inform physician if sore throat, fever, swelling, palpitations, cough, chest pain, difficulty swallowing, swelling of face, vomiting, or diarrhea occurs.
• To reduce hypotensive effect, rise slowly from lying to sitting position and permit legs to dangle from bed momentarily before standing. • Avoid tasks that require alertness, motor skills until response to drug is established (potential for dizziness, drowsiness). • Avoid potassium supplements and salt substitutes.

---

tranylcypromine sulfate

tran-ill-**sip**-roe-meen
(Parnate)

◆ CLASSIFICATION

PHARMACOTHERAPEUTIC: MAOI.
CLINICAL: Antidepressant (see p. 37C).

ACTION

An MAOI that inhibits the activity of the enzyme monoamine oxidase at CNS storage sites, leading to increased levels of the neurotransmitters epinephrine, norepinephrine, serotonin, and dopamine at neuronal receptor sites. **Therapeutic Effect:** Relieves depression.

USES

Treatment of depression in patients refractory to or intolerant of other therapy. **OFF-LABEL:** Post-traumatic stress disorder.

PRECAUTIONS

CONTRAINDICATIONS: CHF, children younger than 16 yr, pheochromocytoma, severe hepatic or renal impairment, uncontrolled hypertension. **CAUTIONS:** Within several hours of ingestion of contraindicated substance (e.g., tyramine-containing food). Cardiac arrhythmias, severe/frequent headaches, hypertension, suicidal tendencies.

 LIFESPAN CONSIDERATIONS: Pregnancy/Lactation: Crosses placenta. Minimally distributed in breast milk. **Pregnancy Category C. Children:** Not recommended for children (increased risk of suicidal ideation). **Elderly:** Increased risk of drug toxicity may require dosage adjustment.

INTERACTIONS

DRUG: Alcohol, other CNS depressants: May increase CNS depressant effects. **Buspirone:** May increase BP. **Caffeine-containing medications:** May increase the risk of cardiac arrhythmias and hypertension. **Carbamazepine, cyclobenzaprine, maprotiline, other MAOIs:** May precipitate hypertensive crisis. **Dopamine, tryptophan:** May cause sudden, severe hypertension. **Fluoxetine, trazodone, tricyclic antidepressants:** May cause serotonin syndrome and neuroleptic malignant syndrome. **Insulin, oral antidiabetics:** May increase the effects of these drugs. **Meperidine, other opioid analgesics:** May produce diaphoresis, immediate excitation, rigidity, and severe hypertension or hypotension, sometimes leading to severe respiratory distress, vascular collapse, seizures, coma, and death. **HERBAL:** None known. **FOOD: Caffeine,**

chocolate, tyramine-containing foods (such as aged cheese): May cause sudden, severe hypertension. **LAB VALUES:** None known.

AVAILABILITY (Rx)

TABLETS: 10 mg.

ADMINISTRATION/HANDLING

◄ **ALERT** ► Make sure at least 14 days elapse between the use of tranylcypromine and a selective serotonin reuptake inhibitor.

INDICATIONS/ROUTES/DOSAGE

DEPRESSION REFRACTORY TO OR INTOLERANT OF OTHER THERAPY
PO: ADULTS, ELDERLY: Initially, 10 mg twice a day. May increase by 10 mg/day at 1- to 3-wk intervals up to 60 mg/day in divided doses.

SIDE EFFECTS

FREQUENT: Orthostatic hypotension, restlessness, GI upset, insomnia, dizziness, lethargy, weakness, dry mouth, peripheral edema. **OCCASIONAL:** Flushing, diaphoresis, rash, urinary frequency, increased appetite, transient impotence. **RARE:** Visual disturbances.

ADVERSE REACTIONS/ TOXIC EFFECTS

Hypertensive crisis occurs rarely and is marked by severe hypertension, occipital headache radiating frontally, neck stiffness or soreness, nausea, vomiting, diaphoresis, fever or chills, clammy skin, dilated pupils, palpitations, tachycardia or bradycardia, and constricting chest pain. Intracranial bleeding has been reported in association with severe hypertension.

NURSING CONSIDERATIONS

BASELINE ASSESSMENT
Perform baseline serum liver/renal function tests. Assess sensitivity to tranylcypromine. Assess for other medical conditions, especially alcoholism, CHF, pheochromocytoma, arrhythmias, cardiovascular disease, hypertension, suicidal tendencies. Question for other medications, including CNS depressants, meperidine, other antidepressants. Do not use in combination with, or within 14 days of taking selective serotonin reuptake inhibitors (SSRIs).

INTERVENTION/EVALUATION
Assess appearance, behavior, speech pattern, level of interest, mood. Supervise suicidal-risk patient closely during early therapy (as depression lessens, energy level improves, increasing suicide potential). Monitor for occipital headache radiating frontally, neck stiffness/soreness (may be first signal of impending hypertensive crisis). Monitor BP diligently for hypertension. Assess skin and temperature for fever. Discontinue medication immediately if palpitations, frequent headaches occur. Monitor weight.

PATIENT/FAMILY TEACHING
• Take second daily dose no later than 4 PM to avoid insomnia. • Antidepressant relief may be noted during first week of therapy; maximum benefit noted within 3 wk. • Report headache, neck stiffness/soreness immediately. • To avoid orthostatic hypotension, change from lying to sitting position slowly and dangle legs momentarily before standing. • Avoid foods that require bacteria/molds for their preparation/preservation, those that contain tyramine (e.g., cheese, sour cream, beer, wine, pickled herring, liver, figs, raisins, bananas, avocados, soy sauce, yeast extracts, yogurt, papaya, broad beans, meat tenderizers), excessive amounts of caffeine (coffee, tea, chocolate), OTC for cold/allergy preparations, weight reduction.

T

trastuzumab 🚩

traz-**two**-zoo-mab

(Herceptin)

◆ CLASSIFICATION

PHARMACOTHERAPEUTIC: Monoclonal antibody. **CLINICAL:** Antineoplastic (see p. 79C).

ACTION

Binds to the HER-2 protein, which is overexpressed in 25%–30% of primary breast cancers, thereby inhibiting proliferation of tumor cells. **Therapeutic Effect:** Inhibits the growth of tumor cells and mediates antibody-dependent cellular cytotoxicity.

PHARMACOKINETICS

Half-life: 5.8 days (range: 1–32 days).

USES

Treatment of metastatic breast cancer patients whose tumors overexpress HER-2 protein and who have received one or more chemotherapy regimens. May be used with paclitaxel without previous treatment for metastatic disease.

PRECAUTIONS

CONTRAINDICATIONS: Preexisting cardiac disease. **CAUTIONS:** Previous cardiotoxic drug or radiation therapy to chest wall, those with known hypersensitivity to trastuzumab.

⏳ **LIFESPAN CONSIDERATIONS: Pregnancy/Lactation:** Unknown if distributed in breast milk. **Pregnancy Category B. Children:** Safety and efficacy not established. **Elderly:** Age-related cardiac dysfunction may require dosage adjustment.

INTERACTIONS

DRUG: Cyclophosphamide, doxorubicin, epirubicin: May increase the risk of cardiac dysfunction. **HERBAL:** None known. **FOOD:** None known. **LAB VALUES:** None known.

AVAILABILITY (Rx)

INJECTION, POWDER FOR RECONSTITUTION: 440 mg.

ADMINISTRATION/HANDLING

📲 **IV**

Reconstitution • Reconstitute with 20 ml bacteriostatic water for injection to yield concentration of 21 mg/ml. • Add calculated dose to 250 ml 0.9% NaCl (do not use D₅W). • Gently mix contents in bag.

Rate of administration • Do not give IV push or bolus. • Give loading dose (4 mg/kg) over 90 min. Give maintenance infusion (2 mg/kg) over 30 min.

Storage • Refrigerate. • Reconstituted solution appears colorless to pale yellow. • Solution is stable for 28 days if refrigerated after reconstitution with bacteriostatic water for injection (if using sterile water for injection without preservative, use immediately; discard unused portions). • Stable for 24 hr in 0.9% NaCl if refrigerated.

⊞ IV INCOMPATIBILITIES

Don't mix trastuzumab with any other medications or with D₅W.

INDICATIONS/ROUTES/DOSAGE

BREAST CANCER

IV: ADULTS, ELDERLY: Initially, 4 mg/kg as a 30- to 90-min infusion, then 2 mg/kg weekly as a 30-min infusion.

SIDE EFFECTS

FREQUENT (greater than 20%): Pain, asthenia, fever, chills, headache, abdominal pain, back pain, infection, nausea, diarrhea, vomiting, cough, dyspnea. **OCCASIONAL (15%–5%):** Tachycardia, CHF, flu-like symptoms, anorexia, edema, bone pain, arthralgia, insomnia, dizziness, paresthesia, depression, rhinitis, pharyngitis, sinusitis. **RARE (less than 5%):** Allergic reaction, anemia, leukopenia, neuropathy, herpes simplex.

ADVERSE REACTIONS/ TOXIC EFFECTS

Cardiomyopathy, ventricular dysfunction, and CHF occur rarely. Pancytopenia may occur.

NURSING CONSIDERATIONS

BASELINE ASSESSMENT

Evaluate left ventricular function. Obtain baseline echocardiogram, EKG, multi-gated acquisition (MUGA) scan. CBC, platelet count should be obtained at baseline and at regular intervals during therapy.

INTERVENTION/EVALUATION

Frequently monitor for deteriorating cardiac function. Assess for asthenia (loss of strength, energy). Assist with ambulation if asthenia occurs. Monitor for fever, chills, abdominal pain, back pain. Offer antiemetics if nausea, vomiting occurs. Monitor pattern of daily bowel activity and stool consistency.

PATIENT/FAMILY TEACHING

• Do not have immunizations without physician's approval (lowers body's resistance). • Avoid contact with those who have recently taken oral polio vaccine. • Avoid crowds, those with infection.

travoprost

(Travatan)
See Antiglaucoma agents (p. 47C)

trazodone hydrochloride

tray-zoe-done
(Apo-Trazodone ✤, Desyrel, Desyrel Dividose, Novo-Trazodone ✤, PMS-Trazodone ✤)
Do not confuse Desyrel with Delsym or Zestril.

◆CLASSIFICATION

CLINICAL: Antidepressant (see pp. 12C, 38C).

ACTION

An antidepressant that blocks the reuptake of serotonin at neuronal presynaptic membranes, increasing its availability at postsynaptic receptor sites. **Therapeutic Effect:** Relieves depression.

PHARMACOKINETICS

Well absorbed from the GI tract. Protein binding: 85%–95%. Metabolized in the liver. Primarily excreted in urine. Unknown if removed by hemodialysis. **Half-life:** 5–9 hr.

USES

Treatment of depression exhibited as persistent, prominent dysphoria (occurring nearly every day for at least 2 wk) manifested by 4 of 8 symptoms: appetite change, sleep pattern change, increased fatigue, impaired concentration, feelings of guilt or worthlessness, loss of interest in usual activities, psychomotor agitation or retardation, suicidal tendencies. **OFF-LABEL:** Treatment of neurogenic pain.

PRECAUTIONS

CONTRAINDICATIONS: None known. **CAUTIONS:** Cardiac disease, arrhythmias.

⧗ LIFESPAN CONSIDERATIONS: **Pregnancy/Lactation:** Drug crosses placenta; minimally distributed in breast milk. **Pregnancy Category C.**

T

Children: Safety and efficacy not established in those younger than 6 yr. **Elderly:** More likely to experience sedative, hypotensive effects; lower dosage recommended.

INTERACTIONS

DRUG: **Alcohol, CNS depression-producing medications:** May increase CNS depression. **Antihypertensives:** May increase the effects of antihypertensives. **Digoxin, phenytoin:** May increase the blood concentration of these drugs. **Indinavir, ketoconazole, ritonavir:** May increase the blood concentration and toxicity of trazodone. HERBAL: **St. John's wort:** May increase the adverse effects of trazodone. FOOD: None known. LAB VALUES: May decrease serum WBC and neutrophil counts.

AVAILABILITY (Rx)

TABLETS: 50 mg (Desyrel), 100 mg (Desyrel), 150 mg (Desyrel Dividose), 300 mg (Desyrel Dividose).

ADMINISTRATION/HANDLING

PO
• Give shortly after snack, meal (reduces risk of dizziness, lightheadedness).
• Tablets may be crushed.

INDICATIONS/ROUTES/DOSAGE

DEPRESSION

PO: ADULTS: Initially, 150 mg/day in equally divided doses. Increase by 50 mg/day at 3- to 4-day intervals until therapeutic response is achieved. **Maximum:** 600 mg/day. ELDERLY: Initially, 25–50 mg at bedtime. May increase by 25–50 mg every 3–7 days. Range: 75–150 mg/day. CHILDREN 6–18 YR: Initially, 1.5–2 mg/kg/day in divided doses. May increase gradually to 6 mg/kg/day in 3 divided doses.

SIDE EFFECTS

FREQUENT (9%–3%): Somnolence, dry mouth, light-headedness, dizziness, headache, blurred vision, nausea, vomiting. **OCCASIONAL (3%–1%):** Nervousness, fatigue, constipation, generalized aches and pains, mild hypotension. **RARE:** Photosensitivity reaction.

ADVERSE REACTIONS/ TOXIC EFFECTS

Priapism, diminished or improved libido, retrograde ejaculation, and impotence occur rarely. Trazodone appears to be less cardiotoxic than other antidepressants, although arrhythmias may occur in patients with pre-existing cardiac disease.

NURSING CONSIDERATIONS

BASELINE ASSESSMENT

For those on long-term therapy, serum liver and renal function tests, blood counts should be performed periodically. Elderly are more likely to experience sedative or hypotensive effects.

INTERVENTION/EVALUATION

Supervise suicidal-risk patient closely during early therapy (as depression lessens, energy level improves, increasing suicide potential). Assess appearance, behavior, speech pattern, level of interest, mood. Monitor WBC, neutrophil count (drug should be stopped if levels fall below normal). Assist with ambulation if dizziness, lightheadedness occurs.

PATIENT/FAMILY TEACHING

• Immediately discontinue medication, consult physician if priapism occurs.
• May take after a meal or snack.
• May take at bedtime if drowsiness occurs. • Change positions slowly to avoid hypotensive effect. • Tolerance to sedative and anticholinergic effects usually develops during early therapy. • Avoid tasks that require alertness, motor skills until response to drug is established. • Photosensitivity to sun may occur. • Dry mouth may be relieved by sugarless gum, sips of tepid

water. • Report visual disturbances. • Do not abruptly discontinue medication. • Avoid alcohol.

treprostinil sodium

tre-**pros**-tin-il
(Remodulin)

CLASSIFICATION

PHARMACOTHERAPEUTIC: Aggregation inhibitor, vasodilator. **CLINICAL:** Antiplatelet.

ACTION

An antiplatelet that directly dilates pulmonary and systemic arterial vascular beds, inhibiting platelet aggregation. **Therapeutic Effect:** Reduces symptoms of pulmonary arterial hypertension associated with exercise.

PHARMACOKINETICS

Rapidly, completely absorbed after subcutaneous infusion; 91% bound to plasma protein. Metabolized by the liver. Excreted mainly in the urine with a lesser amount eliminated in the feces. **Half-life:** 2–4 hr.

USES

As a continuous subcutaneous infusion for the treatment of pulmonary arterial hypertension to diminish symptoms associated with exercise.

PRECAUTIONS

CONTRAINDICATIONS: None known. **CAUTIONS:** Hepatic or renal impairment in those older than 65 yr.

⧗ **LIFESPAN CONSIDERATIONS: Pregnancy/Lactation:** Unknown if distributed in breast milk. **Pregnancy Category B. Children:** Safety and efficacy not

established. **Elderly:** Consider dose selection carefully because of increased incidence of diminished organ function. Concurrent disease; other drug therapy.

INTERACTIONS

DRUG: Anticoagulants, aspirin, heparin, thrombolytics: May increase the risk of bleeding. **Drugs that alter BP, including antihypertensive agents, diuretics, vasodilators:** Reduced BP caused by treprostinil may be exacerbated by these drugs. **HERBAL:** None known. **FOOD:** None known. **LAB VALUES:** None known.

AVAILABILITY (Rx)

INJECTION: 1 mg/ml, 2.5 mg/ml, 5 mg/ml, 10 mg/ml.

ADMINISTRATION/HANDLING

 IV

Reconstitution • Dilute with either sterile water for injection of 0.9% NaCl.

Rate of administration • Give as continuous IV infusion via surgically placed indwelling central venous catheter using an infusion pump. • Calculate infusion rate using the formula: **Step One:** Diluted IV Remodulin concentration (mg/ml) = dose (ng/kg/min) multiplied by weight (kg) multiplied by (0.00006/IV infusion rate (ml/hr). **Step Two:** Amount of Remodulin injection (ml) = diluted IV Remodulin concentration (mg/ml)/Remodulin vial strength (mg/ml) multiplied by total volume of diluted Remodulin solution in reservoir (ml).

Storage • Store at room temperature.

SUBCUTANEOUS

Reconstitution • Intended to be administered without further dilution. • Do not use a single vial for longer

T

than 14 days after initial use. • To avoid potential interruptions in drug delivery, the patient must have immediate access to a backup infusion pump and subcutaneous infusion sets.

Rate of administration • Give as a continuous subcutaneous infusion via a subcutaneous catheter, using an infusion pump designed for subcutaneous drug delivery. • Calculate the infusion rate using following formula: infusion rate (ml/hr) = dose (ng/kg/min) × weight (kg) × (0.00006/treprostinil dosage strength concentration [mg/ml]).

Storage • Store at room temperature.

INDICATIONS/ROUTES/DOSAGE
PULMONARY ARTERIAL HYPERTENSION
CONTINUOUS SUBCUTANEOUS INFUSION, IV INFUSION: ADULTS, ELDERLY: Initially, 1.25 ng/kg/min. Reduce infusion rate to 0.625 ng/kg/min if initial dose cannot be tolerated. Increase infusion rate in increments of no more than 1.25 ng/kg/min per wk for the first 4 wk and then no more than 2.5 ng/kg/min per wk for the duration of infusion.

HEPATIC IMPAIRMENT (MILD TO MODERATE)
ADULTS, ELDERLY: Decrease the initial dose to 0.625 ng/kg/min based on ideal body weight and increase cautiously.

SIDE EFFECTS
FREQUENT: Infusion site pain, erythema, induration, rash. **OCCASIONAL:** Headache, diarrhea, jaw pain, vasodilation, nausea. **RARE:** Dizziness, hypotension, pruritus, edema.

ADVERSE REACTIONS/ TOXIC EFFECTS
Abrupt withdrawal or sudden large reductions in dosage may result in worsening of pulmonary arterial hypertension symptoms.

PATIENT/FAMILY TEACHING
• Offer full, complete instruction of drug administration as delivery occurs via a self-inserted subcutaneous catheter using an ambulatory subcutaneous pump. • Instruct patient on care of subcutaneous catheter and troubleshooting infusion pump problems.

tretinoin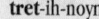

tret-ih-noyn

(Altinac, Avita, Renova, Retin-A, Retin-A Micro, Stieva-A ✤, Vesanoid, Vitamin A Acid ✤)

Do not confuse tretinoin with trientine.

FIXED-COMBINATION(S)
With octyl methoxycinnamate and oxy-benzone, moisturizers, and SPF-12, a sunscreen **(Retin-A Regimen Kit)**.

•CLASSIFICATION
PHARMACOTHERAPEUTIC: Retinoid. **CLINICAL:** Antiacne, transdermal, antineoplastic (see p. 79C).

ACTION
Antiacne: Decreases cohesiveness of follicular epithelial cells. Increases turnover of follicular epithelial cells. Therapeutic Effect: Causes expulsion of blackheads. Bacterial skin counts are not altered. **Transdermal:** Exerts its effects on growth/differentiation of epithelial cells. Therapeutic Effect: Alleviates fine wrinkles, hyperpigmentation. **Antineoplastic:** Induces maturation, decreases proliferation of acute promyelocytic leukemia (APL) cells. Therapeutic Effect: Repopulation of bone marrow, blood by normal hematopoietic cells.

PHARMACOKINETICS

Topical: Minimally absorbed. **PO:** Well absorbed following PO administration. Primarily excreted in urine. Half-life: 0.5–2 hr.

USES

Topical: Treatment of acne vulgaris, especially grades I–III in which blackheads, papules, pustules predominate. **Oral:** Induction of remission in patients with APL. OFF-LABEL: Treatment of disorders of keratinization, including photo-aged skin, liver spots.

PRECAUTIONS

CONTRAINDICATIONS: Sensitivity to parabens (used as preservative in gelatin capsule). **EXTREME CAUTION:** Topical: Eczema, sun exposure. **CAUTIONS:** Topical: Those with considerable sun exposure in their occupation or hypersensitivity to sun. PO: Elevated serum cholesterol/triglycerides.

LIFESPAN CONSIDERATIONS: Pregnancy/Lactation: **Topical:** Use during pregnancy only if clearly necessary. Unknown if excreted in breast milk; exercise caution in breast-feeding mother. **Pregnancy Category C. PO:** Teratogenic, embryotoxic effect. **Pregnancy Category D. Children/Elderly:** Safety and efficacy not established.

INTERACTIONS

DRUG: *Topical:* **Keratolytic agents (e.g., sulfur, benzoyl peroxide, salicylic acid); medicated soaps; shampoos; preparations containing alcohol, menthol, spice, lime (e.g., perfume, cologne, astringents); permanent wave solutions; hair depilatories:** May increase skin irritation. **Photosensitive medication (thiazides, tetracyclines, fluoroquinolones, phenothiazines, sulfonamides):** Augments phototoxicity. *PO:* **Ketoconazole:** May increase tretinoin concentration. HERBAL: None

known. FOOD: None known. LAB VALUES: *PO:* Leukocytosis occurs commonly (40%). May elevate serum hepatic function tests, cholesterol, triglycerides.

AVAILABILITY (Rx)

CAPSULES (VESANOID): 10 mg.
CREAM: 0.02% (Renova), 0.025% (Altinac, Avita, Renova, Retin-A), 0.05% (Altinac, Renova, Retin-A), 0.1% (Altinac, Retin-A). **GEL:** 0.01% (Retin-A), 0.025% (Avita, Retin-A), 0.04% (Retin-A Micro), 0.1% (Retin-A Micro).
LIQUID (RETIN-A): 0.05%.

ADMINISTRATION/HANDLING

PO
• Do not crush/break capsule.

TOPICAL
• Thoroughly cleanse area before applying tretinoin. • Lightly cover only the affected area. Liquid may be applied with fingertip, gauze, cotton, taking care to avoid rubbing onto unaffected skin. • Keep medication away from eyes, mouth, angles of nose, mucous membranes. • Wash hands immediately after application.

INDICATIONS/ROUTES/DOSAGE

ACNE
TOPICAL: ADULTS, CHILDREN 12 YR AND OLDER: Apply once a day at bedtime.

ACUTE PROMYELOCYTIC LEUKEMIA
PO: ADULTS: 45 mg/m²/day given as 2 evenly divided doses until complete remission is documented. Discontinue therapy 30 days after complete remission or after 90 days of treatment, whichever comes first.

REMISSION MAINTENANCE
PO: ADULTS, ELDERLY, CHILDREN: 45–200 mg/m²/day in 2–3 divided doses for up to 12 mo.

SIDE EFFECTS

Topical: Temporary change in pigmentation, photosensitivity. Local

T

inflammatory reactions (peeling, dry skin, stinging, erythema, pruritus) are to be expected and are reversible with discontinuation of tretinoin. **FREQUENT: PO (87%–54%):** Headache, fever, dry skin/oral mucosa, bone pain, nausea, vomiting, rash. **OCCASIONAL: PO (26%–6%):** Mucositis, earache or feeling of fullness in ears, flushing, pruritus, diaphoresis, visual disturbances, hypotension/hypertension, dizziness, anxiety, insomnia, alopecia, skin changes. **RARE (6%):** Change in visual acuity, temporary hearing loss.

ADVERSE REACTIONS/ TOXIC EFFECTS

PO: Retinoic acid syndrome (fever, dyspnea, weight gain, abnormal chest auscultatory findings [pulmonary infiltrates, pleural or pericardial effusions], episodic hypotension) occurs commonly (25%), as does leukocytosis (40%). Syndrome generally occurs during first month of therapy (sometimes occurs after first dose). High-dose steroids (dexamethasone 10 mg IV) at first suspicion of syndrome reduces morbidity, mortality. Pseudotumor cerebri may be noted, especially in children (headache, nausea, vomiting, visual disturbances). **Topical:** Possible tumorigenic potential when combined with ultraviolet radiation.

NURSING CONSIDERATIONS

BASELINE ASSESSMENT

PO: Inform women of childbearing potential of risk to fetus if pregnancy occurs. Instruct on need for use of 2 reliable forms of contraceptives concurrently during therapy and for 1 mo after discontinuation of therapy, even in infertile, premenopausal women. Pregnancy test should be obtained within 1 wk before institution of therapy. Obtain initial serum liver function tests, cholesterol, triglyceride levels.

INTERVENTION/EVALUATION

PO: Monitor serum liver function tests, hematologic and coagulation profiles, cholesterol, triglycerides. Monitor for signs/symptoms of pseudotumor cerebri in children.

PATIENT/FAMILY TEACHING

• **Topical:** Avoid exposure to sunlight, tanning beds; use sunscreens, protective clothing. • Affected areas should also be protected from wind, cold. • If skin is already sunburned, do not use drug until fully healed. • Keep tretinoin away from eyes, mouth, angles of nose, mucous membranes. • Do not use medicated, drying, abrasive soaps; wash face no more than 2–3 times a day with gentle soap. • Avoid use of preparations containing alcohol, menthol, spice, lime, such as shaving lotions, astringents, perfume. • Mild redness, peeling are expected; decrease frequency or discontinue medication if excessive reaction occurs. • Nonmedicated cosmetics may be used; however, cosmetics must be removed before tretinoin application. • Improvement noted during first 24 wk of therapy. • **Antiacne:** Therapeutic results noted in 2–3 wk; optimal results in 6 wk.

triamcinolone
(Aristocort)
triamcinolone acetonide

(Acetocot, Aristocort, Aristocort A, Aristocort Forte, Aristospan Injection, Azmacort, Clinacort, Clinalog, Kenalog, Kenalog in Orabase, Kenalog-10, Kenalog-40, Ken-Jec 40, Nasacort AQ, TriAderm ✦, Triam-A, Triamcot, Triam-Forte,

Triamonide 40, Triderm, Tri-Nasal, U-Tri-Lone)

triamcinolone diacetate

(Amcort, Aristocort Intralesional)

triamcinolone hexacetonide

(Aristospan)

trye-am-**sin**-oh-lone

Do not confuse triamcinolone with Triaminicin or Triaminicol.

FIXED-COMBINATION(S)

Myco-II, Mycolog II, Myco-Triacet: triamcinolone/nystatin (an antifungal): 0.1%/100,000 units/g.

◆ CLASSIFICATION

PHARMACOTHERAPEUTIC: Adrenocortical steroid. **CLINICAL:** Antiinflammatory (see pp. 68C, 84C, 87C).

ACTION

An adrenocortical steroid that inhibits accumulation of inflammatory cells at inflammation sites, phagocytosis, lysosomal enzyme release and synthesis, and release of mediators of inflammation. Therapeutic Effect: Prevents or suppresses cell-mediated immune reactions. Decreases or prevents tissue response to inflammatory process.

USES

Inhalation: Long-term control of bronchial asthma. **Nasal:** Seasonal and perennial rhinitis. **Oral:** Immunosuppressant, relief of acute inflammation. **Topical:** Relief of inflammation and pruritus associated with corticoid-responsive dermatoses.

PRECAUTIONS

CONTRAINDICATIONS: Administration of live virus vaccines, especially smallpox vaccine; hypersensitivity to corticosteroids or tartrazine; IM injection or oral inhalation in children younger than 6 yr; peptic ulcer disease (except life-threatening situations); systemic fungal infection. **Topical:** Marked circulation impairment. **CAUTIONS:** History of tuberculosis (may reactivate disease), hypothyroidism, cirrhosis, non-specific ulcerative colitis, CHF, hypertension, psychosis, renal insufficiency. Prolonged therapy should be discontinued slowly. **Pregnancy Category C (D if used in first trimester).**

INTERACTIONS

DRUG: Amphotericin: May increase hypokalemia. **Digoxin:** May increase the risk of digoxin toxicity caused by hypokalemia. **Diuretics, insulin, oral hypoglycemics, potassium supplements:** May decrease the effects of these drugs. **Hepatic enzyme inducers:** May decrease the effects of triamcinolone. **Live virus vaccines:** May decrease the patient's antibody response to vaccine, increase vaccine side effects, and potentiate virus replication. **HERBAL:** None known. **FOOD:** None known. **LAB VALUES:** May increase blood glucose and serum lipid, amylase, and sodium levels. May decrease serum calcium, potassium, and thyroxine levels.

AVAILABILITY (Rx)

ORAL (TOPICAL PASTE [KENALOG IN ORABASE]): 0.1% or 5 g. **TABLETS (ARISTOCORT):** 4 mg, 8 mg. **INHALATION (ORAL [AZMACORT]):** 100 mcg/actuation. **NASAL SPRAY:** 50 mcg/inhalation (Tri-Nasal), 55 mcg/inhalation (Nasacort AQ). **CREAM:** 50 mcg/inhalation (Tri-Nasal), 55 mcg/inhalation (Nasacort AQ). **OINTMENT (ARISTOCORT A, KENALOG):** 0.025%, 0.1%. **INJECTION (ACETONIDE):** 10 mg/ml (Kenalog-10), 40 mg/ml (Acetocot, Clinalog, Kenalog-40, Ken-Jec 40, Triam-A, Triamcot, Triamonide 40, U-Tri-Lone). **INJECTION**

T

(DIACETATE): 25 mg/ml (Aristocort), 40 mg/ml (Aristocort Forte, Clinacort, Triam-Forte). **INJECTION (HEXACETO-NIDE [ARISTOSPAN INJECTION]):** 5 mg/ml, 20 mg/ml.

ADMINISTRATION/HANDLING

IM
• Do **not** give IV. • Give deep IM in gluteus maximus.

PO
• Give with food, milk. • Single doses given before 9 AM; multiple doses at evenly spaced intervals.

INHALATION
• Shake container well; exhale as completely as possible. • Instruct the patient to place mouthpiece fully into mouth, holding inhaler upright, inhale deeply and slowly while pressing the top of the canister, hold breath as long as possible before exhaling; then exhale slowly. • Wait 1 min between inhalations when multiple inhalations are ordered (allows for deeper bronchial penetration). • Rinse mouth with water immediately after inhalation.

TOPICAL
• Gently cleanse area before application. • Use occlusive dressings only as ordered. • Apply sparingly, rub into area thoroughly.

INDICATIONS/ROUTES/DOSAGE

IMMUNOSUPPRESSION, RELIEF OF ACUTE INFLAMMATION
PO: ADULTS, ELDERLY: 4–60 mg/day.
IM (TRIAMCINOLONE ACETONIDE): ADULTS, ELDERLY: Initially, 2.5–60 mg/day.
IM (TRIAMCINOLONE DIACETATE): ADULTS, ELDERLY: 40 mg/wk.
IM (TRIAMCINOLONE HEXACETO-NIDE): ADULTS, ELDERLY: Initially, 2.5–40 mg up to 100 mg; 2–20 mg.
INTRA-ARTICULAR, INTRALESION-AL: ADULTS, ELDERLY: 5–40 mg.

CONTROL OF BRONCHIAL ASTHMA
INHALATION: ADULTS, ELDERLY: 2 inhalations 3–4 times a day. CHILDREN 6–12 YR: 1–2 inhalations 3–4 times a day. **Maximum:** 12 inhalations/day. Initially, 2.5–60 mg/day.

RHINITIS
INTRANASAL: ADULTS, ELDERLY, CHILDREN 6 YR AND OLDER: Initially, 2 sprays (55 mcg/spray) in each nostril once daily. Maintenance: 1 spray in each nostril once daily.

RELIEF OF INFLAMMATION OR PRURITUS ASSOCIATED WITH CORTICOID-RESPONSIVE DERMATOSES
TOPICAL: ADULTS, ELDERLY: 2–4 times a day. May give 1–2 times a day or as intermittent therapy.

SIDE EFFECTS

FREQUENT: Insomnia, dry mouth, heartburn, nervousness, abdominal distention, diaphoresis, acne, mood swings, increased appetite, facial flushing, delayed wound healing, increased susceptibility to infection, diarrhea or constipation. **OCCASIONAL:** Headache, edema, change in skin color, frequent urination. **RARE:** Tachycardia, allergic reaction (including rash and hives), mental changes, hallucinations, depression. **Topical:** Allergic contact dermatitis.

ADVERSE REACTIONS/ TOXIC EFFECTS

Long-term therapy may cause muscle wasting in the arms or legs, osteoporosis, spontaneous fractures, amenorrhea, cataracts, glaucoma, peptic ulcer disease, and CHF. Abruptly withdrawing the drug following long-term therapy may cause anorexia, nausea, fever, headache, arthralgia, rebound inflammation, fatigue, weakness, lethargy, dizziness, and orthostatic hypotension. Anaphylaxis occurs rarely with parenteral administration. Suddenly discontinuing triamcinolone may be fatal. Blindness has occurred rarely after intralesional injection around face and head.

NURSING CONSIDERATIONS

BASELINE ASSESSMENT

Question for hypersensitivity to any of the corticosteroids or tartrazine (Kenacort). Obtain baselines for height, weight, BP, serum glucose, electrolytes. Check results of initial tests (e.g., tuberculosis [TB] skin test, x-rays, EKG).

INTERVENTION/EVALUATION

Monitor I&O, daily weight, BP, serum glucose, electrolytes. Assess for edema. Check vital signs at least twice a day. Be alert to infection: pharyngitis, fever, vague symptoms. Watch for hypocalcemia (muscle twitching, cramps, positive Trousseau's or Chvostek's signs), hypokalemia (weakness, muscle cramps, paraesthesia [especially in lower extremities], nausea or vomiting, irritability, EKG changes). Assess emotional status, ability to sleep. For oral inhalation, check mucous membranes for signs of fungal infection. Monitor growth in children. Check lab results for blood coagulability, clinical evidence of thromboembolism. Provide assistance with ambulation.

PATIENT/FAMILY TEACHING

• **Oral:** Inform physician if sudden weight gain, facial edema, difficulty breathing, muscle weakness occurs. • Take oral medication with food or after meals. • Inform physician if condition worsens. • Do not stop medication without physician approval. • May cause dry mouth. • Avoid alcohol. • **Inhalation:** Do not take for acute asthma attack. • Rinse mouth to decrease risk of mouth soreness. • Inform physician if mouth lesions, sore mouth occurs (stomatitis). • **Nasal:** Report unusual cough or spasm, persistent nasal bleeding, burning, infection.

triamterene

try-**am**-ter-een
(Dyrenium)
Do not confuse triamterene with trimipramine.

FIXED-COMBINATION(S)

Dyazide, Maxzide: triamterene/hydrochlorothiazide (a diuretic): 37.5 mg/25 mg; 50 mg/25 mg; 75 mg/50 mg.

•CLASSIFICATION

PHARMACOTHERAPEUTIC: Potassium-sparing diuretic. **CLINICAL:** Antiedema (see p. 89C).

ACTION

A potassium-sparing diuretic that inhibits sodium, potassium, ATPase. Interferes with sodium and potassium exchange in distal tubule, cortical collecting tubule, and collecting duct. Increases sodium and decreases potassium excretion. Also increases magnesium, decreases calcium loss. **Therapeutic Effect:** Produces diuresis and lowers BP.

PHARMACOKINETICS

Route	Onset	Peak	Duration
PO	2–4 hr	N/A	7–9 hr

Incompletely absorbed from the GI tract. Widely distributed. Metabolized in the liver. Primarily eliminated in feces via biliary route. **Half-life:** 1.5–2.5 hr (increased in renal impairment).

USES

Treatment of edema, hypertension. **OFF-LABEL:** Treatment adjunct for hypertension, prevention and treatment of hypokalemia.

PRECAUTIONS

CONTRAINDICATIONS: Anuria, drug-induced or preexisting hyperkalemia,

---

T

progressive or severe renal disease, severe hepatic disease.

⌛ LIFESPAN CONSIDERATIONS: **Pregnancy/Lactation:** Drug crosses placenta; is distributed in breast milk. Breast-feeding is not advised. **Pregnancy Category C (D if used in pregnancy-induced hypertension). Children:** Safety and efficacy not established. **Elderly:** May be at increased risk for developing hyperkalemia.

INTERACTIONS

DRUG: **Angiotensin-converting enzyme (ACE) inhibitors (such as captopril), potassium-containing medications, potassium supplements:** May increase the risk of hyperkalemia. **Anticoagulants, heparin:** May decrease the effects of these drugs. **Lithium:** May decrease the clearance and increase the risk of toxicity of lithium. **NSAIDs:** May decrease the antihypertensive effect of triamterene. **HERBAL:** None known. **FOOD:** None known. **LAB VALUES:** May increase urinary calcium excretion; BUN and blood glucose levels; and serum calcium, creatinine, potassium, magnesium, and uric acid levels. May decrease serum sodium levels.

AVAILABILITY (Rx)

CAPSULES: 50 mg, 100 mg.

ADMINISTRATION/HANDLING

PO
• Give with food if GI disturbances occur.• Do not crush, break capsules.

INDICATIONS/ROUTES/DOSAGE

EDEMA, HYPERTENSION
PO: ADULTS, ELDERLY: 25–100 mg/day as a single dose or in 2 divided doses. **Maximum:** 300 mg/day. CHILDREN: 2–4 mg/kg/day as a single dose or in 2 divided doses. **Maximum:** 6 mg/kg/day or 300 mg/day.

SIDE EFFECTS

OCCASIONAL: Fatigue, nausea, diarrhea, abdominal pain, leg cramps, headache. **RARE:** Anorexia, asthenia, rash, dizziness.

ADVERSE REACTIONS/ TOXIC EFFECTS

Triamterene use may result in hyponatremia (somnolence, dry mouth, increased thirst, lack of energy) or severe hyperkalemia (irritability, anxiety, heaviness of legs, paresthesia, hypotension, bradycardia, EKG changes [tented T waves, widening QRS complex, ST segment depression]), particularly in those with renal impairment or diabetes, the elderly or severely ill patients. Agranulocytosis, nephrolithiasis, and thrombocytopenia occur rarely.

NURSING CONSIDERATIONS

BASELINE ASSESSMENT
Assess baseline serum electrolytes, particularly check for hypokalemia. Assess serum renal and liver function tests. Assess for edema (note location, extent), skin turgor, mucous membranes for hydration status. Assess muscle strength, mental status. Note skin temperature, moisture. Obtain baseline weight. Initiate strict I&O. Note pulse rate and regularity.

INTERVENTION/EVALUATION
Monitor BP, vital signs, serum electrolytes (particularly potassium), I&O, weight. Watch for changes from initial assessment (hyperkalemia may result in muscle strength changes, tremors, muscle cramps), altered mental status (orientation, alertness, confusion), cardiac arrhythmias. Weigh daily. Note extent of diuresis. Assess lung sounds for rhonchi, wheezing.

PATIENT/FAMILY TEACHING
• Take medication in the morning.
• Expect increase in volume, frequency

---

of urination. • Therapeutic effect takes several days to begin and can last for several days when drug is discontinued. • Avoid prolonged exposure to sunlight. • Report severe or persistent weakness, headache, dry mouth, nausea, vomiting, fever, sore throat, unusual bleeding/bruising. • Avoid excessive intake of food high in potassium or use of salt substitutes.

triazolam

trye-**ay**-zoe-lam

(Apo-Triazo ✿, Halcion)

Do not confuse Halcion with Haldol or Healon.

◆CLASSIFICATION

PHARMACOTHERAPEUTIC: Benzodiazepine (**Schedule IV**). **CLINICAL:** Sedative-hypnotic (see p. 136C).

ACTION

A benzodiazepine that enhances the action of the inhibitory neurotransmitter gamma-aminobutyric acid, resulting in CNS depression. **Therapeutic Effect:** Induces sleep.

PHARMACOKINETICS

Rapidly and completely absorbed from GI tract. Protein binding: 89%–94%. Metabolized in the liver. Primarily excreted in urine. **Half-life:** 1.5–5.5 hr.

USES

Short-term treatment of insomnia (6 wk or less). Reduces sleep-induction time, number of nocturnal awakenings; increases length of sleep.

PRECAUTIONS

CONTRAINDICATIONS: Angle-closure glaucoma; CNS depression; hypersensitivity to other benzodiazepines; pregnancy or breast-feeding; severe, uncontrolled pain; sleep apnea. **CAUTIONS:** Those with potential for drug abuse.

⧗ **LIFESPAN CONSIDERATIONS: Pregnancy/Lactation:** Drug crosses placenta; is distributed in breast milk. **Pregnancy Category X. Children:** Safety and efficacy not established in children younger than 18 yr. **Elderly:** Initially, small dosage is recommended to avoid excessive sedation, ataxia. May increase dosage gradually.

INTERACTIONS

DRUG: Alcohol, other CNS depressants: May increase CNS depression. **Fluvoxamine, itraconazole, ketoconazole, nefazodone:** May inhibit metabolism and increase serum concentrations of triazolam. **HERBAL: Kava kava, valerian:** May increase CNS depression. **FOOD: Grapefruit, grapefruit juice:** May alter the absorption of triazolam. **LAB VALUES:** None known.

AVAILABILITY (Rx)

TABLETS: 0.125 mg, 0.25 mg.

ADMINISTRATION/HANDLING

PO
• Give without regard to meals.
• Tablets may be crushed. • Grapefruit juice may alter absorption.

INDICATIONS/ROUTES/DOSAGE

INSOMNIA

PO: ADULTS, CHILDREN 18 YR AND OLDER: 0.125–0.5 mg at bedtime.   ELDERLY: 0.0625–0.125 mg at bedtime.

SIDE EFFECTS

FREQUENT: Somnolence, sedation, dry mouth, headache, dizziness, nervousness, light-headedness, incoordination, nausea, rebound insomnia (may occur for 1–2 nights after drug is discontinued). **OCCASIONAL:** Euphoria, tachycardia, abdominal cramps, visual

T

disturbances. **RARE:** Paradoxical CNS excitement or restlessness (particularly in elderly or debilitated patients).

ADVERSE REACTIONS/ TOXIC EFFECTS

Abrupt or too-rapid withdrawal may result in pronounced restlessness, irritability, insomnia, hand tremors, abdominal or muscle cramps, vomiting, diaphoresis, and seizures. Overdose results in somnolence, confusion, diminished reflexes, respiratory depression, and coma.

NURSING CONSIDERATIONS

BASELINE ASSESSMENT

Question for possibility of pregnancy before initiating therapy (Pregnancy Category X). Assess vital signs immediately before administration. Raise bed rails. Provide environment conducive to sleep (back rub, quiet environment, low lighting).

INTERVENTION/EVALUATION

Monitor respiratory, cardiovascular, mental status; hepatic function with prolonged use. Assess sleep pattern of patient. Monitor elderly and debilitated for paradoxical reaction, particularly during early therapy. Evaluate for therapeutic response to insomnia: decrease in number of nocturnal awakenings, increase in length of sleep.

PATIENT/FAMILY TEACHING

• May cause drowsiness. • Avoid tasks that require alertness, motor skills until response to drug is established. • May cause physical or psychological dependence, dry mouth. • Smoking reduces drug effectiveness. • Rebound insomnia may occur when drug is discontinued after short-term therapy. • Avoid alcohol, other CNS depressants. • Inform physician if pregnant or are planning to become pregnant. • May experience disturbed sleep patterns for 1–2 nights after discontinuing triazolam. • Avoid concomitant grapefruit juice.

Tricor, *see fenofibrate*

trifluoperazine hydrochloride

trye-floo-oh-**per**-a-zeen

(Apo-Trifluoperazine ✦, Nono-Trifluzine ✦, PMS-Trifluoperazine ✦, Stelazine)

Do not confuse trifluoperazine with triflupromazine, or Stelazine with selegiline.

CLASSIFICATION

PHARMACOTHERAPEUTIC: Phenothiazine derivative. **CLINICAL:** Antipsychotic, antianxiety (see p. 59C).

ACTION

A phenothiazine derivative that blocks dopamine at postsynaptic receptor sites. Possesses strong extrapyramidal and antiemetic effects and weak anticholinergic and sedative effects. **Therapeutic Effect:** Suppresses behavioral response in psychosis; reduces locomotor activity and aggressiveness.

PHARMACOKINETICS

Readily absorbed following PO administration. Protein binding: 90%–99%. Metabolized in liver. Excreted in urine. **Half-life:** 24 hr.

USES

Treatment of schizophrenia.

PRECAUTIONS

CONTRAINDICATIONS: Angle-closure glaucoma, circulatory collapse,

---

myelosuppression, severe cardiac or hepatic disease, severe hypertension or hypotension. **CAUTIONS:** Seizure disorders, Parkinson's disease.

⚖ **LIFESPAN CONSIDERATIONS:** Pregnancy/Lactation: Drug crosses placenta; is distributed in breast milk. **Pregnancy Category C. Children:** Safety and efficacy not established in children younger than 2 yr. **Elderly:** Higher risk of sedative, anticholinergic, extrapyramidal, hypotensive effects.

INTERACTIONS

DRUG: **Alcohol, other CNS depressants:** May increase CNS and respiratory depression and the hypotensive effects of trifluoperazine. **Antacids:** May inhibit absorption of trifluoperzine if given within 1 hr of drug. **Antithyroid agents:** May increase the risk of agranulocytosis. **Extrapyramidal symptom–producing medications:** May increase extrapyramidal symptoms (EPS). **Hypotension-producing agents:** May increase hypotension. **Levodopa:** May decrease the effects of levodopa. **Lithium:** May decrease the absorption of trifluoperazine and produce adverse neurologic effects. **MAOIs, tricyclic antidepressants:** May increase the anticholinergic and sedative effects of trifluoperazine. **HERBAL:** None known. **FOOD:** None known. **LAB VALUES:** May cause EKG changes.

AVAILABILITY (Rx)

TABLETS: 1 mg, 2 mg, 5 mg, 10 mg. **INJECTION:** 2 mg/ml.

ADMINISTRATION/HANDLING

IM
• Administer deep in large muscle mass.

PO
• May give with food to decrease GI effects.

INDICATIONS/ROUTES/DOSAGE
PSYCHOTIC DISORDERS
PO: ADULTS, ELDERLY, CHILDREN 12 YR AND OLDER: Initially, 2–5 mg once or twice a day. Range: 15–20 mg/day. **Maximum:** 40 mg/day. CHILDREN 6–11 YR: Initially, 1 mg once or twice a day. Maintenance: Up to 15 mg/day.
IM: ADULTS: 1–2 mg q4–6h. **Maximum:** 10 mg/24h. ELDERLY: 1 mg q4–6h. **Maximum:** 6 mg/24h. CHILDREN: 1 mg 2 times/day.

SIDE EFFECTS

FREQUENT: Hypotension, dizziness, and syncope (occur frequently after first injection, occasionally after subsequent injections, and rarely with oral form). **OCCASIONAL:** Drowsiness during early therapy, dry mouth, blurred vision, lethargy, constipation or diarrhea, nasal congestion, peripheral edema, urine retention. **RARE:** Ocular changes, altered skin pigmentation (in those taking high doses for prolonged periods), photosensitivity.

ADVERSE REACTIONS/ TOXIC EFFECTS

EPS appear to be dose-related (particularly high doses) and are divided into 3 categories: akathisia (inability to sit still, tapping of feet), parkinsonian symptoms (such as mask-like face, tremors, shuffling gait, and hypersalivation), and acute dystonias (such as torticollis, opisthotonos, and oculogyric crisis). Dystonic reactions may also produce diaphoresis and pallor. Tardive dyskinesia, marked by tongue protrusion, puffing of the cheeks, and chewing or puckering of the mouth, occurs rarely but may be irreversible. Abrupt withdrawal after long-term therapy may precipitate nausea, vomiting, gastritis, dizziness, and tremors. Blood dyscrasias, particularly agranulocytosis, and mild leukopenia may occur. Trifluoperazine may lower the seizure threshold.

T

NURSING CONSIDERATIONS

BASELINE ASSESSMENT

Assess behavior, appearance, emotional status, response to environment, speech pattern, thought content.

INTERVENTION/EVALUATION

Monitor BP for hypotension. Assess for EPS. Monitor WBC for blood dyscrasias. Monitor for fine tongue movement (may be early sign of tardive dyskinesia); tremors, gait changes; abnormal movement in trunk, neck, extremities. Supervise suicidal-risk patient closely during early therapy (as depression lessens, energy level improves, increasing suicide potential). Monitor target behaviors. Assess for therapeutic response (interest in surroundings, improvement in self-care, increased ability to concentrate, relaxed facial expression).

PATIENT/FAMILY TEACHING

• Do not take antacids within 1 hr of trifluoperazine. • Avoid alcohol. • Avoid excessive exposure to sunlight, artificial light. • Avoid tasks that require alertness, motor skills until response to drug is established (may cause drowsiness). • Rise slowly from lying or sitting position (prevents hypotension).

trihexyphenidyl hydrochloride

try-hex-eh-**fen**-ih-dill

(Apo-Trihex ✤, Artane)

Do not confuse Artane with Altace or Anturane.

◆CLASSIFICATION

PHARMACOTHERAPEUTIC: Anticholinergic. **CLINICAL:** Antiparkinson agent.

ACTION

Blocks central cholinergic receptors (aids in balancing cholinergic and dopaminergic activity). **Therapeutic Effect:** Decreases salivation, relaxes smooth muscle.

USES

Adjunctive treatment for all forms of Parkinson's disease, including postencephalitic, arteriosclerotic, idiopathic types. Controls symptoms of drug-induced extrapyramidal symptoms.

PRECAUTIONS

CONTRAINDICATIONS: Angle-closure glaucoma, GI obstruction, paralytic ileus, intestinal atony, severe ulcerative colitis, prostatic hypertrophy, myasthenia gravis, megacolon. **CAUTIONS:** Hyperthyroidism, renal/hepatic impairment, hypertension, hiatal hernia, tachycardia, arrhythmias, ulcer, esophageal reflux, excessive activity during hot weather or exercise. **Pregnancy Category C.**

INTERACTIONS

DRUG: Alcohol, CNS depressants: May increase sedative effect. **Amantadine, anticholinergics, MAOIs:** May increase anticholinergic effects. **Antacids, antidiarrheals:** May decrease absorption, effects. **HERBAL:** None known. **FOOD:** None known. **LAB VALUES:** None known.

ADMINISTRATION/HANDLING

PO

• Administer with food, water to decrease GI irritation.

AVAILABILITY (Rx)

TABLETS: 2 mg, 5 mg. **ELIXIR:** 2 mg/5 ml.

INDICATIONS/ROUTES/DOSAGE

PARKINSONISM

PO: ADULTS, ELDERLY: Initially, 1 mg on first day. May increase by 2 mg a day at 3- to 5-day intervals up to 6–10 mg a day (12–15 mg a day in patients with postencephalitic parkinsonism).

DRUG-INDUCED EXTRAPYRAMIDAL SYMPTOMS

PO: ADULTS, ELDERLY: Initially, 1 mg a day. Range: 5–15 mg a day in 3–4 divided doses.

SIDE EFFECTS

◀ ALERT ▶ Those over 60 yr tend to develop mental confusion, disorientation, agitation, psychotic-like symptoms. **FREQUENT:** Drowsiness, dry mouth. **OCCASIONAL:** Blurred vision, urinary retention, constipation, dizziness, headache, muscle cramps. **RARE:** Skin rash, seizures, depression.

ADVERSE REACTIONS/ TOXIC EFFECTS

Hypersensitivity reaction (eczema, pruritus, rash, cardiac arrhythmias, photosensitivity) may occur. Overdosage may vary from CNS depression (sedation, apnea, cardiovascular collapse, death) to severe paradoxical reaction (hallucinations, tremor, seizures).

NURSING CONSIDERATIONS

INTERVENTION/EVALUATION

Be alert to neurologic effects: headache, lethargy, mental confusion, agitation. Monitor elderly closely for paradoxical reaction. Assess for clinical reversal of symptoms (improvement of tremor of head/hands at rest, mask-like facial expression, shuffling gait, muscular rigidity).

PATIENT/FAMILY TEACHING

• Take after meals or with food. • Do not stop medication abruptly. • Inform physician if GI effects, palpitations, eye pain, rash, fever, heat intolerance occurs. • Avoid alcohol, other CNS depressants. • May cause dry mouth, drowsiness. • Avoid tasks that require alertness, motor skills until response to drug is established. • Difficulty urinating, constipation may occur (inform physician if they persist).

Trileptal, *see oxcarbazepine*

---

trimethobenzamide hydrochloride

try-meth-oh-**benz**-oh-mide

(Benzacot, Benzocaine-Trimethobenzamide Adult, Benzocaine-Trimethobenzamide Pediatric, Navogan, Tebamide, Tebamide Pediatric, Tigan, Tigan Adult, Tigan Pediatric)

◆ **CLASSIFICATION**

PHARMACOTHERAPEUTIC: Anticholinergic. **CLINICAL:** Antiemetic.

ACTION

An anticholinergic that acts at the chemoreceptor trigger zone in the medulla oblongata. **Therapeutic Effect:** Relieves nausea and vomiting.

PHARMACOKINETICS

Route	Onset	Peak	Duration
PO	10–40 min	N/A	3–4 hr
IM	15–30 min	N/A	2–3 hr

Partially absorbed from the GI tract. Distributed primarily to the liver. Metabolic fate unknown. Excreted in urine. **Half-life:** 7–9 hr.

USES

Control of nausea/vomiting.

PRECAUTIONS

CONTRAINDICATIONS: Hypersensitivity to benzocaine or similar local

---

anesthetics; use of parenteral form in children or suppositories in premature infants or neonates. **CAUTIONS:** Elderly, debilitated, dehydration, serum electrolyte imbalance, high fever.

⏳ **LIFESPAN CONSIDERATIONS: Pregnancy/Lactation:** Unknown if drug crosses placenta or is distributed in breast milk. **Pregnancy Category C. Children/Elderly:** No age-related precautions noted. Avoid parenteral form in children and suppositories in neonates.

INTERACTIONS

DRUG: CNS depressants: May increase CNS depression. **HERBAL:** None known. **FOOD:** None known. **LAB VALUES:** None known.

AVAILABILITY (Rx)

CAPSULES (TIGAN): 250 mg, 300 mg. **INJECTION (BENZACOT, TIGAN):** 100 mg/ml. **SUPPOSITORIES:** 100 mg (Benzocaine-Trimethobenzamide Pediatric, Navogan, Tebamide, Tebamide Pediatric, Tigan Pediatric), 200 mg (Benzocaine-Trimethobenzamide Adult, Tebamide, Tigan Adult, Tigan Pediatric).

ADMINISTRATION/HANDLING

IM
• Give deep IM into large muscle mass.

PO
• Give without regard to meals. • Do not crush, break capsules.

RECTAL
• If suppository is too soft, chill for 30 min in refrigerator or run cold water over foil wrapper. • Moisten suppository with cold water before inserting well into rectum.

INDICATIONS/ROUTES/DOSAGE

NAUSEA AND VOMITING
PO: ADULTS, ELDERLY: 300 mg 3–4 times a day. CHILDREN WEIGHING 30–100 LB: 100–200 mg 3–4 times a day.
IM: ADULTS, ELDERLY: 200 mg 3–4 times a day.

RECTAL: ADULTS, ELDERLY: 200 mg 3–4 times a day. CHILDREN WEIGHING 30–100 LB: 100–200 mg 3–4 times a day. CHILDREN WEIGHING LESS THAN 30 LB: 100 mg 3–4 times a day.

SIDE EFFECTS

FREQUENT: Somnolence. **OCCASIONAL:** Blurred vision, diarrhea, dizziness, headache, muscle cramps. **RARE:** Rash, seizures, depression, opisthotonos, parkinsonian syndrome, Reye's syndrome (marked by vomiting, seizures).

ADVERSE REACTIONS/ TOXIC EFFECTS

A hypersensitivity reaction, manifested as extrapyramidal symptoms (EPS) such as muscle rigidity and allergic skin reactions, occurs rarely. Children may experience paradoxical reactions, marked by restlessness, insomnia, euphoria, nervousness, and tremor. Overdose may produce CNS depression (manifested as sedation, apnea, cardiovascular collapse, and death) or severe paradoxical reactions (such as hallucinations, tremor, and seizures).

NURSING CONSIDERATIONS

BASELINE ASSESSMENT
Assess for dehydration if excessive vomiting occurs.

INTERVENTION/EVALUATION
Check BP, especially in elderly (increased risk of hypotension). Assess children closely for paradoxical reaction. Monitor serum electrolytes in those with severe vomiting. Measure I&O and assess any vomitus. Assess skin turgor, mucous membranes to evaluate hydration status. Assess for EPS (hypersensitivity).

PATIENT/FAMILY TEACHING
• Causes drowsiness. • Avoid tasks that require alertness, motor skills until response to drug is established.

T

- Report visual disturbances, headache.
- Relief from nausea and vomiting generally occurs within 30 min of drug administration. • Inform physician if restlessness, involuntary muscle movements occur.

trimethoprim

trye-**meth**-oh-prim
(Apo-Tremethoprim ✤, Primsol, Proloprim, Trimpex)

FIXED-COMBINATION(S)

Bactrim, Septra: trimethoprim/sulfamethoxazole (a sulfonamide): 16 mg/80 mg/ml (injection); 40 mg/200 mg/5 ml (suspension); 80 mg/400 mg; 160 mg/800 mg (tablets).

CLASSIFICATION

PHARMACOTHERAPEUTIC: Folate antagonist. **CLINICAL:** Urinary tract agent, antibacterial.

ACTION

A folate antagonist that blocks bacterial biosynthesis of nucleic acids and proteins by interfering with the metabolism of folinic acid. **Therapeutic Effect:** Bacteriostatic.

PHARMACOKINETICS

Rapidly and completely absorbed from the GI tract. Protein binding: 42%–46%. Widely distributed, including to CSF. Metabolized in the liver. Primarily excreted in urine. Moderately removed by hemodialysis. **Half-life:** 8–10 hr (increased in impaired renal function and newborns; decreased in children).

USES

Treatment of initial acute uncomplicated UTI. **OFF-LABEL:** Prevention of bacterial UTIs, treatment of pneumonia caused by *Pneumocystis carinii*.

PRECAUTIONS

CONTRAINDICATIONS: Infants younger than 2 mo, megaloblastic anemia due to folic acid deficiency. **CAUTIONS:** Renal or hepatic impairment, patients with folic acid deficiency.

⏳ **LIFESPAN CONSIDERATIONS: Pregnancy/Lactation:** Drug readily crosses placenta; is distributed in breast milk. **Pregnancy Category C. Children:** Safety and efficacy not established. **Elderly:** No age-related precautions noted. May increase incidence of thrombocytopenia.

INTERACTIONS

DRUG: Folate antagonists (including methotrexate): May increase the risk of megaloblastic anemia. **HERBAL:** None known. **FOOD:** None known. **LAB VALUES:** May increase BUN and serum bilirubin, creatinine, AST, and ALT levels.

AVAILABILITY (Rx)

ORAL SOLUTION (PRIMSOL): 50 mg/5 ml. **TABLETS (TRIMPEX, PROLOPRIM):** 100 mg, 200 mg.

ADMINISTRATION/HANDLING

PO
• Space doses evenly to maintain constant level in urine. • Give without regard to meals (if stomach upset occurs, give with food).

INDICATIONS/ROUTES/DOSAGE

ACUTE, UNCOMPLICATED UTI
PO: ADULTS, ELDERLY, CHILDREN 12 YR AND OLDER: 100 mg q12h or 200 mg once a day for 10 days. CHILDREN YOUNGER THAN 12 YR: 4–6 mg/kg/day in 2 divided doses for 10 days.

DOSAGE IN RENAL IMPAIRMENT
Dosage and frequency are modified based on creatinine clearance.

Creatinine Clearance	Dosage Interval
Greater than 30 ml/min	No change
15–29 ml/min	50 mg q12h

T

SIDE EFFECTS

OCCASIONAL: Nausea, vomiting, diarrhea, decreased appetite, abdominal cramps, headache. **RARE:** Hypersensitivity reaction (pruritus, rash), methemoglobinemia (bluish fingernails, lips, or skin; fever; pale skin; sore throat; unusual tiredness), photosensitivity.

ADVERSE REACTIONS/ TOXIC EFFECTS

Stevens-Johnson syndrome, erythema multiforme, exfoliative dermatitis, and anaphylaxis occur rarely. Hematologic toxicity (thrombocytopenia, neutropenia, leukopenia, megaloblastic anemia) is more likely to occur in elderly, debilitated, or alcoholic patients; in patients with impaired renal function; and in those receiving prolonged high dosage.

NURSING CONSIDERATIONS

BASELINE ASSESSMENT

Assess hematology baseline reports and serum renal function tests.

INTERVENTION/EVALUATION

Assess skin for rash. Evaluate food tolerance. Monitor serum hematology reports, renal and liver function test results. Check for developing signs of hematologic toxicity: pallor, fever, sore throat, malaise, bleeding, ecchymoses.

PATIENT/FAMILY TEACHING

• Space doses evenly. • Complete full length of therapy (10–14 days). • May take on empty stomach or with food if stomach upset occurs. • Avoid sun, ultraviolet light; use sunscreen, wear protective clothing. • Immediately report pallor, fatigue, sore throat, bleeding, bruising or discoloration of skin, fever, rash to physician.

trimetrexate glucuronate

try-meh-**trex**-ate

(Neutrexin)

Do not confuse Neutrexin with Neurontin.

CLASSIFICATION

PHARMACOTHERAPEUTIC: Folate antagonist. **CLINICAL:** Anti-infective.

ACTION

Inhibits the enzyme dihydrofolate reductase (DHFR). **Therapeutic Effect:** Disrupts purine, DNA, RNA, protein synthesis, with consequent cell death.

USES

Alternative therapy with concurrent leucovorin administration for treatment of moderate to severe *Pneumocystis carinii* pneumonia (PCP) in immunocompromised patients, including patients with AIDS, who are intolerant of, or are refractory to, trimethoprim-sulfamethoxazole (TMP-SMZ) therapy or for whom TMP-SMZ is contraindicated. **OFF-LABEL:** Treatment of non–small cell lung, prostate, colorectal cancer, head and neck cancer, pancreatic adenocarcinoma.

PRECAUTIONS

CONTRAINDICATIONS: Clinically significant hypersensitivity to trimetrexate, leucovorin, methotrexate. **CAUTIONS:** Fertility impairment, patients with hematologic, renal, hepatic impairment. **Pregnancy Category D.**

INTERACTIONS

DRUG: Acetaminophen, erythromycin, rifampin, rifabutin, ketoconazole, fluconazole: May alter trimetrexate plasma concentration. **Cimetidine:** Reduces trimetrexate metabolism. **Clotrimazole, ketoconazole, miconazole:** May inhibit trimetrexate metabolism. **HERBAL:** None known. **FOOD:** None known. **LAB VALUES:** May increase AST, ALT, BUN, alkaline phosphatase, bilirubin, serum creatinine. May decrease Hgb, Hct, leukocyte, platelet counts.

AVAILABILITY (Rx)

POWDER FOR INJECTION: 25 mg, 200 mg.

ADMINISTRATION/HANDLING

 IV

◄ **ALERT** ► If solution comes in contact with skin/mucosa, wash with soap/water immediately. Use proper cytotoxic disposal technique. Do not reconstitute with solution containing either chloride ion or leucovorin, because precipitate occurs instantly.

Reconstitution • Reconstitute each 25-mg vial with 2 ml D_5W or sterile water for injection to provide concentration of 12.5 mg/ml. • Complete dissolution should occur within 30 sec. • Filter the reconstituted solution before further dilution. • Further dilute with D_5W to yield a final concentration of 0.25–2 mg/ml.

Rate of administration • Give diluted solution by IV infusion over 60–90 min. • Flush IV line thoroughly with at least 10 ml D_5W before and after administering trimetrexate.

Storage • Store vials for parenteral use at room temperature. • After reconstitution, solution is stable for up to 24 hr. • Reconstituted solution appears as pale greenish yellow. • Inspect for particulate matter. Discard if cloudiness or precipitate is present. • Do not freeze reconstituted solution. Discard unused portion after 24 hr.

▩ IV INCOMPATIBILITIES

Foscarnet (Foscavir), indomethacin (Indocin).

INDICATIONS/ROUTES/DOSAGE

◄ **ALERT** ► Even though trimetrexate and leucovorin are given concurrently, they must be administered separately or precipitate will occur; flush IV line thoroughly with 10 ml D_5W between infusions. Dilute leucovorin according to leucovorin instructions and give over 5–10 min q6h.

PCP

IV INFUSION: ADULTS: **(Trimetrexate):** 45 mg/m² once a day over 60–90 min. **(Leucovorin):** 20 mg/m² over 5–10 min q6h for total daily dose of 80 mg/m², or orally as 4 doses of 20 mg/m² spaced equally throughout the day. Round up the oral dose to the next higher 25-mg increment. **Recommended course of therapy:** 21 days trimetrexate, 24 days leucovorin.

◄ **ALERT** ► In event of hematologic, renal, hepatic toxicities, doses of trimetrexate and leucovorin should be modified.

SIDE EFFECTS

OCCASIONAL (8%–2%): Fever, rash, pruritus, nausea, vomiting, confusion. **RARE (less than 2%):** Fatigue.

ADVERSE REACTIONS/ TOXIC EFFECTS

Trimetrexate given without concurrent leucovorin may result in serious or fatal hematologic, hepatic, renal complications, including bone marrow suppression, oral/GI mucosal ulceration, renal/hepatic dysfunction. In event of overdose, stop trimetrexate and give leucovorin 40 mg/m² q6h for 3 days. Anaphylaxis occurs rarely.

NURSING CONSIDERATIONS

BASELINE ASSESSMENT

Leucovorin therapy must extend for 72 hr past the last dose of trimetrexate. CBC, serum liver and renal function tests should be performed twice a wk during

T

therapy. To allow for full therapeutic effect of trimetrexate to occur, zidovudine treatment should be discontinued during trimetrexate therapy.

INTERVENTION/EVALUATION

Closely monitor neutrophil count, platelet count, serum liver/renal function tests for development of serious toxicities. Carefully assess/treat patients with nephrotoxic, myelosuppressive, or hepatotoxic drugs given during trimetrexate therapy.

PATIENT/FAMILY TEACHING

• Use two forms of contraception during therapy (Pregnancy Category D). • Avoid persons with infections. • Immediately contact physician if fever, chills, cough, hoarseness, lower back or side pain, painful urination occurs. • Report any unusual bruising/bleeding, black tarry stools, blood in urine or stools, pinpoint red rash on skin.

triptorelin pamoate

trip-toe-**ree**-linn
(Trelstar Depot, Trelstar LA)

◆ CLASSIFICATION

PHARMACOTHERAPEUTIC: Gonadotropin-releasing hormone analogue. **CLINICAL:** Antineoplastic.

ACTION

A gonadotropin-releasing hormone (GnRH) analogue and antineoplastic agent that inhibits gonadotropin hormone secretion through a negative feedback mechanism. Circulating levels of luteinizing hormone, follicle-stimulating hormone, testosterone, and estradiol rise initially, then subside with continued therapy. **Therapeutic Effect:** Suppresses growth of abnormal prostate tissue.

USES

Treatment of advanced prostate cancer. **OFF-LABEL:** Treatment of endometriosis, growth hormone deficiency, hyperandrogenism, ovarian, pancreatic carcinomas, precocious puberty, uterine leiomyomata.

PRECAUTIONS

CONTRAINDICATIONS: Hypersensitivity to luteinizing hormone-releasing hormone (LHRH) or LHRH agonists, pregnancy. **CAUTIONS:** None known.

⧗ **LIFESPAN CONSIDERATIONS: Pregnancy/Lactation:** Unknown if distributed is breast milk. **Pregnancy Category X. Children:** Safety and efficacy not established. **Elderly:** No age-related precautions noted.

INTERACTIONS

DRUG: Hyperprolactinemic drugs: Reduce the number of pituitary GnRH receptors. **HERBAL:** None known. **FOOD:** None known. **LAB VALUES:** May alter serum pituitary-gonadal function test results. May cause transient increase in serum testosterone levels, usually during first week of treatment.

AVAILABILITY (Rx)

POWDER FOR INJECTION (TRELSTAR DEPOT): 3.75 mg. **POWDER FOR INJECTION (TRELSTAR LA):** 11.25 mg.

INDICATIONS/ROUTES/DOSAGE

PROSTATE CANCER

IM (TRELSTAR DEPOT): ADULTS, ELDERLY: 3.75 mg once q28days.
IM (TRELSTAR LA): ADULTS, ELDERLY: 11.25 mg q84days.

SIDE EFFECTS

FREQUENT (greater than 5%): Hot flashes, skeletal pain, headache, impotence. **OCCASIONAL (5%–2%):** Insomnia, vomiting, leg pain, fatigue. **RARE (less than 2%):** Dizziness, emotional lability, diarrhea, urine retention, UTIs, anemia, pruritus.

ADVERSE REACTIONS/ TOXIC EFFECTS

Bladder outlet obstruction, skeletal pain, hematuria, and spinal cord compression (with weakness or paralysis of the lower extremities) may occur.

NURSING CONSIDERATIONS

INTERVENTION/EVALUATION

Obtain serum testosterone, prostate-specific antigen (PSA), prostatic acid phosphatase (PAP) levels periodically during therapy. Serum testosterone, PAP levels should increase during first week of therapy. Testosterone level then should decrease to baseline level or less within 2 wk, PAP level within 4 wk. Monitor patient closely for worsening signs and symptoms of prostatic cancer, especially during first week of therapy (due to transient increase in testosterone).

PATIENT/FAMILY TEACHING

• Do not miss monthly injections. • May experience increased skeletal pain, blood in urine, urinary retention initially (subsides within 1 wk). • Hot flashes may occur. • Inform physician if tachycardia, persistent nausea or vomiting, numbness of arms or legs, pain or swelling of breasts, difficulty breathing, infection at injection site occurs.

Trizivir, *see abacavir and lamivudine and zidovudine*

---

trospium chloride

trow-spee-um
(Sanctura)

CLASSIFICATION

PHARMACOTHERAPEUTIC: Anticholinergic. **CLINICAL:** Antispasmotic.

ACTION

An anticholinergic that antagonizes the effect of acetylcholine on muscarinic receptors, producing parasympatholytic action. **Therapeutic Effect:** Reduces smooth muscle tone in the bladder.

PHARMACOKINETICS

Minimally absorbed after PO administration. Protein binding: 50%–85%. Distributed in plasma. Excreted mainly in feces and, to a lesser extent, in urine. **Half-life:** 20 hr.

USES

Treatment of overactive bladder with symptoms of urge urinary incontinence, urgency, urinary frequency.

PRECAUTIONS

CONTRAINDICATIONS: Decreased GI motility, gastric retention, uncontrolled angle-closure glaucoma, urine retention. **CAUTIONS:** Renal or hepatic impairment, obstructive GI disorders, ulcerative colitis, intestinal atony, myasthenia gravis, narrow-angle glaucoma, significant bladder obstruction.

⧖ **LIFESPAN CONSIDERATIONS: Pregnancy/Lactation:** Unknown if drug crosses placenta or is distributed in breast milk. **Pregnancy Category C. Children:** Safety and efficacy not established. **Elderly:** Higher incidence of dry mouth, constipation, dyspepsia, UTI, urinary retention in those 75 yr and older.

INTERACTIONS

DRUG: Other anticholinergic agents: Increases the severity and frequency of side effects and may alter the absorption of other drugs because of anticholinergic effects on GI motility. **Digoxin, metformin, morphine, pancuronium, procainamide, tenofovir, vancomycin:** May increase trospium blood concentration. **HERBAL:** None known. **FOOD: High-fat meals:** May reduce trospium absorption. **LAB VALUES:** None known.

AVAILABILITY (Rx)

TABLETS: 20 mg.

ADMINISTRATION/HANDLING

PO
• Store at room temperature. • Do not break or crush glossy-coated tablets. • Give at least 1 hr before meals or on an empty stomach.

INDICATIONS/ROUTES/DOSAGE

OVERACTIVE BLADDER
PO: ADULTS: 20 mg twice a day. ELDERLY (75 YR AND OLDER): Titrate dosage down to 20 mg once a day, based on tolerance.

DOSAGE IN RENAL IMPAIRMENT
For patients with creatinine clearance less than 30 ml/min, dosage reduced to 20 mg once a day at bedtime.

SIDE EFFECTS

FREQUENT (20%): Dry mouth. **OCCASIONAL (10%–4%):** Constipation, headache. **RARE (less than 2%):** Fatigue, upper abdominal pain, dyspepsia, flatulence, dry eyes, urine retention.

ADVERSE REACTIONS/ TOXIC EFFECTS

Overdose may result in severe anticholinergic effects, such as abdominal pain, nausea and vomiting, confusion, depression, diaphoresis, facial flushing, hypertension, hypotension, respiratory depression, irritability, lacrimation, nervousness, and restlessness. Supraventricular tachycardia and hallucinations occur rarely.

NURSING CONSIDERATIONS

BASELINE ASSESSMENT
Assess dysuria, urgency, frequency, incontinence.

INTERVENTION/EVALUATION
Monitor for symptomatic relief. Monitor I&O; palpate bladder for retention. Monitor pattern of bowel activity and stool consistency. Dry mouth may be relieved by sips of tepid water.

PATIENT/FAMILY TEACHING
• Report nausea, vomiting, diaphoresis, increased salivary secretions, palpitations, severe abdominal pain.

tubocurarine chloride

(Tubarine)
See Neuromuscular blockers (p. 112C)

Tygacil, *see tigecycline*

Ultracet, *see acetaminphen and tramadol*

Ultram, *see tramadol*

Unasyn, *see ampicillin/ sulbactam sodium*

valacyclovir

val-a-**sye**-kloe-ver
(Valtrex)

◆CLASSIFICATION
PHARMACOTHERAPEUTIC: Antiviral. **CLINICAL:** Antiherpetic agent (see p. 62C).

ACTION
A virustatic antiviral that is converted to acyclovir triphosphate, becoming part of the viral DNA chain. **Therapeutic Effect:** Interferes with DNA synthesis and replication of herpes simplex virus and varicella-zoster virus.

PHARMACOKINETICS
Rapidly absorbed after PO administration. Protein binding: 13%–18%. Rapidly converted by hydrolysis to the active compound acyclovir. Widely distributed to tissues and body fluids (including cerebrospinal fluid [CSF]). Primarily eliminated in urine. Removed by hemodialysis. **Half-life:** 2.5–3.3 hr (increased in impaired renal function).

USES
Treatment of herpes zoster (shingles) in immunocompetent adults. Episodic treatment of recurrent genital herpes in immunocompetent adults. Prevention of recurrent genital herpes. Treatment of initial genital herpes. Treatment of cold sores. **OFF-LABEL:** To reduce the risk of heterosexual transmission of genital herpes.

PRECAUTIONS
CONTRAINDICATIONS: Hypersensitivity to or intolerance of acyclovir, valacyclovir, or their components. **CAUTIONS:** Bone marrow or renal transplantation, advanced HIV infections, renal or hepatic impairment, dehydration, fluid or electrolyte imbalance, concurrent use of nephrotoxic agents, neurologic abnormalities.

⌛ **LIFESPAN CONSIDERATIONS: Pregnancy/Lactation:** May cross placenta. May be distributed in breast milk. **Pregnancy Category B. Children:** Safety and efficacy not established. **Elderly:** Age-related renal impairment may require dosage adjustment.

INTERACTIONS
DRUG: Cimetidine, probenecid: May increase acyclovir blood concentration. **HERBAL:** None known. **FOOD:** None known. **LAB VALUES:** None known.

AVAILABILITY (Rx)
CAPLETS: 500 mg, 1,000 mg.

ADMINISTRATION/HANDLING
PO
• Give without regard to meals. • Do not crush, break caplets.

INDICATIONS/ROUTES/DOSAGE
HERPES ZOSTER (SHINGLES)
PO: ADULTS, ELDERLY: 1 g 3 times a day for 7 days.

HERPES SIMPLEX (COLD SORES)
PO: ADULTS, ELDERLY: 2 g twice a day for 1 day.

V

INITIAL EPISODE OF GENITAL HERPES

PO: ADULTS, ELDERLY: 1 g twice a day for 10 days.

RECURRENT EPISODES OF GENITAL HERPES

PO: ADULTS, ELDERLY: 500 mg twice a day for 3 days.

PREVENTION OF GENITAL HERPES

PO: ADULTS, ELDERLY: 500–1,000 mg/day.

DOSAGE IN RENAL IMPAIRMENT

Dosage and frequency are modified based on creatinine clearance.

Creatinine Clearance	Herpes Zoster	Genital Herpes
50 ml/min or higher	1 g q8h	500 mg q12h
30–49 ml/min	1 g q12h	500 mg q12h
10–29 ml/min	1 g q24h	500 mg q24h
Less than 10 ml/min	500 mg q24h	500 mg q24h

SIDE EFFECTS

FREQUENT: Herpes zoster (17%–10%): Nausea, headache. **Genital herpes (17%):** Headache. **OCCASIONAL: Herpes zoster (7%–3%):** Vomiting, diarrhea, constipation (50 yr or older), asthenia, dizziness (50 yr and older). **Genital herpes (8%–3%):** Nausea, diarrhea, dizziness. **RARE: Herpes zoster (3%–1%):** Abdominal pain, anorexia. **Genital herpes (3%–1%):** Asthenia, abdominal pain.

ADVERSE REACTIONS/ TOXIC EFFECTS

Thrombotic thrombocytopenic purpura/ hemolytic uremic syndrome (TTP/HUS) has occurred in patients with advanced HIV disease and also in allogenic bone marrow transplant and renal transplant recipients taking valacyclovir at doses of 8 g/day.

NURSING CONSIDERATIONS

BASELINE ASSESSMENT

Question for history of allergies, particularly to valacyclovir, acyclovir. Tissue cultures for herpes zoster, herpes simplex should be done before giving first dose (therapy may proceed before results are known). Assess medical history, especially advanced HIV infection, bone marrow or renal transplantation, hepatic or renal impairment.

INTERVENTION/EVALUATION

Evaluate cutaneous lesions. Monitor serum renal and liver function tests, CBC, urinalysis. Manage herpes zoster with strict isolation. Provide analgesics, comfort measures for herpes zoster (especially exhausting to elderly). Encourage fluids. Keep patient's fingernails short, hands clean.

PATIENT/FAMILY TEACHING

• Drink adequate fluids. • Do not touch lesions with fingers to avoid spreading infection to new site. • **Genital Herpes:** Continue therapy for full length of treatment. • Space doses evenly. • Avoid sexual intercourse during duration of lesions to prevent infecting partner. • Valacyclovir does not cure herpes. • Notify physician if lesions recur or do not improve. • Pap smears should be done at least annually due to increased risk of cervical cancer in women with genital herpes. • Initiate treatment at first sign of a recurrent episode of genital herpes or herpes zoster (early treatment within first 24–48 hr is imperative for therapeutic results).

valerian

Also known as all-heal, amantilla, garden heliotrope, valeriana.

•CLASSIFICATION

HERBAL: See Appendix G.

ACTION

Appears to inhibit enzyme system responsible for catabolism of GABA, increasing GABA concentration and decreasing CNS activity. **Effect:** Produces sedative effects. Has anxiolytic, antidepressant, anticonvulsant effects.

USES

Used as a sedative for insomnia, sleeping disorders associated with anxiety, restlessness. Used for depression and attention deficit hyperactivity disorder (ADHD).

PRECAUTIONS

CONTRAINDICATIONS: Insufficient data on pregnancy or lactation (avoid use); hepatic disease. **CAUTIONS:** None known.

⌛ **LIFESPAN CONSIDERATIONS: Pregnancy/Lactation:** Contraindicated. **Children:** Safety and efficacy not established; avoid use. **Elderly:** No age-related precautions noted.

INTERACTIONS

DRUG: Alcohol, barbiturates, benzodiazepines: May cause additive effect, increase adverse effects. **HERBAL: Chamomile, ginseng, kava kava, melatonin, St. John's wort:** May enhance therapeutic effect/adverse effects. **FOOD:** None known. **LAB VALUES:** None known.

AVAILABILITY (OTC)

CAPSULES. TABLETS. EXTRACT. TEA. TINCTURE.

INDICATIONS/ROUTES/DOSAGE

SEDATION
PO: ADULTS, ELDERLY: (**Extract**): 400–900 mg ½–1 hr before bedtime or 1 cup tea taken several times a day.

SIDE EFFECTS

Headache, hangover, cardiac arrhythmias.

ADVERSE REACTIONS/ TOXIC EFFECTS

Difficulty walking, hypothermia, increased muscle relaxation, excitability, insomnia.

NURSING CONSIDERATIONS

BASELINE ASSESSMENT
Determine whether patient is using other CNS depressants, especially benzodiazepine. Assess baseline serum hepatic function.

valganciclovir hydrochloride

val-gan-**sye**-kloh-veer
(Valcyte)

◆ **CLASSIFICATION**
PHARMACOTHERAPEUTIC: Synthetic nucleoside. **CLINICAL:** Antiviral (see p. 62C).

ACTION

A synthetic nucleoside that competes with viral DNA esterases and is incorporated directly into growing viral DNA chains. **Therapeutic Effect:** Interferes with DNA synthesis and viral replication.

PHARMACOKINETICS

Well absorbed and rapidly converted to ganciclovir by intestinal and hepatic enzymes. Widely distributed. Slowly metabolized intracellularly. Primarily excreted unchanged in urine. Removed by hemodialysis. **Half-life:** 18 hr (increased in impaired renal function).

USES

Treatment of cytomegalovirus (CMV) retinitis in AIDS. Preventative treatment of CMV disease in high-risk, renal, cardiac transplant patients.

V

PRECAUTIONS

CONTRAINDICATIONS: Hypersensitivity to acyclovir or ganciclovir. **CAUTIONS:** Extreme caution in children because of long-term carcinogenicity, reproductive toxicity. Renal impairment, preexisting cytopenias, history of cytopenic reactions to other drugs; elderly (at greater risk of renal impairment).

⌛ **LIFESPAN CONSIDERATIONS: Pregnancy/Lactation:** Effective contraception should be used during therapy; valganciclovir should not be used during pregnancy. Avoid breast-feeding during therapy; may be resumed no sooner than 72 hr after the last dose of valganciclovir. **Pregnancy Category C. Children:** Safety and efficacy not established in those younger than 12 yr. **Elderly:** Age-related renal impairment may require dosage adjustment.

INTERACTIONS

DRUG: Amphotericin B, cyclosporine: May increase the risk of nephrotoxicity. **Bone marrow depressants:** May increase bone marrow depression. **Imipenem and cilastatin:** May increase the risk of seizures. **Probenecid:** Decreases renal clearance of valganciclovir. **Zidovudine (AZT):** May increase the risk of hematologic toxicity. **HERBAL: None** known. **FOOD: All foods:** Maximize drug bioavailability. **LAB VALUES: May** decrease blood Hct and Hgb levels, serum creatinine level, platelet count, and WBC count.

AVAILABILITY (Rx)

TABLETS: 450 mg.

ADMINISTRATION/HANDLING

PO
• Do not break, crush tablets (potential carcinogen). • Avoid contact to skin. • Wash skin with soap and water if contact occurs. • Give with food.

INDICATIONS/ROUTES/DOSAGE

CYTOMEGALOVIRUS (CMV) RETINITIS IN PATIENTS WITH NORMAL RENAL FUNCTION
PO: ADULTS: Initially, 900 mg (two 450-mg tablets) twice a day for 21 days. Maintenance: 900 mg once a day.

PREVENTION OF CMV AFTER TRANSPLANT
PO: ADULTS, ELDERLY: 900 mg once a day beginning within 10 days of transplant and continuing until 100 days post-transplant.

DOSAGE IN RENAL IMPAIRMENT
Dosage and frequency are modified based on creatinine clearance.

Creatinine Clearance	Induction Dosage	Maintenance Dosage
60 ml/min or higher	900 mg twice a day	900 mg once a day
40–59 ml/min	450 mg twice a day	450 mg once a day
25–39 ml/min	450 mg once a day	450 mg every 2 days
10–24 ml/min	450 mg every 2 days	450 mg twice a wk

SIDE EFFECTS

FREQUENT (16%–9%): Diarrhea, neutropenia, headache. **OCCASIONAL (8%–3%):** Nausea, anemia, thrombocytopenia. **RARE (less than 3%):** Insomnia, paraesthesia, vomiting, abdominal pain, fever.

ADVERSE REACTIONS/ TOXIC EFFECTS

Hematologic toxicity, including severe neutropenia (most common), anemia, and thrombocytopenia, may occur. Retinal detachment occurs rarely. An overdose may result in renal toxicity. Valganciclovir may decrease sperm production and fertility.

🖊see color pill atlas   🌿herb   underlined – top prescribed drug

NURSING CONSIDERATIONS

BASELINE ASSESSMENT

Evaluate hematologic, serum chemistry baselines, serum creatinine.

INTERVENTION/EVALUATION

Monitor I&O, ensure adequate hydration (minimum 1,500 ml/24 hr). Diligently evaluate CBC for decreased WBCs, Hgb, Hct, decreased platelets. Question patient regarding vision, therapeutic improvement, complications.

PATIENT/FAMILY TEACHING

• Valganciclovir provides suppression, not cure, of CMV retinitis. • Frequent blood tests are necessary during therapy because of toxic nature of drug. • Ophthalmologic exam q4–6wk during treatment is advised. • It is essential to report any new symptom promptly. • May temporarily or permanently inhibit sperm production in men, suppress fertility in women. • Barrier contraception should be used during and for 90 days after therapy because of mutagenic potential.

---

valproic acid

val-**pro**-ick
(Depakene)

valproate sodium

(Depakene syrup)

divalproex sodium

(Depacon, Depakote, Depakote ER, Depakote Sprinkle)

◆ CLASSIFICATION

CLINICAL: Anticonvulsant, antimanic, antimigraine (see p. 35C).

ACTION

An anticonvulsant, antimanic, and antimigraine agent that directly increases concentration of the inhibitory neurotransmitter gamma-aminobutyric acid. **Therapeutic Effect:** Reduces seizure activity.

PHARMACOKINETICS

Well absorbed from the GI tract. Protein binding: 80%–90%. Metabolized in the liver. Primarily excreted in urine. Not removed by hemodialysis. **Half-life:** 6–16 hr (may be increased in hepatic impairment, the elderly, and children younger than 18 mo).

USES

Prophylaxis of absence seizures (petit mal), myoclonic, tonic-clonic seizure control. Used principally as adjunct with other anticonvulsant agents. Treatment of manic episodes with bipolar disorders, complex partial seizures. Prophylaxis of migraine headaches. **OFF-LABEL:** Prevention of migraine; treatment of behavior disorders in Alzheimer's disease; bipolar disorder; chorea, myoclonic, simple partial, and tonic-clonic seizures; organic brain syndrome; schizophrenia; status epilepticus; tardive dyskinesia.

PRECAUTIONS

CONTRAINDICATIONS: Active hepatic disease, urea cycle disorders. **CAUTIONS:** History of hepatic disease, bleeding abnormalities.

⧗ **LIFESPAN CONSIDERATIONS: Pregnancy/Lactation:** Drug crosses placenta; is distributed in breast milk. **Pregnancy Category D. Children:** Increased risk of hepatotoxicity in those younger than 2 yr. **Elderly:** No age-related precautions, but lower dosages recommended.

V

INTERACTIONS

DRUG: **Alcohol, other CNS depressants:** May increase CNS depressant effects. **Amitriptyline, primidone:** May increase the blood concentration of these drugs. **Anticoagulants, heparin, platelet aggregation inhibitors, thrombolytics:** May increase the risk of bleeding. **Carbamazepine:** May decrease valproic acid blood concentration. **Hepatotoxic medications:** May increase the risk of hepatotoxicity. **Phenytoin:** May increase the risk of phenytoin toxicity and decrease the effects of valproic acid. HERBAL: None known. FOOD: None known. LAB VALUES: May increase serum LDH, bilirubin, AST, and ALT levels. Therapeutic serum level is 50–100 mcg/ml; toxic serum level is greater than 100 mcg/ml.

AVAILABILITY (Rx)

CAPSULES (DEPAKENE): 250 mg. **SYRUP (DEPAKENE):** 250 mg/5 ml. **TABLETS (DELAYED-RELEASE [DEPAKOTE]):** 125 mg, 250 mg, 500 mg. **TABLETS (EXTENDED-RELEASE [DEPAKOTE ER]):** 250 mg, 500 mg. **CAPSULES SPRINKLES (DEPAKOTE SPRINKLE):** 125 mg. **INJECTION (DEPACON):** 100 mg/ml.

ADMINISTRATION/HANDLING
🖐 IV

Reconstitution • Dilute each single dose with at least 50 ml D$_5$W, 0.9% NaCl, or lactated Ringer's.

Rate of administration • Infuse over 5–10 min. • Do not exceed rate of 3 mg/kg/min (5-min infusion) or 1.5 mg/kg/min (10-min infusion). Too rapid infusion increases side effects.

Storage • Store vials at room temperature. • Diluted solutions stable for 24 hr. • Discard unused portion.

PO
• May give with or without regard to food. Do not administer with carbonated drinks. • May sprinkle capsule contents on applesauce and give immediately (do not break, crush sprinkle beads). • Delayed-release and extended-release tablets to be given whole.

🔲 IV INCOMPATIBILITIES
Do not mix valproic acid with any other medications.

INDICATIONS/ROUTES/DOSAGE
SEIZURES
PO: ADULTS, ELDERLY, CHILDREN 10 YR AND OLDER: Initially, 10–15 mg/kg/day in 1–3 divided doses. May increase by 5–10 mg/kg/day at weekly intervals up to 30–60 mg/kg/day. Usual adult dosage: 1,000–2,500 mg/day.
IV: ADULTS, ELDERLY, CHILDREN: Same as oral dose but given q6h.

MANIC EPISODES
PO: ADULTS, ELDERLY: Initially, 750 mg/day in divided doses. **Maximum:** 60 mg/kg/day.

PREVENTION OF MIGRAINE HEADACHES
PO (EXTENDED-RELEASE): ADULTS, ELDERLY: Initially, 500 mg/day for 7 days. May increase up to 1,000 mg/day.
PO (DELAYED-RELEASE): ADULTS, ELDERLY: Initially, 250 mg twice a day. May increase up to 1,000 mg/day.

SIDE EFFECTS
FREQUENT: Epilepsy: Abdominal pain, irregular menses, diarrhea, transient alopecia, indigestion, nausea, vomiting, tremors, weight gain or loss. **Mania (22%–19%):** Nausea, somnolence. **OCCASIONAL: Epilepsy:** Constipation, dizziness, drowsiness, headache, skin rash, unusual excitement, restlessness. **Mania (12%–6%):** Asthenia, abdominal pain, dyspepsia (heartburn, indigestion, epigastric distress), rash. **RARE: Epilepsy:** Mood changes, diplopia, nystagmus, spots before eyes, unusual bleeding or ecchymosis.

ADVERSE REACTIONS/ TOXIC EFFECTS

Blood dyscrasias may occur.

◀ ALERT ▶ Hepatotoxicity may occur, particularly in the first 6 mo of valproic acid therapy. It may be preceded by loss of seizure control, malaise, weakness, lethargy, anorexia, and vomiting rather than abnormal serum liver function test results.

NURSING CONSIDERATIONS

BASELINE ASSESSMENT

Anticonvulsant: Review history of seizure disorder (intensity, frequency, duration, level of consciousness [LOC]). Initiate safety measures, quiet dark environment. CBC, platelet count should be performed before and 2 wk after therapy begins, then 2 wk following maintenance dose. **Antimanic:** Assess behavior, appearance, emotional status, response to environment, speech pattern, thought content. **Antimigraine:** Question patient regarding onset, location, duration of migraine, possible precipitating symptoms.

INTERVENTION/EVALUATION

Monitor serum liver function tests, bilirubin, ammonia, CBC, platelets. **Anticonvulsant:** Observe frequently for recurrence of seizure activity. Monitor serum liver function tests, CBC, platelet count. Assess skin for ecchymoses, petechiae. Monitor for clinical improvement (decrease in intensity/ frequency of seizures). **Antimanic:** Assess for therapeutic response (interest in surroundings, increased ability to concentrate, relaxed facial expression). **Antimigraine:** Evaluate for relief of migraine headache and resulting photophobia, phonophobia, nausea, vomiting. Therapeutic serum level: 50–100 mcg/ml; toxic serum level: over 100 mcg/ml.

PATIENT/FAMILY TEACHING

• Do not abruptly withdraw medication after long-term use (may precipitate seizures). • Strict maintenance of drug therapy is essential for seizure control. • Drowsiness usually disappears during continued therapy. • Avoid tasks that require alertness, motor skills until response to drug is established. • Avoid alcohol. • Carry identification card or bracelet to note anticonvulsant therapy. • Inform physician if nausea, vomiting, lethargy, altered mental status, weakness, loss of appetite, abdominal pain, yellowing of skin, unusual bruising or bleeding occurs.

valrubicin

val-**rue**-bih-sin

(VaHaxan ✧, Valstar, Valtaxin ✧)

Do not confuse valrubicin with valsartan.

CLASSIFICATION

PHARMACOTHERAPEUTIC: Anthracycline antibiotic. **CLINICAL:** Antineoplastic (see p. 79C).

ACTION

An anthracycline antibiotic that inhibits incorporation of nucleosides into nucleic acids after penetrating cells. Therapeutic Effect: Causes chromosomal damage, arresting cells in the G_2 phase of cell division, and interferes with DNA synthesis.

USES

Intravesical therapy of BCG-refractory carcinoma in situ of urinary bladder in patients for whom cystectomy is unacceptable.

PRECAUTIONS

CONTRAINDICATIONS: Perforated bladder, sensitivity to valrubicin, severe

irritated bladder, small bladder capacity, UTI. **CAUTIONS:** None known.

⏳ **LIFESPAN CONSIDERATIONS: Pregnancy/Lactation:** Unknown if drug crosses placenta; breast-feeding not recommended. **Pregnancy Category C. Children:** Safety and efficacy not established. **Elderly:** No age-related precautions noted.

INTERACTIONS

DRUG: None known. **HERBAL:** None known. **FOOD:** None known. **LAB VALUES:** May increase serum glucose levels.

AVAILABILITY (Rx)

SOLUTION FOR INTRAVESICAL INSTILLATION: 40 mg/ml.

INDICATIONS/ROUTES/DOSAGE

BLADDER CANCER
INTRAVESICAL: ADULTS, ELDERLY: 800 mg once weekly for 6 wk.

SIDE EFFECTS

FREQUENT: Local intravesical reaction (10%): Local bladder symptoms, urinary frequency or urgency, dysuria, hematuria, bladder pain, cystitis, bladder spasms. **Systemic (15%–5%):** Abdominal pain, nausea, UTI. **OCCASIONAL: Local intravesical reaction (less than 10%):** Nocturia, local burning, urethral pain, pelvic pain, gross hematuria. **Systemic (5%–2%):** Diarrhea, vomiting, urine retention, microscopic hematuria, asthenia, headache, malaise, back pain, chest pain, dizziness, rash, anemia, fever, vasodilation. **RARE: Systemic (1%):** Flatus, peripheral edema, hyperglycemia, pneumonia, myalgia.

NURSING CONSIDERATIONS

BASELINE ASSESSMENT

Assess if patient is sensitive to valrubicin, is pregnant or breast-feeding (not recommended). Assess other medications, conditions (see Contraindications).

---

valsartan

val-**sar**-tan
(Diovan)

Do not confuse valsartan with Valstan.

FIXED-COMBINATION(S)

Diovan HCT: valsartan/hydrochlorothiazide (a diuretic): 80 mg/12.5 mg; 160 mg/12.5 mg; 160 mg/25 mg.

◆CLASSIFICATION

PHARMACOTHERAPEUTIC: Angiotensin II receptor antagonist. **CLINICAL:** Antihypertensive (see p. 8C).

ACTION

An angiotensin II receptor, type AT_1, antagonist that blocks vasoconstrictor and aldosterone-secreting effects of angiotensin II, inhibiting the binding of angiotensin II to the AT_1 receptors. **Therapeutic Effect:** Causes vasodilation, decreases peripheral resistance, and decreases BP.

PHARMACOKINETICS

Poorly absorbed after PO administration. Food decreases peak plasma concentration. Protein binding: 95%. Metabolized in the liver. Recovered primarily in feces and, to a lesser extent, in urine. Unknown if removed by hemodialysis. **Half-life:** 6 hr.

USES

Treatment of hypertension alone or in combination with other antihypertensives. Treatment of heart failure. Reduce cardiovascular deaths in high risk patients (left ventricular failure, dysfunction) after heart attack. **OFF-LABEL:** Diabetic nephropathy.

PRECAUTIONS

CONTRAINDICATIONS: Bilateral renal artery stenosis, biliary cirrhosis or obstruction, hypoaldosteronism, severe hepatic impairment. **CAUTIONS:** Concurrent use of potassium-sparing diuretics or potassium supplements, mild to moderate hepatic impairment, CHF, unilateral renal artery stenosis, coronary artery disease.

⌛ LIFESPAN CONSIDERATIONS: **Pregnancy/Lactation:** May cause fetal harm. Unknown if distributed in breast milk. **Pregnancy Category C (D if used in second or third trimester). Children:** Safety and efficacy not established. **Elderly:** No age-related precautions noted.

INTERACTIONS

DRUG: **Diuretics:** Produce additive hypotensive effects. HERBAL: None known. FOOD: **All foods:** Decrease peak plasma concentration of valsartan. LAB VALUES: May increase AST, ALT, and serum bilirubin, creatinine, and potassium levels. May decrease blood Hgb and Hct levels.

AVAILABILITY (Rx)

TABLETS: 40 mg, 80 mg, 160 mg, 320 mg.

ADMINISTRATION/HANDLING

PO
• Give without regard to meals.

INDICATIONS/ROUTES/DOSAGE

HYPERTENSION
PO: ADULTS, ELDERLY: Initially, 80–160 mg/day in patients who are not volume depleted. May increase up to a **maximum:** 320 mg/day.

CHF
PO: ADULTS, ELDERLY: Initially, 40 mg twice a day. May increase up to 160 mg twice a day. **Maximum:** 320 mg/day.

POST HEART ATTACK
PO: ADULTS, ELDERLY: Initially, 20 mg twice a day. May increase within 7 days to 40 mg twice a day. May further increase up to target dose of 160 mg twice a day.

SIDE EFFECTS

RARE (2%–1%): Insomnia, fatigue, heartburn, abdominal pain, dizziness, headache, diarrhea, nausea, vomiting, arthralgia, edema.

ADVERSE REACTIONS/ TOXIC EFFECTS

Overdosage may manifest as hypotension and tachycardia. Bradycardia occurs less often. Viral infection and upper respiratory tract infection (cough, pharyngitis, sinusitis, rhinitis) occur rarely.

NURSING CONSIDERATIONS

BASELINE ASSESSMENT
Obtain BP, apical pulse immediately before each dose, in addition to regular monitoring (be alert to fluctuations). If excessive reduction in BP occurs, place patient in supine position, feet slightly elevated. Question for possibility of pregnancy. Assess medication history (especially diuretic). Question for history of hepatic or renal impairment, renal artery stenosis, history of severe CHF. Obtain BUN, AST, ALT, serum creatinine, alkaline phosphatase, bilirubin, Hgb, Hct.

INTERVENTION/EVALUATION
Maintain hydration (offer fluids frequently). Assess for evidence of upper respiratory infection. Monitor serum electrolytes, renal and liver function tests, urinalysis, BP, pulse. Observe for symptoms of hypotension.

PATIENT/FAMILY TEACHING
• Inform female patient regarding consequences of second- and third-trimester exposure to valsartan. • Report pregnancy to physician as soon as

V

possible. • Report any sign of infection (sore throat, fever). • Do not stop taking medication. • Caution against exercising during hot weather (risk of dehydration, hypotension).

Valtrex, *see valacyclovir*

Vancocin, *see vancomycin*

---

vancomycin hydrochloride

van-koe-**mye**-sin

(Lyphocin, <u>Vancocin</u>, Vancocin HCl Pulvules)

◆ **CLASSIFICATION**

CLINICAL: Tricyclic glycopeptide antibiotic.

ACTION

A tricyclic glycopeptide antibiotic that binds to bacterial cell walls, altering cell membrane permeability and inhibiting RNA synthesis. **Therapeutic Effect:** Bactericidal.

PHARMACOKINETICS

PO: Poorly absorbed from the GI tract. Primarily eliminated in feces. **Parenteral:** Widely distributed. Protein binding: 55%. Primarily excreted unchanged in urine. Not removed by hemodialysis. **Half-life:** 4–11 hr (increased in impaired renal function).

USES

Systemic: Treatment of infections caused by staphylococcal and streptococcal species. **PO:** Treatment of antibiotic colitis,

pseudomembranous colitis, antibiotic-associated diarrhea, staphylococcal enterocolitis. **OFF-LABEL:** Treatment of brain abscess, perioperative infections, staphylococcal or streptococcal meningitis.

PRECAUTIONS

CONTRAINDICATIONS: None known. **CAUTIONS:** Renal dysfunction, preexisting hearing impairment, concurrent therapy with other ototoxic or nephrotoxic medications.

⧗ **LIFESPAN CONSIDERATIONS: Pregnancy/Lactation:** Drug crosses placenta. Unknown if distributed in breast milk. **Pregnancy Category B. Children:** Close monitoring of serum levels recommended in premature neonates and young infants. **Elderly:** Age-related renal impairment may increase risk of ototoxicity and nephrotoxicity; dosage adjustment recommended.

INTERACTIONS

DRUG: Aminoglycosides, amphotericin B, aspirin, bumetanide, carmustine, cisplatin, cyclosporine, ethacrynic acid, furosemide, streptozocin: May increase the risk of ototoxicity and nephrotoxicity of parenteral vancomycin. **Cholestyramine, colestipol:** May decrease the effects of oral vancomycin. **HERBAL:** None known. **FOOD:** None known. **LAB VALUES:** May increase BUN level. Therapeutic peak serum level is 20–40 mcg/ml; therapeutic trough serum level is 5–15 mcg/ml. Toxic peak serum level is greater than 40 mcg/ml; toxic trough serum level is greater than 15 mcg/ml.

AVAILABILITY (Rx)

CAPSULES (VANCOCIN HCL PULVULES): 125 mg, 250 mg. **POWDER FOR ORAL SUSPENSION (VANCOCIN):** 1 g (provides 250 mg/5 ml after mixing). **POWDER FOR INJECTION (LYPHOCIN, VANCOCIN HCl):** 500 mg, 1 g, 5 g,

10 g. **INFUSION (PREMIX [VANCOCIN HCI]):** 500 mg/100 ml, 1 g/200 ml.

ADMINISTRATION/HANDLING

 IV

◀ **ALERT** ▶ Give by intermittent IV infusion (piggyback) or continuous IV infusion. Do not give IV push (may result in exaggerated hypotension).

Reconstitution • For intermittent IV infusion (piggyback), reconstitute each 500-mg vial with 10 ml sterile water for injection (20 ml for 1-g vial) to provide concentration of 50 mg/ml. • Further dilute to a final concentration not to exceed 5 mg/ml.

Rate of administration • Administer over 60 min or longer. • Monitor BP closely during IV infusion. • ADD-Vantage vials should not be used in neonates, infants, children requiring less than 500-mg dose.

Storage • After reconstitution, refrigerate and use within 14 days. • Discard if precipitate forms.

PO
• Generally not given for systemic infections because of poor absorption from GI tract; however, some patients with colitis may have effective absorption. • Powder for oral solution may be reconstituted, given by mouth or NG tube. • Oral solution is stable for 2 wk if refrigerated. • Do not use powder for oral solution for IV administration.

▨ IV INCOMPATIBILITIES
Albumin, amphotericin B complex (Abelcet, AmBisome, Amphotec), aztreonam (Azactam), cefazolin (Ancef), cefepime (Maxipime), cefotaxime (Claforan), cefotetan (Cefotan), cefoxitin (Mefoxin), ceftazidime (Fortaz), ceftriaxone (Rocephin), cefuroxime (Zinacef), foscarnet (Foscavir), heparin, idarubicin (Idamycin), nafcillin (Nafcil), piperacillin and tazobactam (Zosyn), ticarcillin and clavulanate (Timentin).

IV COMPATIBILITIES
Amiodarone (Cordarone), calcium gluconate, diltiazem (Cardizem), hydromorphone (Dilaudid), insulin, lorazepam (Ativan), magnesium sulfate, midazolam (Versed), morphine, potassium chloride, propofol (Diprivan), total parenteral nutrition (TPN).

INDICATIONS/ROUTES/DOSAGE
TREATMENT OF BONE, RESPIRATORY TRACT, SKIN AND SOFT-TISSUE INFECTIONS, ENDOCARDITIS, PERITONITIS, AND SEPTICEMIA; PREVENTION OF BACTERIAL ENDOCARDITIS IN THOSE AT RISK (IF PENICILLIN IS CONTRAINDICATED) WHEN UNDERGOING BILIARY, DENTAL, GI, GU, OR RESPIRATORY SURGERY OR INVASIVE PROCEDURES
IV: ADULTS, ELDERLY: 500 mg q6h or 1 g q12h. CHILDREN OLDER THAN 1 MO: 40 mg/kg/day in divided doses q6–8h. **Maximum:** 3–4 g/day. NEONATES: Initially, 15 mg/kg, then 10 mg/kg q8–12h.

STAPHYLOCOCCAL ENTEROCOLITIS, ANTIBIOTIC-ASSOCIATED PSEUDOMEMBRANOUS COLITIS CAUSED BY CLOSTRIDIUM DIFFICILE
PO: ADULTS, ELDERLY: 0.5–2 g/day in 3–4 divided doses for 7–10 days. CHILDREN: 40 mg/kg/day in 3–4 divided doses for 7–10 days. **Maximum:** 2 g/day.

DOSAGE IN RENAL IMPAIRMENT
After a loading dose, subsequent dosages and frequency are modified based on creatinine clearance, the severity of the infection, and the serum concentration of the drug.

SIDE EFFECTS
FREQUENT: PO: Bitter or unpleasant taste, nausea, vomiting, mouth irritation (with oral solution). **RARE: Parenteral:** Phlebitis, thrombophlebitis, or pain at peripheral IV site; dizziness; vertigo; tinnitus; chills; fever; rash; necrosis with extravasation. **PO:** Rash.

ADVERSE REACTIONS/ TOXIC EFFECTS

Nephrotoxicity and ototoxicity may occur. "Red-neck" syndrome (redness on face, neck, arms, and back; chills; fever; tachycardia; nausea or vomiting; pruritus; rash; unpleasant taste) may result from too-rapid injection.

NURSING CONSIDERATIONS

BASELINE ASSESSMENT

Avoid other ototoxic, nephrotoxic medications if possible. Obtain culture, sensitivity test before giving first dose (therapy may begin before results are known).

INTERVENTION/EVALUATION

Monitor serum renal function tests, I&O. Assess skin for rash. Check hearing acuity, balance. Monitor BP carefully during infusion. Evaluate IV site for phlebitis (heat, pain, red streaking over vein). Therapeutic serum level: Peak: 20–40 mcg/ml; trough: 5–15 mcg/ml. Toxic serum level: Peak: over 40 mcg/ ml; trough: over 15 mcg/ml.

PATIENT/FAMILY TEACHING

• Continue therapy for full length of treatment. • Doses should be evenly spaced. • Notify physician in event of tinnitus, rash, signs and symptoms of nephrotoxicity. • Lab tests are important part of total therapy.

---

vardenafil

var-**den**-ah-fill

(Levitra)

Do not confuse Levitra with Lexiva.

CLASSIFICATION

PHARMACOTHERAPEUTIC: Phosphodiesterase inhibitor. **CLINICAL:** Erectile dysfunction adjunct.

ACTION

An erectile dysfunction agent that inhibits phosphodiesterase type 5, the enzyme responsible for degrading cyclic guanosine monophosphate in the corpus cavernosum of the penis, resulting in smooth muscle relaxation and increased blood flow. **Therapeutic Effect:** Facilitates an erection.

PHARMACOKINETICS

Rapidly absorbed after PO administration. Extensive tissue distribution. Protein binding: 95%. Metabolized in the liver. Excreted primarily in feces; a lesser amount eliminated in urine. Drug has no effect on penile blood flow without sexual stimulation. **Half-life:** 4–5 hr.

USES

Treatment of erectile dysfunction.

PRECAUTIONS

CONTRAINDICATIONS: Concurrent use of alpha-adrenergic blockers, sodium nitroprusside, or nitrates in any form. **CAUTIONS:** Renal or hepatic impairment, anatomical deformation of the penis, patients who may be predisposed to priapism (sickle cell anemia, multiple myeloma, leukemia).

⌛ **LIFESPAN CONSIDERATIONS: Pregnancy/Lactation:** Vardenafil is not indicated for use in women, newborns. **Pregnancy Category B. Children:** Vardenafil is not indicated for use in children. **Elderly:** No age-related precautions noted, but initial dose should be 5 mg.

INTERACTIONS

DRUG: Alpha-adrenergic blockers, nitrates: Potentiates the hypotensive effects of these drugs. **Erythromycin, indinavir, itraconazole, ketoconazole, ritonavir:** May increase vardenafil blood concentration. **HERBAL:** None known. **FOOD: High-fat meals:** Delay

---

drug's maximum effectiveness. **LAB VALUES:** None known.

AVAILABILITY (Rx)

TABLETS: 2.5 mg, 5 mg, 10 mg, 20 mg.

ADMINISTRATION/ HANDLING

PO

• May take approximately 1 hr before sexual activity. Do not crush, break film-coated tablets.

INDICATIONS/ROUTES/DOSAGE

ERECTILE DYSFUNCTION

PO: ADULTS: 10 mg approximately 1 hr before sexual activity. Dose may be increased to 20 mg or decreased to 5 mg, based on patient tolerance. Maximum dosing frequency is once daily. ELDERLY, OLDER THAN 65 YR: 5 mg.

DOSAGE IN MODERATE HEPATIC IMPAIRMENT

PO: For patients with Child-Pugh class B hepatic impairment, dosage is 5 mg 60 min before sexual activity.

DOSAGE WITH CONCURRENT RITONAVIR

PO: ADULTS: 2.5 mg in a 72-hr period.

DOSAGE WITH CONCURRENT KETOCONAZOLE OR ITRACONAZOLE (AT 400 MG/DAY), OR INDINAVIR

PO: ADULTS: 2.5 mg in a 24-hr period.

DOSAGE WITH CONCURRENT KETOCONAZOLE OR ITRACONAZOLE (AT 200 MG/DAY), OR ERYTHROMYCIN

PO: ADULTS: 5 mg in a 24-hr period.

SIDE EFFECTS

OCCASIONAL: Headache, flushing, rhinitis, indigestion. **RARE (less than 2%):** Dizziness, changes in color vision, blurred vision.

ADVERSE REACTIONS/ TOXIC EFFECTS

Prolonged erections (lasting over 4 hr) and priapism (painful erections lasting over 6 hr) occur rarely.

NURSING CONSIDERATIONS

BASELINE ASSESSMENT

Assess cardiovascular status before initiating treatment for erectile dysfunction.

PATIENT/FAMILY TEACHING

• Has no effect in the absence of sexual stimulation. • Seek treatment immediately if an erection persists for over 4 hr.

varicella vaccine

(Varivax)
See Appendix N

vasopressin

vay-soe-**press**-in
(Pitressin, Pressyn ♣)
Do not confuse Pitressin with Pitocin.

•CLASSIFICATION

PHARMACOTHERAPEUTIC: Posterior pituitary hormone. **CLINICAL:** Vasopressor, antidiuretic.

ACTION

A posterior pituitary hormone that increases reabsorption of water by the renal tubules. Increases water permeability at the distal tubule and collecting duct. Directly stimulates smooth muscle in the GI tract. **Therapeutic Effect:** Causes peristalsis and vasoconstriction.

PHARMACOKINETICS

Route	Onset	Peak	Duration
IV	N/A	N/A	0.5–1 hr
IM, Sub-cutaneous	1–2 hr	N/A	2–8 hr

Distributed throughout extracellular fluid. Metabolized in the liver and

V

kidney. Primarily excreted in urine.
Half-life: 10–20 min.

USES

Treatment of adult shock-refractory ventricular fibrillation (class IIb). Prevention and control of polydipsia, polyuria, dehydration in patients with neurogenic diabetes insipidus. Stimulates peristalsis in the prevention and treatment of postop abdominal distention, intestinal paresis. Treatment of vasodilatory shock with hypotension unresponsive to fluids or catecholamines. **OFF-LABEL:** Adjunct in treatment of acute, massive hemorrhage.

PRECAUTIONS

CONTRAINDICATIONS: None known. **CAUTIONS:** Seizures, migraine, asthma, vascular disease, renal or cardiac disease, goiter (with cardiac complications), arteriosclerosis, nephritis.

⧗ **LIFESPAN CONSIDERATIONS:** Pregnancy/Lactation: Caution in giving to breast-feeding women. **Pregnancy Category B. Children/Elderly:** Caution due to risk of water intoxication/hyponatremia.

INTERACTIONS

DRUG: **Alcohol, demeclocycline, lithium, norepinephrine:** May decrease the effects of vasopressin. **Carbamazepine, chlorpropamide, clofibrate:** May increase the effects of vasopressin. **HERBAL:** None known. **FOOD:** None known. **LAB VALUES:** None known.

AVAILABILITY (Rx)

INJECTION: 20 units/ml.

ADMINISTRATION/HANDLING
📋 **IV**

Reconstitution • Dilute with D_5W or 0.9% NaCl to concentration of 0.1–1 unit/ml.

Rate of administration • Give as IV infusion.

Storage • Store at room temperature.

IM, SUBCUTANEOUS
• Give with 1–2 glasses of water to reduce side effects.

▦ IV INCOMPATIBILITIES

Amphotericin B complex (Abelcet, AmBisome, Amphotec), diazepam (Valium), etomidate (Amidate), furosemide (Lasix), thiopentothal.

IV COMPATIBILITIES

Dobutamine (Dobutrex), dopamine (Intropin), heparin, lorazepam (Ativan), midazolam (Versed), milrinone (Primacor), verapamil (Calan, Isoptin).

INDICATIONS/ROUTES/DOSAGE

CARDIAC ARREST

IV: ADULTS, ELDERLY: 40 units as a one-time bolus.

DIABETES INSIPIDUS

IV INFUSION: ADULTS, CHILDREN: 0.5 mUnits/kg/hr. May double dose q30min. **Maximum:** 10 mUnits/kg/hr.

IM, SUBCUTANEOUS: ADULTS, ELDERLY: 5–10 units 2–4 times a day. Range: 5–60 unit/day. CHILDREN: 2.5–10 units, 2–4 times a day.

ABDOMINAL DISTENTION, INTESTINAL PARESIS

IM: ADULTS, ELDERLY: Initially, 5 units. Subsequent doses, 10 units q3–4h.

GI HEMORRHAGE

IV INFUSION: ADULTS, ELDERLY: Initially, 0.2–0.4 unit/min progressively increased to 0.9 unit/min. CHILDREN: 0.002–0.005 unit/kg/min. Titrate as needed. **Maximum:** 0.01 unit/kg/min.

VASODILATORY SHOCK

IV: ADULTS, ELDERLY: Initially, 0.04–0.1 unit/min. Titrate to desired effect.

SIDE EFFECTS

FREQUENT: Pain at injection site (with vasopressin tannate). **OCCASIONAL:** Abdominal cramps, nausea, vomiting, diarrhea, dizziness, diaphoresis, pale skin, circumoral pallor, tremors, headache, eructation, flatulence. **RARE:** Chest pain; confusion; allergic reaction, including rash or hives, pruritus, wheezing or difficulty breathing, facial and peripheral edema; sterile abscess (with vasopressin tannate).

ADVERSE REACTIONS/ TOXIC EFFECTS

Anaphylaxis, MI, and water intoxication have occurred. The elderly and very young are at higher risk for water intoxication.

NURSING CONSIDERATIONS

BASELINE ASSESSMENT

Establish baselines for weight, BP, pulse, serum electrolytes, urine specific gravity.

INTERVENTION/EVALUATION

Monitor I&O closely, restrict intake as necessary to prevent water intoxication. Weigh daily if indicated. Check BP, pulse twice a day. Monitor serum electrolytes, urine specific gravity. Evaluate injection site for erythema, pain, abscess. Report side effects to physician for dose reduction. Be alert for early signs of water intoxication (drowsiness, listlessness, headache). Withhold medication and report immediately any chest pain or allergic symptoms.

PATIENT/FAMILY TEACHING

• Promptly report headache, chest pain, shortness of breath, other symptoms. • Stress importance of I&O. • Avoid alcohol.

Vasotec, *see enalapril*

---

vecuronium bromide

(Norcuron)

See Neuromuscular blockers (p. 112C)

---

venlafaxine

ven-la-**fax**een
(Effexor, Effexor XR)

◆CLASSIFICATION

PHARMACOTHERAPEUTIC: Phenethylamine derivative. **CLINICAL:** Antidepressant (see pp. 12C, 38C).

ACTION

A phenethylamine derivative that potentiates CNS neurotransmitter activity by inhibiting the reuptake of serotonin, norepinephrine and, to a lesser degree, dopamine. **Therapeutic Effect:** Relieves depression.

PHARMACOKINETICS

Well absorbed from the GI tract. Protein binding: 25%–30%. Metabolized in the liver to active metabolite. Primarily excreted in urine. Not removed by hemodialysis. **Half-life:** 3–7 hr; metabolite, 9–13 hr (increased in hepatic or renal impairment.

USES

Treatment of depression exhibited as persistent, prominent dysphoria (occurring nearly every day for at least 2 wk) manifested by 4 of 8 symptoms: change in appetite, change in sleep pattern, increased fatigue, impaired concentration, feelings of guilt or worthlessness, loss of interest in usual activities, psychomotor agitation or retardation, or suicidal tendencies. Psychotherapy augments

V

---

therapeutic result. Treatment of generalized anxiety disorder (GAD), social anxiety disorder (SAD). Treatment of panic disorder, with or without agoraphobia. **OFF-LABEL:** Prevention of relapses of depression; treatment of attention-deficit hyperactivity disorder, autism, chronic fatigue syndrome, obsessive-compulsive disorder.

PRECAUTIONS

CONTRAINDICATIONS: Use within 14 days of MAOIs. **CAUTIONS:** Seizure disorder, renal/hepatic impairment, suicidal patients, recent MI, mania, volume-depleted patients, narrow-angle glaucoma, CHF, hyperthyroidism, abnormal platelet function.

⧖ **LIFESPAN CONSIDERATIONS: Pregnancy/Lactation:** Unknown if excreted in breast milk. **Pregnancy Category C. Children:** Children and adolescents are at increased risk of suicidal ideation and behavior or worsening depression, especially during the first few months of therapy. **Elderly:** No age-related precautions noted.

INTERACTIONS

DRUG: MAOIs: May cause neuroleptic malignant syndrome, autonomic instability (including rapid fluctuations of vital signs), extreme agitation, hyperthermia, mental status changes, myoclonus, rigidity, and coma. **HERBAL: St. John's wort:** May increase the sedative-hypnotic effect of venlafaxine. **FOOD:** None known. **LAB VALUES:** May increase BUN level and serum alkaline phosphatase, bilirubin, cholesterol, uric acid, AST, and ALT levels. May decrease serum phosphate and sodium levels. May alter blood glucose and serum potassium levels.

AVAILABILITY (Rx)

CAPSULES   (EXTENDED-RELEASE [EFFEXOR XL]): 37.5 mg, 75 mg, 150 mg. **TABLETS (EFFEXOR):** 25 mg, 37.5 mg, 50 mg, 75 mg, 100 mg.

ADMINISTRATION/HANDLING

PO
• Give without regard to food. Give with food, milk if GI distress occurs. • Scored tablet may be crushed. • Do not crush, chew, or place in water extended-release capsules. • May open, sprinkle on applesauce.

INDICATIONS/ROUTES/DOSAGE

DEPRESSION
PO: ADULTS, ELDERLY: Initially, 75 mg/day in 2–3 divided doses with food. May increase by 75 mg/day at intervals of 4 days or longer. **Maximum:** 375 mg/day in 3 divided doses.

PO (EXTENDED-RELEASE): ADULTS, ELDERLY: 75 mg/day as a single dose with food. May increase by 75 mg/day at intervals of 4 days or longer. **Maximum:** 225 mg/day.

SOCIAL ANXIETY DISORDER, GENERALIZED ANXIETY DISORDER
PO (EXTENDED-RELEASE): ADULTS, ELDERLY: Initially, 37.5–75 mg/day. May increase by 75 mg/day at 4-day intervals up to 225 mg/day.

PANIC DISORDER
PO (EXTENDED-RELEASE): Initially, 37.5 mg/day. May increase to 75 mg after 7 days followed by increases of 75 mg/day at 7-day intervals up to 225 mg/day.

DOSAGE IN RENAL AND HEPATIC IMPAIRMENT
Expect to decrease venlafaxine dosage by 50% in patients with moderate hepatic impairment, 25% in patients with mild to moderate renal impairment, and 50% in patients on dialysis (withhold dose until completion of dialysis).

SIDE EFFECTS

FREQUENT   (greater   than   20%): Nausea, somnolence, headache, dry mouth. **OCCASIONAL (20%–10%):** Dizziness, insomnia, constipation, diaphoresis, nervousness, asthenia, ejaculatory disturbance, anorexia. **RARE (less than 10%):** Anxiety, blurred vision, diarrhea, vomiting, tremor, abnormal dreams, impotence.

ADVERSE REACTIONS/ TOXIC EFFECTS

A sustained increase in diastolic BP of 10–15 mm Hg occurs occasionally.

BASELINE ASSESSMENT

Obtain initial weight, BP. Assess appearance, behavior, speech pattern, level of interest, mood.

INTERVENTION/EVALUATION

Monitor signs/symptoms of depression, BP, weight. Assess sleep pattern for evidence of insomnia. Check during waking hours for somnolence or dizziness, anxiety; provide assistance as necessary. Supervise suicidal-risk patient closely during early therapy (as depression lessens, energy level improves, increasing suicide potential). Assess appearance, behavior, speech pattern, level of interest, mood for therapeutic response.

PATIENT/FAMILY TEACHING

• Take with food to minimize GI distress. • Do not increase, decrease, or suddenly stop medication. • Avoid tasks that require alertness, motor skills until response to drug is established. • Inform physician if breast-feeding, pregnant, or planning to become pregnant. • Avoid alcohol.

Ventolin, *see albuterol*

VePesid, *see etoposide*

---

verapamil hydrochloride

ver-**ap**-a-mill ☙

(Apo-Verap ☙, Calan, Calan SR, Chronovera ☙, Covera-HS, Isoptin, Isoptin I.V., Isoptin SR, Novo-Veramil ☙, Novo-Veramil SR ☙, Verelan, Verelan PM)

Do not confuse Isoptin with Intropin, or Verelan with Virilon, Vivarin, or Voltaren.

FIXED-COMBINATION(S)

Tarka: verapamil/trandolapril (an angiotensin-converting enzyme [ACE] inhibitor): 240 mg/1 mg; 180 mg/2 mg; 240 mg/2 mg; 240 mg/4 mg.

CLASSIFICATION

PHARMACOTHERAPEUTIC: Calcium channel blocker. **CLINICAL:** Antihypertensive, antianginal, antiarrhythmic, hypertropic cardiomyopathy therapy adjunct (see pp. 16C, 69C).

ACTION

A calcium channel blocker and antianginal, antiarrhythmic, and antihypertensive agent that inhibits calcium ion entry across cardiac and vascular smooth-muscle cell membranes. This action causes the dilation of coronary arteries, peripheral arteries, and arterioles. Therapeutic Effect: Decreases heart rate and myocardial contractility and slows SA and AV conduction. Decreases total peripheral vascular resistance by vasodilation.

PHARMACOKINETICS

Route	Onset	Peak	Duration
PO	30 min	1–2 hr	6–8 hr
PO (Extended-release)	30 min	N/A	N/A
IV	1–2 min	3–5 min	10–60 min

Well absorbed from the GI tract. Protein binding: 90% (60% in neonates.) Undergoes first-pass metabolism in the liver to active metabolite. Primarily excreted in urine. Not removed by hemodialysis. Half-life: 2–8 hr.

USES

Parenteral: Management of supraventricular tachyarrhythmias, temporary control of rapid ventricular rate in atrial flutter or fibrillation. **PO:** Management of spastic (Prinzmetal's variant) angina, unstable (crescendo, preinfarction) angina, chronic stable angina (effort-associated angina), hypertension, prevention of recurrent paroxysmal supraventricular tachycardia (PSVT) (with digoxin); control of ventricular resting pulse rate in those with atrial flutter and/or fibrillation. OFF-LABEL: Treatment of bipolar disorder, hypertrophic cardiomyopathy, vascular headaches.

PRECAUTIONS

CONTRAINDICATIONS: Atrial fibrillation or flutter and an accessory bypass tract, cardiogenic shock, heart block, hypotension, sinus bradycardia, ventricular tachycardia. **CAUTIONS:** Sick sinus syndrome, CHF, renal or hepatic impairment, concomitant use of beta-blockers or digoxin.

⧗ LIFESPAN CONSIDERATIONS: **Pregnancy/Lactation:** Drug crosses placenta; is distributed in breast milk. Breast-feeding not recommended. **Pregnancy Category C. Children:** No age-related precautions noted. **Elderly:** Age-related renal impairment may require dosage adjustment.

INTERACTIONS

DRUG: **Beta blockers:** May have additive effect. **Carbamazepine, quinidine, theophylline:** May increase verapamil blood concentration and risk of toxicity. **Digoxin:** May increase

digoxin blood concentration. **Disopyramide:** May increase negative inotropic effect. **Procainamide, quinidine:** May increase risk of QT-interval prolongation. HERBAL: None known. FOOD: **Grapefruit, grapefruit juice:** May increase verapamil blood concentration. LAB VALUES: EKG waveform may show increased PR interval. Therapeutic serum level is 0.08–0.3 mcg/ml.

AVAILABILITY (Rx)

CAPLET (CALAN SR): 120 mg, 180 mg, 240 mg. **CAPSULES (EXTENDED-RELEASE [VERELAN PM]):** 100 mg, 200 mg, 300 mg. **CAPSULES (SUSTAINED-RELEASE [VERELAN]):** 120 mg, 180 mg, 240 mg, 360 mg. **TABLETS (CALAN):** 40 mg, 80 mg, 120 mg. **TABLETS (EXTENDED-RELEASE [COVERA-HS]):** 180 mg, 240 mg. **TABLETS (SUSTAINED-RELEASE [ISOPTIN SR]):** 120 mg, 180 mg, 240 mg. **INJECTION:** 2.5 mg/ml.

ADMINISTRATION/HANDLING
📵 IV

Reconstitution • May give undiluted.

Rate of administration • Administer IV push over 2 min for adults, children; give over 3 min for elderly. • Continuous EKG monitoring during IV injection is required for children, recommended for adults. • Monitor EKG for rapid ventricular rates, extreme bradycardia, heart block, asystole, prolongation of PR interval. Notify physician of any significant changes. • Monitor BP q5–10min. • Patient should remain recumbent for at least 1 hr after IV administration.

Storage • Store vials at room temperature.

PO
• Do not give with grapefruit juice. • Non–sustained-release tablets may be given with or without food. • Swallow extended-release or sustained-released preparations whole; do not chew, crush. • Sustained-release capsules may be

V

opened and sprinkled on applesauce and swallowed immediately (do not chew).

▨ IV INCOMPATIBILITIES

Amphotericin B complex (Abelcet, AmBisome, Amphotec), nafcillin (Nafcil), propofol (Diprivan), sodium bicarbonate.

IV COMPATIBILITIES

Amiodarone (Cordarone), calcium chloride, calcium gluconate, dexamethasone (Decadron), digoxin (Lanoxin), dobutamine (Dobutrex), dopamine (Intropin), furosemide (Lasix), heparin, hydromorphone (Dilaudid), lidocaine, magnesium sulfate, metoclopramide (Reglan), milrinone (Primacor), morphine, multivitamins, nitroglycerin, norepinephrine (Levophed), potassium chloride, potassium phosphate, procainamide (Pronestyl), propranolol (Inderal).

INDICATIONS/ROUTES/DOSAGE

SUPRAVENTRICULAR TACHYARRHYTHMIAS (SVT)

IV: ADULTS, ELDERLY: Initially, 2.5–5 mg over 2 min. May give 5–10 mg 30 min after initial dose. **Maximum initial dose:** 20 mg. CHILDREN 1-15 YR: 0.1–0.3 mg/kg over 2 min. **Maximum initial dose:** 5 mg. May repeat in 15 min. **Maximum second dose:** 10 mg. CHILDREN YOUNGER THAN 1 YR: 0.1–0.2 mg/kg over 2 min. May repeat 30 min after initial dose.

ARRHYTHMIAS, INCLUDING PREVENTION OF RECURRENT PAROXYSMAL SUPRAVENTRICULAR TACHYCARDIA AND CONTROL OF VENTRICULAR RESTING RATE IN CHRONIC ATRIAL FIBRILLATION OR FLUTTER (WITH DIGOXIN)

PO: ADULTS, ELDERLY: 240–480 mg/day in 3–4 divided doses.

VASOSPASTIC ANGINA (PRINZMETAL'S VARIANT), UNSTABLE (CRESCENDO OR PREINFARCTION) ANGINA, CHRONIC STABLE (EFFORT-ASSOCIATED) ANGINA

PO: ADULTS: Initially, 80–120 mg 3 times a day. For elderly patients and those with hepatic dysfunction, 40 mg

3 times a day. Titrate to optimal dose. Maintenance: 240–480 mg/day in 3–4 divided doses.

PO (COVERA-HS): ADULTS, ELDERLY: 180–480 mg/day at bedtime.

HYPERTENSION

PO (IMMEDIATE-RELEASE): ADULTS, ELDERLY: 80 mg 3 times a day. Range: 80–320 mg/day in 2 divided doses.

PO (SUSTAINED-RELEASE): ADULTS, ELDERLY: 120–240 mg/day. Range: 120–360 mg/day as single dose or in 2 divided doses.

PO (EXTENDED-RELEASE [COVERA-HS]): ADULTS, ELDERLY: 120–360 mg once daily at bedtime.

PO (EXTENDED-RELEASE [VERELAN PM]): ADULTS, ELDERLY: 200–400 mg once daily at bedtime.

SIDE EFFECTS

FREQUENT (7%): Constipation. **OCCASIONAL (4%–2%):** Dizziness, light-headedness, headache, asthenia (loss of strength, energy), nausea, peripheral edema, hypotension. **RARE (less than 1%):** Bradycardia, dermatitis or rash.

ADVERSE REACTIONS/ TOXIC EFFECTS

Rapid ventricular rate in atrial flutter or fibrillation, marked hypotension, extreme bradycardia, CHF, asystole, and second- and third-degree AV block occur rarely.

NURSING CONSIDERATIONS

BASELINE ASSESSMENT

Record onset, type (sharp, dull, squeezing), radiation, location, intensity, duration of anginal pain, precipitating factors (exertion, emotional stress). Check BP for hypotension, pulse for bradycardia immediately before giving medication.

INTERVENTION/EVALUATION

Assess pulse for quality, irregular rate. Monitor EKG for cardiac changes, particularly prolongation of PR interval.

V

Notify physician of any significant interval changes. Assist with ambulation if dizziness occurs. Assess for peripheral edema behind medial malleolus (sacral area in bedridden patients). For those taking oral form, check stool consistency, frequency. Therapeutic serum level: 0.08–0.3 mcg/ml; toxic serum level: N/E.

PATIENT/FAMILY TEACHING

• Do not abruptly discontinue medication. • Compliance with therapy regimen is essential to control anginal pain. • To avoid hypotensive effect, rise slowly from lying to sitting position, wait momentarily before standing. • Avoid tasks that require alertness, motor skills until response to drug is established. • Limit caffeine. • Inform physician if angina pain not reduced, irregular heartbeats, shortness of breath, swelling, dizziness, constipation, nausea, hypotension occurs. • Avoid concomitant grapefruit juice.

Versed, *see midazolam*

Viagra, *see sildenafil*

Vidaza, *see azacitidine*

---

*vinBLAStine sulfate ⚑

vin-**blass**-teen
(Velban, Velbe ✽)
Do not confuse vinblastine with vincristine or vinorelbine.

CLASSIFICATION

PHARMACOTHERAPEUTIC: Vinca alkaloid. **CLINICAL:** Antineoplastic (see p. 79C).

ACTION

A vinca alkaloid that binds to microtubular protein of mitotic spindle, causing metaphase arrest. **Therapeutic Effect:** Inhibits cell division.

PHARMACOKINETICS

Does not cross the blood-brain barrier. Protein binding: 75%. Metabolized in the liver to active metabolite. Primarily eliminated in feces by biliary system. **Half-life:** 24.8 hr.

USES

Treatment of disseminated Hodgkin's disease, non-Hodgkin's lymphoma, advanced stage of mycosis fungoides, advanced testicular carcinoma, Kaposi's sarcoma, Letterer-Siwe disease, breast carcinoma, choriocarcinoma. **OFF-LABEL:** Treatment of bladder, head and neck, kidney, or lung carcinoma; chronic myelocytic leukemia; germ cell ovarian tumors; neuroblastoma.

PRECAUTIONS

CONTRAINDICATIONS: Bacterial infection, severe leukopenia, significant granulocytopenia (unless it stems from disease being treated). **CAUTIONS:** Hepatic impairment, neurotoxicity, recent exposure to radiation therapy or chemotherapy.

⧗ **LIFESPAN CONSIDERATIONS: Pregnancy/Lactation:** If possible, avoid use during pregnancy, especially first trimester. Breast-feeding not recommended. **Pregnancy Category D. Children/Elderly:** No age-related precautions noted.

INTERACTIONS

DRUG: Antigout medications: May decrease the effects of these drugs. **Bone marrow depressants:** May

---

* "Tall Man" lettering   𝒮 see color pill atlas   🌿 herb   <u>underlined</u> – top prescribed drug increase myelosuppression. **Live virus vaccines:** May potentiate virus replication, increase vaccine side effects, and decrease the patient's antibody response to the vaccine. HERBAL: None known. FOOD: None known. LAB VALUES: May increase serum uric acid levels.

AVAILABILITY (Rx)

INJECTION: 1 mg/ml. **POWDER FOR INJECTION:** 10 mg.

ADMINISTRATION/HANDLING

‹ ALERT › May be carcinogenic, mutagenic, teratogenic. Handle with extreme care during preparation and administration. Give by IV injection. Leakage from IV site into surrounding tissue may produce extreme irritation. Avoid eye contact with solution (severe eye irritation, possible corneal ulceration may result). If eye contact occurs, immediately irrigate eye with water.

 IV

Reconstitution • Reconstitute 10-mg vial with 10 ml 0.9% NaCl preserved with phenol or benzyl alcohol to provide concentration of 1 mg/ml.

Rate of administration • Inject into tubing of running IV infusion or directly into vein over 1 min. • Do not inject into extremity with impaired or potentially impaired circulation caused by compression or invading neoplasm, phlebitis, varicosity. • Rinse syringe, needle with venous blood before withdrawing needle (minimizes possibility of extravasation). • Extravasation may result in cellulitis, phlebitis. Large amount of extravasation may result in tissue sloughing. If extravasation occurs, give local injection of hyaluronidase and apply warm compresses.

Storage • Refrigerate unopened vials. • Solutions appear clear, colorless. • Following reconstitution, solution is stable for 30 days if refrigerated. • Discard if precipitate forms, discoloration occurs.

IV INCOMPATIBILITIES

Cefepime (Maxipime), furosemide (Lasix).

IV COMPATIBILITIES

Allopurinol (Aloprim), cisplatin (Platinol AQ), cyclophosphamide (Cytoxan), doxorubicin (Adriamycin), etoposide (VePesid), 5-fluorouracil, gemcitabine (Gemzar), granisetron (Kytril), heparin, leucovorin, methotrexate, ondansetron (Zofran), paclitaxel (Taxol), vinorelbine (Navelbine).

INDICATIONS/ROUTES/DOSAGE

USUAL DOSAGE (REFER TO INDIVIDUAL PROTOCOLS)

IV: ADULTS, ELDERLY, CHILDREN: 4–20 mg/m^2 (0.1–0.5 mg/kg) q7–10days or 5 day continuous infusion of 1.5–2 mg/m^2/day or 0.1–0.5 mg/kg/wk.

SIDE EFFECTS

FREQUENT: Nausea, vomiting, alopecia. **OCCASIONAL:** Constipation or diarrhea, rectal bleeding, headache, paraesthesia (occur 4–6 hr after administration and persist for 2–10 hr); malaise; asthenia; dizziness; pain at tumor site; jaw or face pain; depression; dry mouth. **RARE:** Dermatitis, stomatitis, phototoxicity, hyperuricemia.

ADVERSE REACTIONS/TOXIC EFFECTS

Hematologic toxicity is manifested as leukopenia and, less commonly, anemia. The WBC count reaches its nadir 4–10 days after initial therapy and recovers within 7–14 days (21 days with high vinblastine dosages). Thrombocytopenia is usually mild and transient, with recovery occurring in few days. Hepatic insufficiency may increase the risk of toxic drug effects. Acute shortness of breath or bronchospasm may occur, particularly when vinblastine is administered concurrently with mitomycin.

V

NURSING CONSIDERATIONS

BASELINE ASSESSMENT

Nausea, vomiting easily controlled by antiemetics. Discontinue therapy if WBC, thrombocyte counts fall abruptly (unless drug is clearly destroying tumor cells in bone marrow). Obtain CBC weekly or before each dosing.

INTERVENTION/EVALUATION

If WBC falls below 2,000/mm^3, assess diligently for signs of infection. Assess for stomatitis; maintain fastidious oral hygiene. Monitor for hematologic toxicity: infection (fever, sore throat, signs of local infection), unusual bruising or bleeding from any site, symptoms of anemia (excessive fatigue, weakness). Monitor pattern of bowel activity and stool consistency; avoid constipation.

PATIENT/FAMILY TEACHING

• Immediately report any pain or burning at injection site during administration. • Pain at tumor site may occur during or shortly after injection. • Do not have immunizations without physician approval (drug lowers body's resistance). • Avoid crowds, those with infection. • Promptly report fever, sore throat, signs of local infection, unusual bruising or bleeding from any site. • Alopecia is reversible, but new hair growth may have different color, texture. • Contact physician if nausea or vomiting continues. • Avoid constipation by increasing fluids, bulk in diet, exercise as tolerated.

---

*vinCRIStine sulfate ⚑

vin-**cris**-teen
(Oncovin, Vincasar PFS)
Do not confuse vincristine with vinblastine, or Oncovin with Ancobon.

*CLASSIFICATION

PHARMACOTHERAPEUTIC: Vinca alkaloid. **CLINICAL:** Antineoplastic (see p. 79C).

ACTION

A vinca alkaloid that binds to microtubular protein of mitotic spindle, causing metaphase arrest. Therapeutic Effect: Inhibits cell division.

PHARMACOKINETICS

Does not cross the blood-brain barrier. Protein binding: 75%. Metabolized in the liver. Primarily eliminated in feces by biliary system. Half-life: 10–37 hr.

USES

Treatment of acute leukemia, disseminated Hodgkin's disease, advanced non-Hodgkin's lymphomas, neuroblastoma, rhabdomyosarcoma, Wilms' tumor. OFF-LABEL: Treatment of breast, cervical, colorectal, lung, and ovarian carcinomas; chronic lymphocytic and chronic myelocytic leukemias; germ cell ovarian tumors; idiopathic thrombocytopenic purpura; malignant melanoma; multiple myeloma; mycosis fungoides.

PRECAUTIONS

CONTRAINDICATIONS: Demyelinating form of Charcot-Marie-Tooth syndrome, patients receiving radiation therapy through ports that include the liver. **CAUTION:** Hepatic impairment, neurotoxicity, preexisting neuromuscular disease.

⏳ LIFESPAN CONSIDERATIONS: **Pregnancy/Lactation:** If possible, avoid use during pregnancy, especially first trimester. May cause fetal harm. Breastfeeding not recommended. **Pregnancy Category D. Children:** No age-related precautions noted. **Elderly:** More susceptible to neurotoxic effects.

INTERACTIONS

DRUG: Asparaginase, neurotoxic medications: May increase the risk of neurotoxicity. **Antigout medications:** May decrease the effects of these drugs. **Doxorubicin:** May increase the risk of myelosuppression. **Live virus vaccines:** May potentiate virus replication, increase vaccine side effects, and decrease the patient's antibody response to the vaccine. **HERBAL:** None known. **FOOD:** None known. **LAB VALUES:** May increase serum uric acid levels.

AVAILABILITY (Rx)

INJECTION (ONCOVIN): 1 mg/ml.

ADMINISTRATION/HANDLING

 IV

◀ **ALERT** ▶ May be carcinogenic, mutagenic, teratogenic. Handle with extreme care during preparation and administration. Give by IV injection. Use extreme caution in calculating, administering vincristine. Overdose may result in serious or fatal outcome.

Reconstitution • May give undiluted.

Rate of administration • Inject dose into tubing of running IV infusion or directly into vein over 1 min. • Do not inject into extremity with impaired or potentially impaired circulation caused by compression or invading neoplasm, phlebitis, varicosity. • Extravasation produces stinging, burning, edema at injection site. Terminate immediately, locally inject hyaluronidase, apply heat (disperses drug, minimizes discomfort, cellulitis).

Storage • Refrigerate unopened vials. • Solutions appear clear, colorless. • Discard if precipitate forms or discoloration occurs.

⚙ IV INCOMPATIBILITIES

Cefepime (Maxipime), furosemide (Lasix), idarubicin (Idamycin).

IV COMPATIBILITIES

Allopurinol (Aloprim), cisplatin (Platinol AQ), cyclophosphamide (Cytoxan), cytarabine (Ara-C, Cytosar), doxorubicin (Adriamycin), etoposide (VePesid), 5-fluorouracil, gemcitabine (Gemzar), granisetron (Kytril), leucovorin, methotrexate, ondansetron (Zofran), paclitaxel (Taxol), vinorelbine (Navelbine).

INDICATIONS/ROUTES/DOSAGE

ACUTE LEUKEMIA, ADVANCED NON-HODGKIN'S LYMPHOMA, DISSEMINATED HODGKIN'S DISEASE, NEUROBLASTOMA, RHABDOMYOSARCOMA, WILMS' TUMOR
IV: ADULTS, ELDERLY: $0.4–1.4 \text{ mg/m}^2$ once a wk. CHILDREN: $1–2 \text{ mg/m}^2$ once a wk. CHILDREN WEIGHING LESS THAN 10 KG OR WITH A BODY SURFACE AREA LESS THAN 1 M^2: 0.05 mg/kg. **Maximum:** 2 mg.

DOSAGE IN HEPATIC IMPAIRMENT
Reduce dosage by 50% in patients with a direct serum bilirubin concentration more than 3 mg/dl.

SIDE EFFECTS

EXPECTED: Peripheral neuropathy (occurs in nearly every patient; first clinical sign is depression of Achilles tendon reflex). **FREQUENT:** Peripheral paraesthesia, alopecia, constipation or obstipation (upper colon impaction with empty rectum), abdominal cramps, headache, jaw pain, hoarseness, diplopia, ptosis or drooping of eyelid, urinary tract disturbances. **OCCASIONAL:** Nausea, vomiting, diarrhea, abdominal distention, stomatitis, fever. **RARE:** Mild leukopenia, mild anemia, thrombocytopenia.

ADVERSE REACTIONS/ TOXIC EFFECTS

Acute shortness of breath and bronchospasm may occur, especially when vincristine is administered concurrently with mitomycin. Prolonged or high-dose therapy may produce foot or wrist drop,

V

---

difficulty walking, slapping gait, ataxia, and muscle wasting. Acute uric acid nephropathy may occur.

NURSING CONSIDERATIONS

BASELINE ASSESSMENT

Monitor serum uric acid levels, renal and liver function studies, hematologic status. Assess Achilles tendon reflex. Monitor pattern of bowel activity and stool consistency. Monitor for ptosis, diplopia, blurred vision. Question patient regarding urinary changes.

PATIENT/FAMILY TEACHING

• Immediately report any pain or burning at injection site during administration. • Alopecia is reversible, but new hair growth may have different color or texture. • Contact physician if nausea or vomiting continues. • Teach signs of peripheral neuropathy. • Report fever, sore throat, bleeding, bruising, shortness of breath.

---

vinorelbine ⚑

vin-oh-**rell**-bean
(Navelbine)

Do not confuse vinorelbine with vinblastine.

•CLASSIFICATION

CLINICAL: Antineoplastic (see p. 79C).

ACTION

A semisynthetic vinca alkaloid that interferes with mitotic microtubule assembly. **Therapeutic Effect:** Prevents cell division.

PHARMACOKINETICS

Widely distributed after IV administration. Protein binding: 80%–90%. Metabolized in the liver. Primarily eliminated in feces by biliary system. **Half-life:** 28–43 hr.

USES

Single agent or in combination with cisplatin for treatment with unresectable, advanced, non–small-cell lung cancer (NSCLC). **OFF-LABEL:** Treatment of breast cancer, cervical carcinoma, cisplatin-resistant ovarian carcinoma, Hodgkin's disease, non-Hodgkin's lymphoma.

PRECAUTIONS

CONTRAINDICATIONS: Granulocyte count before treatment of less than 1,000 cells/mm^3. **EXTREME CAUTION:** Immunocompromised patients. **CAUTIONS:** Existing or recent chickenpox, herpes zoster, infection, leukopenia, impaired pulmonary function, severe hepatic injury or impairment.

⌛ **LIFESPAN CONSIDERATIONS: Pregnancy/Lactation:** If possible, avoid use during pregnancy, especially during first trimester. May cause fetal harm. Unknown if excreted in breast milk. Breast-feeding not recommended. **Pregnancy Category D. Children:** Safety and efficacy not established. **Elderly:** No age-related precautions noted.

INTERACTIONS

DRUG: Bone marrow depressants: May increase the risk of myelosuppression. **Cisplatin:** Significantly increases the risk of granulocytopenia. **Live virus vaccines:** May potentiate virus replication, increase vaccine side effects, and decrease the patient's antibody response to the vaccine. **Mitomycin:** May produce an acute pulmonary reaction. **HERBAL:** None known. **FOOD:** None known. **LAB VALUES:** May increase total serum bilirubin and AST levels and liver function test results. Decreases granulocyte, leukocyte, thrombocyte, and RBC counts.

---

* "Tall Man" lettering   ✐ see color pill atlas   ✒ herb   underlined – top prescribed drug

AVAILABILITY (Rx)

INJECTION: 10 mg/ml (1-ml, 5-ml vials).

ADMINISTRATION/HANDLING

📋 IV

◀ ALERT ▶ Extremely important that IV needle or catheter is correctly positioned before administration. Leakage into surrounding tissue produces extreme irritation, local tissue necrosis, thrombophlebitis. Handle the drug with extreme care during administration; wear protective clothing per protocol. If solution comes in contact with skin or mucosa, wash immediately and thoroughly with soap, water.

Reconstitution • Must be diluted and administered via a syringe or IV bag.
SYRINGE DILUTION • Dilute calculated vinorelbine dose with D_5W or 0.9% NaCl to a concentration of 1.5–3 mg/ml.
IV BAG DILUTION • Dilute calculated vinorelbine dose with D_5W, 0.45% or 0.9% NaCl, 5% dextrose and 0.45% NaCl, Ringer's or lactated Ringer's to a concentration of 0.5–2 mg/ml.

Rate of administration • Administer diluted vinorelbine over 6–10 min into side port of free-flowing IV closest to IV bag followed by flushing with 75–125 ml of one of the solutions. • If extravasation occurs, stop injection immediately; give remaining portion of the dose into another vein.

Storage • Refrigerate unopened vials. • Protect from light. • Unopened vials are stable at room temperature for 72 hr. • Do not administer if particulate matter is noted. • Diluted vinorelbine may be used for up to 24 hr under normal room light when stored in polypropylene syringes or polyvinyl chloride bags at room temperature.

▨ IV INCOMPATIBILITIES

Acyclovir (Zovirax), allopurinol (Aloprim), amphotericin B (Fungizone), amphotericin B complex (Abelcet, AmBisome, Amphotec), ampicillin (Omnipen), cefazolin (Ancef), cefoperazone (Cefobid), cefotetan (Cefotan), ceftriaxone (Rocephin), cefuroxime (Zinacef), 5-fluorouracil, furosemide (Lasix), ganciclovir (Cytovene), methylprednisolone (Solu-Medrol), sodium bicarbonate.

IV COMPATIBILITIES

Calcium gluconate, carboplatin (Paraplatin), cisplatin (Platinol AQ), cyclophosphamide (Cytoxan), cytarabine (ARA-C, Cytosar), dacarbazine (DTIC-Dome), daunorubicin (Cerubidine), dexamethasone (Decadron), diphenhydramine (Benadryl), doxorubicin (Adriamycin), etoposide (VePesid), gemcitabine (Gemzar), granisetron (Kytril), hydromorphone (Dilaudid), idarubicin (Idamycin), methotrexate, morphine, ondansetron (Zofran), teniposide (Vumon), vinblastine (Velban), vincristine (Oncovin).

INDICATIONS/ROUTES/DOSAGE

UNRESECTABLE, ADVANCED NSCLC (AS MONOTHERAPY OR IN COMBINATION WITH CISPLATIN)
IV: ADULTS, ELDERLY: 30 mg/m² administered weekly over 6–10 min.

DOSAGE ADJUSTMENT GUIDELINES
Dosage adjustments should be based on granulocyte count obtained on the day of treatment, as follows:

Granulocyte count (cells/mm³) on Day of Treatment	Dose
1,500 or higher	30 mg/m²
1,000–1,499	15 mg/m²
Less than 1,000	Do not administer

COMBINATION THERAPY (WITH CISPLATIN)
IV INJECTION: ADULTS, ELDERLY: 25 mg/m² every wk or 30 mg/m² on days 1 and 29, then q6wk.

SIDE EFFECTS

FREQUENT: Asthenia (35%); mild or moderate nausea (34%); constipation (29%); erythema, pain, or vein discoloration at injection site (28%); fatigue (27%); peripheral neuropathy manifested as paraesthesia and hyperesthesia (25%); diarrhea (17%); alopecia (12%). **OCCASIONAL:** Phlebitis (10%), dyspnea (7%), loss of deep tendon reflexes (5%). **RARE:** Chest pain, jaw pain, myalgia, arthralgia, rash.

ADVERSE REACTIONS/ TOXIC EFFECTS

Bone marrow depression is manifested mainly as granulocytopenia, which may be severe. Other hematologic toxicities, including neutropenia, thrombocytopenia, leukopenia, and anemia, increase the risk of infection and bleeding. Acute shortness of breath and severe bronchospasm occur infrequently, particularly in patients with preexisting pulmonary dysfunction and in those receiving mitomycin concurrently.

NURSING CONSIDERATIONS

BASELINE ASSESSMENT

Review medication history. Assess hematology (CBC, platelet count, Hgb, differential) values before giving each dose. Granulocyte count should be at least 1,000 cells/mm^3 before vinorelbine administration. Granulocyte nadirs occur 7–10 days following dosing. Do not give hematologic growth factors within 24 hr before administration of chemotherapy or earlier than 24 hr following cytotoxic chemotherapy. Advise women of childbearing potential to avoid pregnancy during drug therapy.

INTERVENTION/EVALUATION

Diligently monitor injection site for swelling, redness, pain. Frequently monitor for myelosuppression both during and following therapy: infection (fever, sore throat, signs of local infection), unusual bleeding or ecchymoses, anemia (excessive fatigue, weakness). Monitor patients developing severe granulocytopenia for evidence of infection, fever. Crackers, dry toast, sips of cola may help relieve nausea. Assess pattern of bowel activity and stool consistency. Question for tingling, burning, numbness of hands or feet (peripheral neuropathy). Patient complaint of "walking on glass" is sign of hyperesthesia.

PATIENT/FAMILY TEACHING

• Notify nurse immediately if redness, swelling, pain occur at injection site. • Avoid crowds, those with infection. • Do not have immunizations without physician's approval. • Promptly report fever, signs of infection, unusual bruising or bleeding from any site, difficulty breathing. • Avoid pregnancy. • Alopecia is reversible, but new hair growth may have different color, texture.

Viracept, *see nelfinavir*

Viramune, *see nevirapine*

Viread, *see tenofovir*

Vistaril, *see hydroxyzine*

---

vitamin A

vight-ah-myn A

(Aquasol A, Palmitate A)

Do not confuse Aquasol A with Anusol.

CLASSIFICATION

PHARMACOTHERAPEUTIC: Fat-soluble vitamin. **CLINICAL:** Nutritional supplement (see p. 144C).

ACTION

A fat-soluble vitamin that may act as a cofactor in biochemical reactions. Therapeutic Effect: Is essential for normal function of retina, visual adaptation to darkness, bone growth, testicular and ovarian function, and embryonic development; preserves integrity of epithelial cells.

PHARMACOKINETICS

Rapidly absorbed from the GI tract if bile salts, pancreatic lipase, protein, and dietary fat are present. Transported in blood to the liver, where it's metabolized; stored in parenchymal hepatic cells, then transported in plasma as retinol, as needed. Excreted primarily in bile and, to a lesser extent, in urine.

USES

Treatment of vitamin A deficiency (biliary tract or pancreatic disease, sprue, colitis, hepatic cirrhosis, celiac disease, regional enteritis, extreme dietary inadequacy, partial gastrectomy, cystic fibrosis).

PRECAUTIONS

CONTRAINDICATIONS: Hypervitaminosis A, oral use in malabsorption syndrome. **CAUTIONS:** Renal impairment.

⏳ LIFESPAN CONSIDERATIONS: Pregnancy/Lactation: Crosses placenta. Distributed in breast milk. **Pregnancy Category A (X if used in doses above** recommended daily allowance). **Children/Elderly:** Caution with higher dosages.

INTERACTIONS

DRUG: **Cholestyramine, colestipol, mineral oil:** May decrease the absorption of vitamin A. **Isotretinoin:** May increase the risk of toxicity. HERBAL: None known. FOOD: None known. LAB VALUES: May increase BUN and serum cholesterol, calcium, and triglyceride levels. May decrease blood erythrocyte and leukocyte counts.

AVAILABILITY (Rx)

CAPSULES: 10,000 units, 25,000 units. **INJECTION (AQUASOL A):** 50,000 units/ml. **TABLETS (PALMITATE A):** 5,000 units, 15,000 units.

ADMINISTRATION/HANDLING

◄ ALERT ► IM administration used only in acutely ill or patients unresponsive to oral route (GI malabsorption syndrome).

IM
• For IM injection in adults, if dosage is 1 ml (50,000 international units), may give in deltoid muscle; if dosage is over 1 ml, give in large muscle mass. Anterolateral thigh is site of choice for infants, children younger than 7 mo.

PO
• Do not crush, break capsules. • Give without regard to food.

INDICATIONS/ROUTES/DOSAGE
SEVERE VITAMIN A DEFICIENCY

PO: ADULTS, ELDERLY, CHILDREN 8 YR AND OLDER: 500,000 units/day for 3 days; then 50,000 units/day for 14 days, then 10,000–20,000 units/day for 2 mo. CHILDREN 1–7 YR: 5,000 units/kg/day for 5 days, then 5,000–10,000 units/day for 2 mo. CHILDREN YOUNGER THAN 1 YR: 5,000–10,000 units/day for 2 mo.

V

IM: ADULTS, ELDERLY, CHILDREN 8 YR AND OLDER: 100,000 units/day for 3 days; then 50,000 units/day for 14 days. CHILDREN 1–7 YR: 17,500–35,000 units/day for 10 days. CHILDREN YOUNGER THAN 1 YR: 7,500–15,000 units/day.

MALABSORPTION SYNDROME
PO: ADULTS, ELDERLY, CHILDREN 8 YR AND OLDER: 10,000–50,000 units/day.

DIETARY SUPPLEMENT
PO: ADULTS, ELDERLY: 4,000–5,000 units/day. CHILDREN 7–10 YR: 3,300–3,500 units/day. CHILDREN 4–6 YR: 2,500 units/day. CHILDREN 6 MO–3 YR: 1,500–2,000 units/day. NEONATES YOUNGER THAN 5 MO: 1,500 units/day.

SIDE EFFECTS
None known.

ADVERSE REACTIONS/ TOXIC EFFECTS
Chronic overdose produces malaise, nausea, vomiting, drying or cracking of skin or lips, inflammation of tongue or gums, irritability, alopecia, and night sweats. Bulging fontanelles have occurred in infants.

NURSING CONSIDERATIONS

INTERVENTION/EVALUATION
Closely supervise for overdosage symptoms during prolonged daily administration over 25,000 international units. Monitor for therapeutic serum vitamin A levels (80–300 international units/ml).

PATIENT/FAMILY TEACHING
• Foods rich in vitamin A include cod, halibut, tuna, shark (naturally occurring vitamin A found only in animal sources). • Avoid taking mineral oil, cholestyramine (Questran) while taking vitamin A.

vitamin D
vight-ah-myn D

ergocalciferol

(Calciferol, Drisdol, Ostoforet ✦)

CLASSIFICATION
PHARMACOTHERAPEUTIC: Fat-soluble vitamin. **CLINICAL:** Nutritional supplement (see p. 145C).

ACTION
A fat-soluble vitamin that stimulates calcium and phosphate absorption from small intestine, promotes secretion of calcium from bone to blood, and promotes resorption of phosphate in renal tubules; also acts on bone cells to stimulate skeletal growth and on parathyroid gland to suppress hormone synthesis and secretion. **Therapeutic Effect:** Essential for absorption and utilization of calcium and phosphate and normal bone calcification. Reduces parathyroid hormone level. Improves phosphorus and calcium homeostasis in chronic renal failure.

PHARMACOKINETICS
Readily absorbed from small intestine. Concentrated primarily in liver and fat deposits. Activated in the liver and kidneys. Eliminated by biliary system; excreted in urine. **Half-life:** 19–48 hr for ergocalciferol.

USES
Prevention of osteoporosis. Treatment of rickets, hypophosphatemia, hypoparathyroidism. Dietary supplement.

PRECAUTIONS
CONTRAINDICATIONS: Abnormal sensitivity to toxic effects of hypervitaminosis D, hypercalcemia, malabsorption syndrome. **CAUTIONS:** Contrary artery disease, kidney stones, renal impairment.

⌛ **LIFESPAN CONSIDERATIONS:** Pregnancy/Lactation: Unknown if drug crosses placenta. Distributed in breast milk. **Pregnancy Category A (D if used in doses above recommended daily allowance). Children:** May be more sensitive to effects. **Elderly:** No age-related precautions noted.

INTERACTIONS

DRUG: Aluminum-containing antacids (long-term use): May increase aluminum blood concentration and risk of aluminum bone toxicity. **Calcium-containing preparations, thiazide diuretics:** May increase the risk of hypercalcemia. **Magnesium-containing antacids:** May increase magnesium blood concentration. **Mineral oil:** Excessive use of mineral oil decreases vitamin D absorption. **HERBAL:** None known. **FOOD:** None known. **LAB VALUES:** May increase serum cholesterol, calcium, magnesium, and phosphate levels. May decrease serum alkaline phosphatase level.

AVAILABILITY (Rx)

CAPSULES (DRISDOL): 50,000 units (1.25 mg). **INJECTION (CALCIFEROL):** 500,000 units/ml (12.5 mg). **ORAL LIQUID DROPS (CALCIFEROL, DRISDOL):** 8,000 units/ml.

ADMINISTRATION/HANDLING

PO
• Give without regard to food. • Swallow whole; do not crush/chew.

INDICATIONS/ROUTES/DOSAGE

◀ **ALERT** ▶ Oral dosing is preferred. Administer the drug IM only in patients with GI, hepatic, or biliary disease associated with malabsorption of vitamin D.

DIETARY SUPPLEMENT
PO: ADULTS, ELDERLY, CHILDREN: 10 mcg (400 units)/day. NEONATES: 10–20 mcg (400–800 units)/day.

RENAL FAILURE
PO: ADULTS, ELDERLY: 0.5 mg/day. CHILDREN: 0.1–1 mg/day.

HYPOPARATHYROIDISM
PO: ADULTS, ELDERLY: 625 mcg–5 mg/day (with calcium supplements). CHILDREN: 1.25–5 mg/day (with calcium supplements).

NUTRITIONAL RICKETS, OSTEOMALACIA
PO: ADULTS, ELDERLY, CHILDREN: 25–125 mcg/day for 8–12 wk. ADULTS, ELDERLY (WITH MALABSORPTION SYNDROME): 250–7,500 mcg/day. CHILDREN (WITH MALABSORPTION SYNDROME): 250–625 mcg/day.

VITAMIN D–DEPENDENT RICKETS
PO: ADULTS, ELDERLY: 250 mcg–1.5 mg/day. CHILDREN: 75–125 mcg/day. **Maximum:** 1,500 mcg/day.

VITAMIN D–RESISTANT RICKETS
PO: ADULTS, ELDERLY: 250–1,500 mcg/day (with phosphate supplements). CHILDREN: Initially 1,000–2,000 mcg/day (with phosphate supplements). May increase in 250- to 600-mcg increments q3–4mo.

OSTEOPOROSIS PREVENTION
PO: ADULTS, ELDERLY: 400–600 units/day. **Maximum:** 2,000 units/day.

SIDE EFFECTS

FREQUENCY NOT DEFINED: Nausea, constipation, stiffness, weakness, weight loss.

ADVERSE REACTIONS/TOXIC EFFECTS

Early signs and symptoms of overdose are weakness, headache, somnolence, nausea, vomiting, dry mouth, constipation, muscle and bone pain, and metallic taste. Later signs and symptoms of overdose include polyuria, polydipsia, anorexia, weight loss, nocturia, photophobia, rhinorrhea, pruritus, disorientation, hallucinations, hyperthermia, hypertension, and cardiac arrhythmias.

NURSING CONSIDERATIONS

BASELINE ASSESSMENT
Therapy should begin at lowest possible dosage.

INTERVENTION/EVALUATION
Monitor serum and urinary calcium levels, serum phosphate, magnesium, creatinine, alkaline phosphatase, BUN determinations (therapeutic serum calcium level: 9–10 mg/dl). Estimate daily dietary calcium intake. Encourage adequate fluid intake.

PATIENT/FAMILY TEACHING
• Encourage foods rich in vitamin D, including vegetable oils, vegetable shortening, margarine, leafy vegetables, milk, eggs, meats. • Do not take mineral oil while on vitamin D therapy. • If receiving chronic renal dialysis, do not take magnesium-containing antacids during vitamin D therapy. • Drink plenty of liquids.

vitamin E

vight-ah-myn E

(Aqua Gem E, Aquasol E, E-Gems, Key-E, Key-E Kaps)

Do not confuse Aquasol E with Anusol.

◆CLASSIFICATION

PHARMACOTHERAPEUTIC: Fat-soluble vitamin. **CLINICAL:** Nutritional supplement (see p. 145C).

ACTION
An antioxidant that prevents oxidation of vitamins A and C, protects fatty acids from attack by free radicals, and protects RBCs from hemolysis by oxidizing agents. **Therapeutic Effect:** Prevents and treats vitamin E deficiency.

PHARMACOKINETICS
Variably absorbed from the GI tract (requires bile salts, dietary fat, and normal pancreatic function). Primarily concentrated in adipose tissue. Metabolized in the liver. Primarily eliminated by biliary system.

USES
Treatment of vitamin E deficiency. **OFF-LABEL:** Prevention and treatment of Alzhemier's disease, tardive dyskinesia; reduces risk of bronchopulmonary dysplasia or retrolental fibroplasia in infants exposed to high concentrations of oxygen.

PRECAUTIONS
CONTRAINDICATIONS: None   known. **CAUTIONS:** None known.
⧗ **LIFESPAN CONSIDERATIONS: Pregnancy/Lactation:** Unknown if drug crosses placenta or is distributed in breast milk. **Pregnancy Category A (C if used in doses above recommended daily allowance). Children/Elderly:** No age-related precautions noted in normal dosages.

INTERACTIONS
DRUG: Cholestyramine, colestipol, mineral oil: May decrease the absorption of vitamin E. **Iron (large doses):** May increase vitamin E requirements. **HERBAL:** None known. **FOOD:** None known. **LAB VALUES:** None known.

AVAILABILITY (OTC)
CAPSULES: 100 units (E-Gems), 200 units (Aqua-Gem E, Key-E Kaps), 400 units (Aqua-Gem E, Key-E Kaps), 600 units (E-Gems), 800 units (E-Gems), 1,000 units (E-Gems), 1,200 units (E-Gems). **TABLETS (KEY-E):** 100 units, 200 units, 400 units, 800 units.

ADMINISTRATION/HANDLING

PO
• Do not crush, break tablets or capsules. • Give without regard to food.

INDICATIONS/ROUTES/DOSAGE

VITAMIN E DEFICIENCY
PO: ADULTS, ELDERLY: 60–75 units/day.
CHILDREN: 1 unit/kg/day.

SIDE EFFECTS

RARE: Contact dermatitis, sterile abscess.

ADVERSE REACTIONS/ TOXIC EFFECTS

Chronic overdose may produce fatigue, weakness, nausea, headache, blurred vision, flatulence, and diarrhea.

NURSING CONSIDERATIONS

PATIENT/FAMILY TEACHING
• Swallow capsules whole; do not crush, chew. • Toxicity consists of blurred vision, diarrhea, dizziness, nausea, headache, flu-like symptoms. • Encourage foods rich in vitamin E, including vegetable oils, vegetable shortening, margarine, leafy vegetables, milk, eggs, meat.

vitamin K

vight-ah-myn K

phytonadione
(vitamin K₁)

(AquaMEPHYTON, Konakion ✦, Mephyton, Vitamin K1)
Do not confuse Mephyton with melphalan or mephenytoin.

CLASSIFICATION

PHARMACOTHERAPEUTIC: Fat-soluble vitamin. **CLINICAL:** Nutritional supplement, antidote (drug-induced hypoprothrombinemia), antihemorrhagic.

ACTION

A fat-soluble vitamin that promotes hepatic formation of coagulation factors II, VII, IX, and X. **Therapeutic Effect:** Essential for normal clotting of blood.

PHARMACOKINETICS

Readily absorbed from the GI tract (duodenum) after IM or subcutaneous administration. Metabolized in the liver. Excreted in urine; eliminated by biliary system. Onset of action: with PO form, 6–10 hr; with parenteral form, hemorrhage controlled in 3–6 hr and PT returns to normal in 12–14 hr.

USES

Prevention, treatment of hemorrhagic states in neonates; antidote for hemorrhage induced by oral anticoagulants, hypoprothrombinemic states due to vitamin K deficiency. Will not counteract anticoagulation effect of heparin.

PRECAUTIONS

CONTRAINDICATIONS: None known.
CAUTIONS: None known.

⊠ **LIFESPAN CONSIDERATIONS: Pregnancy/Lactation:** Crosses placenta. Distributed in breast milk. **Pregnancy Category C. Children/Elderly:** No age-related precautions noted.

INTERACTIONS

DRUG: Broad-spectrum antibiotics, high-dose salicylates: May increase vitamin K requirements. **Cholestyramine, colestipol, mineral oil, sucralfate:** May decrease the absorption of vitamin K. **Oral anticoagulants:** May decrease the effects of these drugs. **HERBAL:** None known. **FOOD:** None known. **LAB VALUES:** None known.

AVAILABILITY (Rx)

TABLETS (MEPHYTON): 5 mg. **INJECTION (AQUAMEPHYTON, VITAMIN K1):** 1 mg/ 0.5 ml, 10 mg/ml.

ADMINISTRATION/HANDLING

 IV

◀ **ALERT** ▶   Restrict to emergency use only.

Reconstitution • May dilute with preservative-free NaCl or D_5W immediately before use. Do not use other diluents. Discard unused portions.

Rate of administration • Administer slow IV at rate of 1 mg/min. • Monitor continuously for hypersensitivity, anaphylactic reaction during and immediately following IV administration.

Storage • Store at room temperature.

IM, SUBCUTANEOUS
• Inject into anterolateral aspect of thigh or deltoid region.

PO
• Scored tablets may be crushed.

▨ IV INCOMPATIBILITIES
No known incompatibilities for Y-site administration.

IV COMPATIBILITIES
Heparin, potassium chloride.

INDICATIONS/ROUTES/DOSAGE

ORAL ANTICOAGULANT OVERDOSE
PO, IV, SUBCUTANEOUS: ADULTS, ELDERLY: 2.5–10 mg/dose. May repeat in 12–48 hr if given orally and in 6–8 hr if given by IV or subcutaneous route. CHILDREN: 0.5–5 mg depending on need for further anticoagulation and severity of bleeding.

VITAMIN K DEFICIENCY
PO: ADULTS, ELDERLY: 2.5–25 mg/24 hr. CHILDREN: 2.5–5 mg/24 hr.

IV, IM, SUBCUTANEOUS: ADULTS, ELDERLY: 10 mg/dose. CHILDREN: 1–2 mg/ dose.

HEMORRHAGIC DISEASE OF NEWBORN
IM, SUBCUTANEOUS: NEONATE: **Treatment:** 1–2 mg/dose/day. **Prophylaxis:** 0.5–1 mg within 1 hr of birth; may repeat in 6–8 hr if necessary.

SIDE EFFECTS

OCCASIONAL: Pain, soreness, and swelling at IM injection site; pruritic erythema (with repeated injections); facial flushing; unusual taste.

ADVERSE REACTIONS/ TOXIC EFFECTS

Newborns (especially premature infants) may develop hyperbilirubinemia. A severe reaction (cramplike pain, chest pain, dyspnea, facial flushing, dizziness, rapid or weak pulse, rash, diaphoresis, hypotension progressing to shock, cardiac arrest) occurs rarely just after IV administration.

NURSING CONSIDERATIONS

INTERVENTION/EVALUATION
Monitor PT, INR routinely in those taking anticoagulants. Assess skin for ecchymoses, petechiae. Assess gums for gingival bleeding, erythema. Assess urine for hematuria. Assess Hct, platelet count, urine and stool culture for occult blood. Assess for decrease in BP, increase in pulse rate, complaint of abdominal or back pain, severe headache (may be evidence of hemorrhage). Question for increase in amount of discharge during menses. Assess peripheral pulses. Check for excessive bleeding from minor cuts, scratches.

PATIENT/FAMILY TEACHING
• Discomfort may occur with parenteral administration. • **Adults:** Use electric razor, soft toothbrush to prevent bleeding. • Report any sign of red or dark urine, black or red stool, coffee-ground

---

vomitus, red-speckled mucus from cough. • Do not use any OTC medication without physician approval (may interfere with platelet aggregation). • Encourage foods rich in vitamin K_1, including leafy green vegetables, meat, cow's milk, vegetable oil, egg yolks, tomatoes.

Vivelle-DOT, see

estradiol

---

voriconazole

vohr-ee-**con**-ah-zole
(Vfend)

• CLASSIFICATION

PHARMACOTHERAPEUTIC: Triazole derivative. **CLINICAL:** Antifungal.

ACTION

A triazole derivative that inhibits the synthesis of ergosterol, a vital component of fungal cell wall formation. **Therapeutic Effect:** Damages fungal cell wall membrane.

PHARMACOKINETICS

Rapidly and completely absorbed after PO administration. Widely distributed. Protein binding: 98%. Metabolized in the liver. Primarily excreted as a metabolite in urine. **Half-life:** 6 hr.

USES

Treatment of invasive aspergillosis, esophageal candidiasis. Treatment of serious fungal infections caused by *Scedosporium apiospermum* and *Fusarium* spp. Treatment of candidemia in non-neutropenic patients.

PRECAUTIONS

CONTRAINDICATIONS: Concurrent administration of carbamazepine; ergot alkaloids; pimozide or quinidine (may cause prolonged QT interval or torsades de pointes); rifabutin; rifampin; or sirolimus. **CAUTIONS:** Renal or hepatic impairment, hypersensitivity to other antifungal agents.

⧗ **LIFESPAN CONSIDERATIONS:** **Pregnancy/Lactation:** May cause fetal harm. **Pregnancy Category D. Children:** Safety and efficacy not established in those younger than 12 yr. **Elderly:** No age-related precautions noted.

INTERACTIONS

DRUG: **Cyclosporine, omeprazole, phenytoin, rifabutin, sirolimus, tacrilimus, warfarin:** May increase plasma concentrations of these drugs. **Phenytoin, rifabutin, rifampin:** May decrease voriconazole plasma concentration. **HERBAL:** None known. **FOOD:** None known. **LAB VALUES:** May increase serum alkaline phosphatase and ALT levels.

AVAILABILITY (Rx)

TABLETS: 50 mg, 200 mg. **INJECTION POWDER FOR RECONSTITUTION:** 200 mg. **POWDER FOR ORAL SUSPENSION:** 200 mg/5 ml.

ADMINISTRATION/HANDLING

🖫 **IV**

Reconstitution • Reconstitute 200-mg vial with 19 ml sterile water for injection to provide a concentration of 10 mg/ml. Further dilute with 0.9% NaCl or D_5W to provide a concentration of 5 mg or less/ml.

Rate of administration • Infuse over 1–2 hr at a concentration of 5 mg or less/ml.

V

Storage • Store powder for injection at room temperature. • Use reconstituted solution immediately. • Do not use after 24 hr when refrigerated.

PO
• Take 1 hr before or 1 hr after a meal.

PO (ORAL SUSPENSION)

• Do not mix oral suspension or reconstituted oral suspension with any other medication or flavoring agent. • The suspension should not be diluted with water or fluids.

▦ IV INCOMPATIBILITY
Total parenteral nutrition (TPN).

INDICATIONS/ROUTES/DOSAGE
INVASIVE ASPERGILLOSIS, OTHER SERIOUS FUNGAL INFECTIONS CAUSED BY *SCEDOSPORIUM APIOSPERMUM* AND *FUSARIUM* SPECIES
PO: ADULTS, ELDERLY WEIGHING 40 KG AND MORE: Initially, 400 mg q12h for 2 doses on day 1. Maintenance: 200 mg q12h (may increase to 200 mg q12h). ADULTS, ELDERLY WEIGHING LESS THAN 40 KG: Initially, 200 mg q12h for 2 doses on day 1. Maintenance: 100 mg q12h (may increase to 150 mg q12h).

USUAL PARENTERAL DOSAGE
IV: ADULTS, ELDERLY, CHILDREN: Initially, 6 mg/kg/dose q12h for 2 doses, then 4 mg/kg/dose q12h (may decrease to 3 mg/kg/dose if patient is unable to tolerate 4 mg/kg/dose).

CANDIDEMIA IN NON-NEUTROPENIC PATIENTS
PO: ADULTS, ELDERLY: 200 mg q12h.
IV: ADULTS, ELDERLY: Initially, 6 mg/kg/dose q12h for 2 doses, then 3–4 mg/kg/dose q12h.

ESOPHAGEAL CANDIDIASIS
PO: ADULTS, ELDERLY WEIGHING 40 KG AND MORE: 200 mg q12h for minimum of 14 days, then at least 7 days following resolution of symptoms. ADULTS, ELDERLY WEIGHING LESS THAN 40 KG: 100 mg q12h for minimum 14 days, then at least 7 days following resolution of symptoms.

SIDE EFFECTS
FREQUENT (20%–5%): Abnormal vision, fever, nausea, rash, vomiting. **OCCASIONAL (5%–2%):** Headache, chills, hallucinations, photophobia, tachycardia, hypertension.

ADVERSE REACTIONS/ TOXIC EFFECTS
Hepatotoxicity (e.g., jaundice, hepatitis, hepatic failure, acute renal failure) has been observed in severely ill patients.

NURSING CONSIDERATIONS

BASELINE ASSESSMENT
Obtain baseline serum liver and renal function tests.

INTERVENTION/EVALUATION
Monitor serum liver and renal function tests. Monitor visual function (visual acuity, visual field, color perception) for drug therapy lasting longer than 28 days.

PATIENT/FAMILY TEACHING
• Take at least 1 hr before or 1 hr after a meal. • Avoid driving at night. • May cause visual changes (blurred vision, photophobia). • Avoid performing hazardous tasks if changes in vision occur. • Avoid direct sunlight. • Women of childbearing potential should use effective contraception.

warfarin sodium ▷

war-far-in

(Apo-Warfarin ✤, <u>Coumadin</u>, Gen-Warfarin ✤, Jantoven, Tar-Warfarin ✤)

Do not confuse Coumadin with Kemadrin.

◆ CLASSIFICATION

PHARMACOTHERAPEUTIC: Coumarin derivative. **CLINICAL:** Anticoagulant (see p. 30C).

ACTION

A coumarin derivative that interferes with hepatic synthesis of vitamin K–dependent clotting factors, resulting in depletion of coagulation factors II, VII, IX, and X. Therapeutic Effect: Prevents further extension of formed existing clot; prevents new clot formation or secondary thromboembolic complications.

PHARMACOKINETICS

Route	Onset	Peak	Duration
PO	1.5–3 days	5–7 days	N/A

Well absorbed from the GI tract. Metabolized in the liver. Primarily excreted in urine. Not removed by hemodialysis. Half-life: 1.5–2.5 days.

USES

Anticoagulant, including the following: Prophylaxis, treatment of venous thrombosis, pulmonary embolism. Treatment of thromboembolism associated with chronic atrial fibrillation. Adjunct in treatment of coronary occlusion. Prophylaxis and treatment of thromboembolic complications associated with cardiac valve replacement. Reduces risk of death, recurrent MI, stroke, embolization after MI. OFF-LABEL: Prevention of myocardial infarction, recurrent cerebral embolism; treatment adjunct in transient ischemic attacks.

PRECAUTIONS

CONTRAINDICATIONS: Neurosurgical procedures, open wounds, pregnancy, severe hypertension, severe hepatic or renal damage, spinal puncture, uncontrolled bleeding, ulcers. **CAUTIONS:** Active tuberculosis, diabetes, heparin-induced thrombocytopenia, those at risk for hemorrhage, necrosis, gangrene. ⌛ LIFESPAN CONSIDERATIONS: Pregnancy/Lactation: Contraindicated in pregnancy (fetal or neonatal hemorrhage, intrauterine death). Crosses placenta; is distributed in breast milk. **Pregnancy Category D. Children:** More susceptible to effects. **Elderly:** Increased risk of hemorrhage; lower dosage recommended.

INTERACTIONS

DRUG: **Acetaminophen, allopurinol, amiodarone, anabolic steroids, androgens, aspirin, cefamandole, cefoperazone, chloral hydrate, chloramphenicol, cimetidine, clofibrate, danazol, dextrothyroxine, diflunisal, disulfiram, erythromycin, fenoprofen, gemfibrozil, indomethacin, methimazole, metronidazole, oral hypoglycemics, phenytoin, plicamycin, propylthiouracil, quinidine, salicylates, sulfinpyrazone, sulfonamides, sulindac:** Warfarin increases the effects of these drugs. **Alcohol:** May enhance warfarin's anticoagulant effect. **Barbiturates, carbamazepine, cholestyramine, colestipol, estramustine, estrogens, griseofulvin, primidone, rifampin, vitamin K:** Warfarin decreases the effects of these drugs. HERBAL: **American ginseng, St. John's wort:** May decrease the effectiveness of warfarin. **Feverfew,**

✤ Canadian trade name   © see **evolve**   ▷ High Alert drug

W

garlic, ginkgo biloba, ginseng, glucosamine-chondroitin: May increase the risk of bleeding. FOOD: None known. LAB VALUES: None known.

AVAILABILITY (Rx)

TABLETS (COUMADIN, JANTOVEN): 1 mg, 2 mg, 2.5 mg, 3 mg, 4 mg, 5 mg, 6 mg, 7.5 mg, 10 mg.

ADMINISTRATION/HANDLING

PO
• Scored tablets may be crushed. • Give without regard to food. Give with food if GI upset occurs.

INDICATIONS/ROUTES/DOSAGE

ANTICOAGULANT
PO: ADULTS, ELDERLY: Initially, 5–15 mg/day for 2–5 days; then adjust based on INR. Maintenance: 2–10 mg/day. CHILDREN: Initially, 0.1–0.2 mg/kg (**maximum** 10 mg). Maintenance: 0.05–0.34 mg/kg/day.

USUAL ELDERLY DOSAGE (MAINTENANCE)
PO, IV: ELDERLY: 2–5 mg/day.

SIDE EFFECTS

OCCASIONAL: GI distress, such as nausea, anorexia, abdominal cramps, diarrhea. **RARE:** Hypersensitivity reaction, including dermatitis and urticaria, especially in those sensitive to aspirin.

ADVERSE REACTIONS/ TOXIC EFFECTS

Bleeding complications ranging from local ecchymoses to major hemorrhage may occur. Drug should be discontinued immediately and vitamin K or phytonadione administered. Mild hemorrhage: 2.5–10 mg PO, IM, or IV. Severe hemorrhage: 10–15 mg IV and repeated q4h, as necessary. Hepatotoxicity, blood dyscrasias, necrosis, vasculitis, and local thrombosis occur rarely.

NURSING CONSIDERATIONS

BASELINE ASSESSMENT
Cross-check dose with coworker. Determine INR before administration and daily following therapy initiation. When stabilized, follow with INR determination q4–6wk.

INTERVENTION/EVALUATION
Monitor INR reports diligently. Assess Hct, platelet count, urine and stool culture for occult blood, AST, ALT, regardless of route of administration. Be alert to complaints of abdominal or back pain, severe headache (may be signs of hemorrhage). Decrease in BP, increase in pulse rate may also be sign of hemorrhage. Question for increase in amount of discharge during menses. Assess area of thromboembolus for color, temperature. Assess peripheral pulses; skin for ecchymoses, petechiae. Check for excessive bleeding from minor cuts, scratches. Assess gums for erythema, gingival bleeding. Assess urine output for hematuria.

PATIENT/FAMILY TEACHING
• Take medication exactly as prescribed. • Do not take or discontinue any other medication except on advice of physician. • Avoid alcohol, salicylates, drastic dietary changes. • Do not change from one brand to another. • Consult with physician before surgery or dental work. • Urine may become red-orange. • Notify physician if bleeding, bruising, red or brown urine, black stools occur. • Use electric razor, soft toothbrush to prevent bleeding. • Report coffeeground vomitus, blood-tinged mucus from cough. • Do not use any OTC medication without physician approval (may interfere with platelet aggregation).

Wellbutrin, *see* *bupropion*

Wellbutrin SR, *see* *bupropion*

Xanax, *see alprazolam*

Xeloda, *see capecitabine*

Xifaxan, *see rifaximin*

Xigris, *see drotrecogin alfa*

Xopenex, *see levalbuterol*

yohimbe

Also known as aphrodien, corynine, johimbi.

CLASSIFICATION
HERBAL: See Appendix G.

ACTION
Produces genital blood vessel dilation, improves nerve impulse transmission to genital area. Increases penile blood flow, central sympathetic excitation impulses to genital tissues. **Effect:** Improves sexual function, affects impotence.

USES
May be used as an aphrodisiac by some cultures. Used to improve libido, enhance sexual function in male. Also used to manage symptoms associated with diabetic neuropathy, postural hypotension.

PRECAUTIONS
CONTRAINDICATIONS: Pregnancy or lactation (may have uterine relaxant effect, cause fetal toxicity), angina, heart disease, benign prostatic hypertrophy (BPH), depression, renal/hepatic disease. **CAUTIONS:** Anxiety, diabetes mellitus, hypertension, post-traumatic stress disorder (PSTD), schizophrenia.

⧗ **LIFESPAN CONSIDERATIONS: Pregnancy/Lactation:** Contraindicated; avoid use. **Children:** Safety and efficacy not established; avoid use. **Elderly:** Age-related renal/hepatic impairment may require discontinuing.

INTERACTIONS
DRUG: Antihypertensives drugs for diabetes: Yohimbe use may interfere with these drugs. **Clonidine:** Effects may be antagonized. **MAOIs, sympathomimetics, tricyclic antidepressants:** Have additive effects. **HERBAL: Ginkgo biloba, St. John's wort:** Can have additive therapeutic/adverse effects. **FOOD: Tyramine-containing foods (e.g., aged cheese, chianti wine), caffeine-containing products, coffee, tea, chocolate:** May increase

risk of hypertensive crises. **LAB VALUES:** None known.

AVAILABILITY (OTC)
TABLETS: 5 mg. **LIQUID:** 5 mg/5 ml.

INDICATIONS/ROUTES/DOSAGE
IMPOTENCE
PO: ADULTS, ELDERLY: 15–30 mg a day in divided doses.

SIDE EFFECTS
Excitement, tremors, insomnia, anxiety, hypertension, tachycardia, dizziness, headache, irritability, salivation, dilated pupils, nausea, vomiting, hypersensitivity reaction.

ADVERSE REACTIONS/ TOXIC EFFECTS
Paralysis, severe hypotension, irregular heartbeat, cardiac failure. Overdose can be fatal.

NURSING CONSIDERATIONS

BASELINE ASSESSMENT
Assess if patient is pregnant or breast-feeding (contraindicated). Determine other medical conditions, including angina, heart disease, benign prostatic hypertrophy. Assess baseline serum renal/hepatic function, medications (see Interactions).

INTERVENTION/EVALUATION
Monitor serum renal/hepatic function, BP. Assess for hypersensitivity reaction.

PATIENT/FAMILY TEACHING
• Do not use other OTC or prescribed medications before checking with physician. • Inform physician if pregnant or breast-feeding.

zafirlukast
za-**feer**-loo-kast
(Accolate)
Do not confuse Accolate with Accupril or Aclovate.

CLASSIFICATION
PHARMACOTHERAPEUTIC: Leukotriene receptor antagonist. **CLINICAL:** Antiasthma (see p. 68C).

ACTION
An antiasthmatic that binds to leukotriene receptors, inhibiting bronchoconstriction due to sulfur dioxide, cold air, and specific antigens, such as grass, cat dander, and ragweed. Therapeutic Effect: Reduces airway edema and smooth muscle constriction; alters cellular activity associated with the inflammatory process.

PHARMACOKINETICS
Rapidly absorbed after PO administration (food reduces absorption). Protein binding: 99%. Extensively metabolized in the liver. Primarily excreted in feces. Unknown if removed by hemodialysis. Half-life: 10 hr.

USES
Prophylaxis, chronic treatment of bronchial asthma. OFF-LABEL: Exercise-induced bronchospasm.

PRECAUTIONS
CONTRAINDICATIONS: None known. **CAUTIONS:** Hepatic impairment.
⌛ LIFESPAN CONSIDERATIONS: Pregnancy/Lactation: Drug is distributed in breast milk. Do not administer to breast-feeding women. **Pregnancy Category B. Children:** Safety and efficacy not established in those younger than 5 yr. **Elderly:** No age-related precautions noted.

Z

INTERACTIONS

DRUG: **Aspirin:** Increases zafirlukast blood concentration. **Erythromycin, theophylline:** Decreases zafirlukast blood concentration. **Warfarin:** Increases PT. HERBAL: None known. FOOD: None known. LAB VALUES: May increase ALT level.

AVAILABILITY (Rx)

TABLETS: 10 mg, 20 mg.

ADMINISTRATION/HANDLING

PO
• Give 1 hr before or 2 hr after meals.
• Do not crush, break tablets.

INDICATIONS/ROUTES/DOSAGE

BRONCHIAL ASTHMA
PO: ADULTS, ELDERLY, CHILDREN 12 YR AND OLDER: 20 mg twice a day. CHILDREN 5–11 YR: 10 mg twice a day.

SIDE EFFECTS

FREQUENT (13%): Headache. OCCASIONAL (3%): Nausea, diarrhea. RARE (less than 3%): Generalized pain, asthenia, myalgia, fever, dyspepsia, vomiting, dizziness.

ADVERSE REACTIONS/ TOXIC EFFECTS

Concurrent administration of inhaled corticosteroids increases the risk of upper respiratory tract infection.

NURSING CONSIDERATIONS

BASELINE ASSESSMENT

Obtain medication history. Assess serum liver function lab values.

INTERVENTION/EVALUATION

Monitor rate, depth, rhythm, type of respiration; quality, rate of pulse. Assess lung sounds for rhonchi, wheezing, rales. Observe for cyanosis (lips, fingernails appear blue or dusky color in light-skinned patients; gray in dark-skinned patients). Monitor serum liver function tests.

PATIENT/FAMILY TEACHING

• Increase fluid intake (decreases lung secretion viscosity). • Take as prescribed, even during symptom-free periods. • Do not use for acute asthma episodes. • Do not alter or stop other asthma medications. • Do not breast-feed. • Report nausea, jaundice, abdominal pain, flu-like symptoms, worsening of asthma.

zalcitabine

zal-**site**-a-been
(Hivid)

CLASSIFICATION

PHARMACOTHERAPEUTIC: Nucleoside reverse transcriptase inhibitor. CLINICAL: Antiretroviral (see pp. 62C, 103C).

ACTION

A nucleoside reverse transcriptase inhibitor that inhibits viral DNA synthesis. Therapeutic Effect: Prevents replication of HIV-1.

PHARMACOKINETICS

Readily absorbed from the GI tract (absorption decreased by food). Protein binding: less than 4%. Undergoes phosphorylation intracellularly to the active metabolite. Primarily excreted in urine. Removed by hemodialysis. Half-life: 1–3 hr; metabolite, 2.6–10 hr (increased in impaired renal function).

USES

Treatment of HIV infection in combination with other antiretroviral agents.

PRECAUTIONS

CONTRAINDICATIONS: Moderate or severe peripheral neuropathy. EXTREME CAUTION: Those with low CD4 cell counts (risk of peripheral neuropathy is greater), preexisting neuropathy. **CAUTIONS:** Preexisting peripheral neuropathy, diabetes, weight loss, history of hepatic disease, alcohol abuse, renal impairment.

⧖ **LIFESPAN CONSIDERATIONS: Pregnancy/Lactation:** Unknown if drug crosses placenta or is distributed in breast milk. Avoid breast-feeding in HIV-positive women. **Pregnancy Category C. Children:** No age-related precautions in those younger than 6 mo, dosage not established. **Elderly:** Age-related renal impairment may require dosage adjustment.

INTERACTIONS

DRUG: Medications associated with peripheral neuropathy (including cisplatin, disulfiram, phenytoin, vincristine): May increase the risk of neuropathy. **Medications causing pancreatitis (including IV pentamidine):** May increase the risk of pancreatitis. **HERBAL:** None known. **FOOD:** None known. **LAB VALUES:** May increase serum alkaline phosphatase, amylase, bilirubin, lipase, AST, ALT, and triglyceride levels. May decrease serum calcium, magnesium, and phosphate levels. May alter blood glucose and sodium levels.

AVAILABILITY (Rx)

TABLETS: 0.375 mg, 0.75 mg.

ADMINISTRATION/HANDLING

PO

• Best taken on empty stomach (food decreases absorption). • May take with food to decrease GI distress. • Space doses evenly around the clock.

INDICATIONS/ROUTES/DOSAGE

HIV INFECTION (IN COMBINATION WITH OTHER ANTIRETROVIRALS)

PO: ADULTS, CHILDREN 13 YR AND OLDER: 0.75 mg q8h. CHILDREN YOUNGER THAN

13 YR: 0.01 mg/kg q8h. Range: 0.005–0.01 mg/kg q8h.

DOSAGE IN RENAL IMPAIRMENT

Dosage and frequency are modified based on creatinine clearance.

Creatinine Clearance	Dose
10–40 ml/min	0.75 mg q12h
Less than 10 ml/min	0.75 mg q24h

SIDE EFFECTS

FREQUENT (28%–11%): Peripheral neuropathy, fever, fatigue, headache, rash. **OCCASIONAL (10%–5%):** Diarrhea, abdominal pain, oral ulcers, cough, pruritus, myalgia, weight loss, nausea, vomiting. **RARE (4%–1%):** Nasal discharge, dysphagia, depression, night sweats, confusion.

ADVERSE REACTIONS/ TOXIC EFFECTS

Peripheral neuropathy (characterized by numbness, tingling, burning, and pain in the lower extremities) occurs in 17% to 31% of patients. These symptoms may be followed by sharp, shooting pain and progress to a severe, continuous, burning pain that may be irreversible if the drug is not discontinued in time. Pancreatitis, leukopenia, neutropenia, eosinophilia, and thrombocytopenia occur rarely.

NURSING CONSIDERATIONS

BASELINE ASSESSMENT

Monitor CBC, serum triglycerides, amylase levels before and during therapy.

INTERVENTION/EVALUATION

Stop medication, notify physician immediately if signs or symptoms of peripheral neuropathy develop: numbness, tingling, burning, shooting pains of extremities; loss of vibratory sense or ankle reflex. Although rare, be alert to impending potentially fatal pancreatitis: increasing serum amylase, rising serum triglycerides, nausea, vomiting, abdominal pain (withhold medication, notify physician). Assess for therapeutic response: weight gain, increased energy, decreased fatigue. Assess CBC for evidence of blood dyscrasias. Offer emotional support to patient, family.

PATIENT/FAMILY TEACHING

• Zalcitabine is not a cure for HIV, nor does it reduce the risk of transmission to others; patient may continue to contract opportunistic illnesses associated with advanced HIV infection. • Does not preclude the need to continue practices to prevent transmission of HIV. • Report promptly any signs or symptoms of peripheral neuropathy or pancreatitis. • Women of childbearing age should use contraception.

zaleplon

zal-e-plon
(Sonata, Stamoc ✤)

◆CLASSIFICATION

PHARMACOTHERAPEUTIC: Nonbenzodiazepine. **CLINICAL:** Hypnotic (see p. 136C).

ACTION

A nonbenzodiazepine that enhances the action of the inhibitory neurotransmitter gamma-aminobutyric acid. **Therapeutic Effect:** Induces sleep.

PHARMACOKINETICS

Rapidly and almost completely absorbed following PO administration. Protein binding: 60%. Metabolized in liver. Primarily excreted in urine. Partially eliminated in feces. **Half-life:** 1 hr.

USES

Short-term treatment of insomnia (7–10 days). Decreases sleep onset time (no effect on number of nocturnal awakenings, total sleep time).

PRECAUTIONS

CONTRAINDICATIONS: Severe hepatic impairment. **CAUTIONS:** Mild to moderate hepatic function impairment in patients experiencing signs and symptoms of depression, those hypersensitive to aspirin (allergic-type reaction). ⌛ **LIFESPAN CONSIDERATIONS: Pregnancy/Lactation:** Unknown if drug crosses placenta; is distributed in breast milk. **Pregnancy Category C. Children:** Safety and efficacy not established. **Elderly:** May be more sensitive to zaleplon effects.

INTERACTIONS

DRUG: Alcohol, other CNS depressants: May increase CNS depression. **Cimetidine:** May increase the effect of zaleplon. **Rifampin:** Decreases the zaleplon blood concentration. **HERBAL:** None known. **FOOD: High-fat, heavy meals:** May delay onset of sleep by approximately 2 hr. **LAB VALUES:** None known.

AVAILABILITY (Rx)

CAPSULES: 5 mg, 10 mg.

ADMINISTRATION/HANDLING

PO
• Giving drug with or immediately after a high-fat meal results in slower absorption. • Capsules may be emptied and mixed with food.

INDICATIONS/ROUTES/DOSAGE

INSOMNIA
PO: ADULTS, ELDERLY: 10 mg at bedtime. Range: 5–20 mg. ELDERLY: 5 mg at bedtime.

SIDE EFFECTS

EXPECTED: Somnolence, sedation, mild rebound insomnia (on first night after drug is discontinued). **FREQUENT (28%–7%):** Nausea, headache, myalgia, dizziness. **OCCASIONAL (5%–3%):** Abdominal pain, asthenia, dyspepsia, eye pain, paresthesia. **RARE (2%):** Tremors, amnesia, hyperacusis (acute sense of hearing), fever, dysmenorrhea.

ADVERSE REACTIONS/ TOXIC EFFECTS

Zaleplon may produce altered concentration, behavior changes, and impaired memory. Taking the drug while up and about may result in adverse CNS effects, such as hallucinations, impaired coordination, dizziness, and light-headedness. Overdose results in somnolence, confusion, diminished reflexes, and coma.

NURSING CONSIDERATIONS

BASELINE ASSESSMENT
Raise bed rails. Provide environment conducive to sleep (back rub, quiet environment, low lighting).

INTERVENTION/EVALUATION
Assess sleep pattern.

PATIENT/FAMILY TEACHING
• Take right before bedtime or when in bed and not falling asleep. • Avoid tasks that require alertness, motor skills until response to drug is established. • Do not exceed prescribed dosage. • Do not take with or immediately after a high-fat or heavy meal. • Rebound insomnia may occur when drug is discontinued after short-term therapy. • Avoid alcohol, other CNS depressants.

Zanaflex, *see tizanidine*

---

zanamivir

zah-**nam**-ih-vur
(Relenza)

CLASSIFICATION

PHARMACOTHERAPEUTIC: Antiviral. **CLINICAL:** Anti-influenza (see p. 62C).

ACTION

An antiviral that appears to inhibit the influenza virus enzyme neuraminidase, which is essential for viral replication. **Therapeutic Effect:** Prevents viral release from infected cells.

PHARMACOKINETICS

Systemically absorbed, approximately 4%–17%. Protein binding: Low. Not metabolized. Partially excreted unchanged in urine. **Half-life:** 1.6–5.1 hr.

USES

Treatment of uncomplicated acute illness due to influenza virus in adults, adolescents 7 yr and older who have been symptomatic for less than 2 days. Prevention of influenza A and B. **OFF-LABEL:** Influenza prophylaxis.

PRECAUTIONS

CONTRAINDICATIONS: None known. **CAUTIONS:** Chronic obstructive pulmonary disease (COPD), asthma. **LIFESPAN CONSIDERATIONS: Pregnancy/Lactation:** Unknown if drug crosses placenta or is distributed is breast milk. **Pregnancy Category B. Children:** Safety and efficacy not established in children younger than 7 yr. **Elderly:** No age-related precautions noted.

INTERACTIONS

DRUG: None known. **HERBAL:** None known. **FOOD:** None known. **LAB VALUES:** May increase serum creatine kinase (CK) level and liver function test results.

AVAILABILITY (Rx)

POWDER FOR INHALATION: 5 mg/blister.

ADMINISTRATION/HANDLING
INHALATION
• Instruct the patient to use the Diskhaler device provided, exhale

---

completely; then, holding mouthpiece 1 inch away from lips, inhale and hold breath as long as possible before exhaling. • Rinse mouth with water immediately after inhalation (prevents mouth/throat dryness). • Store at room temperature.

INDICATIONS/ROUTES/DOSAGE

INFLUENZA VIRUS
INHALATION: ADULTS, ELDERLY, CHILDREN 7 YR AND OLDER: 2 inhalations (one 5-mg blister per inhalation for a total dose of 10 mg) twice a day (approximately 12 hr apart) for 5 days.

PREVENTION OF INFLUENZA VIRUS
INHALATION: ADULTS, ELDERLY: 2 inhalations once a day for the duration of the exposure period.

SIDE EFFECTS

OCCASIONAL (3%–2%): Diarrhea, sinusitis, nausea, bronchitis, cough, dizziness, headache. **RARE (less than 1.5%):** Malaise, fatigue, fever, abdominal pain, myalgia, arthralgia, urticaria.

ADVERSE REACTIONS/ TOXIC EFFECTS

Neutropenia may occur. Bronchospasm may occur in those with a history of COPD or bronchial asthma.

NURSING CONSIDERATIONS

BASELINE ASSESSMENT
Patients requiring an inhaled bronchodilator at the same time as zanamivir should use the bronchodilator before zanamivir administration.

INTERVENTION/EVALUATION
Provide assistance if dizziness occurs. Monitor pattern of bowel activity and stool consistency.

PATIENT/FAMILY TEACHING
• Instruct on use of delivery device.
• Avoid contact with those who are at high risk for influenza. • Continue treatment for the full 5-day course. • Doses should be evenly spaced. • In patients with respiratory disease, an inhaled bronchodilator should be readily available.

Zantac, *see ranitidine*

Zaroxolyn, *see metolazone*

Zelnorm, *see tegaserod*

Zerit, *see stavudine*

Zestril, *see lisinopril*

Zetia, *see ezetimibe*

---

zidovudine

zye-**dough**-view-deen
(Apo-Zidovudine ✢, AZT, Novo-AZT ✢, Retrovir)

Do not confuse Retrovir with ritonavir.

FIXED-COMBINATION(S)
Combivir: zidovudine/lamivudine (an antiviral): 300 mg/150 mg.

Z

Trizivir: zidovudine/lamivudine/abacavir (an antiviral): 300 mg/150 mg/300 mg.

◆CLASSIFICATION

PHARMACOTHERAPEUTIC: Nucleoside reverse transcriptase inhibitors. **CLINICAL:** Antivirals (see pp. 62C, 103C).

ACTION

A nucleoside reverse transcriptase inhibitor that interferes with viral RNA-dependent DNA polymerase, an enzyme necessary for viral HIV replication. **Therapeutic Effect:** Interferes with HIV replication, slowing the progression of HIV infection.

PHARMACOKINETICS

Rapidly and completely absorbed from the GI tract. Protein binding: 25%–38%. Undergoes first-pass metabolism in the liver. Crosses the blood-brain barrier and is widely distributed, including to cerebrospinal fluid (CSF). Primarily excreted in urine. Minimal removal by hemodialysis. **Half-life:** 0.8–1.2 hr (increased in impaired renal function).

USES

Treatment of HIV infection in combination with other antiretroviral agents. **OFF-LABEL:** Prophylaxis in health care workers at risk of acquiring HIV after occupational exposure.

PRECAUTIONS

CONTRAINDICATIONS: Life-threatening allergic reactions to zidovudine or its components. **CAUTIONS:** Bone marrow compromise, renal or hepatic dysfunction, decreased hepatic blood flow.

⧗ **LIFESPAN CONSIDERATIONS: Pregnancy/Lactation:** Unknown if drug crosses placenta or is distributed in breast milk. Unknown if fetal harm or effects on fertility can occur. **Pregnancy Category C. Children:** No age-related

precautions noted. **Elderly:** Information not available.

INTERACTIONS

DRUG: Bone marrow depressants, ganciclovir: May increase myelosuppression. **Clarithromycin:** May decrease zidovudine blood concentration. **Probenecid:** May increase zidovudine blood concentrations and the risk of zidovudine toxicity. **HERBAL:** None known. **FOOD:** None known. **LAB VALUES:** May increase mean corpuscular volume.

AVAILABILITY (Rx)

CAPSULES (RETROVIR): 100 mg. **SYRUP (RETROVIR):** 50 mg/5 ml. **TABLETS (RETROVIR):** 300 mg. **INJECTION (RETROVIR):** 10 mg/ml.

ADMINISTRATION/HANDLING
🖉 IV

Reconstitution • Must dilute before administration. • Remove calculated dose from vial and add to D₅W to provide a concentration no greater than 4 mg/ml.

Rate of administration • Infuse over 1 hr.

Storage • After dilution, IV solution is stable for 24 hr at room temperature; 48 hr if refrigerated. • Use within 8 hr if stored at room temperature; 24 hr if refrigerated. • Do not use if particulate matter is present or discoloration occurs.

PO
• Keep capsules in cool, dry place. Protect from light. • Food, milk do not affect GI absorption. • Space doses evenly around the clock. • Patient should be in upright position when giving medication to prevent esophageal ulceration.

🕸 IV INCOMPATIBILITIES
None known.

IV COMPATIBILITIES

Dexamethasone (Decadron), dobutamine (Dobutrex), dopamine (Intropin), heparin, lorazepam (Ativan), morphine, potassium chloride.

INDICATIONS/ROUTES/DOSAGE

HIV INFECTION

PO: ADULTS, ELDERLY, CHILDREN OLDER THAN 12 YR: 200 mg q8h or 300 mg q12h. CHILDREN 12 YR AND YOUNGER: 160 mg/m^2/dose q8h. Range: 90–180 mg/m^2/dose q6–8h. NEONATES: 2 mg/kg/dose q6h.

IV: ADULTS, ELDERLY, CHILDREN OLDER THAN 12 YR: 1–2 mg/kg/dose q4h. CHILDREN 12 YR AND YOUNGER: 120 mg/m^2/dose q6h. NEONATES: 1.5 mg/kg/dose q6h.

SIDE EFFECTS

EXPECTED (46%–42%): Nausea, headache. **FREQUENT (20%–16%):** Abdominal pain, asthenia, rash, fever, acne. **OCCASIONAL (12%–8%):** Diarrhea, anorexia, malaise, myalgia, somnolence. **RARE (6%–5%):** Dizziness, paresthesia, vomiting, insomnia, dyspnea, altered taste.

ADVERSE REACTIONS/ TOXIC EFFECTS

Serious reactions include anemia, which occurs most commonly after 4–6 wk of therapy, and granulocytopenia; both effects are more likely to occur in patients who have a low Hgb level or granulocyte count before beginning therapy. Neurotoxicity (as evidenced by ataxia, fatigue, lethargy, nystagmus, and seizures) may occur.

NURSING CONSIDERATIONS

BASELINE ASSESSMENT

Avoid drugs that are nephrotoxic, cytotoxic, myelosuppressive—may increase risk of toxicity. Obtain specimens for viral diagnostic tests before starting therapy (therapy may begin before results are obtained). Check hematology reports for accurate baseline.

INTERVENTION/EVALUATION

Monitor CBC, Hgb, MCV, retriculocyte count, CD4 cell count, HIV RNA plasma levels. Check for bleeding. Assess for headache, dizziness. Determine pattern of bowel activity and stool consistency. Evaluate skin for acne, rash. Be alert to development of opportunistic infections (e.g., fever, chills, cough, myalgia). Monitor I&O, serum renal and liver function tests. Check for insomnia.

PATIENT/FAMILY TEACHING

• Doses should be evenly spaced around the clock. • Zidovudine does not cure AIDS or HIV disease, nor does it reduce risk of transmission to others, but acts to reduce symptoms and slows or arrests progress of disease. • Do not take any medications without physician approval. • Bleeding from gums, nose, rectum may occur and should be reported to physician immediately. • Blood counts are essential because of bleeding potential. • Dental work should be done before therapy or after blood counts return to normal (often weeks after therapy has stopped). • Inform physician if muscle weakness, difficulty breathing, headache, inability to sleep, unusual bleeding, rash, signs of infection occur.

Zinacef, *see cefuroxime*

---

ziprasidone

zye-**pray**-za-done

(Geodon)

CLASSIFICATION

PHARMACOTHERAPEUTIC: Piperazine derivative. **CLINICAL:** Antipsychotic (see p. 59C).

ACTION

A piperazine derivative that antagonizes alpha-adrenergic, dopamine, histamine, and serotonin receptors; also inhibits reuptake of serotonin and norepinephrine. Therapeutic Effect: Diminishes symptoms of schizophrenia and depression.

PHARMACOKINETICS

Well absorbed after PO administration. Food increases bioavailability. Protein binding: 99%. Extensively metabolized in the liver. Not removed by hemodialysis. Half-life: 7 hr.

USES

Treatment of schizophrenia, acute bipolar mania. OFF-LABEL Tourette's syndrome.

PRECAUTIONS

CONTRAINDICATIONS: Conditions that prolong the QT interval, such as congenital long QT syndrome. CAUTIONS: Patients with bradycardia, hypokalemia, hypomagnesemia may be at greater risk for torsades de pointes (atypical ventricular tachycardia).

⧖ LIFESPAN CONSIDERATIONS: Pregnancy/Lactation: Unknown if drug crosses placenta or is distributed in breast milk. Pregnancy Category C. Children: Safety and efficacy not established. Elderly: No age-related precautions noted.

INTERACTIONS

DRUG: Alcohol, other CNS depressants: May increase CNS depression. Carbamazepine: May decrease ziprasidone blood concentration. Ketoconazole: May increase ziprasidone blood concentration. HERBAL: None known. FOOD: All foods: Enhance the bioavailability of ziprasidone. LAB VALUES: May prolong the QT interval.

AVAILABILITY (Rx)

CAPSULES: 20 mg, 40 mg, 60 mg, 80 mg. INJECTION: 20 mg/ml.

ADMINISTRATION/HANDLING
IM

• Store vials at room temperature, protect from light. • Reconstitute each vial with 1.2 ml sterile water for injection to provide a concentration of 20 mg/ml. • Reconstituted solution stable for 24 hr at room temperature or 7 days refrigerated.

PO

• Give with food (increases bioavailability).

INDICATIONS/ROUTES/DOSAGE
SCHIZOPHRENIA

PO: ADULTS, ELDERLY: Initially, 20 mg twice a day with food. Titrate at intervals of no less than 2 days. Maximum: 80 mg twice a day.
IM: ADULTS, ELDERLY: 10 mg q2h or 20 mg q4h. Maximum: 40 mg/day.

MANIA IN BIPOLAR DISORDER

PO: ADULTS, ELDERLY: Initially, 40 mg twice a day. May increase to 60–80 mg twice a day on second day of treatment. Range: 40–80 mg twice a day.

SIDE EFFECTS

FREQUENT (30%–16%): Headache, somnolence, dizziness. OCCASIONAL: Rash, orthostatic hypotension, weight gain, restlessness, constipation, dyspepsia. RARE: Hyperglycemia, priapism.

ADVERSE REACTIONS/ TOXIC EFFECTS

Prolongation of QT interval may produce torsades de pointes, a form of ventricular tachycardia. Patients with bradycardia, hypokalemia, or hypomagnesemia are at increased risk.

Z

NURSING CONSIDERATIONS

BASELINE ASSESSMENT
Assess patient's behavior, appearance, emotional status, response to environment, speech pattern, thought content. An EKG should be obtained to assess for QT prolongation before instituting medication. Blood chemistry for serum magnesium, potassium should be obtained before beginning therapy and routinely thereafter.

INTERVENTION/EVALUATION
Assess for therapeutic response (greater interest in surroundings, improved self-care, increased ability to concentrate, relaxed facial expression). Monitor weight.

PATIENT/FAMILY TEACHING
• Avoid tasks that require alertness, motor skills until response to drug is established.

Zithromax, *see azithromycin*

Zocor, *see simvastatin*

Zofran, *see ondansetron*

Zoladex, *see goserelin*

zoledronic acid

zole-eh-**drone**-ick
(Zometa)

◆CLASSIFICATION
PHARMACOTHERAPEUTIC: Bisphosphonate. **CLINICAL:** Calcium regulator, bone resorption inhibitor.

ACTION
A bisphosphonate that inhibits the resorption of mineralized bone and cartilage; inhibits increased osteoclastic activity and skeletal calcium release induced by stimulatory factors produced by tumors. **Therapeutic Effect:** Increases urinary calcium and phosphorus excretion; decreases serum calcium and phosphorus levels.

USES
Treatment of hypercalcemia, bone metastases of solid tumors. Treatment of multiple myeloma. **OFF-LABEL:** Pre-vention of bone metastases from breast, prostate cancer, treatment of bone diseases.

PRECAUTIONS
CONTRAINDICATIONS: Hypersensitivity to other bisphosphonates, including alendronate, etidronate, pamidronate, risedronate, and tiludronate. **CAUTIONS:** History of aspirin-sensitive asthma, renal impairment, hypoparathyroidism, risk of hypocalcemia.

⧗ **LIFESPAN CONSIDERATIONS: Pregnancy/Lactation:** Unknown if drug crosses placenta or is distributed in breast milk. **Pregnancy Category C. Children:** Safety and efficacy not established. **Elderly:** Age-related renal impairment may require dosage adjustment.

INTERACTIONS
DRUG: Calcium-containing medications, vitamin D: May antagonize the effects of zoledronic acid in treatment of hypercalcemia. **HERBAL:** None known. **FOOD:** None known. **LAB VALUES:** May

decrease serum magnesium, calcium, and phosphate levels.

AVAILABILITY (Rx)

INJECTION POWDER FOR RECONSTITUTION: 4 mg. **INJECTION SOLUTION:** 4 mg/5 ml.

ADMINISTRATION/HANDLING

◀ **ALERT** ▶ Patient should be adequately rehydrated before administration of zoledronic acid.

 IV

Reconstitution • Reconstitute 4-mg vial with 5 ml sterile water for injection. Allow drug to dissolve before withdrawing. • Further dilute with 100 ml 0.9% NaCl or D₅W.

Rate of administration • Adequate hydration is essential in conjunction with zoledronic acid. • Administer as an IV infusion over not less than 15 min (increases risk of deterioration in renal function).

Storage • Store at room temperature. • If not used immediately, reconstituted solution should be refrigerated; time from reconstitution to end of administration should not exceed 24 hr.

▩ IV INCOMPATIBILITIES

Do not mix with other medications.

INDICATIONS/ROUTES/DOSAGE

HYPERCALCEMIA

IV INFUSION: ADULTS, ELDERLY: 4 mg IV infusion given over no less than 15 min. Retreatment may be considered, but at least 7 days should elapse to allow for full response to initial dose.

MULTIPLE MYELOMA, BONE METASTASES OF SOLID TUMORS

IV: ADULTS, ELDERLY: 4 mg q3–4wk.

SIDE EFFECTS

FREQUENT (44%–26%): Fever, nausea, vomiting, constipation. **OCCASIONAL (15%–10%):** Hypotension, anxiety, insomnia, flu-like symptoms (fever, chills,

bone pain, myalgia, and arthralgia). **RARE:** Conjunctivitis.

ADVERSE REACTIONS/ TOXIC EFFECTS

Renal toxicity may occur if IV infusion is administered in less than 15 min.

NURSING CONSIDERATIONS

BASELINE ASSESSMENT
Establish baseline serum electrolytes.

INTERVENTION/EVALUATION
Monitor serum renal function, CBC, Hgb, Hct. Assess vertebral bone mass (document stabilization and improvement). Monitor serum calcium, phosphate, magnesium, creatinine levels. Assess for fever. Monitor food intake, pattern of bowel activity and stool consistency. Check I&O, BUN, serum creatinine in patients with renal impairment.

zolmitriptan

zohl-mih-**trip**-tan

(Zomig, Zomig Rapimelt , Zomig-ZMT)

◆CLASSIFICATION

PHARMACOTHERAPEUTIC: Serotonin receptor agonist. **CLINICAL:** Antimigraine (see p. 57C).

ACTION

A serotonin receptor agonist that binds selectively to vascular receptors, producing a vasoconstrictive effect on cranial blood vessels. **Therapeutic Effect:** Relieves migraine headache.

PHARMACOKINETICS

Rapidly but incompletely absorbed after PO administration. Protein binding: 15%. Undergoes first-pass metabolism in the liver to active metabolite. Eliminated primarily in urine (60%) and, to a lesser extent, in feces (30%). Half-life: 3 hr.

USES

Treatment of acute migraine attack with or without aura.

PRECAUTIONS

CONTRAINDICATIONS: Arrhythmias associated with conduction disorders, basilar or hemiplegic migraine, coronary artery disease, ischemic heart disease (including angina pectoris, history of MI, silent ischemia, and Prinzmetal's angina), uncontrolled hypertension, use within 24 hr of ergotamine-containing preparations or another serotonin receptor agonist, use within 14 days of MAOIs, Wolff-Parkinson-White syndrome. **CAUTIONS:** Mild to moderate renal or hepatic impairment, patient profile suggesting cardiovascular risks, controlled hypertension, history of cerebrovascular accident (CVA).

⧗ LIFESPAN CONSIDERATIONS: **Pregnancy/Lactation:** Unknown if drug is distributed in breast milk. **Pregnancy Category C. Children:** Safety and efficacy not established in those younger than 12 yr. **Elderly:** No age-related precautions noted.

INTERACTIONS

DRUG: **Ergotamine-containing medications:** May produce a vasospastic reaction. **Fluoxetine, fluvoxamine, paroxetine, sertraline:** May produce hyperreflexia, incoordination, and weakness. **MAOIs:** May dramatically increase plasma concentration of zolmitriptan. **Oral contraceptives:** Decrease zolmitriptan clearance and volume of distribution. HERBAL: None known. FOOD: None known. LAB VALUES: None known.

AVAILABILITY (Rx)

TABLETS (ZOMIG): 2.5 mg, 5 mg. **TABLETS (ORALLY-DISINTEGRATING [ZOMIG-ZMT]):** 2.5 mg, 5 mg. **NASAL SPRAY (ZOMIG):** 5 mg/0.1 ml.

ADMINISTRATION/HANDLING

PO
• Give without regard to food.
NASAL
• Instruct the patient to gently blow nose to clear nasal passages. • With head upright, patient should close one nostril with index finger and breathe out gently through mouth. • Instruct patient to insert nozzle into open nostril about ½ inch, close mouth, and while taking a breath through nose, release spray dosage by firmly pressing the plunger. • Have patient remove nozzle from nose, gently breathe in through nose and out through mouth for 15–20 sec. Tell patient to avoid breathing in deeply.

INDICATIONS/ROUTES/DOSAGE

ACUTE MIGRAINE ATTACK
PO: ADULTS, ELDERLY, CHILDREN OLDER THAN 18 YR: Initially, 2.5 mg or less. If headache returns, may repeat dose in 2 hr. **Maximum:** 10 mg/24 hr.
INTRANASAL: ADULTS, ELDERLY: 5 mg. May repeat in 2 hr. **Maximum:** 10 mg/24 hr.

SIDE EFFECTS

FREQUENT (8%–6%): Oral: Dizziness; tingling; neck, throat, or jaw pressure; somnolence. **Nasal:** Altered taste, paresthesia. **OCCASIONAL (5%–3%): Oral:** Warm or hot sensation, asthenia, chest pressure. **Nasal:** Nausea, somnolence, nasal discomfort, dizziness, asthenia, dry mouth. **RARE (2%–1%):** Diaphoresis, myalgia, paresthesia.

ADVERSE REACTIONS/ TOXIC EFFECTS

Cardiac reactions (including ischemia, coronary artery vasospasm, and MI) and noncardiac vasospasm-related reactions (such as hemorrhage and cerebro-vascular accident [CVA]) occur rarely, particularly in patients with hypertension, diabetes, or a strong family history of coronary artery disease; obese patients; smokers; males older than 40 yr; and postmenopausal women.

NURSING CONSIDERATIONS

BASELINE ASSESSMENT

Question for history of peripheral vascular disease or coronary artery disease, renal or hepatic impairment, use of MAOIs. Question patient regarding onset, location, duration of migraine, possible precipitating symptoms.

INTERVENTION/EVALUATION

Monitor for evidence of dizziness. Monitor BP, especially in patients with hepatic impairment. Assess for relief of migraine headache and migraine potential for photophobia, phonophobia (sound sensitivity, light sensitivity, nausea, vomiting).

PATIENT/FAMILY TEACHING

• Take a single dose as soon as symptoms of an actual migraine attack appear. • Medication is intended to relieve migraine, not to prevent or reduce number of attacks. • Lie down in quiet dark room for additional benefit after taking medication. • Avoid tasks that require alertness, motor skills until response to drug is established. • Report chest pain, palpitations, tightness in throat, edema of face, lips, or eyes, rash, easy bruising, blood in urine or stool, pain or numbness in arms or legs.

Zoloft, *see sertraline*

---

zolpidem tartrate ✎

zole-pi-dem
(Ambien, Ambien CR)
Do not confuse Ambien with Amen.

◆ CLASSIFICATION

PHARMACOTHERAPEUTIC: Nonbenzodiazepine. **CLINICAL:** Sedative-hypnotic **(Schedule IV)** (see p. 136C).

ACTION

A nonbenzodiazepine that enhances the action of the inhibitory neurotransmitter gamma-aminobutyric acid. **Therapeutic Effect:** Induces sleep and improves sleep quality.

PHARMACOKINETICS

Route	Onset	Peak	Duration
PO	30 min	N/A	6–8 hr

Rapidly absorbed from the GI tract. Protein binding: 92%. Metabolized in the liver; excreted in urine. Not removed by hemodialysis. **Half-life:** 1.4–4.5 hr (increased in hepatic impairment).

USES

Short-term treatment of insomnia. Reduces sleep-induction time, number of nocturnal awakenings; increases length of sleep; improves sleep quality.

PRECAUTIONS

CONTRAINDICATIONS: None known. **CAUTIONS:** Hepatic impairment, patients with depression, history of drug dependence.

⏳ **LIFESPAN CONSIDERATIONS: Pregnancy/Lactation:** Unknown if drug crosses placenta or is distributed in breast milk. **Pregnancy Category B.**

Children: Safety and efficacy not established. **Elderly:** More likely to experience falls or confusion; decreased initial doses recommended. Age-related hepatic impairment may require dosage adjustment.

INTERACTIONS

DRUG: Alcohol, other CNS depressants: May increase CNS depression. **HERBAL:** None known. **FOOD:** None known. **LAB VALUES:** None known.

AVAILABILITY (Rx)

TABLETS (AMBIEN): 5 mg, 10 mg. **TABLETS (EXTENDED-RELEASE [AMBIEN CR]):** 6.25 mg, 12.5 mg.

ADMINISTRATION/HANDLING

PO
• For faster sleep onset, do not give with or immediately after a meal.

INDICATIONS/ROUTES/DOSAGE

INSOMNIA
PO: ADULTS: 10 mg at bedtime. ELDERLY, DEBILITATED: 5 mg at bedtime.
PO (EXTENDED-RELEASE): ADULTS: 12.5 mg. ELDERLY, DEBILITATED: 6.25 mg.

SIDE EFFECTS

OCCASIONAL (7%): Headache. **RARE (less than 2%):** Dizziness, nausea, diarrhea, muscle pain.

ADVERSE REACTIONS/ TOXIC EFFECTS

Overdose may produce severe ataxia, bradycardia, altered vision (such as diplopia), severe drowsiness, nausea and vomiting, difficulty breathing, and unconsciousness. Abrupt withdrawal of the drug after long-term use may produce asthenia, facial flushing, diaphoresis, vomiting, and tremor. Drug tolerance or dependence may occur with prolonged, high-dose therapy.

NURSING CONSIDERATIONS

BASELINE ASSESSMENT
Assess BP, pulse, respirations. Raise bed rails, provide call light. Provide environment conducive to sleep (back rub, quiet environment, low lighting).

INTERVENTION/EVALUATION
Assess sleep pattern of patient. Evaluate for therapeutic response to insomnia: decrease in number of nocturnal awakenings, increase in length of sleep.

PATIENT/FAMILY TEACHING
• Do not abruptly withdraw medication after long-term use. • Avoid alcohol, tasks that require alertness, motor skills until response to drug is established. • Tolerance or dependence may occur with prolonged use of high dosages.

Zometa, *see zoledronic acid*

Zomig, *see zolmitriptan*

---

zonisamide

zoh-**nis**-a-mide
(Zonegran)

◆CLASSIFICATION
PHARMACOTHERAPEUTIC: Succinimide. **CLINICAL:** Anticonvulsant (see p. 35C).

ACTION

A succinimide that may stabilize neuronal membranes and suppress neuronal hypersynchronization by blocking sodium and calcium channels. **Therapeutic Effect:** Reduces seizure activity.

PHARMACOKINETICS

Well absorbed after PO administration. Extensively bound to RBCs. Protein binding: 40%. Primarily excreted in urine. Half-life: 63 hr (plasma), 105 hr (RBCs).

USES

Adjunctive therapy in the treatment of partial seizures in adults with epilepsy. OFF-LABEL: Treatment of binge eating disorder, bipolar disorder, obesity.

PRECAUTIONS

CONTRAINDICATIONS: Allergy to sulfonamides. CAUTIONS: Renal impairment.

⧖ LIFESPAN CONSIDERATIONS: Pregnancy/Lactation: Unknown if distributed in breast milk. Pregnancy Category C. Children: Safety and efficacy not established in those younger than 16 yr. Elderly: No age-related precautions noted but lower dosages recommended.

INTERACTIONS

DRUG: **Alcohol, other CNS depressants:** May increase zonisamide's sedative effect. **Carbamazepine, phenobarbital, phenytoin, valproic acid:** May increase the metabolism and decrease the effect of zonisamide. HERBAL: None known. FOOD: None known. LAB VALUES: May increase BUN and serum creatinine levels.

AVAILABILITY (Rx)

CAPSULES: 25 mg, 50 mg, 100 mg.

ADMINISTRATION/HANDLING

PO
• May take with or without food.
• Swallow capsules whole. • Do not give to patients allergic to sulfonamides.

INDICATIONS/ROUTES/DOSAGE

PARTIAL SEIZURES

PO: ADULTS, ELDERLY, CHILDREN OLDER THAN 16 YR: Initially, 100 mg/day for 2 wk.

May increase by 100 mg/day at intervals of 2 wk or longer. Range: 100–600 mg/day.

SIDE EFFECTS

FREQUENT(17%–9%): Somnolence, dizziness, anorexia, headache, agitation, irritability, nausea. OCCASIONAL (8%–5%): Fatigue, ataxia, confusion, depression, impaired memory or concentration, insomnia, abdominal pain, diplopia, diarrhea, speech difficulty. RARE (4%–3%): Paresthesia, nystagmus, anxiety, rash, dyspepsia, weight loss.

ADVERSE REACTIONS/ TOXIC EFFECTS

Overdose is characterized by bradycardia, hypotension, respiratory depression, and coma. Leukopenia, anemia, and thrombocytopenia occur rarely.

NURSING CONSIDERATIONS

BASELINE ASSESSMENT

Anticonvulsant: Review history of seizure disorder (intensity, frequency, duration, level of consciousness [LOC]). Initiate seizure precautions. Serum liver function tests, CBC, platelet count should be performed before therapy begins and periodically during therapy.

INTERVENTION/EVALUATION

Observe frequently for recurrence of seizure activity. Assess for clinical improvement (decrease in intensity or frequency of seizures). Assist with ambulation if dizziness occurs.

PATIENT/FAMILY TEACHING

• Strict maintenance of drug therapy is essential for seizure control. • Avoid tasks that require alertness, motor skills until response to drug is established. • Avoid alcohol. • Report if rash, back or abdominal pain, blood in urine, fever, sore throat, ulcers in mouth, easy bruising occurs.

Z

Zosyn, *see piperacillin sodium/tazobactam sodium*

Zovirax, *see acyclovir*

Zyloprim, *see allopurinol*

Zyprexa, *see olanzapine*

Zyrtec, *see cetirizine*

Zyvox, *see linezolid*

Appendixes

CALCULATION OF DOSES

Frequently, dosages ordered do not correspond exactly to what is available and must be calculated.

RATIO/PROPORTION:

A patient is to receive 65 mg of a medication. It is available as 80 mg/2 ml. What volume (ml) needs to be administered to the patient?

STEP 1: Set up ratio.

$$\frac{80 \text{ mg}}{2 \text{ ml}} = \frac{65 \text{ mg}}{x \text{ (ml)}}$$

STEP 2: Cross multiply and divide each side by the number with x to determine volume to be administered.

$$80 \text{ mg} \times (x) \text{ ml} = 65 \text{ mg} \times 2 \text{ ml}$$
$$80 x = 130$$
$$x = \frac{130}{80} = 1.625 \text{ ml}$$

CALCULATIONS IN MICROGRAMS/KILOGRAM PER MINUTE (mcg/kg/min):

A 63-year-old patient (weight 165 lb) is to receive medication A at a rate of 8 mcg/kg/min. Given a solution containing medication A in a concentration of 500 mg/250 ml, at what rate (ml/hr) would you infuse this medication?

STEP 1: Convert to same units. In this problem, the dose is expressed in mcg/kg; therefore, convert weight to kg (2.2 lb = 1 kg) and drug concentration to mcg/ml (1 mg = 1,000 mcg)

$$165 \text{ lb divided by } 2.2 = 75 \text{ kg}$$
$$500 \text{ mg} \times 2 \text{ mg/ml} = 2,000 \text{ mcg/ml} = 250 \text{ ml}$$

STEP 2: Number of mcg/hr.

$$(75 \text{ kg}) \times 8 \text{ mcg/kg/min} = 600 \text{ mcg/min or } 36,000 \text{ mcg/hr}$$

STEP 3: Number of ml/hr.

$$36,000 \text{ mcg/hr divided by } 2,000 \text{ mcg/ml} = 18 \text{ ml/hr}$$

Appendix B

CONTROLLED DRUGS (UNITED STATES)

Schedule I: Medications having no legal medical use. These substances may be used for research purposes with proper registration (e.g., heroin, LSD).

Schedule II: Medications having a legitimate medical use but are characterized by a very high abuse potential and/or potential for severe physical and psychic dependency. Emergency telephone orders for limited quantities of these drugs are authorized, but the prescriber must provide a written, signed prescription order (e.g., morphine, amphetamines).

Schedule III: Medications having significant abuse potential (less than Schedule II). Telephone orders are permitted (e.g., opiates in combination with other substances such as acetaminophen).

Schedule IV: Medications having a low abuse potential. Telephone orders are permitted (e.g., benzodiazepines, propoxyphene).

Schedule V: Medications having the lowest abuse potential of the controlled substances. Some Schedule V products may be available without a prescription (e.g., certain cough preparations containing limited amounts of an opiate.

DRIP RATES FOR CRITICAL CARE MEDICATIONS

Dobutamine

Dopamine

Heparin

Nitroglycerin

Norepinephrine

Propofol

Sodium Nitroprusside

DOBUTAMINE (Dobutrex)
Mix 250 mg in 250 ml of D_5W (1,000 mcg/ml)

	Body Weight														
lb	88	99	110	121	132	143	154	165	176	187	198	209	220	231	242
kg	40	45	50	55	60	65	70	75	80	85	90	95	100	105	110
Dose ordered in mcg/kg/min	*Amount to infuse in mcgtts/min or ml/hr*														
2.5	6	7	8	8	9	10	11	11	12	13	14	14	15	16	17
5	12	14	15	17	18	20	21	23	24	26	27	29	30	32	33
7.5	18	20	23	25	27	29	32	34	36	38	41	43	45	47	50
10	24	27	30	33	36	39	42	45	48	51	54	57	60	63	66
12.5	30	34	38	41	45	49	53	56	60	64	68	71	75	79	83
15	36	41	45	50	54	59	63	68	72	77	81	86	90	95	99
20	48	54	60	66	72	78	84	90	96	102	108	114	120	126	132
25	60	68	75	83	90	98	105	113	120	128	135	143	150	158	165
30	72	81	90	99	108	117	126	135	144	153	162	171	180	189	198
35	84	95	105	116	126	137	147	158	168	179	189	200	210	221	231
40	96	108	120	132	144	156	168	180	192	204	216	228	240	252	264

- Administer 2.5–10 mcg/kg/min initially.
- Increase in increments of 5–10 mcg up to 40 mcg/kg/min as needed.
- Do not mix with sodium bicarbonate.

DOPAMINE (Intropin)
Mix 400 mg in 250 ml of D₅W (1,600 mcg/ml)

Body Weight

lb	88	99	110	121	132	143	154	165	176	187	198	209	220	231
kg	40	45	50	55	60	65	70	75	80	85	90	95	100	105

Dose ordered in mcg/kg/min	Amount to infuse in mcgtts/min or ml/hr														
2.5	4	4	5	5	6	6	7	7	8	8	8	9	9	10
5	8	8	9	10	11	12	13	14	15	16	17	18	19	20
7.5	11	13	14	15	17	18	20	21	23	24	25	27	28	30
10	15	17	19	21	23	24	26	28	30	32	34	36	38	39
12.5	19	21	23	26	28	30	33	35	38	40	42	45	47	49
15	23	25	28	31	34	37	39	42	45	48	51	53	56	59
20	30	34	38	41	45	49	53	56	60	64	68	71	75	79
25	38	42	47	52	56	61	66	70	75	80	84	89	94	98
30	45	51	56	62	67	73	79	84	90	96	101	107	113	118
35	53	59	66	72	79	85	92	98	105	112	118	125	131	138
40	60	68	75	83	90	98	105	113	120	128	135	143	150	158
45	68	76	84	93	101	110	118	127	135	143	152	160	169	177
50	75	84	94	103	113	122	131	141	150	159	169	178	188	197

- Administer 2.5–5 mcg/kg/min initially.
- Increase in increments of 5–10 mcg to 50 mcg/kg/min as needed.
- Do not mix with sodium bicarbonate.

HEPARIN DRIP RATE CHART

ACT (sec)	APTT (sec)	Bolus Dose (ml)	Stop Infusion (min)	Rate Change (ml/hr)	Repeat PTT (hr)	Repeat aPTT (hr)
1–200	1–49	5,000	0	+3 ml/hr (increase by 150 units/hr)	4	4
201–239	50–59	0	0	+2 ml/hr (increase by 100 units/hr)	4	4
240–300	60–85	0	0	0 (no change)	8	8
301–400	86–95	0	0	−1 ml/hr (decrease by 50 units/hr)	8	8
401–500	96–120	0	30	−2 ml/hr (decrease by 100 units/hr)	4	4
500+	120+	0	60	−3 ml/hr (decrease by 150 units/hr)	4	4

NITROGLYCERIN (Tridil)

Dose ordered in mcg/min	50 mg/ 250 cc 100 mg/ 500 cc NTG/D$_5$W	100 mg/ 250 cc 200 mg/ 500 cc NTG/D$_5$W	Dose ordered in mcg/min	50 mg/ 250 cc 100 mg/ 500 cc NTG/D$_5$W	100 mg/ 250 cc 200 mg/ 500 cc NTG/D$_5$W
10	3	—	210	63	32
20	6	3	220	66	33
30	9	5	230	69	35
40	12	6	240	72	36
50	15	8	250	75	38
60	18	9	260	78	39
70	21	10	270	81	41
80	24	12	280	84	42
90	27	14	290	87	44
100	30	15	300	90	45
110	33	17	310	93	47
120	36	18	320	96	48
130	39	19	330	99	50
140	42	21	340	102	51
150	45	23	350	105	53
160	48	24	360	108	54
170	51	26	370	111	56
180	54	27	380	114	57
190	57	29	390	117	59
200	60	30	400	120	60
	Amt to infuse in mcgtts/min or ml/hr			*Amt to infuse in mcgtts/min or ml/hr*	

- Administer at 10–20 mcg/min initially.
- Increase at increments of 6–10 mcg/min every 5–10 min until desired response.

NOREPINEPHRINE (Levophed)
Mix: 4 mg in 250 ml D₅W
Norepinephrine 4 mg in 250 ml D₅W (rate is ml/hr)

mcg/kg/min

kg	0.01	0.02	0.03	0.04	0.05	0.06	0.07	0.08	0.09	0.10	0.20	0.30
50	1.9	3.8	5.7	7.6	9.5	11.4	13.3	15.2	17.1	19.0	38.0	57.0
55	2.1	4.2	6.3	8.4	10.5	12.6	14.7	16.8	18.9	21.0	42.0	63.0
60	2.3	4.6	6.9	9.2	11.5	13.8	16.1	18.4	20.7	23.0	46.0	69.0
65	2.4	4.8	7.2	9.6	12.0	14.4	16.8	19.2	21.6	24.0	48.0	72.0
70	2.6	5.2	7.8	10.4	13.0	15.6	18.2	20.8	23.4	26.0	52.0	78.0
75	2.8	5.6	8.4	11.2	14.0	16.8	19.6	22.4	25.2	28.0	56.0	84.0
80	3.0	6.0	9.0	12.0	15.0	18.0	21.0	24.0	27.0	30.0	60.0	90.0
85	3.2	6.4	9.6	12.8	16.0	19.2	22.4	25.6	28.8	32.0	64.0	96.0
90	3.4	6.8	10.2	13.6	17.0	20.4	23.8	27.2	30.6	34.0	68.0	102
95	3.6	7.2	10.8	14.4	18.0	21.6	25.2	28.8	32.4	36.0	72.0	108
100	3.8	7.6	11.4	15.2	19.0	22.8	26.6	30.4	34.2	38.0	76.0	114

Use: Hypotension, shock

Dose: 2–40 mcg/min or 0.05–0.25 mcg/kg/min doses of greater than 75 mcg/min or 1 mcg/kg/min have been used

Mechanism: Primary α_1 vasoconstriction effect (minor β_1 inotropic)

Elimination: Hepatic   **Half-life:** Minutes

Adverse events: Tachyarrhythmias, hypertension at high doses

PROPOFOL (Diprivan)
Mix: Undiluted (10 mg/ml) 100-ml vial
Propofol 10 mg/ml (premixed) (rate is ml/hr)

mcg/kg/min

kg	10	15	20	25	30	35	40	45	50	55	60	65
50	3	5	6	8	9	11	12	14	15	17	18	20
55	3	5	7	8	10	12	13	15	17	18	20	21
60	4	5	7	9	11	13	14	16	18	20	22	23
65	4	6	8	10	12	14	16	18	20	21	23	25
70	4	6	8	11	13	15	17	19	21	23	25	27
75	5	7	9	11	14	16	18	20	23	25	27	29
80	5	7	10	12	14	17	19	22	24	26	29	31
85	5	8	10	13	15	18	20	23	26	28	31	33
90	5	8	11	14	16	19	22	24	27	30	32	35
95	6	9	11	14	17	20	23	26	29	31	34	37
100	6	9	12	15	18	21	24	27	30	33	36	39

Use: Nonamnestic sedation
Dose: Load 1–2 mg/kg IV push; **do not load if patient is hypotensive or volume depleted**
Maintenance Initial dose of 5–20 mcg/kg/min, may titrate to effect (20–65 mcg/kg/min)
Mechanism: Di-isopropyl phenolic compound with intravenous general anesthetic properties unrelated to opiates, barbiturates, benzodiazepines
Elimination: Hepatic   **Half-life:** 30 minutes
Adverse events: Hypotension, nausea, vomiting, seizures, hypertriglyceridemia, hyperlipidemia.

SODIUM NITROPRUSSIDE (Nipride)
Mix: 50 mg in 250 ml of D₅W (200 mcg/ml)

Body Weight

lb	88	99	110	121	132	143	154	165	176	187	198	209	220	231	242
kg	40	45	50	55	60	65	70	75	80	85	90	95	100	105	110

Dose ordered in mcg/kg/min	*Amount to infuse in mcgtts/min or ml/hr*														
0.5	6	7	8	8	9	10	11	11	12	13	14	14	15	16	17
1	12	14	15	17	18	20	21	23	24	26	27	29	30	32	33
1.5	13	20	23	25	27	29	32	34	36	38	41	43	45	47	50
2	24	27	30	33	36	39	42	45	48	51	54	57	60	63	66
3	36	41	45	50	54	59	63	68	72	77	81	86	90	95	99
4	48	54	60	66	72	78	84	90	96	102	108	114	120	126	132
5	60	68	75	83	90	98	105	113	120	128	135	143	150	158	165
6	72	81	90	99	108	117	126	135	144	153	162	171	180	189	198
7	84	95	105	116	126	137	147	158	168	179	189	200	210	221	231
8	96	108	120	132	144	156	168	180	192	204	216	228	240	252	264
9	108	122	135	149	162	176	189	203	216	230	243	257	270	284	297
10	120	135	150	165	180	195	210	225	240	255	270	285	300	315	330

- Administer 0.5–10 mcg/kg/min initially.
- Increase in increments of 1 mcg/kg/min until desired response.
- Do not leave solution exposed to light.

DRUGS OF ABUSE

Name (Brand)	Class	Signs and Symptoms	Treatment
Acid (see LSD)			
Adam (see MDMA)			
Amphetamine (Adderall, Dexedrine)	Stimulant	Tachycardia, hypertension, diaphoresis, agitation, headache, seizures, dehydration, hypokalemia, lactic acidosis. Severe overdose: hyperthermia, dysrhythmia, shock, rhabdomyolysis, hepatic necrosis, acute renal failure.	Control agitation, reverse hyperthermia, support hemodynamic function. **Antidote:** No specific antidote.
Angel dust (see phencyclidine)			
Apache (see fentanyl)			
Barbiturates (Nembutal, Seconal)	Depressant	Hypotension, hypothermia, apnea, nystagmus, ataxia, hyporeflexia, somnolence, stupor, coma.	Airway management, decontamination, supportive care. **Antidote:** No specific antidote.
Barbs (see barbiturates)			
Benzodiazepines (Xanax, Valium, Librium, Halcion)	Depressant	Respiratory depression, hypothermia, hypotension, nystagmus, miosis, diplopia, bradycardia, nausea, vomiting, impaired speech and coordination, amnesia, ataxia, somnolence, confusion, depressed deep tendon reflexes.	**Antidote:** Flumazenil (Romazicon) is a specific antidote.
Black tar (see heroin)			
Boomers (see LSD)			
Buttons (see mescaline)			
Cactus (see mescaline)			
Candy (see benzodiazepines)			
China girl (see fentanyl)			
China white (see heroin)			

Name (Brand)	Class	Signs and Symptoms	Treatment
Cocaine	Stimulant	Hypertension, tachycardia, mild hyperthermia, mydriasis, pallor, diaphoresis, psychosis, paranoid delusions, mania, agitation, seizures.	Control agitation, seizures, hyperthermia; support hemodynamic function. **Antidote:** No specific antidote.
Codeine	Opioid	Miosis, respiratory depression, decreased mental status, hypotension, cardiac dysrhythmia, hypoxia, bronchoconstriction, constipation, decreased intestinal motility, ileus, lethargy, coma.	Airway management, hemodynamic support. **Antidote:** Naloxone, nalmefene.
Coke (see cocaine)			
Crank (see amphetamine)			
Crank (see heroin)			
Crystal (see amphetamine)			
Crystal meth (see methamphetamine)			
Cubes (see LSD)			
Downers (see benzodiazepines)			
Ecstasy (see MDMA)			
Fentanyl (Sublimaze)	Opioid	Miosis, respiratory depression, decreased mental status, hypotension, cardiac dysrhythmia, hypoxia, bronchoconstriction, constipation, decreased intestinal motility, ileus, lethargy, coma.	Airway management, hemodynamic support. **Antidote:** Naloxone, nalmefene.
Flunitrazepam (Rohypnol)	Depressant	Drowsiness, slurred speech, impaired judgment and motor skills, hypothermia, hypotension, bradycardia, diplopia, blurred vision, nystagmus, respiratory depression, nausea, constipation, depression, lethargy, headache, ataxia, coma, amnesia, incoordination, tremors, vertigo.	Supportive care, airway control. **Antidote:** Flumazenil (Romazicon).
Forget me pill (see flunitrazepam)			

(*continued*)

Name (Brand)	Class	Signs and Symptoms	Treatment
GHB (gamma-hydroxybutyrate)	CNS depressant	Dose-related CNS depression, amnesia, hypotonia, drowsiness, dizziness, euphoria. Other effects: bradycardia, hypotension, hypersalivation, vomiting, hypothermia. Higher dosages: Cheyne-Stokes respiration, seizures, coma, death. Users may become highly agitated.	Supportive care. Severe intoxication may require airway support, including intubation. **Antidote:** No specific antidote.
Gib (see GHB)			
Goodfellas (see fentanyl)			
Grass (see marijuana)			
Hashish (see marijuana)			
Heroin	Opioid	Miosis, coma, apnea, pulmonary edema, bradycardia, hypotension, pinpoint pupils, CNS depression, seizures.	Airway management. **Antidote:** Naloxone, nalmefene.
Horse (see heroin)			
Ice (see amphetamine)			
Ketamine (Ketalar)	Anesthetic	Feeling of dissociation from one's self (sense of floating over one's body), visual hallucinations, lack of coordination, hypertension, tachycardia, palpitations, respiratory depression, apnea, confusion, negativism, hostility, delirium, reduced awareness.	Supportive care, especially respiratory and cardiac function. **Antidote:** No specific antidote.
Keets (see ketamine)			
Kit-kat (see ketamine)			
Liquid ecstasy (see GHB)			
Liquid X (see GHB)			
LSD	Hallucinogen	Diaphoresis, mydriasis, dizziness, muscle twitching, flushing, hyperreflexia, hypertension, psychosis, behavioral changes, emotional lability, euphoria or dysphoria, paranoia, vomiting, diarrhea, anorexia, restlessness, incoordination, tremors, ataxia.	Airway management, control activity associated with hallucinations, psychosis, panic reaction. **Antidote:** No specific antidote.

Name (Brand)	Class	Signs and Symptoms	Treatment
Ludes (see methaqualone)			
Magic mushroom (see psilocybin)			
Marijuana	Cannabinoid	Increased appetite, reduced motility, constipation, urinary retention, seizures, euphoria, somnolence, heightened awareness, relaxation, altered time perception, short-term memory loss, poor concentration, mood alterations, disorientation, decreased strength, ataxia, slurred speech, respiratory depression, coma.	Airway management, supportive care. **Antidote:** No specific antidote.
MDMA (Methylene-dioxymethamphet-amine)	Stimulant	Euphoria, intimacy, closeness to others, loss of appetite, tachycardia, jaw tension, bruxism, diaphoresis.	**Antidote:** No specific antidote.
Mescaline	Hallucinogen	Diaphoresis, mydriasis, dizziness, twitching, flushing, hyperreflexia, hypertension, psychosis, behavioral changes, emotional instability, euphoria or dysphoria, paranoia, vomiting, diarrhea, anorexia, restlessness, incoordination, tremors, ataxia.	Airway management, control activity associated with hallucinations, psychosis, panic reaction. **Antidote:** No specific antidote.
Meth (see methamphetamine)			
Methamphetamine (Desoxyn)	Stimulant	Hypertension, hyper-thermia, hyperpyrexia, agitation, hyperactivity, fasciculation, seizures, coma, tachycardia, dysrhythmias, pale skin, diaphoresis, restlessness, talkativeness, insomnia, headache, coma, delusions, paranoia, aggressive behavior, visual, tactile, or auditory hallucinations.	Airway control, hyperthermia, seizures, dysrhythmias. **Antidote:** No specific antidote.

(continued)

Name (Brand)	Class	Signs and Symptoms	Treatment
Methaqualone (Quaalude)	Depressant	Slurred speech, impaired judgment and motor skills, hypothermia, hypotension, bradycardia, diplopia, blurred vision, nystagmus, mydriasis, respiratory depression, depression, lethargy, headache, ataxia, coma, amnesia, incoordination, hypertonicity, myoclonus, tremors, vertigo.	Airway management, supportive care. **Antidote:** No specific antidote.
Methylphenidate (Ritalin)	Stimulant	Agitation, hypertension, tachycardia, hyperthermia, mydriasis, dry mouth, nausea, vomiting, anorexia, abdominal pain, agitation, hyperactivity, insomnia, euphoria, dizziness, paranoid ideation, social withdrawal, delirium, hallucinations, psychosis, tremors, seizures.	Control agitation, hyperthermia, seizures, support hemodynamic function. **Antidote:** No specific antidote.
Miss Emma (see morphine)			
Mister blue (see morphine)			
Morphine (MS-Contin, Roxanol)	Opioid	Miosis, respiratory depression, decreased mental status, hypotension, cardiac dysrhythmia, hypoxia, bronchoconstriction, constipation, decreased intestinal motility, ileus, lethargy, coma.	Airway management, hemodynamic support. **Antidote:** Naloxone, nalmefene.
Oxy (see oxycodone)			
Oxycodone (OxyContin)	Opioid	Miosis, respiratory depression, decreased mental status, hypotension, cardiac dysrhythmia, hypoxia, bronchoconstriction, constipation, decreased intestinal motility, ileus, lethargy, coma.	Airway management, hemodynamic support. **Antidote:** Naloxone, nalmefene.

Name (Brand)	Class	Signs and Symptoms	Treatment
OxyContin (see oxycodone)			
Peace pill (see phencyclidine)			
Phencyclidine (PCP)	Hallucinogen	Nystagmus, hypertension, tachycardia, agitation, hallucinations, violent behavior, impaired judgment, delusions, psychosis.	Support blood pressure, manage airway, control agitation. **Antidote:** No specific antidote.
Phennies (see barbiturates)			
Pot (see marijuana)			
Propoxyphene (Darvon)	Depressant	Respiratory depression, seizures, cardiac toxicity, miosis, dysrhythmias, nausea, vomiting, anorexia, abdominal pain, constipation, drowsiness, coma, confusion, hallucinations.	Maintain airway, seizures, cardiac toxicity. **Antidote:** Naloxone.
Psilocybin	Hallucinogen	Diaphoresis, mydriasis, dizziness, twitching, flushing, hyperreflexia, hypertension, psychosis, behavioral changes, emotional lability, euphoria or dysphoria, paranoia, vomiting, diarrhea, anorexia, restlessness, incoordination, tremors, ataxia.	Manage airway, control activity associated with hallucinations, psychosis, panic reaction. **Antidote:** No specific antidote.
Purple passion (see psilocybin)			
Quay (see methaqualone)			
Reefer (see marijuana)			
Rock (see cocaine)			
Rocket fuel (see phencyclidine)			
Roofies (see flunitrazepam)			
Rope (see flunitrazepam)			
Rophies (see flunitrazepam)			
Salty water (see GHB)			
Schoolboy (see codeine)			
Scoop (see GHB)			
Snow (see cocaine)			
Special K (see ketamine)			

(*continued*)

APPENDIX D

Name (Brand)	Class	Signs and Symptoms	Treatment
Speed (see amphetamine)			
STP (see MDMA)			
Super acid (see ketamine)			
Super K (see ketamine)			
Tranks (see benzodiazepines)			
Uppers (see amphetamine)			
White girl (see cocaine)			
Yellow jackets (see barbiturates)			
Yellow sunshine (see LSD)			

"CLUB DRUG" WEB SITES

www.drugfreeamerica.org	Partnership for a Drug-Free America
www.clubdrugs.org	Consumer-oriented site sponsored by the National Institute on Drug Abuse
www.health.org	Substance Abuse and Mental Health Services Administration
www.projectghb.org	Independent site devoted to risks and dangers of GHB use
www.nida.nih.gov	National Institute on Drug Abuse
www.dea.gov	Drug Enforcement Administration
www.whitehousedrugpolicy.org	Office of National Drug Control Policy

EQUI-ANALGESIC DOSING

Guidelines for equi-analgesic dosing of commonly used analgesics are presented in the following table. The dosages are equivalent to 10 mg of morphine intramuscularly. These guidelines are for the management of acute pain in the opioid naive patient. Dosages may vary for the opioid-tolerant patient and for the management of chronic pain. Clinical response is the criteria that must be applied for each patient with titration to desired response.

Name	Equi-analgesic Oral Dose	Equi-analgesic Parenteral Dose
Butorphanol (Stadol)	Not available	2 mg q3–4h
Codeine	130 mg q3–4h	75 mg q3–4h
Hydrocodone	5–10 mg q3–4h	Not available
Hydromorphone (Dilaudid)	7.5 mg q3–4h	1.5 mg q3–4h
Meperidine (Demerol)	300 mg q2–3h	75–100 mg q3h
Methadone (Dolophine)	10–20 mg q6–8h	10 mg q6–8h
Morphine	30 mg q3–4h	10 mg q3–4h
Nalbuphine (Nubain)	Not available	10 mg q3–4h
Oxycodone (OxyContin)	20–30 mg q3–4h	Not available
Propoxyphene (Darvon)	65–130 mg q4–6h	Not available

FDA PREGNANCY CATEGORIES

◄ **ALERT** ► Medications should be used during pregnancy only if clearly needed.

A: Adequate and well-controlled studies have failed to show a risk to the fetus in the first trimester of pregnancy (also, no evidence of risk has been seen in later trimesters). Possibility of fetal harm appears remote.

B: Animal reproduction studies have failed to show a risk to the fetus, and there are no adequate/well-controlled studies in pregnant women.

C: Animal reproduction studies have shown an adverse effect on the fetus, and there are no adequate/well-controlled studies in humans. However, the benefits may warrant use of the drug in pregnant women despite potential risks.

D: There is positive evidence of human fetal risk based on data from investigational or marketing experience or from studies in humans, but the potential benefits may warrant use of the drug despite potential risks (e.g., use in life-threatening situations in which other medications cannot be used or are ineffective).

X: Animal or human studies have shown fetal abnormalities and/or there is evidence of human fetal risk based on adverse reaction data from investigational or marketing experience where the risks of using the medication clearly outweigh potential benefits.

HERBAL THERAPIES AND INTERACTIONS

The use of herbal therapies is increasing in the United States. In 1990, an estimated 1 in 3 Americans used at least one form of alternative medicine (of which herbal therapy is part). By 1997, more than $12 billion was spent in the United States for vitamins and minerals, herbals, sports supplements, or specialty supplements (e.g., glucosamine).

Because of the rise in the use of herbal therapy in the United States, the following is presented to provide some basic information on some of the more popular herbs. Please note this is not an all-inclusive list, which is beyond the scope of this handbook.

Name	Uses	Interactions	Precautions
Aloe	**Topical:** Promotes burn/wound healing, treatment of cold sores. **Oral:** Laxative, cathartic.	**Topical:** None. **Oral:** May increase risk of side effects with cardiac glycosides, antiarrhythmics, diuretics.	**Topical:** None. **Oral:** Abdominal pain, diarrhea, reduced serum potassium.
Astaxanthin	**Oral:** Macular degeneration, Alzheimer's disease, Parkinson's disease, stroke, cancer, hypercholesterolemia. **Topical:** Sunburn.	None known.	May cause visual disturbances.
Avocado	Reduce serum cholesterol, stimulate menstrual flow, treatment of osteoarthritis.	May reduce effects of warfarin.	Patients allergic to latex should avoid eating avocado due to possibility of cross sensitivity.
Bilberry	**Topical:** Mild inflammation of mouth/throat. **Oral:** Acute diarrhea, increased visual acuity, angina, atherosclerosis.	May require adjustment of antidiabetic drugs (reduces glucose effect).	May decrease serum glucose, triglycerides.
Bitter orange	Appetite stimulant, treatment of dyspepsia, weight loss, nasal congestion.	Can inhibit cytochrome P450 metabolism of drugs causing increased drug levels, risk of adverse effects [e.g., felodipine (Plendil), indinavir (Crixivan) and midazolam (Versed)].	Contains synephrine and octopamine which may cause hypertension, cardiovascular toxicity. Avoid use in pregnancy when used for medicinal purposes, safe when used orally in amounts found in foods.

(continued)

Name	Uses	Interactions	Precautions
Black cohosh*	Manage symptoms of menopause, hypercholesterolemia, peripheral arterial disease, anti-inflammatory and sedative effects.	May further reduce lipids and/or BP when combined with prescription medications.	Side effects: nausea, dizziness, visual changes, migraine.
Boldo	Mild GI spasms, dyspepsia, anti-inflammatory agent, laxative, gallstones.	May have additive effects when used with anticoagulant or antiplatelet medications.	*Oral:* Seizures. *Topical:* Skin irritation.
Butterbut	Abdominal pain, back pain, gallbladder pain, bladder spasms, tension headache, migraine headaches, asthma.	None known.	May cause headache, itchy eyes, diarrhea, asthma, abdominal discomfort, fatigue, drowsiness.
Capsicum	*Topical:* Postherpetic, trigeminal, diabetic neuralgias; HIV-associated peripheral neuropathy.	None.	Burning, urticaria, irritation to eyes, mucous membranes.
Cat's Claw	Arthritis, peptic ulcer colitis, bone pain.	May increase effect of anti-hypertensives.	Headache, dizziness, vomiting.
Catnip	*Topical:* Arthritis, hemorrhoids. *Oral:* Insomnia, migraine, cold, flu, hives, indigestion, cramping, flatulence.	May be additive with other CNS depressants.	Headache, malaise, vomiting (large doses).
Chamomile*	Antispasmodic, sedative, anti-inflammatory, astringent, antibacterial.	May increase bleeding with anticoagulants. May increase sedative effect with benzodiazepines.	Anaphylactic reaction if allergic; avoid use if allergic to chrysanthemums, ragweed, and/or asters; delays absorption of medications.
Chastberry	*Oral:* Control of menstrual irregularities, painful menstruation.	May interfere with oral contraceptives, hormone replacement therapy, dopamine antagonists (e.g., antipsychotics).	GI disturbances, rash, itching, headache, increased menstrual flow.

*See full herb entry in the A to Z section.

Name	Uses	Interactions	Precautions
Co-Enzyme Q-10	**Oral:** CHF, angina, diabetes, hypertension; reduces symptoms of chronic fatigue; stimulates immune system in those with AIDS.	May decrease effect of warfarin. Statins may decrease effect.	Reduced appetite, gastritis, nausea, diarrhea.
Conjugated linoleic acid	Obesity, bodybuilding, atherosclerosis.	May increase vitamin A storage in liver and breast tissues.	May cause GI upset, diarrhea, nausea, loose stools, dyspepsia, fatigue. Avoid use in pregnancy when used for medicinal purposes, safe when used orally in amounts found in foods.
Cranberry	**Oral:** Prevention, treatment of urinary tract infections; urinary deodorizer.	May increase absorption of vitamin B_{12} in those taking proton pump inhibitors (e.g., Prevacid).	Large doses may cause diarrhea.
Devil's claw	Osteoarthritis, rheumatoid arthritis, gout, myalgia, lumbago, tendonitis.	May increase effect of antihypertensives, warfarin.	Diarrhea, nausea, vomiting, abdominal pain. May cause skin reactions.
DHEA*	Slows aging, boosts energy, controls weight.	None.	Side effects: may increase risk of breast/prostate cancer. Women may develop acne, hair growth on face/body.
Dong quai*	Uterine stimulant, anti-inflammatory, vasodilator, CNS stimulant, immunosuppressant, analgesic, antipyretic.	May increase effects of warfarin.	Diarrhea, photosensitivity, skin cancer; avoid use in pregnancy/lactation; essential oil may contain the carcinogen safrole.
Echinacea*	Prevents/treats colds, flu, bacterial and fungal infections. Immune system stimulator. Aid to wound healing.	May interfere with immunosuppressive therapy.	Not to be used with weakened immune system (e.g., HIV/AIDS, tuberculosis, multiple sclerosis). Habitual or continued use may suppress the immune system (should only be taken for 2–3 mo or alternating schedule of q2–3wk).

(continued)

*See full herb entry in the A to Z section.

Name	Uses	Interactions	Precautions
Elderberry	Treatment of influenza, laxative, diuretic, allergic rhinitis, sinusitis, neuralgia	May interfere with immuno-suppressant therapy [e.g., azathioprine (Imuran), cyclosporine (Neoral), mycophenolate (CellCept)]	Avoid using during pregnancy and lactation. Well tolerated. May cause nausea, vomiting, severe diarrhea.
Emu oil	**Oral:** Hypercholestero-lemia, weight loss, cough syrup. **Topical:** Relief from sore muscles, arthralgia, pain, inflammation, carpal tunnel syndrome.	None known.	None reported.
Evening primrose oil	**Oral:** PMS, symptoms of menopause (e.g., hot flashes), psoriasis, rheumatoid arthritis.	Antipsychotics may increase risk of seizures.	Indigestion, nausea, headache. Large doses may cause diarrhea, abdominal pain.
Fenugreek	Lowered blood glucose, gastritis, constipation, atherosclerosis, elevated serum cholesterol and triglyceride levels.	May have additive effects with antidiabetic, anticoagulant, antiplatelet medications.	Nasal congestion, wheezing. Large doses may cause hypoglycemia.
Feverfew*	Relieves migraine. Treatment of fever, headache, menstrual irregularities.	May increase bleeding time with aspirin, dipyridamole, warfarin.	Side effects: headache, oral ulcers. Should be avoided in pregnancy (stimulates menstruation), nursing mother, children younger than 2 yr.
Fish oils	**Oral:** Hypertension, hyperlipidemia, coronary artery disease, rheumatoid arthritis, psoriasis.	May increase risk of bleeding with antiplatelets, anti-coagulants. Additive effect with antihypertensives.	Belching, heartburn, epistaxis. Large doses may cause nausea, diarrhea.

*See full herb entry in the A to Z section.

Name	Uses	Interactions	Precautions
Garlic*	Reduces serum cholesterol, LDL, triglycerides, increases serum HDL, lowers BP, inhibits platelet aggregation. May possess antibacterial, antiviral, antithrombotic activity.	May increase bleeding time with aspirin, dipyridamole, warfarin.	Side effects: taste, offensive odor. Large doses may cause heartburn, flatulence, other GI distress.
Ginger*	Relieves nausea, effective treatment for motion sickness, anti-inflammatory for arthritis, nausea/vomiting associated with pregnancy. Possesses ability to diminish platelet aggregation; anti-thrombotic properties.	None.	Avoid use during pregnancy when bleeding is a concern. Large overdose could potentially depress the CNS, cause cardiac arrhythmias.
Ginkgo*	Improves memory, concentration; patient may think more clearly. Overcomes sexual dysfunction occurring with SSRI antidepressants. May be able to slow progress of Alzheimer's disease, improve intermittent claudication.	May increase bleeding time with aspirin, dipyridamole, warfarin.	Avoid use in those taking anticoagulants or those hypersensitive to poison ivy, cashews, mangos. Side effects: GI disturbances, headache, dizziness, vertigo.
Ginseng*	Boosts energy, sexual stamina; decreases stress, effects of aging.	May affect platelet adhesiveness/blood coagulation. Use caution with anticoagulants. May increase Hypoglycemia with insulin.	Avoid in patients receiving anticoagulants, medications that increase BP. Side effects: breast tenderness, nervousness, headache, increased BP, abnormal vaginal bleeding.
Glucosamine and chondroitin*	Osteoarthritis.	No known interactions but monitor anticoagulant effects.	None known.

(continued)

*See full herb entry in the A to Z section.

Name	Uses	Interactions	Precautions
Goldenrod	*Oral:* Diuretic, anti-inflammatory, antispasmodic. Prevents urinary tract inflammation, urinary calculi, kidney stones.	May interfere with diuretics.	Allergic reactions.
Goldenseal	*Topical:* Eczema, itching, acne. *Oral:* UTI, hemorrhoids, gastritis, colitis, mucosal inflammation.	May interfere with antacids, sucralfate, H_2 antagonists, proton pump inhibitors.	Constipation, hallucinations. Large doses may cause nausea, vomiting, diarrhea, CNS stimulation, respiratory failure.
Gotu kola	Improves memory, intelligence, venous insufficiency (including varicose veins), wound or burn healing, psoriasis.	None known.	GI upset, nausea, pruritus, photosensitivity.
Grape seed extract	Improves circulation, decreases tissue injury, hemorrhoids. Used as antioxidant to treat hypoxia from atherosclerosis, inflammation.	None.	None reported.
Green tea	*Oral:* Improves cognition function, treats nausea, vomiting, headache, weight loss.	May increase risk of bleeding with antiplatelets.	GI upset, constipation.
Guggul	Lowers serum cholesterol, treatment of acne, skin disease, weight loss.	None known.	May cause headache, nausea, vomiting, loose stools, bloating.
Gymnema	Treatment of diabetes, cough.	May enhance effects of insulin, oral antidiabetics.	None reported.
Hawthorn	Cardiovascular conditions (e.g., atherosclerosis), GI conditions (diarrhea, indigestion, abdominal pain), sleep disorders.	Cardiovascular drugs, digoxin may potentiate or interfere; additive effect with CNS depressants.	Nausea, GI complaints, headache, dizziness, insomnia, agitation.

*See full herb entry in the A to Z section.

Name	Uses	Interactions	Precautions
Hoodia	Appetite suppressant for obesity, weight loss.	None.	None reported.
Horse chestnut	Reduces edema following injury, chronic venous insufficiency including varicose veins, hemorrhoids, phlebitis.	May enhance effects of insulin, oral antidiabetics, antiplatelet medications.	Muscle cramps, pruritus, GI irritation.
Kava kava*	Reduces stress, muscle relaxant, relieves anxiety, induces sleep, counters fatigue.	Increases CNS depression with alcohol, sedatives.	Side effects: GI disturbances, temporary discoloration of skin, hair, nails. Do not use in pregnancy, lactation, endogenous depression. Large doses cause muscle weakness. Chronic use may cause scaly skin resembling psoriasis (reversible). Causes pupil dilation affecting vision (avoid driving, operating heavy machinery). Store in cool, dry place (excess heat/light alters contents).
L-Carnitine	Treatment of primary L-Carnitine deficiency, postmyocardial infarction protection, dementia, angina, congestive heart failure, intermittent claudication.	None known.	Abdominal discomfort, diarrhea, nausea, vomiting, heartburn.
Licorice	*Oral:* Inflammation of upper respiratory tract, mucous membranes, ulcers, expectorant.	May decrease effect of antihypertensives. Thiazides may increase potassium loss.	Large doses may cause pseudoaldosteronism (hypertension, headache, lethargy, edema).
Melatonin*	Aids sleep, prevents jet lag.	Decreases effects of antidepressants.	Side effects: headache, confusion, fatigue. Does not lengthen total sleep time.

(continued)

*See full herb entry in the A to Z section.

Name	Uses	Interactions	Precautions
Milk thistle	Hepatoprotective, antioxidant, hepatic disorders, including poisoning (e.g., mushroom), cirrhosis, hepatitis.	None.	Mild allergic reactions, laxative effect.
MSM (methyl sulfonyl methane)	*Oral/topical:* Chronic pain, arthritis, inflammation, osteoporosis, muscle cramps/pain, wrinkles, protection against windburn or sunburn.	None known.	May cause nausea, diarrhea, headache, pruritus, increase in allergic symptoms.
Omega-6 fatty acid	*Oral:* Coronary artery disease, decreases total serum LDL cholesterol, increases serum HDL.	None.	Increases serum triglycerides.
Policosanol	Hyperlipidemia, intermittent claudication, reducing myocardial ischemia.	Can inhibit platelet aggregation. May increase risk of bruising and bleeding with aspirin, Plavix, NSAIDs, heparin, warfarin.	Usually well tolerated. Avoid using during pregnancy and lactation. May cause erythema, migraines, insomnia, irritability, upset stomach, weight loss, skin rash.
Pome-granate	Increases antioxidant activity. Treatment of hypertension, hyperlipidemia, atherosclerosis, myocardial ischemia.	May have additive effects with ACE inhibitors, antihypertensives. May increase serum levels of calcium channel blockers, protease inhibitiors, benzodiazepines (e.g., Valium).	Avoid using during pregnancy and breastfeeding. May cause allergic reactions, GI disturbances.
Prickly pear cactus	Hypercholesterolemia, obesity, alcohol induced hangover.	None known.	Usually well tolerated. May cause mild diarrhea, nausea, increased stool volume, increased stool frequency, abdominal fullness, headache.

*See full herb entry in the A to Z section.

Name	Uses	Interactions	Precautions
Red clover	**Oral:** Menopausal symptoms, hot flashes, prevention of cancer, indigestion, asthma. **Topical:** Skin sores, burns, chronic skin disease (e.g., eczema, psoriasis).	May increase anticoagulant effects of warfarin. May interfere with hormone replacement therapy, oral contraceptives, tamoxifen.	Rash, myalgia, headache, nausea, vaginal spotting.
SAMe	**Oral:** Depression, heart disease, osteoarthritis, Alzheimer's disease, Parkinson's disease; slows aging process.	May increase adverse effects with antidepressants.	Nausea, vomiting, diarrhea, flatulence; headache.
Saw palmetto*	Eases symptoms of enlarged prostate (frequency, dysuria, nocturia).	None.	Side effects: abdominal discomfort, headache, erectile dysfunction. Does not reduce size of enlarged prostate. Obtain baseline PSA levels before initiating. Large doses can cause diarrhea.
Shark cartilage	**Oral:** Cancer, arthritis, psoriasis, wound healing.	None.	Nausea, vomiting, constipation, dyspepsia, altered taste.
Soy	Menopausal symptoms; prevents osteoporosis and cardiovascular disease in postmenopausal women; hypertension, hyperlipidemia.	May decrease effects of estrogen replacement therapy.	Constipation, bloating, nausea, allergic reaction.
Soybean oil	Lowers total and LDL cholesterol	None known	May cause allergic reactions.
St. John's wort*	Relieves mild to moderate depression, heals wounds.	May cause "serotonin syndrome" (confusion, agitation, chills, fever, diaphoresis, diarrhea, nausea, muscle spasms or twitching), hyperreflexia, tremor with antidepressants, yohimbe.	Side effects: dizziness, dry mouth, increased sensitivity to sunlight. Report symptoms of "serotonin syndrome."

(continued)

*See full herb entry in the A to Z section.

Name	Uses	Interactions	Precautions
Tyrosine	Premenstrual syndrome (PMS), depression, attention deficit disorder (ADD), attention deficit hyperactivity disorder (ADHD), improve alertness	May decrease effects of L-dopa. May have additive effects with thyroid hormone.	May cause nausea, headache, fatigue, heartburn, arthralgia.
Valerian*	Aids sleep, relieves restlessness and nervousness. Does not decrease night awakenings.	None.	Side effects: palpitations, upset stomach, headache, excitability, uneasiness. May cause increased morning drowsiness.
Whey protein	Alternative to milk in those with lactose intolerance, treatment of hyperlipidemia, obesity and weight loss.	May decrease absorption of alendronate (Fosamax), levodopa, quinolone antibiotics (e.g., levofloxacin).	Well tolerated. High doses may cause increased stool frequency, nausea, thirst, bloating, cramps, decreased appetite, fatigue, headache.
Wild yam	**Oral:** Alternative for estrogen replacement therapy, postmenopausal vaginal dryness, premenstrual syndrome, osteoporosis, increases energy/libido, breast enlargement.	None known.	Large amounts may cause vomiting (tincture).
Yohimbe*	Male aphrodisiac. Used to treat impotence, erectile dysfunction, orthostatic hypotension.	Decreases effects of antidepressants, antihypertensives, St. John's wort.	Large doses linked to weakness, paralysis.

*See full herb entry in the A to Z section.

LIFESPAN AND CULTURAL ASPECTS OF DRUG THERAPY

LIFESPAN

Drug therapy is unique to patients of different ages. Age-specific competencies involve understanding the development and health needs of the various age groups. Patients who are pregnant, children, and the elderly represent different age groups with important considerations during drug therapy.

CHILDREN

In pediatric drug therapy, drug administration is guided by the age of the child, weight, level of growth and development, and height. The dosage ordered is to be given either by kilogram of body weight or by square meter of body surface area, which is based on the height and weight of the child. Many dosages based on these calculations must be individualized based on pediatric response.

If the oral route of administration is used, often syrup or chewable tablets are given. Additionally, sometimes medication is added to liquid or mixed with foods. Remember to never force a child to take oral medications because choking or emotional trauma may ensue.

If an intramuscular injection is ordered, the vastus lateralis muscle in the mid-lateral thigh is used, because the gluteus maximus is not developed until walking occurs and the deltoid muscle is too small. For intravenous medications, administer very slowly in children. If given too quickly, high serum drug levels will occur with the potential for toxicity.

PREGNANCY

Women of childbearing years should be asked about the possibility of pregnancy before any drug therapy is initiated. Advise a woman who is either planning a pregnancy or believes she may be pregnant to inform her physician immediately. During pregnancy, medications given to the mother pass to the fetus via the placenta. Teratogenic (fetal abnormalities) effects may occur. Breast-feeding while the mother is taking certain medications may not be recommended due to the potential for adverse effects on the newborn.

The choice of drug ordered for the pregnant women is based on the stage of pregnancy, because the fetal organs develop during the first trimester. Cautious use of drugs in women of reproductive age who are sexually active and who are not using contraceptives is essential to prevent the potential for teratogenic or embryotoxic effects. Refer to the different pregnancy categories (found in Appendix F) to determine the relative safety of a medication during pregnancy.

ELDERLY

The elderly are more likely to experience an adverse drug reaction owing to physiologic changes (e.g., visual, hearing, mobility changes, chronic diseases) and cognitive changes (short-term memory loss or alteration in the thought process) that may lead to multiple medication dosing. In chronic disease states such as hypertension, glaucoma, asthma, or arthritis, the daily ingestion of multiple medications increases the potential for adverse reactions and toxic effects.

Decreased renal or hepatic function may lower the metabolism of medications in the liver and reduce excretion of medications, thus prolonging the half-life of the drug and the potential for toxicity. Dosages in the elderly should initially be smaller than for the general adult population and then slowly titrated based on patient response and therapeutic effect of the medication.

CULTURE

The term *ethnopharmacology* was first used to describe the study of medicinal plants used by indigenous cultures. More recently, it is being used as a reference to the action and effects of drugs in people from diverse racial, ethnic, and cultural backgrounds. Although there are insufficient data from investigations involving people from diverse backgrounds that would provide reliable information on ethnic-specific responses to all medications, there is growing evidence that modifications in dosages are needed for some members of racial and ethnic groups. There are wide variations in the perception of side effects by patients from diverse cultural backgrounds. These differences may be related to metabolic differences that result in higher or lower levels of the drug, individual differences in the amount of body fat, or cultural differences in the way individuals perceive the meaning of side effects and toxicity. Nurses and other health care providers need to be aware that variations can occur with side effects, adverse reactions, and toxicity so that patients from diverse cultural backgrounds can be monitored.

Some cultural differences in response to medications include the following:

African Americans: Generally, African Americans are less responsive to beta-blockers (e.g., propranolol [Inderal]) and angiotensin-converting enzyme (ACE) inhibitors (e.g., enalapril [Vasotec]).

Asian Americans: On average, Asian Americans have a lower percentage of body fat, so dosage adjustments must be made for fat-soluble vitamins and other drugs (e.g., vitamin K used to reverse the anticoagulant effect of warfarin).

Hispanic Americans: Hispanic Americans may require lower dosages and may experience a higher incidence of side effects with the tricyclic antidepressants (e.g., amitryptyline).

Native Americans: Alaskan Eskimos may suffer prolonged muscle paralysis with the use of succinylcholine when administered during surgery.

There has been a desire to exert more responsibility over one's health and, as a result, a resurgence of self-care practices. These practices are often influenced by folk remedies and the use of medicinal plants. In the United States, there are several major ethnic population subgroups (white, black, Hispanic, Asian, and Native Americans). Each of these ethnic groups has a wide range of practices that influence beliefs and interventions related to health and illness. At any given time, in any group, treatment may consist of the use of traditional herbal therapy, a combination of ritual and prayer with medicinal plants, customary dietary and environmental practices, or the use of Western medical practices.

African Americans

Many African Americans carry the traditional health beliefs of their African heritage. Health denotes harmony with nature of the body, mind, and spirit, whereas illness is seen as disharmony that results from natural causes or divine punishment. Common practices to the art of healing include treatments with herbals and rituals known empirically to restore health. Specific forms of healing include using home remedies, obtaining medical advice from a physician, and seeking spiritual healing.

Examples of healing practices include the use of hot baths and warm compresses for rheumatism, the use of herbal teas for respiratory illnesses, and the use of kitchen condiments in folk remedies. Lemon, vinegar, honey, saltpeter, alum, salt, baking soda, and Epsom salt are common kitchen ingredients used. Goldenrod, peppermint, sassafras, parsley, yarrow, and rabbit tobacco are a few of the herbals used.

Hispanic Americans

The use of folk healers, medicinal herbs, magic, and religious rituals and ceremonies are included in the rich and varied customs of Hispanic Americans. This ethnic group believes that God is responsible for allowing health or illness to occur. Wellness may be viewed as good luck, a reward for good behavior, or a blessing from God. Praying, using herbals and spices, wearing religious objects such as medals, and maintaining a balance in diet and physical activity are methods considered appropriate in preventing evil or poor health.

Hispanic ethnopharmacology is more complementary to Western medical practices. After the illness is identified, appropriate treatment may consist of home remedies (e.g., use of vegetables and herbs), use of over-the-counter patent medicines, and use of physician-prescribed medications.

Asian Americans

For Asian Americans, harmony with nature is essential for physical and spiritual well-being. Universal balance depends on harmony among the elemental forces: fire, water, wood, earth, and metal. Regulating these universal elements are two forces that maintain physical and spiritual harmony in the body: the *yin* and the *yang.* Practices shared by most Asian cultures include meditation, special nutritional programs, herbology, and martial arts.

Therapeutic options available to traditional Chinese physicians include prescribing herbs, meditation, exercise, nutritional changes, or acupuncture.

Native Americans

The theme of total harmony with nature is fundamental to traditional Native American beliefs about health. It is dependent on maintaining a state of equilibrium among the physical body, the mind, and the environment. Health practices reflect this holistic approach. The method of healing is determined traditionally by the medicine man, who diagnoses the ailment and recommends the appropriate intervention.

Treatment may include heat, herbs, sweat baths, massage, exercise, diet changes, or other interventions performed in a curing ceremony.

European Americans

Europeans often use home treatments as the front-line interventions. Traditional remedies practiced are based on the magical or empirically validated experience of ancestors. These cures are often practiced in combination with religious rituals or spiritual ceremonies.

Household products, herbal teas, and patent medicines are familiar preparations used in home treatments (e.g., salt water gargle for sore throat).

Appendix I

NORMAL LABORATORY VALUES

HEMATOLOGY/COAGULATION

Test	Specimen	Normal Range
Activated partial thromboplastin time (aPTT)	Whole blood	25–35 sec
Erythrocyte count (RBC count)	Whole blood	M: 4.3–5.7 million cells/mm^3 F: 3.8–5.1 million cells/mm^3
Hematocrit (HCT, Hct)	Whole blood	M: 39%–49% F: 35%–45%
Hemoglobin (Hb, Hgb)	Whole blood	M: 13.5–17.5 g/dl F: 12.0–16.0 g/dl
Leukocyte count (WBC count)	Whole blood	4.5–11.0 thousand cells/mm^3
Leukocyte differential count	Whole blood	
Basophils		0%–0.75%
Eosinophils		1%–3%
Lymphocytes		23%–33%
Monocytes		3%–7%
Neutrophils-bands		3%–5%
Neutrophils-segmented		54%–62%
Mean corpuscular hemoglobin (MCH)	Whole blood	26–34 pg/cell
Mean corpuscular hemoglobin concentration (MCHC)	Whole blood	31%–37% Hb/cell
Mean corpuscular volume (MCV)	Whole blood	80–100 fL
Partial thromboplastin time (PTT)	Whole blood	60–85 sec
Platelet count (thrombocyte count)	Whole blood	150–450 thousand/mm^3
Prothrombin time (PT)	Whole blood	11–13.5 sec
RBC count (see Erythrocyte count)		

CLINICAL CHEMISTRY (SERUM PLASMA, URINE)

Test	Specimen	Normal Range
Alanine aminotransferase (ALT)	Serum	0–55 units/L
Albumin	Serum	3.5–5 g/dl
Alkaline phosphatase	Serum	M: 53–128 units/L F: 42–98 units/L
Anion gap	Plasma or serum	5–14 mEq/L
Aspartate aminotransferase (AST)	Serum	0–50 units/L
Bilirubin (conjugated direct)	Serum	0–0.4 mg/dl
Bilirubin (total)	Serum	0.2–1.2 mg/dl
Calcium (total)	Serum	8.4–10.2 mg/dl
Carbon dioxide (CO_2) total	Plasma or serum	20–34 mEq/L
Chloride	Plasma or serum	96–112 mEq/L
Cholesterol (total)	Plasma or serum	Less than 200 mg/dl
C-Reactive protein	Serum	68–8,200 ng/ml
Creatine kinase (CK)	Serum	M: 38–174 units/L F: 26–140 units/L

(continued)

Test	Specimen	Normal Range
Creatine kinase isoenzymes	Serum	Fraction of total: less than 0.04–0.06
Creatinine	Plasma or serum	M: 0.7–1.3 mg/dl F: 0.6–1.1 mg/dl
Creatinine clearance	Plasma or serum and urine	M: 90–139 ml/min/1.73 m^2 F: 80–125 ml/min/1.73 m^2
Free thyroxine index (FTI)	Serum	1.1–4.8
Glucose	Serum	Adults: 70–105 mg/dl Older than 60 yr: 80–115 mg/dl
Hemoglobin A$_{1c}$	Whole blood	5.6%–7.5% of total Hgb
Homovanillic acid (HVA)	Urine, 24 hr	1.4–8.8 mg/day
17-Hydroxycorticosteroids (17-OHCS)	Urine, 24 hr	M: 3–10 mg/day F: 2–8 mg/day
Iron	Serum	M: 65–175 mcg/dl F: 50–170 mcg/dl
Iron-binding capacity, total (TIBC)	Serum	250–450 mcg/dl
Lactate dehydrogenase (LDH)	Serum	0–250 units/L
Magnesium	Serum	1.3–2.3 mg/dl
Oxygen (O$_2$)	Whole blood, arterial	83–100 mm Hg
Oxygen saturation	Whole blood, arterial	95%–98%
PH	Whole blood, arterial	7.35–7.45
Phosphorus, inorganic	Serum	2.7–4.5 mg/dl
Potassium	Serum	3.5–5.1 mEq/L
Protein (total)	Serum	6–8.5 g/dl
Sodium	Plasma or serum	136–146 mEq/L
Specific gravity	Urine	1.002–1.030
Thyrotropin (hTSH)	Plasma or serum	2–10 mU/ml
Thyroxine (T$_4$) total	Serum	5–12 mcg/dl
Triglycerides (TG)	Serum, after 12-hr fast	20–190 mg/dl
Triiodothyronine resin uptake test (T$_3$RU)	Serum	22%–37%
Urea nitrogen	Plasma or serum	7–25 mg/dl
Urea nitrogen/creatinine ratio	Serum	12/1–20/1
Uric acid	Serum	M: 3.5–7.2 mg/dl F: 2.6–6 mg/dl
Vanillylmandelic acid (VMA)	Urine, 24 hr	2–7 mg/day

ORPHAN DRUGS

The term *orphan drug* refers to either a drug or a biologic that is intended for use in a rare disease or condition. A rare disease or condition is one that affects less than 200,000 people in the United States or, if greater than 200,000 people, in which there is no reasonable expectation that the cost of developing the drug or biologic and making it available would be recovered from the sales of that product.

A drug or biologic becomes an "orphan drug" when it is so designated from the Office of Orphan Products Development (OOPD) at the FDA. Orphan drug designation allows the sponsor of the drug or biologic to receive certain benefits from the government in exchange for developing the drug.

The drug or biologic must go through the FDA approval process like any other drug to evaluate it for both safety and efficacy. Since 1983, over 1,400 drugs and biologics have been designated orphan drugs, with over 250 products approved for marketing. After the orphan drug has been approved by the FDA for marketing, it becomes available through normal pharmaceutical supply channels. If not approved by the FDA, the product may be made available on a compassionate use basis. Contact information can be obtained from the OOPD at the FDA.

Office of Orphan Products Development
Food and Drug Administration
5600 Fishers Lane
Rockville, MD 20857
http://www.fda.gov/orphan/

Examples of orphan drugs include the following:

Drug Name	Proposed Use	Sponsor
90y-Hpama4 (Pancide)	Pancreatic cancer	Immunomedics, Inc.
Alpha-1-acid glycoprotein	Cocaine overdose, tricyclic antidepressant poisoning	Bio Products Laboratory
Ambrisentan	Pulmonary arterial hypertension	Maygen, Inc.
Aplidin	Acute lymphoblastic leukemia	PharmaMar USA, Inc.
Chenodeoxycholic acid (Chenofalk)	Cerebrotendinous xanthomatosis	Dr. Falk Pharma GmbH
Deferitrin	Iron overload	Genzyme Corporation
Depsipeptide	Cutaneous T-cell lymphoma	Glucester Pharmaceuticals, Inc.
Golimumab	Chronic sarcoidosis	Centocor, Inc.
Idebenone	Cardiomyopathy associated with Friedreich's ataxia	Santhera Pharmaceuticals LLC
Lenalidomide (Revimid)	Myelodysplastic syndromes	Celgene Corporation
Nelarabine	Acute lymphoblastic leukemia, lymphoblastic lymphoma	GlaxoSmithKline
Plitidepsin (Aplidin)	Multiple myeloma	PharmaMar USA, Inc.
Rufinamide	Lennox-Gastaut syndrome	Eisai Medical Research, Inc.
Sarsasapogenin	Amyotrophic lateral sclerosis (ALS)	Phytopharm
Sorafenib	Renal cell carcinoma	Bayer Pharmaceutical Corporation.
Suberoylanilide hydroxamic acid	T-cell non-Hodgkin's lymphoma, mesothelioma	Merck & Co., Inc.
Tipifarnib (Zamestra)	Acute myeloid leukemia	Johnson & Johnson Pharmaceutical Research
Trabectedin (Yondelis)	Soft tissue sarcoma	Johnson & Johnson Pharmaceutical Research

P450 (CYP) ENZYMES

Most drugs are eliminated from the body, at least in part, by being changed chemically to a less lipid soluble product (e.g., metabolized), and thus is more likely to be excreted from the body via the kidney or bile. Drugs may go through two different metabolic processes: Phase 1 and Phase 2 metabolism.

In Phase 1 metabolism, hepatic microsomal enzymes found in the endothelium of liver cells metabolizes drugs via hydrolysis and oxidation and reduction reactions. These chemical reactions make the drug more water soluble. In Phase 2 metabolism, large water soluble substances (e.g., glucuronic acid, sulfate) are attached to the drug, forming inactive, or significantly less active, water soluble metabolites. Phase 2 processes include glucuronidation, sulfation, conjugation, acetylation, and methylation.

Virtually any of the Phase 1 and Phase 2 enzymes can be inhibited, and some of these enzymes can be induced by drugs. Inhibiting the activity of metabolic enzymes results in increased concentrations of the drug (substrate) while inducing metabolic enzymes results in decreased concentrations of the drug (substrate).

The term "cytochrome P450" (CYP enzymes) refers to a family of over 100 enzymes in the human body that modulate various physiologic functions. First identified in the 1950s, the CYP enzyme system contains two large subgroups: steroidogenic and xenobiotic enzymes. Only the xenobiotic group is involved in the metabolism of drugs. The xenobiotic group includes 4 major enzyme families: CPP1, CYP2, CYP3, and CYP4. The primary role of these families is the metabolism of drugs. These families are further subdivided into subfamily designated by a capital letter and given a specific enzyme number (1, 2, 3, etc) according to the similarity in amino acid sequence it shares with other enzymes.

The key subfamilies are CYP1A, CYP2A, CYP2B, CYP2C, CYP2D, CYP2E, and CYP3A. CYP enzymes may be responsible for metabolism of 75% of all drugs with the CYP3A subfamily responsible for nearly half of this activity.

The CYP enzymes are found in the endoplasmic reticulum of cells in a variety of human tissue but are primarily concentrated in the liver and intestine. CYP enzymes can be both inhibited and induced, leading to increased or decreased serum concentration of the drug (along with its effects).

The following tables of CYP substrates, inhibitors and inducers provide a perspective on drugs that are affected by, or affect, cytochrome P450 (CYP) enzymes. **CYP substrate** includes drugs reported to be metaboolized, at least in part, by one or more CYP enzymes. **CYP inhibitor** includes drugs reported to inhibit one or more CYP enzymes. **CYP inducer** contains drugs reported to induce one or more CYP enzymes.

P450 ENZYMES: SUBSTRATES, INHIBITORS, INDUCERS

SUBSTRATES	INHIBITORS	INDUCERS
Albuterol	Amprenavir	Aminoglutethimide
Alprazolam	Atazanavir	Carbamazepine
Amiodarone	Clarithromycin	Fosphenytoin

(*continued*)

SUBSTRATES	INHIBITORS	INDUCERS
Amlodipine	Delavirdine	Nevirapine
Amprenavir	Diclofenac	Oxcarbazepine
Atorvastatin	Disulfiram	Phenobarbital
Bromocriptine	Fluconazole	Phenytoin
Budesonide	Fluoxetine	Primidone
Bupropion	Fosamprenavir	Rifampin
Carbamazepine	Ibuprofen	
Citalopram	Indinavir	
Clarithromycin	Isoniazid	
Cyclophosphamide	Itraconazole	
Cyclosporine	Ketoconazole	
Delavirdine	Lidocaine	
Diazepam	Miconazole	
Diltiazem	Nelfinavir	
Docetaxel	Nicardipine	
Doxepin	Omeprazole	
Doxorubicin	Paroxetine	
Enalapril	Pioglitazone	
Esomeprazole	Piroxacim	
Estradiol	Profolol	
Etoposide	Quinidine	
Haloperidol		
Imipramine		
Isosorbide		
Isradipine		
Ketoconazole		
Lansoprazole		
Lidocaine		
Losartan		
Lovastatin		
Midazolam		
Mirtazapine		
Nelfinavir		
Nifedipine		
Ondansetron		
Pacitaxel		
Pioglitazone		
Quetiapine		
Rabeprazole		
Rifampin		
Sildenafil		
Simvastatin		
Tamoxifen		
Tamsulosin		
Theophylline		
Timolol		
Tolterodine		
Trazodone		
Venlafaxine		
Verapamil		
Zolpidem		

POISON ANTIDOTE CHART

Poisoning Agent	Antidote	Indication
Acetaminophen	Acetylcysteine (Acetadote, Mucomyst)	Acute ingestion (more than 7.5 g in adults, more than 150 mg/kg in children); serum level more than 150 mg/L 4 hr postingestion, chronic ingestion of toxic amounts
Anticholinergic agents	Physostigmine	Reverse severe effects, including hallucination, agitation, intractable seizures
Arsenic	Dimercaprol (BAL in oil)	Arsenic poisoning
Benzodiazepines	Flumazenil (Romazicon)	Complete or partial reversal of benzodiazepine effects
Beta blockers	Glucagon	Aid in improving arterial pressure and contractility
Calcium blockers	Glucagon	Aid in improving arterial pressure and contractility
Carbamate pesticides	Atropine	Treatment of cholinergic symptoms due to agents that inhibit acetylcholinesterase activity
Digoxin (Lanoxin)	Digoxin immune FAB (Digibind)	Potentially life-threatening digoxin intoxication (e.g., severe ventricular arrhythmias), ingestion of more than 10 mg in adults or more than 4 mg in children
Ethylene glycol	Fomepizole (Antizol)	Symptomatic patient with suspected ingestion of ethylene glycol
Extravasation vasoconstrictive agents	Phentolamine (Regitine)	Extravasation of vasoconstrictive agents (e.g., epinephrine, norepinephrine)
Heparin	Protamine	Reversal of anticoagulant effect of heparin
Iron	Deferoxamine (Desferal)	Acute iron toxicity, chronic iron overload
Isoniazid	Pyridoxine (vitamin B_6)	Treatment of isoniazid overdose
Lead	Calcium EDTA	Acute and chronic lead poisoning, lead encephalopathy
Lead	Dimercaprol (BAL in oil)	Acute lead poisoning of levels more than 70 mcg/dl when used with calcium EDTA
Lead	Succimer (Chemet)	Lead poisoning in patient with levels more than 45 mcg/dl
Methanol	Fomepizole (Antizol)	Symptomatic patient with suspected ingestion of methanol
Opioids	Naloxone (Narcan)	Complete or partial reversal of narcotic depression including respiratory depresssion

(continued)

Poisoning Agent	Antidote	Indication
Organophosphate pesticides	Atropine	Treatment of cholinergic symptoms due to agents that inhibit acetylcholinesterase activity
Organophosphate pesticides	Pralidoxime (Protopam)	Treatment of severe poisoning in combination with atropine
Warfarin (Coumadin)	Phytonadione (vitamin K)	Excessive anticoagulation induced by warfarin

PREVENTING MEDICATION ERRORS AND IMPROVING MEDICATION SAFETY

Medication safety is a high priority for the health care professional. Prevention of medication errors and improved safety for the patient are important, especially in today's health care environment when today's patient is older and sometimes sicker and the drug therapy regimen can be more sophisticated and complex.

A medication error is defined by the National Coordinating Council for Medication Error Reporting and Prevention (NCC MERP) as "any preventable event that may cause or lead to inappropriate medication use or patient harm while the medication is in the control of the health care professional, patient, or consumer."

Most medication errors occur as a result of multiple, compounding events as opposed to a single act by a single individual.

Use of the wrong medication, strength, or dose; confusion over sound-alike or look-alike drugs; administration of medications by the wrong route; miscalculations (especially when used in pediatric patients or when administering medications intravenously); errors in prescribing and transcription all can contribute to compromising the safety of the patient. The potential for adverse events and medication errors is definitely a reality and is potentially tragic and costly in both human and economic terms.

Health care professionals must take the initiative to create and implement procedures to prevent medication errors from occurring and implement methods to reduce medication errors. The first priority in preventing medication errors is to establish a multidisciplinary team to improve medication use. The goal for this team would be to assess medication safety and implement changes that would make it difficult or impossible for mistakes to reach the patient. Some important criteria in making improved medication safety successful includes the following:

- Promote a nonpunitive approach to reducing medication errors
- Increase the detection and the reporting of medication errors, near misses, and potentially hazardous situations than may result in medication errors
- Determine root causes of medication errors
- Educate about the causes of medication errors and ways to prevent these errors
- Make recommendations to allow organization-wide, system-based changes to prevent medication errors
- Learn from errors that occur in other organizations and take measures to prevent similar errors

Some common causes and ways to prevent medication errors and improve safety include the following:

Handwriting: Poor handwriting can make it difficult to distinguish between two medications with similar names. Also, many drug names sound similar, especially when the names are spoken over the telephone, poorly enunciated, or mispronounced.

- Take time to write legibly.
- Keep phone or verbal orders to a minimum to prevent misinterpretation.

- Repeat back orders taken over the telephone.
- When ordering a new or rarely used medication, print the name.
- Always specify the drug strength, even if only one strength exists.
- Print generic and brand names of look-alike or sound-alike medications.

Zeros and decimal points: Hastily written orders can present problems even if the name of the medication is clear.

- Never leave a decimal point "naked." Place a zero before a decimal point when the number is less than a whole unit (e.g., use 0.25 mg or 250 mcg, **not** .25 mg).
- Never have a trailing zero following a decimal point (e.g., use 2 mg, **not** 2.0 mg).

Abbreviations: Errors can occur because of a failure to standardize abbreviations. Establishing a list of abbreviations that should never be used is recommended.

- Never abbreviate unit as "U," spell out "unit."
- Do not abbreviate "once daily" as OD or QD, or "every other day" as QOD; spell it out.
- Do not use D/C, as this may be misinterpreted as either discharge or discontinue.
- Do not abbreviate drug names; spell out the generic and/or brand names.

Ambiguous or incomplete orders: These types of orders can cause confusion or misinterpretation of the writer's intention. Examples include situations when the route of administration, dose, or dosage form has not been specified.

- Do not use slash marks—they are read as the number one (1).
- When reviewing an unusual order, verify the order with the person writing the order to prevent any misunderstanding.
- Read over orders after writing.
- Encourage that the drug's indication for use be provided on medication orders.
- Provide complete medication orders—do not use "resume preop" or "continue previous meds."

High-alert medications: Medications in this category have an increased risk of causing significant patient harm when used in error. Mistakes with these medications may or may not be more common but may be more devastating to the patient if an error occurs. A list of high-alert medications can be obtained from the Institute for Safe Medication Practices (ISMP) at www.ismp.org.

Technology available today that can be used to address and help to solve potential medication problems or errors include the following:

- Electronic prescribing systems—This refers to computerized prescriber order entry systems. Within these systems is the capability to incorporate medication safety alerts (e.g., maximum dose alerts, allergy screening). Additionally, these systems should be integrated or interfaced with pharmacy and laboratory systems to provide drug–drug and drug–disease interactions alerts and include clinical order screening capability.
- Bar codes—These systems are designed to use bar-code scanning devices to validate identity of patients, verify medications administered, document administration, and provide safety alerts.
- "Smart" infusion pumps—These pumps allow users to enter drug infusion protocols into a drug library along with predefined dosage limits. If a dosage is outside the limits established, an alarm is sounded and drug delivery is halted, informing the clinician that the dose is outside the recommended range.

- Automated dispensing systems–point of use dispensing system—These systems should be integrated with information systems, especially pharmacy systems.
- Pharmacy order entry system—This should be fully integrated with an electronic prescribing system with the capability of producing medication safety alerts. Additionally, the system should generate a computerized medication administration record (MAR), which would be used by a nursing staff while administering medications.

Appendix N

RECOMMENDED CHILDHOOD AND ADULT IMMUNIZATIONS

Recommended Childhood and Adolescent Immunization Schedule UNITED STATES • 2006

Vaccine ▼ Age ▶	Birth	1 month	2 months	4 months	6 months	12 months	15 months	18 months	24 months	4–6 years	11–12 years	13–14 years	15 years	16–18 years
Hepatitis B[1]	HepB	HepB	HepB	HepB[1]		HepB					HepB Series			
Diphtheria, Tetanus, Pertussis[2]			DTaP	DTaP	DTaP		DTaP			DTaP	Tdap		Tdap	
Haemophilus influenzae type b[3]			Hib	Hib	Hib[3]	Hib								
Inactivated Poliovirus			IPV	IPV		IPV				IPV				
Measles, Mumps, Rubella[4]						MMR				MMR		MMR		
Varicella[5]						Varicella					Varicella			
Meningococcal[6]									MPSV4		MCV4		MCV4	MCV4
Pneumococcal[7]			PCV	PCV	PCV	PCV	PCV		PCV		PPV			
Influenza[8]						Influenza (Yearly)				Influenza (Yearly)				
Hepatitis A[9]									HepA Series					

Range of recommended ages   Catch-up immunization   11–12 year old assessment

This schedule indicates the recommended ages for routine administration of currently licensed childhood vaccines, as of December 1, 2005, for children through age 18 years. Any dose not administered at the recommended age should be administered at any subsequent visit when indicated and feasible. Indicates age groups that warrant special effort to administer those vaccines not previously administered. Additional vaccines may be licensed and recommended during the year. Licensed combination vaccines may be used whenever any components of the combination are indicated and other components of the vaccine are not contraindicated and if approved by the Food and Drug Administration for that dose of the series. Providers should consult the respective ACIP statement for detailed recommendations. Clinically significant adverse events that follow immunization should be reported to the Vaccine Adverse Event Reporting System (VAERS). Guidance about how to obtain and complete a VAERS form is available at www.vaers.hhs.gov or by telephone, 800-822-7967.

1. **Hepatitis B vaccine (HepB).** *AT BIRTH:* All newborns should receive monovalent HepB soon after birth and before hospital discharge. **Infants born to mothers who are HBsAg-positive** should receive HepB and 0.5 mL of hepatitis B immune globulin (HBIG) within 12 hours of birth. **Infants born to mothers whose HBsAg status is unknown** should receive HepB within 12 hours of birth. The mother should have blood drawn as soon as possible to determine her HBsAg status; if HBsAg-positive, the infant should receive HBIG as soon as possible (no later than age 1 week). **For infants born to HBsAg-negative mothers,** the birth dose can be delayed in rare circumstances but only if a physician's order to withhold the vaccine and a copy of the mother's original HBsAg-negative laboratory report are documented in the infant's medical record. *FOLLOWING THE BIRTHDOSE:* The HepB series should be completed with either monovalent HepB or a combination vaccine containing HepB. The second dose should be administered at age 1–2 months. The final dose should be administered at age 24 weeks and older. It is permissible to administer 4 doses of HepB (e.g., when combination vaccines are given after the birth dose); however, if monovalent HepB is used, a dose at age 4 months is not needed. **Infants born to HBsAg-positive mothers** should be tested for HBsAg and antibody to HBsAg after completion of the HepB series, at age 9–18 months (generally at the next well-child visit after completion of the vaccine series).

2. **Diphtheria and tetanus toxoids and acellular pertussis vaccine (DTaP).** The fourth dose of DTaP may be administered as early as age 12 months, provided 6 months have elapsed since the third dose and the child is unlikely to return at age 15–18 months. The final dose in the series should be given at age 4 years and older.

   Tetanus and diphtheria toxoids and acellular pertussis vaccine (Tdap—adolescent preparation) is recommended at age 11–12 years for those who have completed the recommended childhood DTP/DTaP vaccination series and have not received a Td booster dose. Adolescents 13–18 years who missed the 11–12-year Td/Tdap booster dose should also receive a single dose of Tdap if they have received the recommended childhood DTP/DTaP vaccination series. Subsequent **tetanus and diphtheria toxoids (Td)** are recommended every 10 years.

3. **Haemophilus influenzae type b conjugate vaccine (Hib).** Three Hib conjugate vaccines are licensed for infant use. If PRP-OMP (PedvaxHIB® or ComVax® [Merck]) is administered at ages 2 and 4 months, a dose at age 6 months is not required. DTaP/Hib combination products should not be used for primary immunization in infants at ages 2, 4 or 6 months, but can be used as boosters after any Hib vaccine. The final dose in the series should be administered at age 12 months and older.

4. **Measles, mumps, and rubella vaccine (MMR).** The second dose of MMR is recommended routinely at age 4–6 years but may be administered during any visit, provided at least 4 weeks have elapsed since the first dose and both doses are administered beginning at or after age 12 months. Those who have not previously received the second dose should complete the schedule by age 11–12 years.

5. **Varicella vaccine.** Varicella vaccine is recommended at any visit at or after age 12 months for susceptible children (i.e., those who lack a reliable history of chickenpox). Susceptible persons aged 13 years and older should receive 2 doses administered at least 4 weeks apart.

6. **Meningococcal vaccine (MCV4).** Meningococcal conjugate vaccine (MCV4) should be given to all children at the 11–12 year old visit as well as to unvaccinated adolescents at high school entry (15 years of age). Other adolescents who wish to decrease their risk for meningococcal disease may also be vaccinated. All college freshmen living in dormitories should also be vaccinated, preferably with MCV4, although **meningococcal polysaccharide vaccine (MPSV4)** is an acceptable alternative. Vaccination against invasive meningococcal disease is recommended for children and adolescents aged 2 years and older with terminal complement deficiencies or anatomic or functional asplenia and certain other high risk groups (see *MMWR* 2005;54 [RR-7]:1–21); use MPSV4 for children aged 2–10 years and MCV4 for older children, although MPSV4 is an acceptable alternative.

7. **Pneumococcal vaccine.** The heptavalent **pneumococcal conjugate vaccine (PCV)** is recommended for all children aged 2–23 months and for certain children aged 24–59 months. The final dose in the series should be given at age 12 months and older. **Pneumococcal polysaccharide vaccine (PPV)** is recommended in addition to PCV for certain high-risk groups. See *MMWR* 2000; 49(RR-9):1–35.

8. **Influenza vaccine.** Influenza vaccine is recommended annually for children aged 6 months and older with certain risk factors (including, but not limited to, asthma, cardiac disease, sickle cell disease, human immunodeficiency virus [HIV], diabetes, and conditions that can compromise respiratory function or handling of respiratory secretions or that can increase the risk for aspiration), healthcare workers, and other persons (including household members) in close contact with persons in groups at high risk (see *MMWR* 2005;54[RR-8]:1–55). In addition, healthy children aged 6–23 months and close contacts of healthy children aged 0–5 months are recommended to receive influenza vaccine because children in this age group are at substantially increased risk for influenza-related hospitalizations. For healthy persons aged 5–49 years, the intranasally administered, live, attenuated influenza vaccine (LAIV) is an acceptable alternative to the intramuscular trivalent inactivated influenza vaccine (TIV). See *MMWR* 2005;54(RR-8):1–55. Children receiving TIV should be administered a dosage appropriate for their age (0.25 mL if aged 6–35 months or 0.5 mL if aged 3 years and older.) Children aged 8 years and younger who are receiving influenza vaccine for the first time should receive 2 doses (separated by at least 4 weeks for TIV and at least 6 weeks for LAIV).

9. **Hepatitis A vaccine (HepA).** HepA is recommended for all children at 1 year of age (i.e., 12–23 months). The 2 doses in the series should be administered at least 6 months apart. States, counties, and communities with existing HepA vaccination programs for children 2–18 years of age are encouraged to maintain these programs. In these areas, new efforts focused on routine vaccination of 1-year-old children should enhance, not replace, ongoing programs directed at a broader population of children. HepA is also recommended for certain high risk groups (see *MMWR* 1999; 48[RR-12]:1–37).

Recommended Adult Immunization Schedule, by Vaccine and Age Group
UNITED STATES, OCTOBER 2005–SEPTEMBER 2006

Vaccine ▼ Age group ▶	19–49 years	50–64 years	65 years and older
Tetanus, diphtheria (Td)[1]*	1-dose booster every 10 yr		
Measles, mumps, rubella (MMR)[2]*	1 or 2 doses	1 dose	
Varicella[3]*	2 doses (0, 4–8 wk)	2 doses (0, 4–8 wk)	
Influenza[4]*	1 dose annually	1 dose annually	
Pneumococcal (polysaccharide)[5,6]	1–2 doses		1 dose
Hepatitis A[7]*	2 doses (0, 6–12 mo, or 0, 6–18 mo)		
Hepatitis B[8]*	3 doses (0, 1–2, 4–6 mo)		
Meningococcal[9]	1 or more doses		

--- Vaccines below broken line are for selected populations

NOTE: These recommendations must be read along with the footnotes.

*Covered by the Vaccine Injury Compensation Program.

For all persons in this category who meet the age requirements and who lack evidence of immunity (e.g., lack documentation of vaccination or have no evidence of prior infection)

Recommended if some other risk factor is present (e.g., based on medical, occupational, lifestyle, or other indications)

This schedule indicates the recommended age groups and medical indications for routine administration of currently licensed vaccines for persons aged 19 years and older. Licensed combination vaccines may be used whenever any components of the combination are indicated and when the vaccine's other components are not contraindicated. For detailed recommendations, consult the manufacturers' package inserts and the complete statements from the ACIP (www.cdc.gov/nip/publications/acip-list.html).

Report all clinically significant postvaccination reactions to the Vaccine Adverse Event Reporting System (VAERS). Reporting forms and instructions on filing a VAERS report are available by telephone, 800-822-7967, or from the VAERS website at www.vaers.hhs.gov.

Information on how to file a Vaccine Injury Compensation Program claim is available at www.hrsa.gov/osp/vicp or by telephone, 800-338-2382. To file a claim for vaccine injury, contact the U.S. Court of Federal Claims, 717 Madison Place, N.W., Washington D.C. 20005, telephone 202-357-6400.

Additional information about the vaccines listed above and contraindications for vaccination is also available at www.cdc.gov/nip or from the CDC-INFO Contact Center at 800-CDC-INFO (232-4636) in English and Spanish, 24 hours a day, 7 days a week.

Footnotes

Recommended Adult Immunization Schedule, UNITED STATES, OCTOBER 2005–SEPTEMBER 2006

1. Tetanus and Diphtheria (Td) vaccination. Adults with uncertain histories of a complete primary vaccination series with diphtheria and tetanus toxoid-containing vaccines should receive a primary series using combined Td toxoid. A primary series for adults is 3 doses; administer the first 2 doses at least 4 weeks apart and the third dose 6–12 months after the second. Administer 1 dose if the person received the primary series and if the last vaccination was received 10 years and longer previously. Consult ACIP statement for recommendations for administering Td as prophylaxis in wound management (www.cdc.gov/mmwr/preview/mmwrhtml/00041645.htm). The American College of Physicians Task Force on Adult Immunization supports a second option for Td use in adults: a single Td booster at age 50 years for persons who have completed the full pediatric series, including the teenage/young adult booster. A newly licensed tetanus-diphtheria-acellular pertussis vaccine is available for adults. ACIP recommendations for its use will be published.

2. Measles, Mumps, Rubella (MMR) vaccination. *Measles component:* adults born before 1957 can be considered immune to measles. Adults born during or after 1957 should receive 1 or more doses of MMR unless they have a medical contraindication, documentation of 1 or more doses, history of measles based on healthcare provider diagnosis, or laboratory evidence of immunity. A second dose of MMR is recommended for adults who 1) were recently exposed to measles or in an outbreak setting, 2) were previously vaccinated with killed measles vaccine, 3) were vaccinated with an unknown type of measles vaccine during 1963–1967, 4) are students in postsecondary educational institutions, 5) work in a healthcare facility, or 6) plan to travel internationally. Withhold MMR or other measles-containing vaccines from HIV-infected persons with severe immunosuppression. *Mumps component:* 1 dose of MMR vaccine should be adequate for protection for those born during or after 1957 who lack a history of mumps based on healthcare provider diagnosis or who lack laboratory evidence of immunity. *Rubella component:* administer 1 dose of MMR vaccine to women whose rubella vaccination history is unreliable or who lack laboratory evidence of immunity. For women of child-bearing age, regardless of birth year, routinely determine rubella immunity and counsel women regarding congenital rubella syndrome. Do not vaccinate women who are pregnant or might become pregnant within 4 weeks of receiving MMR vaccine. Women who do not have evidence of immunity should receive MMR vaccine upon completion or termination of pregnancy and before discharge from the healthcare facility.

3. Varicella vaccination. Varicella vaccination is recommended for all adults without evidence of immunity to varicella. Special consideration should be given to those who 1) have close contact with persons at high risk for severe disease (healthcare workers and family contacts of immunocompromised persons) or 2) are at high risk for exposure or transmission (e.g., teachers of young children; child care employees; residents and staff members of institutional settings, including correctional institutions; college students; military personnel; adolescents and adults living in households with children; nonpregnant women of childbearing age; and international travelers). Evidence of immunity to varicella in adults includes any of the following: 1) documented age-appropriate varicella vaccination (i.e., receipt of 1 dose before age 13 years or receipt of 2 doses [administered at least 4 weeks apart] after age 13 years); 2) born in the United States before 1966; 3) history of varicella disease based on healthcare provider diagnosis or self- or parental report of typical varicella disease for non-U.S.-born persons born before 1966 and all persons born during 1966–1997 (for a patient reporting a history of an atypical, mild case, healthcare providers should seek either an epidemiologic link with a typical varicella case or evidence of laboratory confirmation, if it was performed at the time of acute disease); 4) history of herpes zoster based on healthcare provider diagnosis; or 5) laboratory evidence of immunity. Do not vaccinate women who are pregnant or might become pregnant within 4 weeks of receiving the vaccine. Assess pregnant women for evidence of varicella immunity. Women who do not have evidence of immunity should receive dose 1 of varicella vaccine upon completion or termination of pregnancy and before discharge from the healthcare facility. Dose 2 should be given 4–8 weeks after dose 1.

4. Influenza vaccination. *Medical indications:* chronic disorders of the cardiovascular or pulmonary systems, including asthma; chronic metabolic diseases, including diabetes mellitus, renal dysfunction, hemoglobinopathies, or immunosuppression (including immunosuppression caused by medications or by HIV); any condition (e.g., cognitive dysfunction, spinal cord injury, seizure disorder or other neuromuscular disorder) that compromises respiratory function or the handling of respiratory secretions or that can increase the risk of aspiration; and pregnancy during the influenza season. No data exist on the risk for severe or complicated influenza disease among persons with asplenia; however, influenza is a risk factor for secondary bacterial infections that can cause severe disease among persons with asplenia. *Occupational indications:* healthcare workers and employees of long-term care and assisted living facilities. *Other indications:* residents of nursing homes and other long-term care and assisted living facilities; persons likely to transmit influenza to persons at high risk (i.e., in-home household contacts and caregivers of children birth through 23 months of age, or persons of all ages with high-risk conditions); and anyone who wishes to be vaccinated.

For healthy nonpregnant persons aged 5–49 years without high-risk conditions who are not contacts of severely immunocompromised persons in special care units, intranasally administered influenza vaccine (FluMist®) may be administered in lieu of inactivated vaccine.

5. **Pneumococcal polysaccharide vaccination.** *Medical indications:* chronic disorders of the pulmonary system (excluding asthma); cardiovascular diseases; diabetes mellitus; chronic liver diseases, including liver disease as a result of alcohol abuse (e.g., cirrhosis); chronic renal failure or nephrotic syndrome; functional or anatomic asplenia (e.g., sickle cell disease or splenectomy [if elective splenectomy is planned, vaccinate at least 2 weeks before surgery]); immunosuppressive conditions (e.g., congenital immunodeficiency, HIV infection [vaccinate as close to diagnosis as possible when CD4 cell counts are highest], leukemia, lymphoma, multiple myeloma, Hodgkin disease, generalized malignancy, organ or bone marrow transplantation); chemotherapy with alkylating agents, antimetabolites, or high-dose, long-term corticosteroids; and cochlear implants. *Other indications:* Alaska Natives and certain American Indian populations; residents of nursing homes and other long-term care facilities.

6. **Revaccination with pneumococcal polysaccharide vaccine.** One-time revaccination after 5 years for persons with chronic renal failure or nephrotic syndrome; functional or anatomic asplenia (e.g., sickle cell disease or splenectomy); immunosuppressive conditions (e.g., congenital immunodeficiency, HIV infection, leukemia, lymphoma, multiple myeloma, Hodgkin disease, generalized malignancy, organ or bone marrow transplantation); or chemotherapy with alkylating agents, antimetabolites, or high-dose, long-term corticosteroids. For persons aged 65 years and older, one-time revaccination if they were vaccinated 5 years and older previously and were aged younger than 65 years at the time of primary vaccination.

7. **Hepatitis A vaccination.** *Medical indications:* persons with clotting factor disorders or chronic liver disease. *Behavioral indications:* men who have sex with men or users of illegal drugs. *Occupational indications:* persons working with hepatitis A virus (HAV)-infected primates or with HAV in a research laboratory setting. *Other indications:* persons traveling to or working in countries that have high or intermediate endemicity of hepatitis A (for list of countries, visit www.cdc.gov/travel/diseases.htm#hepa) as well as any person wishing to obtain immunity. Current vaccines should be given in a 2-dose series at either 0 and 6–12 months, or 0 and 6–18 months. If the combined hepatitis A and hepatitis B vaccine is used, administer 3 doses at 0, 1, and 6 months.

8. **Hepatitis B vaccination.** *Medical indications:* hemodialysis patients (use special formulation [40 μg/mL] or two 20-μg/mL doses) or patients who receive clotting factor concentrates. *Occupational indications:* healthcare workers and public-safety workers who have exposure to blood in the workplace; and persons in training in schools of medicine, dentistry, nursing, laboratory technology, and other allied health professions. *Behavioral indications:* injection-drug users; persons with more than one sex partner in the previous 6 months; persons with a recently acquired sexually transmitted disease (STD); and men who have sex with men. *Other indications:* household contacts and sex partners of persons with chronic hepatitis B virus (HBV) infection; clients and staff of institutions for the developmentally disabled; all clients of STD clinics; inmates of correctional facilities; or international travelers who will be in countries with high or intermediate prevalence of chronic HBV infection for longer than 6 months (for list of countries, visit www.cdc.gov/travel/diseases.htm#hepa).

9. **Meningococcal vaccination.** *Medical indications:* adults with anatomic or functional asplenia, or terminal complement component deficiencies. *Other indications:* first-year college students living in dormitories; microbiologists who are routinely exposed to isolates of *Neisseria meningitidis*; military recruits; and persons who travel to or reside in countries in which meningococcal disease is hyperendemic or epidemic (e.g., the "meningitis belt" of sub-Saharan Africa during the dry season [Dec–June]), particularly if contact with the local populations will be prolonged. Vaccination is required by the government of Saudi Arabia for all travelers to Mecca during the annual Hajj. Meningococcal conjugate vaccine is preferred for adults meeting any of the above indications who are aged 55 years and older, although meningococcal polysaccharide vaccine (MPSV4) is an acceptable alternative. Revaccination after 5 years may be indicated for adults previously vaccinated with MPSV4 who remain at high risk for infection (e.g. persons residing in areas in which disease is epidemic).

10. **Selected conditions for which *Haemophilus influenzae* type b (Hib) vaccine may be used.** *Haemophilus influenzae* type b conjugate vaccines are licensed for children aged 6 weeks–71 months. No efficacy data are available on which to base a recommendation concerning use of Hib vaccine for older children and adults with the chronic conditions associated with an increased risk for Hib disease. However, studies suggest good immunogenicity in patients who have sickle cell disease, leukemia, or HIV infection, or have had splenectomies; administering vaccine to these patients is not contraindicated.

Approved by the Advisory Committee on Immunization Practices (ACIP),
the American College of Obstetricians and Gynecologists (ACOG), and the American Academy of Family Physicians (AAFP)

SIGNS AND SYMPTOMS OF ELECTROLYTE IMBALANCE

HYPOGLYCEMIA (excessive insulin)

Tremors, cold/clammy skin, mental confusion, rapid/shallow respirations, unusual fatigue, hunger, drowsiness, anxiety, headache, muscular incoordination, paraesthesia of tongue/mouth/lips, hallucination, increased pulse/blood pressure, tachycardia, seizures, coma.

HYPERGLYCEMIA (insufficient insulin)

Hot/flushed/dry skin, fruity breath odor, excessive urination (polyuria), excessive thirst (polydipsia), acute fatigue, air hunger, deep/labored respirations, mental changes, restlessness, nausea, polyphagia (excessive appetite).

HYPOKALEMIA (potassium level less than 3.5 mEq/L)

Weakness/paraesthesia of extremities, muscle cramps, nausea, vomiting, diarrhea, hypoactive bowel sounds, absent bowel sounds (paralytic ileus), abdominal distention, weak/irregular pulse, postural hypotension, difficulty breathing, disorientation, irritability.

HYPERKALEMIA (potassium level greater than 5.0 mEq/L)

Diarrhea, muscle weakness, heaviness of legs, paraesthesia of tongue/hands/feet, slow/irregular pulse, decreased blood pressure, abdominal cramps, oliguria/anuria, respiratory difficulty, cardiac abnormalities.

HYPONATREMIA (sodium level less than 130 mEq/L)

Abdominal cramping, nausea, vomiting, diarrhea, cold/clammy skin, poor skin turgor, tremors, muscle weakness, leg cramps, increased pulse rate, irritability, apprehension, hypotension, headache.

HYPERNATREMIA (sodium level greater than 150 mEq/L)

Hot/flushed/dry skin, dry mucous membranes, fever, extreme thirst, dry/rough/red tongue, edema, restlessness, postural hypotension, oliguria.

HYPOCALCEMIA (calcium level less than 8.4 mg/dl)

Circumoral/peripheral numbness and tingling, muscle twitching; Chvostek's sign (facial muscle spasm; test by tapping of facial nerve anterior to earlobe, just below zygomatic arch), muscle cramping, Trousseau's sign (carpopedal spasm), seizures, arrhythmias.

HYPERCALCEMIA (calcium level greater than 10.2 mg/dl)

Muscle hypotonicity, incoordination, anorexia, constipation, confusion, impaired memory, slurred speech, lethargy, acute psychotic behavior, deep bone pain, flank pain.

SOUND-ALIKE AND LOOK-ALIKE DRUGS

Generic/Trade Name	Sounds or Looks Like
Accolate	Accutane
Accupril	Accolate, Accutane, Monopril
Acetazolamide	Acetohexamide
Aciphex	Aricept
Adderall	Inderal
Adriamycin	Aredia, Idamycin
Aggrastat	Aggrenox
Akarpine	Atropine
Aldara	Alora
Alkeran	Leukeran
Allegra	Viagra
Alprazolam	Lorazepam
Alupent	Atrovent
Amantadine	Ranitidine, Rimantadine
Ambien	Amen
Amicar	Amikin, Omacor
Anaspaz	Antispas
Aranesp	Aricept
Asparaginase	Pegaspargase
Atarax	Ativan
Atropine	Akarpine
Atrovent	Alupent
Avandia	Prandin
Avapro	Anaprox
Avonex	Avelox
Azithromycin	Erythromycin
Bacitracin	Bactroban
Baclofen	Bactroban
Benadryl	Avandaryl, Bentyl, Benylin
Bentyl	Aventyl
Benylin	Ventolin
Bepridil	Prepidil
Bumex	Buprenex, Permax
Bupropion	Buspirone
Cafergot	Carafate
Calan	Colace
Calciferol	Calcitriol
Captopril	Carvedilol
Carbatrol	Carbitral
Carboplatin	Cisplatin
Cardene	Cardizem
Cardura	Cardene, Ridaura
Carteolol	Carvedilol
Catapres	Combipres
Cefotan	Ceftin
Cefotaxime	Cefuroxime
Ceftazidime	Ceftizoxime
Cefzil	Kefzol, Ceftin

Generic/Trade Name	Sounds or Looks Like
Celebrex	Celexa, Cerebyx
Celexa	Zyprexa, Celebrex
Chlorpromazine	Chlorpropamide, Prochlorperzine
Chlorpropamide	Chlorpromazine
Cirtacal	Citrucel
Clinoril	Clozaril, Oruvail
Clomipramine	Desipramine
Clonazepam	Klonopin, Clorazepate, Lorazepam
Combivir	Combivent, Epivir
Compazine	Chlorpromazine
Covera	Provera
Cozaar	Hyzaar, Zocor
Cycloserine	Cyclosporine
Cytosar	Cytoxan
Cytotec	Cytoxan
Dactinomycin	Daptomycin
Darvon	Diovan
Daunorubicin	Doxorubicin
Deferoxamine	Cefuroxime
Demerol	Detrol, Desyrel
Denavir	Indinavir
depoMedrol	soluMedrol
Desipramine	Clomipramine, Imipramine, Nortriptyline
Desyrel	Zestril
DiaBeta	Zebeta
Diazepam	Ditropam, Lorazepam
Digoxin	Doxepin
Dilantin	Dilaudid
Diovan	Darvon, Dioval, Zyban
Dobutamine	Dopamine
Doxorubicin	Daunorubicin
Dynabac	DynaCirc
Edecrin	Eulexin
Efudex	Eurax
Elavil	Eldepryl, Enalapril, Oruvail
Eldepryl	Enalapril
Elmiron	Imuran
Enalapril	Eldepryl
Epogen	Neupogen
Erythromycin	Azithromycin
Esmolol	Osmitrol
Estraderm	Testoderm
Etidronate	Etomidate, Etretinate
Fioricet	Fiorinal
Flomax	Foxamax, Volmax
Fludarabine	Flumadine
Flumadine	Fludarabine, Flutamide
Folic Acid	Folinic Acid
Furosemide	Torsemide
Gengraf	Prograf
Glimepiride	Glipizide
Glipizide	Glyburide
Glyburide	Glipizide, Glucotrol

(continued)

Generic/Trade Name	Sounds or Looks Like
Guaifenesin	Guanfacine
Herceptin	Perceptin
Humalog, Insulin Human	Humulin, Insulin Human
Hydralazine	Hydroxyzine
Hydromorphone	Morphine
Hydroxyzine	Hydralazine
Imdur	Imuran
Imipramine	Desipramine
Imuran	Inderal
Indanavir	Denavir
Inderal	Adderall, Isordil, Toradol
Invanz	Avinza
Kefzol	Cefzil
Lamictal	Lamisil, Lomotil, Ludiomil
Lamivudine	Lamotrigine
Lanoxin	Levoxine, Lonox
Leucovorin	Leukine, Leukeran
Levbid	Lithobid, Lopid, Larabid
Lithobid	Levbid, Lithostat
Loniten	Lotensin
Lonox	Lanoxin
Lopid	Levbid, Lorabid
Lorabid	Lortab
Lorazapam	Alprazolam, Clonazepam, Diazepam
Lorsartan	Valsartan
Lotensin	Loniten, Lovastatin
Lovenox	Lotronex
Medroxyprogesterone	Methylprednisolone
Melphalan	Myleran
Metolozone	Metoprolol
Metoprolol	Misoprostol
Miacalcin	Micatin
Micro-K	Micronase
Minoxidil	Monopril
MiraLax	Mirapex
Monopril	Minoxidil, Monoket
Myleran	Melphalan, Mylicon
Naprelan	Naprosyn
Nasarel	Nizoral
Navane	Norvasc, Nubain
Neoral	Neurontin, Nizoral
Neurontin	Noroxin
Nicardipine	Nifedipine, Nimodipine
Nicoderm	Nitroderm
Nitrostat	Nilstat
Nizoral	Nasarel, Neoral
Ocufen	Ocuflox, Ocupress
Olanzapine	Olsalazine
Os-Cal	Asacol
Oxycodone	OxyContin
OxyContin	Oxybutynin, Oxycodone
Paclitaxel	Paxil
Parlodel	Pindolol

Generic/Trade Name	Sounds or Looks Like
Paroxetine	Pyridoxine
Paxil	Paclitaxel, Plavix, Taxol
Penicillamine	Penicillin
Pentobarbital	Phenobarbital
Perceptin	Herceptin
Pindolol	Parlodel, Plendil
Platinol	Paraplatin
Plendil	Pindolol, Pletal, Prinivil
Pletal	Plendil
Pravachol	Prevacid, Prinivil, Propranolol
Prednisone	Prednisolone, Primidone
Prepidil	Bepridil
Prilosec	Prozac
Prinivil	Plendil, Prilosec, Proventil
Prochlorperazine	Chlorpromazine
Propranolol	Pravachol, Propulsid
Proscar	ProSom, Prozac
Protonix	Lotronex
Pyridoxine	Paroxetine
Ranitidine	Amatadine, Rimantadine
Ratgam	Atgam
Remegel	Renagel
Remeron	Zemuron
Renagel	Remegel
Retrovir	Ritonavir
Risperidone	Reserpine
Ritonavir	Retrovir
Ropivacaine	Bupivacaine
Sarafem	Serophene
Selegiline	Sertraline
Slobid	Dolobid, Lopid, Lorabid
Sulfadiazine	Sulfasalazine
Sumatriptan	Zolmitriptan
Taxol	Taxotere
Tegretol	Toradol
Tiagabine	Tizanidine
Tiazac	Ziac
Tobradex	Tobres
Topamax	Toprol, Tegretol
Toradol	Tegretol, Torecan, Tramadol
Torsemide	Furosemide
Trandate	Tridate
Trazodone	Tramadol
Trimox	Tylox
Tylox	Tylenol
Ultram	Ultane
Valsartan	Losartan
Vancomycin	Vecuronium
Vantin	Ventolin
VePesid	Versed
Verelan	Virilon
Vexol	VoSol
Viracept	Viramune

(continued)

Generic/Trade Name	Sounds or Looks Like
Vistaril	Restoril, Versed, Zestril
Xanax	Zantac, Zyrtec
Zantac	Xanax, Zyrtec, Zofran
Zebeta	DiBeta
Zemuron	Remeron
Zestril	Desyrel, Vistaril
Ziac	Tiazac
Zocor	Cozaar, Yocon, Zoloft
Zyrtec	Zyprexa

SPANISH PHRASES OFTEN USED IN CLINICAL SETTINGS

TAKING THE MEDICATION HISTORY

Tomando la Historia Médica
(Toh-mahn-doh lah Ees-toh-ree-ah Meh-dee-kah)

- Are you allergic to any medications? (If yes:)
  ¿Es alérgico a algún medicamento? (sí:)
  (Ehs ah-lehr-hee-koh ah ahl-goon meh-dee-kah-mehn-toh) (see:)

- —Which medications are you allergic to?
  ¿A cuál medicamento es alérgico?
  (ah koo-ahl meh-dee-kah-mehn-toh ehs ah-lehr-hee-koh)

- Do you take any over-the-counter, prescription, or herbal medications?
  ¿Toma medicamentos sin receta, con receta, o naturistas (hierbas medicinales)?
  (Toh-mah meh-dee-kah-mehn-tohs seen reh-seh-tah, kohn reh-seh-tah, oh nah-too-rees-tahs [ee-ehr-bahs meh-dee-see-nah-lehs])

  —How often do you take each medication?
  ¿Con qué frequencia toma cada medicamento?
  (Kohn keh freh-koo-ehn-see-ah toh-mah kah-dah meh-dee-kah-mehn-toh)

    Once a day?
    ¿Una vez por día; diariamente?
    (Oo-nah behs pohr dee-ah; dee-ah-ree-ah-mehn-teh)

    Twice a day?   ¿Dos veces por día?
                    (dohs beh-sehs pohr dee-ah)
    Three times a day?   ¿Tres veces por día?
                          (Trehs beh-sehs pohr dee-ah)

    Four times a day?   ¿Cuatro veces por día?
    (Koo-ah-troh beh-sehs pohr-dee-ah)

  —Does the medication make you feel better?
  ¿Le hace sentir mejor el medicamento?
  (Heh ah-seh sehn-teer meh-hohr ehl meh-dee-kah-mehn-toh)

  —Does the medication make you feel the same or unchanged?
  ¿Le hace sentir igual o sin cambio el medicamento?
  (Leh ah-seh sehn-teer ee-goo-ahl oh seen kam-bee-oh ehl meh-dee-kah-mehn-toh)

—Does the medication make you feel worse?
¿Se siente peor con el medicamento?
(Seh see-ehn teh peh-ohr kohn ehl meh-dee-kah-mehn-toh)

PREPARING FOR TREATMENT WITH MEDICATION THERAPY
Preparando para un régimen de medicamento
(Preh-pah-rahn-doh pah-rah oon reh-hee-mehn deh meh-dee-kah-mehn-toh)

MEDICATION PURPOSE
PROPÓSITO DEL MEDICAMENTO
(Proh-poh-see-toh dehl meh-dee-kah-mehn-toh)

This medication will help relieve:
Este medicamento le ayudará a aliviar:
(Ehs-teh meh-dee-kah-mehn-toh leh ah-yoo-dah-rah ah ah-lee-bee-ahr)

abdominal gas
gases intestinales
(gah-sehs een-tehs-tee-nah-lehs)

abdominal pain
dolor intestinal; dolor en el abdomen
(doh-lohr een-tehs-tee-nahl; doh-lohr ehn ehl ahb-doh-mehn)

chest congestion
congestión del pecho
(kohn-hehs-tee-ohn dehl peh-choh)

chest pain
dolor del pecho
(doh-lohr dehl peh-choh)

constipation
constipación; estrenimiento
(kohns-tee-pah-see-ohn; ehs-treh-nyee-mee-ehn-toh)

cough
tos
(tohs)

headache
dolor de cabeza
(doh-lohr deh kah-beh-sah)

muscle aches and pains
achaques musculares y dolores
(ah-chah-kehs moos-koo-lah-rehs ee doh-loh-rehs)

pain
dolor
(doh-lohr)

This medication will prevent:
Este medicamento prevendrá:
(Ehs-teh meh-dee-kah-mehn-toh preh-behn-drah)

blood clots
coágulos de sangre
(koh-ah-goo-lohs deh sahn-greh)

constipation
constipación; estreñimiento
(kohns-tee-pah-see-ohn; ehs-treh-nyee-mee-ehn-toh)

contraception
contracepción; embarazo
(kohn-trah-sehp-see-ohn; ehm-bah-rah-soh)

diarrhea
diarrea
(dee-ah-reh-ah)

infection
infección
(een-fehk-see-ohn)

seizures
convulciónes; ataque epiléptico
(kohn-bool-see-ohn-ehs; ah-tah-keh eh-pee-lehp-tee-koh)

shortness of breath
respiración corta; falta de aliento
(rehs-pee-rah-see-ohn kohr-tah; fahl-tah deh ah-lee-ehn-toh)

wheezing
el resollar; la respiración ruidosa, sibilante
(ehl reh-soh-yahr; lah rehs-pee-rah-see-ohn roo-ee-doh-sah, see-bee-lahn-teh)

This medication will increase your:
Este medicamento aumentará su:
(Ehs-teh meh-dee-kah-mehn-toh ah-oo-mehn-tah-rah soo):

ability to fight infections
habilidad a combatir infecciones
(ah-bee-lee-dahd ah kohm-bah-teer een-fehk-see-oh-nehs)

appetite
apetito
(ah-peh-tee-toh)

blood iron levels
nivel de hierro en la sargre
(nee-behl deh ee-eh-roh ehn lah sahn-greh)

blood sugar
azúcar en la sangre
(ah-soo-kahr ehn lah sahn-greh)

heart rate
pulso; latido
(pool-soh; lah-tee-doh)

red blood cell count
cuenta de células rojas
(koo-ehn-tah deh seh-loo-lahs roh-hahs)

thyroid hormone levels
niveles de hormona tiroide
(nee-beh-lehs deh ohr-moh-nah tee-roh-ee-deh)

urine volume
volumen de orina
(boh-loo-mehn deh oh-ree-nah)

This medication will decrease your:
Este medicamento reducirá su:
(Ehs-teh meh-dee-kah-mehn-toh reh-doo-see-rah soo:)

anxiety
ansiedad
(ahn-see-eh-dahd)

blood cholesterol level
nivel de colesterol en la sangre
(nee-behl deh koh-lehs-teh-rohl ehn lah sahn-greh)

blood lipid level
nivel de lípido en la sangre
(nee-behl deh lee-pee-doh ehn lah sahn-greh)

blood pressure
presión arterial; de sangre
(preh-see-ohn ahr teh-ree-ahl; deh sahn-greh)

blood sugar level
nivel de azúcar en la sangre
(nee-behl deh ah-soo-kahr ehn lah sahn-greh)

heart rate
pulso; latido
(pool-soh; lah-tee-doh)

stomach acid
ácido en el estómago
(ah-see-doh ehn ehl ehs-toh-mah-goh)

thyroid hormone levels
niveles de hormona tiroide
(nee-beh-lehs deh ohr-moh-nah tee-roh-ee-deh)

weight
peso
(peh-soh)

This medication will treat:
Este medicamento sirve para:
(Ehs-teh meh-dee-kah-mehn-toh seer-beh pah-rah)

depression
depresión
(deh-preh-see-ohn)

inflammation
infamación
(een-flah-mah-see-ohn)

swelling
hinchazón
(een-chah-sohn)

the infection in your _____
la infección en su _____
(lah een-fehk-see-ohn ehn soo)

your abnormal heart rhythm
su ritmo anormal de corazón anormal
(soo reet-moh ah-nohr-mahl deh koh-rah-sohn)

your allergy to _____
su alergia a _____
(soo eh-lehr-hee-ah ah)

your rash
su erupción; sarpullido
(soo eh-roop-see-ohn; sahr-poo-yee-doh)

ADMINISTERING MEDICATION
Administrando el Medicamento
(Ahd-mee-nees-trahn-doh ehl meh-dee-kah-mehn-toh)

- Swallow this medication with water or juice.
  Tragüe este medicamento con agua o jugo
  (Trah-geh ehs-teh meh dee-kah-mehn-toh kohn ah-goo-ah oh hoo-goh)

- Do not chew this medication. Swallow it whole.
  No mastique este medicamento. Tragüelo entero.
  (Noh mahs-tee-keh ehs-teh meh-dee-kah-mehn-toh. Trah-geh-loh ehn-teh-roh)

ADMINISTRATION FREQUENCY
FRECUENCIA DE LA ADMINISTRACIÓN
(Freh-koo-ehn-see-ah deh lah Ahd-mee-nees-trah-see-ohn)

English	Spanish	Pronunciation
Once a day	Una vez por día; diariamente	(Oo-nah behs pohr dee-ah; dee-ah-ree-ah-mehn-teh)
Twice a day	Dos veces por día	(Dohs beh-sehs pohr dee-ah)
Three times a day	Tres veces por día	(Trehs beh-sehs pohr dee-ah)
Four times a day	Cuatro veces por día	(Koo-ah-troh beh-sehs pohr dee-ah)
Every other day	Cada tercer día	(Kah-dah tehr-sehr dee-ah)
Once a week	Una vez por semana	(Oo-nah behs pohr seh-mah-nah)
Every 4 hours	Cada cuatro horas	(Kah-dah koo-ah-troh oh-rahs)
Every 6 hours	Cada seis horas	(Kah-dah seh-ees oh-rahs)
Every 8 hours	Cada ocho horas	(Kah-dah oh-choh oh-rahs)
Every 12 hours	Cada doce horas	(Kah-dah doh-seh oh-rahs)
In the morning	En la mañana	(Ehn lah mah-nyah-nah)
In the afternoon	En la tarde	(Ehn lah tahr-deh)
In the evening	En la noche	(Ehn lah noh-cheh)
Before bedtime	Antes de acostarse	(Ahn-tehs deh ah-kohs-tahr-seh)
Before meals	Antes de la comida; Antes del alimento	(Ahn-tehs deh lah koh-mee-dah; Ahn-tehs dehl ah-lee-mehn-toh)
With meals	Con los alimentos; Con la comida	(Kohn lohs ah-lee-mehn-tohs; Kohn lah koh-mee-dah)
After meals	Después de los alimentos; Después de la comida	(Dehs-poo-ehs deh lohs ah-lee-mehn-tohs; Dehs-poo-ehs deh lah koh-mee-dah)
Only when you need it	Solo cuando la necesite	(Soh-loh koo-ahn-doh lah neh-seh-see-teh)
When you have ____ pain	Cuando tiene ____ dolor	(Koo-ahn-doh tee-eh-neh ____ doh-lohr)

50 COMMON SIDE EFFECTS
CINCUENTA EFECTOS SECUNDARIOS COMÚNES
(Seen-koo-ehn-tah Eh-fehk-tohs Seh-koon-dah-ree-ohs Koh-moo-nehs)

English	Spanish	Pronunciation
Abdominal cramps	Retorción abdominal	(Reh-tohr-see-hohn ahb-doh-mee-nahl)
Abdominal pain	Dolor abdominal	(Doh-lohr ahb-doh-mee-nahl)
Abdominal swelling	Inflamación abdominal	(Een-flah-mah-see-ohn ahb-doh-mee-nahl)
Anxiety	Ansiedad	(Ahn-see-eh-dahd)
Blood in the stool	Sangre en el excremento	(Sahn-greh ehn ehl ehx-kreh-mehn-toh)
Blood in the urine	Sangre en la orina	(Sahn-greh ehn la oh-ree-nah)
Bone pain	Dolor de hueso*	(Doh-lohr deh oo-eh-soh)
Chest pain	Dolor de pecho	(Doh-lohr deh peh-choh)
Chest pounding	Palpitación; latidos fuertes en el pecho	(Pahl-pee-tah-see-ohn; lah-tee-dohs foo-ehr-tehs ehn ehl peh-choh)
Chills	Escalofrío	(Ehs-kah-loh-free-oh)
Confusion	Confusión	(Kohn-foo-see-ohn)
Constipation	Constipación, estreñimiento	(Kohns-tee-pah-see-ohn, ehs-treh-nyee-mee-ehn-toh)
Cough	Tos	(Tohs)
Depression, mental	Depresión mental	(Deh-preh-see-ohn mehn-tahl)
Diarrhea	Diarrea	(Dee-ah-reh-ah)
Difficulty breathing	Dificultad al respirar	(Dee-fee-kool-tahd ahl rehs-pee-rahr)
Difficulty sleeping	Dificultad al dormir	(Dee-fee-kool-tahd ahl dohr-meer)
Difficulty urinating	Dificultad al orinar	(Dee-fee-kool-tahd ahl oh-ree-nahr)
Dizziness	Mareos; vahídos	(Mah-reh-ohs; bah-ee-dohs)
Dry mouth	Boca seca	(Boh-kah seh-kah)
Easy bruising	Fragilidad capilar; le salen moretones con facilidad	(Frah-hee-lee-dahd kah-pee-lahr; leh sah-lehn moh-reh-toh-nehs kohn fah-see-lee-dahd)
Faintness	Desvanecimiento; sintió un vahído	(Dehs-bah-neh-see-mee-ehn-toh; seen-tee-oh oon bah-ee-doh)
Fatigue	Fatiga, cansancio	(Fah-tee-gah, kahn-sahn-see-oh)
Fever	Fiebre	(Fee-eh-breh)

English	Spanish	Pronunciation
Frequent urination	Orina frecuente	(Oh-ree-nah freh-koo-ehn-teh)
Headache	Dolor de cabeza	(Doh-lohr deh kah-beh-sah)
Impotence	Impotencia	(Eem-poh-tehn-see-ah)
Increased appetite	Aumento en el apetito	(Ah-oo-mehn-toh ehn ehl ah-peh-tee-toh)
Increased gas	Flatulencia	(Flah-too-lehn-see-ah)
Increased perspiration	Aumento en el sudor	(Ah-oo-mehn-toh ehn ehl soo-dohr)
Indigestion	Indigestión	(Een-dee-hehs-tee-ohn)
Itching	Comezón	(Koh-meh-sohn)
Loss of appetite	Pérdida en el apetito	(Pehr-dee-dah ehn ehl ah-peh-tee-toh)
Menstrual changes	Cambios en la menstruación;	(Kahm-bee-ohs ehn la mehns-truh-ah-see-ohn;
	Cambio en el ciclomenstrual	Kahm-bee-oh ehn ehl see-kloh mehns-truh-ahl)
Mood changes	Cambio en el humor; Cambio en la disposición	(Kahm-bee-oh ehn ehl oo-mohr, Kahm-bee-oh ehn lah dees-poh-see-see-ohn)
Muscle aches	Achaques musculares	(Ah-chah-kehs moos-koo-lah-rehs)
Muscle cramps	Calambre muscular	(kah-lahm-breh moos-koo-lahr)
Muscle pain	Dolores musculares	(Doh-loh-rehs moos-koo-lah-rehs)
Nasal congestion	Congestión nasal	(Kohn-hehs-tee-ohn nah-sahl)
Nausea	Nausea	(Nah-oo-seh-ah)
Ringing in the ears	Zumbido en los oídos	(Soom-bee-doh ehn lohs oh-ee-dohs)
Skin rash	Erupción en la piel	(Eh-roop-see-ohn ehn lah pee-ehl)
Swelling on the hands, legs, or feet	Hinchazón en las manos, piernas, o pies	(Een-chah-sohn ehn lahs mah-nohs, pee-ehr-nahs, oh pee-ehs)
Vaginal bleeding	Sangrado vaginal	(Sahn-grah-doh bah-hee-nahl)
Vision changes	Cambios en la visión; cambios en la vista	(Kahm-bee-ohs ehn lah bee-see-ohn; cahm-bee-ohs ehn lah bees-tah)
Vomiting	Vomitando	(Boh-mee-tahn-doh)
Weakness	Debilidad	(Deh-bee-lee-dahd)
Weight gain	Aumento de peso	(Ah-oo-mehn-toh deh peh-soh)
Weight loss	Pérdida de peso	(Pehr-dee-day deh peh-soh)
Wheezing	Resollar; respiración sibilante	(Reh-soh-yahr; rehs-pee-rah-see-ohn see-bee-lahn-teh)

*h is silent.

TECHNIQUES OF MEDICATION ADMINISTRATION

OPHTHALMIC

Eye Drops

1. Wash hands.
2. Instruct patient to lie down or tilt head backward and look up.
3. Gently pull lower eyelid down until a pocket (pouch) is formed between eye and lower lid (conjunctival sac).
4. Hold dropper above pocket. Without touching tip of eye dropper to eyelid or conjunctival sac, place prescribed number of drops into the center pocket (placing drops directly onto eye may cause a sudden squeezing of eyelid, with subsequent loss of solution). Continue to hold the eyelid for a moment after the drops are applied (allows medication to distribute along entire conjunctival sac).
5. Instruct patient to close eyes gently so that medication is not squeezed out of sac.
6. Apply gentle finger pressure to the lacrimal sac at the inner canthus (bridge of the nose, inside corner of the eye) for 1–2 min (promotes absorption, minimizes drainage into nose and throat, lessens risk of systemic absorption).
7. Remove excess solution around eye with a tissue.
8. Wash hands immediately to remove medication on hands. Never rinse eye dropper.

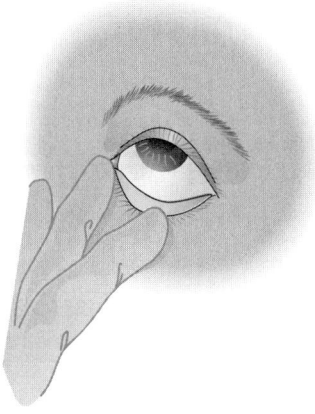

Eye Ointment

1. Wash hands.
2. Instruct patient to lie down or tilt head backward and look up.

3. Gently pull lower eyelid down until a pocket (pouch) is formed between eye and lower lid (conjunctival sac).

4. Hold applicator tube above pocket. Without touching the applicator tip to eyelid or conjunctival sac, place prescribed amount of ointment (¼–½ inch) into the center pocket (placing ointment directly onto eye may cause discomfort).

5. Instruct patient to close eye for 1–2 min, rolling eyeball in all directions (increases contact area of drug to eye).

6. Inform patient of temporary blurring of vision. If possible, apply ointment just before bedtime.

7. Wash hands immediately to remove medication on hands. Never rinse tube applicator.

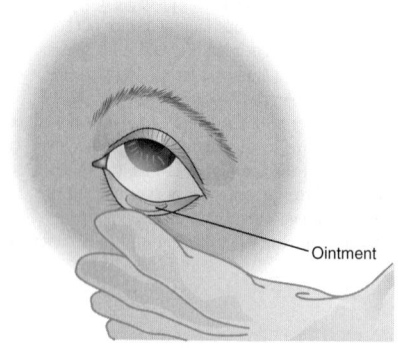

Ointment

OTIC

1. Ear drops should be at body temperature (wrap hand around bottle to warm contents). Body temperature instillation prevents startling of patient.

2. Instruct patient to lie down with head turned so affected ear is upright (allows medication to drip into ear).

3. Instill prescribed number of drops toward the canal wall, not directly on eardrum.

4. To promote correct placement of ear drops, pull the auricle down and posterior in children (A) and pull the auricle up and posterior in adults (B).

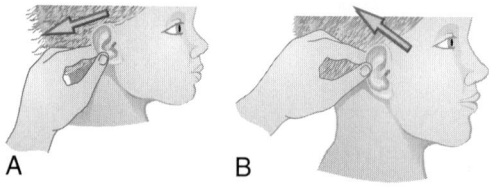

A   B

NASAL

Nose Drops and Sprays

1. Instruct patient to blow nose to clear nasal passages as much as possible.
2. Tilt head slightly forward if instilling nasal spray, slightly backward if instilling nasal drops.
3. Insert spray tip into 1 nostril, pointing toward inflamed nasal passages, away from nasal septum.
4. Spray or drop medication into 1 nostril while holding other nostril closed and concurrently inspire through nose to permit medication as high into nasal passages as possible.
5. Discard unused nasal solution after 3 mo.

INHALATION

Aerosol (Multidose Inhalers)

1. Shake container well before each use.
2. Exhale slowly and as completely as possible through the mouth.
3. Place mouthpiece fully into mouth, holding inhaler upright, and close lips fully around mouthpiece.
4. Inhale deeply and slowly through the mouth while depressing the top of the canister with the middle finger.
5. Hold breath as long as possible before exhaling slowly and gently.
6. When 2 puffs are prescribed, wait 2 min and shake container again before inhaling a second puff (allows for deeper bronchial penetration).
7. Rinse mouth with water immediately after inhalation (prevents mouth and throat dryness).

SUBLINGUAL

1. Administer while seated.
2. Dissolve sublingual tablet under tongue (do not chew or swallow tablet).
3. Do not swallow saliva until tablet is dissolved.

TOPICAL

1. Gently cleanse area prior to application.
2. Use occlusive dressings only as ordered.
3. Without touching applicator tip to skin, apply sparingly; gently rub into area thoroughly unless ordered otherwise.
4. When using aerosol, spray area for 3 sec from 15-cm distance; avoid inhalation.

TRANSDERMAL

1. Apply transdermal patch to clean, dry, hairless skin on upper arm or body (not below knee or elbow).
2. Rotate sites (prevents skin irritation).
3. Do not trim patch to adjust dose.

RECTAL

1. Instruct patient to lie in left lateral Sims position.
2. Moisten suppository with cold water or water-soluble lubricant.

3. Instruct patient to slowly exhale (relaxes anal sphincter) while inserting suppository well up into rectum.

4. Inform patient as to length of time (20–30 min) before desire for defecation occurs or less than 60 min for systemic absorption to occur, depending on purpose for suppository.

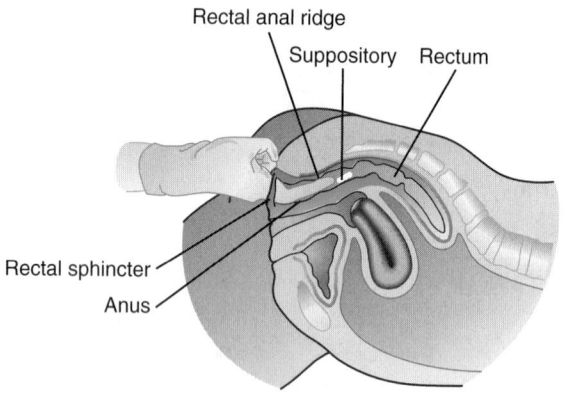

Rectal anal ridge

Suppository   Rectum

Rectal sphincter

Anus

SUBCUTANEOUS

1. Use 25- to 27-gauge, ½- to ⅝-inch needle; 1–3 ml. Angle of insertion depends on body size: 90° if patient is obese. If patient is very thin, gather the skin at the area of needle insertion and administer also at a 90° angle. A 45° angle can be used in a patient with average weight.

2. Cleanse area to be injected with circular motion.

3. Avoid areas of bony prominence, major nerves, blood vessels.

4. Aspirate syringe before injecting (to avoid intra-arterial administration), except insulin, heparin.

5. Inject slowly; remove needle quickly.

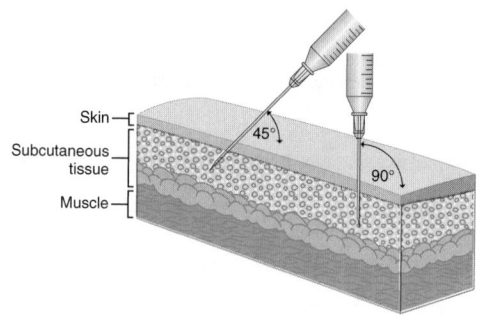

Skin

Subcutaneous tissue

Muscle

45°

90°

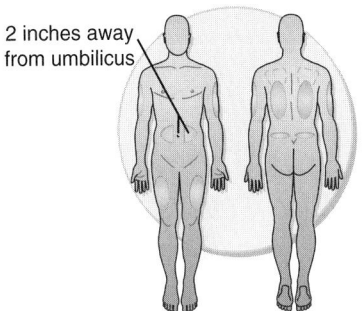

2 inches away
from umbilicus

Subcutaneous injection sites

IM

Injection Sites

Dorsogluteal (upper outer quadrant)

1. Use this site if volume to be injected is 1–3 ml. Use 18- to 23-gauge, 1.25- to 3-inch needle. Needle should be long enough to reach the middle of the muscle.
2. Do not use this site in children younger than 2 yr or in those who are emaciated. Patient should be in prone position.
3. Using 90° angle, flatten the skin area using the middle and index fingers and inject between them.

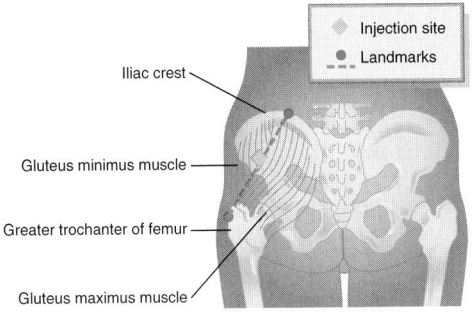

Injection site
Landmarks

Iliac crest

Gluteus minimus muscle

Greater trochanter of femur

Gluteus maximus muscle

Ventrogluteal

1. Use this site if volume to be injected is 1–5 ml. Use 20- to 23-gauge, 1.25- to 2.5-inch needle. Needle should be long enough to reach the middle of the muscle.
2. Preferred site for adults, children older than 7 mo. Patient should be in supine lateral position.
3. Using 90° angle, flatten the skin area using the middle and index fingers and inject between them.

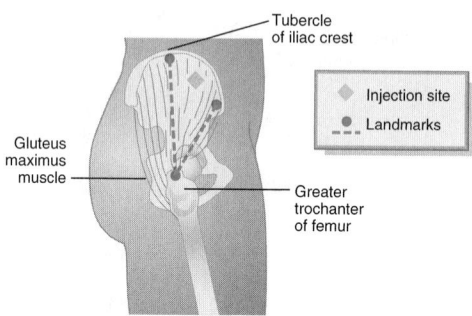

Deltoid

1. Use this site if volume to be injected is 0.5–1 ml. Use 23- to 25-gauge, $\frac{1}{8}$- to $\frac{1}{2}$-inch needle. Needle should be long enough to reach the middle of the muscle.
2. Patient may be in prone, sitting, supine, or standing position.
3. Using 90° angle or angled slightly toward acromion, flatten the skin area using the thumb and index finger and inject between them.

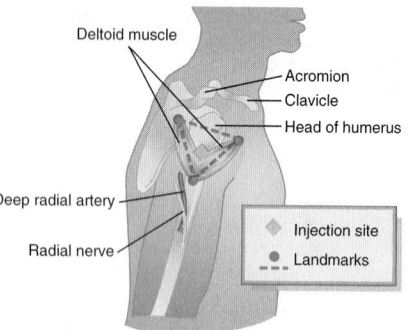

Anterolateral Thigh

1. Anterolateral thigh is site of choice for infants and children younger than 7 mo. Use 22- to 25-gauge, $\frac{5}{8}$- to 1-inch needle.
2. Patient can be in supine or sitting position.
3. Using 90° angle, flatten the skin area using the thumb and index finger and inject between them.

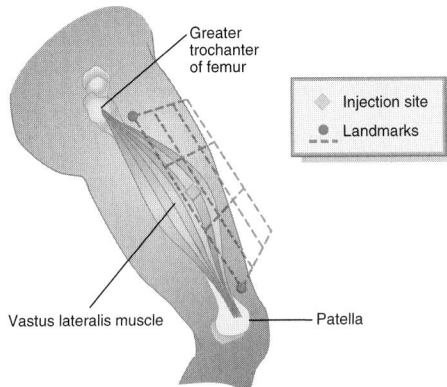

Greater
trochanter
of femur

◆ Injection site
● Landmarks

Vastus lateralis muscle — Patella

Z-TRACK TECHNIQUE

1. Draw up medication with one needle, and use new needle for injection (minimizes skin staining).
2. Administer deep IM in upper outer quadrant of buttock only (dorsogluteal site).
3. Displace the skin lateral to the injection site before inserting the needle.
4. Withdraw the needle before releasing the skin.

IV

1. Medication may be given as direct IV, intermittent (piggyback), or continuous infusion.
2. Ensure that medication is compatible with solution being infused (see IV compatibility chart in this drug handbook).
3. Do not use if precipitate is present or discoloration occurs.
4. Check IV site frequently for correct infusion rate, evidence of infiltration, extravasation.

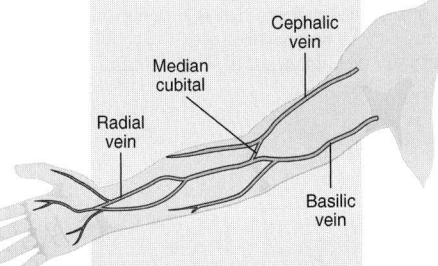

Cephalic
vein

Median
cubital

Radial
vein

Basilic
vein

Intravenous medications are administered by the following:

1. Continuous infusing solution.
2. Piggyback (intermittent infusion).
3. Volume control setup (medication contained in a chamber between the IV solution bag and the patient).
4. Bolus dose (a single dose of medication given through an infusion line or saline lock). Sometimes this is referred to as an IV push.

Adding medication to a newly prescribed IV bag:

1. Remove the plastic cover from the IV bag.
2. Cleanse rubber port with an alcohol swab.
3. Insert the needle into the center of the rubber port.
4. Inject the medication.
5. Withdraw the syringe from the port.
6. Gently rotate the container to mix the solution.
7. Label the IV, including the date, time, medication, and dosage. The label should be placed so that it is easily read when hanging.
8. Spike the IV tubing and prime the tubing.

Hanging an IV piggyback (IVPB):

1. When using the piggyback method, lower the primary bag at least 6 inches below the piggyback bag.
2. Set the pump as a secondary infusion when entering the rate of infusion and volume to be infused.
3. Most piggyback medications contain 50–100 cc and usually infuse in 20–60 min, although larger-volume bags take longer.

Administering IV medications through a volume control setup (Buretrol):

1. Insert the spike of the volume control set (Buretrol, Soluset, Pediatrol) into the primary solution container.
2. Open the upper clamp on the volume control set and allow sufficient fluid into volume control chamber.
3. Fill the volume control device with 30 cc of fluid by opening the clamp between the primary solution and the volume control device.

Administering an IV bolus dose:

1. If an existing IV is infusing, stop the infusion by pinching the tubing above the port.
2. Insert the needle into the port and aspirate to observe for a blood return.
3. If the IV is infusing properly with no signs of infiltration or inflammation, it should be patent.
4. Blood indicates that the intravenous line is in the vein.
5. Inject the medication at the prescribed rate.
6. Remove the needle and regulate the IV as prescribed.

GENERAL INDEX

---

bold – generic drug name   regular type – trade name   ⓔ see **evolve**

---

italics – classification name   **bold page #** – main drug entry

---

bold – generic drug name   regular type – trade name   ℮ see **evolve**

---

bold – generic drug name   regular type – trade name   ℮ see **evolve**

---

bold – generic drug name   regular type – trade name   ℯ see **evolve**

---

italics – classification name   **bold page #** – main drug entry

---

bold – generic drug name   regular type – trade name   *e* see **evolve**

italics – classification name **bold page #** – main drug entry

---

italics – classification name   **bold page #** – main drug entry

---

bold – generic drug name   regular type – trade name   ℮ see *evolve*

---

italics – classification name   **bold page #** – main drug entry

---

bold – generic drug name   regular type – trade name   *e* see **evolve**

---

bold – generic drug name   regular type – trade name   ℮ see **evolve**

---

italics – classification name   **bold page #** – main drug entry

---

bold – generic drug name   regular type – trade name   ⓔ see *evolve*